Zinsser Microbiology

20th edition

Zinsser Microbiology

20th edition

EDITED BY

Wolfgang K. Joklik, D.Phil.
James B. Duke Distinguished Professor
of Microbiology and Immunology and
Chairman, Department of Microbiology
and Immunology
Duke University Medical Center
Durham, North Carolina

Hilda P. Willett, Ph.D.
Professor of Microbiology
Duke University Medical Center
Durham, North Carolina

D. Bernard Amos, M.D.
James B. Duke Distinguished Professor
of Immunology and
Professor of Experimental Surgery
Duke University Medical Center
Durham, North Carolina

Catherine M. Wilfert, M.D.
Professor of Pediatrics and
Professor of Clinical Virology
Duke University Medical Center
Durham, North Carolina

APPLETON & LANGE
Norwalk, Connecticut/San Mateo, California

92 93 94 95 96 / 10 9 8 7 6 5 4 3 2 1

Prentice Hall International (UK) Limited, *London*
Prentice Hall of Australia Pty. Limited, *Sydney*
Prentice Hall Canada, Inc., *Toronto*
Prentice Hall Hispanoamericana, S.A., *Mexico*
Prentice Hall of India Private Limited, *New Delhi*
Prentice Hall of Japan, Inc., *Tokyo*
Simon & Schuster Asia Pte. Ltd., *Singapore*
Editora Prentice Hall do Brasil Ltda., *Rio de Janeiro*
Prentice Hall, *Englewood Cliffs, New Jersey*

Library of Congress Cataloging-in-Publication Data

Zinsser microbiology / edited by Wolfgang K. Joklik ... [et al.].—20th ed.
p. cm.
Includes index.
ISBN 0-8385-9983-4
1. Medical microbiology. I. Zinsser, Hans, 1878–1940.
II. Joklik, Wolfgang K. III. Title: Microbiology.
[DNLM: 1. Microbiology. QW 4 Z7831]
QR46.Z6 1992
616'.01—dc20
DNLM/DLC
for Library of Congress 91-41219

ISBN 0-8385-9983-4

Production Service: CRACOM Corporation
Designer: S. M. Byrum

PRINTED IN THE UNITED STATES OF AMERICA

Contents

Contributors

Wolfgang K. Joklik, D.Phil.
James B. Duke Distinguished Professor of Microbiology and Immunology; Chairman, Department of Microbiology and Immunology, Duke University Medical Center, Durham, North Carolina

Hilda P. Willett, Ph.D.
Professor of Microbiology, Duke University Medical Center, Durham, North Carolina

D. Bernard Amos, M.D.
James B. Duke Distinguished Professor of Immunology and Professor of Experimental Surgery, Duke University Medical Center, Durham, North Carolina

Catherine M. Wilfert, M.D.
Professor of Pediatrics and Professor of Clinical Virology, Duke University Medical Center, Durham, North Carolina

Andrew E. Balber, Ph.D.
Associate Medical Research Professor of Immunology, Duke University Medical Center, Durham, North Carolina

William M. Baldwin III, M.D., Ph.D.
Assistant Medical Research Professor of Pathology, Duke University Medical Center, Durham, North Carolina

Rebecca H. Buckley, M.D.
James B. Sidbury Professor of Pediatrics and Professor of Immunology, Duke University Medical Center, Durham, North Carolina

Thomas R. Cate, Ph.D.
Professor of Microbiology and Immunology, Baylor College of Medicine, Houston, Texas

Peter Cresswell, Ph.D.
Professor of Immunology, Duke University Medical Center
Present position: Professor of Immunobiology, Yale University, New Haven, Connecticut

Jeffrey R. Dawson, Ph.D.
Professor of Immunology, Duke University Medical Center, Durham, North Carolina

Joan L. Drucker, M.D.
Professional Services Division, Burroughs Wellcome Company, Research Triangle Park, North Carolina, and Assistant Consulting Professor of Medicine, Duke University Medical Center, Durham, North Carolina

Robert P. Drucker, M.D.
Associate, Department of Pediatrics, Duke University Medical Center, Durham, North Carolina

Susan P. Fisher-Hoch, M.D.
Deputy Chief, Special Pathogens Branch, Division of Viral Diseases, Center for Infectious Diseases, Centers for Disease Control, Atlanta, Georgia

Donald L. Granger, M.D.
Associate Professor of Medicine and Assistant Professor of Microbiology, Duke University Medical Center, Durham, North Carolina

Laura T. Gutman, M.D.
Associate Professor of Pediatrics and Associate Professor of Pharmacology, Duke University Medical Center, Durham, North Carolina

John D. Hamilton, M.D.
Professor of Medicine and Associate Professor of Microbiology, Duke University Medical Center, Durham, North Carolina

Barton F. Haynes, M.D.
Frederic M. Hanes Professor of Medicine and Professor of Immunology, Duke University Medical Center, Durham, North Carolina

Nancy G. Henshaw, M.P.H., Ph.D.
Assistant Medical Research Professor of Pediatrics, Duke University Medical Center, Durham, North Carolina

Gale B. Hill, Ph.D.
Associate Professor of Obstetrics and Gynecology and Associate Professor of Microbiology, Duke University Medical Center, Durham, North Carolina

Richard L. Hodinka, Ph.D.
Associate Director of Clinical Virology Laboratory, Children's Hospital of Philadelphia, Philadelphia, Pennsylvania

Joyce W. Jenzano, M.S.
Associate Professor of Dental Ecology, University of North Carolina School of Dentistry, Chapel Hill, North Carolina

Samuel L. Katz, M.D.
Wilbert C. Davison Professor of Pediatrics, Duke University Medical Center, Durham, North Carolina

Donna D. Kostyu, Ph.D.
Assistant Research Professor of Immunology, Duke University Medical Center, Durham, North Carolina

Kenneth N. Kreuzer, Ph.D.
Associate Professor of Microbiology, Duke University Medical Center, Durham, North Carolina

Joseph B. McCormick, M.D.
Chief, Special Pathogens Branch, Division of Viral Diseases, Center for Infectious Diseases, Centers for Disease Control, Atlanta, Georgia

Ross E. McKinney, M.D.
Assistant Professor of Pediatrics, Duke University Medical Center, Durham, North Carolina

Thomas G. Mitchell, Ph.D.
Associate Professor of Mycology, Duke University Medical Center, Durham, North Carolina

John D. Moriarty, D.D.S.
Associate Professor of Periodontics, University of North Carolina School of Dentistry, Chapel Hill, North Carolina

Suydam Osterhout, M.D., Ph.D.
Professor Emeritus of Microbiology and Professor Emeritus of Medicine, Duke University Medical Center, Durham, North Carolina

Thomas J. Palker, Ph.D.
Associate Research Professor of Medicine, Duke University Medical Center, Durham, North Carolina

Emilia D. Rivadeneira, M.D.
Fellow, Pediatric Infectious Diseases, Duke University Medical Center, Durham, North Carolina

Wendell F. Rosse, M.D.
Florence McAlister Professor of Medicine, Professor of Immunology, and Professor of Pathology, Duke University Medical Center, Durham, North Carolina

Fred Sanfilippo, M.D., Ph.D.
Professor of Pathology, Professor of Immunology, and Professor of Experimental Surgery, Duke University Medical Center, Durham, North Carolina

David W. Scott, Ph.D.
Dean's Professor of Immunology, University of Rochester School of Medicine, Rochester, New York

Daniel J. Sexton, M.D.
Associate Professor of Medicine, Duke University Medical Center, Durham, North Carolina

Kay H. Singer, Ph.D.
Associate Medical Research Professor of Medicine and Associate Medical Research Professor of Immunology, Duke University Medical Center, and Assistant Dean of Trinity College of Arts and Sciences, Duke University, Durham, North Carolina

Lynn Smiley, M.D.
Head, Clinical Virology Section, Department of Infectious Diseases, Burroughs Wellcome Company, Research Triangle Park, North Carolina

Ralph Snyderman, M.D.
Chancellor, James B. Duke Professor of Medicine and Professor of Immunology, Duke University Medical Center, Durham, North Carolina

Emmanuel B. Walter, M.D.
Associate in Pediatrics, Duke University Medical Center, Durham, North Carolina

Norman F. Weatherly, Ph.D.
Professor Emeritus of Parasitology, University of North Carolina School of Public Health, Chapel Hill, North Carolina

Robert W. Wheat, Ph.D.
Professor of Microbiology and Assistant Professor of Biochemistry, Duke University Medical Center, Durham, North Carolina

Priscilla B. Wyrick, Ph.D.
Professor of Microbiology and Immunology, University of North Carolina School of Medicine, Chapel Hill, North Carolina

Peter Zwadyk, Ph.D.
Associate Professor of Pathology and Associate Professor of Microbiology, Duke University Medical Center, Durham, North Carolina

Preface

With each passing year the term *microbiology* becomes a less satisfactory umbrella for the many disciplines that it attempts to cover. Bacteriology, immunology, virology, mycology, and parasitology have each long since become separate and independent disciplines. They are treated together in a single text simply because they deal with the agents that cause infectious diseases and with the mechanisms by which hosts defend against them.

In spite of the undeniable triumphs of antimicrobial chemotherapy, which has revolutionized the practice of medicine and very likely represents the greatest single triumph of biomedical science, "microbes" are by no means "conquered"; they continue to cause infections that demand a large amount of the physician's time. In fact, knowledge concerning new infectious agents, unsuspected properties of known agents, additional mechanisms for the genesis and persistence of infections, and the behavior of infectious agents at the molecular, cellular, and organismal levels is accumulating at an ever increasing pace. As a result, the scope and complexity of the material presented to students is expanding rapidly, and the compilation of a comprehensive textbook of manageable size is becoming ever more difficult.

This new edition of *Zinsser Microbiology*, the twentieth, is designed for medical students experiencing their first exposure to medical microbiology. To that end, we not only describe the pathogenic infectious agents and the diseases that they cause, but also discuss the basic principles of bacterial physiology and genetics, of molecular and cellular immunology, and of molecular virology. Our overall purpose is to provide a firm basis for growth with the field throughout the student's professional career by presenting not only the principles on which is built the practice of infectious diseases, but also the most important facts, observations, and correlations that led to their establishment. The importance of presenting such background for the purpose of providing an intellectual framework essential for true understanding is illustrated graphically by our recent experience with the human immunodeficiency virus, which causes AIDS. This is a virus, discovered less than a decade ago, that currently kills more than 25,000 persons annually in the United States alone. This country is currently spending more than $1 billion a year on the control of this virus, much of it on basic studies of the mechanisms that control the expression of its genetic information in the various cells in the body that it infects. There is no question that in the course of their professional careers, today's medical students will have to cope with disease caused by this virus, as well as with a new and constantly changing spectrum of infectious agents.

The twentieth edition represents an extensive revision of the nineteenth edition. Many portions of the text have been completely rewritten, and the remainder have been thoroughly updated. The Clinical Virology section in particular has several new contributors who provided completely new chapters on herpesviruses, adenoviruses, papovaviruses, influenza viruses, and retroviruses, as well as on rapid viral diagnosis. In the Basic Virology section the major chapters on virus multiplication cycles, bacteriophages, and tumor viruses have been completely rewritten; these are areas in which a wealth of new information is coming to hand at an ever increasing pace, information embodying new principles concerning the nature of genetic material and of the mechanisms that regulate its expression on the one hand, and the nature of the changes that transform normal cells into cancer cells, on the other. Clearly these are areas of vital importance to medical practitioners. The same applies to the Immunology section, which provides a comprehensive account of both basic and clinical immunology, organized so as to highlight topics currently deemed of maximum relevance to medical students. Finally, all chapters in the Basic Bacteriology, Medical Bacteriology, Medical Mycology, and Parasitology sections have been thoroughly updated, with considerable new material added, especially in the areas of microbial determinants of virulence and host response. Increased emphasis has also been placed on the various organisms commonly associated with opportunistic infections that develop in immunocompromised patients or in patients with prosthetic device implants. In these sections, which like all other sections have been carefully edited by a single editor so as to ensure uniformity of format, emphasis is again placed on correlating the basic and clinical aspects of each infectious agent so that the student may acquire an appreciation of how fundamental research unravels the complexities of host-parasite relationships. Each chapter consists of (1) an introduction to the important biologic properties of the organism, (2) a description of the clinical infection in humans, including a discussion of the mechanisms of pathogenicity, (3) a section on laboratory diagnosis that provides information on modern culture and immunological procedures, and (4) a discussion of the currently recommended treatment.

With regard to the bibliography, we have again elected not to reference specific statements in the text, but to append to each chapter a list of recent reviews and key original papers that will be particularly valuable for instructors. The recent reviews will quickly guide the reader to any specific aspect of microbiology and immunology that he or she wishes to pursue; the original papers provide the detailed considerations and circumstances that have gone into the genesis of the most important discoveries. Many of the papers that are cited already are, or no doubt will soon become, "classics."

We have tried not to increase the size of the book—no

easy task in view of the enormous amount of new information that has accumulated since publication of the last edition in 1988. Obviously, this has entailed the omission of a certain amount of older material; however, we are confident that there are no major gaps and that in our presentation of the newest advances we have not sacrificed careful and logical explanations of fundamental principles.

The list of individuals who have helped to produce this volume extends far beyond the circle of our colleagues who contributed textual material and to whom we are profoundly indebted. We would especially like to thank our many colleagues who permitted us to use illustrative material and who almost invariably supplied us with original photographs, and the many publishers who allowed us to reproduce previously published material. We would also like to thank the artists who did a superb job in drawing the innumerable charts and diagrams, and the many secretaries who cheerfully massaged the text on their word processors again and again. Finally, we wish to express our appreciation to the staff of Appleton & Lange for their efficient cooperation in producing this new edition.

Wolfgang K. Joklik
Hilda P. Willett
D. Bernard Amos
Catherine M. Wilfert

Preface to the First Edition

The volume here presented is primarily a treatise on the fundamental laws and technic of bacteriology, as illustrated by their application to the study of pathogenic bacteria.

So ubiquitous are the bacteria and so manifold their activities that bacteriology, although one of the youngest of sciences, has already been divided into special fields—medical, sanitary, agricultural, and industrial—having little in common, except problems of general bacterial physiology and certain fundamental technical procedures.

From no other point of approach, however, is such a breadth of conception attainable, as through the study of bacteria in their relation to disease processes in man and animals. Through such a study one must become familiar not only with the growth characteristics and products of the bacteria apart from the animal body, thus gaining a knowledge of methods and procedures common to the study of pathogenic and nonpathogenic organisms, but also with those complicated reactions taking place between the bacteria and their products on the one hand and the cells and fluids of the animal body on the other—reactions which often manifest themselves as symptoms and lesions of disease or by visible changes in the test tube.

Through a study and comprehension of the processes underlying these reactions, our knowledge of cell physiology has been broadened, and facts of inestimable value have been discovered, which have thrown light upon some of the most obscure problems of infection and immunity and have led to hitherto unsuspected methods of treatment and diagnosis. Thus, through medical bacteriology—that highly specialized offshoot of general biology and pathology—have been given back to the parent sciences and to medicine in general methods and knowledge of the widest application.

It has been our endeavor, therefore, to present this phase of our subject in as broad and critical a manner as possible in the sections dealing with infection and immunity and with methods of biological diagnosis and treatment of disease, so that the student and practitioner of medicine, by becoming familiar with underlying laws and principles, may not only be in a position to realize the meaning and scope of some of these newer discoveries and methods, but may be in a better position to decide for themselves their proper application and limitation.

We have not hesitated, whenever necessary for a proper understanding of processes of bacterial nutrition or physiology, or for breadth of view in considering problems of the relation of bacteria to our food supply and environment, to make free use of illustrations from the more special fields of agricultural and sanitary bacteriology, and some special methods of the bacteriology of sanitation are given in the last division of the book, dealing with the bacteria in relation to our food and environment.

In conclusion it may be said that the scope and arrangement of subjects treated in this book are the direct outcome of many years of experience in the instruction of students in medical and advanced university courses in bacteriology, and that it is our hope that this volume may not only meet the needs of such students but may prove of value to the practitioner of medicine for whom it has also been written.

It is a pleasure to acknowledge the courtesy of those who furnished us with illustrations for use in the text, and our indebtedness to Dr. Gardner Hopkins and Professor Francis Carter Wood for a number of the photomicrographs taken especially for this work.

P. H. Hiss, Jr.
H. Zinsser
1910

Zinsser Microbiology

20th edition

SECTION I

BACTERIAL PHYSIOLOGY

CHAPTER 1

The Historical Development of Medical Microbiology

The history of the many concepts now embodied in the doctrines of microbiology is an account of attempts to solve the problems of the origin of life, the putrefaction of dead organic materials, and the nature of communicable changes in the bodies of living humans and animals. The visible aspects of these phenomena were as apparent and interesting to ancient observers as they are to modern biologists. In the past, notions of ultimate causes were derived from available factual knowledge colored by the theologic and philosophic tenets of the time. The early history of what has become the science of microbiology is to be found, therefore, in the writings of priests and philosophers.

Infection and Contagion

Among ancient peoples, epidemic and even endemic diseases were regarded as supernatural in origin and sent by the gods as punishment for the sins of humans. The treatment and, more important, the prevention of these diseases were sought by sacrifices and lustrations to appease the anger of the gods. Since humans were thought to be willful and wanton by nature, there was never any difficulty in finding a particular set of sins to justify a specific epidemic.

The concept of contagion and the practice of hygiene were not, however, entirely unknown even then. The Old Testament is often quoted as indicating the belief that leprosy is contagious and can be transmitted by contact. The principle of contagion by invisible creatures was recorded by Varro in the second century BC, and the concept was familiar to Greek, Roman, and Arabic writers. Roger Bacon, in the thirteenth century, more than a millennium later, postulated that invisible living creatures produced disease. In 1546 a Venetian, Fracastorius, wrote from a knowledge of syphilis that communicable disease is transmitted by living germs, *seminaria morbi*, through direct contact or by intermediary inanimate fomites and through air *ad distans*. Fracastorius expressed the opinion that the seeds of disease, passing from one infected individual to another, caused the same disease in the recipient as in the donor. This clear expression of the germ theory of disease was three centuries ahead of its time.

First Observations of Bacteria

Direct observation of microorganisms had to await the development of the microscope. The human eye cannot see objects smaller than 30 μm ($^1/_{1000}$ inch) in diameter, and although knowledge of magnifying lenses reaches back to the time of Archimedes, the science of optics was not initiated until the thirteenth century by the Franciscan monk Roger Bacon. The telescope was invented by Galileo in 1608, followed by the microscope in the same century. The first person known to have made glass lenses powerful enough to observe and

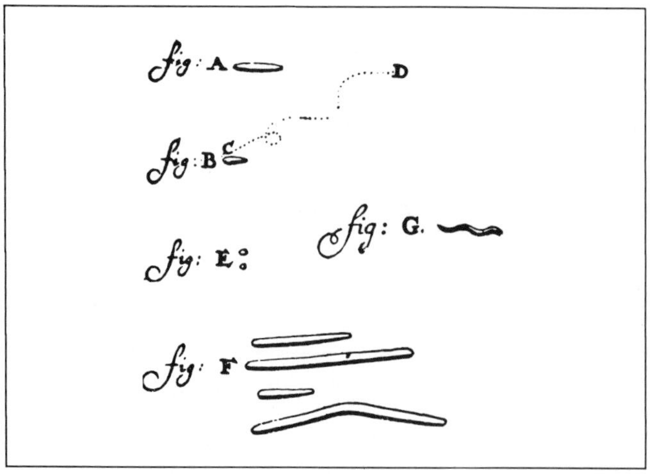

Fig. 1–1. In letters to the Royal Society, Leeuwenhoek described the sizes, shapes, and even the motility of bacteria. These are his drawings of bacteria from the human mouth. **A.** Motile *Bacillus*. **B** to **D.** *Selenomonas sputigena*. **E.** Micrococci. **F.** *Leptothrix buccans*. **G.** Probably *Spirochaeta buccalis*. *(From Dobell: Anton van Leeuwenhoek and his "Little Animals." New York, Harcourt, Brace, 1932.)*

describe bacteria was the amateur lens grinder Anton van Leeuwenhoek (1632–1723) of Delft, Holland. In letters to the Royal Society of London, an experimentalist group, Leeuwenhoek described many "animalcules," including the three major morphologic forms of bacteria (rod, sphere, and spiral), various free-living and parasitic protozoa from human and animal feces, filamentous fungi, and globular bodies we now know as yeasts (Figs. 1–1 and 1–2). His observational reports were enthusiastic and accurate and generated some interest at the time, but unfortunately he did all this as a hobby and left no students to continue his work. However, in 1678, Robert Hooke, who developed the compound microscope, confirmed Leeuwenhoek's discoveries.

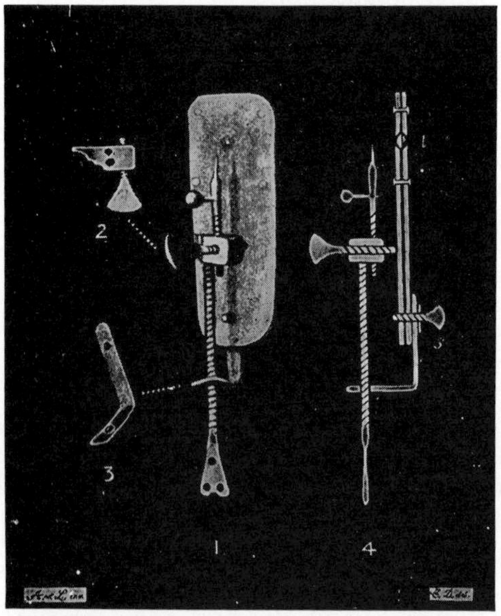

Fig. 1–2. Leeuwenhoek's microscopes consisted of simple biconvex lenses. *(From Dobell: Anton van Leeuwenhoek and his "Little Animals," New York, Harcourt, Brace, 1932.)*

Microorganisms were then occasionally studied by those primarily interested in classifying the various life forms observable with the microscope. These observations lay dormant and were not explored further by those interested in disease. The following 125 to 150 years witnessed the gradual development of knowledge and acceptance of the experimental method, which slowly disseminated throughout the expanding learned centers of the world. Improved microscopes became generally available in the 1800s as a result of the Industrial Revolution, which permitted rapid technologic advances. Even then, no notable advance in microbiology was accomplished until after the scientific world's attention was focused on the role of microbes in the controversies concerning spontaneous generation and the associated phenomenon of fermentation.

Spontaneous Generation

The controversy over the human ability to create life carried over from Greek mythology. Even Aristotle (384–322 BC) thought animals could originate from the soil. Samson, in the Old Testament, and again Virgil, about 40 BC, described recipes for producing bees from honey, and for centuries it was believed that maggots could be produced by exposing meat to warmth in the air. This was not refuted until Francesco Redi (1626–1697) proved that gauze placed over a jar containing meat prevented maggots forming in the meat. Recipes for producing mice and other similar life forms in litter and refuse were gradually disproved and discarded in similar fashion. However, the question was not settled in all minds. When microbes were discovered, their association with putrefaction and fermentation again raised the question of spontaneous generation. John Needham, in 1749, observed the appearance of microorganisms in putrefying meat and interpreted this as spontaneous generation. Spallanzani, however, boiled beef broth for an hour, sealed the flasks, and observed no formation of microbes. Needham and, 100 years later, Pouchet (1859) argued that access of air was necessary for the spontaneous generation of microscopic living beings. Disproof came from several lines of evidence. Franz Schulze (1815–1873) passed air through strong acids and then into boiled broth, while Theodor Schwann (1810–1882) passed air through red hot tubes and observed no growth. About 1850, Schroeder and von Dusch filtered air through cotton filters into broth and observed no growth. Pasteur was able to filter microorganisms from the air and concluded that this was the source of contamination. In 1859, in public controversy with Pouchet, Pasteur prepared boiled broth in flasks with long, narrow, gooseneck tubes that were open to the air. Air could pass, but microorganisms settled in the gooseneck, and no growth developed in any of the flasks. Finally a British physicist, John Tyndall (1820–1893), proved that dust carried germs, and the story was complete.

The Germ Theory of Disease

Empirical Observations

A firm basis for the causal nature of infectious disease was established only in the latter half of the nineteenth century.

One of the first proofs came from Agostino Bassi who, in the early 1800s, proved that a fungus, later named *Botrytis bassiana* in his honor, caused a disease in silkworms called *muscardine* in France and *mal segno* in Italy. In the 1840s, American poet-physician Oliver Wendell Holmes wrote "The Contagiousness of Puerperal Fever," in which he suggested that disease was caused by germs carried from one new mother to another. In 1861, Ignaz Semmelweis, who had drastically decreased childbirth deaths by introducing antiseptic techniques and practices, published his extremely important "The Cause, Concept and Prophylaxis of Childbed Fever." However, the importance of antiseptics in reducing contagious disease was not fully realized until the late 1870s, when Joseph Lister demonstrated the value of spraying operating rooms with aqueous phenol.

Lessons Learned from Fermentation

Further emphasis on microbial activities came from the work of Louis Pasteur from the 1850s to the 1880s. In studies on the diseases of wine, Pasteur demonstrated that alcoholic fermentation of grapes, fruit, and grains was caused by microbes, then called *ferments*. In good wine batches certain types of ferments existed in the vats, while in poor or bad fermentations other types of microbes were found, some of which Pasteur found to be capable of growing anaerobically. He suggested eliminating the bad types of ferments from fresh juices by heating at 63C for one-half hour, then cooling and reinoculating with a culture from the satisfactory vats. Pasteur's success with the problems of the wine industry led the French government to request that he study a disease, pebrine, which was ruining the silkworm industry in Southern France. Pasteur struggled with this problem for several years before he isolated the causative organism.

Observations and Experiments with Animals and Humans

In 1850, Pollender, and Rayer and Davaine, independently observed rod-shaped microorganisms in the blood of animals that had died of anthrax; in 1857 Brauell found anthrax bacilli in the blood of a human and transmitted the disease to sheep. The relationship of another bacterium to disease was demonstrated in 1873 when Obermeier observed spiral forms in the blood of a patient with relapsing fever and reproduced the disease in a human by injecting infected blood.

Importance of Pure Culture Techniques

Through all this time, etiologic research was not based on pure culture work. Pure cultures were obtained largely by accident, and investigators had no way of knowing, except by crude morphologic microscopic examination, when contaminants were present. This resulted in much equivocal thinking and work that hindered progress.

The first pure or axenic culture technique was developed by Joseph Lister in 1878. He made serial dilutions in liquid media to obtain pure cultures of a bacterium that he named *Bacterium* (*Lactobacillus*) *lactis*. Meanwhile, Koch, as a student of Henle who insisted on proof that an organism caused disease, was also developing and refining techniques for the isolation of pure cultures. From the work of others, notably Ehrlich, Koch learned methods for staining bacteria on glass with aniline dyes for microscopic observation. In his early work on anthrax, Koch used sterile aqueous humor of the eyes of animals as a growth medium; later he developed a transparent solid medium by mixing gelatin with Löffler's peptone solution. The gelatin mixture, liquefied on warming, could be heat sterilized and aseptically poured into plates; on cooling, it solidified. Microorganisms streaked on it developed into macroscopic colonies as the result of the growth of a single invisible cell. However, gelatin liquefies at a relatively low temperature (26C), and Koch later switched to agar, the transparent red seaweed extract that solidifies below 43C.

Etiologic Proof of Infectious Agents

Koch was able to isolate the anthrax organism in pure culture by streaking onto his solid media and found that even after many transfers, the organism could still cause the same symptoms and disease when inoculated into animals. On the basis of his experiences, Koch formulated criteria that provided proof that a specific bacterium caused a disease. We now call them Koch's postulates:

1. The organism must always be found in the diseased animal but not in healthy ones.
2. The organism must be isolated from diseased animals and grown in pure culture away from the animal.
3. The organism isolated in pure culture must initiate and reproduce the disease when reinoculated into susceptible animals.
4. The organism should be reisolated from the experimentally infected animals.

Koch's work thus provided impetus for work on and means of proof for the germ theory of disease.

The 20-year period following Koch's work was the Golden Age of Bacteriology. By 1900 almost all major bacterial disease organisms had been described. The list included anthrax (*Bacillus anthracis*), diphtheria (*Corynebacterium diphtheriae*), typhoid fever (*Salmonella typhi*), gonorrhea (*Neisseria gonorrhoeae*), gas gangrene (*Clostridium perfringens*), tetanus or lockjaw (*Clostridium tetani*), dysentery (*Shigella dysenteriae*), syphilis (*Treponema pallidum*), and others.

Viruses

Only with advances in technique and improvement in apparatus is it possible to make fundamental advances through new ideas and observations. The development of bacteriologic filters and the discovery of viruses is a case in point.

Bacteriologic Filters

As an alternative to heat sterilization, unsuccessful efforts to remove bacteria from solutions by filtration through paper and similar materials led Chamberland and Pasteur to test and develop unglazed porcelain as the first successful bacterial filter (1871–1884). The Berkefeld filter of Kieselguhr (diatomaceous earth) was developed shortly thereafter in 1891. Synthetic polymer filters of cellulose nitrate, cellulose acetate, polyester, and so forth have come into common use only since

World War II because of technical advances that allow quality control of pore size. It is of interest to note that these are essentially space-age products developed in part for the rapid removal of microorganisms from jet and rocket fuels.

Discovery of Viruses

There are three major groups of viruses: animal, plant, and bacterial. Since knowledge of each of these groups has accumulated along distinctive lines, extensive specialization has developed. Bacterial viruses are therefore dealt with only briefly in this book, and plant viruses are not considered at all. Yet discoveries made concerning each of these groups of viruses have influenced profoundly our understanding of the nature of each of the others.

The existence of viruses became evident during the closing years of the nineteenth century when, as the result of newly acquired expertise in handling bacteria, researchers were isolating the infectious agents of numerous diseases. For some infectious diseases this proved to be an elusive task until it was realized that the agents causing them were smaller than bacteria. Iwanowski in 1892 was probably the first to record the transmission of an infection (tobacco mosaic disease) by a suspension filtered through a bacteria-proof filter. This was followed in 1898 by similar experiments of Loeffler and Frosch concerning foot-and-mouth disease of cattle. Beijerinck (1898) considered the infectious agents in bacteria-free filtrates to be living but fluid—that is, nonparticulate—and introduced the term *virus* (Latin, poison) to describe them. It quickly became clear, however, that viruses were particulate, and the term "virus" became the operational definition of infectious agents smaller than bacteria and unable to multiply outside living cells. In 1911 Rous discovered a virus that produced malignant tumors in chickens, and during World War I Twort and d'Hérelle independently discovered the viruses that multiply in bacteria, the bacteriophages.

Viruses could not be grown in artificial media, and Koch's criteria could not be specifically applied. Because these pathogens require a living host for propagation, study progressed slowly. As in bacteriology, each new advance had to await the development of appropriate technology. Plant viruses proved easy to obtain in large amounts, which permitted extensive chemical and physical studies. This work led first to the demonstration that plant viruses consist only of nucleic acid and protein and culminated in the crystallization of tobacco mosaic virus by Stanley in 1935. This feat evoked great astonishment, since it cut across preconceived ideas concerning the attributes of living organisms and demonstrated that agents able to reproduce in living cells behaved under certain conditions as typical macromolecules.

Work with bacteriophages concentrated on their clinical application. It was hoped that bacteria could be destroyed inside the body by injecting appropriate bacteriophages. Their activity in vivo, however, never matched their activity in vitro, most probably because they are eliminated efficiently from the bloodstream.

Early work with animal viruses concentrated on the pathogenesis of viral infections and on epidemiology. Throughout this period, fundamental studies on animal cell-virus interactions were severely hampered by the absence of rapid and efficient techniques for quantitating viruses. The only method then available was the expensive and time-consuming serial end-point dilution method, using animals.

About 1940 several breakthroughs occurred. First, the advent of electron microscopy permitted visualization of viruses for the first time. Second, techniques for purifying certain animal viruses were being perfected, and a group of workers at the Rockefeller Institute headed by Rivers carried out some excellent chemical studies on vaccinia virus. Third, Hirst discovered that influenza virus agglutinates chicken red cells. This phenomenon, hemagglutination, was rapidly developed into an accurate method for quantitating myxoviruses, as a result of which this group of viruses became, in the 1940s, the most intensively investigated group of animal viruses. Finally, this period marked the beginning of the modern era of molecular virology. Until then the interaction of bacteriophages with bacteria had been analyzed principally in terms of populations rather than at the level of single virus particles interacting with single cells. This conceptual block was removed by Ellis and Delbrück's study of the one-step growth cycle, as a result of which the bacteriophage-bacterium system became extraordinarily amenable to experimentation. Indeed, many of the major advances in molecular biology have resulted from work in the bacteriophage field.

In animal virology, rapid advances followed the development in the late 1940s of techniques for growing animal cells in vitro. Strains of many types of mammalian cells can now be grown in media of defined composition. As a result, animal cell–virus interactions can now be analyzed with the same techniques that proved so powerful in the case of bacteriophages.

Immunity

Ancient peoples immunized themselves against venomous snakes by introducing small amounts of venom into scratches in the skin. More than 2000 years ago the Chinese used variolation to protect themselves against smallpox. This practice, which involved exposure to dermic lesions from patients who had survived the disease in the hope that it had been caused by a relatively mild virus variant, spread through Asia by trade routes and, in spite of its failure rate of 1% or more, was well accepted in the Middle East and eventually also reached Europe. At the end of the eighteenth century Edward Jenner (1749–1823) noticed that milkmaids who developed cowpox were immune to smallpox and found that he was able to protect susceptible individuals against smallpox by vaccinating them with cowpox. Pasteur developed a chicken cholera vaccine in 1877; he inoculated chickens with old attenuated cultures so that a mild disease rendered the chickens immune to virulent organisms. He called this *vaccination,* after Jenner's procedure. Shortly afterward, in 1881, applying the same concept, Pasteur prepared temperature-attenuated anthrax grown at 42C to 43C and protected sheep by first injecting them with these bacteria before challenging them with virulent anthrax grown at lower temperatures. Salmon and Smith, from 1884 to 1886, used heat-killed cultures of hog cholera bacillus to develop resistance or immunity in swine against challenge by live virulent organisms. Pasteur developed a rabies vaccine in 1886, again using the idea of injecting an attenuated living disease agent. In this case, Pasteur used dried animal spinal cords without, apparently, recognizing the viral form of the disease agent.

Two schools of thought arose in explanation of the

increased resistance following vaccination. In the 1880s Metchnikoff developed the cellular theory of protection; Bordet and others proposed the humoral, or specific, antibody concept of immunity. There is now evidence that both theories are correct. The last several decades have witnessed the isolation and characterization of the major humoral immune proteins, the immunoglobulins, the generation and function of which are currently being studied intensively. Much work is also being devoted to the cellular interactions in immune reactions that occur not only in infectious diseases caused by bacteria, viruses, fungi, and parasites, but also in rejection reactions of tissue and organ transplants, and in cancer.

Antimetabolites

Many antimetabolites, which were pioneered in concept by Ehrlich in the middle to late 1800s, are now accepted household words, e.g., penicillin. The modern era of antibiotics developed only after Domagk reported in 1935 that Prontosil had a dramatic effect on streptococcal infections. It was soon discovered that Prontosil was converted in the body to sulfanilamide, the active chemical agent, which is an analog of the vitamin *p*-aminobenzoic acid. In the 1940s, as the result of the stimulus of World War II, Florey and Chain and their associates reinvestigated Fleming's penicillin, isolated and characterized it, and demonstrated its practical clinical value. As a result of millions of tests with thousands of organisms, we now have numerous other antibiotics active against almost all types of bacteria.

With the recognition of the metabolic and structural differences, at the molecular level, between pathogenic microorganisms and viruses on the one hand and human or animal cells on the other, the rationale for developing new chemotherapeutic agents is now often based on exploiting these differences.

Role of Microbiology in Development of Molecular Biology and Molecular Genetics

The enormous advantages of homogeneous populations of cells for every conceivable type of investigation were soon realized. As a result, many of the epoch-making advances in cell physiology, biochemistry, and genetics have resulted from studies with microorganisms. During the last three or four decades, these advances have led to a precise way of investigating the structure and function of nucleic acids and proteins that has become known as *molecular biology*. For example, the demonstration of the central role of DNA as the repository of genetic information resulted from the studies of Griffith in the 1920s showing that pneumococci could be transformed from one capsular type to another, followed by the demonstration by Avery and associates during the 1940s that the transforming factor was DNA; proof beyond doubt was provided by the demonstration by Hershey and Chase in 1952 that viral nucleic acid itself contained all the information necessary for virus multiplication. At the same time, Watson and Crick developed the double-helix model of DNA structure, which led them to suggest that one of the complementary DNA strands could serve as the template for the synthesis of the other, thus providing a description of self-perpetuating gene replication and continuity.

Demonstration of the transcription from DNA of information in the form of messenger RNA synthesized in complementary sequence to DNA soon followed, again in a microbial system. Messenger RNA was then found to be translated into polypeptides on ribosomes. By the early 1960s Nirenberg, Ochoa, and others had worked out the nature of the triplet RNA base sequences corresponding to the codon signals for all amino acids.

More recently, attention has focused on the arrangement of genetic material, including the nature of genes and the mechanisms that control their expression. This wide area of research also originated in microbiology; it has now become known as *molecular genetics*. While much of this research is still being carried out with microbial systems, cells of higher organisms, particularly mammalian cells, are also being used extensively today. An important factor in this connection has been the development of the technique of tissue culture, which permits animals cells to be grown, cloned, and passaged like microorganisms; in fact, the primary impetus for developing this new technique was the need of virologists to grow and measure viruses. Using this technique, new concepts concerning the regulation of gene expression in cells of higher organisms, and particularly in human cells, are now being developed very rapidly. Among the goals that should be within reach in the foreseeable future are an understanding of the fundamental control mechanisms that operate in both normal and abnormal cell differentiation, including cancer; insight into the mechanisms that control the immune response; and the development of a rational system of antiviral chemotherapy for controlling diseases caused by viruses, just as antibiotics are used to control diseases caused by bacteria.

FURTHER READING

Bulloch W: The History of Bacteriology. London, Oxford University Press, 1938

Dobell C: Anton van Leeuwenhoek and His "Little Animals." New York, Harcourt, Brace, 1932

Dubos RJ: The Professor, the Institute and DNA. New York, Rockefeller University Press, 1976

Dubos RJ: Biochemical Determinants of Microbial Disease. Cambridge, Mass, Harvard University Press, 1954

Dubos RJ: Louis Pasteur, Free Lance of Science. Boston, Little, Brown, 1950

Florey HW: Antibiotics. London, Oxford University Press, 1949

Hughes SS: The Virus: A History of the Concept. New York, Neale Watson Academic Publications, 1977

Marquardt M: Paul Ehrlich. New York, Henry Schuman, 1951

Meleney FL: Treatise on Surgical Infections. London, Oxford University Press, 1948

Tyndall J: Essays on the Floating-Matter of the Air in Relation to Putrefaction and Infection. New York, D Appleton and Co, 1882

CHAPTER 2

The Classification and Identification of Bacteria

Procaryotes and Eucaryotes

Only two types of cells are produced by all living organisms on earth. The procaryote cells (*pro,* or primitive nucleus), do not have a membrane bound nucleus and include all (and only) bacteria. The procaryotes include the eubacteria (true bacteria) and archaebacteria (ancient bacteria) in the kingdom procaryotae. The other type of cell, the eucaryote cell (*eu,* or true nucleus), has a membrane-bound nucleus and is found in all other organisms, including the algae, fungi, protozoa, plants, and animals. Relationships among the eubacteria, archaebacteria, and eucaryotes are shown in Figure 2–1. Because human pathogens are found only among the eubacteria, the eubacteria will be emphasized throughout this book.

Bacteria

General Properties. Bacteria are single-celled organisms that reproduce by simple division, i.e., binary fission. Most are free living and contain the genetic information and energy-producing and biosynthetic systems necessary for growth and reproduction. A few, such as the chlamydiae and rickettsiae, are obligate intracellular parasites. Bacteria differ from eucaryotes in a number of respects. Bacteria do not contain 80S ribosomes or membrane-bound organelles, such as the nucleus, mitochondria, lysosomes, endoplasmic reticulum, or Golgi bodies, and they lack the 9 + 2 fibril flagellum or cilia structure characteristic of eucaryotic cells. Bacteria have 70S ribosomes and a naked, single circular chromosome (nucleoid) composed of double-stranded deoxyribonucleic acid (DNA) that replicates amitotically. The cytoplasmic membrane of eubacteria contains ester-linked lipids and carries out transport, energy-production, and specialized biosynthetic functions. Motility, if it occurs, is often conferred by single-filament flagellar structures. Some bacteria produce external microfibrils (pili or fimbriae) that serve adhesive functions. The mycoplasmas do not possess cell walls, whereas other eubacteria produce envelope structures that contain a chemically similar cell wall peptidoglycan. The cell wall–producing eubacteria (and archaebacteria) may occur as spheres (cocci), rods (bacilli), or curved or spiral-shaped cells. The chemical nature of envelope components and structures imparts useful staining characteristics that permit the eubacteria to be arbitrarily divided into gram-positive, gram-negative, and acid-fast organisms. The archaebacteria may differ from the eubacteria in their ribosome components, presence of ether-linked membrane lipids, the absence of the eubacterial peptidoglycan, and in the possession of different types of metabolism and cofactors.

Bacterial Species and Strains. Bacterial species are defined descriptively (i.e., phenotypically). That is, each kind of bac-

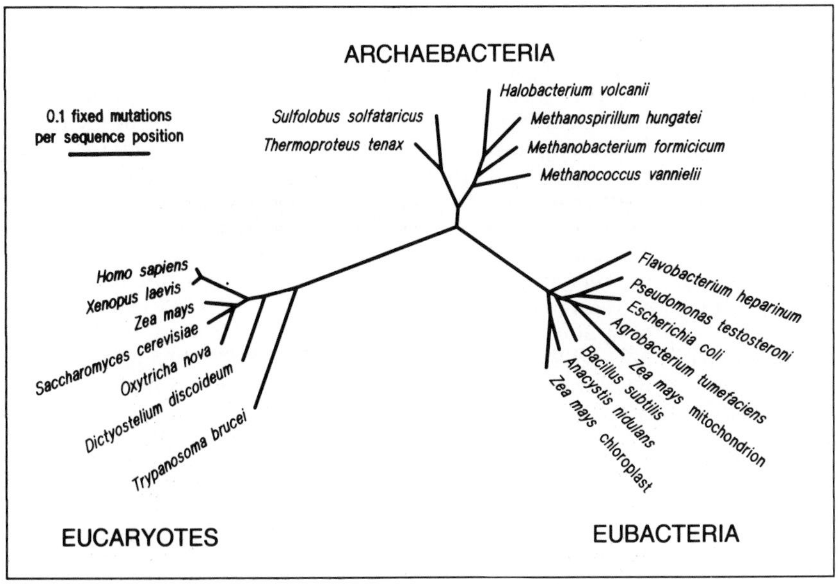

Fig. 2–1. Unrooted phylogenetic tree based on 16S-like ribosomal ribonucleic acid sequences. *(Copyright © Cell Press, from Pace et al: Cell 45:325, 1986.)*

terium may be considered a species, typified as a collection of strains that share many features in common and differ considerably from other strains. A strain is the progeny and subcultures of a single colony isolate in pure culture. Bacterial species are defined by (1) structural traits of shape, size, mode of movement, resting stage, Gram stain reaction, and macroscopic growth, (2) biochemical and nutritional traits, end-products, and other biochemical information on cell components and metabolites, (3) physiologic traits relative to oxygen, temperature, pH, and response to antibacterial agents, (4) ecologic traits, and (5) DNA base composition, homology, and genetic traits.

Species Biotype (Biovar). Bacterial species collections contain strains of interrelated but differing organisms, sometimes known as a *cluster*. The species description includes the main features of the collection. Within each species collection or cluster, a strain is chosen arbitrarily to best represent that species. This strain is known as the *biotype* (or biovar) of that species, and its characteristics will thereafter be used to describe that particular species. Biotype strains are used as "reference strains," available from culture collections such as the American Type Culture Collection (ATCC), Rockville, Maryland, USA.

Biotype strains may not exhibit all the traits of the strains within the species collection. Therefore, subspecies designations, such as serotype (serovar), pathotype (pathovar), morphotypes (morphovars), or phage type (phagovar) are sometimes used to indicate particular modes of strain variation.

The lack of a definitive unifying criterion for species designation in bacteria has understandably resulted in variation in levels at which groups are divided, depending on whether the describing investigator is a splitter or a lumper. In the splitter category are those who have designated each *Salmonella* serotype (serovar) as a species with its own name. The lumpers, on the other hand, have designated individual serotypes as numbered types within a single species of, for example, *Klebsiella* or *Streptococcus*.

Microbial Systematics

Systematics, which encompasses most of microbiology, is the study of the diversity, similarity, and interrelationships of microbes for the purposes of taxonomy. Taxonomy includes classification, nomenclature, and identification. Classification uses the knowledge gained in the study of microbes in an attempt to arrange them in an orderly way into similar or related groups (taxa). Nomenclature is the system of assigning names to the taxonomic groups according to international codes and rules. Identification is the process of ascertaining to which taxonomic group an organism belongs.

Classification would best be based on evolutionary (i.e., phylogenetic) lines of descent. For higher plants and animals this is possible. For bacteria, however, where morphology is generally similar, where sexuality is limited (only a few bacteria conjugate), and where no fossil records exist through time (convincing evidence of 3.5 billion-year-old bacteria came only within the last two decades), a phylogenetic classification has not been possible. Obviously we must work with bacteria as they are today, and much is to be learned of bacterial relatedness. As will be seen, studies of DNA, RNA, proteins, and other information-containing cellular macromolecules (known collectively as *semantides*), their patterns of regulation and of other cellular structures, metabolic systems and components, are thought to offer the best avenue for developing evidence for evolutionary descent and a true phylogenetic classification. At present the conservative trend is to place emphasis on the species and genus, with higher taxonomic levels (e.g., families or orders) being indicated only where genetic evidence is adequate.

Formal Taxonomic Ranks, Nomenclature, and Informal Trivial Names. All procaryotes are placed in the kingdom Procaryotae. A subsequent formal ranking hiarchy of successively smaller, nonoverlapping taxonomic levels may be used to indicate levels of relatedness among various kinds of bacteria. These taxonomic levels are denoted, according to rules of nomenclature, by latinized, italicized names with suffixes to indicate divisions (*-es*), classes (*-aceae*), orders (*-ales*), families (*-aceae*), genera, and species. (Divisions are used for both plants and bacteria, whereas phylum is used for animals.) Generic names (nouns) are capitalized; species names are not. Genus and species names together form the universally known nomenspecies, binomen, or Linnean binomial. All latin names are italicized in print and underlined in script. The first validly published name and description has priority. Since 1980, the description and name of each bacterial species is validated by publication in the *International Journal of Systematic Bacteriology*.

Well-known informal trivial names, such as tubercle bacillus (*Mycobacterium tuberculosis*) and typhoid bacillus (*Salmonella typhi*), often appear in medical literature. When a generic (genus) name is vernacularized in English, such as bacillus, salmonella, or pneumococcus, it is neither capitalized nor italicized.

Classification of Selected Pathogenic Bacteria. In contrast to nomenclature, there is no "official" bacterial classification. This text has followed the approach of *Bergey's Manual of Determinative Bacteriology* through eight volumes preceding, and the current *Bergey's Manual of Systematic Bacteriology*, volumes 1 (1984) and 2 (1986), which is the reference most widely used in the United States. The eighth edition of *Bergey's* dropped the use of higher taxa because of uncertainties about genetic relatedness. The current *Bergey's* recognizes the kingdom Procaryotae as containing four major divisions: I. Gracilicutes, the gram-negative bacteria; II. Firmicutes, the gram-positive bacteria; III. Tenericutes, the cell wall–less bacteria (i.e., the *Mycoplasma* or Mollicutes); and IV. Mendosicutes (Archaeobacteria). Beyond this, the current Bergey's takes a more conservative taxonomic approach, using the neutral and provisional ad hoc term "Section" to indicate groups of similar bacteria without inferring phylogenetic relatedness within the section (except where genetic evidence is available) or between sections. Moreover, the current Bergey's does not accept the kingdom status of the eubacteria, archaebacteria, and eucaryotes as suggested by molecular biologists on the basis of ribosomal RNA sequences (see Fig. 2–1). However, for lack of suitable alternatives we shall refer to the first three divisions recognized in the current Bergey's as eubacteria, since these are the divisions in which human and animal pathogens occur. A selection of some major pathogens is listed in Table 2–1, modified from the "Section" format as used in the current *Bergey's Manual of Systematic Bacteriology*, volumes 1 and 2.

Numerical Taxonomy (Taxometrics). Because of the difficulties in constructing evolutionary (phylogenetic) classifications for bacteria based on only a few arbitrarily weighted characteristics that may or may not reflect evolutionary relationships, descriptive taxonomy and classification of many species has been revised since the 1950s in the form of computerized numerical comparisons of large numbers of phenotypic traits (i.e., descriptive traits without connotation as to genetic origin). First devised by Michel Adanson in the eighteenth century, this system gives equal weight to all traits chosen for comparison. The argument is that if enough (50 to several hundred) phenotypic traits are examined, occurrence of a few variable traits is minimized (e.g., those due to extrochromosomal elements), and objective comparisons result. Numerical taxonomy, then, reveals similarities, resemblances, and differences in bacterial attributes as they exist today (i.e., phenotypic relationships) without reference to genetic origin. Numerical taxonomic comparison of traits between bacteria may be expressed as a Jaccard similarity coefficient (S_J), or as a simple matching coefficient (S_{SM}): the former, S_J, includes only positive features, whereas the latter, S_{SM}, includes both positive and negative features. (Other coefficients may be used for special purposes.) These coefficients express the percentages of traits held in common between organisms. Designations of groups, known as *phenons* or *taxa* (taxospecies or taxogenus), are then made on the basis of the ranges of degrees of similarity. Taxospecies (a cluster of strains of high mutual phenotypic similarity) may or may not include genospecies (capable of gene exchange), whereas both would bear the same binomial name (binomen). The coefficients are as follows:

$$\text{Similarity coefficient} \qquad S_J = \frac{a}{a + b + c}$$

$$\text{Simple matching coefficient} \qquad S_{SM} = \frac{a + d}{a + b + c + d}$$

where a = number of features present in both strains, b = number of features present in first strain only, c = number of features present in strain two only, and d = number of features negative in both strains.

Genetic Basis for Classification. Developments in comparative biochemistry (or molecular biology) indicate that DNA base composition and DNA and ribosomal RNA (rRNA) sequence homology, as well as gene-controlled stable metabolic patterns, cell polymers, organelle structures, and patterns of their regulation, yield information of relatedness of organisms at the genetic level. DNA sequence homology is useful for comparison of closely related strains and species, whereas comparison of rRNA homology affords the most useful criteria of relatedness among diverse organisms. Indeed, it appears that a record of bacterial evolution (i.e., a living, ever-evolving fossil record) may exist in the amino acid sequences of bacterial proteins and in the nucleotide base sequences of bacterial DNA and RNA.

Because these developments are still in progress, a complete phylogenetic correlation with the present classification in Table 2–1 cannot yet be made, although use is made of DNA base composition and DNA homologies. The older empirically developed relationships based on recognition of phenotypic expression of various traits and features are a reflection of gene pool expression and are gradually being modified by molecular approaches that aim at defining relatedness on a genetic basis.

Relatedness Based on Nucleic Acid Homology. Genetic information is encoded in DNA base sequence. Over eons it would be expected that as organisms drift apart by mutation, recombination, and selection in different environments (i.e., evolution), their genomes change in size, nucleotide base composition, and nucleotide base sequence. The approximate sizes of the genomes of several bacteria are listed in Table 2–2. Base composition, constant for each organism, is generally expressed in terms of the mole fraction of guanine (G) plus cytosine (C) (that is, [G + C]/[G + C + A + T] expressed as a percentage). Values of percent G + C for different organisms vary from 25 to more than 75 (Table 2–3). Similar DNA base composition does not guarantee homology in base se-

TABLE 2–1. SELECTED BACTERIA OF MEDICAL IMPORTANCE[a]

Family *Genus species*	Identifying Properties	Clinical Infection
Section 1. The Spirochetes. Gram-Negative Helical Bacteria		
Spirochaetaceae	Slender, flexuous, helically coiled, motile with axial filaments	
Treponema pallidum	Host-associated, tightly coiled, probably microaerophilic	Syphilis
Borrelia hermsii	Host-associated; loose, coarse, irregular coils; microaerophilic	Tick-borne relapsing fever
B. bergdorferi	As above	Tick-borne Lyme disease
Leptospiraceae	Flexible, very tightly coiled motile rods, one or both ends hooked, aerobic	
Leptospira interrogans	Parasitic; other properties as above	Leptospirosis
Section 2. Aerobic/Microaerophilic, Motile, Helical/Vibrioid, Gram-Negative Bacteria		
Campylobacter fetus	Slender, spirally curved rod, microaerophilic, host-associated	Opportunistic septicemic illness
C. jejuni	As above	Enteritis
Helicobacter pylori	As above, grows at 35C	Ulcers
Section 4. Gram-negative Aerobic Rods and Cocci		
Pseudomonadaceae	Straight or curved rods, motile, oxidase (+), respiratory metabolism	
Pseudomonas aeruginosa	Fluorescent pigments produced; other properties as above	Wound, burn, urinary tract infections
Legionellaceae	Motile, difficult to stain, catalase (+), requires special media	
Legionella pneumophila	As above	Pneumonia (Legionnaire's disease)
Neisseriaceae	Biscuit-shaped diplococci, nonmotile, catalase (+), oxidase (+)	
Neisseria meningitidis	Ferments glucose and maltose	Meningitis
N. gonorrhoeae	Ferments glucose	Gonorrhea
Other Genera		
Brucella abortus	Coccobacilli to short rods, nonmotile, facultative intracellular parasite, fastidious growth requirements, catalase (+)	Brucellosis
B. melitensis	As above	Brucellosis
B. suis	As above	Brucellosis
Bordetella pertussis	Minute, nonmotile coccobacilli, mammalian parasites	Pertussis (whooping cough)
Francisella tularensis	Minute, pleomorphic, faintly staining cocci to rods; require enriched media (glucose-cysteine blood agar)	Tularemia
Section 5. Facultative Anaerobic Gram-Negative Rods		
Enterobacteriaceae	Small rods, inhabit intestine, catalase (+), oxidase (−), glucose fermented, nitrates reduced to nitrites; genera and species identified biochemically	
Escherichia coli	Motile, mixed acid fermentation, lactose fermented by most strains, H_2 and CO_2 produced, H_2S(−), citrate not utilized	Opportunistic infections; some strains cause diarrheas
Enterobacter aerogenes	Motile, 2,3-butanediol fermentation, lactose fermented with acid and gas, citrate utilized, ornithine decarboxylated	Opportunistic infections
Shigella dysenteriae	Nonmotile, lactose not fermented, no gas from glucose, H_2S(−)	Dysentery
Salmonella typhi	Motile, lactose not fermented, no gas from glucose, H_2S(+), indole (−), lysine and ornithine decarboxylated	Typhoid fever
S. species	Acid and gas from glucose	Food poisoning
Klebsiella pneumoniae	Nonmotile, encapsulated, lactose fermented with acid and gas, 2,3-butanediol fermentation, citrate utilized, ornithine not decarboxylated	Pneumonia
Proteus mirabilis	Motile, lactose not fermented, urea hydrolyzed	Urinary tract infections

(continued)

TABLE 2–1. SELECTED BACTERIA OF MEDICAL IMPORTANCE (*continued*)

Family *Genus species*	Identifying Properties	Clinical Infection
Section 5. Facultative Anaerobic Gram-Negative Rods (*continued*)		
Serratia marcescens	Motile, lactose not fermented, $H_2S(-)$, lysine decarboxylated, citrate utilized, DNase produced, pigment at R°	Opportunistic infections
Yersinia pestis	Cells ovoid to rod-shaped, nonmotile, lactose not fermented	Bubonic plague
Y. enterocolitica	As above	Gastroenteritis
Vibrionaceae	Rigid rods, straight or curved, polar flagella, oxidase (+), catalase (+), metabolism respiratory and fermentative	
Vibrio cholerae	Lactose not fermented, produces toxin; other properties as above	Cholera
V. parahaemolyticus	Lactose not fermented, halophilic, other properties of family	Gastroenteritis from seafood
Pasteurellaceae	Straight rods, nonmotile, organic N sources required, oxidase (+)	
Pasteurella multocida	Small ovoid rod, bipolar staining, other properties as above	Animal bite infections
Haemophilus influenzae	Small pleomorphic coccobacilli to rods, strict parasite, requires nicotinamide riboside and hematin for growth, most strains oxidase (+)	Meningitis, other pediatric diseases
Section 6. Anaerobic Gram-Negative Straight, Curved, and Helical Rods		
Bacteroidaceae	Straight rod with curved ends, pleomorphic with vacuoles, non-sporeforming, major component of intestinal flora	
Bacteroides fragilis	As above	Opportunistic multiple organism anaerobic abscesses
B. melaninogenicus	Produces dark pigment on blood agar	Opportunistic infections
Fusobacterium sp	Long slender, spindle-shaped rods, present in natural cavities of man	Opportunistic infections
Section 9. Rickettsiae and Chlamydiae, Gram-Negative		
Rickettsiaceae	Small rods, coccoid and diplococcal, usually intracellular parasites associated with arthropods	
Rickettsia rickettsii	Grows intracellularly in cytoplasm and nucleus	Rocky Moutain Spotted Fever (Tick typhus)
R. prowazekii	Grows intracellularly in vacuoles	Epidemic typhus
Coxiella burnetii	Grows preferentially in vacuoles, forms endospores, disseminated by airborne aerosols	Q fever
Chlamydiaceae	Nonmotile, coccoidal, obligately intracellular parasites, developmental cycle in cytoplasm, metabolically limited	
Chlamydia trachomatis	As above	Trachoma, lymphogranuloma venereum
C. psittaci	As above	Psittacosis
Section 10. Mycoplasmas (Cell Wall–Less Bacteria)		
Mycoplasmataceae	Small cell wall–less, highly pleomorphic, gram-negative, require cholesterol for growth, colony has "fried-egg" appearance, penicillin-resistant	
Mycoplasma pneumoniae	Facultatively anaerobic, gliding motility, special structure for attachment to host cell	Primary atypical pneumonia
Ureaplasma urealyticum	Microaerophilic, hydrolyze urea with production of ammonia	Some nongonococcal urethritis
Section 12. Gram-Positive Cocci		
Micrococcaceae	Spherical cells, divide in more than one plane, catalase (+), nonmotile, no endospores	
Staphylococcus aureus	Often occur in grape-like clusters, facultative anaerobe, coagulase (+)	Suppurative abscesses, toxic manifestations
S. epidermidis	Coagulase (−), otherwise as above	Opportunistic infections
S. saprophyticus	As above	Urinary tract infections in young females

(continued)

TABLE 2–1. SELECTED BACTERIA OF MEDICAL IMPORTANCE (*continued*)

Family *Genus species*	Identifying Properties	Clinical Infection
Section 12. Gram-Positive Cocci (*continued*)		
Other Genera		
Streptococcus	Spherical or ovoid cells in pairs or chains, nonmotile, homofermentative metabolism, catalase (−), complex nutritional requirements	
S. pyogenes	β-hemolytic or blood agar, bile-esculin (−)	Pharyngitis, skin infections, acute rheumatic fever
S. agalactiae	Produces CAMP factor, otherwise as above	Neonatal meningitis
S. pneumoniae	α-hemolytic on blood agar, lancet-shaped diplococci or short chains, bile-soluble	Lobar pneumonia
S. faecalis	Grows in 6.5 percent NaCl, withstands 60C, bile-esculin (+)	Oppotunistic infections
Section 13. Endospore Forming Gram-Positive Rods and Cocci		
Bacillus	Cells rod-shaped, often peritrichously flagellated, strict aerobes or facultative anaerobes	
B. anthracis	Non-motile, facultative anaerobe	Anthrax
Clostridium	Cells rod-shaped, anaerobes, motility (±), spores distend cell	
C. botulinum	Motile, produce neurotoxins (7 types)	Botulism
C. perfringens	Nonmotile, stormy fermentation in milk, produces exotoxins	Gas gangrene
C. tetani	Motile, terminal spores, single type of neurotoxin	Tetanus
C. difficile	Motile, produces exotoxin (2 types)	Pseudomembranous colitis
Section 14. Regular, Nonsporing, Gram-Positive Rods		
Lactobacillus sp	Microaerophilic, fermentative lactate producers, catalase (−), no cytochromes	Dental caries (secondary role)
Listeria	Small, short rods, facultatively anaerobic, catalase (+), oxidase (−)	
L. monocytogenes	β-hemolytic	Meningitis
Section 15. Irregular, Nonsporing, Gram-Positive Rods		
Corynebacterium	Straight to slightly curved rods, irregular staining, often produce metachromatic granules, not acid-fast, facultatively anaerobic, produce short chain mycolic acids	
C. diphtheriae	Produces potent exotoxin	Diphtheria
Actinomyces	Nonmotile, nonacid-fast rods, filaments, some branching, facultatively anaerobic, catalase (−), CO_2 required for maximum growth	
A. israelii	As above	Actinomycosis
Section 16. Mycobacteria (Acid-fast Rods)		
Mycobacteriaceae	Slightly curved or straight rods, gram-positive, acid-fast, nonmotile, aerobic, catalase (+), long chain mycolic acids produced	
Mycobacterium tuberculosis	Very slow grower	Tuberculosis
M. avium–M. intracellulare	Properties as for family; one of mycobacterial species other than tuberculosis (MOTT)	Chronic pulmonary disease; disseminated disease in immunocompromised
M. leprae	Cannot be cultured on artificial media	Leprosy
Section 17. Nocardioforms		
Nocardia	Gram-positive, no endospores, nonmotile aerobic bacillus, filaments, fragmentation into rods and cocci; partially acid-fast, produce medium length mycolic acids	
N. asteroides	As above	Nocardiosis

Adapted from Krieg and Holt (eds): Bergey's Manual of Systematic Bacteriology, vol 1, 1984, and Sneath, Mair, Sharpe, Holt (eds): Bergey's Manual of Systematic Bacteriology, vol 2, 1986, Williams & Wilkins.

[a] Only sections have been included that currently contain bacteria of medical importance.

TABLE 2–2. APPROXIMATE DNA CONTENT OF VARIOUS ORGANISMS

Species	Daltons
Mammalian sperm	18×10^{11}
Salmonella typhimurium	28×10^{8}
Escherichia coli	25×10^{8}
Bacillus subtilis	20×10^{8}
Haemophilus influenzae	16×10^{8}
Neisseria gonorrhoeae	9.8×10^{8}
Rickettsia rickettsii	9.8×10^{8}
Chlamydia trachomatis	6.6×10^{8}
Mycoplasma species	5×10^{8}
Coliphage T4	1.3×10^{8}

Data from Kingsbury: J Bacteriol 98:1400, 1969; Muller and Klotz: Biochim Biophys Acta 378:171, 1975; Sober (ed): Handbook of Biochemistry, 1968. Courtesy of Chemical Rubber Co.; Sorov and Becker: J Mol Biol 42:581, 1969.

quence: genomes of vertebrates and bacteria with 44 mole percent GC obviously have heterologous base sequences. DNA sequence homologies of bacteria are quantified by several procedures that determine the extent of formation of hybrid duplexes from separate DNA or DNA and rRNA strands obtained from different bacteria. This approach has been useful in demonstrating the DNA similarity of closely related species, genera, and families of bacteria. Examples are given for the enterobacteria and other groups in Table 2–4. Table 2–4 shows in addition, the lack of DNA homology between dissimilar organisms. DNA homology does not go much beyond the genus or family level. On the other hand, rRNA sequences exhibit more homology among widely dissimilar organisms than does DNA (Table 2–4). Mutational change in RNA sequences has obviously been very low through the ages. Ribosomal RNA homology studies therefore provide extremely interesting information of potential phylogenetic importance. Most startling was the observation that the differences that exist between the eubacteria and the methanogens (see p. 8), halophiles, and thermoplasma in respect to their cell wall and membrane lipids, exotoxin susceptibility, coenzymes, and modes of metabolism correlate with wide differences in their rRNA sequences. These observations resulted in the suggestion that the methanogens, halophiles, and thermoplasma be placed in a separate kingdom known as the Archaebacteria (Fig. 2–1).

TABLE 2–3. NUCLEOTIDE BASE COMPOSITION OF THE DNA OF VARIOUS BACTERIA

Organism	G + C (%)
Clostridium perfringens, C. tetani	24–28
Rickettsia prowezekii, R. ricketsia	29–33
Staphylococcus aureus, Bacillus anthracis	32–36
Streptococcus faecalis, S. agalactiae	34–38
Streptococcus pneumoniae, S. pyogenes	38–40
Haemophilus influenzae, Proteus mirabilis	39
Chlamydia psittici, C. trachomatis, Bacteroides fragilis	41–44
Yersinia pestis, Vibrio cholerae	46–49
Escherichia coli, Shigella dysenteriae, Salmonella spp	48–53
Neisseria meningitidis, N. gonorrhoeae	49–53
Corynebacterium diphtheriae	52–55
Klebsiella pneumoniae	56–60
Pseudomonas aeruginosa	67
Mycobacterium tuberculosis	62–70

Adapted from Krieg and Holt (eds): Bergey's Manual of Systematic Bacteriology, vol 1, 1984, and Sneath, Mair, Sharpe, Holt (eds): Bergey's Manual of Systematic Bacteriology, vol 2, 1986. Williams & Wilkins.

TABLE 2–4. APPROXIMATE PERCENTAGES OF DNA AND REBOSOMAL RNA[a] RELATEDNESS AMONG SOME BACTERIA

	% Homology (to *E. coli*)		
Source of Nucleic Acid	DNA/DNA	DNA/RNA	rRNA
Escherichia coli	100	100	100
Shigella dysenteriae	89		99
Salmonella typhimurium	45		98
Klebsiella pneumoniae	35	75	
Serratia marcescens	25		96
Yersinia pestis	15		
Proteus mirabilis	10	75	94
Pseudomonas aeruginosa	1–3		87
Neisseria meningitidis	1–3		84
Bacillus subtilis	1	16	80
Streptococcus faecalis			79
Clostridium perfringens			79
Mycoplasma pneumoniae			73
Chlamydia trachomatis			75
Bacteroides fragilis			72
Eucaryotes (*Saccharomyces cerevisieae*)			50–55

Data from Brenner: Int J Syst Bacteriol 23:298, 1973; Brenner et al.: J Bacteriol 94:486, 1967; Kingsbury: J Bacteriol 94:879, 1967; McCarthy and Bolton: Proc Natl Acad Sci USA 50:156, 1963; Pace and Campbell: J Bacteriol 107:543, 1971; Krieg and Holt (eds): Bergey's Manual of Systematic Bacteriology, vol 1, 1984, and Sneath, Mair, Sharpe, Holt (eds): Bergey's Manual of Systematic Bacteriology, vol 2, 1986, Williams & Wilkins: CR Woese, personal communication, University of Illinois, Urbana, 1987.

Identification of Bacteria

The primary concern of the medical microbiologist is the isolation and rapid, accurate identification of the disease-causing microorganism and its antibiotic susceptibilities so that adequate specific therapy can be initiated. Rapid identification can be accomplished in most cases.* by pure culture† isolation and determinative procedures that make use of knowledge of specimen source, growth requirements, visible (colony) growth features, microscopic morphology, staining reactions, and biochemical characteristics. Antibiotic susceptibility levels are then determined.

Isolation of Organisms in Pure (Axenic) Culture

The approach used for the isolation of organisms depends on the clinical specimen. Blood and spinal fluid may yield pure bacterial cultures, whereas specimens of sputum, stool, skin, body orifices, and abscesses contain mixtures of organisms. The specimen is generally streaked onto solid agar–containing

* Exceptions occur in the case of exotoxin-producing bacteria. Refer to discussions on botulism, tetanus, and staphylococcal food poisoning.
† Pure in the sense of axenic, i.e., free of other organisms, rather than pure in the genetic sense.

CHAPTER 3

Bacterial Morphology and Ultrastructure

...al Cell

...e a layered cell envelope that includes ... cell wall, and associated proteins and ...bacteria produce capsules or slimes. ...pendages (flagella and pili) may also ... rigid structure that encloses and ...m physical damage and conditions ...ssure. The cell wall also generally ... wide range of environmental ...mprises the naked cytoplasmic ...ternally, bacteria are relatively ... structures include a central ...rounded by an amorphous ... Cytoplasmic inclusion bod... vary in chemical nature ...ts depending on growth ...lasmic structures, such as ... bacteria. Typical gram-positive and gram-negative bacterial cells, which differ primarily in cell envelope organization, are shown in diagram form in Figure 3–1.

Bacterial Size and Form

Pathogenic bacterial species vary from approximately 0.4 to 2 μm in size (Fig. 3–2) and appear under the light or electron microscope as spheres (cocci), rods (bacilli), and spirals (Fig. 3–3). Cocci occur as single spherical cells, in pairs as diplococci, in chains as streptococci, or, depending upon division planes, in tetrads or in grape-like clusters. Bacilli may vary considerably in length, from very short rods (coccobacilli) to long rods that vary in length up to several times their diameter. The ends of bacilli may be gently rounded, as in enteric organisms such as *Salmonella typhi*, or squared, as in *Bacillus anthracis*. Long threads of bacilli that have not separated into single cells are known as *filaments*. Fusiform bacilli, found in the oral and gut cavities, taper at both ends. Curved bacterial rods

medium so as to separate the bacterial population into individual cells which grow as individual colonies (see below). Pathogens present in small numbers in mixtures of organisms may be missed because of overgrowth by other bacteria, or they may be killed by metabolic acids or other products resulting from the growth of nonpathogens. Selective media may be used in such cases. Pathogens may also be missed if their growth requirements are not met. For this reason again, selective culture techniques are employed to establish an environment in which the pathogen has a survival advantage; these include the use of selective media that are of specific pH, ionic strength, or chemical composition, or that contain inhibitors, or that lack nutrients for all but the organism in question. Control of gas phase and temperature of the growth environment must also be considered. Alternatively, for fastidious bacteria, enrichment media are used that contain nutrients ecologically favorable to the organism to be isolated. Such media include chocolate agar, blood agar, and nutrient agar and sometimes include inhibitors, such as found in McConkey's agar. Specific media and growth conditions are discussed in reference to the individual requirements of specific organisms in later chapters under the headings of growth and nutrition. The response of the unknown bacterium to such media is sometimes useful in identification. For example, *Haemophilus influenzae* requires for growth both pyridine nucleotide and hemin, the iron porphyrin derived from hemoglobin, and therefore will grow on chocolate agar (heated to lyse the cells and release the growth factors) but not on blood agar.

Bacterial Colony Morphology

Most bacteria multiply rapidly and form macroscopic, visible masses of growth called colonies when inoculated onto appropriate medium containing 2% agar and incubated 12 to 24 hours in a favorable atmosphere. For some organisms, such as the tubercle bacillus, *M. tuberculosis*, 2 to 8 weeks of incubation is required. Ideally, a colony is composed of the descendents of a single cell, i.e., a clone. In some cases, two or more daughter cells that do not separate are known as a colony-forming unit (CFU). It should be noted, however, that when isolated from sputum, stool, or a similar source, and especially on inhibitor-containing media, a colony may have the gross appearance characteristic of a certain type of bacterium but may contain contaminating organisms and should be restreaked on fresh medium. The gross characteristics of colonies aid in identification, since colonies of different organisms may vary in size, shape, color, odor, texture, and degree of adherence to the medium. Colony morphologic characteristics are related in part to motility or to postfission bacterial movements, which depend on division planes formed by different species. Colonies have been described as loop-forming (wavy edges characteristic of long filaments, such as those of *Bacillus anthracis*), folding and snapping (serrated or crenated edges, such as those formed by *Yersinia pestis* and *Corynebacterium diphtheriae*), and slipping (smooth or lobate edges with spreading smooth growth films, characteristic of *Proteus vulgaris* or *Escherichia coli*).

The serologic characteristics of a bacterium are often correlated with mucoid (M), smooth (S), or rough (R) colony appearance (Figs. 2–2 and 2–3). M or S colonies are characteristic of bacteria recently isolated from natural habitats and are sometimes called "wild-type."

M colonies exhibit a waterlike, glistening, confluent appearance and are characteristic of organisms that form slime or well-developed capsules. Notable examples are *Klebsiella pneumoniae*, *Streptococcus* (*Diplococcus*) *pneumoniae*, *H. influenzae*, and the pathogenic yeast, *Cryptococcus neoformans*. Capsular polymers may be group, species, or strain specific and are usually antigenic for mice and men. The capsule functions as a defense mechanism against phagocytosis, and among pathogenic bacteria, encapsulated organisms are usually more virulent than noncapsulated forms.

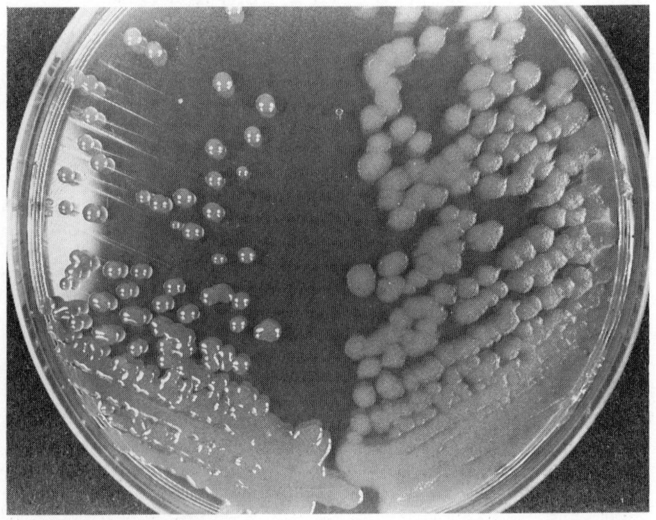

Fig. 2–2. Smooth (S) and rough (R) colonies of *Bacillus anthracis* Pasteur vaccine strain grown on bicarbonate agar in 20% CO_2. Left, wild-type strain 6602; *right*, rough variant R1. *(From Green et al: Infect Immun 49(2):291, 1985.)*

The smooth or S colonies give the appearance of homogeneity and uniform texture without appearing as liquid as mucoid colonies. S colony–forming bacteria are traditionally referred to as colonially or morphologically smooth (i.e., S forms). S forms are characteristic of freshly isolated wild-type organisms, such as the gram-negative enterobacteria (e.g., *Salmonella*, *Shigella*, *E. coli*, *Serratia*, and *Proteus* species), which produce a complete array of surface proteins and the well-known lipopolysaccharide somatic O antigens (Chaps. 3 and 6). For reasons discussed below, the identification of wild-type somatic antigens of S form organisms is sometimes confirmed by serologic tests.

R colonies are granulated and rough in appearance. R colonies are usually produced by mutant strains (R forms) that lack surface proteins or polysaccharides produced by freshly isolated wild-type parent organisms. Intermediate R mutants, detectable only biochemically, serologically, or genetically, may, however, produce morphologically smooth colonies (Chap. 6). Rough forms of enteric bacteria are usually avirulent and more easily killed by phagocytes, in contrast to the more resistant parent or wild-type S colony bacteria. However, with some organisms, such as the anthrax bacillus and the human and bovine types of tubercle bacilli, the R forms are more virulent.

L colonies were first associated with certain bacilli, notably *Streptobacillus moniliformis*, but have also been isolated from *H. influenzae* and various enteric bacteria. The rigid cell wall that is characteristic of bacteria is absent in L forms. Exposure to

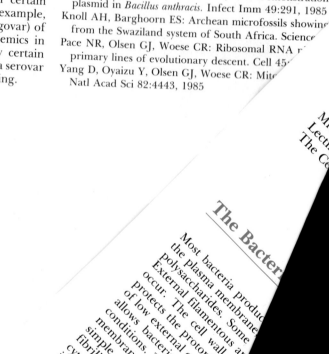

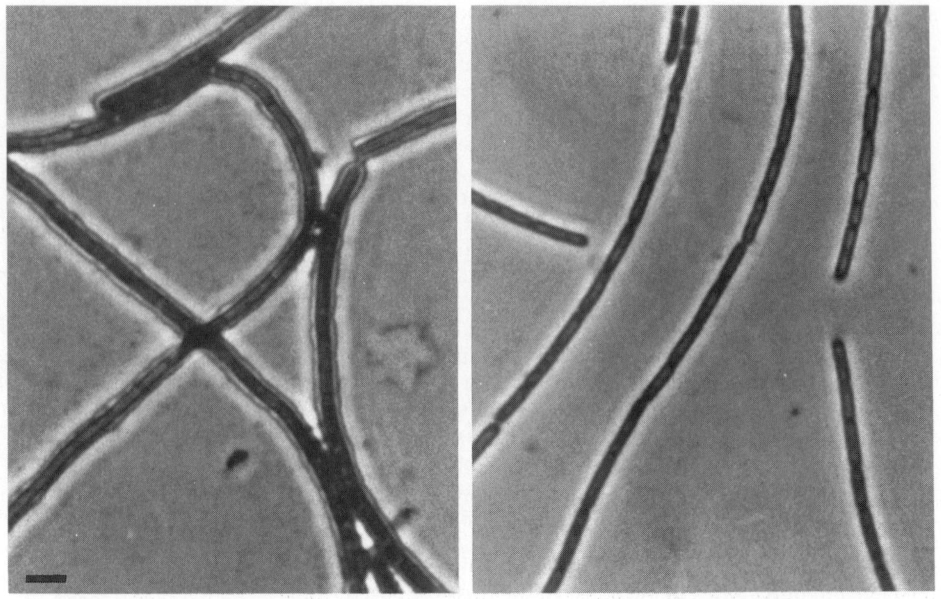

Fig. 2–3. Phase-contrast photomicrography of smooth (S), *left*, and rough (R), *right*, of cells of *Bacillus anthracis* Pasteur vaccine strain grown on bicarbonate agar in 20% CO_2. Note capsule around S cells on left. *(From Green et al: Infect Immun 49(2):291, 1985.)*

penicillin and other drugs and growth in osmotically supportive media facilitates L colony formation. Small coccoid and filamentous forms are observed, as well as large globoid forms, which also contain the minute forms. L forms induced in this manner normally resynthesize a cell wall once the penicillin or other drug is removed.

Microscopic Morphology and Staining Reactions

Light microscopic examination of gram-stained preparations with the oil immersion lens and without a coverslip is routinely used to determine the shape of bacteria. Common shapes are cocci (spherical), bacilli (rodlike), and spiral forms. The Gram stain also provides a check on contamination by noting morphologic and staining homogeneity. Depending on source and growth features, other differential stains may be used, as in the case of acid-fast staining of sputum smears or cultures. Special stains may also be used to detect capsules, flagella, spores, or intracellular inclusion bodies.

The Gram Stain. A heat-fixed bacterial smear on a glass slide is treated with the basic dye, crystal violet. All organisms take up the dye. The smear is then covered with Gram's iodine solution (3% iodine–potassium iodide in water or a weak buffer, pH 8.0, to neutralize acidity formed from iodine on standing). After a water rinse and decolorization with acetone, the preparation is washed thoroughly in water and counterstained with a red dye, usually safranin. The stained preparation is then rinsed with water, dried, and examined under oil with the light microscope.

Bacteria can be differentiated into two groups by this stain, devised in the early 1800s by the Danish bacteriologist Christian Gram. Gram-positive organisms stain blue, while about one third of the cocci, one half of the bacilli, and all spiral organisms stain red and are said to be gram-negative. Animal cells also stain gram-negative, and the gram stain procedure can therefore be used to detect large gram-positive bacteria, such as *Nocardia asteroides*, in tissues.

The mechanism of the Gram stain appears to be generally related to the thickness of the cell wall, pore size, and permeability properties of the intact cell envelope. Gram-positive bacteria stain gram-negative if they lose osmotic integrity by rupture of the plasma membrane. Autolyzed, old, or dead gram-positive cells and isolated cell envelopes stain gram-negative. A unique bacterial cell wall chemical composition does not appear to explain the Gram stain, since thick-walled yeast cells, which also stain gram-positive, have a chemical composition and structure different from gram-positive bacteria.

The Acid-fast Stain. The mycobacteria are lipophilic and difficult to stain, but once stained, they are resistant to destaining. Typically, a sputum or culture smear on a glass slide is stained with carbolfuchsin. The phenol appears to aid penetration of the dye through the mycobacterial lipid. The slide is then rinsed with water, destained with acid alcohol, and counterstained briefly with methylene blue. When examined under the light microscope, mycobacteria appear as bright red bacilli against a light blue background. Alternatively, the organisms may be stained by lipophilic fluorescent dyes which are detected by ultraviolet microscopy.

Biochemical Characteristics

Various strains, species, and genera of organisms exhibit characteristic patterns of substrate utilization, metabolic product formation, and sugar fermentation. Some 60% or more of common pathogens are identified by metabolic tests. The choice of traits most useful for development of specific test patterns for the identification of particular pathogenic species is greatly aided by correlation of taxometric phenotypic analyses, DNA base composition and DNA homology information.

A number of commercial kits are now available that make use of a battery of some 20 or more biochemical tests in combination with taxometric analyses for identification of enterobacteria. It is also notable that specific DNA "probes" for rapid hybridization identification of certain species have been introduced commercially.

Antibiotic Susceptibility

Equally as important as the identification of a clinical isolate is the determination of antibiotic susceptibility for purposes of treatment. Antibiotics vary in their effect on different bacterial species and on strains of even the same species. Each pathogen must be tested for sensitivity to various concentrations of effective chemotherapeutic agents to determine the concentration level at which its growth is inhibited. The dosage necessary to obtain the blood level required for adequate therapy can then be established.

Epidemiology: Phage Typing and Serotyping

Epidemiologists have found bacteriophage or serologic typing to be useful in tracing the source of outbreaks for certain bacterial diseases. These approaches include, for example, determining the bacteriophage typing patterns (phagovar) of specific strains of *S. aureus,* which may cause epidemics in hospital wards and show lysis susceptibility to only certain bacteriophage. Serotyping is sometimes used to trace a serovar as a source of an outbreak of *Salmonella* food poisoning.

FURTHER READING

Books and Reviews

Amato I: Ticks in the tocks of molecular clocks. Science News 131:74, 1987

Gray MW, Doolittle WF: Has the endosymbiont hypothesis been proven? Microbiol Rev 46:1, 1982

Johnson JL: Genetic characterization. In Gerhardt P, Murray RGE, Costilow RN, et al (eds): Manual of Methods for General Bacteriology. Washington DC, American Society for Microbiology, 1981, p 450

Krieg NR, Holt JG (eds): Bergey's Manual of Systematic Bacteriology, vol 1. Baltimore, Williams & Wilkins, 1984

Sneath PHA, Mair NS, Sharpe ME, Holt JG (eds): Bergey's Manual of Systematic Bacteriology, vol 2. Baltimore, Williams & Wilkins, 1986

Woese CR: Bacterial Evolution. Microbiol Rev 51:221, 1987

Selected Papers

Darnell JE, Doolittle WF: Speculations on the early course of evolutio[n] Proc Natl Acad Sci 83:1271, 1986

Green BD, Battisti L, Koehler TM, et al: Demonstration of a ... plasmid in *Bacillus anthracis.* Infect Imm 49:291, 1985

Knoll AH, Barghoorn ES: Archean microfossils showin[g] ... from the Swaziland system of South Africa. Science ...

Pace NR, Olsen GJ, Woese CR: Ribosomal RNA ... primary lines of evolutionary descent. Cell 45...

Yang D, Oyaizu Y, Olsen GJ, Woese CR: Mit... Natl Acad Sci 82:4443, 1985

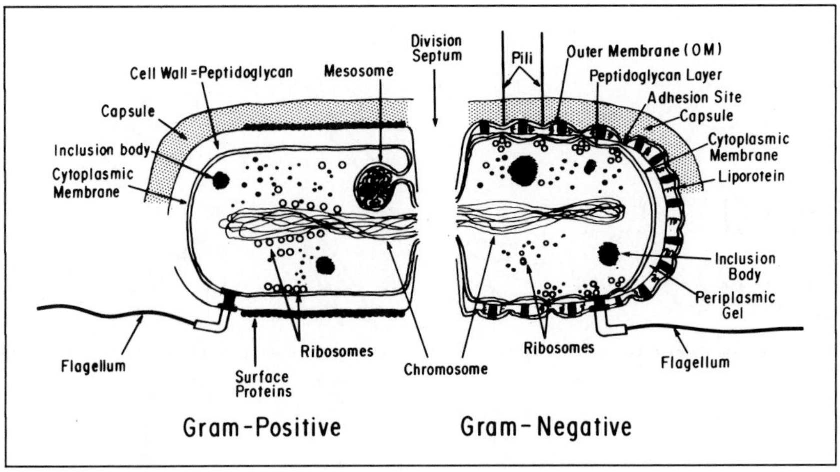

Fig. 3–1. Diagram of sections through idealized typical bacterial cells, showing similarities and cell envelope differences.

vary from small, comma-shaped or mildly helical organisms with only a single curve, such as *Vibrio cholerae,* to the longer spirochete forms, such as *Borrelia, Treponema,* and *Leptospira,* which have multiple coils.

Microscopy

The Light Microscope

Brightfield Microscopy. The human eye cannot resolve objects much less than 0.1 to 0.2 mm or detect an object less than about one-thousandth inch (30 μm) in diameter. The light microscope must therefore be used to see bacteria, which often range from 0.5 to 2 μm in size. Detection of such small objects depends on resolving power (R), which is the ability to distinguish between two adjacent points. Resolving power of the compound light microscope is determined by the wavelength of light (λ) and a characteristic of the objective lens, the numerical aperture (NA). This relationship, expressed as $R = \lambda/NA$, becomes $R = \lambda/2NA$ when the microscope is equipped with a condenser. Numerical aperture is determined by the product of the refractive index (n) of the medium, usually air ($n = 1$) or oil ($n \cong 1.5$), between the lens and the object examined and the sine of half the angle (θ) formed by light rays entering the lens from a point on the object examined when centered under the lens. Numeric aperture is then calculated as $NA = n \sin \theta/2$. Because the range of visible light is fixed (0.4 to 0.7 μm), resolution with the oil immersion objective (NA usually 1.25) at best becomes 0.4 μm/(2 × 1.25), or 0.16 μm. Because green light at about 0.55 μm is best detected by the human eye, the usual limit of light microscopy resolution is approximately 0.3 μm. In brightfield microscopy, objects appear dark in a brightly lighted field. Bacterial cells are not easily seen unless suspended in glycerol or nonaqueous solutions that enhance differences in refractive index or unless the cells are stained. Capsules can be stained or visualized as halos around cells suspended in india ink. Flagella and pili are below the limit of resolution and must be specially stained with dyes.

Phase Contrast Microscopy. The phase contrast light microscope enhances small differences in refraction caused by cellular substructures but reveals only gross details of internal bacterial structure. Capsules, endospores, cytoplasmic particles, and cell wall can be observed.

Phase contrast is achieved by causing beams of partly out-of-phase light waves to interact (after passing through the

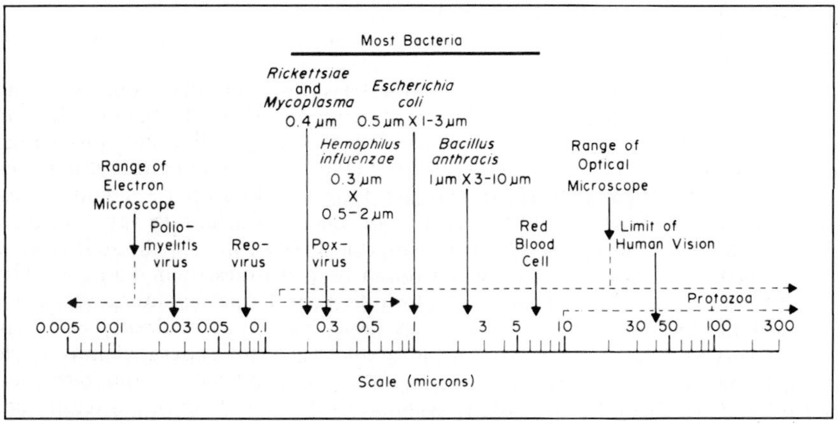

Fig. 3–2. Relative sizes of bacteria.

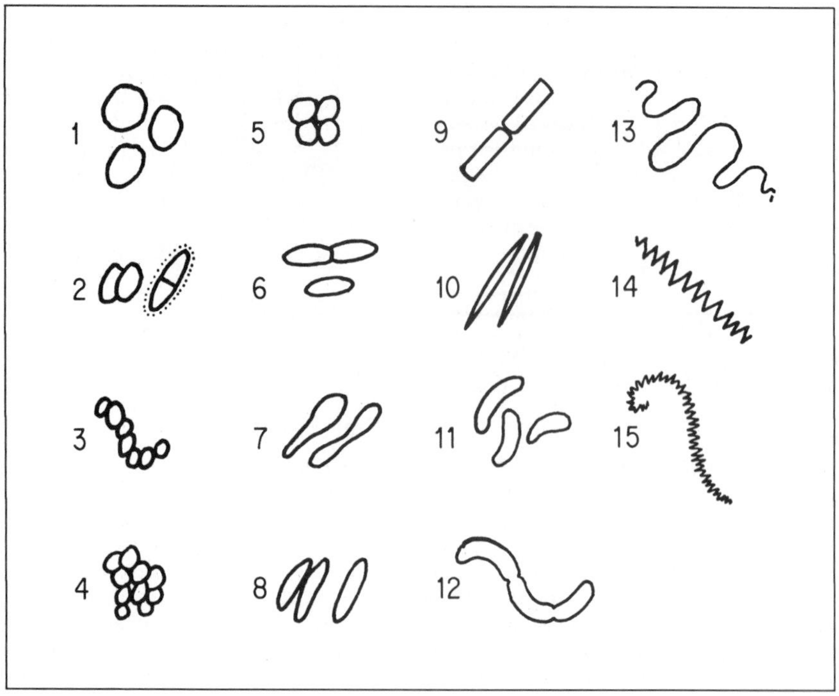

Fig. 3–3. Morphology. 1. Single cocci. 2. Cocci in pairs. 3. Cocci in chains. 4. Cocci in clusters. 5. Cocci in tetrads. 6. Coccobacilli. 7. Club-shaped bacilli. 8. Bacilli with rounded ends. 9. Bacilli with square ends. 10. Fusiform bacilli. 11. Vibrios. 12. *Spirillum*. 13. *Borrelia*. 14. *Treponema*. 15. *Leptospira*.

object) to yield increases in light wave amplitude when in phase or decreases (darkness) when out of phase. The phase contrast system is essentially composed of two annular rings, one in the condenser diaphragm and the other in the objective lens. The annular diaphragm allows only a ring of light to pass through the condenser and specimen on a glass slide to the objective lens. The objective lens contains a phase disk made of optically clear glass that has on it a phase ring of dielectric material. Incident light from the phase condenser normally passes through this phase ring in the objective lens, resulting in a phase shift of one-quarter wavelength, that is, $\lambda/4$. However, when the incident light from the condenser passes through a specimen, substructures of different densities and thickness reflect, refract, or diffract light rays that pass through them. Refracted rays passing through the optically clear portion of the objective lens phase disk interact with light waves that passed through the phase rings. The result is a range of enhanced brightness (i.e., increased wave amplitude), where the two are in phase, to enhanced darkness, where the two waves are out of phase and interfere (i.e., decreased wave amplitude), hence the term *phase contrast*.

Interference Microscopy. Interference microscopes based on dual-beam optical systems generally achieve slightly less resolution but more depth and dimensional effect than the phase contrast microscope. They can also be used as an extremely accurate optical balance for the measurement of cellular components (usually of eucaryotes) down to 1×10^{-14} g, based on the well-known change in refractive index of 0.0018 per 1% change dry weight of substance in solution.

Darkfield Microscopy. This technique produces a black background against which objects appear brightly. A special condenser blocks direct illumination and directs light at an angle such that no incident light reaches the objective lens. If a specimen scatters light by reflection or refraction, light will enter the objective lens. The specimen appears brilliantly illuminated against the black background. This technique is valuable in examination of unstained organisms in fluid suspensions and has been effectively used to demonstrate the very thin spirochete that causes syphilis, *Treponema pallidum*.

Confocal Laser Scanning Microscopy. This system combines conventional microscope optics with a laser light source and sophisticated computer-controlled mechanical and electronic devices to develop images at different planes chosen within an object. The high-energy laser light source passes through conventional optics and a mechanical beam splitter in an *X-Y* scanning plane and interacts with the specimen at the first plane of focus. The plane of focus is controlled as in conventional microscopy, or by computer. The lower energy fluorescent light emitted by the object returns through the microscope optics and scanner and onto a pinhole aperture at the second related point of focus necessary for confocal microscopy. Light signals detected are processed electronically to form an image of the scanned area. A computer controls all mechanical and electronic operations in addition to image storage and processing. This allows development of serial sections for three-dimensional reconstruction as well as vertical cross-sections.

The Electron Microscope

Bacterial ultrastructure was demonstrated only after the development of the transmission electron microscope (TEM), which has a resolving power of about 0.001 μm, or some 200 times that of the light microscope. Transmission electron microscopy develops an image resulting from the variable electron density (stopping power) of the specimen interposed in the electron beam. Specimens must be fixed, stained, and dried. Improved techniques of fixation, embedding, and thin sectioning have gradually allowed better definition of structural components. The fine detail of flagella and pili, as well as of the cell envelope, membrane, and the internal cell fine structure, can be visualized by either shadow casting, (i.e., deposition of an electron-dense metal film at an angle) or negative staining procedures. The scanning electron microscope (SEM) has a practical limit of resolution of about 0.005 μm, or five-fold less than that of the TEM. The SEM produces a three-dimensional image by detection at a 90-degree angle of secondary electrons emitted from the specimen surface as a result of bombardment by the primary electron beam.

NEGATIVE STAINING. This technique for observing ultrafine structure uses electron-dense heavy metal salt solutions, such as phosphotungstate, phosphosilicate, or ammonium molybdate, to interface with the surface of the sample to reveal a delicate, finely detailed outline of components.

THIN SECTIONS. Thin sections of 0.1 μm or less, as compared to the usual 2 to 7 μm sections used in light microscopy, allow resolution and study of structures by electron microscopy without interference from other components present in thick sections.

FREEZE ETCHING. This technique involves freezing of specimens in situ with dry ice or liquid nitrogen. The specimen surface is then barely shaved or scratched with a microtome, followed by surface replication with carbon or metal. These preparations allow examination of surface layer and inner membrane structures.

Bacterial Ultrastructure

Flagella and Axial Filaments

Flagella (singular, flagellum) are helical protein filaments of uniform length and diameter responsible for the rapid free swimming motility of many pathogenic bacteria (Fig. 3–4). The flagellum is composed of three parts: the filament, the hook, and the basal body (Figs. 3–5 and 3–6). The basal body, anchored in the plasma membrane, is composed of a rod and two or more sets of encircling rings contiguous with the plasma membrane, peptidoglycan, and, in the case of gram-negative bacteria, the outer membrane of the cell envelope (Fig. 3–6).

Pseudomonads may have either one polar flagellum (monotrichous), a tuft of several polar flagella (lophotrichous), or flagella at both poles (amphitrichous). By contrast, motile enterobacteria (e.g., *Salmonella*) or *Bacillus* species may have flagella distributed over the entire cell surface and are said to be "peritrichous." Flagella may vary in number from a few, as in some *Escherichia coli,* up to several hundred per cell, as is observed on *Proteus* species. Flagellated *Proteus* species sometimes swarm as a thin film of growth on agar media surfaces. This phenomenon gave rise to the term *H antigen* (flagellar antigen), derived from the German word *Hauch,* indicating a spreading film of growth, like breath condensing on a cold glass surface. In contrast, the term *O* for the somatic O surface antigen of nonflagellated forms derives from the German term *Ohne Hauch* (without film), indicating a nonspreading type of growth.

Bacterial motility can be observed microscopically in fluid suspensions (in a hanging drop or under a coverslip), by spread of bacterial growth as a film over agar, or as turbidity spreading through soft (e.g., 0.5%) semisolid agar. Flagella may be detected by darkfield or phase contrast microscopy and in stained preparations by light and electron microscopy. Flagellated cells react with specific flagella antisera to give a typical, loose, flocculent agglutination, especially useful in diagnostic identifications. Serologic agglutination is used in the identification of *Salmonella* species that alternately produce one of two flagellar filament antigens specified by separate structural genes (the *H* genes) by a process known as *phase variation.*

Flagella are not required for viability. Flagella are removed by shaking with glass beads or by agitation in a blender. The cells remain viable and regain motility as the flagella regrow. Newly synthesized flagellin monomers appear at the distal tip of the growing flagellum. Flagella production is controlled by nutritional need or physiologic energy charge level. Cells of *E. coli* grown in the presence of glucose are inhibited from producing flagella by catabolite repression (Chap. 4). Flagellated cells, on the other hand, are able either to search for nutrients or to avoid poisons by following a gradient either toward a chemoattractant or away from a repellent.

Flagella propel the cell by spinning around their long axis, like a propeller. Flagellar rotation is powered by proton current. Flagellar function is governed by chemotactic responses, indicating a sensory feedback regulation system. Multiple flagella rotate counterclockwise to form a coordinated bundle and effect cell movement generally in the direction of a nutrient (i.e., positive chemotaxis). In the presence of a repellent, coordination is lost, the flagellar bundle becomes disorganized, and the cell tumbles and tends to move away from the repellent. Coordination of flagellar function involves chemoreceptors, known as "periplasmic binding proteins," that interact in membrane transport and at the methylation level of a specific plasma membrane protein. In the presence of chemoattractants, the methylation level of this protein is increased, whereas in the presence of a repellent, the methylation level is decreased or nil.

Axial Filaments. The spirochetes, i.e., the treponemes, leptospires, and borrelia, move by a traveling helical wave, a type of motion that allows penetration of viscous media. These bacteria produce flagellum-like axial filaments around which the cell is coiled (Fig. 3–7). These filaments occur in the periplasmic space between the inner and outer membranes of the cell (Fig. 3–8). *Treponema microdentium* produces two filaments per cell, *Treponema reiteri* produces six to eight, and some species produce many more. The filaments do not run from one pole of the cell to the other; instead, they originate at opposite poles of the cell and overlap at the center with no obvious connection. Axial filaments are suggested to mimic planetary drive gears by rotating against the cell body, imparting to it a twisting screwlike motion opposite in rotation to that of axial filament spin.

Microfibrils: Fimbriae and Sex Pili (Adhesins, Lectins, Evasins, and Aggressins)

Fimbriae, also called pili or common pili, are hairlike microfibrils of 0.004 to 0.008 μm, observable by electron microscopy on the surface of various bacteria (Fig. 3–4). They are straighter, thinner, and shorter than flagella. Like flagella,

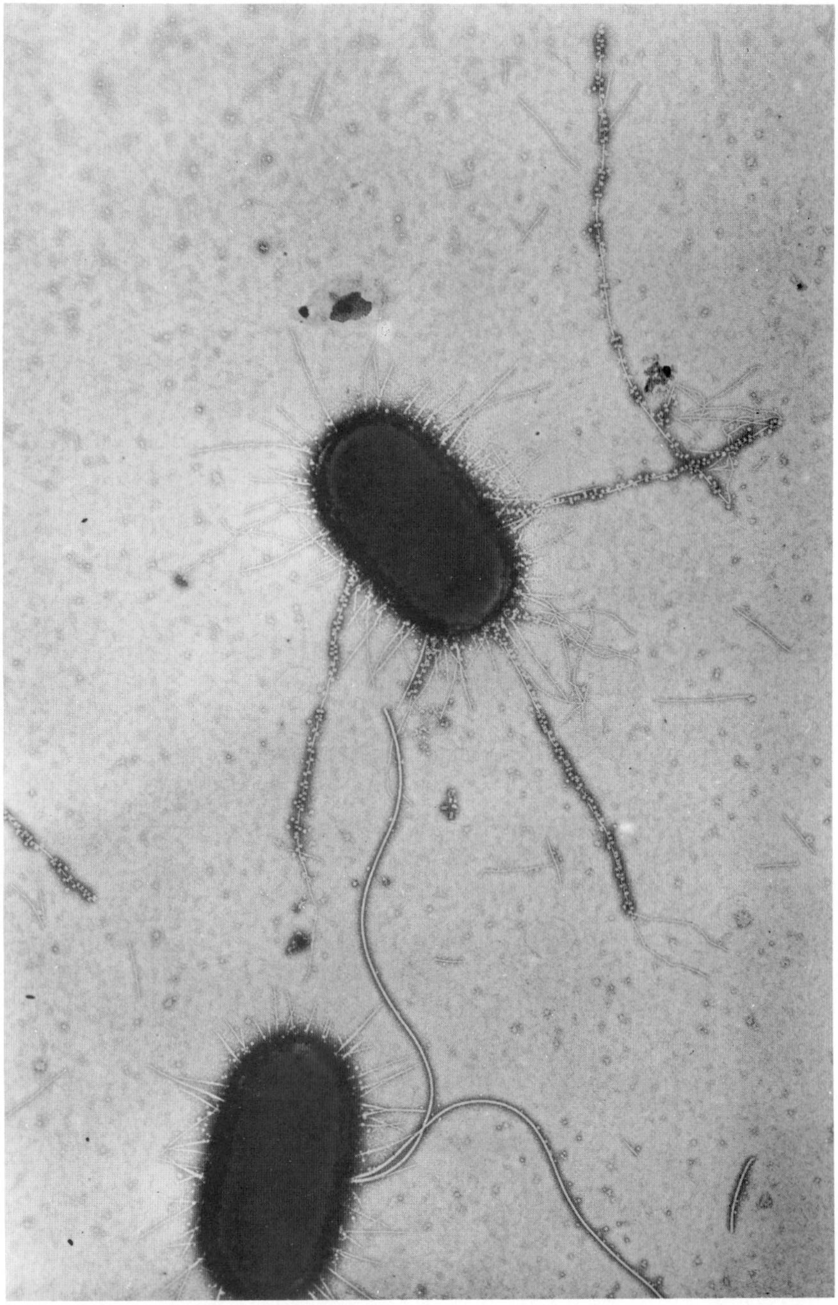

Fig. 3–4. Transmission electron microscopy of negatively stained *E. coli* K12 Hfr Cavalli. Note two long, large flagella, F-type sex pili with round RNA bacteriophage adsorbed to their sides and filamentous DNA bacteriophage adsorbed to their tips, and phage-free, short common pili. *(Courtesy of Dr. Charles C. Brinton.)*

fimbriae are composed of self-aggregating monomers, forming strands that originate in the plasma membrane. One of the best sources of richly piliated bacteria is the infected urinary tract.

Fimbriated cells adhere to interfaces, hydrophobic surfaces, and specific receptors. Fimbriae are, therefore, thought to afford bacteria survival advantagese in host-parasite interactions. Fimbriae, among other bacterial surface components, may therefore be categorized according to functional activities as adhesins, lectins, evasins, aggressins, or sex pili. In infectious disease organisms, fimbriae and other cell surface components may act as specific adherence factors, called adhesins, in host-parasite interactions. Fimbrial adherence specificity may allow a bacterium to adhere to and colonize specific host tissue cells. For example, the 987P, K88, and K99 fimbriae of enteropathogenic (i.e., diarrheal) *E. coli* strains are important in the colonization by this organism of the intestines of piglets and of calves. Moreover, only fimbriated *Neisseria gonorrhoeae* (Kellogg types 1 and 2) are infectious.

The group A *Streptococcus pyogenes* M protein, a known virulence factor, serves as an adherence factor (adhesin) in colonization of the pharynx and, unless neutralized with specific antiserum, also prevents phagocytosis (acts as an evasin) and, finally, is leukocidal (acts as an aggressin or toxin). Fimbriae may also fall into a category of proteins known as *lectins,* also found in plants and animals, that bind to specific

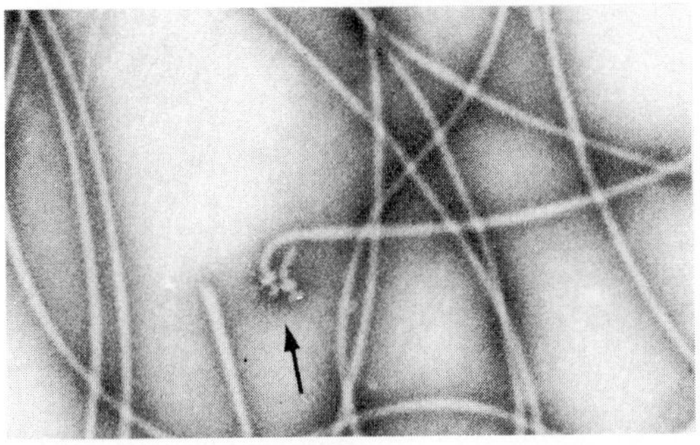

Fig. 3–5. Isolated basal body-hook complex and flagellar filaments from *E. coli*. *(From DePamphlis and Adler: J Bacteriol 105:384, 1971.)*

sugars on cell surfaces. For example, the adhesion of *Shigella flexneri* and *E. coli* fimbriae to red blood cells and tissues (e.g., intestinal cells) is specifically inhibited by D-mannose and α-D-methylmannoside. In a similar manner, fimbriae specific for binding α-methyl-D-galactose (*Pseudomonas aeruginosa*), D-galactose (*S. pyogenes*), L-fucose or D-mannose (*V. cholerae*), and a β-D-galactose-containing oligosaccharide (*N. gonorrhoeae*) have been reported.

Fimbriae of different strains of *N. gonorrhoeae* show great antigenic variation. This occurs because of variation of fimbrial monomer units that are comprised of variable antigenic terminal peptide domains and a common nonantigenic, conserved, peptide domain: the latter is antigenic only when isolated by chemical means. The antigenic variability of gonococcal fimbriae thus appears to be another type of the phenomenon of host immune system evasion by parasite antigenic variation. On this basis, gonococcal fimbriae could be called *evasins*.

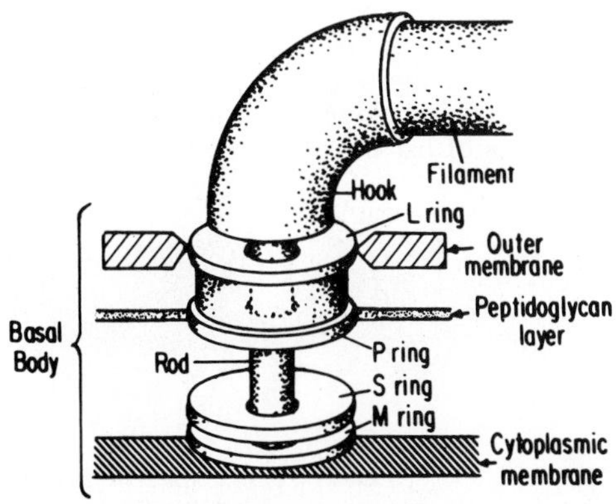

Fig. 3–6. Idealized interpretive diagram of hook–basal body ring structures and integration into the cell envelope of *E. coli*. The top pair of rings are connected near their periphery and resemble a closed cylinder. The individual rings are referred to as the *L ring* (for attachment to outer-lipopolysaccharide-O-antigen complex membrane of the cell wall), the *P ring* (for its association with the peptidoglycan layer of the cell wall), the *S ring* (for supramembrane, which appears to be located just above the cytoplasmic membrane), and the *M ring* (for its attachment to the cytoplasmic membrane). *(Adapted from DePamphlis and Adler: J Bacteriol 105:396, 1971.)*

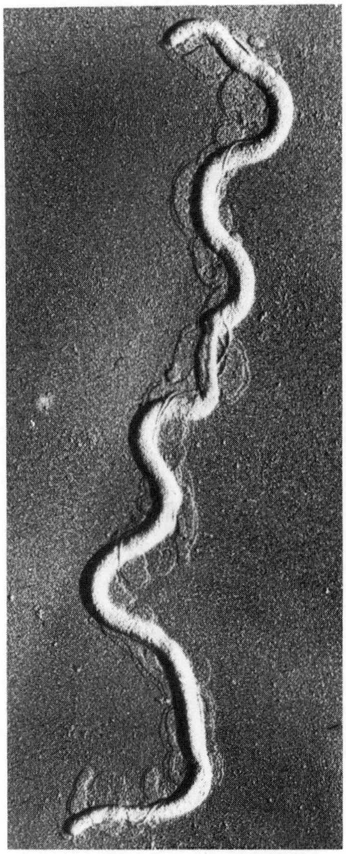

Fig. 3–7. Axial filaments of *Treponema zuelzera* after treatment with distilled water to disrupt outer envelope. Shadowed with gold-palladium. A single axial filament originates at each pole. In the region of overlap, the two filaments have separated from each other and from the cell. × 15,000. *(From Barrier et al: J Bacteriol 105:413, 1971.)*

Microfibrils of gram-negative bacteria are often referred to as common pili (fimbriae) or as sex pili, according to function. They may occur independently or simultaneously on the same cell (Fig. 3–4). Some 100 to 200 ordinary fimbriae may be evenly distributed over the cell surface of *E. coli*, compared to only 1 to 4 sex pili found at random sites. Sex pili function in cell-to-cell adhesion in bacterial conjugation. Sex pili are detected by the ability of cells to donate genes to recipients, by the presence of specific sex pilus antigen, or by the ability of the suspected pilus-bearing bacteria to inactivate certain bacteriophages, which attach specifically to sex pili. Specific RNA phages attach along the sex pilus filament, whereas filamentous DNA phages attach to the pilus tips (Fig. 3–4).

Microfibrillar structures have also been implicated in the gliding and slow twitching motion of nonflagellated bacteria (surface translocation).

The Cell Envelope

The bacterial cell envelope includes the plasma membrane, the overlying cell wall, specialized proteins or polysaccharides,

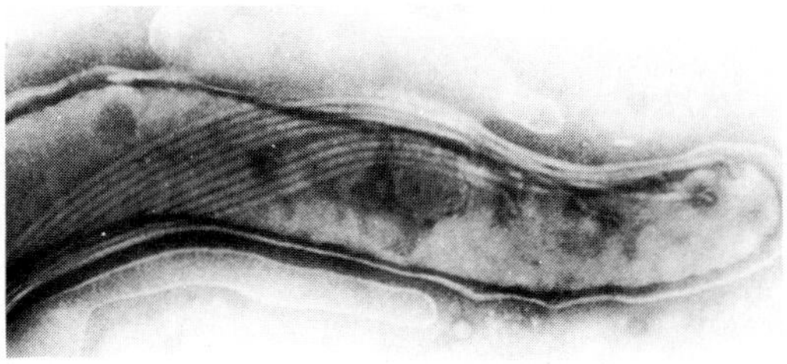

A

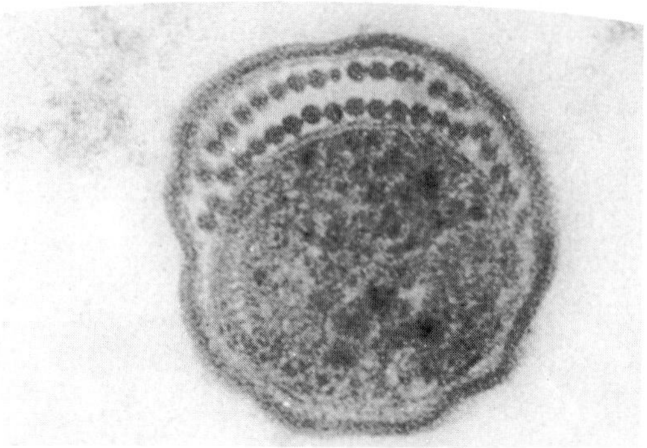

B

Fig. 3–8. Axial filament of spirochetes from the mouth. **A.** End of a negatively stained cell showing multifibrilla axial filament. Insertion points of two fibrils are visible at the ple of the cell. × 60,000. **B.** Cross-section of a spirochete showing location of axial fibrils between outer membrane and cytoplasmic membrane. × 185,000. *(From Listgarten and Socransky: J Bacteriol 88:1087, 1964.)*

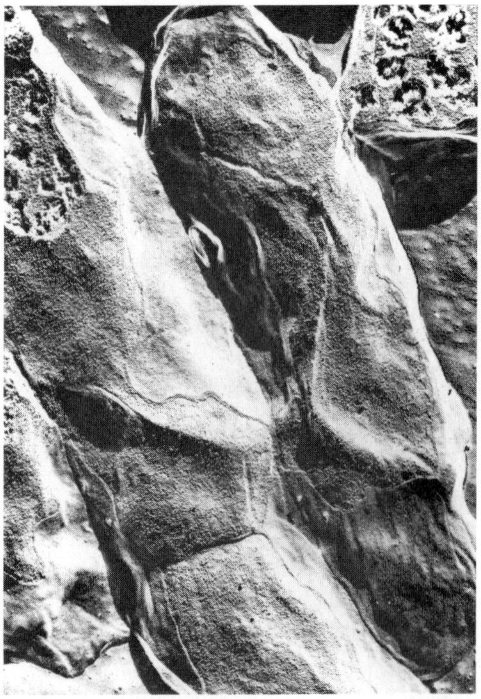

Fig. 3–9. Structure of *Escherichia coli* after freeze etching. The cell on the left is dividing. Areas of intact cell surface can be seen on either side of the centrally exposed cytoplasmic membrane, which is studded with particles. Two distinct envelope layers can be seen at the cut surfaces above the plasma membranes and are especially visible on the cell on the right. At the upper left and right, the cells have been transected, showing granular cytoplasm and holes that contain some fibrillar material, presumably DNA. *(From Bayer and Remsen: J Bacteriol 101:304, 1970.)*

and any outer adherent materials. This multilayered organelle (Fig. 3–9) of the procaryotic cell comprises some 20% or more of the cell dry weight. The bacterial cell envelope contains transport sites for nutrients and receptor sites for bacterial viruses and bacteriocins, influences host-parasite interactions, is the site of antibody and complement reactions, and often contains components toxic to the host.

Capsules and Slimes

Virulence of pathogens often correlates with capsule production. Virulent strains of pneumococci produce capsular polymers that protect the bacteria from phagocytosis. These bacteria form watery mucoid (M) or smooth (S) colonies on solid media in contrast to non-capsule-forming rough (R) strains. Loss of capsule-forming ability by S to R mutation correlates with loss of virulence and increased ease of destruction by phagocytes but does not affect viability.

Capsules form gels that tend to adhere to the cell, whereas slimes and extracellular polymers are more easily washed off. Capsules are easily visualized by negative staining. A capsule appears as a halo of light surrounding a cell suspended in india ink (Fig. 3–10) under the microscope. Capsules may also be specially stained. If cells produce no visually demonstrable capsule and still react serologically with anticapsule sera, they are said to produce microcapsules.

The Cell Wall

The cell wall, found in all free-living pathogenic bacteria except *Mycoplasma,* protects the cell from bursting in low osmotic pressure environments and maintains cell shape. This can be demonstrated by plasmolysis, by isolation of the particulate envelope after mechanical disruption of the bacterial cell, or by lysozyme digestion. The isolated cell wall retains the shape of the cell: envelopes of cocci resemble grape hulls, whereas envelopes of bacilli appear as long deflated balloons

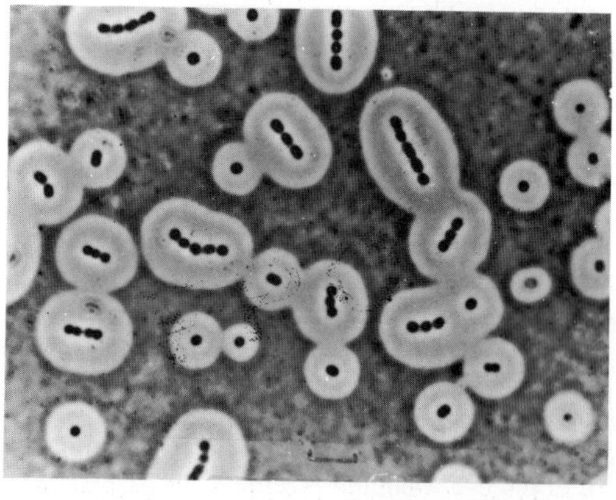

Fig. 3–10. Demonstration of capsules of *Acinetobacter calcoaceticus* (*Bacterium anitratum*) cells suspended in india ink and observed by phase contrast microscopy. *(From Juni and Heym: J Bacteriol 97:461, 1964.)*

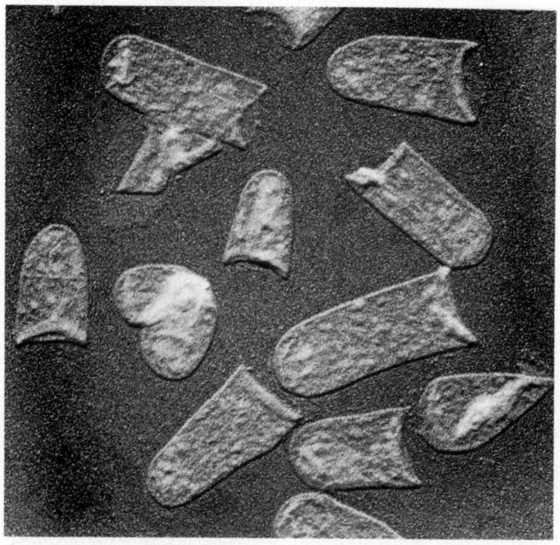

Fig. 3–11. Electron micrograph of cell envelopes of *Mycobacterium tuberculosis*. × 22,000. *(From Ribi et al: Proc Soc Exp Biol Med 100:647, 1959.)*

(Fig. 3–11). If whole cells or isolated envelopes are treated with lysozyme, the particulate cell walls of eubacteria (but not archaebacteria) characteristically dissolve.

Differences Between Gram-Positive and Gram-Negative Cell Envelopes

Gram-Positive Cell Envelope. Medically important and other gram-positive eubacteria characteristically produce specific surface polysaccharides and proteins associated with the peptidoglycan. The better-known polysaccharides include teichoic acids, many of the pneumococcal capsular substances, and the streptococcal group polysaccharides. Poly-D-glutamic acid polymers are produced by some *Bacillus* species, and the M protein of the group A streptococcus is a virulence factor. Under electron microscopy, thin cross-sections of gram-positive cells reveal a relatively thick, contiguous cell wall layer overlying the plasma membrane, which is lysozyme sensitive. Both protein and polysaccharide may contribute to the layered wall substructure. The serologic type–specific M protein of the group A streptococcus forms a diffuse, thick, externally fimbriate wall layer, which can be removed by trypsin without destroying cell viability.

Gram-Negative Cell Envelope. Gram-negative bacteria exhibit three envelope layers (Fig. 3–12). These are the outer membrane (OM), a middle dense layer which is the cell wall or murein layer, and the inner plasma membrane. The periplasmic space between the outer and cytoplasmic membranes is filled with a gel, known as the periplasmic gel. Both plasma and outer membranes are about 0.0075 μm (75 Å) thick. Both exhibit the typical bileaflet-trilayered sandwich structure seen by transmission electron microscopy of membrane cross-sections: that is, two hydrophilic lamina (layers), 2.5 nm (25 Å) each, sandwich an inner hydrophobic 2.5 nm lamina usually composed of fatty acid alkyl chains (Fig. 3–12). A helical lipoprotein, one third of which is covalently linked at one end to the outer surface of the peptidoglycan, inserts its lipid end into the outer membrane, anchoring the outer membrane to the cell. The envelope can be isolated free of soluble cytoplasm by cell rupture and differential centrifugation. The inner membrane may be dissolved with mild nonionic detergent, leaving the outer membrane bound to insoluble peptidoglycan. The outer membrane can be disrupted by EDTA, strong ionic detergent, aqueous phenol, or butanol extraction.

OUTER MEMBRANE (OM). The outer membrane (Fig. 3–12) contains lipopolysaccharide (LPS) (also known as the somatic O surface antigen or endotoxin), phospholipids, and unique proteins that differ from those of the plasma membrane. The inner and outer leaflets of the outer membrane are also uniquely asymmetrical. In enteric bacteria (e.g., *Salmonella*), phosphatidylethanolamine occurs almost entirely in the inner leaflet (cell side), whereas the anionic, hydrophilic lipopolysaccharide occurs only in the outer leaflet of the outer membrane. In *Neisseria* and *Haemophilus* species, phospholipid occurs in both the OM inner and outer leaflets. Proteins known as porins which occur in the outer membrane form transmembrane diffusion channels. Porins serve as channels for small-molecular-weight water-soluble substances or as bacteriophage (virus) receptors.

ADHESION SITES (BAYER JUNCTIONS). In gram-negative cells, points of connection between inner and outer membranes are known as adhesion sites or Bayer junctions, (Fig. 3–13). The Bayer junctions are physiologically active. On the outside they are sites of bacteriophage attachment–DNA injection and complement-mediated lysis. Internally, adhesion sites appear to be growth zones (as sites of periannular septa), and they serve as sites for translocation of secretory protein, outer membrane proteins, lipopolysaccharides, and capsular polysaccharides and as emergence sites for sex pili and flagella.

Protoplasts and Spheroplasts

Bacteria ordinarily lyse in water or serum when the rigid cell wall peptidoglycan layer of the cell envelope is dissolved by lysozyme or other agents. However, if stabilized by hypertonic solutions of sucrose or salts (0.2 to 0.5 M, depending on the organism), a wall-less, osmotically sensitive spherical body called a *protoplast* is liberated. If envelope components are retained, the osmotically sensitive body is called a *spheroplast*. Gram-positive bacteria generally yield protoplasts, whereas gram-negative organisms yield spheroplasts since some outer membrane components inevitably are retained. Spheroplasts can also be produced by growth in hypertonic environments in the presence of cell wall synthesis inhibitors, such as penicillin (Fig. 3–14).

Periplasm

Periplasm, which occurs in the space between the plasma inner membrane and the outer membrane, may readily be observed in gram-negative bacteria (Fig. 3–15), but not at all or only with difficulty in gram-positive bacteria. This may be explained by the high internal osmotic pressures of gram-positive bacteria (0.05 to 0.2 Pa [5 to 20 atm]) compared to those of gram-negative bacteria (0.03 to 0.05 Pa [3 to 5 atm]). The periplasmic gel space of gram-negative bacteria varies with growth conditions and among individual bacteria. The gel is quite viscous and may be highly ordered in structure. The gel surrounds and is interspersed with the porous peptidoglycan. The periplasmic gel contains membrane-derived oligosaccharides

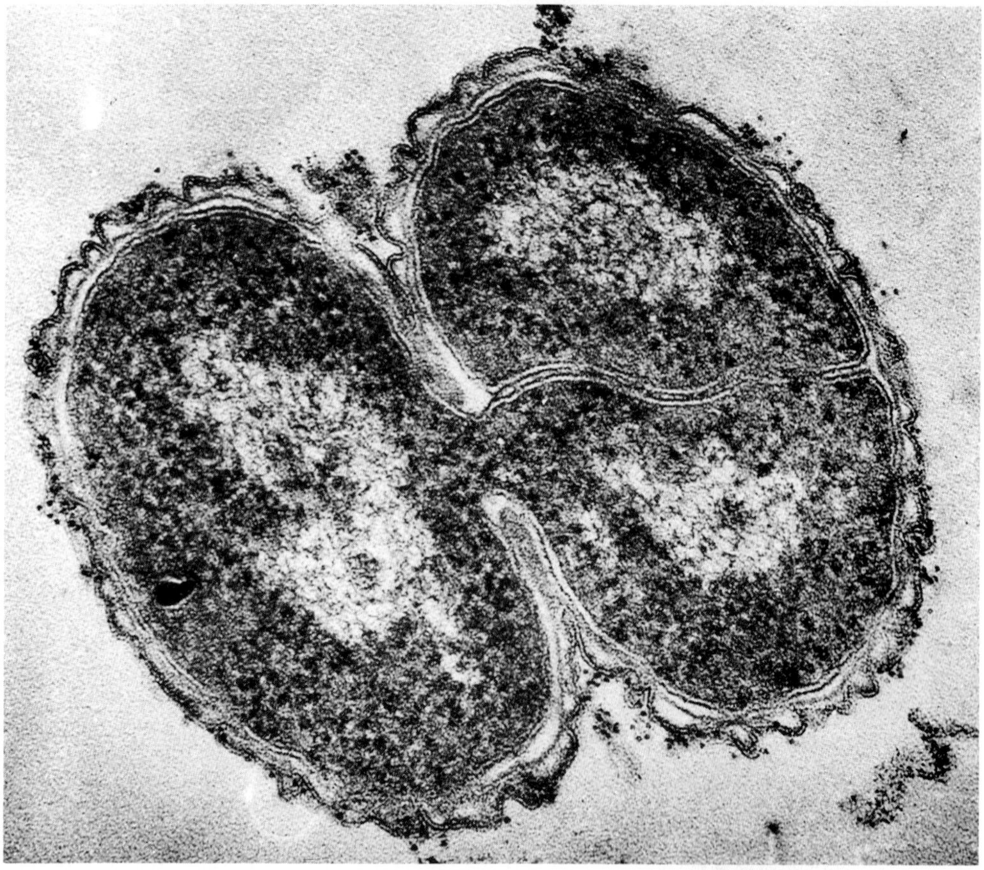

Fig. 3–12. Transverse thin section of *Veillonella parvula.* The layered structure of the gram-negative cell envelope includes a convoluted outer unit membrane, a middle dense layer, and the plasma unit membrane. Note formation of division septa and fibrillar chromatin network in the cell interior. Dark spots of ferritin-labeled O-specific antibody are found primarily on the outside surface of the outer membrane. *(From Bladen and Mergenhagen: Ann NY Acad Sci 2:288, 1966.)*

(MDO) that occur in inverse proportion to the osmolarity of the growth medium, various hydrolytic enzymes such as phosphatases, nucleases, plasmid-controlled β-lactamases (penicillinases), and proteins that specifically bind sugars, transport materials, amino acids, and inorganic ions. These can be released from the cell by osmotic shock, i.e., rapid dilution of hypertonic (0.5 M sucrose) cell suspensions, after EDTA treatment.

The Plasma Membrane

Beneath the rigid cell wall layer and in close association with it is the delicate cytoplasmic membrane, vitally important to the cell. In thin sections the plasma membrane shows a typical trilaminar sandwich structure of dark-light-dark layers by electron microscopy (Fig. 3–12).

Membrane as Osmotic Barrier. Although bacteria are regarded as extremely tolerant of osmotic changes in their external environment, their protoplasts undergo either plasmolysis (shrinkage) or plasmoptysis (swelling) when placed in appropriate media. Placing cells in hypertonic solutions results in plasmolysis, that is, shrinkage of the membrane and cytoplasm from the cell wall (Fig. 3–13). Gram-negative cells are more easily plasmolyzed than are gram-positive cells, which correlates with their relative internal osmotic pressures.

The osmotic barrier in bacteria is indicated by their ability to concentrate certain amino acids against gradients. In gram-positive bacteria, a gradient of 300- to 400-fold may exist across the surface layers. Phosphate esters, amino acids, and other solutes contribute to the internal osmotic pressure. Osmotic activity is also indicated by selective permeability toward various compounds.

Membrane Components. Membranes account for some 30% or more of the cell weight. Membranes contain 60% to 70% protein, 30% to 40% lipid, and small amounts of carbohydrate. Phosphatidylethanolamines (75%), phosphatidylglycerol (20%), and glycolipids are found as major constituents. Choline, sphingolipids, polyunsaturated fatty acids, inositides, and steroids are generally absent. Pathogenic mycoplasma incorporate steroids from the environment into their plasma membranes. Glycolipids include diglycosyldiglycerides, found primarily in gram-positive bacterial membranes, which also contain lipoteichoic acids. A 55-carbon polyisoprenoid alcohol known as undecaprenol or bactoprenol occurs in small amounts.

Various enzymic activities are associated with membrane proteins. These include the energy-producing bacterial cytochrome and oxidative phosphorylation system, the membrane permeability systems discussed in later chapters, and various polymer-synthesizing systems. An ATPase has been isolated from knoblike membrane structures similar to those found in

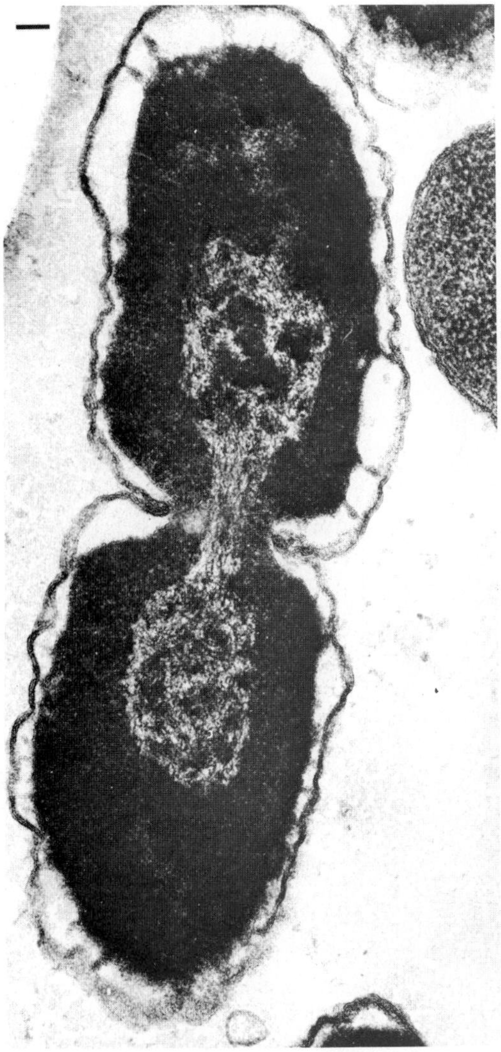

Fig. 3–13. Plasmolyzed dividing cell of *Escherichia coli* B in an almost longitudinal section. Note adhesion sites (Bayer junctions) between outer and inner cytoplasmic membranes and division of nuclear material in the central portion. Bar equals 0.1 μm. *(From Bayer: J Gen Microbiol 53:395, 1968.)*

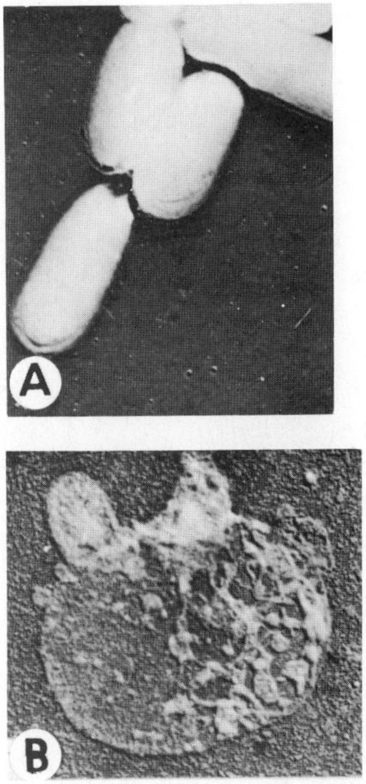

Fig. 3–14. Spheroplast of *E. coli* W 173-25. **A.** Untreated cells. **B.** Cell treated for 90 minutes with 500 units of penicillin. (× 9000.) *(From Schwarz et al: J Mol Biol 41:419, 1969.)*

eucaryotic mitochondria. Up to 90% of the ribosomes may be isolated as a membrane-polyribosome-DNA aggregate.

Mesosomes. Mesosomes are usually seen as membrane-associated cytoplasmic sacs in gram-positive cells that contain lamellar, tubular, or vesicular structures; these are often associated with division septa (Fig. 3–16). Attachment of mesosomes to both DNA chromatin and membrane has been demonstrated by thin-section electron microscopy.

Cytoplasmic Structures

The Nuclear Body. Bacterial DNA can be detected as nucleoids or chromatin bodies by light microscopy using Feulgen staining. It is difficult to demonstrate chromatin bodies by direct staining because of the high concentration of RNA, which can be removed by pretreatment with ribonuclease. Chromatin bodies can then be seen at all stages of the growth cycle.

Electron microscopy of stained thin sections reveals nuclear material as an irregular, thin, fibrillar (DNA) network, which frequently runs parallel to the axis of the cell (Fig. 3–13). A direct attachment to the membrane is sometimes

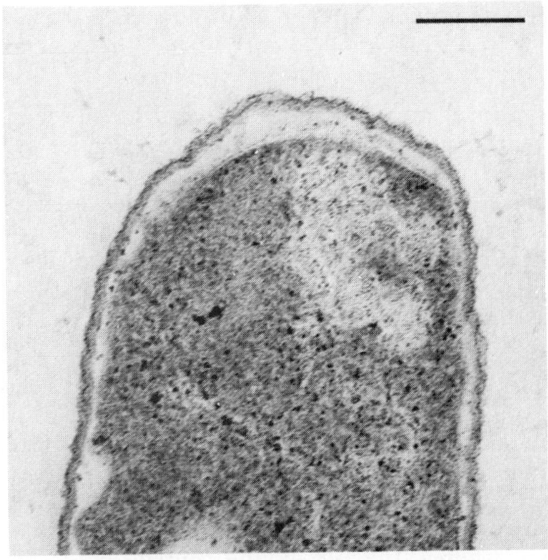

Fig. 3–15. Periplasmic space of *Citrobacter freundii* shown in thin section. Bar equals 0.2 μm. *(Courtesy of Dr. Sara Miller.)*

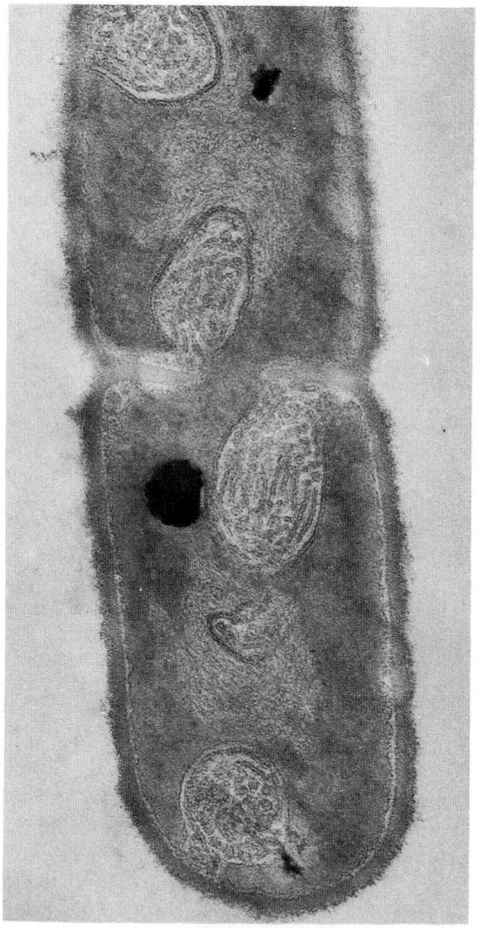

Fig. 3–16. Dividing cell of *Lactobacillus plantarum,* showing prominent mesosomes associated with a newly forming cross-wall. The immature type of mesosome seen at the bottom is not associated with nucleoplasm, in contrast to the upper mature mesosomes, which are surrounded by a triple-layered boundary and are continuous with the nucleoplasm. The black bodies are inclusion granules. × 94,300. *(From Kakefuda et al: J Bacteriol 93:474, 1967.)*

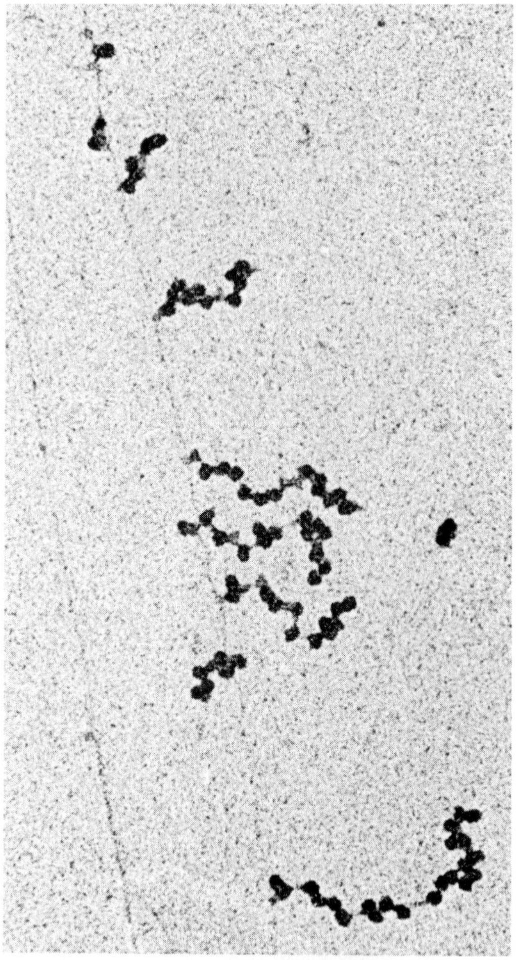

Fig. 3–17. Electron photomicrograph of polyribosomes from *E. coli.* The central long vertical strand is DNA. The wavy lines extending from it are molecules of mRNA to which ribosomes are attached (i.e., polysomes). The gradual increase in length of mRNA from top to bottom indicates that transcription was proceeding in that direction. × 76,350. *(From Hamkalo and Miller: Annu Rev Biochem 42:379, 1973.)*

obvious. During multiplication, bacterial DNA remains as a diffuse chromatin network and never aggregates to form a well-defined chromosome during cell division, in contrast to eucaryotic chromosomes. When bacterial cells are very gently lysed, the bacterial chromosome may be visualized by radioautography as a circular molecule. Although bacterial DNA represents only 2% to 3% of the cell weight, it occupies 10% or more of the cell volume.

Ribosomes. Negatively stained thin sections allow resolution by electron microscopy of small cytoplasmic particles that correspond to the ribosomes present in pellets after lysed protoplasts or disrupted bacterial cells are centrifuged at 100,000 *g*. The 70S bacterial ribosome of about 800,000 Da dissociates into 30S and 50S subunits. The 30S subunit contains 16S RNA, whereas the 50S subunit contains both 23S and 5S RNA. Polyribosome-membrane aggregates contain all components of the protein-synthesizing system; polyribosomes are chains of 70S ribosomes (monomers) attached to messenger RNA (Fig. 3–17). Ribosome numbers vary according to growth conditions: rapid-growing cells in rich medium contain many more ribosomes than do slow-growing cells in poor medium.

Histonelike proteins have only recently been found in small amounts in association with *E. coli* DNA. The occurrence of polyamines, such as putrescine and spermidine, in bacteria is well known.

Cytoplasmic Granules. Granules, identified by appropriate staining procedures, indicate accumulation of food reserves, including polysaccharides, lipids, or polyphosphates (Fig. 3–16). Granules vary with the type of medium and the functional state of the cells. Glycogen is the major storage material of enteric bacteria (40% of the weight of some species). Similarly,

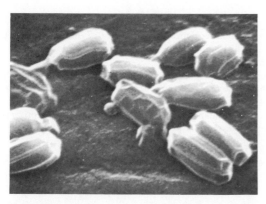

Fig. 3–18. *Bacillus polymyxa* endospores examined in a scanning electron microscopy. Both parallel ribbing and random reticulation of the surface structure are exhibited. × 4800. *(From Murphy and Campbell: J Bacteriol 98:727, 1969.)*

some *Bacillus* and *Pseudomonas* species accumulate 30% or more of their weight as poly-β-hydroxybutyrate. Finally, polyphosphates, also known as metachromatically staining Babès-Ernst or volutin granules, occur in *Corynebacterium diphtheriae*, the plague bacillus (*Yersinia pestis*), mycobacteria (e.g., *Mycobacterium tuberculosis*), and others. Volutin granules stain in various colors, varying from red to blue (i.e., metachromatically), with toluidine blue and methylene blue.

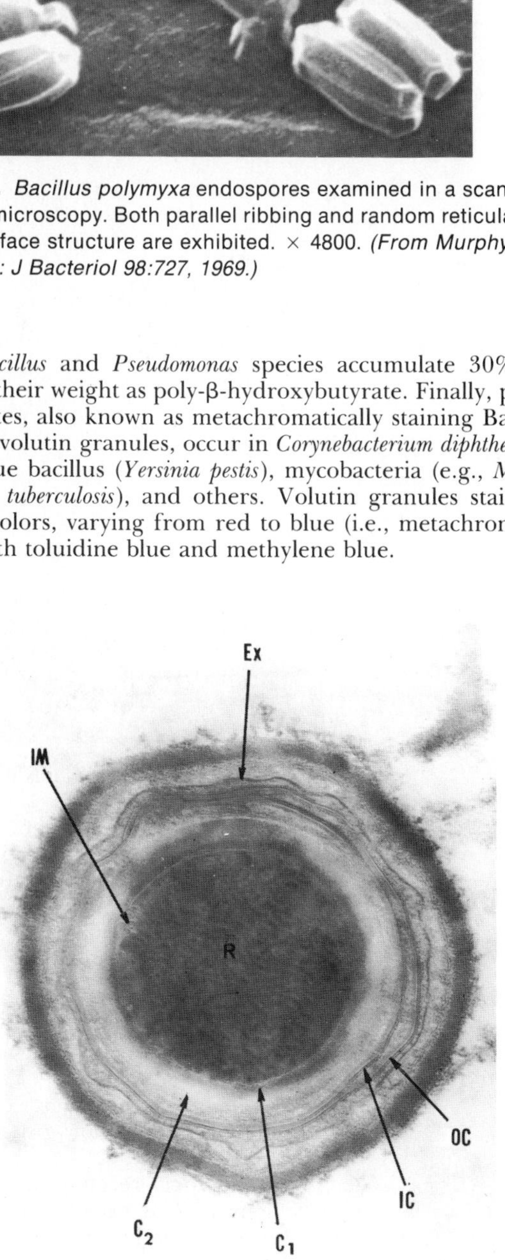

Fig. 3–19. Cross-section of a *Bacillus cereus* endospore before release from parent cell, showing various spore coats and layers. Ex, exosporium; IM, inner membrane; R, ribosomal aggregates; OC, outer coat; IC, inner coat; C_1, inner dense cortical layer; C_2, less dense cortical layer. Note that parent cell still surrounds the exosporium. × 75,000. *(From Ellar and Lundgren: J Bacteriol 92:1748, 1966.)*

Bacterial Endospores

Endospores are notably produced by the aerobic genus *Bacillus* and the anaerobic genus *Clostridium*. Endospores resist adverse environmental conditions of dryness, heat, and poor nutrient supply. The true endospore is a highly refractile body formed within the vegetative bacterial cell. The size, shape, and position of the spore in the mother cell are relatively constant characteristics of a given species (Fig. 3–18). Spore coats include a rigid peptidoglycan layer, which differs in composition from that of the parent vegetative cell. Spore surface antigens usually differ from those of vegetative bacilli (Fig. 3–19).

FURTHER READING

Books and Reviews

Beachey EH: Bacterial adherence: Adhesin-receptor interactions mediating the attachment of bacteria to mucosal surfaces. J Infect Dis 143:325, 1981

Clegg S, Gerlach GF: Enterobacterial fimbriae. Mini Reviews. J Bacteriol 169:934, 1987

Gaastra W, de Graaf FK: Host-specific fimbrial adhesins of noninvasive enterotoxigenic *Escherichia coli* strains. Microbiol Rev 46:129, 1982

Hancock RE: Role of porins in outer membrane permeability. Mini Reviews. J Bacteriol 169:929, 1987

Korhonen TK, Dawes EA, Mäkelä (eds): Enterobacterial Surface Antigens. Methods for Molecular Characterization. New York, Elsevier, 1985

Lindberg AA: Specificity of fimbriae and fimbrial receptors. In Schlessinger D (ed): Microbiology 1982. Washington DC, American Society for Microbiology, 1982, p 317

McNab RM, Aizawa S-I: Bacterial motility and the bacterial flagella motor. Annu Rev Biophys Bioeng 13:51, 1984

Nikaido H, Vaara M: Molecular basis of outer membrane permeability. Microbiol Rev 49:1, 1985

Schoolnik GK, Tal JYT, Gotschlich EC: Receptor binding and antigenic domains of gonococcal pili. In Schlessinger D (ed): Microbiology 1982. Washington DC, American Society for Microbiology, 1982, p 312

Schockman GD, Wicken AJ (eds): Chemistry and Biological Activities of Bacterial Surface Amphiphiles. New York, Academic Press, 1981

Selected Papers

Berg HC: Dynamic properties of bacterial flagellar motors. Nature 249:77, 1974

Berg HC: How spirochetes may swim. J Theor Biol 56:269, 1976

Brass JM, Higgins CF, Foley M, et al.: Lateral diffusion of proteins in the periplasm of *Escherichia coli*. J Bacteriol 165:787, 1986

Cook WR, MacAlister TJ, Rothfield LI: Compartmentalization of the periplasmic space at division sites in gram-negative bacteria. J Bacteriol 168:1430, 1986

Freudl R, Schwarz H, Degen M, Henning U: The signal sequence suffices to direct export of outer membrane protein OmpA of *Escherichia coli* K-12. J Bacteriol 169:66, 1987

Godwin SL, Fletcher M, Burchard RP: Interference reflection microscopic study of sites of association between gliding bacteria and glass substrata. J Bacteriol 171:4589, 1989

Jones CJ, Homma M, MacNab RM: Identification of proteins of the outer (L and P) rings of the flagellar basal body of *Escherichia coli.* J Bacteriol 169:1489, 1987

Jones CJ, MacNab RM: Flagellar assembly in Salmonella typhimurium: analysis with temperature-sensitive mutants. J Bacteriol 172:1327, 1990

MacAlister TJ, MacDonald B, Rothfield LI: The periseptal annulus: an organelle associated with cell division in gram-negative bacteria. Proc Natl Acad Sci USA 80:1372, 1983

Morgan RL, Isaacson RE, Moon HW, et al: Immunization of suckling pigs against enterotoxigenic *Escherichia coli*–induced diarrheal disease by vaccinating dams with purified 987 or K99 pili: Protection correlates with pilus homology of vaccine and challenge. Infect Immun 22:771, 1978

Nikaido H, Rosenberg EY: Porin channels in *Escherichia coli:* Studies with liposomes reconstituted from purified proteins. J Bacteriol 153:241, 232, 1983

Yoshimura F, Zalman LS, Nikaido H: Purification and properties of *Pseudomonas aeruginosa* porin. J Biol Chem 258:2308, 1983

CHAPTER 4

Energy Metabolism

Sources of Energy and Carbon

Bacterial cells, like the cells of all living organisms, accomplish work. For continued viability they require a source of energy. Although the wide variety of substances that serve as a source of energy for microorganisms is almost limitless, there is remarkable simplicity in the basic metabolic patterns by which this energy is transformed into a useful form. Many of these systems are fundamentally similar to those found in mammalian and plant cells, but superimposed on these basic mechanisms are examples of differentiation unique to the bacterial world.

Bacteria can be divided into two large groups on the basis of their carbon requirement, the autotrophic (lithotrophic) bacteria and the heterotrophic (organotrophic) organisms (Table 4–1). The autotrophic bacteria can utilize carbon dioxide as the sole source of carbon and synthesize from it

TABLE 4–1. CLASSIFICATION OF BACTERIA ACCORDING TO SOURCE OF CARBON AND ENERGY

Type	Carbon Source	Energy Source	Electron Donor	Examples
Photolithotrophs	CO_2	Light	Inorganic compounds (H_2S, S)	Green and purple sulfur bacteria
Photoorganotrophs	Organic compounds (in addition to CO_2)	Light	Organic compounds	Purple nonsulfur bacteria
Chemolithotrophs	CO_2	Oxidation-reduction reactions	Inorganic compounds (H_2, S, H_2S, Fe, NH_3)	Hydrogen, sulfur, iron, and denitrifying bacteria
Chemoorganotrophs	Organic compounds	Oxidation-reduction reactions	Organic compounds (glucose)	Most bacteria

the carbon skeletons of all their organic metabolites. They require only water, inorganic salts, and CO_2 for growth. Their energy is derived either from light or from the oxidation of one or more inorganic substances.

Heterotrophic bacteria are unable to utilize CO_2 as the sole source of carbon but require it in an organic form, such as glucose. For the heterotrophic organism, a portion of the organic compound that serves as an energy source is also used for the synthesis of organic compounds required by the organism. All of the bacteria that cause disease in humans are found in this group.

Energy-yielding Metabolism

The systems in bacteria that transform chemical and radiant energy into a biologically useful form include respiration, fermentation, and photosynthesis. In respiration, molecular oxygen is the ultimate electron acceptor, whereas in fermentation, the foodstuff molecule is usually broken down into two fragments, one of which is then oxidized by the other. In photosynthesis, light energy is converted into chemical energy. In all types of cells, however, and regardless of the mechanism used to extract useful energy, the reaction is accompanied by the formation of adenosine triphosphate (ATP). ATP is a common intermediate of both energy-mobilizing and energy-requiring reactions, and its formation provides a mechanism by which the available energy may be channeled into the energy-requiring biosynthetic reactions of the cell.

The metabolic activity of bacteria is very high, as manifested by very high rates of cell division and catabolism. The evolution of heat associated with these processes is much greater than for other organisms. Since the heat produced during metabolism is unavailable for the performance of work, bacteria in general are less efficient as converters of free energy than are organisms with a slower metabolic rate.

Bioenergetics

Principles of Thermodynamics

Fundamentally, the bacterial cell is a physicochemical system whose activities occur in large part by the flow of chemical energy. The same laws of thermodynamics that deal with energy and its transformation also hold in the biologic world. The most useful of these concepts is that of free energy. Knowledge of the free energy change (ΔG) of a reaction tells us whether a reaction may proceed spontaneously or whether it must be driven by other reactions.

The standard free energy change ΔG^{o} for any reaction may be calculated as the difference between the standard free energy of the products and the standard free energy of the reactants:

$$\Delta G^{o}s0 = \Sigma^{o}_{products} - \Sigma G^{o}_{reactants}$$

For the reaction to proceed spontaneously as written, ΔG^{o} must be negative, that is, the products must be lower on the free energy scale than the reactants. Thus, reactions only go downhill energetically, from compounds of higher to those of lower free energy. Reactions that have a positive ΔG^{o} do not occur spontaneously but must be supplied with free energy greater than ΔG^{o} from another source if they are to proceed. In the bacterial cell where work is performed under isothermal conditions, a large fraction of the system's energy cannot be made to perform in the manner required of work. This energy is regarded as unavailable or lost to entropy, and heat is given up by the system to the surroundings.

The free energy change of chemical reactions can in principle be quite accurately measured. Since the equilibrium reached in a chemical reaction is a function of the drive toward minimum free energy of the reaction components, the equilibrium constant is a mathematical function of the free energy change of the components of the reaction. Thus for the reaction

$$A + B \rightleftharpoons C + D$$

the free energy change is

$$\Delta G = G^{o\prime} + RT \ln \frac{[C][D]}{[A][B]}$$

where R is the gas constant, T is the absolute temperature, and the brackets denote initial molar concentrations of reactants and products. The symbol $\Delta G^{o\prime}$ designates the standard free energy change of the reaction. It is a fixed constant for any given chemical reaction and is a measure of the decrease in free energy of the reaction at 25C, at a pH of 7.0, as 1 mole of reactant is converted to 1 mole of product.*

At equilibrium, there is no free energy change, and $\Delta G = 0$. Also,

$$K'_{eq} = \frac{[C][D]}{[A][B]}$$

* The standard free energy change at pH 7.0 is designated by $G^{o\prime}$; that at pH 0.0 by G^{o}.

TABLE 4–2. RELATIONSHIP BETWEEN THE EQUILIBRIUM CONSTANT AND THE STANDARD FREE ENERGY CHANGE AT 25C

K'_{eq}	$\Delta G^{o\prime}$ (cal mol^{-1})
0.001	+4089
0.01	+2726
0.1	+1363
1.0	0
10.0	−1363
100.0	−2726
1000.0	−4089

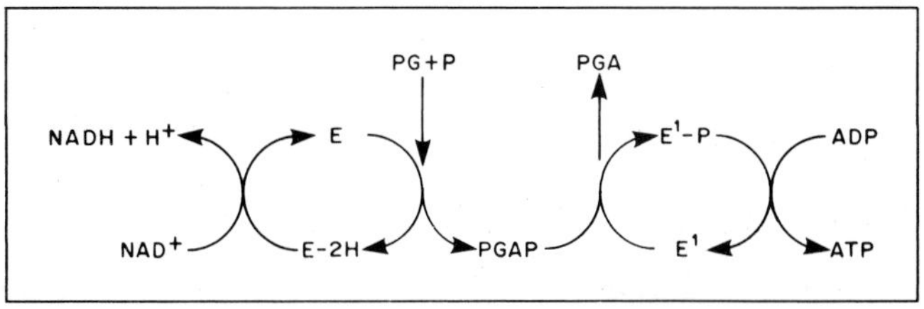
PG+P
PGA
NADH + H+
E
E'-P
ADP
NAD+
E-2H
PGAP
E'
ATP

Fig. 4–1. Primary chemical coupling between the phosphorylation of ADP and the NAD-linked oxidation of 3-phosphoglyceraldehyde (PG) to 3-phosphoglycerate (PGA) via 1,3-diphosphoglycerate (PGAP). E/E-2H and E′/E′-P stand for 3-phosphoglyceraldehyde dehydrogenase and 3-phosphoglycerate kinase, respectively.

By substituting the equilibrium constant K'_{eq} in the above reaction:

$$\Delta G^{o\prime} = -RT \ln K'_{eq}$$

The standard free energy change of any chemical reaction can thus be calculated from its equilibrium constant. Table 4–2 shows the relationship between the equilibrium constant and the standard free energy change. When the equilibrium constant is high, the reaction tends to go to completion, and the standard free energy change is negative. Such a reaction is an exergonic or downhill reaction and proceeds with a decline of free energy. When the equilibrium constant is low, the reaction does not go far in the direction of completion, the free energy change is positive, and energy must be put into the system. Such processes are endergonic or uphill reactions.

Energy from Organic Compounds

The heterotrophic bacterial cell ultimately derives its energy from the chemical energy stored in the molecules of its carbon substrate. The complete oxidation of glucose releases 686 kcal per mole. In *Escherichia coli* about 50% of the glucose is oxidized to CO_2. This results in enough ATP to convert the remaining 50% of the substrate into cell material.

In biologic oxidations as well as in chemical ones, the essential characteristic is the removal of electrons from the substance being oxidized. Since the majority of biologic oxidations involve a dehydrogenation, biologic oxidations may be expressed more simply in terms of the transfer of hydrogen if it is remembered that such a transfer actually involves a loss of electrons. In the transfer of hydrogen from the substrate to a final hydrogen acceptor, reducing equivalents are removed, two at a time, and passed via a graded series of oxidation-reduction systems such that the derivatives en route are alternately reduced and oxidized. The occurrence of several reversible oxidation-reduction reactions between the initial substrate and final oxidant makes for a smoother release of energy, providing a system whereby oxidations involving large amounts of energy resulting from the complete oxidation of a carbohydrate are split into several integrated partial reactions, and the energy is stored or liberated in smaller packets. In this sequence of reactions, chemical energy is transferred from one reaction to another by means of a common intermediate or coupling factor. An example of this common intermediate principle is the coupling between the oxidation of one substrate (AH_2) and the reduction of another (B) by the appropriate AH_2 and BH_2 dehydrogenases in the presence of the specific coupling factor (NAD), which is alternately reduced and oxidized:

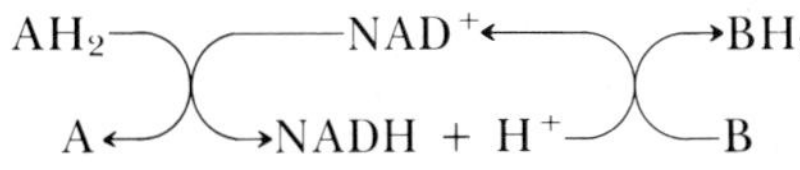
AH2
NAD+
BH2
A
NADH + H+
B

The most important common intermediate, however, in the transfer of chemical energy is ATP. It effectively links or couples enzymatic reactions involving the transfer of phosphate groups (Fig. 4–1).

Free Energy Changes of Oxidation-Reduction Reactions

The calculation of free energy changes for oxidation-reduction reactions is based on the oxidation-reduction potential, a quantitative measure of the ability of the system to accept or donate electrons reversibly with reference to the standard hydrogen electrode. In biologic systems, the normal potential of any two oxidation-reduction systems enables one to predict the direction of interaction. A system with a more positive normal oxidation-reduction potential than another system has a greater tendency to take up electrons, i.e., it is a stronger oxidizing agent. The standard free energy change of oxidative reactions in calories per mole may be calculated from equilibrium data. Some electrode potentials of biochemical interest are shown in Table 4–3.

Key Position of Adenosine Triphosphate

In both aerobic and anaerobic cells, all of the usable energy released by oxidation is transformed to ATP for use in driving the various energy-requiring reactions involved in the biosynthesis of cell material. The amount of ATP available from a particular substrate depends upon whether the organism employs a fermentative type of metabolism or whether the compound is completely oxidized to CO_2 and H_2O (p. 34).

ATP occurs in all types of cells. In the intact cell at pH 7.0, the molecule is completely ionized and exists as a complex with Mg^{2+} (Fig. 4–2). Its free energy of hydrolysis is significantly higher than that of simple esters, glycosides, and many phosphorylated compounds. Molecules, such as ATP, that are characterized by a free energy of hydrolysis at pH 7 more negative than 7 kcal per mole are classified as high-energy compounds. These energy-rich compounds include a number

TABLE 4–3. STANDARD OXIDATION-REDUCTION POTENTIALS OF SOME CONJUGATE REDOX PAIRS

System (pH 7.0)	E'_o, V
$\frac{1}{2}O_2/H_2O$	0.82
NO_3^-/NO_2^-	0.42
Fe^{3+} cytochrome *a*/Fe^{2+}	0.29
Fe^{3+} cytochrome *c*/Fe^{2+}	0.22
Ubiquinone ox/red (pH 7.4)	0.10
Fe^{3+} cytochrome *b*/Fe^{2+} (pH 7.4)	0.07
Fumaric acid/succinic acid	0.03
FMN old yellow enzyme/$FMNH_2$	−0.12
Oxaloacetic acid/malic acid	−0.17
Pyruvic acid/lactic acid	−0.19
Acetaldehyde/ethanol	−0.20
$NAD^+/NADH + H^+$	−0.32
Ferredoxin ox/red (*Clostridium pasteurianum*) (pH 7.5)	−0.42
$H^+/\frac{1}{2}H_2$	−0.42
Acetic acid/acetaldehyde	−0.60

of other important molecules: acetylphosphate, aminoacyladenylates, phosphoenolpyruvate, and the esters of coenzyme A and lipoic acid, all of which serve as a driving force for the various endergonic reactions of the cell.

The standard free energies of hydrolysis of various phosphate compounds are shown in Table 4–4. Compounds with the more negative values have a higher equilibrium constant than those lower in the scale. This scale is thus a quantitative measure of the affinity of the compound for its phosphoryl group. Those high in the scale tend to lose their phosphate groups, and those lower in the scale tend to hold on to their phosphate groups. ATP is unique because its free energy of hydrolysis occupies the midpoint of this thermodynamic scale of phosphorylated compounds. The direction of enzymatic phosphate group transfer is specified by this thermodynamic scale. Phosphate groups are transferred only from compounds of high potential to acceptors of low potential, i.e., down the scale.

The ATP-ADP system functions as an intermediate carrier of phosphate groups. ADP serves as a specific acceptor of phosphate groups from cellular phosphate compounds of very high potential formed during the oxidation of substrate by the cell:

$$\text{Phosphoenolpyruvate} + \text{ADP} \rightleftharpoons \text{Pyruvate} + \text{ATP}$$

The ATP so formed then donates its terminal phosphate group enzymatically to phosphate acceptor molecules, such as

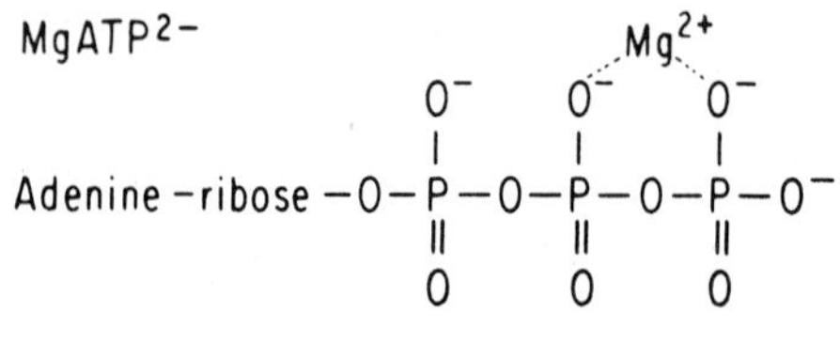

Fig. 4–2. Magnesium complex of ATP.

TABLE 4–4. STANDARD FREE ENERGY OF HYDROLYSIS OF PHOSPHORYLATED COMPOUNDS

	$\Delta G^{o\prime}$ (kcal)	Direction of Phosphate Group Transfer
Phosphoenolpyruvate	−14.8	↓
1,3-Diphosphoglycerate	−11.8	
Acetylphosphate	−10.1	
ATP	−7.3	
Glucose 1-phosphate	−5.0	
Fructose 6-phosphate	−3.8	
Glucose 6-phosphate	−3.3	

glucose, transforming them to phosphate derivatives with a higher energy content:

$$\text{ATP} + \text{D-Glucose} \rightleftharpoons \text{ADP} + \text{D-Glucose 6-phosphate}$$

Generation of ATP. Bacteria utilize two fundamentally different classes of reactions to make energy available. One class consists of those reactions that generate ATP and other energy-rich compounds by substrate-level phosphorylation. Included in this group are ATP-yielding reactions of the glycolytic pathway, arginine fermentation, and a number of bizarre ATP-yielding processes characteristic of clostridia. In these reactions, a part of the energy that is released is initially conserved in energy-rich compounds formed in dehydrogenase (or lyase) reactions and then transferred to the ATP system by kinase reactions (Fig. 4–1). The second general class of reactions for the synthesis of ATP in bacteria includes oxidative phosphorylation and photophosphorylation. In these reactions, during the flow of electrons from the first electron carrier to the final electron acceptor in a catabolic redox sequence, ATP is generated via the mechanism of electron transport phosphorylation.

Energy-yielding Heterotrophic Metabolism

Fermentation and Respiration

Although all heterotrophic microorganisms ultimately obtain their energy from oxidation-reduction reactions, the amount of energy obtained and the mechanisms by which they extract it vary. Two basic mechanisms are employed—fermentation and respiration.

In fermentation, electrons are passed from the electron donor, an intermediate formed in the breakdown of the substrate molecule, to an electron acceptor, which is some other organic intermediate in the fermentation process. Fermentation results in the accumulation of a mixture of end products, some more oxidized and some more reduced than the substrate. The average oxidation level of the end products in a fermentation, however, is always identical to that of the initial substrate. Fermentations are carried out by both obligate and facultative anaerobes (p. 55).

Respiration is a process in which molecular oxygen usually serves as the ultimate electron acceptor. When oxygen is the ultimate acceptor the process is referred to as "aerobic respiration" to distinguish it from anaerobic respiration, in which an inorganic compound, such as nitrate, sulfate, or carbonate, is used.

Fermentation is a less efficient mechanism than respiration for extracting energy from the substrate molecule. When organisms ferment glucose, only a small amount of the energy potentially available in the glucose molecule is released. Most of the energy is still locked up in the product of the reaction, e.g., lactate. When organisms oxidize glucose completely to CO_2 and H_2O, all of the available energy of the glucose molecule is released:

$$\text{Glucose} \rightarrow 2\ \text{Lactate} \qquad \Delta G^{o\prime} = -47.0\ \text{kcal mol}^{-1}$$

$$\text{Glucose} + 6\ O_2 \rightarrow 6\ CO_2 + 6\ H_2O \qquad \Delta G^{o\prime} = -686.0\ \text{kcal mol}^{-1}$$

Among the microorganisms that carry out aerobic respiration are the obligate aerobes and facultative anaerobes. In addition, some of the facultative anaerobes can also employ nitrate as their terminal electron acceptor. However, organisms that use sulfate or carbonate as electron acceptors in anaerobic respiration are obligate anaerobes. A more complete discussion of aerobes and anaerobes is found on p. 55.

Dissimilation of Glucose. Glucose occupies an important position in the metabolism of most biologic forms, and its dissimilation provides a metabolic pathway common to most forms of life. The ability to utilize a sugar or related compound of a configuration different from glucose is the result of the organism's ability to convert the substrate to intermediates common to the pathways for glucose fermentation.

Entry into Cell. The utilization of a specific monosaccharide by an organism also depends on the presence of specific carrier systems for the transport of the sugar across the cell membrane. A diversity of systems of this type occurs. Some of these utilize ATP generated by electron transport. In *E. coli,* the phosphotransferase system derives its energy directly from phosphoenolpyruvate (PEP) rather than from ATP, and phosphorylation of the sugar occurs during transport. Transport systems present in bacteria are discussed on p. 55.

Glycolytic Pathway

Three central routes of intermediary carbohydrate metabolism are present in bacteria—glycolysis, the pentose phosphate pathway, and the Entner-Doudoroff pathway. For most cells, however, the major route of glucose catabolism is glycolysis. In this pathway the glucose molecule is degraded to two molecules of lactic acid without the intervention of molecular oxygen. The basic concepts of glycolysis are incorporated in the 11 enzymatic reactions of the Embden-Meyerhof-Parnas (EMP) scheme, shown in Figure 4–3. Although the basic pathway is the same for all cell types, the properties of certain of the enzymes in the pathway are not uniform in all species or cell types. Such variations have apparently been introduced for purposes of cellular differentiation and control of specific steps in the pathway.

Glycolysis consists basically of two major phases. In the first, glucose is phosphorylated either by ATP or PEP, depending on the organism, and cleaved to form glyceraldehyde 3-PO_4. In the second phase, this three-carbon intermediate is converted to lactic acid in a series of oxidoreduction reactions that are coupled to the phosphorylation of ADP. A mechanism is thus provided for the conservation of the energy originally present in the glucose molecule.

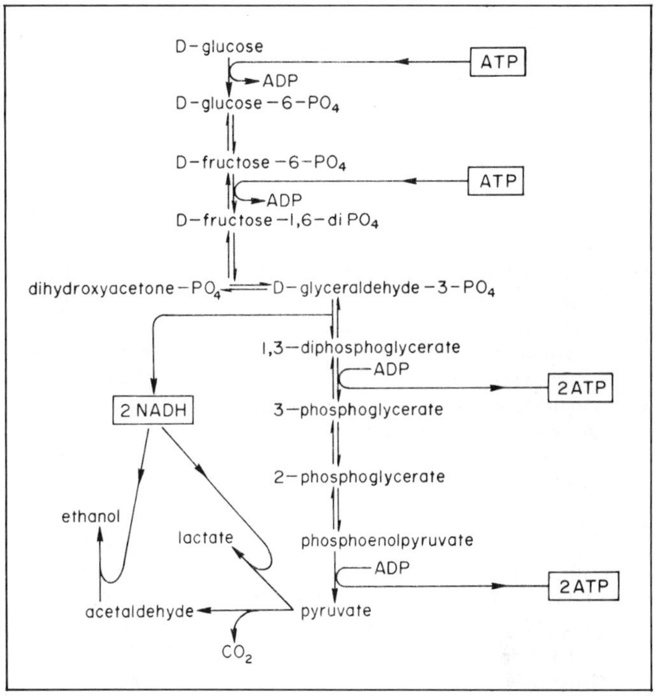

Fig. 4–3. The Embden-Meyerhof-Parnas glycolytic scheme.

Phase I of Glycolysis

The conversion of glucose to glyceraldehyde 3-PO_4 proceeds as follows:

$$\text{Glucose} + \text{ATP} \rightarrow \text{Glucose 6-}PO_4 + \text{ADP} \quad (1)$$

$$\text{Glucose 6-}PO_4 \rightleftharpoons \text{Fructose 6-}PO_4 \quad (2)$$

$$\text{Fructose 6-}PO_4 + \text{ATP} \rightleftharpoons \text{Fructose 1,6-bis}PO_4 + \text{ADP} \quad (3)$$

$$\text{Fructose 1,6-bis}PO_4 \rightleftharpoons \text{Glyceraldehyde 3-}PO_4 + \text{Dihydroxyacetone } PO_4 \quad (4)$$

Reaction 3, the phosphorylation of D-fructose to fructose 1,6-bisphosphate, occupies a strategic position in the glycolytic pathway. Alternate pathways of hexose metabolism diverge from the other hexose phosphates in the earlier part of the pathway. This reaction may be regarded as the first one characteristic of the glycolytic sequence proper and thus constitutes a very important branch and control point, subject to strong metabolic regulation. Phosphofructokinase, the enzyme catalyzing this pathway, is an allosteric enzyme responding to fluctuations in adenine nucleotide levels (p. 50). Control at this point ensures that when an abundant supply of ATP is available, as occurs when lactate and pyruvate are oxidized to CO_2 via the citric acid cycle, glycolysis will be essentially blocked and glucose synthesis will be favored. The reverse is also true. When glycolysis is absolutely required for energy generation, glycolysis will be favored and carbohydrate synthesis turned off.

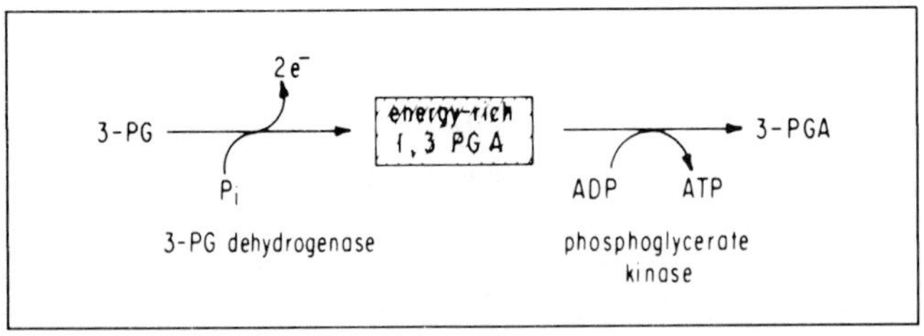

Fig. 4–4. Substrate-level phosphorylation during glycolysis. These two consecutive reactions comprise one of the most important sequences of the glycolytic pathway. In these reactions the energy of oxidation of the aldehyde group in 3-phosphoglyceraldehyde (3-PG) to the carboxylate group in 3-phosphoglycerate (3-PGA) is conserved in the form of ATP. 1,3-Diphosphoglycerate is an energy-rich intermediate in the sequence.

Reaction 4, the cleavage of fructose 1,6-bisphosphate to glyceraldehyde 3-PO_4 and dihydroxyacetone PO_4, is catalyzed by aldolase. Different types of aldolases are produced by different cell types. In bacteria, fungi, and blue-green algae, the aldolases are of class II and differ from the animal class I enzyme in a number of their properties. The products of this reaction are interconvertible by an enzyme, triose phosphate isomerase, that directs most of the dihydroxyacetone phosphate into the central stream of glycolysis. Whereas most of this compound is metabolized via glyceraldehyde 3-phosphate, it has an alternate fate that is essential to lipid metabolism, the formation of glycerol phosphate.

Phase II of Glycolysis

During the second stage of glycolysis, the two molecules of glyceraldehyde 3-PO_4 formed from one molecule of glucose are oxidized in a two-step reaction that leads to the synthesis of ATP:

$$\text{Glyceraldehyde 3-}PO_4 + NAD^+ + P_i \rightleftharpoons \text{1,3-Diphosphoglycerate} + NADH + H^+ \quad (5)$$

$$\text{1,3-Diphosphoglycerate} + ADP \rightleftharpoons \text{3-Phosphoglycerate} + ATP \quad (6)$$

In the first of these reactions, the aldehyde group of glyceraldehyde 3-phosphate is oxidized to the oxidation level of a carboxyl group. The other important component of the reaction is the oxidizing agent nicotinamide adenine dinucleotide (NAD), which accepts electrons from the aldehyde group of glyceraldehyde 3-PO_4. The electrons are then carried to pyruvate that is formed later in the glycolytic pathway.

In the second reaction, the 1,3-diphosphoglycerate that was formed in reaction 5 transfers a phosphate group to ADP, with the resultant formation of 3-phosphoglycerate. As a result of these two reactions, the energy derived from the oxidation of an aldehyde group has been conserved as the phosphate bond energy of ATP.

These two reactions are a prototype example of substrate-level oxidative phosphorylation. In these reactions, the phosphorylation of ADP is coupled to the NAD-linked oxidation of 3-phosphoglyceraldehyde, as shown in Figure 4–4. In this type of coupling, hydrogen is transferred from an initial donor to a final acceptor via transitional intermediates and via intermediate carrier compounds. The intermediate, 1,3-diphosphoglycerate, is the common covalent intermediate in the above reactions.

The dehydration of 2-phosphoglycerate to phosphoenolpyruvate, as shown in Figure 4–3, is the second reaction of the glycolytic sequence in which a high-energy phosphate bond is generated. The formation of this bond involves an internal rearrangement of a phosphorylated molecule, leading to the conversion of a phosphoryl group of low energy into one of high energy. In the subsequent reaction the phosphate group from phosphoenolpyruvate is transferred to ADP, yielding ATP and pyruvate.

Energy Yield

In the glycolytic pathway, a total of 4 moles of ATP are formed per mole of glucose used. Since 2 moles of ATP are used in the initial steps, the net ATP yield is 2 moles per mole of glucose fermented. The stoichiometry observed in the production of pyruvate from hexoses is

$$C_6H_{12}O_6 + 2\,NAD^+ + 2\,ADP + 2\,P_i \rightarrow 2\,CH_3COCOO^- + 2\,NADH + 2\,ATP$$

$$\Delta G^{\circ}y' = 15 \text{ kcal mol}^{-1}$$

Only a very small proportion of the total free energy potentially derivable from the breakdown of a hexose molecule is actually made available via this pathway. This is because of the inherent inefficiency of the system and because the reaction products are compounds in which carbon is still at a relatively reduced level. The ultimate fate of the key metabolite, pyruvate, depends on the means employed for the regeneration of NAD^+ from NADH. For this purpose microorganisms have evolved a variety of pathways (p. 37).

Pentose Phosphate Pathway (Phosphogluconate Pathway)

Whereas the EMP scheme is the major pathway in many microorganisms, as well as in animal and plant tissues, it is not the only available pathway for carbohydrate metabolism. The pentose phosphate pathway, also known as the *phosphogluconate pathway,* is a multifunctional pathway that may be used in the fermentation of hexoses, pentoses, and other carbohydrates (Fig. 4–5). For some organisms, such as the heterolactic fermentors, this is their major energy-yielding pathway. For most organisms, however, its principal use is to generate NADPH, which provides reducing power for biosynthetic reactions. It also provides pentoses for nucleotide synthesis, and a mechanism for the oxidation of pentoses by the glycolytic sequence. Because of its multifunctional use, in contrast to glycolysis, it cannot be visualized as a consecutive set of reactions leading directly from glucose and always ending in its complete oxidation to six molecules of CO_2.

The point of departure of this route from the EMP system is the oxidation of glucose 6-phosphate to 6-phosphogluconate, which is in turn decarboxylated and further oxidized to D-ribulose 5-phosphate. The dehydrogenases catalyzing these reactions, glucose 6-phosphate dehydrogenase and 6-phosphogluconate dehydrogenase, require $NADP^+$ as an electron acceptor. The overall equation for the pathway to this stage is

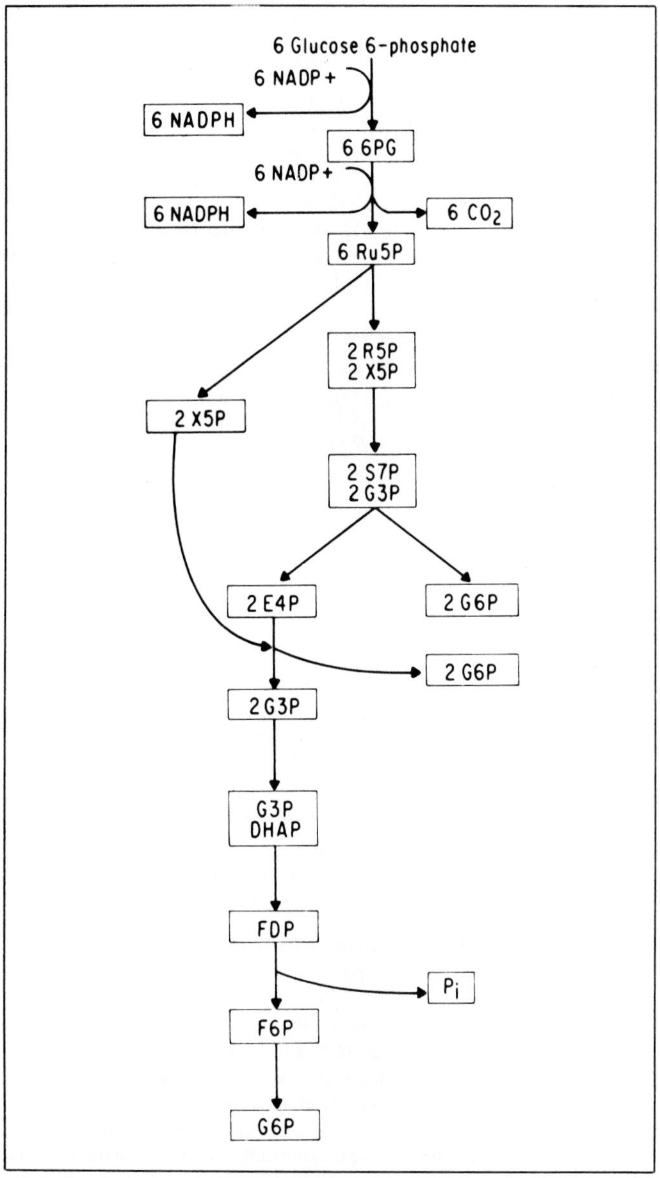

Fig. 4–5. Phosphogluconate pathway. Complete oxidation of glucose 6-phosphate to CO_2.

$$\text{Glucose 6-PO}_4 + 2\ \text{NADP}^+ + H_2O \rightleftharpoons \text{D-Ribose 5-PO}_4 + CO_2 + 2\ \text{NADPH} + 2\ H^+$$

The D-ribose 5-phosphate produced results from the reversible isomerization of D-ribulose 5-phosphate.

In some organisms or metabolic circumstances, the phosphogluconate pathway proceeds no further. In others, the pool of ribose and ribulose 5-phosphates is converted to xylulose 5-phosphate, which is the starting point for a series of transketolase and transaldolase reactions, leading ultimately to the initial compound of the pathway, glucose 6-phosphate. By a complex sequence of reactions in which six molecules of glucose 6-phosphate are oxidized to six molecules each of ribulose 5-phosphate and CO_2, the pentose phosphate pathway can also bring about the complete oxidation of glucose 6-phosphate to CO_2:

$$\text{Glucose 6-PO}_4 + 12\ \text{NADP}^+ + 7\ H_2O \rightarrow 6\ CO_2 + 12\ \text{NADPH} + 12\ H^+ + P_i$$

The complete oxidative pathway is operative only when the demand for NADPH is high, such as occurs in organisms actively engaged in lipid biosynthesis.

Heterolactic fermenting microorganisms utilize this pathway instead of glycolysis for the fermentation of glucose and the pentoses. These organisms lack the glycolytic enzymes, phosphofructokinase, aldolase, and triose phosphate isomerase, but possess the key enzyme, phosphoketolase, which cleaves xylulose 5-phosphate to acetylphosphate and glyceraldehyde 3-phosphate. The use of this pathway provides an explanation for the source of ethanol in these organisms (Fig. 4–6). In addition to the heterolactic fermenters, other organisms also using this pathway include *Brucella abortus* and species of *Acetobacter*.

When glucose is fermented through the pentose phosphate pathway, the net yield of ATP is half that characteristic of the EMP pathway. This lower energy yield is characteristic of a pathway of dehydrogenation before cleavage.

Entner-Doudoroff Pathway

This is a major dissimilatory pathway for glucose by obligate aerobes that lack the enzyme phosphofructokinase and thus cannot synthesize fructose 1,6-bisphosphate. Among the organisms for which it is functional are *Pseudomonas, Azotobacter,* and *Neisseria* species. The pathway diverges at 6-phosphogluconate from the pentose phosphate pathway. In this sequence, 6-phosphogluconate is dehydrated and then cleaved to yield one molecule of glyceraldehyde 3-PO_4 and one molecule of pyruvate, from which ethanol and CO_2 are formed via the same series of reactions as in the alcoholic fermentation by yeast (Fig. 4–6). As in the pentose phosphate pathway, only one molecule of ATP is produced per molecule of glucose fermented.

Fate of Pyruvate Under Anaerobic Conditions

The fermentation of glucose takes place in the cell cytosol after its phosphorylation to glucose 6-PO_4. The pyruvic acid to which glucose 6-PO_4 is converted is a key intermediate in the fermentative metabolism of all carbohydrates. In its formation, NAD is reduced and must be reoxidized in order to achieve a final oxidation-reduction balance. This reoxidation characteristically occurs in the terminal step reactions and is accompanied by the reduction of a product derived from pyruvic acid.

Bacteria differ markedly from animal tissues in the manner in which they dispose of pyruvic acid. In mammalian physiology, the main course of respiration is such that substrates are oxidized to CO_2 and H_2O, oxygen being the ultimate hydrogen acceptor. Among the bacteria, however, incomplete oxidation is the rule rather than the exception, and the products of fermentation may accumulate to an extraordinary degree. The final product in certain organisms is either alcohol or lactic acid. In others, the pyruvic acid is

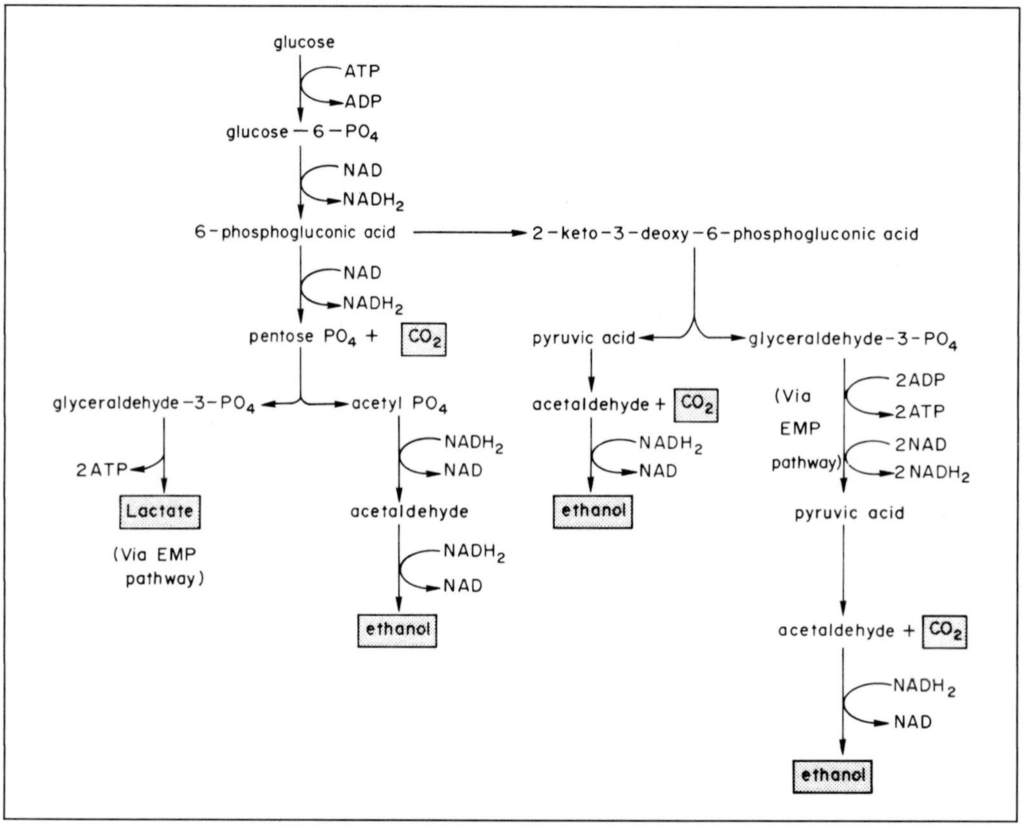

Fig. 4–6. Alternate pathways of glucose fermentation in certain bacteria. The pentose phosphate pathway used in heterolactic fermentation is shown on the left. A variation of this pathway, the Entner-Doudoroff pathway, on the right, results in the alcoholic fermentation of glucose.

further metabolized to such products as butyric acid, butyl alcohol, acetone, and propionic acid. Bacterial fermentations are of practical importance because they provide products of industrial value and are useful in the laboratory in the identification of bacterial species (Fig. 4–7).

Alcoholic Fermentation. The oldest known type of fermentation is the production of ethanol from glucose. In yeasts that carry out an almost pure alcoholic fermentation, the alcohol arises from the decarboxylation of pyruvic acid by pyruvate decarboxylase, the key enzyme of alcoholic fermentation. The free acetaldehyde formed is then reduced to ethanol by alcohol dehydrogenase, and the NADH is reoxidized. Although a number of bacteria produce alcohol, it is produced via other pathways (Fig. 4–6).

Homolactic Fermentation. All members of the genera *Streptococcus* and *Pediococcus* and many species of *Lactobacillus* ferment glucose predominantly to lactic acid with no more than a trace accumulation of other products. In the dissimilation of glucose by the homofermenters, pyruvate is reduced to lactic acid by the enzyme lactic dehydrogenase, with NADH acting as the hydrogen donor. The homofermentative mechanism owes its characteristically high yields of lactic acid to the action of aldolase, which cleaves the hexose diphosphate into two equal parts, both of which form pyruvate and hence lactate. The same fermentation occurs in animal muscle (see Fig. 4–3).

Heterolactic Fermentation. In addition to the production of lactic acid, some of the lactic acid bacteria (*Leuconostoc* and certain *Lactobacillus* species) produce a mixed fermentation in which only about half the glucose is converted to lactic acid, the remainder appearing as CO_2, alcohol, formic acid, or acetic acid. The heterolactic fermentation differs fundamentally from the homolactic type in that the pentose phosphate pathway rather than the EMP scheme is employed. The release of carbon 1 of glucose as CO_2 is characteristic of glucose fermentations by all heterolactic organisms. Also significant is the finding that the energy yield as measured by growth is one-third lower per mole of glucose fermented than that observed for homolactic organisms.

Propionic Acid Fermentation. Propionate is a major end-product of fermentations carried out by some of the anaerobic bacteria. The pathway is characteristic of the genus *Propionibacterium,* anaerobic gram-positive non-spore-forming rods closely related to the lactobacilli. The propionic acid produced by these organisms from glucose or from lactic acid contributes to the characteristic taste and smell of Swiss cheese. The ability of the propionic acid bacteria to ferment lactic acid, an end product of other fermentations, is significant in that it enables these organisms to net an additional ATP.

In the fermentation of hexose, the early stages of the glycolytic pathway are employed. Part of the pyruvate, derived either from hexose or from lactic acid, is further oxidized to CO_2 and acetyl-CoA, thus accounting for the presence of acetate and CO_2 among the reaction products. The energy-rich bond of acetyl-CoA is used for the synthesis of ATP.

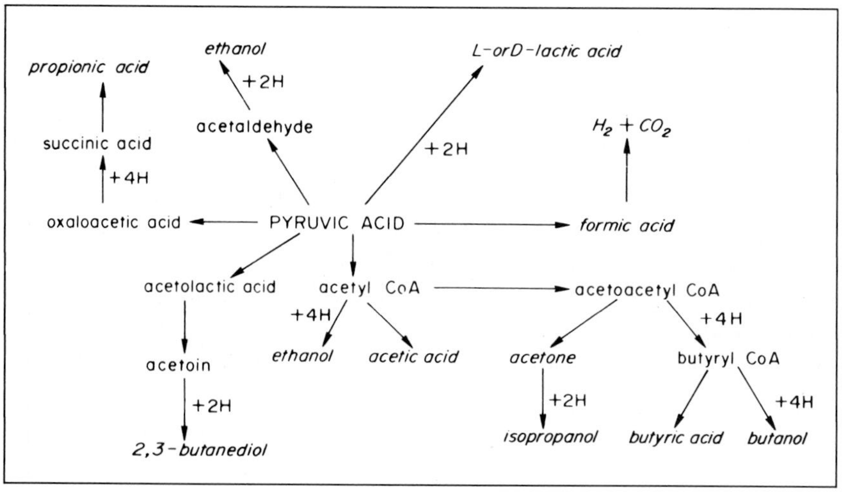

Fig. 4–7. Fate of pyruvate in major fermentations by microorganisms.

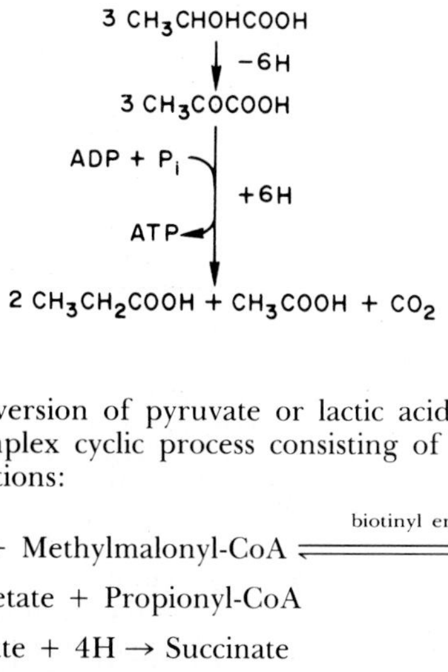

The conversion of pyruvate or lactic acid to propionic acid is a complex cyclic process consisting of the following series of reactions:

$$\text{Pyruvate} + \text{Methylmalonyl-CoA} \xrightleftharpoons{\text{biotinyl enzyme}} \text{Oxaloacetate} + \text{Propionyl-CoA} \quad (1)$$

$$\text{Oxaloacetate} + 4\text{H} \rightarrow \text{Succinate} \quad (2)$$

$$\text{Succinate} + \text{Propionyl-CoA} \rightleftharpoons \text{Succinyl-CoA} + \text{Propionate} \quad (3)$$

$$\text{Succinyl-CoA} \rightleftharpoons \text{Methylmalonyl-CoA} \quad (4)$$

The first step in the sequence is a unique CO_2 transfer reaction, catalyzed by a biotin-containing enzyme that acts as both CO_2 acceptor and donor. Propionyl-CoA, one of the products of this reaction, gives rise to propionate.

Mixed Acid Fermentation. This type of fermentation is characteristic of most of the Enterobacteriaceae. Organisms within the genera *Escherichia, Salmonella,* and *Shigella* ferment sugars via pyruvate to lactic, acetic, succinic, and formic acids. In addition, CO_2, H_2, and ethanol are produced. The nature and quantitative relationships of these products vary with the organism and degree of anaerobiosis. All of the enterobacteria produce formate, which either accumulates or, under acid conditions, is converted by formic hydrogenlyase to molecular hydrogen and carbon dioxide. The formic acid produced in this fermentation is derived from pyruvate in a cleavage involving coenzyme A to yield acetyl-CoA and formate. The enzyme catalyzing the reaction in equation 1, pyruvate formate-lyase, is a key enzyme in governing the fermentation route. Its catalytic activity is very high, and it is tightly controlled at both the transcriptional and posttranslational level. The acetyl CoA formed in reaction 1 is rapidly converted to acetyl PO_4. The combined reaction whereby formate and acetate are produced from pyruvate is known as the phosphoroclastic split. This reaction sequence represents the backbone of the cellular machinery for the anaerobic life of *E. coli* and other members of this family:

$$\text{Pyruvate} + \text{CoA} \rightleftharpoons \text{Acetyl-CoA} + \text{Formate} \quad (1)$$

$$\text{Acetyl-CoA} + P_i \rightleftharpoons \text{CoA} + \text{Acetyl } PO_4 \quad (2)$$

$$\text{Acetyl } PO_4 + \text{ADP} \rightleftharpoons \text{ATP} + \text{Acetate} \quad (3)$$

The conversion of formate to CO_2 and H_2 is catalyzed by formic hydrogenlyase, an inducible enzyme complex whose formation is inhibited by aerobiosis. Fermentations by *E. coli* and most *Salmonella* are characterized by CO_2 and H_2 production, but in *Shigella* and *Salmonella typhi,* no CO_2 and H_2 are produced and an equivalent amount of formic acid accumulates. The inability of *S. typhi* and *Shigella* to cleave formate is useful in the clinical microbiology laboratory:

$$\text{HCOOH} \rightarrow H_2 + CO_2$$

The overall fermentation of glucose by *E. coli* is as follows:

$$2\ \text{Glucose} + H_2O \rightarrow 2\ \text{Lactate} + \text{Acetate} + \text{Ethanol} + 2\ CO_2 + 2\ H_2$$

The ethanol produced by *E. coli* comes from acetyl-CoA via acetaldehyde and its subsequent reduction. The lactic acid is produced via the EMP scheme.

Butanediol Fermentation. Several groups of organisms, including *Enterobacter, Bacillus,* and *Serratia,* produce 2,3-butanediol in fermentations that are otherwise of the mixed acid type. Two molecules of pyruvate, the precursor of acetoin (acetylmethylcarbinol), are decarboxylated in the formation of one molecule of the neutral acetoin, which is then reduced to 2,3-butanediol:

$$2\ CH_3COCOOH \rightarrow CH_3\text{—}C(OH)(COCH_3)COOH + CO_2$$

(pyruvic acid) → (acetolactic acid)

$$CH_3CHOHCHOHCH_3 \xleftarrow{(2H)} CH_3CHOHCOCH_3 + CO_2$$

(2,3-butanediol) ← (acetoin)

This reduction is slowly reversible in air, and when made strongly alkaline is the basis for the Voges-Proskauer reaction, a test for acetoin.

The diversion of part of the pyruvate to 2,3-butanediol greatly reduces the amount of acid produced relative to the mixed acid fermentation and is responsible for the positive methyl red reaction often used in the differentiation of *Escherichia* and *Enterobacter*.

Butyric Acid Fermentation. Among the distinctive primary products of carbohydrate fermentation by many species of *Clostridium* are butyric acid, acetic acid, CO_2, and H_2. The clostridia employ phosphotransferase systems for sugar uptake and the EMP pathway for degradation of hexose phosphates to pyruvate. The conversion of pyruvate to acetyl-CoA is catalyzed by the pyruvate-ferredoxin oxidoreductase system. In this reaction sequence, the two hydrogens are not transferred to NAD as in the pyruvate dehydrogenase reaction (described below) but are used to reduce ferredoxin. Ferredoxin has a very low redox potential, which at pH 7.0 is about the same as that of the hydrogen electrode. Therefore, when clostridia ferment carbohydrates, reduced ferredoxin can transfer electrons to hydrogenase and hydrogen can be evolved.

The key reaction in the butyric acid fermentation is the formation of acetoacetyl CoA by the condensation of two molecules of acetyl-CoA derived from acetate or from pyruvate:

$$2\ CH_3CO\text{–}SCoA \rightleftharpoons CH_3COCH_2CO\text{–}SCoA + HSCoA$$

This C_4 compound is the key to all of the C_4-forming reactions of the clostridia. Its subsequent reduction and conversion to butyric acid permit ATP formation. In some organisms, the primary acidic products of the fermentation are reduced, resulting in the accumulation of neutral end products: butanol, acetone, isopropanol, and ethanol. The end products of clostridial fermentations can thus be very numerous and vary with the species.

Generally, only obligate anaerobes form butyrate as a primary fermentation product. In addition to several species of *Clostridium,* members of the genera *Fusobacterium, Butyrivibrio,* and *Eubacterium* also produce butyric acid.

Fermentation of Nitrogenous Organic Compounds. Some anaerobes are not primarily butyric acid producers. Amino acids, derived from proteins by extracellular proteases, and purine and pyrimidine bases are fermented by a variety of organisms. Single amino acids can serve as major energy sources for selected species. For proteolytic clostridia, however, such as *Clostridium sporogenes, Clostridium difficile,* and *Clostridium botulinum* types A and B, the most characteristic type of amino acid fermentation is the Stickland reaction, a coupled oxidation-reduction involving a pair of amino acids, one of which serves as the electron donor and the other as the electron acceptor. An example of this type of reaction is the fermentation of alanine and glycine:

$$\text{Alanine} + 2\text{Glycine} + 2H_2O \rightarrow 3\text{Aceticacid} + 3NH_3 + CO_2$$

The degradation of amino acids in a protein hydrolysate is very complex. The process always involves oxidation and reduction reactions between one or more amino acids or nonnitrogenous compounds derived from amino acids. The oxidation reactions are usually similar to corresponding reactions in aerobic organisms, i.e., oxidative deaminations, transaminations, and α-keto acid oxidations. The reduction reactions are more distinctive and utilize such electron acceptors as amino acids, α- and β-keto acids, α and β unsaturated acids, or their coenzyme A thiolesters, and protons. The ultimate reduction products include a variety of short-chain fatty acids, succinic acid, δ-aminovaleric acid, and molecular hydrogen.

Aerobic Respiration

In aerobic cells, energy is obtained from the complete oxidation of the substrate, with molecular oxygen usually serving as the ultimate hydrogen acceptor. In respiration the large amount of energy set free in the formation of water is made available to the process. The pathways of aerobic dissimilation are exceedingly complex. They consist of many enzymes and a large number of biochemical reactions. The most important respiratory mechanism for terminal oxidation is the tricarboxylic acid (TCA) cycle of Krebs, which together with the known reactions of glycolysis, can account for the complete oxidation of glucose. This cycle is unique in that it provides the cell not only with an energy source but also with carbon skeletons for the synthesis of cellular material.

Tricarboxylic Acid Cycle

Oxidative Decarboxylation of Pyruvate. In aerobic cells, the pyruvate formed from the glycolytic pathway is enzymatically oxidized by the pyruvate dehydrogenase complex to a two-carbon compound, acetyl CoA:

$$CH_3COCOOH + NAD + CoA\text{–}SH \rightarrow CH_3CO\text{–}S\text{–}CoA + CO_2 + NADH$$

The electrons accepted from pyruvate by NAD are carried in the form of NADH to the respiratory chain.

Oxidation of Acetyl CoA. The TCA cycle carries out the oxidation of the acetyl moiety of acetyl CoA to CO_2 with transfer of the reducing equivalents to NAD, NADP, and FAD. Acetyl CoA enters the cycle via the citrate synthase reaction, in which oxaloacetate and acetyl CoA are condensed to form citric acid (Fig. 4–8). In one turn of the cycle this six-carbon molecule is then decarboxylated and oxidized to regenerate the four-carbon oxaloacetate and liberate two carbon atoms as CO_2. In so doing, four pairs of electrons are enzymatically extracted from the intermediates of the cycle. Anything capable of generating acetyl CoA can be oxidized via the cycle. Important synthetic mechanisms utilize reactants

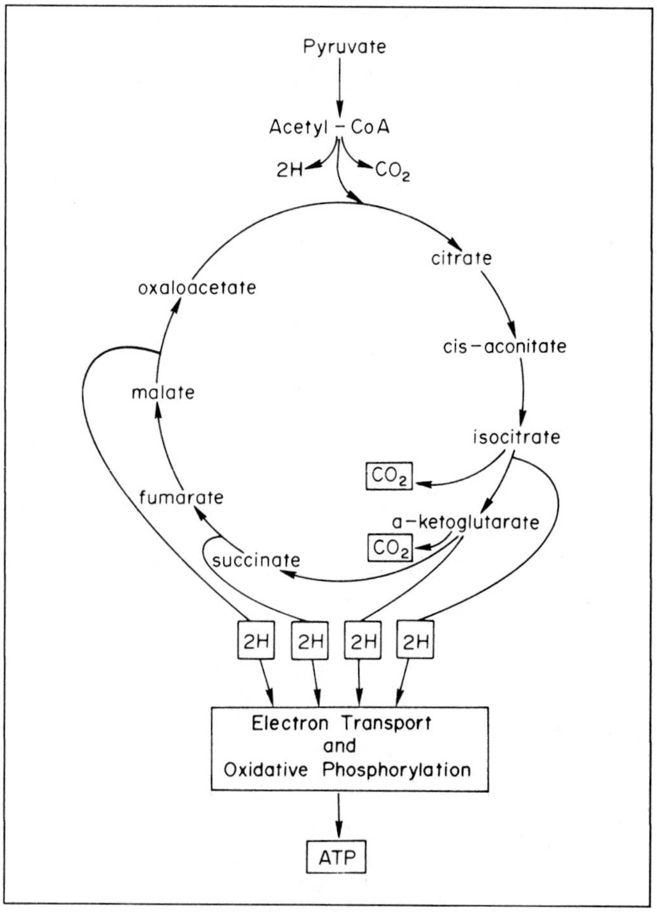

Fig. 4–8. The tricarboxylic acid cycle. The four pairs of H atoms liberated are fed into the respiratory chain.

of the cycle to provide a common meeting ground for carbohydrate, lipid, and protein metabolism.

Anaplerotic Reactions

Under normal conditions, the reactions by which the TCA cycle intermediates are formed and drained away remain in balance. This is made possible by enzymatic mechanisms for replenishing the TCA cycle intermediates as they are diverted into biosynthetic pathways.

Phosphoenolpyruvate (PEP)–Carboxylase Reaction. The most important of these anaplerotic (filling-up) reactions is the enzymatic carboxylation of pyruvate to oxaloacetate:

$$\text{Phosphoenolpyruvate} + CO_2 + P_i \rightarrow \text{Oxaloacetate} + P_i$$

The reaction is catalyzed by pyruvate carboxylase, an allosteric enzyme containing biotin. The rate of the forward reaction is low unless acetyl CoA, the fuel of the TCA cycle, is present in excess.

Glyoxylate Cycle. When microorganisms are grown on fatty acids or acetate as a sole carbon source, acetyl CoA is formed without the intermediate formation of pyruvic acid. Under such circumstances there is no mechanism for the generation

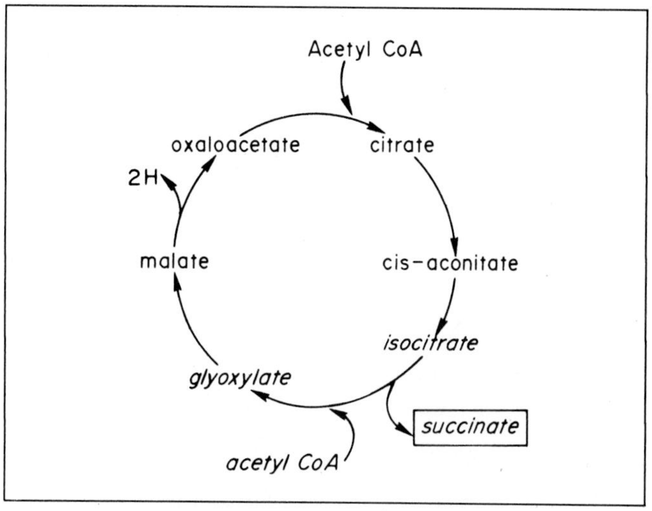

Fig. 4–9. The glyoxylate cycle. This cycle provides both energy and 4-carbon intermediates for biosynthetic purposes. In each turn of the cycle, two molecules of acetyl-CoA enter, and one molecule of succinate is formed. The reactions in the pathway between isocitrate and malate are catalyzed by auxiliary enzymes. All of the others are reactions of the TCA cycle.

of oxaloacetate from pyruvate by the PEP carboxylase reaction. Growth on acetate, however, induces the synthesis of two enzymes, isocitrate lyase and malate synthase, which together with some of the enzymes of the TCA cycle carry out a modification of the TCA cycle, the glyoxylate cycle. This cycle bypasses the CO_2-evolving steps of the TCA cycle. The succinate formed can be converted by reactions of the TCA cycle to oxaloacetate, which may then condense with acetyl CoA to start another turn of the cycle, or alternatively the oxaloacetate may be used for biosynthetic purposes (Fig. 4–9).

Electron Transport

Components of System. In procaryotic organisms the redox carriers and enzymes involved in electron transport are located in the plasma membrane. Although the same basic types of carriers are present as occur in the mitochondria of higher organisms, considerable diversity also exists, especially in the number and properties of the cytochrome components.

The major components that participate in the transport of electrons from an organic substrate to oxygen are pyridine and flavin-linked dehydrogenases, iron-sulfur proteins, quinones, and cytochromes.

PYRIDINE-LINKED DEHYDROGENASES. Nicotinamide adenine dinucleotide (NAD^+) is the coenzyme most frequently employed as an acceptor of electrons from the substrate (Fig. 4–10). It functions in five of the six oxidative steps in the oxidation of glucose. NADP-linked dehydrogenases serve primarily to transfer electrons from intermediates of catabolism to intermediates of biosynthesis. The pyridine nucleotides are relatively loosely bound to the enzyme protein by noncovalent bonds. They are therefore not fixed prosthetic groups but substrates that can serve as dissociable carriers of electrons.

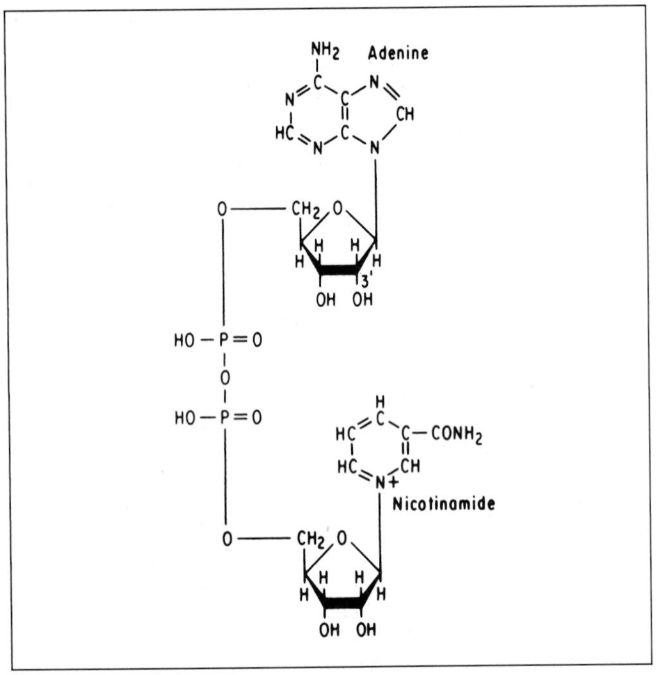

Fig. 4–10. Nicotinamide adenine dinucleotide (NAD). In nicotinamide adenine dinucleotide phosphate (NADP) the 3′ hydroxyl group is esterified with phosphate.

FLAVIN-LINKED DEHYDROGENASES. These enzymes contain the vitamin riboflavin, either as flavin mononucleotide (FMN) or flavin adenine dinucleotide (FAD) (Fig. 4–11). Unlike the pyridine-linked dehydrogenases, in the flavin-linked dehydrogenases the flavin nucleotide is tightly bound. Among the most important of the flavoproteins is NADH dehydrogenase, which catalyzes the transfer of electrons from NADH to the next component of the electron transport chain. Some of the flavoproteins, such as succinic dehydrogenase, are active in primary dehydrogenations. Another class of flavin-linked enzymes, the flavin oxidases, are reoxidized by molecular oxygen to yield hydrogen peroxide (p. 45). Among the numerous enzymes in this group are D-amino acid oxidase and xanthine oxidase. In addition to flavin nucleotide, some of the flavoproteins contain metals (iron and molybdenum) that are essential for catalytic activity.

IRON-SULFUR PROTEINS. These proteins contain iron and an equimolar amount of acid-labile sulfur. They apparently function as electron carriers by undergoing reversible Fe(II)–Fe(III) transitions. A number of different iron-sulfur proteins have been described from a variety of sources. These vary in the number of iron-sulfur centers per molecule and oxidation-reduction potential. Among the best studied are the ferredoxins from the anaerobic nitrogen-fixing *Clostridium pasteurianum* and from the photosynthetic bacterium *Chromatium*. Their precise role in electron transport is unknown.

QUINONES (COENZYME Q). Also participating in electron transport are lipid-soluble quinones that function with their hydroquinone as a redox couple (Fig. 4–12). The quinones are not bound to specific proteins but are present as a small pool in the liquid phase of the membrane, where they serve

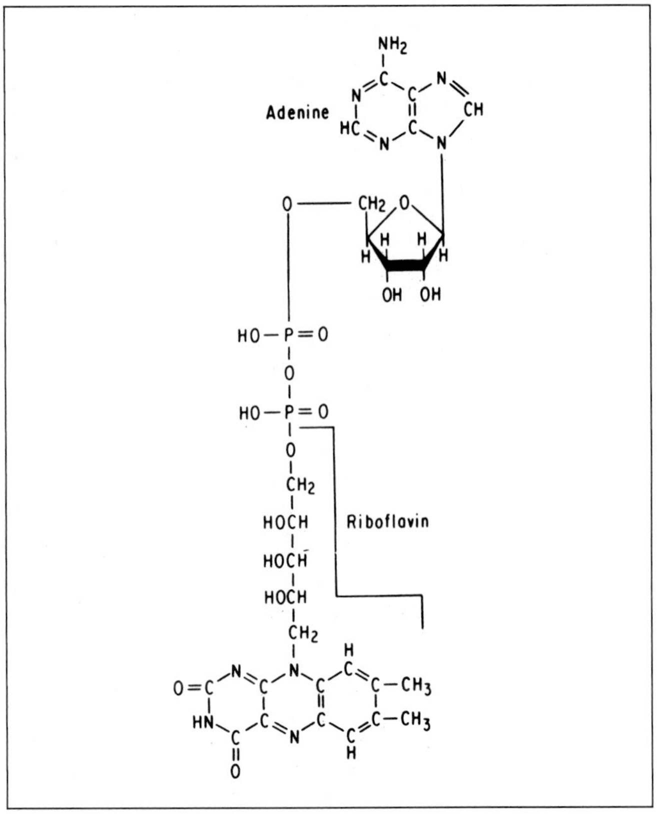

Fig. 4–11. Flavin adenine dinucleotide (FAD).

as an electron acceptor for one group of enzymes and an electron donor to the next component of the chain. As a mobile liquid-soluble substrate, they are available to enzymes more rigidly locked into position in the membrane.

Although ubiquinone is ubiquitous in its occurrence and

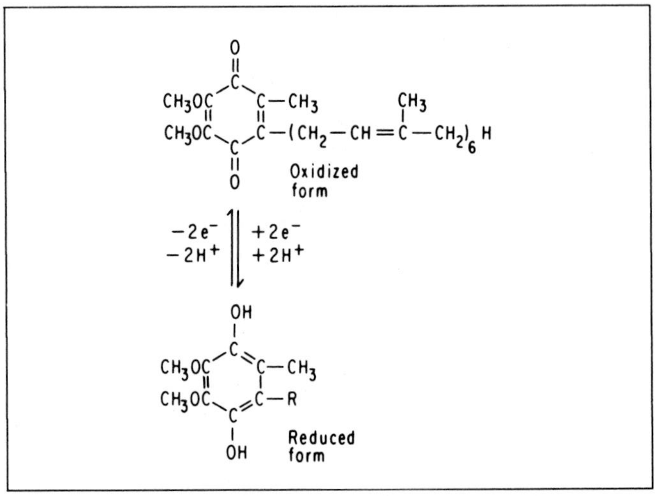

Fig. 4–12. Ubiquinone (coenzyme Q), a carrier of electrons in gram-negative microorganisms. In most gram-positive species it is replaced by menaquinone.

is the major quinone of the electron transport system of mitochondria, additional quinones play a role in bacterial electron transport. In most gram-positive organisms, menaquinone replaces ubiquinone, and in many of the Enterobacteriaceae, both quinones are present. The ratio of the two quinones in *E. coli* membranes is variable. Under conditions of high aeration and in logarithmic phase, ubiquinone-8 predominates over menaquinone-8 by a ratio of 22:1. In an 18-hour aerobic stationary phase culture, the ratio was 1.5:1, and in an anaerobic stationary phase culture, ubiquinone-8 was undetectable, whereas menaquinone-8 was at relatively high concentrations. In *Mycobacterium phlei* the naphthoquinone vitamin K_9 occurs and has been shown to act between the flavoprotein and cytochrome b.

CYTOCHROMES. The cytochromes are iron-porphyrin components of the electron transport chain. During their catalytic cycle, they undergo reversible Fe(II)–Fe(III) valence changes and act sequentially to carry electrons toward molecular oxygen. Although basically similar to the mammalian cytochromes, the bacterial cytochromes are more diverse and possess properties not encountered in mammalian systems. Four broad classes of bacterial cytochromes have been identified on the basis of their characteristic absorption spectra. Among the various species, there is considerable diversity in the classes of cytochromes present, as well as in their structure, functions, and conditions for existence.

Some bacteria have more than one autooxidizable cytochrome of the α class. Many contain cytochrome *o*, a widely distributed heme protein resembling cytochrome *c* that appears to serve as a terminal oxidase. The conditions under which a bacterium is grown markedly affect both the total and relative amounts of the cytochrome components in the organism. Oxygen deprivation tends to cause the replacement of cytochrome oxidase $\alpha\alpha_3$ by *o* in *Paracoccus denitrificans* and the enhanced synthesis of cytochrome oxidase *d* relative to *o* (*E. coli, Haemophilus parainfluenzae*). Such changes reflect attempts by the organism to compensate for oxygen deficiency by the increased synthesis of higher concentrations of alternate oxidases that have an increased affinity for oxygen or that exhibit higher turnover numbers. Whereas mammalian cytochromes function primarily as members of a respiratory electron transport chain, bacterial cytochromes also transport electrons to nonoxygen acceptors (Fig. 4–13). In *E. coli*, for example, cytochromes function as part of the nitrate reductase system (p. 46). They also play a role in photosynthesis (p. 48).

Electron Transport Chain. In each revolution of the TCA cycle, there are four dehydrogenations. In three of these, NAD serves as the electron acceptor, and in the fourth, the electron acceptor is FAD. The reoxidation of these reduced coenzymes is accomplished by passing of the electrons through a series of intermediate carriers, capable of undergoing freely reversible oxidation and reduction. The last carrier in the series reacts with oxygen in a reaction mediated by a terminal oxidase (Fig. 4–14). The series of carriers that link the dehydrogenation of an oxidizable substrate with the reduction of molecular oxygen to water, is termed the "electron transport chain." The carriers participate in a series of reactions of gradually increasing E_0' values. Thus electrons will tend to pass from the more negative carrier NAD, shown in Figure 4–15, to the more positive carrier above it on the scale. A decline in free energy is associated with each electron transfer and is directly related to the magnitude of the drop in electron pressure. The decline in free energy during the passage of the pair of electrons from NADH to molecular oxygen is large enough to make possible the synthesis of ATP from ADP and P_i.

The typical electron transport sequence of

$$\text{Flavoprotein} \rightarrow \text{Cyt } b \rightarrow \text{Cyt } c \rightarrow \text{Cyt } a \rightarrow O_2$$

found in mammals is also found in bacteria. However, the

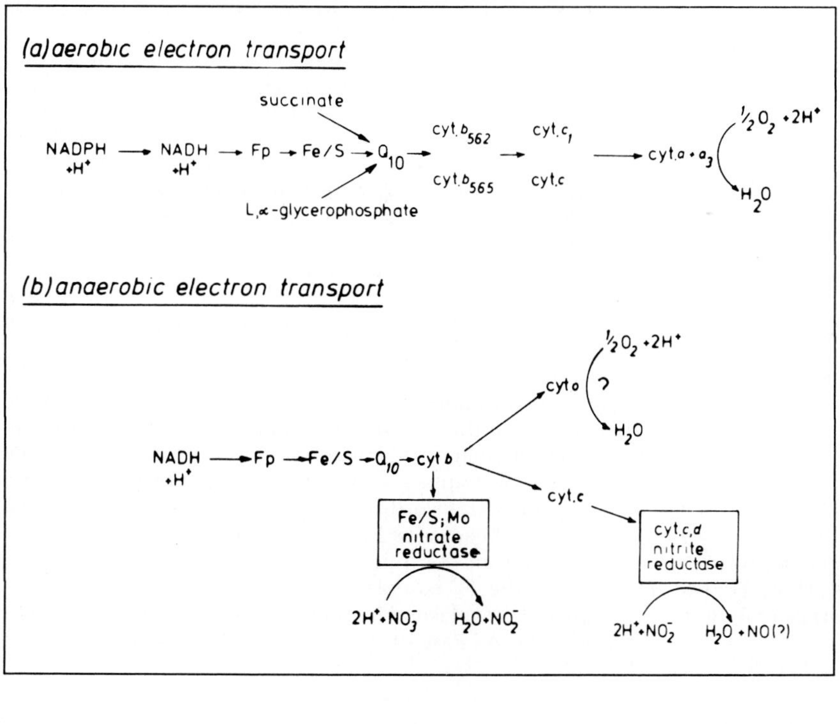

Fig. 4–13. Electron transport chains in *P. denitrificans*, illustrating the linear sequence of redox carriers associated with aerobically grown cells as compared with anaerobically grown cells in the presence of NO_3^-. *(From Haddock and Jones: Bacteriol Rev 41:47, 1977.)*

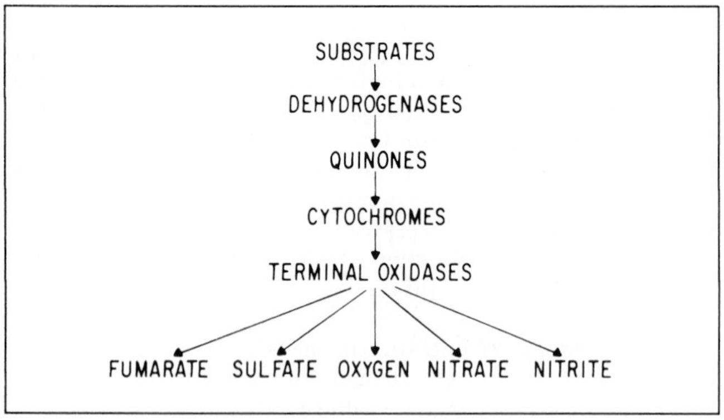

Fig. 4–14. Generalized scheme of electron transport systems in bacteria.

structure of the electron transport chain in bacteria appears to be more complex, in that a number of transport chain systems may exist. The flavoprotein dehydrogenases may be inputs to a number of the chain systems, and the chains may be more branched in structure than is found in mammalian systems. A bacterial respiratory chain should be conceptualized as a three-dimensional model, with each member having possibly more than one input and output, rather than as a two-dimensional linear and almost unbranched chain, as is often done in representations of the mammalian respiratory chain (Fig. 4–16).

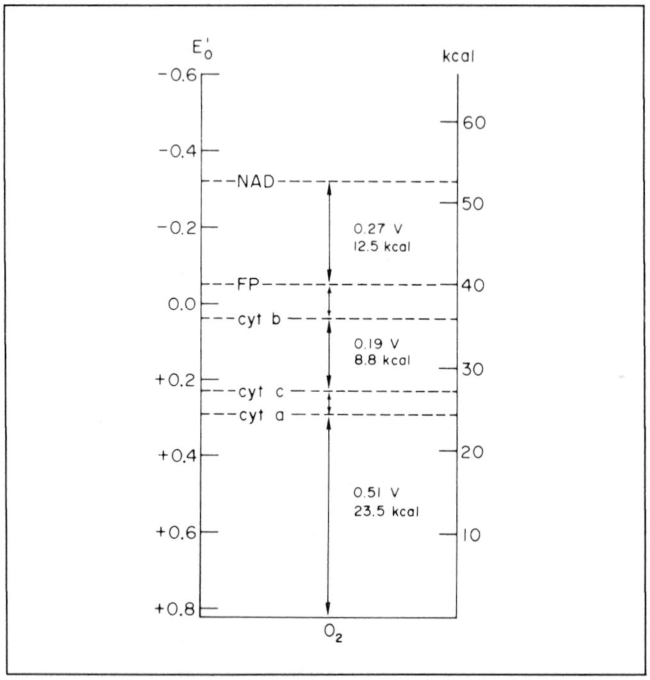

Fig. 4–15. Release of free energy as a pair of electrons passes down the respiratory chain to oxygen. Sufficient energy is generated in three of the segments for the formation of a molecule of ATP: between NAD and FP, between cyt *b* and cyt *c*, and between cyt *a* and O_2.

Oxidative Phosphorylation. The movement of electrons down the respiratory chain of carriers is coupled with the production of energy-rich phosphate bonds as a result of oxidative phosphorylation. The multiplicity of catalysts in the chain provides a device for bleeding off the energy in convenient packets. Oxidative phosphorylation is thus a process whereby the large amount of free energy liberated during the complete oxidation of metabolites via the citric acid cycle can be utilized to drive the synthesis of ATP.

The mechanism by which respiratory chain or photosynthetic oxidoreductions are coupled to ATP synthesis is best explained by the attractive but highly complex chemiosmotic hypothesis. This model is based on the assumption that a protonmotive force consisting of a pH gradient (ΔpH) and an electrical potential difference ($\Delta\Psi$) can be generated by the redox reactions of electron transport, and that this protonmotive force drives the synthesis of ATP. The essence of this hypothesis, as shown in Figure 4–17, emphasizes the role of the membrane as the site in which electron transport and phosphorylation are coupled, and which is impermeable to protons and hydroxyl ions.

According to the chemiosmotic mechanism, the electron carriers are so arranged in the membrane that electron transfer from centers of low to high redox potential is coupled obligatorily with the transport of protons across the membrane from the inside to the outside of the cell (Fig. 4–18). As a consequence of this electrogenic proton transport, protons are delivered to the outside at high electrochemical potential and return to their starting side by traveling through a proton channel in the membrane leading to an ATPase complex. The ATPase system couples the hydrolysis of ATP with the translocation of protons through the channel away from the ATPase. Since this reaction is reversible, the passage of protons toward the ATPase is coupled with the synthesis of ATP, and the ATPase functions as an ATP synthase.

The number of ADPs phosphorylated per atom of oxygen is frequently expressed as the P:O ratio. In the mitochondrial chain it is 3 when NADH is the electron donor and 2 for $FADH_2$ as electron donor. The bacterial respiratory chain is exquisitely sensitive to isolation procedures but data obtained by the use of vesicle preparations of whole cells indicate that at least some aerobic bacterial species have P:O ratios of 3. In many bacteria, however, it appears that there are only one or two energy conservation sites. Loss of these sites and the presence of nonphosphorylative electron transport bypass reactions, both of which have been demonstrated, may account for the lower P:O ratios observed in most bacteria. For *E. coli*, the P:O ratio is probably 2, and the sites of ATP formation are the dehydrogenation of NADH and the oxidation of one of the cytochromes. The ATP yield in many bacteria is thus lower than the 36 moles generated in the complete oxidation of one mole of glucose by mitochondria.

Microbial ATPases may be visualized in photomicrographs of membranes as knob-shaped structures that stud the inner surface of the membrane and project into the cytoplasm. The molecular structure and composition of the bacterial ATPase complex appear to be similar to that of mitochondria and chloroplasts. Two distinct regions comprise the enzyme complex: the headpiece F_1, which contains the catalytic site and is located on the inner surface of the cytoplasmic membrane, and the F_0 basepiece of the enzyme, which extends through the cytoplasmic membrane and contains the proton channel. The ATPase of *E. coli* consists of eight subunits.

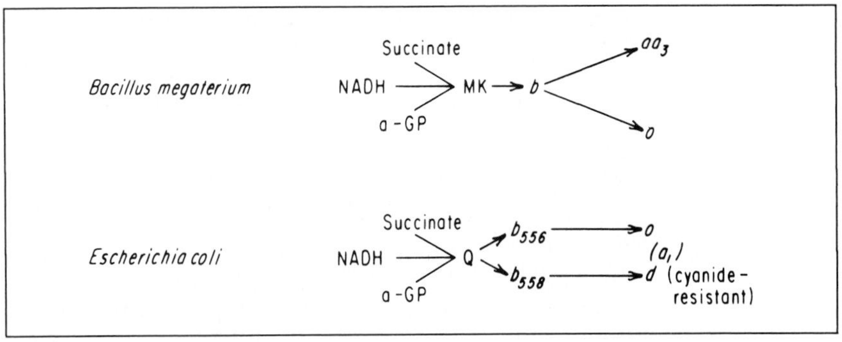

Fig. 4–16. Bacterial respiratory chains with terminal pathways that are branched either before or at the cytochrome oxidase level. *(From Jones: In Haddock and Hamilton (eds): Microbial Energetics, Cambridge University Press, 1977.)*

PYRIDINE-NUCLEOTIDE TRANSHYDROGENASE. Transhydrogenases have been detected in bacteria that catalyze the exchange of reducing equivalents between the nucleotide pools:

$$NADPH + NAD^+ \rightleftharpoons NADP^+ + NADH$$

The reaction makes possible the utilization of the reducing equivalents of NADPH by the electron transport chain. In aerobic organisms, however, when excess ATP is present, the reverse reaction allows reduction of $NADP^+$ for biosynthetic purposes. Although the molecular mechanism of the transhydrogenase reaction is unclear, the enzyme is an integral membrane protein and the reaction has the earmarks of a process dependent upon the energized state of the membrane.

Flavin-mediated Reactions

Although electron transport accounts for the great bulk of oxygen utilization in microbial systems, a number of other enzymes also catalyze reactions with oxygen. Many of these are inducible enzymes produced in large quantities by the organism when it is grown on various aromatic compounds as the sole carbon source. Some of these enzymes, such as the D- and L-amino acid oxidases, are flavoproteins, autooxidizable by molecular oxygen. The reaction with oxygen is accompanied by the formation of hydrogen peroxide, which is highly toxic if allowed to accumulate:

$$FPH_2 + O_2 \rightarrow FP + H_2O_2$$

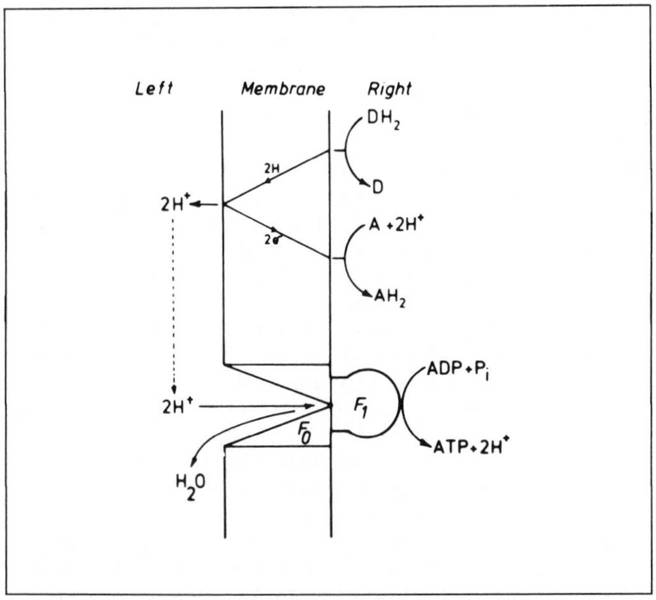

Fig. 4–17. Schematic representation of a proton-translocating oxidoreduction segment of the electron transport chain and of a proton-translocating ATPase. Two protolytic reactions, involving the oxidation of a donor (DH_2) and the reduction of an acceptor (A), are catalyzed by an enzyme complex, comprising an alternating sequence of a hydrogen carrier and an electron carrier, arranged across the membrane to form a proton-translocating oxidoreduction loop. *(From Haddock and Jones: Bacteriol Rev 41:47, 1977.)*

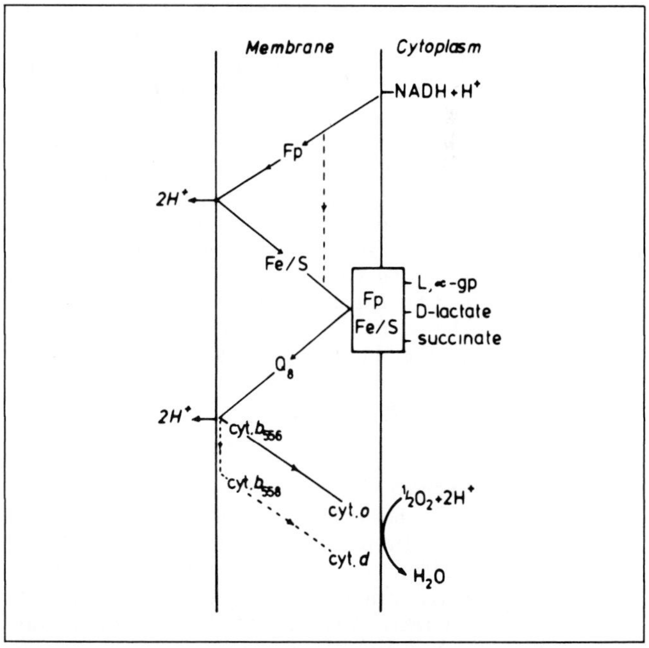

Fig. 4–18. Proposed functional organization of the redox carriers responsible for aerobic electron transport in *E. coli.* The scheme includes the various routes for aerobic electron transport in *E. coli,* with the dashed lines indicating alternative pathways for reducing equivalents. L-α-gp, L-α-glycerophosphate. *(From Haddock and Jones: Bacteriol Rev 41:47, 1977.)*

Aerobic organisms produce catalase, an enzyme that breaks down the hydrogen peroxide to water and oxygen:

$$2\ H_2O_2 \rightarrow 2\ H_2O + O_2$$

The streptococci are facultative anaerobes that grow readily in the presence of air although they lack cytochromes and catalase. These organisms contain a peroxidase that destroys any peroxide produced by flavoprotein enzymes. The destruction of hydrogen peroxide by this mechanism requires the action of two enzymes, a flavoprotein NADH oxidase and a peroxidase:

$$NADH + H^+ + O_2 \xrightarrow{\text{NADH oxidase}} NAD^+ + H_2O_2$$

$$NADH + H^+ + H_2O_2 \xrightarrow{\text{peroxidase}} NAD^+ + 2\ H_2O$$

$$\text{Sum: } 2\ NADH + 2\ H^+ + O_2 \rightarrow 2\ NAD^+ + 2\ H_2O$$

Most anaerobic organisms lack both catalase and peroxidase.

Superoxide Dismutase

The reduction of oxygen results in the production of free radical intermediates that are very toxic to the bacterial cell. Among the most important of these is the superoxide anion O_2^-. Superoxide is generated during electron transport to molecular oxygen as well as in the autooxidation of hydroquinones, leukoflavins, ferredoxins, and flavoproteins. The catalytic actions of several enzymes (e.g., xanthine oxidase) also evolve O_2^-.

All aerobic and aerotolerant bacteria possess the enzyme superoxide dismutase, which scavenges the superoxide radical in a very bizarre enzymatic reaction:

$$O_2^- + O_2^- + 2H^+ \xrightarrow{\text{superoxide dismutase}} H_2O_2 + O_2$$

The presence of catalase in these organisms prevents the accumulation of the noxious H_2O_2 formed from O_2^-.

Superoxide dismutases are metalloenzymes. The same basic type of enzyme is found in bacteria and in eucaryotic mitochondria. Both contain Mn^{2+} and exhibit a high degree of homology of their amino acid sequence. A second type of enzyme found in the cytoplasm of eucaryotes contains Cu^{2+} and Zn^{2+} and has a significantly different structure.

The absence of catalase, peroxidase, and superoxide dismutase in anaerobic organisms provides at least a partial explanation for the oxygen toxicity in these organisms. The inhibitory role of other highly toxic radicals, such as singlet oxygen and the hydroxyl radical generated by the reduction of oxygen, remains to be explored.

Anaerobic Electron Transport

In obligately aerobic bacteria, oxygen is the only terminal electron acceptor, and cytochromes of the *a*, *d*, and *o* types can function as terminal oxidases. In facultatively anaerobic organisms, however, a wide variety of other electron acceptors may be used. When these organisms are grown under aerobic conditions, they contain a functional respiratory chain, whereas under anaerobic conditions, their electron transport systems may be coupled to electron acceptors other than oxygen (Fig. 4–14). Anaerobic electron transport systems have also been demonstrated in some obligate anaerobes.

ATP generation can be coupled to many of these electron-accepting, hydrogen-consuming reactions in both facultatively and obligately anaerobic organisms. There is also evidence that some of the systems are coupled to active transport of metabolites in a manner comparable to that of the aerobic electron transport chain. Systems in which the reductive processes are coupled with phosphorylation are shown in Table 4–5.

TABLE 4–5. REDUCTIVE PROCESSES COUPLED WITH PHOSPHORYLATION

Reaction[a]	kcal/Electron Equivalent from H_2
CO_2 reduction to methane	3.9
Sulfate reduction to sulfide	4.5
Fumarate reduction to succinate	10.3
Nitrate reduction to nitrite	19.5
Nitrite reduction to N_2	31.7
O_2 reduction to H_2O (for comparison)	28.3

[a] CO_2, CH_4, H_2, N_2, NO, and N_2O in the gaseous state; all other substances in aqueous solution.

From Thauer et al: Bacteriol Rev 41:118, 1977.

Nitrate and Nitrite Reduction. The best characterized of the anaerobic electron transport systems is nitrate respiration, in which nitrate is used as the terminal electron acceptor. Nitrate respiration occurs in a wide range of bacterial species, including strictly aerobic, anaerobic, and facultatively anaerobic organisms:

$$NO_3^- + H_2 \rightarrow NO_2^- + H_2O$$

The reduction of nitrate to nitrite is catalyzed by a membrane-associated electron transport system consisting of dehydrogenases, electron carriers, and nitrate reductase (Fig. 4–19). In general, the dehydrogenases are inducible enzymes. In *E. coli* grown anaerobically in the presence of nitrate, formate is the most effective electron donor. Other substrates that may also function as electron donors for nitrate reduction include lactate, succinate, and NADH.

The reduction product of nitrate respiration, nitrite, is highly toxic, and growth of most organisms is limited. In a few organisms, however, such as *Bacillus* and *Pseudomonas*, nitrate can be reduced beyond the level of nitrite to molecular nitrogen by a series of anaerobic respiratory processes that in sum are called *denitrification*. The one physiologic property characteristic of most denitrifying organisms is their ability to produce nitrogen gas by respiratory nitrate reduction:

$$2\ NO_2^- + 3\ [H_2] + 2\ H^+ \rightarrow N_2 + 4\ H_2O$$

Nitric oxide (NO) and nitrous oxide (N_2O) are intermediates in the reduction process (Fig. 4–20).

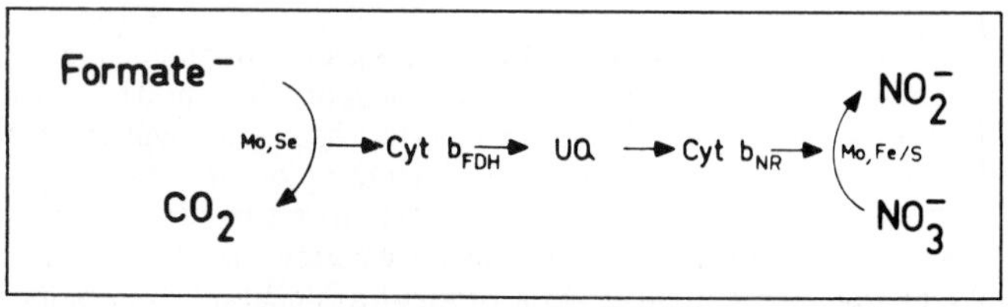

Fig. 4–19. Scheme of the electron flow from formate to nitrate in *E. coli. (From Thauer et al: Bacteriol Rev 41:100, 1977.)*

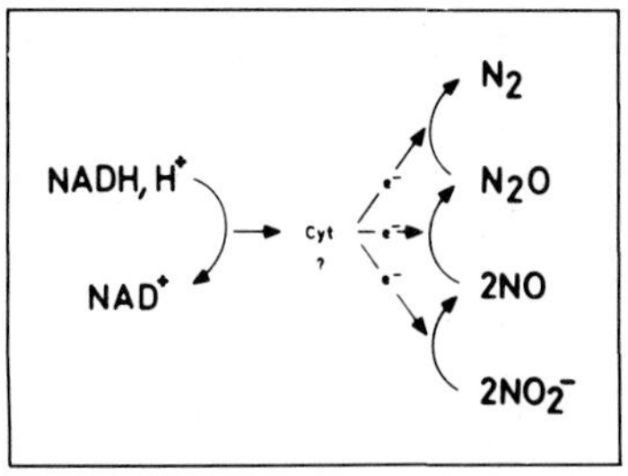

Fig. 4–20. Scheme of the electron transport system involved in nitrite reduction to N_2. *(According to Payne: Bacteriol Rev 37:409, 1973; from Thauer et al: Bacteriol Rev 41:100, 1977.)*

Fumarate Reduction. A number of bacteria, including both strict and facultative anaerobes, use fumarate as an electron acceptor (Fig. 4–21):

$$\text{Fumarate}^{2-} + 2\,H_2 \rightarrow \text{Succinate}^{2-}$$

Fumarate can easily be formed from a wide range of carbon sources, such as malate, aspartate, and pyruvate, and thus is readily available to the organisms as an electron acceptor. The standard redox potential of the fumarate-succinate couple ($E_0' = +33$ mV) is greater than that of most of the other redox couples of metabolism, which makes it useful in the oxidation of various hydrogen donors (e.g., NADH, lactate, formate).

Energy-yielding Autotrophic Metabolism

During the past decade, our concept of autotrophy has become increasingly blurred as we have gained a better understanding of the biochemistry of the organisms previously classified unequivocally as autotrophs or heterotrophs. At present, the unique property that may be considered to be common to all autotrophs is their ability to obtain the major part of their biosynthetic carbon from carbon dioxide or the metabolism of a one-carbon compound. They obtain their energy from light (phototrophs), from the oxidation of inorganic compounds (chemolithotrophs), or from the oxidation of methyl groups attached to atoms other than carbon (methylotrophs) (Table 4–6).

Chemolithotrophs

These organisms are widely distributed in nature, where they play an important role in the maintenance of the nitrogen, carbon, and sulfur cycles. A variety of inorganic compounds can serve as their energy source. There is, however, no shared mechanism of inorganic chemical oxidation among the members of the group. The different substrates (H_2, S^{2-}, NH_4^+, NO_2^-, Fe^{2+}) are all oxidized by different enzyme complexes and pathways, and the oxidation of a reduced inorganic compound is not a unique property restricted to autotrophs (Table 4–6).

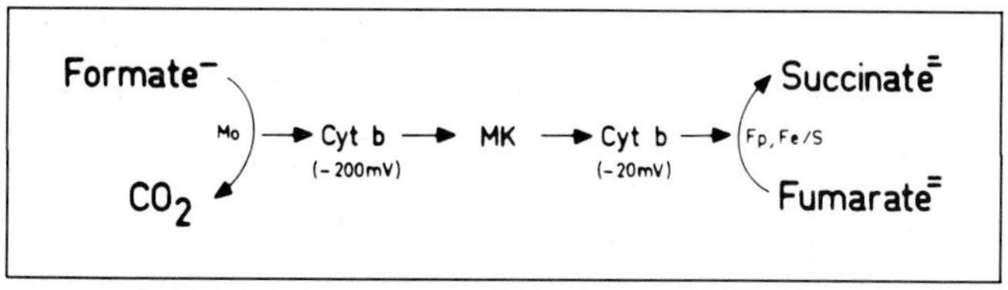

Fig. 4–21. Scheme of the electron flow from formate to fumarate in *Vibrio succinogenes. (According to Kröger: 27th Symposium Society General Microbiology; from Thauer et al: Bacteriol Rev 41:100, 1977.)*

Hydrogen Bacteria. These are aerobic organisms, most of which can utilize compounds in addition to hydrogen as an energy source. They possess the enzyme hydrogenase, which activates molecular hydrogen:

$$H_2 \xrightleftharpoons{\text{hydrogenase}} 2\,H^+ + 2e$$

The acceptors that function subsequent to the primary step vary with the kinds of coupling reactions that exist between the hydrogenase and the final electron acceptor. In some members of the group, a coupling with pyridine nucleotides and the electron transport chain occurs, with oxygen serving as the ultimate electron acceptor. An example of this type of coupling is found in *P. denitrificans,* which contains a membrane-bound respiratory chain very similar to that of mitochondria (Fig. 4–13). It has been speculated that the mitochondrion probably evolved from the plasma membrane of an ancestor of *P. denitrificans* via endosymbiosis.

Nitrifying Bacteria. In the nitrifying bacteria *Nitrosomonas* and *Nitrobacter,* the E_0' values for the oxidations involved do not permit a coupling with the reduction of NAD. In *Nitrobacter,* the electrons enter the transport chain at the level of cytochrome α_1:

$$\textit{Nitrosomas}\ NH_3 + 1\tfrac{1}{2}\,O_2 \rightarrow NO_2^- + H_2O + H^+$$

$$\textit{Nitrobacter}\ NO_2^- + \tfrac{1}{2}\,O_2 \rightarrow NO_3^-$$

Most of the nitrifying bacteria are obligate anaerobes, incapable of using organic substrates as an energy source.

Methanogenic Bacteria. Methane is the most reduced organic compound, and its formation is the terminal step in an anaerobic food chain. Methane is generated mainly from acetate, CO_2, and H_2 by the methanogens, a specialized group of anaerobic bacteria that inhabit anaerobic environments where organic matter is being decomposed. Methanogenic bacteria have the most stringent anaerobic requirements among anaerobes and carry out methanogenesis only where the redox potential is lower than -330 mV. They thus occupy a very narrow ecologic niche.

The biodegradation of organic compounds to methane in anaerobic habitats involves a microbial metabolic food chain, the complexity of which depends on the habitat. In the absence of nitrate, sulfate, or elemental sulfur, carbon dioxide becomes a major electron sink for anaerobic respiration, permitting obligate proton-reducing bacteria to carry out the oxidation of fatty acids and alcohols in such environments. By rapidly oxidizing and removing hydrogen from the anaerobic habitat, conditions thermodynamically favorable for the more complete anaerobic oxidation of carbon skeletons are produced.

The reduction of CO_2 to CH_4 proceeds stepwise, but the intermediates (formate, formaldehyde, and methanol) remain firmly bound to carriers that have not been completely identified. One carrier, coenzyme M, has been identified as 2-

TABLE 4–6. SOME ORGANISMS EXPLOITING UNCONVENTIONAL SOURCES OF ENERGY

Group	Energy Source	Heterotrophic Growth	
		+[a]	–[b]
Phototrophs	Light	*Rhodospirillum rubrum*	*Chromatium okenii*
Lithotrophs	H_2	*Alcaligenes eutrophus* *Paracoccus denitrificans*	*Methanobacterium thermoautrophicum*
	S^{2-}	*Thiobacillus acidophila* *Thiobacillus intermedius*	*Thiobacillus denitrificans* *Thiobacillus thiooxidans*
	NH_4^+	None	*Nitrosomonas europaea* *Nitrosospira briensis*
	NO_2^-	*Nitrobacter agilis*	*Nitrobacter* sp. *Nitrococcus mobilis*
Methylotrophs	CH_4 and other [CH_3—] compounds	Methylotroph strain XX	*Methylobacter* sp. *Methylomonas methanooxidans*
	[CH_3—] compounds other than CH_4	*Arthrobacter* 2B2 *Pseudomonas* 3A2	Methylotroph 4B6 Methylotroph C2A1

Adapted from Smith and Hoare: Bacteriol Rev 41:419, 1977.
[a] Growth on organic compounds in the absence of the specific energy source (versatile strains).
[b] No growth on organic compounds in the absence of the specific energy source (specialist strains).

mercaptoethanesulfonic acid. Methylcoenzyme M is probably the direct precursor of methane:

$$HCO_3^- + H_2 \rightarrow HCOO^- + H_2O$$

$$HCOO^- + H_2 + H_2 \rightarrow CH_2O + H_2O$$

$$CH_2O + H_2 \rightarrow CH_3OH$$

$$CH_3OH + H_2 \rightarrow CH_4 + H_2O$$

$$HCO_3^- + H^+ + 4H_2 \rightarrow CH_4 + 3H_2O$$

$$\Delta G^{o\prime} = -32.4 \text{ kcal}$$

The formation of methane from CO_2 and H_2 cannot be coupled to ATP synthesis by substrate-level phosphorylation. It thus appears that methanogenic bacteria gain ATP by electron transport phosphorylation.

Methylotrophs

This group of organisms is able to fulfill their energy requirement by the oxidation of methyl groups attached to atoms other than carbon. Some of these are obligate methylotrophs, growing only at the expense of compounds containing no carbon-carbon bonds (methane, methanol). Others are facultative methylotrophs, capable of growing on a variety of carbon sources, including C_1-compounds. The oxidation of methane to carbon dioxide proceeds via a series of two-electron oxidation steps. In the metabolism of methane, formaldehyde occupies a key position, since it is at this level that the carbon is both assimilated into biomass and dissimilated to carbon dioxide to provide energy.

Phototrophs

These organisms derive their energy for growth from light by the process of photosynthesis. Mechanistically this is the most complex mode of energy-yielding metabolism. Although the overall reaction is basically the same in all photosynthetic organisms, bacteria possess an evolutionarily more primitive mechanism.

Photosynthesis. Photosynthesis consists of an oxidation-reduction sequence in which carbon dioxide is reduced to the level of carbohydrate at the expense of a variety of hydrogen donors activated by light reactions.

$$2\ H_2A + CO_2 \rightarrow (CH_2O) + H_2O + 2\ A$$

The nature of the compound H_2A varies with the organism, and it is this property that distinguishes bacterial photosynthesis from that present in green plants. In plants that can grow aerobically in the light, H_2A can be water, and oxygen is liberated in the reaction. In bacteria, however, photosynthesis proceeds only under anaerobic conditions, no oxygen is evolved, and H_2A must be supplied as reduced sulfur, molecular hydrogen, or organic compounds. The photosynthetic bacteria are typically aquatic species and include the green and purple sulfur bacteria and the purple nonsulfur bacteria. The cyanobacteria, until recently classified as blue-green algae, are typical prokaryotes but are aerobic and carry out an oxygenic photosynthesis like green plants.

PHOTOSYNTHETIC APPARATUS. Photosynthesis occurs within specialized membrane systems, either in deeply invaginated membranes (thylakoids) or in enclosed vesicles. Within these structures are the components of the photosynthetic apparatus—bacteriochlorophylls, carotenoids, electron carriers, and proteins. These are oriented in the membrane systems in such a way that light can be absorbed by the bacteriochlorophylls and carotenoid pigments and the energy used to generate a protonmotive force across the membrane.

PHOTOSYNTHETIC ELECTRON TRANSPORT. Plants have two distinct photochemical reaction centers, whereas bacteria have only one. The primary photochemical event is initiated when a molecule of chlorophyll absorbs a quantum of light and transfers it to a reaction center buried within the membrane. The chlorophyll serves in some manner to effect a photochemical separation of oxidizing and reducing power, resulting in a flow along two transport systems. One of these systems accepts the electron delivered to the acceptor, and the other replaces it (Fig. 4–22).

In a photosynthetic bacterium, such as *Rhodospirillum*

rubrum, a nonheme-iron center complexed with quinone serves as the immediate electron acceptor and a cytochrome *c*-like protein as the electron donor to the activated chlorophyll. The flow of electrons is accompanied by the generation of ATP. The coupling mechanism is similar in principle to the coupling mechanisms employed in respiratory chain phosphorylation.

The fixation of the CO_2 into carbohydrate requires a supply of both NADPH and ATP. This relationship may be summarized in the following general statement:

$$H_2A + NAD(P)^+ + yADP + yP_i \xrightarrow{mh\nu} A + NAD(P)H + H^+ + yATP$$

For photosynthetic bacteria, the H_2A may be an inorganic substance, such as H_2S, or an organic compound, such as succinate. The energy of absorbed photons drives this reaction. In this event, the flow of electrons is open or noncyclic. In the absence of oxidizable substrate, however, light-induced electron flow occurs along a circular path (see Fig. 4–22). The electrons that come from the excited chlorophyll molecule may quite simply return to it again after they have traveled a circular route around the closed chain of electron carriers. This circuitous flow of electrons is a device to conserve some of the energy of the high-energy electrons that leave the excited chlorophyll. Cyclic photophosphorylation may represent the most primitive form of photosynthesis, useful to organisms in an environment rich in organic compounds and requiring only ATP.

DARK PHASE OF PHOTOSYNTHESIS. The formation of glucose in photosynthesis is a dark process that begins with the reduced NADP and ATP generated by light. The mechanism by which CO_2 fixation occurs in all photosynthesizing organisms is cyclic in nature and occurs in both eucaryotic and procaryotic organisms. This complex series of reactions is known as the

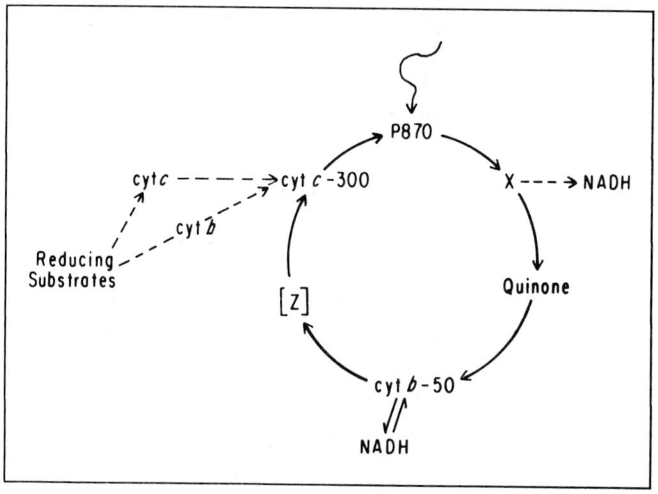

Fig. 4–22. A generalized scheme for photosynthetic electron flow in photosynthetic bacteria. Electrons lost from the cyclic electron flow system during the formation of NADH are replaced by electron transport from reduced substrates. X is probably an iron protein or an iron-quinone complex; Z is an intermediate suggested by kinetic data. *(From Jones OTG: In Haddock and Hamilton (eds): Microbial Energetics, Cambridge University Press, 1977.)*

Calvin cycle, the initial reaction of which is the synthesis of ribulose 1,5-diphosphate from ribulose 5-phosphate.

$$\text{Ribulose 5-PO}_4 + \text{ATP} \rightarrow \text{Ribulose 1,5-PO}_4 + \text{ADP}$$

$$\text{Ribulose 1,5-PO}_4 + CO_2 \rightarrow 2\ \text{3-Phosphoglyceric acid}$$

These two reactions are specific for organisms that use CO_2 as a sole carbon source and are not found in organisms that have a heterotrophic metabolism. The reduction of the two molecules of 3-phosphoglycerate occurs at the expense of NADPH and ATP formed in the light reaction. The two molecules of 3-phosphoglycerate occurs at the expense of NADPH and ATP formed in the light reaction. The two molecules of 3-phosphoglyceraldehyde thus formed are then converted into glucose essentially by reversal of the reactions of glycolysis.

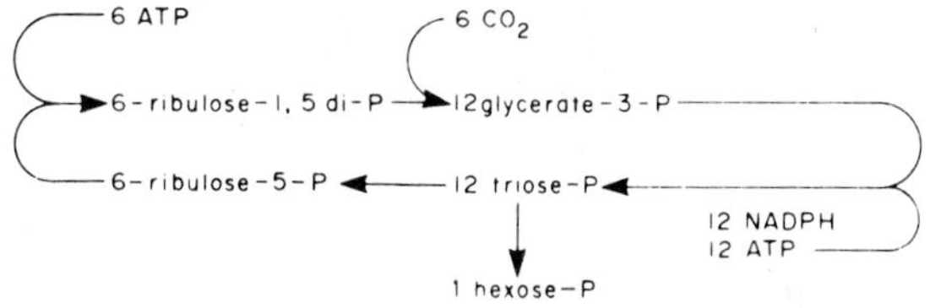

Control of Energy Metabolism

If a microorganism is to function efficiently, the rate of metabolism along the various branching and anastomosing metabolic pathways must be regulated in such a way that optimal use is made of the available substrates. For this purpose, the microbial cell has evolved an extremely sophisticated system of controls, some of which regulate its energy-supplying processes. Regulation of the energy-yielding metabolism is tightly controlled and takes place on different levels: by altering the rates of transcription and translation, by posttranslational modification, and by finely tuned feedback loops that regulate enzymatic activity in response to changes in substrate and product levels, and to culture conditions.

Genetic Regulation

In its natural habitat, the cell is confronted with a variety of potential energy sources. The survival of a particular species in its highly competitive environment has resulted from the ability of that species to adapt to new experiences in its environment. In so doing, the enzymatic machinery for the degradation of a wide variety of organic compounds is produced. Although the potential for the dissimilation of different substrates is great, the enzymes for such activities are produced (induced) only when needed. Controls of this type, induction and repression, are exceedingly common in microorganisms and are examples of genetic regulatory mechanisms. In general, induction exerts effective control of catabolic sequences involving carbon and energy sources, where the synthesis of enzymes catalyzing a particular sequence is turned on or off, depending on the demands for that specific sequence. The classic example of genetic regulation is the utilization of the disaccharide lactose by *E. coli.* The molecular biology of the lactose operon is discussed on p. 115.

Catabolite Repression. This type of control is frequently observed when organisms are grown on glucose or some other rapidly metabolizable energy source. Often called the *glucose effect,* catabolite repression results in a repression of synthesis of enzymes that would metabolize the added substrate less rapidly than glucose. When the *lac* system is induced, the rate of synthesis of β-galactosidase is considerably reduced in cultures growing upon glucose, compared with cells for which some other metabolite is provided as the carbon source. Glucose elicits catabolite repression by depressing the level of 3′-5′-cyclic AMP (cAMP) in the cell. The addition of cAMP to cultures overcomes glucose repression by stimulating transcription of the inducible enzyme, β-galactosidase. The level of cAMP in the cell varies with conditions of growth and reflects the energetic needs of the cell. The level is low when the available energy exceeds the biosynthetic requirement for energy, and the level of cAMP rises when the organism's carbon supply is depleted. The molecular aspects of catabolite repression are discussed in Chapter 8.

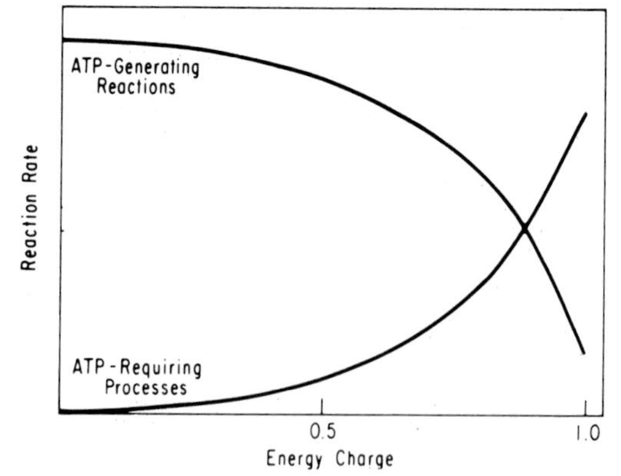

Fig. 4–23. Generalized response to the adenylate energy charge expected from enzymes involved in regulation of ATP-regenerating and ATP-utilizing sequences. *(From Atkinson: Biochemistry 7:4030, 1968.)*

Metabolic Regulation

Adenylate Energy Charge. The adenine nucleotides (ATP, ADP, and AMP) are metabolic energy modulators strategically placed to regulate the entire metabolic economy of the cell. In general, catabolic sequences contain regulatory enzymes that are activated by ADP or AMP or inhibited by ATP. Degradation of the substrate, therefore, proceeds maximally only when there is a need for ATP.

In its role as a primary metabolic coupling agent, the adenylate system has been compared with a storage battery in its ability to accept, store, and supply chemical energy. The term *adenylate energy charge* defines the relative amount of energy stored in the system and may be expressed on a linear scale by the equation

$$\text{Energy charge} = \frac{\text{ATP} + \frac{1}{2}\text{ADP}}{\text{ATP} + \text{ADP} + \text{AMP}}$$

The catalytic properties of a number of enzymes are modified by changes in the energy charge. As the energy charge increases, adenylate-regulated enzymes in ATP-regenerating sequences decrease in activity. The adenylate system is poised to run optimally in a steady state in which the energy charge is between 0.8 and 0.9 and strongly resists deviations from this range (Fig. 4–23). In view of the very rapid turnover rate of ATP in growing bacteria (1 to 10 s^{-1}), the tight stabilization of the energy charge is indicative of very sensitive and fast controls.

Modulation of the Glycolytic Pathway

PASTEUR EFFECT. In facultative organisms the fermentative capacity of the cell is blocked in the presence of oxygen, and the energy is supplied almost exclusively by respiration. As a result, less glucose is consumed, and the accumulation of lactate is decreased. This phenomenon, first recognized by Pasteur in fermenting yeast, is known as the *Pasteur effect.* The benefits of this effect are obvious in terms of the energy gain realized in switching from an anaerobic metabolism to an aerobic one. Anaerobic glycolysis releases only about 8% of the energy that is obtained from the complete breakdown of glucose. Therefore, if oxygen is available and the glucose is oxidized to CO_2 and H_2O without the accumulation of lactic acid, the energy needs of the cell can be met by the utilization of less glucose.

Several factors may be responsible for the Pasteur effect, but the major determinant is the key enzyme phosphofructokinase, which plays a central role in the regulation of glycolysis (p. 35). In the generation of ATP via the respiratory pathways, increased levels of ATP relative to ADP inhibit phosphofructokinase, thereby decreasing the flow of glucose into the glycolytic pathway.

The inhibition of phosphofructokinase activity by ATP is illustrative of regulation of an allosteric enzyme by a negative effector. The reaction catalyzed by phosphofructokinase, the formation of fructose 1,6-bisphosphate from fructose 6-phosphate, is a critical control point subject to strong metabolic regulation (Fig. 4–3). It is exquisitely sensitive to changes in the adenylate energy charge (Fig. 4–23), ensuring that whenever a plentiful supply of ATP is available, as when pyruvate is metabolized aerobically to CO_2 via the TCA cycle, glycolysis will be essentially blocked. The reverse is also true. When glycolysis is absolutely required for the generation of energy, that is, when the ATP drops to low levels and ADP or AMP accumulates, glycolysis will be favored.

In addition to ATP, other products of respiration can modulate glycolytic activity. The need for additional controls stems from the dual function of glycolysis as an amphibolic pathway. The glycolytic rate must respond to the need for supplying synthetic intermediates as well as the need for regenerating ATP. Phosphofructokinases from various bacterial species exhibit many similar, though not identical, regulatory properties. In general, activators of phosphofructokinase, such as AMP, ADP, P_i, and fructose 1,6-bisphosphate, are those that tend to accumulate during anaerobic conditions, whereas inhibitors of the enzyme, such as ATP and citrate, are those that tend to increase with transition from anaerobic to aerobic conditions.

Regulatory inputs that are also important either generally or in specific cases are the charges of the nicotinamide adenine nucleotides ($NADH/NADH + NAD^+$) and ($NADPH/NADPH + NADP^+$) and positive feed-forward effects (stimulation of a reaction by precursors one or more steps earlier in the sequence).

PYRUVATE DISSIMILATION CONTROL. For anaerobic metabolism in *E. coli,* which has a mixed-acid pattern of fermentation, the key enzyme in the central metabolic step of pyruvate to acetyl-CoA conversion is pyruvate formate-lyase. Pyruvate formate-lyase is a homodimeric protein subject to posttranslational interconversion. It occurs in an inactive form, E_i, and an active form, E_a. The latter form carries a free radical which is extremely sensitive to destruction by oxygen. In *E. coli* cells during aerobic growth in glucose medium, pyruvate formate-lyase is totally arrested in the inactive form. Triggered by either a changed redox potential or a possibly elevated cytoplasmic pyruvate concentration, a shift to strict anaerobiosis immediately results in posttranslational processing of the aerobically presynthesized E_i form to E_a. During strict anaerobiosis, the possible fermentation route to lactate is completely bypassed by the high activity of pyruvate formate-lyase.

FURTHER READING

Books and Reviews

Atkinson DE: Adenine nucleotides as stoichiometric coupling agents in metabolism and as regulatory modifiers: The adenylate energy charge. In Vogel HJ (ed): Metabolic Regulation. Metabolic Pathways. New York, Academic Press, 1971, vol 5, p 1

Atkinson DE: Cellular Energy Metabolism and Its Regulation. New York, Academic Press, 1977

Bédard C, Knowles R: Physiology, biochemistry, and specific inhibitors of CH_4, NH_4, and CO oxidation by methanotrophs and nitrifiers. Microbiol Rev 53:68, 1989

Barker HA: Amino acid degradation by anaerobic bacteria. Annu Rev Biochem 50:23, 1981

Brown CM, Macdonald-Brown DS, Meers JL: Physiological aspects of microbial inorganic nitrogen metabolism. Adv Microb Physiol 15:1, 1977

Chapman AG, Atkinson DE: Adenine nucleotide concentrations and turnover rates. Their correlation with biological activity in bacteria and yeast. Adv Microb Physiol 15:253, 1977

Colby J, Dalton H, Whittenbury R: Biological and biochemical aspects of microbial growth on C_1 compounds. Annu Rev Microbiol 33:481, 1979

Dawes EA: Microbial Energetics. Glasgow, Blackie & Son, Ltd, 1986

Drews G: Structure and functional organization of light-harvesting complexes and photochemical reaction centers in membranes of phototrophic bacteria. Microbiol Rev 49:59, 1985

Fridovich I: Superoxide dismutases. Annu Rev Biochem 44:147, 1975

Futai M, Kanazawa H: Structure and function of proton-translocating adenosine triphosphatase (F_0F_1): biochemical and molecular biological approaches. Microbiol Rev 47:285, 1983

Gottschalk G: Bacterial Metabolism, 2nd ed. New York, Springer-Verlag, 1986

Gottschalk G, Andreesen JR: Energy metabolism in anaerobes. Int Rev Biochem 21:85, 1979

Gunsalus IC, Stanier RY (eds): The Bacteria. New York, Academic Press, 1961, vol 2

Haddock BA, Hamilton WA (eds): Microbial Energetics. London, Cambridge University Press, 1977

Haddock BA, Jones CW: Bacterial respiration. Bacteriol Rev 41:47, 1977

Hooper AB, DiSpirito AA: In bacteria which grow on simple reductants, generation of a proton gradient involves extracytoplasmic oxidation of substrate. Microbiol Rev 49:140, 1985

Ingledew WJ, Poole RK: The respiratory chains of *Escherichia coli.* Microbiol Rev 48:222, 1984

Jones CW: Aerobic respiratory systems in bacteria. In Haddock BA, Hamilton WA (eds): Microbial Energetics. London, Cambridge University Press, 1977, p 23

Jones CW: Energy metabolism in aerobes. Int Rev Biochem 21:49, 1979

Jones OTG: Electron transport and ATP synthesis in the photosynthetic bacteria. In Haddock BA, Hamilton WA (eds): Microbial Energetics. London, Cambridge University Press, 1977, p 151

Kaback HR: Membrane vesicles, electrochemical ion gradients and active transport. Curr Top Memb Transp 16:393, 1982

Kondratieva EN: Interrelation between modes of carbon assimilation and energy production in phototrophic purple and green bacteria. Int Rev Biochem 21:117, 1979

Konings WN, Boonstra J: Anaerobic electron transfer and active transport in bacteria. In Bronner F, Kleinzeller A (eds): Curr Top Memb Transp 9:177, 1977

Lehninger AL: Bioenergetics, 2nd ed. New York, Benjamin, 1971

Lehninger AL: Biochemistry, 2nd ed. New York, Worth Publishers, 1975

Mah RA, Ward DM, Baresi L, et al: Biogenesis of methane. Annu Rev Microbiol 31:309, 1977

Mitchell P: Vectorial chemiosmotic processes. Annu Rev Biochem 46:996, 1977

Moloney PC: Coupling between H^+ entry and ATP synthesis in bacteria. Curr Top Memb Transp 16:175, 1982

Neidhardt FC, Ingraham JL, Low KB, et al: *Escherichia coli* and *Salmonella typhimurium.* Washington, Am Soc Microbiology, 1987

Nunn WD: A molecular view of fatty acid catabolism in *Escherichia coli.* Microbiol Rev 50:179, 1986

Pastan I, Adhya S: Cyclic adenosine 5′-monophosphate in *Escherichia coli.* Bacteriol Rev 40:527, 1976

Quayle JR, Ferenci T: Evolutionary aspects of autotrophy. Microbiol Rev 42:251, 1978

Ramaiah A: Pasteur effect and phosphofructokinase. Curr Top Cell Regul 8:297, 1974

Rosen BP: Ion Transport in Prokaryotes. San Diego, Academic Press, 1987

Smith AJ, Hoare DS: Specialist phototrophs, lithotrophs, and methylotrophs: A unity among a diversity of procaryotes. Bacteriol Rev 41:419, 1977

Stanier RY, Doudoroff M, Adelberg EA: The Microbial World. 4th ed. Englewood Cliffs, NJ, Prentice-Hall, 1976

Stouthamer AH: The search for correlation between theoretical and experimental growth yields. Int Rev Biochem 21:1, 1979

Thauer RK, Jungermann K, Decker K: Energy conservation in chemotrophic anaerobic bacteria. Bacteriol Rev 41:100, 1977

Trumpower BL: Cytochrome bc_1 complexes of microorganisms. Microbiol Rev 54:101, 1990

Wolfe RS, Higgins IJ: Microbial biochemistry of methane—a study in contrasts. Int Rev Biochem 21:267, 1979

Zeikus JG: The biology of methanogenic bacteria. Bacteriol Rev 41:514, 1977

Zeikus JG: Chemical and fuel production by anaerobic bacteria. Annu Rev Microbiol 34:423, 1980

Selected Papers

Anderson KB, von Meyenburg K: Charges of nicotinamide adenine nucleotides and adenylate energy charge as regulatory parameters of the metabolism in *Escherichia coli.* J Biol Chem 252:4151, 1977

Archibald FS, Fridovich I: Manganese, superoxide dismutase, and oxygen tolerance in some lactic acid bacteria. J Bacteriol 146:928, 1981

Bragg PD: The ATPase complex of *Escherichia coli.* Can J Biochem Cell Biol 62:1190, 1985

Cross AR, Anthony C: The electron-transport chains of the obligate methylotroph *Methylophilus methylotrophus.* Biochem J 192:429, 1980

DiGuiseppi J, Fridovich I: Oxygen toxicity in *Streptococcus sanguis.* The relative importance of superoxide and hydroxyl radicals. J Biol Chem 257:4046, 1982

Graham A, Boxer DH: The organization of formate dehydrogenase in the cytoplasmic membrane of *Escherichia coli.* Biochem J 195:627, 1981

Jamieson DJ, Higgins CF: Two genetically distinct pathways for transcriptional regulation of anaerobic gene expression in *Salmonella typhimurium.* J Bacteriol 168:389, 1986

Jamieson DJ, Sawers RG, Rugman PA, et al: Effects of anaerobic regulatory mutations and catabolite repression on regulation of hydrogen metabolism and hydrogenase isoenzyme composition in *Salmonella typhimurium.* J Bacteriol 168:405, 1986

Kashket ER: Effects of aerobiosis and nitrogen source on the proton motive force in growing *Escherichia coli* and *Klebsiella pneumoniae* cells. J Bacteriol 146:377, 1981

Klionsky DJ, Brusilow WSA, Simoni RD: In vivo evidence for the role of the subunit as an inhibitor of the proton-translocating ATPase of *Escherichia coli.* J Bacteriol 160:1055, 1984

Krasna AI: Regulation of hydrogenase activity in enterobacteria. J Bacteriol 144:1094, 1980

Krinsky NI: Singlet oxygen in biological systems. Trends Biochem Sci 2:35, 1977

McCord JM, Keele BB Jr, Fridovich I: An enzyme-based theory of obligate anaerobiosis: The physiological function of superoxide dismutase. Proc Natl Acad Sci USA 68:1024, 1971

Mitchell CG, Dawes EA: The role of oxygen in the regulation of glucose metabolism, transport and the tricarboxylic acid cycle in *Pseudomonas aeruginosa.* J Gen Microbiol 128:49, 1982

Moody CS, Hassan HM: Mutagenicity of oxygen free radicals. Proc Natl Acad Sci USA 79:2855, 1982

Neidhardt FC, Ingraham JL, Low KB, Magasanik B, Schaechter M, Umbarger HE (eds): *Escherichia coli* and *Salmonella typhimurium.* Cellular and Molecular Biology. Washington DC, Am Soc Microbiology, 1987, vol 1

Reddy TLP, Weber MM: Solubilization, purification, and characterization of succinate dehydrogenase from membranes of *Mycobacterium phlei.* J Bacteriol 167:1, 1986

Sunnarborg A, Klumpp D, Chung T, LaPorte DC: Regulation of the glyoxylate bypass operon: cloning and characterization of *icl R.* J Bacteriol 172:2642, 1990

Winkelman JW, Clark DP: Anaerobically induced genes of *Escherichia coli.* J Bacteriol 167:362, 1986

Wong KK, Suen KL, Kwan HS: Transcription of *pfl* is regulated by anaerobiosis, catabolite repression, pyruvate, and oxrA: *pfl::*Mμ dA operon fusions of *Salmonella typhimurium.* J Bacteriol 171:4900, 1989

Yerkes JH, Casson LP, Honkanen AK, Walker GC: Anaerobiosis induces expression of *ant,* a new *Escherichia coli* locus with a role in anaerobic electron transport. J Bacteriol 158:180, 1984

CHAPTER 5

Physiology of Bacterial Growth

Requirements for Growth

Growth may be defined as the orderly increase of all chemical constituents of the cell. It is a process that entails the replication of all cellular structures, organelles, and protoplasmic components from the nutrients present in the surrounding environment. In order for bacteria to grow, they must be provided with all the substances essential for the synthesis and maintenance of their protoplasm, with a source of energy, and with suitable environmental conditions.

As a group, bacteria are extremely versatile organisms. They exhibit tremendous capabilities for the utilization of quite diverse food materials, ranging from completely inorganic substrates to highly complex organic compounds. Many species also have learned to grow in a wide diversity of ecologic niches with extremes in temperature, acidity, and oxygen tensions. The ability of bacteria to exist under such circumstances is proof of their tremendous adaptability and reflects their capacity to respond successfully to a stimulus that is completely foreign to their past history.

Nutrient Requirements

Carbon. Two basic patterns characterize the nutritional requirements of bacteria and reflect their metabolic capabilities (see Table 4–1). At one end of the spectrum are the autotrophic bacteria (lithotrophs) that require only water, inorganic salts, and carbon dioxide for growth. These organisms synthesize a major portion of their essential organic metabolites from carbon dioxide. At the other end of the spectrum are the heterotrophic bacteria (organotrophs) that require an organic form of carbon for growth. Although glucose is extensively used as the organic source of carbon in routine laboratory practice, a wide variety of other substances also can be used as an exclusive or a partial source of carbon by different species of bacteria. Among the most versatile bacteria are the pseudomonads, some of which can utilize more than 100 different organic compounds as the sole carbon and energy source.

Nitrogen. The nitrogen atoms of amino acids, purines, pyrimidines, and other biomolecules come from NH_4^+. The flow of nitrogen into these compounds starts with the reduction of atmospheric N_2 to NH_4^+ by nitrogen-fixing microorganisms. NH_4^+ is then assimilated into amino acids by way of glutamate and glutamine, the two pivotal molecules in nitrogen metabolism (Fig. 5–1).

NITROGEN FIXATION. Higher organisms depend on certain nitrogen-fixing species of bacteria and blue-green algae to convert N_2 into the organic form. Because of the strength of the N≡N bond, nitrogen-fixation is highly energy demanding, requiring adenosine triphosphate (ATP) and a powerful reductant. The process is catalyzed by a complex enzyme, the nitrogenase complex, composed of two kinds of iron-sulfur proteins. In most nitrogen-fixing organisms, reduced ferredoxin is the source of electrons:

$$N_2 + 6e^- + 12\ ATP + 12\ H_2O \rightarrow 2\ NH_4^+ + 12\ ADP + 12\ P_i + 4\ H^+$$

Among the systems that have been extensively studied are those of the anaerobe *Clostridium pasteurianum* and the aerobes *Azotobacter vinelandii* and *Klebsiella pneumoniae.*

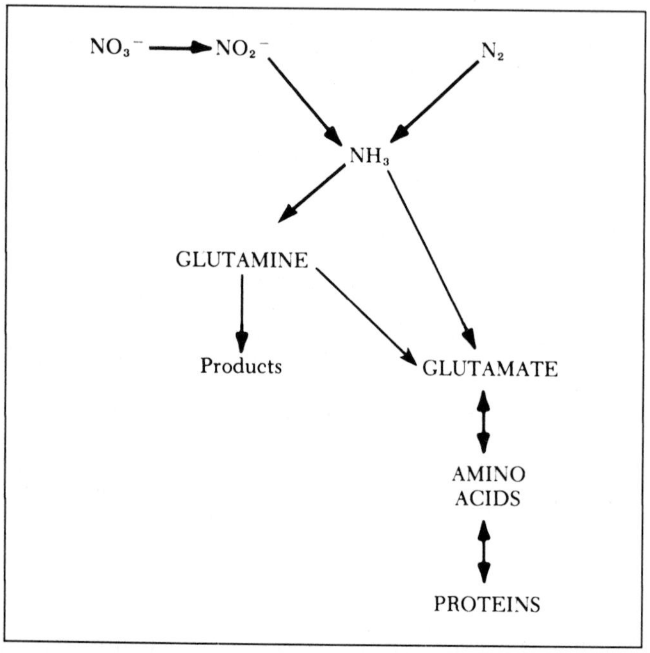

Fig. 5–1. Inorganic nitrogen assimilation in microorganisms.

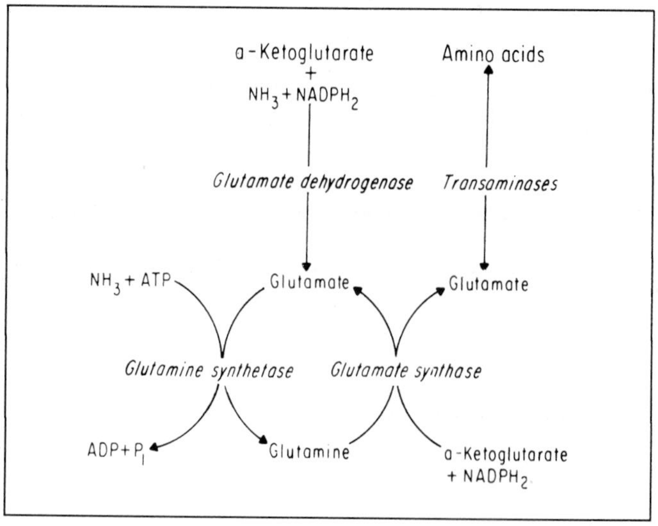

Fig. 5–2. Pathways of ammonia assimilation in procaryotic organisms. *(Adapted from Brown et al: Adv Microb Physiol 15:1, 1977.)*

NITRATE REDUCTION. Nitrate reduction may be accomplished by two distinct physiologic mechanisms: (1) assimilatory nitrate reduction, a process in which nitrate is reduced via nitrite and probably hydroxylamine to ammonia, which is then assimilated, and (2) dissimilatory nitrate reduction in which nitrate serves as an alternative electron acceptor to oxygen (i.e., anaerobic respiration, p. 46), with N_2 and NO_2 being the usual products. Nitrate assimilation is quite widespread in microorganisms, but dissimilatory nitrate reduction is common only in anaerobic bacteria and in facultatively anaerobic organisms growing at low oxygen tensions. Assimilatory nitrate reduction is catalyzed by two enzymes, nitrate reductase and nitrite reductase, both of which are distinct from the dissimilatory reductases.

AMMONIA ASSIMILATION. Ammonia occupies a central position in the metabolism of organisms grown on organic sources of nitrogen. Its assimilation by procaryotic organisms is accomplished by three major pathways (Fig. 5–2).

The first of these, the formation of glutamic acid from ammonia and α-ketoglutaric acid by l-glutamate dehydrogenase, is the primary pathway for the formation of α-amino acids directly from ammonia. The versatility of glutamic acid as amino-group donor in a number of transamination reactions permits the introduction of α-amino groups into most of the other amino acids.

$$NH_3 + \alpha\text{-Ketoglutarate} + NADPH + H^+ \xrightleftharpoons{\text{Glutamate dehydrogenase}} \text{Glutamate} + NADP^+ + H_2O$$

Glutamate dehydrogenase has a high K_m for ammonia and functions efficiently only when the environmental ammonia concentration is high. When the concentration of ammonia is low, the two enzymes, glutamine synthetase and glutamate synthase, together provide an alternate route for the incorporation of ammonia.

$$\text{Glutamate} + NH_3 + \text{ATP} \xrightleftharpoons{\text{Glutamine synthetase}} \text{Glutamine} + \text{ADP} + P_i$$

$$\text{Glutamine} + \alpha\text{-ketoglutarate} + \text{NADPH} + H^+ \xrightleftharpoons{\text{Glutamate synthase}} 2\ \text{glutamate} + \text{NADP}^+$$

Glutamine synthetase exerts strong regulatory control over the synthesis of enzymes responsible for the formation of glutamate from ammonia (see Chap. 7).

Growth Factors. Many of the heterotrophic bacteria are unable to grow unless supplied with one or more specific growth factors. These substances, usually provided in the culture medium in the form of yeast extract or whole blood, include the B-complex vitamins, amino acids, purines, and pyrimidines. The B-complex vitamins play a catalytic role within the cell either as components of coenzymes or as prosthetic groups of enzymes. Organisms that do not require an exogenous source of a given growth factor are capable of synthesizing their own. They are referred to as *prototrophic* in respect to that trait in order to distinguish them from *auxotrophic* mutants that require the addition of the growth factor to culture media in order for growth to occur.

Inorganic Ions. Small amounts of a number of inorganic ions are required by all bacteria. In addition to nitrogen, sulfur, and phosphorus, which are present as constituents of important biologic compounds, potassium, magnesium, and calcium occur in bacteria functionally associated with certain anionic polymers. Magnesium functions to stabilize ribosomes, cell membranes, and nucleic acids and is required for the activity of many enzymes. Potassium also is required for the activity of a number of enzymes, and in gram-positive organisms its concentration in the cell is influenced by the teichoic acid content of the cell wall. A requirement for iron, manganese, zinc, copper, and cobalt also has been shown in most organisms, and for others, molybdenum and selenium are essential. The need for others is more difficult to assess because of the minute amounts required and the presence of trace amounts as contaminants in constituents of media.

Trace elements play an important role in host-parasite interactions. In the animal host, powerful iron-binding proteins in the body fluids function to withhold iron from microbial invaders. The successful microbial invader has developed its own powerful iron chelators that vigorously extract iron from a variety of environments. A number of these iron compounds (siderophores) have been recognized in different bacterial species. Their existence emphasizes the essential role of iron for the organism, as well as the evolutionary significance of systems that ensure that the organism can compete successfully with the host for essential nutrients that may be present in limited amounts. For a further discussion of iron-binding proteins, see page 60.

Oxygen. The oxygen requirement of a particular bacterium reflects the mechanism employed for satisfying its energy needs. On the basis of their oxygen requirements, bacteria may be divided into five groups:

1. Obligate anaerobes that grow only under conditions of high reducing intensity and for which oxygen is toxic
2. Aerotolerant anaerobes that are not killed by exposure to oxygen
3. Facultative anaerobes that are capable of growth under both aerobic and anaerobic conditions
4. Obligate aerobes that require oxygen for growth
5. Microaerophilic organisms that grow best at low oxygen tensions, high tensions being inhibitory

In the obligate and aerotolerant anaerobes, the metabolism is strictly fermentative. In the facultative anaerobe, however, a respiratory mode of metabolism is employed when oxygen is available, but in its absence fermentation occurs. When organisms are grown in the presence of air, a number of enzymatic reactions occur that result in the production of hydrogen peroxide and the superoxide radical, O_2^-. In aerobes and the aerotolerant and facultative anaerobes, the enzyme superoxide dismutase prevents the accumulation of the superoxide ion, but in the obligate anaerobe this enzyme is absent:

$$2\ O_2^- + 2\ H^+ \xrightarrow{\text{Superoxide dismutase}} O_2 + H_2O_2$$

The hydrogen peroxide formed in the dismutase reaction is rapidly destroyed by the enzyme catalase, which is present in the aerobic and facultative anaerobes. Although some aerotolerant organisms, such as the lactic acid bacteria, lack catalase, they possess peroxidases that catalyze the destruction of H_2O_2, thereby enabling the organism to grow in the presence of oxygen (p. 46). An explanation of the requirement of microaerophilic organisms for a reduced oxygen tension appears to vary considerably, even within a single genus. For some, however, increased susceptibility to toxic forms of oxygen is associated with the absence of catalase or superoxide dismutase, or both. Possible targets for damage by H_2O_2 and O_2^- include specific outer membrane proteins, redox active components of the cytoplasmic membrane, and enzymes in the periplasmic space. In *Treponema pallidum,* oxygen sensitivity is related to H_2O_2-associated damage to DNA.

Carbon Dioxide. In addition to the chemolithotrophic and photolithotrophic bacteria that use CO_2 as the principal source of cellular carbon, chemoorganotrophs also have a requirement for an adequate supply of CO_2 for heterotrophic CO_2 fixation and for the synthesis of fatty acids. Because carbon dioxide normally is produced during the catabolism of organic compounds, it usually does not become a limiting factor. Some organisms, however, such as *Neisseria* and *Brucella,* presumably have one or more enzymes with a low affinity for CO_2 and require for growth a higher concentration (10%) of CO_2 than usually is present in the atmosphere (0.03%). This need must be considered in the isolation and culture of these organisms.

Physical Requirements

Oxidation-Reduction Potential. The oxidation-reduction potential (E_h) of the culture medium is a critical factor in determining whether growth of an inoculum will occur when transferred to a fresh medium. For most media in contact with air, the E_h is about +0.2 to +0.4 V at pH 7. Obligate anaerobes are unable to grow unless the E_h is at least as low as −0.2 volt. In order to establish anaerobic conditions in a culture, oxygen may be excluded by the use of anaerobic culture systems or by the addition of sulfhydryl-containing compounds, such as sodium thioglycollate (mercaptoacetate). During growth of both aerobic and anaerobic bacteria, there is a progressive decrease in the E_h of the environment, an observation that is of clinical importance in wound infections, in which a mixed population of aerobic and anaerobic organisms is capable of setting up an infection in an initially aerobic setting (see Chap. 44).

Temperature. For each bacterium there is an optimal temperature at which the organism grows most rapidly and a range of temperatures over which growth can occur. Cellular division is especially sensitive to the damaging effects of high temperature; very large and bizarre forms often are observed in cultures grown at a temperature higher than that supporting the most rapid division rate.

Bacteria are divided into three groups on the basis of the temperature ranges through which they grow: psychrophilic, −5 to 30C, optimum at 10 to 20C; mesophilic, 10 to 45C, optimum at 20 to 40C; and thermophilic, 25 to 80C; optimum at 50 to 60C. The optimum temperature usually is a reflection of the normal environment of the organism. Thus, bacteria pathogenic for humans usually grow best at 37C. One practical example of the importance of temperature on the growth of microorganisms in vivo is found in studies with *Mycobacterium leprae*. Growth of this organism in vivo is temperature-dependent, as reflected by the distribution of lesions in clinical cases of leprosy. The skin usually shows the most obvious lesions, whereas the internal organs are not involved. Under ordinary circumstances laboratory animals are not susceptible to infection with leprosy bacilli, but by inoculation of the foot pads of mice, a site with a reduced body temperature, successful passage of the organism can be obtained.

Hydrogen Ion Concentration. The pH of the culture medium also affects the growth rate, and here also there is an optimal pH with a wider range over which growth can occur. For most pathogenic bacteria the optimal pH is 7.2 to 7.6. Although a given medium may be initially suitable for growth, subsequent growth may be severely limited by metabolic products of the organisms themselves.

Bacteria possess extremely effective mechanisms for maintaining tight regulatory control over their cytoplasmic pH (pH_i). In many organisms, the pH_i varies by only 0.1 units per pH unit change in external pH. This is achieved by control of the activity of ion transport systems that facilitate proton entry. The diverse systems that have evolved reflect the wide range of pH_i values exhibited by the various bacteria. Thus, acidophiles have pH_i values in the range of pH_i 6.5 to 7.0, neutrophiles have pH_i values of 7.5 to 8.0, and alkalophiles have values of 8.4 to 9.0. Fermentative organisms exhibit a greater range of pH_i values over which growth occurs than do organisms that use respiratory pathways. In these organisms the production of acidic fermentation products and their accumulation results in failure of pH homeostasis and curtailment of growth. Some organisms have evolved compensatory mechanisms to avert the toxic effects of high concentrations of accumulated acidic products. Two well-known examples of the induction of a new metabolic pathway for this purpose are the production of the neutral product butanol from butyrate by *Clostridium acetobutylicum* and of butanediol from acetate by *Klebsiella aerogenes* (p. 39).

Osmotic Conditions. The concentration of osmotically active solutes inside a bacterial cell is, in general, higher than the concentration outside the cell. Except for the mycoplasmas and other cell wall–defective organisms, the majority of bacteria are unusually osmotically tolerant and have evolved complex transport systems and osmotic sensor-regulating devices for the maintenance of constant osmotic conditions within the cell.

A hitherto unrecognized class of cell constituents, the membrane-derived oligosaccharides (MDO), has been found in *Escherichia coli*. In *E. coli* and other gram-negative bacteria, there are two distinct aqueous compartments, the cytoplasm contained within the inner membrane and the periplasmic space contained between the inner and outer membranes. When the organisms are grown in a medium of low osmolarity, the cytoplasmic membrane, which has little mechanical rigidity, will swell unless prevented from doing so by an osmolarity of the periplasmic space, similar to that found in the cytoplasm. In cells grown in a medium of low osmolarity, MDO is the principal source of fixed anion in the periplasmic space and thus acts to maintain the high osmotic pressure and Donnan membrane potential of the periplasmic compartment. These unique oligosaccharides are structurally well suited for their regulatory role. They have molecular weights in the range of 2200 to 2600 and are thus impermeable to the outer membrane, a property essential for their specific function. They consist of 8 to 10 glucose units in a highly branched structure, multiply substituted with membrane-derived phosphoglycerol and succinate residues, which allow them to maintain a high anionic charge. Cells grown in a medium of low osmolarity synthesize MDO at a maximum rate, the rate of synthesis apparently being regulated at the genetic level in response to changes in osmolarity of the medium.

Uptake of Nutrients

Bacteria, in common with all living organisms, are surrounded by a semipermeable membrane that restricts the entry of most molecules into the cell. Highly specialized systems have evolved for the transport of small molecules across the membrane barrier. The large molecules found in the organism's natural environment, however, cannot be used unless the organism produces enzymes and exports them from their site of synthesis in the cytoplasm to the various extracytoplasmic compartments.

Secreted Enzymes

A large number of different types of proteins are located outside the cytoplasmic membrane in both gram-positive and gram-negative bacteria. All of these are exported proteins in the sense that they must cross the cytoplasmic membrane to reach their final destination. Many of these are exoenzymes secreted in large amounts into the growth medium, very little remaining cell-associated. These enzymes have tremendous survival value for the organism in its natural habitat where it usually finds accessible sources of carbon, nitrogen, and other nutrients rate-limiting for growth. In fact, the capability of microorganisms to degrade complex macromolecules of high molecular weight is so enormous that it is always possible, by looking in the right place and in the proper way, to find some organism that can break down any selected naturally occurring substance. This hypothesis is the basis for the enrichment culture technique used in isolating organisms specifically for this purpose.

Some of the exoenzymes are virulence factors of the organisms excreting them. A number of the more invasive pathogenic bacteria, especially gram-positive species such as *Streptococcus pyogenes, Staphylococcus aureus,* and certain *Clostridium* species, elaborate a variety of exoenzymes that destroy vital components of the body tissues and thus contribute to the overall pathogenesis of infection.

Although some gram-negative bacteria such as *Pseudomonas* species and *Vibrio cholerae* do excrete many proteins into the extracellular environment, except for certain specialized proteins such as toxins and hemolysins, excretion through both the inner and outer membranes and into the surrounding media is not a general property of many gram-negative bacteria, including *E. coli.* For these organisms, most of the secreted enzymes remain localized in the periplasmic compartment. For certain enzymes, such as alkaline phosphatase and β-lactamase, gram-positive organisms may compensate for the absence of a periplasmic storage compartment by anchorage of these proteins to the plasma membrane. They also may be able to achieve effective local concentrations in the surrounding medium by regulating the amount of membrane-bound or secreted molecules in response to various stimuli.

Synthesis. Exoenzymes may be constitutive or inducible, and in most cases the rate of synthesis appears to be regulated by end-product inhibition and catabolite repression. No universal statement can be made concerning the stage of the growth cycle during which exoenzymes are produced. Although many are formed toward the end of the logarithmic phase of growth, such as the lecithinase of *Clostridium perfringens* and the hyaluronidase of *S. aureus,* others, including the nicotinamide adenine dinucleotidase of *S. pyogenes* and the proteinase of *Clostridium botulinum,* are formed in approximately equivalent proportions during most of the growth cycle.

The study of protein export into or across membranes is currently one of the most active areas of cell biology research. As a result of the rapid advances being made, we have a much better although still incomplete understanding of how periplasmic enzymes and exoenzymes are synthesized and secreted. It now appears that almost all procaryotic-secreted proteins are made initially in a precursor form with an amino-terminal signal (leader) sequence of 20 to 40 amino acids. These leader sequences are enriched in hydrophobic residues and are thought to initiate protein export. Data on translocation per se are limited, but in *E. coli* the same protein can be translocated both cotranslation and posttranslation. Signal peptidase, an integral membrane protein, removes the signal peptides during or shortly after translocation across the cytoplasmic membrane. This processing, or removal of the signal sequence, is necessary for proper localization and activity of secreted proteins. In gram-negative bacteria, as well as in eucaryotic cells, removal of the signal sequence by signal peptidase yields essentially the mature protein. In gram-positive bacilli, however, the putative cleavage sites are followed by long stretches (up to 200 residues) of amino acids that contain multiple processing sites. In bacteria, the energy required for transport appears to be provided by the membrane potential.

Membrane Transport

Growth and survival of an organism depend on its ability to transfer solutes from the external milieu into the cytoplasm. This transfer is not a matter of selective permeability, as is often inferred in the definition of the cytoplasmic membrane, but of transport. With only a few exceptions, such as water and ammonia, which enter the cell by passive diffusion in response to a concentration gradient, the passage of metabolites is accomplished by specific transport or carrier systems. During the course of bacterial evolution, a large number of highly diverse transport systems have evolved for the capture of nutrients. The substrates for these systems range from the trace metals, vitamins, and major nutrients to the precursors of extracellular macromolecules. For these nutrients, translocation across the membrane constitutes the first step in metabolism.

Transport Systems

Porin and Maltose Channels. Although most of the specific transport systems of bacteria are energy-dependent, a few do not require metabolic energy. In this latter category are two systems located in the outer membrane of *E. coli,* the porin channel (p. 25) and the maltose channel (lambda receptor). The porin channel is relatively nonspecific and allows the passage of hydrophilic solutes with a molecular weight of 600 daltons or less. There are multiple species of porin in enteric bacteria, each existing in the cell as trimers of porin protein. The LamB protein (phage λ receptor) of *E. coli* is involved with the passage of maltose and maltodextrins through the outer membrane. Physical interaction of the LamB protein with the maltose-binding protein of the periplasmic space confers specificity on this outer membrane channel.

In the cytoplasmic membrane of *E. coli,* there also is at least one energy-independent transport system, the glycerol facilitator. With this exception, most bacterial transport systems are geared to the performance of osmotic work and allot a considerable fraction of their energy supply to the work of transport.

Facilitated Diffusion. This simple mode of transport is typified by the process of glycerol uptake. In *E. coli* a single membrane-associated protein facilitates the rapid equilibrium of substrate across the cell membrane (Fig. 5–3). Functioning in tandem with a cytoplasmic ATP-dependent kinase, it effects the capture of glycerol from the medium. Once phosphorylated, the glycerol is trapped inside the cell. Glycerol kinase is an effective scavenger and pacemaker of carbon source consumption and has properties suitable for this role, a high affinity for substrate and susceptibility to remote feedback inhibition. The glycerol facilitator behaves in many ways as a membrane channel.

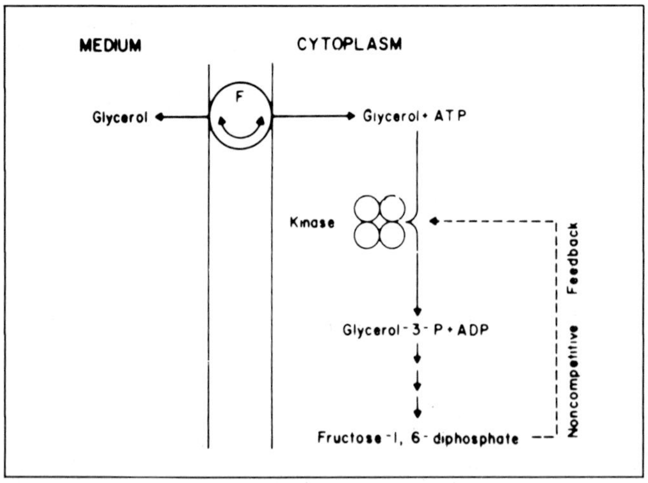

Fig. 5–3. Facilitated diffusion of glycerol. A membrane-associated facilitator protein functions in tandem with a cytoplasmic kinase for the capture of glycerol from the medium. *(From Andrews and Lin: Fed Proc 35:2185, 1976.)*

Phosphoenolpyruvate: Sugar Phosphotransferase System (PTS). This transport system mediates group translocation, a vectorial pathway in which metabolic sequences are oriented across the membrane so as to catalyze transport and chemical transformation concurrently. The sugars apparently are phosphorylated as they are translocated across the cell membrane.

COMPONENTS OF THE SYSTEM. The phosphotransferase system is a multiprotein complex consisting of four proteins, as shown in Figure 5–4. Two of these proteins are general proteins of the system required for the phosphorylation of all sugar substrates, whereas the other two proteins are sugar specific, a given pair being required for the transport of a particular sugar.

The two nonspecific components of the system, enzyme I and HPr, are soluble proteins and are produced constitutively. Enzyme I catalyzes the transfer of the energy-rich phosphoryl group from phosphoenolpyruvate (PEP) to HPr, a low molecular weight, histidine-containing protein. Enzyme I itself is phosphorylated during the transfer reaction (reaction 1).

$$\text{PEP} + \text{Enzyme I} \rightleftharpoons \text{Phosphoenzyme I} + \text{Pyruvate} \quad (1)$$
$$\text{Phosphoenzyme I} + \text{HPr} \rightleftharpoons \text{Enzyme I} + \text{Phospho-HPr} \quad (2)$$
$$\text{Phospho-HPr} + \text{Enzyme II} \rightleftharpoons \text{HPr} + \text{Phosphoenzyme II} \quad (3)$$
$$\text{Phosphoenzyme II} + \text{Carbohydrate}_{out} \rightarrow \text{Enzyme II} + \text{Carbohydrate phosphate}_{in} \quad (4)$$

In a number of cases, phospho-HPr transfers its phosphoryl group directly to the substrate specific, membrane-bound enzyme II. In some cases, however, transfer occurs instead to enzyme III, a third soluble protein in the system, which acts as the immediate phosphoryl carrier. Substrate specificity, however, always is restricted to enzyme II, which spans the membrane and catalyzes the binding and translocation of substrates through the membrane.

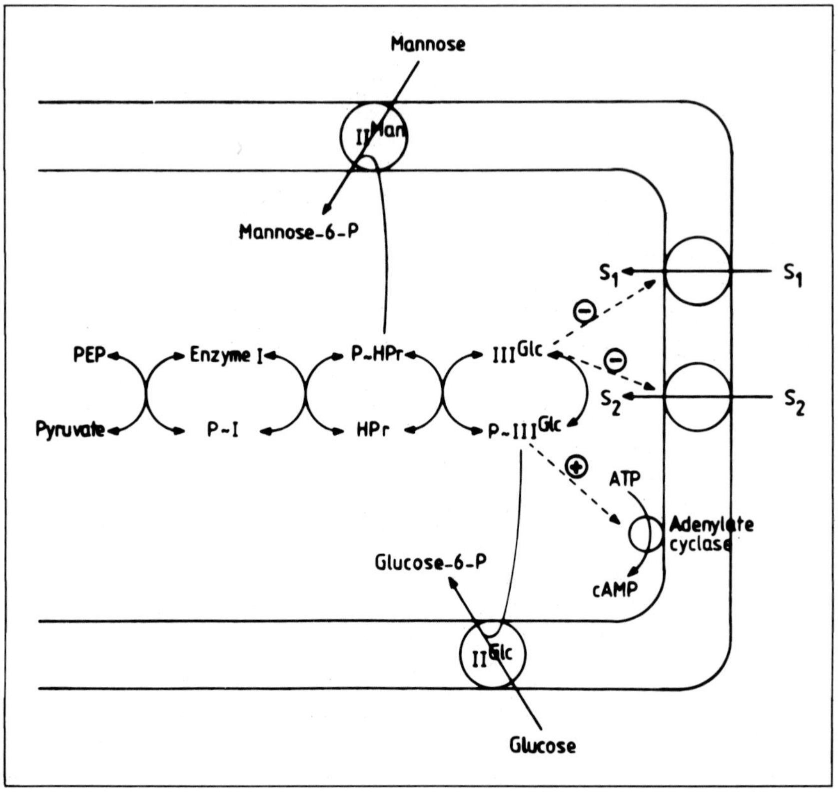

Fig. 5–4. Model for the regulation of substrate uptake by PTS. In addition to the general proteins of the PTS, two enzymes II are shown, specific for mannose (II^{Man}) and glucose (II^{Glc}). Activation (+) of adenylate cyclase by phosphorylated III^{Glc}($P \sim III^{Glc}$) and inhibition (−) of two different non-PTS uptake systems by III^{Glc} are indicated. S_1 and S_2 represent lactose, melibiose, maltose, or glycerol. *(From Postma and Lengeler: Microbiol Rev 49:232, 1985.)*

The PTS is widespread among microorganisms, being generally present in facultative aerobes and anaerobic organisms but not in the obligate aerobes. The intracellular accumulation of the corresponding sugar phosphate concomitant to translocation and phosphorylation is an energetically favorable pathway, permitting the uptake of an external sugar and its conversion to the first catabolic product in a single step. For sugars such as galactose that are not taken up via the PTS, two energy-requiring steps are essential. The sugar phosphate product of PTS translocation is trapped and accumulates within the cell.

In addition to catalyzing the transport and phosphorylation of its sugar substrates, PTS is involved in a number of other processes. The proteins of the PTS function as a chemoreceptor system, permitting the organisms to recognize sugar substrates of the PTS in the extracellular environment and to swim up concentration gradients of these compounds. Another major function of PTS is to regulate the utilization of certain non-PTS substrates, such as glycerol, maltose, and melibiose in *Salmonella typhimurium* and also lactose in *E. coli.* In culture media containing both a PTS and a non-PTS sugar, the PTS sugar is utilized before induction of the catabolic systems for the non-PTS sugar. This regulatory function, known as the *glucose effect* or *diauxic* growth, has been intensely studied for many years. It involves both the inhibition of uptake of the non-PTS sugar (inducer exclusion) and regulation of adenylate cyclase. The inhibition occurs directly at the level of the functional permease and is effected by a direct interaction between that transport protein and one or more PTS components (Fig. 5–4).

In addition to the PTS, bacteria also contain other transport systems that operate via group translocation. Adenine is glycosylated to adenosine monophosphate in a vectorial reaction catalyzed by a membrane-bound enzyme. During transport fatty acids are converted to acyl coenzyme A (CoA) by the acyl-CoA synthetase.

Active Transport (Substrate Translocation). Active transport resembles facilitated diffusion in that it also requires the participation of specific membrane-associated transport proteins. Active transport of solute, however, occurs at the expense of metabolic energy. A source of energy is required because the cell must do work in moving the substance through the cell membrane against a concentration gradient. Within the bacterial cell, concentrations of solutes may be several thousand times as great as those outside the cell (e.g., 10^5 in the case of maltose). The substrate molecule is not altered during transport but appears in the cytoplasm in a chemically unchanged form.

Substrate translocation in bacteria is mediated by two distinct mechanisms. One of these requires only membrane-associated components. The second class of mechanisms, found in gram-negative organisms and utilized for the transport of a wide range of substrates, requires the participation of soluble-binding proteins present in the periplasmic space.

β-GALACTOSIDE PERMEASE. This is the archetypal substrate translocation system (Fig. 5–5). It is a system by which lactose is transported by a carrier into the cell and accumulated to a concentration many times that in the medium. A single membrane protein or permease (M protein) coded for by the *y* gene of the *lac* operon is responsible for the recognition and translocation of substrate. The carrier demonstrates typical Michaelis-Menten kinetics. Under conditions of energy abundance the binding site of the M protein has a high affinity for the substrate when it is oriented externally and a low affinity when it is internally oriented. This results in the energetically uphill movement of substrate into the cell. When the cell is deprived of energy, the function of the M protein is reduced to the role of facilitating diffusion of the substrate to a transmembrane equilibrium.

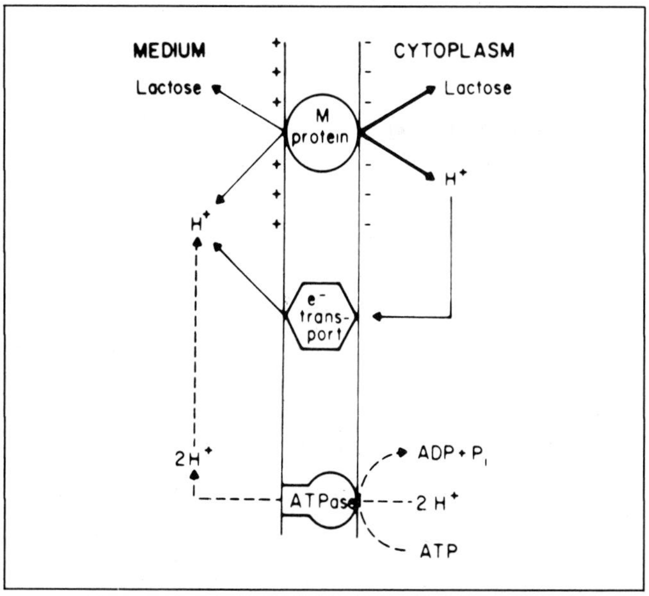

Fig. 5–5. β-Galactoside permease system. A single membrane protein (M protein) is responsible for the recognition and translocation of substrate. *(From Andrews and Lin: Fed Proc 35:2185, 1976.)*

The energy-coupling mechanisms employed in active transport are best interpreted by the chemiosmotic theory of transport and metabolism proposed by Mitchell (p. 44). According to this concept the accumulation of solutes is brought about by coupling solute movement to proton movement down the electrochemical gradient. The electrochemical gradient or proton motive force can be generated by either oxidation or ATP hydrolysis.

PERIPLASMIC BINDING PROTEINS. In gram-negative organisms a number of active transport systems are associated with binding proteins localized in the periplasmic space. These may be released by cold osmotic shock treatment, which damages the outer layer of the cell wall and releases proteins in the periplasmic space. After osmotic shock and loss of these proteins, the uptake of a number of metabolites is impaired. The binding proteins are low molecular weight, water-soluble proteins that bind the metabolite with high affinity and specificity but have no known enzymatic activity. They are thus believed not to carry the substrate across the membrane but to function as efficient scavengers in the recognition of substrate, which is then transported by a membrane-bound transport system. The energetics of the periplasmic transport systems is not fully understood, but it appears to differ considerably from that of the β-galactoside system.

Among the wide variety of transport systems for which binding proteins are essential are maltose, ribose, sulfate, phosphate, oligopeptides, glutamine, and several amino acids. One of the best characterized of these is the maltose transport

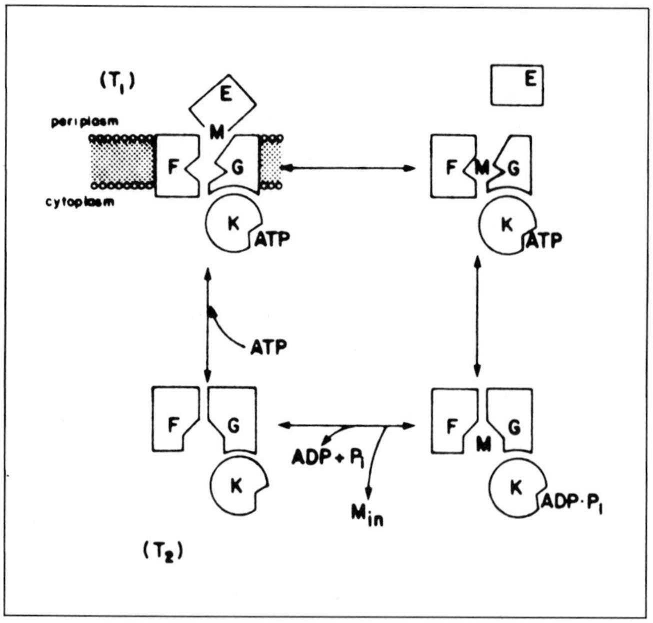

Fig. 5–6. Model for the accumulation of maltose across the cytoplasmic membrane. In this model, the *mal F*, *mal G*, and *mal K* gene products form a complex in the cytoplasmic membrane. The *mal E* gene product, maltose-binding protein, interacts with this complex from the external periplasmic side of the membrane. *M* indicates a molecule of substrate, maltose, or longer maltodextrin. *(From Shuman: J Biol Chem 257:5455, 1982.)*

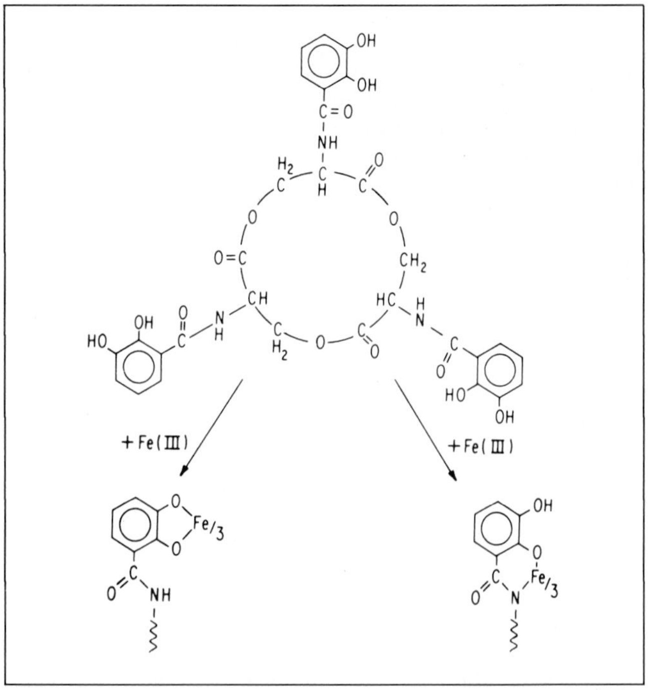

Fig. 5–7. Enterobactin, the cyclic triester of 2,3-dihydroxy-N-benzoyl-l-serine, a phenolic iron transport compound. Two possible coordination geometries with Fe^{3+} are given. *(After Anderson et al: Nature 262:722, 1976.)*

system, the only system in *E. coli* that is able to transport maltose across the cytoplasmic membrane. In this organism the accumulation of maltose requires five proteins, including an outer membrane protein (LamB), a periplasmic maltose-binding protein, and three plasma membrane proteins. The outer membrane protein also serves as the receptor for bacteriophage λ. The membrane-bound proteins appear to consist of both integral and peripheral membrane proteins that are present in smaller amounts than the corresponding periplasmic component. According to the model depicted in Figure 5–6, accumulation of substrate occurs as a result of a cycle of conformational changes of membrane proteins.

In the galactose system, the galactose-binding protein also acts as a signal receptor for chemotaxis, but there does not appear to be a general correlation between the presence of periplasmic binding proteins and chemotaxis.

Iron Uptake and Transport. Iron is a universally required nutrient. In aerobic environments and at neutral pH, however, the concentration of soluble iron is too low to achieve maximum growth rates. Under these conditions it is present in its ferric state (Fe^{3+}) as highly insoluble hydroxides, carbonates, and phosphates. Microorganisms have evolved multiple systems to obtain an adequate amount of this essential element. A low affinity system is present in most bacteria, permitting the organism to utilize the polymeric forms of iron in spite of the profound insolubility of Fe^{3+}. For this pathway, relatively high levels of iron are required to achieve maximum growth rates, and no specific solubilizing and transporting compounds or membrane receptors are required.

SIDEROPHORES. The high-affinity iron assimilation system is comprised of two parts, the siderophore and the matching membrane-associated receptors and transport apparatus. Siderophores are relatively low molecular weight (500 to 1000), virtually ferric-specific ligands whose function is to supply iron to the cell. They are viewed as the evolutionary response to the appearance of oxygen in the atmosphere and concomitant oxidation of Fe^{2+} to Fe^{3+}. Although considerable structural variation exists among the many siderophores that have been characterized, most are of two general structural types: catechols, of which enterobactin (Fig. 5–7) is the best characterized, and hydroxamates (Fig. 5–8), typified by ferri-

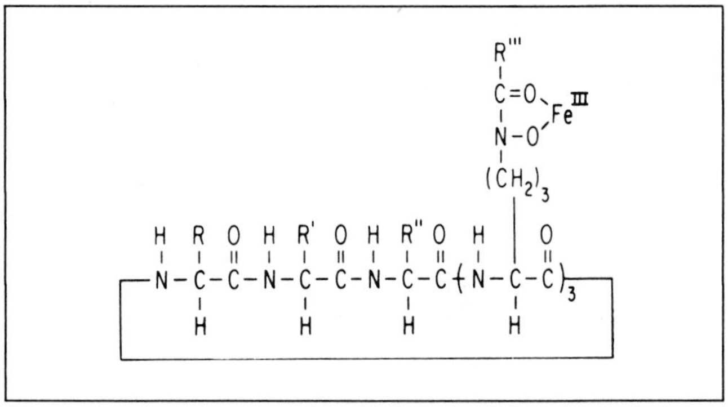

Fig. 5–8. General structure of a hydroxamate siderophore. In ferrichrome, a hydroxamate produced by fungi, R = R[1] = R[2] = H; R[3] = CH_3.

chrome, which are produced by certain fungi. Citrate also functions in some organisms as a high affinity carrier, but its receptor on the outer membrane is induced only by growth of the organism in the presence of substrate.

Enterobactin is a powerful chelating agent produced rapidly by *E. coli* under conditions of iron stress and secreted into the medium. The organism also has developed a scavenger ability to utilize siderophores, such as ferrichrome produced by other species, and possesses efficient transport systems for this purpose.

MEMBRANE RECEPTORS. In gram-negative bacteria, specific receptor proteins for the siderophores are present in the outer membrane. From there the complexes are channeled to system-specific receptors on the cytoplasmic membrane. In *E. coli* there are four different Fe^{3+}-chelator transport systems specific for Fe^{3+}-ferrichrome, Fe^{3+}-enterochelin, Fe^{3+}-citrate, or Fe^{3+}-aerobactin. The synthesis of these receptors and of enterobactin appears to be regulated coordinately by the intracellular iron concentration. Assimilation of the Fe^{3+}-siderophore complex implicates reduction of the metal iron and release into the cell after enzymatic hydrolysis of the ligand moiety. Uptake strongly depends on an energized membrane state.

In addition to their role in iron transport, the Fe^{3+}-siderophore receptors serve as receptors for certain bacteriophages and colicins. Mutants lacking a specific receptor are phage resistant and insensitive to the specific colicins and are simultaneously defective in iron transport.

Bacterial Chemotaxis

Motile bacteria have a well-developed sensory system that allows them to compete successfully in their natural environment. The system enables the organism to detect changes in concentration of certain chemicals and to move either toward (positive chemotaxis) or away (negative chemotaxis) from the substance, depending on its nature. Bacteria are attracted to many different kinds of chemicals, most of which can serve as nutrients. There is, however, no correlation between the metabolism of a substance and its ability to attract bacteria. Although most of the repellents that cause negative chemotaxis are toxic, toxicity is not essential for a negative response.

Chemotactic Response. Elegant quantitative methods have been used to follow the motion of bacteria by microscopic and photomicrographic techniques. In the absence of a stimulus a bacterium swims in a straight line for a few seconds and then turns abruptly, appearing to tumble head over tail for a fraction of a second before swimming off in a new direction. The bacterium responds to chemical stimuli by modification of this normal pattern of swimming. Bacteria tumble less frequently when they encounter increasing concentrations of attractant, and they tumble more frequently when the concentration decreases. This sensing of change in concentration is temporal; that is, the organism has some kind of memory that allows it to compare the environment of its past with that of its present and to interpret this signal.

Sensory Apparatus

CHEMORECEPTORS. The component of the sensory system that recognizes the chemical and measures the change in concentration is a chemoreceptor located either in the plasma membrane or in the periplasmic space. Receptors are protein molecules specifically designed to receive signals only from those molecules or physical conditions that the apparatus needs to sense. In *E. coli,* there are approximately 20 attractant receptors and 10 repellent receptors. Most of the receptors are specific for one or two chemicals at high affinities, but they usually exhibit a limited range of substances with which they will react, some with appreciably lower affinity. The total environment sensed by the bacterium is, thus, a product of the specificity of each individual receptor multiplied by the repertoire of receptors present on its surface. A few of the receptors, such as those for aspartate and serine, are constitutive, but most, especially for the sugars, are induced by growth on a particular substrate. These receptors are present in substantial concentration. There are about 10,000 molecules of periplasmic galactose, ribose, and maltose receptors per cell when fully induced and about 5000 molecules of aspartate and serine receptors per cell. For such sugars as maltose, ribose, and galactose, the chemoreceptor is a small soluble protein located in the periplasmic space. These are the same binding proteins active in the uptake of the corresponding sugar, although uptake is not necessary for taxis. Other chemoreceptors are integral membrane proteins, as in the case of amino acids and those sugars transported into the cell via the phosphotransferase system. Transport and chemotaxis are thus very closely related.

TRANSDUCER PROTEINS. Four transducer proteins, or methyl-accepting chemotaxis proteins (MCPs), play central roles in the processing of transmembrane signals, acting as the comparator in the sensory system and relaying information to the flagellar apparatus about changes in the concentration of chemoeffectors (Fig. 5–9). These integral membrane proteins are products of the *tsr* (MCP I), *tar* (MCP II), *trg* (MCP III), and *tap* (MCP IV) genes, and each is specific for mediating signals from a different set of stimuli. The transducer proteins receive signals from the chemoreceptors, which presumably induce a conformational change in the transducer proteins. As a result, posttranslational methylation of a glutamyl residue by methyltransferase and the methyl donor, *S*-adenosylmethionine, occurs. The degree of methylation reflects the cell's environment and increases until it reaches a plateau level that is a function of the receptor occupancy. Adaptation to the stimulus is complete, and prestimulus behavior is resumed when methylation reaches the plateau and protein methyltransferase activity is balanced by the activity of a protein methylesterase. There is thus a dynamic process of methylation and demethylation occurring constantly. Control of these processes is the mechanism that permits response and adaptation.

Information from the four transducer proteins converges on the switch of the flagellar motor, producing an immediate effect upon flagellar rotation. The switch consists of a complex of three proteins (FlaA11.2, FlaQ, and FlaN) that determine the rotational sense, either counterclockwise or clockwise, of the motor and also participate in the conversion of proton energy into mechanical work of rotation. This switch complex probably is mounted to the base of the flagellar basal body. In a free-swimming cell, all the flagella come together to form a synchronously rotating bundle of filaments that drives the cell through the medium. During smooth swimming, the flagella are all rotated counterclockwise. A reversal of rotation of one or more filaments disrupts the flagellar bundle and

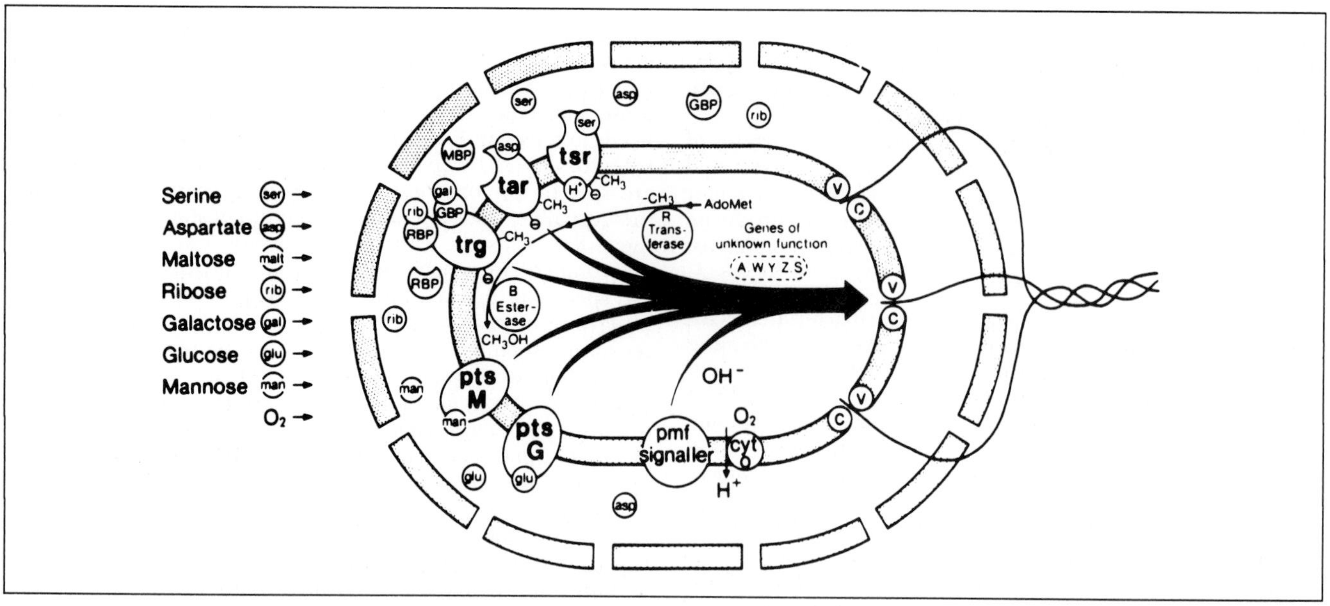

Fig. 5–9. Schematic representation of sensory transduction in chemotaxis in *E. coli* and *S. typhimurium.* The chemoeffectors (e.g., serine, aspartate) can cross the outer membrane and bind to receptors in the periplasmic space (RBP, GBP, MBP) or in the membrane (e.g., pts M, trg). For signals processed through MCPs (tsr, tar, trg), adaptation depends on methylation or on demethylation catalyzed by protein methyltransferase (R) or protein methylester (B), respectively. For signals processed through other signaling proteins (pts M, pts G, pmf signaler), adaptation may be independent of the activity of R. All sensory transduction pathways converge prior to C and V, which represent the switch on the flagellar motor. A, W, Y, Z, S are chemotaxis gene products with unassigned functions in signal processing. *(From Niwano and Taylor: Proc Natl Acad Sci USA 79:11, 1982.)*

leads to tumbling. The chemotactic response that stems from the regulation of tumble frequency thus arises as a result of the regulation of flagellar reversal. Addition of an attractant results in suppression of tumbling by causing counterclockwise rotation of the bacterial flagella, whereas addition of a repellent causes increased tumbling, a result of clockwise rotation.

Growth of Bacterial Populations

Measurement of Bacterial Growth

When placed in a nutritionally complete medium, a bacterial cell grows larger and eventually divides to form two cells. This continues, with the production of a population of vegetative, undifferentiated cells. In the development of a bacterial culture, there is an increase both in cell mass and in number of organisms, but there is no constant relationship between the two parameters. In quantitative studies dealing with cell growth, it is therefore necessary to distinguish between cell concentration, or the number of cells per unit volume of culture, and bacterial density, defined as total protoplasm per unit volume.

Determination of Bacterial Mass. Cell mass can be determined directly in terms of dry weight. This method, although time-consuming, is especially useful for reference in isolation and purification work and in the basic calibration of other methods. The most widely used method for estimating total biomass in suspension is the measurement of optical density of a broth culture in a spectrophotometer. Turbidimetric techniques are especially useful in determining mass of cells during growth, as in the evaluation of the effects of antibacterial agents on bacteria. Other methods, such as nitrogen determination and measurement of cell volume after centrifugation, are useful when problems are encountered with the clumping of cells or with light absorption by colored materials in the turbidimetric assay. In permeability studies, data on packed cell volume have proved useful.

Determination of Cell Number. The number of organisms in a culture may be determined either by total direct count or by indirect viable count. Total count of both living and dead organisms may be made by use of a bacterial counting chamber, such as the Petroff-Hauser counter, or more conveniently by the Coulter counter, an electronic particle counter that measures both the distribution of sizes and the numbers in bacterial suspensions.

For determination of viable numbers, it is necessary to plate out a sample of the culture. The microbial population is diluted in a nontoxic diluent, and an aliquot of the diluted population is dispersed in or on a suitable solid medium, so that after incubation each viable unit forms a colony. The number of viable individuals or clusters originally present is determined from the colony count and the dilution. Samples containing fewer than 100 microorganisms per milliliter, such as urine or clear natural water, often require concentration rather than dilution before counting. This is done by passing the sample through a sterile membrane filter of pore size capable of retaining all the bacteria, then transferring the membrane to an absorbent pad saturated with a nutrient broth.

Bacterial Culture Systems

Closed Systems

As bacteria usually are grown in the laboratory in batch culture, the conditions approximate that of a closed system. If a suitable medium is inoculated with bacteria and small samples are taken at regular intervals, a plotting of the data will yield a characteristic growth curve (Fig. 5–10). The changes of slope on such a graph indicate the transition from one phase of development to another. Usually logarithmic values of the number of cells are plotted rather than arithmetic values. Logarithms to the base 2 are the most useful, since each unit on the ordinate represents a doubling of population. The bacterial growth curve can be divided into four major phases: lag phase, exponential growth phase, stationary phase, and phase of decline. These phases reflect the physiologic state of the organisms in the culture at that particular time.

LAG PHASE. After inoculation, there is an increase in cell size at a time when little or no cell division is occurring. During this phase, there is a marked increase in macromolecular components, metabolic activity, and susceptibility to physical and chemical agents. The lag phase is a period of adjustment necessary for the replenishment of the cell's pool of metabolites to a level commensurate with maximum cell synthesis. By taking a large inoculum from a logarithmic phase culture, the lag phase may be essentially eliminated. When inocula are taken from the period of decline, however, hours may elapse before cell division occurs.

EXPONENTIAL GROWTH PHASE. In the exponential or logarithmic phase, the cells are in a state of balanced growth. During this state, the mass and volume of the cell increase by the same factor in such a manner that the average composition of the cells and the relative concentrations of metabolites remain constant. During this period of balanced growth, the rate of increase can be expressed by a natural exponential function. The cells are dividing at a constant rate determined both by the intrinsic nature of the organism and environmental conditions. There is a wide diversity in the rate of growth of the various microorganisms. The doubling time for a broth culture of *E. coli* at 37C is approximately 20 minutes, as compared with a minimum doubling time of approximately 10 hours for mammalian cells at the same temperature.

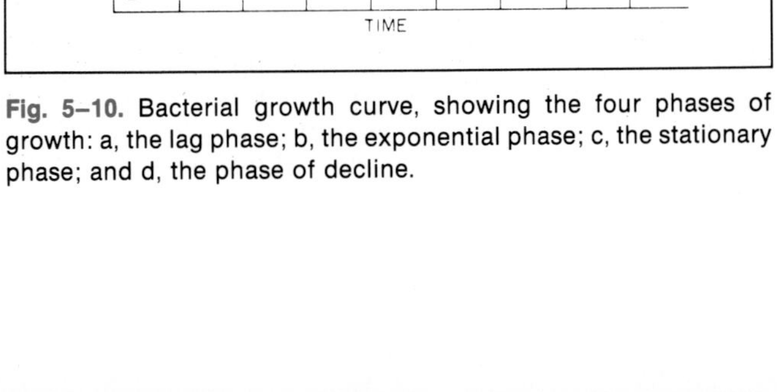

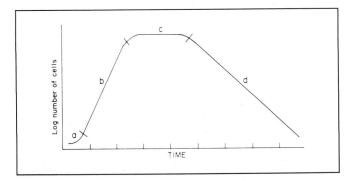

Fig. 5–10. Bacterial growth curve, showing the four phases of growth: a, the lag phase; b, the exponential phase; c, the stationary phase; and d, the phase of decline.

STATIONARY PHASE. When routine culture conditions are used, the accumulation of waste products, exhaustion of nutrients, change in pH, and other obscure factors exert a deleterious effect on the culture, resulting in a decreased growth rate. During the stationary phase, the viable count remains constant for a variable period, depending on the organism, but eventually gives way to a period of decreasing population. In some cases the cells in dying cultures become elongated, abnormally swollen, or distorted, a manifestation of unbalanced growth.

Growth Rate and Doubling Time. Knowledge of the growth rate is important in determining the state of the culture as a whole. If one assumes the doubling of the initial mass M_i in time g, the final concentration of microorganisms M is

$$M = M_i 2^n \qquad (1)$$

where n is the number of cell divisions in time t. The equation

$$g = \frac{t}{n} \qquad (2)$$

expresses the doubling time or mean generation time. The term *doubling time* represents the average generation time of the culture as a whole, usually determined by doubling of the microbial mass in the culture. The doubling time g is best determined by calculation. To accomplish this, the increase of cell mass is determined in a known time interval and the generation time is calculated from the values obtained. Rearranging equation (2) to the form

$$n = \frac{t}{g}$$

which is substituted into equation (1), we have

$$M = M_i 2^{t/g} \qquad (3)$$

By conversion to the logarithmic form and rearranging, we obtain

$$g = \frac{\ln 2\, t}{\ln M - \ln M_i} = \frac{0.69t}{\ln M - \ln M_i} \qquad (4)$$

Equation (4) is the formula for calculating the doubling time from two measurements that give the increase of the mass in time t. Measurements must be performed under constant conditions, and the amount of microorganisms is best determined as dry weight.

For calculating the specific growth rate or exponential growth rate of an organism, the logarithmic form of equation (3) is used:

$$\ln M = t\frac{\ln 2}{g} + \ln M_i \qquad (5)$$

For the exponential phase of growth, the expression $(\ln 2)/g$

is a constant. Therefore, in equation (5) we can substitute μ. The resulting equation:

$$\ln M = \mu t + \ln M_i \quad (6)$$

which expresses the increase of mass within a certain time, is the equation of a straight line. When the values of t are plotted on the abscissa and the values of $\ln M$ on the ordinate, a straight line is obtained, and the constant μ is the slope of this straight line. It determines the growth rate of the bacterial mass as a function of time. It is, therefore, called the *specific growth rate* or *instantaneous growth rate* constant. Its value can be determined either graphically, by calculation:

$$\mu = \frac{\ln 2}{g} = \frac{0.69}{g} \quad (7)$$

or it can be calculated directly from equation (6):

$$\mu = \frac{\ln M - \ln M_i}{t} \quad (8)$$

where the time t is the interval $t_1 - t_2$ during which the bacterial mass M_i increases to the value of M.

The instantaneous growth rate μ is specific for every organism and culture medium. It is governed primarily by such factors as the growth capacity of the organism but also is affected by the environment. In order to express the real maximum value, the value corresponding to the exponential phase of the growth curve, the culture must grow under optimal environmental conditions in an unrestricted medium with substrate and growth factors in excess, so that the growth rate is independent of these.

Continuous Culture

In many types of investigative work, it is advantageous to use organisms that are in their exponential phase of growth. With use of the routine batch culture techniques, it is impossible to maintain the culture at a steady state over a long period of time. Continuous culture techniques circumvent this problem and permit a bacterial population of fixed size to be grown for many generations under constant conditions and at a selected growth rate.

One of the most widely used continuous system cultivators is the chemostat (Fig. 5–11). This is an open-system apparatus consisting of a culture tube in which the population of organisms is maintained at a constant size by continuous dilution. This is accomplished by the admission of fresh nutrient medium into the culture tube at a defined and constant rate, with simultaneous removal by overflow of an equal volume of the bacterial suspension. In the chemostat the most important factor that controls growth of the organisms is the rate at which fresh medium is added to the culture tube. The ratio of the rate at which fresh medium is added to the culture (f), to the operating volume of the culture (V), is referred to as the dilution rate (D):

$$D = f/V$$

The dilution rate is the number of volumes of medium that pass through the culture vessel in 1 hour. Its reciprocal, $1/D$, is the mean residence time of an organism in the culture tube.

In a chemostat, the organisms are growing, but they also are being washed out of the culture tube. The net change in the number of organisms with time therefore is determined by the relative rates of growth and washout:

$$\frac{dN}{dt} = \mu N - \frac{f}{V} \quad (9)$$

Thus:

$$\frac{dN}{dt} = \mu N - DN \quad (10)$$

where μ is the instantaneous growth rate constant and N is the number of organisms per milliliter. For the size of the population to remain constant in the culture tube, it is necessary that

$$\frac{dN}{dt} = 0 \quad (11)$$

and

$$\mu = D \quad (12)$$

If the dilution rate is constant, the concentration of all of the components of the cell becomes constant and a steady state is established that may be maintained for an extended period of time.

The key to an understanding of the mode of action of the chemostat lies in the way in which the growth rate depends on the concentration of a limiting growth factor in the culture medium. In a batch culture, substrate is consumed as the organisms grow. As a result, the substrate concentration continually decreases, accompanied by a parallel decrease in the growth rate. In a chemostat, however, the continued addition of fresh medium fixes the substrate concentration and the growth rate at some predetermined value that is less than the maximum growth rate. The nutrient medium is so constituted that it contains a large excess of all except a single required nutrient, which now becomes the growth-limiting factor. As long as the growth rate exceeds the dilution rate, the number of organisms increases with time. However, because an increase in the number of organisms in the culture tube results in a continuous decrease in the concentration of the growth-limiting factor in the tube, a decrease in the bacterial growth rate eventually results. The growth rate continues to fall until it is equal to the dilution rate, at which time the concentration of organisms in the culture tube stabilizes and remains at a constant level.

At very low nutrient concentrations, the specific growth rate is directly proportional to the concentration (c) of the

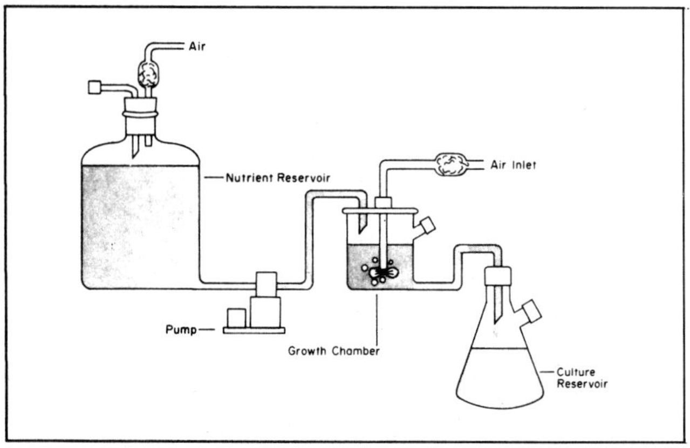

Fig. 5–11. Simplified diagram of a chemostat.

TABLE 5–1. EFFECT OF GROWTH RATE ON CELL SIZE AND COMPOSITION OF *SALMONELLA TYPHIMURIUM*

Medium	Growth Rate (μ^a)	Dry Weight per Cell ($g \times 10^{-15}$)	Nucleoids per Cell	RNA per Nucleoid ($g \times 10^{-15}$)
Lysine salts	0.6	240	1.1	22
Glucose salts	1.2	360	1.5	31
Nutrient broth	2.4	840	2.4	65
Heart infusion	2.8	1090	2.9	84

From Schaechter et al: J Gen Microbiol 19:608, 1958.
[a] Growth rate expressed as generations per hour.

nutrient. This relationship may be expressed in equation (10) so that

$$\frac{dN}{dt} = \mu(c)\,N - D \qquad (13)$$

and in the steady state, in which

$$\frac{dN}{dt} = 0 \qquad (14)$$

$$\mu(c) = D \qquad (15)$$

The chemostat has been especially useful in the study of population genetics and of regulatory mechanisms that control the flow of material into the major classes of macromolecules.

Effect of Growth Rate on Bacterial Structure and Composition. The structure and chemical composition of bacteria vary markedly with changes in the growth rate. Some of these changes are shown in Table 5–1, in which the growth rate of *S. typhimurium* was controlled by providing different carbon and nitrogen sources. The size of the cell and the average number of nucleoid bodies per cell are both directly related to the organism's growth rate. The most sensitive indicator, however, of a change in growth rate is the ribosomal RNA. Except at very low growth rates, the number of ribosomes per milligram of protein is proportional to the growth rate.

The response of RNA to changes in growth rate can be demonstrated by the use of shift experiments, either a shift up if the change of medium leads to an increase in growth rate or a shift down if there is a decrease (Fig. 5–12). In both types of experiments, the first process to respond to the change in environment is the synthesis of RNA. When bacteria growing on one medium at 37C under conditions of balanced growth are transferred to another medium that will support a higher growth rate, the transition is characterized by an instantaneous increase in the rate of RNA synthesis, followed more slowly by corresponding changes in the rates of protein and DNA synthesis. The slower increase in the rate of protein synthesis after a shift to a richer medium is closely correlated with an increase in total RNA per cell, which regulates the capacity of the translational apparatus. According to current ideas, one of the early physiologic effects of such a nutritional shift up is a greater extent of transfer RNA (tRNA) charging with amino acids, which reduces ribosome idling and thus synthesis of guanosine tetraphosphate. A low concentration of this nucleotide is presumed to increase the expression of ribosomal RNA (rRNA) and ribosomal protein genes, thereby stimulating ribosome synthesis. A more detailed discussion of the stringent response and metabolic growth rate control is found on page 117.

Synchronous Growth

As bacteria are usually grown, cell division occurs at random, producing a mixture of cells representing all phases of the division cycle. Studies on such cultures yield average values only. Techniques are available, however, for synchronizing division and inducing all the cells in the culture to divide simultaneously. By withdrawing cells representing a single age class, a sample is obtained that is large enough for analysis by standard biochemical techniques. Two fundamentally differ-

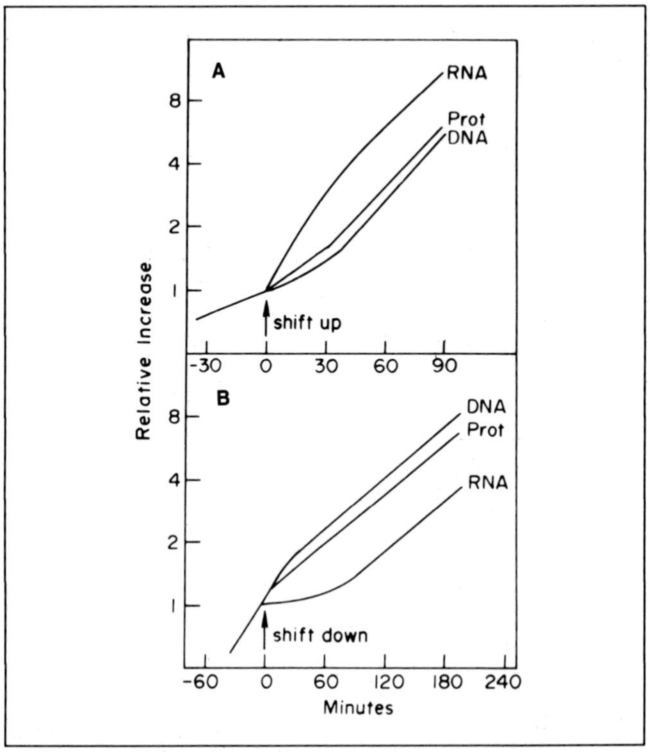

Fig. 5–12. Relative rate of RNA, DNA, and protein synthesis in *E. coli* after a shift in medium. **A.** Cells are shifted up from a glucose-salts medium to a nutrient broth. **B.** Cells growing in nutrient broth are shifted down to a glucose-salts medium. The value of each component is normalized to 1.0 at 0 time.

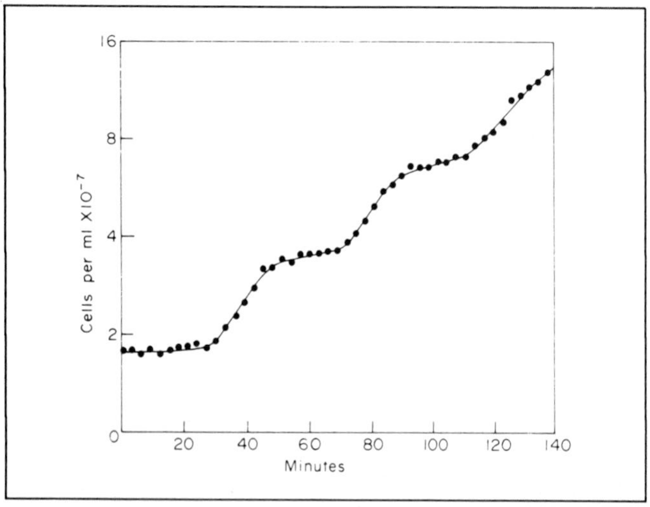

Fig. 5–13. Cells of *E. coli* synchronized by the selection of newly formed cells eluted from membrane filter. *(Adapted from Helmstetter: In Norris and Ribbons (eds): Methods in Microbiology, vol 1. Academic Press, 1969.)*

ent approaches have been employed. In the first the cells are sorted out according to age or size, whereas in the second, synchrony is induced by manipulating environmental conditions.

Selection by Size and Age

MEMBRANE ELUTION. This method for obtaining synchronously dividing populations selects cells of uniform age by passing a population of growing cells through a membrane filter. The filter is of pore size small enough to bind all the bacteria irreversibly on its surface. When the filter is then inverted and medium is passed through, the only cells appearing in the eluted medium are the unbound sister cells, the youngest cells in an exponential phase culture. Under the proper conditions, new daughter cells can be removed from the population growing on the surface and, when incubated, will grow in a synchronous manner (Fig. 5–13). This technique has been highly useful in studying the biochemical events accompanying the bacterial division cycle.

FILTRATION. Another useful technique for synchronization of bacteria is based on size selection by filtration. This method takes advantage of the cyclic changes in size that accompany the division cycle. A culture is filtered through a stack of filter papers that retains the larger cells near the top of the pile and allows the small cells to pass through and to be collected in the filtrate. The cells in the filtrate, or those obtained by eluting selected papers, grow synchronously during subsequent incubation.

VELOCITY SEDIMENTATION. The use of velocity sedimentation for the separation of exponentially growing cell populations into different age classes on the basis of size and density differences is a less reliable approach; currently it is not recommended.

Induction Techniques. Some techniques for obtaining synchronized cells have used shock treatments, such as temperature, starvation, and illumination. Although synchronized growth is induced by these techniques, and the degree of synchrony usually is as good as or better than that achieved by size and age selection techniques, induction techniques often introduce physiologic abnormalities. The use of temperature for synchronization is based on the assumption that the processes that occur during cell division are differentially sensitive to temperature. If the temperature of an exponentially growing culture is reduced from 37C to 25C for 15 minutes and then returned to 37C, cell division of most of the cells is synchronized.

The phasing of cell division that occurs in cultures of a thymine-requiring mutant following withdrawal and readdition of thymine to the cultures is an example of synchronization by starvation.

Bacterial Cell Cycle

Cells that are growing are destined to divide. Their growth rate, and thus the frequency at which they divide, depends on the species and environmental conditions. Within a short period, often as short as 20 minutes, a bacterium can create a complete duplicate of itself, which then in turn is capable of duplicating. In exponentially growing cultures, the organisms divide after each doubling of their cell volume. In rod-shaped organisms, the doubling of cell volume between successive divisions takes place entirely by a doubling of cell length.

Bacteria do not exhibit the characteristic cell cycle observed in eucaryotic organisms. Whereas in eucaryotic cells DNA synthesis is confined to the S phase of the cell cycle, in exponentially growing bacteria DNA synthesis occurs virtually throughout the entire division cycle (Fig. 5–14). In bacteria

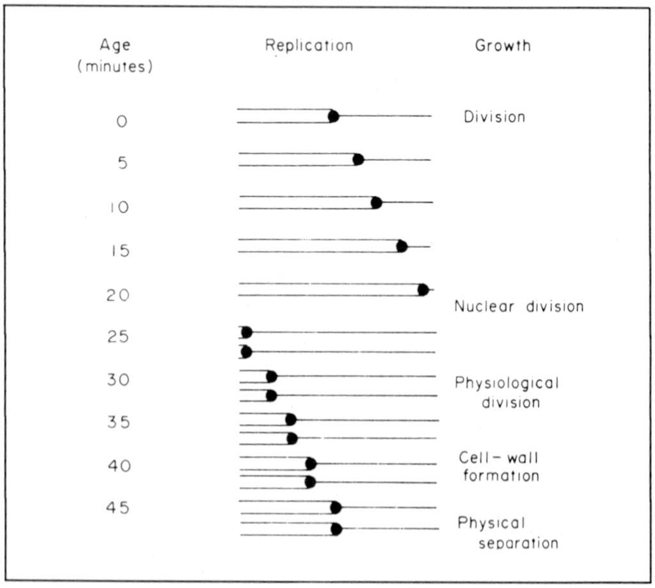

Fig. 5–14. DNA replication in *E. coli* growing with a doubling time of 45 minutes. Newborn cells at 0 time possess half-replicated chromosomes. The end of a round occurs at 20 to 25 minutes. Nuclear division occurs, and a new round of replication begins. At the time of division, cells contain two half-replicated chromosomes. *(Adapted from Clark: J Bacteriol 96:1223, 1968.)*

the duplication sequences do not necessarily follow one after the other but overlap, the amount of overlapping depending on the culture medium.

Bacterial Cell Division

The number of chromosomes per cell and the extent of their replication are determined by the physiologic state and age of the cell. Chromosomes of very slow-growing cells have a single replication origin. In such cells, replication occupies only part of the cell cycle, and gaps in DNA synthesis occur. Cells in rapidly growing cultures, however, contain multiple replication origins. Because replication occurs simultaneously at several points along these chromosomes, the entire chromosome can be replicated in a fraction of the time that would be required if there were but a single replication fork. Genetic material thus can be duplicated at rates that otherwise could not be attained.

In bacteria, cell division and DNA replication are closely coordinated to ensure that each daughter cell receives an equal portion of the chromosome. The control of DNA replication in bacteria is concerned primarily with the control of initiation of rounds of replication.

Chromosome Replication. In bacteria, chromosome replication is a bidirectional process involving two replication forks that move in opposite directions around the chromosome. In *E. coli* with a generation time of 60 minutes, approximately 40 minutes is required for one of these replication forks to travel one half the length of the chromosome. Because of the simultaneous movement of the two forks, a complete doubling of the DNA molecule is accomplished during this 40-minute period. Cell division takes place about 20 minutes after the completion of each round of replication. During this 20-minute period there is no further replication of the chromosome. Replication is initiated at 60 minutes when the cell has attained twice its initial unit mass, that is, when the ratio of number of unit mass equivalents to number of chromosome origins reaches 1 (Fig. 5–15).

An understanding of the relationship between DNA replication and the cell division cycle is provided by the Helmstetter-Cooper model. According to this model, two events of fixed duration make up the division cycle: *C*, which is the time required for the completion of one round of DNA replication after initiation at the origin, and *D*, which is the time interval between completion of a round of replication and cell division.

For *E. coli* growing under conditions providing a generation time of 60 minutes or less, *C* and *D* are 40 and 20 minutes, respectively. In cells with a generation time of 30 minutes, which can be obtained by the use of a richer medium, growth is twice as fast, with a doubling of mass every 30 minutes. In such cells the first round of chromosome replication is initiated at zero time, and the first replication forks meet at the terminus 40 minutes later. By 30 minutes, however, the cell will have doubled its mass and will start new rounds of replication at the two copies of the chromosome origin that were formed as soon as the first round of replication began. The result is that between 30 and 40 minutes, there are three pairs of replicating forks on the chromosome. Therefore, in media in which the mass doubling time is less than 40 minutes, successive rounds of chromosome replication will overlap to give a dichotomously replicating chromosome (Fig. 5–15).

In summary, as presently conceptualized, a duplication sequence begins with the initiation of DNA synthesis at a unique site on the chromosome, the replication origin, known as *oriC*. Initiation of chromosome replication requires protein synthesis and takes place when the ratio of cell mass to the number of initiation sites reaches a critical value. Chromosome replication begins when a fixed amount of initiator proteins (DnaA and possibly other proteins) has accumulated regardless of the position of other replication forks on the chromosome. Thus, in a given culture medium, the rate of cell division is determined by the time required for accumulation of the initiator substances. Initiation is not influenced by the presence, absence, position, or rate of movement of replication forks on the chromosome.

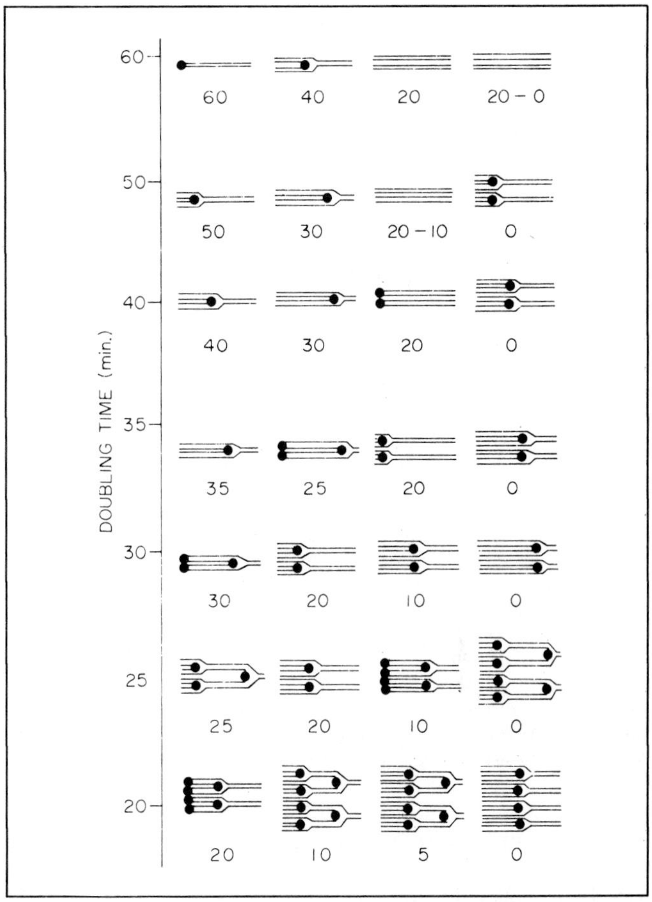

Fig. 5–15. Relationship between chromosome replication and the division cycle in *E. coli* B/r growing at different rates. The time required for a replication point to proceed from the original to the terminus of the genome is 40 minutes; the time between the end of a round of chromosome replication and cell division is 20 minutes. The dot indicates a replication point, and the numbers indicate the time in minutes before cell division. *(Adapted from Cooper and Helmstetter: J Mol Biol 31:521, 1968.)*

Role of Cell Membrane in Chromosome Separation. Electron microscopy has failed to show any bacterial structure equivalent to the mitotic apparatus of eucaryotic cells. It is evident, however, that there must be some mechanism for ensuring equitable separation of chromosomes after each replication. For a number of years the replicon model of Jacob and associates has provided the best explanation of how this might be achieved. According to this model, the circular DNA is attached to the cytoplasmic membrane, where replication occurs by passage of the DNA through an enzyme complex in the membrane. The replicated daughter chromosomes attached to the membrane would be separated by zonal insertion of newly synthesized membrane between the points of attachment. Coordination of growth and division thus would be mediated by the membrane, with the position of the chromosome playing a critical role in determining the site of growth. Although membrane attachment of the chromosome has been documented, because of the fluidity of the plasma membrane, it is uncertain whether a stable distribution of chromosomes could be mediated solely by cytoplasmic membrane proteins. It is more likely that conserved portions of the cell wall, that is, the poles, are involved in the segregation process, as well as in the centering of the septum. In both *Bacillus subtilis* and *E. coli*, a cell wall–chromosome attachment has been demonstrated.

Terminal Steps in Cell Division. In the commonly invoked model for the timing of some of the events leading to cell division in *E. coli*, two parallel sequences of events, initiated at the same time in the cell cycle, are required. It is assumed that both sequences occur throughout most of the cell cycle but that completion of DNA synthesis is required to produce a positive signal (a protein) that permits the final stages of septation. A 40-minute period of protein synthesis is followed by a final process that takes about 20 minutes to complete. Inasmuch as neither RNA, DNA, nor protein synthesis is required during the 20-minute period that follows the 40-minute period of protein synthesis, it is assumed that assembly of preformed components of the septum occurs at this time. The final stages of septation, however, require the participation of a terminal protein that is synthesized immediately after the completion of chromosome duplication at 40 to 55 minutes. According to this model, the rate-limiting process for division in the bacterial cell cycle is the completion of events in the temporal division sequence and not completion of chromosome replication.

SEPTUM FORMATION. Compartmentalization or physiologic division of the cell occurs before the actual physical separation of the daughter cells. This is the time at which the cytoplasmic events at one end of the cell become independent of cytoplasmic events occurring at the opposite end. The end of a round of replication occurs well in advance of this compartmentalization. This stage of growth is characterized by the biosynthesis of septal murein and the development of a weak septum, followed by the formation of a strong crosswall. At least 12 different genes are required specifically for septum formation in *E. coli*. One of these codes for penicillin-binding protein 3 (PBP3), a membrane protein that has both transpeptidase and transglycosidase activity and that is involved in the synthesis of septal murein. The β-lactam antibiotic cephalexin binds to *E. coli* PBP3 with high affinity and specifically inhibits septation in growing cells, but it has no effect on cell elongation.

CELL WALL GROWTH. During balanced growth, a greater surface area normally is required to cover a greater volume. In some organisms such as *Streptococcus faecalis*, this is accomplished by growth of the wall from discrete and well-defined equatorial zones, or wall bands, that mark the site of the future septum. Each unit cell splits its wall band as it initiates cell division, forming two new bands that mark the junction between old and new wall. The bands are formed at the beginning of a growth cycle and can be used as morphologic markers to monitor cell cycle–related events (Fig. 5–16).

In bacilli there is no clear-cut picture of how walls are assembled. There is evidence for both zonal and a totally diffuse pattern of growth. Present conceptions of wall assembly in bacilli, however, suggest that the surface enlarges by a process of inside-to-outside growth, thus conferring some degree of mobility on nascent wall constituents (Fig. 5–17). Coupling of nucleoid extension with increase of cell length is envisaged to occur through an exponentially increasing number of DNA-surface attachment sites occupying most of the available cell surface. In *E. coli* the various PBPs play different enzymatic roles in peptidoglycan metabolism, and different ones appear to be required specifically for lateral wall synthesis during elongation and for septum formation. Bacterial rod shape is assumed to depend on the balance of these two specific systems.

SEPARATION OF BACTERIA. Separation of the two daughter cells takes place some time after the completion of the transverse septum. The separation begins with a constriction between the daughter cells and a thickening of the cell wall in the constriction region. Further thickening of the wall accompanies constriction between the cells until the pole of the cell assumes its characteristic rounded shape. The normal thickness of the cell wall is achieved only after constriction is complete and the two daughter cells have separated. Separation of the daughter cells is mediated by murein hydrolases

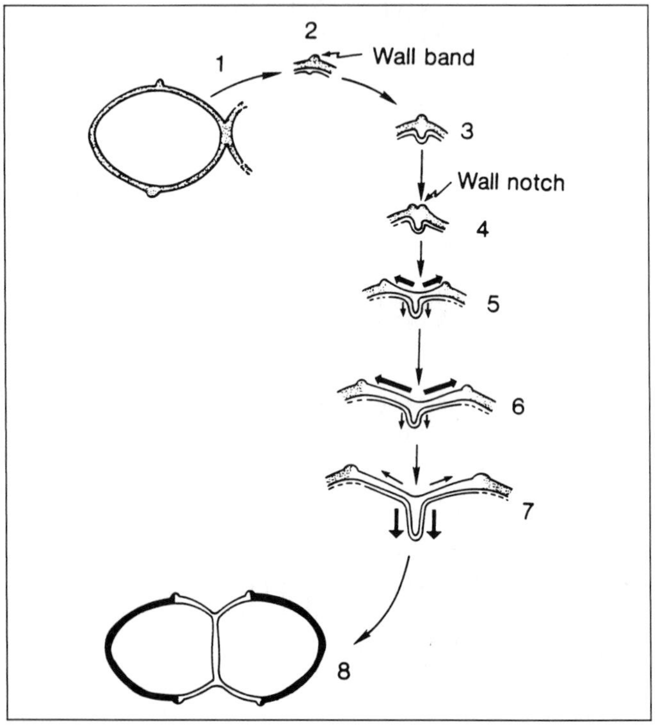

Fig. 5–16. Sequence of events during surface enlargement of *Enterococcus hirae. (From Shockman et al: Ann NY Acad Sci 235:161, 1974, as modified by Harold: Microbiol Rev 54:381, 1990.)*

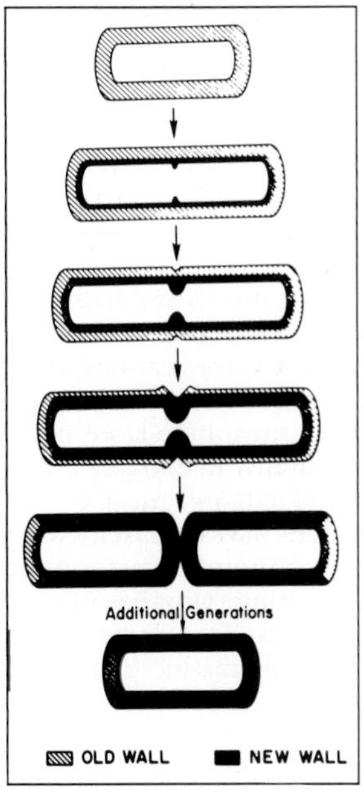

Proposed model for cell wall assembly in *Bacillus subtilis.* *(From Doyle and Koch: Crit Rev Microbiol 15:169, 1987.)*

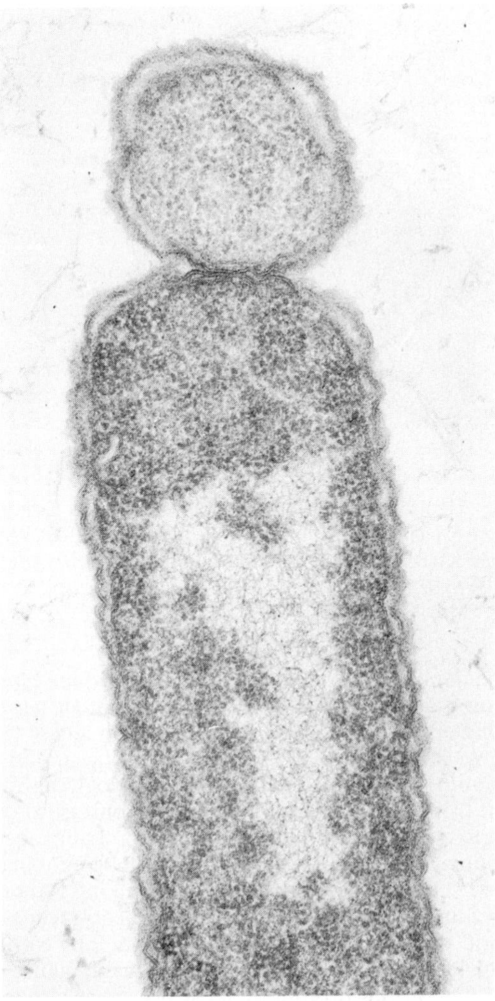

Fig. 5–18. Thin section of an *E. coli* minicell-producing cell (× 925) dividing to yield a minicell. × 49,140. Electron micrograph taken by D. P. Allison. *(From Frazer and Curtiss: Curr Top Microbiol Immunol 69:1, 1975.)*

that are localized at the site of septum formation and are latent in nondividing cells.

Asymmetric Cell Division. Regulation of the site at which cell division occurs is under genetic control. In rod-shaped organisms, division sites normally arise in an equatorial position, partitioning the daughter genomes into cells of approximately the same length. A number of bacterial mutants have been described, however, in which the division site location is abnormal (Fig. 5–18). The most extensively studied of these are the minicells of *E. coli.* These are tiny, spherical cells produced from the ends of the parent, rod-shaped cells. *E. coli* minicells lack host chromosomes although they may contain plasmid DNA. Minicells lacking DNA are unable to synthesize any polymer whose synthesis is DNA-dependent.

Differentiation in Bacterial Cells

Sporulation

A unique property of certain bacteria (e.g., *Bacillus* and *Clostridium*) is their ability to form endospores. At some point in the vegetative cell cycle of spore-forming organisms, growth is arrested and the cell undergoes progressive changes that result in the formation of an endospore (Fig. 5–19). A spore is a dormant structure capable of surviving for prolonged periods and endowed with the capacity to reestablish the vegetative stage of growth under appropriate environmental conditions. The process involved in sporulation, as well as the breaking of the spore's dormancy and subsequent emergence of a vegetative cell, represents a primitive example of unicellular differentiation.

Properties of Endospores

Endospore formation occurs during the stationary phase of growth after depletion of certain nutrients in the culture medium or environment. A single spore is produced within a vegetative cell and differs from the parent cell in its morphology and composition, increased resistance to adverse environments, and absence of detectable metabolic activity. Although the thermal resistance of spores is of primary concern to the medical microbiologist, the increased resistance of spores to desiccation, freezing, radiation, and deleterious chemicals is of greater importance in their natural environment. The primary selective value of the spore lies in its longevity in the soil coupled with its ability to germinate under the proper environmental conditions.

Basis of Spore Resistance. In the sporulating cell, resistance to various chemical and physical agents appears at different stages, concomitant with changes in the physiochemical composition of the cell. Resistance to radiation, drying, and toxic chemicals appears after the cell becomes refractile and depends, at least in part, on the properties of the cystine-rich, keratin-like spore coat proteins. Thermal resistance is attributed to the very low water content of the protoplast,

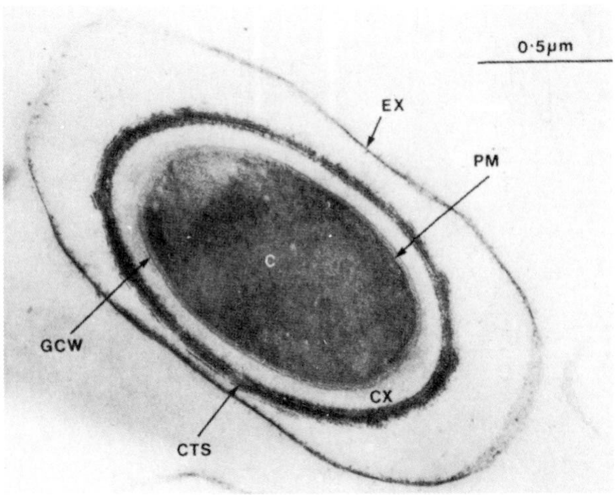

Fig. 5–19. Electron micrograph of spore of *Bacillus cereus* showing the core (C), plasma membrane (PM), germ cell wall (GCW), cortex (CX), coats (CTS), and exosporium (EX). *(From Warth: Adv Microb Physiol 17:1, 1978.)*

which renders the proteins and nucleic acids more resistant to denaturation. This reduction in water content occurs late in sporulation at the time of cortex formation and at the time that the spore first appears as a refractile object. The major component of the cortex is a unique peptidoglycan radically different from that of vegetative cells. In contrast to cell wall peptidoglycan in which there is extensive cross-linkage of the tetrapeptides, cross-linkage in the cortical polymer is markedly decreased. This reduced degree of cross-linking is thought to play a significant role in the compressive contraction of the cortex and dehydration during sporulation. The cortex is in itself capable of and necessary for the maintenance of the resistant state of the protoplast. Heat resistance also is correlated with the concentration of calcium in the spore and with the massive synthesis during this stage of the spore-specific component, dipicolinic acid (Fig. 5–20). Dipicolinic acid is a chelating agent present as the calcium salt in the protoplast of the spore and accounts for as much as 10% of the dry weight of the mature spore. The dipicolinate chelate intercalates within the helical structure of DNA, thus displacing intramolecular water. It also binds different RNA species.

Biochemistry of Sporulation

At some period in the development of a cell, the metabolism is irreversibly channeled in the direction of sporulation. There is no single point of commitment for the sporulation process as a whole but a separate point of commitment for each new specific macromolecule. Accompanying these physiologic changes is an ordered series of cytologic and structural changes (Fig. 5–21). During sporulation, certain storage polymers, such as poly-β-hydroxybutyrate, accumulate and are later utilized. Extensive turnover of macromolecules occurs, and some enzyme levels change drastically. New and characteristic spore structures are synthesized, and previously existing structures are degraded.

The pools of small molecules found in spores are distinctly different from those of vegetative cells. In addition to dipicolinic acid, there is an accumulation of divalent cations, and high levels of L-glutamic acid. The predominant component of the drastically reduced acid-soluble phosphate pool is 3-phosphoglyceric acid instead of ATP, which is a major component of vegetative cells.

During sporulation many differences may be observed in the pattern of enzyme activities. Some of these are associated with mechanisms related to spore formation, whereas others are specific components of the spore itself. A heat-stable catalase found in spores is immunologically distinct from the vegetative cell enzyme, and certain enzymes, such as glucose dehydrogenase, a ribonuclease, and spore lytic enzymes are present solely in the spore. One of the most characteristic events of the onset of sporulation is the production and secretion of peptide antibiotics and various exoenzymes, especially proteases. Proteases play an important role in the intracellular turnover of protein, but the reason for the correlation between sporulation and antibiotic production is unknown. Also synthesized during sporulation is a family of small acid-soluble spore proteins (SASP), which are stored in the mature spore, rapidly degraded to free amino acids during germination, and reutilized for protein synthesis. Two of these proteins also have been shown to play a key role in the dormant spore's resistance to heat and UV radiation.

Initiation of Sporulation

Sporulation is a response to nutritional deprivation, especially of an available carbon and a nitrogen source. The regulation of spore formation is negative: the cell makes a repressor from some ingredient in the medium that prevents the initiation of sporulation. When this ingredient is exhausted, inhibition is released and sporulation begins. A metabolizable supply of both carbon and nitrogen is required to inhibit sporulation. If there is a deficiency in the supply of either of these, inhibition will be relieved and sporulation initiated.

The specific factor that regulates the initiation of sporulation is guanosine triphosphate (GTP). A decrease in the GTP pool of growing cells suffices to initiate sporulation in *B. subtilis.* All conditions of nutritional deficiency known to initiate sporulation cause a GTP decrease at the time at which sporulation begins. Two types of nutritional deprivation are responsible for GTP decreases under conditions of nutrient limitation: (1) a decrease in the purine precursor, P-ribosyl-PP, caused by a limited carbon supply, and (2) the stringent response to amino acid deprivation, which is correlated with an increase in the concentration of the highly phosphorylated guanine nucleotides, ppGpp and pppGpp (p. 17). Under sporulation conditions, ppGpp inhibits the function of inosine 5′-monophosphate (IMP) dehydrogenase, the first enzyme in the synthesis, thus explaining the decrease of guanine nucleotides. There is little definitive information on the role this nucleotide plays in the repression of sporulation, although it has been postulated that a GTP-binding protein could be involved in the signal transduction mechanism.

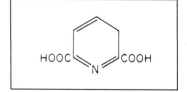

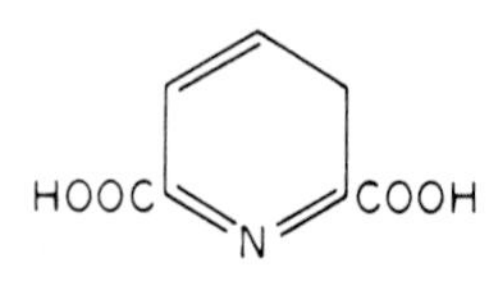

Fig. 5–20. Dipicolinic acid (pyridine 2,6-dicarboxylic acid.)

STAGE	MORPHOLOGIC EVENT	BIOCHEMICAL EVENT
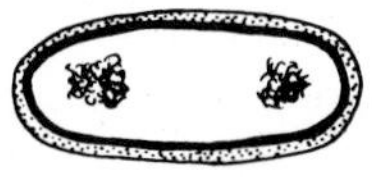	Vegetative cell	
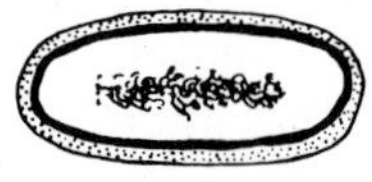	Chromatin filament	Exoenzymes Antibiotic
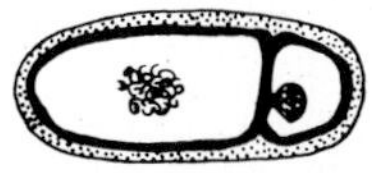	Spore septum	Alanine dehydrogenase
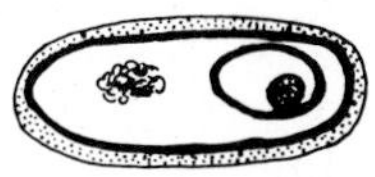	Spore protoplast	Alkaline phosphatase Glucose dehydrogenase Aconitase Heat-resistant catalase
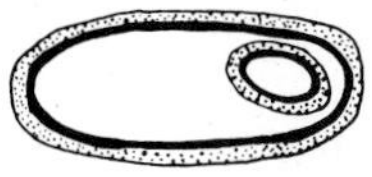	Cortex formation (refractility)	Ribosidase Adenosine deaminase Dipicolinic acid
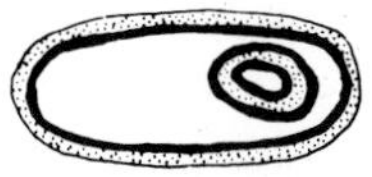	Coat formation	Cysteine incorporation Chemical resistance
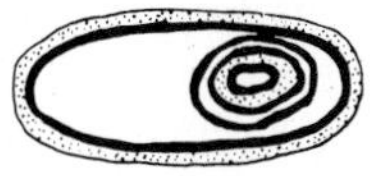	Maturation	Alanine racemase Heat resistance

Fig. 5–21. Morphologic and biochemical events associated with sporulation in *Bacillus subtilis.* The process is timed from the end of exponential growth at t_0 when each vegetative cell contains two chromosomes, and at hourly periods thereafter. *(Adapted from Mandelstam: Microbial Growth. Cambridge University Press, 1969.)*

Genetic Regulation of Sporulation

Most of our current knowledge of the molecular genetics of sporulation has been obtained from studies in *B. subtilis.* By use of asporogenous mutants blocked at different stages of the developmental cycle and transformation and transduction techniques, a linkage map has been constructed that shows the position of many genetic loci for sporulation. The location of spore genes on the linkage map reveals a complex mechanism of expression inasmuch as the sequence of spore genes on the chromosome does not correspond with the time of gene expression.

Sporulation and germination genetic loci are not confined to one segment of the genome but are clustered in distinct and widely dispersed regions of the chromosome. The clustering of developmental genes occurs in about five chromosomal segments, in regions distinct from essential functions. There are approximately 50 of these clusters (operons), but the number of genes within each genetic locus is unknown. The loci are expressed in a specific temporal sequence during the 8 to 10 hours required for development of the endospore.

Gene Expression During Sporulation. Transition from vegetative growth to the first morphologically distinct stage of sporulation, the formation of the spore septum, requires seven genes. One of these codes for DNA-binding protein is SpoOA, which is part of the sporulation sensory mechanism. Its activation appears to be a key step in the initiation of sporulation. The SpoOA protein is the master regulator of most late growth processes, including antibiotic and extracellular protease synthesis, the SOS response (p. 132), and the expression of several early sporulation genes.

With the formation of the forespore septum, the cell becomes a compartmentalized structure. In the compartment developing into the forespore, DNA replication is inhibited, and the substances synthesized include some spore-specific products. In the second compartment, the sporangium, replication of vegetative DNA continues, and products of the vegetative cell continue to be produced. Thus, in the sporulating cell both the vegetative and spore genomes are transcribed. The messenger RNA (mRNA) contains some of the same mRNA molecules as derepressed cells transferred from a rich medium to a poor one but, in addition, molecules specific to sporulation. There is no evidence that the mRNA produced late in sporulation is stable and retained in the spore for protein synthesis during outgrowth.

Role of RNA Polymerases. The changes that occur during sporulation result from the turnoff of certain vegetative genes and the expression of new classes of genes. This temporal control of gene expression is believed to be caused by the appearance of novel sigma factors that are associated with the DNA-dependent RNA polymerase of the differentiating cells. This mechanism can account at least in part for the simultaneous activation and silencing of large groups of genes even though they are scattered on the chromosome.

In *B. subtilis,* nine sigma factors have been identified (Table 5–2). When associated with the core polymerase (α^2, β, β'), the sigma factors give rise to multiple forms of RNA polymerase, each having specific promoter recognition sequences that permit it to transcribe only certain regions of DNA at specific times during growth or sporulation, or both. In vegetative cells of *B. subtilis,* σ^A is the most abundant factor. It probably directs transcription of most of the genes needed during growth, as well as some during the early stages of sporulation. Thus far, five sigma factors have been identified that are required for sporulation but not for growth.

σ^H, a secondary sigma factor present in exponentially growing cells, is necessary for the initiation of sporulation. The best characterized of the sporulation-specific sigma factors that are transcribed only during sporulation is σ^E. σ^E appears about 2 hours after the onset of sporulation and disappears about 3 hours later. The synthesis of σ^E is complex and highly regulated. In addition to developmental control at the level of transcription, the primary translation product is a precursor protein that requires processing into its sigma factor form for activation. It is likely that the activation of σ^E leads to the sequential transcription of a specific set of genes; only a few of these have been identified. It also is probable that additional regulatory factors interact with the sigma factors during sporulation to fine-tune the temporal expression and compartmentalization of specific genes.

TABLE 5–2. SIGMA FACTORS IN *BACILLUS SUBTILIS*

Sigma Factor	Previous Designations	Gene	Functions
σ^A	σ^{55}, σ^{43}	*rpoD*	Housekeeping
σ^B	σ^{37}	*sigB*	Unknown
σ^C	σ^{32}	*sigC*	Unknown
σ^D	σ^{28}	*sigD*	Flagellar synthesis
σ^E	σ^{29}	*sigE, spoIIGB*	Sporulation
σ^F	$\sigma^{spoIIAC}$	*sigF, spoIIAC*	Sporulation
σ^G		*sigG, spoIIIG*	Sporulation: forespore specific
σ^H	σ^{30}	*sigH, spoOH*	Sporulation
σ^K	σ^{27}	*spoIVCB, spoIIIC*[a]	Sporulation: mother cell specific

From Moran: In Smith, Slepecky, Setlow (eds): Regulation of Procaryotic Development. American Society for Microbiology, 1989
[a] These two genes must be fused during sporulation to encode σ^K.

Germination and Outgrowth

Simultaneous structural and physiologic changes also are manifested during the transformation of a dormant spore into a vegetative cell. The process of spore germination consists of three sequential phases: (1) an activation stage that conditions the spore to germinate in a suitable environment, (2) a germination stage, during which the characteristic properties of the dormant spore are lost, and (3) an outgrowth stage during which the spore is converted into a new vegetative cell.

Activation is a reversible process that is essential for spore germination. Spores do not germinate or germinate very slowly unless activated either by heat or by various chemical treatments. Activation probably involves the reversible denaturation of a specific but presently undefined macromolecule. Germination is an irreversible process triggered by the exposure of activated spores to a wide range of nutrient and nonnutrient stimulants. L-Alanine is the most common nutrient germinant; others include several amino acids, nucleosides, and glucose. Germination is the stage during which the dormant stage is ended. During the early stages of germination there is a loss of refractility, swelling of the cortex, and appearance of fine nuclear fibrils. Accompanying these changes is a loss of resistance to deleterious physical and chemical agents, an increase in the sulfhydryl level of the spore, a release of spore components, and an increase in metabolic activity. The germination of spores is not inhibited by antibiotics that perturb protein and nucleic acid synthesis, indicating that the enzymes responsible for germination are already present in the spore.

Although it is unclear at present whether a single model can be proposed to encompass the germination response of most organisms, a model based on the findings with *Bacillus megaterium* has been proposed. According to this model, heat shock activates the L-alanine receptor, which because of its stereospecific properties is a protein that is activated allosterically. Upon triggering by L-alanine, the receptor has proteolytic activity that converts the proenzyme of a germination-specific cortex lytic enzyme (GSLE) to an active heat-sensitive enzyme. Commitment may represent either the triggering of the receptor by L-alanine or the conversion of the cortex-lytic proenzyme to the active lytic form. Cortex hydrolysis permits uptake of water and all the other downstream germination events. GSLE is a crucial component of this model.

During outgrowth there is de novo synthesis of proteins and structural components that are characteristic of vegetative cells. During this stage the spore core membrane develops into the cell wall of the vegetative cell. Outgrowth is a period of active biosynthetic activity and is markedly inhibited by interference with the energy supply or by antibiotics that inhibit cell wall, protein, or nucleic acid synthesis.

If heat-activated spores are germinated under suitable conditions, a high degree of synchrony is obtained. Such a synchronous population provides a model system for the study of the initiation of transcriptional and translational events occurring during differentiation. Since the dormant spore is devoid of functional mRNA, the conversion of the spore to a vegetative cell during outgrowth requires transcription and de novo synthesis of gene products. The appearance of these gene products is ordered, determined by the time of transcription of particular genes. Ribosome synthesis starts early, vegetative cell wall synthesis begins later, and DNA synthesis begins just before division of the cell. During a stepwise doubling of cell number for several generations, the initiation of certain enzymes occurs at a specific time during each division cycle and results in a doubling of each enzyme during only a fraction of the total cycle.

FURTHER READING

Books and Reviews

Adler J: Chemotaxis in bacteria. Annu Rev Biochem 41:341, 1975

Ames GF-L: Bacterial periplasmic transport systems: Structure, mechanism, and evolution. Annu Rev Biochem 55:397, 1986

Ames GF-L, Joshi AK: Energy coupling in bacterial periplasmic permeases. J Bacteriol 172:4133, 1990

Benson SA, Hall MN, Silhavy TJ: Genetic analysis of protein export in *Escherichia coli* K12. Annu Rev Biochem 54:101, 1985

Booth IR: Regulation of cytoplasmic pH in bacteria. Microbiol Rev 49:359, 1985

Brass JM: The cell envelope of gram-negative bacteria: New aspects of its function in transport and chemotaxis. Curr Top Microbiol Immunol 125:1, 1986

Bremer H, Dennis PP: Modulation of chemical composition and other parameters of the cell by growth rate. In Neidhardt FC, Ingraham JL, Low KB, et al (eds): *Escherichia coli* and *Salmonella typhimurium:* Cellular and Molecular Biology. Washington, DC, American Society for Microbiology, 1987, p 1527

Brown MRW, Williams P: The influence of environment on envelope properties affecting survival of bacteria in infections. Annu Rev Microbiol 39:527, 1985

Carlberg DM: Determining the effects of antibiotics on bacterial growth by optical and electrical methods. In Lorian V (ed): Antibiotics in Laboratory Medicine, 2nd ed. Baltimore, Williams & Wilkins, 1986, p 64

Crosa JH: Genetics and molecular biology of siderophore-mediated iron transport in bacteria. Microbiol Rev 53:517, 1989

Donachie WD, Begg KJ, Sullivan NF: Morphogenes of *Escherichia coli.* In Losick R, Shapiro L (eds): Microbial Development. Cold Spring Harbor, NY, Cold Spring Harbor Laboratory, 1984, p 27

Donachie WD, Robinson AC: Cell division: Parameter values and the process. In Neidhardt FC, Ingraham JL, Low KB, et al (eds): *Escherichia coli* and *Salmonella typhimurium:* Cellular and Molecular Biology. Washington, DC, American Society for Microbiology, 1987, p 1578

Doyle RJ, Koch AL: The functions of autolysins in the growth and division of *Bacillus subtilis.* Crit Rev Microbiol 15:169, 1987

Dworkin M: Spores, cysts, and stalks. In Gunsalus IC, Sokatch JR, Ornston LN (eds): The Bacteria, vol 7. New York, Academic Press, 1979, p 1

Furlong CE: Osmotic-shock-sensitive transport systems. In Neidhardt FC, Ingraham JL, Low KB, et al (eds): *Escherichia coli* and *Salmonella typhimurium:* Cellular and Molecular Biology. Washington, DC, American Society for Microbiology, 1987, p 768

Guirard BM, Snell EE: Nutritional requirements of microorganisms. In Gunsalus IC, Stanier RY (eds): The Bacteria, vol 4. New York, Academic Press, 1962, p 33

Hancock REW: Alterations in outer membrane permeability. Annu Rev Microbiol 38:237, 1984

Harold FM: Membrane and energy transduction in bacteria. Curr Top Bioenergetics 6:83, 1977

Harold FM: To shape a cell: An inquiry into the causes of morphogenesis of microorganisms. Microbiol Rev 54:381, 1990

Helmstetter CE: Timing of synthetic activities in the cell cycle. In Neidhardt FC, Ingraham JL, Low KB, et al (eds): *Escherichia coli* and *Salmonella typhimurium:* Cellular and Molecular Biology. Washington, DC, American Society for Microbiology, 1987, p 1594

Higgins ML, Shockman GD: Prokaryotic cell division with respect to wall and membranes. CRC Crit Rev Microbiol 1:29, 1971

Ingraham J: Effect of temperature, pH, water activity, and pressure on growth. In Neidhardt FC, Ingraham JL, Low KB, et al (eds): *Escherichia coli* and *Salmonella typhimurium:* Cellular and Molecular Biology. Washington, DC, American Society for Microbiology, 1987, p 1543

Jensen KF, Pedersen S: Metabolic growth rate control in *Escherichia coli* may be a consequence of subsaturation of the macromolecular biosynthetic apparatus with substrates and catalytic components. Microbiol Rev 54:89, 1990

Koshland DE Jr: Bacterial chemotaxis. In Gunsalus IC, Sokatch JR, Ornston LN (eds): The Bacteria, vol 7. New York, Academic Press, 1979, p 111

Krieg NR, Hoffman PS: Microaerophily and oxygen toxicity. Annu Rev Microbiol 40:107, 1986

Leive L, Wu HC: Molecular aspects of protein secretion and membrane assembly. In Leive L, Wu HC (eds): Microbiology—1986. Washington, DC, American Society for Microbiology, 1986, p 233

Lloyd D, Poole RK, Edwards SW: The Cell Division Cycle. Temporal Organization and Control of Cellular Growth and Reproduction. New York, Academic Press, 1982

Losick R, Youngman P: Endospore formation in *Bacillus.* In Losick R, Shapiro L: Microbial Development. Cold Spring Harbor, NY, Cold Spring Harbor Laboratory, 1984, p 63

Maaløe O, Kjeldgaard NO: Control of Macromolecular Synthesis. New York, Benjamin, 1966

Macnab RM: Motility and chemotaxis. In Neidhardt FC, Ingraham JL, Low KB, et al (eds): *Escherichia coli* and *Salmonella typhimurium:* Cellular and Molecular Biology. Washington, DC, American Society for Microbiology, 1987, p 732

Malek I, Fenel Z: Theoretical and Methodological Basis of Continuous Culture of Microorganisms. New York, Academic Press, 1966

Maurizi MR, Switzer RL: Proteolysis in bacterial sporulation. Curr Top Cell Regul 16:163, 1980

Neidhardt FC, Ingraham JL, Schaechter M: Physiology of the Bacterial Cell. A Molecular Approach. Sunderland Mass, Sinauer Associates, 1990

Neilands JB: Microbial envelope proteins related to iron. Annu Rev Microbiol 36:285, 1982

Nikaido H, Vaara M: Molecular basis of bacterial outer membrane permeability. Microbiol Rev 49:1, 1985

Nomura M, Gourse RL, Baughman G: Regulation of the synthesis of ribosomes and ribosomal components. Annu Rev Biochem 53:75, 1984

Oliver D: Protein secretion in *Escherichia coli.* Annu Rev Microbiol 39:615, 1985

Ordal GW: Bacterial chemotaxis: Biochemistry of behavior in a single cell. CRC Crit Rev Microbiol 12:95, 1985

Postma PW, Lengeler JW: Phosphoenolpyruvate: Carbohydrate phosphotransferase system of bacteria. Microbiol Rev 49:232, 1985

Saier MH Jr: Protein phosphorylation and allosteric control of inducer exclusion and catabolite repression by the bacterial phosphoenolpyruvate: Sugar phosphotransferase system. Microbiol Rev 53:109, 1989

Schlessinger D (ed): Bacilli: Biochemical genetics, physiology, and industrial applications. In Microbiology—1976. Washington, DC, American Society for Microbiology, 1976, p 1

Simon M, Silverman M, Matsumura P, et al: Structure and function of bacterial flagella. In Stanier RY, Rogers HJ, Ward JB (eds): Relationship Between Structure and Function in the Prokaryotic Cell. London, Cambridge University Press, 1978, p 271

Smith AJ, Hoare DS: Specialist phototrophs, lithotrophs, and methylotrophs: A unity among a diversity of procaryotes. Bacteriol Rev 41:419, 1977

Smith I, Slepecky RA, Setlow P (eds): Regulation of Procaryotic Development. Structural and Functional Analysis of Bacterial Sporulation and Germination. Washington, DC, American Society for Microbiology, 1989

Snow GA: Mycobactins: Iron-chelating growth factors from mycobacteria. Bacteriol Rev 34:99, 1970

Stanier RY, Ingraham JL, Wheelis ML, Painter PR: The Microbial World, 5th ed. Englewood Cliffs, NJ, Prentice-Hall, 1986

Stock JB, Ninfa AJ, Stock AM: Protein phosphorylation and regulation of adaptive responses in bacteria. Microbiol Rev 53:450, 1989

Stolp H, Starr MP: Principles of isolation, cultivation, and conservation of bacteria. In Starr MP, Stolp H, Trüper HC, et al (eds): The Prokaryotes. New York, Springer-Verlag, 1981, vol I, p 135

Tipper DJ, Pratt I, Guinand M, et al: Control of peptidoglycan synthesis during sporulation in *Bacillus sphaericus*. In Schlessinger D (ed): Microbiology—1977. Washington, DC, American Society for Microbiology, 1977, p 50

von Meyenburg K, Hansen FG: Regulation of chromosome replication. In Neidhardt FC, Ingraham JL, Low KB, et al (eds): *Escherichia coli* and *Salmonella typhimurium:* Cellular and Molecular Biology. Washington, DC, American Society for Microbiology, 1987, p 1555

Wu HC, Tai PC (eds): Protein secretion and export in bacteria. Curr Top Microbiol Immunol 125:1, 1986

Selected Papers

Adler J, Hazelbauer GL, Dahl MM: Chemotaxis toward sugars in *Escherichia coli.* J Bacteriol 115:824, 1973

Bechtel DB, Bulla LA Jr: Ultrastructural analysis of membrane development during *Bacillus thuringiensis* sporulation. J Ultrastruct Res 79:121, 1982

Begg KJ, Donachie WD: Cell shape and division in *Escherichia coli:* Experiments with shape and division mutants. J Bacteriol 163:615, 1985

Begg KJ, Takasuga A, Edwards DH, et al: The balance between different peptidoglycan precursors determines whether *Escherichia coli* cells will elongate or divide. J Bacteriol 172:6697, 1990

Blasco B, Pisabarro AG, de Pedro M: Peptidoglycan biosynthesis in stationary-phase cells of *Escherichia coli.* J Bacteriol 170:5224, 1988

Brass JM, Higgins CF, Foley M, et al: Lateral diffusion of proteins in the periplasm of *Escherichia coli.* J Bacteriol 165:787, 1986

Bukau B, Walker GC: Cellular defects caused by deletion of the *Escherichia coli dnaK* gene indicate roles for heat shock protein in normal metabolism. J Bacteriol 171:2337, 1989

Chiaramello AE, Zyskind JW: Coupling of DNA replication to growth rate in *Escherichia coli:* A possible role for guanosine tetraphosphate. J Bacteriol 172:2013, 1990

Clark DJ: Regulation of deoxyribonucleic acid replication and cell division in *Escherichia coli* B/r. J Bacteriol 96:1214, 1968

Cooper S: Rate and topography of cell wall synthesis during the division cycle of *Salmonella typhimurium.* J Bacteriol 170:422, 1988

Cooper S, Helmstetter CE: Chromosome replication and the division cycle of *Escherichia coli* B/r. J Mol Biol 31:519, 1968

Cummings CW, Haldenwang WG: Characteristics of an RNA polymerase population isolated from *Bacillus subtilis* late in sporulation. J Bacteriol 170:5863, 1988

D'Ari R, Jaffé A, Bouloc P, Robin A: Cyclic AMP and cell division in *Escherichia coli.* J Bacteriol 170:65, 1988

Dix DD, Helmstetter CE: Coupling between chromosome completion and cell division in *Escherichia coli.* J Bacteriol 115:786, 1973

Donachie WD, Begg KJ: Cell length, nucleoid separation, and cell division of rod-shaped and spherical cells of *Escherichia coli.* J Bacteriol 171:4633, 1989

Donachie WD, Begg KJ, Vincente M: Cell length, cell growth and cell division. Nature 264:328, 1976

Eisenbach M, Constantinou C, Aloni H, Shinitzky M, et al: Repellents for *Escherichia coli* operate neither by changing membrane fluidity nor by being sensed by periplasmic receptors during chemotaxis. J Bacteriol 172:5218, 1990

Gibson CW, Daneo-Moore L, Higgins ML: Analysis of initiation of sites of cell wall growth in *Streptococcus faecium* during a nutritional shift. J Bacteriol 160:935, 1984

Goodell EW: Recycling of murein by *Escherichia coli.* J Bacteriol 163:305, 1985

Groat RG, Schultz JE, Zychlinsky E, et al: Starvation proteins in *Escherichia coli:* Kinetics of synthesis and role in starvation survival. J Bacteriol 168:486, 1986

Haldenwang WG, Losick R: Novel RNA polymerase σ factor from *Bacillus subtilis.* Proc Natl Acad Sci USA 77:7000, 1980

Heller KB, Lin ECC, Wilson TH: Substrate specificity and transport properties of the glycerol facilitator of *Escherichia coli.* J Bacteriol 144:274, 1980

Helmstetter CE, Krajewski CA: Initiation of chromosome replication in *dna* A and *dna* C mutants of *Escherichia coli* B/rF. J Bacteriol 149:685, 1982

Herbert D, Elsworth R, Telling RC: The continuous culture of bacteria: A theoretical and experimental study. J Gen Microbiol 14:601, 1956

Ingham C, Buechner M, Adler J: Effect of outer membrane permeability on chemotaxis in *Escherichia coli.* J Bacteriol 172:3577, 1990

Jacob F, Brenner S, Cuzin F: On the regulation of DNA replication in bacteria. Cold Spring Harbor Symp Quant Biol 28:329, 1963

Jones THD, Kennedy EP: Characterization of the membrane protein component of the lactose transport system of *Escherichia coli.* J Biol Chem 244:5981, 1969

Kennedy EP: Osmotic regulation and the biosynthesis of membrane-derived oligosaccharides in *Escherichia coli.* Proc Natl Acad Sci USA 79:1092, 1982

Kihara M, Homma M, Kutsukake K, Macnab RM: Flagellar switch of *Salmonella typhimurium:* Gene sequences and deduced protein sequences. J Bacteriol 171:3247, 1989

Koch AL, Mobley HLT, Doyle RJ, Streips UN: The coupling of wall growth and chromosome replication in gram-positive rods. FEMS Microbiol Lett 12:201, 1981

Kubitschek HE: Cell volume increase in *Escherichia coli* after shifts to richer media. J Bacteriol 172:94, 1990

Lai JS, Sarvas M, Brammar WJ, et al: *Bacillus licheniformis* penicillinase synthesized in *Escherichia coli* contains covalently linked fatty acid and glyceride. Proc Natl Acad Sci USA 78:3506, 1981

Lampel KA, Uratani B, Chaudhry GR, et al: Characterization of the developmentally regulated *Bacillus subtilis* glucose dehydrogenase gene. J Bacteriol 166:238, 1986

Lleo MM, Canepari P, Satta G: Bacterial cell shape regulation: Testing of additional predictions unique to the two-competing-sites model for peptidoglycan assembly and isolation of conditional rod-shaped mutants from some wild-type cocci. J Bacteriol 172:3758, 1990

Loewen PC, Switala J: Multiple catalases in *Bacillus subtilis.* J Bacteriol 169:3601, 1987

Lopez JM, Dromerick A, Freese E: Response of guanosine 5′-triphosphate concentration to nutritional changes and its significance for *Bacillus subtilis* sporulation. J Bacteriol 146:605, 1981

Mason JM, Setlow P: Essential role of small, acid-soluble spore proteins in resistance of *Bacillus subtilis* spores to UV light. J Bacteriol 167:174, 1986

McIntosh MA, Earhart CF: Coordinate regulation by iron of the synthesis of phenolate compounds and three outer membrane proteins in *Escherichia coli.* J Bacteriol 131:331, 1977

Mitchell C, Vary JC: Proteins that interact with GTP during sporulation of *Bacillus subtilis.* J Bacteriol 171:2915, 1989

Mitchell WM, Misko TP, Roseman S: Sugar transport by the bacterial phosphotransferase system. Regulation of other transport systems (lactose and melibiose). J Biol Chem 257:14553, 1982

Mobley HLT, Koch AL, Doyle RJ: Insertion and fate of the cell wall in *Bacillus subtilis.* J Bacteriol 158:169, 1984

Mukherjee A, Donachie WD: Differential translation of cell division proteins. J Bacteriol 172:6106, 1990

Nelson SO, Scholte BJ, Postma PW: Phosphoenolpyruvate: Sugar phosphotransferase system-mediated regulation of carbohydrate metabolism in *Salmonella typhimurium.* J Bacteriol 150:604, 1982

Norris TE, Koch AL: Effect of growth rate on the relative rates of synthesis of messenger, ribosomal and transfer RNA in *Escherichia coli.* J Mol Biol 64:633, 1972

Ochi K, Kandala J, Freese E: Evidence that *Bacillus subtilis* sporulation induced by the stringent response is caused by the decrease in GTP or GDP. J Bacteriol 151:1062, 1982

Panzer S, Losick R, Sun D, Setlow P: Evidence for an additional temporal class of gene expression in the forespore compartment of sporulating *Bacillus subtilis.* J Bacteriol 171:561, 1989

Philson SB, Llinas M: Siderochromes from *Pseudomonas fluorescens:* Isolation and characterization. J Biol Chem 257:8081, 1982

Pierucci O: Dimensions of *Escherichia coli* at various growth rates: Model for envelope growth. J Bacteriol 135:559, 1978

Pierucci O, Rickert M, Helmstetter CE: DnaA protein overproduction abolishes cell cycle specificity of DNA replication from *oriC* in *Escherichia coli.* J Bacteriol 171:3760, 1989

Ray GL, Haldenwang WG: Isolation of *Bacillus subtilis* genes transcribed in vitro and in vivo by a major sporulation-induced, DNA-dependent RNA polymerase. J Bacteriol 166:472, 1986

Reizer J, Panos C: Regulation of β–galactoside phosphate accumulation in *Streptococcus pyogenes* by an expulsion mechanism. Proc Natl Acad Sci USA 77:5497, 1980

Ryals J, Little R, Bremer H: Control of RNA synthesis in *Escherichia coli* after a shift to higher temperature. J Bacteriol 151:1425, 1982

Ryter A: Association of the nucleus and the membrane of bacteria: A morphological study. Bacteriol Rev 32:39, 1968

Schwarz U, Asmus A, Frank H: Autolytic enzymes and cell division of *Escherichia coli.* J Mol Biol 41:419, 1969

Seligman SJ: Cell division in staphylococci: A clue to the three-dimensional structure of peptidoglycan. J Infect Dis 155:423, 1987

Shapiro JA, Hsu C: *Escherichia coli* K-12 cell-cell interactions seen by time-lapse video. J Bacteriol 171:5963, 1989

Shepherd N, Churchward G, Bremer H: Synthesis and function of ribonucleic acid polymerase and ribosomes in *Escherichia coli* B/r after a nutritional shift-up. J Bacteriol 143:1332, 1980

Shockman GD, Daneo-Moore L, Higgins ML: Problems of cell wall and membrane growth, enlargement and division. Ann NY Acad Sci 235:161, 1974

Shuman HA: Active transport of maltose in *Escherichia coli.* J Biol Chem 257:5455, 1982

Smit J, Nikaido H: Outer membrane of gram-negative bacteria. 18. Electron microscopic studies on porin insertion sites and growth of cell surface of *Salmonella typhimurium.* J Bacteriol 135:687, 1978

Smith WP, Tai P-C, Davis DB: *Bacillus licheniformis* penicillinase: Cleavages and attachment of lipid during cotranslational secretion. Proc Natl Acad Sci USA 78:3501, 1981

Sonnenfeld EM, Koch AL, Doyle RJ: Cellular location of origin and terminus of replication in *Bacillus subtilis.* J Bacteriol 163:895, 1985

Springer MS, Goy MF, Adler J: Sensory transduction in *Escherichia coli:* Two complementary pathways of information processing that involve methylated proteins. Proc Natl Acad Sci USA 74:3312, 1977

Springer WR, Koshland DE Jr: Identification of a protein methyltransferase as the *che R* gene product in the bacterial sensing system. Proc Natl Acad Sci USA 74:533, 1977

Stock JB, Waygood EB, Meadow ND, et al: Sugar transport by the bacterial phosphotransferase system. The glucose receptors of the *Salmonella typhimurium* phosphotransferase system. J Biol Chem 257:14543, 1982

Todd JA, Roberts AN, Johnstone K: Reduced heat resistance of mutant spores after cloning and mutagenesis of the *Bacillus subtilis* gene encoding penicillin-binding protein 5. J Bacteriol 167:257, 1986

Tormo A, Almirón M, Kolter R: *sur A*, an *Escherichia coli* gene essential for survival in stationary phase. J Bacteriol 172:4339, 1990

Trempy JE, Morrison-Plummer J, Haldenwang WG: Synthesis of σ^{29}, an RNA polymerase specificity determinant is a developmentally regulated event in *Bacillus subtilis.* J Bacteriol 161:340, 1985

Tso W-W, Adler J: Negative chemotaxis in *Escherichia coli.* J Bacteriol 118:560, 1974

Tuomanen E, Tomasz A: Induction of autolysis in nongrowing *Escherichia coli.* J Bacteriol 167:1077, 1986

Uratani-Wong B, Lopez JM, Freese E: Induction of citric acid cycle enzymes during initiation of sporulation by guanine nucleotide deprivation. J Bacteriol 146:337, 1981

Warth AD: Molecular structure of the bacterial spore. Adv Microb Physiol 17:1, 1978

Weigand RA, Vinci KD, Rothfield LI: Morphogenesis of the bacterial division septum: A new class of septation-defective mutants. Proc Natl Acad Sci USA 73:1882, 1976

Weis RM, Koshland DE Jr: Chemotaxis in *Escherichia coli* proceeds efficiently from different initial tumble frequencies. J Bacteriol 172:1099, 1990

Wong S-L, Doi RH: Peptide mapping of *Bacillus subtilis* RNA polymerase σ factors and core-associated polypeptides. J Biol Chem 257:11932, 1982

Yamaguchi S, Aizawa S-I, Kihara M, et al: Genetic evidence for a switching and energy-transducing complex in the flagellar motor of *Salmonella typhimurium.* J Bacteriol 168:1172, 1986

Young CC, Alvarez JD, Bernlohr RW: Nutrient-dependent methylation of a membrane-associated protein of *Escherichia coli.* J Bacteriol 172:5147, 1990

CHAPTER 6

Composition, Structure, and Biosynthesis of Bacterial Cell Envelope and Energy Storage Polymers

Bacterial Envelope

Gross Composition

The structure and chemical nature of eubacterial envelopes correlate with whether a bacterium stains gram-positive, gram-negative, or acid-fast. The three groups of organisms differ considerably in envelope lipids, polysaccharides, proteins, and ultrastructural arrangement. These differences are most notable in the occurrence of an outer membrane on gram-negative bacteria, which is not found on gram-positive and acid-fast bacteria, and in the presence in both gram-positive and acid-fast bacteria of polysaccharides linked to peptidoglycan, a pattern not found in gram-negative cells. In addition, acid-fast and related organisms produce a variety of unique complex lipids not found in other organisms. The different types of envelope components produced by the three groups of organisms are summarized in Table 6–1.

Cell Wall Peptidoglycan

The rigid component of the cell wall of pathogenic eubacteria is a single bag-shaped giant macromolecule, or sacculus,

TABLE 6–1. COMPARISON OF CHARACTERISTIC TYPES OF BACTERIAL ENVELOPE COMPONENTS

Gram-positive Bacteria	Acid-fast Bacteria	Gram-negative Bacteria
Peptidoglycan 0.02–0.06 nm (multilayer)	Peptidoglycan 0.01 nm (trilayer)	Peptidoglycan 0.01 nm (bilayer or trilayer)
Proteins	Polypeptides	Lipoproteins
Lipoteichoic acids	Mycolic acid–glycolipids	Outer membrane
Teichoic acids	Arabinogalactans Arabinomannans	Lipopolysaccharide
Teichuronic acids	Cord factor	Proteins
Polysaccharides	Sulfolipids Mycosides Lipooligosaccharides	Polysaccharides

composed of a network of cross-linked peptidoglycan. It is synonomously called *peptidoglycan, murein,* or *cell wall.* Murein and associated components account for 2% to 40% of the cell dry weight. The glycan component is invariably constituted of the two amino sugars, glucosamine and muramic acid. These occur as alternate β-1,4-linked *N*-acetyl-D-glucosamine (GlcNAc) and *N*-acetyl-D-muramic acid [3-0-(1′-D-carboxyethyl)-*N*-acetyl-D-glucosamine] (i.e., MurNAc) residues (Fig. 6–1). Chains vary from <10 to >170 disaccharide units. The glycan and peptide units are linked through the lactic acid carboxyl group of MurNAc to the amino terminus of a tetrapeptide. The glycotetrapeptides are cross-linked through the tetrapeptide units, forming a continuous framework. The invariant feature of the tetrapeptide component is the presence of D-alanine, which is always the linkage unit between peptidoglycan chains.

Peptide Structure and Variations

As shown in Figure 6–1, the muramic acid–linked peptide component of many bacteria is the tetrapeptide -L-Ala-D-*iso*-Glu-*meso* DAP (or L-Lys)-D-Ala, which may be generalized as a–b–c–d. Cross-linkage between two peptidoglycan chains may be established directly (Fig. 6–2A) or through an interposed peptide bridge (Fig. 6–2B). *Escherichia coli* and all gram-negative eubacteria are of type A (Fig. 6–2A), whereas *Staphylococcus aureus,* the streptococci, and other gram-positive eubacteria accomplish cross-linkage through an interposed peptide bridge that may be composed of one or many amino acid residues (Fig. 6–2B). The *E. coli* direct cross-linkage may occur through -D-Ala-DAP- or -DAP-DAP-, whereas in gram-positive organisms, cross-linkage occurs through D-Ala-(amino acid)$_n$-L-Lys-cross-bridge but may, in some organisms, also include cross-linking through diamine bridges through *iso*glutamic acid, vis, *iso*-D-Glu(NH-diamine-NH)-D-Ala.

Further peptide modifications include the in vivo removal of terminal D-alanine residues from tetrapeptides (e.g., Fig. 6–2A) as in *E. coli,* or the removal of whole peptide units from the glycan chain. This happens in *E. coli* and *Micrococcus luteus,* in which half or more of the glycan chains are not cross-linked and may be free of part or all of the tetrapeptide units. Cross-linkage of peptidoglycan in these organisms, therefore, may approach only 30% to 70%. In contrast, *S. aureus* glycan retains all its tetrapeptide units, which are completely cross-linked (Fig. 6–2B). In addition to variations in cross-linkages, variation occurs in the presence of peptidoglycan-bound polypeptides, polysaccharides, or proteins. In *E. coli* and other gram-negative bacteria, a lipoprotein is attached covalently to the ε-amino group of diaminopimelic acid of the peptidoglycan. In gram-positive bacteria, various polysaccharides are found in covalent linkage with the peptidoglycan.

Cell shape is determined by the cell division machinery, not by peptidoglycan chemical structure, inasmuch as rod-

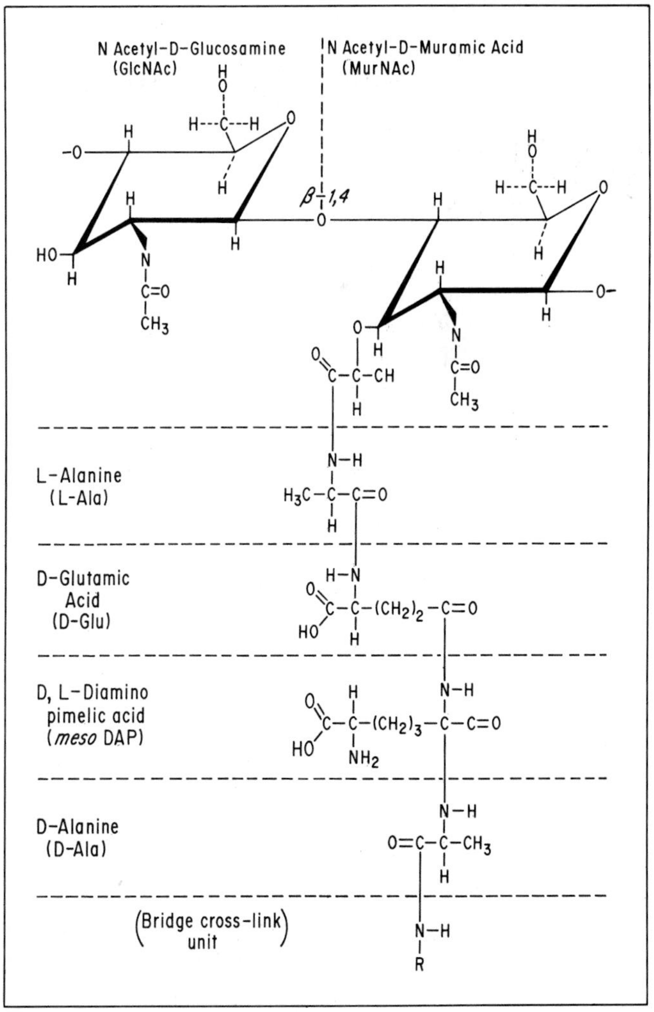

Fig. 6–1. Structure of the eubacterial peptidoglycan repeating unit.

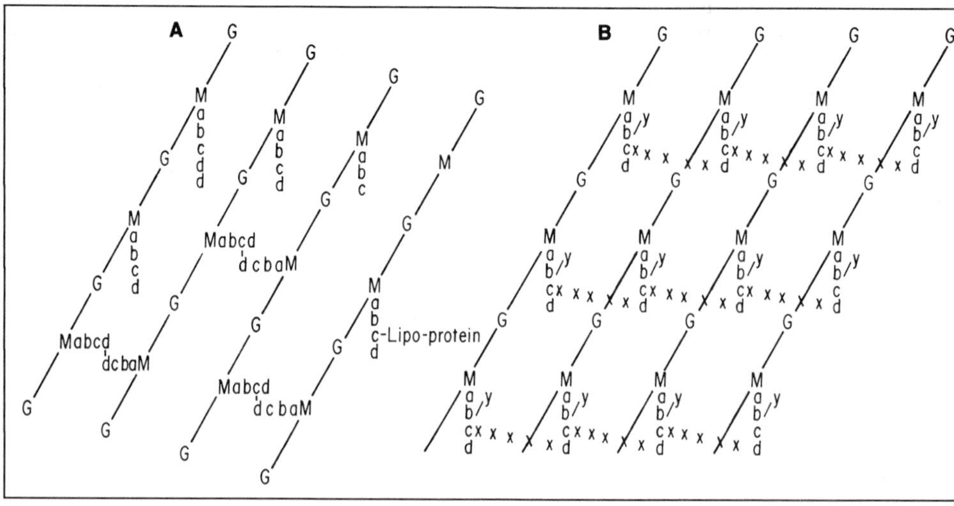

Fig. 6–2. A. Schematic generalization of *E. coli* peptidoglycan structure. **B.** Schematic generalization of *S. aureus* H peptidoglycan structure. M (*N*-acetylmuramic acid); G (*N*-acetylglucosamine); a (L-alanine); b (D-glutamic acid); c (either *meso*-diaminopimelic acid, in **A,** or L-lysine, in **B**); d (D-alanine); X (pentaglycine bridge); Y (-NH_2).

shaped and spherical *E. coli* yield chemically similar peptidoglycan. The glycan chains tend to be aligned circumferentially around the cell, in contrast to a longitudinal orientation of the cross-linked tetrapeptide units (Fig. 6–3). *E. coli* contains 10^6 repeating disaccharide-tetrapeptide units, or enough for two to three layers of peptidoglycan. A gram-positive cell may contain 20 times as much peptidoglycan, or enough for 40 layers or more.

Cell Wall Lytic Enzymes

Lytic enzymes fall into three major groups: (1) endo-β-1,4-*N*-acetylhexosaminidases, which cleave the glycan strands either between *N*-acetylmuramic acid and *N*-acetylglucosamine (e.g., the muramidases or lysozymes of egg white, tears, and white blood cells) or between the alternative acetylglucosamine-muramic acid glycoside linkages; (2) endopeptidases, many of which attack D-alanine at the bridge peptide cross-linkage, whereas others may specifically hydrolyze the interpeptide bridge linkages (e.g., lysostaphin, which splits glyclyglycine bonds in the pentaglycine bridge of *S. aureus* [Fig. 6–2B]); and (3) amidases, which cleave the glycan-peptide junction between *N*-acetylmuramic acid and L-alanine, thereby separating the glycan strands from the interlocking peptides. Because of their D-amino acid content, peptidoglycans are not susceptible to L-proteases.

The lytic enzymes described above also are found as bacterial autolysins. A notable example is the *N*-acetylmuramyl-L-alanine amidase found in *Streptococcus pneumoniae,* which is activated by low pH or bile salts.

Biologic Activities of Muramylpeptides

Adjuvants are substances that enhance the immune response in a nonspecific manner, making it possible to boost responses to specific immunogens. Long studied because of this property, mycobacterial cell wall products initially were thought to be active because of their peculiar lipids. Investigation of mycobacterial adjuvant components, however, led to the unexpected discovery that water-soluble peptidoglycan components common to many bacteria effect adjuvant responses. The smallest adjuvant active cell wall fragment is *N*-acetylmuramyl-L-alanyl-D-isoglutamine, known as muramyldipeptide or MDP (Fig. 6–1). MDP recently was discovered also to have the peculiar properties of being a pyrogen (fever-causing agent) and a somnagen (sleep-inducing factor). In addition, cell wall muramyl peptides compete with serotonin for receptors on macrophages. Moreover, cell wall fragments that contain covalently linked peptidoglycan-polysaccharides, such as the group A polysaccharide of *Streptococcus pyogenes,* may cause a variety of responses in experimental animals, the nature of the response being dependent on the animal's genetic background. Such responses include induction of endogenous pyrogens (e.g., interleukin-1 [IL-1]) by macrophages, inflam-

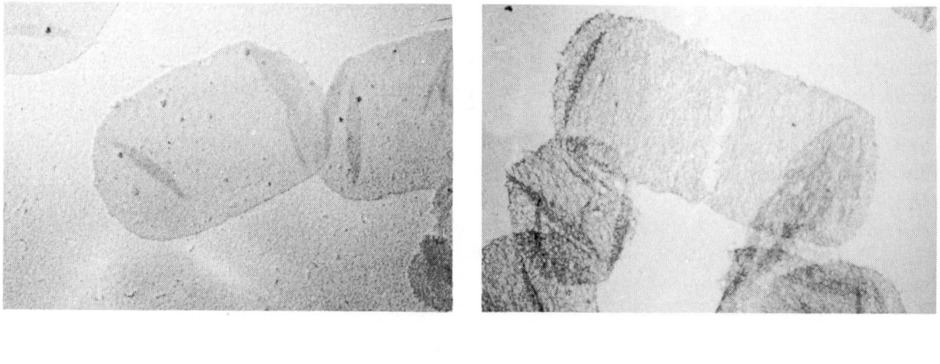

Fig. 6–3. Orientation of *E. coli* wall peptidoglycan. **Left.** *E. coli* cell wall after SDS and trypsin treatment. **Right.** After limited endopeptidase digestion of peptide cross-linkages, the glycan components appear to be oriented perpendicular to the long axis of the cell, indicating that the dissolved peptide cross-links were oriented with the long axis of the cell. *(From Verwer et al: J Bacteriol 136:723, 1978.)*

matory arthritic joint disease, granulomatis liver disease, stimulation of hematopoietic stem cells, and a Crohn's disease–like chronic inflammatory bowel disease.

Nonpeptidoglycan Components

Envelope Proteins

Both gram-positive and gram-negative cells produce envelope proteins that may influence host-parasite interaction. These include, among others, the M proteins of the group A streptococci, the *S. aureus* protein A (Table 6–2), and the fimbriae, lipoprotein, and porins of *E. coli* and other gram-negative organisms.

Envelope Polysaccharides: Capsular Polysaccharides

A variety of chemically diverse capsule and surface polymers are produced by both gram-positive and gram-negative bacteria. Among the best known capsular polymers are the soluble specific substances (SSS) or acidic polysaccharides produced by the pneumonia-causing organisms—the gram-positive *Streptococcus pneumoniae* and the gram-negative *Klebsiella pneumoniae*—and hyaluronic acid, which is produced by the gram-positive group A *Streptococcus pyogenes.* These polymers are composed of repeating oligosaccharide units of two to four monosaccharides, one of which is usually a uronic acid. The *Klebsiella* polymers may contain acetic and pyruvic acids and sometimes the methyl ethers of hexoses. Examples of some types of capsules are listed in Table 6–2.

Capsules are dispensable. Loss of the ability to produce capsules has no effect on viability. Capsule production is markedly influenced by environment and cultural conditions such as large amounts of nutrient carbohydrate, the restrictive growth conditions of low nitrogen, sulfur, or phosphorus, low temperature, or high salt concentration. A high CO_2 concentration is necessary for production of the *Bacillus anthracis* polypeptide capsule, composed of D-glutamic acid linked through γ-carboxyl groups (see Fig. 2–3). Other factors also may affect capsule production. For example, the hyaluronic acid capsule of groups A and C streptococci can be demonstrated only very early in the growth of hyaluronidase-producing strains.

Several different types of genetically determined capsular polysaccharides may be produced by subgroups of a single species. These often can be differentiated serologically, hence the terms *serovar* (serologic variant), *serogroup,* and *serotype.* For example, more than 70 immunologically distinct capsular polysaccharide serotypes of *S. pneumoniae* have been defined. Other organisms such as *Klebsiella, Escherichia,* and *Haemophilus,* also produce a variety of type-specific capsular polysaccharides. Differences in capsular types are detected by an antigen-antibody reaction known as Neufeld's quellung reaction, in which cells are mixed with specific anticapsule serum. If the appropriate capsular antigen is present, brightfield microscopy reveals an optically refractive "swelling" around the cell.

Although capsular polysaccharides may be washed off bacterial cells, small amounts often remain cell-bound and are detectable by sensitive serologic procedures. In the case of the pneumococci, many of the capsular polysaccharides have the chemical structure of teichoic acid–like polymers (see below). However, because of the ease with which the pneumococci autolyze, it sometimes is difficult to know whether the easily removed capsular materials are in fact excreted as extracellular polysaccharides, released by autolysis as originally cell wall-bound teichoic acids, or whether they are easily extractable lipoteichoic acids anchored by lipophilic groups in the cytoplasmic membrane. In the case of gram-negative cells, covalent linkage of polysaccharides to peptidoglycan is unknown.

Capsular polysaccharides may serve as bacteriophage receptors. These bacteriophages produce specific depolymerases, which dissolve the capsule at the site of attachment in order to allow the virus access to the cell.

Envelope of Gram-positive Bacteria

Cell wall polysaccharides of gram-positive bacteria contribute 10% to 50% of the mass of the cell wall, and, as indicated above, in many instances these polymers appear to be covalently linked to peptidoglycan.

TABLE 6–2. VARIOUS BACTERIAL SURFACE POLYMERS

Bacterium	Surface Polymer	Components
Yersinia pestis	Protein	Protein
Staphylococcus aureus	Teichoic acid	Ribitol-1,5-phosphodiester, *N*-acetylglucosamine, D-alanine
	Protein A	Protein
Streptococcus pyogenes	Hyaluronic acid capsule	[-*N*-acetyl-D-glucosamine-β-1,4D-glucuronic acid-β-1,3-]1_n
	M (virulence) antigens (fimbriae)	Proteins
	Group A polysaccharide	Polyrhamnan, *N*-acetyl-D-glucosamine
Streptococcus faecalis	Lipoteichoic acid (group D)	Glycerol-1,3-phosphodiester
Streptococcus pneumoniae	Type II	D-Glucose, L-rhamnose, D-glucuronic acid
	Type III	D-Glucose, D-glucuronic acid
	Type XVIII (teichoic acid–like)	[D-Glucose, D-galactose, L-rhamnose, glycerol-PO_4, O-acetyl]$_n$
Haemophilus influenzae	Type b capsule	Polyribose–ribitol phosphate
Klebsiella pneumoniae	Type I capsule	D-Glucose, fucose, glucuronic acid, pyruvic acid
Neisseria meningitidis	Serogroup B antigen	[*N*-Acetylneuraminic acid]$_n$
	Serogroup C antigen	[*N*-Acetyl,O-acetylneuraminic acid]$_n$
Pseudomonas aeruginosa	Capsule	Alginic acid

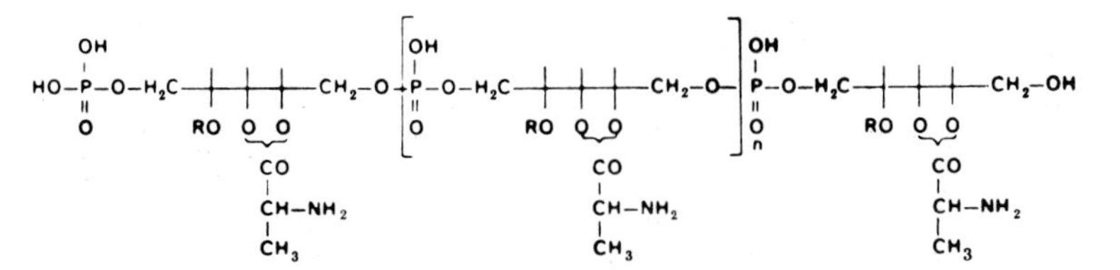

Fig. 6–4. Ribitol teichoic acids. *Bacillus subtilis:* R = β-glucosyl, n = 7; *S. aureus* H: R = α- and β-*N*-acetylglucosaminyl, n = 6; *Lactobacillus arabinosus* 17-5: R = α-glucosyl, alternate ribitol residues also have α-glucosyl at the 3-position, n = 4.5. *(From Baddiley: Endeavour 23:33, 1964.)*

Teichoic Acid, Teichoic Acid–like Polymers, and Teichuronic Acids

Teichoic acids (from the Greek *teichos,* for wall) are polymers of repeating anionic phosphodiester-linked polyols (Fig. 6–4). Cell wall teichoic acids (CWTA) usually contain ribitol or occasionally, glycerol, and are covalently linked to peptidoglycan through substituted phosphodiester groups on the C-6-hydroxyl of *N*-acetylmuramic acid residues. Up to 50% of the peptidoglycan may be combined with teichoic acids in the bacilli and staphylococci. Membrane or lipoteichoic acids (LTAs) are glycerophosphate polymers that terminate in glycolipid (Figs. 6–5, 6–6, and 6–11), which is anchored in the cytoplasmic membrane. The enterococcal group D polysaccharide is a lipoteichoic acid. The lipoteichoic acids are amphiphiles (Fig. 6–11), are excreted as vesicles thought to be involved in protein secretion, and exhibit at higher concentrations many of the less toxic properties of the gram-negative endotoxins discussed below (Table 6–3).

Teichoic acids are specifically modified in different bacteria by addition to the polyol units of ester-linked D-alanine, D-lysine, or O-glycoside–linked glucose, galactose, or *N*-acetylhexosamines. The substituted teichoic acids are important as specific cell surface antigens of *Staphylococcus, Streptococcus, Lactobacillus,* and *Bacillus* species. For example, most human strains of *S. aureus* produce galactosamine- or glucosamine-substituted ribitol cell wall teichoic acids, whereas *Staphylococcus epidermidis* produces glucose-substituted glycerol teichoic acids.

Many teichoic acid–like polymers also occur in a variety of bacteria. These polymers are composed of phosphodiester-linked oligosaccharides. A notable example is the teichoic acid–like C polysaccharide of *S. pneumoniae* that is composed of phosphate, *N*-acetyl-D-galactosamine, D-glucose, *N*-acetyl-2,4-diamino-2,4,6-trideoxyhexose, ribitol, and choline.

Teichuronic acids (TAs) are polymers composed of *N*-acetylgalactosamine (GalNAc) and glucuronic acid (GlcUA), linked as the disaccharide repeating unit (GlcUA → 1,3 → GalNAc)$_n$. TAs contain no phosphate, but they still serve as acidic polyanionic polymers because of the carboxyl of the uronic acids. TAs are linked through an *N*-acetylglucosamine-1-phosphodiester to the C-6 hydroxyl group of muramic acid. Teichuronic acids may be found in the same cell together with teichoic acids: teichuronic acids are synthesized when cells are deprived of phosphate with which to make teichoic acids.

Other Cell Wall Polysaccharides

Nonteichoic acid polysaccharides are usually, but not always, specific for each species or strain. For example, a characteristic highly branched cell wall–bound L-rhamnose polymer substituted with D-glucosamine and D-galactose occurs as the groups B and group G streptococcal-specific polysaccharides, whereas the L-rhamnose polymer is substituted with *N*-acetyl-D-glucosamine in group A streptococci and with *N*-acetyl-D-galactosamine in group C organisms. These organisms also may produce teichoic acids different from the group polysaccharides (Fig. 6–6).

Envelope of Acid-fast and Related Bacteria

Members of the genus *Mycobacterium* and some *Nocardia* species, which characteristically stain red with carbolfuchsin and

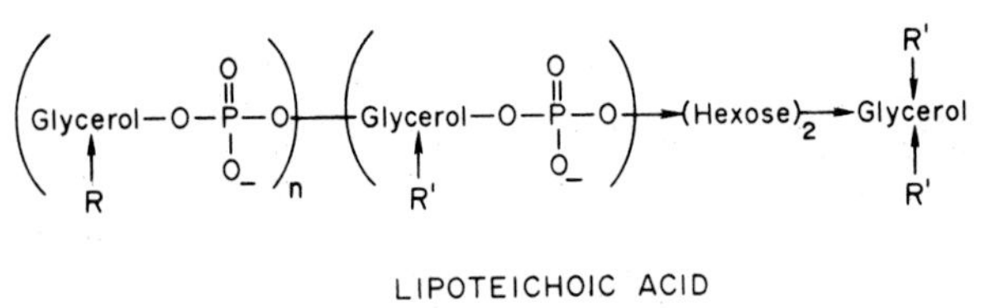

Fig. 6–5. Postulated structure of lipoteichoic (membrane teichoic) acid includes possibility of fatty acid (R′) substituted glycerophosphate interposed between glycerol teichoic acid chain and glycolipid. R-H or glycosyl; R′-H or esterified fatty acid residue; hexose disaccharide may be either α-1,2- or β-1,6-glucosylglucose or α-1,2-galactosylglucose; n > 28. *(Adapted from Knox and Wicken: Bacteriol Rev 37:215, 1973.)*

TABLE 6–3. SELECTED BIOLOGIC PROPERTIES OF BACTERIAL AMPHIPHILES

Property	Endotoxin	Lipoteichoic Acid
Lethal toxicity	+	−
Pyrogenicity	+	−
Shwartzman reaction	+	+
Mitogenicity	+	+
Immunogenicity	+	+
Eucaryote membrane binding	+	+
Complement activation	+	+
Hypersensitivity reactions	+	+
Stimulation of nonspecific immunity	+	+
Limulus lysate assay	+	+

Adapted from Wicken and Knox: Biochim Biophys Acta 604:1, 1980.

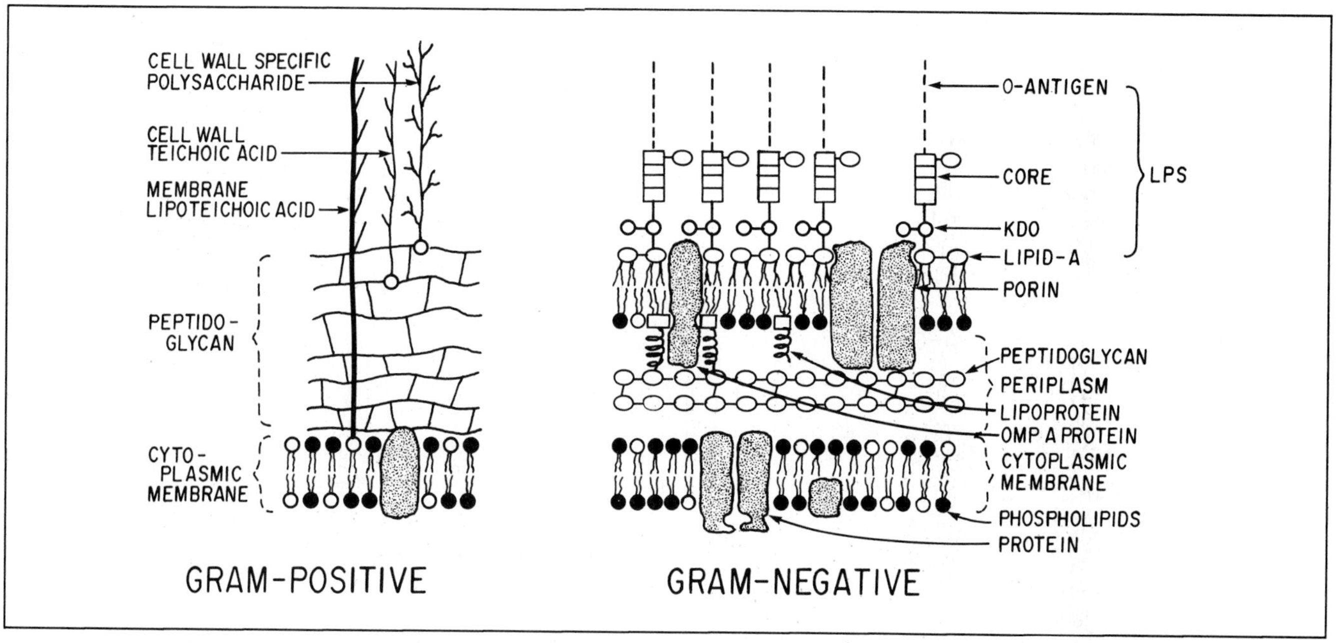

Fig. 6–6. Diagram comparing some major envelope structures of gram-positive and gram-negative eubacterial cells. The peptidoglycan layer of typical gram-positive cells is much thicker than that of gram-negative cells. Gram-positive cells often have polysaccharides covalently linked to peptidoglycan (represented by straight lines ending at peptidoglycan layer), as well as lipoteichoic acids that penetrate the peptidoglycan layer from the cytoplasmic membrane (represented by single feathered lines). Gram-positive bacteria do not have an OM. In contrast, gram-negative cells do have an OM and often exhibit a periplasmic space between the cytoplasmic membrane and the OM, in which is found the relatively thin peptidoglycan layer. Helical lipoproteins, covalently linked to the peptidoglycan anchor the OM. No polysaccharides are bound to the peptidoglycan of gram-negative bacteria. Lipopolysaccharides are found in the outer leaflet of the OM. Transmembrane proteins (OmpA and porins) occur only in OM.

resist decolorization with acid-alcohol, are said to be *acid-fast.* This staining property correlates with the presence of mycolic acids in the cell wall of the intact bacterium. Mycolic acids (Fig. 6–7) are α-substituted, β-hydroxy fatty acids that occur in mycobacteria as esters bound to cell wall polysaccharides and as components of extractable (i.e., free) glycolipids sometimes known as *cord factors.* Mycolic acid–producing corynebacteria, nocardiae, and mycobacteria are known as the CNM group of bacteria. The CNM group produces mycolic acids that increase in chain length from corynemycolic acids (C_{30}), through the nocardic acids (C_{50}) and the mycolic acids (C_{90}). Only the nocardiae and mycobacteria produce cell wall–bound mycolic acids.

Cell Wall. The cell wall of *Mycobacterium tuberculosis* contains approximately equal amounts of peptidoglycan, arabinans, and lipid. More than 50% of the lipid components are esterified mycolic acids, whereas some 25% are normal fatty acids. Peptidoglycan-linked poly-L-glutamic acid also occurs in *M. tuberculosis.* The basic peptidoglycan structure of *Corynebacterium diphtheriae, Nocardia* species, and *M. tuberculosis* is represented in Figure 6–2A. Muramic acid 6-phosphate is the primary linkage between cell wall–bound arabinogalactans, arabinomannans, and peptidoglycan. Cell wall–bound mycolic acids are esterified through the C-5-hydroxyl of D-arabinose residues of the neutral arabinogalactans. A second major cell

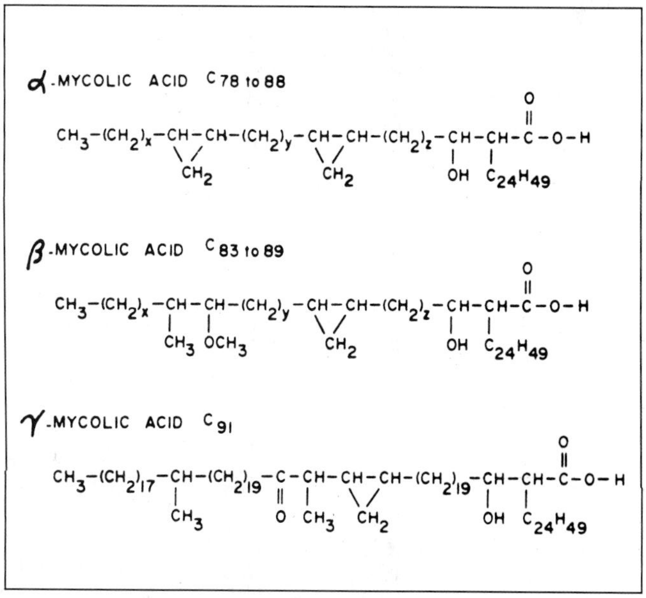

Fig. 6–7. Structures of selected α, β, and γ mycolic acids. *(Data from Toubiana et al: Cancer Immunol Immunother 2:189, 1977; Ribi et al: Cancer Immunol Immunother 3:171, 1978.)*

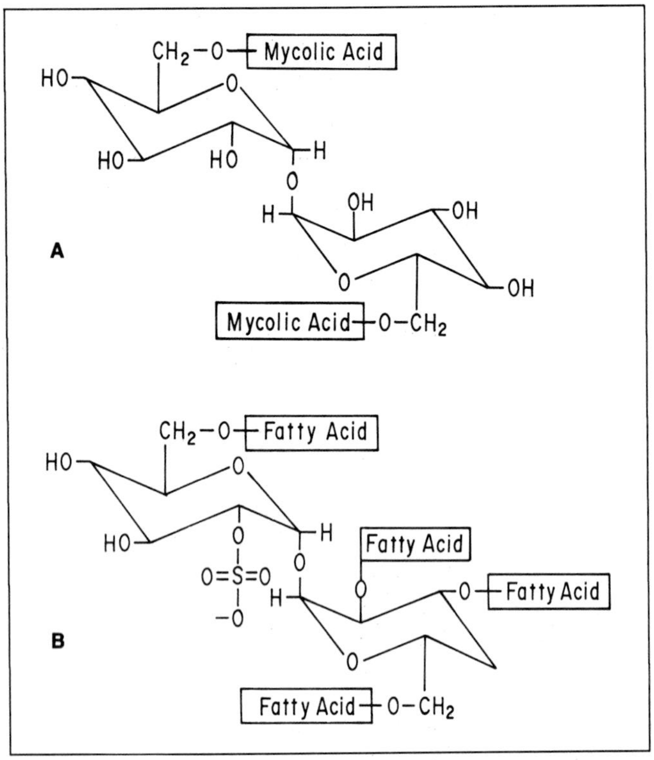

Fig. 6–8. **A.** Cord factors, 6,6′-dimycolyltrehalose. **B.** Sulfolipids 2,3,6,6′-tetraacyltrehalose-2-sulfate, in which R groups are different fatty acids. *(Adapted from Goren: Bacteriol Rev 36:33, 1972.)*

wall polymer, arabinomannan, is highly acidic, being succinylated and esterified with inositol-1-phosphate residues.

Glycolipids. Several unusual glycolipids occur in the acid-fast and related bacteria that are not cell wall bound. These include trehalose mycolates, sulfolipids, and lipooligosaccharides, mycosides, and lipopolysaccharides.

TREHALOSE MYCOLATES. Trehalose mycolates are 6,6′-dimycolyl esters of the α,α′-1,1′-linked glucose disaccharide, trehalose (Fig. 6–8A), and are found throughout the corynebacteria, nocardiae, and mycobacteria. *C. diphtheriae* produces trehalose esterified with the C_{32} acids, corynemycolic acids, and corynemycolenic acid. In some *Nocardia* species, only nocardic acids are found, but in *Nocardia asteroides,* a mixture of nonwall C_{28} to C_{36} trehalose-linked corynemycolic acids occur, and the cell wall is esterified with C_{50} to C_{56} nocardic acids. The trehalose mycolates of *M. tuberculosis* contain a series of mycolic acids ranging in size from C_{78} to C_{90} and characteristically containing a methyl group, a methoxyl group, and cyclopropane rings (Fig. 6–7).

Mycobacterial trehalose dimycolates disrupt mitochondria, decreasing respiration and oxidative phosphorylation; they induce production of tumor necrosis factor (TNF, also known as cachectin) in macrophages, as well as cachexia and antitumor activity in mice.

TREHALOSE SULFOLIPIDS. Sulfolipids are peripherally located within the envelope and are responsible for the neutral-red staining properties of cord-forming mycobacteria. In *M. tuberculosis,* the production of sulfolipids appears to correlate with virulence. The principal sulfatide of *M. tuberculosis* has been identified as 2,3,6,6′-tetraacyltrehalose-2′-sulfate (Fig. 6–8B).

TREHALOSE LIPOOLIGOSACCHARIDES. In addition to mycolic acid derivatives, trehalose-based lipooligosaccharides (LOSs) occur as alkali-labile mycobacterial lipid antigens. These antigens, which occur in the "rough" organism, *Mycobacterium smegmatis,* contain trehalose as part of a tetraglucose core to which various other unusual sugars may be linked (as in *Mycobacterium kansasii*) in analogy with the enterobacterial *rough* lipopolysaccharide (e to a) core mutants described in Figure 6–12.

MYCOSIDES. Some 34 or more specific antigens known generally as *mycosides* occur peripherally as a capsular electron transparent zone of fibrils on the cell surface of "mycobacteria other than *M. tuberculosis,*" sometimes referred to as "MOTT." These include the two apolar phenolic mycosides A of *M. kansasii* and *Mycobacterium leprae,* the mycoside B of *Mycobacterium bovis,* and the 31 polar alkali stable peptidoglycolipids, or mycosides C of the MAIS complex, that is, *M. avium* (types 1 to 3), *M. intracellulare* (types 4 to 28), and *M. scrofulaceum* (types 41 to 43). More polar mycosides C undoubtedly will be found. Chemically, the mycosides contain a variety of unusual compounds. These include O-methylated sugars and uronic acid, deoxysugars, amino sugars, and in the case of the mycosides C, D-amino acid derivatives (e.g., Fig. 6–9), which form an acylated tetrapeptidyldimethoxy-L-rhamnoside core. The apolar mycosides A and B contain various O-methyl sugars as part of glycosylphenolic phthiocerol diesters. These compounds are thought to show some promise as diagnostic antigens for leprosy. Also, phthiocerols, C_{30} to C_{34} branched chain alcohols, have been found as dimycolates in lepromatous tissue.

PHOSPHOLIPIDS AND LIPOPOLYSACCHARIDES. These components probably are membrane-associated, although their exact location within the cell is unknown. Mycobacterial phospholipids include, among others, diphosphatidyglycerol (cardiolipin) and phosphatidylethanolamine. In addition, the mycobacteria produce phosphatidylinositol monosaccharides and oligosaccharides, such as tetracylated phosphatidylinositol pentamannosides.

Lipoglycans (lipopolysaccharides) also have been described in the mycobacteria. *M. tuberculosis* and *Mycobacterium phlei* produce a branched-chain polymer composed of 11 6-0-methyl-D-glucose and seven D-glucose residues in α-1,4 linkage. The reducing terminus is linked to acylated glycerol.

Envelope of Gram-negative Bacteria

The gram-negative bacterial cell envelope encompasses everything from the cytoplasmic membrane to the outer surface of the cell. Structurally, the cell envelope consists of a periplasmic gel sandwiched between the inner cytoplasmic membrane and the overlying outer membrane (OM) (Fig. 6–6; see also Figs. 3–12, 3–13, 3–15). The periplasmic gel includes proteins and membrane-derived oligosaccharides (MDOs). The periplasmic gel proteins include substrate-binding proteins that allow concentration of substrates against a gradient and various

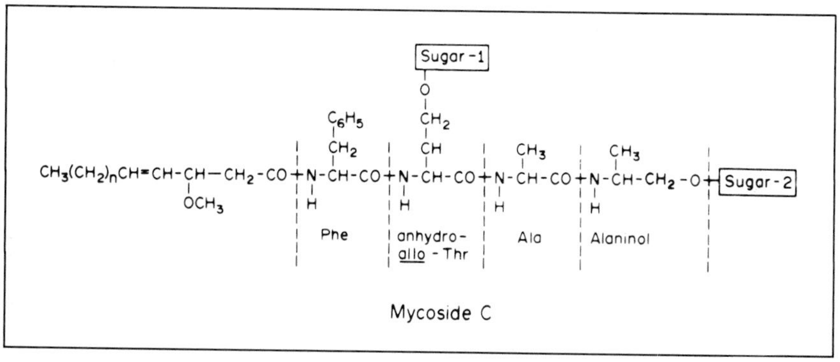

Fig. 6–9. Mycoside C. The tetrapeptide is composed of unusual D-amino acids or derivatives. Sugar 1 can be diacetyl-5-deoxytalose or an oligosaccharide that contains a variety of unusual sugars, aminosugars, and a uronic acid. *(Adapted from Brennan PJ: In Lieve and Schlessinger (eds): Microbiology—1984. American Society of Microbiology, 1985, p 366.)*

hydrolytic (digestive) enzymes. MDOs fluctuate inversely with external medium ionic strength, and MDOs thereby help regulate cellular osmolarity.

Outer Membrane

The OM is unique to gram-negative bacteria. The OM contains phospholipids, lipopolysaccharides (LPS), and a variety of proteins, of which pore proteins (porins) and lipoprotein are the most prominent (Fig. 6–6). In enteric bacteria the OM is asymmetric in that all the LPS occurs in the outer leaflet, whereas phospholipid is found in the inner leaflet of the OM (Fig. 6–6). The outer surface of enteric bacteria is about 40% LPS and 60% protein. In contrast, phospholipid may occur in both inner and outer leaflets of the OM of nonenteric bacteria.

The OM serves as a sophisticated physiologically active organelle. It (1) forms a barrier to hydrophobic compounds, (2) functions as a molecular sieve for water-soluble molecules, (3) presents sites for host cell and bacteriophage attachment and bacterial conjugation, (4) may contain proteases and other enzymes, aggressins, evasins and toxins for host cells in instances of pathogenesis, (5) encloses and protects from environmental poisons and lysins the cell wall peptidoglycan, periplasmic gel components, and plasma membrane, (6) releases vesicular blebs of LPS and protein that may serve secretory functions, and (7) possesses LPS and proteins that contain molecular signals sensed by animal cells.

Barrier Effect. This effect is seen most clearly in enteric bacteria that must cope with bile salts, chemicals, and digestive enzymes. Enteric bacteria are enclosed by the tightly fitting polyanionic and hydrophilic LPS, metal ligands, and water-filled pore proteins of the OM outer surface, which form a size exclusion barrier for hydrophilic molecules and a hydrophilic barrier against hydrophobic molecules. Many antibiotics, chemicals, macromolecules, enzymes, and detergents are excluded. The effectiveness of the barrier is disrupted by treatment with EDTA, which removes divalent metal ions, LPS, and protein. Mutations that result in loss of LPS O-polysaccharide and core components, as well as proteins, also decrease the barrier effect. The barrier effect is less obvious in the nonenteric *Neisseria* and *Haemophilus* species in which phospholipid occurs in both the inner and outer leaflets of the OM. Organisms of these genera also are more susceptible to antibiotics than enteric bacteria.

Porins. Porins are stable trimeric OM proteins that facilitate diffusion of small molecules across the OM into the cell. Porins are found uniquely in the OM of gram-negative bacteria and mitochondria of eucaryotes (a fact that intrigues students of evolution). Each monomer within the porin trimer contains a pore formed from 19 transmembrane β-sheet peptides that form a rather large channel except for inner peptide units that constrict the channel like the "eye of the needle." Porins exhibit specific and nonspecific pore activity. They allow passage of relatively small water-soluble molecules such as maltose and vitamin B_{12}. Enterobacterial porins generally exclude molecules >0.6 kilodaltons (kDa), whereas *Pseudomonas aeruginosa* and gonococcal porins exhibit tenfold higher cutoff ranges (e.g., 3 to 9 kDa). Most porins are nonspecific, but some porins, such as the specific maltose transport LamB porin of *E. coli,* are regulated environmentally by presence or absence of substrate, whereas low phosphate induces PhoE, which specifically transports anions. *E. coli* porins OmpF, OmpC, and PhoE are over 60% homologous, with limited homology to LamB. The OM protein A (OmpA) is a 35 kDa transmembrane protein that aids in stabilizing the OM and serves as the F-pilus receptor in conjugation but that has low pore activity. Both porins and LPS activate tumoricidal activity by macrophages, indicating that mammalian host systems are geared to detect surface components of potentially infectious organisms. "Endotoxin (LPS) associated" proteins, probably porins and lipoproteins that are known to bind tightly with LPS in the presence of Mg^{2+}, have been reported to exhibit IL-1 activity.

Peptidoglycan (Murein) and Lipoprotein

The peptidoglycan of gram-negative eubacteria corresponds to the type A structure of Figure 6–2. Covalently linked lipoprotein molecules appear by means of electron microscopy to be spaced every 10 to 12 nm on the outer surface of the peptidoglycan structure. The insoluble murein accounts for 1% to 2% of the cell dry weight after trypsin digestion to remove the relatively large amount of lipoprotein (>4% cell dry weight). One third of the total lipoprotein is covalently linked at its carboxy terminus through the trypsin-sensitive sequence, Lys-Tyr-Arg-Lys, to *meso*-diaminopimelic acid (DAP) units of the peptidoglycan. At the *N*-terminus, because of covalently linked saturated (e.g., palmitic) and unsaturated (e.g., palmitoleic and vaccenic) fatty acids inserted into the lipid bilayer of the OM, the lipoprotein is strongly lipophilic and anchors the OM to the cell wall (Fig. 6–6). The lipoprotein also associates with the OmpA protein. Mutants that lack either OmpA or lipoprotein leak periplasmic proteins and

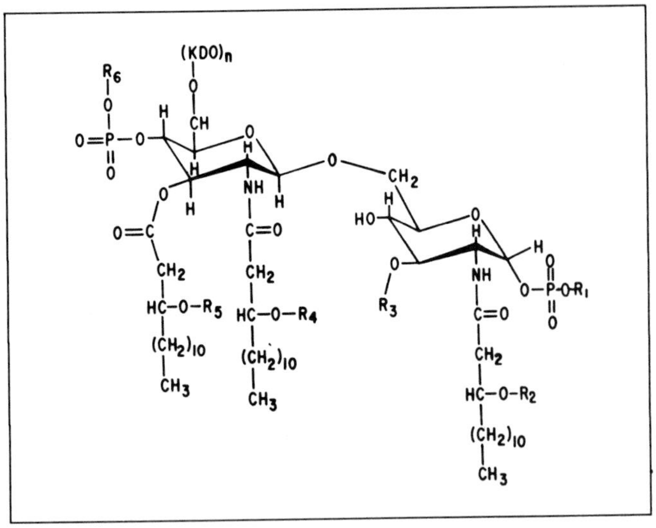

Fig. 6–10. Structure of naturally occurring KDO-lipid A, from the Re mutant of *Salmonella typhimurium.* The glucosamine disaccharide is linked β(1-6), and both are *N*-acyl substituted with β-hydroxymyristic acid groups. R_1 = H, phosphate, or phosphorylethanolamine; R_2 = H (may be palmitic acid in *S. minnesota*); R_3 = β-hydroxymyristic acid; R_4 = lauric acid; R_5 = double ester, two β-hydroxy myristic acids; R_6 = H, or 4 amino-4 deoxy-L-arabinose in α-1-phosphate linkage; n = 2 or 3. *(Adapted from Takayama et al: J Biol Chem 258:7379, 1983.)*

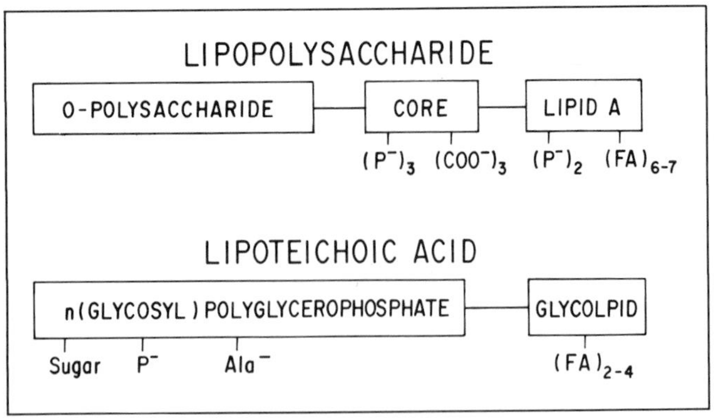

Fig. 6–11. Eubacterial amphiphiles (one end is hydrophilic, the other lipophilic). These long-chain polysaccharide molecules have different structures but have some similar properties. They occur at the cell surface with the lipophilic end anchored in the cytoplasmic membrane of gram-positive cells (lipoteichoic acids) or in the outer layer of the OM of gram-negative cells (lipopolysaccharides).

shed OM vesicles. The lipoprotein contains no histidine, proline, phenylalanine, or tryptophan. Lipoproteins are the major surface antigens of the two spirochetes, *Borrelia burgdorferi* (agent of Lyme disease) and *Treponema pallidum* (agent of syphilis), as well as the cell wall–less *Mycoplasma pneumoniae* (a cause of pneumonia). A recombinant lipoprotein from *P. aeruginosa* has been used as a protective antigen in experimental studies in mice.

Lipopolysaccharide Lipid A/Endotoxin

Endotoxin (ET) is a term used before the discovery of the identity of endotoxin as the lipid A component of LPS (Figs. 6–6 and 6–10). For almost 100 years endotoxin has described a heat-stable, cell-associated pyrogenic (fever causing), and potentially lethal toxin of gram-negative bacteria in contrast to heat-labile protein exotoxins, for example, tetanus toxin, which are found outside the cell in culture filtrates. Some 50 years ago, LPS was isolated and found to contain the endotoxic activity. Subsequently, the lipid A component of LPS of endotoxic gram-negative bacteria was shown to be identical in basic structure and to be responsible for endotoxic activities.

Lipopolysaccharide Structure. LPS is an amphiphile (one end hydrophilic, the other end hydrophobic) (Fig. 6–11) with three regions: O-specific polysaccharide (region I), core polysaccharide (region II), and lipid A (region III). Some bacteria, for example, *Neisseria* and *Haemophilus* species, which do not produce region I polysaccharides, produce shorter polymers called *lipooligosaccharides* (LOS) that correspond to region II. Serologic specificity resides primarily in region I, also sometimes in region II, and the bioactive center, or endotoxin, in region III. Lipid A, with fatty acids at one end and phosphate groups at the other, also is an amphiphile. The general structure of lipopolysaccharides is indicated in Figures 6–6 and 6–11. As amphiphiles, isolated LPS and lipid A form biologically active, self-aggregating complexes, or micelles, of molecular weights ranging from 10^5 to 10^8.

O-SPECIFIC POLYSACCHARIDE (REGION I). Bacterial colonies that produce O antigen polysaccharide (i.e., wild type) appear visually as smooth (S) on agar surfaces. Constituents of O-specific polysaccharide vary among species and even among strains. The O antigen polysaccharide chain contains 10 to 100 or more repeating oligosaccharide units composed of three to four monosaccharides. Lower chain lengths may occur under environmental stress conditions such as high, almost limiting growth temperatures, low pH, low phosphate, low magnesium, or high salt. Monosaccharides, including various pentoses, 4-aminopentose, hexoses, 2-aminohexoses, 6-deoxyhexoses, 3,6-dideoxyhexoses, 6-deoxy sugars with amino groups at the C-2, C-3 and C-4 positions, aminohexose uronic acids, heptoses, and others have been isolated from the region I polymers of various bacteria. Amino groups of sugars usually are *N*-acetylated. Within the enteric bacteria, organisms that produce O antigens with high hydrophobic group content (e.g., dideoxy-sugars) tend to be more pathogenic than those that do not. The LPS of the enterobacteria, that is, *Salmonella, Escherichia, Shigella, Citrobacter,* and related genera, often contain similar O antigen monosaccharides and can be grouped into a limited number of similar chemotypes on the basis of O antigen sugar composition: however, different sugar sequences, linkage groups, and other substituents (e.g., acetyl groups) on repeating oligosaccharide units will cause differences in O-antigenic (serologic) and bacteriophage specificities. Several thousand different serologic combinations have been found in salmonellae alone.

CORE POLYSACCHARIDE (REGION II). This region is less variable among genera and species than is region I. Region II is arbitrarily separated into inner and outer core areas. Inner core contains heptose, phosphate, and 2-keto-3-deoxy-

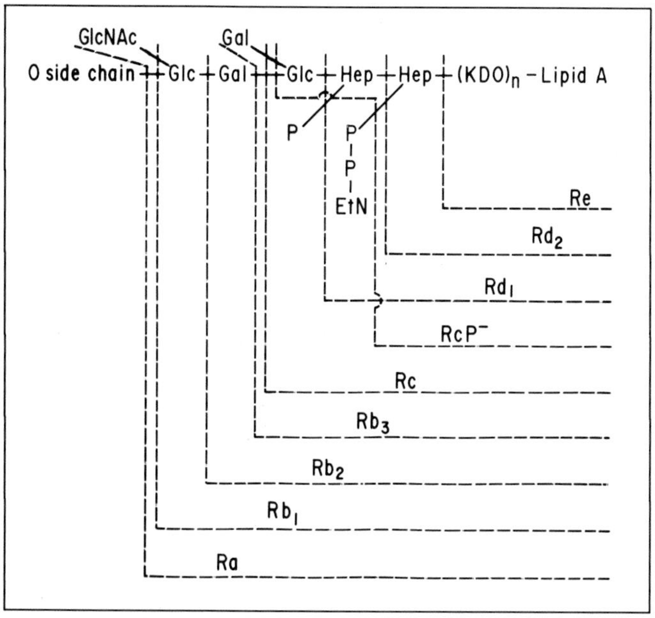

Fig. 6–12. Core mutant structures of *Salmonella typhimurium* lipopolysaccharide. Loss of capability to add O side chains to core yields Ra mutants. Loss of capability to add *N*-acetylglucosamine results in an Rb_1 mutant, and so on. Mutants incapable of making the Re glycolipid are incapable of growth. *(Adapted from Nikaido and Vaara: Microbiol Rev 49:1, 1985.)*

octulosonic acid (KDO). Formation of ligands among phosphate, KDO, and divalent metal cations results in stabilizing the OM. KDO is bound to lipid A by an acid-labile ketosidic linkage. Of unknown significance is the occurrence of KDO in plant cell walls, the only other place KDO is found. The outer core of enteric bacteria is composed of the hexoses, glucose, galactose, and *N*-acetylglucosamine (Fig. 6–12). All *Salmonella* share a common core polysaccharide that differs from those of *Shigella* or *Escherichia* species. *E. coli,* which may produce several core sequence structures different from those of salmonellae, also may produce a rhamnose oligomer linked to KDO.

Core mutants, Ra to Re (Fig. 6–12), incapable of completing biosynthesis of O antigen polysaccharide or various steps in the biosynthesis of core polysaccharide, are called *rough* or *R-form mutants* because they tend to form visually rough colonies on agar surfaces. Mutants unable to synthesize KDO are nonviable; the Re mutant is the last viable LPS mutant. Purified Ra and Re LPS have been crystallized. Colonies of Ra and Rb mutants may be visually similar to smooth (S) "wild type" colonies that make complete LPS, but differences between various LPS R-form mutants can be detected chemically, serologically, or by susceptibility to specific bacteriophages.

LIPID A (REGION III). Region III is highly conserved among eubacteria: lipid A basic structure is common to gram-negative bacteria, including the enterobacteria, neisseriae, the pseudomonads, and others that exhibit endotoxic properties.

Basic Structure. Lipid A of enterobacteria (Fig. 6–10), composed of a β-1,6-linked D-glucosamine disaccharide substituted at positions 4′ and 1 by phosphomonoester groups, is known as *diphospholipid A* (DPLA): the C1-position phosphate is esterified as an α-glucosamine-1-phosphate. The hydroxyl group at C6′ serves as the attachment site of KDO and to the latter, the core polysaccharide. Fatty acids linked to the hydroxyl and amino groups of the glucosamine disaccharide confer hydrophobic properties to the lipid A molecule. Amide and ester-linked D-3-hydroxy fatty acids, which consist of 14 carbons (β-hydroxymyristic acid), characteristically are found in the lipid A of enterobacteria, and the C3-OH positions of these unusual fatty acids may be further esterified with saturated fatty acids.

Microheterogeneity. Some degree of lipid A structural microheterogeneity occurs among genera and species with retention of biologic activity. For example, *Neisseria* species produce 12 (instead of 14) carbon 3-hydroxy fatty acids, the degree of substitution with saturated fatty acids varies, and the C′4-phosphoglucosamine disaccharide position may be substituted with 4-amino-L-arabinose in salmonellae and *P. aeruginosa* but not in *E. coli* nor *Shigella.* In some cases the C1 position phosphomonoester group is further diesterified with phosphoethanolamine: neither amino nor hydroxyl groups of these secondary substituents are acylated. Finally, the number of fatty acid substituents may vary within the LPS isolated from a single culture. These differently substituted lipid A molecules have been separated, characterized, derivatives prepared, chemically synthesized, and bioactivity studied. Some derivatives show little toxicity while retaining useful biologic activities, which indicates that minor variations in the lipid A structure modify its biologic signals. For example, the most potent lipid A molecule was found to be substituted with six fatty acids, that is, the hexaacyl-1,4′-diphospholipid A (hexaacyl-1,4′-DPLA), whereas a lipid A with one more or one less fatty acid is less toxic, as are tetraacyl and decreasingly acylated lipid A derivatives. Removal of all fatty acids results in complete loss of biologic activity. Also, absence of only one of the phosphate groups (either at C1 or C′4; Fig. 6–10) again results in significant loss of toxicity without loss of adjuvant activity.

Biologic Activities of Lipopolysaccharide Lipid A/Endotoxin. Endotoxin (LPS lipid A) is a potent pleiotropic (multiple effect) biomodifier that causes many of the pathophysiologic effects associated with gram-negative bacterial infection and bacteremia. Response to LPS depends on animal species, dose, site, or route and rapidity of release into the circulatory system. Small, nonlethal doses of LPS cause dramatic changes in body temperature, the hematologic, immune, and endocrinologic systems, and metabolism. Lethal doses of endotoxin may result in hypotension, disseminated intravascular coagulation (DIC), irreversible shock, and death.

FEVER INDUCTION. In most animals (e.g., rabbits, dogs, and monkeys) injected intravenously with nonlethal doses of LPS (0.1 to 100 μg), neutropenia develops rapidly, followed within 30 minutes by fever and hypotension. The fever curve develops within 20 to 30 minutes and shows a biphasic response that peaks at about 1 hour, followed by a small drop and then a higher fever peak at about 3 hours, after which temperature falls slowly over the next several hours. Dose response is proportional only if the area under the temperature curve is measured, and as dose is increased, a maximum temperature is reached. If injected intracerebrally, only a thousandth the

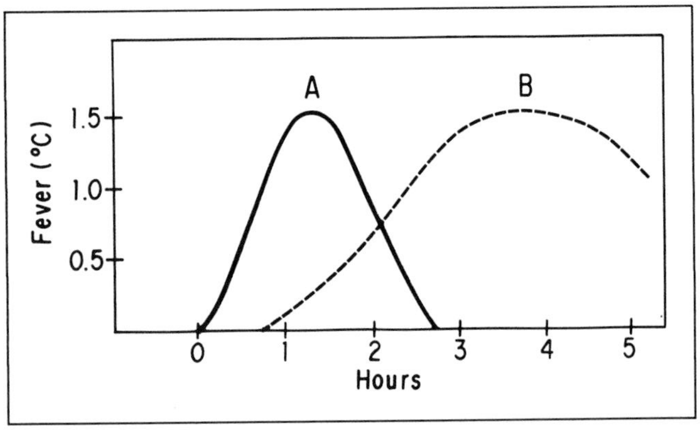

Fig. 6–13. Pyrogenic effect of endotoxin. Fever curve produced in humans after injection of small amount of endogenous pyrogen (A) or endotoxin (B) at 0 time. Note time lag for endotoxin curve resulting from LPS induction of leukocytes to synthesize endogenous pyrogens. *(Adapted from Petersdorf et al: J Exp Med 106:787, 1957.)*

dose is needed, indicating that the temperature control center in the brain is more directly affected. In rats and mice, however, hypothermia instead of fever may develop.

The human being is the animal most sensitive to endotoxin (about tenfold more sensitive than are rabbits): about 2 ng LPS/kg from *Salmonella abortus equi* (not purified to obtain the most active molecular species) induces granulocytosis (i.e., increase of circulating neutrophils, basophils, and eosinophils), a 7-hour fever of about 2C maximal temperature rise, and an increase in plasma cortisol level (Fig. 6–13). In humans, development of fever is slower than in animals, the fever curve is monophasic, and with development of endotoxin tolerance (see below) fever disappears completely. Neutropenia is not often observed because the human response curve to LPS is very steep, and the higher LPS concentrations withstood by animals in eliciting this response cannot be used in humans. A dose of 100 μg LPS is estimated to be lethal in humans.

ENDOTOXIN TOLERANCE. Tolerance to endotoxin is a classic phenomenon seen as a diminishing or absence of fever response to subsequent successive injections of LPS. In animals, the biphasic temperature response is replaced with a diminishing monophasic fever response, whereas in humans the monophasic response entirely disappears. Injection of endogenous pyrogens does not invoke tolerance; however, repeated successive injections of endogenous pyrogens (EP) yield immediate and equivalent responses, which allow differentiation between LPS and endogenous pyrogens. Early tolerance occurs within 12 hours, peaks at about 3 days, and persists for some 7 to 8 days, whereas late tolerance appears gradually over several weeks as a result of development of circulating antibody to LPS. The mechanism of early tolerance is unknown.

HEMATOLOGIC CHANGES. Changes observed in blood in response to LPS injection reflect changes in immune cells, the endocrine system, and metabolism. These may include, among others, the presence of cytokines, including IL-1, tumor necrosis factor (TNF), and IL-6, leukocytosis, a rise in plasma cortisol, hypoferremia, hypozincemia, hypertriglyceridemia, hypoglycemia, production of colony-stimulating growth factor (G-CSF), changes in liver enzymes and protein synthesis (e.g., appearance of serum amyloid A [SAA]), presence of fibrin polymers, and other changes. These changes are associated with the acute-phase response to inflammation produced by infection or tissue injury.

HYPOTENSION. Although a drop in blood pressure may be seen in animals given small doses of endotoxin to produce fever, larger doses are necessary to produce sustained hypotension and shock. In lethal endotoxicosis in the rabbit, marked hypotension occurs about 30 minutes after intravenous administration of LPS. Preceding this is a rise in pulmonary artery pressure that occurs because of acute resistance in the pulmonary veins. A fall in cardiac output follows, and reduced oxygen perfusion to tissues results. Cardiac failure, arterial pressure drop, and death follow (Fig. 6–14). Gram-negative bacteremia and shock are estimated to account for tens of thousands of human deaths every year, primarily in elderly persons.

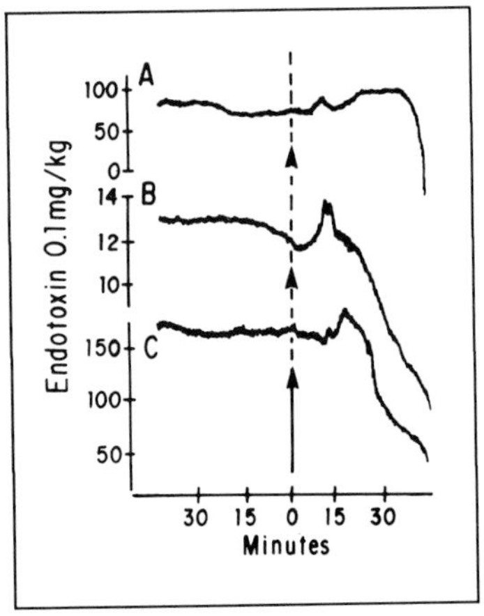

Fig. 6–14. Early phase of endotoxin shock in the rabbit. The fall in cardiac output occurs before blood pressure drops. Upper curve, arterial pressure, mm Hg; middle curve, oxygen uptake, ml/kg/min; lower curve, cardiac output, ml/kg/min. *(Adapted from Neuhof: In Urbaschek et al (eds): Gram-Negative Bacterial Infections. Springer-Verlag, 1975, p 259.)*

SHWARTZMAN REACTIONS. Massive release of endotoxin into the circulatory system may result in DIC. The local and general Shwartzman reactions are classic examples of the results of clotting in response to endotoxin. Both reactions require two injections of LPS about 18 to 24 hours apart, and these reactions are easily demonstrated in a rabbit model. The dermal or local Shwartzman reaction is induced by an initial intradermal injection with a small dose of LPS (e.g., 0.25 mg), followed about 24 hours later by a tenfold lower intravenous dose. Within 2 to 6 hours, an area of hemorrhagic necrosis occurs at the site of the original intradermal injection. The general Shwartzman reaction is developed by two intravenous injections of LPS about 24 hours apart at the same dose levels as in the local Shwartzman reaction: the response is bilateral cortical hemorrhagic necrosis of the kidney. Both Shwartzman reactions are caused by occlusion of small vessels by circulating fibrin polymers induced by intravenous injection of LPS, followed by inflammation, tissue damage, and necrosis. The mechanisms suggested are the following. In the local Shwartzman reaction, many of the fibrin polymers induced by the second intravenous injection of LPS are trapped in the small skin vessels injured at the inflammatory site of the first LPS injection, or they are cleared by the reticuloendothelial system (RES) and do not occlude the kidney. In the general Shwartzman reaction, the first intravenous injection of LPS initiates coagulation and production of circulating fibrin polymers, whereas the second injection blocks the RES with the result that fibrin is filtered out by the kidney.

POTENTIATION OF ENDOTOXIN. Increased sensitivity of animals to endotoxin (reduced lethal dose) by a hundredfold to several thousandfold can be achieved by several procedures, including pretreatment with actinomycin D, lead acetate, thorium dioxide, colloidal iron saccharate, trypan blue, a high molecular weight polygalactose (carrageenan), or galactosamine. Blockage of the RES may be in part responsible, but the complete mechanism is unclear.

LIMULUS ASSAY FOR LPS. A useful biologic activity of endotoxins is the induction of clotting of horseshoe crab (*Limulus* spp) amebocyte lysates at 10^{12} or greater dilution of endotoxin. This provides a highly sensitive assay for the presence of endotoxin in biologic fluids. The assay is not completely specific, but it is fast and sensitive and has been used to detect LPS in spinal fluid in cases of meningitis.

HOST MODIFICATION OF LPS. Little is known of LPS metabolism by mammalian systems. LPS is reversibly detoxified by forming a complex with proteins as it passes through the hepatic portal circulation. The protein, thought to be lipoprotein, forms a reversible complex with LPS. Formation of the complex appears to be regulated in part by protein(s) formed by macrophages in response to prior exposure to LPS. Human peripheral blood monocytes and neutrophils partially deacylate lipid A by a specific acyloxyacyl hydrolase that removes normal fatty acids esterified to β-hydroxymyristic acid at the C3-O position (e.g., R_2, R_4, and R_5 in Fig. 6–10), but does not hydrolyze β-hydroxymyristic acid esters (e.g., R_3 in Fig. 6–10). Deacylation results in a hundredfold decrease in toxic activity of the LPS molecule as measured by the dermal Shwartzman reaction and in ability to induce TNF, although some degree of adjuvant activity (nonspecific enhancement of immune response) and capability to modulate further "toxic" responses to LPS is retained.

PREVENTION OF ENDOTOXIC SHOCK. Although polymyxin B is somewhat toxic, it is a valued research tool because it forms a complex with LPS and prevents endotoxic activity. Of more clinical potential is the observation that monoclonal antibody to TNF can prevent lethal endotoxicosis in mice and baboons: recombinant TNF alone can reproduce most of the symptoms of endotoxicity. Also, patients with gram-negative bacteremia with high antibody titers to the R-mutant core-lipid A components of LPS have a higher recovery rate (lower rate of gram-negative bacteremic shock and death) than do patients who have little or no antibody levels. Some success in using R-mutant vaccines to produce protective antibody in persons at risk from gram-negative bacteremia and shock has been achieved, and either vaccination or the use of monoclonal human antibody promises to be of clinical value. This is especially important in elderly persons inasmuch as some tens of thousands of patients are estimated to die annually of gram-negative bacteremic shock.

MECHANISM OF LPS FEVER INDUCTION. LPS (or lipid A)—that is, endotoxin—has little direct bioactivity, but it is a molecular signal that induces macrophages to produce endogenous pyrogens, which in turn induce production of mediators, such as prostaglandins (e.g., PGE_2) that act directly on the temperature control centers in the brain. Endogenous pyrogens include IL-1, TNF-α (also called *cachechtin*), IL-6, macrophage inflammation factor-1-alpha (MIF-1-α) and MIF-1-β. The first three cytokines induce fever through induction of synthesis of prostaglandins (e.g., PGE_2), which act directly on the fever centers in the hypothalamus: prostaglandin synthesis (and fever) are blocked by aspirin or indomethacin. (Prostaglandins also can cause increased vascular permeability, decreased cardiac output, and contraction of smooth muscles.) More than one fever-producing pathway is involved, however, because indomethacin does not block fever production by MIF-1. Endogenous pyrogens are hormonelike mediator proteins of overlapping functions known collectively as *cytokines,* which are produced in the acute-phase inflammatory response to tissue injury and damage. For example, IL-6 is an endogenous pyrogen but is also a primary mediator of the hepatic acute phase response to infection and inflammation.

ENDOTOXIC ACTIVITY: SUMMARY. LPS can induce the production of a variety of cytokines, including interferon (IFN α and β), IL-1, IL-6, TNF, MIF-1 (α and β), and possibly others. Most endotoxic effects result from LPS-triggered cytokine mediated responses, although clotting and complement activation are independent of cytokines. Thus the multiplicity of LPS effects can largely be explained through the pleiotropy of responses of various cytokines, cells, and tissues. That is, LPS-induced cytokines are multifunctional, may overlap in functions, and may mediate different host responses and regulate multiple target cells so that in one instance they may act as a beneficial initiator or enhancer and in another case as a suppressor or even as a mediator of toxic effects. For example, LPS-induced IL-1 not only is an endogenous pyrogen but also induces IL-6, which is a mediator for late, acute-phase hepatic response (e.g., synthesis of serum amyloid A). IL-1 also may be a key mediator of inflammation and tissue damage in inflammatory bowel disease in rabbits with immune complex–induced colitis, as shown by use of a recombinant IL-1-specific receptor blocking protein that reduced inflammation and necrosis.

Thus some responses to LPS, such as potential lethality, are deleterious, whereas others, such as the adjuvant effect (nonspecific enhancement of immune response), induction of growth factor production (e.g., LPS induces IL-1, which induces IL-2), increase of nonspecific resistance to infections, increase in radiation protection, and tumor necrosis activities are beneficial (Table 6–3). Overall, many negative effects attributed to LPS appear to result from overstimulation of normally beneficient systems.

Biosynthesis of Intracellular Storage Polymers

Glycogen. Bacterial glycogen, an intracellular α-1,4-linked polyglucan with α-1,6 branch points, is synthesized from adenosine diphosphate glucose by a variety of organisms, including *E. coli, Enterobacter aerogenes, Micrococcus luteus, Rhodopseudomonas,* and *Mycobacterium.* Its rate of production varies inversely with the growth rate, and it accumulates most readily in media rich in carbohydrate and poor in nitrogen or sulfur,

$$ADP-Glucose + (Glycogen)_n \longrightarrow$$
$$(Glycogen)_{n+1} + ADP$$

Fig. 6–15. Glycogen synthesis in bacteria.

$$^-O-\overset{\overset{O}{\|}}{\underset{\underset{O_-}{|}}{P}}-O-\left(\overset{\overset{O}{\|}}{\underset{\underset{O_-}{|}}{P}}-O\right)_n +ATP \xrightarrow{Mg^{2\oplus}} ADP + {}^-O-\overset{\overset{O}{\|}}{\underset{\underset{O_-}{|}}{P}}-O-\left(\overset{\overset{O}{\|}}{\underset{\underset{O_-}{|}}{P}}-O\right)_{n+1}$$

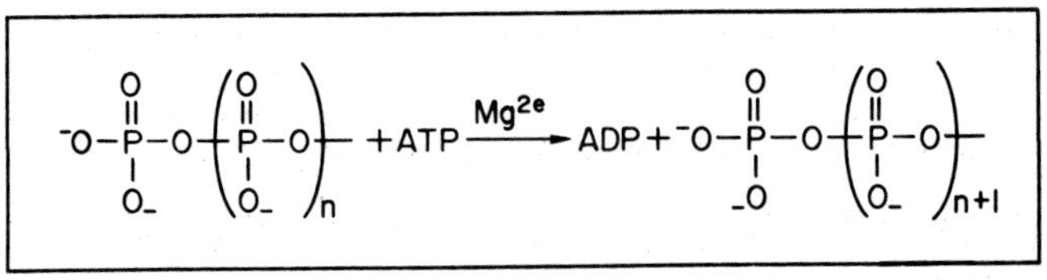

Fig. 6–17. Polyphosphate biosynthesis.

conditions that restrict growth but not metabolism. Glycogen synthesis occurs by transfer of glucose from adenosine diphosphate (ADP)–glucose to the terminal nonreducing end groups of the glycogen polymer (Fig. 6–15). As in the animal system, branching is achieved by the action of an amylo-α-1,4 to α-1,6-transglucosylase.

Poly-β-Hydroxybutyric Acid (PHB). Some *Bacillus* species are capable of producing this polymer in amounts ranging from 7% to more than 40% of the dry cell weight. The polymer is encased in a thin layer of protein that is assumed to contain the enzymes involved in its metabolism (Fig. 6–16). The polymer is depleted during active growth and again accumulates during the stationary phase or under restrictive conditions of growth.

Polyphosphate. Babès-Ernst, or volutin granules, are polymetaphosphates and have been identified in a wide variety of organisms, including *E. coli*, *E. aerogenes*, *C. diphtheriae*, *Mycobacterium*, and *Saccharomyces cerevisiae*. During active growth, only minute amounts of polyphosphates are detectable, whereas amounts equivalent to 1% to 2% of the dry cell weight accumulate under conditions of restrictive growth in media poor in nitrogen or sulfur. Synthesis of polyphosphate in *E. coli* proceeds as shown in Figure 6–17.

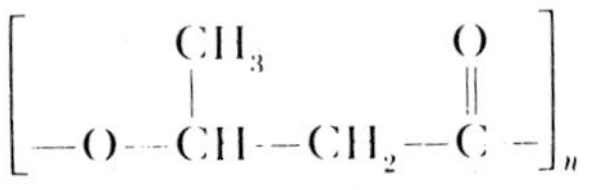

Biosynthesis of Cell Envelope Polymers

Bacterial envelope polymers are synthesized by membrane-bound enzymes from nucleotide-sugar precursors that are synthesized in the cytoplasm. A membrane-bound cofactor, generally known as *glycosylphosphate lipid carrier*, is involved in the biosynthesis of peptidoglycan and the O-specific polysaccharide chain of lipopolysaccharides. The carrier lipid is a phosphomonoester of the C_{55}-polyisoprenoid alcohol, undecaprenol (Fig. 6–18). This substance was first named *bactoprenol* before it was known that analogous lipid cofactors also are found in eucaryotic cells. The membrane-bound carrier forms glycosylpyrophospholipid oligosaccharide intermediates, which then are transferred to form polymers. Similar membrane lipid-linked oligosaccharide derivatives are involved in the biosynthesis of membrane-bound mannan in *M. luteus* (*lysodeikticus*) and capsular polysaccharides in *E. aerogenes*.

Teichoic Acid and Teichuronic Acid Biosynthesis

Polyolphosphodiester polymers, or teichoic acids, are formed by particulate enzyme systems from cytidine diphosphate (CDP)–glycerol or CDP-ribitol. The newly made teichoic acid chains are added to nascent peptidoglycan chains during the synthesis of both polymer units in the membrane. The teichoic acid then is transferred as a unit to the growing cell wall peptidoglycan.

Peptidoglycan Biosynthesis

There are five stages in the biosynthesis of bacterial peptidoglycan: (1) the biosynthesis of soluble precursors in the cytoplasm (Fig. 6–19), (2) transfer of precursors to membrane-bound carrier lipid (phosphoundecaprenol) and the formation of disaccharide pentapeptide units, (3) transfer of the disaccharide pentapeptide to the cell wall, thereby extending the peptidoglycan backbone polymer, (4) formation of cross-links between peptidoglycan polymers (Fig. 6–21), and (5) regeneration of monophosphocarrier lipid.

$$\left[-O-\overset{\overset{CH_3}{|}}{CH}-CH_2-\overset{\overset{O}{\|}}{C}-\right]_n$$

1. $2\ Acetyl{\sim}SCoA \rightleftharpoons$
 $Acetoacetyl{\sim}SCoA + HSCoA$

2. $Acetoacetyl{\sim}SCoA + NADH \rightleftharpoons$
 $\beta\text{-}OH\text{-}butyryl{\sim}SCoA + NAD^+$

3. $(PHB)_n + CoA\text{-}S\text{-}\overset{\overset{O}{\|}}{C}\text{-}CH_2\text{-}CHOH\text{-}CH_3 \rightleftharpoons$
 $(PHB)_{n+1} + HSCoA$

Fig. 6–16. Poly-β-hydroxybutyric acid biosynthesis.

$$^-O-\overset{\overset{O}{\|}}{\underset{\underset{O_-}{|}}{P}}-O-\left(CH_2-CH=\overset{\overset{CH_3}{|}}{C}-CH_2\right)_{11}-H$$

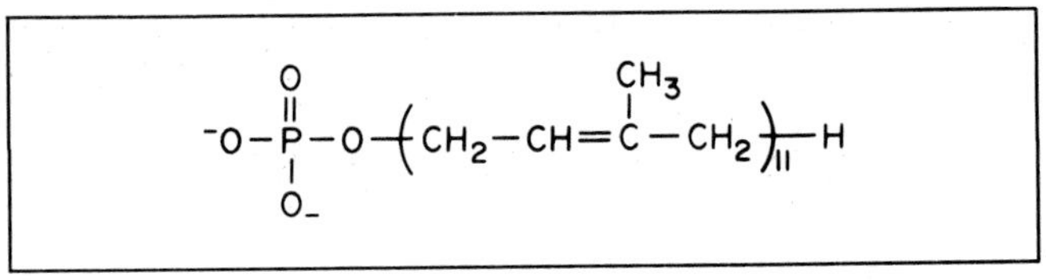

Fig. 6–18. Phosphoundecaprenol.

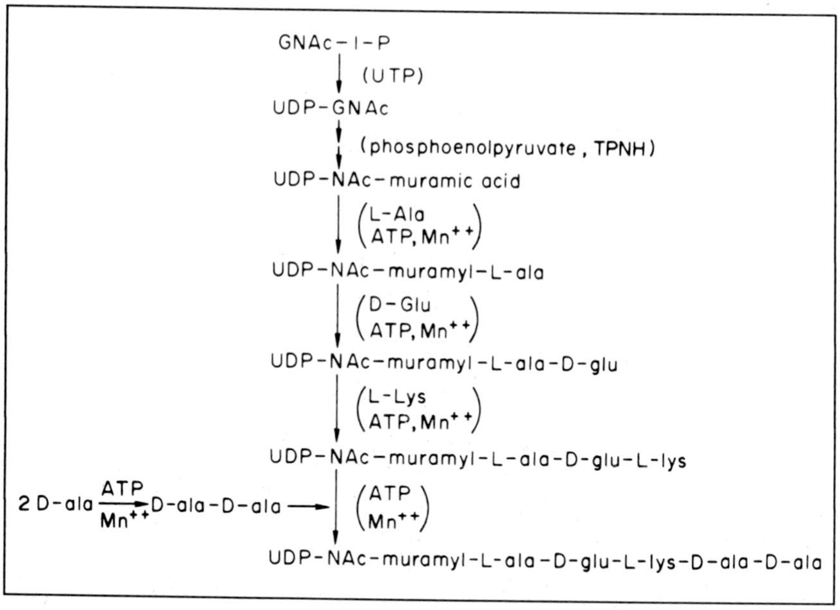

Fig. 6–19. Biosynthesis of the UDP-*N*-acetylglucosamine-*N*-acetylmuramic and pentapeptide precursor of cell wall peptidoglycan.

1. The first stage of peptidoglycan synthesis involves formation of uridinediphospho-*N*-acetylmuramic acid (UDP-MurNAc) from uridinediphospho-*N*-acetylglucosamine (UDP-GlcNAc) by soluble cytoplasmic enzymes. First, the enolpyruvic acid group is transferred from phosphoenolpyruvic acid to the acetylglucosamine carbon-3-hydroxyl group, which is followed by its enzymic reduction by means of nicotinamide adenine dinucleotide phosphate (NADPH) to a 3-0-lactic acid group. The amino acids of the pentapeptide then are added to the lactyl carboxyl group of UDP-MurNAc in stepwise fashion (Fig. 6–19) by separate soluble enzymes that require adenosine triphosphate (ATP) and a divalent cation, either Mg^{2+} or Mn^{2+}. The last two amino acids are added as the dipeptide, D-alanyl-D-alanine, by a reaction that also requires ATP and divalent cation. The D-alanine is produced from L-alanine by a racemase.
2. A series of steps then occurs in the particulate membrane fraction (Fig. 6–20). First, the phosphoacetylmuramyl-pentapeptide group is transferred to the membrane-bound carrier lipid, with formation of a pyrophosphate bridge and release of uridine monophosphate (UMP) (Fig. 6–20, step 1). Then β-1,4-linked disaccharide-pentapeptide-pyrophospho carrier lipid is formed by addition of acetylglucosamine from UDPGlcNAc to the C-4 hydroxyl of the muramic acid component (Fig. 6–20, step 2). Various modification steps may follow, depending on the species; for example, in *S. aureus* the α-carboxyl group of glutamic acid is amidated, and a pentaglycine bridge peptide is formed by addition of glycine to the ε-amino group of the muropeptide L-lysine residues. This latter reaction is mediated by a special 4-thiouridine-containing transfer RNA (tRNA), which differs from the glycyl-tRNA involved in protein biosynthesis (Fig. 6–20, steps 3 and 4).
3. The third stage, extension of the peptidoglycan backbone, occurs by transglycosylation (translocation) of the disaccharide-pentapeptide unit from the carrier lipid to the cell wall acceptor peptidoglycan backbone (Fig. 6–20, step 5), thereby releasing the pyrophospho carrier lipid, from which phosphatase regenerates the monophospho carrier lipid by removal of phosphate (Fig. 6–20, step 6).
4. The cell wall polymer formed at this stage is a non–cross-linked peptidoglycan with pentapeptide units terminating in D-Ala-D-Ala-COOH. Closure of the peptide bridge linkages by transpeptidation to form the cross-linked murein polymer finishes the biosyn-

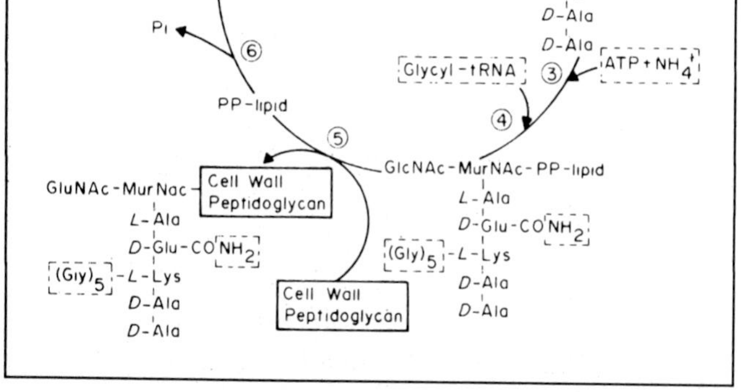

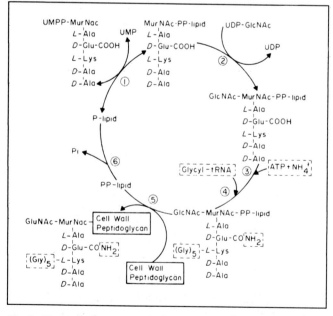

Fig. 6–20. Biosynthesis of peptidoglycan: membrane-involved carrier lipid reactions.

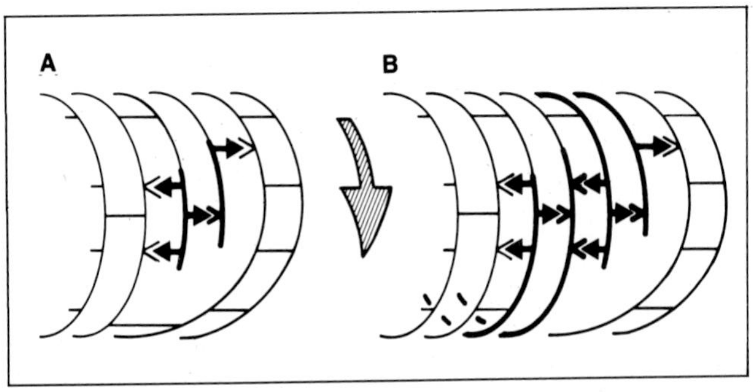

Fig. 6–21. Cell elongation in *E. coli*. **A.** Two strands of peptidoglycan (heavy lines) are inserted between preexisting strands (thin vertical lines). **B.** The new strands have circled the periphery of the cell and are establishing new cross-linked peptidoglycan. The arrows and V represent cross-links. *(From Burman and Park: Proc Natl Acad Sci USA 81:1844, 1984.)*

thetic sequence. In *S. aureus* this is accomplished by a reaction in which the penultimate D-alanine carboxyl group is linked to the free amino group of the pentaglycine bridge peptide of a neighboring peptidoglycan chain with concomitant release of the terminal D-alanine.

This sequence of reactions is essentially similar in all bacteria studied so far. Differences known include the species-specific substitution of alternative amino acids during pentapeptide synthesis (e.g., *meso*-DAP instead of L-lysine) and various peptide and bridge peptide modification reactions. In addition, some bacteria, including *E. coli, Bacillus subtilis, Lactobacillus casei,* and others, control the extent of interpeptidoglycan cross-linkage. Removal of whole peptides may occur by action of the autolysin MurNAc-L-Ala amidase, as in the case of *M. luteus,* in which 30% to 70% of the glycan chains are not cross-linked. In addition, one or both D-alanines may be removed from soluble UDP-MurNAc-pentapeptide precursors or non–cross-linked pentapeptidoglycan by carboxypeptidase. This explains the occurrence of tripeptides and tetrapeptides, as in *E. coli* (Fig. 6–2). Further, cell elongation occurs by a different mechanism (Fig. 6–21) than does cell septum formation leading to division. Little is known of the latter process.

Lipopolysaccharide Biosynthesis

Lipid A, LPS core, and side chain are synthesized in the membrane in several stages. Lipid A (region III) is synthesized (Fig. 6–22) and serves as an acceptor for the stepwise addition of core polysaccharide units (region II) (Fig. 6–23), followed by the addition of preassembled O-specific polysaccharide units (region I) (Fig. 6–24). The completed LPS then is rapidly and irreversibly translocated into the OM. Translocation occurs at adhesion sites between inner and outer membranes. Randomization of newly synthesized lipopolysaccharide in OM occurs within several minutes of growth.

Lipid A Biosynthesis (Region III). The pathway of lipid A biosynthesis, as far as is known on the basis of temperature-sensitive mutants, is shown in Figure 6–22. UDP-GlcNAc is first acylated with β-hydroxymyristic acid at the C-3 hydroxyl

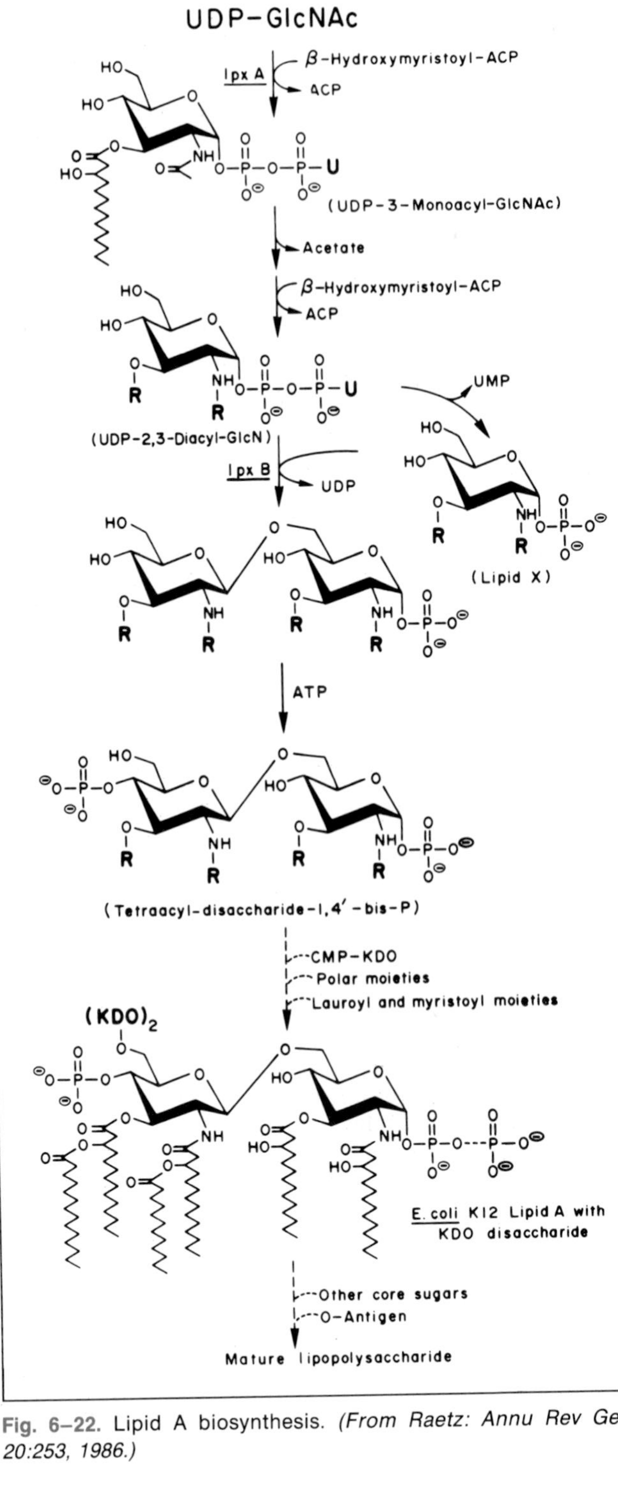

Fig. 6–22. Lipid A biosynthesis. *(From Raetz: Annu Rev Genet 20:253, 1986.)*

group, followed by *N*-deacetylation and *N*-acylation with another β-hydroxymyristic acid molecule to yield the UDP-2,3-diacylglucosamine intermediate. Another similar molecule is used to form the tetraacyldiglucosamine-α-1-phosphate, that is, the β(1-6)-linked disaccharide intermediate. This is then

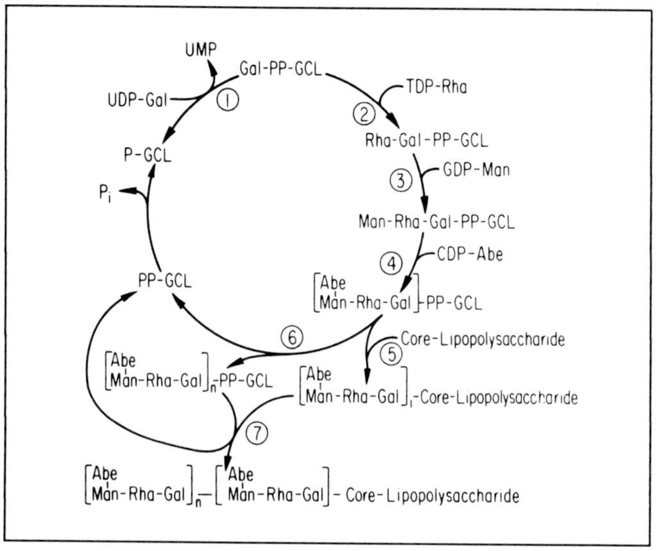

Fig. 6–23. Biosynthesis of lipopolysaccharide: cytoplasmic membrane-involved glycosyl carrier lipid reactions. P-GCL, membrane phospho carrier lipid; UDP-, uridine diphosphate; UMP-, uridine monophosphate; PP-GCL, diphospho carrier lipid; P$_i$, phosphate; Gal-, galactosyl; Rha-, rhamnosyl; Man-, mannosyl. Note that different transferases add the initial single and subsequent polymerized oligosaccharide repeating units to the growing lipopolysaccharide chain.

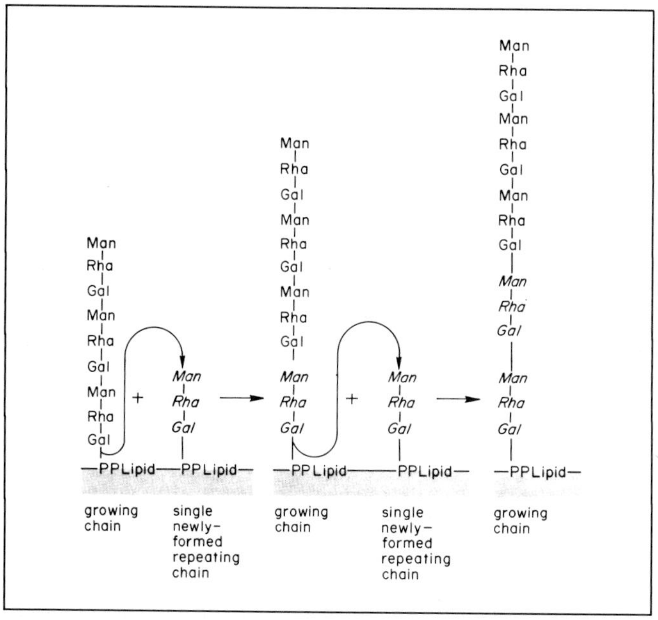

Fig. 6–24. Polymerization of preassembled repeating units during the biosynthesis of O antigen. Mechanism allows extension of growing polysaccharide side chain into external environment without requiring movement of biosynthesis machinery.

phosphorylated at the C′4 hydroxyl position to give the diphosphoryl compound. Addition of two molecules of KDO at the C′6 position, 4-amino-L-arabinose to the C′4 phosphate, further polar (e.g., phosphate) groups to the C1 α-phosphate, and further fatty acids follows to give the product known as the *Re glycolipid* (Fig. 6–14). The Re glycolipid is the first of the various lipid A products found in the OM in normal Re mutants. Apparently, cells cannot grow if they cannot at least make the Re glycolipid.

Core Polysaccharide Biosynthesis (Region II). The basic mechanism of core polysaccharide synthesis involves membrane-associated enzymes that catalyze the stepwise addition of monosaccharides from nucleotide sugar intermediates to the nonreducing terminus of the growing core polymer (Fig. 6–14). Inner core units (KDO, heptose, phosphate, and ethanolamine) are added stepwise, followed by the outer core hexose units (glucose, galactose, and *N*-acetyl-D-glucosamine). The sequence of addition is ordered by specific enzyme recognition of both acceptor and activated nucleotide-sugar donor.

Much of the knowledge of core polymer structure and biosynthesis has been made possible by the availability of a series of *Salmonella* R or rough form mutants (Fig. 6–14). Such mutants are defective in their ability to synthesize nucleotide sugar precursors, such as UDP-galactose, or they lack one or more of the necessary nucleotide sugar transferases or O polymer transferases. By use of cell envelope preparations from appropriate mutant organisms, the stepwise addition of each core component in sequence was demonstrated.

O Antigen Biosynthesis (Region I). The synthesis of the O antigen polysaccharide hapten is basically similar to that of peptidoglycan, in that soluble nucleotide sugars are utilized by membrane enzymes to synthesize carrier lipid–O antigen repeating oligosaccharide unit intermediates, which are then polymerized. The biosynthetic sequence in particulate cell envelope membrane preparations occurs in four stages: (1) preassembly of O antigen repeating units as oligosaccharide-pyrophosphate carrier lipid intermediates, (2) polymerization of the preassembled repeating units, (3) transfer of the O-chain polymer to LPS core polysaccharide, and (4) regeneration of monophospho carrier lipid (Fig. 6–23).

1. In *Salmonella typhimurium* the first step in synthesis of the oligosaccharide repeating unit involves the transfer of galactose-1-phosphate from UDP-galactose (UDPGal) to membrane-bound phospho carrier lipid to form galactosyl-pyrophospho carrier lipid with release of UMP. Transfer of L-rhamnose from thymidine diphosphorhamnose (TDPRha), mannose from guanosine-diphosphomannose (GDP-Man), and abequose from cytidine diphosphoabequose (CDPAbe) follow to complete the tetrasaccharide repeating unit intermediate (Fig. 6–23).
2. This step involves the transfer of the proximal ends of growing chains from membrane-attached PP-lipid to single, newly formed oligosaccharide repeating units, which are themselves linked to membrane-bound PP-lipid (Fig. 6–24). This is exactly the opposite of the mechanisms of intracellular biosynthesis of cytoplasmic polymers, such as glycogen, in which each new repeating unit is added to the distal ends of growing polymer chains.

3. Transfer of O antigen oligosaccharide repeating units to the core polysaccharide involves two steps. First, a single repeating unit is transferred, and then a different enzyme transfers the polymerized O antigen polysaccharide (Fig. 6–24).
4. Monophosphopolyisoprenol, the P-lipid carrier, is regenerated from the corresponding pyrophosphate by phosphatase action, as described above for peptidoglycan synthesis (Fig. 6–23).

FURTHER READING

Books and Reviews

Adams DO, Johnson SP, Uhing RJ: Early gene expression in the activation of mononuclear phagocytes. Curr Top Membrane Transport 35:587, 1990

Alving CR, Morrison DC (eds): Molecular concepts of lipid A. Rev Infect Dis 6:427, 1984

Arai KI, Lee F, Miyajima A, et al: Cytokines: Coordinators of immune and inflammatory responses. Annu Rev Biochem 59:783, 1990

Beutler B, Cerami A: Tumor necrosis, cachexia, shock, and inflammation: A common mediator. Annu Rev Biochem 57:508, 1988

Barksdale L, Kim K-S: Mycobacterium. Bacteriol Rev 41:217, 1977

Brook I: Encapsulated anaerobic bacteria in synergistic infections. Microbiol Rev 50:452, 1986

Chedid L (ed): Muramyl peptides as modulators of sleep, temperature, and immune responses. Fed Proc 45:2531, 1986

Davatelis G, Wolpe SD, Sherry B, et al: Macrophage inflammatory protein-1: A prostaglandin-independent endogenous pyrogen. Science 243:1006, 1990

Dinarello CA: Interleukin-1 and its biologically related cytokines. Adv Immunol 44:153, 1989

DiRienzo JM, Nakamura K, Inouye M: The outer membrane proteins of gram-negative bacteria: Biosynthesis, assembly, and functions. Annu Rev Biochem 47:481, 1978

Ghuysen JM: Use of bacteriolytic enzymes in determination of wall structure and their role in cell metabolism. Bacteriol Rev 32:425, 1968

Goren MB: Mycobacterial lipids. Bacteriol Rev 34:33, 1972

Greenblatt CL: Molecular mimicry and the carbohydrate language of parasitism. ASM News 49:488, 1983

Hancock REW: Role of porins in outer membrane permeability. J Bacteriol 169:929, 1987

Inouye M (ed): Bacterial Outer Membranes: Biogenesis and Functions. New York, Wiley, 1979

Karnovsky ML: Muramyl peptides in mammalian tissues and their effects at the cellular level. Fed Proc 45:2556, 1986

Munford RS, Erwin AL, Riedo FX, et al: Lipopolysaccharide signal modification by acyloxyacyl hydrolase, a leukocyte enzyme. In Ayoub EM, Cassell GH, Branche WC, et al: Microbial Determinants of Virulence in Host Response. Washington, DC, American Society for Microbiology, 1990, p 271

Nikaido H: Outer membrane barrier as a mechanism of antimicrobial resistance. Antimicrob Agents Chemother 33:1831, 1989

Nikaido H, Vaara M: Molecular basis of bacterial outer membrane permeability. Microbiol Rev 49:1, 1985

Quereshi N, Takayama K: Structure and function of lipid A. In Gunsalus IC, Sokatch JR, Ornston LN (eds): The Bacteria, vol 11: Iglewski B, Clark VL (eds): Molecular Basis of Bacterial Pathogenesis. New York, Academic Press, 1990, p 319

Raetz CRH: Biochemistry of endotoxins. Annu Rev Biochem 59:129, 1990

Rothfield LI, MacAlister TJ, Cook WR: Murein-membrane interactions in cell division. In Inouye M (ed): Bacterial Outer Membranes as Model Systems. New York, John Wiley & Sons, 1986

Smith KA: Interleukin-2. Sci Am 262:50, 1990

Tipper DJ, Wright A: The structure and biosynthesis of bacterial cell walls. In Sokatch J (ed): The Bacteria, vol 7. New York, Academic Press, 1979

Tracey KJ, Cerami A: Review: Cachectin/TNF in the cachexia of infection. In Parasites: Molecular Biology, Drug and Vaccine Design. New York, Wiley-Liss, 1990, p 401

Ulrich JT, Cantrell JL, Gustafson GL, et al: The adjuvant activity of monophosphoryl lipid A. In Spriggs DR, Koff WC (eds): Topics in Vaccine Adjuvant Research. Boca Raton, Fla, CRC Press, 1991

Vogel SN, Hogan MM: Role of cytokines in endotoxin mediated host responses. In Oppenheim JJ, Shevach E (eds): Immunophysiology: Role of Cells and Cytokines in Immunity and Inflammation. New York, University of Oxford Press, 1990, p 238

Ward JB: Teichoic and teichuronic acids: Biosynthesis, assembly, and location. Microbiol Rev 45:211, 1981

Westphal O, Westphal U, Sommer T: The history of pyrogen research. In Schlessinger D (ed): Microbiology—1977. Washington, DC, American Society for Microbiology, 1978, p 221

Wicken AJ, Knox KW: Bacterial cell surface amphiphiles. Biochim Biophys Acta 604:1, 1980

Wolff SM: Biological effects of bacterial endotoxins in man. In Kass E, Wolff SM (eds): Bacterial Lipopolysaccharides, J Inf Dis 128(suppl 1):251, 1973

Selected Papers

Beutler B, Cerami A: Cachechtin: More than a tumor necrosis factor. N Engl J Med 316:379, 1987

Beutler B, Krochin N, Milsark IW, et al: Control of cachectin (tumor necrosis factor) synthesis: Mechanisms of endotoxin resistance. Science 232:977, 1986

Bjornson BH, et al: Endotoxin-associated protein: A potent stimulus for human granulocytopenic activity which may be accessory cell dependent. Infect Immun 56:1602, 1988

Burman LG, Park JT: Molecular model for elongation of the murein sacculus of *Escherichia coli.* Proc Natl Acad Sci USA 81:1844, 1984

Chetty C, Klapper DG, Schwab JH: Soluble peptidoglycan-polysaccharide fragments of the bacterial cell wall induce acute inflammation. Infect Immun 38:1010, 1982

Cominelli F, Nast CC, Clark BD, et al: Interleukin 1 (IL-1) gene expression, synthesis, and effect of specific IL-1 receptor blockade in rabbit immune complex colitis. J Clin Invest 86:972, 1990

Crowell DN, Anderson MS, Raetz CRH: Molecular cloning of the genes for lipid A disaccharide synthase and UDP-*N*-acetylglucosamine acyltransferase in *Escherichia coli.* J Bacteriol 168:152, 1986

DeMaria A, Johns MA, Berbich H, et al: Immunization with rough mutants of *Salmonella minnesota:* Initial studies in human subjects. J Infect Dis 158:301, 1988

Dinarello CA, Cannon JG, Wolff SM, et al: Tumor necrosis factor (cachechtin) is an endogenous pyrogen and induces production of interleukin 1. J Exp Med 163:1433, 1986

Gassner GT, Dickie JP, Hamerski DA, et al: Teichuronic acid reducing terminal *N*-acetylglucosamine residue is linked by phosphodiester to peptidoglycan of *Micrococcus luteus.* J Bacteriol 172:2273, 1990

Johns MA, Sipe JD, Melton LB, et al: Endotoxin-associated protein: Interleukin-1–like activity on serum amyloid A synthesis and T-lymphocyte activation. Infect Immun 56:1593, 1988

Johnson GL, Hogen JH, Ratnayake JH, et al: Characterization of the intermediates in the biosynthesis of teichuronic acid of *Micrococcus luteus.* Arch Biochem Biophys 235:679, 1984

Kato N, et al: Crystallization of R-form lipopolysaccharides from *Salmonella minnesota* and *Escherichia coli*. J Bacteriol 172:1516, 1990

Knutton S, Baldini MM, Kaper JB, et al: Role of plasmid-encoded adherence factors in adhesion of enteropathogenic *Escherichia coli* to HEp-2 cells. Infect Immun 55:78, 1987

Krueger JM, Pappenheimer JR, Karnovsky ML: The composition of sleep-promoting factor isolated from human urine. J Biol Chem 257:1664, 1982

Krueger JM, Pappenheimer JR, Karnovsky ML: Sleep-promoting effects of muramyl peptides. Proc Natl Acad Sci USA 79:6102, 1982

Qureshi N, Takayama K, Ribi E: Purification and structural determination of nontoxic lipid A obtained from the lipopolysaccharide of *Salmonella typhimurium*. J Biol Chem 257:11808, 1982

Ribi E: Beneficial modification of the endotoxin molecule. J Biol Response Mod 3:1, 1984

Scherrer R, Gerhardt P: Molecular sieving by the *megaterium* cell wall and protoplast. J Bacteriol 107:718, 1971

Silva CL, Faccicioli LH: Tumor necrosis factor (cachectin) mediates induction of cachexia by cord factor from mycobacteria. Infect Immun 56:3067, 1988

Simpson SA, Lerch RA, Cleland DR, et al: Effect of acetylation on arthropathic activity of group A streptococcal peptidoglycan-polysaccharide fragments. Infect Immun 55:16, 1987

Takada H, Galanos C: Enhancement of endotoxin lethality and generation of anaphylactoid reactions by lipopolysaccharides in muramyl-dipeptide–treated mice. Infect Immun 55:409, 1987

Takahashi I, Kotani S, Takada H, et al: Requirement of a properly acylated β(1-6)-D-glucosamine disaccharide triphosphate structure for efficient manifestation of full endotoxic and associated activities of lipid A. Infect Immun 65:57, 1987

Takayama K, Qureshi N, Mascagni P, et al: Fatty acyl derivatives of glucosamine-1-phosphate in *Escherichia coli* and their relation to lipid A. J Biol Chem 258:7379, 1983

Warren HS, Riveau GR, Deckker FA, et al: Control of endotoxin activity and interleukin-1 production through regulation of lipopolysaccharide-lipoprotein binding by a macrophage factor. Infect Immun 56:204, 1988

Weinberg JB, Ribi E, Wheat RW: Enhancement of macrophage-mediated tumor cell killing by bacterial outer membrane proteins (porins). Infect Immun 42:219, 1983

Yin ET, Galanos C, Kinsky S, et al: Picogram-sensitive assay of endotoxin: Gelation of *Limulus polyphemus* blood cell lysate induced by purified lipopolysaccharides and lipid A from negative bacteria. Biochim Biophys Acta 261:284, 1972

Zinner SH, McCabe WR: Effects of IgM and IgG antibodies in patients with bacteremia due to gram-negative bacilli. J Infect Dis 133:37, 1976

CHAPTER 7

Molecular Basis of Genetics and Metabolic Regulation

The preceding chapters have summarized many of the important properties of the bacterial life cycle, including metabolic pathways, structural features, and growth characteristics. From these discussions, it should be clear that bacterial species are highly evolved; many are capable of rapid growth and efficient adaptation to a variety of environmental conditions. The complex developmental processes of sporulation and germination allow survival of certain bacterial species in some of the most extreme environmental conditions that any organism is likely to encounter.

To understand the remarkable adaptability of bacterial cells, the molecular mechanisms of DNA replication, transcription, and translation must be considered. The bacterial chromosome contains essentially all the information necessary for the regulated expression of metabolic pathways, the duplication of all cellular components during growth, and the structural differentiation that occurs during such processes as sporulation. The many complexities that will be encountered in this and the subsequent chapter should be viewed in perspective; they are required to achieve an economical regulation of metabolic activities and a rapid but very accurate duplication of cellular components during growth. This chapter summarizes our current state of knowledge concerning the mechanisms by which this duplication and transfer of information occur.

Structure of Bacterial Genome

The essential genetic information of a bacterial cell is contained in a single circular duplex DNA molecule with a typical size of a few million base pairs. Ancillary genetic elements called plasmids, which often carry determinants such as antibiotic resistance, are also circular duplex DNA but are much smaller than the chromosome. Important structural features of DNA will be described before such processes as replication and gene expression are considered.

Primary Structure of DNA

DNA is a polymer composed of 2′-deoxyribonucleosides linked by phosphodiester bonds between the 3′- and 5′- positions of adjacent sugar residues. The asymmetry of the phosphodiester bond gives each DNA strand a polarity (either 3′ → 5′ or 5′ → 3′), and duplex DNA is composed of two strands that are *antiparallel* with respect to this polarity. The complementary interactions between bases on the opposite strands of a duplex are absolutely required for both the duplication and the transfer of information. Each base pair is composed of one purine and one pyrimidine; guanine and cytosine pair with three hydrogen bonds, whereas adenine and thymine pair with two bonds (Fig. 7–1). These pairs are almost exactly the same size and shape, giving duplex DNA a constant diameter. The hydrogen bonding between base pairs determines the precise sequence of the complementary bases on

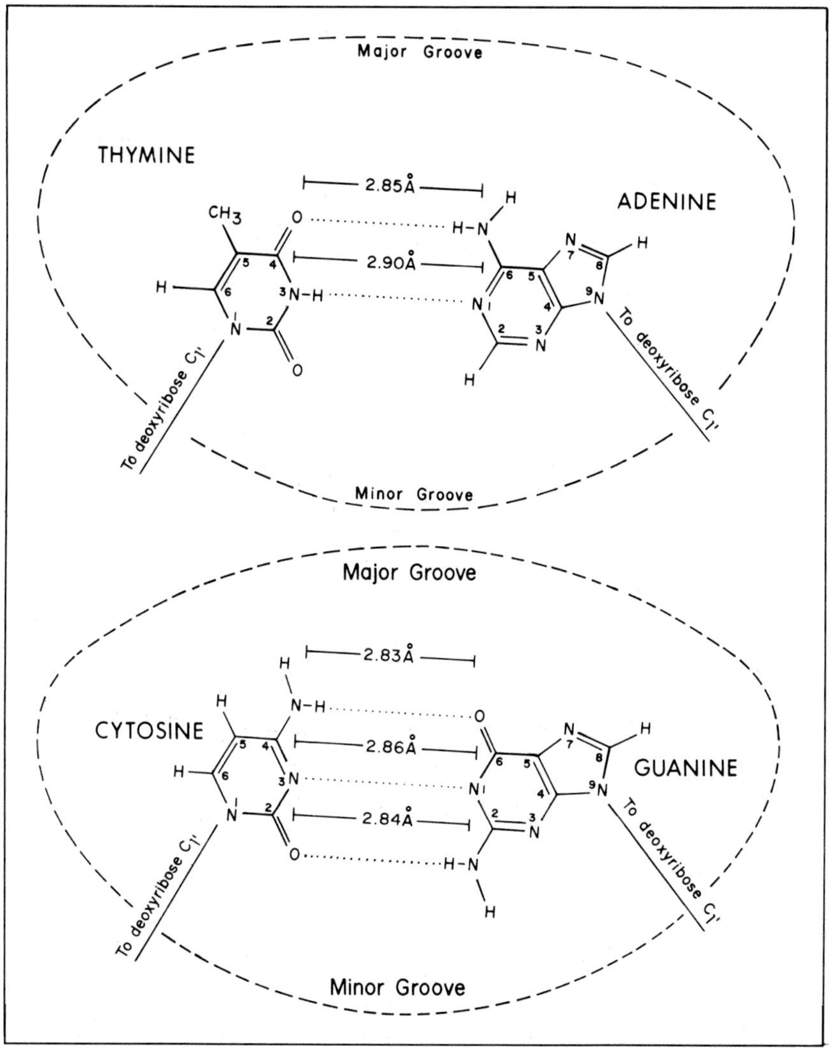

Fig. 7–1. Purine-pyrimidine base pairs. The two arcs represent the minor and major groove orientation of the bases in B DNA.

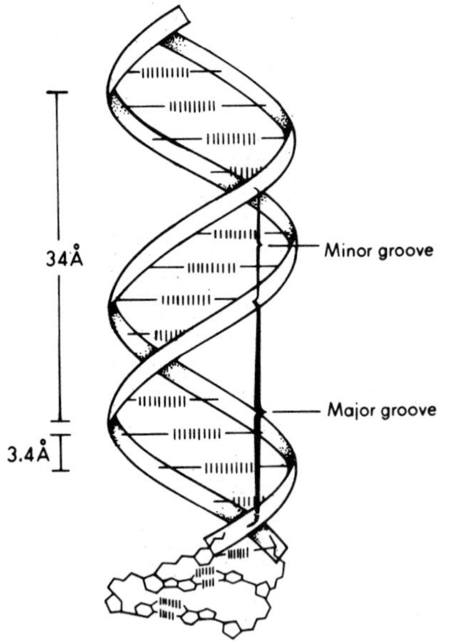

Fig. 7–2. A model of B form DNA. *(From Kornberg: DNA Replication. W. H. Freeman, 1980.)*

the two strands of the double helix. However, the stability of the double helix is primarily the result of hydrophobic interactions between adjacent base residues stacked one on top of the other. These stacking interactions are maximal between sets of properly paired residues, and they counteract the repulsive electrostatic force between the negatively charged phosphate groups. Within a cell, the phosphate anions are also neutralized by divalent cations and the multivalent polyamines and by a variety of proteins (see below).

In spite of the structural constraints implicit in base pairing and stacking, duplex DNA can adopt a variety of structures. The classic B structure of DNA was proposed by Watson and Crick on the basis of fiber diffraction data of Franklin and Wilkins, and it has since been shown to be the predominant form of DNA both within and outside the cell. In B form DNA, the sugar-phosphate backbones form right-handed helices wound around each other, with an average repeating period of about 10.6 base pairs (Fig. 7–2). There is much microheterogeneity within B form DNA, and these variations may be important in the specific binding of proteins and drugs to DNA. Depending on the exact nucleotide sequence, B form DNA contains significant variations in the helical parameters and in the conformation of nucleotide residues. In addition, certain sequences cause a sharp bend in the three-dimensional path of the double helix. The binding of proteins can also induce bending and/or looping of DNA, with important consequences for the regulation of gene expression (see below).

There are several minor forms of duplex DNA that may have physiologic significance. Perhaps the most radical of these is the recently discovered Z structure. Z-DNA is characterized by a left-handed helix and alternating sugar-base conformations; this results in a zigzag course of the sugar-phosphate backbone (hence the designation Z). Particular proteins that recognize Z-DNA have been found, and certain alternating purine-pyrimidine sequences can form a Z structure under physiologic conditions. Furthermore, the existence of Z-DNA within bacterial cells has been demonstrated, although the physiologic functions of Z-DNA remain to be determined. The so-called A structure of polynucleotides is important because it appears to be the predominant form of RNA duplexes and RNA-DNA hybrids; aggregated or dehydrated duplex DNA can also adopt the A structure.

Higher-order Structure

A major problem faced by all cells is how to maintain the enormous amount of information contained in their genomes. The chromosome of the relatively simple bacterium *Escherichia coli* contains about 4.5 million base pairs. This constitutes a DNA molecule about 1 mm long, whereas the bacterial cell is only 1 or 2 μm in length. Much of the compaction necessary to fit the bacterial chromosome into the cell is achieved by formation of a higher-order structure that involves the coiling of the axis of the double helix upon itself. After the nature of this *supercoiled* (or *superhelical*) DNA is described, the mechanisms used by bacteria to maintain this structure are explored.

As mentioned above, normal B form DNA has about one helical twist (as the two strands wind around each other) for every 10.6 base pairs. This is the structure adopted by DNA with ends that are free to rotate, and therefore this represents an energetically unstrained configuration. However, closed circular DNA isolated from cells is found to be underwound by about one turn every 200 base pairs, compared to unstrained DNA. The underwinding of circular duplex DNA can take two forms. The first is a toroidal coil, which is illustrated by the winding of a telephone cord. The second form of coiling is the interwound form, which is illustrated in the supercoiled DNA depicted in Figure 7–3B. These two forms are topologically equivalent, and both serve to compact any molecule (or telephone cord) in which they are found.

The tertiary structure of DNA can be analyzed in precise topologic terms. Closed circular duplex DNA has no free ends in either of the two strands. Therefore, the number of times that the two strands wind around each other cannot change unless one of the strands becomes broken (at least transiently). This is the linking number of the molecule, and can most easily be visualized by counting the number of times one strand winds around the other when the latter is forced to lie in a plane. For example, if an unstrained circular DNA (B form) of 370 base pairs is considered (most natural DNA molecules are much larger), the linking number would be 370 divided by the helical repeat of 10.6, or 35 (Fig. 7–3A). A real population of unstrained DNA would form a Gaussian distribution of linking numbers around this value. When this same DNA is isolated from a cell it is in a strained configuration, being underwound by about one turn every 200 base pairs. Because the linking number is decreased (the molecule is *under*wound), this molecule is negatively supercoiled, with an average linking number of about 33 (Fig. 7–3B). In a topologic sense, the underwinding implicit in negative superhelicity is equivalent to an unwinding of a segment of double helix into the single-stranded form. In the 370–base pair DNA, the unwinding (or *denaturation*) of a segment of about 21 base pairs would remove two helical twists of the strands around each other, and this would thereby relieve the two negative superhelical turns (Fig. 7–3C). The linking number

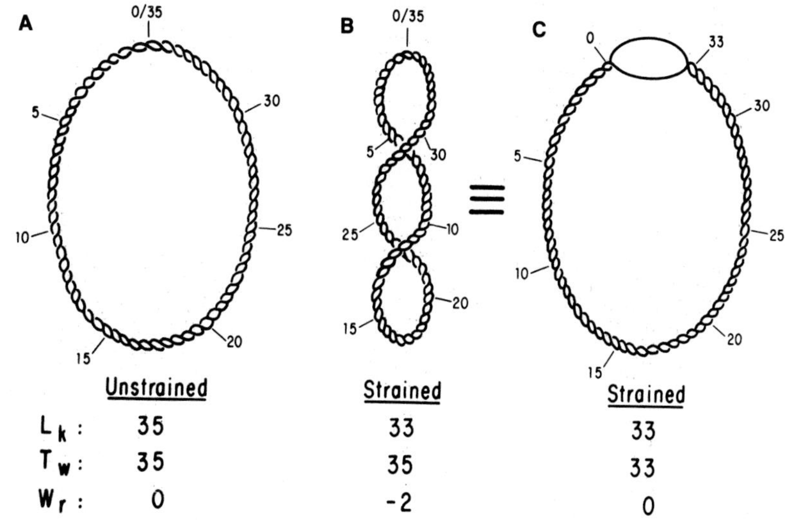

Fig. 7–3. Circular DNA. A small, covalently closed, circular DNA composed of 370 base pairs is depicted in **A.** Each turn (twist or T_w) of the helix (approximately 10.6 base pairs per turn) results in a single linkage (L_k) of the interwound strands, and therefore both T_w and L_k have a value of 35 in **A.** The molecule depicted in **B** is identical except that it is underwound by two turns; this is the superhelical form generally isolated from cells. In this molecule, the number of turns of the double helix is identical to that in **A;** therefore, $T_w = 35$. The deficiency of two turns in this underwound molecule ($L_k = 33$) is reflected in a value of -2 in the writhing number (W_r). The writhing number describes the twisting of the helix upon itself, and for any covalently closed circle, $L_k = T_w + W_r$. The molecule depicted in **C** has the same linking number as that in **B,** but the underwinding is now accommodated by a denaturation of two turns of the double helix. Therefore the twist of the helix is identical to the linking number ($T_w = L_k = 33$), and there is no writhing of the helix upon itself ($W_r = 0$). Because the linking number of a duplex DNA molecule is a discrete topologic property describing the total number of times one strand winds around the other, L_k cannot change unless one or both of the strands are transiently broken. Transient strand breakage is therefore required to interconvert the molecules in **A** and **B** but not to interconvert those in **B** and **C.** *(Adapted from Kornberg: DNA Replication. W. H. Freeman, 1980.)*

in this molecule would still be 33 (because neither strand has been broken), but all of those linkages would now result directly from the helical twisting of one strand around the other in the remaining duplex part of the molecule.

In addition to its propensity to make DNA compact, negative superhelicity has several other important ramifications, all of which derive from the fact that superhelicity is a form of stored energy that is used in a variety of processes. First, negative superhelicity facilitates the energetically unfavorable unwinding of the two strands during such processes as DNA replication and transcription. Second, the binding of many proteins is directly facilitated, either because they unwind a short stretch of DNA or because they bind a coiled segment of duplex. A third important consequence is that of enhanced binding of intercalating drugs, which are planar aromatic compounds that slide in between adjacent base pairs. Because the phosphodiester bond has a given length and the phosphodiester backbones rotate around each other in the double helix, drug intercalation unwinds the helix and increases the length of duplex DNA.

The considerations discussed above pose a potentially serious problem. Because the circular DNA of *E. coli* has about 4.5 million base pairs, it should be underwound by more than 20,000 turns (once every 200 base pairs). This level of superhelicity represents a tremendous energy potential that, in principle, could be lost every time either of the phosphodiester backbones is broken (because the strands are then free to rotate). DNA can be broken by a variety of processes inside the cell, most notably by repair and recombination reactions (Chap. 8). So how is this potentially devastating loss of energy prevented? Various experiments show that the bacterial chromosome is organized into a series of loops, each of which is a topologically independent domain. Breaking a single domain of the *E. coli* chromosome releases only about 2% of the total superhelicity, implying that the chromosome has about 50 such domains. The nature of the mechanism that holds these loops in place is not yet clear. All that is required is that the two segments of DNA that constitute the base of the loop be held so that they cannot rotate with respect to each other. The organization of the chromosome into topologic domains also aids in the overall compaction of the chromosome, because the bases of the loops are close to each other.

DNA-binding Proteins

The binding of particular proteins to DNA can have profound effects on DNA structure. As discussed above, the coiling of DNA in the toroidal form is one way to organize supercoils (similar to a telephone cord). Toroidal coiling can occur when DNA is bound on the surface of proteins, in which case the DNA is said to be wrapped around the protein. From an energetic point of view, the free energy of superhelicity within the DNA facilitates the binding of the protein; once bound, that energy is restrained in the protein-DNA complex. In eucaryotic cells, DNA is wrapped around histone proteins in the nucleosomes, and this wrapping accounts for most or all of the negative superhelicity of eucaryotic DNA (see Chap. 53). In contrast, only a small amount of the negative superhelicity in procaryotic DNA appears to be dependent on wrapping around proteins. Bacteria have proteins that apparently correspond to the histones of eucaryotic cells, and nucleosome-like particles can be visualized on bacterial DNA, but they are not as important to DNA structure in procaryotes as in eucaryotes.

Single-stranded DNA is an important intermediate in such processes as replication, repair, and recombination, and all cells have proteins that bind this intermediate. The single-strand binding proteins stabilize the denatured form of DNA and also participate in many genetic processes directly. This kind of protein binding also has a direct effect on the tertiary structure of DNA, because the denaturation of a segment of DNA relieves negative superhelical turns (see above).

Enzymatic Alterations in DNA Structure

It should be clear at this point that the precise structure of DNA inside a cell is quite dynamic. Negative superhelicity can be converted into denatured segments of DNA, and proteins that bind either single-stranded or double-stranded segments of the DNA can strongly influence this denaturation. Furthermore, the negative superhelicity can take a variety of forms within the duplex segments, such as wrapping on a protein surface and both toroidal and interwound supercoils in space. We now turn our attention to a set of proteins that directly regulate these processes of supercoiling and denaturation by virtue of their enzymatic activities.

The most important class of enzymes that alter DNA structure are the DNA topoisomerases. These are enzymes that enzymatically alter the linking number of DNA, either introducing or removing superhelical turns. As might be expected, the topoisomerases are carefully controlled to provide the bacterial cell with an optimal level of supercoiling.

DNA Gyrase. The bacterial enzyme DNA gyrase introduces negative superhelical turns into duplex DNA, using the energy of adenosine triphosphate (ATP) hydrolysis to drive the reaction. This is the crucial enzyme that maintains the negative superhelical tension of the bacterial chromosome. Bacterial cells also contain one or more enzymes that remove negative superhelical turns, and it is actually the balance of these competing activities that determines the overall linking number of a functional bacterial chromosome (see below). DNA gyrase is implicated in several important processes and is also the physiologic target for a series of antibiotics.

Because the linking number of DNA is invariant as long as both strands are intact (see above), topoisomerases must break either one or both of the phosphodiester backbones to change the linking number. Enzymes of both types exist. Type I topoisomerases break one strand of the helix (see below), whereas type II enzymes such as DNA gyrase break both strands. A current model of the reaction mechanism of DNA gyrase is shown in Figure 7–4. A transient double-strand break is introduced into one segment of the DNA, with the enzyme becoming covalently attached to both newly formed ends of the broken DNA. The crucial change in linking number then occurs by means of the passage of another segment of duplex DNA through the transient break. After DNA passage, the broken phosphodiester bonds are reformed as the covalent DNA-protein bonds are broken. The DNA break and the covalent DNA-protein bonds are important

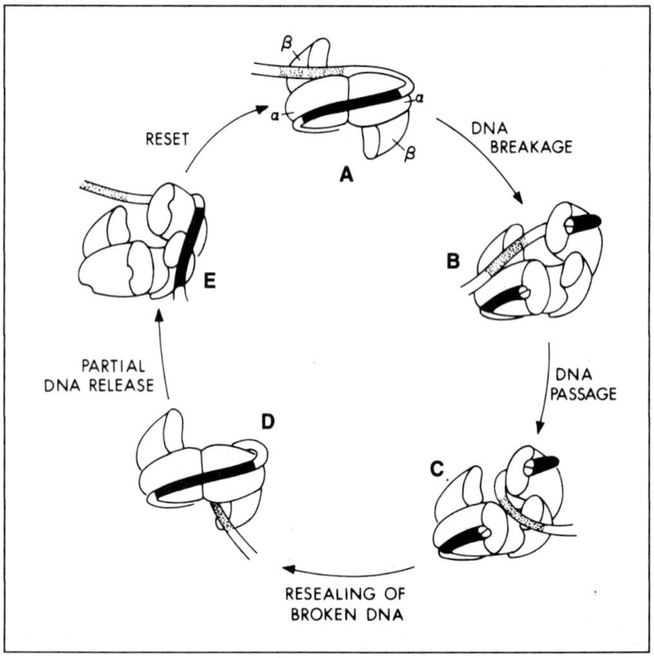

Fig. 7–4. Model for the action of DNA gyrase. In **A** the $\alpha_2\beta_2$ gyrase molecule is shown with a section of DNA wrapped around the enzyme. The solid DNA represents the region within which a double-stranded scission occurs. The transiently formed gap is a passageway for the stippled section of DNA. Steps **B** through **D** depict this DNA passage and result in the conversion of a right-handed loop of DNA into a left-handed loop. The conformational changes in the enzyme that allow these gymnastics require the binding of the energy cofactor, ATP, to the β subunit of the enzyme. The hydrolysis of the cofactor is required only for turnover of the enzyme, allowing repeated reaction cycles by the enzyme. *(From Morrison and Cozzarelli: Proc Natl Acad Sci USA 78:1461, 1981.)*

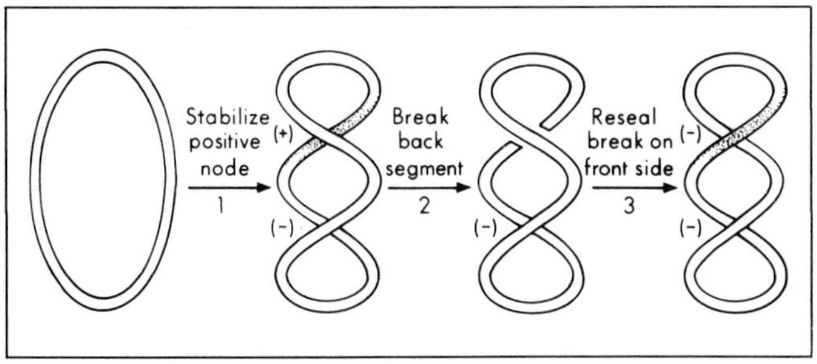

Fig. 7–5. The sign-inversion mechanism for DNA gyrase. See text for details. *(From Brown and Cozzarelli: Science 206:1082, 1979.)*

components of a transient intermediate in the DNA gyrase reaction cycle.

The covalent linkage of topoisomerase to the broken DNA has at least two important functions. First, this linkage guarantees that the broken DNA ends do not dissociate from each other; they are both covalently attached to the same enzyme. Second, the covalent protein-DNA bond is a high-energy phosphotyrosine; the protein-DNA bond thereby stores the energy from the initial phosphodiester bond cleavage for use in the reformation of the phosphodiester bond at the completion of the reaction cycle. Hydrolysis of the high-energy cofactor ATP is required by DNA gyrase for recycling during successive rounds of supercoiling; a nonhydrolyzable analogue of ATP allows only a single cycle of supercoiling by the enzyme.

A visual inspection of the gyrase reaction model shown in Figure 7–5 offers a surprising prediction, namely, that the linking number of DNA should change by two with every reaction cycle of a type II topoisomerase. This prediction has been confirmed and provides clear evidence for the proposed mechanism.

DNA gyrase is the physiologic target for two groups of antibiotics. First, the quinolones appear to block specifically the re-formation of the phosphodiester bond in the gyrase reaction cycle. Thus when DNA gyrase reactions are conducted in the presence of a quinolone, a large proportion of the enzyme is converted into the form of the covalent DNA-protein reaction intermediate. Most of the studies on DNA gyrase have been conducted with the prototype quinolone, nalidixic acid. However, a very large number of new quinolone derivatives, particularly fluoroquinolones such as norfloxacin and ciprofloxacin, have much higher potency and a broader spectrum of antibacterial action (Chap. 9). The second group of DNA gyrase inhibitors is exemplified by novobiocin, which blocks supercoiling by competitively inhibiting the binding of ATP to DNA gyrase. *E. coli* mutants resistant to the two groups of drugs provided important evidence of the subunit structure of the enzyme: drug resistance is controlled by two genes (*gyrA* and *gyrB*), which are the structural genes for the two subunits of the enzyme. Mutations in the *gyrA* gene can result in resistance to the quinolones, whereas novobiocin resistance is conferred by mutations in the *gyrB* gene.

Topoisomerase I. In contrast to DNA gyrase, which introduces negative superhelical turns into DNA, most topoisomerases catalyze the opposite reaction. In *E. coli,* an enzyme called topoisomerase I provides the major activity counteracting DNA gyrase. Topoisomerase I is a single-subunit enzyme that removes negative superhelical turns with no dependence on an exogenous energy source and is encoded by a gene called *topA*. This enzyme is a type I topoisomerase and therefore acts by making a transient break in only one of the two strands of the double helix. Passage of the complementary single strand through this break then results in a topologic change in the DNA, but this time the quantum of change in linking number is one rather than two.

Helicases. A second important class of enzymes that alter DNA structure catalyzes the denaturation of duplex DNA into its complementary single strands. These are called DNA helicases, and they function in a variety of processes where duplex DNA needs to be denatured. There are several DNA helicases in bacterial cells, and each requires an energy source such as ATP to catalyze the energetically unfavorable reaction. The helicases should not be confused with the single-strand binding proteins discussed above; the latter facilitate DNA denaturation by binding to and thereby stabilizing single-stranded DNA, whereas helicases actively denature a duplex in an enzymatic reaction involving nucleotide cofactor hydrolysis.

Replication of Bacterial Genome

A fundamental difference between procaryotic and eucaryotic DNA replication is in the relationship of replication to the cell-division cycle. Eucaryotic cells traverse distinct phases in the cell cycle, and one of these—the S phase—is a discrete period for chromosome replication (Chap. 52). In contrast, rapidly growing bacterial cells replicate their DNA continuously throughout the cell-division cycle. As discussed in more detail in Chapter 5, a single bacterial cell can even have multiple rounds of replication occurring on the same chromosome at one time.

A second important difference between procaryotic and eucaryotic DNA replication is related to the initiation process. Chromosome replication in procaryotes begins at a single origin of replication on the DNA molecule, whereas replication of even a single eucaryotic chromosome begins at multiple replication origins along the DNA. A general concept used to dissect these events is that of the replicon, which is a discrete unit of replication containing an origin where replication begins and a terminus where it ends. The chromosome of a bacterial cell is a single replicon, whereas each eucaryotic chromosome contains multiple replicons that function together during the S phase. The organization of the bacterial chromosome into a single replicon has an important consequence, namely, that the entire replicative process can be controlled by actions at a single site on the chromosome. Once replication is initiated at the origin, the entire bacterial chromosome will be replicated in an orderly manner.

The orderly replication of the bacterial chromosome first became obvious with the classic density-shift experiment (Fig. 7–6). This analysis demonstrated that replication is semiconservative: each daughter molecule contains *exactly* one strand from the parental DNA molecule and one newly synthesized strand. Semiconservative replication stresses the importance of complementarity in DNA structure, as each strand of the parental DNA must contain all of the information in the genome. However, complementarity does not demand a semi-

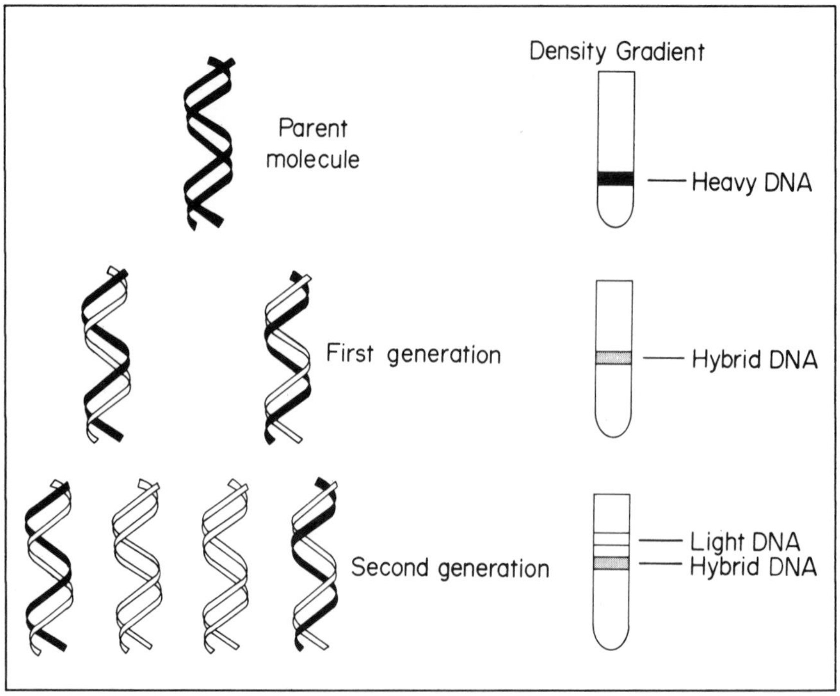

Fig. 7–6. The semiconservative replication of the bacterial chromosome; the classic Meselson and Stahl experiment. Cells of *E. coli* that had grown for several generations in medium containing the heavy isotope ^{15}N were transferred to medium containing ^{14}N, and the distribution of the isotopes in the DNA was monitored after subsequent generations. The left side of the figure depicts the distribution of uniformly labeled heavy (^{15}N) DNA following 0, 1, and 2 generations, respectively, in light (^{14}N) medium. The right side of the figure depicts the location at equilibrium in a cesium chloride gradient of heavy, hybrid, and light DNA. These results are consistent with the semiconservative replication of DNA. The results also illustrate another very significant aspect of DNA replication, namely, that it occurs in a continuous and sequential fashion, as shown by the fact that all of the heavy DNA becomes hybrid prior to the appearance of light DNA.

conservative mechanism, and several additional consequences of semiconservative replication will become obvious when the enzymology and the fidelity of replication are considered (below and Chap. 8, respectively).

A most impressive aspect of DNA replication is its rapidity. The 4.5 million–base pair chromosome of *E. coli* is replicated in toto in about 45 minutes. As discussed in Chapter 5, *E. coli* can divide every 20 minutes only because it is capable of multiple simultaneous rounds of replication. During each round, the replication origin of *E. coli* assembles two functioning replication complexes, which travel in opposite directions until they meet in a region about 180 degrees around the circular chromosome. This is called bidirectional replication. Because these two complexes replicate a 4.5 million–base pair DNA molecule in 45 minutes, each complex replicates almost 1000 base pairs of DNA per second. This number becomes even more impressive when the fidelity of replication is considered—spontaneous mutation frequencies are in the range of only one in every 10^7 to 10^{11} base pairs replicated (Chap. 8).

Genetic and Biochemical Approaches to DNA Replication

One of the most fruitful approaches for understanding the mechanism of DNA replication has been the isolation of mutants blocked in the process. A mutation that completely inactivates some protein required for replication cannot be detected, because any bacterial cell with such a mutation will never grow. This problem was circumvented by isolation of *conditional lethal* mutants, which carry mutations that render some essential protein nonfunctional only under certain conditions. For example, temperature-sensitive mutants can grow normally at low temperatures, which constitute *permissive* conditions, but are unable to grow at high temperatures, which constitute *restrictive* conditions. Among conditional lethal mutants of *E. coli* and other bacteria, two kinds of DNA replication mutants were found. *Fast-stop* mutants immediately cease DNA replication when shifted to the restrictive condition. These contain mutations in genes whose products are essential for the continuous functioning of the replication complex. *Slow-stop* mutants, on the other hand, are conditionally defective only in the process of initiation of replication. The rate of DNA synthesis in these mutants decays slowly, because replication complexes that are already initiated at the time of shift can continue functioning until the chromosome is completely duplicated.

The reconstitution of partial and complete replication reactions in vitro has led to the clearest picture of replication mechanisms. These in vitro systems have been used, in conjunction with the conditional lethal mutants described above, to purify and characterize most of the essential replication proteins of *E. coli.* The experimental details are neglected in the following description of replication, but it is important to appreciate the above-mentioned strategies that allowed a successful dissection of DNA replication mechanisms.

Three Phases of Replication

Initiation. Chromosomal replication initiates near or within a small (245–base pair) region of the *E. coli* genome, called *oriC.* This same segment of DNA can drive the replication of other circular DNA molecules, and in practice small plasmid derivatives containing *oriC* are used to study the mechanism of initiation. The DNA sequences of replication origins from a large number of gram-negative bacteria show strong homology with each other (Fig. 7–7), demonstrating an evolu-

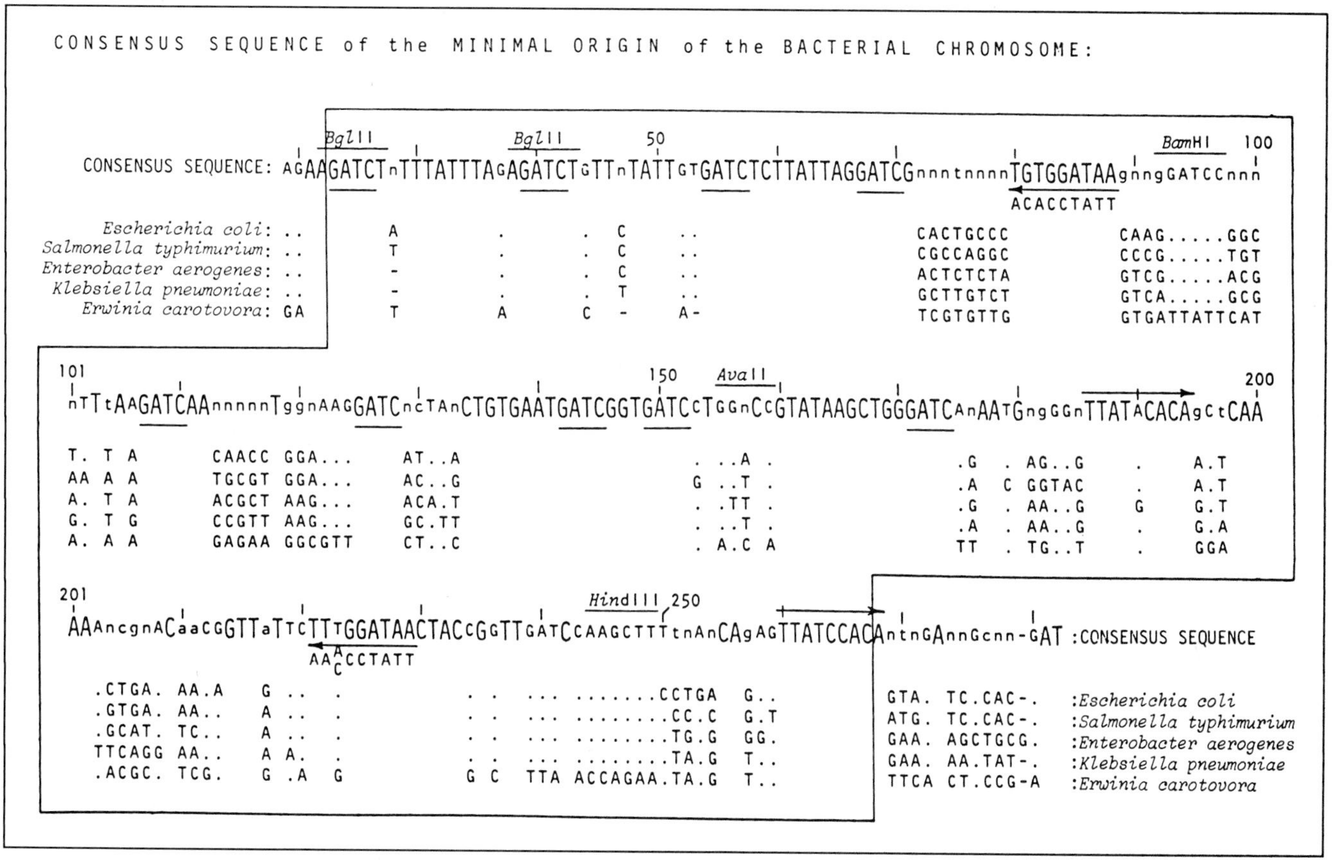

Fig. 7–7. Consensus sequence of enteric bacterial replication origins. The consensus sequence is derived from the nucleotide sequences of the origins of five enteric bacterial species. The consensus sequence residues are as follows: large capital letters represent identical nucleotides in the five origins; small capital letters represent nucleotides that are identical in four of the five origin sequences; lowercase letters indicate nucleotides present in three of the five origins, with only two different nucleotides present at that site; and the letter n is used in all other cases. In the individual origin sequences, the sequences that differ from the consensus are shown. A dash means a deletion of that base with respect to the consensus sequence, and a period indicates that the nucleotide residue is identical to the consensus sequence. The repeated GATC sequences found in bacterial replication origins are underlined, and a series of representative restriction enzyme cleavage sites are shown. The four related nine-base pair repeats indicated by arrows have been shown to be the binding sites for a critical initiation protein, the product of gene *dnaA;* the complementary 5′ to 3′ sequence is shown below two of the arrows. The minimal origin sufficient for replication in *E. coli* is enclosed within the box. *(Courtesy of Dr. Judith W. Zyskind and Dr. Douglas W. Smith.)*

tionary conservation in the mechanism of replication. The initiation of DNA replication from *oriC* has been duplicated in vitro with the use of highly purified components. Although the precise molecular mechanism of initiation is not entirely clear, many of the important features of the initiation reaction have been elucidated.

One key protein, the product of the *dnaA* gene, acts as a positive activator of replication from *oriC*. The earliest intermediate detectable in the in vitro initiation reaction is a large nucleoprotein complex consisting of multiple copies of the *dnaA* protein bound to a series of five closely related sequences in *oriC*. The assembly of *dnaA* protein on the origin facilitates the binding of additional proteins, including the product of the *dnaB* gene. The *dnaB* protein is a helicase that unwinds DNA in and near the origin, a reaction that is necessary for subsequent replication. However, before DNA replication can begin, a primer for extension by DNA polymerase must be provided. Every known DNA polymerase has an absolute requirement for a preexisting primer containing a 3′-hydroxyl group. A specialized RNA polymerizing complex called the primosome provides the short RNA primer to begin nucleic acid synthesis at the origin. The primosome of *E. coli* is a large complex composed of seven different proteins. One protein, the product of the *dnaG* gene, synthesizes the RNA primer and is thus called primase. The other six proteins are required for the proper assembly and functioning of the *dnaG* primase. After primer synthesis, DNA polymerase begins the incorporation of nucleotide residues into DNA (see below).

The initiation mechanisms used by some simpler replicons are understood in even greater detail. Bacterial plasmids and viruses use a variety of mechanisms to initiate DNA synthesis (Chaps. 8 and 60). Depending on the system, the initial primer for extension by DNA polymerase is provided by one or more of the following means: (1) a short RNA primer is synthesized by primase; (2) an RNA primer is synthesized by the RNA polymerase that is normally used in transcription; (3) a specific break in one DNA strand provides a free 3′ end; and (4) a specialized protein is covalently linked to a nucleotide, onto which the newly synthesized DNA is polymerized. Some of these same mechanisms are encountered in the replication of animal virus genomes (Chap. 55).

As in most biosynthetic pathways, the regulation of replication is at the beginning of the pathway, during the initiation step. When growing bacteria are shifted into media without essential nutrients, they immediately stop initiating replication forks but allow those forks already started to continue through termination. In addition, the frequency of initiation is precisely regulated so that it coincides with the rate of growth, but the speed of replication fork movement is quite constant. As described above, the *dnaA* protein is intimately involved in regulation of replication. However, the nature of the coupling of *dnaA* activity to the growth rate of the cell is not currently understood. The same general problem is central to an understanding of development and neoplasia in eucaryotic systems.

Elongation. The result of the initiation reaction is the assembly of two functional replication complexes that traverse the genome in opposite directions, duplicating the genetic information of the bacterial cell. The two complexes are essentially equivalent in a functional sense, and we will now proceed to dissect one such complex.

The chemical reaction central to all DNA replication is quite simple and can be catalyzed by a single enzyme, DNA polymerase. Every known DNA polymerase adds nucleotide residues in the overall 5′ → 3′ direction for chain growth and requires a template, primer, and activated deoxyribonucleoside triphosphates (Fig. 7–8). The rules of base complementarity are used to insert the correct base at each position; for example, a deoxythymidylate residue is inserted opposite a deoxyadenylate residue in the template strand. The chemical reaction central to DNA synthesis is a nucleophilic substitution, with the 3′-hydroxyl of the growing DNA chain attacking the α-phosphate of the incoming nucleoside 5′-triphosphate. This liberates pyrophosphate from the nucleoside triphosphate and results in formation of the appropriate phosphodiester bond.

Bacterial cells such as *E. coli* actually contain at least three DNA polymerases. The enzyme that synthesizes the bulk of the DNA is polymerase III, encoded by the *polC* gene. DNA polymerase I plays a role in repair of gaps (see below), while polymerase II appears to play an important role in DNA repair (the enzymes were named according to their order of discovery). In addition to the *polC* protein, the replicative DNA polymerase III complex contains at least 6 (perhaps as many as 12) additional proteins that are important for its activity; this complete assembly is referred to as the DNA polymerase III *holoenzyme*. The associated proteins markedly affect the properties of DNA polymerase III. Not only do they keep the polymerase from frequently falling off the template; they also increase the speed of polymerization and probably the fidelity of replication. The gram-positive bacterium, *Bacillus subtilis*, also has three DNA polymerases with properties quite similar to those of *E. coli*. This provides

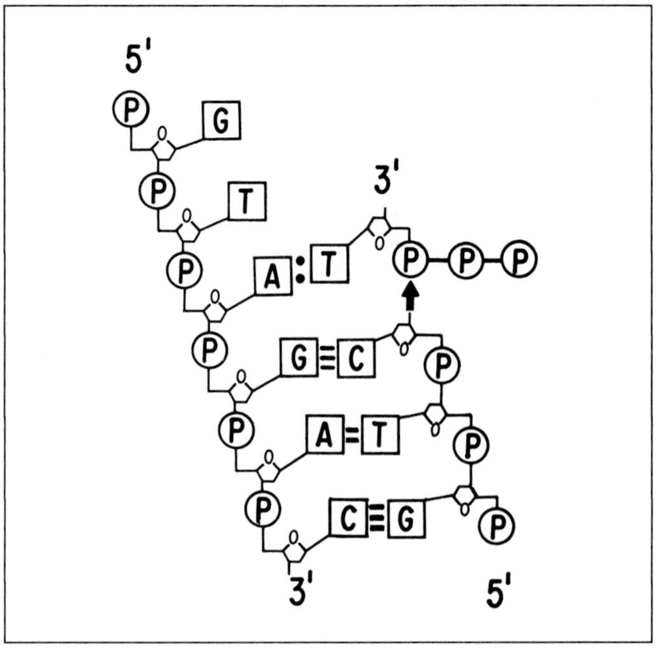

Fig. 7–8. DNA synthesis reaction mechanism. The template-directed addition of a deoxythymidylate residue into a daughter strand is depicted. The base portion of each nucleotide residue is indicated by letters A, G, C, and T, and each phosphate group by the letter P.

additional evidence that replication mechanisms in diverse bacteria are similar. However, one notable difference is that DNA polymerase III from some (but not all) gram-positive bacteria is sensitive to a class of antimicrobial agents called arylazopyrimidines. These compounds apparently bind to the active site of the enzyme in a manner that blocks the binding of the incoming nucleoside triphosphate.

Because DNA polymerase can synthesize DNA only in the 5′ → 3′ direction and the two parental DNA strands are antiparallel, somewhat different mechanisms must be used to copy the two strands at each replication fork. One of the parental strands can be copied continuously in *leading strand* synthesis, with a single daughter strand extending (5′ → 3′) from the site of initiation to the site of termination. The other parental strand (the *lagging strand*) must be copied in discontinuous retrograde patches, called *Okazaki fragments* (Fig. 7–9). These fragments are generally 1000 to 2000 bases long and are spliced together after the replication complex passes.

The continuous DNA synthesis on the leading strand can proceed through the entire DNA molecule with only the single primer provided during the initiation reaction. However, because all DNA polymerases require a preexisting primer, each of the Okazaki fragments on the lagging strand must be initiated by another mechanism. A primosome complex that had been loaded onto the DNA during initiation at *oriC* travels along the lagging strand of the template molecule and provides an RNA primer for Okazaki fragment synthesis every 1000 to 2000 nucleotides (Fig. 7–9).

Recent evidence indicates that the lagging strand is folded around in such a way that the polymerase complexes on both the leading and the lagging strands are associated and syn-

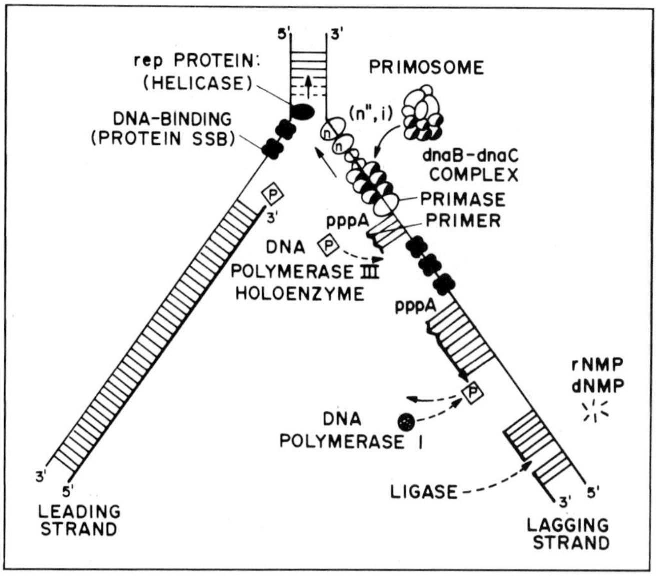

Fig. 7–9. A scheme for DNA chain growth at a replication fork of the *E. coli* chromosome. The roles of many of the indicated proteins are explained in the text. At least one DNA polymerase III holoenzyme complex (P) is required for each of the leading and lagging strands, and the primosome complex is required to synthesize the ribonucleotide primers on the discontinuously synthesized lagging strand. *(From Kornberg: Supplement to DNA Replication. W. H. Freeman, 1982.)*

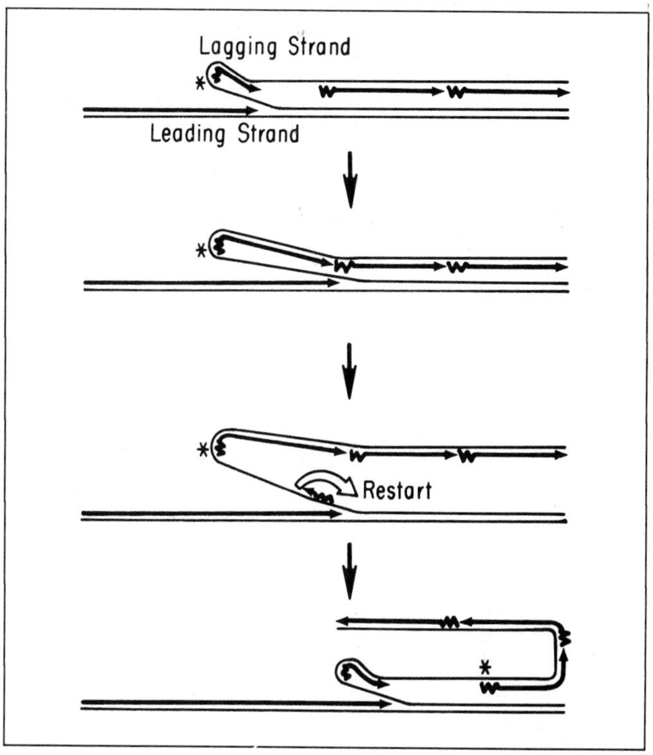

Fig. 7–10. A model for the coordination of leading and lagging strand DNA synthesis. The completion of one particular Okazaki fragment is shown in the first step, with the lagging strand folded so that both leading and lagging strand polymerase complexes are associated. The asterisk indicates the site at which that Okazaki fragment was initiated with the synthesis of a short RNA primer. The second step depicts the reorganization proposed to occur between the synthesis of each subsequent Okazaki fragment. The folded loop is first released, and a new loop is re-formed upon synthesis of the next RNA primer (wavy line). The replication fork at the bottom is equivalent to that at the top, except that one additional Okazaki fragment has been completed. *(Adapted from Alberts et al: Cold Spring Harbor Symp Quant Biol 47:655, 1983.)*

thesizing DNA in the same direction in space (Fig. 7–10). At the completion of each Okazaki fragment, the lagging-strand DNA can rearrange while the lagging-strand polymerase complex remains associated with the leading-strand polymerase complex. Without this elegant mechanism, a new polymerase complex would have to associate with the DNA to synthesize each Okazaki fragment.

The Okazaki fragments on the lagging strand must be linked together after synthesis to provide an intact daughter molecule. In this step, DNA polymerase I extends each Okazaki fragment by inserting several deoxyribonucleotide residues while removing the short RNA primer at the 5′ end of the next Okazaki fragment (Fig. 7–9). Once the ribonucleotide residues have been replaced with deoxyribonucleotides, an enzyme called DNA ligase splices the two Okazaki fragments together. DNA ligase can join any two adjacent DNA fragments, as long as one has a 3′-hydroxyl and the other a 5′-phosphate. On a practical level, DNA polymerases and ligases are widely used in current recombinant DNA research (Chap. 8).

The unwinding of the parental DNA at the replication fork is required to allow synthesis of the two new complements. All of the elements that facilitate this unwinding were introduced above. Negative superhelicity makes an energetic contribution, specific DNA helicases (including the *dnaB* protein) enzymatically drive open the helix, and single-strand binding protein stabilizes the transient single-stranded regions of DNA at the fork. An important topologic problem arises from the unwinding of the parental strands. A swivel on the parental helix is required to counteract the rapid unwinding and prevent the two daughter molecules from becoming hopelessly tangled. DNA gyrase appears to provide this swivel by maintaining a negative superhelical tension ahead of the replication fork.

Termination. After the two forks have each traversed half the chromosome in opposite directions, they meet in the terminus region of the genome. Termination must allow the orderly completion of replication by the opposing forks and is presumably coupled to the segregation of the two product DNA molecules into daughter cells. At present, the events that occur during termination are understood in only sketchy detail.

The terminus region contains four identical DNA sequences that act as blocks to the progress of replication forks. One important feature of the termination sequences is that they are directional—they block replication forks going in one direction but not in the other. Two termination sequences are located at each end of the terminus, with orientations such that forks can enter, but not leave, the intervening terminus region. This arrangement ensures that all replication will terminate in this small region of the chromosome, even if the two replication forks do not arrive at the same time. Restricting termination to this small region presumably facilitates the segregation of product molecules away from each other and into the daughter cells.

A major problem in termination is that the two parental strands are interwound about once every 10.6 base pairs. The swivel discussed above relieves this interwinding during elongation. However, because the swivel must act in *front* of the replication fork, it cannot relieve all interwinding as the two forks approach each other during termination. Therefore the daughter molecules should be topologically linked together in the form of a multiply intertwined catenane after replication (Fig. 7–11). There is now direct evidence that such catenanes can be the immediate product of replication in both procaryotic and eucaryotic cells. Once again, DNA gyrase and related type II topoisomerases turn out to be important in solving this topologic problem. As described above, type II topoisomerases change the topologic state of a single DNA molecule by passing one segment of double helix through a transient break elsewhere in the molecule. The enzymes are almost equally adept at passing a duplex segment of one molecule through a transient break in a second molecule and thus can separate catenated DNA circles with high efficiency (compare Fig. 7–5 and Fig. 7–11). DNA gyrase plays an important role in the resolution of the products of bacterial chromosome replication, because conditional-lethal gyrase mutants accumulate daughter chromosomes that are topologically linked under restrictive conditions.

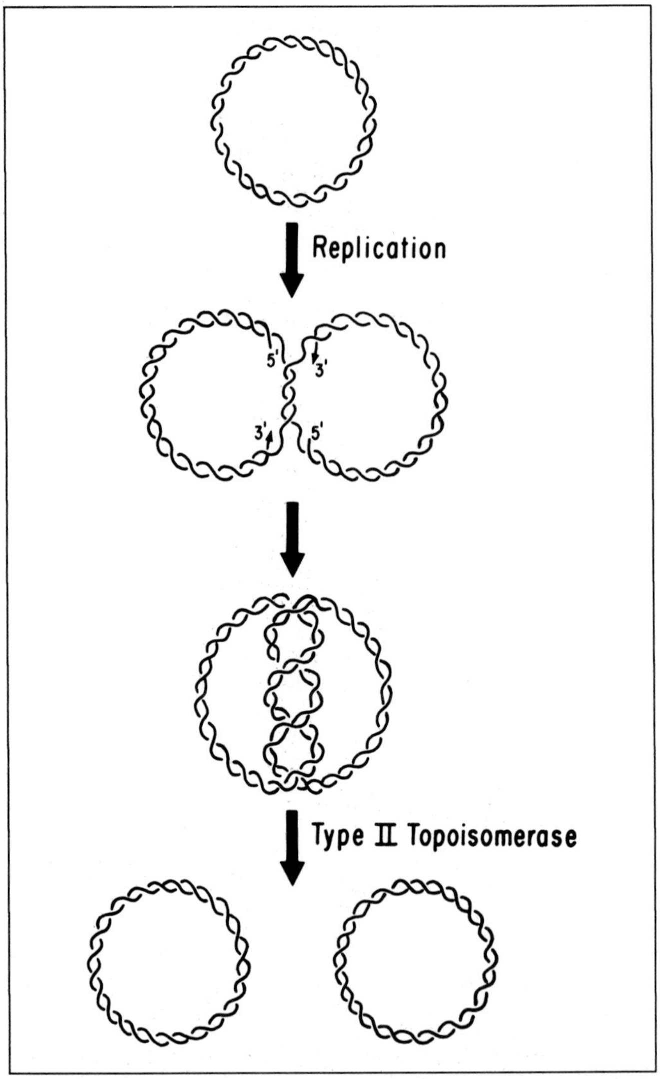

Fig. 7–11. Resolution of catenated DNA circles after replication. The final stages of replication of a circular molecule result in interlocked daughter molecules because of the winding of the two parental strands about each other. DNA gyrase and other type II DNA topoisomerases resolve these interlocked daughter molecules by a simple variant of the double-strand DNA passage mechanism discussed above.

Transcription

Gene expression in all cells depends on the sequential processes of transcription and translation. Together, these transmute the nucleotide sequence of a gene into the amino acid sequence of the corresponding protein gene product. During transcription, the rules of base-pairing are used by RNA polymerase to synthesize an RNA product that is complementary to one strand of the gene. The three major types of RNA produced are messenger RNA (mRNA), ribosomal RNA (rRNA), and transfer RNA (tRNA). Translation is the process whereby rRNA, tRNA, and numerous proteins participate in *reading* the nucleotide triplet code encrypted by the mRNA and *writing* the appropriate amino acid sequence of the protein.

RNA synthesis is much simpler in procaryotes than in eucaryotes. Bacteria contain only a single RNA polymerase (excluding the primase discussed above), whereas higher cells have at least three specialized enzymes. Messenger RNA in eucaryotic cells is capped, spliced, and transported to the cytoplasm before it can be translated. In contrast, bacterial mRNA is generally translated as it is being transcribed, with no requirements for posttranscriptional modification or transport. A third major difference is the relative simplicity of transcription start signals in procaryotes compared with those in eucaryotes. From an evolutionary standpoint, it is quite interesting that the RNA polymerase from archaebacteria more closely resembles eucaryotic than eubacterial polymerase. (The same relationship is observed for ribosomal RNA sequences.)

The diversity of RNA molecules, even in simple procaryotic cells, includes on the order of a few thousand mRNA species, roughly 50 to 60 species of tRNA, and three different rRNA molecules. The majority of the RNA isolated from a cell consists of rRNA and tRNA, but this does not accurately reflect the rates of synthesis of RNA species. The explanation of this disparity is that both rRNA and tRNA are very stable, whereas mRNA turns over rapidly. The differential stabilities of RNA species are quite logical. Ribosomal RNA and tRNA are structural components of the translation machinery that do not need to be replaced frequently. On the other hand, the rapid turnover of mRNA allows for rapid regulation of the protein composition of a cell by mechanisms operating at the level of transcription. After a discussion of the machinery of transcription and translation, the variety and power of such regulatory mechanisms are described.

RNA Polymerase

The transcription machinery of all (eubacterial) procaryotes appears to be quite similar. The DNA-dependent RNA polymerase of *E. coli* has been the most extensively studied and is considered here as a prototype. The simplest form of the enzyme with some catalytic activity is the *core*, which is composed of four subunits in the form $\alpha_2\beta\beta'$. The β subunit is involved in binding of the nucleotide substrate, whereas β′ has been shown to be involved in template DNA binding. Several antibiotics, including rifampicin and streptolydigin, block RNA polymerase by binding to the β subunit; bacterial mutants resistant to these compounds have an altered β subunit. Core RNA polymerase is a large enzyme, with a total molecular weight of just under 379,000. This form of RNA polymerase is able to synthesize RNA complementary to a DNA template, but it does so at random locations on the template and only when the template is single stranded. The core enzyme clearly has a functional active site for polymerizing nucleotide residues with the correct complementarity but is incapable of recognizing the natural transcription start sites on duplex DNA. These transcription start sites, called promoters, consist of variants of a particular nucleotide sequence (see below).

To achieve proper recognition of natural promoters, the σ subunit (M_r = 70,236) must be added. This reconstitutes the complete or holoenzyme form of RNA polymerase. The holoenzyme binds to a region of about 75 base pairs containing an acceptable promoter sequence, and then the enzyme-DNA complex undergoes a series of conformational changes leading to the initiation of RNA chain growth (see below). Only one strand of the double helix is used as a template for any particular transcript, but the template strand is different for various genes throughout the genome. In addition to this predominant σ subunit, several alternative σ subunits are used to activate transcription of a small number of specialized genes. These are described in more detail when the mechanisms of regulation are considered (see below).

Promoter Recognition. Many bacterial promoters are recognized properly in reactions containing only the RNA polymerase holoenzyme, which then initiates transcription. This is in striking contrast to transcriptional initiation in eucaryotes, where complex collections of proteins are necessary to achieve transcriptional initiation.

Based on the DNA sequences of more than 100 functional *E. coli* promoters, a *consensus sequence* for RNA polymerase recognition has been identified (Fig. 7–12). The consensus sequence contains two conserved stretches of nucleotides, 5′-TTGACA-3′ centered at position −35 with respect to the start of transcription and 5′-TATAAT-3′ centered at −10. The concept of a consensus sequence is well illustrated here: no known *E. coli* promoter has exactly the consensus sequence under discussion, but all promoters have some variant of that sequence. In general, the closer the sequence is to consensus, the better the promoter. It is estimated that the *E. coli* genome has on the order of 2000 functional promoters, but these differ greatly in transcriptional strength.

A series of discrete steps in promoter recognition has been elucidated and clarifies some of the problems that RNA polymerase encounters in initiating transcription. The first step (Fig. 7–13A) involves nonspecific binding to any duplex

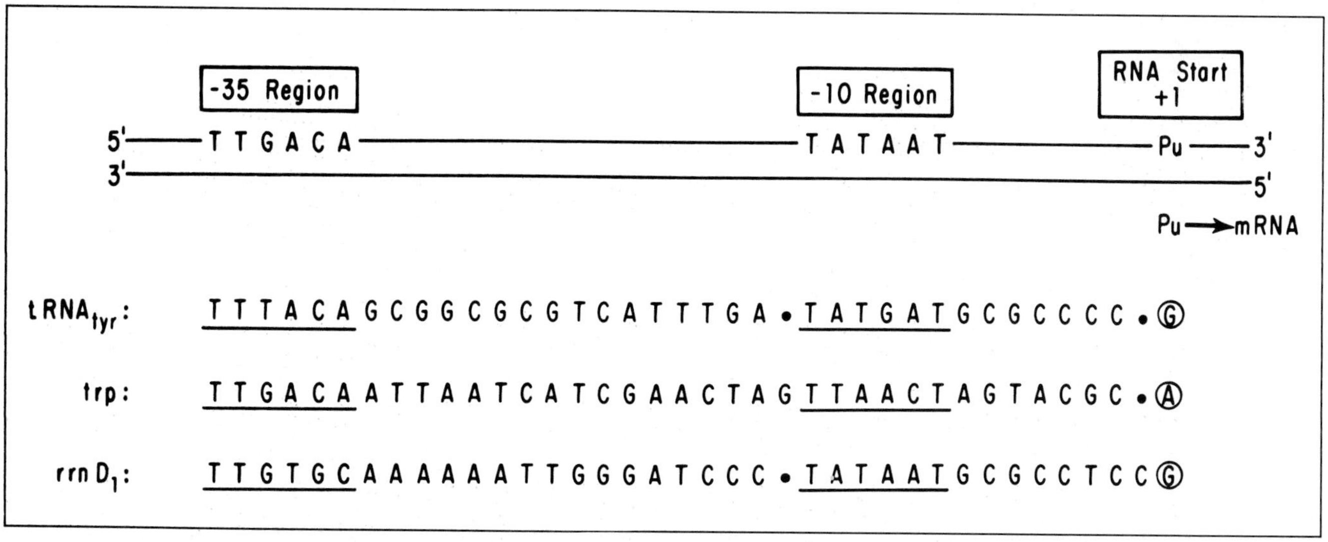

Fig. 7–12. The consensus sequence of bacterial promoters. The conserved sequences in the "−35" and "−10" regions of bacterial promoters are shown on top, with the RNA start site indicated at the right. Most promoters show a spacing of 15 to 19 nucleotides between the −35 and −10 regions and 5 to 7 nucleotides between the −10 region and the RNA start. No known natural *E. coli* promoter has exactly the consensus sequence in both the −35 and −10 regions. The sequences of three representative promoters are shown, with the −35 and −10 regions underlined. The RNA start site of each is circled, and a period indicates a base missing from the spacing that is shown. *(Adapted from Rosenberg and Court: Annu Rev Genet 13:323, 1979.)*

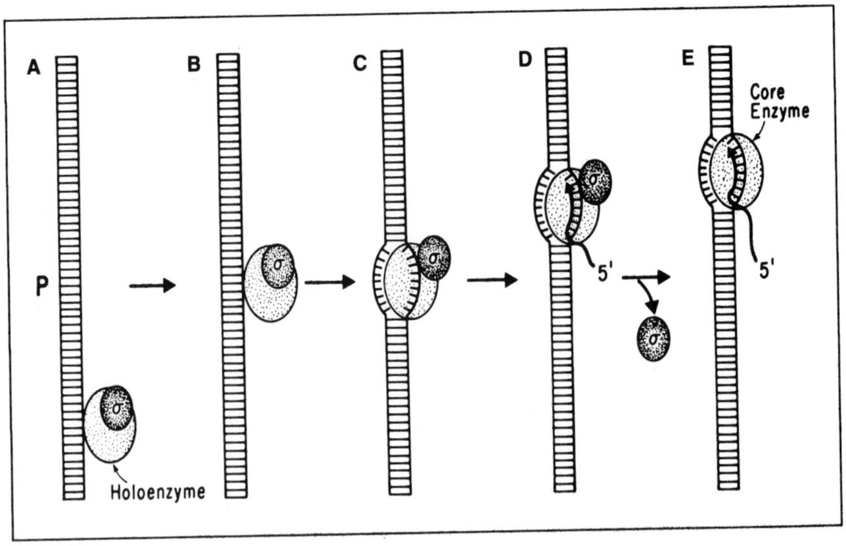

Fig. 7–13. Promoter recognition by RNA polymerase. The steps involved in the recognition and utilization of a promoter (P) are depicted. RNA polymerase holoenzyme binds nonspecifically to DNA in **A**, which facilitates its subsequent specific binding to the promoter sequence in **B**. The protein-DNA complex in **B** is referred to as the closed complex, and this converts into the open complex in **C** upon denaturation of DNA within the promoter. After the synthesis of a short stretch of RNA (step **D**), the σ subunit is released; all subsequent RNA is polymerized by the core enzyme devoid of σ (step **E**). *(Adapted from Kornberg: DNA Replication. W. H. Freeman, 1980.)*

DNA, followed by a search for proper promoter sequences somewhere within the DNA molecule. The search mechanism probably involves a linear diffusion of the protein along the DNA; this appears to be a general strategy whereby site-specific DNA binding proteins find their recognition sites in DNA. When a correct promoter sequence is found by the enzyme, the first detectable complex is called the *closed complex* (Fig. 7–13B). The promoter DNA within the closed complex is completely duplex, and therefore RNA polymerase must recognize features of the base pairs that extend into the minor or major groove of the double helix. A major transition occurs next: the DNA helix is unwound by about 540 degrees, and the region of −9 to +3 nucleotides on the DNA becomes sensitive to single-strand-specific reagents. This unwinding of the helix is absolutely required if RNA polymerase is to synthesize RNA complementary to the template DNA strand and signals the formation of the *open complex* (Fig. 7–13C). There is some evidence that the conversion of the closed to the open complex is actually a series of steps, and undoubtedly there are major conformational changes in the enzyme as well as in the DNA. The next step is the actual initiation of transcription, with the formation of the first phosphodiester bond. In a large majority of promoters, the first residue of the RNA chain is a purine, complementary to position +1 of the DNA template. Because the transcribing complex contains protein, DNA, and nascent RNA, it is termed a *ternary complex* (Fig. 7–13D). Shortly after formation of the ternary complex, the σ subunit is released by the transcribing RNA polymerase (Fig. 7–13E), and thus the role of σ is limited to only the promoter recognition and initiation steps.

Elongation and Termination. Once transcription has started, the addition of each subsequent base (elongation) involves the binding of a ribonucleoside triphosphate substrate, phosphodiester bond formation and release of pyrophosphate, and translocation of the polymerase by one base on the DNA template. This sequence of events occurs 20 to 50 times per second, but certain sequences cause significant pausing and/or termination of transcription (see below). Physical studies of the active ternary complex indicate that a region of about 18 base pairs of DNA is denatured at any time, with about 12 bases of the denatured template strand base pairing with the 3′ end of the nascent RNA. The DNA duplex must be denatured ahead of the enzyme as elongation proceeds and then re-formed behind the enzyme as the product RNA is dissociated from the template DNA strand. How RNA polymerase activates these various denaturation and renaturation reactions is currently unknown. There are also serious topologic problems inherent in producing a long RNA transcript from a double-helical DNA template, particularly when the nascent transcript has functional ribosomes attached. A recent proposal suggests that topoisomerases may provide a dual swivel on both sides of the transcription complex, allowing rapid rotation by the DNA template rather than by the RNA polymerase and nascent transcript.

The mechanisms of pausing and termination by RNA polymerase are related. For unknown reasons, the enzyme pauses when the nascent RNA behind it forms an appropriate stem-loop structure by internal base pairing (Fig. 7–14). At this point, the enzyme can either resume synthesis of the same transcript (with some lag time) or terminate transcription. The latter occurs whenever the actual site of transcription is within a series of 4 to 8 uridine residues (Fig. 7–14). This is thought to reflect the denaturation of the RNA-DNA hybrid just behind the polymerase, because an rU-dA hybrid is unusually weak.

A second mechanism of transcription termination is dependent on a specific protein, the product of the *rho* gene. ρ-Dependent termination also occurs at sites of pausing by RNA polymerase, but in this case the sequence of tandem uridine residues is not essential. The ρ protein is thought to bind to the nascent transcript and then travel along the RNA in the 5′→3′ direction, toward the transcribing RNA polymerase. In this model, once ρ reaches a paused RNA polymerase, it denatures the short region of RNA:DNA hybrid and thereby releases the nascent transcript.

There are also protein factors that block termination. The best-studied example is the antitermination factor N induced by bacteriophage λ. When RNA polymerase passes special sites in the phage λ DNA template (called *nut* or *N-utilization* sites), the phage-induced gene *N* protein and one or more host proteins bind to the transcribing polymerase,

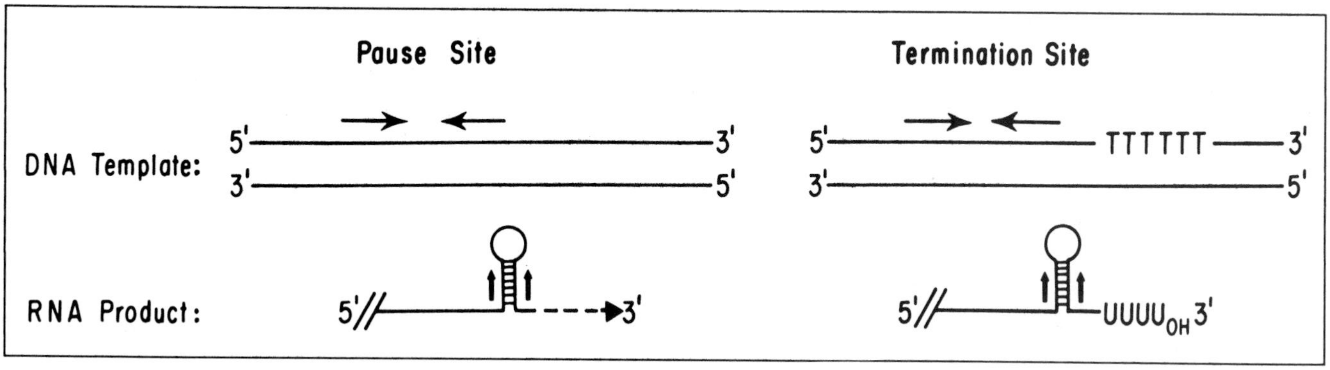

Fig. 7–14. Transcriptional pause and termination sites. The sites at which RNA polymerase pauses and terminates contain inverted complementary sequences (arrows), resulting in a partially duplex region in the nascent RNA product. Termination requires both the inverted sequences and a stretch of T residues in the template DNA strand. A second mechanism of termination is described in the text.

modifying it so that termination sites are no longer recognized. This antitermination mechanism has a profound impact on the transcriptional program of phage λ development (Chap. 60). The fact that several host proteins are involved in this phage regulatory pathway suggests that host transcription may also use similar antitermination mechanisms.

Translation

The elucidation of the triplet genetic code during the early 1960s represents one of the triumphs of modern biology. Most of the crucial evidence for the code was derived from experiments with bacterial systems, but it turns out that precisely the same genetic code is used in plant and animal cells. Translation is the general process whereby this nucleotide triplet code in mRNA is used to direct the sequence of amino acids in protein molecules.

Machinery of Translation

Translation is a complex process that requires the participation of a variety of protein and RNA species. The *workbench* for protein synthesis is the ribosome, whereas the crucial adaptor molecules that read the nucleotide code are the tRNA molecules. In addition, several soluble protein factors are required for ribosome function, and a class of enzymes called tRNA synthetases are responsible for charging the tRNA molecules with the correct amino acids.

Ribosomes. The ribosome is probably the most extensively studied macromolecular complex. The *E. coli* ribosome is composed of three structural RNA molecules and 53 protein species, and the primary (nucleotide or amino acid) sequence of each of these is known. Ribosomes are designated according to their sedimentation coefficients—the bacterial ribosome is a 70S particle composed of two subparticles, the 50S (large) and the 30S (small). The relative positions of many of the proteins in the ribosome have been mapped by a variety of techniques, including direct visualization of antibody-bound ribosomes in the electron microscope (Fig. 7–15).

The 50S (large) subunit is concerned primarily with peptide bond formation and contains the 23S and 5S rRNA molecules. It is now agreed that the large subunit contains 32 proteins. Because two numbers (L8 and L26) were misassigned, the proteins in the 50S subunit are designated L1 through L34. Protein L7 and L12 have identical amino acid sequences and differ only in that L7 has an acetyl modification at the amino terminal end. The remaining 30 proteins have distinct amino acid sequences. Each of the RNA and protein components of the large subunit is present in a single copy, with the exception of proteins L7 and L12 (which have four copies each). The total mass of the 50S subunit is about 1.5 million Da, which should give a suitable impression of its complexity. The precise path of a nascent protein through the 50S particle is not yet clear. Peptide bond formation occurs near the interface with the small subunit, whereas the newly synthesized protein exits almost 15 nm (150 Å) away, on the opposite face of the 50S subunit (Fig. 7–16).

The 30S subunit is involved primarily with decoding the mRNA and thereby contains the binding sites for activated tRNA molecules. In addition, the small subunit has a major role in the initiation of translation, with both *i*nitiation *f*actor (IF3) and mRNA binding to the 16S rRNA (see below). The 30S subunit contains one copy each of 16S rRNA and 21 different proteins, named S1 through S21, and has a total mass of about 900,000 Da.

The assembly of the ribosome has been studied by in vitro reconstitution experiments. All three rRNA molecules are initially transcribed as a single precursor molecule. A processing enzyme called RNase III cleaves the precursor to generate individual precursors of each of the three rRNA molecules. RNase III recognizes regions of duplex RNA that form in self-complementary regions of the large precursor, between the domains of the three rRNAs. Each of the cleaved portions is then capable of associating with certain of the ribosomal proteins to begin the process of ribosome assembly. For example, about two thirds of the small subunit proteins bind to pre-16S rRNA to form a 21S complex, which can then rearrange to form a more compact 26S complex when heated to 37C. The remaining proteins then bind to form the complete small subunit. Many of the ribosomal proteins bind

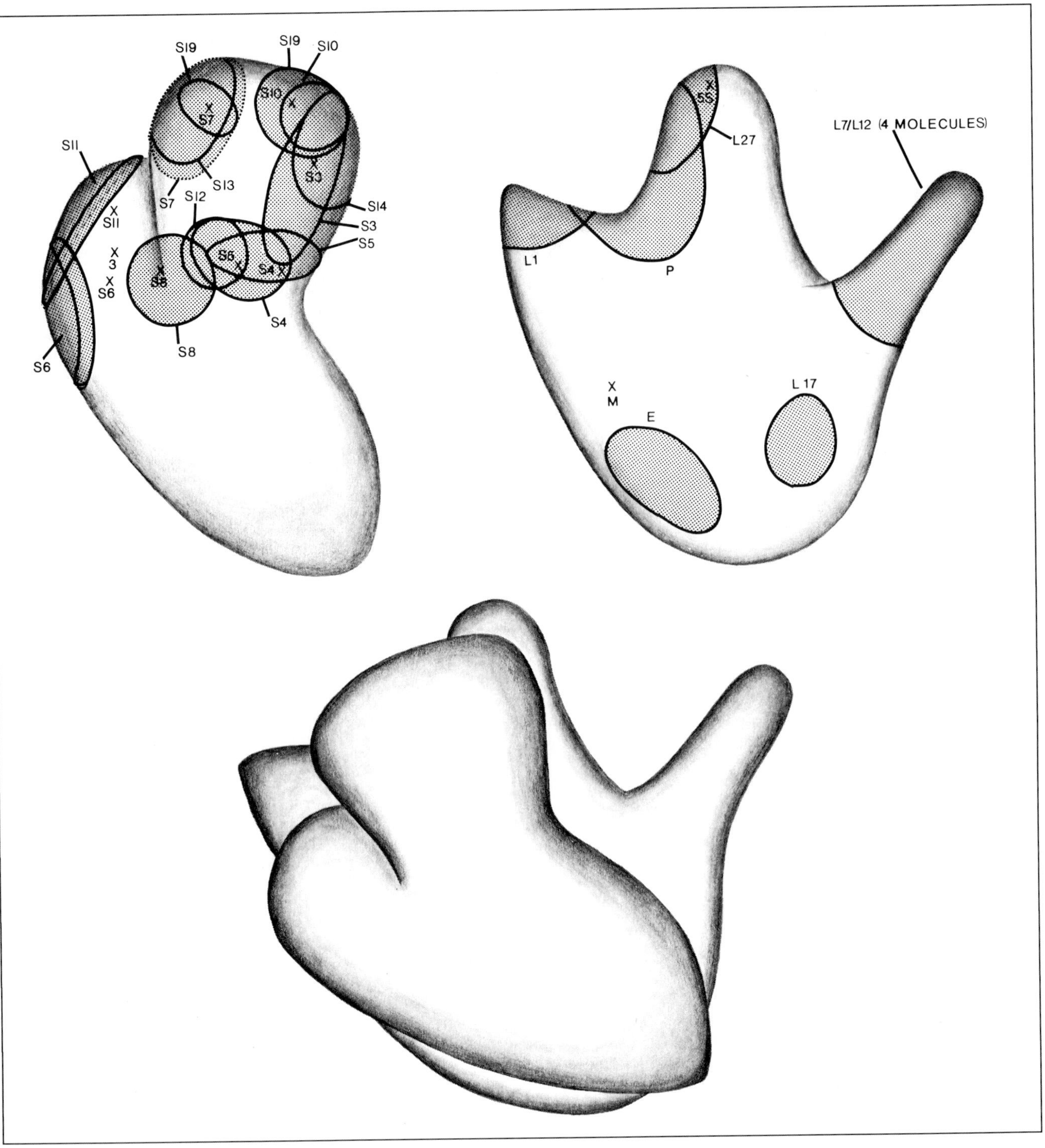

Fig. 7–15. The shapes of ribosome subunits and map of ribosome proteins. The 30S subunit is on the left, above, and the 50S subunit is on the right, above. The patches were mapped by immunoelectron microscopy. The crosses were mapped by neutron diffraction. Five additional sites are shown. They are M, the site at which the ribosome can be anchored to intracellular membrane; 5S, the location of 5S RNA, a part of the large subunit; 3′, an end of the 16S ribosomal RNA; P, the site at which successive amino acids are linked to make a polypeptide chain; and E, the site where the newly synthesized polypeptide chain emerges from the ribosome. *(Adapted from Lake: Sci Am 245:84, 1981.)*

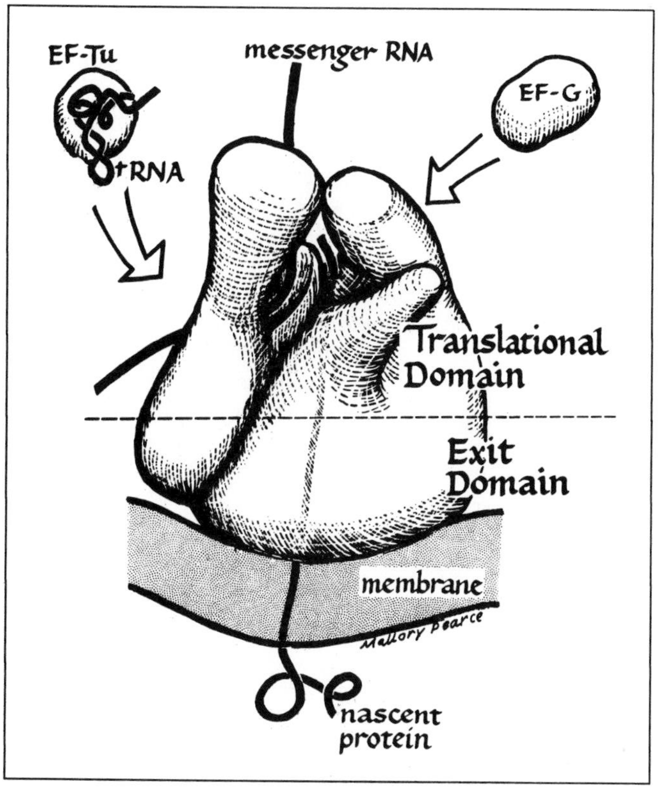

Fig. 7–16. The domains of a functioning ribosome. The translational and exit domains of the ribosome are distinct, with the exit domain located in the region of membrane binding. The transport of certain proteins through membranes is facilitated by the binding of the exit domain to the membrane. *(From Lake: Annu Rev Biochem 54:507, 1985.)*

to specific sites on the rRNA, with target regions of from 50 to 500 bases. During protein assembly, other ribonucleases perform a final trimming of both 16S and 23S rRNA to produce the native molecule found in mature ribosomes. An interesting aspect of assembly is the role of L20 and L24; these two proteins are required only to assemble the large subunit and are dispensable once the correct assembly is accomplished.

Early studies of ribosome structure and function indicated that rRNA has relatively little role in translation, because most antibiotic-resistant mutants of bacteria contain altered ribosomal proteins. This conclusion is now being reassessed. Each of the ribosomal proteins is encoded by single-copy genes, whereas rRNA molecules are generally encoded by multiple genes, and this introduced a bias against finding mutations in the rRNA genes. In fact, most antibiotic-resistance mutations in mitochondria with single-copy rRNA genes are in these and not the ribosomal protein genes. In addition, the catalyzing potential of RNA has gained acceptance with the discovery of an RNA species as an enzyme subunit (RNase P) and self-splicing RNA in both procaryotes and eucaryotes. On the basis of these considerations, the rRNA molecules may perform a fundamental role in the mechanics of translation, with the ribosomal proteins enhancing and modifying this function. There is currently no clear picture of how the ribosome coordinates all the various reactions it must perform, which include binding and release of tRNAs, transpeptidation, and concerted movements of mRNA template and protein product (see below). With an increasingly sophisticated knowledge of ribosome structure, however, the precise conformational changes and relative movements of ribosomal components are now being directly approached.

tRNA and tRNA Synthetases. The ribosomes depend on soluble tRNA molecules to aid in the decoding process. The tRNA family plays the role of adaptors in protein synthesis—they are responsible for reading the nucleotide triplets in mRNA and translating this code into an amino acid sequence. The crucial experiment that proved the adaptor role of tRNA used an in vitro translation system reading an RNA with a sequence of repeating $(UG)_n$, which codes for alternating valine and cysteine in the polypeptide product (see below). When the cysteinyl-tRNA was modified by chemically removing the –SH group to produce alanine-tRNA, alanine instead of cysteine was incorporated into the polypeptide. This result demonstrates that during translation the messenger RNA specifies a particular tRNA species; if a wrong amino acid happens to be esterified to the tRNA, a translational mistake will occur.

All tRNA species must be recognized by the ribosome during translation, and therefore they share a similar overall structure. They range in size from 73 to 93 nucleotides and contain numerous modified bases (Table 7–1). Each tRNA folds into a compact structure because of self-complementary regions; the structure is often presented as a cloverleaf, but x-ray diffraction analysis shows that the overall shape is more like an L (Fig. 7–17). The anticodon (AC) of each tRNA is in a strictly conserved location, and all tRNA molecules contain a 3′-terminal CCA sequence to which the appropriate amino acid is added.

The addition of amino acids to tRNA molecules is performed by a remarkable class of enzymes called aminoacyl-tRNA synthetases. The synthetases are ultimately responsible for the fidelity of protein synthesis, because a tRNA with the wrong amino acid results in a translational mistake (see above). The tRNA synthetases catalyze a two-step transfer reaction in which a free amino acid is first activated by covalent attachment to adenosine monophosphate (AMP) (Fig. 7–18). The nucleotide substrate for this reaction is ATP, and pyrophosphate is released as the amino acid is activated. The aminoacyl-AMP is then competent for the second transfer step, this time to one of the free hydroxyl moieties of the 3′-terminal adenine residue of tRNA.

Because of the redundant nature of the genetic code (see below), there can be several tRNA *isoaccepting* species for a given amino acid. However, there is only a single aminoacyl-tRNA synthetase for each amino acid, and therefore some of the synthetases can recognize and charge several isoaccepting tRNA molecules. The exquisite discriminatory abilities of the synthetases can now be appreciated—each must recognize only one out of the 20 natural amino acids and also a distinct set of isoaccepting tRNA molecules out of all tRNA molecules in the cell (in spite of the conserved structure of all tRNA molecules; see above).

The fidelity of tRNA charging conferred by the forward reaction of the synthetases is quite high, but apparently not high enough to prevent crucial mistakes in protein synthesis. To counteract this low level of mischarging, each synthetase is also competent to perform the reverse reaction on tRNA molecules that are mischarged. For example, isoleucyl-tRNA

TABLE 7–1. MODIFIED NUCLEOSIDES[a]

I	Inosine	s^4U	4-thiouridine
m^1I	1-methyl inosine	s^2m^5U	2-thio-5-methyl uridine
m^1A	1-methyl adenosine	V	5-oxyacetic acid uridine
m^2A	2-methyl adenosine	s^2am^5U	2-thio-5-acetic acid methyl ester uridine
m^6A	N^6-methyl adenosine	s^2cm^5U	2-thio-5-carboxymethyl uridine
i^6A	N^6-isopentenyl adenosine	cmm^5U	5-carboxymethyl uridine methyl ester
ms^2i^6A	2-methylthio-N^6-isopentenyl adenosine	cm^5U	5-carboxymethyl uridine
t^6A	N^6-(N-threonylcarbonyl) adenosine	Um	2′-O-methyl uridine
m^1G	1-methyl guanosine	ψm	2′-O-methyl pseudouridine
		mam^5s^2U	5-methylaminomethyl-2-thiouridine
m^2G	N^2-methyl guanosine	X	3-(3-amino-3-carboxypropyl) uridine
m^2G	N^2-dimethyl guanosine	s^2m^5C	2-thio-5-methyl cytidine
m^7G	N^7-methyl guanosine	s^2C	2-thiocytidine
Gm	2′-O-methyl guanosine	Cm	2′-O-methyl cytidine
T	(ribo) Thymidine	ac^4C	N^4-acetyl cytidine
ψ	Pseudouridine (5-ribofuranosyl uracil)	m^3C	N^3-methyl cytidine
D or hU	5,6-dihydrouridine	m^5C	5-methyl cytidine

Modified from Kim: Prog Nucleic Acid Res Mol Biol 17:181, 1976.
[a] Modified nucleosides found as minor components in tRNA molecules. The biologic role of most of these modifications is unknown.

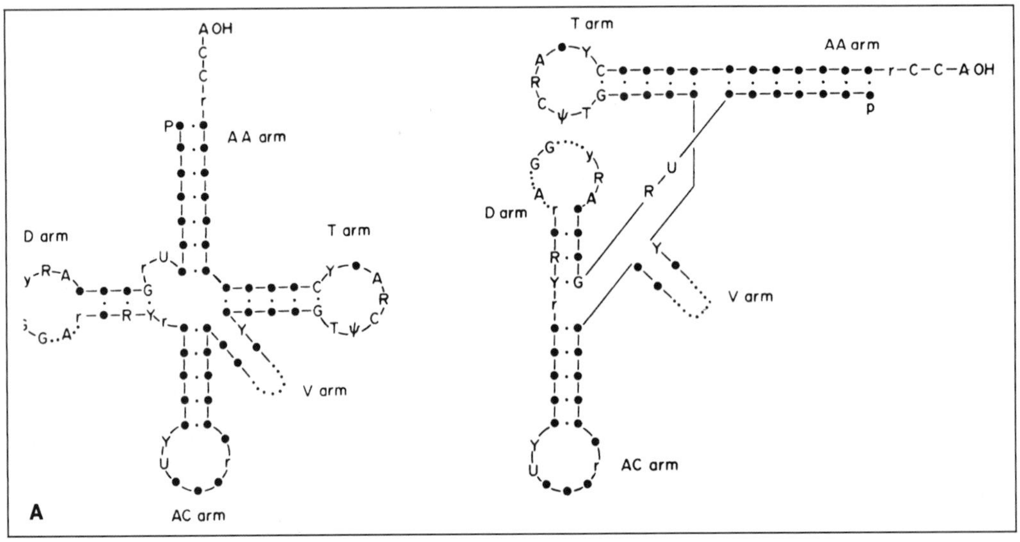

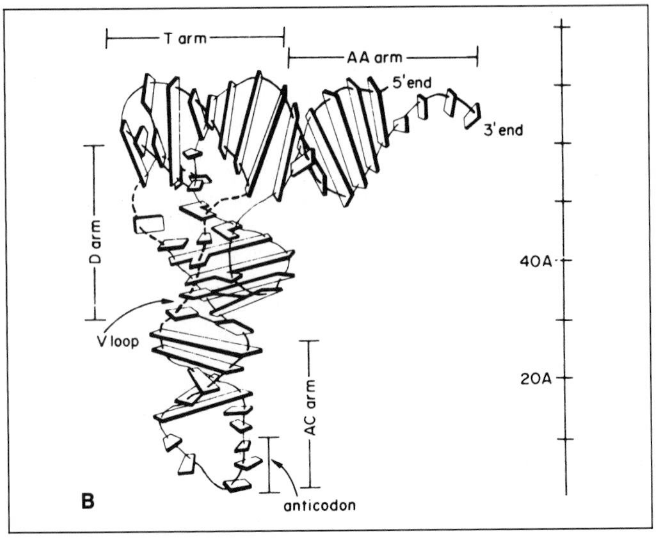

Fig. 7–17. The structure of transfer RNA. **A.** Sequence analysis of tRNA shows that the molecule can possess secondary structure maintained by intramolecular hydrogen bonding; the clover-leaf configuration is depicted above. The solid circles in the figure represent nucleotides that are generally variable among various tRNA molecules; the letters r and y indicate positions that are usually occupied, respectively, by purine and pyrimidine; R and Y indicate positions invariably occupied, respectively, by purine and pyrimidine; H indicates the position usually occupied by a modified nucleoside. **B.** X-ray crystallographic studies reveal additional structure and suggest the rearrangement of the relative position of the domains as depicted at the left. A three-dimensional representation of the tRNA molecule is shown. *(Courtesy of Dr. S. H. Kim.)*

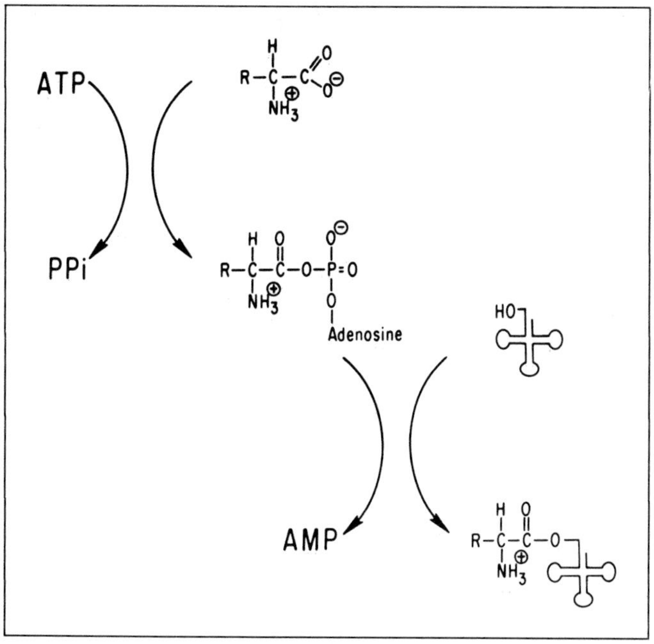

Fig. 7–18. Formation of aminoacyl-tRNA. The aminoacylation of tRNA molecules occurs in two steps, with an aminoacyl-AMP intermediate.

synthetase rapidly deacylates a valine esterified to $tRNA^{Ileu}$ to yield free valine and $tRNA^{Ileu}$. The combination of discriminatory abilities in the forward and reverse reactions of the tRNA synthetases yields a translation system that makes very few errors.

Genetic Code

A triplet code using four nucleotides can generate 64 (4^3) possible codons (Table 7–2). Three codons—UAA, UGA, and UAG—serve as termination signals and are referred to as *nonsense* codons (because they specify no amino acid). This leaves 61 codons for 20 amino acids. In spite of the fact that 61 codons must be recognized in a sensible way, fewer than 61 tRNA species are required for translation. This is because some tRNA molecules can recognize more than one codon, using the so-called *wobble* in the 3′ base of the codon. Table 7–3 lists the allowable base-pairing interactions between the 5′ base of the anticodon in tRNA and the 3′ base of the codon in mRNA. Included in Table 7–3 are two modified bases (inosine and 5-oxyacetic acid uridine) found in the anticodon of certain tRNAs. Like other modified bases in tRNA, these are produced enzymatically after transcription of the tRNA precursor. According to the wobble rules, a cell would require a minimum of 32 tRNAs to recognize the 61 codons for amino acids.

The wobble at the 3′ position of the codon does not decrease translational fidelity, because of the precise pairing required in the first two positions of the codon. An inspection of the genetic code in Table 7–2 reveals that the third position is relatively unimportant in amino acid coding. Evolution has found an economical way of using 64 possible codons to signal only 21 distinct instructions (20 different amino acids and *stop*). A two-base codon system could signal only 16 (4^2) different instructions and, therefore, would not be sufficient.

The rules of codon recognition do not eliminate the possibility that a single nucleotide sequence could contain overlapping (out-of-phase) reading frames for different proteins. In fact, exactly this situation is observed in numerous instances. In general, the regions of overlap are very small because of the obvious constraints on evolution when a single sequence codes for two proteins. The most extensive use of overlapping reading frames is found exactly where it would be expected—in certain bacterial viruses that need to conserve a very small size for successful reproduction (Chap. 60).

TABLE 7–2. NUCLEOSIDE SEQUENCES OF RNA CODONS AND CORRESPONDING AMINO ACIDS

1st Base	2nd Base: U	C	A	G	3rd Base
U	Phe	Ser	Tyr	Cys	U
	Phe	Ser	Tyr	Cys	C
	Leu	Ser	Ochre[a]	Opal[a]	A
	Leu	Ser	Amber[a]	Trp	G
C	Leu	Pro	His	Arg	U
	Leu	Pro	His	Arg	C
	Leu	Pro	Gln	Arg	A
	Leu	Pro	Gln	Arg	G
A	Ileu	Thr	Asn	Ser	U
	Ileu	Thr	Asn	Ser	C
	Ileu	Thr	Lys	Arg	A
	Met	Thr	Lys	Arg	G
G	Val	Ala	Asp	Gly	U
	Val	Ala	Asp	Gly	C
	Val	Ala	Glu	Gly	A
	Val	Ala	Glu	Gly	G

From Crick: Cold Spring Harbor Symp Quant Biol 31:1, 1966.
[a] Nonsense codon.

Three Phases of Translation

Initiation. As in the processes of replication and transcription, the initiation step in translation is the control point that modulates the overall efficiency of the process. Different mRNA molecules of *E. coli* can vary by more than 1000-fold

TABLE 7–3. CODON-ANTICODON BASE PAIRING PERMITTED BY WOBBLE AND EFFECT OF BASE MODIFICATION ON WOBBLE

5′ Base of Anticodon	3′ Base of Codon
A	U
C	G
U	A or G
G	C or U
I	U, C, or A
O^5U (5-oxyacetic acid uridine)	A, G, or U

in their efficiencies of translation, and thus the rate of synthesis of various proteins does not strictly correlate to the levels of their corresponding mRNA templates. This variation in translation efficiencies is dependent on complementary base pairing between the mRNA and the 3′ end of the 16S rRNA within the small ribosomal subunit. The 16S rRNA contains the sequence 5′-ACCUCC-3′, whereas the mRNA contains the complementary sequence, 5′-GGAGGU-3′. The latter is referred to as the *Shine-Dalgarno* sequence (after its discoverers) or ribosome binding site. An mRNA with the Shine-Dalgarno

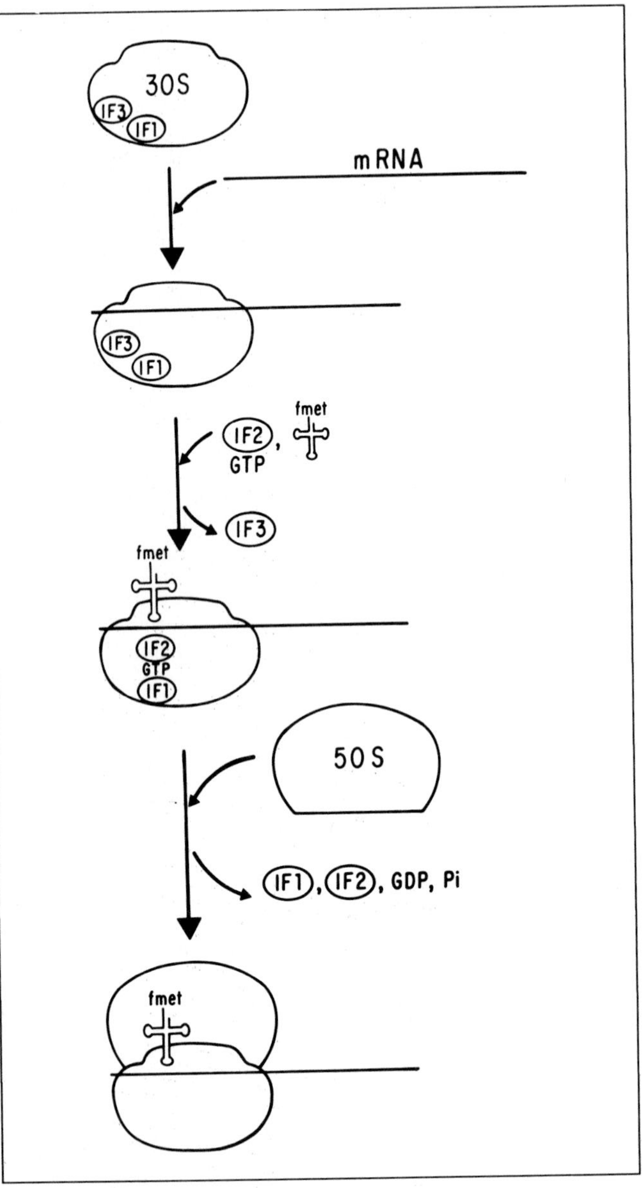

Fig. 7–19. Formation of a translation initiation complex. In the first step, the binding of mRNA to the 30S ribosomal subunit is dependent on IF3 and the ribosome binding site within the mRNA. IF2 promotes the binding of the initiator tRNA to the growing complex in the second step, and the initiation complex is then completed by the acquisition of the 50S ribosomal subunit.

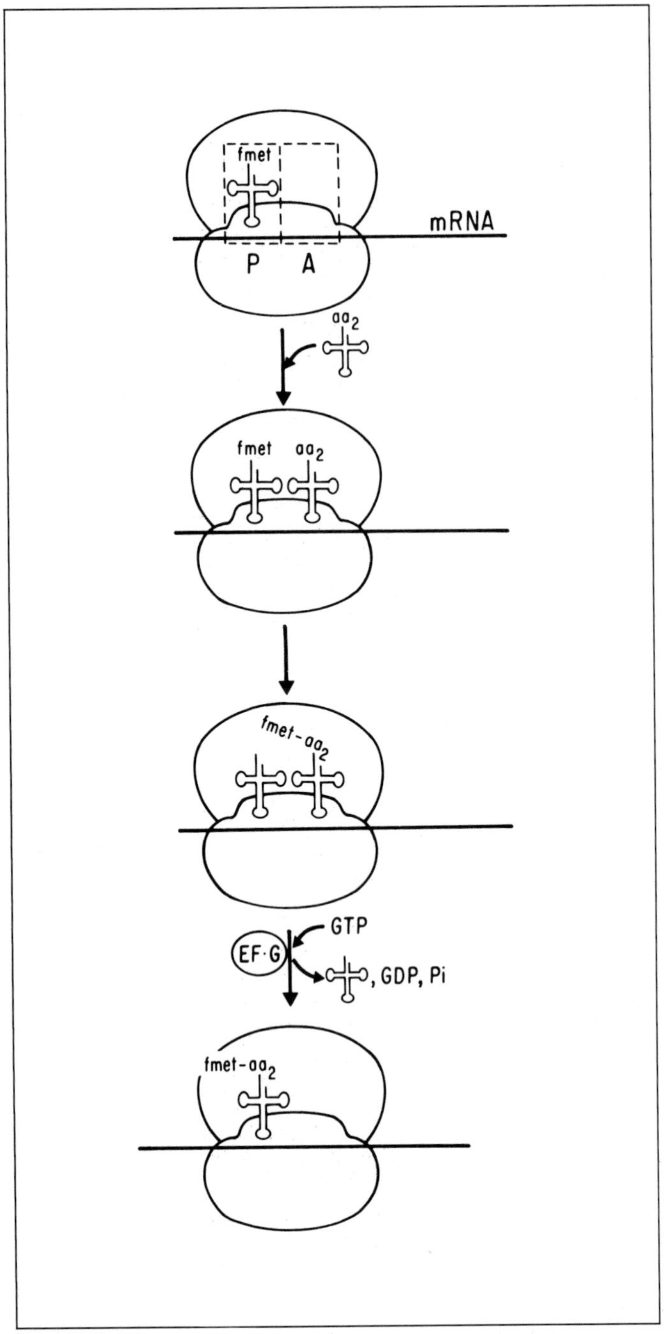

Fig. 7–20. The elongation cycle of translation. The ribosome has (at least) two tRNA binding sites, here denoted P and A (see text). After formation of the initiation complex (Fig. 7–19), the structure depicted at the top is obtained. The first step in the elongation cycle is the binding of the second aminoacyl-tRNA, corresponding to the second codon in the particular mRNA being translated. This binding is dependent on elongation factors Tu and Ts (Fig. 7–21). The growing polypeptide chain is transferred from the tRNA at the P site to that at the A site by a peptidyl transferase reaction. The last step involves the translocation of peptidyl-tRNA and mRNA with respect to the ribosome, and is dependent on elongation factor G and GTP hydrolysis. Repeated cycles of peptide bond formation occur by a repetition of this series of steps.

sequence located about seven bases upstream from an initiation codon is optimally recognized and translated with high efficiency. The large variation in mRNA translation efficiencies is generally dependent on sequence deviations that reduce complementarity to the 16S rRNA and on variations in the spacing between the Shine-Dalgarno sequence and the initiator codon. Other factors also influence the efficiency of translation of a particular message, but these are less well understood at present.

Protein synthesis in bacteria is initiated with a special amino acid, *N*-formylmethionine (fmet), which is specified by the codon AUG (and occasionally GUG). The specialized initiator tRNA ($tRNA_f^{Met}$) is first charged with methionine and then *N*-formylated by a specific transformylase that uses N^{10}-formyltetrahydrofolate as donor.

The assembly of mRNA and initiator tRNA into a functional translation complex occurs by the series of steps outlined in Figure 7–19. The initiation factor IF3 plays a direct role in the binding of mRNA to the 30S ribosomal subunit (step 1) and also maintains the 30S subunit free of the 50S until initiation is under way. Factor IF2 plays a crucial role in promoting the binding of charged $tRNA_f^{Met}$ to the 30S complex, and the binding (but not hydrolysis) of guanosine triphosphate (GTP) is required for this step (step 2). The IF2-dependent binding of initiator tRNA is aided by IF1 and results in the release of IF3. The final step in initiation is the association of the growing complex with the 50S ribosomal subunit. This results in the hydrolysis of the bound GTP by IF2 and then release of the remaining initiation factors (IF1 and IF2). The assembled complex after step 3 contains both 30S and 50S ribosomal subunits, mRNA, and initiator tRNA and is competent for elongation.

Elongation. Once the above initiation complex is formed, growth of the polypeptide chain occurs by the repetitive addition of amino acids in the elongation cycle. There are at least two binding sites on the ribosome for activated tRNA molecules, and these sites must be considered in the elongation cycle. The site from which the growing chain is transferred is called the P (peptidyl or donor) site, and the site for the incoming aminoacyl-tRNA, to which the chain is transferred, is called the A (acceptor) site (Fig. 7–20). At the beginning of each cycle, the P site contains either initiator fmet-tRNA (the first cycle) or peptidyl-tRNA (all subsequent cycles). The first step of the cycle is the binding of the incoming aminoacyl-tRNA to the A site. As soon as the two sites are appropriately occupied, transpeptidation transfers the peptidyl residue from the P site onto the aminoacyl-tRNA at the A site (step 2). Finally, translocation of the new peptidyl-tRNA from the A to the P site completes the cycle (step 3). This step involves several important movements: the deacylated tRNA must be ejected from the P site, and then both the mRNA and peptidyl-tRNA must translocate relative to the ribosome so that the next codon in the mRNA is available at the now vacant A site (Fig. 7–20). Each of these three steps is now considered in more detail.

The transfer of the incoming aminoacyl-tRNA to the A site of the ribosome (Fig. 7–20, step 1) is facilitated by elongation factors Tu and Ts (the designation T refers to *t*ransfer, while u and s refer to *u*nstable and *s*table to heat inactivation, respectively). These soluble factors participate in the cycle shown in Figure 7–21, with the overall objective of simply transferring the charged tRNA onto the ribosome. The native Tu-Ts complex is dissociated by the binding of GTP, and the nucleotide then remains associated with Tu.

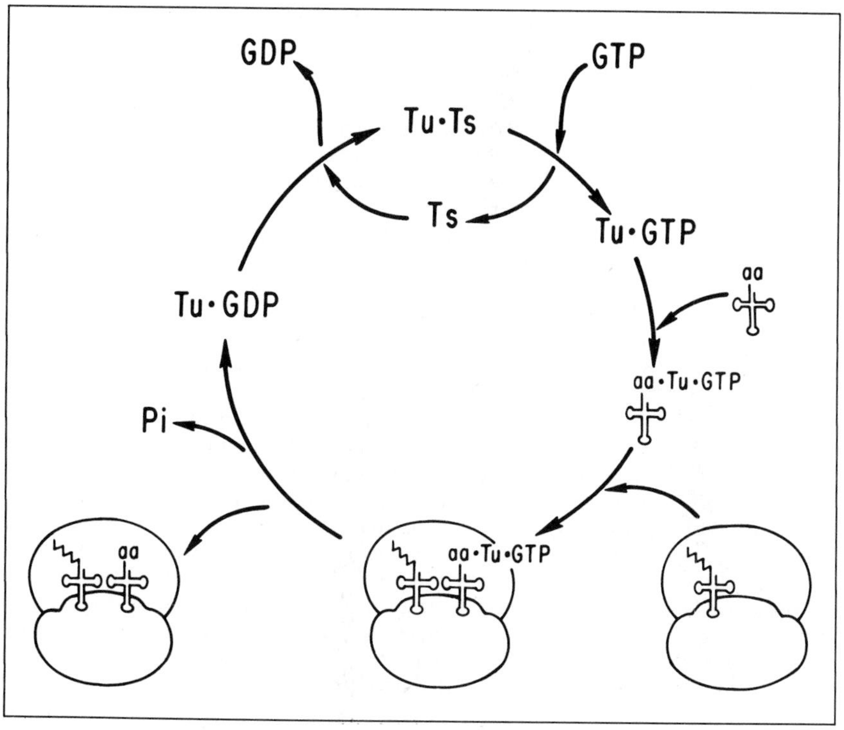

Fig. 7–21. Binding of aminoacyl-tRNA to the A site of the ribosome. During every cycle of elongation, elongation factor Tu facilitates the binding of the incoming aminoacyl tRNA to the ribosome (also see Fig. 7–20). The role of elongation factor Ts is to regenerate the active Tu-GTP complex from the inactive Tu-GDP complex.

The Tu-GTP complex is now competent to bind aminoacyl-tRNA, and this ternary complex then binds to the A site on the ribosome. Next, the hydrolysis of GTP allows dissociation of Tu from the ribosome in the form Tu-GDP. To complete the cycle, Ts displaces GDP to regenerate the native Tu-Ts complex for the next round. The only role of Ts is in the recycling of Tu; Ts does not effect the formation or cleavage of any covalent bonds and can be replaced in vitro with enzymes that directly phosphorylate Tu-GDP to Tu-GTP.

The peptidyl transferase activity (Fig. 7–20, step 2) is localized on the 50S ribosomal subunit, and no soluble factors are required for transpeptidation. Peptide bond formation occurs by uncoupling the carboxyl end of the growing polypeptide chain from the tRNA at the P site and joining it to the aminoacyl group linked to the tRNA at the A site.

The translocation that occurs in the third step (Fig. 7–20) requires the energy source GTP and a soluble protein, elongation factor G (for *G*TPase). The hydrolysis of the nucleotide to GDP and phosphate by elongation factor G is coupled to the various movements in an unknown manner. Notice that once translocation is complete, the translating complex is exactly equivalent to that at the beginning of step 1 (Fig. 7–20), except that the peptidyl-tRNA has been elongated by one amino acid residue and the mRNA has moved by one codon. All subsequent amino acids can therefore be added by a sequential repetition of the same steps in the elongation cycle.

Termination. Termination of polypeptide chain synthesis occurs when one of the nonsense codons in the mRNA comes into register with the A site on the ribosome. There is no tRNA for nonsense codons; instead they are recognized by RF1 and RF2 (*r*elease *f*actors). With the assistance of a third factor (RF3), these cause the peptidyl transferase activity to become a hydrolase, transferring the nascent chain from the peptidyl-tRNA at the P site to water. The completed protein is now free to leave the ribosome, and translation is complete.

Antibiotics and the Ribosome

The mechanism of action of antibiotics that block translation are considered in detail in Chapter 9, but several points that relate directly to ribosome structure and function are worth considering here. The ribosome is the target for the largest group of antibiotics, and most of these compounds block only the procaryotic ribosome. This alone implies that there are significant differences between the ribosomes of procaryotes and eucaryotes, even though a great part of the machinery and mechanisms of translation is quite highly conserved. In addition, certain antibiotics are effective only against either gram-positive or gram-negative organisms because of differences in ribosome structure even within the eubacterial kingdom. The ribosomes of eucaryotic mitochondria are more similar to procaryotic than to eucaryotic cytoplasmic ribosomes, presumably reflecting the evolutionary origin of mitochondria. As might be expected, the antibiotic sensitivities of mitochondrial ribosomes also resemble that of bacteria. It is possible that some of the side effects of antibiotic (e.g., chloramphenicol) therapy reflect an inhibition of mitochondrial translation in particular cell types.

The mechanism of one translational inhibitor deserves special mention here because it was instrumental in deciphering the mechanism of translation. Puromycin is an analogue of the terminal aminoacyl-adenosine portion of activated tRNA and competes with aminoacyl-tRNA for binding to the A site of the ribosome (Chap. 9). Once bound to the A site, puromycin becomes the acceptor for the peptidyl residue from the P site, and translation is thereby terminated. The action of puromycin provided the first evidence for two distinct binding sites on the ribosome. This compound illustrates well the structural analogue concept of antimetabolite action.

Regulation of Gene Expression

Bacteria use a stunning variety of mechanisms to control the expression of their several thousand genes. To a good first approximation, a particular gene product is produced only when it is needed, and in roughly the amount that is optimal for growth. Essentially every bacterial gene product studied is regulated at some step in its synthesis, and many are regulated by multiple mechanisms. Significant controls operate by altering the rates of transcription, mRNA stability, and translation. In addition, posttranslational regulation is achieved by modulating the processing, stability, and activity of proteins. As should become clear from the examples described below, regulatory mechanisms generally take advantage of low-molecular-weight compounds that signal the physiologic or environmental state of the cell. In addition, many regulatory mechanisms involve finely tuned feedback loops that provide only the amount of product necessary for a given condition.

Control of Transcription Initiation

Regulation of the extent of transcription is perhaps the most important level of control exerted in bacterial systems. As described in detail above, the extent of transcription is generally dependent on the initiation stage, namely, the recognition and utilization of promoter sequences by RNA polymerase holoenzyme. The most common form of transcriptional control is exerted by specific regulatory proteins that bind near or within the promoter sequence. Negative regulatory proteins block promoter usage, whereas positive regulatory proteins enhance promoter usage. Two specific elements in the genome are required for any such mechanism. First, there must be a gene coding for the regulatory protein. This element is said to be *trans*-acting, because the gene need not be near the promoter that it controls or even on the same DNA molecule. The second element is the specific nucleotide sequence to which the regulatory protein binds. This element must be in a particular location near or within the promoter that is being controlled, and thus it is called a *cis*-acting element. The formalization of these two elements was instrumental in approaching control mechanisms, because mutations that destroyed a particular form of control could be easily classified into one of the two categories.

Operons

Negative Regulation in *lac* Operon. The term *operon* was first coined by Jacob and Monod to describe a group of adjacent genes of related function that are coordinately regulated. They were studying three genes that encode enzymes involved in the utilization of lactose, namely, β-galactosidase, galactoside permease, and galactoside transacetylase. The simultaneous control of these three products is achieved by having all three genes organized into one transcription unit, with a polygenic mRNA and a single promoter (Fig. 7–22). The *cis*-acting element of the *lac* operon is called the *lac* operator, and it overlaps the *lac* promoter sequence. The *trans*-acting element is the *lac* repressor, coded for by the nearby *lacI* gene. The repressor responds to a series of compounds related to lactose, including several synthetic derivatives that are experimentally useful. These compounds, called inducers, bind to the *lac* repressor and change its affinity for the operator. In the absence of inducer, the repressor binds to the operator in a site-specific manner. This blocks the activity of RNA polymerase at the *lac* promoter, probably by preventing RNA polymerase binding (Fig. 7–22). In the presence of inducer, the repressor can no longer bind to the operator, and transcription of the *lac* operon occurs. This mechanism ensures that the *lac* operon will be transcribed only when lactose or a related compound is present, and the economy of this arrangement is obvious. A second important control that operates on the *lac* operon is described below in the section on Global Regulatory Networks.

In the case of the *lac* operon, the lactose-related compounds that bind to repressor comprise the physiologic signals that mediate gene control. The binding of a signal molecule causes the *lac* repressor to lose its affinity for the operator. This arrangement is well suited for a catabolic pathway, where the presence of the relevant compound should induce the pathway. However, in anabolic pathways, the presence of the end product would be a convenient signal to turn the pathway off rather than induce it. This is accomplished by inverting the function of the intracellular signal. For example, the tryptophan biosynthetic operon is controlled (in part) by a repressor that binds to the operator only when the repressor is complexed with the signal, tryptophan. Thus synthesis of the enzymes needed to produce more tryptophan occurs only when tryptophan is limiting, and the pathway is turned off when tryptophan is in excess (also see below).

Negative Regulation by DNA Looping. The model for *lac* operon regulation described above is conceptually pleasing; the repressor protein simply binds to an operator site that overlaps the promoter, and the presence of bound repressor prevents binding of RNA polymerase to the promoter. However, several well-studied repressors cannot act in this simple way because they exert their action by binding to sites that do not overlap the promoter. Recent analyses of these systems have thereby challenged an overly simplistic view of negative regulation.

Genetic and physical studies of the *gal* operon of *E. coli* have revealed not one but two operators that are important for repressor action. One site is located just upstream of the promoter region, whereas the second is centered more than 50 base pairs *downstream* from the start of transcription. In spite of these locations, a mutation that destroys either repressor-binding site prevents negative regulation. How can these two sites, separated from each other by more than 100 base pairs, cooperate to repress transcription of the *gal* operon? A partial answer was provided by the finding that *gal* repressor molecules bound at the two sites interact to form a stable DNA loop. The approximately 100–base pair DNA loop, which represents a distinct topologic domain, includes the *gal* promoter region. The constraints of bending the DNA around into a tight loop alters the structure of the intervening DNA, and this altered structure is probably responsible for repression. Perhaps surprisingly, the binding of *gal* repressor and formation of the DNA loop do not prevent RNA polymerase binding to the promoter region. Although the mechanism of repression is not currently understood, it appears that transcription is repressed by blocking some step after polymerase binding. For example, the altered DNA structure referred to above may prevent open complex formation, or it may inhibit the movement of RNA polymerase as it begins transcription in the promoter region.

Repression of several other *E. coli* operons, including *ara* and *deo,* is also dependent on multiple repressor binding sites and DNA looping. Even the prototype for negative regulation, the *lac* operon, contains two additional operator sequences downstream of the *lac* promoter. These two sites bind repressor rather weakly and are not absolutely required for repres-

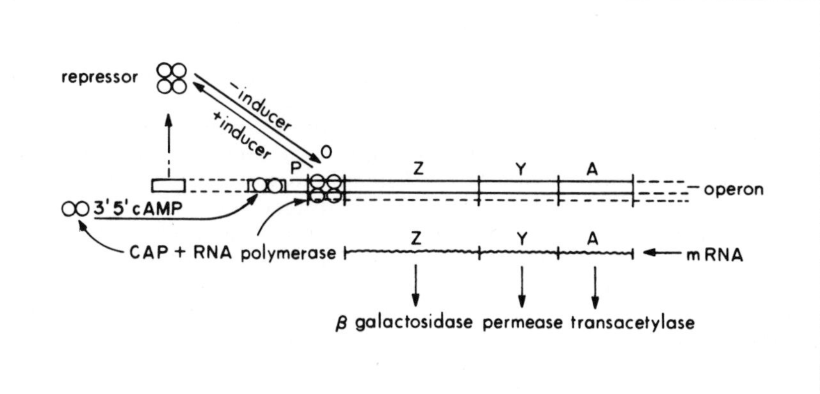

Fig. 7–22. The lactose operon. The structural genes for β-galactosidase, galactoside permease, and galactoside transacetylase are *lacZ, lacY,* and *lacA* (Z, Y, and A, respectively). *lacP* (P) is the promoter, the binding site for RNA polymerase. *lacO* (O) is the operator region, the binding site for the repressor, which is encoded by gene *lacI.* CAP is the catabolite activator protein, which in the cAMP-liganded form is required for the maximal expression of the *lac* operon.

sion, but nonetheless they appear to contribute to the efficiency of repression. The formation of DNA loops by the binding of regulatory proteins to nonadjacent sites may well be a general and important aspect of regulation in bacterial systems. Similar DNA looping is likely involved in the action of enhancers and silencers in eucaryotic systems, where regulatory sites can be thousands of base pairs from the promoters that they affect.

Positively Controlled Operons. The mechanisms discussed above are negative in the sense that a particular repressor protein blocks transcription of an operon under a given condition. This is probably the most common form of control of gene expression in bacteria, but positive control mechanisms also exist. One example is in the regulation of the *mal* operons, which code for seven proteins involved in maltose uptake and catabolism. In this system, the control protein (the product of the *malT* gene) directly stimulates transcription by RNA polymerase, but only when maltose is present. The *malT* gene product is therefore called an activator protein. Some regulatory proteins can act both as an activator and as a repressor; the *araC* protein controls the arabinose operon (*araBAD*) in this way. Other important examples of positive control function in global regulatory networks (see below).

A Survey of Bacterial Operons. The concept of the operon has now been extended to include both monogenic and polygenic arrangements, regardless of the functions of the gene products. Like the operons described above, many polygenic *E. coli* operons encode proteins of closely related function. For example, the *his* operon specifies nine enzymes involved in histidine biosynthesis, whereas the *ilv* operon encodes four enzymes involved in the isoleucine-valine synthetic pathway. As in the case of the *lac* operon, a single control mechanism can modulate several products in a given biochemical pathway.

Some other operons contain genes whose functions are not as closely related. The streptomycin operon encodes two (small subunit) ribosomal proteins and two translation elongation factors, and all four products are involved in the mechanism of translation. The β operon encodes four (large subunit) ribosomal proteins and two of the subunits of RNA polymerase, and its products are involved in both transcription and translation. Similarly, the σ operon encodes a crucial protein for each of the processes of translation (S21), replication (DNA primase), and transcription (σ). These two mixed-function operons presumably coordinate the cells' overall levels of macromolecular synthesis. The σ operon seems particularly interesting in this context, because each of the three products acts at a very early stage in their respective pathways. A general lesson of this chapter is that biologic processes are regulated at these early stages, and thus the expression of the σ operon seems particularly important in coordinating DNA, RNA, and protein synthesis. In spite of attempts to rationalize the relatedness of the functions of a given operon, some other collections of genes within an operon may be nothing more than evolutionary accidents.

Many operons contain multiple promoters, increasing the possible number of regulatory mechanisms. In certain cases, an additional promoter is even found between genes of an operon. This allows a subset of the genes in the operon to be expressed independently of the others, extending the regulatory possibilities even further.

Global Regulatory Networks

The organization of genes into operons is a common mechanism used by bacteria to coordinate production of a set of gene products. At a higher level, the expression of a series of operons is often coordinated by a common control mechanism; such a collection of operons is called a regulon. Many regulons include genes for only a single metabolic pathway. The *araC* regulatory protein is required for expression of at least three operons involved in the uptake and utilization of arabinose. All that is necessary for such a regulon is that the same *cis*-acting control sequence (e.g., the operator) be used in the promoter region of each of the relevant operons. Because the regulatory protein is freely diffusible, its gene need not be duplicated for the protein to operate on multiple operons.

A most important subset of regulons contains operons with gene products that function in several different pathways; these are called global regulons. The value of a global regulon is that it can coordinate a unified response to a gross change in environmental conditions or cellular physiology. Several important global regulons are now described in some detail.

Catabolite Activation. Perhaps the best understood global regulon is the catabolite activation system. When *E. coli* is grown in the presence of glucose or other sugars that can be efficiently metabolized, it will not synthesize enzymes for the catabolism of sugars that are used with lower efficiency (lactose, galactose, arabinose, etc.). This system is dependent on the catabolite activator protein (CAP), which is a positive activator that is required for the transcription of a series of operons involved in utilization of these other sugars. For example, the *lac* and *ara* operons that were discussed above both require activation by CAP for efficient transcription. For historical reasons, the catabolite system is often called catabolite repression, even though it is primarily a positive control system.

As with the other regulatory proteins discussed, CAP responds to a specific chemical signal, in this case 3′,5′-cyclic AMP (cAMP). In the presence of cAMP, the CAP protein binds to the appropriate control sequences near the promoters that it regulates and, in so doing, enhances transcription by RNA polymerase. (See Fig. 7–22 for an example in the *lac* operon.) In the absence of cAMP, CAP is unable to bind to these promoters and transcription is reduced or absent. The crystal structure of CAP complexed with cAMP shows that the nucleotide binds in the amino-terminal domain of the protein, whereas site-specific DNA binding is effected by the carboxy-terminal domain. The DNA-binding region contains a structure that is used by many regulatory proteins to bind DNA in a sequence-specific manner: two α-helices separated by a tight turn. When the protein binds to DNA, the first α-helix sits above and the second within the major groove of DNA at the recognition site. Hydrogen bonds between the second α-helix and the edges of the base pairs facing the major groove are crucial for the sequence recognition.

The CAP binding site is located at various distances upstream of CAP-regulated promoters. In a manner that may be related to these variable distances, CAP appears to play different roles in stimulating transcription from these promoters. There is evidence that in certain cases CAP directly interacts with RNA polymerase by means of protein-protein contacts. In other cases, CAP appears to change the local DNA structure (for example, helping RNA polymerase to denature the promoter DNA during the closed- to open-complex transition).

As noted above, the intracellular signal that is required for CAP action is cAMP. The concentration of cAMP is modulated by the metabolism of the cell. When glucose (or another very efficient energy source) is available, the concentration of cAMP is low so that other catabolic operons are not expressed. Conversely, when glucose becomes depleted, cAMP levels rise; this allows operons for the catabolism of poorer energy sources to be induced by CAP action. Superimposed on the CAP system are the specific regulatory systems described above. For example, the *lac* operon is maximally active when lactose is present (to inactivate the *lac* repressor) and glucose is absent (to increase cAMP and thereby activate CAP) (Fig. 7–22). The modulation of cAMP levels by glucose appears to be by inhibition of the enzyme adenyl cyclase, which converts ATP to cAMP.

Alternate σ Subunits. Several important global regulatory networks employ a very direct strategy, namely, the replacement of a subunit of RNA polymerase. Recall that the σ subunit has a crucial role in the recognition and utilization of promoter sequences (see above). When the standard vegetative σ subunit is replaced with a novel one, an entirely different set of promoter sequences are recognized by RNA polymerase. Replacement of σ subunit is involved in several important physiologic responses, including sporulation (studied in *Bacillus subtilis*), the heat-shock response, and nitrogen metabolism. In addition, several bacteriophage regulate the expression of their genes by replacing the host σ subunit with one of their own (Chap. 60).

Vegetative cells of *B. subtilis* contain at least five different σ factors. The predominant form, called σ^A, directs RNA polymerase recognition of promoter sequences indistinguishable from those used by *E. coli* RNA polymerase. The four minor σ factors present in vegetative cells direct RNA polymerase to alternate promoters and appear to have a variety of functions. One of these, σ^H, is required for the expression of certain sporulation-specific genes early in the developmental process of sporulation.

Following the action of σ^H, the expression of sporulation genes is guided, in part, by the function of four additional σ factors found only in sporulating cells. These four proteins are produced sequentially, directing an orderly program of gene expression. Interestingly, two of the σ factors are produced only in particular locations: σ^K directs transcription of spore coat proteins in the mother-cell compartment, whereas σ^G directs gene expression in the forespore.

The *heat-shock* response is another example of a global regulon that uses a replacement σ subunit. On exposure to high temperature or certain other noxious conditions, *E. coli* induces a set of at least 17 different proteins involved in diverse pathways of cellular physiology. Although the detailed molecular mechanism of induction is not known, the heat-shock response is mediated by the product of gene *htpR* (also called *rpoH*), which is the replacement σ subunit. One protein induced by the heat-shock response, the product of the *dnaK* gene, is also involved in regulation of the response. The *dnaK* protein is one of the most conserved elements in all of biology—the corresponding protein in *Drosophila* or human cells is about 50% homologous to that of *E. coli.* In addition, the heat-shock response itself is highly conserved throughout the biologic world. The full significance of the heat-shock response for cell survival is not clear at present, but the remarkable conservation implies that the response is of fundamental importance.

Signal Transduction in Bacteria. Signal transduction by means of protein phosphorylation has recently been shown to be an important regulatory mechanism in bacteria. Although the details have not been fully worked out in each system, signal transduction plays an important role in nitrogen and phosphate deprivation, response to osmolarity changes, chemotaxis, sporulation, and expression of certain virulence genes. In each case, two regulatory proteins have been identified. One is a *sensor protein* that evaluates the physiologic environment, either directly or with the participation of other proteins. Under the appropriate conditions, the sensor protein acts as a specific protein kinase, phosphorylating the *effector protein.* In most of the systems, phosphorylation of the effector protein converts it into a positive activator of transcription for a collection of appropriate promoters. The diverse systems were first linked together by means of protein homologies: the sensor proteins all share regions of strong homology, as do the effector proteins.

Perhaps the best-studied case involves the regulation of genes for nitrogen assimilation. Submillimolar concentrations of ammonia result in the transcriptional activation of several genes, including *glnA.* This gene encodes glutamine synthetase, which is the major enzyme for assimilating ammonia at these low concentrations. The regulation of *glnA* and other genes in the regulon is achieved by an intricate mechanism involving several proteins. Focusing on only the signal transduction involved in nitrogen regulation, the product of the *ntrB* gene is the sensor protein and the product of the *ntrC* gene is the effector. The *ntrB* protein phosphorylates the *ntrC* protein under conditions of nitrogen depletion, but it dephosphorylates the same protein when nitrogen is plentiful. Thus, the *ntrB* protein acts as both a protein kinase and a protein phosphatase. Two additional proteins are involved in sensing nitrogen availability and modulating the activity of the *ntrB* kinase/phosphatase. The *ntrC* effector protein is a positive activator of transcription only when it is phosphorylated, and therefore it is functional only when nitrogen is limiting. The *ntrC* protein binds to and activates transcription from a collection of sites that are upstream of the regulated *glnA* promoter. These binding sites thereby resemble eucaryotic transcriptional *enhancers,* which also allow activation of transcription from a distance.

Transcriptional activation of *glnA* and other nitrogen-regulated genes also involves an alternative σ subunit. As in the other cases of σ subunit replacement discussed above, nitrogen-regulated promoters have unique sequences recognized by RNA polymerase associated with the alternate σ subunit.

Stringent Response. The last global regulatory network to be considered is the so-called *stringent* response. When wild-type *E. coli* is starved for amino acids, numerous cellular activities are altered in a complex manner. Perhaps most notably, the rate of rRNA and tRNA synthesis decreases and the synthesis of many amino acid biosynthetic enzymes is induced. Thus, the stringent response prevents the accumulation of translational machinery, which is not needed in the absence of amino acids, and increases the production of amino acids by the induced biosynthetic enzymes. Once enough amino acids are produced, the stringent response ceases and normal vegetative levels of transcription resume.

The intracellular signal for the stringent response is the unusual nucleotide 3′-diphosphate 5′-diphosphate guanosine (ppGpp). Amino acid starvation results in the production of ppGpp by an enzyme called the stringent factor, which is the product of gene *relA*. The stringent factor is ribosome-associated and its activity is triggered by the binding of uncharged tRNA to the translation machinery; this is the basis for its ability to sense amino acid starvation. An additional protein, the product of gene *spoT*, degrades ppGpp so that the stringent response can be terminated when amino acids become available. The synthesis of rRNA and tRNA is also modulated by the growth rate of the cell, but it is not yet clear whether this modulation also involves ppGpp and stringent factor.

During the stringent response, the guanosine nucleotide can modulate the activity of RNA polymerase in either a positive or a negative sense, depending on the promoter sequence. Promoters for rRNA and tRNA, which are negatively regulated, contain a GC-rich region between the −10 consensus sequence of the promoter and the transcription start site (+1). On the other hand, positively controlled promoters also appear to have unique features, such as the lack of a consensus A residue in the fourth position of the −10 sequence (5′-TATAAT-3′). In spite of these hints from the promoter sequences, there is currently no clear understanding of how ppGpp modulates RNA polymerase activity at these various promoters.

Control of Transcription Termination

The regulatory mechanisms considered above modulate the frequency of transcription initiation, but transcription termination is also used as a point of regulation. As described above (in the discussion on Transcription), RNA polymerase terminates synthesis at two classes of specific nucleotide sequences, ρ-dependent and ρ-independent terminators. Important regulatory mechanisms that prevent recognition of terminator sequences have been documented for a variety of operons. The best understood examples, involving amino acid biosynthetic operons, use a unique mechanism called *attenuation*. Interestingly, some of the operons that are subject to attenuation are also regulated by repression of transcription initiation, providing dual control over expression.

Attenuation. Antitermination of amino acid biosynthetic operons depends strictly on the fact that transcription and translation are coupled in bacterial systems. The example of the tryptophan operon is described here, but several other amino acid biosynthetic operons are controlled by analogous mechanisms.

The transcript synthesized from the *trp* promoter contains a short leader region that precedes the enzyme-coding portion of the transcript. The control elements for attenuation are all contained in this leader region (Fig. 7–23). The first element is a short coding sequence for a peptide of 14 amino acids with two consecutive tryptophan codons in a critical location. As described below, translation of this leader polypeptide is central to the switch that determines whether attenuation will occur. The other elements necessary for attenuation are a series of complementary sequences that can participate in alternative stem-loop structures in the mRNA. Four related sequences, designated 1 through 4, can base pair to form stem loops 1:2, 2:3, and 3:4 (Fig. 7–23). The transcription terminator consists of stem loop 3:4, along with a series of U residues that immediately follows segment 4. Thus, the terminator has exactly the structure of a ρ-independent transcription terminator.

During the initial stages of transcription, RNA polymerase synthesizes until it reaches the end of segment 2 (Fig. 7–24, top). The formation of stem loop 1:2 in the nascent transcript then causes RNA polymerase to pause temporarily. Pausing at stem loop 1:2 is critical for attenuation, because it allows a period of time for a ribosome to recognize the ribosome binding site of the nascent transcript. As the ribosome subsequently synthesizes the leader peptide, it enters segment 1 and thereby disrupts stem loop 1:2. This disruption eliminates the pause structure, and therefore RNA poly·erase can now proceed to synthesize the transcript, with the riuosome following close behind.

When tryptophan is in excess (Fig. 7–24, bottom right), the leader peptide is efficiently translated and the ribosome traverses the entire leader peptide region. This results in formation of the transcription terminator (stem loop 3:4), and therefore ıranscription of tl·e *trp* operon is aborted. Formation

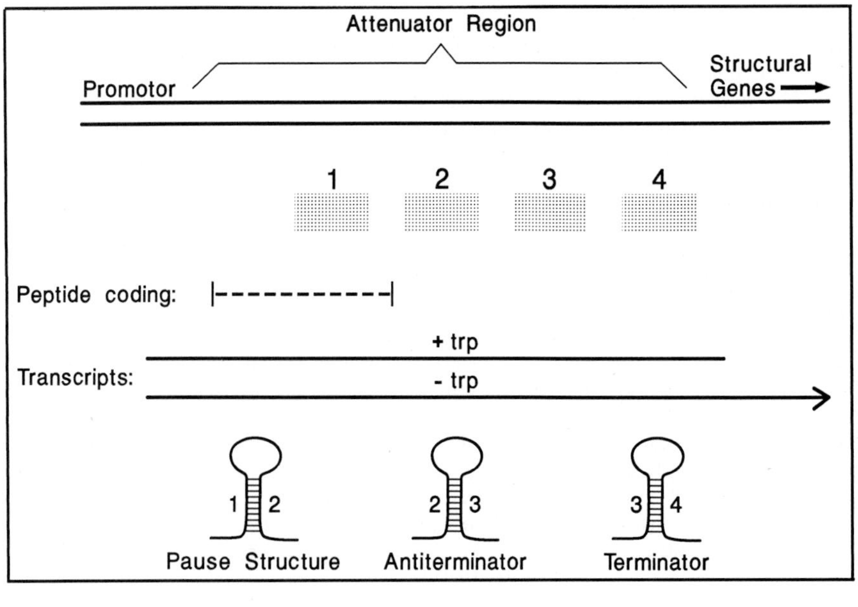

Fig. 7–23. The *trp* operon attenuator region. Transcription of the *trp* operon is regulated by the function of the attenuator region just downstream from the promoter. The attenuator region contains four related sequences, labelled *1* through *4*, which can base-pair in three alternative configurations (the pause structure, the antiterminator, and the terminator). The peptide-coding region (dashed line) overlaps sequence *1*. The mRNA transcripts formed in the presence or absence of tryptophan (+*trp* and −*trp*, respectively) are also shown. *(Adapted from Landick and Yanofsky: In Neidhardt et al (eds):* Escherichia coli *and* Salmonella typhimurium. *Cellular and Molecular Biology. American Society for Microbiology, 1987.)*

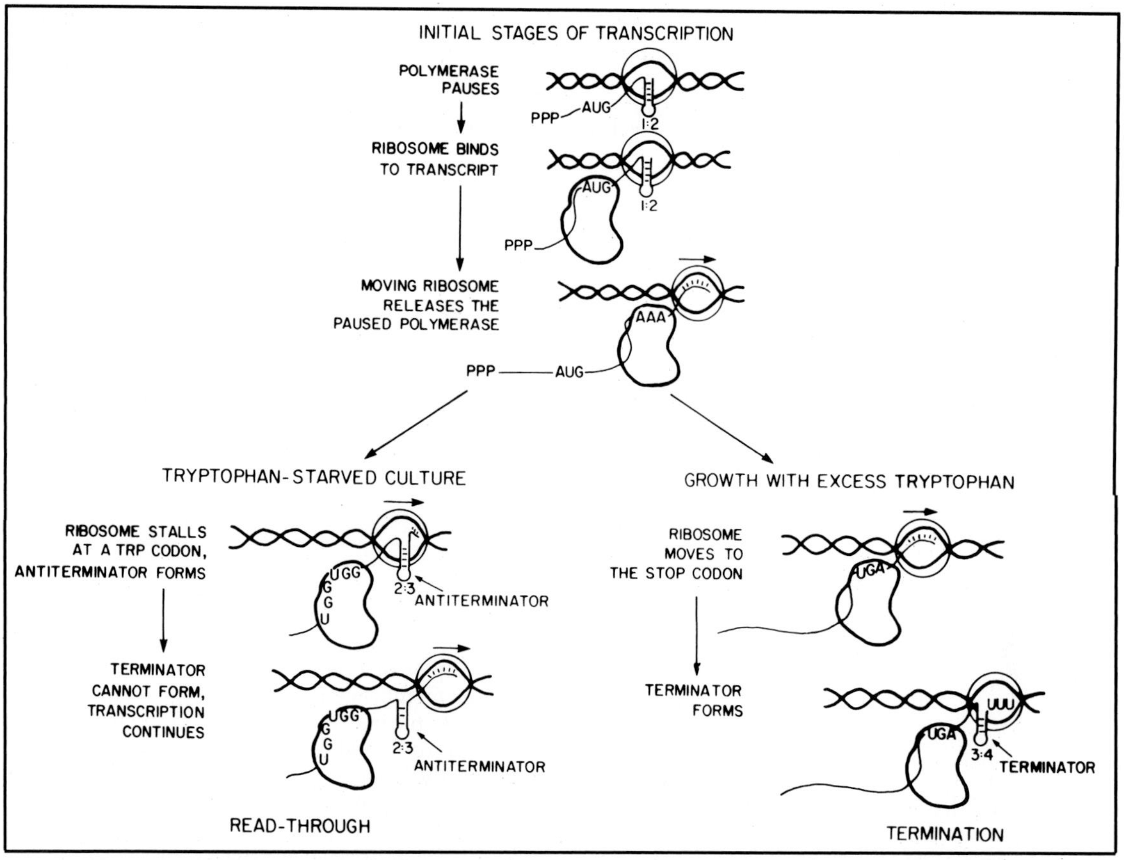

Fig. 7–24. Model for attenuation of *trp* operon transcription. *(From Landick and Yanofsky: In Neidhardt et al (eds):* Escherichia coli *and* Salmonella typhimurium. *Cellular and Molecular Biology. American Society for Microbiology, 1987.)*

of the terminator structure may be promoted by either of two configurations. First, when the ribosome is located at the translational stop codon, it covers part of segment 2 and thereby blocks formation of 2:3, which in turn allows formation of 3:4. Second, when the ribosome dissociates from the nascent transcript, the combination of both stem loops 1:2 and 3:4 can form, which is energetically favored over formation of just stem loop 2:3.

When tryptophan is the limiting amino acid (Fig. 7–24, bottom left), the ribosome stalls when it reaches the consecutive tryptophan codons in the leader peptide sequence. These codons are arranged so that the stalled ribosome occludes only segment 1. Stem loop 2:3, the antiterminator, probably forms even before segment 4 is transcribed by RNA polymerase. The formation of stem loop 2:3 prevents formation of the terminator 3:4, and the terminator is therefore inactive. Transcription of the remainder of the operon occurs, and tryptophan biosynthetic enzymes are produced in response to the shortage of tryptophan.

Other amino acid biosynthetic operons controlled by attenuation function in much the same manner as the *trp* operon, except that the leader peptide is rich in codons for the appropriate amino acid. This provides the requisite specificity so that a shortage of one particular amino acid leads to induction of biosynthetic enzymes for only that compound. The nature of the specificity has been demonstrated directly. Replacement of four leucine codons with threonine codons in the *Salmonella typhimurium leu* operon attenuator leads to regulation of the operon by threonine deprivation.

Control of Translation

As described above, the intrinsic rate of translation of different coding sequences can vary more than 1000-fold depending on the quality of the ribosome binding site in the message. In several well-documented situations, regulation of the efficiency of translation of a given mRNA constitutes an important mechanism for control of gene expression. The unifying characteristic of translational control appears to be occlusion of the ribosome binding site, either by specific protein binding or by base-pairing with another segment of RNA.

Feedback Regulation of Ribosomal Protein Synthesis. An important example of translational control is the repression of ribosomal protein synthesis. Many of the ribosomal proteins bind to particular regions of ribosomal RNA during the assembly of ribosomes. For each of the operons encoding ribosomal proteins, one of the proteins encoded by that operon is a translational repressor for the entire operon. The mechanism of repression involves the binding of repressor to a region of the mRNA that includes the ribosome binding site. Once the repressor is bound, that particular mRNA is no longer translated. The basis for repressor binding to mRNA is quite elegant—the mRNA binding site closely resembles the

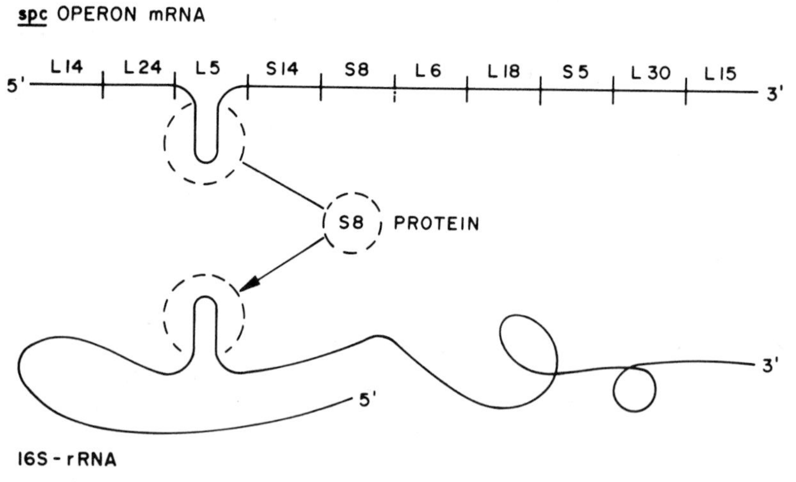

Fig. 7–25. Feedback regulation of ribosomal protein synthesis in *E. coli.* The competition of mRNA and 16S rRNA for protein S8 governs the rate of translation of the L5 and all downstream genes of the *spc* operon. It is not known whether the upstream L14 and L24 genes are regulated by a similar mechanism.

binding site for that protein on ribosomal RNA (Fig. 7–25). The repressor prefers binding to rRNA, and thus in the presence of free rRNA translation is not repressed. Once all free rRNA is complexed with ribosomal protein, repression ensues and production of ribosomal proteins is blocked. This mechanism guarantees that ribosomal proteins will be produced only when there is free ribosomal RNA to allow ribosome assembly, and thereby the synthesis of ribosomal proteins is coupled to that of rRNA. In those operons with multiple ribosomal protein genes, translational repression of the first gene is sufficient to regulate all downstream genes. This is due (at least in part) to a tight coupling between translation of adjacent genes in the operon. A ribosome traveling down the mRNA translates each of the genes and does not dissociate until it reaches the 3′ end of the polygenic mRNA.

Inducible Resistance to Erythromycin. The control of translational efficiency by alternate secondary structures in the mRNA has been documented in bacteriophage systems (Chap. 60) and in the induction of erythromycin resistance in *Staphylococcus aureus* and *B. subtilis.* The latter case resembles the mechanism of attenuation described above, except that it is strictly a translational phenomenon. As in attenuation, a leader peptide and alternative secondary structures are present at the 5′ end of the mRNA. When the leader peptide is efficiently translated, the secondary structure of the mRNA occludes ribosome binding to the initiator region of the drug-resistance coding sequence. However, when low levels of erythromycin are present, the ribosomes stall within the leader peptide region. This prevents the base-pairing associated with occlusion of the ribosome binding site, and thus the drug-resistance protein is translated. The net result is that erythromycin resistance is inducible by erythromycin.

Regulation by Antisense RNA. A novel set of regulatory phenomena has recently been uncovered in which the translation of a particular bacterial protein is efficiently and specifically repressed by RNA molecules that are complementary to the mRNA for that protein. A useful example to illustrate the principles of regulation by *antisense RNA* is that of the *E. coli* outer membrane porins. The *E. coli* chromosome encodes two major porins, the products of genes *ompC* and *ompF.* Although the total amount of outer membrane porin is constant, the relative proportions of the *ompC* and *ompF* gene products vary considerably, depending on the osmolarity of the growth medium. The inverse relationship between expression of *ompC* and *ompF* is effected by an antisense RNA that inhibits translation of the *ompF* mRNA. The antisense RNA is complementary to the 5′ end of the *ompF* mRNA and inhibits *ompF* translation by base pairing with the ribosome binding site of that message. The inverse correlation between production of *ompC* and *ompF* proteins is the result of coordinate expression of *ompC* mRNA and the *ompF*-antisense RNA. These two RNAs are synthesized (in opposite directions) from the same region of DNA, and their levels of transcription are coordinated by a complex regulatory pathway. When *ompC* transcription is induced, the *ompF*-antisense RNA is produced in large amounts and effectively represses translation of *ompF.* The important principle is that an RNA molecule with a sequence complementary to a particular mRNA can block translation of that message.

There are now several other well-documented cases of regulation by antisense RNA, including the control of Tn*10* transposase protein, autoregulation of the synthesis of catabolite activator protein, and control of DNA replication in certain bacterial plasmids. In addition to its intrinsic interest, the discovery of antisense RNA has led to much excitement regarding the development of artificial systems. With the use of modern recombinant DNA methods (Chap. 8), the complement of virtually any mRNA can be fused to promoter sequences to produce an artificial antisense RNA for that particular gene. Transcription of the antisense RNA in vivo can effectively block translation of the corresponding mRNA. This creates the potential for regulating the activity of any gene product, and this potential is now being realized in both procaryotic and eucaryotic cells. The possible adaptations of antisense RNA systems to provide immunity to infecting viruses, and as a general tool in future gene therapy, holds great promise.

Posttranslational Regulation

All the regulatory mechanisms described above alter the concentration of particular gene products in response to changing conditions. The combination of these regulatory schemes makes macromolecular synthesis quite economical—most proteins are produced in roughly the amounts required for optimal growth. However, these mechanisms are limited in several important ways. First, they cannot provide a fine level of control over metabolic pathways, particularly when several pathways overlap or branch. If one enzyme is used in the production of two important compounds, regulation of only the synthesis of that enzyme cannot differentially modulate production of the two compounds. Second, regulation of synthesis of enzymes can result in a sluggish response because most proteins are relatively long-lived. When bacteria are growing in the absence of some amino acid, they will contain all the biosynthetic enzymes for that pathway. If the amino acid suddenly becomes available, the synthesis of those enzymes will cease, but the preexisting enzymes will remain until they are either diluted out by growth or destroyed by proteolysis. During the intervening time, the cells would needlessly continue to synthesize the amino acid. All living cells have developed elaborate mechanisms to avoid these and other problems by directly modulating the activities of enzymes after their synthesis. These posttranslational mechanisms are particularly important in regulating the flow of the numerous overlapping biochemical pathways, both anabolic and catabolic. The following section provides a brief overview of such mechanisms; more complete accounts can be found among the references listed at the end of this chapter.

Protein Degradation

The mechanisms of regulation of intracellular proteases are largely unknown, but they presumably contribute to posttranslational control. *E. coli* cells contain at least eight different proteases, including the *lon* protease, an ATP-dependent enzyme that apparently degrades abnormal proteins (including damaged and mutant proteins). Judging from the limited information currently available, these proteases probably play many important roles in the regulation of gene expression.

A few cases of protease induction have been examined in some detail. The first is the induction of protease activities during the heat-shock response. One of the conditions that can trigger this response is the production of abnormal proteins, and high temperatures may generally lead to denaturation of cellular proteins. Thus degradation of abnormal and denatured proteins may be an important function of the heat-shock response. The *lon* protease is induced to a high level during the heat-shock response, although it is also produced at a lower level in normal growing *E. coli* cells. In addition, several other proteins induced by the heat-shock response are involved in protein degradation by a pathway independent of the *lon* protease.

A second example occurs during sporulation of *B. subtilis*. The process of endospore formation requires the synthesis of many new proteins and a drastic change in the overall protein composition of the cell (Chap. 5). To accomplish this massive replacement, induced proteases degrade a large fraction of the vegetative cellular proteins.

A third case involves the SOS response, which is triggered by a posttranslational mechanism. As will be described in more detail in Chapter 8, the *recA* protein of bacterial cells is a very specific protease that is active only when the cells have sustained DNA damage. The protease activity appears to be induced by the binding of short DNA oligomers and results in the destruction of a crucial repressor. The inactivation of the repressor, in turn, results in the transcriptional induction of a variety of cellular proteins that repair DNA damage and inhibit cell division to allow time for repair functions. Some of these proteins must be destroyed when the repair is complete, or the cell could not return to normal growth. Interestingly, the *lon* protease participates in this step, degrading some of the induced proteins to terminate the SOS response.

Covalent Modification of Proteins

The strategy of altering enzyme activity by covalent modification is used extensively in eucaryotic cells; phosphorylation by protein kinases is only one of several classes of regulatory mechanisms. In contrast, bacterial cells have thus far presented only a few examples of enzyme regulation by covalent modification, but many others may be waiting to be uncovered.

As described above in the section on Signal Transduction in Bacteria, the synthesis of glutamine synthetase is regulated at the level of transcription initiation by covalent modification of a regulatory protein. In addition, the activity of glutamine synthetase is modulated by means of covalent modification in response to nitrogen availability. When nitrogen is readily available, glutamine synthetase is inactivated by the adenylylation of a specific tyrosine residue of the enzyme. Adenylylation is controlled by an enzyme that catalyzes both the forward and the reverse (de-adenylylation) reactions, and this enzyme is regulated by nitrogen availability.

Feedback Regulation of Enzyme Activity

The feedback regulation of enzyme activity represents a very important mechanism in the integration of the myriad of metabolic reactions occurring within bacterial cells (Chap. 4 to 6). Virtually every biochemical pathway is controlled, at least in part, by feedback regulation of one type or another. Moreover, most branching and intersecting pathways display multiple levels of control to allow the balanced synthesis or utilization of the substrates and products of each branch. Several important principles and relevant examples of feedback regulation are considered.

Allosteric Mechanisms. A fundamental principle for metabolic regulation is *allostery*. An allosteric protein is one that has two separable binding sites, one being the active site for the corresponding enzyme activity and the other a binding site for an effector molecule. The enzyme can exist in (at least) two alternate conformations, one of which is less active or completely inactive. The role of effector binding is to trap the enzyme in one of these conformations, thus modulating enzyme activity. The binding of an effector may block activity by promoting a conformation in which the active site of the enzyme is disturbed. Alternatively, the binding of an effector may be required to induce the active conformation of the enzyme. Thus, allosteric effectors can be either negative or positive regulators of enzyme activity.

Allosteric proteins were discussed earlier in this chapter. The transcriptional control proteins described above respond to their respective effector molecules by an alteration in affinity for DNA binding. The *lac* repressor loses its affinity for *lac* operator DNA as a result of effector binding, and CAP requires a bound effector for site-specific DNA binding. In the case of CAP, the DNA-binding and effector-binding activities of the protein reside in two different domains (see above), demonstrating that allosteric sites need not be close to active sites. The binding of an effector to one particular site of a protein can alter the conformation of the protein at any arbitrary distance from the effector binding site.

The effector binding site of an allosteric enzyme need not even be in the same polypeptide chain. Aspartate transcarbamylase is composed of six each of two different kinds of subunits. One type of subunit contains the catalytic site, whereas the other is a regulatory subunit that binds the effector, CTP. Allosteric regulation of the enzyme is lost when the regulatory subunit is removed, but enzyme activity is retained. If the regulatory subunit is added back to the depleted enzyme, regulation is restored.

Feedback Inhibition. Perhaps the simplest form of metabolic regulation is the feedback inhibition of a pathway with a single end product, of which there are numerous examples. Historically, one of the most important of these is the inhibition by isoleucine of threonine deaminase, the first enzyme in the isoleucine biosynthetic pathway. This example also illustrates a nearly universal principle of metabolic regulation, that control is exerted at the first step (or the first step following a branch point) of the pathway. Regulation at any other point of the pathway would be uneconomical and lead to accumulation of useless intermediates.

Most biochemical pathways have multiple branches, overlaps, or both, and thus the example shown in Figure 7–26 is more typical. This is the biosynthetic pathway for synthesis of the aspartate family of amino acids, including lysine, methionine, and threonine. The isoleucine pathway described above follows from the threonine branch of this more complex pathway. The first point worth noting is that feedback inhibition again occurs at the first step of the pathway, and also at every step immediately following a branch. A total of five enzymatic conversions are feedback-inhibited. The first step in the pathway is the phosphorylation of aspartate by aspartokinase. In *E. coli,* this step is catalyzed by three separate enzymes, named aspartokinase I, II, and III. Enzyme I is inhibited by threonine, whereas enzyme III is inhibited by lysine, providing control by two of the three end products. Aspartokinase II does not appear to be feedback-inhibited by an end product but is repressed at the transcriptional level by methionine. Thus each of the three enzymes is controlled by one of the three end products.

In certain bacteria (e.g., *Bacillus polymyxa*) a single aspartokinase catalyzes the first step in this pathway. The single enzyme is allosterically inhibited by both threonine and lysine, which act in a synergistic fashion. Numerous enzymes show such feedback inhibition (or activation) by multiple substances. The details of these multivalent effector mechanisms are quite varied, and the inhibitors do not always act in a synergistic fashion.

The first unique step in the synthesis of threonine and methionine (conversion of aspartate semialdehyde to homoserine) is catalyzed by homoserine dehydrogenase. As with aspartokinase, this step is catalyzed by multiple enzymes in *E. coli.* Homoserine dehydrogenase I is inhibited by threonine, and homoserine dehydrogenase II is not feedback inhibited.

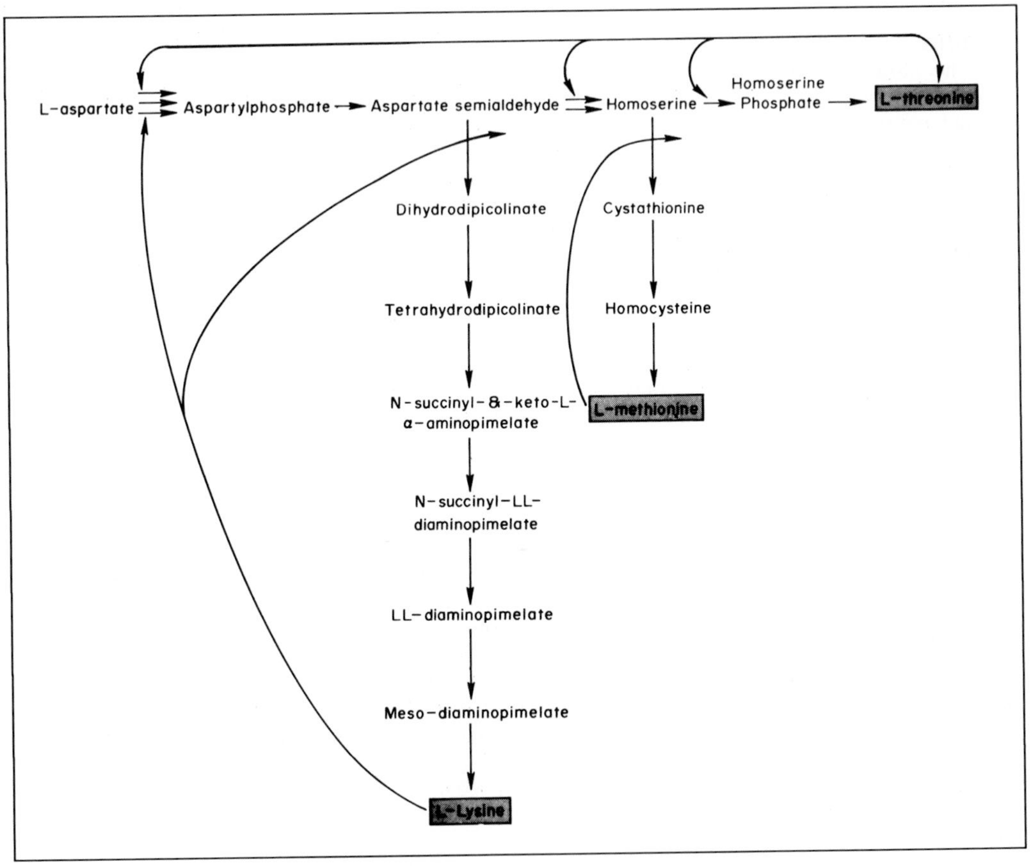

Fig. 7–26. Pathways for synthesis of the aspartate family of amino acids. The enzymes inhibited by the end products are indicated. End product inhibition provides for efficient control of carbon flow through this highly branched pathway.

The ultimate in metabolic integration is achieved with these sets of enzymes: aspartokinase I and homoserine dehydrogenase I reside in the same protein, and aspartokinase II and homoserine dehydrogenase II are also a single protein.

Each of the branch points that lead uniquely to one of the three products is regulated by the respective end product (Fig. 7–26). This, together with the complex regulation of aspartokinase, allows the pathway to synthesize almost any combination of end products. In the presence of excess threonine, aspartokinase I is blocked by feedback inhibition, but aspartokinase II and III are active. Thus, the total aspartokinase activity is reduced in response to the reduced demand on the entire pathway. The excess threonine also blocks the branch unique to the synthesis of threonine (phosphorylation of homoserine) but allows the methionine and lysine branches to continue.

The examples considered above involve biosynthetic pathways that are inhibited by their end products, an obviously economical arrangement. Many pathways are also controlled by metabolites that are not strictly their end products, but such effectors make sense when viewed in a larger context. Catabolic pathways are ultimately concerned with energy production, and the first enzyme in many catabolic pathways is feedback-inhibited by ATP.

A property that is characteristic of many allosteric enzymes is that the reaction velocity changes in a sigmoidal fashion as the substrate or effector concentration is increased. Invariably, such enzymes are multisubunit proteins. Every model to explain such higher-order kinetic patterns involves the interactions of the subunits within the oligomer, with a conformational change in one subunit inducing the corresponding change in each of the other subunits. This property can have at least two important physiologic consequences. First, it can amplify small changes in substrate/effector concentrations. If the intracellular concentration of the metabolite is near the inflection point of the curve, a quite small change in metabolite concentration can have a large effect on reaction velocity. Second, a sigmoidal response can assure the maintenance of a finite intracellular pool of the reaction substrate. In the pathways described above, threonine serves as a precursor to isoleucine, but threonine must also be maintained as a direct amino acid precursor for protein synthesis. A sigmoidal response of threonine deaminase to threonine concentration virtually blocks deaminase activity when the threonine concentration is low (Fig. 7–27). Isoleucine also inhibits threonine deaminase by an allosteric mechanism (again in a sigmoidal fashion), and the combination of these regulatory effects maintains a proper balance of threonine and isoleucine under a wide variety of conditions.

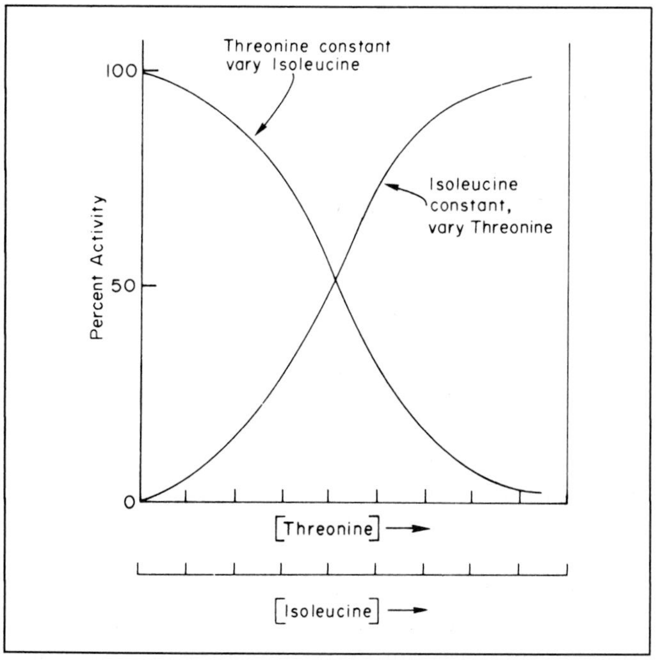

Fig. 7–27. The reciprocal effects of threonine and isoleucine on the activity of threonine deaminase. Threonine is the substrate for the enzyme, and isoleucine is an allosteric inhibitor of enzyme activity. Isoleucine induces cooperativity with respect to enzyme activity, and threonine induces cooperativity with respect to isoleucine inhibition.

FURTHER READING

Books and Reviews

Adhya S: Multipartite genetic control elements: Communication by DNA loop. Annu Rev Genet 23:227, 1989

Adhya S, Garges S: How cyclic AMP and its receptor protein act in *Escherichia coli*. Cell 29:287, 1982

Albright LM, Huala E, Ausubel FM: Prokaryotic signal transduction mediated by sensor and regulator protein pairs. Annu Rev Genet 23:311, 1989

Bauer WR, Crick FHC, White JH: Supercoiled DNA. Sci Am 243:118, 1980

Cozzarelli NR: DNA gyrase and the supercoiling of DNA. Science 207:953, 1980

Drlica K: Biology of bacterial deoxyribonucleic acid topoisomerases. Microbiol Rev 48:273, 1984

Gellert M: DNA topoisomerases. Annu Rev Biochem 50:879, 1981

Gold L, Pribnow D, Schneider T, et al: Translational initiation in procaryotes. Annu Rev Microbiol 35:365, 1981

Gottesman S: Bacterial regulation: Global regulatory networks. Annu Rev Genet 18:415, 1984

Green PJ, Pines O, Inouye M: The role of antisense RNA in gene regulation. Annu Rev Biochem 55:569, 1986

Holmes WM, Platt T, Rosenberg M: Termination of transcription in *E. coli*. Cell 32:1029, 1983

Jacob F, Monod J: Genetic regulatory mechanisms in the synthesis of protein. J Mol Biol 3:318, 1961

Kolter R, Yanofsky C: Attenuation in amino acid biosynthetic operons. Annu Rev Genet 16:113, 1982

Kornberg A, Baker TA: DNA Replication, ed 2. New York, WH Freeman, 1992

Kozak M: Comparison of initiation of protein synthesis in procaryotes, eucaryotes, and organelles. Microbiol Rev 47:1, 1983

Kucherlapati R, Smith GR (eds): Genetic Recombination. Washington, DC, American Society for Microbiology, 1988

Kuempel PL, Pelletier AJ, Hill TM: Tus and the terminators: The arrest of replication in prokaryotes. Cell 59:581, 1989

Lake JA: Evolving ribosome structure: Domains in archaebacteria, eubacteria, eocytes and eucaryotes. Annu Rev Biochem 54:507, 1985

Lehninger AL: Principles of Biochemistry. New York, Worth, 1982

Losick R, Chamberlin M (eds): RNA Polymerase. Cold Spring Harbor, NY, Cold Spring Harbor Laboratory, 1976

Losick R, Youngman P, Piggot PJ: Genetics of endospore formation in *Bacillus subtilis*. Annu Rev Genet 20:625, 1986

Low KB (ed): The Recombination of Genetic Material. San Diego, Academic Press, 1988

Maitra U, Stringer EA, Chauduri A: Initiation factors in protein biosynthesis. Annu Rev Biochem 51:869, 1982

McClure WR: Mechanism and control of transcription initiation in procaryotes. Annu Rev Biochem 54:171, 1985

Miller JH, Reznikoff WS (eds): The Operon. Cold Spring Harbor, NY, Cold Spring Harbor Laboratory, 1978

Monod J, Wyman J, Changeux JP: On the nature of allosteric transitions: A plausible model. J Mol Biol 12:88, 1965

Neidhardt FC, Ingraham JL, Low KB, et al (eds): *Escherichia coli* and *Salmonella typhimurium*. Cellular and Molecular Biology. Washington, DC, American Society for Microbiology, 1987

Neidhardt FC, van Bogelen RA, Vaughn V: The genetics and regulation of heat-shock proteins. Annu Rev Genet 18:295, 1984

Noller HF: Structure of ribosomal RNA. Annu Rev Biochem 53:119, 1984

Nomura M, Gourse R, Baughman G: Regulation of the synthesis of ribosomes and ribosomal components. Annu Rev Biochem 53:75, 1984

Pabo CO, Sauer RT: Protein-DNA recognition. Annu Rev Biochem 53:293, 1984

Pettijohn DE: Structure and properties of the bacterial nucleoid. Cell 30:667, 1982

Raibaud O, Schwartz M: Positive control of transcription initiation in bacteria. Annu Rev Genet 18:173, 1984

Reznikoff WS, Siegele DA, Cowing DW, et al: The regulation of transcription initiation in bacteria. Annu Rev Genet 19:355, 1985

Rosenberg M, Court D: Regulatory sequences involved in the promotion and termination of RNA transcription. Annu Rev Genet 13:319, 1979

Schimmel PR, Söll D: Aminoacyl-tRNA synthetases: General features and recognition of transfer RNAs. Annu Rev Biochem 48:601, 1979

Simons RW, Kleckner N: Biological regulation by antisense RNA in prokaryotes. Annu Rev Genet 22:567, 1988

Smith I, Slepecky RA, Setlow P (eds): Regulation of Procaryotic Development. Washington, DC, American Society for Microbiology, 1989

Umbarger HE: Amino acid biosynthesis and its regulation. Annu Rev Biochem 47:533, 1978

von Hippel PH, Bear DG, Morgan WD, et al: Protein-nucleic acid interactions in transcription: A molecular analysis. Annu Rev Biochem 53:389, 1984

Wang JC: DNA topoisomerases. Annu Rev Biochem 54:665, 1985

Watson JD, Hopkins NH, Roberts JW, et al: Molecular Biology of the Gene, ed 4. New York, Benjamin/Cummings, 1987

Weissbach H, Pestka S (eds): Molecular Mechanisms of Protein Biosynthesis. New York, Academic Press, 1977

Wittmann HG: Components of bacterial ribosomes. Annu Rev Biochem 51:155, 1982

Wittmann HG: Architecture of procaryotic ribosomes. Annu Rev Biochem 52:35, 1983

Zimmerman SB: The three-dimensional structure of DNA. Annu Rev Biochem 51:395, 1982

Selected Papers

Adams JM, Capecchi MR: *N*-formylmethioninyl-sRNA as the initiator of protein synthesis. Proc Natl Acad Sci USA 55:147, 1966

Baker TA, Sekimizu K, Funnell BE, et al: Extensive unwinding of the plasmid template during staged enzymatic initiation of DNA replication from the origin of the *Escherichia coli* chromosome. Cell 45:53, 1986

Brennan CA, Dombrowski AJ, Platt T: Transcription termination factor rho is an RNA-DNA helicase. Cell 48:945, 1987

Brown PO, Cozzarelli NR: A sign inversion mechanism for enzymatic supercoiling of DNA. Science 206:1081, 1979

Burgess RR, Travers AA, Dunn JJ, et al: Factor stimulating transcription by RNA polymerase. Nature 22:43, 1969

Burton ZF, Gross CA, Watanabe KK, et al: The operon that encodes the sigma subunit of RNA polymerase also encodes ribosomal protein S21 and DNA primase in *E. coli* K12. Cell 32:335, 1983

Crick FHC: Codon-anti-codon pairing: The wobble hypothesis. J Mol Biol 19:548, 1966

Crick FHC, Barnett L, Brenner S, et al: General nature of the genetic code for proteins. Nature 192:1227, 1961

DeCrombrugghe B, Chem B, Gottesman M, et al: Regulation of *lac* mRNA synthesis in a soluble cell-free system. Nature (New Biol) 230:37, 1971

Gilbert W, Müller-Hill B: The *lac* operator is DNA. Proc Natl Acad Sci USA 58:2415, 1967

Jacob F, Brenner S, Cuzin F: On the regulation of DNA replication in bacteria. Cold Spring Harbor Symp Quant Biol 28:329, 1963

Liu LF, Wang JC: Supercoiling of the DNA template during transcription. Proc Natl Acad Sci USA 84:7024, 1987

Meselson M, Stahl FW: The replication of DNA in *Escherichia coli*. Proc Natl Acad Sci USA 44:671, 1958

Mizuno T, Chou M-Y, Inouye M: A unique mechanism regulating gene expression: Translational inhibition by a complementary RNA transcript (micRNA). Proc Natl Acad Sci USA 81:1966, 1984

Nirenberg MW, Leder P: RNA and protein synthesis: The effect of trinucleotides upon the binding of sRNA to ribosomes. Science 145:1399, 1964

Nordheim A, Rich A: The sequence $(dC\text{-}dA)_n \cdot (dG\text{-}dT)_n$ forms left-handed Z DNA in negatively supercoiled plasmids. Proc Natl Acad Sci USA 80:1821, 1983

Pardee AB, Jacob F, Monod J: The genetic control and cytoplasmic expression of "inducibility" in the synthesis of β-galactosidase by *E. coli*. J Mol Biol 1:165, 1959

Roberts JW: Termination factor for RNA synthesis. Nature 224:1168, 1969

Silhavy TJ, Shuman HA, Beckwith J, et al: Use of gene fusions to study outer membrane protein localization in *Escherichia coli*. Proc Natl Acad Sci USA 74:5411, 1977

Silverstone AE, Magasanik B, Reznikoff WS, et al: Catabolite sensitive site of the *lac* operon. Nature 221:1012, 1969

Steitz JA, Jakes K: How ribosomes select initiator regions in mRNA: Base pair formation between the 3′ terminus of 16S rRNA and the mRNA during initiation of protein synthesis in *Escherichia coli*. Proc Natl Acad Sci USA 72:4734, 1975

von Ehrenstein G, Weisblum B, Benzer S: The function of sRNA as amino acid adapter in the synthesis of hemoglobin. Proc Natl Acad Sci USA 49:669, 1963

Watson JD, Crick FHC: A structure for deoxyribose nucleic acid. Nature 171:737, 1953

Yanofsky C, Carlton BC, Guest JR, et al: On the collinearity of gene structure and protein structure. Proc Natl Acad Sci USA 51:266, 1964

CHAPTER 8

Genetic Variation and Exchange

The chemical structure of DNA is subject to a wide variety of changes, some of which occur at a relatively high frequency. The vast majority of these alterations are corrected by DNA repair mechanisms, but those that escape correction can result in heritable mutations that provide genetic diversity. Common types of mutation encountered in microbiology affect easily recognizable properties, such as nutritional requirements, morphology, and resistance to antibiotics or to bacteriophage. The importance of these mutationally derived traits is accentuated by several common mechanisms that allow the rearrangement, exchange, and dissemination of bacterial genes.

Mutation

Because the frequency of mutation is generally very low, only microorganisms can easily achieve numbers high enough to permit the detection of spontaneous mutational events. For this and related reasons, bacterial systems have played a major role in our understanding of the mechanisms of mutation. The knowledge of these simple systems is quite applicable to other cell types, because the chemical and enzymatic reactions in which DNA participates are very similar throughout the biologic world.

Early studies of mutation concentrated on characters that could be directly selected, such as resistance to bacteriophage. A resistant bacterial mutant can be obtained simply by exposing a culture of (sensitive) bacteria to the appropriate bacteriophage; only the resistant mutant can survive. Most mutations do not provide their carriers with such a growth advantage and are therefore more difficult to obtain. Many mutations have a detrimental effect on cell growth (for example, by destroying the activity of an enzyme important in some biochemical pathway). Many of these types of mutation can be recognized because they result in a new nutritional requirement or an inability to catabolize some common sugar. Numerous genetic tricks have been developed over the last several decades to facilitate the isolation of mutants defective in virtually any bacterial gene. The ability to isolate diverse mutants has been instrumental in the progress of molecular biology.

Types of Mutation

A classification of mutations at the primary level is quite simple—a mutation changes the sequence of bases in the DNA molecule. *Deletion* and *insertion* mutations can alter the base sequence by any number of base pairs and include major disruptions of the genome. These large deletions and insertions are generally caused by transpositional mechanisms and are discussed later in the chapter. Mutations that change one base into another are subdivided into *transitions* and *transversions.* Considering one strand of the helix, a transition mutation changes one purine into the other (adenine ↔ guanine) or one pyrimidine into the other (thymine ↔ cytosine). Conversely, a transversion interconverts a purine with a pyrimidine. These classifications at the molecular level are useful because they provide insight into the mechanism of mutation.

Functional Consequences of Mutation

There are many ways of classifying mutations at the functional level. For mutations within the coding sequence of genes, several generic terms describe the mutational consequence in terms of the coding properties. A *missense* mutation is one that changes one amino acid codon into another, resulting in a simple amino acid substitution in the resultant protein. Missense mutations are all transitions or transversions at the DNA sequence level. Because of the redundancy of the genetic code, some transition or transversion mutations have no consequence for the protein sequence. Many of these *silent* mutations occur in the third position of the codon (Chap. 7). Another possible consequence of a transition or transversion is the generation of a *nonsense* mutation. These are mutations that change an amino acid codon into one of the *stop* signals (Chap. 7) and, therefore, result in premature polypeptide chain termination.

Deletion and insertion mutations can affect a small number of bases within a gene coding sequence. Because of the triplet nature of the genetic code, only mutations that add or remove a multiple of three bases will correspondingly insert or delete a number of amino acids. All others will change the reading frame at all points distal to the mutation, and these are called *frameshift* mutations. Because the distal reading frame is shifted, it will contain an essentially random sequence of codons. This has two consequences. First, the distal amino acid sequence of a frameshift mutant protein will bear no obvious relationship to the wild-type protein. Second, one of the nonsense codons will often be put into register a short distance from a frameshift mutation, resulting in a truncated protein.

The effects of each of these kinds of mutation can also be analyzed in terms of the effect on protein function. Missense mutations can have a wide variety of possible consequences. Mutations that cause drastic amino acid substitutions (e.g., basic to acidic residue) at the active site of an enzyme are likely to result in complete inactivation of the enzyme. On the other hand, many possible amino acid substitutions in a peripheral region of a protein have little or no effect on activity. Between these two extremes, a mutation can alter the function of a protein in almost countless ways. The kinetic properties or allosteric interactions of an enzyme can be changed in subtle ways. Other missense mutations affect the ability of a polypeptide to form complexes, either with itself or with other proteins. Very rare missense mutations actually improve a protein in some way, and these are of obvious importance in evolution.

A special class of missense mutations are those that destroy protein function only under particular conditions. Among the most commonly isolated *conditional lethal* mutations are those that result in a thermolabile protein. These are often caused by amino acid substitutions that distort the secondary or tertiary structure of the protein. The elevated temperatures may induce conformational changes that are incompatible with function, or they may block the normal folding pathway that occurs during and immediately after translation.

Nonsense mutations cause the premature termination of a polypeptide chain and therefore usually cause complete inactivation of the gene product. Most bacterial genes are organized into polycistronic operons, and it has been observed that many nonsense mutations also reduce or eliminate expression of downstream genes of the operon. These *polar* effects generally relate to the mechanism of transcription termination. ρ-Dependent terminators (Chap. 7) occur within many structural genes but are not functional when the messenger RNA (mRNA) is covered with translating ribosomes. Presumably, ρ protein normally binds to nascent mRNA only when the message is free of ribosomes. Because nonsense mutations result in ribosome dissociation, any ρ-dependent terminator downstream of the nonsense mutation will cause transcriptional termination, blocking transcription of downstream genes. Nonsense mutations are thereby often *pleiotropic,* meaning that a single mutation has more than one phenotypic effect.

Mechanisms of Suppression

Many mutations that produce a defective gene product can be counteracted by a second mutational event. If the second mutation is the exact reversal of the first, the normal wild-type gene sequence is restored. Very often, however, the second mutation is not a simple reversal of the first. A second mutation elsewhere in the genome, called a *suppressor,* can nullify the effect of the original mutation by a variety of interesting mechanisms.

Suppression of Missense Mutations. Missense mutations are often suppressed by an intragenic mechanism. If the primary mutation causes an altered protein conformation, a second amino acid substitution elsewhere in the protein can sometimes restore a conformation close to that of the wild type. Often either mutation alone produces an inactive protein. These types of suppressor mutations can be useful in the analysis of protein structure. A second class of missense suppressors are extragenic, and these can operate by any of several mechanisms. If two (or more) polypeptides interact to form a functional complex, a mutation in one can sometimes counteract a mutation in the other by restoring suitable protein-protein contacts. In addition, a blockage in one biochemical pathway can sometimes be suppressed by altering a second preexisting pathway or by inducing some new pathway that was previously not expressed.

Suppression of Frameshift Mutations. The suppression of frameshift mutations generally occurs by means of a second compensating frameshift close to the site of the first. If the original mutation involved the deletion of one base, the addition of one base in a nearby region can obviously restore the correct reading frame for the remainder of the protein. There would be a garbled region of protein between the two frameshift mutations, but this is sometimes compatible with protein function. The suppression of frameshift mutations is not limited to the exact opposite numerical change. Because the genetic code is triplet, numerous combinations can restore the correct reading frame. For example, a deletion of two or of five bases can suppress a nearby deletion of one base because the total change is a multiple of three.

Suppression of Nonsense Mutations. The suppression of nonsense mutations is, in many ways, the most interesting and important form of suppression. When the translational machinery encounters one of the nonsense codons (UAG, UAA, and UGA), there is no corresponding transfer RNA (tRNA) to recognize that codon. Nonsense suppressors are mutations that allow a particular tRNA to recognize one of the nonsense codons. The outcome of this situation is that some amino acid will be incorporated, and translation will not terminate at the nonsense codon. The inserted amino acid will probably not be identical to the original amino acid in the wild-type protein; as stated above, however, many amino acid substitutions do not have a significant effect on protein structure or function.

The availability of bacterial strains with nonsense suppressors has allowed the isolation of nonsense mutations in many hundreds of genes. A nonsense mutation in an essential gene is considered a conditional lethal mutation, because only cells containing a nonsense suppressor can survive with the mutation. Nonsense mutations have been of particular importance in identifying genes required for survival, even when the exact function of the corresponding gene product is not known.

Figure 8–1 summarizes the generation of a suppressor tRNA mutation in the *supF* gene of *E. coli.* The wild-type *supF* gene specifies a tyrosine tRNA with an anticodon of 5′-GUA-3′. Because base pairing with the codon is antiparallel, this tRNA recognizes the tyrosine codon 5′-UAC-3′. The first mutational event shown is the generation of a nonsense codon in some protein-coding sequence. This changes a tyrosine codon (UAC) into a stop signal (UAG). The second mutation is the suppressor, which alters the anticodon of the tyrosine tRNA so that it now base pairs with the nonsense codon. The charging of the tRNA with tyrosine is not affected, and therefore tyrosine is inserted when the nonsense codon comes into register. In the example shown, the original mutation (of the codon) is exactly the converse of the suppressor mutation (in the anticodon). This need not be the case, as many different codons can be mutated into this nonsense codon (e.g., the leucine codon UUG can become UAG by a single transversion; see the genetic code in Table 7–2).

This explanation of suppression by *supF* is incomplete in one important aspect. If the tRNA that recognizes the tyrosine

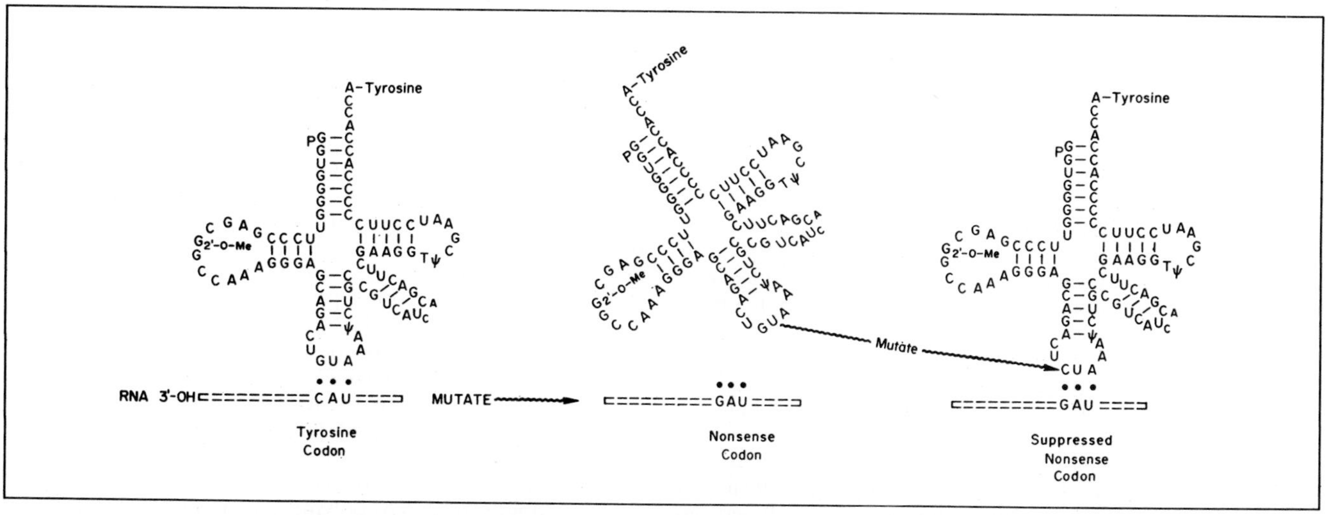

Fig. 8–1. Reading of a nonsense codon by a suppressor tRNA. The product of the *supF* gene of *E. coli* is a tyrosine-accepting tRNA. A mutation affecting the anticodon region of this tRNA allows it to read the nonsense codon 5′-UAG-3′.

codon UAC has mutated so that it now recognizes UAG, what happens to translation of any mRNA with normal UAC codons? The answer is that *E. coli* has two genes for this particular tyrosine tRNA, and only one of them has become mutant. All other UAC codons are decoded normally by the second (nonmutant) tRNA. This mechanism of suppression is thereby limited to multiple-copy tRNA genes.

A slightly different mechanism of suppression exists for single-copy tRNA genes. As discussed previously (Chap. 7), some ambiguity in the third position of the codon is allowed by the *wobble* rules. A suppressor mutation in the tryptophan tRNA gene of *E. coli* increases the wobble of the third position so that the tRNA can recognize both UGG (codon for tryptophan) and UGA (stop codon). The mutation that increases wobble in tryptophan tRNA is far removed from the anticodon loop, so the effect on wobble is presumably due to a change in the overall conformation of the tRNA.

Suppression by alteration in the information-transfer machinery is not limited to nonsense codons. Mutations within tRNA genes can also generate suppressors of missense and frameshift mutations by similar mechanisms. For example, an additional nucleotide in the anticodon loop of a phenylalanine tRNA produces a frameshift suppressor that reads UUUC instead of UUU as the codon for phenylalanine.

A different form of suppression can be induced by treatment with certain antibiotics. Sublethal concentrations of streptomycin and related compounds cause a low level of misreading of the genetic code by the translational machinery, resulting in the suppression of both nonsense and missense mutations (Chap. 9). This *phenotypic suppression* operates at a relatively low efficiency; therefore only genes whose products are needed in small amounts can be effectively suppressed. Because the misreading is at a low frequency, the detrimental effects on nonmutant proteins are relatively benign.

Spontaneous Mutation

The simplest method of isolating bacterial mutants is to plate a large number of cells on Petri dishes where the wild type cannot grow but the desired mutant can. For example, when 10^9 bacterial cells are spread onto a plate seeded with a large number of bacteriophage, several phage-resistant bacterial colonies will be observed after an overnight incubation. In this case, the selective condition is the presence of the bacteriophage, but any number of conditions (presence of antibiotics or some unusual nutritional provisions) could be used. It is not clear a priori whether the selective condition is just allowing preferential growth of the mutant or whether it might actually be responsible for the induction of the mutation. One of the seminal experiments in the early history of molecular biology answered this question unambiguously and indicated that bacterial mutants arise in a Darwinian rather than a Lamarckian fashion.

The fluctuation test of Luria and Delbrück is designed to determine whether phage-resistant bacteria exist before the selection is imposed or are generated as a result of exposure to the bacteriophage. When a series of plates are each seeded with 10^9 bacterial cells from the same culture, a narrow fluctuation in the number of resistant colonies is observed. The distribution is consistent with expectations based on random chance. If, instead of just one culture, a series of independent cultures of the same bacterial strain is used in the plating, a very different result is obtained: there is a huge fluctuation in the number of resistant colonies (Fig. 8–2). This is precisely the result that would be expected if the bacterial mutants arose before the plating with bacteriophage, because the mutation to resistance would occur at different times before plating in the independent cultures. Those few cultures that happen to generate a phage-resistant mutant relatively early have very large numbers of the clonal descendents by the time of plating under selective conditions. This experiment shows that bacterial mutants are generated spontaneously, with no necessary influence of the selective condition. How do these spontaneous mutations in the bacterial genome occur?

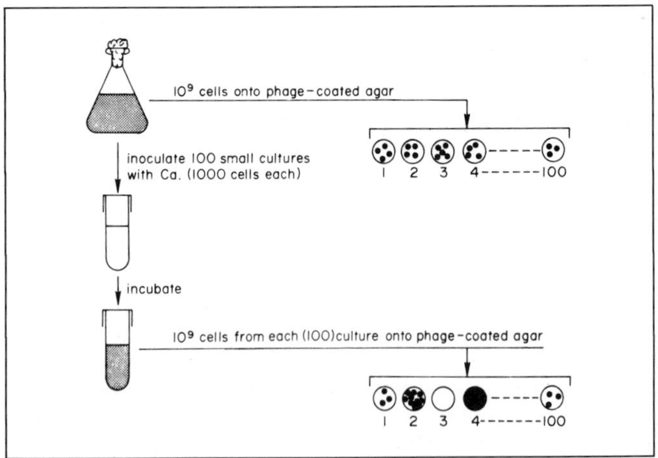

Fig. 8–2. A fluctuation test. The results of this experiment show that phage-resistant mutants appear spontaneously before exposure to phage. The number of resistant mutants in each sample from a single culture is relatively constant. When several cultures are sampled, however, the number of mutants varies over a wide range, indicating that the mutants arise at different times in the course of the growth of the individual cultures. The time between the appearance of the mutant and sampling governs the number of resistant organisms per culture.

Replication Errors

A significant source of spontaneous mutation is the replication machinery itself. The error frequency for the replicative DNA polymerase complex is in the range of 10^{-7} to 10^{-11} per base pair replicated. Thus less than one mistake occurs on average during one cycle of replication of the *E. coli* genome. The most striking fact is not that replication makes an occasional mistake but, rather, that the mistakes are so infrequent. If free nucleotides are mixed with polynucleotides and allowed to associate spontaneously, the best discrimination for proper base pairing with no added proteins is only about 100-fold. Furthermore, the bases in DNA can undergo tautomeric shifts that should generate *incorrect* base pairs at a frequency of about 10^{-4}. Procaryotic DNA polymerases have apparently bypassed these chemical limitations by at least two means. These enzymes achieve more accuracy than expected during the initial incorporation, and they are also able to *proofread* the newly replicated DNA and to make corrections.

The ability of DNA polymerase to make fewer errors than expected during polymerization is not understood in detail but must reflect the nature of the polymerase-DNA-nucleotide complex. Presumably the base pairing between the incoming nucleotide and the template is constrained by the surrounding DNA polymerase to reduce the frequency of incorrect base pairs. This argument is supported by the observation that different DNA polymerases show nucleotide-specific differences in their error frequencies on exactly the same template (in the absence of proofreading).

The ability of DNA polymerase to proofread its product is dependent on an associated exonuclease activity that senses incorrect base pairs. Whenever the nucleotide just incorporated into the product strand does not pair properly with the template, the exonuclease is activated to remove that nucleotide residue. The exonuclease activity is clearly important in the overall mutation frequency of an organism, because mutations that destroy the nuclease (but maintain polymerization ability) result in much higher spontaneous mutation frequencies. Interestingly, mutations that increase the exonuclease relative to the polymerase activity show the opposite, namely, reduced frequencies of spontaneous mutation. The fact that the spontaneous mutation frequency can be either increased or decreased by a simple (mutational) change in DNA polymerase suggests that organisms evolve optimal mutation frequencies. If mutations occur too frequently, essential genes would be destroyed in most progeny, whereas a very low mutation frequency may prevent mutational adaptation to environmental challenges.

Mismatch Repair

Another mechanism that prevents replication errors from becoming mutations operates after the replication machinery has passed and is called mismatch repair. In this process, newly replicated DNA is scanned for base mismatches, which signal the replicative insertion of an incorrect base. The strand of newly synthesized DNA, including the incorrect base, is then excised and replaced by resynthesis. *E. coli* mutants deficient in mismatch repair exhibit spontaneous mutation frequencies about 100-fold higher than the wild type, indicating that this process corrects 99% of the errors made by the replication machinery.

The critical feature of mismatch repair is that the repair enzyme system can recognize which of the DNA strands in a duplex is the newly synthesized daughter strand and thereby preferentially restore the wild-type sequence using the parental strand as template. In *E. coli,* this recognition is based on the methylation of adenines in the sequence 5′-GATC-3′, which occurs throughout the genome. A specific methylase, the product of the *E. coli dam* gene, recognizes and methylates GATC sequences some time after DNA synthesis. At the start of a round of replication, all GATC sequences in both parental strands are methylated. During replication, the GATC sequences in each daughter strand are unmethylated for a short period of time before the *dam* methylase modifies them. This delay in daughter strand methylation allows the mismatch repair enzyme system a chance to recognize the unmethylated strand as being newly replicated. When a base mismatch is encountered, a segment of this unmethylated strand is excised, and the methylated (parental) strand is used as the template during resynthesis to correct the error.

Spontaneous DNA Lesions

Nonreplicating DNA is also subject to mutational lesions. The *N*-glycosidic bond between the sugar and the base is particularly susceptible, resulting in the occurrence of spontaneous depurination and depyrimidization at appreciable frequencies. Another common lesion is the deamination of cytosine into uracil, which can lead to a C to T transition mutation. There are numerous other spontaneous lesions in DNA that can lead to mutation, and some are even promoted by normal intracellular metabolites. *S*-adenosylmethionine, an important methyl donor in the cell, can apparently alkylate DNA to form a premutational lesion. The vast majority of these and other DNA lesions are corrected by a remarkable set of DNA repair reactions that are discussed below, but those lesions that escape repair account for a significant fraction of spontaneous mutations.

Induced Mutagenesis

A great variety of physical and chemical agents can cause mutation by damaging DNA. A complete description of the action of any one of these agents can be quite complex. In addition to determining the DNA lesion that causes mutation, the possibilities of metabolic activation, repair of damage, and induction of lethal but nonmutagenic lesions all need to be considered. The discussion in this chapter is confined to the mechanism of mutation and repair.

Radiation Damage

Among the physical agents, ultraviolet light is the most extensively studied mutagen. The major photoproducts induced by UV light are pyrimidine dimers, but other lesions can also be detected. The dimerization of adjacent pyrimidines occurs by a reaction involving the unsaturated 5,6(carbon-carbon) bonds, with conversion to a four-member cyclobutane ring (Fig. 8–3). Thymine is the preferred reactive base, with about 50% T-T, 40% T-C, and only 10% C-C dimers observed. The mutations induced by UV light are generated by a complex mechanism involving one of the repair pathways that correct UV-induced damage (see below).

Ionizing radiations have greater penetrance than UV radiation and produce free radicals that can cause DNA strand scission. Ligation of DNA broken at two different positions

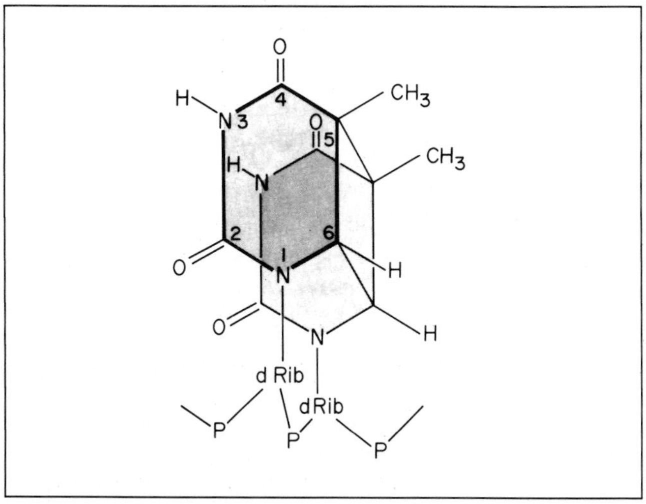

Fig. 8–3. Pyrimidine dimer.

by this mechanism apparently results in many deletion and rearrangement mutations.

Chemical Mutagenesis

A great deal of experimental study has been invested in the mechanisms of chemical mutagenesis. The known chemical mutagens can be classified into three general categories: (1) agents that cause covalent modification of the DNA bases, (2) agents that interact noncovalently with DNA, generally intercalating between the base pairs, and (3) base analogues that are incorporated during replication.

Alkylating agents such as ethylmethane sulfonate and nitrosoguanidine are potent mutagens that covalently modify DNA bases. Most of the oxygens and nitrogens in DNA can be alkylated, but mutagenicity is correlated with modification of the O^6 position of guanine. This modified guanine base can mispair with thymine, resulting in GC to AT transitions. A second common mechanism of covalent base modification is deamination—for example, by hydroxylamine or nitrous acid. These two agents frequently deaminate cytosine into uracil, which can result in a CG to TA transition. Deamination of adenine into hypoxanthine can also lead to a transition mutation.

Another important class of base-modification mutagens do not cause mispairing but, rather, completely block base pairing. These agents include many important carcinogens, such as benzo[a]pyrene and aflatoxin B_1, that commonly modify purines with *bulky lesions.* As in the case of UV damage, the relevant DNA repair pathway is intimately involved with the generation of mutations (see below). There are several important parallels between bulky-lesion and UV damage, which can be rationalized by considering the pyrimidine dimer as a form of bulky lesion that blocks base pairing.

The most important mutagens that interact noncovalently with DNA to cause mutation are the intercalating agents, such as proflavine and acridine orange. These compounds contain planar aromatic rings that intercalate between the stacked bases of DNA, distorting the DNA structure. The majority of mutations caused by these agents are frameshifts involving the addition or deletion of a small number of base pairs. There are many different intercalating agents, and their mechanisms of growth inhibition and mutagenesis appear to vary significantly. Some have found important use as antitumor or antimalarial agents, and others have significant antiviral activity.

The third general class of mutagens are the base analogues. These are compounds that resemble the normal bases of DNA but can base pair with two alternative residues to cause mutation. For example, 5-bromouracil in its usual keto form is an analogue of thymine and thus pairs with adenine. However, rare tautomerization to the enol form allows base pairing with guanine. Therefore, replication of an A:5-BU base pair can lead to G:C, with G:5-BU as an intermediate (Fig. 8–4).

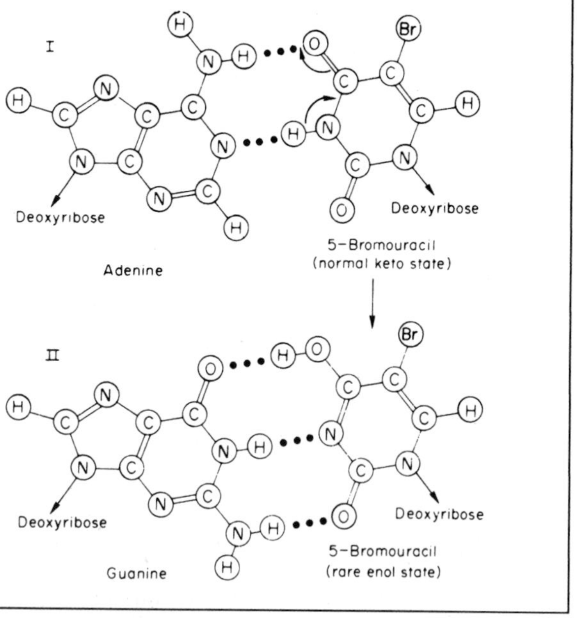

Fig. 8–4. Proper and spurious base pairing with the tautomers of 5-bromouracil. 5-Bromouracil is a thymine analogue, which, when in its normal keto state, pairs with adenine but, when in its rarer enol state, pairs with guanine. Replication of 5-bromouracil–containing DNA is occasionally accompanied by the mispairing of the analogue with guanine, with the result that mutant daughter DNA molecules are produced.

Correlation of Mutagenesis and Carcinogenesis

One of the strongest indications that cancer often arises as a result of mutational events is that most carcinogens are also mutagens. This observation has led to an economical and efficient method of testing compounds for their carcinogenic potential. Ames and his collaborators have developed sensitive mutagenicity tests using the reversion of histidine auxotrophs of *Salmonella typhimurium.* A battery of specific his^- mutants are exposed to the suspected mutagen, and the induction of his^+ revertants is measured. Each his^- mutant can revert to his^+ only by a particular mutation at the DNA level, allowing a quick survey for any potential mutagenic lesion. Because numerous compounds require metabolic activation that *S. typhimurium* cannot perform, a sterile microsomal extract from mammalian tissues can be added to the mutagenesis test. The Ames test for mutagenesis is quicker, easier, and far more economical than direct carcinogenesis tests with animals, and thus it is often used as the first screen for potentially carcinogenic compounds.

An observation that naively seems to be an antithesis of the above is that many antitumor agents are also mutagens. Strong alkylating (e.g., nitrogen and sulfur mustards) and intercalating compounds (e.g., aminoacridines and anthracyclines) are among the best antitumor agents available today. Although there is no case in which the precise mechanism of therapeutic action is clear, it is presumed that these agents preferentially attack rapidly growing cells. They may interfere with important aspects of replication or gene expression, or may induce additional mutations that inactivate tumor cells, or do both. Clearly, insight into the mechanisms of mutation is central to an understanding of both the genesis and the destruction of cancer cells.

Repair of DNA Damage

As implied above, most DNA lesions are repaired before they have a chance to become heritable genetic mutations. The

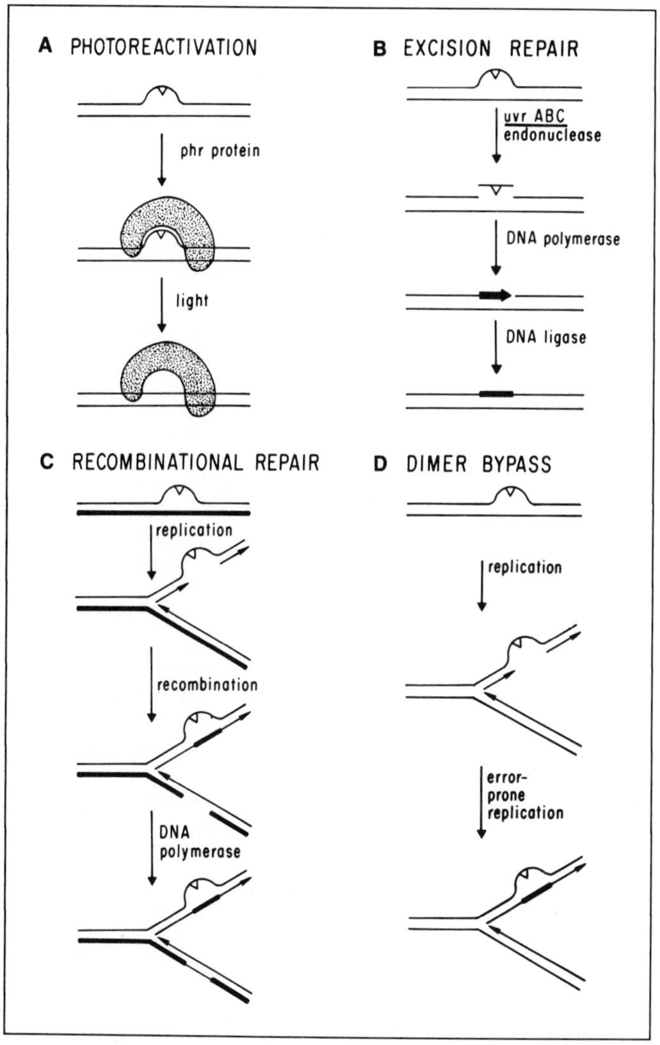

Fig. 8–5. The repair of pyrimidine dimer-containing DNA. Current models for the four known pathways of pyrimidine dimer repair are shown. In **B** and **D** the heavy line represents newly synthesized DNA, whereas in **C** the heavy line represents one of the two parental strands. See text for details of the repair reactions. *(Adapted from Kornberg: DNA Replication. WH Freeman, 1980.)*

human disease xeroderma pigmentosum is caused by a deficiency in one specific repair pathway; this deficiency results in a large incidence of skin tumors due to unrepaired DNA lesions from the UV component of sunlight. The same DNA lesions occur in the skin cells of normal persons, but the efficient repair system removes the lesions and thereby prevents a high incidence of neoplasia. All organisms, including bacteria, have quite complex and efficient pathways to correct the various lesions that occur in DNA. Whereas wild-type *E. coli* can efficiently survive very high UV doses, mutants without the ability to repair UV-induced damage are killed by a single pyrimidine dimer. The repair of these dimers serves to illustrate the general strategies of the major DNA repair pathways, which are now considered (summarized in Fig. 8–5). Before we proceed to the particulars, it is worth noting that most repair pathways are possible only because of the double-helical nature of DNA. The complement of the damaged strand is generally used to recover the information that was lost during DNA damage.

Direct Reversal of Damage

There are two well-understood pathways to repair DNA damage directly by a simple reversal mechanism. One of these, photoreactivation, involves a flavoprotein called photolyase that converts a cyclobutane dimer back to its constituent pyrimidines (Fig. 8–5A). The action of photolyase requires light, and thus this pathway can be blocked by incubating bacteria in the dark. The photolyase of *E. coli* is encoded by the *phr* gene, and similar activities have been detected in some other organisms.

The second direct reversal mechanism acts on alkyl-substituted DNA and is catalyzed by a class of enzymes called methyltransferases. The *E. coli ada* gene encodes a protein that can accept methyl groups directly from DNA, thereby reversing at least three different kinds of alkylation damage (including O^6-methylguanine, the major premutagenic lesion discussed above). The methyl groups are transferred to one of two cysteine residues in the protein. Strikingly, the methylated cysteine residues cannot be reversed, and thus the methyltransferase acts in a suicidal fashion.

The *ada* protein also controls the *adaptive response,* a regulatory network involved in repairing alkylation damage. The alkylation of one of the cysteine residues converts the *ada* protein into a positive regulator that activates transcription of at least three operons. One of the operons encodes *ada,* and therefore alkylation of *ada* protein results in the synthesis of more *ada* protein. A second operon includes a methylated-base-specific DNA glycosylase that feeds lesions into an excision repair pathway (see below). At least two pathways of alkylation repair are thereby induced by the adaptive response, leading to a large increase in survival after treatment with alkylating agents.

Excision Repair

Excision repair pathways are prevalent in all organisms studied and constitute the most important general mechanism of DNA repair. The overall process of excision repair involves cleavage of one strand of the DNA near the damage, excision of a portion of that strand containing the damaged base, resynthesis through the gap, and then ligation to restore an intact double helix (Fig. 8–5B). This complex series of reactions requires the participation of many of the same proteins that are involved in genome replication, with DNA polymerase I usually performing the replacement synthesis in *E. coli* (Chap. 7). The focus here is on the reactions that initiate excision repair, and these are catalyzed by any of several protein complexes that recognize a particular form of damage.

The process of excision repair of UV-induced cyclobutane dimers in *E. coli* is initiated by the action of a complex endonuclease encoded by three genes, *uvrA, uvrB,* and *uvrC.* The nuclease recognizes the DNA lesion, incises the damaged strand on each side of the lesion, and thereby excises an oligonucleotide of 12 or 13 bases that contains the lesion. Resynthesis using the complementary strand as template and final ligation complete the repair process. Recent evidence indicates that these enzymes probably function together, with coordinated incision and resynthesis reactions. The *uvrABC* nuclease recognizes both UV-induced damage and covalently attached bulky lesions, probably by sensing a gross pertubation in DNA structure. As discussed above, the repair of bulky lesions is particularly relevant in preventing carcinogenesis; the pathway defective in xeroderma patients is probably the analogue of the *uvrABC* pathway of *E. coli.* In contrast to the UV and bulky-lesion pathway, most excision repair of mutagen-damaged DNA is initiated by a two-step process. Every cell has a series of enzymes, called DNA glycosylases, that cleave the *N*-glycosidic bond connecting a damaged base to the sugar-phosphate backbone. Each DNA glycosylase recognizes a particular form of damage, but otherwise the enzymes are similar. Removal of the damaged base leaves an apurinic or apyrimidinic site, which is then recognized by endonucleases that cleave nearby. The subsequent sequence of events is similar to that in the *uvrABC* pathway, namely, removal of the segment of DNA containing the lesion, resynthesis using the complement as template, and resealing by DNA ligase.

The versatility of this form of excision repair is conferred by the variety of DNA glycosylases. There are glycosylases for several alkylated bases, deaminated bases such as hypoxanthine and uracil (see the discussion on Induced Mutagenesis above), and bases that have suffered ring-opening reactions. In addition to repairing mutagen-induced damage, some of the glycosylases are important for the correction of spontaneous damage. As described above, both deamination and alkylation occur without mutagen treatment, and specific glycosylases trigger excision repair of these lesions.

The most common spontaneous damage to DNA is hydrolysis of the *N*-glycosidic bond. The resulting apurinic and apyrimidinic sites are identical to the product of DNA glycosylase action and are similarly substrates for the specific endonucleases mentioned above. Once again, repair is completed by excision of a segment of DNA containing the damaged (abasic) site, resynthesis using the complement as template, and ligation into an intact duplex.

Bypass Repair and SOS System

A special set of repair reactions are carried out by proteins that are specifically induced in response to certain forms of DNA damage. Before the nature of the repair reactions is described, the regulatory network that includes these repair pathways is summarized.

SOS Regulon

In response to DNA damage, *E. coli* induces a global regulon (Chap. 7) that affects diverse processes including DNA repair, mutagenesis, recombination, and cell division. The two key regulatory elements in this SOS regulon are the products of genes *recA* and *lexA* (Fig. 8–6). The *recA* protein is a multifunctional enzyme that participates in several important reactions involving DNA and also functions as a protease when it senses DNA damage. The induced proteolysis serves to degrade the *lexA* protein, which is normally the repressor of all operons in the SOS regulon. One of the genes controlled by *lexA* is *recA* itself, and therefore the synthesis of *recA* protein is induced by DNA damage in a feedback loop. The activation of the protease function of *recA* protein is not completely understood. Recent evidence indicates that any of several possible signals are sufficient, and these include certain DNA lesions (such as UV photoproducts), short DNA oligonucleotides that result from DNA repair, and single-stranded DNA that results from inhibition of chromosome replication. This would account for the fact that the SOS response is induced both by a variety of mutagenic treatments and by nonmutagenic conditions that block replication.

The proteins that are induced in the SOS regulon are involved in a variety of processes that enhance survival in extreme environmental conditions. Some of the proteins are involved in excision repair (the products of *uvrABC*) and two novel repair pathways (see below) and thereby directly counteract damage to the chromosome. One of these pathways creates frequent mutations, and this may increase genetic variability in the face of extreme environmental pressure (see below). An inhibitor of cell division is also induced, presumably giving the cell a chance to correct all lesions before it attempts to propagate.

Recombinational Repair. One of the induced repair pathways is called recombinational or daughter-strand-gap repair and is thought to operate as follows (Fig. 8–5C). When the normal replication machinery reaches the site of DNA damage (e.g., a pyrimidine dimer), it simply skips that segment of DNA and starts synthesizing again farther down the template. This leaves a gap of single-stranded DNA (parental strand) that includes the DNA lesion. Because cell division is inhibited, the two chromosomes produced by replication are still contained in the same cell, and daughter-strand-gap repair involves splicing the completed regions of each of these together

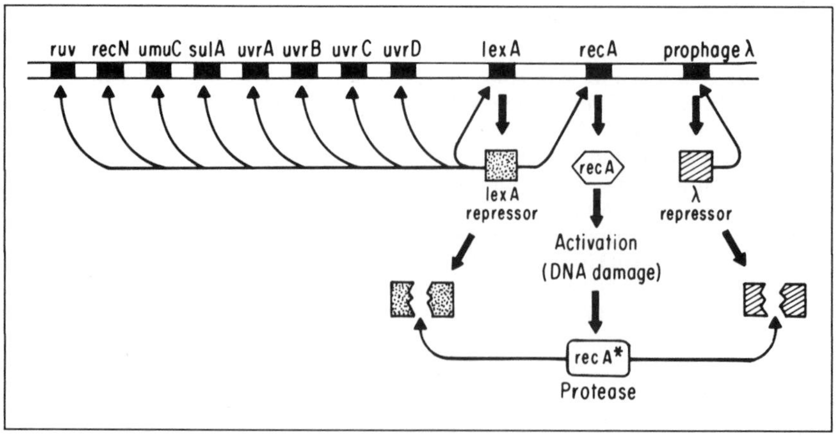

Fig. 8–6. The SOS regulon of *E. coli.* DNA damage or inhibition of chromosomal DNA replication can result in the activation of the protease activity of the *recA* protein. The *recA* protease is very specific, inactivating the *lexA* repressor; the protease also destroys the repressor of prophage λ, if the affected cell is lysogenic for that phage (Chap. 60). The *lexA* protein is a transcriptional repressor for a variety of genes, only some of which are shown here. Inactivation of the *lexA* protein by proteolysis thereby results in the derepression of all genes in the SOS regulon. *(Adapted from Kornberg: Supplement to DNA Replication. WH Freeman, 1982.)*

to form one nondamaged chromosome. This repair pathway is, therefore, a special form of recombination and, like other recombination reactions, depends critically on the *recA* protein (see below).

Error-prone Repair. The second induced pathway is remarkable because of its inherent mutagenesis and is therefore called error-prone repair. Although the mechanistic details of error-prone repair are uncertain, the process probably generates mutations by replicating damaged template DNA with little or no attention to the normal rules of base pairing. Most of the mutations so generated occur at the site of the lesion (targeted mutagenesis), and thus the lesion itself appears to trigger the relaxed specificity of replication. Recent evidence indicates that the multifunctional *recA* protein binds preferentially at the site of UV damage in single-stranded DNA, and numerous studies show that *recA* is required for induced mutagenesis. In the simplest model, *recA* protein, bound at the site of damage, modifies one of the DNA polymerases into a form with relaxed specificity (Fig. 8–5D). As implied above, DNA polymerases normally do not replicate through a damaged region of DNA.

Error-prone repair pathways are not limited to bacteria, because even animal cells show clear evidence of induction of both DNA repair and mutagenesis. The widespread occurrence of these pathways has led to many interesting speculations. Bacterial mutagenesis is induced by a wide variety of conditions that damage DNA and also by conditions that simply block replication. Therefore the induced mutagenesis can be viewed as a mechanism for generating genetic diversity in times of extreme stress. Very rapid speciation (saltatory evolution) has been inferred from a variety of genetic and paleobiologic approaches, and it is possible that pathways of induced mutagenesis play a role. The error-prone repair pathway of mammalian cells could also play some important role in carcinogenesis, particularly because many of the same mutagens that induce error-prone repair (in bacteria) are among the strongest carcinogens.

Genetic Recombination

Recombination is a collection of processes whereby genetic information is reassorted between chromosomes. The major form of recombination during gene transfer involves exchange reactions between two homologous DNA molecules, so that there is no change in the order of particular genes along the chromosome. However, if the two participating chromosomes contain different mutations in their genes, novel combinations of these mutations will result from recombination. For example, a chromosome with a lac^- mutation can recombine with a chromosome containing a trp^- mutation, producing both lac^- trp^- and lac^+ trp^+ recombinants. Virtually every known pathway of gene transfer requires homologous recombination at one or more steps, and recombination mechanisms are therefore important for an understanding of gene transmission. After a consideration of the mechanics of homologous recombination, the processes by which bacteria exchange genetic information will be described.

Mechanisms of Homologous Recombination

Models of the way DNA molecules recombine with each other were first based on purely genetic approaches. By analyzing patterns of segregation, geneticists were able to generate remarkably detailed models explaining the behavior of DNA during acts of recombination. By modifying minor aspects of the models, recombination in bacteria and their viruses, fungi, and fruit flies could all be consolidated. More recently, molecular biologic and enzymologic techniques have been applied to recombination mechanisms with great success. Certain idealized reactions can now be performed in vitro with only a few highly purified proteins, and important general features of recombination have thus become clear.

Analyses of recombination mechanisms have been guided by two related models, the first proposed by Holliday and the second by Meselson and Radding. It is important to realize at the outset that no single model can accommodate every recombination reaction; some of the variations on a theme will be mentioned below. However, the Meselson-Radding model does serve to illustrate many important principles of recombination (Fig. 8–7).

In this model, recombination is initiated by endonucleolytic cleavage of one of the participating DNAs (the *donor* molecule), followed by limited replication of one strand using the newly generated 3′ end as a primer (Fig. 8–7A). DNA synthesis serves to displace a single-stranded region of the donor DNA molecule, which then proceeds to invade the homologous region of the *recipient* DNA molecule (Fig. 8–7B). Because the incoming donor strand pairs only with its complement, one strand of the recipient molecule is displaced into a single-stranded loop, which is then postulated to be digested by nucleases (Fig. 8–7C). The process has now generated a heteroduplex in only one of the two helices and is therefore called asymmetric strand transfer.

The only exchange of genetic information in the preceding steps is the donation of the single strand into the heteroduplex region of the recipient molecule. This would not lead to recombination for genetic markers outside the region of heteroduplex. The crucial step required for exchange of outside markers is called isomerization (Fig. 8–7D). To visualize this step, simply imagine a 180-degree rotation of the two duplex segments on the far right around each other, with the left ends kept stationary. Isomerization brings the newly synthesized 3′ end of the donor into close proximity with the broken 5′ end of the homologous strand of the recipient, and therefore DNA ligase can seal this (and any other) nick to create an intact fused molecule (Fig. 8–7E).

Genetic evidence indicates that the two recombinant molecules can each contain heteroduplex regions in the vicinity of the exchange site. This is accounted for by a process called branch migration, in which the location of the cross-strand structure moves one way or the other with respect to the DNA sequence (Fig. 8–7F). Branch migration is an efficient and rapid process in vitro, and requires only rotary diffusion of the participating DNA duplexes (Fig. 8–8). Notice that there is a conservation of base-pairing during branch migration: every region of base-pairing disrupted in the parental molecules is re-formed in the heteroduplex regions of the product molecules. Because both molecules now contain heteroduplex regions, this phase of the reaction is designated as symmetrical. The final steps in this recombination model are cleavage of the cross-strand exchange followed by resealing, to generate two free duplex DNAs (Fig. 8–7G).

The heteroduplex regions generated in the vicinity of crossovers deserve special comment. If the two participating DNAs are exactly homologous (i.e., have precisely the same sequence), the region of heteroduplex DNA has no genetic

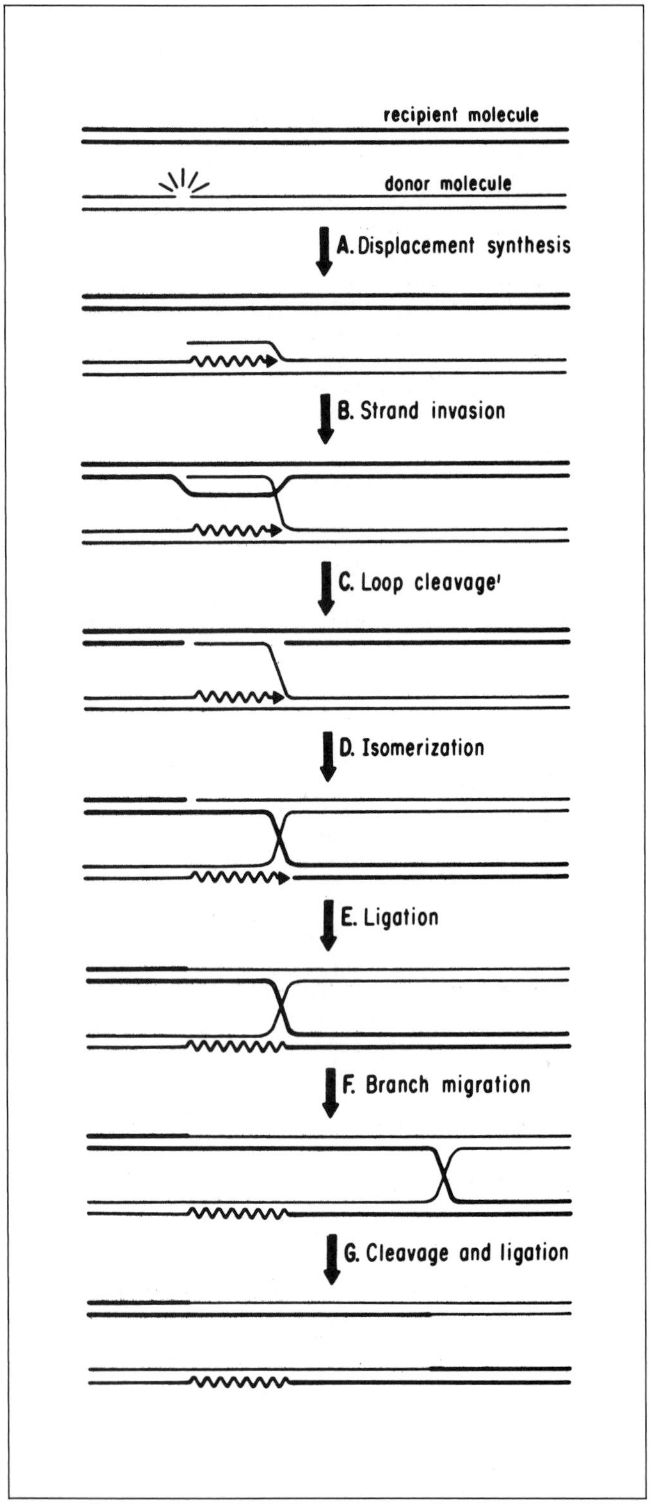

Fig. 8–7. The Meselson-Radding model for homologous genetic recombination. The individual steps in the recombination model are described in detail in the text. The isomerization (step **D**) involves the rotation of the right ends of the two duplexes by 180 degrees with respect to each other, with the left ends fixed. For clarity, the top and bottom strands within each duplex region have been inverted in this diagram during the isomerization step. *(Adapted from Radding: Annu Rev Biochem 47:847, 1978.)*

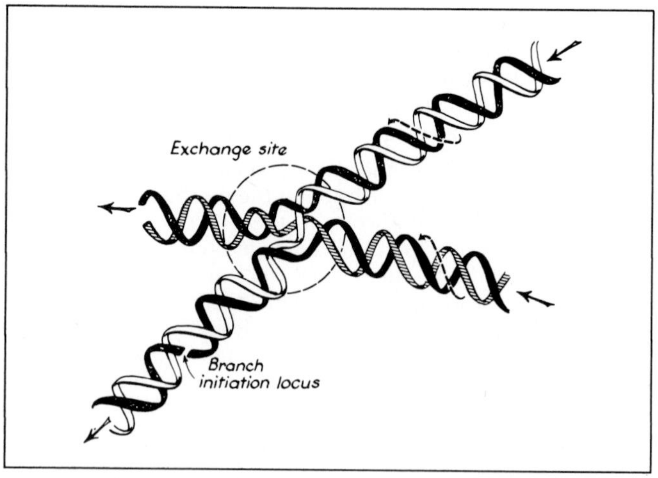

Fig. 8–8. Migration of a cross-strand exchange by rotary diffusion. Heteroduplex DNA can be formed on both DNA molecules by rotating each participating duplex in the same sense. *(Courtesy of Dr. T. Broker.)*

consequence for the progeny. However, when one DNA molecule has a mutation while the other is wild-type in sequence, the heteroduplex will contain a mispaired region where the sequences differ. The site of mispairing can be acted on by DNA repair mechanisms (see above), resulting in conversion of the heteroduplex into a homoduplex with no mismatch. In general, the conversion can occur to either the wild-type or the mutant sequence, and often the nature of the particular base mismatch determines which strand is excised and resynthesized. Whenever this correction of mismatches within heteroduplex regions does not occur, the resulting progeny will be a mixed population of wild-type and mutant, because replication of a heteroduplex results in one daughter molecule of each type.

This pathway for recombination should not be viewed as the single correct mechanism but, rather, as a useful model that can be adapted to explain various recombination events. The pathway contains steps that are clearly important for most homologous recombination, such as isomerization, branch migration, and cross-strand cleavage. Furthermore, proteins that have been shown to be important in recombination can catalyze many of the steps (see below). However, many recombination events do not use exactly this pathway; for example, transformation involves recombination between one single-stranded and one double-stranded DNA. Even pathways that use two duplex participants show distinctive features, such as the length of heteroduplex regions.

One of the major unsolved problems in understanding recombination is the mechanism of initiation. There are indications that the generation of single-stranded regions is crucial, and there are specific sites (called recombination *hot spots*) in most or all genomes that stimulate recombination in their vicinity. Some hot spots could function by providing the initial nick shown in Figure 8–7A (see below).

Genetics and Enzymology of Homologous Recombination

recA **Protein.** Mutations that block genetic recombination have been instrumental in our understanding of the process.

In *E. coli,* mutations in the *recA* gene can reduce the frequency of recombination more than 1000-fold, and the role of the *recA* protein in recombination has been elucidated by in vitro approaches. The major activity of *recA* protein is to facilitate the exchange of homologous DNA strands, but *recA* protein by itself is unable to break or reseal any phosphodiester bonds in DNA.

The strand exchange catalyzed by *recA* protein is a formidable reaction. In bacterial cells such as *E. coli,* any segment of DNA that undergoes recombination must find its complement among the 4.5 million base pairs of the genome. This search is even more difficult in eucaryotic cells, given their larger genome sizes. Furthermore, because at least one of the participating DNA molecules is generally duplex, the two complementary strands need to be separated to permit formation of a heteroduplex with invading DNA.

One of the most useful model reactions catalyzed by *recA* protein is the strand exchange shown in Figure 8–9. In this reaction, a single-stranded DNA circle invades a homologous duplex linear molecule, displacing the appropriate linear single strand in the process. The first step in strand exchange is the binding of *recA* protein to the single-stranded circle, which activates all other activities of the protein. Once in the activated form, *recA* protein can bind to and denature duplex DNA, the latter being dependent on the energy of adenosine triphosphate (ATP) hydrolysis. The ability of *recA* protein to catalyze ATP-dependent DNA denaturation categorizes it as a DNA helicase (Chap. 7). Coincident with the denaturation of the duplex, a search for homology is conducted between the incoming single-stranded circle and the newly denatured linear strands. Once homologous sequences come into register, the *recA* protein drives the formation of longer regions of heteroduplex, leading to complete strand exchange in the model reaction. One of the major unanswered questions is how the *recA* protein organizes itself and the various DNA strands during its search for homology.

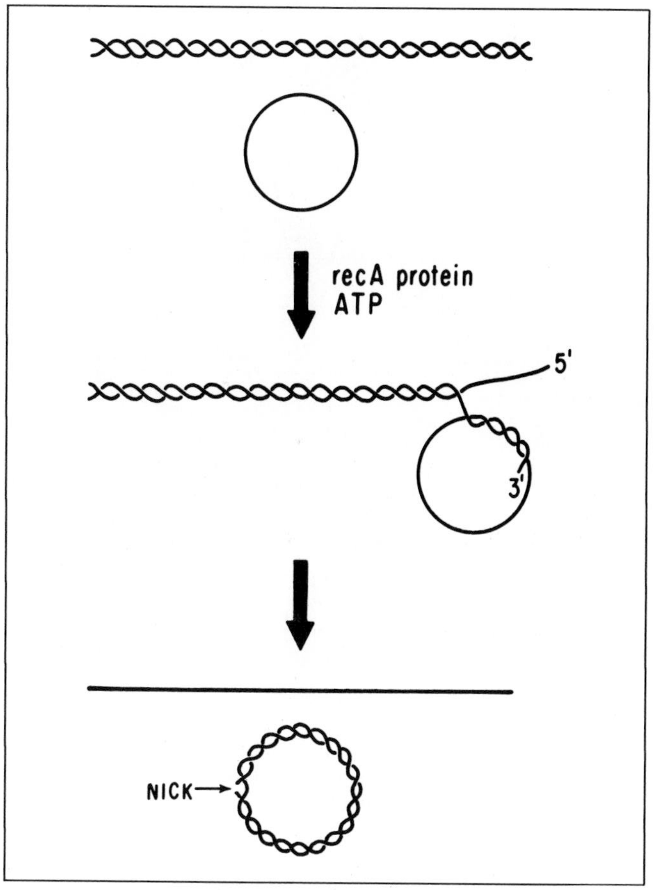

Fig. 8–9. Strand exchange catalyzed by the *recA* protein. One strand of a linear duplex is assimilated into a circular molecule by the action of the *recA* protein. In the first step, synapsis is accomplished by a *recA*-promoted search for homology between the participating DNA molecules. Once a homologous region is encountered, *recA*-promoted branch migration completes the exchange of strands, resulting in a single-stranded linear and a nicked duplex circular molecule. Strand exchange catalyzed by the *recA* protein is directional, as shown, because of the polar nature of the *recA*-promoted branch migration. *(Adapted from Kornberg: Supplement to DNA Replication. WH Freeman, 1982.)*

The *recA* protein can catalyze many distinct strand exchange reactions in addition to the one shown in Figure 8–9. The major requirement is the provision of at least one single-stranded region for the initial binding of the protein, but this can be provided by even a short gap in an otherwise duplex molecule. The electron micrographs in Figure 8–10 show the *recA* protein complexed with linear single-strand and circular duplex DNA, with homologous pairing limited to the central region of the linear substrate. An impressive filament of protein assembled on the single strand extends into the three-stranded region where homologous joining has occurred.

The versatility of the *recA* protein can be appreciated when one considers the numerous reactions it must perform in genetic recombination and in DNA repair (see above). The binding of single-stranded segments of DNA converts the *recA* protein into an adenosine triphosphatase (ATPase), a duplex-DNA binding protein, a DNA helicase, a DNA synaptase, and a protease. In addition, *recA* protein appears to play a direct (though currently ill-defined) role in replication past pyrimidine dimers (see above). The ability of a rather modestly sized (M_r = 38,000) protein to perform all of these functions is surely one of the wonders of evolution.

Other Proteins Involved in Homologous Recombination. The *recA* protein is aided in strand exchange by several other proteins. Single-strand binding protein dramatically improves the efficiency of in vitro reactions and is probably important for recombination in vivo. The topoisomerases are likely to play pivotal roles in recombination, allowing the intertwining of duplex molecules (type I topoisomerases) and providing a driving energy for strand assimilation from the negative superhelicity of participating DNAs (DNA gyrase).

As exemplified in the Meselson-Radding model, DNA replication is often intimately involved in recombination. Therefore, DNA polymerases and related proteins must also function in many recombination reactions. The enzyme that catalyzes cleavage of the cross-strand exchange has been isolated from bacteriophage T4, and other organisms presumably have similar activities. The final sealing of the broken cross-strand exchange must generally be catalyzed by DNA ligase.

Because *recA* protein requires single-stranded DNA for activation, the question of how recombination is initiated might be rephrased into a question of how appropriate single-stranded regions of DNA are generated. A second important class of recombination-deficient mutants of *E. coli* has helped

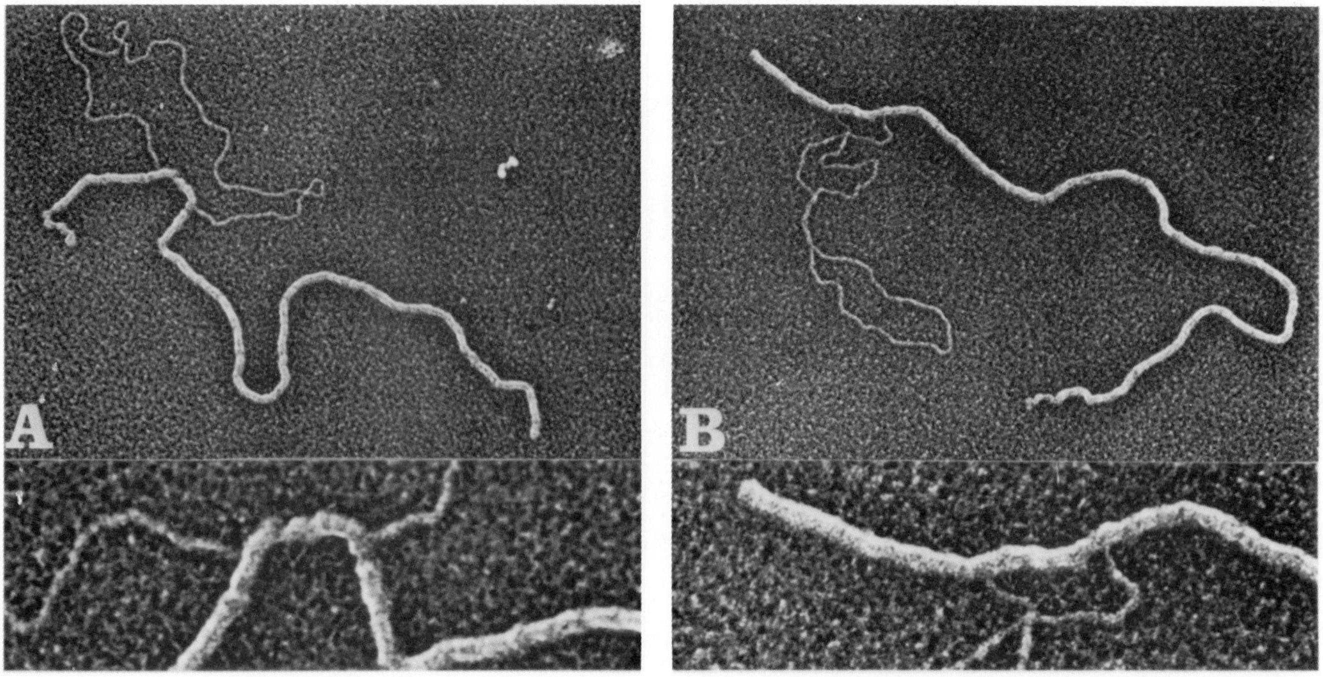

Fig. 8–10. Electron micrographs of the *recA* protein complexed with DNA. Single-stranded linear DNA molecules coated with *recA* protein (thick rods) are seen in synaptic complexes with duplex circles. The higher magnifications are enlargements of the regions of joining; synapsis occurs within homologous sequences of the two DNA molecules. *(From Christiansen and Griffith: Proc Natl Acad Sci USA 83:2066, 1986.)*

illuminate this problem. Mutations in any of three genes, called *recB, recC,* and *recD,* inactivate another multifunctional protein involved in recombination. The *recBCD* nuclease (also called exonuclease V) has at least two activities that appear to be important for recombination. First, the protein acts as a DNA helicase by transiently denaturing the duplex at the expense of ATP hydrolysis. This helicase activity cannot begin within an intact segment of duplex DNA; it functions only when the duplex contains either a short single-stranded gap or a broken end. The denaturation catalyzed by *recBCD* nuclease presumably provides single-stranded regions for the assembly of *recA* protein. A second activity that appears to play a role in recombination is endonucleolytic cleavage of DNA. During the course of the helicase reaction, the nuclease activity of the *recBCD* complex is activated whenever it passes a specific octanucleotide sequence, 5′-GCTGGTGG-3′. The enzyme then cleaves one strand of the helix, and the newly broken ends apparently become a powerful substrate for recombination promoted by *recA* protein. These special sites were first uncovered as recombination hot spots in bacteriophage λ and were subsequently found to occur about once in every 10,000 base pairs in the *E. coli* genome.

Mutations that inactivate the *recBCD* nuclease reduce recombination only about 100-fold. Alternate pathways must exist to account for the residual 1% recombination observed in *recBCD* mutants. These have also been dissected by applying the genetic approach, and other cellular nucleases play critical roles in these alternate pathways. This again reinforces the critical roles of DNA breaks and single-stranded regions in initiating the process of homologous genetic recombination.

Mechanisms of Gene Transfer

There are three major pathways by which bacteria exchange genetic information. *Transformation* involves the uptake and assimilation of naked DNA and occurs naturally with only certain bacterial species. *Transduction* is a process whereby a bacterial virus serves as a vector for gene transmission, carrying bacterial genes from one cell to another. The most sophisticated mechanism of genetic exchange available to bacteria is the process of *conjugation,* where one cell directly transmits part or all of its genetic information to a suitable recipient. In each of these processes, DNA introduced into the recipient cell can undergo recombination with the resident genome of the recipient, giving rise to a new combination of genetic characters. The three routes of gene transfer are unidirectional in character, with DNA passing only from a donor to a recipient cell.

Transformation

The process of transformation played an important part in the development of molecular biology. In 1944 Avery, MacLeod, and McCarty demonstrated that purified DNA was the active principle that allowed the transfer of a gene involved in encapsulation in *Pneumococcus,* and this was the first demonstration of DNA as the genetic material. The emphasis in this section is on the natural transformation that occurs in several important gram-positive and gram-negative species. Other bacterial species are not capable of natural transformation but can be artificially induced to accept DNA. For example, many *E. coli* strains can incorporate exogenous DNA after treatment with calcium chloride, and even eucaryotic cells can be persuaded to assimilate DNA given the proper treatment. These latter two examples of artificial transformation are critical for current recombinant DNA methods.

Transformation is perhaps the most important mechanism of genetic exchange for certain bacterial species, notably *Streptococcus pneumoniae, Streptococcus sanguis, Bacillus subtilis, Haemophilus influenzae*, and *Neisseria gonorrhoeae*. The common steps in transformation involve binding of exogenous DNA to the cell surface, transport of DNA into the cell, and then recombination with the resident genome. In general, virtually any segment of DNA can be assimilated during transformation; the lysis of a bacterial cell can provide all segments of the genome for uptake by a second cell.

Transformation in Gram-Positive Organisms

Bacterial cells in a state that allows transformation are said to be *competent*. In the gram-positive organisms the competent state is obtained only under particular physiologic conditions. Cultures of the streptococci reach competence late in their growth, usually when the cell density has increased to 10^7 or 10^8/mL. The development of competence is due to an extracellular signal, called competence factor (CF), that accumulates in the growth media. Each streptococcal species has its own specific CF, which are all small (5,000 to 10,000 Da) peptides. The precise mechanism by which CF induces competence is not yet clear, but it apparently involves specific receptors that bind CF and the induction of about 10 new proteins involved in the transformation process.

Given a competent gram-positive cell, the next step in transformation is the binding of DNA to the outside surface of the cell (Fig. 8–11). The details of this binding reaction differ in various species, but it usually involves a loose, reversible binding of duplex DNA, followed by a tighter binding in which the bound DNA cannot be washed off the cell surface. In both conditions, the transforming DNA is still sensitive to exogenously added DNase. The transforming DNA becomes resistant to DNase only when it is transported into the cell. Transport of the DNA into the cell requires the association of DNA with a special protein found only in competent cells; this is one of the proteins described above that are induced by CF. The uptake of DNA into the cell is also associated with a drastic change in DNA structure. During the course of binding and penetration into the cell, the DNA is broken into smaller pieces and denatured, with only one of the two strands entering the cell. The complementary strand is generally degraded and released back into the medium.

The single-stranded pieces that enter the cell by this route are now poised for recombination with the resident genome. In general, only DNA that shares significant sequence homology with the genome is capable of recombination (see above). Therefore most foreign DNA without homology to the resident chromosome will not integrate (but is nonetheless transported into the cell by the above mechanism). Recombination of homologous DNA is very efficient, with as much as 50% of the transported DNA becoming integrated into the chromosome. The transforming single strand replaces one of the two strands in the appropriate region of the chromosome, forming a heteroduplex in the region of homology. As de-

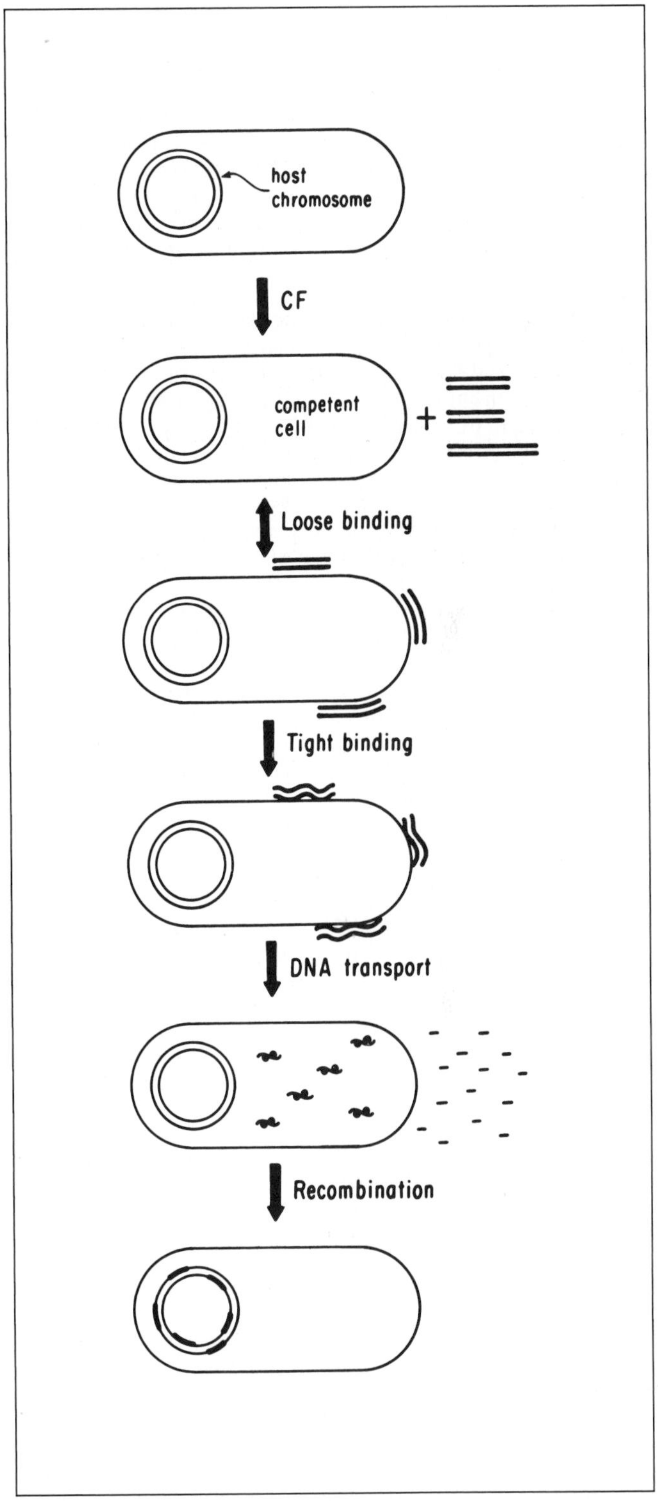

Fig. 8–11. Model for the transformation of *Streptococcus*. Competence factor (CF) is required for the induction of the competent state. Duplex DNA binds to competent cells in at least two distinct steps, referred to as loose and tight binding. Transport of single-strand fragments results in intracellular protein-DNA complexes and subsequent recombination of the fragments into the host chromosome.

scribed above, the heteroduplex has genetic consequence only if its constituent strands differ by at least one base at some position, as would be the case if one strand contained a mutant sequence for some gene. The base mismatch can be corrected so that the progeny is either purely mutant or purely wild-type, or the mismatch may escape correction, resulting in a mixed progeny. The details of mismatch correction need not be of concern here; they may result in one particular genetic marker being transferred at a higher efficiency than another, but all markers are capable of transfer at some frequency.

Transformation in Gram-Negative Organisms

Natural transformation in gram-negative organisms has several important differences from that described above for gram-positive organisms. First, there is a large variation in the mechanism of competence induction, and none of the gram-negative organisms appear to rely on an extracellular signal. Some, such as *Acinetobacter,* become competent only in the stationary phase, whereas others, such as *Neisseria gonorrhoeae,* are competent only if they are a piliated variety. A second significant difference is that many of the gram-negative organisms will bind and transport DNA only if it is from a closely related species. The mechanism appears to be a sequence-dependent DNA binding, with particular nucleotide sequences appearing frequently in the genomes of the closely related species. A third difference relates to the transport mechanism. During transformation of *H. influenzae,* the transforming DNA cannot be detected in the intracellular single-stranded form described above. Duplex donor DNA first enters membrane-bound vesicles called *transformasomes.* The donor DNA apparently does not leave the transformasome until recombination with recipient DNA is under way. As one strand of the donor DNA exits the vesicle and forms a heteroduplex with the recipient chromosome, the other donor strand is degraded. Among both the gram-positive and the gram-negative species, it seems to be generally true that only one strand of transforming DNA is incorporated into the resident genome. This presumably prevents transformation by DNA that does not have a high degree of homology.

Transduction

The process of transduction involves two distinct mechanisms whereby a bacteriophage (a bacterial virus) can carry bacterial genes from one cell to another. The first mechanism, called *generalized transduction,* allows the transfer of virtually any bacterial gene, whereas the second, called *specialized transduction,* can operate only on particular genes but does so with a relatively high efficiency.

The details of transduction by any particular bacteriophage depend on the life cycle of the virus. (For descriptions of life cycles, see Chap. 60.) Many bacteriophage can grow by only the *virulent* mode, in which every infected cell is taken over by the virus. The infecting virus converts the cell into a factory for producing more virus particles, and within a short time (often as little as 20 minutes) the cell lyses and releases hundreds or thousands of progeny virus particles.

Generalized Transduction

The process of generalized transduction arises from this virulent mode of bacteriophage growth. Each bacteriophage has a mechanism for packaging its genome into a proteinaceous capsid, and some bacteriophage occasionally package fragments of host DNA instead. This aberrant packaging usually occurs randomly with respect to the host sequences that are packaged, and therefore any bacterial gene can be transferred. The amount of host DNA that can be transferred is limited by the size of the phage capsid, because DNA packaging stops when the capsid is full (Chap. 60). The packaged DNA is contained in a capsid that is fully competent for binding to a second cell and DNA injection. Subsequent recombination between the injected DNA and the resident genome can result in the transmission of whatever genetic information was contained in the packaged DNA. Because the transducing particle with bacterial DNA does not carry any of the genetic information of the bacteriophage, the recipient cell is able to survive this pseudoinfection.

Lysogeny and Specialized Transduction

A second important mode of growth for certain bacteriophage involves a benign relationship with the host, called *lysogeny.* In the lysogenic state, the genome of a bacteriophage such as λ is integrated at a particular location in the bacterial chromosome (Chap. 60). While in the lysogenic state, most of the viral genes are repressed, and therefore the lysogenic phage has little effect on bacterial growth. However, a variety of stimuli can induce the lysogenic phage into its virulent mode of growth. When this occurs, the genome of the virus is excised from the host genome and undergoes repeated replication, viral gene expression, and finally packaging into phage capsids.

The process of specialized transduction depends on the lysogenic state of the bacteriophage genome. A bacteriophage genome is excised from the bacterial chromosome by a special recombination mechanism that generally results in precise excision of the phage genome. This recombination mechanism is not perfect, however. Occasionally, excision occurs in such a way that a nearby bacterial gene is included in the excised DNA, and this can lead to specialized transduction of that gene. The interesting feature of specialized transduction is that, once this aberrant excision occurs, the bacterial gene becomes part of the phage genome for all subsequent infections. The novel phage strain produced in this manner can be stably propagated and is called a specialized transducing phage. If that particular transducing phage enters into a lysogenic relationship with a second cell sometime in the future, the second cell will have gained bacterial genes from the previous host and is therefore a transductant.

Sometimes a transductant also arises during a subsequent infection by a mechanism involving normal homologous recombination between the infecting (specialized transducing) phage genome and the bacterial chromosome. Recombination occurs only between the homologous bacterial genes in the phage genome and in the host chromosome, and the genes of the bacteriophage do not integrate into the chromosome. In this way, some transductants generated by a specialized transducing phage are not lysogenic but have gained only the bacterial gene in question.

Most lysogenic bacteriophage genomes integrate at particular locations, called attachment sites, in the bacterial chromosome. This limits the bacterial genes that can be gained in specialized transduction to those that are near the attachment sites. For example, bacteriophage λ integrates between the *gal* and *bio* operons of *E. coli* and forms specialized transducing phage carrying either of these operons.

Conjugation

The sexuality of bacteria was discovered in 1946 by Lederberg and Tatum. They found that genetic markers could be transferred from one strain of *E. coli* to another in a process that required direct contact between the two cells and a special fertility (F) factor in the donor cell. Since that time, numerous conjugation systems have been investigated and found to be more or less similar to the F system. In this section, gene transfer mediated by the F factor is described in some detail, and the other conjugal systems are summarized below (in the discussion on Bacterial Plasmids).

Transfer of the F Factor

The simplest form of the F factor is a 94,500–base pair plasmid that carries genes involved in its own replication and conjugal transfer. *E. coli* donors that carry F (called F^+) can transfer the factor to suitable recipients, thereby converting an F^- recipient into an F^+ exconjugant. Conjugal transfer is a replicative process, and therefore the donor remains an F^+ cell after conjugation.

The process of conjugation is critically dependent on the production of a specialized appendage, the F pilus, present only on cells containing the F factor. The F pilus apparently binds to recipient (F^-) cells and then retracts to bring the conjugal pair in close proximity. Contact between the cell walls of the pair appears to be necessary to allow DNA transfer, but the mechanism of DNA passage is not yet clear. The F pilus is composed predominantly of repeating units of a single protein subunit, F pilin, but several other proteins are required for the correct assembly and function of the pilus. F pilin and the proteins required for pilus assembly are all encoded by genes within the F factor (see genetic map in Fig. 8–12). Nearly all of these genes and others required for DNA transfer are arranged in one large transcription unit, the 30,000–base pair *tra* (transfer) operon.

The F factor contains two distinct replication systems—one that is operational during vegetative growth and one that is used only during conjugation. F replication during normal vegetative growth of the cell is initiated at *oriV* and requires the plasmid-encoded gene, *repE*. In addition, many of the host replication proteins encoded by the bacterial chromosome are necessary for plasmid replication (Chap. 7). The plasmid also encodes a partitioning system that functions, in fashion similar to a eucaryotic centromere, to ensure that each daughter cell receives at least one copy of the element. The combination of the vegetative replication and partitioning systems makes the F plasmid very stable: even during rapid growth, the plasmid is rarely lost.

The replication origin for conjugal transfer, *oriT*, is used to initiate the transfer and replication of the element during conjugation (Fig. 8–13). The first step, which occurs only after formation of a stable mating pair, is a single-strand cleavage event at a particular location in *oriT*. The 5′ end of the broken strand is then passed into the recipient cell, requiring unwinding of the parental helix in the donor cell. In general, the unwinding of the parental DNA occurs concomitantly with replication to replace the transferred single strand.

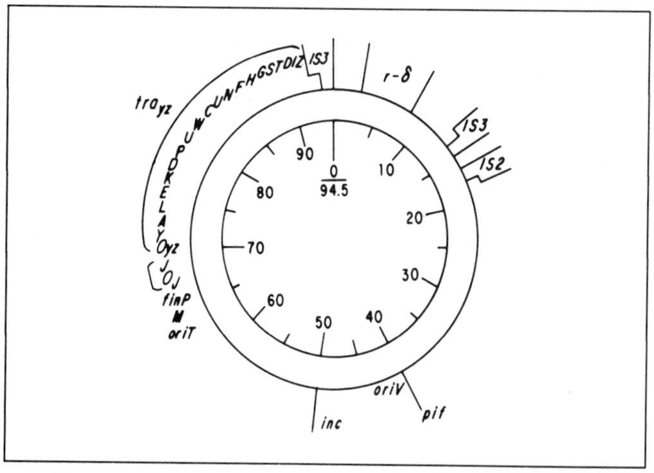

Fig. 8–12. Genetic map of *E. coli* fertility (F) factor. The inner circle represents physical distance in kilobases. *traA, L, E, K, B, V, W, C, U, F, H,* and *G* are involved in the synthesis of pilin and pilus assembly. *finP* is a fertility-inhibition function. *traN* and *traG* are involved in stabilization of mating pairs. *traMYGDIZ* are involved in conjugal DNA metabolism. *traS* and *T* are part of a surface exclusion system involving membrane proteins that reduce the ability of F-bearing cells to act as recipients in conjugation. *pif* renders F-bearing cells resistant to certain phages (viz., coliphage T7, which consequently is a female-specific phage). *inc* governs incompatibility, that is, the inability of related plasmids to coexist with F. *oriV* is the origin of vegetative replication of F, and *oriT* is the origin of replication for conjugal transfer of F. γ-δ, IS*2*, and IS*3* are insertion sequences through which F is integrated into the chromosome to form Hfr cells.

Replacement synthesis of the transferred strand explains why the donor cell remains an F^+ after conjugation. This replication is not, however, required for transfer of the single strand into the recipient. The driving force for single-strand DNA transfer is not entirely clear. Because the process is inhibited by nalidixic acid, the supercoiling provided by DNA gyrase is probably required for strand transfer. Two significant events must occur in the recipient cell to allow establishment of the plasmid. The single strand that is received must be converted into a stable duplex form, and this is accomplished by discontinuous DNA replication. The DNA must also be religated to form a circle, and this reaction might be performed by the same enzyme that performs the single-strand cleavage (encoded by the plasmid). Neither of these two reactions is understood in detail.

Transfer of Chromosomal Genes by the F Factor

The F factor was first recognized by its ability to effect the transfer of chromosomal genes. Any chromosomal gene can be transferred, with a frequency of approximately 10^{-5} to 10^{-6} per F^+ donor cell. The recipient cell must be recombination-competent (*recA*$^+$) to incorporate the transferred chromosomal genes into its own genome. The nature of chromosomal gene transfer by an F^+ is not completely understood, but at least some of it depends on the ability of the F factor to integrate into the bacterial chromosome. The integration of F into the chromosome occurs at a rate of about 10^{-5} per

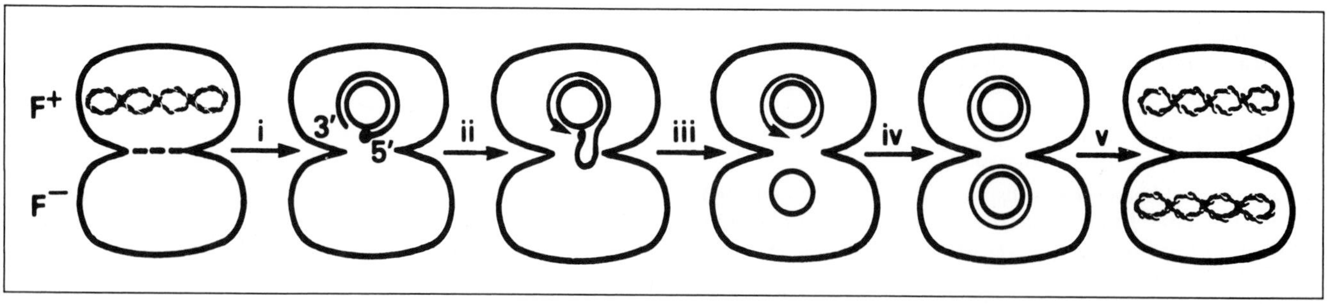

Fig. 8–13. Model for the transfer of F factor DNA. Site-specific cleavage at *oriT* produces a 3′ end that is used as the primer for initiation of replication. The newly replicated strand is maintained in the donor cell, whereas the nicked parental strand is transferred to the recipient. A second single-strand break, followed by ligation, allows the transfer of a single-stranded, monomeric DNA circle. The transferred single strand is converted into duplex form by replication in the recipient cell. *(From Kornberg: DNA Replication. WH Freeman, 1980.)*

cell division, and therefore all F^+ cultures of reasonable density contain cells with integrated F. Such cells can be isolated and show the novel property of high-frequency recombination in the transfer of chromosomal markers, and they are therefore called Hfr (Fig. 8–14).

The transfer of chromosomal genes from an Hfr occurs by exactly the same mechanism as transfer of the autonomous F by an F^+ cell. Because the F factor is integrated in the chromosome of an Hfr, the cleavage and single-stranded DNA transfer described above results in transfer of segments of both F factor sequence and chromosomal DNA. The F factor integrates at a variety of locations to form many different types of Hfr strain, and each strain has its own characteristics for gene transfer during conjugation. As described above, transfer is initiated by a single-strand break and then proceeds in a directional manner starting from the 5′ end at the break. This results in a directionality of the chromosomal genes transferred by any particular Hfr.

The practical value of this arrangement is that it provides

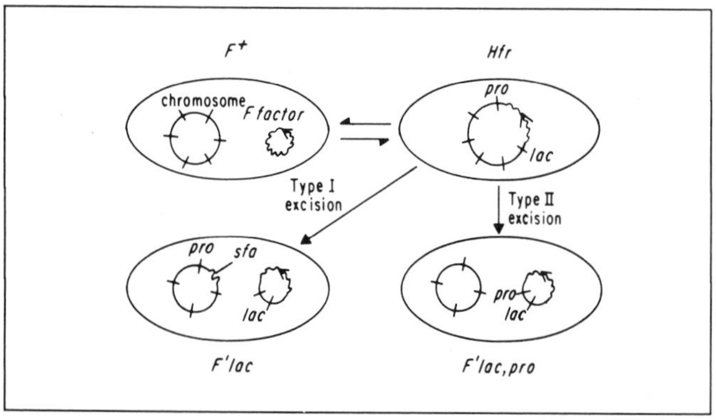

Fig. 8–14. The formation of Hfr and F′ cells. The integration of the fertility factor occurs by a reciprocal recombination event between the circular factor and the circular chromosome. Disintegration of the fertility factor also occurs by reciprocal recombination. The site of recombination governs the chromosome-derived material that will be present in the F′. Type 1 excision, as shown, frequently results in a portion of the fertility factor remaining in the chromosome, creating a sex factor affinity locus.

a powerful method for mapping the genes in the bacterial chromosome. Conjugating pairs can be disrupted by violent agitation, and therefore chromosome transfer can be interrupted as a function of time. When particular genetic markers are tested for their time of entry in this interrupted mating experiment, the order of genes along the chromosome is detected (Fig. 8–15). In the example shown, the F factor is integrated between the *his* and *trp* operons of *E. coli,* with transfer occurring in the counterclockwise direction. Transfer

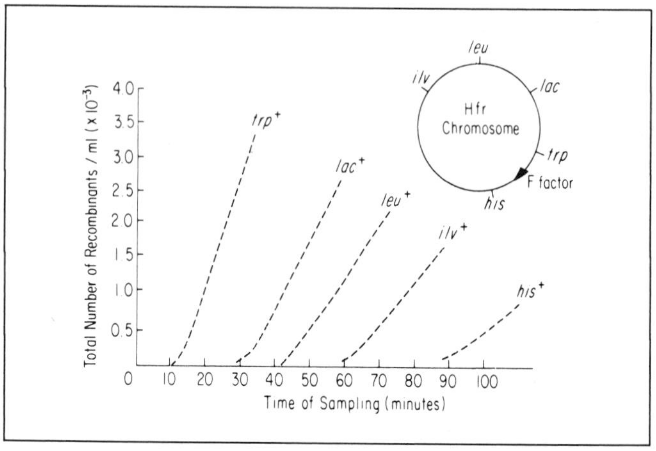

Fig. 8–15. Interrupted mating experiment. Hfr strain of *E. coli* with the fertility factor integrated at the position shown is mixed with an F^- strain that is auxotrophic for the indicated amino acids. Samples are removed from the mating mixture at the times shown, subjected to moderate shear forces, and plated on medium that is selective for the desired recombinants and that prevents growth of the Hfr. The relative time of appearance of recombinants reflects the time of entry of the relevant region of the Hfr chromosome and, therefore, represents the position of the various loci relative to the fertility factor. The decrease in the slopes of the lines representing the frequency of recombinants for late-entering loci is caused by the smaller number of zygotes formed that contain the relevant genetic loci. This smaller number is the result of accidental separation of mating pairs during the course of the linear, polarized transfer of the Hfr chromosome.

of a single strand of the entire chromosome (4.5×10^6 bases) takes about 100 minutes at 37C, and therefore the rate of DNA transfer is about 750 bases per second. Hfr strains with F integrated at other locations transfer different bacterial genes first, but the relative order is always a simple permutation. Chromosome transfer can occur in either direction, depending on the orientation of the inserted F with respect to the chromosome. Because of the nature of the integration event, the *tra* operon of the F plasmid itself is transferred only after the bacterial genome. Random pertubations generally disrupt a mating pair before that time, and thus the recipients in an Hfr $\times$ F^- cross often remain F^-.

The formation of Hfr from F^+ cells (and the reverse event) is dependent on the existence of insertion sequences throughout both the plasmid and the chromosome (see below). In *recA*$^+$ cells, homologous recombination between these identical sequences results in a simple integration event. However, integration can also occur in the absence of homologous recombination using the site-specific recombination systems of the insertion sequences (see discussion on Transpositional Recombination below). These same homologous and site-specific recombination events give rise to a third significant cell type, called an F′ (Fig. 8–14). F′ cells contain an autonomously replicating plasmid that consists of part or all of the F plasmid coupled to a segment of the bacterial chromosome. The F′ factor arises during excision of F from the chromosome of an Hfr—for example, by an excisive recombination event that occurs between an insertion sequence in the F factor and another far removed in the bacterial chromosome. The significance of the F′ factors is that they represent the permanent incorporation of bacterial genes in a transmissible plasmid replicon. This is probably analogous to the acquisition of antibiotic-resistance genes by plasmids (see below).

Transpositional Recombination

The rearrangements of the F factor described above are critically dependent on the existence of insertion sequences in procaryotic DNA. Insertion sequences and other mobile genetic elements participate in transpositional recombination events that use specific DNA sites in one or both DNA molecules as the basis of recognition. Site-specific recombination events are responsible for the movement of insertion sequences and transposons, the integration and rearrangement of various replicons, and the generation of large deletion and insertion mutations. This form of recombination plays a crucial role in the evolution of antibiotic-resistance plasmids and is probably of great importance for mechanisms of evolution in general. Such recombination events are found throughout the biologic world; important examples in eucaryotic systems include immunoglobulin gene rearrangements (Chap. 12), integration of retroviruses (Chap. 59), and antigenic variation in the trypanosomes (Chap. 87).

Each procaryotic site-specific recombination system involves a specific enzyme that catalyzes the strand-exchange reaction; the proteins involved in homologous recombination (*recA* and *recBCD* proteins) are generally not required. Some site-specific systems use specific sequences on both DNAs, whereas others use a particular sequence on only the donor DNA, recombining with recipient DNA at essentially random locations. Important examples of both classes are discussed below.

Mobile Genetic Elements

The simplest of the mobile genetic elements are the insertion sequences (IS elements). The IS elements were first recognized as novel insertion mutations that inactivate the *gal* operon of *E. coli;* virtually all large insertion mutations are caused by the action of IS elements. Most IS elements have a similar structure, containing about 1000 base pairs of duplex DNA and a single gene within the confines of the element (Fig. 8–16A). The gene codes for an enzyme called transposase, which is essential for transposition of the IS element. The transposases are specific to each IS family; for example, the transposase encoded by IS*1* only induces transposition of members of IS*1*. The genomes of bacteria contain numerous IS elements; various isolates of *E. coli* have as many as 40 copies of one IS element or another.

A related class of element is of paramount importance in the generation of antibiotic-resistant bacteria. Transposons are mobile genetic elements that carry a wide variety of genes, notably those involved in drug resistance. Virtually every antibiotic used clinically is rendered ineffective by one or another transposon, and transposons that carry as many as six antibiotic-resistance genes are known. Most of these transposons are contained in plasmids that can be passed between bacterial species, allowing the rapid spread of drug resistance (see the discussion on Drug-Resistance Plasmids below).

The simplest types of transposons are closely related to the IS elements, being just two copies of an IS element surrounding some ancillary gene(s). Thus, Tn*10* is a 9300-base pair element composed of two (inverted) copies of IS*10* that bracket a gene for tetracyline resistance (Fig. 8–16B). The properties of these composite transposons are very similar to those of the IS elements of which they are composed. Transposition occurs at the ends of an IS element, and the IS element and transposon have exactly the same sequence at their respective ends.

A second type of transposon does not contain repeated IS elements at the two ends like the composite transposons above. This class is typified by Tn*3*, a 4700–base pair transposon that carries a β-lactamase (penicillinase) gene (Fig. 8–16C). A distinguishing feature of the Tn*3* family of transposons is that they encode two proteins involved in transposition. In addition to transposase, an enzyme called resolvase is produced to catalyze the resolution of fused replicons (see below).

Mechanism of Transposition

The mechanism of transposition has been the subject of intensive study during the last 15 years. The DNA sequence of the IS and Tn elements and surrounding DNA provided important clues concerning the mechanism. First, each element was found to have inverted complementary repeat sequences of about 10 to 40 base pairs at the two ends (Fig. 8–16). These repeats are unique to each particular element and provide a site at each end of the element for recognition by the transposase. The combination of a specific transposase and particular nucleotide sequences at each end of the element explains the specific nature of the recombination events; a

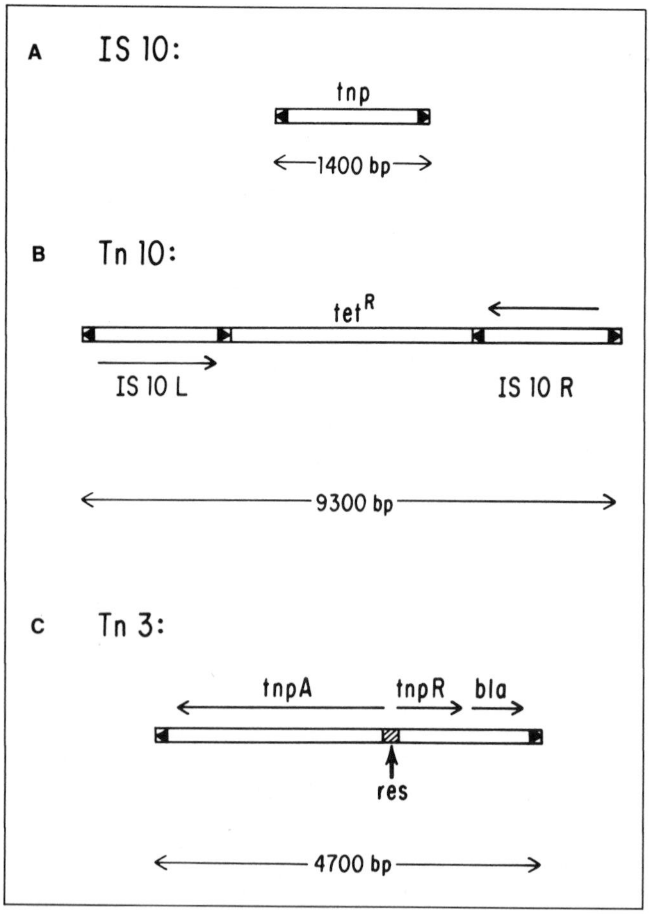

Fig. 8–16. Procaryotic mobile genetic elements. The structures of three representative elements are depicted, with the small enclosed arrows indicating the inverted terminal repeats. **A.** The insertion sequence IS*10* encodes only an IS*10*-specific transposase (*tnp*). **B.** Transposon Tn*10* is composed of two (nearly identical) copies of IS*10* bracketing a gene for tetracycline resistance (*tetR*). Both IS*10* L (left) and IS*10* R (right) contain the IS*10* transposase gene; however, the protein specified by IS*10* L has reduced activity due to several mutations. **C.** Transposon Tn*3* is one member of a large family of related elements that encode resistance to a variety of antibiotics. Tn*3* itself contains genes for β-lactamase (*bla*), transposase (*tnpA*) and resolvase (*tnpR*). Resolvase is responsible for the site-specific recombination event that resolves cointegrate structures formed by the initial transposition event (see text).

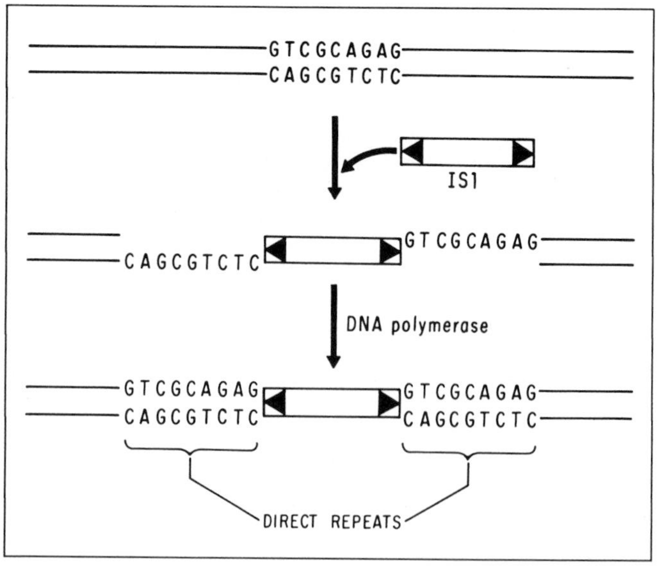

Fig. 8–17. Generation of target-site duplications during transposition. The duplication of a nine–base pair segment of the *lacI* gene of *E. coli* as a result of IS*1* transposition is depicted. The precise details of the transposition reaction are not entirely clear (see text). However, the only simple mechanism capable of generating such target-site duplications is the staggered cleavage of the target DNA, followed by element insertion and limited DNA synthesis. Two different pathways incorporating variations of this mechanism are shown in Figures 8–18 and 8–19. *(Adapted from Calos et al: Cell 13:411, 1978.)*

given IS element or transposon can induce transposition of only itself or elements that have the same end sequence.

A second clue from DNA sequence analysis concerns the nature of the DNA just outside the confines of the element. The DNA surrounding an element invariably contains a directly repeated sequence of a small number of base pairs. The direct repeats are not part of the element but, rather, are generated from the target DNA on insertion of the IS element. A simple mechanism for generating such duplications is by a staggered cleavage of the target DNA, followed by insertion of the element and repair synthesis to fill the short gaps (Fig. 8–17). In this way, whatever sequence is at the initial site of insertion becomes duplicated, with one copy appearing just outside each end of the element. Each particular mobile element invariably generates the same number of base pairs duplicated at every site of insertion. For example, IS*1* generates 9–base pair duplications, while Tn*3* duplicates five base pairs during transposition. Because the nature of the duplication is determined by the element itself, the element-encoded transposase is thought to be responsible for the staggered cleavage of the target DNA.

There are two models for transposition that incorporate the above features. The first is simple transposition, in which the element is cleaved out of the donor DNA molecule by transposase and inserted into the target DNA by the steps described above (Figs. 8–17 and 8–18). Simple transposition apparently accounts for the majority of the transposition events of the composite transposons and their constituent IS elements. Simple transposition results in the transfer of the element from one DNA to another; the donor DNA molecule is probably destroyed in the process.

The Tn*3* family of transposons uses a more sophisticated method of transposition involving duplication of the element. Duplicative transposition results in the appearance of a new copy of Tn*3* at some location, as well as the maintenance of the original copy in its native location. The outline of a current model for duplicative transposition is shown in Figure 8–19. The first steps involve staggered cleavage of both the donor (AB) and target (CD) molecules. The two single-strand cleavages of donor DNA occur at the opposite ends of the element, but the element is not cleaved away from the rest of the donor

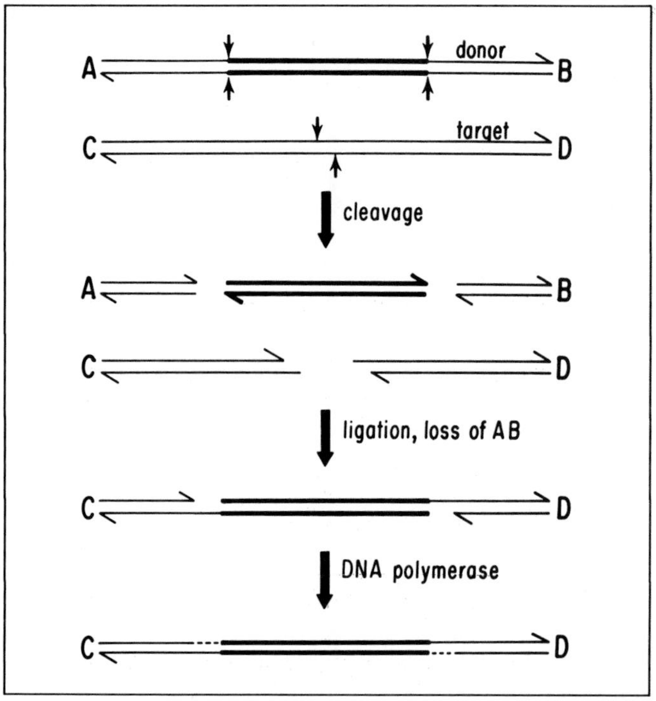

Fig. 8–18. Proposed mechanism for simple transposition. The transposition of an IS element (or composite transposon) from a donor molecule, AB, to a target molecule, CD, is depicted. The first step involves staggered cleavage of the target molecule and the formation of (nonstaggered) double-strand breaks at each end of the element within the donor molecule. Ligation of the element to the staggered breaks in the target is as shown in Figure 8–17, with the loss of the remainder of the donor molecule. Because bacterial cells generally contain several copies of any particular replicon, the loss of one copy of the donor molecule would be of little consequence.

DNA. The target DNA is cleaved by transposase at a (more or less) random location, with a short staggered break. The cleaved donor and target DNAs are next joined together to form a molecule with an unusual structure (Fig. 8–19, step 3). This joint molecule contains two 3′ ends that serve as primers for replication, resulting in the observed duplication of the transposable element (Fig. 8–19, step 4). The product of this replication is a special molecule called a cointegrate, in which donor, target, and two copies of the element are contained. (Note that the two segments AD and CB in Fig. 8–19 must belong to the *same* molecule, if the original donor and target were each circular.)

The last step in duplicative transposition is the resolution of the cointegrate into two autonomous replicons (Fig. 8–19, step 5). Resolution is catalyzed by a second site-specific recombination system, involving specific resolution sites (*res*) within the transposon and the resolvase protein. Resolution is a simple *cut-and-paste* process in which both resolution sites are cleaved (again with staggered breaks), exchanged into the recombinant configuration, and ligated to produce the resolved products. The resolvase reaction has been reconstituted in vitro with highly purified protein, and the mechanism of resolution is closely related to the mechanism of topoisomerase

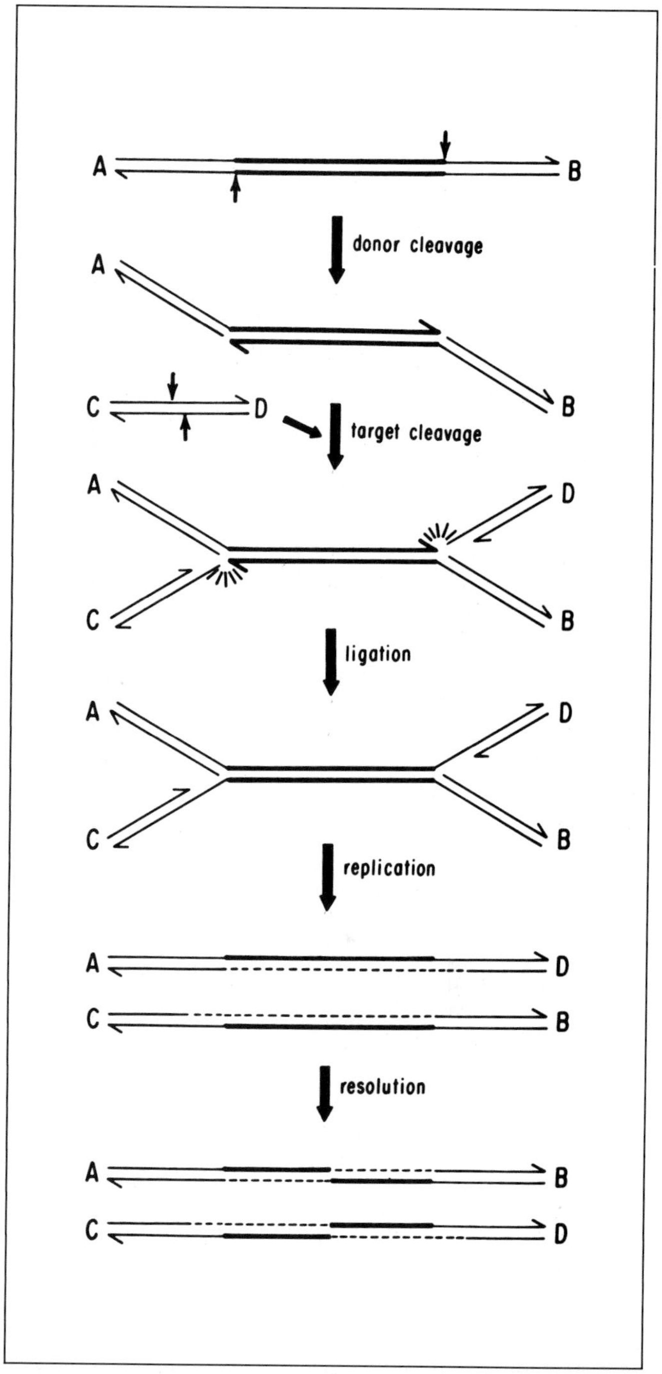

Fig. 8–19. Proposed mechanism for duplicative transposition. The steps involved in this current model for duplicative transposition are described in the text. For the sake of clarity, the donor molecule is rearranged after cleavage. Note that the two halves of the target attach to opposite ends of the transposable element during ligation. Replication through the entire transposable element results in its duplication (newly replicated strands indicated by dashed lines). Subsequent site-specific recombination (resolution) regenerates the donor (AB) and target (CD) molecules, each containing the transposable element. *(Adapted from Shapiro: Proc Natl Acad Sci USA 76:1933, 1979.)*

action (Chap. 7). Mutants of Tn*3* without a functional resolvase gene have been isolated. These mutants are competent for transposition but always produce cointegrates as their final product.

The models for simple and duplicative transposition have been generated from studies with several well-characterized IS elements and transposons. As the transposition reactions are reconstituted in vitro, confirmation and refinements in these models are likely. It is worth pointing out that many transposons have not been studied in as much depth, and novel mechanisms of transposition may therefore await discovery.

Genetic Consequences of Transposition

A wide variety of genetic alterations are caused by the action of mobile genetic elements. The simplest consequence of transposition is the inactivation of a gene into which the element transposes. As mentioned above, insertions of a mobile genetic element into the *gal* operon resulted in the discovery of insertion sequences in bacteria. These insertion mutations were polar in nature, inactivating the downstream genes of the operon as well as the gene that suffered the insertion event. This is explained by the finding that many IS elements have both termination codons and transcription termination sites.

Certain mobile genetic elements are also able to activate bacterial genes. IS*2*, IS*3*, and several other elements carry functional promoters (or parts of promoters) near or at their ends. When such an element inserts just upstream of an inactive (or poorly transcribed) gene, transcription of that gene can commence. If insertion occurs upstream of a polycistronic operon, several proteins that carry out related functions may be affected.

A different class of genetic consequences of mobile elements results from their repetitive nature. Because many different bacterial DNA molecules contain one or more copy of any given IS element, homologous recombination can occur between the different elements. This can lead to the fusion of replicons, the resolution of one replicon into two, and various other rearrangements of DNA. This homologous recombination occurs by the standard *recA*-dependent pathways discussed above, and reflects a role of IS elements as *portable regions of homology*. These are precisely the events that lead to the interconversions of F^+, Hfr, and F' strains (see the section on Conjugation above). Because transpositional recombination can also give rise to and resolve cointegrates, several distinct pathways for rearrangement exist.

IS elements also play an important role in the generation of large deletion mutations in bacterial chromosomes. Many large deletions are found to have one end point at the end of an IS element, implicating a transpositional event in their generation. One way in which this might occur is by means of a two-step process. If an IS element is located at position A, and a second IS element (of the same type) transposes into position B, all DNA between points A and B can be deleted by either homologous recombination or resolution between the two identical elements.

Perhaps the most important rearrangement with respect to antibiotic resistance is the generation of composite transposons from isolated IS elements and drug-resistance genes. Given a drug-resistance gene in some bacterial cell, there is a finite probability that an IS element will transpose into the

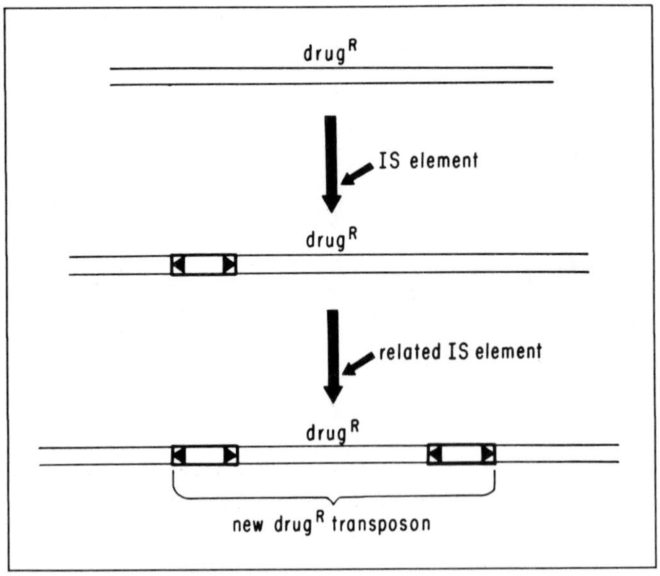

Fig. 8–20. The genesis of a new transposon. The generation of a new antibiotic-resistance transposon from isolated IS elements and an antibiotic-resistance gene is depicted. Two simple transposition events result in the bracketing of the antibiotic-resistance gene by copies of the same IS element, thereby creating the composite transposon.

adjoining DNA (Fig. 8–20, step 1). A second transposition event, involving either the same or a related element, can then introduce an IS element on the other side of the drug-resistance gene (Fig. 8–20, step 2). Each of these transposition events may occur at a low frequency, but the large numbers that bacterial cells easily achieve make the entire sequence quite plausible. The critical point is that a new transposon for the drug-resistance gene has been created. This new transposon is fully capable of transposing into other replicons, and some of these can be transferred between different bacterial species (see the discussion on Bacterial Plasmids below). This general mechanism for creating new transposons has been demonstrated in laboratory cultures of bacteria.

Conjugative Transposons in *Streptococcus*

A special class of transposons confers antibiotic resistance in the genus *Streptococcus*. The conjugative transposons have the remarkable property of inducing conjugation between two cells and subsequently transposing from the chromosome of the donor to that of the recipient. The precise mechanism of transfer is not known, but it may involve a circular intermediate generated by excision of the transposon from the donor chromosome. It is important to note that only the transposon itself is transferred during the conjugative event; the transfer of other chromosomal markers is not detectable. Recipients of a conjugative transposon are found to have the transposon inserted at any of numerous sites around the chromosome, and these recipients themselves become competent for subsequent transfer of the element to another cell. These results imply that element transfer is indeed a transpositional event and also that the element encodes critical functions necessary for conjugation.

The prototype of the conjugative transposons is Tn*916*, a 16,400–base pair tetracycline-resistance element originally isolated from *Enterococcus faecalis*. Tn*916* induces conjugative transfer of itself at frequencies ranging from 10^{-8} to 10^{-5} per donor, depending on the precise location of the element in the donor chromosome. Most of the suspected conjugative transposons include a tetracycline-resistance determinant similar to that of Tn*916*, but some carry additional antibiotic-resistance genes.

The conjugative transposons are thought to play a major role in antibiotic resistance in the streptococci. In many clinically important strains, conjugative antibiotic-resistance transposons appear to be more common than antibiotic-resistance plasmids. The dissemination of conjugative transposons may be increased by their ability to transpose onto various plasmids, some of which are themselves conjugative. Recent studies suggest that conjugative transposons are not limited to the genus *Streptococcus*. Conjugative antibiotic resistance (with no detectable plasmid vector) has been detected in *Clostridium difficile* and in *Bacteroides fragilis*.

Invertible DNA Segments

Certain properties of bacterial cells change at a frequency that is much higher than that expected on the basis of spontaneous mutation. The affected properties include several of medical importance, relating to antigenicity, virulence, and adhesion. The molecular mechanisms controlling many of these unstable phenotypes have not yet been elucidated. However, several operate by a site-specific inversion mechanism that was first elucidated in the *phase variation* system of *Salmonella typhimurium*.

Phase variation was discovered as a switch between two alternate serologic forms and was shown to depend on the production of two discrete flagellar antigens, called H1 and H2. Molecular analysis has shown that the gene encoding the H2 flagellar protein is adjacent to a 970–base pair segment of DNA that can exist in either of two alternate orientations with respect to the *H2* gene (Fig. 8–21). In one orientation (*ON*), a promoter within this DNA segment allows transcription of the *H2* gene and a contiguous gene, *rh1*. The *rh1* gene encodes a repressor that blocks transcription of the *H1* gene, and therefore the *ON* orientation results in production of only the H2 flagellar antigen. In the alternate orientation (*OFF*), the promoter is reversed with respect to the *H2* and *rh1* genes, and thus neither is transcribed. This results in transcription of the *H1* gene (because the repressor of *H1* is not present), and therefore only the H1 flagellar antigen is produced. The two alternate orientations of the 970–base pair DNA segment thus result in a genetic *flip-flop* between H1 and H2 antigen production. At frequencies of roughly 10^{-4} per cell division, the DNA segment inverts to interconvert the two antigenic serotypes.

The mechanism of DNA inversion is closely related to the process of transposon cointegrate resolution described above. The 970–base pair DNA segment contains a gene, *hin*, the product of which catalyzes site-specific recombination between the two ends of the segment. The sites of recombination at the ends are a pair of inverted complementary repeat sequences, and recombination thereby inverts the intervening DNA. (In the resolution of cointegrates during transposition, the two recombining sites are directly repeated, and thus the outcome is resolution rather than inversion). The similarity between these two classes of site-specific recombination events is not superficial. The *hin* protein of *S. typhimurium* shares significant sequence homology with the resolvase protein of Tn*3*, indicating that the two systems are related in an evolutionary sense.

Several bacteriophage use nearly identical flip-flop systems for altering the range of host bacterial cells that can be infected. The site-specific recombinases induced in these bacteriophage systems are very closely related to the *hin* protein and can even catalyze inversion of the *S. typhimurium* invertible segment. An interesting analogy between these invertible segments is that they control properties related to the interaction of an organism with its environment. The relatively rapid switching of invertible DNA segments provides an efficient mechanism for successful adaptation to rapidly changing environments. Bacterial pathogens may generally use this and related strategies to evade the host immune response.

Bacterial Plasmids

Plasmids are ancillary genetic elements of bacteria that generally replicate as duplex DNA circles independent of the bacterial chromosome. Many, like the F plasmid, are capable of self-transmission by virtue of plasmid-encoded proteins that allow bacterial conjugation. These *conjugative* plasmids can also allow the transfer of nonconjugative plasmids, and thus virtually every plasmid can be disseminated at some frequency. Plasmids range in size from fewer than 1000 to more than 400,000 base pairs and can carry a wide variety of genes between bacteria of the same or different species. From a

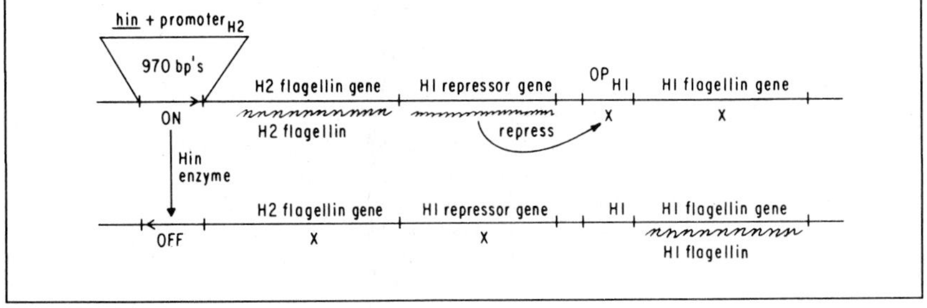

Fig. 8–21. The basis for the control of flagellar phase variation in *S. typhimurium*. Other details are given in the text.

medical standpoint, plasmids confer most of the antibiotic-resistance properties of bacteria, several important cases of pathogen virulence, and systems for the production of some antibiotics.

Classification of Plasmids

The genetic content of various plasmids forms the basis of one classification system. Thus the drug-resistance (R) plasmids carry antibiotic-resistance genes, often with several resistance genes carried by a single R plasmid. The *colicinogenic* (Col) plasmids encode small proteins (colicins) that kill a variety of enteric bacteria related to the producing organism. Each plasmid also encodes an immunity protein so that the cell producing the colicin does not commit suicide. Antibacterial proteins are also specified by streptococcal and staphylococcal plasmids; members of this general category of proteins are called bacteriocins. *Virulence* plasmids encode various proteins involved in the pathogenic properties of bacteria. The most striking examples involve the production of toxins, such as tetanus, anthrax, and enterotoxins. Some virulence plasmids encode proteins that are important for colonization (e.g., factors that allow adherence of bacteria to cells in the small intestine). Another large class of plasmids affects the metabolic activities of bacteria, and some of these play important ecologic roles. Several *Pseudomonas* plasmids allow their hosts to degrade and thereby detoxify organic chemicals such as toluene, octane, and naphthalene. In addition, nitrogen fixation by *Rhizobium* species depends on a series of plasmids that are important for both the nodulation of roots by the bacteria and the actual fixation of nitrogen that occurs within the nodules.

Many plasmids isolated from nature fit into one or another of these categories in a simple way, but others do not. Certain large conjugative plasmids encode multiple colicins, along with antibiotic-resistance and virulence factors. The combination of virulence and antibiotic-resistance genes on single plasmids has obvious medical consequences. The rearrangement of genes into such complex plasmids is considered below in the context of antibiotic resistance.

A second useful classification system for plasmids is that of *compatibility*. Two plasmids are said to be compatible if they can stably coexist in the same bacterial cell and incompatible if they cannot. Incompatibility is always observed with two distinguishable versions of the same plasmid, and it is often observed with closely related plasmids. Conversely, plasmids that are not related to each other in any way are usually compatible. Incompatibility is a consequence of the replication and segregation of plasmids, but precise molecular details are, for the most part, still lacking. Approximately 25 different incompatibility groups have been observed among the enterobacterial plasmids; the F plasmid is a member of incompatibility group FI.

These and other methods of classification can be used not only for understanding relationships between plasmids but also as epidemiologic tools. A particular outbreak of dysentery may show a preponderance of *Shigella* with one particular plasmid, and the nature of the plasmid can be used to trace the infection. If the plasmid carries a particular combination of drug-resistance genes, the information is also of obvious importance in deducing the correct treatment for the pathogen (also see below).

Conjugative Plasmids in Gram-Negative Organisms

Although plasmids can be transferred between bacteria by transformation and transduction, the most important route of transmission is generally through plasmid-encoded conjugation systems. The most extensively studied system is that of the F factor described above. Other gram-negative plasmids encode a conjugation system that is quite homologous to that of F, and these are closely related to F in an evolutionary sense. F-related plasmids have been found to be important in certain cases of antibiotic resistance and in the production of some colicins.

Several other conjugative systems with some similarities to that of F have been described. The plasmid ColI (and related plasmids) carry the I conjugation system. Like the F plasmid, these encode a pilin protein that forms sex pili, but the protein is antigenically distinct from that of F. Although studied in less detail, these other conjugative systems probably function in a manner analogous to that of F.

Many conjugative plasmids are restricted to just a few gram-negative species, limiting their importance in gene transmission. Other plasmids have a very broad host range, being able to propagate and promote conjugation in virtually any gram-negative bacterium. Examples of broad-host-range plasmids include the antibiotic-resistance plasmids RP4 and R68.45 (incompatibility group PI). The critical importance of broad-host-range plasmids is that they allow gene transfer between many unrelated bacterial cells. An antibiotic-resistance plasmid in a nonpathogen can be transferred into a pathogenic bacterial strain, threatening antibiotic therapy against the pathogen.

The importance of conjugative plasmids is accentuated by their ability to effect the transfer of nonconjugative plasmids. Many plasmids that do not encode conjugation systems can nevertheless enjoy transmission in a process called *plasmid mobilization.* Mobilization does not generally require any recombination between the two plasmids, and sometimes only the nonconjugative plasmid is transferred in a particular mating pair. The details of plasmid mobilization can be quite complex; for example, certain combinations of plasmids demonstrate mobilization in only some bacterial hosts. In spite of this, plasmid mobilization can be a very efficient process, leading to the dissemination of nonconjugative plasmids throughout the gram-negative organisms. The combination of plasmid mobilization and broad-host-range plasmids essentially provides many of the gram-negative organisms with a common gene pool that allows rapid evolution in the face of environmental pressures (such as antibiotics).

Conjugative Plasmids in Gram-Positive Organisms

In contrast to the ubiquity of conjugative plasmids in the gram-negative organisms, only a few gram-positive organisms are known to possess such plasmids. (However, see the discussion on Conjugative Transposons in *Streptococcus* above.) Conjugative plasmids have been found in *Streptococcus, Streptomyces, Clostridium,* and *Bacillus,* and each of these is quite different from the gram-negative systems described above.

None of the gram-positive conjugation systems described

to date depend on sex pili but, rather, use other mechanisms to bring mating pairs into close contact. The streptococcal R plasmid pAMβ1 is transferred very inefficiently in liquid culture (only about one conjugation event per 10^6 donors) but can transfer quite efficiently (as many as 1 per 10^2 donors) when the cells are brought together on a filter. Presumably, this plasmid encodes no system to attract mating partners but depends instead on accidental associations of mating pairs.

Other streptococcal plasmids, such as pAD1, transfer at high frequency in liquid culture by way of an induced aggregation of donor and recipient cells. Recipient cells without the plasmid secrete a small peptide that functions as a *sex pheromone,* causing donor cells to become adherent and form stable mating pairs with the recipients. The pheromone interacts with donor cells by means of a cell surface receptor to induce the synthesis of a special aggregation substance known as adhesin. On acquisition of the plasmid, the synthesis of the pheromone becomes repressed, and the cell is no longer able to induce clumping in other cells containing pAD1. Several pheromones exist, however, and each appears to be specific for a given plasmid. Therefore a cell containing pAD1 still secretes pheromones that affect donor cells containing other plasmids, and the presence of pAD1 does not block transfer of these other plasmids.

Drug-resistance Plasmids

The phenomenon of transmissible drug resistance was first recognized in Japan during the late 1950s. A strain of *Shigella flexneri* was isolated during an epidemic of dysentery and was found to be resistant to four different antibiotics: chloramphenicol, tetracycline, streptomycin, and sulfonamides. This particular strain harbored a plasmid specifying all four resistance traits, and the plasmid soon became widespread. The same R plasmid was found in *E. coli* strains isolated from affected patients, implying that the plasmid could be transferred between different bacterial species. The biochemical nature of the drug-resistance mechanisms specified by this and other R plasmids is discussed in Chapter 9.

Virtually every antibacterial drug in use can be rendered ineffective by one R plasmid or another, and many of these plasmids contain multiple drug-resistance determinants. The potential of such plasmids for dispersal is evidenced by the isolation of plasmids R1, R100, and R6 from samples in London, Japan, and Austria, respectively. Each of these plasmids carries the F conjugation system, and the three plasmids are quite closely related to each other. The effective dissemination of these plasmids is related to their conjugal nature. However, as described above, even nonconjugative plasmids can be mobilized for transfer. Roughly one half of the enterobacteria isolated from nature carry conjugative plasmids (some of which do not specify drug resistance themselves), and in many cases these conjugative plasmids mobilize nonconjugative R plasmids.

Rapid Evolution of R Plasmids

R plasmids have been found in many different incompatibility and conjugative groups, and the same drug-resistance gene is often found on plasmids that are otherwise unrelated. These and other results indicate that R plasmids are quite plastic, evolving rapidly under the selective pressure of antibiotic treatments. This view is supported by an analysis of the structure of R plasmid DNAs. Figure 8–22 presents a schematic diagram of a typical conjugative R plasmid, R1. All of the drug-resistance genes are clustered in a region of the plasmid called the *r-determinant,* while the genes involved in conjugal transfer are clustered in another region called the *resistance transfer factor* (RTF). The RTF can be viewed as the

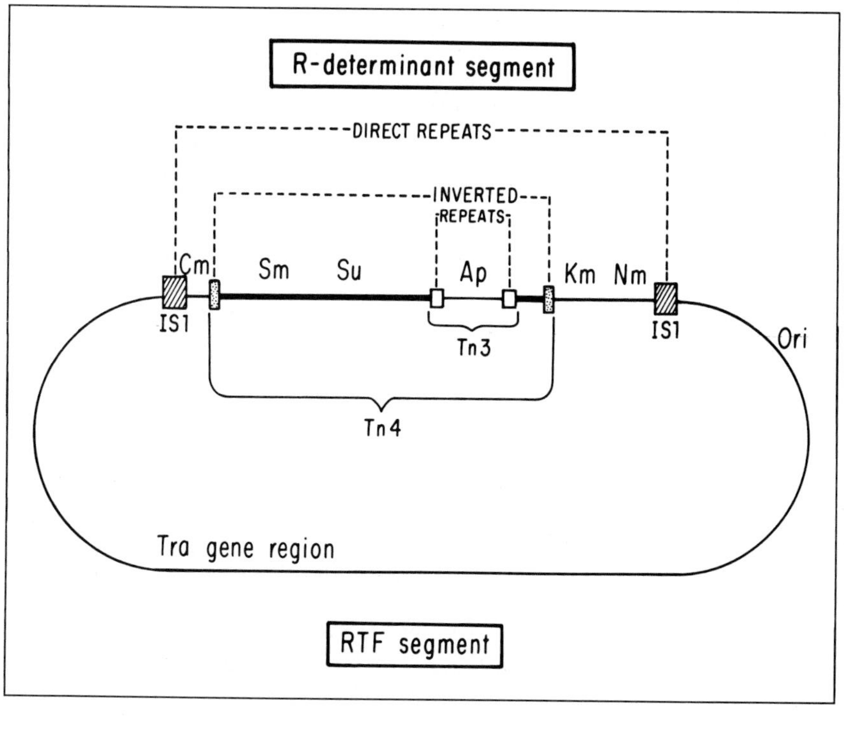

Fig. 8–22. Structure of resistance plasmid R1. Plasmid R1 encodes resistance to chloramphenicol (Cm), streptomycin (Sm), sulfonamide (Su), ampicillin (Ap), kanamycin (Km), and neomycin (Nm). The locations of the replication origin (ori) and the genes for conjugal transfer (Tra) are also indicated. *(Adapted from Cohen: In Bukhari et al (eds): DNA Insertion Elements, Plasmids, and Episomes. Cold Spring Harbor Laboratory, 1977.)*

remnant of a primordial conjugative plasmid that acquired drug-resistance genes (the r-determinant) by transpositional events. The r-determinant is clearly a complex collection of mobile genetic elements. A large central Tn*4* transposon encodes resistance to streptomycin and sulfonamides, and a Tn*3* element with its ampicillin resistance gene is contained within the Tn*4*. The entire r-determinant is flanked by directly repeated copies of IS*1*, and genes specifying chloramphenicol and kanamycin resistance are also included. The complexity of the r-determinant is easy to understand after the discussion of the activities of transposable elements and insertion sequences (see above). Virtually any plasmid in nature can acquire a drug-resistance transposon at some frequency. The generation of multiple-drug-resistance transposons and plasmids is also exemplified in the structure of the R1 plasmid. The Tn*4* shown in Figure 8–22 contains an ampicillin-resistance gene as the result of transposition of Tn*3* into Tn*4*.

The r-determinants of R plasmids are often flanked by repeats of IS elements, as in the R1 plasmid under discussion. This direct repeat of IS*1* allows a significant rearrangement, namely, the dissociation of the r-determinant and the RTF. With directly repeated IS elements, this dissociation results from a simple act of homologous recombination between the repeated segments (Fig. 8–23A). This recombination event can interconvert a conjugative and a nonconjugative R plasmid. Perhaps more important, the r-determinant itself can move onto another completely distinct plasmid. Many plasmids contain one or more copies of IS*1* (and other IS elements), and therefore the dissociated r-determinant can integrate into another plasmid via homologous recombination between the IS elements (Fig. 8–23B). Another route for R plasmid rearrangement is transpositional. As discussed in the context of transposition (see above), any stretch of DNA surrounded by functional IS elements becomes a larger mobile genetic element, transposing by means of the repeated IS elements at the ends. Therefore the r-determinant of many R plasmids can transpose en masse onto another plasmid or a bacterial chromosome, with consequences identical to those shown in Figure 8–23B. A third significant rearrangement of R plasmids is the amplification of drug-resistance genes, which can provide bacterial cells with increased resistance to certain antibiotics (Fig. 8–23C).

In summary, the repeated sequences contained in bacterial plasmids allow many rearrangements by homologous recombination acts, and these repeated sequences themselves are also capable of transpositional recombination. These events endow bacterial plasmids with a remarkable plasticity, a plasticity that itself must be understood in assessing the medical problems associated with antibiotic resistance.

Origin and Preponderance of R Plasmids

Several studies strongly indicate that R plasmids predate the modern era of antibiotic therapy. Some R plasmids may be the result of selection by naturally occurring antibiotics, which are quite ubiquitous in the environment (Chap. 9). However, it is clear that the widespread use of antibiotics greatly increases the prevalence and diversity of such plasmids. In patients given oral tetracycline, the predominant fecal *E. coli* isolates carry tetracycline-resistance R plasmids within 1 week. On a larger scale, the percentage of drug-resistant pathogens isolated from the population increases dramatically with the use of the corresponding antibiotic. Antibiotics are also used widely as growth promoters in livestock, and drug-resistant bacteria have been shown to transfer readily from animals to humans. These various increases in prevalence are the result of the selection of those bacteria that can survive in a given environment, a simple case of *survival of the fittest.* When such

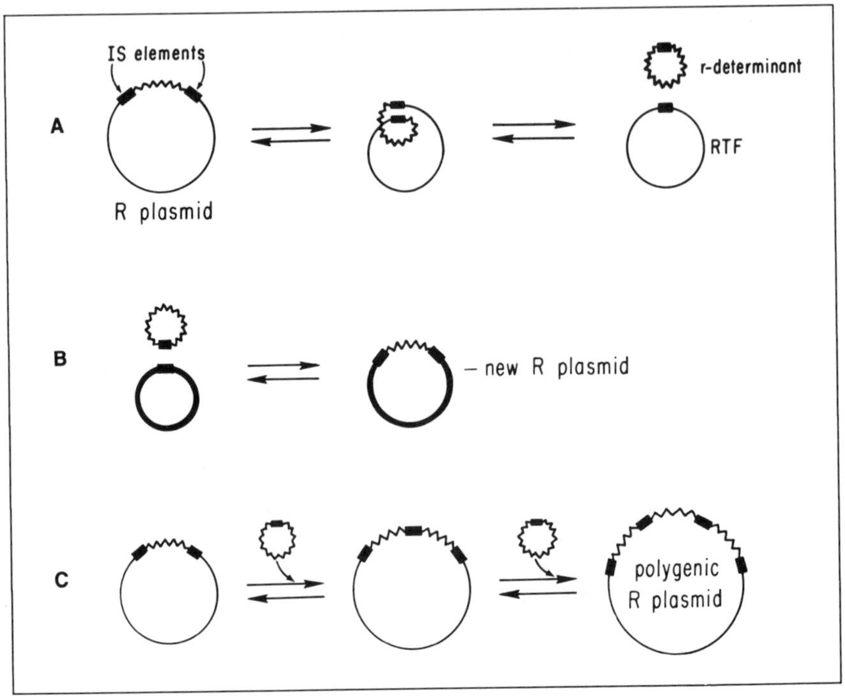

Fig. 8–23. Common rearrangements of the R plasmids. **A.** Recombination between directly repeated IS elements results in the dissociation of the R plasmid into two circular molecules, the *r-determinant* (containing all or most of the antibiotic-resistance genes) and the *resistance transfer factor* (RTF) (containing all genes necessary for conjugal transfer). **B.** The recombination of an isolated r-determinant with a different plasmid can generate a novel R plasmid. This recombination can occur either by recombination between an IS element in the r-determinant and a homologous element in the plasmid, or by transposition of the r-determinant segment of an R plasmid. **C.** Polygenic R plasmids are generated by iterative recombination events in which exogenous r-determinants are incorporated into an R plasmid. The multiple copies of the antibiotic-resistance genes can provide resistance to higher drug concentrations than a simple R plasmid. *(Adapted from Cohen: Nature 263:731, 1976.)*

powerful selective pressures are combined with the plasticity and mobility of plasmids, it is not surprising that novel R plasmids are frequently encountered in various pathogens. It is also worth noting that treatment with one antibiotic may simultaneously select for several drug-resistance traits, because many R plasmids contain multiple antibiotic-resistance determinants.

Restriction-Modification Systems

The foregoing discussion of gene transfer in bacteria may give the impression that different bacterial species exchange genetic information in a completely promiscuous fashion. This is not true. Several significant barriers exist to reduce, but not abolish, the transfer of genes between different species. One barrier that has already been described relates to the nature of conjugal transfer. Although broad-host-range plasmids exist, most plasmids cannot survive in more than a few species. Furthermore, conjugal acts between different species are presumably quite inefficient.

A second significant barrier to gene transfer is the existence of restriction-modification systems, which generally destroy incoming DNA unless it has the *fingerprint* of a closely related bacteria. Restriction of foreign DNA is not complete but, rather, reduces transfer about 1000-fold. The combination of these barriers to gene transfer strongly tempers the promiscuous exchange of genes between bacterial species. The fact that such exchange is still significant again relates to the tremendous cell densities that bacterial cultures can reach. Even two barriers, each of 1000- or 10,000-fold efficiency, cannot block exchange when cell numbers exceed 10^8.

Biologic Aspects of Restriction-modification

The bacterial restriction-modification systems are interesting in their own right and have also led to the burgeoning field of recombinant DNA methodology and modern molecular genetics. Several hundred systems have been described in different bacteria, and virtually all these systems operate by a similar mechanism. Each consists of two enzymes—an endonuclease and a DNA methylase—that recognize the same short sequence in DNA. For example, the *Eco*RI system, encoded on plasmid R1, recognizes the sequence 5'-GAATTC-3' (Table 8–1). The fingerprint mentioned above is the existence of methyl group modifications of the DNA at that particular sequence. These methyl groups are added by the *Eco*RI methylase and block cleavage by the *Eco*RI restriction endonuclease.

The methylase enzyme protects the endogenous DNA of a cell against self-digestion. Every GAATTC site in the DNA of a cell containing plasmid R1 is methylated and therefore not a substrate for *Eco*RI endonuclease. However, foreign DNA entering the cell will not contain these specific methyl groups unless it also originated from a bacterium with the *Eco*RI system. Therefore foreign DNA is generally cleaved by the endonuclease and subsequently degraded. If it happens that the foreign DNA has no GAATTC sequences, it will survive restriction. However, most DNA molecules contain the sequence simply by random chance.

TABLE 8–1. TYPE II RESTRICTION-MODIFICATION RECOGNITION SITES[a]

Specificity Designation	Enzyme	Substrate ↓ = Hydrolysis • = Methylation					
*Eco*RI:	Endonuclease	G↓A	A	T	T	C	
		C	T	T	A	A↑G	
				•			
	Methylase	G	A	A	T	T	C
		C	T	T	A	A	G
					•		
*Hind*III:	Endonuclease	A↓A	G	C	T	T	
		T	T	C	G	A↑A	
			•				
	Methylase	A	A	G	C	T	T
		T	T	C	G	A	A
							•
*Taq*I:	Endonuclease	T↓C	G		A		
		A	G	C	↑T		
				•			
	Methylase	T	C	G	A		
		A	G	C	T		
			•				

[a] The nucleotide sequence specificities of three restriction modification systems are indicated; more than 150 different nucleotide sequence specificities for restriction endonucleases have been discovered. In each duplex DNA sequence, the top strand is given in the 5' to 3' direction and the bottom strand in the 3' to 5' direction. The nomenclature for restriction-modification systems is given in Smith and Nathans: J Mol Biol 81: 419, 1973.

An important biologic aspect of restriction-modification systems is the fate of replicating DNA. Given a cell with methylated GAATTC sites in its chromosome, DNA replication should produce daughter molecules that are deficient in methylation. These are not subject to self-digestion, for the following reason. Every methylation system provides one methylated base on each of the two strands of DNA; the *Eco*RI sites are methylated at the second A residue on each of the strands (Table 8–1). Because DNA replication is semiconservative (Chap. 7), each of the two newly replicated daughter molecules contains exactly one methylated strand (hemimethylated DNA). Hemimethylated DNA is a good substrate for the methylase but not for the restriction enzyme. Therefore, the two daughter molecules become fully methylated before the restriction enzyme has a chance to act.

As mentioned above, restriction systems are not completely efficient, and some incoming DNA molecules escape restriction. This presumably occurs when the methylase enzyme manages to reach the critical recognition sequences before the restriction enzyme. An interesting feature of this arrangement is that those few foreign DNA molecules that do become methylated are now recognized by the cell as *self* rather than as foreign. If these molecules can replicate, their hemimethylated daughter molecules will become fully methylated, just as occurs after replication of the endogenous chromosome. Thus certain DNA molecules that penetrate the restriction barrier propagate indefinitely in the recipient cell.

Restriction Enzymes

The restriction and modification enzymes have been the subject of intense investigation. These enzyme systems are encoded by genes within bacterial chromosomes, a large number of plasmids, and lysogenic phage genomes. A given bacterial strain may have several such systems and thus cleave foreign DNA at several different sequences. Each restriction-modification system recognizes a particular DNA sequence, generally of four or six base pairs, but these sequences differ widely with different systems (see Table 8–1 for examples). Most restriction enzymes are relatively simple, cleaving the DNA within or very close to the recognition site. For historical reasons, these are called type II restriction enzymes. Type I and III enzymes are more complex (and correspondingly less useful)—for example cleaving DNA at random sites quite far from the recognition site. Most (but not all) recognition sites for restriction systems show dyad symmetry; that is, the sequence of each strand, read $5' \rightarrow 3'$, is identical. This is a fairly common theme among proteins that bind specific sites on DNA and is not limited to the restriction-modification enzymes.

Recombinant DNA Methods

The type II restriction enzymes are essential for modern recombinant DNA research. Because most enzymes recognize different sequences that occur in essentially all DNAs, restriction enzymes can be used to generate a physical map of any DNA molecule. The locations of enzyme cleavage sites for a variety of enzymes are compared, and these are then calibrated with whatever genetic information is available. Using one or a combination of enzymes, a segment of DNA encoding a particular gene can then be cleaved from a given genome and purified on the basis of its size or other properties.

Many restriction enzymes cleave DNA in a staggered fashion, leaving either 3′- or 5′-overhanging termini (Table 8–1). The importance of these overhanging termini is that every restriction site for a particular enzyme will always generate exactly the same end structure, whether the DNA is from a human chromosome or a bacterial plasmid. Furthermore, these overhanging ends can base pair with each other and are therefore called *sticky ends*. The action of DNA ligase (Chap. 7) can seal these sticky ends together; if the participating fragments arose from different genomes, an artificial

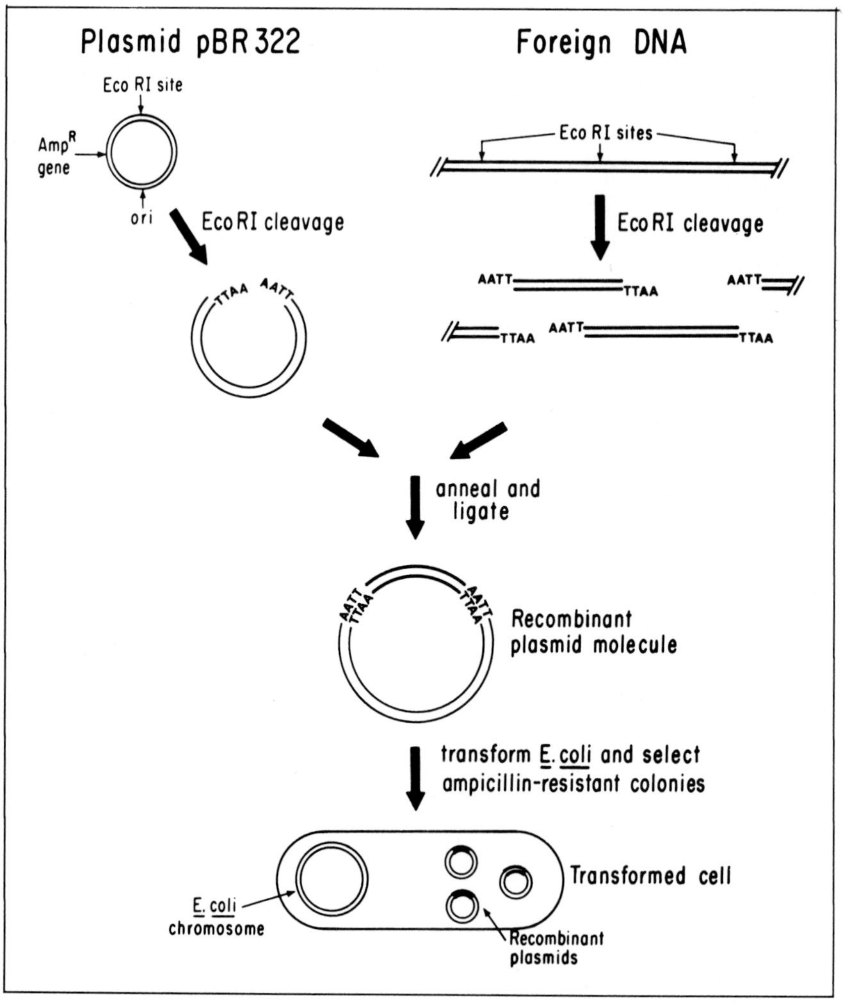

Fig. 8–24. Cloning of foreign DNA into a bacterial plasmid vector. The bacterial plasmid pBR322 and a sample of foreign (e.g., human) DNA are each cleaved with restriction enzyme *Eco*RI, and recombinant molecules are produced by the action of DNA ligase. A collection of ligated products are transformed into competent cells of *E. coli*, and plasmid-bearing strains are isolated by selection of ampicillin-resistant colonies. See text for further details.

recombinant DNA molecule has been produced. Figure 8–24 presents a schematic of such a simple construction. Plasmid pBR322 is cleaved at its single *Eco*RI site, and fragments of foreign DNA are cleaved and then ligated to the linearized pBR322. A collection of different ligated products, including circles that have a single copy of the plasmid and one inserted fragment of foreign DNA, is produced. This mixture is then used to transform a special strain of *E. coli* to propagate the DNA molecules (see the section on Transformation above). The *E. coli* strain contains no restriction-modification systems, and therefore the transforming DNA is not destroyed. Plasmid pBR322 contains an ampicillin-resistance gene, and thus the desired transformants can be obtained simply by selection with ampicillin. Only bacterial cells that have been transformed with the pBR322 DNA will be ampicillin resistant, because the starting *E. coli* strain is sensitive to the drug. With this procedure, up to 10^8 bacterial transformants can be obtained with only 1 μg of plasmid DNA.

Each bacterial colony produced from these manipulations contains a particular recombinant plasmid, and a foreign gene on the plasmid can now be propagated and studied as if it were a bacterial gene. The most important consequence is that very large quantities of the DNA can be obtained, because bacterial cultures can easily be grown to high densities. The complete DNA sequence of the cloned fragment can be determined with the use of either chemical or enzymatic methods for DNA sequencing. Furthermore, genes encoding previously rare eucaryotic proteins can be cloned in such a way that they are transcribed and translated efficiently by the bacterial machinery. This has led to the production of large quantities of human proteins, such as insulin and growth hormones.

Many other enzymes that have been introduced here and in Chapter 7 also have important roles in recombinant DNA research. DNA and RNA polymerases are used to synthesize particular fragments of nucleic acids, various nucleases (in addition to the restriction enzymes) cleave nucleic acids in useful ways, and the various DNA binding proteins can be used to manipulate DNA and RNA molecules. This brief summary is meant only to introduce the subject; several manuals with detailed descriptions of recombinant DNA methods and results are given in the references.

FURTHER READING

Books and Reviews

Berg DE, Howe MM (eds): Mobile DNA. Washington, DC, American Society for Microbiology, 1989

Bukhari AI, Shapiro JA, Adhya SL (eds): DNA Insertion Elements, Plasmids and Episomes. Cold Spring Harbor, NY, Cold Spring Harbor Laboratory, 1977

Clewell DB, Gawron-Burke C: Conjugative transposons and the dissemination of antibiotic resistance in streptococci. Annu Rev Microbiol 40:635, 1986

Cohen SN: Transposable genetic elements and plasmid evolution. Nature 263:731, 1976

Cox MM, Lehman IR: Enzymes of general recombination. Annu Rev Biochem 56:229, 1987

Dressler D, Potter H: Molecular mechanisms in genetic recombination. Annu Rev Biochem 51:727, 1982

Ferretti JJ, Curtis R III (eds): Streptococcal Genetics. Washington, DC, American Society for Microbiology, 1987

Franklin TJ, Snow GA: Biochemistry of Antimicrobial Action, ed 3. New York, Chapman and Hall, 1981

Goodgal SH: DNA uptake in *Haemophilus* transformation. Annu Rev Genet 16:169, 1982

Gorini L: Informational suppression. Annu Rev Genet 4:107, 1970

Grindley NDF, Reed R: Transpositional recombination in procaryotes. Annu Rev Biochem 54:863, 1985

Helinski DR: Plasmid-determined resistance to antibiotics: Molecular properties of R factors. Annu Rev Microbiol 27:437, 1973

Kleckner N: Transposable elements in procaryotes. Annu Rev Genet 15:341, 1981

Kornberg A, Baker TA: DNA Replication, ed 2. New York, WH Freeman, 1992

Kucherlapati R, Smith GR (eds): Genetic Recombination. Washington, DC, American Society for Microbiology, 1988

Levy SB, Clowes RC, Koenig EL (eds): Molecular Biology, Pathogenicity and Ecology of Bacterial Plasmids. New York, Plenum Press, 1981

Lindahl T: DNA repair enzymes. Annu Rev Biochem 51:61, 1982

Loeb LA, Kunkel TA: Fidelity of DNA synthesis. Annu Rev Biochem 51:429, 1982

Low KB (ed): The Recombination of Genetic Material. San Diego, Academic Press, 1988

Miller JH: Mutational specificity in bacteria. Annu Rev Genet 17:215, 1983

Modrich P: DNA mismatch correction. Annu Rev Biochem 56:435, 1987

Neidhardt FC, Ingraham JL, Low KB, et al (eds): *Escherichia coli* and *Salmonella typhimurium*. Cellular and Molecular Biology. Washington, DC, American Society for Microbiology, 1987

Radding CM: Homologous pairing and strand exchange in genetic recombination. Annu Rev Genet 16:405, 1982

Radman M, Wagner R: Mismatch repair in *Escherichia coli*. Annu Rev Genet 20:523, 1986

Sambrook J, Fritsch EF, Maniatis T: Molecular Cloning: A Laboratory Manual, ed 2. Cold Spring Harbor, NY, Cold Spring Harbor Laboratory, 1989

Shapiro JA (ed): Mobile Genetic Elements. New York, Academic Press, 1983

Silhavy TJ, Berman ML, Enquist LW: Experiments With Gene Fusions. Cold Spring Harbor, NY, Cold Spring Harbor Laboratory, 1984

Smith HO, Danner DB, Deich R: Genetic transformation. Annu Rev Biochem 50:41, 1981

Smith I, Slepecky RA, Setlow P (eds): Regulation of Procaryotic Development. Washington DC, American Society for Microbiology, 1989

Walker GC: Inducible DNA repair systems. Annu Rev Biochem 54:425, 1985

Walker GC, Marsh L, Dodson LA: Genetic analyses of DNA repair: Inference and extrapolation. Annu Rev Genet 19:103, 1985

Waring MJ: DNA modification and cancer. Annu Rev Biochem 50:159, 1981

Watson JD, Hopkins NH, Roberts JW, et al: Molecular Biology of the Gene. Menlo Park, California, Benjamin/Cummings, 1987

Whitehouse HLK: Genetic Recombination. New York, Wiley, 1982

Willetts N, Skurray R: The conjugation system of F-like plasmids. Annu Rev Genet 14:41, 1980

Selected Papers

Avery OT, MacLeod CM, McCarty M: Induction of transformation by a deoxyribonucleic acid fraction isolated from pneumococcus type III. J Exp Med 79:137, 1944

Bender J, Kleckner N: Genetic evidence that Tn10 transposes by a nonreplicative mechanism. Cell 45:801, 1986

Calos MP, Johnsrud L, Miller JH: DNA sequence at the integration sites of the insertion element IS1. Cell 13:411, 1978

Cavalli S, Sforza LL, Lederberg J, et al: An infective factor controlling sex compatibility in *Bacterium coli.* J Gen Microbiol 8:89, 1953

Christiansen G, Griffith J: Visualization of the paranemic joining of homologous DNA molecules catalyzed by the RecA protein of *Escherichia coli.* Proc Natl Acad Sci USA 83:2066, 1986

Craigie R, Mizuuchi K: Mechanism of transposition of bacteriophage Mu: Structure of a transposition intermediate. Cell 41:867, 1985

Franke A, Clewell DB: Evidence for conjugal transfer of a *Streptococcus faecalis* transposon (Tn916) from a chromosomal site in the absence of plasmid DNA. Cold Spring Harbor Symp Quant Biol 45:77, 1980

Goodman HM, Abelson J, Landy A, et al: Amber suppression: A nucleotide change in the anticodon of tyrosine transfer RNA. Nature 217:1019, 1968

Holloman WK, Wiegand R, Hoessli C, et al: Uptake of homologous single-stranded fragments by superhelical DNA: A possible mechanism for initiation of genetic recombination. Proc Natl Acad Sci USA 72:2394, 1975

Horinouchi S, Weisblum B: Posttranscriptional modification of mRNA conformation: Mechanism that regulates erythromycin-induced resistance. Proc Natl Acad Sci USA 77:7079, 1980

Kier LD, Yamasaki E, Ames BN: Detection of mutagenic activity in cigarette smoke condensates. Proc Natl Acad Sci USA 71:4159, 1974

Kopecko DJ, Brevet J, Cohen SN: Involvement of multiple translocating DNA segments and recombinational hotspots in the structural evolution of bacterial plasmids. J Mol Biol 108:333, 1976

Lacey RW, Richmond MH: The genetic basis of antibiotic resistance in *S. aureus:* The importance of gene transfer in the evolution of this organism in the hospital environment. In Yotis WW (ed): Recent Advances in Staphylococcal Research. Ann NY Acad Sci 236:395, 1974

Lederberg J, Tatum EL: Gene recombination in *Escherichia coli.* Nature 158:558, 1946

Luria S, Delbrück M: Mutation of bacteria from virus sensitivity to virus resistance. Genetics 28:491, 1943

Meselson MS: Formation of hybrid DNA by rotary diffusion during genetic recombination. J Mol Biol 71:795, 1971

Meselson MS, Radding CM: A general model for genetic recombination. Proc Natl Acad Sci USA 72:358, 1975

Meselson MS, Yuan R: DNA restriction enzyme from *E. coli.* Nature 217:110, 1968

Meyer TF, Mlawer N, So M: Pilus expression in *Neisseria gonorrhoeae* involves chromosomal rearrangement. Cell 30:45, 1982

Morrow JS, Cohen S, Chang A, et al: Replication and transcription of eucaryotic DNA in *Escherichia coli.* Proc Natl Acad Sci USA 71:1743, 1974

Novick RP, Khan SA, Murphy E, et al: Hitchhiking transposons and other mobile genetic elements and site-specific recombination systems in *Staphylococcus aureus.* Cold Spring Harbor Symp Quant Biol 45:67, 1980

Scott JR, Kirchman PA, Caparon MG: An intermediate in the transposition of the conjugative transposon Tn916. Proc Natl Acad Sci USA 85:4809, 1988

Setlow RB, Carrier WL: The disappearance of thymine dimers from DNA: An error correcting mechanism. Proc Natl Acad Sci USA 51:226, 1964

Shapiro JA: Molecular model for the transposition and replication of bacteriophage Mu and other transposable elements. Proc Natl Acad Sci USA 76:1933, 1979

Sigal N, Alberts B: Genetic recombination: The nature of a crossed strand exchange between two homologous DNA molecules. J Mol Biol 71:789, 1972

Simon M, Zieg J, Silverman M, et al: Phase variation: Evolution of a controlling element. Science 209:1370, 1980

Teo I, Sedgwick B, Kilpatrick MW, et al: The intracellular signal for induction of resistance to alkylating agents in *E. coli.* Cell 45:315, 1986

Zinder ND, Lederberg J: Genetic exchange in *Salmonella.* J Bacteriol 64:679, 1952

CHAPTER 9

Antimicrobial Agents

One of the major triumphs of medical science in the twentieth century has been the virtual eradication of many infectious diseases by the use of specific antimicrobial agents. Two important discoveries marked the beginning of a new era in chemotherapy and revolutionized the therapy of infectious diseases. The first of these was the discovery in 1935 of the curative effect of the red dye Prontosil on streptococcal infections. Prontosil was the forerunner of the sulfonamides, and although the intact molecule has no antibacterial activity in vitro, in the body it releases its active component, *p*-aminobenzenesulfonamide (sulfanilamide). The second important discovery, the one that ushered in the "golden age" of antimicrobial therapy, was the discovery and development of penicillin from culture filtrates of the fungus *Penicillium notatum*. Although the discovery of penicillin had been made by Fleming in 1929, it was Florey, Chain, and their associates at Oxford University who in 1940 demonstrated and published an account of its tremendous potency and the feasibility of its extraction from culture fluids. A few of the useful antibiotics, such as penicillin, were entirely fortuitous discoveries, but from the discovery of streptomycin in 1944 to the present, the search for such agents has been a highly planned, scientifically designed effort.

Chemotherapeutic Agents

Desirable Properties. A number of properties characterize the ideal antimicrobial used for chemotherapeutic purposes. (1) Selective toxicity is an essential property of a chemotherapeutic agent; it must inhibit or destroy the pathogen without injury to the host. (2) The ideal chemotherapeutic agent is bactericidal rather than bacteriostatic in its action. Bactericidal agents kill the organisms against which they are used, whereas bacteriostatic agents are only inhibitory and rely on host defense mechanisms for final eradication of the infection. This distinction between bactericidal and bacteriostatic agents is especially important when host defenses are compromised. (3) The ideal chemotherapeutic agent is one to which susceptible organisms do not become genetically or phenotypically resistant. (4) It is desirable that the agent be effective against a broad range of microorganisms commonly encountered in clinical practice; however, problems often arise as a consequence of the use of such broad-spectrum drugs. (5) The ideal agent should not be allergenic; nor should continued administration of large doses cause adverse side effects. (6) It should remain active in the presence of plasma, body fluids, or exudates. (7) The agent should be water soluble and stable, and bactericidal levels in the body should be rapidly reached and maintained for prolonged periods.

Antibiotics. As originally defined, an antibiotic was a chemical substance produced by various species of microorganisms that was capable in small concentrations of inhibiting the growth of other microorganisms. The advent of synthetic methods, however, has resulted in a modification of this definition. The term *antibiotic* now refers to a substance produced by a microorganism or to a similar substance produced wholly or partially by chemical synthesis, which in low concentrations inhibits the growth of other microorganisms.

Microorganisms that produce the various antibiotics are widely distributed in nature, where they play an important role in regulating the microbial populations of soil, water, sewage, and compost. The chemical, physical, and pharmacokinetic properties of the antibiotics are quite varied, as are their antimicrobial spectra and mechanisms of action. There is thus little or no relationship between the various antibiotics other than their ability to affect adversely the life processes of certain microorganisms. Of the several hundred naturally produced antibiotics that have been purified, only a few have been sufficiently nontoxic to be of use in medical practice. Those that are currently of greatest use have been derived from a relatively small group of microorganisms belonging to the genera *Penicillium, Streptomyces, Cephalosporium, Micromonospora,* and *Bacillus.*

Mechanisms of Action. The inhibitory activity of chemotherapeutic agents is targeted at a number of vulnerable sites in the cell. They interfere with (1) cell wall synthesis, (2) membrane function, (3) protein synthesis, (4) nucleic acid metabolism, and (5) key enzymatic reactions. One must keep in mind, however, that there may be a number of stages between the initial or primary effect of the drug and the eventual death of the cell that results. Also, some agents may have more than one primary site of attack or mechanism of action.

Cell Wall Inhibitors

The bacterial cell is surrounded by a rigid cell wall that protects the protoplasmic membrane from osmotic and mechanical trauma. The assimilation in the cell of low-molecular-weight soluble substances from the external environment creates an osmotic pressure within the cell that is many times that of the surrounding medium. Any substance that destroys the wall or that prevents the synthesis or incorporation of the wall polymers in growing cells leads to the development of osmotically sensitive cells and death. Since the bacterial cell wall is unique, and the mechanism for its biosynthesis is absent in eucaryotic cells, agents that interfere at this site are highly specific and are more likely to be low in toxicity. Among the antibiotics whose primary action is on cell-wall biosynthesis are the β-lactam antibiotics (e.g., penicillins, cephalosporins), cycloserine, vancomycin, and bacitracin. Species of eubacteria that lack a cell wall (i.e., mycoplasmas) are not inhibited by these agents.

The component of the wall that confers rigidity is the peptidoglycan layer. This substance consists of polysaccharide chains composed of alternating units of *N*-acetylglucosamine and *N*-acetylmuramic acid. Short peptides linked to the carboxyl group of muramic acid are covalently cross-linked with peptides of neighboring polysaccharide chains (p. 77).

Peptidoglycan Synthesis. The biosynthesis of peptidoglycan consists of three stages, each of which occurs at a different site in the cell (Fig. 9–1): (1) In the first stage, which occurs in the cytoplasm, the recurring units of the backbone structure of murein, *N*-acetylglucosamine and *N*-acetylmuramylpentapeptide, are synthesized in the form of their UDP derivatives. D-Cycloserine interferes with this stage of peptidoglycan synthesis by inhibiting reactions involving the incorporation of D-alanine into the pentapeptide. (2) The second stage of synthesis takes place on the inner surface of the cytoplasmic

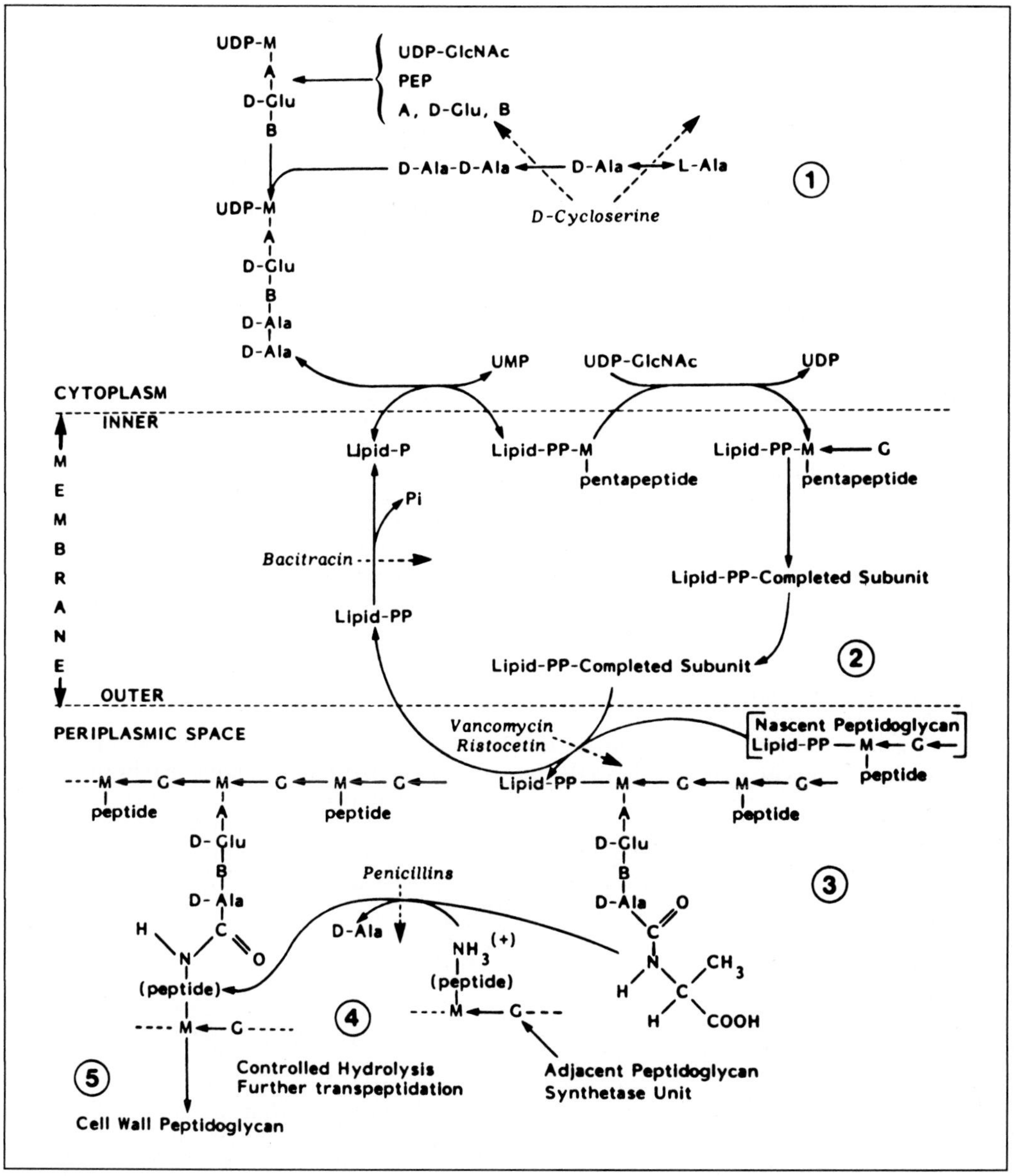

Fig. 9–1. Biosynthesis of peptidoglycan showing the site of action of various cell wall inhibitors. *(From Tipper: In Queener, Webber, Queener (eds): Beta-Lactam Antibiotics for Clinical Use. Marcel Dekker, 1986.)*

membrane, where *N*-acetylmuramylpentapeptide is transferred from UDP to a carrier lipid and is then modified to form a complete nascent peptidoglycan subunit. The nature of the modification depends on the organism. This stage terminates with translocation of the completed subunit to the exterior of the cytoplasmic membrane. (3) The third stage of synthesis begins with the polymerization of peptidoglycan by transglycosylation. The lipid-PP released in the reaction recycles through the membrane and is hydrolyzed to the lipid-P acceptor. The cell wall inhibitor bacitracin interferes with this recycling by inhibiting the pyrophosphatase reaction. Vancomycin and ristocetin inhibit the transglycosylase by binding to the D-alanyl-D-alanine peptide termini of its substrates. Stage 3 of biosynthesis continues with transpeptidation and the binding of soluble un-cross-linked, nascent peptidoglycan to the preexisting, cross-linked, insoluble cell wall peptidoglycan matrix (Fig. 9–1, reaction 4). In some organisms modification by D,D-carboxypeptidases may be an alternative at this stage, resulting in the removal of the terminal D-alanine residue without transpeptidation. Stage 3 of cell wall synthesis is the phase during which inhibition by penicillin and the other β-lactams occurs.

β-Lactam Antibiotics

All the antibiotics in this group contain a unique four-member β-lactam ring. The penicillins (penams) and cephalosporins (cephems) are the two largest and best-known subgroups of this family of compounds. Included in the group, however, are newer agents with novel β-lactam structures, such as the penems, carbapenems, and monobactams (Fig. 9–2). Although

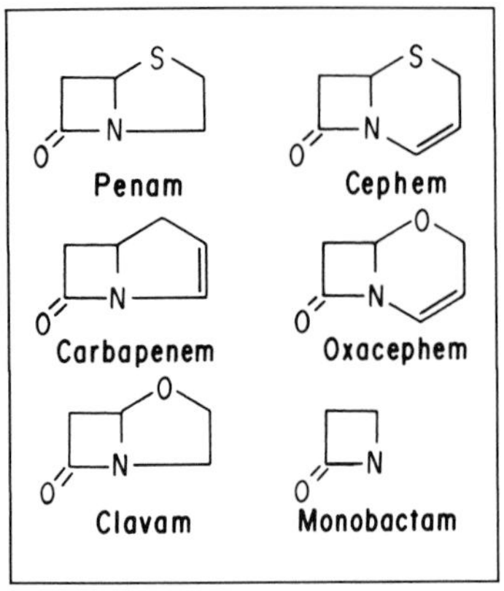

Fig. 9–2. Structural nuclei of major β-lactam agents. Penicillin is a penam; cephalosporin and cephamycin are cephens; thienamycin and imipenem are carbapenems; moxalactam is an oxacephem; clavulanic acid has a clavam nucleus; and aztreonam is a monobactam.

penicillin has been the most extensively studied, all β-lactam antibiotics are believed to share basically the same mechanism of action.

Mechanism of Action

The β-lactams are bactericidal agents. The bacterial response after exposure to these agents is complex and varies with respect to the organism and to the particular antibiotic. This is a reflection of the interaction with specific targets in the membrane, the penicillin-binding proteins, and of events occurring during normal cell wall growth. The precise molecular mechanism, however, by which these agents exert their lethal effect remains elusive.

The last stage in cell wall synthesis has been identified as the phase during which inhibition occurs. The peptidoglycan cross-linking enzyme system, considered as a whole, is the target specifically inhibited by penicillin. During this stage the linear peptidoglycan strands are cross-linked by a transpeptidation step in which a peptide bridge is formed between two adjacent strands with the elimination of the terminal D-alanine. When bacteria are grown in the presence of penicillin, un-cross-linked uridine nucleotide intermediates of cell wall synthesis accumulate, and new walls cannot be formed.

Penicillin inhibits not only the transpeptidases responsible for the cross-linking but also, and reversibly, D-alanine carboxypeptidases, which specifically remove D-alanine from a pentapeptide side chain (Chap. 6, p. 77). These enzymes are especially important in the final stages of cell wall synthesis in gram-negative bacilli, where there is usually only a single cross-link between one peptide side chain and another.

A structural analogy between penicillin and the D-alanyl-D-alanine end of the pentapeptide in the un-cross-linked precursor of the cell wall has been invoked to explain the molecular basis for the antibacterial action of penicillin (Fig. 9–3). The labile CO—N bond in the β-lactam ring of penicillin lies in the same position as the peptide bond involved in the transpeptidation. It has thus been proposed that penicillin, acting as a substrate analogue of the normal transpeptidation substrate, combines with the transpeptidase and thereby irreversibly inactivates it. Antibiotics containing a β-lactam ring behave chemically as acylating agents, reacting to produce penicilloyl derivatives. The action of penicillin on these enzymes might therefore involve acylation of the enzymically active site with formation of a rather stable inactive complex (Fig. 9–4).

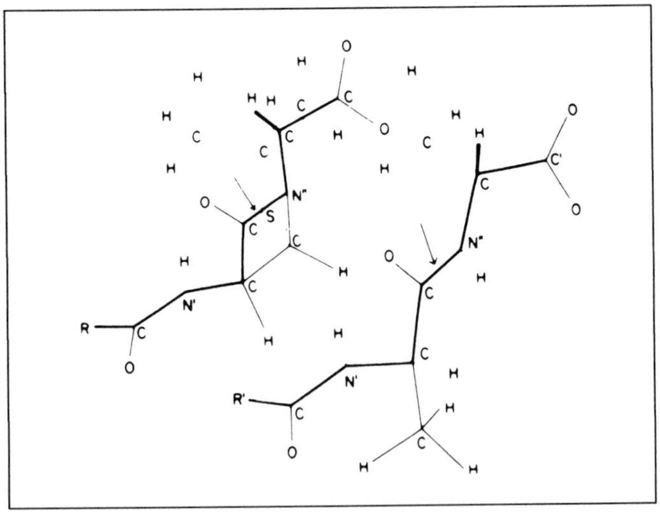

Fig. 9–3. Stereomodels of penicillin (left) and of the D-alanyl-D-alanine end of the peptidoglycan strand (right). Arrows indicate the position of the CO—N bond in the β-lactam ring of penicillin and of the CO—N bond in D-alanyl-D-alanine at the end of the peptidoglycan strand. *(From Blumberg and Strominger: Bacteriol Rev 38:291, 1974.)*

Penicillin-binding Proteins. The inhibition of biosynthesis reactions by β-lactam drugs is accompanied by distinctive morphologic changes. The nature of these changes depends on the specific organism, the antibiotic used, and the concentration. The morphologic differences observed are due to the particular penicillin-binding protein (PBP) that is affected. These proteins, which are present in the membranes of all eubacteria except *Mycoplasma,* are the enzymes that catalyze the last steps of peptidoglycan biosynthesis. In *Escherichia coli* there are seven PBPs that bind covalently to β-lactam antibiotics. These are numbered by decreasing molecular weight: PBPs 1a, 1b, and 2 to 6. The higher-molecular-weight PBPs (1a, 1b, 2, and 3) are essential to the cell and are the killing sites for β-lactam antibiotics. PBPs 1a and 1b are involved in cell elongation and are the major transpeptidases of the cell. PBP 2 maintains the rod shape of the organism, and PBP 3 functions in septum formation in organisms undergoing division. The low-molecular-weight PBPs are carboxypeptidases and are not essential for cell viability. Some of the β-lactam antibiotics have binding affinities toward only one or two specific penicillin-binding proteins of *E. coli.* Each of these agents elicits a distinct morphologic response in the organism, such as lysis, filamentation, or ovoid cell formation. For example, cephalothin and benzyl penicillin produce lytic effects on *Staphylococcus aureus,* cephalexin causes filamentation of *E. coli,* and mecillinam (amdinocillin) tends to produce osmotically fragile round forms.

The effects of the β-lactams are observed only in growing organisms. If growth is prevented by the omission of a nutrient or by the addition of a bacteriostatic agent, penicillin is without effect. The specific response also depends on the concentration. If staphylococci are exposed to concentrations of penicillin above the minimum inhibitory concentration (MIC), the septum loses its density, the cell wall becomes thinner, there is rapid loss of viability, and the cell lyses. At sub-MICs, however, the cell wall remains normal but the septum becomes

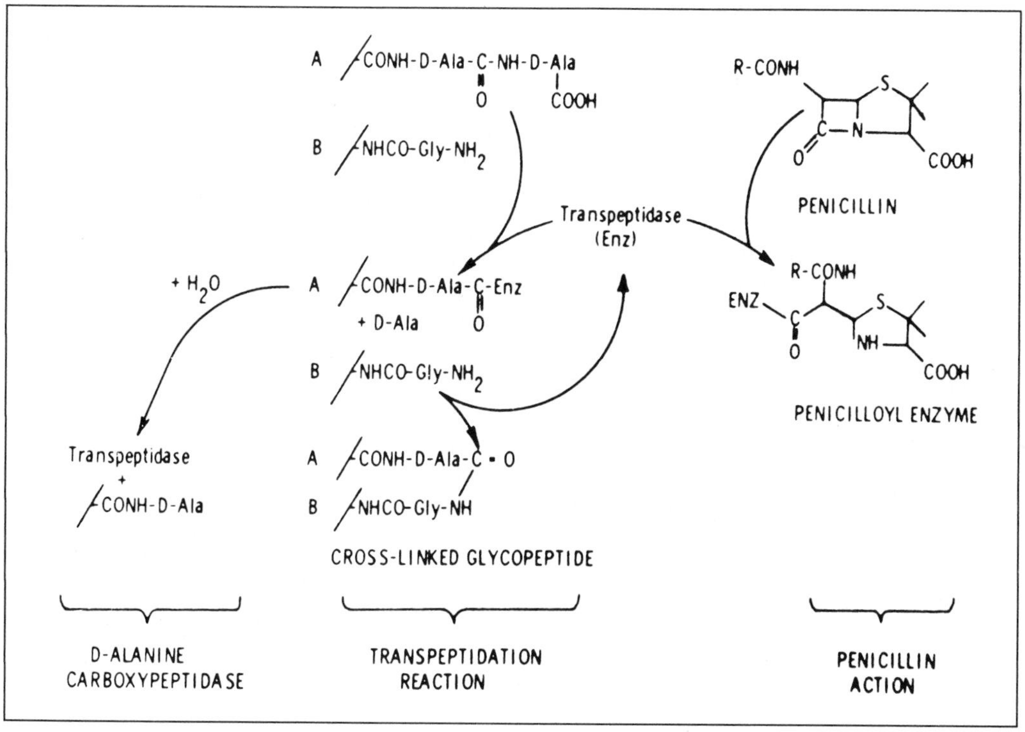

Fig. 9–4. Proposed mechanism of transpeptidation and its relationship to penicilloylation and D-alanine carboxypeptidase activity. **A.** The end of the main peptide chain of the glycan strand. **B.** The end of the pentaglycine substituent from an adjacent strand. If the acyl enzyme intermediate can react with water instead of the acceptor (left), the enzyme would be regenerated and the substrate released. The overall reaction would be the hydrolysis of the terminal D-alanine residue of the substrate (D-alanine carboxypeptidase activity). *(From Blumberg and Strominger: Bacteriol Rev 38:291, 1974.)*

much thicker. Gram-negative bacilli exposed to sub-MICs of β-lactam antibiotics become elongated and, in the absence of septation, form long filamentous cells. Elongation is inhibited by high concentrations of these agents, and the bacilli form large osmotically fragile globular forms that lyse unless the medium is osmotically stabilized.

The lytic effect of penicillin is the result of unbalanced cell growth and involves autolysins, the endogenous peptidoglycan hydrolyzing enzymes that normally participate in the turnover of cell-wall material and separation of bacteria after cell division. In gram-positive organisms, penicillin also causes the release of lipids and teichoic acids, an event that has been linked with the onset of autolytic activity, which is normally regulated by these compounds.

Cells that are not undergoing multiplication can survive in the presence of penicillin because their peptidoglycan is unbroken and there is no reparative cross-linking activity for the penicillin to block. Such organisms are "persisters" and may be responsible for recurrence of infection after penicillin treatment has been discontinued.

Resistance to β-Lactam Antibiotics

Biochemical resistance to the β-lactam antibiotics may be attributed to three distinct mechanisms: (1) inactivation of the drug, (2) alteration of the target site, and (3) blocking of transport of the drug into the cell. The major basis for bacterial resistance to penicillin, whether occurring naturally or acquired in vivo, is the inactivation of the drug by β-lactamases. These enzymes split the β-lactam ring of the penicillins and cephalosporins between the C and N atoms to form inactive compounds.

β-Lactamases are found in both gram-positive and gram-negative organisms and are responsible for many highly resistant strains, including penicillin-resistant staphylococci obtained from patients. In the development of semisynthetic penicillins and cephalosporins, one of the primary goals was to find compounds that are insensitive to β-lactamase activity. The β-lactamases of gram-positive bacteria are inducible and have a very high affinity for their substrates. They are extracellular and are produced in relatively large amounts. The production of β-lactamases in gram-positive organisms is mediated by both chromosomal and plasmid genes. However, as in the case of *S. aureus,* the gene on the plasmid can be derived from that on the chromosome via a transposon. In *S. aureus,* penicillinase production is mediated mainly by a plasmid gene that can be easily transferred to other susceptible organisms by bacteriophages.

The β-lactamases from gram-negative organisms are different in many respects from the enzymes of gram-positive species. They are usually constitutive and are cell bound, whether they are mediated by R-factor plasmids or by chromosomes. They are produced in smaller amounts and have a much lower affinity for their substrates. The release by gram-positive species of large amounts of β-lactamase into the immediate environs results in a population effect. By contrast, localization of the enzyme in the periplasmic space of gram-negative species restricts access of the drug to the membrane target sites only after the drug has penetrated the cell-wall layer. In these organisms, penicillinase resistance cannot be attributed to β-lactamase activity alone but is due to a complex interaction between β-lactamase and a permeability barrier in the outer membrane.

The second mechanism of resistance to the β-lactam drugs is due to an alteration in either the amounts of PBPs or the affinities of the PBPs for the antibiotic. Methicillin resistance in *S. aureus,* and penicillin resistance in *Streptococcus pneumoniae* and *Neisseria gonorrhoeae* are associated with altered PBPs. In some gram-negative organisms, resistance to certain cephalosporins is also related to reduced affinity for the target.

Before the β-lactam antibiotics can inhibit growth, they must be able to reach the susceptible target site(s) on the membrane. In gram-positive organisms the cell wall is not a major barrier to entry of these drugs. Gram-negative bacteria, however, have a complex outer membrane that retards the entry of the anionic β-lactam antibiotics. Penicillin G has more difficulty penetrating the outer membrane of gram-negative bacilli than do ampicillin and the cephalosporins. Most gram-negative organisms are therefore relatively resistant to penicillin G. *Pseudomonas aeruginosa* provides a good example of the role of permeability and other mechanisms in resistance. Wild-type strains of *Pseudomonas* are intrinsically resistant to most β-lactam antibiotics through (1) the ability of the outer membrane to restrict entry of the antibiotic molecules and (2) the inactivation of those that do enter by periplasmically located β-lactamases. Altered PBPs have also been described in these organisms. Acquired penicillin resistance due to changes in permeability and outer membrane protein has been described in *N. gonorrhoeae*. Further discussion of penicillin resistance, its genetics, epidemiology, and clinical importance is found on page 184 of this chapter and in Chapters 8 and 23.

Penicillins

Penicillin is still the most widely used antibiotic for general therapeutic use. In the years since the first crude product was obtained from *P. notatum*, the penicillin molecule has been chemically manipulated, and numerous natural and semisynthetic congeners have been produced. Several of these are useful therapeutically. By greater attention to cultural conditions that provide the chemical precursors of the antibiotic and by substitution of a high-yielding mutant of *Penicillium chrysogenum*, penicillin production has been enhanced manyfold. The term *penicillin* is generic for the entire group of natural and semisynthetic penicillins. The basic structure consists of a thiazolidine ring joined to a β-lactam ring, to which is attached a side chain that determines many of the antibacterial and pharmacologic properties of a particular type of penicillin (Fig. 9–5).

Natural Penicillins. Of the natural penicillins, benzylpenicillin or penicillin G is clinically the most useful. Its almost exclusive formation is ensured by the addition to the culture medium of the appropriate precursor, phenylacetic acid. Penicillin G is effective against most gram-positive organisms and gram-negative cocci (Table 9–1). It remains the drug of choice for treatment of *Streptococcus pyogenes* and *Streptococcus pneumoniae* infections, regardless of the site of infection. Among the least susceptible of the gram-positive cocci are the enterococci and penicillinase-producing strains of *S. aureus*. In general, gram-positive bacteria inhibited by the natural penicillins are more susceptible to these penicillins than to the semisynthetic congeners. Therefore, in the nonallergenic person, penicillin should usually be the drug of choice to treat infections caused by susceptible organisms.

The chemical modification of the penicillin molecule has extended its range of activity and has counteracted some of its undesirable properties. The major disadvantages of penicillin G are that (1) it is inactivated by the acid pH of the gastric juice, (2) it is destroyed by β-lactamases, bacterial enzymes that split the β-lactam ring, and (3) its use is sometimes associated with hypersensitivity reactions, which range in severity from a rash to immediate anaphylaxis.

Penicillin V is a side chain variant of penicillin G with a similar antimicrobial spectrum. Its sole advantage is that it is more stable in an acid medium and thus is better absorbed from the gastrointestinal tract.

Semisynthetic Penicillins. The penicillin nucleus itself, 6-aminopenicillanic acid, is the primary structural requirement for biologic activity. It can be prepared in quantity from benzyl or other natural penicillins by treatment with an amidase derived from a number of microbial species (Fig. 9–5). Once this penicillin nucleus is available, various side chains can be attached, and an almost unlimited number of semisynthetic penicillins can be produced. These may be divided into three

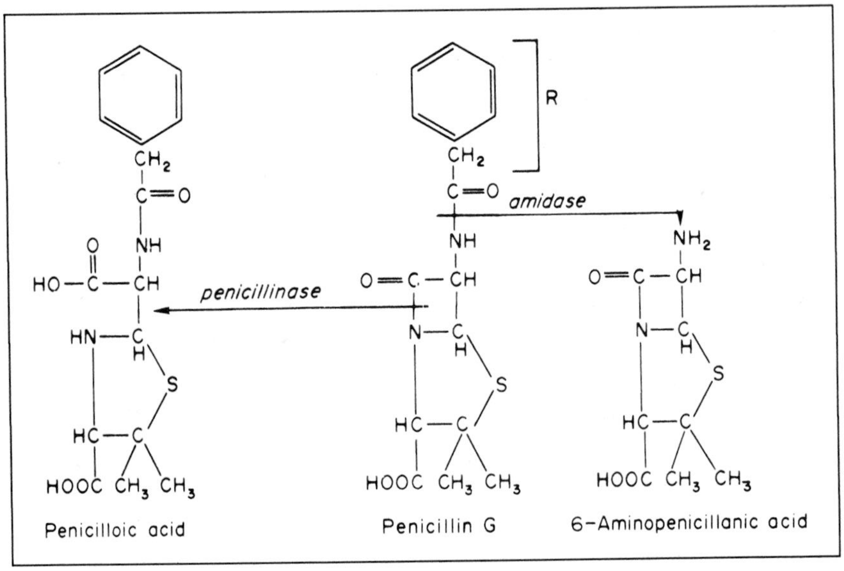

Fig. 9–5. Benzylpenicillin (penicillin G) and products of its enzymatic hydrolysis. Penicilloic acid is inactive. 6-Aminopenicillanic acid is the starting point for semisynthetic penicillins.

TABLE 9–1. ANTIMICROBIAL AGENTS OF CHOICE

Organism	Antimicrobial of Choice	Alternative Therapy
Gram-positive Cocci		
Staphylococcus aureus		
Nonpenicillinase-producing	Penicillin G	A cephalosporin,[a] vancomycin, imipenem, or erythromycin
Penicillinase-producing	Penicillinase-resistant penicillin[b]	As above
Streptococcus pneumoniae	Penicillin G	A cephalosporin,[a] erythromycin, chloramphenicol
Streptococcus pyogenes	Penicillin G	A cephalosporin,[a] erythromycin, vancomycin
Streptococcus (viridans group)	Penicillin G	A cephalosporin,[a] vancomycin, or erythromycin
Enterococcus faecalis		
Endocarditis	Penicillin G (or ampicillin) plus gentamicin or streptomycin	Vancomycin plus gentamicin or streptomycin
Urinary tract infection	Ampicillin or amoxicillin	Ciprofloxacin or nitrofurantoin
Gram-negative Cocci		
Neisseria meningitidis	Penicillin G	Chloramphenicol, a sulfonamide
Neisseria gonorrhoeae		
Penicillin-sensitive	Penicillin G	Spectinomycin, ceftriaxone
Penicillin-resistant	Ceftriaxone	Spectinomycin, cefuroxime or cefoxitin, ciprofloxacin
Gram-positive Bacilli		
Actinomyces israelii	Penicillin G, ampicillin	A tetracycline, erythromycin, clindamycin
Bacillus anthracis	Penicillin G	A tetracycline or erythromycin
Corynebacterium diphtheriae	Penicillin G	Erythromycin
Listeria monocytogenes	Ampicillin or penicillin G	Erythromycin
Nocardia species	A sulfonamide	Trimethoprim-sulfamethoxazole
Gram-negative Bacilli		
Enterobacteriaceae		
Enterobacter species	A cephalosporin (G3),[a] gentamicin or tobramycin[c]	Carbenicillin, mezlocillin, piperacillin, amikacin, aztreonam, imipenem
Escherichia coli		
Uncomplicated urinary tract infection	Trimethoprim-sulfamethoxazole or ampicillin	A cephalosporin,[a] ciprofloxacin
Systemic infection	Ampicillin, a cephalosporin (G3)[a]	An aminoglycoside, aztreonam or a penicillin + penicillinase inhibitor
Klebsiella pneumoniae	A cephalosporin[a]	Cephalosporin (G3),[a] cefotaxime, moxalactam, amikacin, chloramphenicol
Proteus mirabilis	Ampicillin	Gentamicin or tobramycin, a cephalosporin[a]
Proteus (other than *P. mirabilis*)	Gentamicin or tobramycin,[c] a cephalosporin (G3)[a]	Carbenicillin, piperacillin, amikacin, aztreonam, imipenem
Salmonella typhi	Chloramphenicol	Ampicillin or trimethoprim-sulfamethoxazole
Salmonella (nontyphi species)	Ampicillin	Chloramphenicol, trimethoprim-sulfamethoxazole, ciprofloxacin
Serratia marcescens	A cephalosporin (G3),[a] imipenem	Carbenicillin, mezlocillin, aztreonam, gentamicin (or amikacin)
Shigella	Ciprofloxacin	Trimethoprim-sulfamethoxazole, ampicillin, chloramphenicol
Yersinia pestis	Streptomycin	Tetracycline, chloramphenicol
Yersinia enterocolitica	Trimethoprim-sulfamethoxazole	A cephalosporin (G3)[a], an aminoglycoside
Other Gram-negative Bacilli and Vibrios		
Bordetella pertussis	Erythromycin	Tetracycline, chloramphenicol
Brucella species	Tetracycline + rifampin	Chloramphenicol (± gentamicin)
Campylobacter species	Erythromycin	Tetracycline, gentamicin, ciprofloxacin
Francisella tularensis	Streptomycin	Tetracycline, chloramphenicol
Haemophilus influenzae		
Meningitis	Chloramphenicol, a cephalosporin (G3)[a]	Ampicillin
Other infections	Ampicillin	Trimethoprim-sulfamethoxazole, cefaclor, cefuroxime, ciprofloxacin
Pasteurella multocida	Penicillin G	A tetracycline, a cephalosporin[a]

(*continued*)

TABLE 9–1. ANTIMICROBIAL AGENTS OF CHOICE (*continued*)

Organism	Antimicrobial of Choice	Alternative Therapy
Other Gram-negative Bacilli and Vibrios (*continued*)		
Pseudomonas aeruginosa	Tobramycin or gentamicin (± carbenicillin, azlocillin, mezlocillin, or piperacillin)[c]	Amikacin, ceftazidime, aztreonam, imipenem
Vibrio cholerae	Tetracycline	Trimethoprim-sulfamethoxazole
Anaerobic Organisms		
Anaerobic streptococci	Penicillin G	A cephalosporin,[a] clindamycin, erythromycin, chloramphenicol
Bacteroides fragilis	Clindamycin Metronidazole	Chloramphenicol, metronidazole, cefoxitin, cefotetan, ticarcillin-clavulanate
Bacteroides (non-*fragilis* species)	Penicillin G	Clindamycin, metronidazole, cefoxitin, cefotetan, chloramphenicol
Clostridium species	Penicillin G	Clindamycin, chloramphenicol, metronidazole, a cephalosporin (G3)[a]
Acid-fast Bacilli		
Mycobacterium tuberculosis	Isoniazid + rifampin + pyrazinamide	Isoniazid + rifampin + ethambutol
Mycobacterium leprae	Dapsone + rifampin	Clofazimine
Spirochetes		
Treponema pallidum	Penicillin G	Ceftrixone, tetracycline
Borrelia burgdorferi	Penicillin G	Ceftrixone, tetracycline
Leptospira	Penicillin G	Tetracycline
Miscellaneous Bacteria		
Chlamydia species	Tetracycline	Erythromycin
Legionella species	Erythromycin	Rifampin
Mycoplasma pneumoniae	Erythromycin	Tetracycline
Rickettsia species	Tetracycline	Chloramphenicol

[a] The term *cephalosporin* refers to a first-generation cephalosporin; *cephalosporin (G3)* refers to a third-generation cephalosporin.
[b] See Table 9–2.
[c] If an aminoglycoside is given before speciation of organism, a shift to a less toxic agent is recommended if susceptibility data permit.

major groups on the basis of their antibacterial activity (Table 9–2).

PENICILLINASE-RESISTANT PENICILLINS. In the penicillinase-resistant group of semisynthetic penicillins an alteration has been made in the side chain, which protects the β-lactam ring from the action of β-lactamase without removing its antibacterial activity. Such penicillins include methicillin and nafcillin, which are acid labile, and the isoxazolyl penicillins (oxacillin, cloxacillin, and dicloxacillin), which combine resistance to β-lactamase with resistance to acid (Fig. 9–6). At present, semisynthetic penicillinase-resistant penicillins are the drugs of choice only for penicillin-resistant *S. aureus* and *Staphylococcus epidermidis.* Their use in some parts of the United States is now limited, however, by the emergence of resistant strains of these organisms. Methicillin resistance in staphylococci is not due to β-lactamase activity but to altered PBPs.

EXTENDED-SPECTRUM PENICILLINS. The most striking change brought about by chemical manipulation of the penicillin side chain is an increase of activity against gram-negative organisms. Among the most clinically useful of these broad-spectrum compounds are the aminopenicillins, ampicillin and amoxicillin, which are acid-stable but β-lactamase-sensitive (Fig. 9–7). The presence of the amino group enhances the penetration of these agents through the outer membrane of gram-negative organisms. They are highly active against *Haemophilus influenzae, E. coli, Proteus mirabilis, Salmonella,* and *Shigella,* but an increasing percentage of these organisms are now resistant.

Amdinocillin, formerly called mecillinam, is the most active of the amidinopenicillanic derivatives. It has unusual antibacterial properties for a penicillin. It is extremely active against *E. coli,* but for an equal effect on gram-positive organisms a concentration more than 60 times greater is required. In contrast to ampicillin, it is active against many strains of *Klebsiella* and *Enterobacter.* Amdinocillin does not inhibit *Pseudomonas,* and its action on *Proteus* is variable.

ANTI-*PSEUDOMONAS* PENICILLINS. The development of carboxy and ureido derivatives of ampicillin has led to the introduction of agents with increased activity against *P. aeruginosa* (Fig. 9–8). The carboxy penicillins (carbenicillin, ticarcillin) are also more active against strains of *Enterobacter, Serratia,* and certain strains of *Proteus* that are not susceptible to the earlier penicillins (Table 9–1). This expanded spectrum against gram-negative bacilli was accomplished at the expense of diminished activity against gram-positive organisms. The

TABLE 9–2. CLASSIFICATION OF PENICILLINS

Type and Generic Name	Acid Resistance
Natural Penicillins	
Benzylpenicillin (G)	−
Phenoxymethyl penicillin (V)	+
Semisynthetic Penicillins	
Penicillinase-resistant	
Methicillin	−
Nafcillin	+
Isoxazolyl penicillins	
Cloxacillin	+
Dicloxacillin	+
Oxacillin	+
Extended-spectrum penicillins	
Ampicillin	+
Amoxicillin	+
Amdinocillin (mecillinam)	a
Antipseudomonas penicillins	
Carbenicillin	a
Azlocillin	a
Mezlocillin	a
Piperacillin	a
Ticarcillin	a

a Not well absorbed from gut; must be given parenterally.

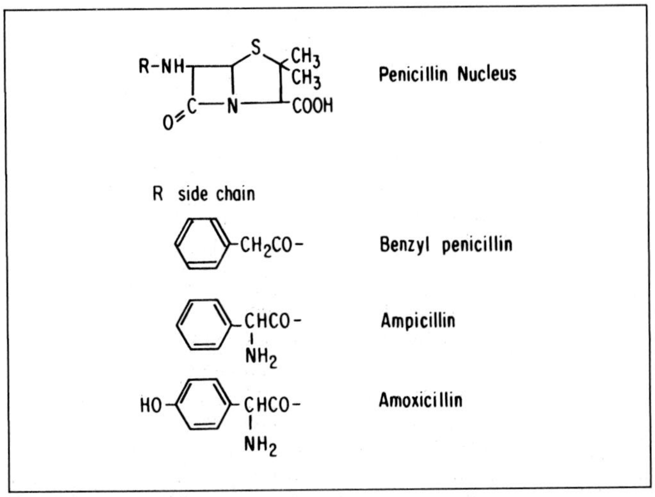

Fig. 9–7. Benzyl penicillin (penicillin G) and the aminopenicillins. The aminopenicillins are more active than penicillin G against group D streptococci and a number of gram-negative species. They are not stable to β-lactamases of either gram-positive or gram-negative organisms.

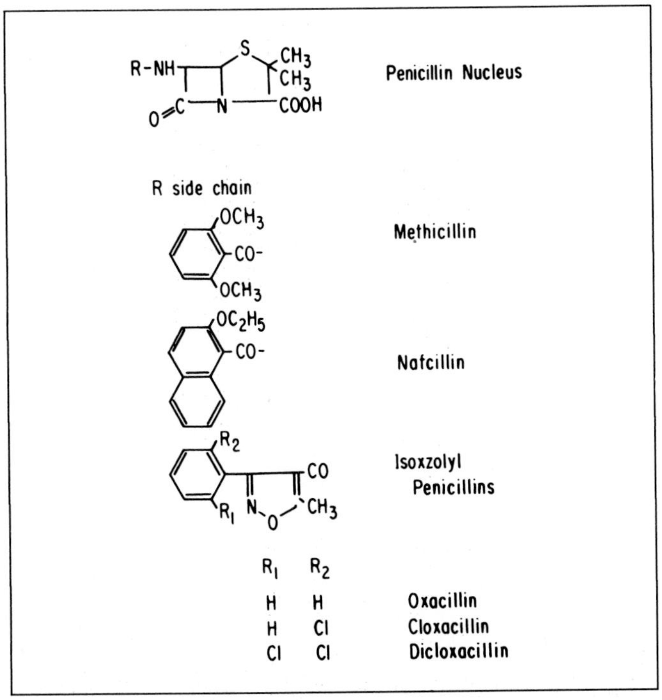

Fig. 9–6. Penicillinase-resistant penicillins. These semisynthetic penicillins are especially useful in the treatment of penicillin G–resistant staphylococcal infections. They are inactive against gram-negative bacilli.

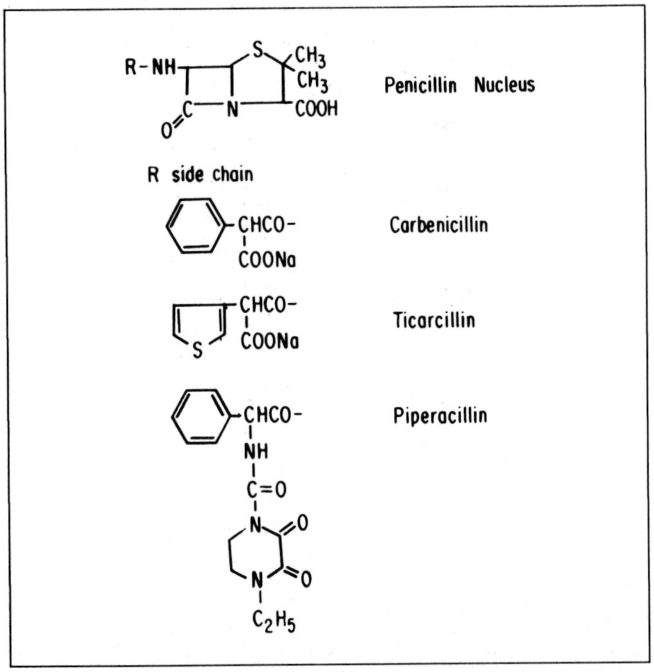

Fig. 9–8. Anti-*Pseudomonas* penicillins. The principal advantage of carbenicillin and ticarcillin is in their activity against *P. aeruginosa* and indole-positive *Proteus* species. Piperacillin has an extended spectrum, similar to ampicillin for gram-positive species and to carbenicillin for gram-negative species. Its activity against *Pseudomonas* is greater than that of carbenicillin.

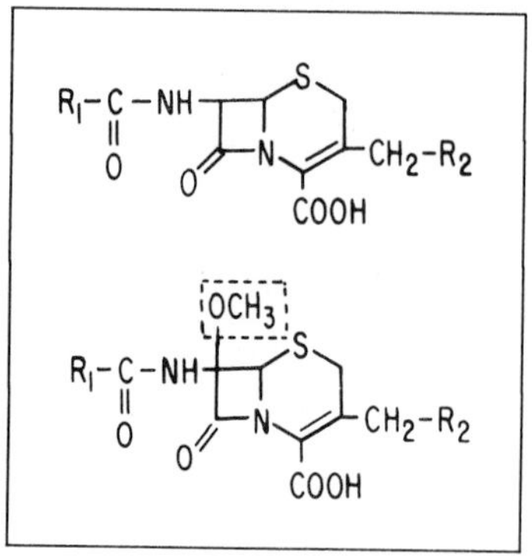

Fig. 9–9. Basic structure of the cephalosporins (top) and cephamycins (bottom). In the cephamycins a methoxyl group replaces the hydrogen at the 7 position of 7-aminocephalosporanic acid. This confers unusually high resistance to the β-lactamases. Substitutions at the R_1 and R_2 positions have yielded clinically useful derivatives.

ureido penicillins (azlocillin, mezlocillin, piperacillin) are even more inhibitory for *P. aeruginosa* than the carboxy derivatives, and their activity against streptococci is similar to that of ampicillin.

Cephalosporins

The major fermentation product of the fungus *Cephalosporium* is cephalosporin C. This antibiotic, which resembles penicillin in structure and mode of action, is the basis for the newer cephalosporins. It has a β-lactam ring that is fused with a six-member dihydrothiazine ring instead of the five-member thiazolidine ring characteristic of the penicillins. The cephem nucleus (7-aminocephalosporanic acid) obtained by acid hydrolysis, lends itself to modifications that alter both microbiologic activity and pharmacologic properties (Fig. 9–9). All cephalosporins have a sulfur atom at position 1 of the dihydrothiazine ring with the exception of moxalactam, which has an oxygen atom. Substitutions at position 7 or nearby affect stability against β-lactamases, and further changes in the acyl side chain can alter both antibacterial and pharmacologic properties (Fig. 9–10). Substitutions at position 3 of the ring usually affect pharmacologic properties to a greater degree than microbiologic activity.

The cephamycin antibiotics are similar in structure to the cephalosporins, but they are derived from species of *Streptomyces*. The best known of the cephamycin derivatives is cefoxitin.

Spectrum of Activity. The cephalosporins are widely used antibiotics. They are active against most organisms susceptible to the penicillins and have been useful alternatives in patients who are allergic to penicillin. They are often classified into groups or generations based on general features of antimicrobial activity (Table 9–3). All the older first-generation cephalosporins have very similar activity in vitro. They are bactericidal against most gram-positive cocci and many of the common gram-negative bacilli of clinical importance. However, *Enterobacter* species, indole-positive *Proteus* strains, and *Pseudomonas* species are resistant to these older agents (Table 9–4). Of the first-generation cephalosporins currently marketed in the United States, cephalothin, cefazolin, and cephalexin are the most useful.

The second-generation cephalosporins are more resistant to the action of cephalosporinases produced by gram-negative organisms. They have improved activity against gram-negative bacilli but are generally less active than the first-generation agents against gram-positive organisms. The major advantage

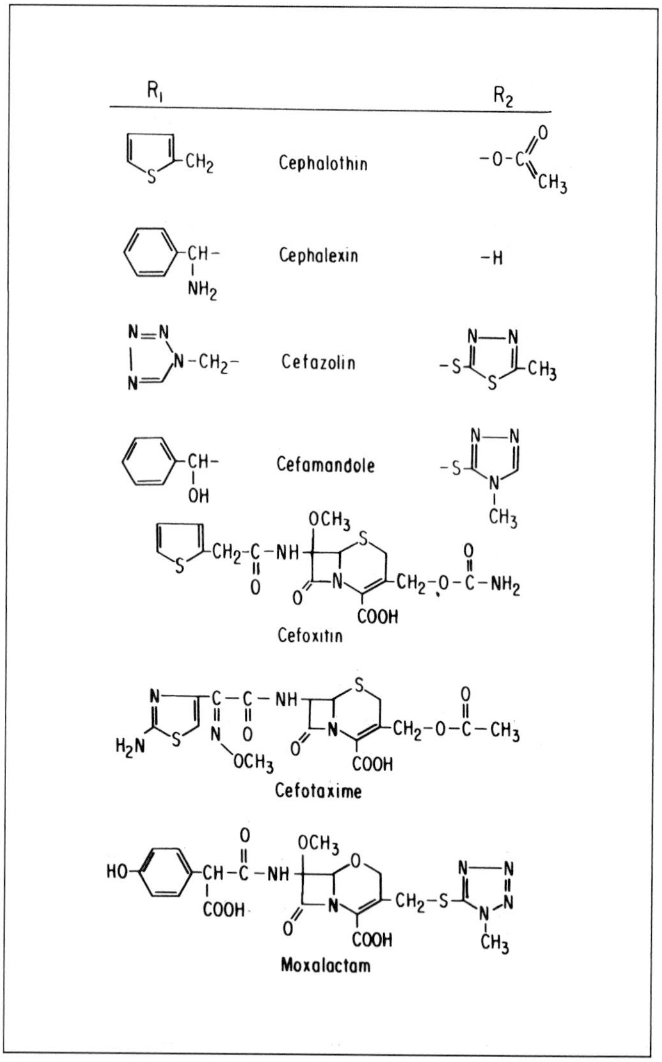

Fig. 9–10. Cephalosporins and cephamycins. All are derivatives of the active nucleus of the natural product, cephalosporin C, except cefoxitin, which is a cephamycin derivative (see Fig. 9–9).

TABLE 9–3. CLASSIFICATION OF SOME CEPHALOSPORINS AND CEPHAMYCINS

First Generation	Second Generation	Third Generation
Cephalothin	Cefamandole	Cefotaxime
Cephapirin	Cefoxitin[b]	Ceftizoxime
Cephalexin[a]	Cefuroxime	Ceftriaxone
Cephradine[a]	Cefaclor[a]	Ceftazidime[c]
Cefazolin	Cefonicid	Cefoperazone[c]
Cefadroxil[a]	Cefotetan[b]	Moxalactam[bd]
	Ceforanide	

[a] Oral agents.
[b] Cephamycin.
[c] Good activity against *Pseudomonas*.
[d] Not recommended for clinical use because of toxicity.

TABLE 9–4. IN VITRO ACTIVITY OF REPRESENTATIVE CEPHALOSPORINS AGAINST GRAM-NEGATIVE BACTERIA

Organism	MIC (μg/ml)		
	Cephalothin[a]	Cefamandole[a]	Moxalactam[a]
Escherichia coli	4	0.5	0.06
Enterobacter aerogenes	4	1	0.125
Enterobacter cloacae	>128	8	0.25
Proteus morganii	>128	8	1
Serratia marcescens	>128	64	1
Pseudomonas aeruginosa[b]	>128	>128	16 (range 8–32)

From Webber and Yoshida: Rev Infect Dis 4(suppl):S496,1982.
[a] Cephalothin and cefamandole are first- and second-generation cephalosporins. Moxalactam is a third-generation agent.
[b] Mean MIC values for three strains.

of cefamandole is its increased activity for *Enterobacter*, indole-positive *Proteus*, and *Haemophilus*. Compared with cefamandole, cefoxitin is active against a broader range of gram-negative organisms, including *N. gonorrhoeae*, *Serratia*, and *Bacteroides fragilis*.

As a rule, the third-generation cephalosporins are less active than the older cephalosporins against gram-positive cocci but are much more active against the Enterobacteriaceae, including multiply resistant isolates. A subset of the third-generation agents also exhibits marked activity against *P. aeruginosa* (cefoperazone, ceftazidime, cefpiramide, cefpirome). Because of the variation in spectrum of activity among these agents, susceptibility of a given isolate must be determined to each specific agent.

The cephalosporins are relatively nontoxic, but they may elicit hypersensitivity reactions in a small proportion of persons.

Other β-Lactam Antibiotics

Monobactams. The monobactams constitute a unique family of β-lactams with a monocyclic nucleus (Fig. 9–2). The naturally occurring monobactams, produced by a number of soil bacteria, exhibit weak antibacterial activity, but some synthetic derivatives such as aztreonam are highly active. Aztreonam does not bind to the penicillin-binding proteins in gram-positive and anaerobic bacteria, and thus it has no appreciable antibacterial activity against these species. However, it exhibits excellent activity against a broad spectrum of aerobic gram-negative organisms, such as the Enterobacteriaceae, *P. aeruginosa*, *N. gonorrhoeae*, and *H. influenzae*, including β-lactamase-producing strains of *H. influenzae* and gonococci.

Thienamycins. The thienamycins are carbapenem compounds (Fig. 9–2) that are stereochemically different from penicillin and the cephalosporins. They are in a *trans* configuration, and the ring sulfur atom is replaced by a methylene group, with the sulfur atom adjacent to a more strained bicyclic ring system. Imipenem, the *N*-formimidoyl derivative, is the thienamycin in clinical use. It has an extremely broad spectrum of activity and is the first β-lactam to exhibit marked activity against virtually all medically important species, including organisms frequently resistant to other β-lactams, such as *Staphylococcus*, *Streptococcus faecalis*, *P. aeruginosa*, multiply-resistant Enterobacteriaceae, *B. fragilis*, and β-lactamase-producing strains of *H. influenzae* and *N. gonorrhoeae*.

β-Lactamase Inhibitors. Several β-lactams that function as β-lactamase inhibitors have been developed. Such agents have little intrinsic antibacterial activity, but, when combined with a β-lactam that is susceptible to hydrolysis, they protect the susceptible β-lactam from degradation and allow it to exert its lethal effect. For a β-lactamase-inhibiting compound to be effective, it must have a β-lactam ring that can undergo normal enzymatic attack to form an acyl enzyme intermediate that hydrolyzes at a relatively slow rate (Fig. 9–2). It is also essential that the β-lactam compound have the ability to pass readily through porin channels in gram-negative organisms so that sufficiently high concentrations are attained in the periplasmic space to inhibit the β-lactamases and thus allow the protected β-lactam to inactivate the penicillin-binding proteins before it is hydrolyzed.

CLAVULANIC ACID AND SULBACTAM. Clavulanic acid and sulbactam act primarily as suicide inhibitors of certain plasmid- and chromosome-mediated β-lactamases of both gram-positive and gram-negative organisms. They act synergistically with amoxicillin, ampicillin, piperacillin, mezlocillin, and cefoperazone, all of which can be destroyed by β-lactamase-producing strains of *S. aureus*, Enterobacteriaceae, and other gram-negative bacilli. The combinations of amoxicillin-clavulanic acid, ticarcillin-clavulanic acid, and ampicillin-sulbactam have proved clinically effective in various infections—lower respiratory tract, urinary tract, skin, and soft tissue, among others. Selective and restrictive situations for their use, however, remain to be clarified.

Cycloserine

Cycloserine is a broad-spectrum antibiotic that has found clinical use only in the treatment of tuberculosis. Even here, because of central nervous system toxicity, its use is limited to re-treatment in drug-resistant cases, where it is administered as one of a three-or-more drug combination.

Cycloserine is an inhibitor of peptidoglycan synthesis. The molecular basis for its bactericidal activity lies in its structural similarity to D-alanine (Fig. 9–11). Cycloserine is a competitive inhibitor of two sequential reactions in the syn-

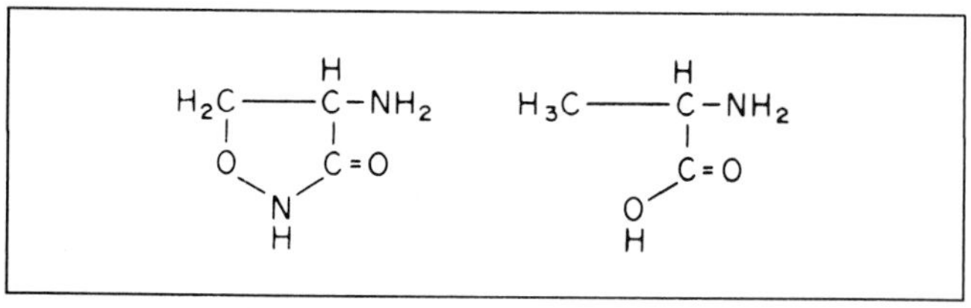

Fig. 9–11. Structural relationship between cycloserine (left) and D-alanine (right).

thesis of peptidoglycan in which D-alanine is incorporated: alanine racemase and D-alanyl-D-alanine synthetase. The synthetase has two binding sites for cycloserine, the donor and acceptor sites. The donor site is believed to be the primary site of antibiotic action. The effectiveness of cycloserine as a competitive enzyme inhibitor can be attributed to a significantly higher affinity than the natural substrate D-alanine for both of the D-alanine reacting sites of the D-alanyl-D-alanine synthetase.

Resistance of cycloserine may be attributed to two different mechanisms. In *E. coli* and *S. faecalis* the antibiotic is effective only if a transport system for D-alanine is present. Loss of the alanine transport system protects the organism against D-cycloserine activity. In other mutants, resistance is attributed to elevated levels of both alanine racemase and D-alanyl-D-alanine synthetase.

Vancomycin

Vancomycin is a narrow-spectrum, bactericidal antibiotic active against many species of gram-positive cocci. Although its toxicity has limited its clinical usefulness, it remains valuable as alternative therapy for a number of serious infections in patients who are allergic to the β-lactam agents and for serious infections caused by methicillin-resistant *S. aureus* or multiply resistant pneumococci. It is the treatment of choice for antibiotic-associated colitis caused by *Clostridium difficile* and, in combination with gentamicin, for *Enterococcus faecalis* endocarditis in patients who are allergic to penicillin. The development of resistance during clinical use of vancomycin has not been a problem. However, clinically significant vancomycin-resistant enterococci have now been isolated and may foretell problems in the future.

Vancomycin is a complex glycopeptide with a molecular weight of about 1450 (Fig. 9–12). It interferes with peptidoglycan biosynthesis by binding very rapidly and irreversibly to the acyl-D-alanyl-D-alanine terminus of a membrane-bound peptidoglycan precursor. In the presence of sufficient vancomycin both glycan chain extension and incorporation of new chain by transpeptidation are curtailed.

Bacitracin

Bacitracin is a polypeptide antibiotic produced by a specific strain of *Bacillus subtilis.* It is bactericidal for many gram-positive organisms and pathogenic *Neisseria* (Fig. 9–13), but its toxicity limits its clinical usefulness to topical administration only. Resistance to the drug does not readily develop.

Bacitracin interferes with the third stage of peptidoglycan biosynthesis. In the last step of this stage, the pyrophosphate form of the phospholipid (undecaprenyl pyrophosphate) is dephosphorylated to yield inorganic phosphate and regenerated phospholipid.

$$C_{55}\ \text{isoprenyl-PP} \rightleftharpoons C_{55}\ \text{isoprenyl-P} + P_i$$

Bacitracin binds to the pyrophosphate and specifically blocks this reaction. It thus inhibits peptidoglycan synthesis by preventing reentry of the lipid carrier into the reaction cycle.

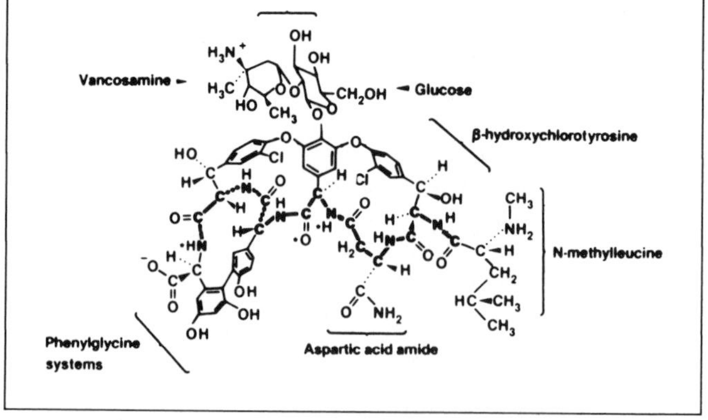

Fig. 9–12. Vancomycin, a glycopeptide. The structure consists of a disaccharide (vancosamine and glucose), two β-hydroxychlorotyrosine units, three substituted phenylglycine systems, *N*-methylleucine, and aspartic acid amide. The peptide backbone is shown in heavier type. The atoms involved in hydrogen bonding with acetyl-D-alanyl-D-alanine are indicated by asterisks. *(From Pfeiffer: Rev Infect Dis 3[Suppl]:S205, 1981.)*

Cell Membrane Inhibitors

The cell membrane plays a vital role in the cell. It poses an osmotic barrier to free diffusion between the internal and external environments. It effects the concentration of metabolites and nutrients within the cell and serves as a site for respiratory and certain biosynthetic activities. Several antibiotics impair one or more of these functions, resulting in major disturbances in the viability of the cell. The action of agents whose primary target is the cell membrane is independent of

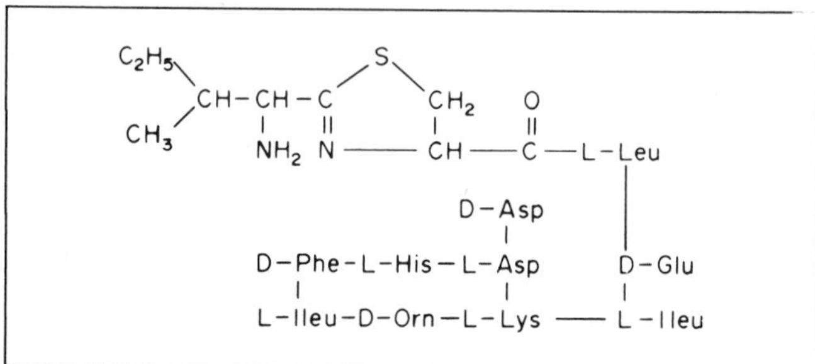

Fig. 9–13. Bacitracin A, one of a group of polypeptide antibiotics containing a thiazoline ring structure.

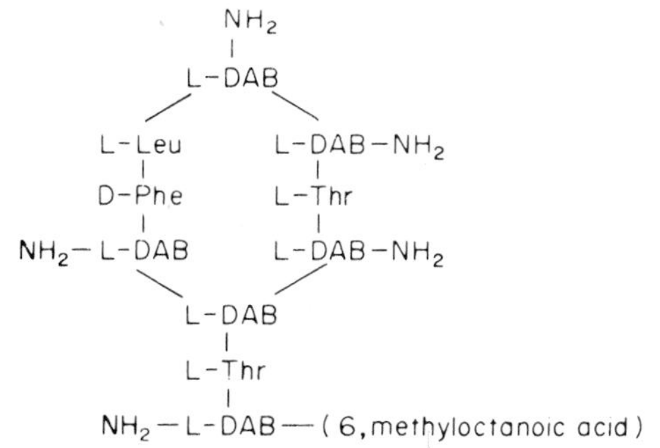

Fig. 9–14. Polymyxin B. DAB is α, γ-diaminobutyric acid, a component that is present together with L-threonine and D-6-methyloctanoic acid in all polymyxins.

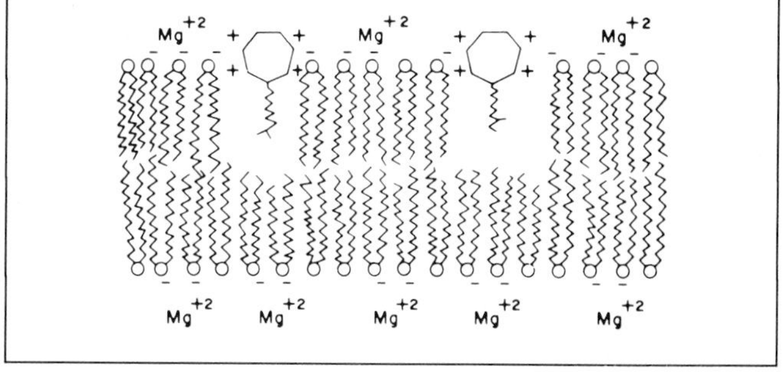

Fig. 9–15. Hypothetical model for interaction of polymyxin with a phospholipid bilayer. It is proposed that the fatty acid tail of the peptide penetrates the hydrophobic domain of the bilayer, with the peptide amino groups interacting electrostatically with phospholipid phosphates. *(From Storm et al: Annu Rev Biochem 46:723, 1977.)*

growth and begins immediately when cells and antibiotic come together. Unlike inhibitors that interfere with cell-wall biosynthesis and that are relatively innocuous for mammalian tissues, antibiotics that attack the cell membrane distinguish less successfully between microorganisms and host tissues. Because of their toxicity, few have found a place in clinical medicine.

Polymyxins

The polymyxins are produced by *Bacillus polymyxa.* They consist of a family of relatively simple polypeptides characterized by poor diffusibility and significant toxicity. Members of this group are designated by the letters A, B, C, D, and E, but of these only polymyxin B and polymyxin E (colistin) are currently of clinical use (Fig. 9–14). The polymyxins are decapeptides that contain a high percentage of 2,4-diaminobutyric acid (DAB), a fatty acid, and a mixture of D- and L-amino acids. The activity of polymyxin is restricted to gram-negative organisms. Because of severe adverse reactions, polymyxin is usually reserved for serious *P. aeruginosa* infections when the organism is resistant to other antibiotics or the patient is intolerant of the preferred drug.

Polymyxin binds specifically to the outer surface of cell membranes, altering their structure and osmotic properties. There is a leakage of metabolites and inhibition of a number of biochemical processes secondary to membrane damage. Damage to the membrane is attributed to an electrostatic binding and disruption of the structure of the phospholipid and lipopolysaccharide components, probably by competitively displacing Mg^{2+} or Ca^{2+} from negatively charged phosphate groups on membrane lipids (Fig. 9–15).

Polyenes

The polyenes are macrolide antibiotics, the most important of which are the antifungal agents amphotericin B and nystatin. All polyene agents have a large lactone ring containing a flexible hydroxylated portion and a rigid hydrophobic system of unsubstituted conjugated double bonds. In amphotericin B and nystatin there is also an amino sugar mycosamine (Fig. 9–16).

Amphotericin B remains the cornerstone of antifungal therapy. It is active against most fungi that cause deep-seated infections. It does, however, produce a number of serious side effects, including nephrotoxicity. Nystatin is also clinically useful, but its toxicity prevents parenteral use. Its most important use is in the treatment of cutaneous or superficial infections caused by *Candida.*

The polyenes selectively inhibit organisms whose membranes contain sterols. They are active against yeast, fungi, and other eucaryotic cells but are not inhibitory for procaryotic organisms. The selectivity of both amphotericin B and nystatin for fungi is attributable to the drugs' preferential binding to ergosterol, the sterol present in all fungus membranes. Since some interaction does occur, however, with the cholesterol present in mammalian membranes, the use of these agents is often associated with severe dose-related adverse reactions in the host. Interaction of the polyenes with ergosterol molecules leads to the formation of lethal pores that span the membrane, resulting in an increase in the permeability of the membrane and loss of a variety of small metabolites vital to the cell.

Mechanisms for drug-induced resistance to the polyenes include (1) a decrease in the membrane ergosterol content and (2) a modification of the membrane sterol content to include sterols that bind less efficiently to polyenes.

Azoles

Imidazoles: Ketoconazole, Miconazole, and Clotrimazole. Of the imidazole derivatives currently available, these

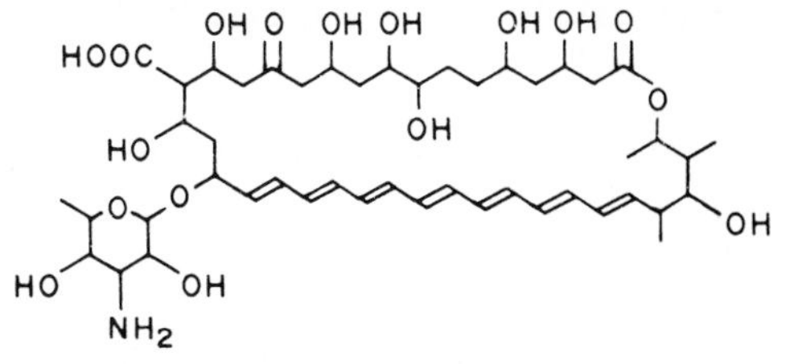

Fig. 9–16. Amphotericin B, a polyene antibiotic with selective activity for fungi.

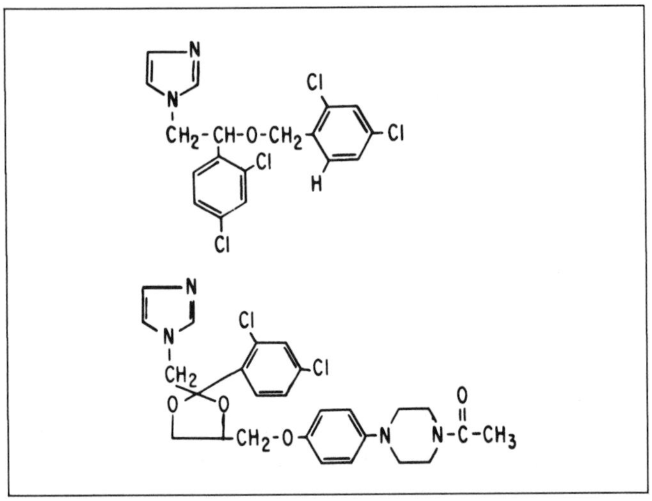

Fig. 9–17. Chemical structure of miconazole (top) and ketoconazole (bottom), imidazole derivatives useful in antifungal chemotherapy.

agents are clinically the most useful (Fig. 9–17). They are broad-spectrum antifungal agents active against dermatophytes, dimorphic fungi, and yeasts, as well as some bacteria and protozoa. Because of the adverse side effects when they are administered parenterally, the use of miconazole and clotrimazole is limited to topical application. They are especially useful in the treatment of cutaneous and vaginal candidiasis. Ketoconazole, however, is efficacious when given orally for a broad spectrum of superficial and deep mycotic infections in humans and when administered parenterally causes few adverse reactions. The inhibitory effects of the imidazoles are due to their interference with ergosterol synthesis by the fungus cell. These agents block demethylation at the C14 site of the ergosterol precursor, lanosterol. This results in the accumulation of lanosterol-like sterols in the cell, altered properties of the cell membrane, and leakage of potassium ions and phosphorus-containing compounds.

Triazoles: Itraconazole and Fluconazole. These azoles are *N*-substituted imidazoles with an antifungal spectrum and a mechanism of action similar to that of the imidazoles. They are better tolerated when administered orally than the imidazoles and promise to be effective in the treatment of some deep mycoses and opportunistic infections.

Inhibitors of DNA Function

A number of antimicrobial agents specifically interfere with the structure and function of DNA, but few of these drugs have shown a selective toxicity that would make them acceptable for clinical use. They have been useful, however, as biochemical tools and have contributed significantly to studies in the area of molecular biology. The structure of the DNA molecule is intimately related to its two primary roles, duplication and transcription. Any agent that disturbs the structure of the organized double helix of DNA is potentially capable of causing profound effects on all phases of cell growth and metabolism. Among the mechanisms employed by antimicrobial agents for altering the structure or function of DNA are cross-linking and intercalation between the stacked bases of the double helix.

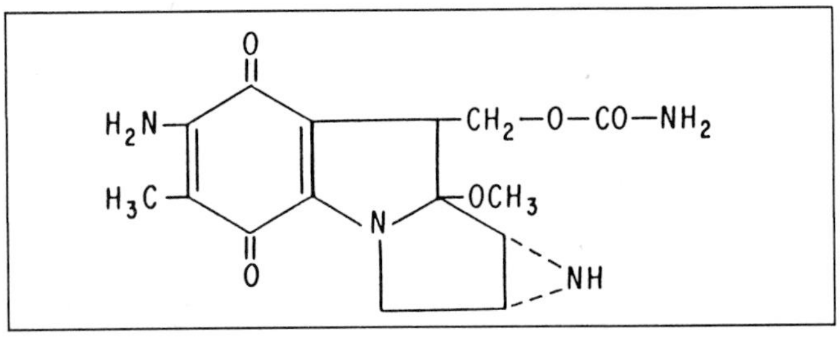

Fig. 9–18. Mitomycin C, an antibiotic that cross-links with DNA.

Mitomycin

The addition of mitomycin to growing bacterial cells results in inhibition of cell division with the formation of long filamentous forms, bacteriostasis, and death (Fig. 9–18). The bactericidal effect coincides with inhibition of DNA synthesis and usually is accompanied by massive degradation of the preexisting DNA.

Before its inhibitory effects are expressed in vivo, mitomycin is converted enzymatically to a highly reactive hydroquinone derivative that acts as a bifunctional alkylating agent. This reactive, short-lived species readily cross-links with DNA by bonding to two sites, one on each of the complementary strands. Guanine residues in DNA are the most probable sites for alkylation. The formation of covalent cross-links in DNA prevents separation of the complementary strands, thereby inhibiting progress of the replicating fork and causing a blockage of DNA synthesis. Cross-link formation is not the only mechanism by which mitomycin damages the cell. Monoalkylated sites on a single strand of DNA occur with a ten times greater frequency than cross-links. The DNA degradation that follows treatment with mitomycin is due to the excision of the cross-linked zones and to endonucleolytic breaks in the damaged DNA at the monoalkylated sites. The appearance of nucleases is associated with lysogenic phages induced by mitomycin.

Mitomycin exhibits some selectivity in the cross-linking of DNA. Under certain conditions it blocks the synthesis of host cell DNA but permits viral DNA synthesis. The reason for the relative resistance of viral DNA is not clear, but the finding has been useful in studies of viral DNA synthesis in the absence of DNA synthesis by the host cell.

Since mitomycin fails to distinguish between the DNA of the infecting organism and that of the host, its toxicity prohibits clinical use.

Quinolones

All agents in the quinolone class of antibacterial agents are synthetic products; they are similar in structure and have a unique mechanism of action (Fig. 9–19). Nalidixic acid, the first of this group to be introduced, is a derivative of 1,8-naphthyridine. Previously used for the clinical management of uncomplicated urinary tract infections, nalidixic acid and

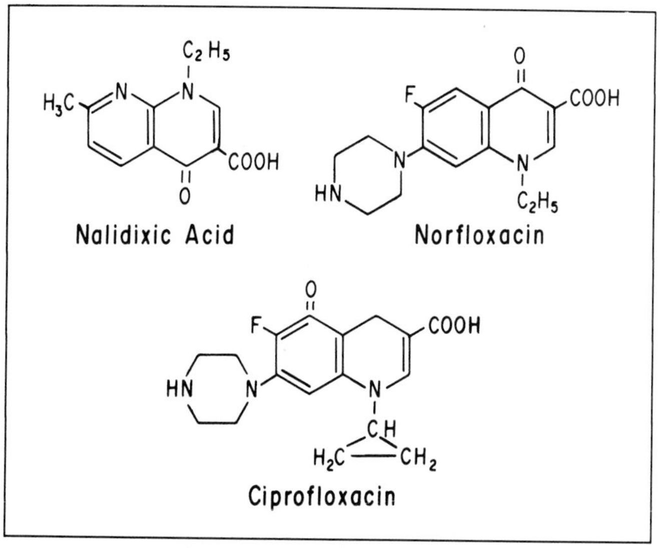

Fig. 9–19. Quinolones, synthetic agents used in the treatment of urinary tract infections.

the older quinolones have now been largely replaced by the newer quinolones that have a broadened antibacterial spectrum and activities 1000 times that of nalidixic acid.

Nalidixic acid and related quinolones selectively and reversibly block DNA replication in susceptible bacteria but exhibit no demonstrable mutagenicity. They inhibit the A subunit of DNA gyrase and induce the formation of a relaxation complex analogue. Complex formation, unlike the introduction of supertwists into closed circular DNA, is insensitive to novobiocin, another drug that also inhibits gyrase activity. Nalidixic acid, but not novobiocin, inhibits the nicking-closing activity of the swivelase component of DNA gyrase that relieves the positive winding stress on the supercoiled DNA. In nalidixic acid mutants, mutation at the *nal A* gene locus confers resistance to high levels of nalidixic acid but not to novobiocin.

Norfloxacin and Ciprofloxacin. Of the newer quinolones the fluorinated compounds norfloxacin and ciprofloxacin have been the most useful. The spectrum of norfloxacin includes enterococci and staphylococci as well as *Pseudomonas*. Ciprofloxacin is the most potent of the quinolones. It is active against most strains of gram-negative and gram-positive bacteria that cause urinary tract infections at concentrations that are readily attained in the urine. Promising results have also been obtained with the oral use of these fluorinated quinolones in the treatment of infections of the respiratory tract, gastrointestinal tract, skin, and bone and in the prophylactic selective decontamination of the intestine in neutropenic patients. Although the frequency of spontaneous resistance to the new quinolones is lower than that observed with nalidixic acid, the emergence of fluroquinolone resistance in clinical isolates of *S. aureus* threatens their usefulness in the treatment of methicillin-resistant infections. DNA gyrase A subunit mutations have been implicated in resistance to ciprofloxacin in *S. aureus*.

Metronidazole

Metronidazole is an effective antimicrobial agent for the treatment of infections with anaerobic bacteria and certain protozoa. It has little or no effect on facultative and aerobic organisms.

Metronidazole is a synthetic 5-nitroimidazole derivative of low molecular weight. A key feature of its antimicrobial activity is the reduction of its nitro group, which requires a redox potential more negative than the −350 mV normally attainable during the growth of aerobic organisms. Reduction of the drug decreases the intracellular concentration of unchanged drug, thereby maintaining a gradient for continued uptake. Reduction of metronidazole results in the production of toxic short-lived intermediates or free radicals that damage the DNA and rapidly inhibit replication.

Novobiocin

Novobiocin is bactericidal for a variety of bacteria, especially gram-positive organisms. Although a number of biosynthetic processes in vivo are inhibited by novobiocin, its primary inhibitory effect is on the replication of DNA. It inhibits the supercoiling of DNA by DNA gyrase (p. 98). The target site for novobiocin is the subunit B component of DNA gyrase, rather than subunit A, as in the case of nalidixic acid. This accounts for some of the observed differences between the action of these two agents.

At present there are no valid indications for the therapeutic use of novobiocin.

Inhibitors of Protein Synthesis and Assembly

Protein synthesis is the end result of two major processes: (1) DNA-dependent ribonucleic acid synthesis (transcription) and (2) RNA-dependent protein synthesis (translation). An antibiotic that inhibits either of these processes will inhibit protein synthesis. Although the antibiotics that primarily inhibit translation have been the most useful clinically, the agents that inhibit transcription have been useful in characterizing the steps involved in protein synthesis.

Inhibitors of Transcription

During transcription, the genetic information in DNA is transferred to a complementary sequence of RNA nucleotides by the RNA polymerase, a complex enzyme composed of four subunits: β, β′, α, α. Associated with this core polymerase that forms the internucleotide linkages is the sigma factor, a dissociable component that acts catalytically in the accurate initiation of RNA chains. Antibiotics that either alter the structure of the template DNA or inhibit the RNA polymerase will interfere with the synthesis of RNA and, consequently, with protein synthesis.

Actinomycin. Actinomycin D is a bright red oligopeptide that is active against many gram-positive and gram-negative organisms as well as mammalian cells (Fig. 9–20). Actinomycin forms complexes specifically with DNA, thereby impairing DNA function. Binding is dependent on guanine residues and helical secondary structure. The action of actinomycin is attributed to the planar character of its chromophoric ring,

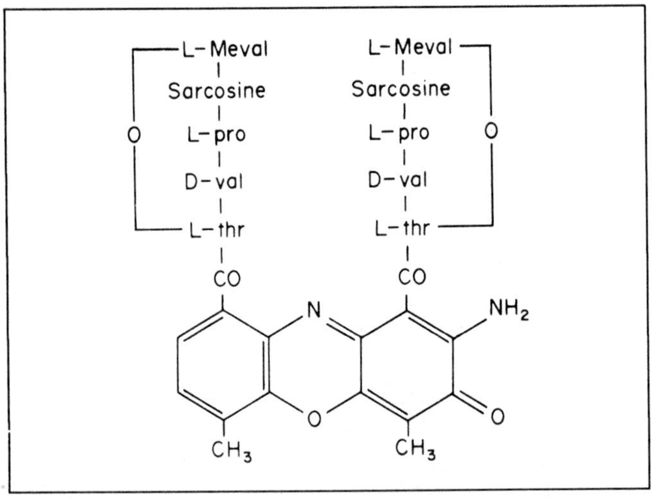

Fig. 9–20. Actinomycin D. This agent forms complexes with DNA by binding to deoxyguanosine residues.

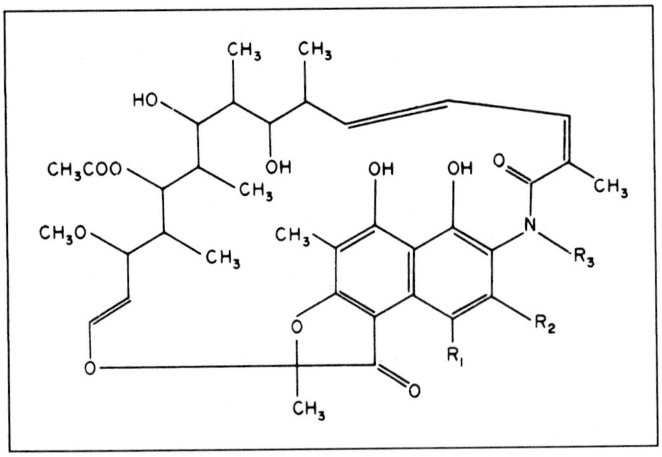

Fig. 9–21. Basic structure of the rifamycins. Various derivatives are substituted in the R_1, R_2, and R_3 positions. In rifampin, R_1 is —OH; R_2 is —CH=N—N⬡N—CH_3; R_3 is H.

which permits it to intercalate between the adjacent stacked basepairs of the double helix. To permit this insertion, there is a preliminary local unwinding of the double helix to produce spaces into which the planar chromophore can move. The actinomycin molecule is stabilized internally by hydrogen bonding between its two cyclic pentapeptides, which lie in the minor groove of the double helix, and by bonding of guanine residues with the L-threonines of one of the peptide rings. Since the normal progression of RNA polymerase is along the minor groove of the DNA template, the presence of cyclic pentapeptide rings in the groove blocks polymerase movement. Although actinomycin also inhibits DNA synthesis, DNA-dependent RNA synthesis is inhibited at much lower concentrations.

Actinomycin has been used extensively as an investigative tool, but its toxicity prevents its clinical use.

Rifampin. The rifamycins are ansa compounds, that is, compounds that contain an aromatic ring system spanned by a long aliphatic bridge. Some members of the group occur in nature, but most are semisynthetic derivatives (Fig. 9–21). One of the most useful members of the group is rifampin. Rifampin has a wide antibacterial spectrum and is especially effective against gram-positive organisms and mycobacteria. It is a major drug for the treatment of tuberculosis and leprosy and for meningococcal meningitis prophylaxis.

Rifampin inhibits protein synthesis by selectively inactivating the DNA-dependent RNA polymerase. In the first step of transcription the polymerase is bound to a specific initiation site on the DNA template, followed by the binding to the enzyme of the first nucleoside 5′-triphosphate. To this initiation complex, the second nucleoside 5′-triphosphate is added, and the first phosphodiester bond is formed. Rifampin binds noncovalently to the β-subunit of RNA polymerase and blocks RNA chain initiation after formation of the first phosphodiester bond. The binding by rifampin apparently induces an isomerization or conformational change of the enzyme, which is responsible for its inactivation. Only the initiation of RNA synthesis is arrested; there is no effect on chain elongation. Rifampin is inactive on DNA-directed RNA polymerases from eucaryotic nuclei. Its effect on mammalian DNA viruses and oncogenic viruses is discussed in Chapter 56.

Resistance to rifampin, which develops rapidly both in vitro and in vivo, is caused by a mutation that results in a change in structure of the β subunit of RNA polymerase.

Inhibitors of Translation

In bacterial cells, the translation of mRNA into protein can be divided into three major phases: initiation, elongation, and termination of the peptide chain. Protein synthesis starts with the association of mRNA, a 30S ribosomal subunit, and formylmethionyl-tRNA (fMet-tRNA) to form a 30S initiation complex. The formation of this complex also requires guanosine triphosphate (GTP) and protein initiation factors. The codon AUG is the initiation signal in mRNA and is recognized by the anticodon of fMet-tRNA. A 50S ribosomal subunit is subsequently added to form a 70S initiation complex, and the bound GTP is hydrolyzed.

In the elongation phase of protein synthesis, amino acids are added one at a time to a growing polypeptide in a sequence dictated by mRNA. It is this phase that is most susceptible to inhibition by a number of antibiotics (Fig. 9–22). For many of these the ribosome is the target site. There are two binding sites on the ribosome, the P (peptidyl or donor) site and the A (aminoacyl) site. At the end of the initiation stage the fMet-tRNA molecule occupies the P site, and the A site designated for a tRNA molecule is empty. In the first step of the elongation cycle an aminoacyl-tRNA is inserted into the vacant A site on the ribosome. The particular species inserted depends on the mRNA codon that is positioned in the A site. Protein elongation factors and GTP are required for polypeptide chain elongation.

In the next step of the elongation phase the formylmethionyl residue of the fMet-tRNA located at the peptidyl donor site is released from its linkage to tRNA and is joined with a peptide bond to the α-amino group of the aminoacyl-tRNA in the acceptor site to form a dipeptidyl-tRNA. The enzyme catalyzing this peptide formation is peptidyl transferase, which is part of the 50S ribosomal subunit.

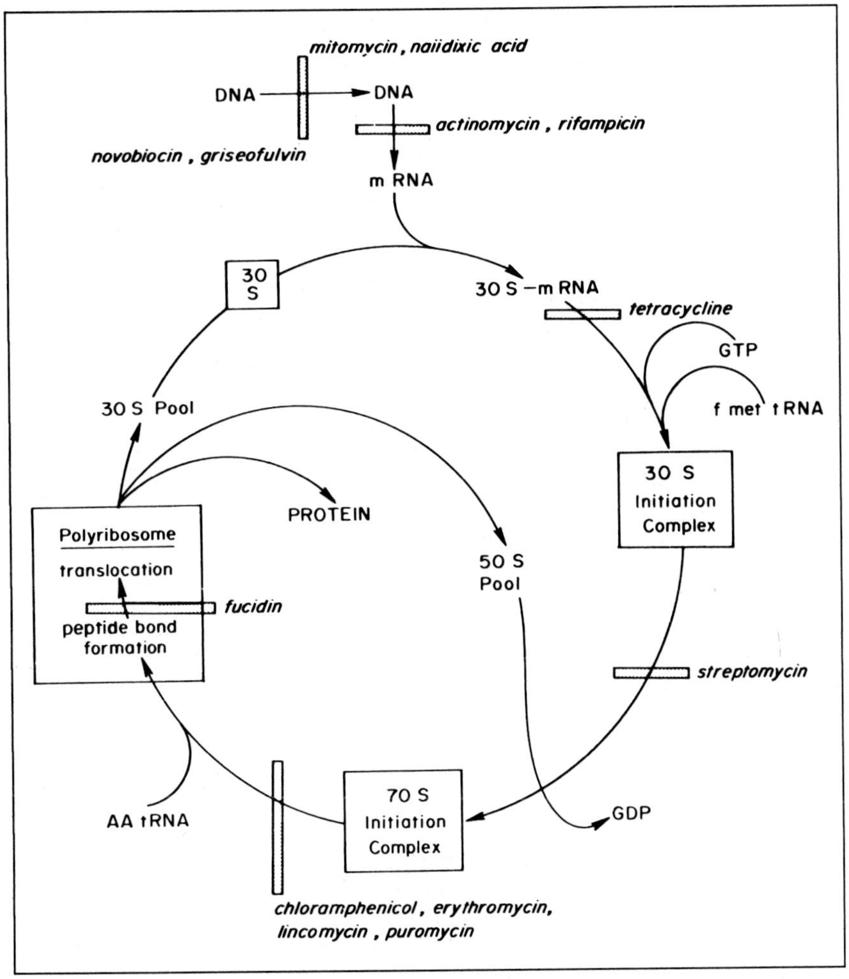

Fig. 9–22. Site of action of antibiotics that inhibit DNA, RNA, and protein synthesis.

After the formation of a peptide bond an uncharged tRNA occupies the P site, and a dipeptidyl tRNA occupies the A site. The final phase of the elongation cycle is translocation, catalyzed by elongation factor EF-G and requiring GTP. It consists of three movements: (1) removal of the discharged tRNA from the P site, (2) movement of fMet-aminoacyl-tRNA from the acceptor site to the peptidyl donor site, and (3) movement or translocation of the ribosome along the mRNA from the 5′ toward the 3′ terminus by the length of three nucleotides. After translocation the stage is prepared for the binding of the next aminoacyl residue to the fMet-AA-tRNA, each addition requiring aminoacyl-tRNA binding, peptide bond formation, and translocation. Peptidyl-tRNAs replace the fMet-tRNA in the second cycle and in all subsequent cycles.

The polypeptide chain grows from the amino terminal toward the carboxyl terminal amino acid and remains linked to tRNA and bound to the mRNA-ribosome complex during elongation of the chain. When completed, it is released during chain termination. Termination is triggered when a chain termination signal (UAA, UAG, or UGA) is encountered at the A site of the ribosome. Protein release factors bind to the terminator codons triggering hydrolysis by the peptidyl transferase. The polypeptide is released, and the messenger-ribosome-tRNA complex dissociates.

Several medically important antibiotics owe their selective antimicrobial action to a specific attack on the 70S ribosomes of bacteria; mammalian 80S ribosomes are unaffected. A subdivision of antibiotics into major classes has been made on the basis of whether they bind to the 30S or 50S ribosomal subunits, with the assumption that the site of fixation provides presumptive evidence of its site of action.

Inhibitors of the 30S Ribosomal Subunit

As noted above, 30S ribosomal subunits provide attachment sites for mRNA and move relative to it during translation. The 30S subunit also provides a binding site for fMet-tRNA and aminoacyl-tRNA. Inhibition of protein synthesis on the 30S subunit could result if (1) mRNA is prevented from attaching, (2) movement of mRNA relative to the 30S subunit is impaired, or (3) the aminoacyl acceptor site is blocked. Among the antibiotics that act at the level of the 30S ribosomal subunit are the aminoglycosidic aminocyclitol antibiotics and the tetracyclines.

Aminoglycosidic Aminocyclitol Antibiotics. Among the

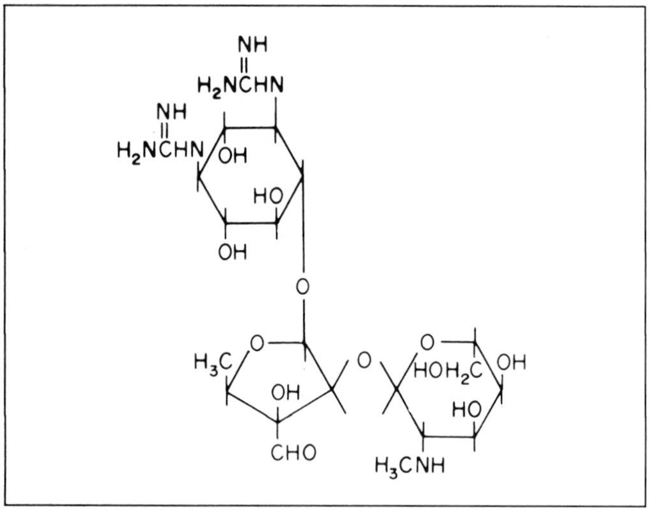

Fig. 9–23. Streptomycin. The streptidine moiety (upper ring structure) is an inositol substituted with two guanido groups linked to the streptobiosamine moiety by a glycosidic bond.

aminoglycosidic aminocyclitol antibiotics are such important antimicrobial agents as streptomycin, neomycin, kanamycin, gentamicin, tobramycin, and amikacin (Fig. 9–23). The unique aminocyclitol ring structure that forms the backbone of each of these compounds is a derivative of inositol in which various hydroxyl groups have been replaced with amino groups or substituted amino groups (Fig. 9–24). Kasugamycin is the simplest of these compounds and consists of an amino-containing sugar joined by a glycosidic linkage to inositol itself. Streptidine is the aminocyclitol component of streptomycin, and 2-deoxystreptamine provides the backbone for kanamycin, gentamicin, tobramycin, and amikacin (Fig. 9–25). To this aminocyclitol ring, two amino sugars are attached by a glycosidic linkage, hence the name aminoglycosidic aminocyclitol. Spectinomycin, an antibiotic usually included in discussions of this group, contains an aminocyclitol ring structure but lacks an amino sugar residue (Fig. 9–26). Unlike the other members of this group, it has a bacteriostatic rather than a bactericidal action.

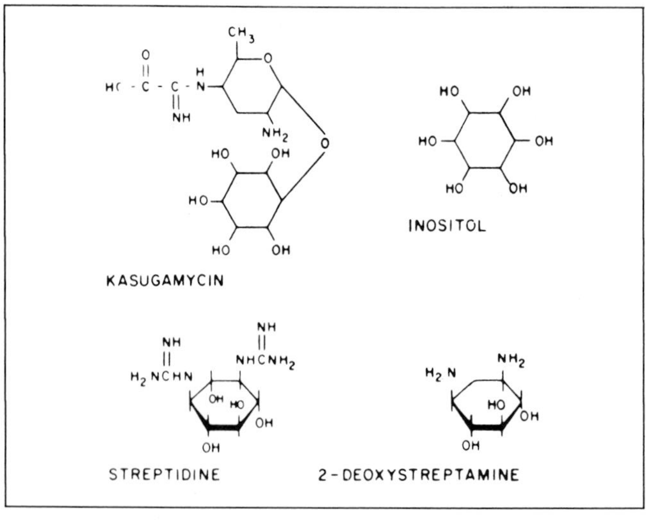

Fig. 9–24. Structural formulas of components of various aminoglycosidic aminocyclitol antibiotics. *(From Moellering: Med J Aust(spec suppl)2:4, 1977.)*

The pharmacokinetic properties of the group are attributable to their polarity as polycations. They are poorly absorbed orally, penetrate poorly into the cerebrospinal fluid, and are rapidly excreted by the kidney. A number of adverse reactions are associated with their use; among the most serious are neuromuscular paralysis, ototoxicity, and nephrotoxicity.

STREPTOMYCIN. Streptomycin is bactericidal for a wide variety of gram-positive and gram-negative species and for *Mycobacterium tuberculosis*. Clinically, the chief merit of streptomycin lies in its ability to attack certain organisms that are not affected by penicillin (Table 9–5). However, the introduction of newer agents with a broader antibacterial spectrum has limited the current indications for streptomycin. It remains the drug of choice for *Francisella tularensis* and *Yersinia pestis* infections. It is also useful in combination with penicillin or vancomycin in the treatment of endocarditis caused by *S. faecalis* or *Streptococcus viridans*, and in combination with other agents in the management of tuberculosis.

The rapid development of resistance to high levels of streptomycin has been a major factor in limiting its clinical usefulness. Plasmid-mediated resistance to the aminoglycoside antibiotics is frequently seen in clinical strains and is responsible for most of the resistance to this group of antibiotics. The biochemical mechanisms of streptomycin resistance are discussed on page 184.

Mechanism of Action. In spite of the enormous amount of attention that streptomycin has received since its introduction in the mid-1940s, its precise mechanism of action has remained elusive. Streptomycin clearly inhibits protein synthesis. Whereas this inhibition of protein synthesis appears to be an essential component of the bactericidal effect, it does not in itself provide a complete and adequate explanation for the antimicrobial's lethal activity.

When streptomycin is added to in vitro polypeptide-synthesizing systems, it has two major effects: (1) It markedly inhibits polypeptide synthesis, and (2) it causes misreading of the synthetic polynucleotide messengers. If ribosomes from streptomycin-resistant strains are used, both of these effects are abolished or greatly reduced.

Inhibition of Protein Synthesis. Streptomycin binds irreversibly to the 30S ribosomal subunit, drastically interrupting the ribosome cycle at the initiation of protein synthesis. It does not inhibit the formation of the initiation complex but inhibits the initiation of peptide chains on the complex (Fig. 9–22). When streptomycin is added to an in vitro polypeptide-synthesizing system employing viral RNA, a natural messenger, polypeptide synthesis in progress on polysomes is slowed down, but ribosomes are allowed to leave mRNA either prematurely or at the termination signal. On release, they dissociate into subunits but subsequently reassociate at the normal initiation sites on mRNA to form streptomycin monosomes, irreversibly inactivated initiation complexes that contain stabilized mRNA. These modified complexes cannot form peptide bonds. Their movement along the mRNA is impeded, thereby blocking the ribosome cycle at an early stage in the initiation of protein synthesis. These effects on initiation and

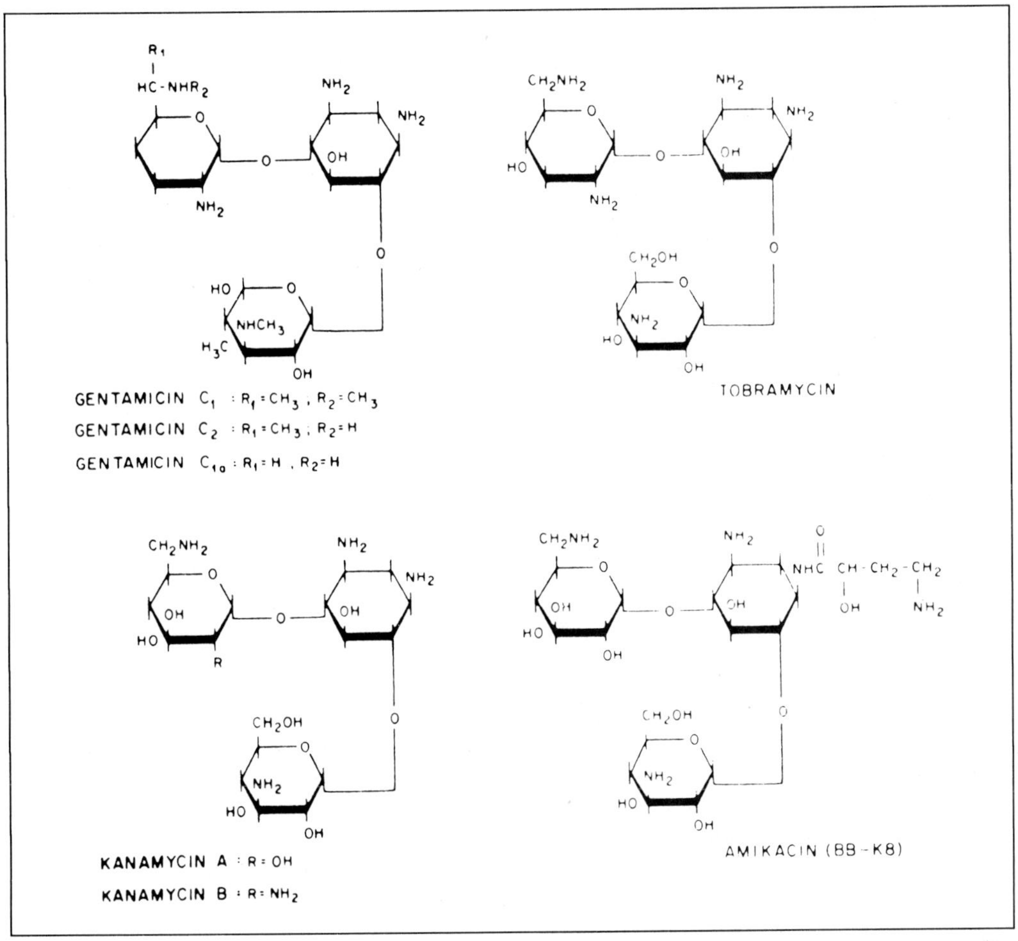

Fig. 9–25. Structural formulas of the gentamicins, tobramycin, the kanamycins, and amikacin. *(From Moellering: Med J Aust(spec suppl)2:4, 1977.)*

elongation are attributed to conformational changes by streptomycin at both acceptor and donor sites.

Interaction of streptomycin with the 30S subunit is complex. A single protein in the 30S ribosomal subunit, S12, is the ultimate target of streptomycin, but for binding of the antibiotic at least four additional ribosomal proteins—S3, S5, S9, and S14—are required. Binding to 16S RNA may also be involved.

Streptomycin-induced Misreading. One of the effects produced by streptomycin when added to an in vitro polypeptide-synthesizing system is misreading of the messenger. Streptomycin can inhibit the incorporation of certain synthetic polymer-directed incorporations and can stimulate the incorporation of amino acids not coded for. The extensive misreading provides an explanation for the ability of streptomycin to suppress mutations in a class of mutants that are conditionally streptomycin-dependent (CSD). Such mutants can grow in the absence of their specific growth requirement, provided streptomycin is present in the medium. This behavior apparently is due to a misreading of the genetic message by streptomycin. The wrong message of the mutant is not corrected physically but is read differently in the presence of streptomycin. The net result of this misreading of an incorrect message is the synthesis of a functional protein. In strains that permit correction by streptomycin, streptomycin mimics the action of a suppressor, a mutation at a second distinct site that reverses the mutant phenotype. Unlike the genetic suppression, however, the correction produced by streptomycin is phenotypic and is not heritable.

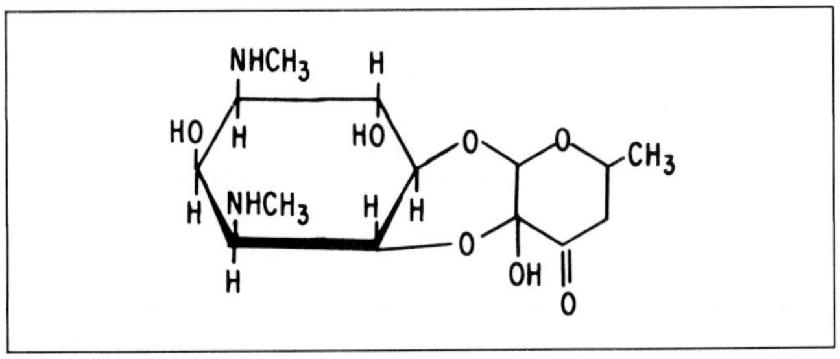

Fig. 9–26. Spectinomycin, a bacteriostatic aminocyclitol antibiotic that differs from the aminoglycoside group in that it lacks an amino sugar residue.

Although it is difficult to assess the in vivo significance of misreading of the code, an apparent relationship does exist between misreading, killing action, and phenotypic suppression. The streptamine or deoxystreptamine moiety of the aminoglycoside is the chemical structure responsible for misreading. Aminocyclitol drugs such as spectinomycin that lack

TABLE 9–5. CLINICALLY USEFUL AMINOCYCLITOL ANTIBIOTICS

Agent[a]	Source	Major Clinical Use
Streptomycin	*Streptomyces griseus*	Tularemia, plague, brucellosis
Neomycin	*Streptomyces fradiae*	Superficial skin infections, bacterial conjunctivitis, preoperative suppression of bowel flora
Kanamycin	*Streptomyces kanamyceticus*	Preoperative suppression of bowel flora
Gentamicin	*Micromonospora purpurea*	Infections by susceptible gram-negative rods; in combination with penicillin for enterococcal infections
Tobramycin	*Streptomyces tenebrarius*	Systemic *Pseudomonas* infections; alternative to gentamicin for gram-negative rod infections
Amikacin	Semisynthetic	Reserved for treatment of severe gram-negative rod infections resistant to other aminoglycosides
Netilmicin	Derivative of sisomicin	Gram-negative rod infections (not *Pseudomonas, Serratia*), especially gentamicin-resistant strains that produce adenylylating enzymes
Spectinomycin	*Streptomyces spectabilis*	Penicillinase-producing gonococcal infections and in patients allergic to penicillin

[a] All of the agents listed are aminoglycosidic aminocyclitols except spectinomycin. Their activity is primarily directed against aerobic gram-negative bacilli and *Staphylococcus aureus.*

this moiety cause no misreading and are bacteriostatic only in their action.

The biochemical basis for all of the in vivo effects of streptomycin is unknown, but the major effects observed (i.e., inhibition of protein synthesis, misreading, and phenotypic suppression) have been attributed to the irreversible binding of streptomycin to the 30S ribosomal subunit. This binding produces a conformational change at the aminoacyl-tRNA binding site, resulting in an interference with both the binding of aminoacyl-tRNA and the fidelity of translation. One of the key steps in ensuring fidelity of protein biosynthesis, the selection of aminoacyl-tRNA by the ribosome, involves two recognition steps, one involving the ternary complex of aminoacyl-tRNA, EFTu, and GTP and the other occurring after GTP hydrolysis and involving only the aminoacyl-tRNA. Streptomycin inhibits exclusively the latter recognition step, known as proofreading. When the ability to reject an error is impaired, streptomycin-induced misreading results.

Streptomycin Resistance. In a bacterium, three phenotypically distinct responses to streptomycin are possible: sensitivity, resistance, or dependence. These responses are determined by multiple alleles of a single genetic locus, the *str* locus that codes for protein S12 of the 30S subunit. This protein determines the sensitivity of the entire 30S ribosomal particle to streptomycin. A mutation to resistance would result if this site were eliminated or if it were altered in such a manner that the bound drug could no longer exert its effect. There is evidence of the existence of single-step, high-level mutations to resistance of both of these types. Resistance conferred by mutations in protein S12 can be suppressed by mutations in protein S4 and S5 of the 30S subunits.

The amount of misreading observed in a cell-free polypeptide synthesizing system containing ribosomes from a str^r mutant is tenfold less than that observed with ribosomes from str^s strains, even in the absence of streptomycin. This observation may explain the finding that mutations to streptomycin resistance often introduce other phenotypic effects.

Streptomycin Dependence. When a population of streptomycin-sensitive organisms is plated on a medium containing a high level of streptomycin, a number of the survivors require streptomycin for growth. These mutants are streptomycin dependent and arise from the str^s wild-type strain in a single step. The str^d phenotype is determined by a mutation allelic with or very close to the str^r locus. The genetic basis for streptomycin dependence in these mutants is thus quite different from the CSD phenotype discussed above (p. 171).

As with streptomycin resistance, mutation to dependence also exhibits pleiotropic effects. Unlike streptomycin resistance, however, where phenotypic suppression is restricted, in str^d strains phenotypic suppression is enhanced. In these strains most of the nonsense and missense mutations that normally occur are weakly suppressed, and ambiguity in translation is introduced. The absolute requirement for streptomycin for growth by str^d mutants can be satisfied by certain other agents that also cause misreading.

Bacterial resistance that emerges after the clinical use of streptomycin and the other aminoglycosides is usually mediated by plasmids that code for aminoglycoside-modifying enzymes. This type of resistance is discussed on page 184.

OTHER AMINOGLYCOSIDE ANTIBIOTICS. In addition to streptomycin the aminoglycoside antibiotics that have been used clinically are neomycin, kanamycin, gentamicin, tobramycin, and amikacin (Table 9–5). Compared with the β-lactam antibiotics, the margin between toxic and therapeutic doses is very narrow for all of these agents. However, some have retained their place in the treatment of various infections, especially infections acquired in the hospital setting. At present, gentamicin, tobramycin, and amikacin are clinically the most useful and can be used interchangeably. They are active against a broad spectrum of gram-negative bacteria, including *Pseudomonas.* With the exception of *S. aureus,* gram-positive organisms are generally resistant to all of these drugs. Gentamicin is widely used for serious gram-negative bacillary infections, but its use in nosocomial infections is becoming more limited because of an increase in gentamicin-resistant organisms in the hospital environment. Tobramycin has superior activity against *P. aeruginosa* and is the drug of choice for the treatment of bacteremia, pneumonia, and osteomyelitis caused by this organism. Amikacin is a semisynthetic aminoglycoside that is resistant to most of the bacterial enzymes that inactivate the other aminoglycosides. It is the preferred initial treatment for serious nosocomial gram-negative bacillary infections in hospitals where gentamicin and tobramycin resistance have become a problem. It has been recommended that its use be restricted to such situations to avoid the emergence of resistant strains.

Because of its toxicity, the current clinical use of neomycin is restricted to the preoperative suppression of intestinal flora. Kanamycin is active against most gram-negative bacteria with the exception of *Pseudomonas,* but now it has limited clinical usefulness because of its toxicity and the emergence of resistant strains.

Mechanism of Action. All of the aminoglycosides inhibit protein synthesis at the level of the 30S ribosomal subunit, and most of them also produce ambiguity in translation. The level of misreading produced by neomycin, kanamycin, and gentamicin is much greater than that produced by streptomycin. As expected, those aminoglycosides that cause translational errors are also capable of phenotypic suppression of nonsense and missense mutations. In contrast to streptomycin, which has a single ribosomal binding site, neomycin, kanamycin, and gentamicin have at least two binding sites each. These sites appear to be different from the streptomycin binding site.

AMINOCYCLITOL ANTIBIOTIC: SPECTINOMYCIN. This antibiotic lacks the amino sugar residue that characterizes members of the aminoglycoside group. Its clinical use is restricted to the treatment of uncomplicated gonorrhea in patients who are allergic to penicillin. Resistance to spectinomycin is rarely seen in *N. gonorrhoeae.*

Spectinomycin inhibits protein synthesis at the level of the messenger-ribosome interaction but causes no misreading. Also, since the structure responsible for misreading, the streptamine nucleus, is replaced in spectinomycin by a stereoisomer, not only is the misreading property lost but its lethality as well.

Tetracyclines.

The tetracyclines are a family of broad-spectrum antibiotics with activity against a wide range of gram-positive and gram-negative species, mycoplasmas, rickettsiae, and chlamydiae. Included in the group are the parent compound tetracycline, several natural products (chlortetracycline, oxytetracycline, demethylchlortetracycline), and a number of semisynthetic derivatives (doxycycline, minocycline) (Fig. 9–27). The antibacterial spectrum of the tetracycline group is very broad and overlaps that of penicillin, streptomycin, and chloramphenicol. The tetracyclines inhibit only rapidly multiplying organisms and are bacteriostatic.

The antimicrobial, pharmacologic, and therapeutic properties of the older fermentation-derived tetracyclines are similar. The semisynthetic derivatives have significantly improved therapeutic properties as a result of improved pharmacokinetics. One of the most undesirable side effects associated with the administration of the natural tetracyclines is superinfections, caused by incomplete oral absorption and resulting in inhibition of the normal intestinal flora. Such infections are caused by the outgrowth of drug-resistant indigenous bacteria or fungi that normally are kept in check by the drug-sensitive members of the intestinal flora. The two semisynthetics—doxycycline and minocycline—are more lipophilic than the natural antibiotics. They are almost completely absorbed from the intestine and, therefore, are less inhibitory for the normal gut flora. Another major adverse reaction associated with the tetracyclines results from deposition of the drug in calcified tissue, which causes staining and impairment of the structure of bone and teeth. This effect also is diminished with use of the more lipophilic semisynthetic derivatives.

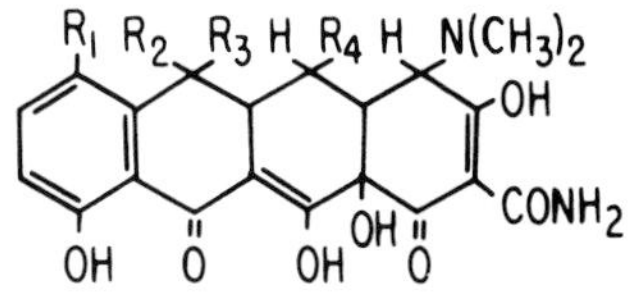

	R_1	R_2	R_3	R_4
Tetracycline	H	OH	CH_3	H
Oxytetracycline	H	OH	CH_3	OH
Chlorotetracycline	Cl	OH	CH_3	H
Demeclocycline	Cl	OH	H	H
Doxycycline	H	H	CH_3	OH
Minocycline	$N(CH_3)_2$	H	H	H

Fig. 9–27. Structural formulas for tetracycline and some of its analogues.

Unfortunately, with excessive use of the natural tetracyclines, a high level of drug resistance has developed, especially in the hospital environment. With the exception of minocycline, organisms that have become insensitive to one tetracycline exhibit approximately the same level of resistance to other members of the group.

Although the tetracyclines are broad-spectrum antibiotics with relatively low host toxicity, at present they are secondary in importance to the broad-spectrum penicillins and cephalosporins. They are reserved primarily for specific indications, such as the treatment of brucellosis, cholera, infections caused by chlamydiae, rickettsiae, and *Mycoplasma pneumoniae,* and urinary tract infections caused by sensitive gram-negative species. They also remain an important group of reserve drugs for ampicillin- and cephalosporin-resistant organisms. Tetracycline, the least expensive of the group, is generally the preferred drug.

MECHANISM OF ACTION. Unlike the aminoglycoside antibiotics, the tetracyclines inhibit protein synthesis of both procaryotic and eucaryotic cells. They are, however, much more effective inhibitors of protein synthesis in intact procaryotic cells than in eucaryotic cells. This selective activity is due primarily to the suicidal ability of bacteria to accumulate these drugs by an energy-dependent transport system that is not present in eucaryotic cells. The tetracyclines are transported across the membrane as a complex with magnesium ions. Within the cell, they bind to phosphate residues of the 30S ribosomal subunit by chelation with magnesium. This binding of tetracycline interferes with the binding of aminoacyl-tRNA to the acceptor site on the ribosome and thus inhibits protein synthesis. Tetracycline binds specifically to the S4 and S18 proteins of intact 70S ribosomes, with secondary binding to proteins S7, S13, and S14.

Bacteria develop resistance to the tetracyclines primarily

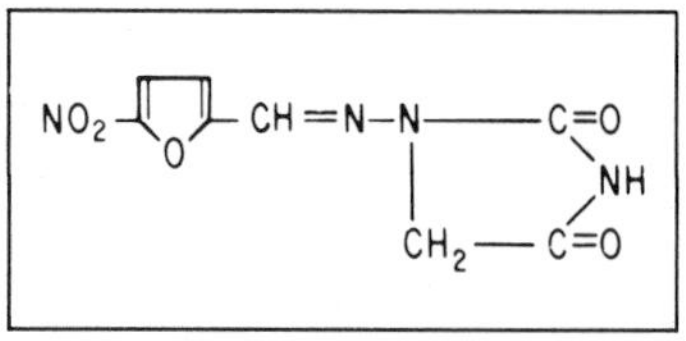

Fig. 9–28. Furadantin, a nitrofuran, is a clinically useful synthetic antimicrobial agent. Nitrofurans are derivatives of the furans, 5-membered ring sugars, and possess a nitro group in the 5-position.

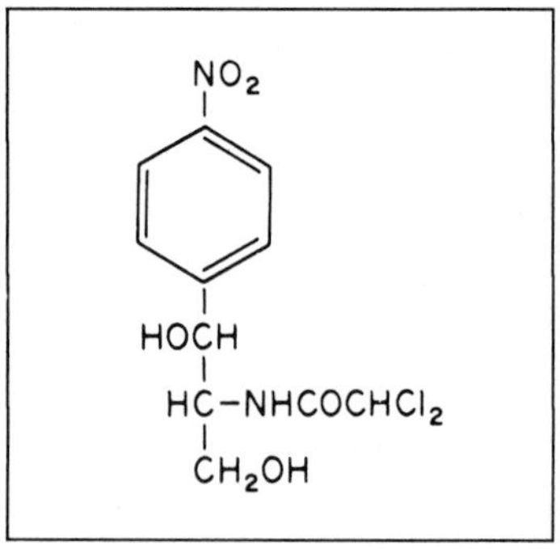

Fig. 9–29. Chloramphenicol, an antibiotic that inhibits peptide bond formation.

by becoming less permeable to the antibiotic. The biochemical, genetic, and epidemiologic aspects of tetracycline resistance are discussed on page 183.

Nitrofurans. One of the best known of this group of synthetic antibacterials is nitrofurantoin, which has been used clinically in the treatment of urinary tract infections, especially in patients who are unable to tolerate sulfonamides. All nitrofurans possess a nitro group in the 5 position of the furan ring. The activity spectrum is wide and includes both gram-positive and gram-negative organisms (Fig. 9–28). It is most active against *E. coli* and some strains of *Klebsiella, Enterobacter,* and *S. faecalis.* At present it is recommended only for uncomplicated urinary tract infections.

The nitrofurans inhibit protein synthesis both in vitro and in vivo. They appear to inhibit preferentially the synthesis of inducible enzymes by blocking the initiation of translation. The unique feature of this inhibition is that it apparently discriminates among various mRNAs. At concentrations sufficient to inhibit the translation of mRNAs of inducible enzymes, such as those of the lactose and galactose operons, it has almost no effect on the translation of other types of mRNA, such as mRNA from the tryptophan operon or coliphage RNA.

Inhibitors of the 50S Ribosomal Subunit

In the synthesis of protein, the 50S ribosomal subunit provides an attachment site for peptidyl-tRNA. It also contains the active center for catalyzing the peptide bond-forming reaction of protein synthesis. Inhibition of protein synthesis at the 50S ribosomal subunit could result (1) if attachment of peptidyl-tRNA is prevented, (2) if there is an interference with peptide bond formation, or (3) if the translocation step is inhibited (i.e., the movement of peptidyl-tRNA and the ribosome relative to each other). Among the antibiotics that act at the level of the 50S ribosomal subunit are chloramphenicol, lincomycin, and the macrolide group of agents.

Chloramphenicol. Chloramphenicol is a bacteriostatic agent active against a wide range of gram-positive and gram-negative bacteria, rickettsiae, and chlamydiae (Fig. 9–29). It is rapidly and completely absorbed from the gastrointestinal tract and penetrates well into all tissues, including the brain and cerebrospinal fluid. Its clinical use, however, demands caution because of its associated toxic effects, the most important of which is bone marrow suppression. Currently its primary use is in the treatment of *H. influenzae* meningitis, anaerobic infections, and typhoid fever (Table 9–1); however, if equally effective but potentially less toxic drugs than chloramphenicol are available, they should be used instead.

MECHANISM OF ACTION. Chloramphenicol inhibits growth of bacteria by interfering with protein synthesis. It binds exclusively to the 50S subunit. The binding is stereospecific, and a 1:1 equivalence exists between the number of ribosomes present and the number of chloramphenicol molecules bound. Other antibiotic inhibitors of the 50S subunit, such as erythromycin and lincomycin, compete with chloramphenicol for this binding.

Chloramphenicol inhibits peptide bond formation. It has no effect on the initiation of protein synthesis since polyribosome formation continues in the absence of protein synthesis. An understanding of the mechanism of inhibition by chloramphenicol has been provided by the use of a model system, the "puromycin reaction," in which peptidyl transfer is uncoupled from other reactions of protein synthesis, making possible the identification of inhibitors that act specifically on the peptidyl transferase. When puromycin is added to a system synthesizing peptides, it is incorporated into the growing peptide chain instead of the next incoming amino acid, and peptidyl puromycin (i.e., an incomplete peptide chain terminated by puromycin) is released from the ribosome. Chloramphenicol prevents the formation of peptidyl puromycin at concentrations that inhibit protein synthesis in vivo. This inhibition results from the binding of chloramphenicol to a site on the 50S subunit in the vicinity of but not identical with the site that binds the aminoacyl end of aminoacyl-tRNA in the peptidyl transferase catalytic center.

Several proteins have been identified that are thought to form the binding site(s) of chloramphenicol. The most important of these appears to be L16, which is concerned in the peptidyl transferase activity and also forms part of the acceptor site. The interaction of chloramphenicol with 70S ribosomes is rapidly reversible and is highly specific. Chloramphenicol is completely inactive against 80S ribosomes.

RESISTANCE. Chloramphenicol and the macrolide antibiotics, erythromycin and lincomycin, compete for binding at the chloramphenicol binding site on the 50S subunit. Since they bind to or near the same unique site on the ribosome in a 1:1 ratio and are mutually exclusive, a ribosome to which erythromycin is bound is resistant to chloramphenicol. This type of resistance is important in the effective clinical use of antibiotics whose activity is related to inhibition of 50S subunit function. Since the simultaneous use of a competitive pair of these agents results in the therapeutic effects of a single agent, there would be no advantage to the simultaneous administration of two or more of the 50S inhibitors.

Resistance to chloramphenicol may be mutational (chromosomal) or mediated by plasmids. In some organisms, mutation to chloramphenicol resistance may be attributed to an

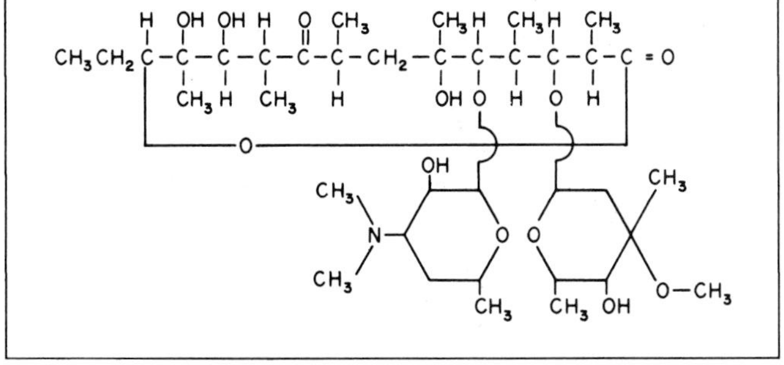

Fig. 9–30. Erythromycin, a macrolide antibiotic.

alteration of the 50S ribosomal subunit resulting in a decreased affinity for the drug. Ribosomes from such mutants have low activity in cell-free protein synthesis and are able to bind labeled chloramphenicol, erythromycin, or lincomycin.

Resistance to chloramphenicol is not infrequently accompanied by resistance to the tetracyclines. This cross-resistance phenomenon is largely confined to the Enterobacteriaceae and is mediated by plasmids. The phenomenon involves the intraspecies or interspecies transfer of plasmids that carry, among other genetic properties, genes determining multiple drug resistance, including resistance to chloramphenicol (p. 185). In this type of resistance the biochemical basis is either acquisition of the ability to degrade the antibiotic or altered membrane permeability. High-level resistance is usually associated with the presence of the enzyme chloramphenicol acetyltransferase, which inactivates the drug by catalyzing its O-acetylation in the presence of acetyl-CoA. In gram-negative organisms the enzyme is constitutive. R factor–mediated resistance by this mechanism has been responsible for widespread epidemics of chloramphenicol-resistant typhoid fever and *Shigella* dysentery.

The second mechanism of resistance, altered permeability, is encountered less frequently and is inducible. It has been detected both in enteric bacteria and in *P. aeruginosa.*

Erythromycin. Erythromycin is the most important of the macrolide antibiotics, a group characterized chemically by a macrocyclic lactone ring of 12 to 22 carbon atoms to which one or more sugars are attached (Fig. 9–30, Table 9–1). Although primarily bacteriostatic, it may be bactericidal for some organisms if sufficiently high concentrations are used.

Erythromycin may be used as the primary drug in the treatment of *Mycoplasma pneumoniae* and *Legionella pneumophila* infections, diphtheria, and pertussis. It is also useful in patients allergic to penicillin who have infections caused by group A streptococci or pneumococci. Bacteria readily develop resistance to erythromycin both in vitro and in vivo, but at present most clinical isolates are sensitive to this agent.

MECHANISM OF ACTION. The 50S ribosomal subunit is the target site of erythromycin, but the mechanistic details of its action on protein synthesis remain ill-defined. Although chloramphenicol and erythromycin compete for a binding site on the 50S subunit, they appear to bind to different but interacting sites. In the 70S ribosome, L15 protein has both erythromycin binding and peptidyl transferase activity, both functions being modulated by interaction with protein L16, to which chloramphenicol binds.

In intact bacteria, erythromycin blocks the translocation step by specifically interfering with the release of the charged tRNA bound to the donor site (P site) of the ribosome after peptide bond formation. Persistence of deacylated tRNA at this site interferes with the translocation of peptidyl-tRNA from the acceptor site back to the donor site. It is unclear whether the peptidyl-tRNA is immobilized at the acceptor site or whether it binds to a site closely adjacent to the donor site that does not allow proper positioning for peptide bond formation.

RESISTANCE. Resistance to erythromycin is a genetically controlled property of ribosomes and may be either mutational or plasmid-mediated. Ribosomes from mutants highly resistant to erythromycin have a reduced affinity for erythromycin and are less active in in vitro polypeptide synthesis. These differences can be correlated with an altered 50S ribosomal subunit protein component, either protein L4 or L12, the conformation of which is less favorable for erythromycin binding. This one-step high-level resistance is the result of chromosomal mutation. A second mechanism of resistance found in clinical isolates involves an alteration in the 23S RNA of the 50S subunit. This type of resistance is plasmid-mediated and may be either constitutive or inducible. It is due to the dimethylation of a specific adenine residue in the 23S subunit, thereby reducing its affinity for erythromycin. The modified ribosomes are cross-resistant to lincomycin and to other macrolide antibiotics.

Lincomycin and Clindamycin. The activity spectrum of lincomycin and clindamycin is similar to that of erythromycin, but they are chemically unrelated (Fig. 9–31). They are especially active against group A streptococci, pneumococci, and penicillinase-producing staphylococci.

Clindamycin is the chloroderivative of lincomycin and is superior to the parent compound in its activity and absorption properties. It shows significantly greater activity against most clinically significant anaerobic bacteria, especially *B. fragilis.* Clindamycin is usually administered clinically as its phosphate ester, which is inactive in vitro but in vivo is hydrolyzed to the parent compound by lipases present in the intestinal tract. Its antibacterial range, low toxicity, and clinical efficacy make it a suitable substitute for penicillin in the treatment of infections where penicillin is contraindicated. It should be reserved primarily, however, for the treatment of infections caused by *B. fragilis* or for other anaerobic infections in persons allergic to penicillin.

MECHANISM OF ACTION. Lincomycin binds exclusively to the 50S ribosomal subunit and competes with chloramphenicol for its binding site on the ribosome. It does not bind to the 60S subunit of mammalian 80S ribosomes. Qualitatively, at least, the mode of action of lincomycin is similar to that of chloramphenicol. Lincomycin, like chloramphenicol, blocks the peptide bond–forming step. Unlike chloramphenicol, however, in whose presence polyribosomes are completely preserved by high concentrations of the drug, in the presence of lincomycin an extensive and rapid breakdown of polyribosomes occurs at all drug concentrations, and the majority of the ribosomes dissociate to 50S and 30S ribosomal subunits. This breakdown of polyribosomes by lincomycin apparently results from selective inhibition of a very early phase of polypeptide synthesis and is caused by an interference with

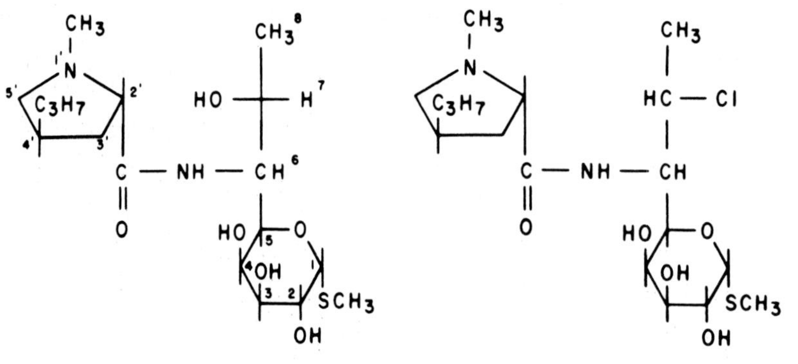

Fig. 9–31. Structural formulas for lincomycin (left) and clindamycin (right). The replacement of the 7-hydroxy group in lincomycin by chlorine, with inversion of configuration, yields a drug with significantly more activity and very efficient absorption. *(From Lewis: Fed Proc 33:2303, 1974.)*

the correct positioning of aminoacyl-tRNA and peptidyl-tRNA at the acceptor and donor sites.

RESISTANCE. Lincomycin-resistant strains emerge during the course of therapy. Some of these strains are resistant only to lincomycin and erythromycin, while others show the dissociated type of resistance characteristic of the macrolides; that is, strains sensitive to lincomycin when tested in the absence of erythromycin are resistant to lincomycin when tested in its presence. This type of resistance involving inhibitors of the 50S ribosomal subunit is due to the induction by erythromycin of a RNA methylase that dimethylates an adenine moiety on the 23S RNA. Binding of lincomycin to the altered subunit is inhibited (p. 175).

Puromycin. This antibiotic provides an excellent example of the structural analogue concept of antimetabolite action (Fig. 9–32). It is structurally analogous to the terminal aminoacyl adenosine portion of tRNA and, therefore, inhibits protein synthesis by terminating the growth of polypeptide chains. As a result, growth of the cells is prevented.

Because puromycin inhibits protein synthesis at a step that is present in all living cells, it inhibits growth of both procaryotic and eucaryotic species. As a result, it is not clinically useful but is included in this discussion because it is helpful in elucidating the reactions involved in peptide bond formation.

MECHANISM OF ACTION. As mentioned previously, there are two binding sites on the ribosome, the peptidyl-tRNA donor site (P site), which is the site where the peptidyl group of peptidyl-tRNA is donated to the incoming tRNA or to puromycin, and the aminocyl-tRNA acceptor site (A site), which accepts aminoacyl-tRNA during chain elongation. When peptidyl-tRNA is on the P site and the A site is vacant, puromycin can bind at the A site, with subsequent formation of a covalent peptidyl-puromycin derivative. The peptidyl-puromycin then dissociates from the ribosome. Growth of the peptide chain is reinitiated at frequent intervals as the ribosome moves along the mRNA molecule, resulting in the abortive synthesis of a collection of oligopeptides with random *N*-terminal amino acids. Puromycin also causes an increase in the rate of subunit exchange, suggesting that the release of peptide chains is accompanied by the release of 50S subunits bearing tRNA, while only 30S subunits remain associated with mRNA, which subsequently recombines with 50S subunits to form initiation complexes.

Fusidic Acid. A steroidal antibiotic with a rather narrow antibacterial spectrum, fusidic acid inhibits the growth of gram-positive bacteria but has no significant activity against gram-negative species. Fucidin, the sodium salt of fusidic acid and the clinically useful form, has been used successfully in the treatment of a variety of serious staphylococcal infections. Although it is little used at present, fucidin provides a useful addition to the antistaphylococcal armamentarium.

MECHANISM OF ACTION. Unlike 50S ribosomal subunit inhibitors, fusidic acid neither binds to the ribosomes nor inhibits chloramphenicol binding. The specific site of attack of fusidic acid is the translocation reaction, the last composite step in peptide bond formation. In the presence of fusidic acid, elongation factor EF-G and GTP form a stable complex with ribosomes. The antibiotic freezes the EF-G~GDP~ribosome complex and prevents the release of EF-G from the ribosome, a process required for the next round of translocation and GTP hydrolysis. In systems containing 80S ribosomes, fusidic acid also blocks protein synthesis by the same mechanism.

Inhibitor of Protein Assembly

Griseofulvin. A fungistatic agent specific for fungi whose walls contain chitin (Fig. 9–33), griseofulvin has no effect on fungi with cellulose cell walls or on bacteria, yeasts, or yeast protoplasts. Its clinical use is limited to the management of dermatophyte infections, for which it is standard therapy. After oral administration, griseofulvin is delivered to the stratum corneum by the sweat or by deposition in keratinocytes.

Treatment of growing cells with griseofulvin causes morphologic abnormalities, such as swelling and branching in the growing tip, whereas old cells distant from the growing point are not affected. It inhibits mitosis in the metaphase, causing multipolar mitosis and abnormal nuclei. The molecular basis for the antimitotic action of griseofulvin is attributed to an interference with the assembly process of tubulin into microtubules. Griseofulvin binds to proteins involved in tubulin assembly. Cell processes that depend on microtubule function, such as the movement of chromosomes during mitosis, are thus inhibited by the drug.

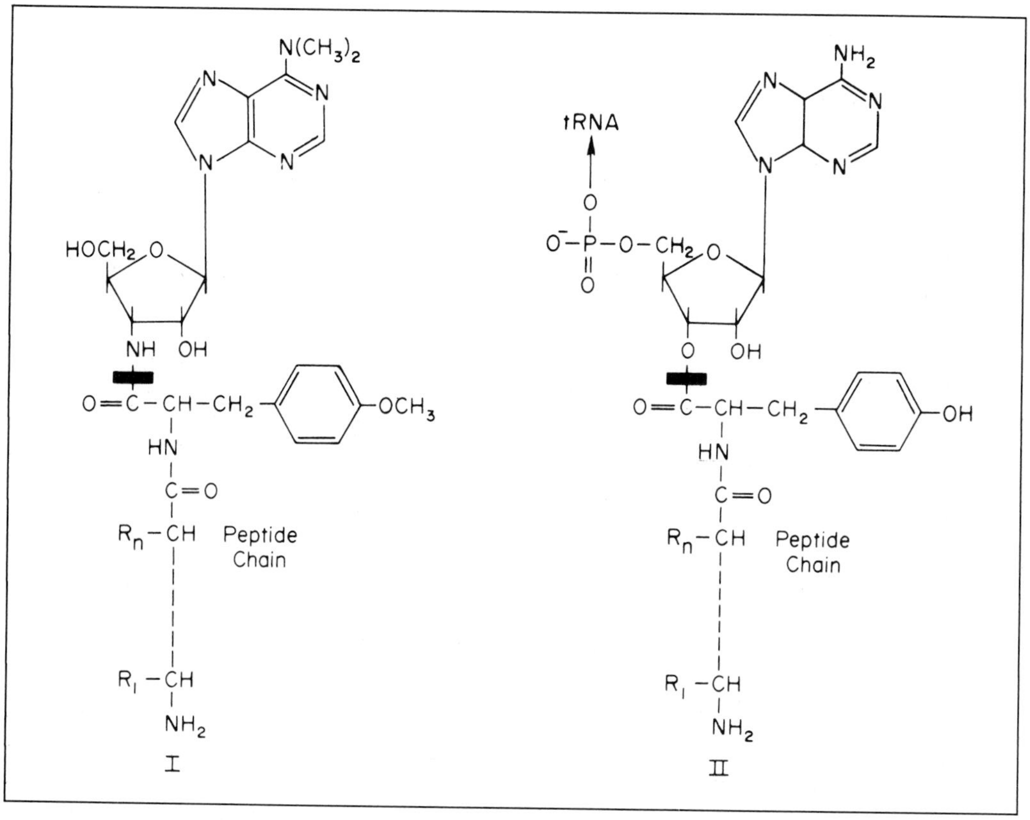

Fig. 9–32. Mechanism of action of puromycin, showing its structural similarity to the terminal AMP residue of aminoacyl-tRNA. I is peptidyl-puromycin, II is peptidyl-tRNA. The crossbar marks the bond that is normally cleaved during extension of the peptide chain but that cannot be cleaved in peptidyl-puromycin.

Metabolite Analogues

Enzymes are often inhibited by compounds possessing a structure similar to the natural substrate. Such inhibitors combine with the enzyme in such a manner as to prevent the normal substrate-enzyme combination and subsequent catalytic reaction. Many inhibitors of this type are analogues of the bacterial growth factors, organic factors required by all bacteria for growth. Such growth factors include the B-complex vitamins, amino acids, purines, and pyrimidines.

Competitive Versus Noncompetitive Inhibition. Antimetabolites that inhibit enzymatic reactions are of two major types, competitive and noncompetitive. Competitive inhibition can be overcome by increasing the substrate concentration, whereas noncompetitive inhibition cannot be reversed by the substrate.

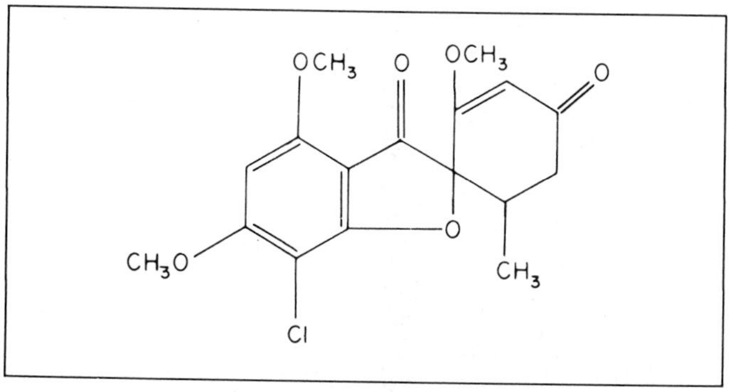

Fig. 9–33. Griseofulvin, a selectively toxic antibiotic for fungi whose walls contain chitin.

In the competitive type of inhibition, both inhibitor (I) and substrate (S) compete for the same enzyme site:

$$E + S \rightleftharpoons ES \rightarrow E + P$$

$$E + I \rightleftharpoons EI$$

The EI complex yields no reaction products, and although the formation of EI is reversible, the continuing competition with substrate reduces the effective free enzyme concentration. In inhibitions of this type, the percentage of inhibition of the enzyme is a function of the ratio of the concentrations of inhibitor and substrate rather than a function of the absolute concentration of the inhibitor alone.

In noncompetitive inhibition, inhibition depends only on the concentration of the inhibitor and is not reversed by increasing the substrate concentration. In contrast with the competitive type of inhibition, the inhibitor binds at a locus on the enzyme other than the substrate binding site. It may bind to the free enzyme, to the ES complex, or to both, resulting in the formation of inactive EI and ESI complexes:

$$E + I \rightleftharpoons EI$$

$$ES + I \rightleftharpoons ESI$$

The rate of conversion of S → P is slowed but not stopped. The effect exerted may be on the affinity of the enzyme for substrate or on the rate of the reaction.

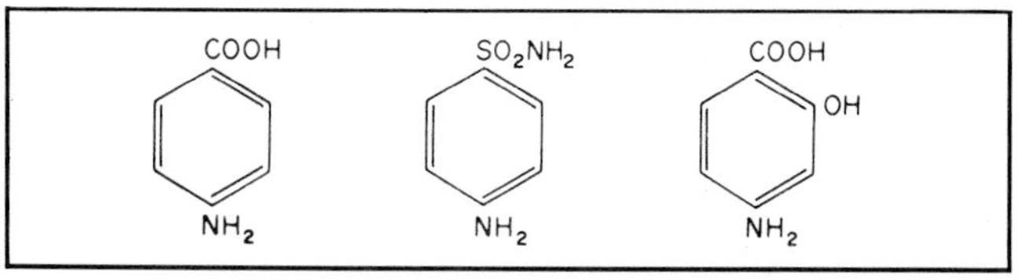

Fig. 9–34. Structural relationship between *p*-aminobenzoic acid (left), sulfanilamide (center), and *p*-aminosalicylic acid (right).

Usefulness of Competitive Inhibitors in Chemotherapy. After introduction of the therapeutic agent sulfanilamide, attention focused on the potential value of metabolite analogues as new chemotherapeutic agents. Although thousands of analogues of the essential metabolites have been designed, many of which have been effective inhibitors in vitro, with the exception of analogues of *p*-aminobenzoic acid (PABA), most have lacked the requisite selectivity necessary for clinical use. The basis for this lack of selectivity lies in the similarity of most of the enzymatic reactions present in bacterial and mammalian cells. Also, although a compound may strongly inhibit an isolated, purified enzyme in vitro, such defined conditions are nonexistent in vivo. For structural analogues to be successful antimicrobial agents, either they must have a much higher affinity for the enzyme than the natural substrate has or they must function as something more than simple competitive inhibitors. Most of the competitive inhibitors that have been studied have a lower affinity for the target enzyme. An exception is the antibiotic cycloserine, which is an analogue of D-alanine (p. 163). This drug binds to D-alanyl-D-alanine synthetase 100 times more effectively than the natural substrate, which may account for its clinical efficacy.

Whereas structural analogues that inhibit by competing at the substrate binding site of an enzyme are usually only transient inhibitors, these inhibitors may be quite effective when they function as end-product inhibitors or repressors. In such cases they mimic the effect of the essential metabolite and inhibit the activity or the synthesis of new enzymes. Their action is thus to reduce the availability of the natural analogues.

Inhibitors of Tetrahydrofolate Synthesis

Sulfonamides

The term *sulfonamide* is a generic name for derivatives of *p*-aminobenzene-sulfonamide or sulfanilamide. First administered in 1935 by Domagk as the red dye Prontosil, sulfanilamide was the first effective chemotherapeutic agent to be used systemically for the prevention and cure of bacterial infections in humans. In vitro, Prontosil is inactive against bacteria, but in the body it is broken down to *p*-aminobenzenesulfonamide, the chemotherapeutic moiety of the molecule.

Since the introduction of sulfanilamide, numerous derivatives have been synthesized and tested for their clinical value in various types of infection. The minimal structural requirement for antibacterial action is that the sulfur be linked directly to the benzene ring and that the NH_2 group in the *para* position be either retained as such or replaced only by radicals that can be converted in the tissues to a free amino group (Fig. 9–34). Of the thousands of derivatives synthesized, fewer than 25 are clinically useful. Although the advent of the antibiotics detracted from the popularity and usefulness of the sulfonamides, they continue to play an important but smaller role in the control of infectious diseases.

Antibacterial Spectrum. Sulfonamides exhibit inhibitory activity against a broad spectrum of gram-positive and gram-negative species as well as *Nocardia, Chlamydia,* and certain protozoa, such as *Pneumocystis* and *Plasmodium.* Although there is usually a direct correlation between in vitro and in vivo efficacy of the sulfonamides, the presence in tissues of such substances as PABA, methionine, and the purines can neutralize their inhibitory activity. Since bacteria are impermeable to folic acid, its presence in tissues does not interfere with efficacy of the drug. In vivo usefulness is also conditioned by the extent of protein binding of the drug after absorption, since the conjugate is therapeutically inactive.

Current Clinical Use. At present, sulfonamides are used primarily in the treatment of uncomplicated urinary tract infections caused by susceptible strains of *E. coli.* They are also effective in the treatment of *Nocardia asteroides* infections, in the prophylaxis of recurrent attacks of rheumatic fever in patients who are allergic to penicillin, and in the prophylaxis of close contacts of patients with sulfonamide-sensitive *Neisseria meningitidis.* For presurgical sterilization of the gut, some of the poorly absorbed sulfonamide derivatives in combination with neomycin have been used extensively. Some of the clinically useful sulfonamides and their major uses are shown in Table 9–6.

Sulfonamides are also used in combination with antifolate drugs to potentiate their activity and to prevent the development of resistance. Since the antifolates block the same metabolic pathway as the sulfonamides but at a different site, the combination of a sulfonamide and an antifolate drug, such as trimethoprim, is synergistic.

A number of adverse reactions have been attributed to the various sulfonamides; the most frequent are nausea, vomiting, diarrhea, and a serum sickness–like syndrome. More serious adverse reactions include blood dyscrasias and significant hypersensitivity reactions.

TABLE 9–6. SULFONAMIDES OF CLINICAL IMPORTANCE

Drug	Properties	Clinical Use
Sulfadiazine	Rapidly absorbed and excreted	Meningitis prophylaxis
Sulfisoxazole (Gantrisin)	Rapidly absorbed and excreted	Urinary tract infections
Sulfamethoxazole (Gantanol)	Rapidly absorbed and excreted	Urinary tract infections
Sulfacytine (Renoquid)	Rapidly absorbed and excreted	Urinary tract infections
Sulfasalazine (Azaline, azulfidine)	Poorly absorbed	Treatment of ulcerative colitis and regional enteritis

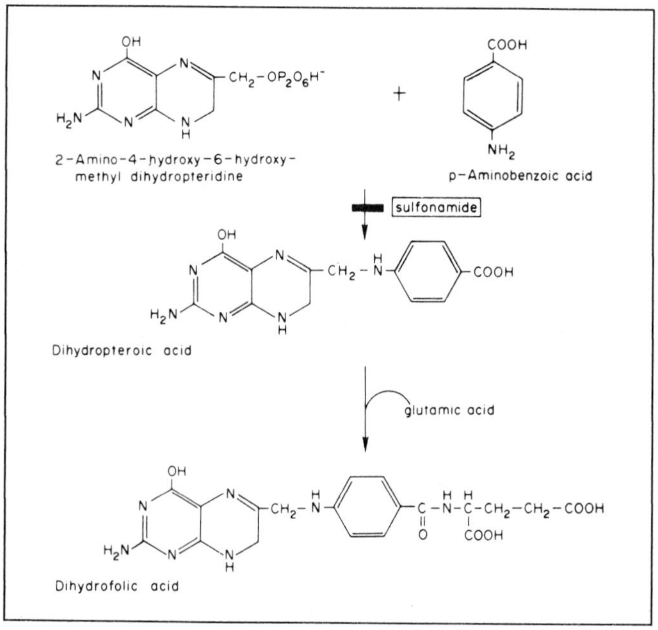

Fig. 9–35. Inhibition of dihydropteroic acid synthesis by the sulfonamides.

Mechanism of Action. The sulfonamides are structural analogues of PABA, a precursor of folic acid (pteroylglutamic acid). The biologically active form of folic acid is tetrahydrofolic acid (FH_4), a coenzyme important in the transfer and reduction of 1-carbon fragments. Tetrahydrofolate serves as the acceptor of the β-carbon atom of serine when it is cleaved to yield glycine. This reaction is of special significance as a source of active 1-carbon units required in the synthesis of methionine, thymine, and the purines.

Sulfonamides interfere with the synthesis of folic acid by inhibiting the condensation of PABA with 2-amino-4-hydroxy-6-dihydropteridinylmethyl pyrophosphate to form dihydropteroic acid. The sulfonamides compete with PABA in this reaction, not simply by occupying the active site on the enzyme but by acting as alternative substrates for dihydropteroate synthetase (Fig. 9–35).

Organisms that synthesize folic acid are sensitive to sulfonamides, whereas those that have a requirement for preformed folic acid are insensitive because they lack the sulfonamide-inhibited reaction. The addition of PABA to a system in which growth has been inhibited by the sulfonamides neutralizes the inhibitory effect. Certain metabolites involved in folic acid coenzyme-requiring reactions (i.e., methionine, serine, thymine, and the purines) also overcome inhibition produced by these drugs.

Humans, like certain microorganisms, require preformed folic acid for growth and cannot synthesize it from PABA. The successful use of the sulfonamide drugs in therapy, in spite of the presence of folic acid in human tissues, is due to the impermeability of the bacterial cell to folic acid as it occurs in the tissues.

Resistance. The emergence of drug-resistant strains has limited the clinical usefulness of the sulfonamides. This has been a serious problem, especially in the treatment of bacillary dysentery and meningococcal meningitis, infections for which the sulfonamides were previously very useful. Resistance to one sulfonamide results in cross-resistance to other members of the group. The major mechanism responsible for this increased resistance is mediated by plasmids and is due to the production of a target enzyme with diminished affinity for the drug. Other mechanisms of resistance are listed in Table 9–7, on p. 180, and on p. 185.

Other Analogues of *p*-Aminobenzoic Acid

Sulfones. Derivatives of 4,4′-diaminodiphenylsulfone (dapsone) form a group of agents that display marked specificity, primarily against the genus *Mycobacterium* (Fig. 9–36). Although previously used in the treatment of tuberculosis, their present use is limited to the management of leprosy. Dapsone is the agent most useful clinically and, when employed in the early stages of leprosy, is successful in halting progression of the disease. A number of toxic reactions accompany its use, including hemolytic anemia, peripheral neuropathy, dermatitis, and erythema nodosum. Sulfones interfere with the metabolism of PABA, which neutralizes the drug's activity in vitro.

***p*-Aminosalicylic Acid (PAS).** The antimicrobial activity of PAS is highly specific for *M. tuberculosis.* It is a bacteriostatic agent structurally similar to PABA and is antagonized by PABA in vitro (Fig. 9–34). At present it is used primarily as a second-line drug in chemotherapy for tuberculosis.

Inhibitors of Dihydrofolate Reductase

Trimethoprim. An antifolic acid agent, trimethoprim is a potent and selective inhibitor of bacterial dihydrofolate reductase (Fig. 9–37). Its spectrum of activity is similar to that of the sulfonamides and includes most gram-positive cocci and gram-negative rods. Although sulfonamides are bacteriostatic even at high concentrations, trimethoprim may be bactericidal. For clinical use, trimethoprim is combined with the sulfonamide sulfamethoxazole, with which it acts synergistically. The trimethoprim-sulfamethoxazole combination (co-trimoxazole) has proved especially useful in the management of recurrent or chronic urinary tract infections and *Pneumocystis* infections. It is also effective in the treatment of patients with bronchitis, shigellosis, and typhoid fever resistant to both chloramphenicol and ampicillin. Trimethoprim causes the same adverse reactions as the sulfonamides do.

MECHANISM OF ACTION. The inhibitory action of trimethoprim is based on its ability to reduce the pool of tetrahydrofolate cofactors in the bacterial cell to a level that is inadequate for growth (Fig. 9–38). The tetrahydrofolates function in a battery of biosynthetic reactions in which they serve as carriers of 1-carbon fragments. In one of these reactions, the synthesis of thymine by thymidylate synthetase, tetrahydrofolate reverts to the dihydro state. This must be converted to the more reduced form for growth to continue. The enzyme that catalyzes this reaction, dihydrofolate reductase, is the enzyme that is inhibited by trimethoprim. Depletion of the tetrahydrofolate pool interferes with the synthesis of purines, pyrimidines, several amino acids, pantothenate, and *N*-formylmethionyl-tRNA, resulting in cessation of growth and ultimately death. The highly selective activity of trimethoprim for bac-

TABLE 9–7. MAJOR MECHANISMS OF ANTIMICROBIAL RESISTANCE

Mechanism	Agents	Organisms
Failure to enter cell[a]	β-Lactams	*Pseudomonas aeruginosa, Enterobacter*
	Aminoglycosides	*P. aeruginosa, Serratia, Enterococcus faecalis*
	Chloramphenicol, trimethoprim	*P. aeruginosa*
Decreased uptake		
Alterations in outer-membrane proteins	β-Lactam antibiotics, chloramphenicol, quinolones, tetracycline	Enterobacteriaceae
Enzymatically modified drug not transported	Aminoglycosides	Enterobacteriaceae, *Pseudomonas*
Enzymatically modified drug poorly transported	Chloramphenicol	*Pseudomonas*
Membrane not energized	Aminoglycosides	Anaerobes
Active efflux		
New membrane-transport system	Tetracyclines, erythromycin, quinolones	Enterobacteriaceae, *Streptococcus epidermidis*
Enzymatic inactivation of drug		
β-Lactamase	β-Lactams	*Staphylococcus aureus,* Enterobacteriaceae, *Pseudomonas, Haemophilus influenzae*
Chloramphenicol acetyltransferase	Chloramphenicol	*S. aureus*, Enterobacteriaceae
Acetylation, phosphorylation, nucleotidylation	Aminoglycosides	*S. aureus, Streptococcus,* Enterobacteriaceae, *Pseudomonas*
Alteration of target		
Methylation of 23S RNA	Erythromycin, clindamycin	*S. aureus*
Altered DNA gyrase	Quinolones	Enterobacteriaceae
Altered RNA polymerase	Rifampin	Enterobacteriaceae
Penicillin-binding proteins	Penicillin	*Neisseria gonorrhoeae, Streptococcus pneumoniae, Enterococcus faecalis, S. aureus,* Enterobacteriaceae
Altered S12 protein of 30S ribosome	Streptomycin	Enterobacteriaceae
New drug-insensitive dihydrofolate reductase	Trimethoprim	Enterobacteriaceae
New drug-insensitive dihydropteroate synthetase	Sulfonamides	Enterobacteriaceae, *S. aureus*

[a] Intrinsic resistance.

terial reductases and the low toxicity for mammals are due to its extremely high affinity for bacterial enzymes and weak binding to mammalian reductases.

The use of trimethoprim in combination with sulfamethoxazole exploits the biochemical differences between humans and bacteria to selectively damage the parasite. Since both drugs block the folic acid pathway but at different points, the double blockage is effective in cutting off completely the supply of tetrahydrofolate to the bacteria.

RESISTANCE. At the present time, the resistance levels of clinical isolates to trimethoprim or to trimethoprim-sulfamethoxazole are still fairly low (4% to 11%), although there is concern that plasmid-encoded resistance may eventually compromise the clinical effectiveness of the agents. Several mechanisms of trimethoprim resistance have been described, but the major cause of significant resistance among clinical isolates is the production of a plasmid-encoded trimethoprim-resistant form of dihydrofolate reductase.

Other Metabolite Analogues

Isoniazid

Isoniazid, the hydrazide of isonicotinic acid, is highly specific for *M. tuberculosis* (Fig. 9–39). It is effective in low concentrations and is bactericidal only for actively growing organisms. Isoniazid does not inhibit growth immediately but only after the organisms undergo one or two divisions. Tubercle bacilli exposed to the drug lose their acid-fast staining property. Isoniazid penetrates cells with ease and, unlike streptomycin,

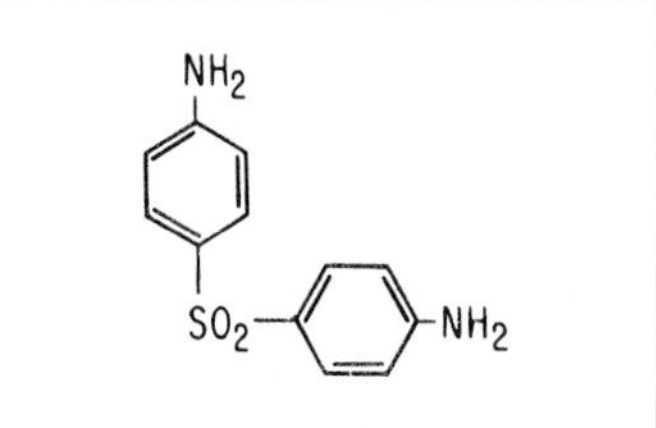

Fig. 9–36. Dapsone (4,4′-diaminodiphenyl sulfone), the basic therapeutic agent for *Mycobacterium leprae* infections.

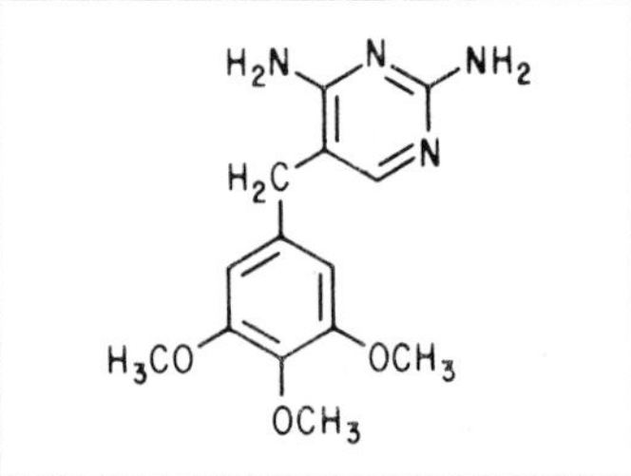

Fig. 9–37. Trimethoprim, the most active and selective agent of a series of synthetic inhibitors of dihydrofolate reductase.

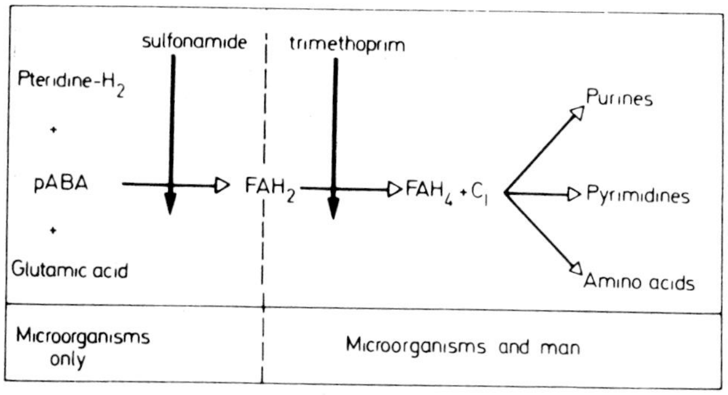

Fig. 9–38. The folic acid pathway: loci of trimethoprim and sulfonamide inhibition. *(From Burchall: In Corcoran and Hahn (eds): Antibiotics III. Mechanism of Action of Antimicrobial and Antitumor Agents. Springer-Verlag, 1975.)*

is as effective against bacilli within monocytes as against extracellular organisms.

Isoniazid remains the keystone of initial treatment of pulmonary tuberculosis and is highly effective, well absorbed, and of low toxicity. Drug resistance, however, may emerge within large bacterial populations, such as those present in pulmonary or renal cavities. This can be largely circumvented by the simultaneous use of one or more companion drugs (ethambutol or rifampin). At present, this combination therapy represents the mainstay in the treatment of tuberculosis. The most important side effects of isoniazid are related to its hepatotoxicity and toxicity for the peripheral and central nervous systems. Of these, hepatitis is the most significant and is thought to be secondary to the conversion of isoniazid to acetylhydrazine. Symptoms of vitamin B_6 deficiency, such as peripheral neuritis and seizures, may also occur.

Mechanism of Action. In spite of extensive studies, there is no convincing evidence that pinpoints any single mechanism as the primary site of attack by isoniazid. Its structural similarity to both niacin and pyridoxal suggests that the drug might act as an antimetabolite against either of these vitamins. Interference with either would have pleiotropic effects because of their importance in many aspects of metabolism. A number of hypotheses have been proposed to explain the effects observed on lipid and nucleic acid biosynthesis and on glycolysis. The most widely accepted mechanism advanced is that the action of isoniazid is due to an inhibition of the synthesis of mycolic acid. This mechanism could provide a possible explanation for the exquisite sensitivity of isoniazid for mycobacteria, but it is unlikely that it is the primary lethal event. Especially difficult to evaluate at present is the significance of the structural relationship of isoniazid to nicotinamide adenine dinucleotide (NAD). Isoniazid has been found to reduce the NAD supply of the cell. This is done by activating NADase, an enzyme normally present in an inactive form in the membrane of the intact cell. Isoniazid activates NADase by altering the conformation of a protein inhibitor with which the enzyme is normally associated, resulting in the rapid breakdown of NAD and depletion of the cell's supply.

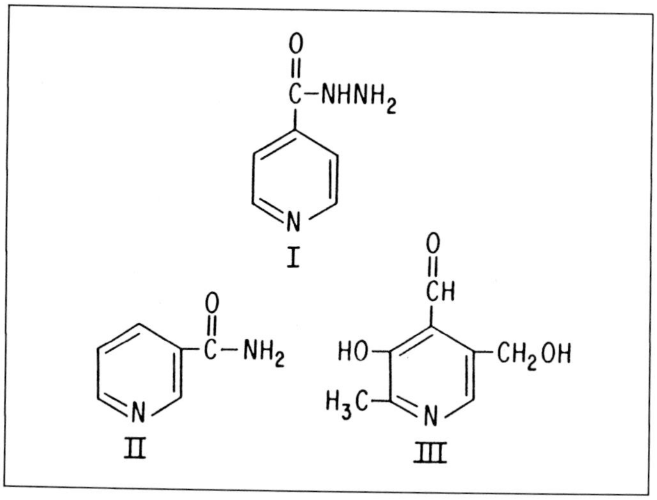

Fig. 9–39. Structural relationships among I, isoniazid (isonicotinic acid hydrazide); II, nicotinamide; and III, pyridoxal.

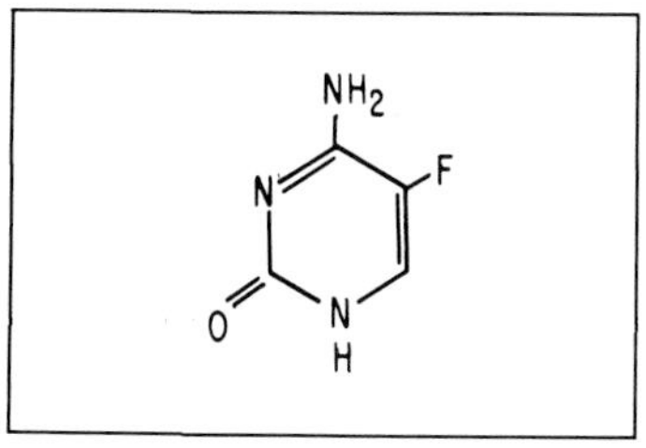

Fig. 9–40. Flucytosine (5-fluorocytosine), a fluorine analogue of cytosine, useful in the treatment of cryptococcosis, candidiasis, torulopsosis, and chromomycosis.

Flucytosine (5-Fluorocytosine)

Flucytosine, the fluorine analogue of cytosine, is the only antifungal agent in clinical use that is a true antimetabolite (Fig. 9–40). It is useful in the systemic treatment of some deep-seated fungal infections in humans, particularly candidiasis, cryptococcosis, and chromomycosis. Only in chromomycosis, however, is it the drug of choice. Since flucytosine-resistant strains may emerge rapidly if the drug is used alone, it is used primarily in combination with amphotericin B, especially in cryptococcal meningitis.

Mechanism of Action. Flucytosine enters the cell via the cytosine permease. It is first deaminated to 5-fluorouracil by cytosine deaminase and subsequently is phosphorylated and incorporated into RNA. Another pathway for 5-fluorouracil involves the formation of 5-fluorodeoxyuridine monophosphate, a noncompetitive inhibitor of thymidylate synthetase. This interferes with DNA synthesis and leads to defective cell division. At present, no definitive statement can be made as to whether impaired DNA synthesis or the dysfunction of fungal RNA leading to disturbed protein synthesis is the primary cause of the drug's antifungal activity.

Resistance to flucytosine can be attributed to many mechanisms. Resistant mutants may have either deficient enzyme systems involved with the metabolism of the drug, increased de novo synthesis of competing pyrimidines, or compensating mechanisms for the abnormal RNA function. The plurality of mechanisms of resistance to flucytosine, most of which are independent of each other and result from one-step mutation, explains the high frequency of resistance to this agent.

Drug Resistance

The introduction of the sulfonamides and penicillin opened a new era in clinical medicine and stimulated a wave of optimism in the fight against infectious diseases. Early in the use of these drugs, however, it was realized that even though devastating epidemics had been curbed, disease caused by infectious organisms remained a serious problem. One of the major factors contributing to the persistence of infectious diseases is the tremendous capacity of microorganisms for circumventing the action of inhibitory agents. The ability of many microorganisms to develop resistance to the various antimicrobial agents offers a serious threat to their future usefulness and demands both resourcefulness and ingenuity in meeting and counteracting this problem.

Origin of Drug-resistant Strains

There are two major mechanisms by which increased resistance to antibiotics and other drugs used in clinical practice may arise: (1) by mutation (chromosomal) and (2) by genetic exchange.

Selection of Drug-resistant Mutants. In the past the origin of drug-resistant strains of microorganisms aroused much controversy. Considerable effort was directed toward determining whether resistant cells result from phenotypic adaptation induced by some interaction of the drug with the organism or whether they are mutants that arise independently of the antibiotic. It is now firmly established that drug resistance arises by the latter mechanism, that is, by a random mutation that results in an altered susceptibility to the drug, with the drug serving only as a selective agent favoring the survival of resistant over sensitive organisms once the genetic alteration has taken place and has been expressed phenotypically.

Mutations generally occur at a frequency of about 1 in 10^5 to 10^{10} cell divisions. Knowledge of the mutation rate for a particular organism as well as the site of attack of a specific drug is important for a rational approach to chemotherapy. The successful use of combination treatment in the management of tuberculosis provides such an example. The exceedingly large numbers of tubercle bacilli present within the tuberculous lesion provide an opportunity for the rapid emergence of resistant strains if a single drug is administered. By the use of combined therapy, however, the likelihood of an organism mutating to resistance to two drugs administered simultaneously is about 1 in 10^{15} cell divisions.

Resistance Mediated by Genetic Exchange. Genetic information that controls bacterial drug resistance occurs both in the bacterial chromosome and in the DNA of extrachromosomal plasmids. The resistance trait may be transmitted from these loci by the transfer of genetic material from a resistant cell to a sensitive one by transformation, conjugation, or transduction. Under natural conditions, bacteria rarely, if ever, exchange their chromosomal genes. Plasmids, however, constitute a very efficient and powerful means for the dissemination and rearrangement of genetic information. The host range of some plasmids is quite broad, for example, R (resistance) plasmids residing in certain *Pseudomonas* species that can be transmitted by conjugation into certain soil bacteria, photosynthetic bacteria, and *Neisseria* (Fig. 9–41).

Plasmids may be classified into two major types: conjugative or nonconjugative. Conjugative plasmids are self-transmissible from one cell to another and have a region concerned with conjugation and the synthesis of a sex pilus. The plasmids that are associated with the transference of drug-resistance markers by conjugation are referred to as R plasmids. They consist of two distinct components: (1) the resistance transfer factor (RTF), which initiates and controls the conjugation process, and (2) the r-determinant, a series of one or more linked genes that confer resistance to specific antimicrobial agents. The r-determinants and the RTFs are independent replicons, each of which is capable of replicating and operating on its own in the bacterial cell. The r-determinants confer resistance only in the cell possessing them unless the RTF is also present to mediate conjugation.

Infectious drug resistance of this kind is especially im-

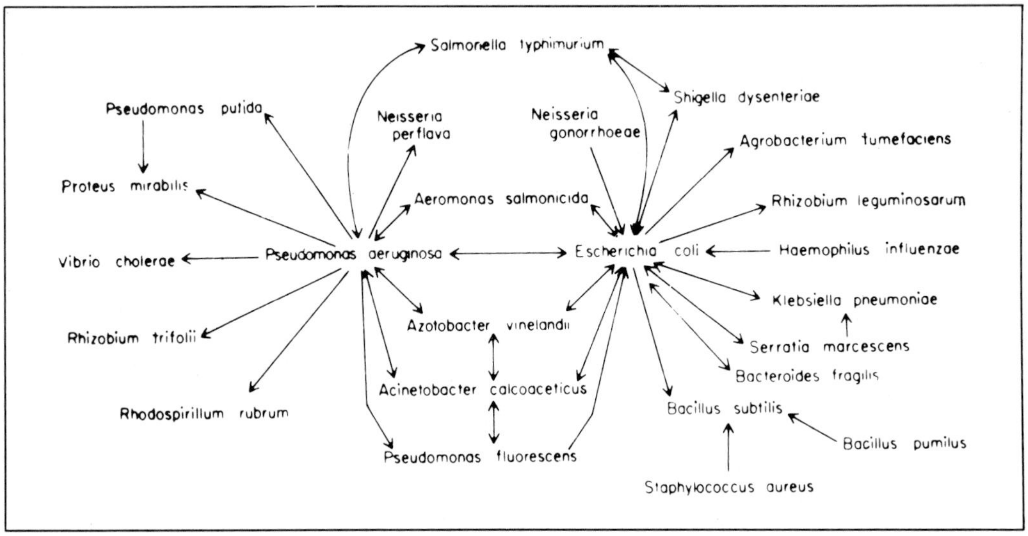

Fig. 9–41. Flow of plasmids among organisms by DNA-mediated transformation or conjugation. Arrows indicate the flow of genetic information from donor to recipient. *(From Young and Mayer: Rev Infect Dis 1:55, 1979.)*

portant among gram-negative bacilli and has far-reaching epidemiologic implications. It was first recognized in Japan in 1957 during an epidemic of bacillary dysentery, when strains of *Shigella dysenteriae* became simultaneously resistant to chloramphenicol, streptomycin, sulfanilamide, and tetracycline. Multiple drug resistance is now very common in many countries throughout the world, complicating and in some cases precluding the successful treatment of many bacterial infections. Environmental exposure of the normal intestinal flora to antibiotics favors the growth of organisms that carry R plasmids. When persons with such organisms in the gut become infected with pathogenic species, the drug-resistant saprophytes can transmit the R plasmids to the sensitive pathogen, which may then, if antibiotics are used in treatment, completely replace the initially drug-sensitive organism. There is clear-cut clinical evidence that transfer of drug resistance of this type occurs within the human intestinal tract.

Nonconjugative plasmids are unable to initiate self-transfer and do not encode for a sex pilus. They are smaller in mass (about 5×10^6 Da) than conjugative plasmids (40×10^6 to 200×10^6 Da) and rarely encode for more than two antibiotic-resistance genes. Their transfer is mediated by co-resident conjugative plasmids by the process of mobilization. This mechanism of transfer occurs in *N. gonorrhoeae,* where nonconjugative R plasmids are transmitted from gonococcus to gonococcus.

Nonconjugative as well as conjugative plasmids can also be transmitted by transduction or transformation. In staphylococci, all plasmids are nonconjugative, including the penicillinase plasmid, and dissemination is solely by transduction. The staphylococcal penicillinase plasmids contain the determinants for the enzyme β-lactamase (p. 184). Genetic markers, such as resistance to erythromycin and to a number of inorganic ions, may also be located on this plasmid, but resistance to streptomycin, tetracycline, chloramphenicol, and the macrolides, which can also be transduced, are located on different plasmids.

The acquisition of genetic material by plasmids and chromosomes is not limited by the classic recombination processes. Many drug-resistance genes reside on transposons, DNA sequences that have the capacity for excising themselves from one genome and inserting into another. The resistance genes can transpose from plasmid to plasmid, from plasmid to chromosome, or from plasmid to bacteriophage. Genes that specify resistance to a number of our most useful antibiotics, including ampicillin, chloramphenicol, tetracycline, kanamycin, streptomycin, and trimethoprim, are found on transposons, thus providing a possible explanation for the rapid evolution of R plasmids that possess a wide variety of antibiotic-resistance determinants. A more detailed discussion of drug-resistance plasmids is found on page 147.

Biochemical Mechanisms of Drug Resistance

Resistance is due to genetically controlled peculiarities of the metabolism or the structure of the cell that enable it to escape the action of the drug. Among the biochemical mechanisms by which microorganisms resist the inhibitory effect of an antimicrobial agent are (1) decreased permeability of the organism to the drug, (2) inactivation of the inhibitor by enzymes produced by the resistant organism, (3) modification of the properties of the drug receptor site, and (4) increased synthesis of an essential metabolite that is antagonistic for the drug (Table 9–7).

Among clinical isolates, chromosomal drug resistance usually causes changes in cellular structures that make the organism impermeable to the antibiotic or that render the specific target site indifferent to the presence of the drug. R plasmid–mediated resistance usually involves either a decrease in the permeability of the cell or enzymatic inactivation of the inhibitor.

Decreased Cell Permeability

Altered permeability to antimicrobial agents may involve changes in specific receptors for the drug, loss of capacity for active transport through the cell membrane, or structural changes in one or more components of the cell envelope that influence permeability in a relatively nonspecific manner.

The lipid-containing outer membrane of gram-negative bacteria provides an effective barrier to the entry of many antibiotics into the cell. Penetration by hydrophilic compounds occurs through water-filled porin channels that discriminate on the basis of gross physicochemical properties of the solute (e.g., molecular size, hydrophobicity, electrical charge). This restrictive sieving mechanism provides intrinsic resistance to both vancomycin and bacitracin, preventing their entry and thus limiting the spectrum of these agents to gram-positive bacteria. The permeability barrier is not constant for all species of gram-negative organisms. For example, *H. influenzae* and *N. gonorrhoeae* are generally susceptible to a wide variety of β-lactams; the gram-negative enteric organisms are intermediate in susceptibility, and *P. aeruginosa* is resistant to all but specific antipseudomonal β-lactams. This is attributed to the presence in all isolates of both β-lactamase and a significant permeability barrier to the drugs. In some clinical isolates, alterations in outer membrane permeability is responsible for resistance to some of the newer β-lactam antibiotics. This resistance, unlike that associated with induction of β-lactamase, involves cross-resistance between β-lactams and aminoglycosides and is associated with a change in outer membrane porin.

Decreased cell permeability is the most commonly encountered mechanism of resistance to the tetracyclines and is a cause in some cases for sulfonamide resistance. The impermeability mechanism is specific for each drug, since loss of either sulfonamide or tetracycline resistance in strains resistant to both agents does not impair resistance to the other. Bacterial resistance to tetracycline is caused by at least five different determinants carried on plasmids in the host bacterial cell. In gram-negative organisms the genes that determine tetracycline resistance are often, but not always, found on transposon 10, which is a component of several R plasmids. In most cases, resistance is inducible by subinhibitory concentrations of tetracycline, and for some plasmids it can reach 200 times the resistance of sensitive cells. Coincident with the appearance of induced resistance in *E. coli* is the synthesis of new cell membrane proteins that are thought to be components of a new transport system that limits tetracycline uptake and accumulation by the cell. In tetracycline-sensitive cells, there are two transport systems for tetracycline, only one of which is energy-dependent. Both of these systems are altered in resistant organisms. The energy-dependent component of uptake is replaced in resistant cells by a non-energy-requiring uptake at a lower rate, and the energy-independent rate is decreased. This decrease in accumulation of tetracycline is attributed to an active efflux of the drug.

Enzymatic Inactivation of the Drug

This type of resistance, commonly observed among clinical isolates of resistant organisms, is the primary mechanism of resistance to penicillin, chloramphenicol, and the aminoglycoside antibiotics. Specific inactivating enzymes for these agents occur in a number of bacteria carrying R factors and other plasmids (Table 9–7).

Inactivation of β-Lactam Antibiotics. From a clinical standpoint, the most important and widespread of the degradative enzymes that attack the β-lactam antibiotics are the β-lactamases. These enzymes form a covalent acyl enzyme intermediate via the carbonyl of the β-lactam ring, resulting in an opening of the β-lactam ring and inactivation of the drug. The primary role of the β-lactamases is not to protect bacteria from β-lactam antibiotics but, rather, to break bonds in transitory intermediates of β-lactam structure in peptidoglycan biosynthesis. The β-lactamases of gram-positive organisms are usually plasmid encoded. There are four minor variants of staphylococcal penicillinase (types A to D), all of which are predominantly penicillinases, hydrolyzing penicillin and ampicillin at high rates. Because of steric interference, they hydrolyze methicillin, oxacillin, and cloxacillin poorly and show little activity against cephalosporins. With the exception of the type D enzyme, high levels are produced only after induction, with most of the activity being extracellular.

The complex cell envelope of gram-negative organisms makes them intrinsically less sensitive than gram-positive species to many of the β-lactam antibiotics, and significant differences exist between the properties of the lactamases of the two groups. In contrast to gram-positive organisms, gram-negative bacteria produce a plethora of β-lactamases that exhibit a range of hydrolytic activities against both penicillins and cephalosporins. β-Lactam resistance in gram-negative bacteria can be determined by either chromosomal or plasmid genes, but in clinical isolates, resistance is usually mediated by genes on R plasmids. In the enteric bacteria, the β-lactamases are produced constitutively in small amounts and remain bound to the cells. They prevent access of β-lactam antibiotics to the membrane-associated target sites by destroying the antibiotics as they pass through the cell envelope. Plasmid-mediated β-lactamases have been divided into three broad groups: (1) broad-spectrum penicillinases, (2) oxacillinases, and (3) carbenicillinases. The most important β-lactamase, TEM-1, which has a broad activity range against penicillins and cephalosporins, is carried on a transposon (Tn4), which undoubtedly accounts for its wide distribution.

Chromosomally encoded β-lactamases are produced by virtually all gram-negative bacilli and are responsible for most of the resistance to cephalosporins and the newer β-lactam antibiotics. Although normally present at low levels in most wild-type strains of *Enterobacter, Serratia, Proteus,* and *Pseudomonas,* high levels of cephalosporinases are produced in the presence of certain β-lactam drugs. Cefoxitin is one of the most efficient inducers of cephalosporinases and, when used with third-generation cephalosporins or carbenicillin, will result in their inactivation.

Inactivation of Aminoglycoside Antibiotics. In clinical isolates of gram-negative organisms, resistance to the aminoglycoside antibiotics is due to the production of enzymes that specifically modify the antibiotic so that it can no longer gain entry into the cell. The genes for the aminoglycoside-modifying enzymes are carried on R plasmids, and several of the genes have been found on transposons.

These enzymes inactivate the drug by acetylation of amino groups, phosphorylation of hydroxyl groups, or adenylylation of hydroxyl groups (Table 9–8). Thirteen enzymes that inactivate the aminoglycoside antibiotics have been identified. Five of these are phosphorylating enzymes, three are acetylating enzymes, and five adenylylate some of the antibiotics. They are produced constitutively and are located near the cell surface, probably in the periplasmic space. Except for the streptomycin- and spectinomycin-inactivating enzymes, one enzyme can inactivate a number of different aminocyclitol antibiotics, and one antibiotic can be inactivated by more than one enzyme or mechanism. The primary effect of the enzymatic modification of the drug is to interfere with the transport of the antibiotic into the cell. The modified compound is apparently unable to induce the transport system needed for entry.

A number of semisynthetic derivatives of the aminoglycoside antibiotics have been synthesized in an attempt to find agents that are resistant to the aminoglycoside-modifying enzymes. One of these derivatives, amikacin, is resistant to all but one of the enzymes capable of inactivating the amino-

TABLE 9–8. AMINOCYCLITOL-INACTIVATING ENZYMES

	Acetyltransferases (AAC)			Phosphotransferases (APD)					Adenylyltransferases (AAD)				
Antibiotic	2′	6′	3	3′	2″	3″	6	5″	2″	4′	3″(a)	6	9
Kanamycins	+	+	+	+	(+)	−	−	−	+	+	−	−	−
Tobramycin	+	+	+	−	(+)	−	−	−	+	+	−	−	−
Amikacin	−	+	−	+	(+)	−	−	−	−	+	−	−	−
Gentamicin	+	+	+	−	+	−	−	−	+	−	−	−	−
Sisomicin	+	+	+	−	+	−	−	−	+	−	−	−	−
Netilmicin	+	+	(+)	−	+	−	−	−	−	−	−	−	−
Neomycin	+	+	+	+	−	−	−	(+)	−	+	−	−	−
Streptomycin	−	−	−	−	−	+	+	−	−	−	+	−	−
Spectinomycin	−	−	−	−	−	−	−	−	−	−	+	−	+

+ = normal substrate; (+) = substrate for some forms of the enzyme; − = nonsubstrate for enzyme.

glycosidic aminocyclitol antibiotics. This explains the enhanced activity spectrum of amikacin against organisms resistant to kanamycin, gentamicin, and tobramycin.

Inactivation of Chloramphenicol. In the majority of drug-resistant clinical isolates of gram-positive and gram-negative species, resistance is mediated by a plasmid coding for an inactivating enzyme, chloramphenicol acetyltransferase. The enzyme is found intracellularly and is synthesized constitutively in gram-negative organisms. In *S. aureus*, however, the enzyme is induced in the presence of the drug. Like the β-lactamases, the chloramphenicol acetyltransferases of gram-positive and gram-negative species appear to constitute a family of immunologically related but electrophoretically distinguishable proteins.

Modification of Drug Receptor Site

Penicillin Resistance. The most important example of resistance caused by an altered target site is that seen in methicillin-resistant *S. aureus*. In all clinical isolates examined to date, methicillin resistance is due to the production of a new 78,000-molecular-weight penicillin-binding protein, PBP 2a or PBP 2′, with a low affinity for methicillin. Resistance is encoded by an acquired chromosomal gene (*mec A*) that is absent from organisms susceptible to methicillin. The spread of staphylococcal clones carrying the PBP 2a gene has resulted in the worldwide dissemination of methicillin-resistant staphylococci. At present, however, a complete understanding of the phenotypic expression of methicillin resistance is lacking. Although the ability to produce PBP 2a is essential for resistance, the MICs for resistant strains vary widely, from 3.1 to more than 400 μg/mL. Additional genes appear to be required for the homogeneous expression of high-level resistance.

The *mec A* is confined to the *Staphylococcus*, but low-affinity PBPs are also responsible for the development of β-lactam resistance in certain other organisms. Among the most important of these is penicillin-resistant *S. pneumoniae*, first isolated in South Africa. These strains are found in the United States, but their prevalence is low. Also, although resistance is usually low with MICs of 0.1 to 2.0 μg/mL, it is sufficient to cause treatment failures in cases of meningitis. Higher levels of resistance have been associated with therapy failures in pneumonia and bacteremia. In penicillin-resistant pneumococci, there are several PBPs with decreased penicillin-binding affinity. Each of these contributes incrementally to resistance. Sequencing analyses have shown that a resistant PBP gene has a mosaic structure with segments similar to those of a sensitive PBP alternating with segments that are so different from the sensitive strain that they are thought to have come from another organism, presumably another type of *Streptococcus*.

Altered PBPs have also been detected in clinical isolates of *N. gonorrhoeae*, *N. meningitidis*, and *H. influenzae* that were penicillin-resistant but did not produce β-lactamase.

Streptomycin Resistance. Resistance controlled by chromosomal genes is usually due to changes in enzymes or active sites involved in essential metabolic reactions in the cell. An example of this mechanism is resistance to streptomycin where differences exist between the ribosomes of streptomycin-resistant and streptomycin-sensitive organisms. As discussed on page 170, streptomycin binds to a specific site on the ribosome, thereby deranging protein synthesis. Any mutation that deletes this site or alters it in such a manner that the drug cannot exert its effect results in streptomycin resistance. The binding site that is modified in streptomycin mutants involves a single amino acid replacement in the S12 protein on the 30S ribosomal subunit coded for by the *strA* gene. Following exposure of cultures of *E. coli* to high levels of streptomycin, survivors generally are all mutants in this gene. This mechanism of resistance, however, is less significant clinically than is plasmid-mediated enzymatic inactivation.

Kasugamycin Resistance. Kasugamycin is an aminoglycoside antibiotic that acts on the 30S subunit of 70S ribosomes. It inhibits protein synthesis but does not cause misreading or phenotypic suppression. Mutation to resistance causes an alteration, not in the ribosomal protein but in the 16S ribosomal RNA. Kasugamycin resistance is associated with a failure to methylate two adenine residues in the sequence AACCUG near the 3′ end of the 16S RNA. This alteration prevents binding of the drug to the ribosome.

Erythromycin Resistance. Resistance to erythromycin is associated with an altered 50S ribosomal subunit. In *E. coli* and a number of other species, the alteration is in a specific protein of the 50S subunit (L4 or L12), resulting in reduced affinity of the ribosome for erythromycin. In *S. aureus*, however, binding of the drug in resistant strains is blocked by dimethylation of a specific adenine sequence in the 23S ribosomal RNA. A plasmid-mediated ribosomal RNA methylase is responsible for this type of erythromycin resistance in *S. aureus* and is either inducible or constitutive.

Rifampin Resistance. Mutants resistant to rifampin have an RNA polymerase with an altered β subunit. Alteration of the β subunit is accompanied by failure of the core enzyme to bind the antibiotic and is the result of a chromosomal mutation.

Synthesis of Resistant Pathway

Sulfonamide and Trimethoprim Resistance. Resistance to the sulfonamides may be mutational or plasmid mediated and may involve more than one mechanism. The major cause of significant sulfonamide resistance among clinical isolates, however, is the plasmid-mediated production of an altered dihydropteroate synthetase, which is 1000 times less sensitive to the drug than the wild-type enzyme. Similarly, trimethoprim resistance is mediated by R plasmids that code for a trimethoprim-resistant dihydrofolate reductase (DHFR). Two types of plasmid-encoded DHFR are known; both are several thousand times more resistant to trimethoprim than the chromosomal enzyme of the wild type. The synthesis of a plasmid-encoded replacement enzyme that is selectively refractory to the antimicrobial agent provides a mechanism for bypass of the blocked reaction.

FURTHER READING

Books and Reviews

Acar JF, Neu HC (eds): Gram-negative aerobic bacterial infections: A focus on directed therapy, with special reference to aztreonam. Rev Infect Dis 7(suppl 4):S537, 1985

Allan JD, Eliopoulos GM, Moellering RC Jr: The expanding spectrum of beta-lactam antibiotics. Adv Intern Med 31:119, 1986
Atkinson BA, Amaral L: Sublethal concentrations of antibiotics, effects on bacteria and the immune system. CRC Crit Rev Microbiol 1982, p 101
Cozzarelli NR: The mechanism of action of inhibitors of DNA synthesis. Annu Rev Biochem 46:641, 1977
Demain AL, Solomon NA (eds): Antibiotics Containing the Beta-Lactam Structure. I. Handbook of Experimental Pharmacology 67/I. New York, Springer-Verlag, 1983
Elwell LP, Falkow S: The characterization of R plasmids and the detection of plasmid-specified genes. In Lorian V (ed): Antibiotics in Laboratory Medicine, ed 2. Baltimore, Williams & Wilkins, 1986, p 683
Finland M, Kass EH, Platt R: Trimethoprim-sulfamethoxazole revisited. Rev Infect Dis 4:185, 1982
Geddes AM, Stille W (eds): Imipenem: The first thienamycin antibiotic. Rev Infect Dis 7(suppl 3):S353, 1985
Hancock REW: Aminoglycoside uptake and mode of action—with reference to streptomycin and gentamicin. I. Antagonists and mutants. J Antimicrob Chemother 8:249, 1981
Handwerger S, Tomasz A: Antibiotic tolerance among clinical isolates of bacteria. Rev Infect Dis 7:368, 1985
Hay RJ, Dupont B, Graybill JR (eds): First international symposium on intraconazole. Rev Infect Dis 9(suppl 1):S1, 1987
Jacoby GA, Archer GL: New mechanisms of bacterial resistance to antimicrobial agents. N Engl J Med 324:601, 1991
Kropp H, Gerckens L, Sundelof JG, Kahan FM: Antibacterial activity of imipenem: The first thienamycin antibiotic. Rev Infect Dis 7(suppl 3):S389, 1985
Lode H, Kass EH (eds): Enzyme-mediated resistance to β-lactam antibiotics: A symposium on sulbactam/ampicillin. Rev Infect Dis 8(suppl 5):S465, 1986
Lorian V (ed): Antibiotics in Laboratory Medicine, ed 2. Baltimore, Williams & Wilkins, 1986
Lyon BR, Skurray R: Antimicrobial resistance of *Staphylococcus aureus:* Genetic basis. Microbiol Rev 51:88, 1987
Mandell GL, Douglas RG Jr, Bennett JE: Principles and Practice of Infectious Diseases, ed 3. New York, Wiley, 1990, Chap 15–33
Norrby SR, Bergan T, Holm SE, Normark S (eds): Evaluation of new β-lactam antibiotics. Rev Infect Dis 8(suppl 3):S235, 1986
Pestka S: Insights into protein biosynthesis and ribosome function through inhibitors. Prog Nucleic Acid Res Mol Biol 17:217, 1976
Queener SF, Webber JA, Queener SW (eds): Beta-Lactam Antibiotics for Clinical Use. New York, Marcel Dekker, 1986
Rubinstein E, Adam D, Moellering R Jr, Waldvogel F: International symposium on new quinolones. Rev Infect Dis 10(suppl 1):S1, 1988
Rubinstein E, Adam D, Moellering R Jr, Waldvogel F: Second international symposium on new quinolones. Rev Infect Dis 11(suppl 5):S897, 1989
Sanders CC, Wiedemann B (eds): New developments in resistance to β-lactam antibiotics among nonfastidious gram-negative organisms. Rev Infect Dis 10:677, 1988
Storm DR, Rosenthal KS, Swanson PE: Polymyxin and related peptide antibiotics. Annu Rev Biochem 46:723, 1977
Symposium: Fluconazole: A novel advance in therapy for systemic fungal infections. Rev Infect Dis 12(suppl 3):S263, 1990
Tipper DJ (ed): Antibiotic Inhibitors of Bacterial Cell Wall Biosynthesis. New York, Pergamon Press, 1987
Tomasz A: New and complex strategies of β-lactam antibiotic resistance in pneumococci and staphylococci. In Ayoub EM, Cassell GH, Branche WC Jr, Henry TJ (eds): Microbial Determinants of Virulence and Host Response. Washington DC, Am Soc Microbiol, 1990
Washington JA II: The effects and significance of subminimal inhibitory concentrations of antibiotics. Rev Infect Dis 1:781, 1979
Wehrli W: Rifampin: Mechanisms of action and resistance. Rev Infect Dis 5(suppl 3):S407, 1983
Weisblum B: Inducible resistance to macrolides, lincosamides and streptogramin type B antibiotics: The resistance phenotype, its biological diversity, and structural elements that regulate expression—A review. J Antimicrob Chemother 16(suppl A):63, 1985
Wise RI, Kory M (eds): Reassessments of vancomycin—a potentially useful antibiotic. Rev Infect Dis 3(suppl):S200–S300, 1981

Selected Papers

Barbas JA, Díaz J, Rodríguez-Tébar, Vázquez D: Specific location of penicillin-binding proteins within the cell envelope of *Escherichia coli.* J Bacteriol 165:269, 1986
Bryant DW, McCalla DR: Nitrofuran-induced mutagenesis and error prone repair in *Escherichia coli.* Chem Biol Interact 31:151, 1980
Burdett V: Streptococcal tetracycline resistance mediated at the level of protein synthesis. J Bacteriol 165:564, 1986
Dekker AW, Rozenberg-Arska M, Verhoef J: Infection prophylaxis in acute leukemia: A comparison of ciprofloxacin with trimethoprim-sulfamethoxazole and colistin. Ann Intern Med 106:7, 1987
Dougherty TJ: Intrinsic resistance: penicillin target alterations and effects on cell wall synthesis. In Leive L, Schlessinger D (eds): Microbiology—1984. Washington DC, American Society for Microbiology, 1984, p 398
Eccles SJ, Chopra I: Biochemical and genetic characterization of the *tet* determinant of *Bacillus* plasmid pAB124. J Bacteriol 158:134, 1984
Eliopoulos GM: In vitro activity of new quinolone antimicrobial agents. In Leive L (ed): Microbiology—1986. Washington DC, American Society for Microbiology, 1986, p 219
Farrar WE: Antibiotic resistance in developing countries. J Infect Dis 152:1103, 1985
Garvin RT, Biswas DK, Gorini L: The effects of streptomycin or dihydrostreptomycin binding to 16S RNA or to 30S ribosomal subunits. Proc Natl Acad Sci USA 71:3814, 1974
Gellert M, Mizuuchi K, O'Dea MH, et al: Nalidixic acid resistance: A second genetic character involved in DNA gyrase activity. Proc Natl Acad Sci USA 74:4772, 1977
Greenberg RN, Reilly PM, Luppen KL, et al: Treatment of serious gram-negative infections with aztreonam. J Infect Dis 150:623, 1984
Gutmann L, Kitzis MD, Billot-Klein D, et al: Plasmid-mediated β-lactamase (TEM-7) involved in resistance to ceftazidime and aztreonam. Rev Infect Dis 10:860, 1988
Hartman BJ, Tomasz A: Low-affinity penicillin-binding protein associated with β-lactam resistance in *Staphylococcus aureus.* J Bacteriol 158:513, 1984
Herrlich P, Schweiger M: Nitrofurans, a group of synthetic antibiotics, with a new mode of action: Discrimination of specific messenger RNA classes. Proc Natl Acad Sci USA 73:3386, 1976
Higgins ML, Ferrero M, Daneo-Moore L: Relationship of shape to initiation of new sites of envelope growth of *Streptococcus faecium* cells treated with β-lactam antibiotics. J Bacteriol 167:562, 1986
Horinouchi S, Weisblum B: Posttranscriptional modification of mRNA conformation: Mechanism that regulates erythromycin-induced resistance. Proc Natl Acad Sci USA 77:7079, 1980
Karp JE, Merz WG, Hendricksen C, et al: Oral norfloxacin for prevention of gram-negative bacterial infections in patients with acute leukemia and granulocytopenia. Ann Intern Med 106:1, 1987
Luzzatto L, Apirion D, Schlessinger D: Polyribosome depletion and blockage of the ribosome cycle by streptomycin in *Escherichia coli.* J Mol Biol 42:315, 1969

McCoy EC, Petrullo LA, Rosenkranz HS: Non-mutagenic genotoxicants: novobiocin and nalidixic acid, 2 inhibitors of DNA gyrase. Mutat Res 79:33, 1980

McMurray L, Petrucci RE Jr, Levy SB: Active efflux of tetracycline encoded by four genetically different tetracycline resistance determinants in *Escherichia coli.* Proc Natl Acad Sci USA 77:3974, 1980

Mendelman PM, Caugant DA, Kalaitzoglou G, et al: Genetic diversity of penicillin G-resistant *Neisseria meningitidis* from Spain. Infect Immun 57:1025, 1989

Modolell J, Davis BD: Rapid inhibition of polypeptide chain extension by streptomycin. Proc Natl Acad Sci USA 61:1279, 1968

Murakami K, Tomasz A: Involvement of multiple genetic determinants in high-level methicillin resistance in *Staphylococcus aureus.* J Bacteriol 171:874, 1989

Neu HC: Relation of structural properties of beta-lactam antibiotics to antibacterial activity. Am J Med 79(suppl 2A):2, 1985

Nozawa Y, Kitajima Y, Sekiya T, et al: Ultrastructural alterations induced by amphotericin B in the plasma membrane of *Epidermophyton floccosum* as revealed by freeze-etch electron microscopy. Biochim Biophys Acta 367:32, 1974

Pattishal KH, Acar J, Burchall JJ, et al: Two distinct types of trimethoprim-resistant dihydrofolate reductase specified by R plasmids of different compatibility groups. J Biol Chem 252:2319, 1977

Pestka S: Translocation, aminoacyl-oligonucleotides, and antibiotic action. Cold Spring Harbor Symp Quant Biol 34:395, 1969

Polak A, Scholer HJ: Mode of action of 5-fluorocytosine and mechanisms of resistance. Chemotherapy 21:113, 1975

Sanders CC, Sanders WE Jr: Microbial resistance to newer generation β-lactam antibiotics: Clinical and laboratory implications. J Infect Dis 151:399, 1985

Sanders CC, Sanders WE Jr: Type I β-lactamases of gram-negative bacteria: interactions with β-lactam antibiotics. J Infect Dis 154:792, 1986

Sandler P, Weisblum B: Erythromycin-induced ribosome stall in the *ermA* leader: A barricade to 5′- to 3′ nucleolytic cleavage of the *ermA* transcript. J Bacteriol 171:6680, 1989

Sheldrick GM, Jones PG, Kennard O, et al: Structure of vancomycin and its complex with acetyl-D-alanyl-D-alanine. Nature 271:223, 1978

Siegenthaler WE, Bonetti A, Luthy R: Aminoglycoside antibiotics in infectious diseases: An overview. Am J Med 80(suppl 6B):2, 1986

Siewert G, Strominger JL: Bacitracin: an inhibitor of the dephosphorylation of lipid pyrophosphate, an intermediate in biosynthesis of the peptidoglycan of bacterial cell walls. Proc Natl Acad Sci USA 57:767, 1967

Sokol-Anderson ML, Brajtburg J, Medoff G: Amphotericin B-induced oxidative damage and killing of *Candida albicans.* J Infect Dis 154:76, 1986

Speer BS, Salyers AA: Novel aerobic tetracycline resistance gene that chemically modifies tetracycline. J Bacteriol 171:148, 1989

Sreedharan S, Oram M, Jensen B, et al: DNA gyrase *gyrA* mutations in ciprofloxacin-resistant strains of *Staphylococcus aureus:* Close similarity with quinolone resistance mutations in *Escherichia coli.* J Bacteriol 172:7260, 1990

Sugino A, Peebles CL, Kreuzer KN, et al: Mechanism of action of nalidixic acid: Purification of *Escherichia coli nal A* gene product and its relationship to DNA gyrase and a novel nicking-closing enzyme. Proc Natl Acad Sci USA 74:4767, 1977

Tai P-C, Wallace BJ, Davis BD: Selective action of erythromycin on initiating ribosomes. Biochemistry 13:4653, 1974

Tai P-C, Wallace BJ, Davis BD: Streptomycin causes misreading of natural messenger by interacting with ribosomes after initiation. Proc Natl Acad Sci USA 75:275, 1978

Tuomanen E: Newly made enzymes determine ongoing cell wall synthesis and the antibacterial effects of cell wall synthesis inhibitors. J Bacteriol 167:535, 1986

Uno J, Shigematsu ML, Arai T: Primary site of action of ketoconazole on *Candida albicans.* Antimicrob Agents Chemother 21:912, 1982

Waring MJ: Drugs which affect the structure and function of DNA. Nature 219:1320, 1968

Weber DA, Sanders CC, Bakken JS, Quinn JP: A novel chromosomal TEM derivative and alterations in outer membrane proteins together mediate selective ceftazidime resistance. J Infect Dis 162:460, 1990

Wehland J, Herzog W, Weber K: Interaction of griseofulvin with microtubules, microtubule protein and tubulin. J Mol Biol 111:329, 1977

Yarbrough LR, Wu Y-H, Wu C-W: Molecular mechanism of the rifampicin-RNA polymerase. Biochemistry 15:2669, 1976

Yoshida H, Bogaki M, Nakamura S, et al: Nucleotide sequence and characterization of the *Staphylococcus aureus norA* gene, which confers resistance to quinolones. J Bacteriol 172:6942, 1990

CHAPTER 10

Sterilization and Disinfection

An understanding of the basic principles of sterilization and disinfection is fundamental to the intelligent practice of medicine. New techniques of sterilization and disinfection are continually being introduced, but we still use some of the same agents and procedures that were introduced centuries before there was any concept of infection. Although most of the simple chemical agents once used in therapy have been replaced by more specific chemotherapeutic agents, many of this group have retained their importance as effective antiseptics or disinfectants in the destruction of microorganisms in the nonliving environment.

Definitions. The following terms are useful in describing the damaging effects of certain chemical and physical agents on microorganisms. The term *sterilization* is an absolute one that implies the total inactivation of all forms of microbial life in terms of the organism's ability to reproduce. The suffix *-cide* is added when a killing action is implied, while *-stasis* is added when the organism is merely inhibited in growth or prevented from multiplying. A *bactericide* destroys bacteria; a *germicide* or *disinfectant* is an agent that kills microorganisms capable of producing an infection. A *bacteriostatic* agent is a substance that prevents the growth of bacteria. An *antiseptic* opposes sepsis or putrefaction either by killing microorganisms or by preventing their growth. This term is commonly used for agents that are applied topically to living tissues.

The selection of an appropriate procedure or agent is determined by the specific situation and by whether it is necessary to kill all microorganisms or only certain species. For example, the complete destruction of all microorganisms present in or on any material is essential in surgical procedures, in the preparation of all media and glassware used in the microbiology laboratory, and in the canning of nonacid high-protein foods. In the care of persons with communicable diseases, the destruction of the pathogen is necessary to prevent spread of the infection to susceptible persons. For this purpose a disinfectant is adequate and is usually employed in the cleaning-up process.

Dynamics of Sterilization and Disinfection

Death Rate of Microorganisms. Information concerning the kinetics of death of a bacterial population is essential for an understanding of the basis of sterilization by lethal agents. For microorganisms, the only valid criterion of death is the irreversible loss of the ability to reproduce. This is usually

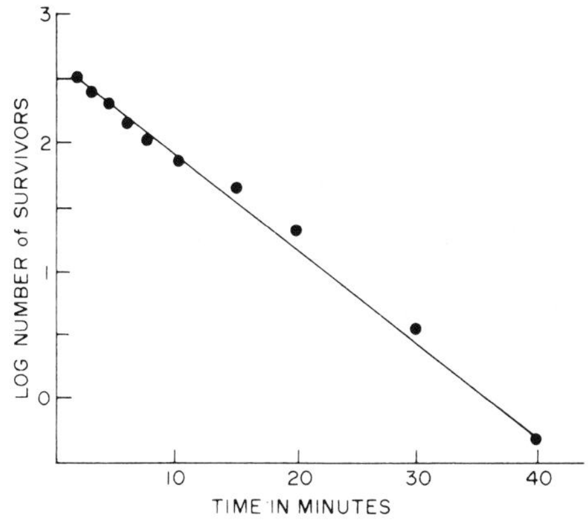

Fig. 10–1. Death rate of *Escherichia coli* when exposed to 0.5% phenol at 20C. *(From Chick: J Hyg (Camb) 10:237, 1910.)*

determined by plating techniques that quantitate by colony count the number of survivors.

When a bacterial population is exposed to a lethal agent, there is with time a progressive reduction in the number of survivors. The kinetics of death of a microbial population are usually exponential: the number of survivors decreases with time. If the logarithm of the number of survivors is plotted as a function of the time of exposure, a straight line is obtained (Fig. 10–1), the negative slope of which defines the death rate. The death rate, however, tells only what fraction of the initial population survives a given period of exposure to the antibacterial agent. To determine the actual number of survivors, one must also know the initial population size. This relationship is expressed mathematically by the formula

$$K = \frac{1}{t} \log \frac{B}{b}$$

where B is the initial number of organisms and b is the number remaining after time t.

Although the logarithmic curve is mathematically convenient and approximately correct when relatively high concentrations of a disinfectant are used, with lower concentrations the disinfection curve is sigmoidal, the rate being slow in the early stages, then proceeding rapidly for most of the disinfection process, and finally slowing down at the end. The flattening of the slope toward the end of the process is extremely important from the standpoint of sterilization, resulting in the requirement for more prolonged or intense treatment to destroy the resistant survivors that are more likely to be present in an initially large microbial population. Practical experience has shown that under no circumstances can one extrapolate the exponential death rate to zero and assume that the time of exposure thus indicated will guarantee sterility.

Because of the exponential form of the survivor-time curve, the larger the initial number of cells to be killed, the more intense or prolonged is the treatment required for sterilization. In addition, as might be expected, the rate of disinfection varies with the concentration of disinfectant. The effect of concentration on rate, however, is not constant but varies with the different disinfectants, as discussed below.

Antimicrobial Chemical Agents

Factors Affecting Disinfectant Potency. In contrast with chemotherapeutic agents that exhibit a high degree of selectivity for certain bacterial species, disinfectants are highly toxic for all types of cells. The effectiveness of a particular agent is determined to a great extent by the conditions under which it operates.

CONCENTRATION OF AGENT. Many agents are lethal for bacteria only when used in extremely high concentrations. Others in very low concentrations may stimulate, retard, or even kill the organism. The concentration required to produce a given effect, however, as well as the range of concentrations over which a given effect is demonstrable, varies with the disinfectant, the organism, and the method of testing. A close relationship exists between the concentration of drug employed and the time required to kill a given fraction of the population. This relationship is shown in the expression

$$C^n t = K$$

where C is the drug concentration, t is the time required to kill a given fraction of the cells, and n and K are constants. With phenolic compounds, a change in the concentration of the disinfectant has a pronounced effect on the disinfection rate; for example, reducing the concentration by one half increases approximately 64-fold the time required for sterilization. With most disinfectants, however, the effect is much less dramatic.

TIME. When bacteria are exposed to a specific concentration of a bactericidal agent, even in excess, not all the organisms die at the same time; rather, there is a gradual decrease in the number of living cells. Disinfection is usually considered a process in which bacteria are killed in a reasonable length of time, but there are varying opinions about what this should be (Fig. 10–1).

pH. The hydrogen ion concentration influences bactericidal action by affecting both the organism and the chemical agent. When suspended in a culture medium of pH 7, bacteria are negatively charged. An increase of pH increases the charge and may alter the effective concentration of the chemical agent at the surface of the cell. The pH also determines the degree of ionization of the chemical. In general, the nonionized form of a dissociable agent passes through the cell membrane more readily than the relatively inactive ionic forms.

TEMPERATURE. The killing of bacteria by chemical agents increases with an increase in temperature. At low temperatures, for each 10C temperature increment, there is a doubling of the death rate. With some agents, such as phenol, the rate is increased five to eight times, suggesting a more complex reaction and the interplay of additional factors.

NATURE OF THE ORGANISM. The efficacy of a particular agent depends on properties of the organism against which it is tested. The most important of these are the species of organism, the growth phase of the culture, the presence of special structures, such as spores or capsules, the previous

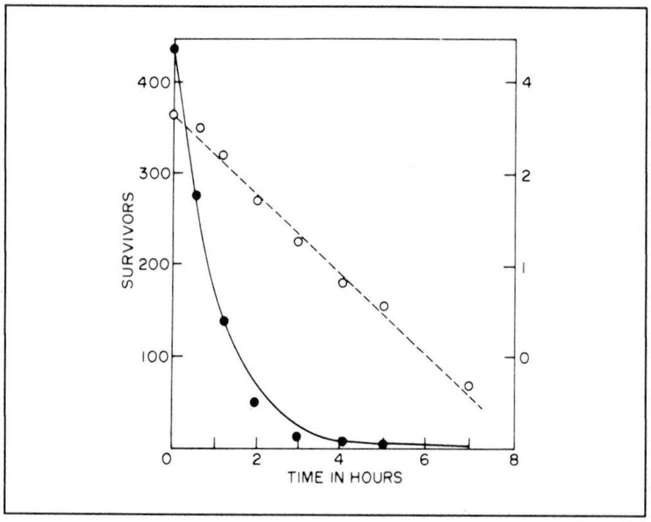

Fig. 10–2. Death rate of anthrax spores treated with 5% phenol at 33.3C. Number of surviving spores is plotted on an arithmetic scale and on a logarithmic scale. *(From Chick: J Hyg (Camb) 8:92, 1908.)*

history of the culture, and the number of organisms in the test system (Fig. 10–2).

PRESENCE OF EXTRANEOUS MATERIALS. The presence of organic matter, such as serum, blood, or pus, influences the activity of many disinfectants and renders inert substances that are highly active in their absence. These foreign materials alter disinfectant activity in a number of ways: surface absorption of the disinfectant by protein colloids, formation of a chemically inert or less active compound, and binding of the disinfectant by active groups of the foreign protein. Among the disinfectants whose inhibitory activity is greatly diminished by organic material with a high protein content are the aniline dyes, mercurials, and cationic detergents. The mercurials are markedly inhibited by compounds containing sulfhydryl groups, and the quaternary ammonium compounds are inhibited by soaps and lipids.

Evaluation of Disinfectants. In the United States the evaluation of disinfectants is the responsibility of the Environmental Protection Agency. A number of protocols, referred to as the Association of Official Analytical Chemists (AOAC) methods, are approved for evaluation purposes. Among these is the classic phenol coefficient test, which employs phenol as the standard reference material. The method is based on a tube dilution procedure designed to determine the ratio of the highest dilution of the germicide that will kill the test organism within a specified time to the greatest dilution of phenol showing the same result. The official method specifies standardized conditions for the testing against strains of *Salmonella typhi, Staphylococcus aureus,* and *Pseudomonas aeruginosa.*

Of wider use and applicability at the present time is the AOAC use-dilution method, a carrier inoculum method to measure bactericidal activity against *S. aureus, Salmonella choleraesuis,* and *P. aeruginosa.* This method involves testing of pure cultures that are dried either on surgical threads or in small stainless steel cylinders against a specific chemical germicide at a controlled contact time and temperature. The assay procedure is based on growth or no growth of surviving organisms after exposure. These methods, which confirm phenol coefficient results, are designed for determining bactericidal activity in practical disinfection.

Mechanisms of Antimicrobial Action. The mechanisms by which drugs kill or inhibit the growth of microorganisms are varied and complex. Sequential or simultaneous changes often occur and make it difficult to differentiate primary from secondary effects. In general, however, all of the observable effects of chemical agents on bacteria are the result of changes in its macromolecular components. Some of these changes damage the cell membrane, some irreversibly inactivate proteins, and others induce extensive nucleic acid damage.

Agents That Damage the Cell Membrane

The structural integrity of the membrane depends on the orderly arrangement of the proteins and lipids of which it is composed. Organic solvents and detergents disrupt this structural organization, resulting in an interference with normal membrane function. The net effect is the release of small metabolites from the cell and interference with active transport and energy metabolism.

Surface-active Disinfectants. Substances that alter the energy relationships at interfaces, producing a reduction of surface or interfacial tension, are referred to as surface-active agents. Surface-active agents are compounds that possess both water-attracting (hydrophilic) and water-repelling (hydrophobic) groups. The interface between the lipid-containing membrane of a bacterial cell and the surrounding aqueous medium provides a susceptible target site for agents of this type. The hydrophobic portion of the molecule is a fat-soluble, long-chain hydrocarbon, while the hydrophilic portion may be either an ionizable group or a nonionic but highly polar structure. Included in the surface-active agents are cationic, anionic, nonionic, and amphoteric substances (Table 10–1). Of these, the cationic and anionic compounds have been the most useful antibacterial agents.

CATIONIC AGENTS

Quaternary Ammonium Compounds. The most important antibacterial surface-active agents are the cationic compounds in which a hydrophobic residue is balanced by a positively charged hydrophilic group, such as a quaternary ammonium nucleus (Fig. 10–3). When bacteria are exposed to agents of this type, the positively charged group associates with phosphate groups of the membrane phospholipids, while the nonpolar portion penetrates into the hydrophobic interior of the membrane. The resulting distortion causes a loss of membrane semipermeability and leakage from the cell of nitrogen- and phosphorus-containing compounds. The agent itself may then enter the cell and denature its proteins. The activity of quaternary ammonium compounds is greatest at an alkaline pH. Although these compounds are bactericidal for a wide range of organisms, gram-positive species are more susceptible. Antibacterial activity is reduced in the presence of organic matter.

ANIONIC AGENTS. Among the anionic detergents are soaps and fatty acids that dissociate to yield a negatively charged

TABLE 10–1. SURFACE-ACTIVE AGENTS

Trade Name	Type of Compound	Structure
Zephiran	Cationic	Alkyldimethylbenzyl ammonium chloride
Triton K-12	Cationic	Cetyldimethylbenzyl ammonium chloride
Ceepryn chloride	Cationic	Cetylpyridinium chloride
Duponol LS	Anionic	Sodium oleyl sulfate
Triton W-30	Anionic	Sodium salt of alkylphenoxyethyl sulfonate
Carbowax 1500 dioleate	Nonionic	Oleic acid ester of polymerized polyethylene glycol
Tween 80	Nonionic	Sorbitan monooleate polyoxyalkylene derivative

ion. These agents, most active at an acid pH, are effective against gram-positive organisms but are relatively ineffective against gram-negative species because of their lipopolysaccharide outer membrane. By combining an anionic agent with acid, very effective acid-anionic surfactant sanitizers that are synergistic and display very rapid bactericidal action (within 30 seconds) have been devised.

The anionic detergents cause gross disruption of the lipoprotein framework of the cell membrane. The primary injury of the bile salts, long used by microbiologists to lyse pneumococci, is dissociation of the cell membrane, permitting autolytic enzymes to act on substrates from which they are restricted in the intact cell. When used together, the cationic and anionic detergents neutralize each other.

Phenolic Compounds. At low concentrations these compounds are rapidly bactericidal, causing leakage of cell contents and irreversible inactivation of membrane-bound oxidases and dehydrogenases. At present, use of the parent compound phenol (carbolic acid) is limited primarily to the testing of new bactericidal agents (p. 190). It has been replaced as a practical disinfectant by less caustic and toxic phenol derivatives.

The antibacterial activity of phenol is greatly increased by various substitutions in the phenol nucleus; the compounds of greatest importance are the alkyl- and chloro- derivatives and the diphenyls. Not only do many of these derivatives have a very high antibacterial activity; they are considerably less toxic than phenol. Because most phenolic disinfectants have a low solubility in water, they are formulated with emulsifying agents, such as soaps, which also increase their antibacterial action.

CRESOLS. The simplest of the alkyl phenols are the cresols. *Ortho-*, *meta-*, and *para*cresol are appreciably more active than phenol and are usually employed as a mixture (tricresol). Cresols, obtained industrially by the distillation of coal tar, are emulsified with green soap and sold under the trade names of Lysol and Creolin.

DIPHENYL COMPOUNDS. The halogenated diphenyl compounds exhibit unique antibacterial properties. Of these compounds, the most important is the chlorinated derivative, hexachlorophene, which is highly effective against gram-positive organisms, especially staphylococci and streptococci. Hexachlorophene is bactericidal if used in sufficiently high concentrations and, unlike many disinfectants, retains its antimicrobial potency when mixed with soaps or when added to various cosmetic preparations. It has been used in a wide variety of products, such as germicidal soaps and antiperspirants. Absorption through the skin, however, can cause neurotoxicity, especially in infants, and its use is now severely restricted.

Alcohols. Alcohols provide an insight into the interaction of organic solvents with lipid membranes. They disorganize lipid structure by penetrating into the hydrocarbon region. Short-chain alcohols produce quantitatively greater changes in membrane organization than do the higher homologues. In addition to their effect on the cell membrane, alcohols and other organic solvents also denature cellular proteins.

The aliphatic alcohols, especially ethanol, have been widely employed as skin disinfectants because of their bactericidal action and ability to remove lipids from skin surfaces. Their action as disinfectants, however, is severely restricted by their inability at normal temperatures to kill spores; for this reason, they should not be relied on for the sterilization of instruments.

Ethanol is used extensively to sterilize the skin prior to cutaneous injections (Fig. 10–4). It is also used for the disinfection of clinical thermometers and is very effective, provided a sufficient period of contact is allowed. It is active against gram-positive, gram-negative, and acid-fast organisms and is most effective at a concentration of 50% to 70%.

The bactericidal activity of isopropyl alcohol is slightly greater than that of ethanol, and it is less volatile. For these reasons, it has been recommended as a replacement for ethanol for the sterilization of thermometers. The toxic effects of isopropyl alcohol, however, are greater and longer lasting than those produced by ethanol. Narcosis may result from

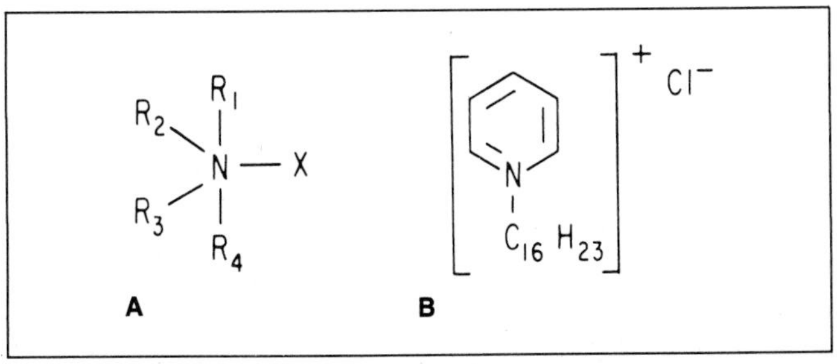

Fig. 10–3. **A.** Basic formula of the quaternary ammonium compounds. R_1, R_2, R_3, R_4 are alkyl groups that may be alike or different. The nitrogen atom has a valency of 5, and X is usually a halogen. For marked antibacterial activity, one of the four radicals must have 8 to 18 carbon atoms. **B.** Cetylpyridinium chloride (Ceepryn), a quaternary.

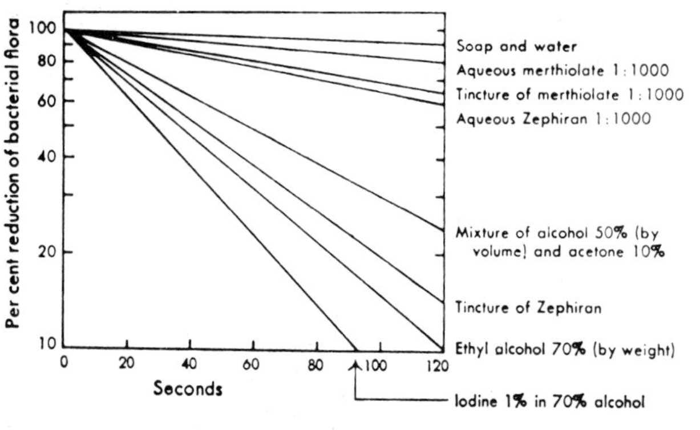

Fig. 10–4. Comparative effects of various antiseptics on the resident bacterial flora of the hands and arms. *(From Altemeier: In Block (ed): Disinfection, Sterilization, and Preservation, ed 3. Lea & Febiger, 1983.)*

the absorption of isopropyl alcohol vapors through the lungs during alcohol sponge baths.

Agents That Denature Proteins

In its native state, each protein has a characteristic conformation that is required for its proper functioning. Agents that alter the conformation of the protein by denaturation cause an unfolding of the polypeptide chain so that the chains become randomly and irregularly looped or coiled. Among the chemical agents that denature cellular proteins are the acids, alkalies, alcohols, acetone, and other organic solvents. The organic solvents have already been discussed in the previous section, since their primary target appears to be the cell membrane.

Acids and Alkalies. Acids and alkalies exert their antibacterial activity through their free H^+ and OH^- ions, through the undissociated molecules, or by altering the pH of the organism's environment. The strong mineral acids and strong alkalies have disinfectant properties proportional to the extent of their dissociation in solution. Some hydroxides, however, are more effective than their degree of dissociation would indicate, suggesting that the metallic cation also exerts a direct toxic action on the organism.

The intact molecule of the organic acids is responsible for their antibacterial activity. Although the extent of their dissociation in solution is less than that of mineral acids, they are sometimes more potent disinfectants. Benzoic acid, widely used as a food preservative, is approximately seven times as effective as hydrochloric acid, showing that both the whole molecule and the organic radical have disinfectant activity. Other organic acids that have been used extensively as food preservatives to extend the storage life of food products include lactic, acetic, citric, and propionic acids.

Agents that Modify Functional Groups of Proteins and Nucleic Acids

The catalytic site of an enzyme contains specific functional groups that bind the substrate and initiate the catalytic events. Inhibition of enzyme activity results if one or more of these functional groups is altered or destroyed. Important functional groups of the cell wall, membrane, and nucleic acids are also susceptible to inactivation.

Compounds containing mercury or arsenic combine with sulfhydryl groups; formaldehyde, anionic detergents, and acid dyes react with amino and imidazole groups; basic dyes, quaternary ammonium compounds, and cationic detergents react with acidic groups, such as hydroxyl or phosphoric acid residues. The presence of organic matter and other substances containing free reactive groups markedly reduces the effectiveness of agents whose toxicity results from combination with reactive groups of cell components.

Heavy Metals. Soluble salts of mercury, arsenic, silver, and other heavy metals poison enzyme activity by forming mercaptides with the sulfhydryl groups of cysteine residues. The initial reaction is reversible, and if extraneous-SH groups are provided in the form of glutathione or sodium thioglycollate, most of the cells recover. The binding ability of the mercurials extends to a broad range of ligands other than SH-containing groups (e.g., carboxylates, phosphates, hydroxyl, amines, imidazoles, and indoles).

MERCURIALS. Various forms of mercury have been employed in medicine for many years. Mercuric chloride, once popular as a disinfectant, is very toxic and at present has limited use. Organic mercurials, such as Metaphen, Merthiolate, and Mercurochrome, are less toxic and, although unreliable as skin disinfectants, are useful antiseptic agents. The phenylmercury salts are among the most efficient inhibitors of gram-positive and gram-negative bacteria, fungi, yeasts, and algae. They have been especially useful in the control of pseudomonads and other microbial contaminants in pharmaceutical, ophthalmic, and cosmetic preparations. The development of resistance to both organic and inorganic mercurials has been widespread and has been the result of the universal distribution of metal from natural sources as well as from industrial, agricultural, and medical usages. Commonly, antibiotic and mercury resistances are found on a single bacterial plasmid, together with other heavy metal resistances.

SILVER COMPOUNDS. Silver compounds are widely used as antiseptics, either as soluble silver salts or as colloidal preparations. The inorganic silver salts are efficient bactericidal agents, but their practical value is restricted by their irritant and caustic effects. The most commonly employed of the silver salts is silver nitrate, which is highly bactericidal for the gonococcus and is routinely used in a 1% solution, as legally required in many areas, for the prophylaxis of ophthalmia neonatorum in newborn infants. Colloidal silver compounds in which an insoluble, poorly ionized silver salt is combined with a protein, and from which silver ions are slowly released, have been extensively used as antiseptics, especially in ophthalmology. These compounds are primarily bacteriostatic, however, and are relatively poor disinfectants. The most recent application of silver compounds has been in the handling of burn patients. Topical application of silver nitrate or silver sulfadiazine in cream has significantly reduced the mortality in these patients. Thousands of burn patients have been successfully treated, but the increase in incidence of Ag^+-resistant organisms in the hospital environment has discouraged its use as the exclusive treatment.

Oxidizing Agents. The most useful antimicrobial agents in this group are the halogens and hydrogen peroxide. They inactivate enzymes by converting functional —SH groups to the oxidized S—S form. The stronger agents also attack amino groups, indole groups, and the phenolic hydroxyl group of tyrosine.

HALOGENS. Chlorine and iodine are among our most useful disinfectants. For certain purposes—iodine as a skin disinfectant and chlorine as a water disinfectant—they are unequaled. They are unique among disinfectants in that their activity is almost exclusively bactericidal and in that they are effective against sporulating organisms.

Iodine. Iodine exists principally in the form of I_2 at pH values below 6, where maximal bactericidal action is manifested. The rate of killing decreases as the pH is increased above 7.5. The iodide ion, I^-, formed as a result of iodine hydrolysis in aqueous solutions, has no significant bactericidal effect; the triiodide ion, I_3^-, also present in aqueous solutions, has minimal activity. Iodine tincture (USP XX) contains 2% iodine and 2.4% sodium iodide in aqueous alcohol (1:1). The principal use of iodine is in the disinfection of the skin; for this purpose it is probably superior to any other agent. Mixtures of iodine with various surface-active agents that act as carriers for the iodine are known as iodophors. The carriers are neutral polymers that serve not only to increase the solubility of the iodine but also to provide a sustained-release reservoir of the halogen. The best known iodophor and the compound of choice is povidone-iodine (Betadine), a compound of 1-vinyl-2-pyrrolidinone polymer with iodine, with not less than 9% and not more than 12% available iodine. In human medicine, iodophors have replaced aqueous and tincture iodine solutions to a considerable extent because they cause fewer unwanted side effects.

Chlorine. In addition to chlorine itself, there are three types of chlorine compound—the hypochlorites and the inorganic and organic chloramines. The disinfectant action of all chlorine compounds is due to the liberation of free chlorine. When elemental chlorine or hypochlorites are added to water, the chlorine reacts with water to form hypochlorous acid, which in neutral or acidic solution is a strong oxidizing agent and an effective disinfectant.

$$Cl_2 + H_2O \rightarrow HOCl + H^+ + Cl^-$$

$$Ca(OCl)_2 + H_2O \rightarrow Ca^{2+} + H_2O + 2\ OCl^-$$

$$Ca(OCl)_2 + 2\ H_2O \rightarrow Ca(OH)_2 + 2\ HOCl$$

$$HOCl \rightleftharpoons H^+ + OCl^-$$

The dissociation of hypochlorous acid depends on pH, which determines the disinfection efficiency.

The activity of chlorine is markedly influenced by the presence of organic matter. Therefore, in the disinfection of water, to compensate for the presence of any substances capable of combining with chlorine, it is necessary to determine the chlorine demand. It is customary to add sufficient chlorine to the water supply to satisfy the chlorine demand of the water and, at the same time, to provide enough residual for complete disinfection. In the case of swimming-pool water, however, a wide spectrum of organisms is being constantly introduced, and the contact time with chlorine may be very short. A concentration of 0.6 to 1.0 ppm of free chlorine residual should be maintained to assure rapid kill (15 to 30 seconds). Chlorine and chlorinated compounds have also been recommended for the sanitation of spas and hot tubs. To satisfy the large chlorine demand of the water and to provide a residual of available chlorine to render the water safe, a level of 1 to 3 ppm of free available chlorine must be continuously maintained.

Hypochlorites are the most useful of the chlorine compounds and are available in liquid or powder form as salts of calcium, lithium, and sodium. Hypochlorites are widely used in the food and dairy industries for sanitizing dairy and food-processing equipment. They are employed as sanitizers in most households, hospitals, and public buildings and are marketed under such popular labels as Clorox and Purex bleach.

HYDROGEN PEROXIDE. In a 3% solution, hydrogen peroxide is a harmless but very weak antiseptic whose primary clinical use is in the cleansing of wounds. When hydrogen peroxide is applied to tissues, oxygen is rapidly released by the tissue catalases, and the germicidal action is brief. Although the antibacterial action of hydrogen peroxide is usually attributed to its oxidizing ability, it is probable that the formation of the more toxic free hydroxyl radical ($^{\cdot}OH$) from the peroxide in an iron-dependent reaction accounts for most of this activity.

$$Fe^{2+} + H_2O \rightarrow Fe^{3+} + {}^{\cdot}OH + OH$$

At low nonlethal levels under aerobic conditions, hydrogen peroxide directly incises DNA, causing damage which is repaired by an incision repair pathway that requires DNA polymerase I. As a disinfectant of inanimate materials, hydrogen peroxide is a very useful and effective agent. It has been used increasingly in the last 10 years, especially for the disinfection of medical-surgical devices and soft plastic contact lenses (Table 10–2).

Dyes. Some of the coal-tar dyes, especially the triphenylmethanes and the acridines, not only stain bacteria but are inhibitory at very high dilutions. Within the usual pH range the basic dyes are the most effective. They exhibit a marked affinity for the acidic phosphate groups of nucleoproteins and other cell components, and they are inactivated by serum and other proteins. Their current medical use is limited primarily to the treatment of dermatologic lesions.

TRIPHENYLMETHANE DYES. Of the aniline dyes, derivatives of triphenylmethane, especially brilliant green, malachite green, and crystal violet, have had many uses. They are highly selective for gram-positive organisms and have been used in the laboratory in the formulation of selective culture media. The activity of triphenylmethane dyes is a property of the pseudobase formed on ionization of the dye (Fig. 10–5). The pseudobase is more lipid-soluble than the cation, and it is probably in this form that it gains access to the interior of the cell.

The specific mode of action of most of the dyes in this group remains ill defined. The action of crystal violet is attributed to its interference with the synthesis of the peptidoglycan component of the cell wall, where it blocks the conversion of UDP-acetylmuramic acid to UDP-acetylmuramylpeptide. In gram-negative organisms, lipopolysaccharide in the outer membrane provides a major penetration barrier for the uptake of the dye and accounts for the selectivity of gentian violet for gram-positive organisms.

TABLE 10–2. LENS DISINFECTION WITH 3 PERCENT HYDROGEN PEROXIDE SOLUTION

	Time Required for Disinfection[a]
Neisseria gonorrhoeae	0.3
Haemophilus influenzae	1.5
Pseudomonas aeruginosa	2.2
Bacillus subtilis (vegetative)	2.7
Propionibacterium acnes	3.0
Escherichia coli	3.0
Proteus vulgaris	3.1
Bacillus cereus (vegetative)	5.5
Proteus mirabilis	6.0
Streptococcus pyogenes	8.0
Staphylococcus epidermidis	9.7
Staphylococcus aureus	12.5
Herpes simplex	12.8
Serratia marcescens	20.5
Candida albicans	21.2
Fusarium solani	26.1
Aspergillus niger	45.3
Candida parapsilosis	96.9

From Favero: In Block (ed): Disinfection, Sterilization, and Preservation, ed 3. Lea & Febiger, 1983.
[a] Minutes of exposure required to reduce organisms in inoculum to 0.5/ml.

ACRIDINE DYES. The acridine dyes, often referred to as "flavines" because of their yellow color, exert a bactericidal and bacteriostatic effect on a number of organisms. Among the compounds of clinical use are proflavine and acriflavine, which have been employed in wound antisepsis. Unlike the aniline dyes, antimicrobial activity is retained in the presence of serum or pus.

The acridine dyes interfere with the synthesis of nucleic acids and proteins in both bacterial and mammalian cells. They are planar heterocyclic molecules that interact with double-stranded helical DNA by intercalation (Fig. 10–6). Because of its flat hydrophobic structure, acridine is inserted between two successive bases in DNA, separating them physically (Fig. 10–7). When the chain is replicated, an extra base is inserted into the complementary chain opposite the intercalated drug. When the latter chain is then replicated, the new chain will also contain an extra base.

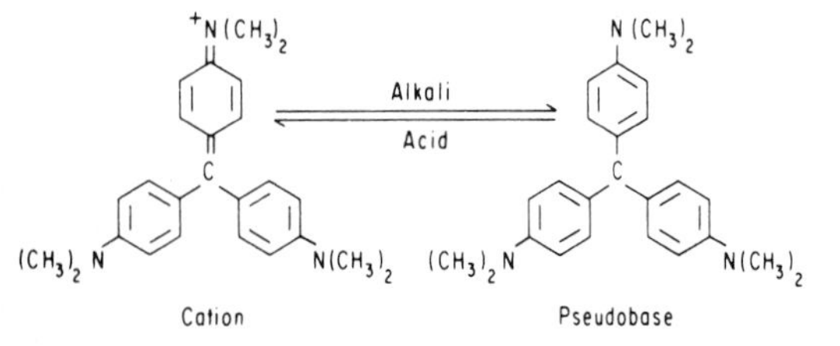

Fig. 10–5. Crystal violet, a triphenylmethane dye. Activity of these dyes is a property of the pseudobase.

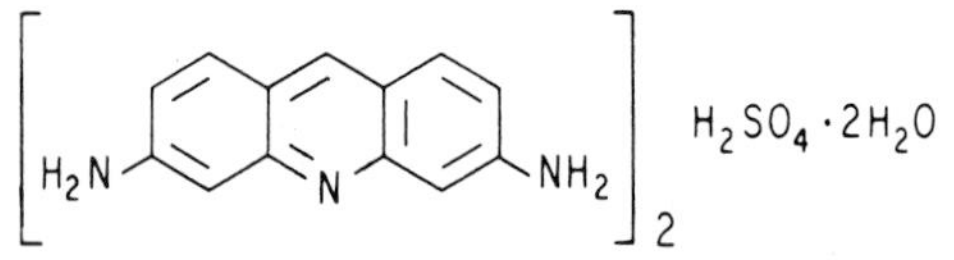

Fig. 10–6. Proflavine (3,6-diaminoacridine hemisulfate), an acridine dye.

Alkylating Agents. The lethal effects of formaldehyde, ethylene oxide, and glutaraldehyde result from their alkylating action on proteins. Inhibition produced by such agents is irreversible, resulting in enzyme modification and inhibition of enzyme activity.

FORMALDEHYDE. Formaldehyde (Fig. 10–8) is one of the least selective agents acting on proteins. Carboxyl, hydroxyl, or sulfhydryl groups are alkylated by direct replacement of a hydrogen atom with a hydroxymethyl group. Its reaction with a sulfydryl group of an enzyme protein is as follows:

$$E{-}SH + H{-}\overset{H}{\overset{|}{C}}{=}O \rightarrow E{-}S{-}\underset{H}{\underset{|}{\overset{H}{\overset{|}{C}}}}{-}OH$$

Formaldehyde is commercially available in aqueous solutions containing 37% formaldehyde (formalin) or as paraformaldehyde, a solid polymer that contains 91% to 99% formaldehyde. Formalin is used for preserving fresh tissues and is the major component of embalming fluids. When used at a sufficiently high concentration, it destroys all organisms, including spores. Formalin has been used extensively to inactivate viruses in the preparation of vaccines, since it has little effect on their antigenic properties. Generally, from 0.2% to 0.4% formalin has been used for this purpose. As a gas, formaldehyde has been used for years to decontaminate rooms, buildings, fabrics, and instruments.

GLUTARALDEHYDE. Within the last few years, glutaraldehyde,

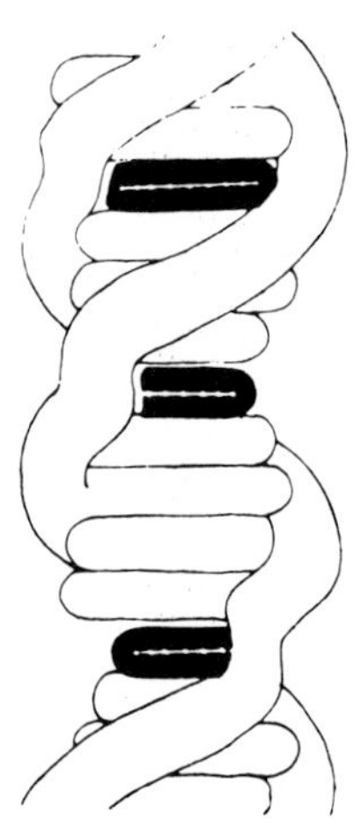

Fig. 10–7. Diagrammatic representation of the secondary structure of DNA containing intercalated proflavine molecules. *(From Lerman: J Cell Comp Physiol 64(suppl1):1964.)*

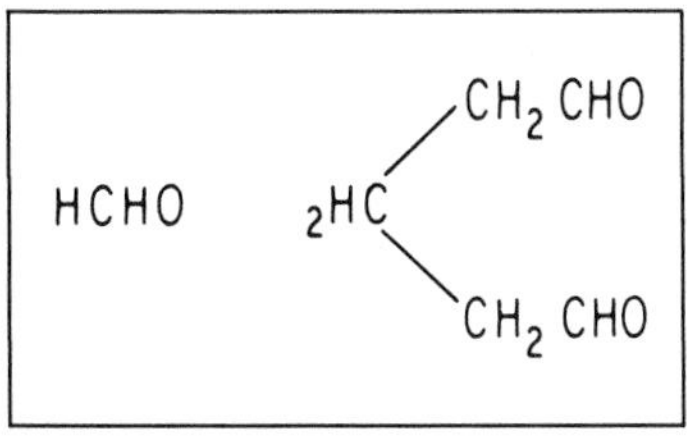

Fig. 10–8. Aldehyde disinfectants. **Left.** Formaldehyde. **Right.** Glutaraldehyde.

a saturated 5-carbon dialdehyde, has been used increasingly as a cold sterilant for surgical instruments (Table 10–3). It is the most commonly used disinfectant for endoscopic equipment, and at present it is the only available highly effective cold chemical sterilant recommended by the United States Centers for Disease Control for use on respiratory therapy equipment. It has a broad spectrum of activity and a rapid bactericidal rate. Glutaraldehyde is 10 times more effective than formaldehyde as a bactericidal and sporicidal agent and is considerably less toxic. Its bactericidal effectiveness is not diminished by protein-containing materials.

The mode of action of glutaraldehyde has been attributed to its binding of sulfhydryl or amino groups, but the specific target in the cell has not been defined (Fig. 10–8).

ETHYLENE OXIDE. Ethylene oxide is an alkylating agent extensively employed in gaseous sterilization. It is active against all types of bacteria, including spores and tubercle bacilli, but its action is slow. Its greatest applicability lies in the sterilization of materials that would be damaged by heat, such as polyethylene tubing, electronic and medical equipment, biologicals, and drugs. It has been especially useful in the sterilization of heart-lung machines and endoscopic equipment.

TABLE 10–3. DISINFECTION LEVELS OF SELECTED GERMICIDES

Class	Use Concentration
Gas	
Ethylene oxide	450–800mg/L[a]
Liquid	
Glutaraldehyde, aqueous	2%
Formaldehyde + alcohol	8% + 70%
Formaldehyde, aqueous	3% to 8%
Iodine + alcohol	0.5% + 70%
Alcohols	70%
Chlorine compounds	0.1% to 0.5%[b]
Phenolic compounds, aqueous	0.5% to 3%[c]
Iodine, aqueous	1%
Iodophors	0.007% to 0.015%[d]
Quaternary ammonium compounds	0.1% to 0.2% aqueous
Hexachlorophene	1%
Mercurial compounds	0.1% to 0.2%

From Turner: In Block (ed): Disinfection, Sterilization, and Preservation, ed 3. Lea & Febiger, 1983.

[a] In autoclave-type equipment at 55C to 60C.

[b] Chlorine.

[c] Dilution of concentrate.

[d] Available iodine.

The alkylating action of ethylene oxide is responsible for its bactericidal activity. It is an epoxy compound with the formula

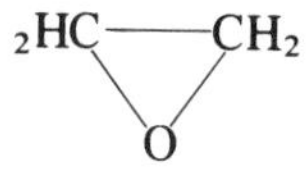

The ethylene oxide ring opens in the presence of a labile hydrogen and forms a hydroxy ethyl radical (CH_2CH_2OH), which then attaches to the position in the protein formerly occupied by the hydrogen. A labile hydrogen is available in carboxyl, amino, sulfhydryl, hydroxyl, and phenolic groups of proteins. Irreversible death of the cell results from blockage of these reactive groups. In addition to its action on protein, ethylene oxide also reacts with DNA and RNA, possibly by esterification of phosphate groups or reaction with the ring nitrogen of purines and pyrimidines. It is mutagenic for bacteria. Its use as a disinfectant involves some hazard of potential toxicity for humans, including mutagenicity and carcinogenicity.

Antimicrobial Physical Agents

Most pathogenic bacteria have limited tolerance to extreme variations in their physical environment and have little ability to survive outside the living body. Others, however, produce spores that are highly resistant to deleterious physical conditions in the environment and endow the organism with an increased survival value. In the discussion that follows, attention will be focused primarily on those physical agents that are useful as sterilizing agents.

Heat

Heat is the most reliable and universally applicable method of sterilization and, whenever possible, should be the method of choice. As with other types of disinfection, the sterilization of a bacterial population by heat is a gradual process, and the kinetics of death are exponential. The first-order inactivation by heat means that a constant fraction of the organisms undergoes an inactivating chemical change in each unit of time and that one such change is sufficient to inactivate an organism.

The time required for sterilization is inversely related to the temperature of exposure. This relationship may be expressed by the term *thermal death time,* which refers to the minimum time required to kill a suspension of organisms at a predetermined temperature in a specified environment. Because of the high temperature coefficients involved in heat sterilization, a minimal change in temperature significantly alters the thermal death time. In accordance with the law of mass action, the sterilization time is directly related to the number of organisms in the suspension.

MECHANISM OF THERMAL INJURY. Heat inactivation of bacteria cannot be defined in simple biochemical terms. Although the lethal effect of moist heat above a particular temperature is usually attributed to the denaturation and coagulation of protein, the pattern of thermal damage is quite complex, and

TABLE 10–4. MINIMUM TIMES REQUIRED FOR STERILIZATION BY MOIST AND DRY HEAT AT VARIOUS TEMPERATURES

	Moist Heat		Dry Heat
Temperature	Time (min)	Pressure	Time (min)
121C	15	15	—
126C	10	20	—
134C	3	30	—
140C	—	—	180
150C	—	—	150
160C	—	—	120
170C	—	—	60

From Meynell and Meynell: Theory and Practice in Experimental Bacteriology, Cambridge University Press, 1970.

coagulation undoubtedly masks other more subtle changes induced in the cell before coagulation becomes apparent.

The production of single-strand breaks in DNA may be the primary lethal event. The loss of viability of cells exposed to mild heat can be correlated with the introduction of these breaks. Damage to the DNA appears to be enzymatic in nature and is a consequence of nuclease activation. The ability of the cell to repair this damage and to recover viability depends on the physiologic state and genetic makeup of the organism.

Heat also causes a loss of functional integrity of the membrane and leakage of small molecules and 260 nm absorbing material. This material is of ribosomal origin and apparently results from degradation of the ribosomes by ribonucleases activated by the heat treatment. There appears to be a correlation between the degradation of ribosomal RNA and the loss of viability of cells exposed to high temperatures.

The mechanism by which organisms are destroyed by dry heat is different from that of moist heat. The lethal effects of dry heat, or desiccation in general, are usually ascribed to protein denaturation, oxidative damage, and toxic effects of elevated levels of electrolytes. In the absence of water, the number of polar groups on the peptide chain decreases, and more energy is required to open the molecules; hence the apparent increased stability of the organism.

Moist Heat. Objects may be sterilized either by dry heat applied in an oven or by moist heat provided as steam (Table 10–4). Of the two methods, moist heat is preferred because of its more rapid killing. Exposure of most mesophilic non-spore-forming bacteria to moist heat at 60C for 30 minutes is sufficient for sterilization. Among the exceptions are *S. aureus* and *Enterococcus faecalis,* which require an exposure time of 60 minutes at 60C. Exposure to a temperature of 80C for 5 to 10 minutes destroys the vegetative form of all bacteria, yeast, and fungi. Among the most heat-resistant cells are the spores of *Clostridium botulinum,* an anaerobic organism that causes food poisoning. Spores of this organism are destroyed in 4 minutes at 120C, but at 100C it takes 5.5 hours.

The application of moist heat in the destruction of bacteria may take several forms: boiling, live steam, and steam under pressure. Of these, steam under pressure is the most efficient because it makes possible temperatures above the boiling point of water. Such temperatures are necessary because of the extremely high thermal resistance of bacterial spores.

Steam sterilization is carried out in a pressure chamber called an autoclave. The basic essential in this type of sterilization is that the whole of the material to be sterilized shall be in contact with saturated steam at the required temperature for the necessary period of time. For sterilizing small objects, an exposure of 20 minutes at 121C (15 pounds of steam pressure per square inch) is used and provides a substantial margin of safety.

For the sterilization of certain liquids or semisolid materials that are easily destroyed by heat, a fractional method of sterilization is employed. This process, often called tyndallization, consists of heating the material at 80C or 100C for 30 minutes on three consecutive days. The rationale for this fractional type of sterilization is that vegetative cells and some spores are killed during the first heating and that the more resistant spores subsequently germinate and are killed during either the second or the third heating. The method is useful in sterilizing heat-sensitive culture media containing such materials as carbohydrates, egg, or serum.

PASTEURIZATION. As indicated above, most vegetative bacteria can be killed by relatively short exposures to temperatures of 60C to 65C. The most important application of temperatures in this range is in the pasteurization of milk and preparation of bacterial vaccines. Although originally devised by Pasteur as a means of destroying microorganisms that cause spoilage of wine and beer, the pasteurization process is now used primarily to make food and beverages safe for consumption. The application of this treatment to the pasteurization of milk consists of heating to a temperature of 62C for 30 minutes, followed by rapid cooling. This temperature does not sterilize the milk, but it does kill all disease-producing bacteria commonly transmitted by milk.

Dry Heat. Sterilization by dry heat requires higher temperatures and a longer period of heating than does sterilization with steam. Its use is limited primarily to the sterilization of glassware and such materials as oils, jellies, and powders that are impervious to steam. The lethal action results from the heat conveyed from the material with which the organisms are in contact and not from the hot air that surrounds them; this emphasizes the importance of uniform heating of the entire object to be sterilized. The most widely used type of dry heat is the hot-air oven. Sterilizing times of 2 hours at 180C are required for the killing of all organisms, including the spore formers. Other useful forms of dry heat include incineration of disposable objects and passage of bacteriologic needles, coverslips, or small instruments through the flame of a Bunsen burner.

Freezing

Although many bacteria are killed by exposure to cold, freezing is not a reliable method of sterilization. Its primary use is in the preservation of bacterial cultures. Repeated freezing and thawing are much more destructive to bacteria than is prolonged storage at freezing temperatures. In the freezing of bacteria, the formation of ice crystals outside the cell causes the withdrawal of water from the cell interior, resulting in an increased intracellular electrolyte concentration and a denaturation of proteins. The cell membrane is damaged, and a leakage of intracellular organic compounds ensues. The leakage material contains inorganic phosphorus, ribose, peptides, and nucleotides that arise as a consequence of the activation of latent ribonucleases and peptidases.

When bacteria are frozen rapidly to temperatures below

−35C, ice crystals form within the cell and produce a lethal effect during defreezing. If, however, cultures are dried in vacuo from the frozen state by the process of *lyophilization* or freeze-drying, the initial mortality is greatly diminished. This method is widely used for the preservation of bacterial cultures.

Radiation

Sunlight has appreciable bactericidal activity and plays an important role in the spontaneous sterilization that occurs under natural conditions. Its disinfectant action is due primarily to its content of ultraviolet rays, most of which, however, are screened out by glass and by the presence of ozone in the outer atmosphere. Other electromagnetic rays of shorter wavelength, such as x-rays and γ-rays, as well as rays produced by radioactive decay and by ion accelerators, also exert a pronounced effect when absorbed by bacteria (Fig. 10–9).

Effects of Radiation. Only absorbed light promotes photochemical reactions. As a molecule absorbs light, it receives energy in the form of discrete units termed "quanta." The energy of a quantum is inversely related to its wavelength. In the primary reaction, only 1 quantum of light is absorbed by each molecule of absorbing substance. The number of quanta absorbed by a biologic system is proportional to the product of the duration and intensity of the radiation as well as to the absorption coefficient of the irradiated material. The absorption of a quantum by an electron in an atom results in activation of the molecule, which then either uses the extra energy for chemical changes, such as decomposition and internal rearrangements, or loses it entirely as heat or fluorescence.

Radiation may have sufficient energy to remove an electron completely from an atom and produce an electrical charge (ionization) or only enough energy to raise electrons to states of higher energy (excitation). Energy equivalent to 10 electron volts is required to pull an electron completely out of an atom. This is provided by x-rays and γ-rays that ionize atoms by the ejection of electrons from any atom through which the radiation passes.

In the visible and UV range, although the quantum energy absorbed by the molecule cannot remove an electron completely, the excitation produced often leads to photochemical changes. In the infrared range of the spectrum, the energy is inadequate to initiate a chemical change in biologic material, and the absorbed energy is dissipated as heat.

Ultraviolet Radiation

MECHANISM OF ULTRAVIOLET RADIATION INJURY. The effectiveness of UV light as a lethal and mutagenic agent is closely correlated with its wavelength. The most effective bactericidal wavelength is in the 240 to 280 nm range, with the optimum at about 260 nm, which corresponds with the absorption maximum of DNA. The major mechanism of the lethal effect of UV light on bacteria is attributed to this absorption by, and resultant damage to, the DNA. Ultraviolet radiation leads to the formation of covalent bonds between pyrimidine residues adjacent to each other in the same strand, resulting in the formation of cyclobutane-type pyrimidine dimers. These dimers distort the shape of the DNA and interfere with normal base pairing. This results in an inhibition of DNA synthesis and secondary effects, such as inhibition of growth and respiration. UV light is also mutagenic. The mutagenic effect is dependent on induction by the cyclobutane dimer of the SOS response, a coordinately regulated group of negatively repressed operons (p. 132). Other effects are also produced by UV radiation, such as photohydration of cytosine and cross-linkage of complementary strands of DNA, but the extremely high dose required rules them out as major mechanisms for UV damage to cells.

Repair Mechanisms. If, after treatment with UV light, cells are immediately irradiated with visible light in the 300 to 400 nm range, both the mutation frequency and the bactericidal effect of UV light are greatly reduced. This phenomenon is known as "photoreactivation" and results from the activation by light of an enzyme that hydrolyzes the pyrimidine dimers. Another mechanism also exists in some cells for the repair of light-damaged DNA. This is a dark-repair mechanism that invokes the activity of an efficient set of enzymes for the excision of the UV-induced dimers and repair of the damaged strand. Excision-repair is probably the primary cause of an enhanced resistance to UV light in some strains of bacteria.

PRACTICAL APPLICATIONS. Ultraviolet radiation can be produced artificially by mercury vapor lamps. The unit of radiation energy is measured in terms of microwatts per unit area per unit of time. A 15-watt UV light delivers 38 $\mu W/cm^2/s$ of radiation at a distance of 1 m. UV radiation is equally effective against gram-positive and gram-negative organisms. The lethal dose for most of the common, non-spore-forming bacteria varies from 1800 $\mu W/cm^2$ to 6500 $\mu W/cm^2$. Bacterial spores require up to 10 times this dose.

Although the bactericidal properties of UV radiation are indisputable, UV radiation cannot be properly classified as a sterilizing agent because of the many uncertainties surrounding its use. Unlike ionizing radiation, the energy of UV radiation is low, and its power of penetration is poor. It does

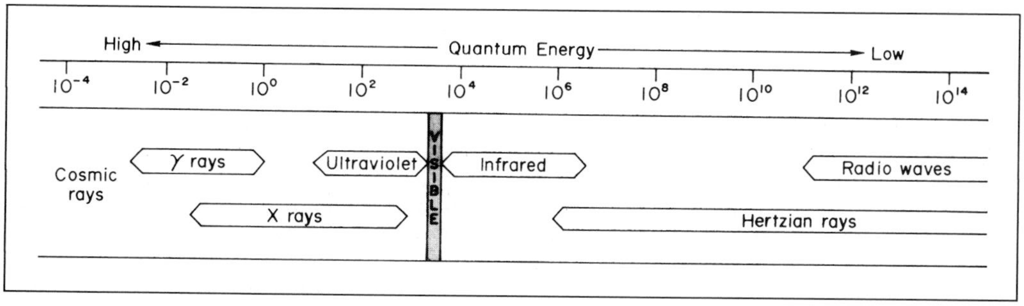

Fig. 10–9. The electromagnetic spectrum. The wavelength in nanometers is plotted on an exponential scale.

not penetrate into solids, and it penetrates into liquids only slightly. For this reason, UV rays have no effect on organisms shielded or protected from the incident beams.

The primary application of UV irradiation is in the control of airborne infection, where it is used for the disinfection of enclosed areas, such as hospital wards and operating rooms.

Ionizing Radiations

PROPERTIES OF IONIZING RADIATIONS. Ionizing radiations are classified into two major categories according to their physical properties: (1) those that have mass and that may be either charged or uncharged and (2) those that are energy only. Some of the ionizing radiations are products of radioactive decay (α-, β-, γ-rays), and others are produced in an x-ray machine, by particle bombardment, or by nuclear reactors. The ionizing radiations of greatest practical value for purposes of sterilization are the electromagnetic x-rays and γ-rays and the particulate cathode rays (artificially accelerated electrons). These radiations have a much higher energy content than UV radiation and thus a much greater capacity to produce lethal effects.

The penetrating power of ionizing radiations contributes to their effectiveness as sterilizing agents. Although cathode rays, because of their particulate nature, have a greater intrinsic energy and, consequently, the greater power of penetration, x-rays and γ-rays have a relatively greater penetrating ability. Because of the nature of the mechanisms involved, optimum activity never occurs at the surface of the material being treated. With γ-rays it occurs just below or inside the surface; with cathode rays it occurs a few centimeters deeper.

RADIATION UNITS. The effect of ionizing radiations on living systems depends on the amount of energy absorbed. The amount of radiation to which a system is exposed is the exposure dose. For x-rays or γ-rays the exposure dose is measured in roentgens and is equivalent to an energy absorption of about 83 ergs/g of air. That portion of the exposure dose that is actually absorbed by the biologic system (the absorbed dose) is the biologically effective dose, the unit of which is the rad. The rad is based on an energy absorption of 100 ergs/g of air. For practical purposes, the Mrad equal to 10^6 rad, is used because this is the dose required for sterilization.

LINEAR ENERGY TRANSFER. In the passage of ionizing radiations through matter, the energy of the protons is transferred by collisions with an orbital electron in an atom of the absorbing medium. After such a collision, an electron is ejected from the atom with high energy and at great speed. As this electron moves through the medium, it will ionize and excite atoms with which it interacts. The energy given to it will be dissipated as it moves through the medium.

RADIOLYSIS OF WATER. Ionizing radiation has both direct and indirect effects on the macromolecules of the cell. The direct effect is exerted by the initial transfer of energy within a limited vital or sensitive area, according to the target theory. However, since biologic systems are composed of large amounts of water, the primary mechanism for the lethal effect of ionizing radiation is an indirect one. As ionizing radiations pass through water, they cause the water molecules to ionize:

$$H_2O \xrightarrow[\text{Quantum}]{\text{Energy}} H_2O^+ + e^-$$

The resulting positive ion reacts with un-ionized water to yield another species of charged water molecule and the free hydroxyl radical:

$$H_2O^+ + H_2O \rightarrow H_3O^+ + {}^{\cdot}OH$$

The ejected electron can also react with un-ionized water to give an OH^- ion and a free hydrogen radical:

$$e^- + H_2O \rightarrow OH^- + H^{\cdot}$$

The hydroxyl radical is a strong oxidizing agent, and the hydrogen radical is a powerful reducing agent. The hydroxyl radical is highly reactive with macromolecules, especially DNA, and ruptures it by effecting a break in both of the constituent chains.

The presence of oxygen in cells at the time of irradiation enhances the magnitude of the irradiation effect. The increased effect results from the interaction of oxygen with radiation-produced free radicals, drawing these radicals into destructive auto-oxidative chain reactions. The presence of oxygen during irradiation also promotes the formation of hydrogen peroxide and organic peroxides:

$$H^{\cdot} + O_2 \rightarrow {}^{\cdot}HO_2$$

$$2\ {}^{\cdot}HO_2 \rightarrow H_2O_2 + O_2$$

Chemical compounds that contain sulfhydryl groups protect biologic systems from the damaging effects of ionizing radiation by diverting the absorbed energy.

LETHAL EFFECTS. Most pathogenic non-spore-forming bacteria are relatively sensitive to ionizing radiation. Among the nonspore formers gram-positive organisms are generally more resistant than gram-negative species, and spores are among the most radiation-resistant microorganisms known.

The death of microorganisms exposed to ionizing radiation is usually exponential throughout the sterilization period, although in some cases it tends to be sigmoidal. The slope of the time-survivor curve is determined by the intensity of the irradiation, but in terms of dose against percentage killed, the relationship is always exponential. Toward the end of the process, however, a tailing effect may become prominent, emphasizing the importance of ensuring that the full dose has been given.

PRACTICAL APPLICATIONS. Although the sterilizing dose is dependent on the initial level of contamination, a dose of 2.5 Mrad of ionizing radiation has been accepted as the sterilizing dose. This dose is sufficient to kill the most resistant microorganisms and also provides an adequate margin of safety under conditions of practical use.

The main areas in which ionizing radiations have been applied for purposes of sterilization are in pharmacy and medicine. They are especially suitable for sterilizing such articles as catgut and nylon sutures and disposable surgical and medical supplies.

Ultrasonic and Sonic Vibrations

Sound vibrations at high frequency, in the upper audible and ultrasonic range (20 to 1000 kc), provide a useful technique for disrupting cells. The sound wave generators that are widely employed for this purpose operate in the frequency range of 9 to 100 kc/s. No specific frequency has been found to be uniquely effective, but generally ultrasonic waves are more effective as the frequency is increased.

The passage of sound through a liquid produces alternating pressure changes, which, if the sound intensity is sufficiently great, cause cavities to form in the liquid. The cavities, which are about 10 μm in diameter, grow in size until they collapse violently with the production of high local velocities and pressures of the order of 1000 atmospheres. During this violent-collapse stage, the cell disintegrates. In addition to disintegrating cells, cavitation produces a number of chemical and physical changes in the suspending medium, which may be deleterious to certain enzymes. Among the most important of these is the formation of hydrogen peroxide when cavitation takes place in a liquid containing dissolved oxygen. Ultrasonic vibrations have also been shown to cause a depolymerization of macromolecules and intramolecular regroupings. Double-strand breaks are produced in transforming DNA by sonic vibration, and integration into the host genome is inhibited.

Microorganisms vary markedly in their sensitivity to sonic and ultrasonic vibrations. The most susceptible are the gram-negative rods, and among the most resistant are the staphylococci, which require long periods of exposure. Although sonic vibrations are lethal to many members of the exposed bacterial population, there are numerous survivors. Consequently, treatment with sonic vibrations is of no practical value in sterilization and disinfection.

Filtration

The principal method used in the laboratory for the sterilization of heat-labile materials is filtration. Although mechanical sieving plays a role in all filtration processes, electrostatic and absorption phenomena and the physical construction of the filter also exert a pronounced effect. A number of different types of filter have been employed for the purpose of sterilization. Most of the older types (Berkefeld, Chamberland, Seitz) have been replaced by membrane filters consisting of porous disks of biologically inert cellulose esters. They absorb little of the fluid being filtered and thus are useful for the sterilization of certain materials that cannot tolerate, without deterioration, the high temperatures used in heat sterilization.

Membrane Filters. Membrane filters are available in pore sizes of 14 to 0.023 μm. The 0.22 μm filter is the most widely used for sterilization purposes because the pore size is smaller than that of bacteria. It should always be used for sterilizing solutions containing serum, plasma, or trypsin where species of *Pseudomonas* or other small bacteria are often present.

Membrane filters act essentially as two-dimensional screens, retaining all particles that exceed the pore size. In liquid filtration, a large number of particles somewhat smaller than the pore size are retained by van der Waals forces, by random entrapment in the pores, and by buildup on previously retained particles. However, the important characteristic of the membrane filter is that all particles larger than the pore size are positively retained on the filter surface.

FURTHER READING

Books and Reviews

Allwood MC, Russell AD: Mechanisms of thermal injury in nonsporulating bacteria. Adv Appl Microbiol 12:89, 1970

Bennett EO: Factors affecting the antimicrobial activity of phenols. Adv Appl Microbiol 1:123, 1959

Block SS (ed): Disinfection, Sterilization, and Preservation, ed 3. Philadelphia, Lea & Febiger, 1983

Chambers CW, Clarke NA: Control of bacteria in nondomestic water supplies. Adv Appl Microbiol 8:105, 1966

Él'piner IE: Action of ultrasonic waves on microorganisms, viruses, and bacteriophages. In Ultrasound: Its Physical, Chemical, and Biological Effects. New York, Consultants Bureau, 1964, chap 9

Farrell J, Rose AH: Low-temperature microbiology. Adv Appl Microbiol 7:335, 1965

Favero MS: Chemical disinfection of medical and surgical materials. In Block SS (ed): Disinfection, Sterilization, and Preservation, ed 3. Philadelphia, Lea & Febiger, 1983, p 469

Gray TRG, Postgate JR (eds): The Survival of Vegetative Microbes. 26th Symposium of the Society for General Microbiology. Cambridge, Cambridge University Press, 1976

Harold FM: Antimicrobial agents and membrane function. Adv Microb Physiol 4:45, 1970

Heckly RJ: Preservation of bacteria by lyophilization. Adv Appl Microbiol 3:1, 1961

Hugo WB (ed): Inhibition and Destruction of the Microbial Cell. New York, Academic Press, 1971

MacLeod RA, Calcott PH: Cold shock and freezing damage to microbes. In Gray TRG, Postgate JR (eds): The Survival of Vegetative Microbes. 26th Symposium of the Society for General Microbiology. Cambridge, Cambridge University Press, 1976, p 81

McDade JJ, Philips GB, Sivinski HD, et al: Principles and applications of laminar-flow devices. In Norris JR, Ribbons DW (eds): Methods in Microbiology, vol 1. New York, Academic Press, 1969, p 137

Meynell GG, Meynell E (eds): Theory and Practice in Experimental Bacteriology, ed 2. Cambridge, Cambridge University Press, 1970

Mulvany JG: Membrane filter techniques and microbiology. In Norris JR, Ribbons DW (eds): Methods in Microbiology, vol 1. New York, Academic Press, 1969, p 205

Petrocci AN: Surface-active agents: Quaternary ammonium compounds. In Block SS (ed): Disinfection, Sterilization, and Preservation, ed 3. Philadelphia, Lea & Febiger, 1983, p 309

Pizzarello DJ, Witcofski RL: Basic Radiation Biology. Philadelphia, Lea & Febiger, 1967

Reddish GF (ed): Antiseptics, Disinfectants, Fungicides, and Chemical and Physical Sterilization, ed 2. Philadelphia, Lea & Febiger, 1957

Sykes G: Methods and equipment for sterilization of laboratory apparatus and media. In Norris JR, Ribbons DW (eds): Methods in Microbiology, vol 1. New York, Academic Press, 1969, p 77

Turner FJ: Hydrogen peroxide and other oxidant disinfectants. In Block SS (ed): Disinfection, Sterilization, and Preservation, ed 3. Philadelphia, Lea & Febiger, 1983, p 240

Selected Papers

Brash DE, Haseltine WA: Photoreactivation of *Escherichia coli* reverses *umu* C induction by UV light. J Bacteriol 163:460, 1985

Chick H: An investigation of the laws of disinfection. J Hyg(Camb) 8:92, 1908

Chick H: The process of disinfection by chemical agents and hot water. J Hyg (Camb) 10:237, 1910

Fried VA, Novick A: Organic solvents as probes for the structure and function of the bacterial membrane: Effects of ethanol on the wild type and an ethanol-resistant mutant of *Escherichia coli* K12. J Bacteriol 114:239, 1973

Gustafsson P, Nordström K, Normark S: Outer penetration barrier of *Escherichia coli* K12: Kinetics of the uptake of gentian violet by wild-type and envelope mutants. J Bacteriol 116:893, 1973

Hagensee ME, Moses RE: Repair response of *Escherichia coli* to hydrogen peroxide DNA damage. J Bacteriol 168:1059, 1986

Horiuchi H, Takagi M, Yano K: Relaxation of supercoiled plasmid DNA by oxidative stresses in *Escherichia coli.* J Bacteriol 160:1017, 1984

Imlay JA, Linn S: Bimodal pattern of killing of DNA-repair-defective or anoxically grown *Escherichia coli* by hydrogen peroxide. J Bacteriol 166:519, 1986

Knapp HR, Melly MA: Bactericidal effects of polyunsaturated fatty acids. J Infect Dis 154:84, 1986

Laipis PJ, Ganesan AT: In vitro repair of x-irradiated DNA extracted from *Bacillus subtilis* deficient in polymerase I. Proc Natl Acad Sci USA 69:3211, 1972

Repine JE, Fox RB, Berger EM: Hydrogen peroxide kills *Staphylococcus aureus* by reacting with staphylococcal iron to form hydroxyl radical. J Biol Chem 256:7094, 1981

Schnaitman CA: Solubilization of the cytoplasmic membrane of *Escherichia coli* by Triton X-100. J Bacteriol 108:545, 1971

Shew CW, Freese E: Lipopolysaccharide layer protection of gram-negative bacteria against inhibition by long-chain fatty acids. J Bacteriol 115:869, 1973

SECTION II

IMMUNOLOGY

CHAPTER 11

Introduction to Immunity

General Features of Immune System

When a small child becomes infected with a pathogenic microorganism such as *Corynebacterium diphtheriae,* there is a high probability of sickness and a possibility of death. When a child previously vaccinated with diphtheria-pertussis-tetanus (DPT) vaccine (Chap. 28) subsequently encounters the organism, the chances of an infection are slight and the probability of death from diphtheria negligible, although the risk of other infectious diseases such as measles is unchanged.

This example represents immunization with a noninfectious form of an organism and illustrates some of the best-known attributes of the immune system. The unimmunized child is at risk because the immune system has not been forearmed. Vaccinated, the child becomes specifically immunized against foreign (non-self) products of the diphtheria organism known as antigens. The child who is immune to diphtheria will have no increased immunity to measles (specificity), but the state of immunity to diphtheria will persist for years (immunologic memory). Any subsequent exposure will not only reinforce the immunity, but capacity to respond will also be faster and more vigorous (anamnestic response).

Less well known are the ways in which the immune system orchestrates the cellular responses of the individual and the subtle ways in which the immune system integrates with many diverse physiologic processes. Immunology is a rapidly changing science, and exciting new discoveries are constantly being made.

The most convenient indicator of immunity is antibody; antibodies are the best known of the many products of the immune system. Antibodies are globular proteins produced in the lymph nodes and the spleen. When a small mononuclear cell (lymphocyte) arising in the lymphoid organs encounters its appropriate antigen, two events are triggered: (1) a series of lymphocyte divisions to form a clone of responding cells and then (2) the production of effector molecules by cells of this clone. Antibody is the effector molecule of a subclass of lymphocytes called B cells that give rise to plasma cells; the T cell receptor is the effector of the other great subclass. Some of the numerous ways of detecting antibodies are described in Chapter 12. Antibody-containing serum from an immune individual will, for example, aggregate (agglutinate) suspensions of bacteria or neutralize the adverse effects of injurious toxins so that they can no longer kill a person or an experimental animal. Such events can easily be observed.

Procedures for measuring antibodies were first developed nearly 100 years ago. Methods for detecting antibodies have been modified, improved, and given great precision since then (Chap. 12). Immunologists thus have many exquisitely sensitive, specific, and efficient ways of measuring the antibody response to the carbohydrates, proteins, and glycolipids, which are recognized as foreign and which constitute the vast majority of microbial antigens. Antibody is only one of several different effectors of immunity; indeed, some antibodies such as antibody to the flagellar antigen of typhoid have little protective effect, and antibodies alone would provide a very inadequate defense.

Of at least equal importance in protection is the cellular immune response (Chaps. 12 and 13) mediated by a different subset of lymphocytes called T cells. Arising in the thymus, T cells circulate in the bloodstream and lymphatic vessels; T cells also migrate through the extracellular spaces. A well-known measure of the cellular response is the reaction to tuberculin, an extract of tubercle bacilli. This response is called the tuberculin reaction (Chaps. 13 and 17), also known as delayed hypersensitivity. The most prominent feature of tuberculin hypersensitivity is the effusion of lymphocytes into the tissues and especially into the areas adjacent to small vessels—the perivascular cuffing so typical of cellular immune responses. This type of inflammatory response is observed only in persons who already have been immunized. The tiny fraction of T cells (less than 1 in 10,000) reactive to tuberculin proliferates to form a clone of reactive cells after the initial exposure. This tuberculin-specific clone releases a multitude of effector molecules to produce a detectable reaction on subsequent exposure, another example of clonal expansion and immunologic memory (anamnestic or secondary response).

The vascular network of the immune system is comprised of lymph vessels, which are thin-walled structures with valves, the lymph capillaries. These are analogous to blood capillaries, but the lymphatics are freely permeable to tissue fluids (lymph) and to migrating lymphocytes and macrophages. The lymph fluid and cells are pumped by contractions of the skeletal muscles through the lymph vessels into the thoracic duct and then into the vena cava, where they rejoin the blood. The lymph nodes, which are placed at strategic locations, interrupt the returning lymph and filter it through fine sinusoids lined with dendritic cells that trap particulate matter and expose it to phagocytic cells and lymphocytes (Chap. 13). Antibodies and primed lymphocytes are released into the efferent lymph.

Although the immunologist is mainly concerned with the proteins and cells of the lymph, the physician and surgeon are concerned with the integrity of the lymph channels; the lymphatic circulation is indispensable for the homeostasis of the circulatory system. If the lymphatics draining the peritoneum are blocked, ascites fluid collects. Blockage of the peripheral lymphatics results in edema of the affected limb. Edema of the upper extremities is a frequent complication of radical mastectomy, whereas elephantiasis can occur when deposits of parasites of metastatic tumor cells block the ilial or femoral lymphatics.

Response to infection is the most obvious function of the immune system. Patients in whom immunity is impaired characteristically suffer and often die from chronic infection. The most devastating deficiency is called, appropriately, severe combined immunodeficiency syndrome (SCID). The "boy in the bubble" who died from infection when brought into contact with microorganisms in the outside world was an example of a patient with SCID. This patient, whose life was dramatized in a movie, remained healthy indefinitely, provided he was maintained constantly in a germfree environment. He was given a bone marrow transplant in an attempt to provide him with a functional immune system and was brought out of the isolation room. Unfortunately, the marrow transplant was not successful, and he died from sepsis; other children treated with a bone marrow transplant have been more fortunate (Chap. 18). Acquired immunodeficiency syndrome (AIDS) is another example of an immunodeficiency disease with a devastatingly high mortality rate from infection. The increased risk of death from infection extends even to organisms such as *Pneumocystis,* which normally are not regarded as dangerous. However, as will become apparent, defense against infection is by no means the only function of the immune system, although this function is understood best.

The keystone of immune responsiveness is the ability to discriminate between molecules found within the individual (self) and those foreign to the individual. Foreign molecules are recognized as non-self or altered self. Altered self can take many forms. The development of immunity to altered self leads to the autoimmune destructive lesions of lupus erythematosus, rheumatism, and many other autoaggressive diseases of varying severity (Chap. 17). Conversely, reactions against altered self are essential for the removal of dead or dying cells, including red blood cells that change chemically as they age. A tumor cell can be regarded as altered self and although tumors can acquire many evasive defenses, immunity against tumors may slow their growth or, under some circumstances, paradoxically enhance it (Chap. 20). To the mother, her fetus is part self and part non-self. The non-self triggers an immune response. Why this response does not lead to spontaneous abortion is one of the most fascinating topics in immunology (Chap. 14). Knowledge of the concepts of self and non-self and of clonal responsiveness is essential for understanding the intricacies of the immune system.

States of Immunity. Immunity can be active, adoptive, or passive. Active immunity follows exposure to antigen as explained previously. Adoptive immunity is a term used to describe immunity that results when lymphoid cells are transferred from an immune to a nonimmune host, and passive immunity results from the transfer of serum or colostrum (the early secretions of the mammary gland after parturition) from an immune to a nonimmune subject. The human infant is passively immunized by the transplacental passage of immunoglobulins, mainly IgG, in utero. Many domestic animals, notably the pig, goat, and sheep, are born agammaglobulinemic because their placentation is such that globulins cannot pass to the fetal circulation. The newborn is achlorhydric, and antibodies from the colostrum pass through the gut within a few hours of birth, raising the immunoglobulin level to maternal levels. The importance of passive immunity can be demonstrated by depriving piglets of colostrum; such piglets die of overwhelming infections within 48 hours if they are not fed colostrum or if they are not protected in a germfree environment. The importance of colostrum to humans is controversial because human infants receive transplacental IgG, but there is a consensus that milk has a protective role against enteric organisms in the gut. Active immunity develops as the individual is exposed to environmental antigens. Active immunity is the method of choice for the protection of an individual. The therapeutic transfer of passive immunity, for example, to tetanus, was once an important and sometimes lifesaving procedure. It is now little used because (1) it is of short duration because the transferred antibody is soon metabolized and is not replaced; (2) the serum used was frequently from immune animals, and the recipient soon produced antibody to the animal serum and developed serum sickness if treatment with that serum were repeated; and (3) much more is known about the production of highly effective vaccines. Passive immunization with human globulin is still of value, especially in patients with B cell deficiencies or when protection is required against a threatened epidemic, for example, of hepatitis. Very little is known about adoptive immunity except in the experimental animal, where it has been invaluable for analyzing cellular immune processes. A certain number of maternal lymphocytes can be identified in the infant for 24 to 48 hours after birth, but the maternal cells then disappear from the circulation, and their function, if any, is not known.

Natural Immunity and Cross-Reactivity. Active immunity is acquired through environmental exposure, for example, to *Escherichia coli* ingested orally or to a harmless derivative of the toxin of *Clostridium tetani* by injection. Although the immunity developed is specific for the immunogen, the individual often produces antibodies that may also react with antigens from similar, and sometimes even from very different, sources. A person with group O or A blood who is exposed to *E. coli* will not only develop antibodies to components of the coliform organisms (species-specific antigens) but will also have antibodies reacting with red cells from a donor with group B blood because some of the carbohydrates of *E. coli* resemble those found on the group B red cell. This phenomenon is called cross-reactivity. It is the primary basis for natural immunity since humans are exposed to many endemic organisms. That is, natural immunity is a broad range of active immunity to environmental antigens not deliberately administered. Cross-reactivity also has been exploited for purposes of diagnosis; a subject exposed to typhus develops antibodies that cross-react with antigens of a subline (X19) of *Proteus vulgaris* (it has been easier to use *Proteus* than *Rickettsia* in laboratory diagnostic procedures). Cross-reactivity is also in part responsible for the important phenomenon of herd immunity. When a group of people or animals is exposed to a pathogen causing an epidemic, some individuals will become infected, whereas others will escape. Differences in genetic control of immune responsiveness and previous environmental exposure (natural immunity) act to protect certain individuals who have not been specifically immunized and form the basis for herd immunity. The genetics of regulation of the immune response are discussed in Chapters 14 and 19.

Components of Immune System

Antibodies

General Properties. Antibodies are globular proteins, also referred to as immunoglobulins (Ig). Their basic structure is built around the union of a heavy (H) glycoprotein chain with a light (L) chain. There are five main classes of H chain, α, γ, μ, ϵ, δ, which give the designations of IgA, IgG, IgM, IgE, and IgD to the corresponding complete antibody. There are two main classes of L chain, the κ and λ light chains. Each H and each L chain has a distinctive peptide sequence. Extensive amino acid substitution is a special feature of the peptides adjacent to the amino (N) terminus. This part of the H or L chain is called the variable (V) region. Short sequences within the V region, called hypervariable sequences, determine the physicochemical forces that cause the antibody to bind specifically with antigen (Chap. 12). Thousands of different hypervariable binding sequences are made by the many millions of cells of every individual, with each binding sequence or specificity being faithfully reproduced by the clone of descendants of the progenitor stem, or cell. By contrast, the region closest to the carboxyl terminus is relatively invariable for each class of H or L chain from a given individual, so this portion of the molecule is called the constant (C) region. Although there is great homology between the C regions of all immunoglobulins, certain amino acid sequences in the C region are characteristic of each major class (e.g., δ, μ, α). Limited substitutions characterize subclasses or isotypes (e.g., γ_1, α_2) of the H chain of IgG and IgA of all members of a species. Other limited substitutions of different amino acid residues of the constant region occur only in the κ chains or the γ_1H chains of an individual. These individual specific markings are called allotypes: the Km and Gm allotypes. The function of the V regions is to confer antibody specificity; the function of the C regions, especially of the H chains, is to confer different biologic properties on the immunoglobulin molecule.

As mentioned previously, each complete immunoglobulin molecule has two or more H chains, each with its complementary L chain. Each molecule of IgG, IgD, and IgE typically has two homologous H chains and two homologous L chains. This is known (confusingly) as the monomeric form. IgA occurs in two forms, a lower-molecular-weight monomeric form and a higher-molecular-weight polymeric form with four H and L chains. This doublet is formed by the union of the C regions of two molecules of IgA by means of a J (joining) chain (Chap. 12). Another molecule called the secretory piece is added to the polymeric form whenever IgA-producing lymphocytes pass through mucous membranes. Polymeric IgA typically is found only in secretions in which the glycoprotein secretory piece provides protection against proteolytic digestion (Chap. 18). IgM occurs in three forms. On the surface of lymphocytes it is monomeric; IgM in solution is polymeric and has multiple chains (10 H and 10 L). A third, recently discovered, form has 12 H and 12 L chains. In every case the H and L chains are paired. The H chains (with their attendant L chains) are also bound by disulfide bonds and a single J chain. IgM is usually referred to as a pentamer, even though it has 10 H and 10 L chains, just as secretory IgA, which has four H and four L chains, is called dimeric. This is because the functional valency of IgM is usually 5 and of IgA, 2.

Antibody Production. As mentioned earlier, the immunoglobulins are produced by lymphocytes of a restricted lineage, called B lymphocytes (B cells), and by their direct descendants, known as plasma cells. Approximately 10% of the blood lymphocytes and 5% of thoracic duct lymphocytes are B cells; most B cells and almost all plasma cells, however, reside in specialized structures known as the peripheral lymphoid organs. The peripheral lymphoid organs are the spleen, the lymph nodes, and various lymphoid aggregates such as tonsils, adenoids, Peyer's patches, and the appendix. B cell precursors are present in the yolk sac, fetal liver, and bone marrow (Chap. 13). Birds possess a unique central lymphoid organ, the bursa of Fabricius, in which B cell differentiation occurs. In mammals there is no bursa, and the bone marrow and peripheral lymphoid organs appear to have taken over many of its functions in regulating differentiation.

Immature or pre-B lymphocytes do not secrete immunoglobulins. They do, however, synthesize them and are recognizable as B cell precursors. The scanty cytoplasm of pre-B cells of man or mouse can be stained by fluoresceinated anti-immunoglobulin obtained by immunizing an animal from a different species, often a goat or a rabbit, with purified Ig or L chains from a human or a mouse. As B cells mature, more Ig is formed. One form of IgM has an additional hydrophobic sequence that becomes inserted into the plasma membrane as surface immunoglobulin (sIg) (Chaps. 12 and 13). sIg acts as the membrane receptor for antigen on B cells. Although the first sIg to appear in ontogeny is IgM, as the B cell matures, sIgD is also found. At about this stage the mature B cell can be stimulated by antigen in the presence of various accessory molecules to secrete immunoglobulin into the environment. Even though IgM remains the predominant sIg of a B cell, the antibody it secretes may be of another class because of molecular rearrangements that join the V-region gene of the H chain to different C-region genes during maturation. The modification that occurs as B cells mature is called class switching. With maturation the antibody retains its original specificity, but it has a different C region; hence it has different biologic properties (Chap. 12).

Although the cell has two sets of V-region genes (alleles), only one allele is active; one cell makes only one immunoglobulin (allelic suppression). When the cell switches from IgM production to, for example, IgA, the cell-surface immunoglobulin usually remains IgM and is not replaced. Because no further rearrangement of the V-region genes can occur, the specificity of binding of the original IgM remains unchanged, and the IgA formed after class switching (new IgA) has the same specificity as that of the IgM.

Up to this stage the B cell is capable of mitosis and, in dividing, forms a clone of cells making the same antibody (clonal expansion). When the B cell reaches the final stage of differentiation as a plasma cell, it rapidly secretes many thousands of Ig molecules. The plasma cell carries very little sIg, and there are changes (losses and gains) in the production of several cell-surface glycoproteins. These membrane-associated (or membrane-inserted) glycoproteins are referred to as differentiation antigens (Chap. 13). The fully differentiated plasma cell rarely divides or enters the bloodstream. Exceptions occur in the rare plasma cell malignancy, multiple myeloma, and in some very severe infections.

Antibody Distribution and Function. The size of the molecule is one of the factors determining the tissue distribution of an immunoglobulin. IgG is found in the blood and tissue spaces. IgM, being larger, is unable to pass through capillary walls easily and is mainly restricted to the bloodstream. It does not cross the placenta. The healthy newborn infant has no IgM unless the placenta has become inflamed as in congenital measles or syphilis (Chap. 18). IgA is, in its multimeric form, the immunoglobulin of mucous surfaces and in its monomeric form is a minor immunoglobulin in the blood. IgG, IgM, and IgA all have protective functions against microorganisms or their products. IgE is present in very low concentration in the bloodstream and tends to be bound, through its Fc, by IgE receptors on the surface of two related and highly specialized granular cells known as tissue mast cells and blood basophils. When IgE bound to a mast cell reacts with its appropriate antigen, the cell releases histamine and other permeases from its granules; thus IgE is the immunoglobulin responsible for allergic or anaphylactic reactions (Chap. 17). No function is yet known for IgD other than as a membrane receptor, and this immunoglobulin might have remained unknown but for the rare uncontrolled proliferation of IgD-producing plasma cells in IgD myelomas. Because it is found on the surface of maturing B lymphocytes, IgD is believed to play a role in preventing immunologic tolerance (Chap. 13).

A typical immune response results in the stimulation of many different lymphocytes; some form antibody, and others do not. Those that do not are described below under "Cellular Aspects of Immunity." Even those cells that form antibody have different lineages. Whereas the descendants of single lymphocyte form a clone, conventional antibody responses stimulate to a greater or lesser extent a large number of B cells of somewhat differing specificity.

Most natural-product antigens are large and complex molecules, so the response to these molecules is typically polyclonal and includes many antibody molecules that differ in binding affinities. Of particular importance for diagnostic, therapeutic, and investigational purposes are those exceptional antibodies that are formed by a single clone of antibody-producing cells. These are called monoclonal antibodies. Monoclonal antibodies are excessively rare in the natural state but are produced in the laboratory by fusing a single antibody-producing lymphocyte to a myeloma cell to form a hybrid. The hybrid can proliferate to form a cell line called a hybridoma (Chap. 12). The myeloma cell used for fusion is usually a doubly deficient mutant unable to secrete myeloma protein and lacking thymidine kinase (tk^-). Normal untransformed B lymphocytes do not proliferate in vitro but can supply tk^- to the tk^- fusion partner. Production of specific immunoglobulin and the ability to survive in the absence of thymidine are then controlled by the B cell partner of the fusion; the myeloma partner contributes an unlimited capacity to proliferate. A conventional antibody can be likened to the white light of a searchlight and a monoclonal antibody to the monochromatic light of a laser beam. Antibodies formed as a consequence of immunization are focused to a considerable extent but do not approach the exquisite specificity of monoclonal antibody produced in the laboratory.

Molecular Genetics: The Generation of Diversity

Antibody diversity is generated by gene rearrangements that affect a cluster of H-chain genes on the twelfth (human) chromosome. The cluster of H chain genes can be called a haplotype. The H-chain haplotype includes four classes of gene called V (for variability), D (for diversity), J (for joining), and C (for constant) region genes. In the germline state the genes are quite far apart, and they remain that way in the liver and other nonlymphoid tissues. In the B lymphocyte one of several hundred V genes, together with its leader sequence, is translocated to lie close to one of about a dozen D genes and one of four J genes to form a VDJ complex. This complex constitutes the immunologic profile of the H chain of that B cell and its progeny. In the early B cell the VDJ complex lies close to the μ constant region gene, but by excision of portions of the C region, it may be translocated to lie next to a δ, γ, ε, or α C region gene (Chap. 12). The transcribed RNA is processed to splice out the intervening sequences, and the polyadenylated RNA is translated to make the immunoglobulin H chain. Only one such transcription to an RNA occurs in each cell; the daughter cells of a clone behave in the same way. Cells from two clones that select the same V segment may use a different D or J. This gives an H chain of somewhat different binding affinity. Under the influence of accessory factors, the VDJ sequence of the H chain can be translocated to a different C_H gene as the response matures in an irreversible process. Most of the amino acids of the H chain come from the C-region genes. These code for the amino acids of three or four C_H domains, D codes for only three amino acids, and J codes for 12 amino acids. Although isolated H chains can bind antigen, the affinity is greatly augmented by the acquisition of a κ or λ L chain that has been generated by a similar genetic mechanism. The L-chain genes, however, lack D segments; thus the number of combinations is smaller, and the specificity is of necessity different.

Similar genetic mechanisms govern the generation of the α- and β-receptor genes of the T cell. The Ig genes remain in the germline (unrearranged) configuration in T cells and in all other somatic cells; conversely, the T cell receptor genes rearrange in maturing T cells, but the Ig genes remain in the germline state in non-B cells. These processes, which are unique to the immune system, are described in detail in Chapters 12 and 13.

Antigens

Antigen is the traditional name given to a molecule that can be bound by the combining site of an antibody; diphtheria toxin is an antigen in the classic sense (Chap. 12). However, because the combining site of an antibody molecule forms a relatively small cavity that can only encompass a structure not much larger than a pentapeptide, it is obvious that the whole toxin is bigger than a single antigen. Various terms have been coined for that part of an antigenic molecule that is actually bound. Antigenic site, ligand, and epitope are terms that have frequently been used. Furthermore, although an antigen is defined as a structure that is capable of being recognized by an antibody, some antigenic substances (immunogens) can stimulate immunity, whereas others (haptens) cannot. A hapten, which by itself is not immunogenic, can become an immunogen when combined with another molecule called a carrier. Haptens are small and can be of any chemical class (from azobenzene arsenate to nucleotide, to peptide, to fucose). Most carriers are large proteins, commonly having a molecular weight of more than 10,000, although polysaccharides and peptides can also be carriers. In addition, a simple chemical may bind to the lysine, cysteine, or tyrosine of a protein; thus the body's own proteins can become carriers. This feature becomes especially important in the contact hypersensitivity to allergens such as the urushiols of poison ivy or the simple chemicals such as dinitrobenzene or formaldehyde. In a person with contact hypersensitivity the carrier protein is in the skin, but other proteins on red cells or platelets, for example, can also serve as carriers.

Certain portions of a protein or glycoprotein molecule may be more highly charged or may be more accessible than others. These portions are sometimes called the immunodominant loops or sites; this term is also being replaced by the term *epitope*. Myoglobin has at least five separate oligopeptide epitopes, and albumin has a similar number; the epitope of a blood group antigen may consist of four or five monosaccharides or amino sugars forming a complex with a protein, and more than one such epitope may be part of a linear array. In a protein with a tertiary structure the component molecules need not be sequential members of a peptide chain to be recognized by B cells (Chap. 17). T cells, however, do usually recognize linear sequences. Thus it is apparent that the fine specificities of B cells differ from those of T cells, although both "see" the same molecule.

Consequences of the Combination of Antibody with Antigen

Antibody-antigen reactions are exothermic and occur almost instantaneously. The rate of reaction is influenced by temperature and concentration and by the binding constant for each antibody, according to the laws of mass action. However, the gross manifestation of antibody-antigen reactions, through which antibody-antigen reactions are usually observed, involves steps other than simple binding; it takes minutes to hours to appear and may involve many intermediates. One example already cited is the release of histamine from a tissue mast cell after the reaction of IgE with antigen. Other consequences are the activation of a complex series of blood proteins known collectively as the complement cascade (Chap. 15) or the release of powerful mediators called lymphokines (Chap. 17). Some of the lymphokines or accessory factors are described below.

The increased uptake by phagocytic cells of microorganisms in the presence of antibody is called opsonization. This process, one of the first activities of antibodies to be detected, is of fundamental importance in the defense against infection. Only complement and low concentrations of antibodies are needed, and the rate of uptake of bacteria by granular cells in the blood and by monocytes and polymorphonuclear neutrophils (PMNs) can be increased 100-fold.

Another important feature of antibody is its ability to form large complexes with soluble antigen. This occurs when both antibody and antigen are multivalent and when neither is present in great excess. Because even the smallest of the antibodies (e.g., IgG) is divalent and the same epitope may be present several times in a large molecule of antigen, a lattice forms. In vitro the lattice becomes so large that the complexes precipitate from solution. Antibodies with this property therefore are known as precipitins. In vivo the complexes can be trapped during filtration through the kidney's glomerulus. The trapped complexes can fix complement and can also be chemotactic for PMNs. In either event damage to the glomerular basement membrane triggers that form of glomerulonephritis found in patients with serum sickness. Immune complexes can also form in the joints and in other locations and are responsible for many autoimmune or autoaggressive diseases (Chap. 17).

The Complement Cascade

Complement is the collective term used to describe a family of proteins and glycoproteins with nearly 20 members. It has two main branches: the classic and the alternative (or alternate) pathways. The classic pathway usually is activated when two or more molecules of certain classes of antibody lie close to each other as they bind to antigen. The antigens can be identical repeating units or, when the antibody is polyvalent, dissimilar epitopes of a complex molecule. In the presence of calcium three proteins, C1q, r, and s, combine to form the first component, C1, which binds to the adjacent constant portions of the bound antibodies. The bound C1 displays enzymatic activity and cleaves the next component, unfortunately named C4 (because the components were named in the order of their discovery and not in their sequence of activation), to a fragment, C4b. The C4b binds to the cell surface if the antigen is on a red cell membrane and then can bind and cleave C2 to reveal its enzymatically active site, C2a. The complex C4b2a, which is called C3 convertase, then cleaves C3 to the enzymatically active C3b. Activated C3b can trigger the so-called late components, and a C567 complex soon forms, setting the stage for C8 and C9, which together are known as the attack complex because they are capable of forming a lesion in the surface of a cell (Chap. 15).

The critical third component can also be activated by many other agents, including cobra venom, yeast cell walls, and bacterial endotoxin. This is called the alternative pathway in which C3 is enzymatically activated by an alternative pathway C3 convertase without the need for antibody binding or the C1, C4, and C2 activation sequence. It became notorious not only because it could lead to non-antibody-mediated cytolysis but because during investigations of this initially controversial process several previously unknown molecules with biologically active properties were found to have been released. Best known of these are C5a and C3a, which are chemotactic and inflammatory. More recently, it has been found that C4a fixed during activation of the classic pathway has some similar but weaker biologic effects. The intricate enzymatic processes, the varied activities of the released peptides, and the system of checks and balances that normally inhibit the indiscriminate activation of these powerful agents are described in Chapters 15 and 17. Although complement usually is measured by the lysis of sheep red cells coated with limiting amounts of antibody, the most important biologic activities are probably those mediated by C3a and C5a and include immune adherance, chemotaxis, and opsonization.

Cellular Aspects of Immunity

Up to this point the antibodies formed by the B lymphocytes and the plasma cells have been considered the primary agents of immunity. Reactions carried out by antibodies are called humoral immune reactions. These topics were dealt with first because they are relatively straightforward. However, the intervention of the other great lineage of cells, the thymus-derived (or T) lymphocytes, is required for most immune responses. T cells, one of the most primitive and most fundamental of the body's defenses, interact with B cells for the production of antibody against most antigens. The antigens that require the intervention of T cells to trigger antibody production by B cells are called T-dependent antigens. The activities of T cells, other lymphoid cells called natural killer (NK) cells, and macrophages are known collectively as cellular immunity. The cellular and humoral defense systems interdigitate and regulate each other in an intricate manner (Chap. 13).

Thymus, Other Lymphoid Organs, and the T Cell. During development the thymus develops as an outgrowth from the third and fourth pharyngeal pouches. Although the anatomy of the thymus differs considerably in different species, it basically consists of a mass of tightly packed mononuclear cells forming a cortex around a looser medulla rich in epithelial elements. The epithelial cells are responsible for the differentiation and maturation of lymphocytes. The thymus is regarded as a central lymphoid organ, as opposed to the spleen and lymph nodes, which are regarded as peripheral lymphoid organs. Unlike B cells, mature T cells do not carry surface immunoglobulins, but they do express T cell receptors (TCRs) with idiotypes that can be recognized through binding studies with the appropriate monoclonal antibodies. T cells have the special property of recognizing antigens only when these antigens are presented together with certain self-antigens, products of the major histocompatibility complex (MHC) (Chaps. 13 and 14), whereas B cells can "see" antigen directly.

T Cell Maturation and Proliferation, Clonal Selection. Animals and birds deprived of their thymus at birth or genetically lacking a thymus are immunodeficient. They cannot reject grafts of foreign tissue, and they are subject to infections, especially viral infections (Chap. 18). An animal that has been immunocompetent can be converted experimentally to immunodeficiency by thymectomy combined with irradiation. An intact thymus and an adequate number of T lymphocytes are essential to health. With increasing age, the thymus atrophies, and its lymphocyte output decreases but does not cease. Nonetheless, by adulthood, sufficient numbers of mature T lymphocytes with a wide spectrum of reactivities have been seeded into the peripheral lymph nodes (T cell memory).

T cell precursors, like B cell precursors, are formed early in embryonic life and arise from primitive stem cells in the fetal yolk sac and liver. The maturation of T cells can be followed through changes in surface markers. The primitive T cells migrate to the thymus and are found in the superficial layers of the cortex. Called double-negative cells because they lack the CD4 and CD8 markers of more mature cells, they do express the CD3 pan–T cell receptor. Thymic cells multiply rapidly and progress through the cortex to the medulla, and the majority then carry both the CD4 and CD8 markers (double positive). Mature T cells in the periphery and 5% to 10% of the cells in the thymus carry the CD4 or CD8 marker. Maturation within the thymus depends on complex interactions with thymic epithelial cells in which certain cell surface markers called lymphocyte function antigen (LFA) 2 and LFA3 interact. LFA2 found on the T cell and LFA3 on the epithelium bind; their interaction appears to be essential for T cell maturation. This rapidly evolving area of immunology is dealt with in Chapter 16, which also describes the properties of some of the many T cell differention markers so far reported.

The processes of T cell maturation baffled immunologists until recently. One peculiarity recognized in early studies was the extraordinary wastage that occurs; 95% of cells in the thymus never leave it. Burnet attempted to explain this by assuming that random genetic rearrangements (mutations) that occur during lymphoid maturation before birth would give rise to large numbers of autoreactive cells that underwent self-destruction. He believed that after birth the mutation rate fell and that stimulation by exogenous antigen then caused a nonharmful clonal proliferation. This was the basis for Burnet's clonal selection hypothesis. The clonal selection theory has been valuable in promoting experiments to prove or disprove its validity. The theory led immunologists to explore the idiopathic avoidance of autoimmunity but did not provide a complete explanation for a phenomenon Ehrlich named "horror autotoxicus." It is now known that production of immature cells continues after birth and that T cells, while in the thymus, can still rearrange their cell receptor into adult life. The reason why the vast majority of thymic lymphocytes die while still in the thymus remains unknown. Jerne has suggested that the trigger is provided by an encounter with autologous histocompatibility antigen.

The thymus is regarded as one of several privileged sites that are shielded from antigen under normal conditions. (The brain, the testes, and the anterior chamber of the eye are also privileged sites.) Thus the immature T cell rarely, if ever, encounters environmental antigens. When it reaches the periphery, it meets exogenous antigen for the first time, usually in the paracortical areas of the lymph node, where proliferation and final maturation occur.

Antigen Presentation, Accessory Molecules

The activation of both T and B lymphocytes requires two signals or triggers. Most antibody (B cell) responses are T dependent. In the case of the T-dependent B cell response, one signal is usually provided by the combination of sIg with its homologous antigen. The second signal may be provided by a helper T cell primed to the antigen or by one of several B cell–activating factors produced by activated T cells. These factors include a variety of cytokines (IL2, IL4, IL5, and IL6). T-independent antigens are usually characterized by repetitive sequences on the antigen. This repetitive sequence can cross-link two sIg molecules directly and thus activate the B cell directly. For T cell activation, one signal is provided by a suitably processed antigen offered by an antigen-presenting cell (APC). The APC must express the same class II major histocompatibility complex (MHC) molecule (see below) as is found on the responding cell (MHC restriction). Many different cell types can act as an APC. The B cell is believed to be the most efficient at low antigen concentrations, but because of the great diversity of specificities, only a few B cells of the appropriate specificity may be present. Macrophages and related cells, including dendritic cells and Langerhans' cells of the skin, are less effective in presentation but act nonspecifically; thus there are more of these cells to present. Macrophages also process antigens. Processing involves internalization of antigen and may include its partial digestion to peptides. It is probable that the antigenic peptide is brought into a cleft in the class II molecule during this internalization in the endosomes of the APC. The class II molecule, at this stage, forms a complex with a heavy glycosylated carrier molecule called an I chain, which is then destroyed by proteolysis as the peptide–class II complex is transported to the surface.

During helper T cell (T_h) activation, numerous accessory factors or lymphokines are produced. Best known are the interleukins (IL). Interleukin 1 (IL-1), produced by macrophages and other cells during antigen processing, can act as a second signal for T cells. IL-2, produced by various subsets of T cells, is a growth factor for T cells and may act in B cell differentiation. IL-3 induces the differentiation of a diversity of stem cells. Several other factors (e.g., for eosinophils) have also been described. The corresponding receptors for these and other molecules serve as differentiation markers and are designated as a cluster of differentiation antigens (CD). These are described in the appropriate chapters (e.g., Chaps. 12, 13, 16, and 17).

During or after the activation of T_h, suppressor T cells (T_s) are also activated. It is believed that T_s produce their effects by releasing T-suppressor substances, but these substances have not yet been adequately characterized. Whereas T_h usually carry the cell-surface marker CD4 (formerly T4), T_s usually, but not invariably, carry the marker CD8 (T8), as do cytotoxic T cells. Clinically, the T4:T8 ratio often is used to assess the immune status of immunosuppressed patients after organ transplantation or in various immunodeficiency states. Because CD8 is also a marker for cytotoxic or effector T cells (T_c), a low CD4 number is taken as inadequate help, and low CD8 numbers indicate inadequate effector cell function.

Cell-Cell Collaboration and the Major Histocompatibility Complex

The major histocompatibility complex (MHC) is a collection of highly polymorphic genes grouped in two or more clusters on an autosome. These genes code for cell surface recognition molecules. This array is known as a histocompatibility complex because it was first recognized through the part it plays in the rejection of transplants. There are many transplantation antigens (in the mouse well over 100 have been detected), but the MHC stood out from all the other histocompatibility antigens because transplants from donors differing from the recipient at the MHC were rapidly rejected, and the rejection was difficult to control with immunosuppressive drugs or X-irradiation. The rejection due to incompatibility for other H antigens was slower, weaker, and easier to suppress, so these were called minor H antigens. It is now known that the MHC is involved in the presentation of protein antigens and in the recognition of self and nonself. The MHC probably plays a major part in almost every immunologic reaction.

The human MHC is called HLA and that of the mouse, H-2; every mammalian and avian species so far tested has an MHC. Most of the MHC antigens of other species resemble the intensively studied representatives HLA and H-2 very closely, although there are differences in organization and degree of polymorphism. These differences might be expected considering the millions of years of separation from a primitive common ancestor.

The most conspicuous MHC antigens are cell surface glycoproteins found on virtually every cell and tissue of the body and designated class I antigens. These are heterodimers of an H chain that is noncovalently bound to a small, highly conserved (invariable) molecule called $\beta 2$ microglobulin. The class I H-chain genes on the MHC haplotype have a leader sequence and exons for three extracellular domains, $\alpha 1$, $\alpha 2$, and $\alpha 3$. Typically $\alpha 1$ and $\alpha 2$ differ markedly from individual to individual within the species; they are highly polymorphic. Because they differ from individual to individual, the molecules are also called alloantigens. The H chain also carries one or two carbohydrate side chains and has a molecular weight of approximately 45,000 daltons. The HLA system of man has six separate class I products. Of these, HLA-A and HLA-B are highly polymorphic, and HLA-C is less so. So-called nonclassic genes, HLA-E, HLA-F, and HLA-G, are also expressed; they have only one known allele each in man, but variants of HLA-E and HLA-F, differing by approximately six amino acids, occur in primates.

The tertiary structure of the intact class I molecule is of

extreme interest. A series of beta sheets and two alpha helices form a groove. This groove is frequently occupied by a peptide. Current evidence suggests that the groove in the MHC molecule presents the antigenic peptide to a T cell.

Another series of MHC antigens called class II is controlled by the corresponding class II region of the MHC haplotype. The class II antigens are heterodimers of a heavy (α) and a light (β) chain. Like those molecules in class I, the two molecules are not covalently bound, but unlike those in class I most of the polymorphism in the HLA class II antigens is in the β chain. Class II antigens are not expressed on all classes of cells; they are present on B cells, macrophages, and dendritic cells. They frequently are present on endothelial cells, some melanoma (tumor) cells, and activated T cells. They are present transiently on other cell types during rapid cell division. The human class II antigens are HLA-DP, HLA-DQ, and HLA-DR. A fourth representative originally was called DO-DX. The genes for DO, now called DNA, and DX, now called DOB, are separate from each other, and as might be anticipated, very little is known about DO-DX. Only one α chain gene is expressed for DP, DR, and DO, but there may be two or three expressed DRβ chain genes. There are numerous pseudogenes in both class I and class II. The three-dimensional structure of class II is very similar to that of class I, but the peptides presented and the manner of presentation are different. The functioning of the class II molecules is detailed in Chapter 14.

The MHC of man is part of the short arm of chromosome 6. The class II genes lie closest to the centromere, and HLA-A is the most distal. The class II and class I regions are separated by a chromosomal segment carrying a number of immunologically important genes, including genes for complement components C2, C4 and factor B. Also present on this segment—sometimes called the class III region—are two genes for tumor necrosis factors α and β and two genes for the enzyme 21-hydroxylase.

The MHC haplotype of the mouse, H-2, also carries these genes; it also has one set of nonclassic class I–like MHC genes called Qa and another set called TL. These genes are expressed only on some cell types and often only during certain stages of differentiation (differentiation antigens). TL, for example, is so named because it is present on cells in the thymus and on a subset of T cell leukemias. A different set, called BG, which is expressed on red cells and lymphocytes, is linked to the chicken MHC. These antigens all resemble those in class I in having an H chain bound to β2m. It is believed that the MHC complex and class I, class II, and the nonclassic MHC genes arose from a single immunoglobulin-like gene that underwent repeated duplication and modification. The polymorphism appears to be due to a special form of mutation called gene conversion, which is a common feature of this gene family. Gene conversion is a basic genetic mechanism, which was first described in yeasts and fungi, and may be important for maintaining polymorphism. This hypothesis suggests that short DNA sequences of some of the invariable genes, including HLA-E in man, H-2L in the mouse, and, perhaps, some of the pseudogenes, can be shuffled and translocated into the sequences of the major polymorphic genes. In mammals, genetic variability is essential for the ability to distinguish self from non-self. A mouse or a man can sense that a virally modified protein or a chemically modified protein is non-self. Then T cell immunity against the modified protein can be developed, and it can destroy the tumor cell or the virally transformed cell carrying the foreign message. MHC variability, especially class II variability, is therefore an integral part of the repertoire of T cell responsiveness and of T-dependent antibody formation.

Perversions of the immune response to infection are autoimmunity and allograft rejection. A persistent virus, other microorganisms, or even smaller fragments of microbial invaders can modify body cells and thus fuel a persistent T cell and antibody response responsible for many degenerative autoaggressive processes (Chap. 17). The part played by the MHC in graft rejection has been thoroughly established through genetic studies. Grafts of skin, spleen, ovary, tumor, heart, kidney, and bone marrow were exchanged in the mouse, and grafts of skin, kidney, cornea, and bone marrow were used in man. In the mouse, grafts taken from one genetically homozygous, uniform, inbred strain were transplanted to a second inbred strain or to various hybrids between the two strains. From these studies were derived the "laws" of transplantation. Although this type of experiment could not be done in man, comparable studies have been carried out in nuclear human families. Because the HLA gene cluster, or haplotype, is inherited as a gametic unit, each parent can possess only two HLA haplotypes: a and b or c and d. A parent can pass on only one of these haplotypes to each child, so each child inherits a and c, a and d, b and c, or b and d. Siblings who inherit the same pair of haplotypes (e.g., ac and ac) are called HLA identical. Siblings who inherit the same haplotype from one parent but different haplotypes from the other parent (e.g., ac and ad) are called haploidentical; and two who inherit different pairs of haplotypes (e.g., ac and bd) are haplodistinct. In a series of more than 600 interfamilial skin grafts the median survival time of HLA identical skin grafts was 23 days; haploidentical graft survival, 15 days; and haplodistinct graft survival, 11 days. This series of graft exchanges proved the importance of HLA in skin grafting. The fact that HLA identical grafts were rejected at all showed the independent inheritance (segregation) of minor histocompatibility antigens. Kidney grafts behaved similarly. These studies are considered in Chapter 14, which also discusses the role of HLA in febrile transfusion reactions.

Clinical and Applied Immunology

Information about the clinical problems encountered by patients with immunodeficiency, designated "experiments of nature" by Robert Good, have provided most of the information we have about the functioning of the human immunologic defenses. The chapter on immunologic deficiencies (Chap. 18) should be read in conjunction with the chapters on immunopathology (Chap. 17), infection (Chap. 19), and tumors (Chap. 20) because these topics are closely interrelated.

T Cell Function and Immunopathologic States

The suppressor and helper functions of the corresponding subsets of T cells have been clearly defined in clinical and in experimental situations. A number of lymphocytic leukemias, for example, represent clones of T cells frozen in their differentiation stages by the oncogenic process. Some leukemic lymphocytes carry out normal functions; Sézary cell leukemia can provide a source of pure suppressor cells. The role of T-effector cells and of another subset of lymphocyte, the null or NK cell, has been established by in vitro experiments. The demonstration of their role in killing tumor cells in vivo has been inferred by observations of patients with depressed T cell function; these subjects have an increased incidence of leukemia. Infants with congenital absence of the thymus (DiGeorge's syndrome) who have normal immunoglobulin levels but impaired T cell function (Chap. 18) reject skin grafts slowly, have absent or weak cutaneous hypersensitivity responses to the *Candida* antigen or dinitrochlorobenzene (both of which measure T cell function), and are unduly susceptible to infection from a wide range of infectious agents. Transplant patients are treated with immunosuppressive agents to minimize the risk of rejection. One price such patients may pay for retaining their transplanted kidney or heart is an increased risk of lymphoma or leukemia (Chap. 17). A more frequent threat is chronic infection (Chap. 19). Cytomegalovirus is a common invader of the lungs of kidney transplant recipients. Pregnancy often results in a subtle impairment of T cell function (Chap. 20), but fortunately the infections of pregnancy may be no more serious than oral or vaginal candidiasis. Infection is common in all subjects with impaired T cell reactivity; resistance to infection develops when the subjects are successfully reconstituted with thymic tissue.

Although the precise manner in which T cells protect against microorganisms is not known, three cellular functions that are easily demonstrated in vitro may operate in vivo: antibody-dependent cell-mediated cytotoxicity (ADCC), natural killing (NK), and cell-mediated lympholysis (CML) (Chap. 19). ADCC depends on the ability of mononuclear cells from nonimmune subjects to lyse sensitive target cells in the presence of even minute traces of antibody; NK is the lytic capacity of a special subset of nonimmune lymphocytes to lyse other target cells in the absence of antibody; and CML is a cytolytic function of T_c from previously immunized subjects against antigens (usually of the MHC) of the donor. ADCC has been described as a normal mechanism for eliminating effete red cells, and NK and CML are thought to have a role in the elimination of virally infected cells or of some tumor cells.

Immunodeficiency, Infection

Chapters 18 and 19 provide some detailed links between the disciplines of immunology and microbiology. Chapter 18, Abnormal Development of the Immune System, details the severe, often fatal consequences not only of the failure of the system to develop because of abnormal thymic development but also of single component deficiencies. Even abnormally high levels of Ig can disturb host defenses. Abnormally high IgE (and IgD) with normal IgG, IgM, and IgA is a laboratory finding in some patients with recurrent staphylococcal abcesses and pneumonia. Patients with IgA deficiencies demonstrate the importance of this immunoglobulin to the defense of mucous surfaces and are liable to infections of the respiratory, gastrointestinal, and urinary systems. Even the inability to produce secretory component has led to severe diarrhea.

Defects in T cells are associated with a wide spectrum of diseases, including viral and protozoan infections. Infections associated with the failure of expression of the MHC antigens illustrate the dependence of T cells on the MHC for the recognition of foreignness. Chapter 18 also illustrates the interdependence of different systems as illustrated by the Wiscott-Aldrich syndrome, which is due to a gene on the X chromosome. Patients with this syndrome have abnormal platelets and a bleeding tendency. They have abnormal skin responses and severe atopic dermatitis and suffer from infections, especially with encapsulated organisms, deficient humoral responses, and increased rates of turnover of all classes of immunoglobin. These and other immunodeficient patients show clear indications of the importance of a fully functional immune system to prevent tumor growth. More than 10% of patients with Wiscott-Aldrich syndrome die from their malignancies. Even more complex interactions are apparent in patients with ataxia-telangiectasia, which affects the cerebellum, the skin, T cell function, and DNA repair. The gene is on chromosome 11, but break points are often found on chromosomes 7 and 14, involving the genes for T cell receptors and the immunoglobulin genes.

The clinical importance of adhesion molecules (Chap. 16) is manifested by patients with leukocyte adhesion deficiency (LAD) (Chap. 18). Cytotoxic lymphocyte function is decreased, and these patients develop severe bacterial and fungal infections; rather surprisingly, viral infections are not prominent. The manner in which all of the immune systems are brought together for the protection of the individual against bacterial, viral, and rickettsial fungal and parasitic diseases is presented in Chapter 19.

Autoimmunity

Excessive or uncontrolled reactivity of any of the components of the immune system has grave consequences. Whereas a low level of responsiveness to self antigens is constantly required for self-surveillance, augmented levels lead to autoaggressive disease. The list of diseases from known or suspected immunologic reactivity against self antigens is steadily expanding. Hashimoto's thyroiditis, lupus erythematosus, and rheumatoid arthritis are but a few of the known autoaggressive diseases discussed in Chapter 17. The list of suspected autoimmune diseases is much longer and includes many cases of immune complex disease. In some instances (e.g., Goodpasture's syndrome) the complexes fix complement and can be visualized by indirect fluorescence microscopy. Many chronic lupuslike syndromes are probably sustained by the release of viral or microbial antigens, but unless the antigen is known, the diagnosis may be difficult to make. In many instances it is possible to produce the disease experimentally. The experimental disease produced by injecting tissue or a tissue extract, usually with an adjuvant to intensify the response, tends to be self-curing and represents a major distinction from the natural disease, which is more frequently progressive. A series of postulates drawn up by Witebsky and comparable to Koch's postulates for microbial infection set rules for the determination of autoimmunity. It is frequently difficult to satisfy Witebsky's postulates for human disease; hence many diseases for which immune cells, antibodies, complement components, and their inhibitors are probably responsible must still be regarded as being of doubtful etiology. This is one of the major areas in which our knowledge of diseases will develop a surer foundation in the future.

Transfusion and Reactions Against Red Cells

Red blood cells carry a rich variety of individual specific antigens. Some of them, although highly immunogenic, are so frequent (public) or so rare (private) that they are seldom involved in untoward reactions, although they can be responsible for immunizing against a fetus or against transfused cells. Severe transfusion reactions usually are due to incompatibility for the antigens of the ABO blood group system. These antigens are often oligosaccharides, usually carried by a protein core. Individuals of blood group O have fucose as the terminal sugar; blood group A persons have an added *N*-acetyl-galactosamine, whereas those of group B have galactose. The glycosyl transferases are expressed in a codominant manner, so persons with glycosyl transferases for galactosamine and galactose have both A and B antigens. Because these sugars are commonly found in bacteria and in foodstuffs, natural antibodies, usually IgM, are frequently formed. Persons of group O usually have natural anti-A and anti-B antibodies, persons of group A have anti-B antibody, and persons of group B have anti-A antibody. Transfusion of incompatible blood into recipients with preformed antibodies leads to agglutination, rapid destruction of the transfused cells, and to the excretion of breakdown products in the urine. Oliguria is a serious sequel (Chap. 17).

Antigens of the Rh system are sometimes responsible for less severe transfusion reactions for individuals with autoimmune hemolytic anemia. The Rh antigens are proteins and are rarely encountered in the environment, so preformed antibodies are rare. The Rh antigens appear to be the product of a complex of structural genes. One allelic form, frequently designated RhD, is present in about 85% of the U.S. population. Formerly of great concern, the inheritance of RhD from the father when the mother was Rh negative could lead to sensitization of the mother and to the transplacental transfer of antibodies, leading to the condition of hemolytic disease of the newborn. A triumph of immunoprophylaxis, the passive administration of high-titered anti-Rh antiserum to the mother during pregnancy before active immunization can occur, has almost abolished this complication.

Summary

In this brief presentation the major components of the immune system, the central and peripheral lymphoid organs, the cells, accessory cells, and their products have been introduced. The wonderfully intricate way in which the system is self-regulated and the grave consequences that result from imbalances in immune function have been mentioned. Some of the ways in which knowledge of the immune system has been used to prevent and correct a variety of diseases have been discussed. Thus the stage is set for a more complete understanding of basic and applied immunology.

Abbreviations and Terms Commonly Used in Immunology

Acquired Immunity. immunity that develops as a result of exposure to a foreign substance or organism.

ADCC. antibody-dependent cell-mediated cytotoxicity; ability of nonsensitized cells (i.e., cells from an unimmunized animal) to lyse other cells that have been coated by specific antibody.

Adjuvant. any of many foreign materials introduced with an antigen to enhance its immunogenicity; includes killed bacteria (*Bordetella pertussis*, mycobacteria) or bacterial products (endotoxin) in emulsions (Freund's adjuvant), precipitates (alum), or fine particulate clay (bentonite).

Adoptive Transfer. transfer of the ability to respond to antigen by transplanting immunocompetent cells into a host previously made immunoincompetent, usually by irradiation, or genetically unable to respond.

Affinity. equilibrium constant that defines the interaction of two molecules; usually the binding of an antibody with its corresponding antigenic determinant.

Ag. antigen; molecule bound by antibodies or lymphocytes.

Allergy. hypersensitive state acquired through exposure to a specific (environmental) allergen.

Allogeneic. originating from a genetically different individual or inbred cell line of the same species; hence alloantibody, alloantigen, etc.

Allotype. antigenic determinants on immunoglobulin molecules coded at one genetic locus and inherited as alleles in different members of the same species.

Alternative Pathway. mechanism of complement activation that does not involve the binding of C1, C2, or C4 by antigen-antibody complexes.

Anamnestic Response. see secondary immune response.

Anaphylaxis. systemic immediate hypersensitivity reaction from administration of allergen to a sensitized subject, resulting in respiratory distress or vascular collapse.

Anaphylatoxin. small fragment of C3 (C3a) or C5 (C5a) capable of degranulating mast cells and liberating vasoactive amines.

Antibody (Ab). immunoglobulin molecule capable of combining specifically with a known antigen.

APC. antigen-presenting cell; usually a B lymphocyte or reticuloendothelial cell.

Arthus Reaction. local immediate hypersensitivity reaction mediated by IgG-antigen complexes; if severe, it results in vascular injury and local lymphadenenopathy.

Atopy. genetic tendency to develop sudden hypersensitivity states such as allergic asthma or hay fever.

Autoimmunity. immunity to one's own body constituents or tissues.

Avidity. an imprecise measurement of the strength of binding of antibody and antigen molecules; usually involves multiple different molecular interactions.

β_2 Microglobulin. 12,000 Da polypeptide found in association with histocompatibility antigens on the surface of cells.

B Lymphocyte (B Cell). subclass of lymphocyte with rearranged immunoglobulin chains that is capable of synthesizing a single species of antibody.

Blood Groups. antigens present at the surface of red blood cells that vary between individuals of the same species; ABO and Rh are important blood groups in man.

BSA. bovine serum albumin; a commonly used antigenic substance and carrier.

Bursa of Fabricius. lymphoid organ in the hindgut of birds that influences B cell development.

C Complement. series of serum proteins with numerous biologic activities; individual components are numbered in order of their discovery (e.g., C1, C2).

C3 Receptor. site on the surface of B cells and phagocytes able to bind activated C3.

CAM. cell adhesion molecules; a series of receptors, including leukocyte adhesion molecules (e.g., LFA-1).

Capping. coordinated movement of membrane molecules to one region of the cell surface after binding by a multivalent ligand such as an antibody or an antigen.

Carrier. molecule to which haptens are bound; usually an immunogenic protein.

Central Lymphoid Organs. thymus, bursa of Fabricius (in birds), bone marrow; important in lymphopoiesis and lymphocyte differentiation.

CD. cluster determinant; a cell surface marker, usually a receptor.

CFA. complete Freund's adjuvant; an aqueous emulsion of *Mycobacterium,* oil, and wax.

CFU. colony forming unit; a stem cell and its progeny, usually specified (e.g., CFUG, a granulocyte forming unit).

CH_{50}. 50% lysis; a measure used in the measurement of complement activity.

C_H Region. carboxyterminal region of the heavy chain of immunoglobulins.

C_L Region. carboxyterminal region of the light chain of immunoglobulins.

Classic Pathway. mechanism of complement activation by antigen-antibody complexes involving the binding of C1, C4, and C2 to activate C3.

Clone. family of cells derived from a single cellular ancestor and therefore genetically identical.

CML. cell-mediated lymphocytotoxicity; ability of T cells from an immunized individual to lyse target cells.

CMV. cytomegalovirus; an opportunistic virus.

Con A. concanavalin A; a plant lectin used as a mitogen for lymphocytes.

CSF. colony stimulating factor.

CTL (T_c). cytotoxic lymphocyte; a committed T lymphocyte.

D Region. diversity region; diversity-generating sequence of Ig or TCR gene.

Delayed Hypersensitivity (DTH). specific T cell–mediated inflammatory immune reaction elicited by antigen in the skin of immune individuals.

Determinant. that part of the structure of antigen that binds to an antibody-combining site or a specific lymphocyte cell–surface receptor.

DNP. dinitrophenol; commonly used as a hapten.

EBV. Epstein-Barr virus.

ECM. extracellular matrix proteins that stimulate adhesion and migration.

ELAM. endothelial leukocyte adhesion molecule.

Endotoxin. lipopolysaccharide that has multiple biologic effects derived from cell walls of gram-negative organisms.

Enhancement. prolongation of allograft or tumor survival by specific antibodies against the foreign tissue.

Epitope. an antigenic determinant; usually one that occurs many times on the same antigen.

E-Rosettes. cluster of sheep red blood cells around a human T cell; used to define the human T cell population.

Fab Fragment. product of papain digestion of immunoglobulins; consists of one light chain and part of one heavy chain.

$F(ab')_2$ Fragment. product of pepsin digestion of immunoglobulin consisting of two intact light chains and parts of two heavy chains; has two combining sites for antigen.

Fc Fragment. product of papain digestion of immunoglobulin with the constant regions of two heavy chains and no combining sites for antigen.

Fc Receptor. site on the surface of most lymphocytes and phagocytes able to bind the Fc portion of immunoglobulins.

Follicle. circumscribed region in lymphoid tissue, usually in the superficial cortex of lymph nodes, containing mostly B cells and dendritic macrophages.

GAG. glycosaminoglycan; cross-linked to protein to form proteoglycans.

Gamma Globulin. globulin with slow electrophoretic mobility; includes most immunoglobulins.

Globulin. any of a large number of serum proteins (distinct from albumin) insoluble at high salt concentrations.

GVH. graft-vs-host reaction; the pathologic reaction caused by transplantation of immunocompetent T lymphocytes to an incompetent host.

H chain. heavy chain of Ig.

H-2. major histocompatibility complex in the mouse; the main loci are H-2K and H-2D, H-2IA and H-2IE.

Hapten. chemically defined determinant that binds antibody but in itself is not capable of stimulating antibody production unless in a complex with a carrier such as BSA.

Haplotype. set of genetic determinants coded by closely linked genes on a single chromosome.

HAT. hypoxanthine, aminopterin, thymidine; selective medium.

HBSS. Hanks' balanced salt solution.

Heavy Chain (H chain). the higher molecular weight polypeptide chain in an immunoglobulin molecule and the one determining the class of the immunoglobulin.

Helper Cells. subpopulation of specific T cells that are necessary to "help" B cells produce antibody to thymus-dependent antigens; may also provide help in T cell–mediated responses (e.g., killing).

HEPES. *N*-2-hydroxyethylpiperazine-*N*′-2-ethanesulfonic acid; used in buffers.

Histocompatibility Antigen. cell-surface antigen characteristic of an individual or an inbred line that stimulates the rejection of tissue allografts.

HIV. human immunodeficiency virus.

HLA. the major histocompatibility complex (MHC) in man; HLA-A, HLA-B, HLA-DP, HLA-DQ, and HLA-DR are the main components.

HLA-D. region of the MHC of man coding HLA-DP, HLA-DQ, and HLA-DR; HLA-D region antigens are expressed primarily on B cells, where they stimulate allogeneic T cells.

Humoral Immunity. immune phenomenon involving the production of specific antibody.

Hypersensitivity. state, existing in a previously immunized individual, in which an inflammatory reaction results from the immune reaction to a further dose of antigen.

Hypervariable Region. defined portion of the variable region of either heavy or light immunoglobulin chains; the antibody-combining site.

Ia. histocompatibility antigen found primarily on B cells but also on some macrophages, activated human T cells, and skin; it is encoded by the I region of H-2 or the D region of HLA.

ICAM. intracellular adhesion molecule.

ICFA (Incomplete Freund's Adjuvant). Freund's adjuvant with mycobacteria.

Id. idiotype; a specific conformation.

Idiotype. antigenic determinant on a specific antibody that is characteristic of that antibody.

IFN. interferon (e.g., IFN-β).

Ig. immunoglobulin or antibody; globular protein with the basic structure of two heavy chains and two light chains.

IL. interleukin (e.g., IL-2).

Immediate Hypersensitivity. specific immune reaction that takes place in minutes to hours after the administration of antigen and is mediated by IgE (immediate anaphylactic hypersensitivity) or IgG (Arthus type hypersensitivity).

Immunogen. molecule that elicits an immune response; part of the molecule acts as hapten and part as carrier.

Ir. immune response as in Ir genes.

Ir Gene. gene located in the I region of the MHC that controls the ability to develop specific immune responses to thymus-dependent antigens.

I-A, I-B, I-C, I-E, I-J. subregions of the I region of the mouse H-2 complex.

Isologous. originating from the same individual or a member of the same inbred strain; hence isogeneic.

Isotype. class or subclass of an immunoglobulin common to all members of that species.

J Chain. small polypeptide found in IgM and IgA polymers and responsible for maintaining the polymeric form of the immunoglobulins.

J Gene Segment. genetic locus encoding a small segment that joins a variable region gene segment to a constant region gene segment.

J region. joining region of Ig or T cell receptor for antigen.

K Cell. mononuclear cell able to mediate ADCC.

Killer Cells. same as cytotoxic lymphocytes.

Kinin System. activity in serum responsible for many biologic effects of antibodies and composed of many proteins acting in sequence.

L Chain. light chain of Ig.

LAK Cell. lymphokine-activated killer cell.

LAM. leukocyte adhesion molecule.

LEC-CAM. lymphocyte endothelial cell–cell adhesion molecule.

Lectin. any of a number of plant products that bind to cells, usually by nature of a combining site for specific sugars.

Leukocyte. any of the white cells of the blood.

LFA. lymphocyte function antigen.

Light Chain (L Chain). lower-molecular-weight polypeptide chain present in all immunoglobulin molecules.

LPS (lipopolysaccharide). active component of endotoxin derived from bacterial cell walls; a B cell mitogen for mouse lymphocytes.

Lymphokine. biologically active molecule produced by lymphocytes.

Lyt. older term for a system of antigens found on T cells that distinguish different functional classes of T cells; now renamed CD.

mAb. monoclonal antibody.

Macrophage. ubiquitous nonlymphoid phagocytic cell found in tissues; an important accessory cell in immune responses; see also monocyte.

Medulla. central region of lymph node consisting of lymphatic sinuses and medullary cords.

2-ME. 2-mercaptoethanol.

MEM. minimum essential medium.

Memory. ability of the immune system to mount a specific secondary response to an immunogen that was previously introduced.

MHC (Major Histocompatibility Complex). large region of genetic material containing genes coding for histocompatibility antigens, immune response genes, and lymphocyte surface antigens and responsible for the rapid rejection of allografts (H-2 in mouse, HLA in man).

MIF (Migration Inhibition Factor). protein produced by lymphocytes upon interaction with antigens that inhibits the motility of macrophages in culture; now called IL-1.

Mitogen. substance that stimulates lymphocytes to proliferate independently or any specific antigen.

MLR or MLC (Mixed Lymphocyte Reaction or Culture). proliferative response of allogeneic lymphocytes when cocultured.

Monocyte. phagocytic blood leukocyte, the precursor of most tissue macrophages; monocytes originate from cells in the bone marrow.

Mononuclear Leukocytes. monocytes and lymphocytes.

mRNA. messenger RNA.

m.w. (molecular weight). expressed in daltons.

Myeloma. plasma cell tumor producing a characteristic immunoglobulin (paraprotein); a plasmocytoma.

NK Cell (Natural Killer Cell). natural killing mediated by large granular lymphocytes.

Nonadherent Cells. those cells in suspension of spleen and other lymphoid tissue that do not adhere to plastic or glass (in contrast to macrophages); usually includes lymphocytes.

Nude Mouse. congenitally athymic mouse.

Null Cell. class of lymphocyte that does not bear markers for either T cells or B cells; includes NK cells.

Opsonization. enhancement of phagocytosis of a particle or a cell (especially bacteria) by virtue of its being covered by antibody and complement.

OVA. ovalbumin; like BSA, a commonly used antigen.

PAGE. polyacrylamide gel electrophoresis.

Passive Immunity. temporary and partial immunity conferred on a naive host by the injection of antibody.

PBL. peripheral blood lymphocyte.

PBS. phosphate-buffered saline.

PCA (Passive Cutaneous Anaphylaxis). induction of a local, immediate-type immune reaction by injecting antibody into the skin and later injecting antigen intravenously or locally.

PFC (Plaque-Forming Cell). cell-secreting antibody visualized as a clear plaque in a layer of red cells in the presence of complement.

PG. prostaglandin.

PHA (Phytohemagglutinin). plant lectin that agglutinates red and white cells and stimulates lymphocytes, mostly T cells, to proliferate.

Plasma Cell. cell of the B cell lineage actively secreting large amounts of immunoglobulin; an end cell that no longer divides.

PMA. phorbol myristate acetate; a powerful mitogen.

Primary Immune Response. response occurring on first exposure to an immunogen.

Primary Lymphoid Organs. thymus, bursa of Fabricius (in birds), bone marrow.

Properdin. component of the alternative pathway.

PWM (Pokeweed Mitogen). plant substance that stimulates B lymphocytes to proliferate.

R. receptor (e.g., IL-2R).

RFLP. restriction fragment length polymorphism.

RIA. radioimmunoassay.

RNA. ribonucleic acid.

RNase. ribonuclease.

S. Svedberg unit of sedimentation coefficient.

Secondary Immune Response. response occurring on the second and subsequent exposure to an immunogen (memory).

Secretory Component. polypeptide synthesized by epithelial cells and added to IgA (and some IgM) in secretion of these immunoglobulins (transport piece).

SEM. standard error of the mean.

Serum. liquid part of blood remaining after cells and fibrin have been removed.

Serum Sickness. syndrome resulting from the localization of circulating immune complexes in small vessels and especially the kidney glomeruli.

SLE (Systemic Lupus Erythematosus). autoimmune disease characterized by the production of autoantibodies to different autoantigens and especially to DNA.

Specificity. ability of antibodies or lymphocytes to distinguish between different determinants.

SRBC (Sheep Red Blood Cells). common antigen used in experimental work.

SRS-A (Slow-Reacting Substance of Anaphylaxis). molecule released immunologically and responsible for some of the effects of anaphylaxis.

Subclass. immunoglobulins of the same class but differing in electrophoretic mobility or in an antigenic determinant detectable in the constant heavy chain region (e.g., IgG1, IgG2, IgG3, IgG4).

Suppressor Cells. poorly characterized subpopulation of T cells that are able to suppress the immune response to an antigen; there are specific and nonspecific suppressor cells.

SV40. simian virus 40.

T Cell. class of lymphocytes that differentiate in the thymus; they are capable of responding to thymus-dependent antigens and MHC gene products.

T_c Cell. cytotoxic T cell.

TCR. T cell receptor for antigen.

T-Dependent Antigen. immunogen that requires T cell participation to elicit an antibody response.

T_h Cell. T helper cell.

Thymocyte. thymic lymphocyte.

Thymus-Dependent Area. region of peripheral lymphoid tissue (e.g., lymph nodes and spleen) containing mostly T cells.

Thymus-Independent Area. region within peripheral lymphoid tissue (e.g., follicles of lymph nodes found in the superficial cortex) containing mostly B cells.

TL. system of mouse T cell antigens originally found on T cell leukemia cells and expressed in some mouse strains on normal thymocytes; a differentiation alloantigen.

TLC. thin layer chromatography.

TNF. tumor necrosis factor.

TNP. trinitrophenol.

Tolerance. failure of the immune system, as the result of previous contact with antigen, to respond to the same antigen, although it is capable of responding to others.

Transport Piece. polypeptide found associated with secreted IgA but not with serum IgA (secretory component).

TRIS. tris(hydroxymethyl)aminomethane.

T_s Cell. T suppressor cell.

TSTA (Tumor-Specific Transplantation Antigen). antigen found on the cell membrane of tumors against which tumor rejection reactions are directed.

TAA. tumor-associated antigens.

UV. ultraviolet.

V Region. variable region of Ig.

VCAM (Vascular Cellular Adhesion Molecule). ligand for VLA-4.

V_H Region. variable amino acid sequence region of the heavy chain.

V_L Region. variable amino acid sequence region of the light chain.

VLA. very late antigen of activated T cells.

Xenogeneic. originating from a different species.

Definitions and abbreviations are adapted from the following:

Benacerraf B, Unanue ER: Textbook of Immunology. Baltimore, Williams & Wilkins Co, 1979

Golub ES: The Cellular Basis of the Immune Response. Sunderland, Mass, Sinauer Associates, 1977

Task Force on Immunology and Disease: Immunology: Its role in disease and health. U.S. Dept of Health, Education and Welfare, DHEW Pub, NIH, 75-940, 1976

Standard abbreviations. Information for contributors. J Immunol 147:ii, 1991

FURTHER READING

Austrian R: Life with the Pneumococcus. Philadelphia, University of Pennsylvania Press, 1985

Beveridge WIB: The Art of Scientific Investigation. New York, WW Norton, 1957

de Kruif P: Microbe Hunters Blue Ribbon Books. New York, 1926

Landsteiner K: The Specificity of Serological Reaction. New York, Dover, 1962

Thomas L: Late Night Thoughts on Listening to Mahler's Ninth Symphony. New York, Viking Press, 1983

Thomas L: The Lives of a Cell. New York, Viking Press, 1974

CHAPTER 12

Immunogens (Antigens) and Antigen-binding Molecules and Their Detection

In the first part of this chapter the discussion centers on the types of molecules that initiate an immune response (immunogens) and the nature of those distinct sites (antigenic determinants) that are reactive with cells and cell products of the immune system (e.g., antigen-presenting cells [APC], antigen-specific T and B lymphocytes, and humoral antibodies). The central discussions of this chapter cover the molecular structure and function of antigen-binding molecules, that is, antibodies and the T cell receptor (TCR) complex, and the generation of immunoglobulin and TCR diversity through gene rearrangements and somatic mutation. The final sections are devoted to antigen-antibody reactions and how antibody- and cell-based determinations are performed.

Immunogens

General Properties

An immunogen (or antigen) is defined as any substance that induces a specific immune response in the individual exposed to it. The term *antigen* may also be used to define a substance that reacts with preformed products of the immune response (e.g., antigen binding to antibody) but is not necessarily immunogenic, that is, it does not induce or initiate a new immune response on its own.

The immune response to a bacterium or virus is very complex because these organisms present a multitude of distinct macromolecular immunogens, including proteins, glycoproteins, phospholipids, glycolipids, polysaccharides (carbohydrates), and nucleic acids, each of which may be recognized independently during the course of an immune response. Many of the isolated proteins, glycoproteins, and large, complex polysaccharides are strongly immunogenic alone, whereas in general the phospholipids, glycolipids, and smaller, less complex carbohydrates are not. Immune responses to native nucleic acids are usually difficult to demonstrate experimentally, but antibodies are frequently present in the sera of patients and animals with autoimmune diseases, and, experimentally, antibodies can be elicited readily to nucleic acids and oligonucleotides or to individual nucleotide bases when they are used as haptens in hapten-carrier conjugates (see below).

One reason large macromolecules are strong immunogens is that the B cells and T cells of the immune system are capable of recognizing a number of distinct antigenic determinants on a single molecule (Fig. 12–1). There are also immunogens that contain many repeating copies of the same antigenic determinant. For example, the flagellar organelles of *Salmonella adelaide* consist of higher-order polymers of a single polypeptide unit, or monomer. Each monomer expresses a limited number of strong (immunodominant) B and T cell antigenic determinants and additional weaker ones; the organelle represents an array of these repeating determinants. The immune response to flagella is, in large part, characterized by the response to a limited number of immunodominant determinants.

On the other hand, nonpolymeric, macromolecular im-

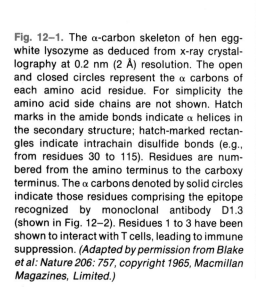

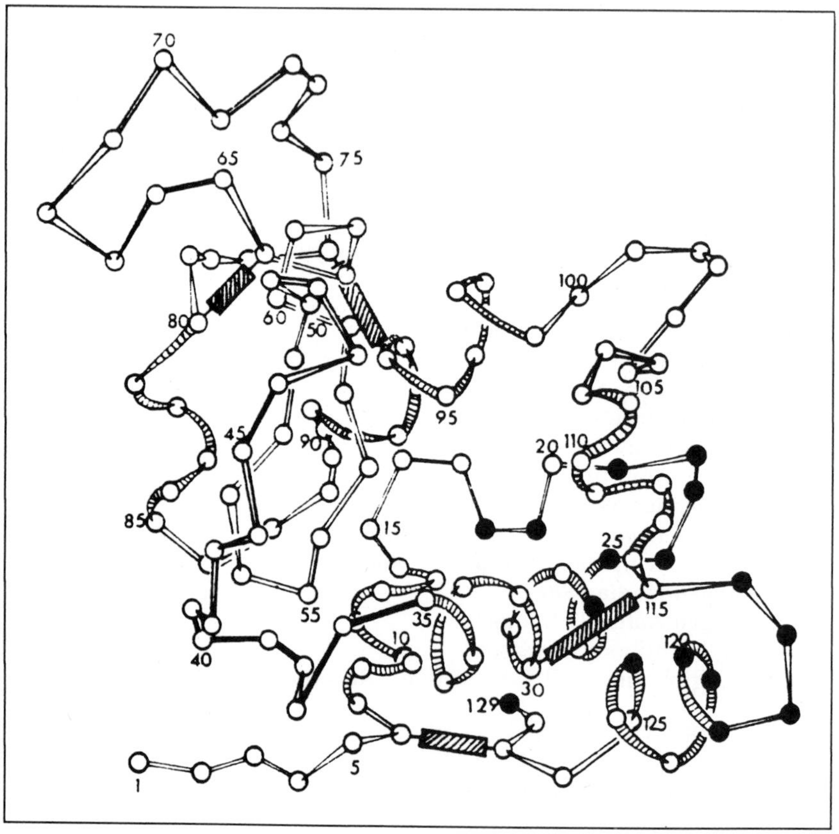

Fig. 12–1. The α-carbon skeleton of hen egg-white lysozyme as deduced from x-ray crystallography at 0.2 nm (2 Å) resolution. The open and closed circles represent the α carbons of each amino acid residue. For simplicity the amino acid side chains are not shown. Hatch marks in the amide bonds indicate α helices in the secondary structure; hatch-marked rectangles indicate intrachain disulfide bonds (e.g., from residues 30 to 115). Residues are numbered from the amino terminus to the carboxy terminus. The α carbons denoted by solid circles indicate those residues comprising the epitope recognized by monoclonal antibody D1.3 (shown in Fig. 12–2). Residues 1 to 3 have been shown to interact with T cells, leading to immune suppression. *(Adapted by permission from Blake et al: Nature 206: 757, copyright 1965, Macmillan Magazines, Limited.)*

munogens such as lysozyme (Fig. 12–1) may express several, nonidentical, immunodominant B cell antigenic determinants (or epitopes) as well as a few immunodominant T cell epitopes. As a consequence of multiple cellular recognition of distinct epitopes, the immune response to lysozyme, as an example of a typical protein antigen, is necessarily complex, consisting of distinct subsets of lymphocytes and antibodies, each of which interacts with one of several, nonidentical epitopes.

Since the B cell immune response (as measured by antibody) to even well-characterized protein antigens such as lysozyme may be very complex, it has been very difficult for the experimentalist to use antigens of this type to detail specific aspects of the immune response. In many cases it has been desirable to examine the recognition at the level of the antigen-specific lymphocyte and its response to well-defined antigenic determinants. Although it has been possible to isolate a few intact determinants recognized by B cells (B cell epitopes) from protein antigens, this has not been the general case. Most B cell epitopes are conformation dependent (see below), and in the process of their isolation, reactivity with antibodies is often lost irreversibly. Thus experimentalists have resorted to techniques pioneered by Karl Lansteiner and his contemporaries. Their approach was to create a new B cell epitope from a small, well-characterized molecule (hapten) and to complex it chemically to a suitable macromolecular carrier (usually a protein or a synthetic polypeptide) for immunization. A hapten (e.g., 2,4-dinitrophenol [DNP]) is not immunogenic alone but functions as an immunodominant determinant when complexed to a larger immunogenic carrier such as poly-L-lysine (PLL) and presented to the immune system as hapten-carrier conjugate. Antibodies specifically produced to the haptenic determinant can be readily purified from immune serum (antiserum) by affinity chromatography or adsorption methods (immunoadsorption), using the original hapten coupled to an inert matrix as a solid phase support. The hapten-carrier technique has been used to produce antibodies specific for a variety of small molecules (e.g., penicillin, certain steroids, hormones, lipids, and individual nucleotides).

A number of naturally occurring, small-molecular-weight components of complex organisms, such as membrane glycolipids not immunogenic on their own, function as haptens when they are administered as part of an immunogenic complex. Thus the Forssman hapten, a glycolipid consisting of *N*-acetyl-galactosamine, galactose, galactose, and glucose covalently coupled to a ceramide lipid, is nonimmunogenic in purified form. In its native plasma membrane environment, it is a strong epitope (hapten). Since it is a membrane component of wide and diverse tissue and species distribution (a heterophilic antigen), immunization of a Forssman-negative species with Forssman-positive tissue or cells often results in the production of Forssman-specific antibodies.

Requirements for Immunogenicity

Foreignness

The mature immune system can distinguish between self and nonself. Antigenic differences between species (xenoantigens) are those recognized during natural infection (or environmental exposure); these differences form the basis of most planned immunization (vaccination). Many studies have shown that the immune response is directed at epitopes on an immunogen that differ structurally from host self components. One of the best examples of this relationship is the response of one species to the cytochrome *c* molecule derived from another. Cytochrome *c* is common to all eukaryotes, and the amino acid residues related to its function are highly conserved. Margoliash and coworkers have shown that the immune response to foreign cytochrome *c* is directed at determinants (amino acids) that differ between the species. In general, the greater the phylogenetic distance from the host, the more immunogenic the molecule will be.

However, there are also very strong antigenic differences among individuals within a species. The best examples are the ABO blood group antigens and the major histocompatibility complex antigens (Chap. 14). Exposure to these antigens through transfusion or transplantation can result in very strong immune responses. These antigenic differences relate to alternative genes (alleles) at identical loci and their respective gene products (alloantigens).

Within an individual an immune response to the host's own tissue, an autoimmune response, may also occur infrequently. The reason for these antiself responses may include responses to self-antigens normally sequestered from the immune system but exposed during injury or disease, breakdown in a regulatory mechanism (especially with advancing age), or part of a normal idiotype-antiidiotype regulatory response (Chaps. 13 and 17). These responses may be tissue damaging (hypersensitivities) or relatively benign.

Charge, Size, and Shape

The charge of a molecule does not appear to influence immunogenicity; however, the charge expressed by an antigen may have an effect on the overall charge of antibodies made in response to it. Likewise, the shape of a molecule does not determine its immunogenicity; proteins and polypeptides with globular, rodlike, and random coil configurations can be equally immunogenic. Molecular size, on the other hand, does affect immunogenicity; the smaller the molecule, the less immunogenic it is likely to be. For example, bovine and porcine insulin (about 6000 Da) are poor immunogens, but if insulin is polymerized by chemical methods or is heat aggregated, it may become immunogenic. Similarly, the H antigen of *S. adelaide* (the flagellar protein antigen described earlier) can be prepared in various stages of polymerization: as intact organelles (flagella), as 38,500 Da monomers (flagellin, or MON), or as repolymerized flagellin (POL) (prepared by aggregating monomers). The flagella are more immunogenic than POL, and POL more so than MON. In general, polymerization (or aggregation) increases immunogenicity of the antigen.

The minimum size for immunogenicity appears to be about 500 to 1000 Da. For example, angiotensin II (1031 Da), a native polypeptide hormone; α-dinitrophenyl-hepta-L-lysine (1200 Da), a conjugate of hapten with a synthetic polypeptide; and a synthetic compound of 450 Da (*p*-azobenzene arsonate-*N*-acetyl tyrosineamide) have been shown to be immunogenic on their own in guinea pigs. Smaller compounds that apparently are immunogenic, such as the urushiols from poison ivy (120 to 320 Da) and penicillin (in certain individuals), are only immunogenic by virtue of their chemical reactivity with self-proteins and lipids, thereby creating hapten-carrier conjugates. Penicillin is an example of a highly reactive hapten that complexes with normal cell membrane proteins, which then function as natural carriers. As a general rule, the number of antigenic determinants that a molecule expresses is directly related to its size, and this may be a critical factor in determining the relative immunogenicity of the molecule.

Complexity and Composition

Synthetic polypeptides have been used effectively to study the effect of complexity and composition of immunogenicity. Linear homopolymers such as poly-L-lysine or poly-L-glutamic acid are usually not immunogenic alone. If they are used as conjugated haptens with a suitable protein carrier, specific antibody responses can be detected. Linear random copolymers, on the other hand, are immunogenic. For example, poly-L-($glu_{60}lys_{40}$), where the subscripts denote the mole percent concentrations of the initial reactants, is immunogenic in rabbits but not in man, whereas poly-L-($glu_{50}lys_{30}ala_{20}$) is immunogenic in both species. Increasing complexity and host genetic factors contribute to a molecule's immunogenicity. The amino acid composition of the copolymers is also important in that addition of aromatic amino acids such as tyrosine to random copolymers leads to dramatic increases in immunogenicity. Incorporation of amino acids such as cysteine, lysine, alanine, and glutamic acid leads to more modest increases in immunogenicity.

Branched copolymers like (T,G) A-L, in which short side chains of poly-DL-ala ending in short mixed polymers of poly-L-(tyr,glu) are synthesized off the epsilon amino groups of a poly-L-lys polypeptide backbone, are extremely potent immunogens. The (T,G) A-L polymer has also been used to demonstrate that the immunodominant groups (T,G) must be readily accessible (on the surface exposed to the solvent) for immune recognition to take place. Similar branched polymers have been used extensively in studies elucidating genetic control over a number of immune responses (Chaps. 14 and 17).

T-Dependent and T-Independent Immunogens

Certain immunogens appear to require only stimulation of specific B cells for humoral antibodies to be formed (T cell–independent immunogens) (Chap. 13). More often, however, an immunogen requires specific recognition by B cells (through B cell antigenic determinants expressed by the immunogen) and T helper (T_h cells, through distinct antigenic determinants, or T cell epitopes). Although antigen-specific T_h cells do not produce any detectable antibody, they do regulate the activation and differentiation of B cells in the immune response. Additional details are in Chapter 13.

Role of Immune Response Genes

As noted previously, the immune response to some immunogens may show species dependence. Further, within a species there are differences in reactivity between individuals. This is most easily demonstrated in inbred strains of mice or guinea pigs (Chaps. 13 and 14). Some outbred guinea pigs are responders to the hapten-carrier conjugate α-dinitrophenyl-poly-L-lysine. Responders express the product of a specific immune response (Ir) gene necessary for efficient recognition of the poly-L-lys carrier, whereas the nonresponders lack this gene. This gene has been identified as a major histocompatibility complex (MHC) class II gene (Chap. 14). Both responders and nonresponders are capable of responding to the hapten (DNP) conjugated to a different carrier. Inbred guinea pigs of strain 2 carry the appropriate Ir gene, and all strain 2 animals respond. No member of a second inbred line, strain 13, responds. The F1 hybrid between strains 2 and 13 does respond, so the capacity to respond is dominant. By appropriate backcross experiments with the F1 and a parental strain, it was possible to show that immune responsiveness to PLL mapped to a single gene.

Immunization Protocol

The dose of antigen administered, the route of injection, the timing between booster injections, and the use of adjuvants may also influence the quantity and type of immune response an animal makes. Indeed, immune paralysis or a tolerant state, as opposed to an immune response, can be induced by varying these conditions (Chap. 13). The use of adjuvants with immunization results in dramatic increases in immunogenicity. Common adjuvants include water-in-oil emulsions such as Freund's incomplete adjuvant (mineral oil, water, and an emulsifying agent such as lanolin), fine particulate suspensions (alum precipitates), and silica or bentonite particles. Complete Freund's adjuvant contains, in addition to the emulsion, heat-killed mycobacteria; their inclusion results in an intense, local inflammatory reaction and augmentation of the immune response. The exact mechanism of action varies from one adjuvant to another, but some adjuvants are thought to protect the antigen from rapid elimination and catabolism, slowly releasing antigen over extended periods of time.

B Cell and T Cell Antigenic Determinants

As mentioned before, antigenic determinants (or epitopes) are those discrete sites on an immunogen to which antibodies, B cells, and T cells are specifically directed. The chemical and physical properties of these sites have in some cases been detailed through the use of specific antibodies, specific, responding T cells, or both.

Size of Antigenic Determinants Recognized by B Cells

The size of B cell antigenic determinants has been estimated by determining the minimum size of a fragment of an antigen that can combine with a specific antibody. The assay commonly used is inhibition of the reaction between the intact antigen and its antibodies by antigenic fragments of the original immunogen. For example, a dextran-antidextran reaction can be inhibited by small polymers of glucose, whereas polypeptide-antipolypeptide reactions can be inhibited by oligopeptides. The extended size of the antigenic determinant appears to be about $3 \times 1.5 \times 0.7$ nm ($30 \times 15 \times 7$Å). This estimate compares favorably with that calculated from the size of the interacting surfaces between an antibody and one epitope on lysozyme (3×2 nm [30×20 Å]; Fig. 12–2). Although this approach has worked for antigens in which the determinants can be approximated with simple, linear oligosaccharides or oligopeptides, it has not been as successful for B cell epitopes that have a defined conformation (tertiary structure) determined by the native structure of the whole immunogen. The conformation of the epitope often is altered in attempts to isolate it by fragmentation of the protein immunogen.

Isolation and Characterization of B Cell Antigenic Determinants

In a few cases it has been possible to isolate an intact epitope from a complex protein antigen by controlled proteolytic

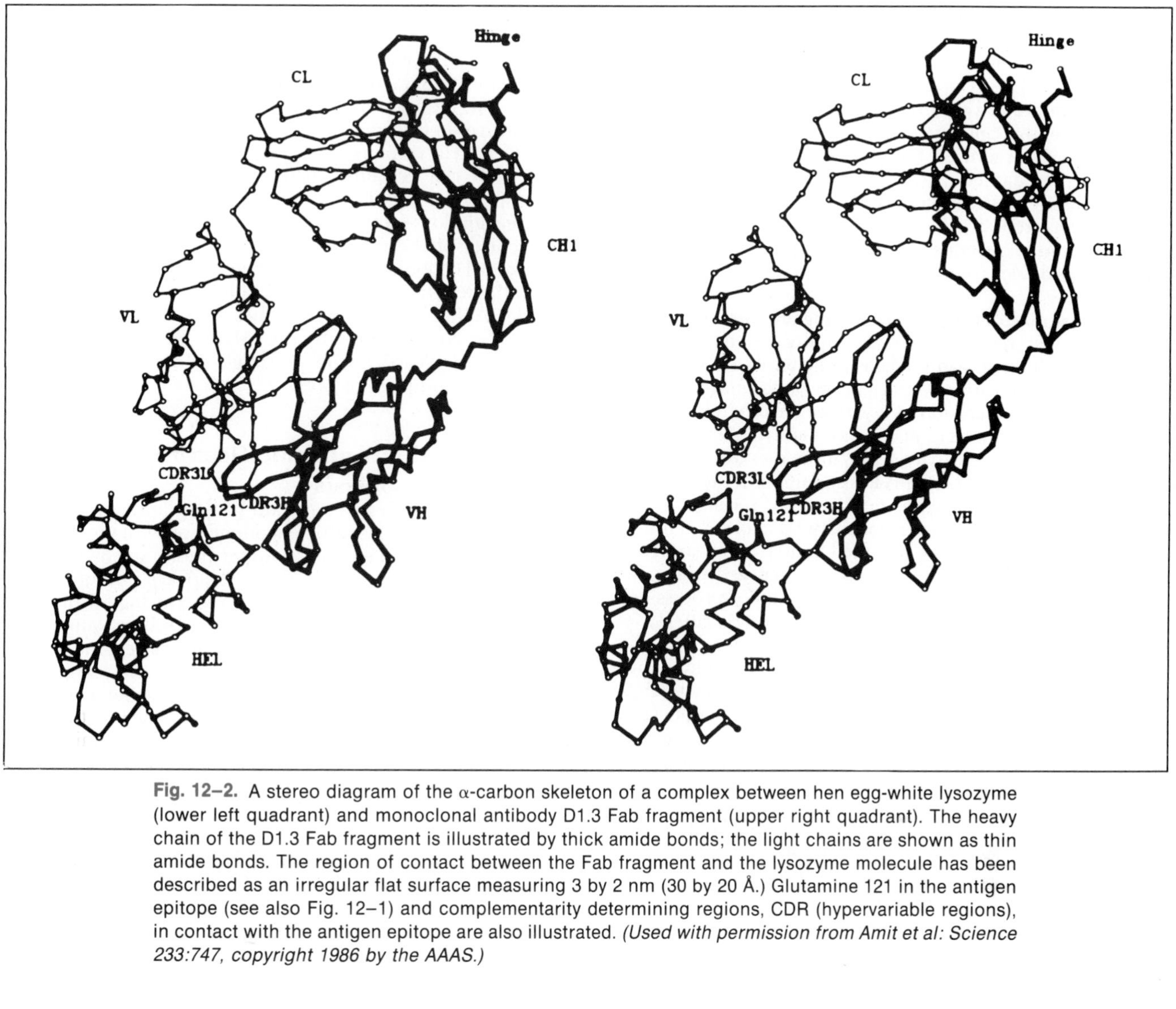

Fig. 12–2. A stereo diagram of the α-carbon skeleton of a complex between hen egg-white lysozyme (lower left quadrant) and monoclonal antibody D1.3 Fab fragment (upper right quadrant). The heavy chain of the D1.3 Fab fragment is illustrated by thick amide bonds; the light chains are shown as thin amide bonds. The region of contact between the Fab fragment and the lysozyme molecule has been described as an irregular flat surface measuring 3 by 2 nm (30 by 20 Å.) Glutamine 121 in the antigen epitope (see also Fig. 12–1) and complementarity determining regions, CDR (hypervariable regions), in contact with the antigen epitope are also illustrated. *(Used with permission from Amit et al: Science 233:747, copyright 1986 by the AAAS.)*

digestion. A 6600 Da fragment derived from bovine serum albumin contains a single epitope capable of binding a specific subpopulation of antibodies from an antiserum raised to the intact albumin. Although this epitope escapes degradation, much of the antigenic activity of the whole albumin molecule is lost after this procedure because other epitopes are destroyed. Similarly, a particular antibody response against tobacco-mosaic virus coat protein subunits is directed against a single oligopeptide that can be isolated from the intact immunogen.

The polypeptide hormone glucagon, 29 amino acids in length, has been partially digested into several fragments with trypsin. Antibodies raised to intact glucagon in guinea pigs are directed primarily at the amino terminus of the hormone, whereas cell-mediated immune recognition sites for T cells (T cell epitopes) are confined largely to the carboxy terminus.

The entire surface of a protein may consist of overlapping B cell antigenic determinants. These determinants often consist of hydrophilic and highly motile residues, widely separated in the primary amino acid sequence of the molecule but brought into juxaposition in the final three-dimensional folding. Thus these surface B cell epitopes consist of a three-dimensional array of amino acids, often associate with loops and turns, that will not survive disruption of the native structure of the protein by protease digestion or denaturation.

Characterization of T Cell Determinants

The function of the protein carrier in conferring T cell immunogenicity on coupled haptens has been studied intensively by conjugating haptens such as 2,4-dinitrophenol (DNP) to various immunogenic carriers such as bovine serum albumin (BSA), bovine gamma globulin (BGG), ovalbumin (OVA), and keyhole-limpet hemocyanin (KLH). Animals primed with DNP-BGG conjugates and challenged later with DNP-BGG respond vigorously with an antibody specific for DNP (and to other surface B cell epitopes expressed by both the unsubstituted and hapten-conjugated carrier). Priming establishes immunologic memory in cells specific for both the hapten (presumably B cells) and the carrier (both B and T cells). If, instead, DNP-BGG-primed animals are challenged with DNP on a different carrier such as DNP-KLH, only a small antibody response to the hapten is observed. Although there are sufficient memory B cells specific for the hapten in the primed animal, the number of cells specific for the new carrier is greatly limited. The recognition of carrier-specific determinants in an immune response to a hapten is a reflection of cooperation at the cellular level. T cell responses to carrier determinants are required for there to be significant B cell responses to the hapten (as well as to other carrier epitopes). A coordinated response by both B cells and T cells to distinctive epitopes expressed by the immunogen is required in the antibody immune response to most immunogens. Antigens requiring this dual recognition are referred to as T-dependent antigens.

Although conformation of the antigenic determinants is critical in antigen recognition by B lymphocytes, determinants recognized by T_h cells (and T cells in general) are much less dependent on the native conformation of the molecule. For example, after denaturation of lysozyme and chemical reduction of its disulfide bonds (and carboxy-methylation to prevent their reformation), reactivity with antibodies to the native structure is lost. In contrast, T cell recognition of the modified lysozyme remains unaltered as measured by T cell proliferation assays and delayed hypersensitivity reactions (Chaps. 13 and 17). Indeed, it is now accepted that protein antigenic determinants recognized by T cells are exposed only after denaturation or partial enymatic degradation ("processing") by the antigen-presenting cell (macrophage or B cell).

T cells preferentially recognize sequential (vs conformational) antigenic determinants. When exogenous, soluble protein antigens are taken up by antigen-presenting cells, these sequential determinants become exposed after endocytosis and subsequent partial degradation in a lysosomal compartment. The surviving peptide fragments of the exogenous antigen are bound, in this case, in the peptide-binding groove of MHC class II molecules (Chap. 14). When reexpressed at the antigen-presenting cell surface, this complex of MHC class II molecules with bound antigenic peptides is recognized by the appropriate antigen-specific $CD4^+$ T cells.

Foreign antigens synthesized within the cell (e.g., viral antigens synthesized in the infected cell) are handled slightly differently. The endogenously synthesized antigens are degraded (or unfolded) in, as yet, an unidentified compartment and are bound to the peptide-binding groove of MHC class I molecules. This complex, when expressed at the infected cell surface, is recognized by the appropriate antigen-specific $CD8^+$ T cells (Chap. 14).

Several experiments suggest that T cells recognize an epitope consisting of a minimum of seven to nine amino acids. Maximum stimulation occurred with peptides of ≤ 15 amino acids. This size range suggests that either a specific conformation of the T cell epitope (such as an α-helix) is stabilized or the extra amino acids, although not recognized by the T cell receptor, contribute to the affinity of the ternary complex of MHC molecule, antigenic peptide, and TCR.

Two models have been proposed as characterizing T cell epitopes. The first hypothesizes that T cell determinants form amphipathic α-helices; that is, a helix with hydrophilic amino acid side chains on one face and hydrophobic side chains on the other. Several T cell epitopes have been successfully predicted from the sequence of a protein antigen with this model. Not all predicted epitopes stimulate a response in a given animal since the T cell response depends on expression of the appropriate MHC class II molecule (Ir gene product) and the presence of appropriate TCR genes in the repertoire. The second model is based on the analysis of all known T cell epitopes for a common structural motif. A short sequence characterized by one charged amino acid (or glycine) followed by two hydrophobic amino acids is common to these T cell epitopes. This model, too, has been used to predict successfully T cell epitopes in previously uncharacterized protein antigens.

The T cell response to a single epitope is, like the analogous B cell response, heterogeneous. Several distinct antigen-specific T cells can be stimulated to respond. Because T cell recognition involves a ternary complex of molecules, heterogeneity of the responding cells may represent heterogeneity of MHC molecules (due to heterozygosity) and differences in the way the peptide is bound to the MHC-presenting molecule. A heterogeneous response may also represent a difference in conformation by the MHC's bound peptide, or heterogeneous TCRs' having a range of affinities for the MHC-peptide complex, or both.

B Cell and T Cell Antigenic Determinants: A Unifying Hypothesis

Although macrophages will and do present antigens, B cells are required for the most efficient antigen presentation. Since these cells are most likely to encounter immunogens in their native conformation, it follows that cell-surface immunoglobulins of B cells must be capable of recognizing distinctive epitopes in their native conformation. Hence B cell antigenic determinants are largely conformational and reflect the native structure of the antigen. After endocytosis of the antigen by B cells (or macrophages) and processing, peptide determinants recognized by T cells are expressed at the B cell (or macrophage) surface as MHC class II–peptide complexes. T cells are, in the strictest sense, only capable of recognizing altered self-molecules.

Role of Host in Response to Particular T and B Cell Determinants

Although the surface of a protein immunogen consists of a continuum of possible B cell epitopes, only a subset of these determinants is recognized in a given animal (or inbred strain of animal). Likewise, a number of potential T cell epitopes are expressed by the immunogen, but only a subset is recognized by a given animal (or inbred strain of animals). The particular subset of determinants recognized depends on many different host-related factors, including structural differences between the antigen and tissue antigens of the host, the repertoire of possible antigen-specific immunoglobulin and TCR binding sites, a variety of regulatory mechanisms including Ir gene effects (usually MHC class I and class II gene effects), and the effects of specific suppressor T cells (T_s cells) (Chap. 13). Presentation and recognition of certain epitopes may preferentially lead to the generation of T cell suppression rather than T cell help. Thus the response to an immunogen has been characterized as the response to a multideterminant regulatory model.

Specificity and Cross-Reactivity of Antigenic Determinant Recognition

Both the initial recognition of the immunogen at the level of the responding cell and the response phase (e.g., the effector T cell or secreted antibody) are specific for the challenging

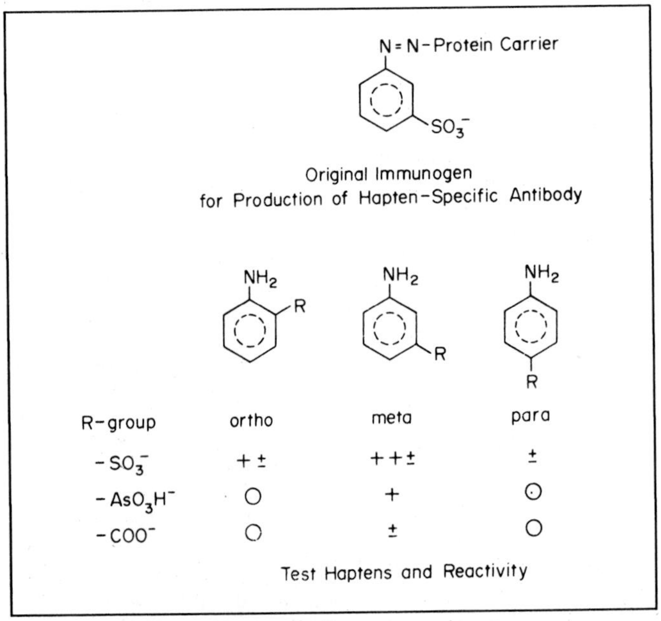

Fig. 12–3. Specificity of antibodies produced to the meta-sulfonyl aminobenzene hapten. The hapten was coupled through an azo intermediate (via the available amino group) to a protein carrier. The resulting antibodies were tested with the homologous hapten and with several structural analogues coupled to different protein carriers. The extent of precipitation was scored 0, ∓, +, +∓, ++, in order of increasing reaction. *(Adapted from Landsteiner: The Specificity of Serological Reactions. Dover Publications, 1962.)*

immunogen. In a humoral response the antibodies elicited to a single epitope are complementary to that particular determinant. The classic contributions of Lansteiner and his contemporaries demonstrated the specifity of antibodies produced to hapten-protein conjugates. One example of these exquisite studies is shown in Figure 12–3. The antibody was produced in rabbits to a meta-sulfonyl aminobenzene hapten conjugated to horse serum proteins. A change in the position of the sulfonyl group from meta to para or ortho in the test hapten resulted in complete or partial loss of antibody recognition. Slight and extremely subtle changes in the chemistry of the side group from sulfonyl to arsenyl or carboxyl also had dramatic effects on antibody binding. Thus the immune system can discriminate on a fine scale; the specificity of binding can be precise.

In many cases an antibody specific for one antigen may display significant cross-reactivity for an apparently unrelated antigen. Cross-reactivity has two primary causes. The first is chemical similarity of the antigenic determinant. This is illustrated by the example just given in which antibody to the *meta*-sulfonyl aminobenzene hapten partially reacts with the *ortho*- and *para*-sulfonyl haptens. Anti-*meta*-sulfonyl aminobenzene antibody also cross-reacts with *meta*-arsenyl or carboxyl substitutions of the aminobenzene group. The second cause of cross-reactivity is the presence of the same antigenic determinant in two otherwise dissimilar antigens. For example, rabbit antisheep red cell antisera cross-react with the red blood cell membranes of many animal species and the membranes of certain bacteria because all contain the Forssman hapten and anti-Forssman antibody is a major component of the antiserum. Cross-reactivity of this type is often quite unpredictable unless the molecular structures are known.

Immunoglobulins (Antibodies)

General Properties

Antibodies as Globular Proteins

Animals immunized with killed microorganisms can withstand later challenge with live, virulent organisms or with toxins produced by them. Serum from an immune animal can be transferred to a healthy animal and will protect it against a challenge (passive immunization). To characterize the substances in serum having protective capacity (antibodies), several approaches have been used. One has been to sequentially precipitate proteins from serum with salts, especially with ammonium or sodium sulfate. High-molecular-weight proteins such as fibrinogen precipitate readily with no interference with the protective activity of the serum. Increasing the salt concentration precipitates both the serum globulins and the protective activity but leaves the major serum protein (albumin) in solution. A more sophisticated approach became possible when Tiselius introduced electrophoresis and found that different serum proteins moved at characteristic mobilities in an electric field. Kabat and Tiselius then electrophoresed a potent precipitating antiserum and compared the patterns given by whole antiserum to serum that had been exposed to (absorbed by) antigen (Fig. 12–4). After absorption the slow-moving γ-globulin (immunoglobulin G, or IgG) peaks showed a marked depletion, indicating that the precipitating antibody was predominantly of γ-mobility. More modern methods of characterization have given greater precision to the definition of the immunoglobulins, have permitted their subdivision into

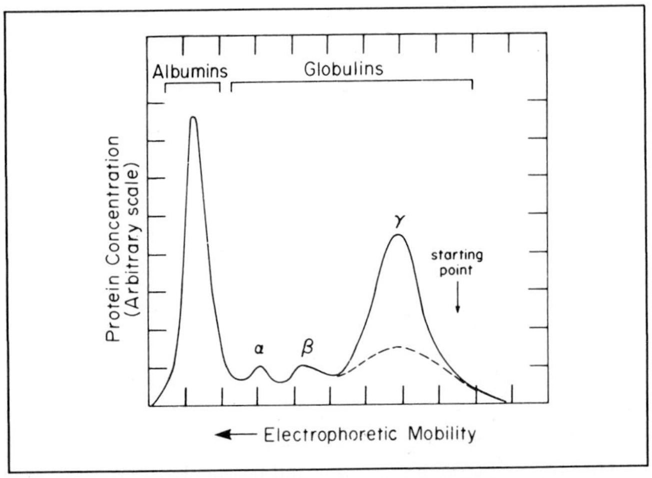

Fig. 12–4. Free-zone electrophoresis of rabbit serum after hyperimmunization with ovalbumin. Data were obtained before (—) and after (- - -) absorption of the serum with the immunizing antigen. Albumin is the most prominent and fastest moving serum protein. Subsequent serum protein peaks (α, β, and γ) were named for their characteristic electrophoretic mobilities. *(Adapted from Tiselius and Kabat: J Exp Med 69:119, 1939.)*

subclasses (e.g., IgG1), and have identified additional classes of immunoglobulin (Table 12–1).

Immunoglobulin Classes

In humans five major classes of immunoglobulins have been described: IgG, the major serum component; IgM, or macroimmunoglobulin; IgA, the predominant immunoglobulin in extracellular secretions; IgD, a minor serum component but an important B cell antigen receptor; and IgE, the immunoglobulin implicated in anaphylactic hypersensitivity (Chap. 17). Some of the physiocochemical, biologic, and physiologic properties associated with these distinct classes of immunoglobulins are illustrated in Table 12–1.

Although electrophoretic analyses could distinguish between some immunoglobulin classes, there is extensive heterogeneity even within a single class of immunoglobulin. For example, IgG separated by ammonium sulfate precipitation and ion exchange chromatography from immune serum is electrophoretically heterogeneous (Table 12–1). This electrophoretic heterogeneity relates, in part, to further subclassification of IgG. Human serum IgG consists of four subclasses (Table 12–2). Subclasses also have been described for IgA (Table 12–1). The subclass distinctions are based on slight amino acid composition differences in the heavy (H) chains, which often can be distinguished serologically with anti-isotypic antibodies (see below).

Complete characterization of an immunoglobulin requires sequence analyses of homogeneous protein, a condition that cannot be met with immunoglobulins isolated from normal sera. Serum IgG3, for example, consists of many IgG3 molecules having distinct antigen specificities and, hence, distinct amino acid sequences (see below).

Significance of Serum Paraproteins

Neoplastic and proliferative diseases of antibody-forming cells (e.g., plasma cell tumors, myeloma) result in an excess of a serum immunoglobulin, reflecting the product of these malignant cells—the serum paraprotein. The serum paraprotein from a single myeloma patient is electrophoretically homogeneous, implying a single component. The plasma cell tumor in a myeloma patient produces the characteristic serum paraprotein and, often, a low-molecular-weight protein (Bence Jones protein), which is excreted in urine and consists of free light (L) chains or their catabolic fragments. Myeloma paraproteins of every immunoglobulin class (except IgM) and subclass have been described in the literature. In certain plasma cell tumors with a distinct clinical syndrome including serum hyperviscosity, Waldenström's macroglobulinemia, an

TABLE 12–1. PHYSICAL, PHYSIOLOGIC, AND BIOLOGIC PROPERTIES OF HUMAN SERUM IMMUNOGLOBULINS

Property	IgG	IgA	IgM	IgD	IgE
Physical Properties					
Sedimentation coefficient, $S_{20\omega}$	6.8–7.0	6.6–14.0	18.0–19.0	7.0	7.9
Molecular weight in kilodaltons	14.3–16.0	15.9–44.7	90.0	17.7–18.5	18.8–20.0
Electrophoretic mobility[a]	γ^2–α^1	γ^2–β^2	γ^1–β^1	γ^1	γ^1
Carbohydrate content, %(w/w)	2.3	7.5	7–11	13	11–12
Number of four-chain units per molecule	1	1–3	5–6	1	1
Heavy chains	γ	α	μ	δ	ϵ
Heavy-chain allotypes	Gm	Am	—	—	—
Heavy-chain subclasses	$\gamma1$, $\gamma2$, $\gamma3$, $\gamma4$	$\alpha1$, $\alpha2$	—	—	—
Heavy-chain molecular weight in kilodaltons	50–55	62	65	70	75
Light-chain molecular weight or κ, λ in kilodaltons	23	23	23	23	23
Physiologic Properties					
Normal adult serum concentration (mg/ml)	8–16	1.4–4.0	0.4–2.0	0.03	ng amounts
Percent total serum immunoglobulin	80	13	6	1	0.002
Synthetic rate, mg/kg/d	26	27	5.7	0.4	0.003
Catabolic rate in serum, %/d (half-life in days)	6 (23)	25 (6)	15 (5)	37 (3)	70–90 (<3)
Intravascular distribution, %	48	41	76	75	51
Biologic Properties					
Agglutinating capacity	±	++	++++	—	—
Complement-fixing capacity	+	—[b]	++++	—	—
Anaphylactic hypersensitivity	—	—	—	—	++++
Guinea pig anaphylaxis (heterologous skin)	+	—	—	—	—
Fixation to homologous mast cells and basophils	—	—	—	—	++++
Placental transport to fetus	+	—	—	—	—
Rheumatoid-factor binding	+	—	—	—	—
Present in external secretions	+	++++	±	—	++

[a] Various immunoglobulins exhibit from α^1 to γ^2 electrophoretic mobilities (see Figs. 12–4 and 12–22).

[b] Aggregated IgA can initiate the alternative complement activation pathway.

TABLE 12–2. PROPERTIES ASSOCIATED WITH SUBCLASSES OF HUMAN IgG

Properties of IgG Subclasses	IgG1	IgG2	IgG3	IgG4
Percent of total serum IgG	65–75	15–23	7	3
Synthetic rate, mg/kg/d in serum	25	?	3.4	?
Catabolic rate, %/d, in serum (half-life, d)	8 (23)	6.9 (23)	16.8 (7)	6.9 (23)
Intravascular distribution, %	51	53	64	54
Allotypic markers (Gm types)	1, 2, 3, 4, 17	23	5, 6, 10, 11, 13, 14, 21	?
Complement-fixing capacity	+	+	+	—
Heterologous skin-binding capacity	+	—	+	+
Placental transport to fetus	+	±	+	+

excess of a homogeneous IgM serum paraprotein is detected. No two paraproteins of the same class and subclass from different myeloma (or Waldenström) patients are completely identical, and with the exceptions of rare double myelomas, paraproteins show none of the electrophoretic heterogeneity of conventional immunoglobulins. This homogeneity led to the supposition that a single cell becomes neoplastic and from this cell a clone develops, the cells of which all produce an identical immunoglobulin with a single amino acid sequence.

The paraproteins, because of their high concentrations, are readily purified in quantity from patient sera. They have been important in elucidating both structural and functional attributes of immunoglobulins (Tables 12–1 and 12–2). Antisera to myeloma proteins produced in goats or rabbits can distinguish the various classes and subclasses of human immunoglobulins (anti-isotypic antisera).

Plasmacytomas are preferentially produced in two inbred strains of mice, BALB/C and NZB. Intraperitoneal injections of mineral oil frequently induce the formation of these tumors. As in the human disease, mouse myelomas produce a characteristic serum paraprotein and may produce a urinary Bence Jones protein. These tumors may be passaged in mice of the same inbred strain or may be adapted to tissue culture.

Köhler and Milstein and Sharff and coworkers have described methods by which cultured murine myeloma tumor cell lines (producing an immunoglobulin of unknown specificity) can be fused with splenic lymphocytes from mice immunized with a defined antigen. They further described techniques whereby hybrid cell lines (hybridomas) can be selected that secrete a monoclonal immunoglobulin with distinct antigenic specificity (determined by the immune spleen cell population) while retaining the growth characteristics of the parent tumor cell line (see below). Virtually every antibody with any desired antigen specificity can be immortalized. Thus it is now possible to determine structure-function relationships for monoclonal antibodies having a defined amino acid sequence and antigenic specificity.

Characterization of Antibodies

Most of the early physicochemical studies were with heterogeneous IgG purified from rabbit, horse, and human sera. Important structural features of IgG were predicted from these studies long before amino acid sequences and x-ray diffraction studies were reported. The molecular weight of IgG was calculated from sedimentation and diffusion studies. It was predicted from its viscosity parameters that the molecule would be asymmetric. Its unique proteolytic fragmentation pattern suggested the molecule consisted of enzyme-resistant globular domains covalently linked by protease-sensitive regions.

Functional studies also suggested distinct regions. Hapten-specific antibodies express two specific hapten-binding sites per IgG molecule. The existence of a third functional domain was suggested from complement component activation subsequent to antigen binding, which was not dependent on the specificity of the antibody. Thus these early studies predicted a minimum of three functional and structural domains. This concept has been abundantly verified.

Polypeptide Structure of IgG

Classic studies by Edelman and his coworkers showed by zone electrophoresis under denaturing and reducing conditions that human and rabbit IgG consists of H and L polypeptide chains. Porter and coworkers demonstrated by gel filtration under similar denaturing and reducing conditions that rabbit IgG consists of H chains (50,000 to 53,000 Da) and L chains (22,000 to 25,000 Da) and that the mass ratio of H to L was 2:1. From these and other data a four-chain structure (two H plus two L) was postulated.

Porter and coworkers also digested rabbit IgG with the proteolytic enzyme papain and chromatographed the resulting subunits on cation-exchange columns. A fragment containing a univalent binding site for hapten or antigen (Fab) was isolated, as was a fragment that contained no hapten-binding site but was readily crystallizable (the Fc fragment) in low ionic strength buffer. The intact IgG was characterized by a sedimentation coefficient of 7S, whereas the sedimentation coefficient of both the Fab and the Fc was 3.5.

Digestion of rabbit IgG with pepsin resulted in a bivalent fragment $F(ab')_2$ and a smaller pFc fragment. If reducing agents such as β-mercaptoethanol were added to the $F(ab')_2$ fragment, a critical disulfide bond was reduced, and two Fab′ fragments were produced. Extensive reduction of Fab′ or Fab with β-mercaptoethanol yielded an Fd′ or Fd fragment, respectively, and a free L chain. Taken together, these studies led to the proposed structure for rabbit IgG shown in Fig. 12–5.

Subsequent studies with the different human Ig classes and subclasses have shown that they all possess the same fundamental four-chain structure. The differences mainly reside in the number of four-chain units per Ig molecule and the appearance of additional accessory polypeptides. For example, IgM and often IgA (Fig. 12–6) contain a j chain

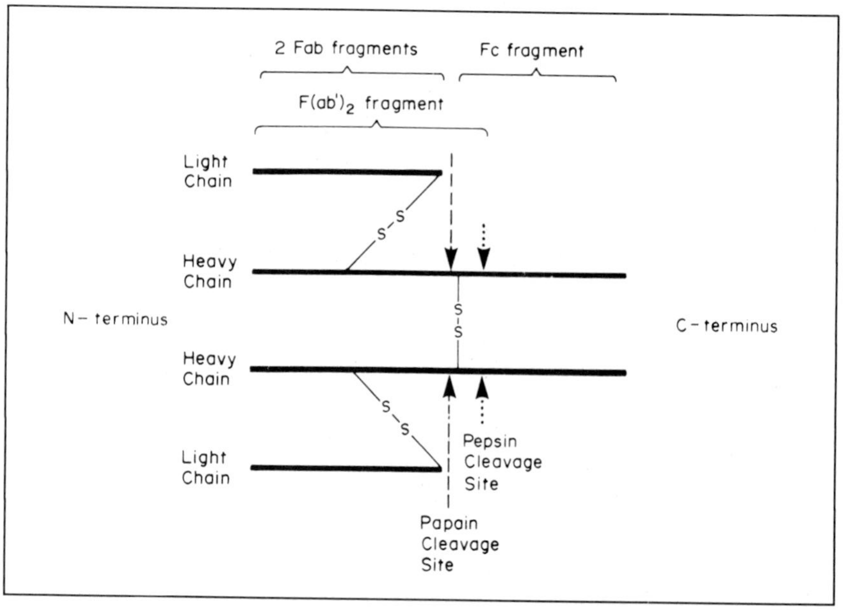

Fig. 12–5. Proposed structure for rabbit IgG showing the four-chain basic structure, important disulfide bonds, and probable sites of enzymatic cleavage by papain or pepsin. The enzyme papain cleaves the heavy chains on the amino terminal side of the single interheavy chain disulfide bond, whereas multiple pepsin cleavage sites are to the carboxyl terminal side of this disulfide bond. Reduction of the light-heavy chain disulfide bonds in the presence of denaturants results in the separation of light chains and heavy chains or heavy chain fragments.

(15,000 Da) produced by the immunoglobulin-secreting cell that initiates and stabilizes higher polymerization of these immunoglobulins through disulfide bonds. Secreted IgA (and sometimes IgM) can also contain an associated secretory component (60,000 Da), produced as a cell-surface IgA receptor by a proximal epithelial cell, that enhances IgA secretion into extracellular compartments.

Characterization of Immunoglobulin Domains

The formation of certain intrachain disulfide bonds confers a repeating domain structure on immunoglobulin H and L chains (Fig. 12–7). Loops of 60 to 80 amino acids are generated in each 110–amino acid segment. For the H chains of IgG, IgA, and IgD (440 to 470 amino acids in length), each of four 110–amino acid segments contains a disulfide-bonded loop of 60 to 80 amino acids. For L chains there are two 110–amino acid segments, each containing a 60 to 80 amino acid loop. This 110–amino acid domain containing a disulfide-bonded loop is characteristic of immunoglobulin H and L chains and all other member proteins of the immunoglobulin superfamily (such as the T cell receptor).

The differences in the molecular weights of the major immunoglobulin classes are largely due to differences in the number and size of H chains: the H chains for IgM (μ) and IgE (ε) are longer than the IgG (γ) chain by approximately 110 amino acids and contain one additional domain. The two classes of L chain (κ or λ and subtypes of λ) are shared by all classes and subclasses of the H chains.

Peptide Mapping and Sequence Studies

Bence Jones proteins are either intact or fragmented homogeneous L chains and represent catabolic products of the serum paraprotein. Clonally derived, they are chemically identical from a given individual and are therefore ideal for structure determination. They can be readily purified, characterized by tryptic peptide mapping, and sequenced. When several different L chains had been characterized in this manner, it became apparent first that there were at least two major classes of L chain (κ and λ). Second, all L chains possessed two distinct regions: a variable (V) amino terminal end (no two Bence Jones proteins have identical V regions) and a constant (C) carboxyl terminal end. The C_κ region of all κ Bence Jones proteins possesses 95% to 100% sequence homology in residues 111 to 214 and little homology with C_λ regions. C_κ regions are encoded by a single gene that exists in three allelic forms; two of the alleles (Km1 and Km1,2) encode a leucine at residue 191, whereas Km3 encodes a valine at this position. Km1 and Km1,2 can be further distinguished by a single amino acid difference at position 153. The amino acid differences attributed to the Km genetic markers, or allotypes, can also be detected by specific antisera. Individuals and families can be typed serologically with respect to the Km marker. In a heterozygote (Km1,2 or Km 3) a single Ig molecule carries L chains derived from a single allotype (Km1,2 or Km 3) and never both. No allotypic markers have been demonstrated for human λ chains. Five tandemly arranged genes encode five distinct human λ chains (λ subtypes). All five gene products can be expressed in any individual. All individuals produce the same five λ subclasses, but a single immunoglobulin contains only two copies of a single subtype.

Amino acid sequence studies of many Bence Jones proteins have shown the amino terminal half of the molecule is variable (the V region) and have implicated this region in antigen binding, with the variability reflecting individual antibody specificities. However, the first 22 to 23 amino acids of the V region exhibit much less heterogeneity, and based on the available sequences in this first framework region, κ chains can be subgrouped (κI, κII, κIII) (Fig. 12–8), and λ L chains can be subgrouped similarly (λI, λII, λIII, λIV, λV). Therefore sequencing an unknown Bence Jones protein through the first 22 to 23 amino acids is often sufficient for isotyping (κ or λ), subtyping (λ subtypes), and V-region subgrouping since V_κ is always found with C_κ (and V_λ with C_λ).

When the H chains from homogeneous myeloma proteins were similarly characterized, an analogous structural relation-

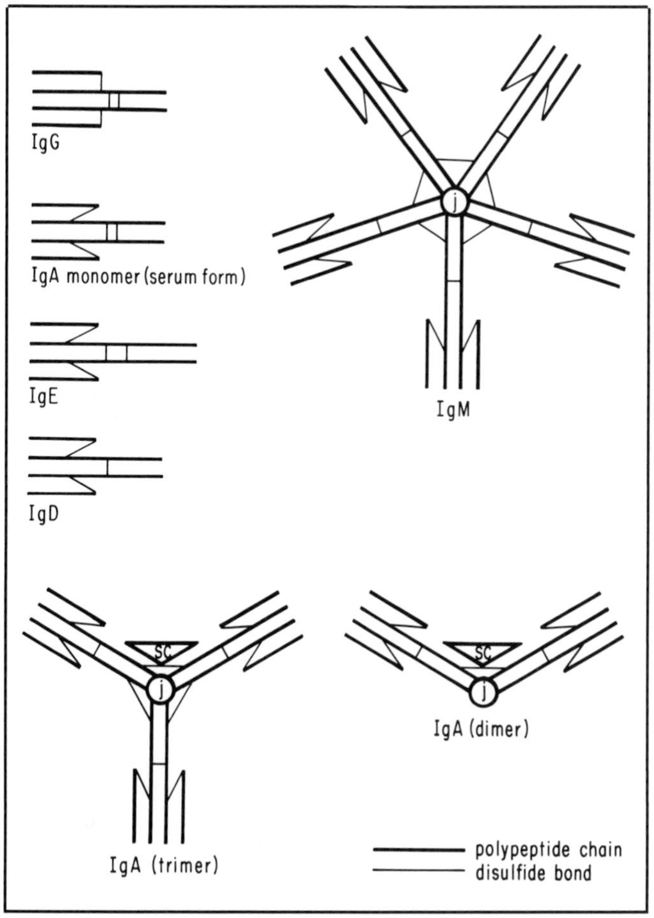

Fig. 12–6. Representative structures for the major human immunoglobulin classes. Each contains the basic four-chain unit, and some may exist as polymers (e.g., serum IgM and secreted IgA). The accessory polypeptides j chain (j) and secretory component (SC) may also be present in the polymeric forms. All immunolglobulin classes have an alternative, hydrophobic heavy chain carboxy terminus when used as a B cell surface antigen receptor (see Fig. 12–14).

ship became apparent (see Fig. 12–7). In all cases the amino terminal 110–amino acid segment contained variable sequences (V_H), and the remaining segments were constant (C_H) except for a few amino acid changes that accounted for H chain allotypic markers. Alleles exist for all the IgG subclass genes and the IgA2 subclass gene (encoding Gm and Am2 allotypes, respectively). For example, all IgG1 myeloma H chains (γ1) share a largely identical amino acid sequence from residue 111 to the carboxy terminal end with the exception of amino acid differences encoded by one of several alleles. Like the Km allotypes of κ light chains, Gm and Am2 allotypes can be distinguished serologically. IgG1 H chain constant regions show very distinct amino acid sequence differences from the H chains of other IgG subclasses (γ2, γ3, γ4). Each subclass, in turn, has its own unique constant regions and Gm allotypic markers (see Table 12–2). The Gm allotypic markers can, in some cases, be defined by sequence studies, and in the case of Gm1 (or Gma) of IgG1 H chains, this is due to amino acid changes in two residues (Table 12–3). The IgA2 allotype $Am2^+$ has no H-L interchain disulfide bond, whereas the $Am2^-$ allotype does.

The amino terminal 22 amino acids in the V regions of the H chains of several human paraproteins have been compared, and by analogy with the L chains, the amino terminal 22 amino acids fall into four subgroups (V_{HI}, V_{HII}, V_{HIII} and V_{HIV}), but in contrast to the class (κ or λ) association for L chains, the H-chain V_H subgroups apparently are shared by all H-chain classes and subclasses. Exceptional myeloma patients produce more than one class of paraprotein (e.g., IgG and IgA paraproteins), each of which shares the identical amino acid sequence in the H-chain V region and the identical pair of L chains. Thus the same V_H subgroup (and H-chain V region) is associated with two distinct H-chain constant regions. These observations first suggested that separate genes control the synthesis of variable and constant regions of immunoglobulins.

An additional important domain, unique to the H chains, was suggested from both hydrodynamic studies and electron microscopy—the hinge region. Sequence studies have confirmed the existence of a hinge region between the Fab arms of an immunoglobulin and its Fc region. This region contains a highly flexible glycine doublet flanked by two relatively inflexible proline-rich sequences (Fig. 12–9).

Control of the effector activities of immunoglobulin molecules appears to center exclusively in the Fc regions. For example, fixation of C1q, the first component of complement (Chap. 15), depends on the availability of defined Fc subunit sites in IgM, IgG1, IgG2, and IgG3. Limited proteolysis of immunoglobulins resulted in unique fragments that maintained C1q binding sites. When these fragments were sequenced, the C1q recognition sites for IgG mapped to the CH2 domain and for IgM, to the CH3-CH4 domain. A variety of effector cells express surface Fc receptors for IgG (FcR[γ] on lymphocytes, macrophages, polymorphonuclear neutrophils [PMNs], and eosinophils), IgM (FcR[μ] on lymphocytes), or IgE (FcR[ε] on mast cells and basophils). The recognition sites for these receptors map to the Fc regions. Finally, certain physiologic properties of immunoglobulins, including biologic half-life, placental transport, seromucosal secretion, and intestinal absorption of immunoglobulins, are in large part dictated by the nature of the Fc region.

Antigen-binding Site

The amino terminal V regions of H and L chains are directly involved in antigen binding. Rabbit antisera directed at the binding sites of hapten-specific antibodies produced in other rabbits (anti-idiotype antibodies) have been highly informative. Donor and recipient animals were matched for rabbit immunoglobulin allotypes so that the specificity detected could be ascribed only to differences in the V regions (idiotypes). Anti-idiotypic antibodies may block the hapten-specific binding of the donor antibody, and anti-idiotypic immunoglobulins only react with intact donor immunoglobulin or the isolated Fab or $F(ab')_2$ fragments and never with Fc fragments. Therefore the idiotypic specificity must reside in, or be proximal to, the antigen-binding site. It is most likely that the idiotype is in the V regions of the H and L chains.

Proteolytic fragments Fab and $F(ab')_2$ contain antigen-specific binding sites. More extensive pepsin digestion of the Fab fragments from a mouse IgA myeloma protein (with significant DNP-lysine specificity) yielded a fragment (Fv)

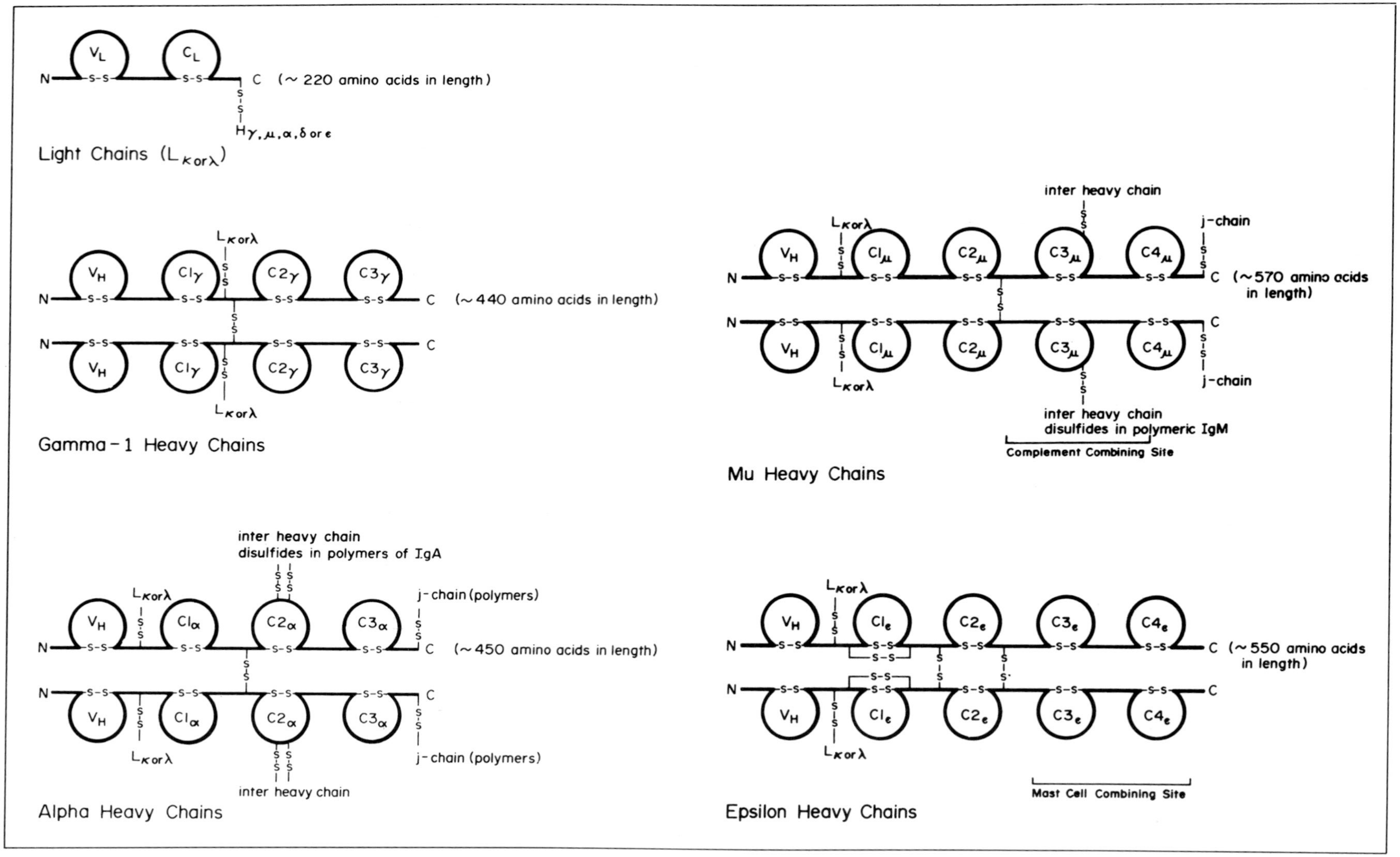

Fig. 12–7. Detailed description of the light and heavy chains for various human immunoglobulins. A single schematic representation of a light chain is shown, illustrating variable (V_L) and constant (C_L) region domains of 60 to 80 amino acids each and the position of the light-to-heavy chain disulfide bond. Heavy chain dimers are illustrated for $\gamma 1$, α, μ, and ϵ chains, respectively. The variable and constant region domains in each are marked, and positions of the light-to-heavy disulfide bonds and various other stabilizing bonds are shown. The carboxyl terminal disulfide bonds in α and μ chains may be covalently linked to j chain in the polymeric forms. Physiologic properties of the immunoglobulins (Tables 12–1 and 12–2) are largely controlled by the constant region domains. *(For further details see Winkelhake: Immunochemistry 15:695, 1978.)*

AMINO ACID RESIDUE POSITION FROM AMINO TERMINUS

		10 20		CODE
VκI Subgroup			A	alanine
	ROY	DIQMTSSRSSLSASVGDRVTITC	B	asparaginyl (D or N)
	EU	BIZMTZSPSTLSASVGBRVTITC	C	cysteine
	OU	DIQMTZSPSSLSASVGBRVTITC	D	aspartic acid
	DAV	DIQMTQSPSTLSTVVGDRVTITC	E	glutamic acid
VκII Subgroup			F	phenylalanine
	TEW	DIVMTQSPLSLPVTPGEPASISC	G	glycine
	MIL	DIVLTQSPLSLPVTPGEPASISC	H	histidine
	MAN	DIVMTQSPLSLPVTPGEPASISC	I	isoleucine
VκIII Subgroup			K	lysine
	Ti	EIVLTQSPGTLSLSPGERATLSC	L	leucine
	B6	ZIVLTZSPGTLSLSPGZRAALSC	M	methionine
	DIL	EIVLTQSPGTLSLSPGDRATLSC	N	asparagine
			P	proline
			Q	glutamine
			R	arginine
			S	serine
			T	threonine
			V	valine
			W	tryptophan
			Y	tyrosine
			Z	glutamyl (E or Q)

Boxed residues indicate subgroup typing residues and cysteine 23, the beginning of the first disulfide loop.

Fig. 12–8. The subtyping of human κ chains based on sequence analyses of the first 23 amino acids of the amino terminus. Five groups of κ chains can be distinguished in this manner by examination of the amino acids in positions 9 and 13; three groups are illustrated here. For example, the $V_{\kappa II}$ subgroup is characterized by leucine at position 9 and valine at 13. *(Data and the one-letter amino acid code adapted from Hood and Prahl: Adv Immunol 14:291, 1971.)*

containing only the V_H region of the H chain and the V region of the L chain. This Fv fragment was capable of binding DNP-lysine.

Largely because of the work of Singer and coworkers, important residues in the region of the binding site were defined by the affinity-labeling technique. In this technique, antibody with affinity for a hapten is reacted with an analogue of the hapten containing a chemically reactive group. During recognition and binding, a covalent bond may be formed between the reactive hapten and an amino acid at or near the binding site (usually tyr or lys). The reactive residue can then be identified by limited-sequence analysis of tryptic digests. These studies have implicated tyr residues at positions 24 to 34, 50 to 75, and 90 to 114 and lys residues at position 54 of H chains as important for binding. Significant labeling of tyr 33, 34, and 86 and lys 54 were noted for L chains.

TABLE 12–3. RELATED SEQUENCE CHANGES IN THE Gm1 (OR α) ALLOTYPIC MARKER IN HUMAN IgG1 HEAVY CHAINS

Gm Type	Amino Acid Residues Involved	Residue Positions
1+	-Asn-Glu-Leu-	356–357–358
1−	-Glu-Glu-Met-	

Data from Waxdal et al: Biochemistry 7:1967, 1968; Frangione et al: Nature 221:145, 1969; Burton and Deutsch: Immunochemistry 7:145, 1970

Further evidence that the V region comprises the antigen-binding site derives from the studies of Wu and Kabat and of Capra and Kehoe. The amino acid sequences of V regions of both paraprotein L and H chains were analyzed for the extent of variation in each residue. Wu and Kabat studied the variability in human κ chains ($V_{\kappa I}$, $V_{\kappa II}$, $V_{\kappa III}$) and described three hypervariable regions (residues 24 to 34 [L1], 50 to 56 [L2], and 89 to 97 [L3]) irrespective of their subgroup. Certain residues were invariant and were presumably structurally important (e.g., cys 23 and 88, tyr 35, gly 99, and gly 101). By comparing the sequences of only $V_{\kappa I}$ L chains, the first hypervariable region (L1) could be narrowed to residues 30 to 32. The hypervariable regions (or complementarity-determining regions, CDR) are believed to be direct-contact residues with antigen, whereas areas of minimum variability in the V region (framework regions such as the first 22 or 23 amino acids) are necessary for a certain basic tertiary structure and for intersubunit interactions (such as V_L and V_H union).

The H-chain V regions were similarly studied for a limited number of available H chains. Regions of hypervariability are currently assigned to three regions (residues 31 to 35 [H1], 50 to 56 [H2], and 95 to 102 [H3]). Again the cys residues 22 and 92, responsible for the V region loop, were invariant, as were trp 36, arg 38, pro 41, gly 41, trp 47, ala 88, tyr 90, gly 106, val 111, and ser 112.

Several of the paraproteins from BALB/C and NZB mice have been extensively studied by sequence analysis throughout the L- and H-chain V regions. These studies suggest that not

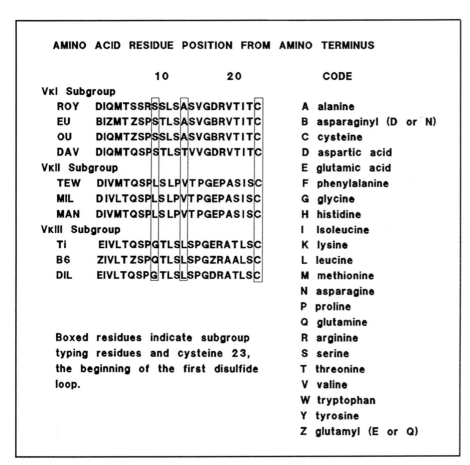

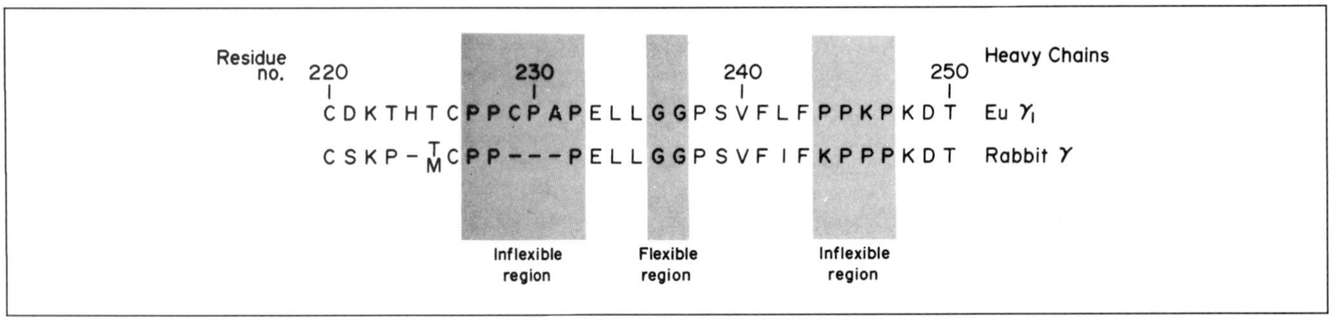

Fig. 12–9. Structural analysis of the immunoglobulin hinge region. Partial sequences in the region of the proposed hinge region are shown for rabbit IgG and the human IgG1 paraprotein Eu. The hinge regions for the two immunoglobulins are not equal in length; residues were matched for best fit, and the dashes represent the insertion of artificial gaps in the rabbit γ chain. Note that relatively stiff, proline-rich, conserved sequences are found to either side of a flexible, double-glycine region. The one-letter amino acid code of Figure 12–8 has been used. *(Adapted from Day: Advanced Immunochemistry. Williams & Wilkins, 1972.)*

only is the variation of amino acids in the hypervariable regions important in determining antibody specificity, but the size of hypervariable regions may vary. This change in length has the effect of changing the structural shape of the antibody-binding site to form long crevices and pockets of varying depths. Most V-region sequence and length variability concentrates in the H3 (CDR3) hypervariable region.

The three-dimensional structure for the paraprotein IgG, New, which has affinity for the γ-hydroxyl derivative of vitamin K_1, has been reported. Crystals of the Fab fragments were prepared, and through a combination of amino acid sequencing and x-ray crystallography, the three-dimensional structure was determined. X-ray crystallography of the Fab–vitamin K complex is shown in Figure 12–10 (see also Fig. 12–2). The complete three-dimensional structure of an IgG molecule (the human myeloma Dob) is shown in Figure 12–11.

Antigen-Antibody Complexes

X-ray crystallographic structural data are available for a number of antigen–Fab antibody fragment complexes. These data can be used to determine the details of complex formation. In every case examined, the fit between the binding site and its ligand is so complementary that water molecules are virtually excluded from the interface. Questions do remain regarding changes in the conformation of either the interacting ligand or the antibody-binding site. In the case of the New protein complexed to the vitamin K_1 ligand (Fig. 12–10), the complex is best described by the lock-and-key model—an exact fit with no induced conformational changes in the antibody-binding site. Since the native conformation of the ligand is not known, no conclusions can be made about induced conformational changes of the vitamin ligand. A recent report by Stanfield and others documents the association of a peptide ligand with the B1312 monoclonal antibody Fab′ fragment; in this case the association induces a significant change in the conformation of the peptide ligand with little change in the conformation of the antibody-binding site. The peptide ligand was a synthetic partial peptide of a naturally occurring protein, myohemerythrin. The native conformation of this peptide in the intact molecule is known from structural studies and differs significantly from the induced structure bound to the antibody. In a report by Bhat and others the interaction of lysozyme with the monoclonal antibody D1.3 Fab fragment (Fig. 12–2) has been studied in more detail. The D1.3 Fab fragment and its lysozyme epitope interact over a broad area; at several points the side chains of each interdigitate. A small but significant alteration in the conformation of both the antibody-binding site and the lysozyme epitope does occur in this complex. Whether any or all of these model interactions can be generalized to other antigen-antibody associations is not known; too few have been examined to draw any strong conclusions.

What is apparent is that the fit between the surface of the antibody-binding site and the surface of the antigen epitope is extremely close. The exclusion of water molecules (a favorable change in entropy) and closeness of interacting side chains from both molecules (favorable enthalpic contributions) contribute to the high association constants typical of these reactions (see below). The additional observation that the amino acid residues of an antigenic determinant are characterized as highly motile is in keeping with the slight to dramatic conformational changes induced in the epitope when bound to antibody.

Origin of Antibody Diversity

Since an individual may have the capacity to respond to as many as 10^8 or more different antigenic determinants, the mechanism for generating this huge number of unique antibodies has received special attention. The requirements are simplified in one respect since it is assumed that any given L chain can combine with any given H chain; 10^3 different L-chain V regions and 10^3 different H-chain V regions could therefore generate 10^6 different antibodies.

In recent years there have been rapid and spectacular advances in the understanding of immunoglobulin gene structure. Relatively accurate assessments of the number of copies of immunoglobulin V and constant (C) region genes have been made by molecular hybridization. The specific messenger RNA for a given unique L or H chain isolated from a plasmacytoma is transcribed into radioactively labeled DNA

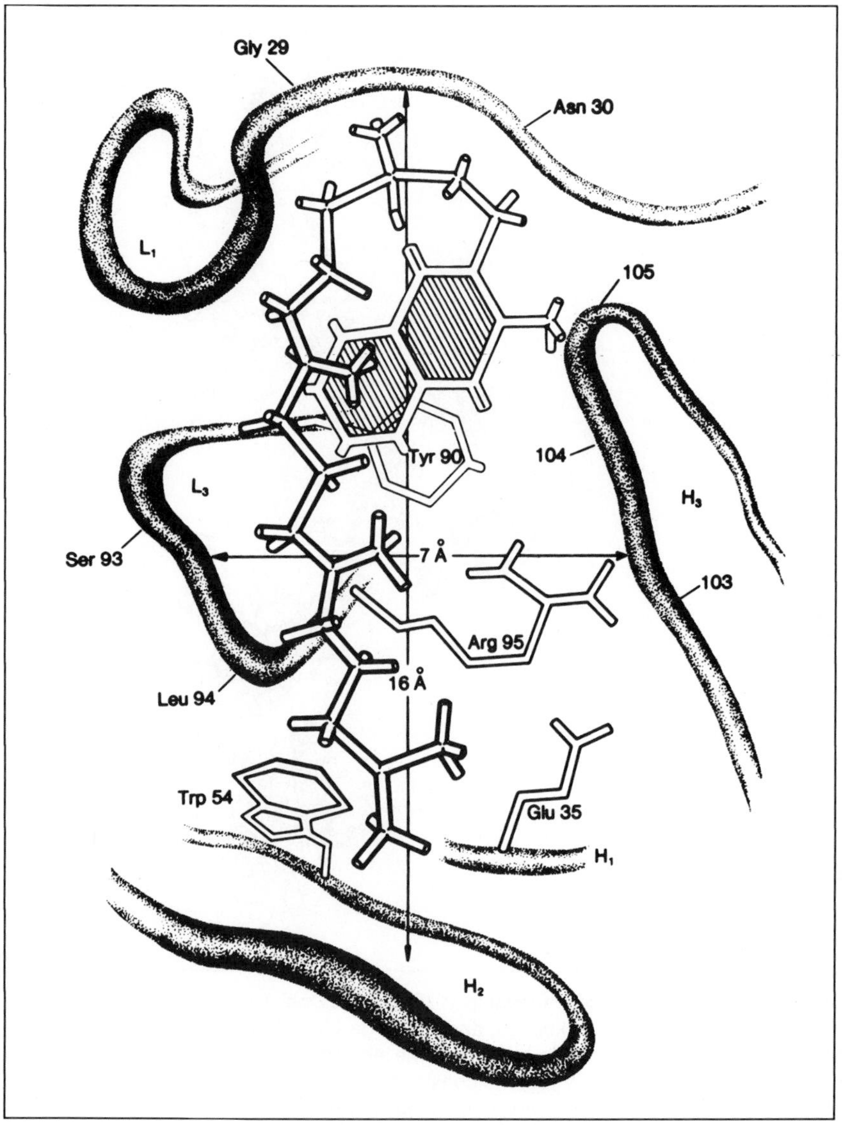

Fig. 12–10. The antibody-combining site of the human IgG1 paraprotein New as determined by x-ray diffraction studies. The position of the hapten, a derivative of vitamin K, has also been determined. Two of the light chain hypervariable regions (L_1, L_3) and three of the heavy chain hypervariable regions (H_1, H_2, H_3) can be seen in this representation. The aromatic rings of vitamin K_1 (striped centers) are in proximity to light chain tyrosine residue 90. The aliphatic chain of vitamin K_1 extends from one side of the antibody-binding site (L_1, Gly 29) to the other (H_2, Trp 54). *(From Amzel et al: Proc Natl Acad Sci USA 71:1427, 1974.)*

(cDNA) using reverse transcriptase (Chap. 69). The rate with which this labeled DNA probe hybridizes with the genome of the plasmacytoma cell or embryonic DNA is then measured. The faster it hybridizes, the more the DNA that specifies L or H chains is present in the cell, that is, the more gene copies it contains. The results indicate that both in the mouse and human there are very few C-region genes. In the mouse the number of V_λ-region genes has been estimated at one to five copies per genome, whereas a similar estimate of V_κ-gene copies runs as high as 350. L-chain V regions are constructed from two initially separate genetic elements, V and J, on the same chromosome. V_κ genes (Fig. 12–12) code for a 22-amino acid leader sequence, initially translated but ultimately cleaved from the κ chain before secretion, and amino acids 1 to 95 of the completed κ chain. The coding region for the leader sequence is split by an intervening sequence of 175 base pairs. Amino acids 96 to 108 of the classically defined V region are coded for by one of four functional J_κ genes. One V_κ gene is translocated by an unknown mechanism to a position 5′ to the selected J_κ gene to make a functional V_κ-region gene. These two rearranged gene segments remain separated from the C_κ gene by an intervening sequence of 2.5 to 4 kilobases. The entire V-region gene, together with the C_κ gene, is transcribed into RNA, the intervening sequences are removed by the splicing processes common in eukaryotes, and the result is a polyadenylated mRNA coding for an intact κ chain.

Murine λ chains derive from only two V_λ genes, which are similar in construction to V_κ genes, each of which can translocate to a position where it is transcribed together with one of two J_λ—C_λ sets. However, $V_{\lambda 2}$ uses only one of the alternative J_λ—C_λ sets. Subsequent to the translocation event, the transcription of the V_λ-J_λ-C_λ complex and subsequent RNA processing and translation are identical to the steps described for κ chains.

The formation of murine H chain V regions is more like that of the V_κ region than the V_λ region in that multiple sequentially ordered V_H genes exist (Fig. 12–13), each coding for a leader sequence and amino acids 1 to 97 of the V_H

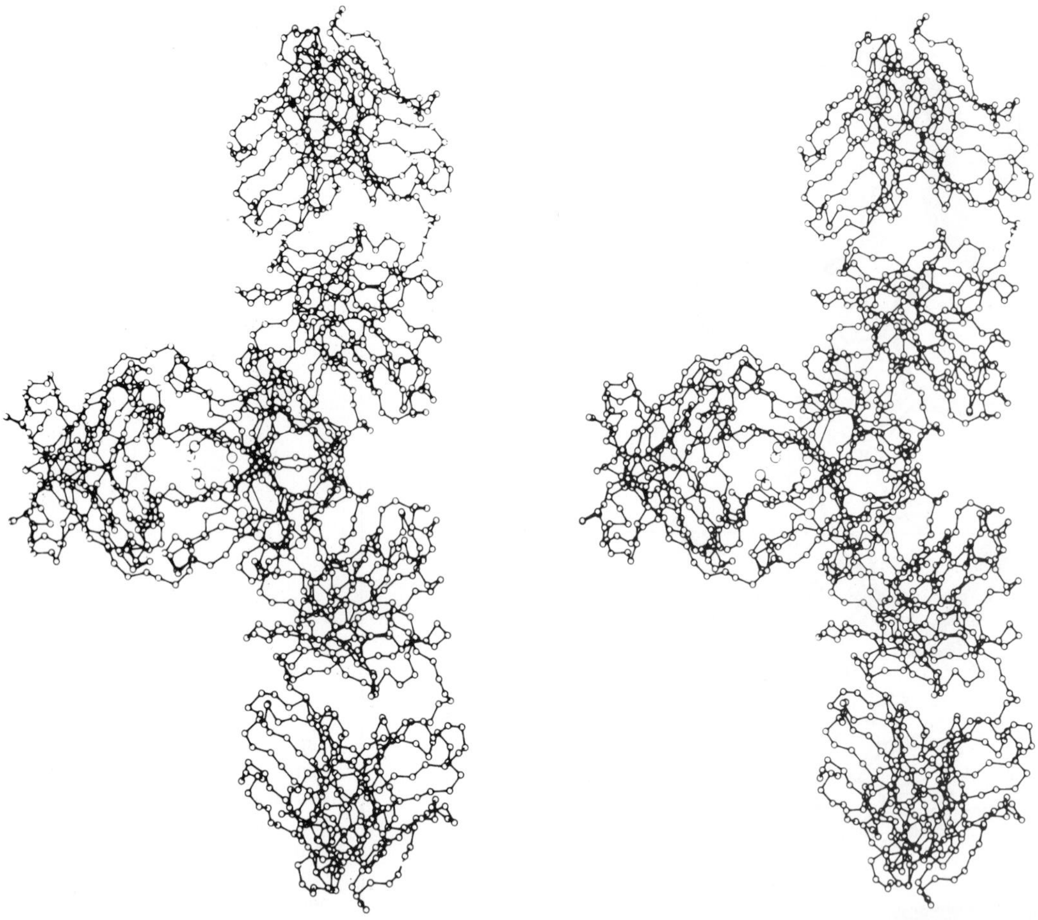

Fig. 12–11. Stereoview of the three-dimensional structure of a human IgG1 (κ) protein Dob. The small circles represent the α-carbon atoms of the polypeptide backbones, and the large circles in the Fc region of the molecule denote carbohydrate units. The Fc region is oriented to the left of center, whereas the Fab regions are at the top and bottom of the figure. The V regions consist of two domains (H and L), showing β-pleated sheet structures in two dimension; they are connected by open stretches of linear polypeptide to the C_L-C_{HI} domains. The Fc domains show a prominent central groove in which much of the covalently coupled carbohydrate resides. The antibody-binding sites lie at the very top and bottom ends of the molecule. (Many individuals can visualize three-dimensional stereograms by staring at the two figures. A third image will appear in the center field in three dimensions.) *(From Silverton et al: Proc Natl Acad Sci USA 74:5140, 1977.)*

region. An additional order of variability is introduced by additional genes, the D_H genes. To form a functionally active V_H region, one of a number of D_H genes (10 to 15) first is translocated to a position adjacent to one of four J_H segments. A second translocational event juxtaposes the rearranged D_HJ_H segment and one of several hundred V_H genes to code for a complete V_H region. An intervening sequence of 6.5 kilobases separates the J_H cluster from C_μ, the μ-chain C region gene. Transcription of the VDJ segment, together with C_μ, gives rise to a precursor RNA that ultimately is spliced and processed to yield an mRNA coding for an intact μ chain.

Antibody-binding site diversity can be attributed to this recombination of gene segments in the middle of the third hypervariable region (H3, or CDR3). In addition, variation in the codons encoding the precise junction of these gene segments and a mechanism for adding exogenous nucleotides at these sites (N-terminal nucleotide transferase activity) significantly increase the level of variability in CDR3. During immunoglobulin class switching (see below), significant somatic mutation accounts for much of the variability in the remaining regions of hypervariability (CDR1 and CDR2).

An additional property of the H-chain gene cluster not shared by the L-chain systems is the potential for class switching. The newly assembled H-chain VDJ gene set can be translocated to a position immediately 5′ to any of the H-chain C region genes (δ, γ3, γ1, γ2b, γ2a, ϵ, or α), forming a functional set that can code for an intact chain of the appropriate class or subclass and that shares the V_H region initially

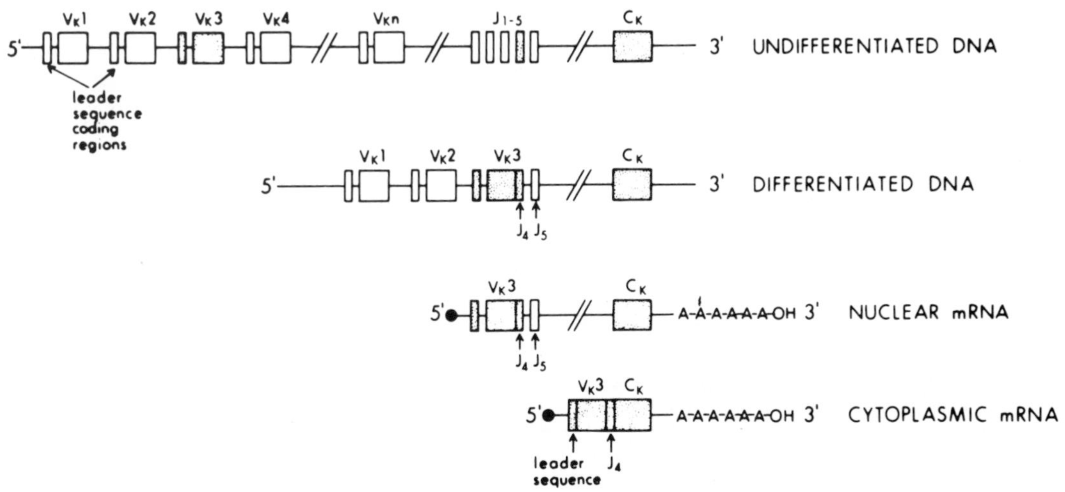

Fig. 12–12. Construction of a murine κ light chain mRNA. In this schematic representation of the genome the boxes represent coding regions (exons), and lines separating the boxes are intervening sequences. Multiple V_κ genes exist, each consisting of two gene segments coding for the leader sequence and the N-terminal sequence of the mature κ chain, separated by an intervening sequence. In undifferentiated cells V_κ genes, J genes, and the C_κ gene are well separated on the chromosome. Plasma cell differentiation and commitment to the production of a single κ chain involve translocation of a V_κ gene ($V_{\kappa 3}$ above) to a position 3′ to a selected J gene (J_4 above). Nuclear mRNA is transcribed from this configuration. Processing of the precursor mRNA involves loss of intervening sequences (including the J_5 sequence above), modification of the 5′ terminus, and addition of polyadenylic acid to the 3′ terminus. The precursor form of the κ light chain is translated from the cytoplasmic mRNA on membrane-associated ribosomes. The leader sequence of the protein is removed in the rough endoplasmic reticulum to give mature κ chains.

present in the μ chain. Thus the phenomenon of two immunoglobulins of different classes sharing a common binding site and idiotype can be explained at molecular level.

The precise mechanism of the class switch has not been elucidated, but particular regions of the DNA between the C region genes are involved. They are known as switch regions (S regions) and consist of tandem repetitive sequences, which appear to provide recognition sites for the translocation process, postulated as a homologous recombination (i.e., recombination between genes on the same chromosome). The S_μ region, for example, which lies between the J_H cluster and C_μ gene, has the nucleotide sequence $[(GAGCT)_n\ (GGGGT)]_m$ where n varies between 1 and 7, and m is on the order of 150.

The individual H-chain C-region genes are organized in a fashion remarkably reminiscent of the organization of the ultimately translated protein. Each domain is encoded by an exon, which is separated by an intron or intervening sequence from an exon coding for the adjacent domain. The hinge region of C_γ genes is encoded by a small exon between those coding for C_{H1} and C_{H2} of the γ1 chain. Intervening sequences are removed from transcribed RNA before translation as described above.

Membrane IgM, which acts as the antigen receptor of B lymphocytes, is attached to the membrane by a sequence of 26 hydrophobic amino acids at the C-terminal end of the μ-chain (see below). The hydrophobic sequence is encoded by the region M, which is 3′ to the last exon encoding the C_μ region (Fig. 12–14). The synthesis of the membrane form of the μ chain appears to be regulated at the RNA-splicing level. For soluble μ chains the C_μ DNA region up to the 3′ terminus of the exon coding for the fourth C domain is transcribed. For membrane μ chains an entire transcript that includes the M region is modified at the splicing level; RNA coding for the C-terminal 20 residues of the soluble μ chains is removed; and the M region, coding for 41 amino acids, which include the 16 amino acid hydrophobic stretch, is retained. This mechanism (which is also used by other immunoglobulin classes and subclasses in a similar, although not identical, fashion) is consistent with the fact that B cells can simultaneously express surface IgM and also secrete IgM.

The genetic mechanisms described for murine immunoglobulin gene rearrangements are, in all essential characteristics, identical in humans. Perhaps the major difference is that there are multiple V_λ genes in the human. As a consequence, λ L chains are much more commonly used in generating functional human immunoglobulins. In the mouse approximately 99% of circulating immunoglobulins contain κ chains.

Immunoglobulins As B Cell Antigen Receptors

The transmembrane polypeptide sequence of 26 hydrophobic amino acids of cell-surface IgM are thought to form an

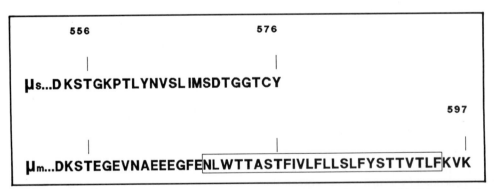

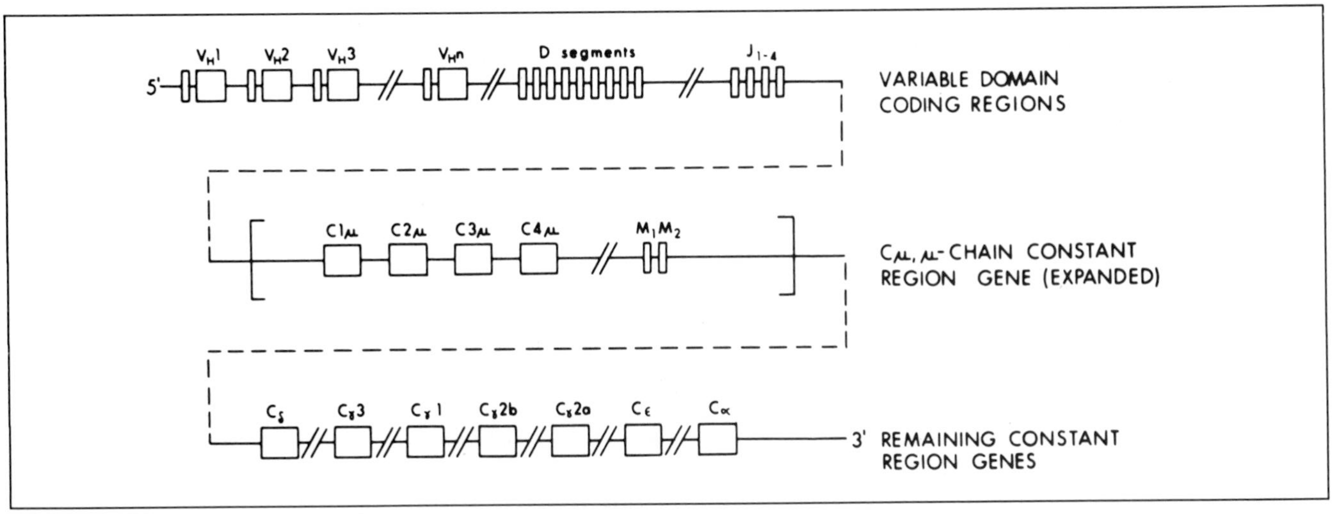

Fig. 12–13. Schematic representation of the heavy chain gene complex of the mouse in undifferentiated cells. During differentiation to an IgM-producing plasma cell one of the D_H genes is translocated to a position adjacent to one of the 4J segments. A further translocation associates the V_HD coding sequence with one of the H genes to yield a complete variable region gene. This gene is coexpressed with the C_μ gene, expanded above to show the exons that code for the individual C_μ domains (see Fig. 12–7), and the M exons coding for the membrane integration sequence at the C-terminus of membrane-associated μ chains. Further differentiation—to an IgG-secreting cell, for example—would involve the translocation of the V_HDJ transcription unit to a position immediately 5′ to the $C_\gamma1$ gene. Individual C-region genes are organized in a similar way to the C gene represented above, with individual exons coding for separate domains.

inverted α-helix, with hydrophobic side chains oriented outward. The short, highly charged cytoplasmic tail (lys, val, lys) may communicate with cytoskeletal elements. Equivalent, although not identical, transmembrane domains and cytoplasmic tails (some much longer than membrane IgM) are associated with the alternative membrane forms of all other classes of immunoglobulin.

The first antigen-specific receptor expressed by B cells is membrane IgM. This IgM is not further polymerized by the addition of j chain and exists as a basic four-chain (two H and two L chains) unit at the cell surface. Immature B cells express surface IgM alone. Mature B cells coexpress surface IgM and IgD, with each sharing the identical L chain and the identical H-chain VDJ region sequence. They share the same immu-

556 576

μs...DKSTGKPTLYNVSLIMSDTGGTCY

597

μm...DKSTEGEVNAEEEGFE[NLWTTASTFIVLFLLSLFYSTTVTLF]KVK

Fig. 12–14. The alternative carboxy terminal amino acid sequences for secreted IgM heavy chain (μ_S) and membrane IgM heavy chain (μ_M). The sequences for each are identical through the fourth heavy chain domain to residue 556 and change dramatically thereafter. The μ_M chain terminus contains a transmembrane, hydrophobic region (boxed) that is thought to form an inverted α helix, with its hydrophobic side chains oriented outward and into the lipid bilayer. The μ_M chain terminates in a short, highly charged, cytoplasmic tail, KVK. Other classes of immunoglobulin also have alternative carboxy termini for the membrane forms; the exact sequence of the transmembrane section and the sequence and length of the cytoplasmic tail may differ appreciably from μ_M. *(Adapted from Rogers et al: Cell 20:303, 1980.)*

noglobulin idiotype and the same antigenic specificity. These receptors differ only in the C region of the H chain. In mature B cells a single long, nuclear message is transcribed, which reads through the rearranged VDJ gene region and both the μ and δ constant gene regions. This single, nuclear mRNA is processed to alternative mRNAs encoding the secreted and membrane forms of IgM and IgD, with the ratio of secreted to membrane forms depending on the stage of B cell differentiation. Memory B cells and mature, virgin B cells in special anatomic compartments (such as the mucosal tracts) may express different isotypes of cell-surface immunoglobulin (e.g., a preponderance of membrane IgA in mucosal B lymphocytes).

Recently, additional membrane molecules associated with cell-surface immunoglobulin have been implicated in signal transduction. For example, the B cell receptor complex for exogenous antigen may include membrane, antigen-specific immunoglobulin, and perhaps an associated, GTP-binding protein (or G protein) important in receptor-ligand signal transduction. This antigen-immunoglobulin receptor complex may also undergo endocytosis and pass through a lysosomal compartment where the complex and bound intact antigen are degraded. Degraded antigenic peptides may associate with MHC class II molecules in this compartment and may eventually be reexpressed at the cell surface as a complex for T cell recognition.

Antigen-specific T Cell Receptor

Polypeptide Structure of the T Cell Receptor

The basic structure of immunoglobulins has been known for several years. However, the nature of the antigen-specific receptor of T cells eluded investigators until comparatively recently. Both cytotoxic (largely CD8$^+$) and helper (largely CD4$^+$) T lymphocytes recognize fragments of foreign antigens in association with MHC antigens at the cell surface. CD8$^+$ T cells are generally restricted to MHC class I antigens, and CD4$^+$ T cells to MHC class II antigens (Chaps. 13 and 14). The TCR must therefore recognize a complex of foreign antigen peptide bound in the peptide-binding cleft of an MHC molecule.

Elucidation of the structure of the TCR began with the development of monoclonal antibodies exhibiting idiotypic specificity for functional T cell lines propagated in vitro. Antibodies capable of inhibiting the function of helper and cytotoxic T cells that had no effect on the function of other T cell lines with a different MHC-restricted specificity were produced. In both murine and human systems the antibodies reacted with a cell-surface heterodimeric glycoprotein, which was the antigen-specific TCR.

Figure 12–15 shows schematically the structure of the TCR ($\alpha\beta$). It consists of two integral membrane glycoprotein subunits, α and β, covalently linked by a disulfide bond. Each of the subunits has a similar domain structure, remarkably reminiscent of the structure of an immunoglobulin L chain. Both polypeptides subsequently have been classified as members of the immunoglobulin superfamily, based on this structural similarity. In the mouse, both chains have molecular weights of approximately 43,000. In the human the α chain is slightly larger, 45,000 to 50,000 Da, whereas the β chain has a molecular weight of 40,000. In both species the core proteins have molecular weights of approximately 30,000, with the additional size resulting from the addition of N-linked oligosaccharides. Each chain consists of an extracytoplasmic region, a transmembrane region, and a short carboxy terminal cytoplasmic region. The extracytoplasmic region consists of two domains, an N-terminal V-region domain and a C-region domain. These domains exhibit sequence homology to the equivalent immunoglobulin V and C domains and contain the classic disulfide loop of approximately 60 amino acids. Variations in the amino acid sequence of the V_α and V_β regions are responsible for the antigenic specificity of the receptor.

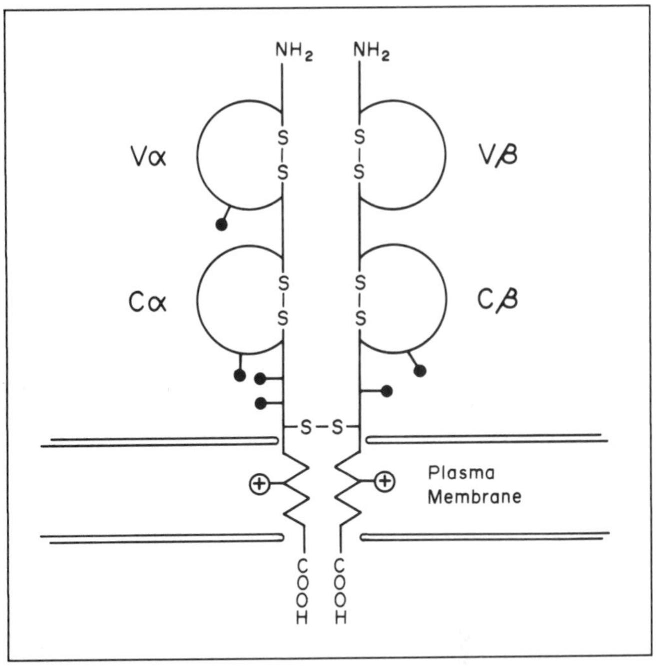

Fig. 12–15. Schematic representation of the antigen-specific, MHC-restricted, T cell receptor. The basic heterodimeric structure involving disulfide-linked α and β subunits has been demonstrated at the protein level. Additional features such as the number and position of asparagine-linked carbohydrate structures (●) and the presence of positively charged lysine or arginine residues in the otherwise hydrophobic transmembrane region (⊕) are inferred from cDNA sequences. The positively charged transmembrane residues are believed to associate via salt-bridge formation with similarly placed acidic aminoacid residues in the transmembrane regions of the δ and ϵ components of the CD3 complex. The α subunit of the human T cell receptor consists of 248 amino acids, and the β subunit contains 282.

Origin of T Cell Receptor Diversity

The genetic mechanisms involved in generating the diversity of TCR are essentially the same as those used by immunoglobulin genes. The α and β chains are the products of two unlinked genetic systems on chromosomes 14 and 7, respectively, in humans (14 and 6 in the mouse). Multiple V_α and V_β genes exist, each of which encodes the majority of the V domain plus a leader sequence of 20 or so amino acids that is removed with the insertion of nascent protein into the endoplasmic reticulum of the T cell. The gene region encoding TCR α chains is analogous to immunoglobulin L-chain genes, that is, intact α chains are encoded by rearranged gene segments V_α, J_α, and C_α. The β chains are encoded by a group of genes analogous to immunoglobulin H chains, that is, β chains derive from transcription of rearranged V_β, D_β, J_β, and C_β gene segments. The first of these TCR genes to rearrange in T cell development is the β-chain gene. Translocation of an individual D_β-region gene immediately 5′ to a J_β segment is followed by a second translocation to one of a number of V_β segments and generates a functional unit (VDJ) encoding the total V region domain of a β chain. The β-chain C region gene, 3′ to the J segment and separated from it by an intervening sequence, encodes the extra cytoplasmic C domain, a short connecting peptide, the transmembrane region, and cytoplasmic tail. In the case of murine and human C_β genes, these protein domains are encoded by separate exons. There are, in addition, two C_β genes, either of which can be used. The subsequent rearrangement of α-chain gene segments initiates, with a V_α to J_α gene, translocation analogous to that of immunoglobulin L chains. Current evidence suggests that only one C_α gene exists. The rearranged VDJ-C (β) or VJ-C (α) segment constitutes a functional transcriptional unit. The same α- and β-chain genes are used to generate the antigen-specific receptor of both T_h and T_c cells.

TCR diversity is largely junctional diversity built into the equivalent of an immunoglobulin CDR3 region in the α and β chains. Additional junctional diversity is built into this region through the use of alternate triplet codons in the splice sites and addition of exogenous nucleotides in a manner analogous, if not identical, to the generation of diversity in the immunoglobulin CDR3 site. Indeed, the CDR3-equivalent regions of the TCR polypeptide chains are hypothesized to make direct contact with the foreign peptide in the groove of the MHC molecule. The highly conserved CDR1 and CDR2-equivalent regions of the TCR α and β chains may make direct contact with allele-specific regions (restricting elements) on the α-helices of the MHC-presenting molecule (Chap. 14). There is no evidence for additional TCR V-region diversity generated by subsequent somatic mutation and selection (as seen for the immunoglobulin CDR1 and CDR2 hypervariable regions).

T Cell Receptor–CD3 Complex

Associated with the heterodimer in the plasma membrane are a number of other proteins and glycoproteins that together are known as the CD3, or T3, complex. For insertion of newly synthesized and complexed TCR α and β chains in the T cell plasma membrane, the CD3 family of molecules must be expressed and added to the receptor complex. The CD3 subunits (γ, δ, ε, and ζ or η) do not exhibit somatic variability and were originally defined by monoclonal antibodies reactive with all peripheral blood human T lymphocytes. Certain antibodies to CD3 epitopes are directly mitogenic for T cells, leading to the hypothesis that the CD3 complex is also involved in transmembrane signaling. Activation of T cells through the CD3 complex leads to elevated intracellular calcium levels and phosphorylation of various CD3 subunits.

The current view of antigen recognition by T cells is that a ternary complex of TCR, antigen-presenting cell MHC molecule, and processed foreign peptide antigen is formed, with peptide bridging the two different, but interacting antigen-binding molecules. The functions of the MHC molecule, the antigen-building molecule on the antigen-presenting cell, are not completely understood but may include some selective aspect of peptide binding (MHC allele dependent), protection of this bound peptide from further degradation in intracellular compartments, and presentation of this peptide at the surface of the antigen-presenting cell. The function of the T cell antigen-binding molecule (the TCR heterodimer) and its associated CD3 complex is recognition of a specific peptide in the appropriate MHC-restricting element and transduction of a signal across the T cell membrane. It is this signal that initiates the T cell function (e.g., the release of cytokines such as interleukin-2 [IL-2] by a helper T cell or activation of the lytic machinery of a cytotoxic T cell).

T Cells Expressing the Alternative γδ Receptor

Although the vast majority of T cells express the αβ heterodimeric receptor, a small population of T cells express a different receptor, which also is a heterodimer. One subunit (γ) has a structure very similar to the α chain described above and is the product of a similar genetic complex with multiple V_γ genes and two sets of J_γ genes, each with a corresponding C_γ gene. The γ-chain gene complex in the human resides on chromosome 7 (13 in the mouse). The second subunit (δ) maps in the middle of the TCR α-chain gene complex in both man and mouse (chromosome 14 in both species). The δ-chain genes differ from the linked α-chain genes in that the δ region contains additional diversity genes, D_δ, and is more like the TCR β-chain gene complex.

Although the true function of the T cell subset bearing the γδ receptor is unknown, there have been some interesting recent observations. For example, $\gamma\delta^+$ T cells carry the CD3 marker like the more common T cell bearing the αβ receptor, but they lack CD4 and CD8. As a consequence, those $\gamma\delta^+$ that are cytotoxic to certain types of tumor cell lines appear to be non-MHC restricted. These cells probably arise in the thymus before $\alpha\beta^+$ T cells. They constitute a small minority of peripheral blood T cells but are highly enriched in the epidermis of the skin and in various epithelia (as intraepithelial T cells). Some $\gamma\delta^+$ T cells may recognize stress proteins such as the heat shock proteins expressed on epidermal or epithelial cell surfaces.

Antigen-Antibody Reactions

Thermodynamics

Theoretically, if an antigen-antibody reaction is truly reversible, it should obey the law of mass action:

$$Ag + Ab \rightleftharpoons AgAb \text{ complex} \qquad (1)$$

It follows that at equilibrium, the following relationship should apply:

$$K_a = \frac{[AgAb]}{[Ag][Ab]} \qquad (2)$$

where the values in brackets reflect the molar concentrations of reactants and the product at equilibrium. Once the equilibrium constant has been determined, the change in the standard free energy, $-\Delta G^0$, can be calculated (the free energy of a reaction taking place under standard conditions of 1 mol/L concentrations of reactants):

$$-\Delta G^0 = RT \ln K_a \quad (3)$$

where R is the universal gas constant (1.986×10^{-3} kcal/°K/mole) and T is the absolute temperature (in degrees Kelvin). If the equilibrium constant K_a is measured at two or more temperatures, the enthalpy, ΔH^0, can be calculated.

$$\frac{d(\ln K_a)}{dT} = \frac{\Delta H^0}{RT^2} \quad (4)$$

Alternatively, the ΔH^0 can be measured directly by microcalorimetry. The entropy change, ΔS^0, can be calculated with the measured values of $-\Delta G^0$ and ΔH^0.

$$-\Delta G^0 = -\Delta H^0 + T\Delta S^0 \quad (5)$$

Since antigens may be multideterminant and antibodies are at least bivalent, it is difficult to obtain quantitative data for most antigen-antibody complex precipitates; the reactants and product are not in a true state of equilibrium. However, if the reactions are carried out in extreme antigen excess where the complexes are soluble, valid data can be obtained.

Hapten-Antibody Reactions

It is relatively easy to treat hapten-antibody reactions quantitatively when the hapten is univalent and the antibody is at least bivalent. The reaction of an antibody site rm) with a free hapten (H) can be written as follows:

$$H + S \underset{k_r}{\overset{k_f}{\rightleftharpoons}} HS \quad (6)$$

where the equilibrium constant K_a is defined by the ratio of the forward-to-reverse rate constants ($K_a = k_f/k_r$). Although the rate constants can in some cases be measured, more often K_a is measured directly by equilibrium dialysis. The technique involves the dialysis of a mixture of free hapten and specific antibody in which only the free hapten can pass easily through dialysis membrane. By knowing the initial concentration of hapten and the concentration of free hapten at equilibrium, the amount of bound hapten, the association constant (K_a), and the valence of the antibody (the number of binding sites per molecule of antibody) can be determined.

If r = moles of bound hapten divided by total moles of antibody (calculated), c = moles of free hapten at equilibrium (measured), n = valence of antibody (or number of sites divided by antibody molecule (calculated), and K_a = equilibrium constant (or affinity constant) (calculated), the mass action formula (eq 6) can be rewritten and rearranged according to the method of Scatchard:

$$r/c = nK_a - rK_a \quad (7)$$

By plotting r/c against r, K_a can be obtained from the slope and n from the intercept on the abscissa. In practice, several different concentrations of hapten are dialyzed in individual experiments, with a fixed concentration of antibody to generate the points in Figure 12–16. Curvature in this type of data presentation reflects heterogeneity in the binding affinities of a population of antibodies in the serum. Antisera are generally heterogeneous and contain antibodies of varying affinity for the antigens to which they are produced. The average association constant can be obtained by measuring the value of r/c at which half of the sites are filled (Fig. 12–16). The extent of heterogeneity can be estimated by several methods, one of which assumes a Sips distribution of equilibrium constants; thus

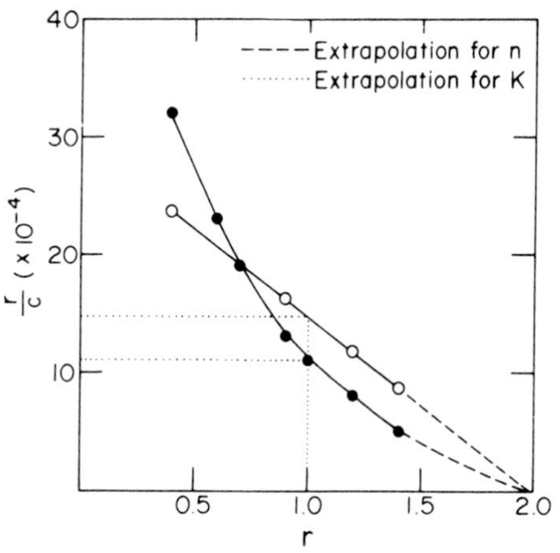

Fig. 12–16. Scatchard plots for two hypothetical hapten-antibody systems. The linear relationship reflects a homogeneous antibody response to the haptenic determinant. The nonlinear relationship reflects a heterogeneous antibody response. Both sets of data can be used to obtain values for n and K (or K_0) by the proper extrapolations.

$$(cK_{avg})^a = \frac{r}{n - r} \quad (8)$$

where a is a power function reflecting the dispersion of equilibrium constants about an average constant, K_{avg}. If a = 1, the expression reduces to that of equation 7. By plotting the log of equation 8,

$$\log \frac{r}{n - r} = a \log c + a \log K_{avg} \quad (9)$$

a straight line may be obtained (Fig. 12–17), the slope of which can be used to calculate a. For homogeneous binding (a single affinity constant) a = 1, and for a heterogeneous mixture of hapten-binding antibodies $a < 1$. When a is determined, the average K_{avg} can be calculated.

Reactions of Antibodies With Multivalent Antigens

Several methods can be used for measuring in vitro antibody-antigen reactions, such as precipitation, complement fixation, agglutination, and radioimmune assay. These techniques are described later in this chapter. For quantitative measurement of association constants (or affinity), antigen-antibody reactions must be studied in the region of antigen excess (where the complexes are soluble) or through the binding of univalent

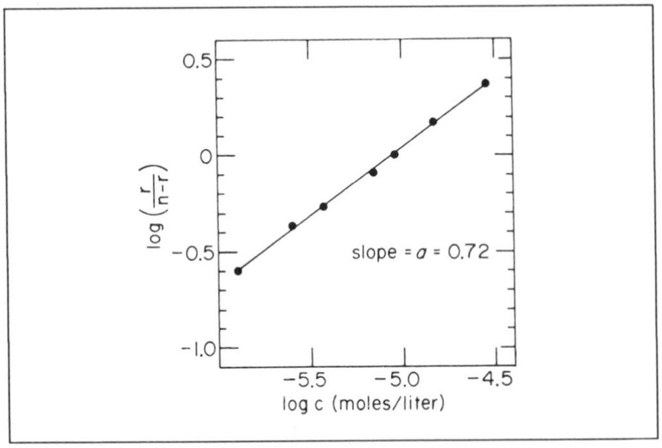

Fig. 12–17. Sips analysis of the nonlinear data illustrated in Figure 12–16. The value of the Sips constant (*a*) can be obtained, and an average affinity constant can be recalculated from Equation 9.

Fab fragments with multivalent antigens. Both techniques can be used to obtain association constants.

Affinity is strictly defined by the experimentally determined equilibrium constant. The term *avidity* often is used semiquantitatively to describe the overall combining properties of an antiserum with a multivalent antigen. The avidity of a particular antiserum depends on the number of different antibodies directed at distinct antigenic determinants on the antigen and their intrinsic association constants. If, in addition, an antigen possesses two or more identical antigenic determinants in close proximity (e.g., viral capsid proteins), the binding of a single antibody to two adjacent determinants results in a large increase in the observed association constant. For example, the primary immune response to an infectious agent such as a bacterium or a virus is characterized by IgM. Although the intrinsic binding affinity of an isolated IgM Fab subunit might be characterized as weak, multideterminant binding by pentameric IgM with a multivalent infectious agent(s) would result in very efficient recognition at a critical time in the infection. This latter phenomenon is known as monogamous bivalent binding. A combination of some or all of these factors determines the avidity of a particular antiserum and also complicates the exact determination of intrinsic affinity constants.

One of the peculiar aspects of the humoral immune response is that it is usually heterogeneous, even to simple chemically defined haptenic determinants. For example, if an animal is immunized with the hapten-protein conjugate DNP-BSA and the resulting antibodies specific for the hapten (DNP) are isolated by immunoadsorption techniques, they will demonstrate a range of intrinsic affinity constants from very low to very high. In other words, in this population of DNP-specific antibodies there are subpopulations with unique affinities for the hapten. Each one of these has a unique antibody-binding site and, therefore, a unique V region amino acid sequence (or idiotype). These observations are consistent with their production by clones of cells derived from single parent cells.

Implicit in this hypothesis is that a single antibody-forming cell (and its precursor) is capable of synthesizing an antibody of a single restricted specificity. During antigenic challenge, cells with both high and low affinities for the antigen may be stimulated to proliferate and transform to antibody-producing plasma cells. Heterogeneous antibodies therefore reflect a heterogeneous response. It is possible to manipulate this response. If very small amounts of antigen are used in the immunization schedule, only precursor cells (B cells) with high-affinity receptor molecules (cell-surface immunoglobulins) will respond, and antibodies of high affinity will be produced. In more conventional immunizations when excess antigen is administered repeatedly, the affinity of the antibodies rises as the residual quantity of antigen wanes after elimination or catabolism, and clones of high-affinity precursor cells compete for antigen and continue to expand in preference to cells of lower affinity.

Methods of Detecting and Quantitating Antigen and Antibody Reactions

Since it is important for the clinician to understand the processes used in the clinical immunology laboratory, this section and the following one are concerned with various in vitro methods of detecting and quantitating antigen-antibody interactions and assessing the number or function of antigen-specific T lymphocytes. The techniques used for detecting antigens with antibodies (this discussion) differ, depending on whether the antigen in question is soluble or cell bound. Accordingly, the following section is divided into two subsections about these areas. This discussion is not intended to be a detailed exposition of the methods but to give an explanation of the principles used. The appropriate detailed sources are indicated in the bibliography.

Soluble Antigens

Quantitative Precipitation

Most techniques examining the reactions of soluble antigens with their antibodies depend on precipitation. Precipitation follows the reaction of divalent IgG antibody with a multivalent antigen. Precipitation depends on the formation of large, insoluble lattices of interconnected antigen and antibody molecules. A typical quantitative precipitin curve is shown in Figure 12–18. Increasing amounts of carbohydrate antigen are added to constant volumes of antiserum. The precipitates are washed and the total protein determined for each point. The amount of antibody precipitated with increasing antigen is linear initially, eventually reaching a peak (the equivalence point). With antigen excess, the amount of antibody precipitated usually falls since adequate cross-linking for the formation of large complexes no longer occurs. An antiserum characterized in this way can subsequently be used to determine the amount of antigen in unknown samples, always working in the linear portion of the quantitative precipitin curve (i.e., in antibody excess).

Ouchterlony Analysis

Ouchterlony analysis is a powerful yet simple technique that allows qualitative detection of antigens in solution and permits

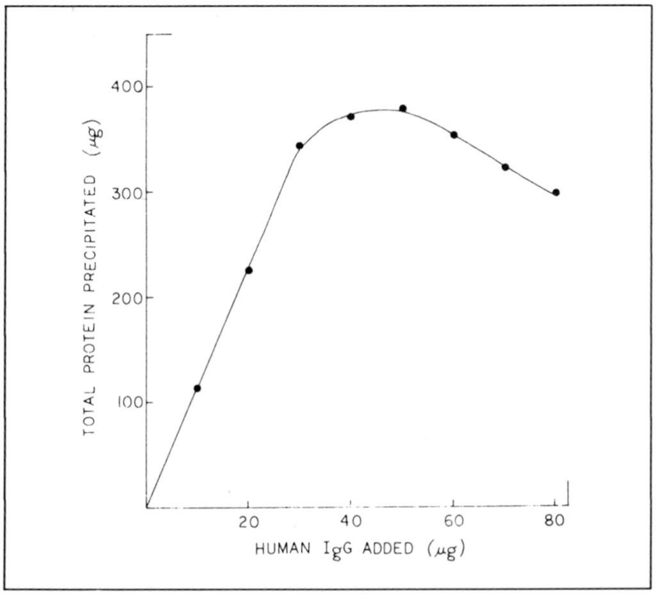

Fig. 12–18. A quantitative precipitin assay with goat antiserum to human IgG, with human IgG as antigen.

the determination of antigenic relationships between different antigens. A 2% (w/v) solution of hot agar in isotonic saline solution is poured into a Petri dish or onto a microscope slide. With a special punch, various patterns of circular holes are cut in the agar layer after it cools. A commonly used pattern consists of six holes in a hexagonal arrangement surrounding a central hole that contains antiserum. When an antiserum and its corresponding antigen in solution are placed in adjacent wells, both diffuse through the agar layer and eventually meet and combine. A band of precipitated antigen forms between the wells. Typical precipitation patterns observed when using related and unrelated antigens with a polyspecific serum are shown in Figure 12–19. If the two antigens, A and B, are identical (Fig. 12–19A), a continuous precipitin line is formed between the two antigen wells and the antiserum well. Two unrelated antigens produce the result shown in Figure 12–19B, where the line produced with one antigen completely crosses that produced with the other. This result also implies that the antiserum contains two unrelated populations of antibodies specific for antigen A and for antigen B, respectively. An interesting pattern is seen when A and B have some antigenic determinants in common. In Figure 12–19C the antiserum primarily reacts with antigen B, but some of the antigenic determinants are shared by A. The result is a "spur" of precipitation with antigen B, resulting from diffusion of antibodies that fail to react with A through the zone of precipitation given by A, and the subsequent reaction with B.

Radial Immunodiffusion

In the radial immunodiffusion method molten agar is premixed with antiserum and is poured onto a plate as in the Ouchterlony method, and wells are cut, usually as two lines of holes. Dilutions of an antigen solution are introduced into each well. Circular zones of precipitation form around the well as the antigen diffuses into the agar and reacts with the antibody. The greater the amount of antigen, the larger the zone of precipitation. For a fixed volume of antigen solution, the square of the diameter of the zone of precipitation is proportional to the antigen concentration. Radial immunodiffusion plates are commercially available for the quantitation of levels of various human serum proteins. Standards containing known amounts of the protein in question are placed in the same plate as the unknown sample (e.g., a patient's serum) and a standard curve constructed. Figure 12–20 shows a radial immunodiffusion plate for the determination of human IgG.

Electroimmunodiffusion

In this quantitative technique of immunoprecipitation devised by Laurell, antiserum is incorporated into the agar layer as described previously. However, instead of relying on diffusion to establish zones of precipitation, antigen migration is induced electrophoretically. Agarose (ion-free agar) is substituted for agar to reduce the cathodal migration of incorporated IgG.

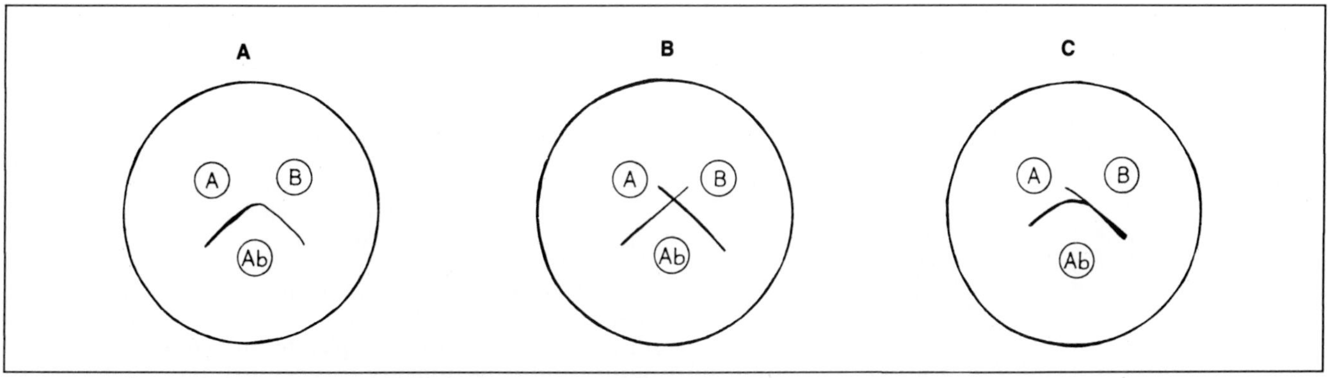

Fig. 12–19. Ouchterlony analysis of a precipitating antiserum (Ab) to two antigens, A and B. **A.** A and B are antigenically identical, and the antiserum reacts equally well with both, showing a line of identity. **B.** A and B are antigenically unrelated, and separate crossed lines of precipitation are produced with the antiserum. **C.** A and B are antigenically related, with antigen A possessing only a portion of the antigenic determinants of B, resulting in a spur of precipitation with B.

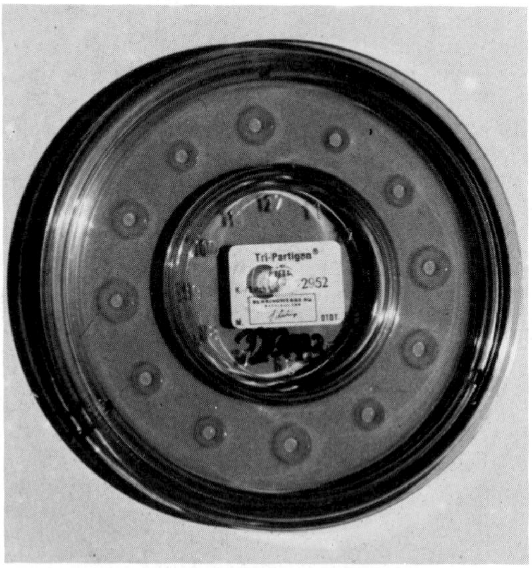

Fig. 12–20. Radial immunodiffusion used to determine human IgG levels. The outer annulus of the plate contains agarose with incorporated goat antiserum to human IgG. In the wells are samples containing various amounts of IgG. Circular areas of precipitation can be seen around each well. *(Courtesy of A. G. Hoechst.)*

The samples (1 to 3 μL) are introduced into wells cut into the plate, and electrophoresis is performed with a potential gradient of 3 to 4 V/cm. Cooling the plate during electrophoresis is usually necessary. "Rocket-shaped" precipitin lines are formed, the height of which is proportional to the antigen concentration under standard conditions. Figure 12–21 shows examples of the kinds of patterns produced.

Immunoelectrophoresis

The immunoprecipitation method of Ouchterlony gives a confusion of lines when a complex antiserum and a complex antigen mixture (e.g., human serum and rabbit or goat anti-whole human serum) are placed in adjacent wells. The immunoelectrophoresis technique of Grabar and Williams overcomes this problem by separating the complex antigen mixture electrophoretically before antiserum is added. Figure 12–22 shows the result of a typical immunoelectrophoretic analysis.

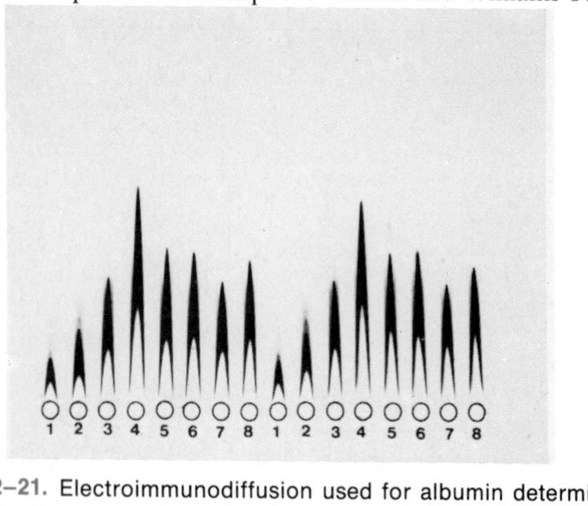

Fig. 12–21. Electroimmunodiffusion used for albumin determination. Duplicate samples (1 to 8) containing varying amounts of human albumin were subjected to electrophoresis through agarose containing goat antiserum to human albumin. *(Courtesy of A. G. Hoechst.)*

A 2% agar solution is allowed to solidify on a microscope slide. A special die then cuts the pattern shown in Figure 12–22. Wells for the sample are adjacent to a trough for antiserum. A sample (2 to 5 μL) is then introduced into the sample well, and electrophoresis is performed for about 45 minutes at 6 V/cm to separate the different components. Subsequently, the antiserum (40 to 50 μL) is introduced into the trough. Diffusion of separated antigens and the antiserum gives rise to the arcs of precipitation visible in Figure 12–22. Some 30 different human serum proteins can be differentiated by this method. By using antisera to individual proteins, any arc of questionable identity usually can be unambiguously identified. Immunoelectrophoresis is a frequently used diagnostic tool in medicine, useful in the detection of monoclonal gammopathies (paraproteins) (e.g., by an enormously enlarged and distorted IgM precipitin line in cases of Waldenström's macroglobulinemia), in the detection of Bence Jones proteins (L chain dimers) in serum or urine, and in the identification of many other serum protein deficiencies or disorders.

Two-Dimensional Immunoelectrophoresis

Two-dimensional immunoelectrophoresis is a combination of the electrophoretic separation method used in conventional immunoelectrophoresis and electroimmunodiffusion. Initially, the antigen mixture is separated in agarose electrophoretically as described for immunoelectrophoresis. A "strip" of agarose containing the separated antigens is placed on a second slide, and an antibody-containing agarose solution is allowed to solidify adjacent to it. Electrophoresis as described for electroimmunodiffusion is then performed at right angles to the original electrophoretic separation, giving rise to peaks such as those shown in Figure 12–23. Quantitation is possible with this technique by comparing the surface area of the precipitated arcs with those given by known amounts of standard antigens.

Radioimmunoassays and Enzyme-Linked Immunosorbent Assays

Some of the most sensitive techniques used in clinical and basic science laboratories are the various kinds of radioimmunoassays for the detection and quantitation of diverse substances from hormones to immunoglobulin allotypes. The principle of quantitation used is that of inhibition. Binding of a radioactively labeled antigen to its antibody is inhibited by known amounts of unlabeled antigen to generate a standard curve; unknown samples are compared to this.

The quantitation of bound labeled antigen can be accomplished in various ways. Systems have been devised using electrophoretic separation of antibody-bound and unbound labeled antigen, separation of the immune complex from free antigen on the basis of size by gel filtration, and precipitation of the antigen-antibody complex by an anti-immunoglobulin serum or by the addition of saturated ammonium sulfate. However, the most convenient is the solid-phase radioimmunoassay. In this technique, antibody is covalently attached to an insoluble matrix, commonly agarose beads that have been "activated" to bind protein amino groups using cyanogen bromide. A mixture of labeled standard antigen and unlabeled test material is then added. Antibody-bound radioactively

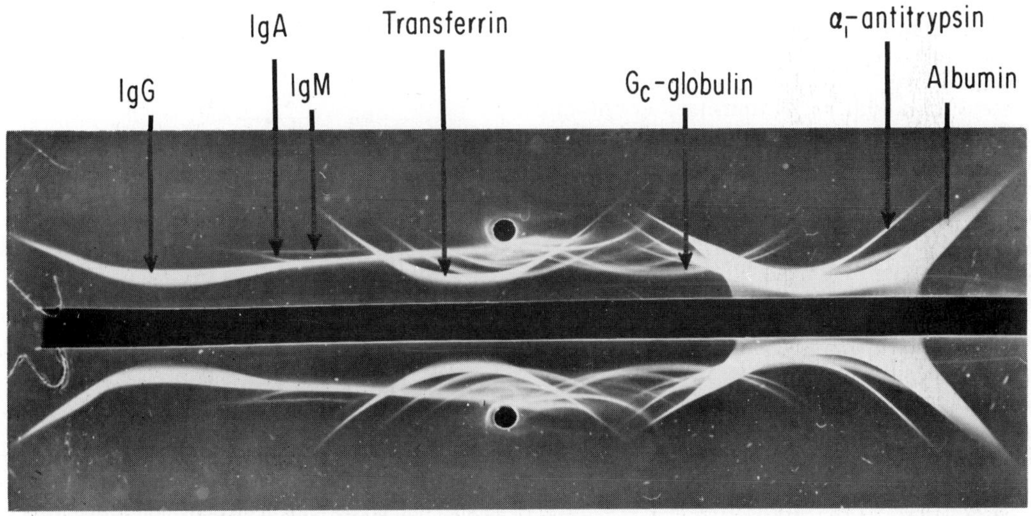

Fig. 12–22. Immunoelectrophoresis of normal human serum. The electrophoretic separation and precipitation with a goat antiserum to whole human serum were performed as described in the text. The precipitin arcs corresponding to some serum proteins are indicated. *(Courtesy of A. G. Hoechst.)*

labeled antigen can then be separated from free antigen by centrifugation or filtration. The greater the recovery of free label, the higher the concentration of the unknown. An example of the kind of data obtained in a solid-phase radioimmunoassay is shown in Figure 12–24.

Technical problems with radioimmunoassay techniques are the decay of isotope used to label the antigen (commonly iodine 125, with a half-life of 60 days) and the general dangers inherent in handling radioactive substances. An alternative method that circumvents these problems is the enzyme-linked immunosorbent assay, often abbreviated ELISA. In this approach the antigen standard in question is conjugated to an enzyme such as alkaline phosphatase or horseradish peroxidase. Glutaraldehyde is often used for the coupling. In the solid-phase variation of the technique, antibody again is attached to an insoluble matrix, and binding of enzyme-linked antigen to the antibody is inhibited by standard amounts of unlabeled antigen or by the unknown samples. After the washing the amount of enzyme-linked antigen coupled to the insoluble antibody is quantitated, using a chromogenic substrate for the enzyme such as *p*-nitrophenyl phosphate in the case of alkaline phosphatase.

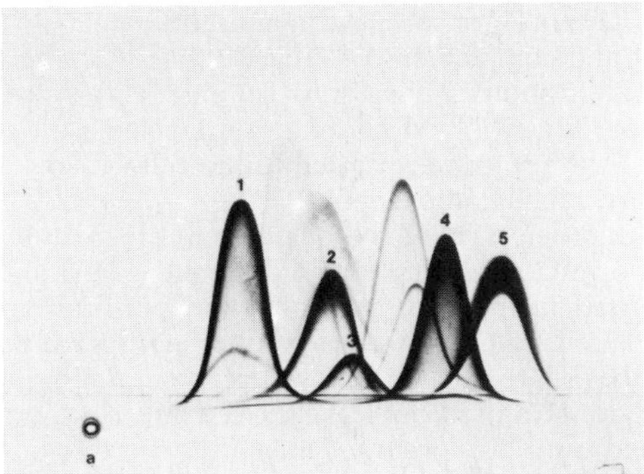

Fig. 12–23. Two-dimensional immunoelectrophoresis. The application well (a) of the first dimension (electrophoresis from left to right) contained normal human serum. The agarose gel of the second dimension (from bottom to top) contained an oligospecific antiserum. The numbered precipitates belong to the following proteins: (1) transferrin, (2) α_2-macroglobulin, (3) ceruloplasmin, (4) α_1-antitrypsin, and (5) α_1-acid glycoprotein. *(Courtesy of A. G. Hoechst.)*

Complement-Fixation Tests

Complexes of antibodies and antigens, both soluble and cell-bound, have the ability to fix serum complement (Chap. 15). Thus measurements of complement fixation can be used to

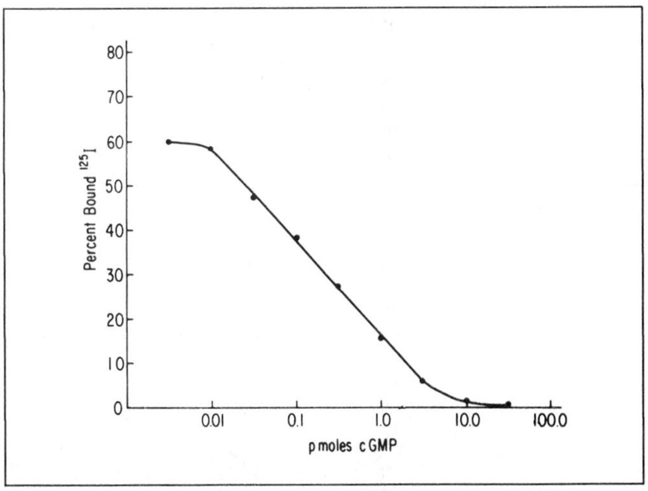

Fig. 12–24. A solid-phase radioimmunoassay for guanosine 3′-5′-cyclic monophosphate (cyclic-GMP). Shown is a standard curve obtained by measurement of the binding of a radioactive derivative of cyclic-GMP (^{125}I-succinyl-cyclic-GMP-tyrosine methyl ester) to agarose beads with covalently attached rabbit antibody to cyclic-GMP in the presence of known amounts of unlabeled cyclic-GMP. Unknown samples are quantitated by comparison with this standard curve.

determine the presence of immune complexes and therefore antigens or antibodies.

Complement levels usually are measured by adding sheep erythrocytes presensitized with rabbit antisheep erythrocyte antibodies to aliquots of the complement (normally from guinea pigs). During incubation at 37C, hemolysis occurs and can be quantitated by centrifuging the samples and estimating the hemoglobin released into the supernatant by visible absorption spectroscopy.

The complement-fixation protocol for a soluble antigen involves incubating dilutions of antigen with its antiserum in the presence of guinea pig complement. After incubation, usually at 4C for periods up to 18 hours, sensitized sheep erythrocytes are added, and hemolysis is measured after 1 hour at 37C. If complement has been fixed by antigen-antibody complexes, hemolysis is reduced. The protocol for cellular antigens is the same, except the antigen-antibody-complement complexes (i.e., cells) can be removed by centrifugation before the sensitized sheep erythrocytes are introduced. By comparison with known, standard, amounts of antigens, unknown samples of antigen can be quantitated.

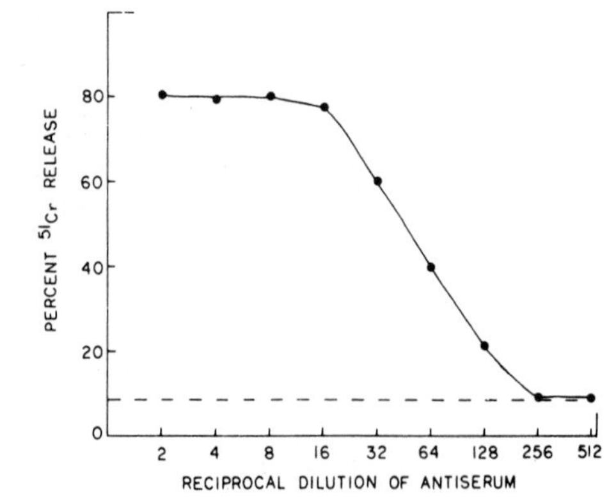

Fig. 12–25. A titration of a cytotoxic anti-HLA-A2 alloantiserum against human peripheral blood lymphocytes from an HLA-A2-positive individual, using the ^{51}Cr-release assay. The dashed line indicates the background release of ^{51}Cr by cells in the absence of antiserum but with added complement.

Cellular Antigens

Agglutination Reactions

The adherence of red blood cells to each other in the direct and indirect agglutination procedures is used in immunohematology and blood banking. The process of agglutination can be modified to detect other antigens. One such modification is called passive agglutination. Erythrocyte membranes are modified by soluble antigens bound to their surface. The method of attachment depends on the nature of the antigen. Bacterial lipopolysaccharides bind to red blood cells during simple incubation, as do some proteins. Reactive haptens such as trinitrobenzene sulfonic acid will attach covalently to red blood cell membranes. Red blood cells treated with tannic acid will bind protein antigens and are more easily agglutinable than untreated red blood cells. Bifunctional cross-linking agents such as bisdiazobenzidine or 1, 3-difluoro-4, 6-dinitrobenzene also can be used to bind a variety of antigens to erythrocytes. Cells with bound antigen form a convenient method of detecting and assaying antibodies to almost any hapten or soluble antigen. Inhibition of passive agglutination also can be used to quantitate haptens or antigens in solution.

Other assays based on the general principles of hemagglutination include mixed hemabsorption and leukoagglutination. Both of these assays were at one time used for the detection of antigens of leukocyte membranes (Chap. 14), but both present many technical difficulties, and leukocyte antigens are currently almost always determined by the cytotoxicity test.

Cytotoxicity Assays

Lymphocytes for human leukocyte antigen (HLA) typing can be easily prepared from heparinized blood by Ficoll-Hypaque gradient centrifugation. Ficoll is a commercial high-molecular-weight polysaccharide that induces spontaneous red blood cell agglutination. Hypaque is a radiopaque dye used to vary the density of the Ficoll-Hypaque solution in water. The density of the mixture is adjusted to 1.078 g/cm^3, a density at which granulocytes and agglutinated erythrocytes sink and lymphocytes float. By simply layering diluted defibrinated blood on the Ficoll-Hypaque solution and centrifuging, lymphocytes can be isolated from the interface.

For HLA typing the lymphocytes are incubated in small typing trays with human alloantisera or mouse monoclonal antibodies specific for the different HLA antigens. Following a wash step to remove unbound antibody, rabbit complement is added to effect lysis. To differentiate between live and dead cells, a vital dye, commonly trypan blue, is added. Such dyes penetrate the membrane of cells lysed by complement but fail to stain living cells. By testing lymphocytes with a battery of sera, unambiguous HLA typing usually can be achieved. Similar procedures are used for detecting the presence of antigens present only in certain stages of development of animal and human cells.

A more quantitative measure of cytotoxicity is the chromium 51 (^{51}Cr) release assay. Lymphocytes are prelabeled by incubating with $Na_2^{51}CrO_4$, which is rapidly incorporated but released from a viable cell at a rate of approximately 5% per hour. A cell that has suffered membrane damage caused by antibody and complement will release the ^{51}Cr label rapidly. Figure 12–25 shows a titration of an anti-HLA antiserum on human peripheral blood lymphocytes labeled with ^{51}Cr. Dilutions of the serum were added to the cells, followed by the addition of rabbit complement.

Yet another assay of cell death by antibody and complement involves adding fluorescein diacetate (FDA) to the cells. FDA is itself membrane permeable and nonfluorescent. On entering a cell, natural esterases convert FDA into fluorescein, causing the cells to become visibly fluorescent under ultraviolet light. Fluorescein itself can leave the cell only slowly, and most is retained until lysis occurs. Thus, after a cytotoxicity assay, dead cells are nonfluorescent and live cells fluorescent. This assay currently is performed in special microtiter trays that can be read and analyzed by machine, and the technique is a particularly powerful method for screening hybridoma supernatants for the presence of specific monoclonal antibodies (see below). An additional generation of fluorescent dyes with different excitation and emission characteristics has been developed in the application of this new technology.

Immunofluorescence

Immunofluorescence is a sensitive technique for the detection of cellular antigens, whether they are cytoplasmic, nuclear, or plasma membrane bound. Direct immunofluorescence requires an antibody that is conjugated to a fluorescent dye such as fluorescein or rhodamine. The isothiocyanate derivatives of the dyes are used to bind them covalently to IgG preparations of the antisera. Intact or sectioned cells are then incubated with the fluorescent antibodies, washed, and examined through a microscope with an ultraviolet light source. Cells that have bound the antibody are brightly fluorescent and easily visible. The site of intracellular localization can be determined in tissue sections. The sensitivity of the technique can be increased dramatically by using indirect immunofluorescence. In this case the fluorescent dye is conjugated to IgG from an anti-immunoglobulin serum. The cells under study are first incubated with antigen-specific antiserum, washed, and incubated with the fluorescent-conjugated anti-immunoglobulin serum. Stained cells are again detected by observation through an ultraviolet microscope. Examples are shown in Figure 12–26.

Flow cytofluorimetry has been developed for analyzing cells within a population that bind fluorescent antibodies (express a given antigen) from those that do not and for separating these cells based on quantitative differences in the level of antigen expressed by individual cells. The method uses a machine called a "fluorescence-activated cell sorter" (FACS). A suspension of cells is passed through the FACS as a stream of positively charged microdroplets, each containing a single cell on average. Illumination of the droplets with laser light allows discrimination of those containing fluorescent cells from those containing nonfluorescent cells. Microdroplets containing fluorescent cells can be selectively deviated by briefly exposing them to a negative charge, and they can be collected separately. Cell populations that differ in intensity of fluorescence rather than being absolutely positive and negative, respectively, can also be separated by the FACS.

More frequently the technique of flow cytofluorimetry is used for analysis of cell populations without subsequent separation. For example, FACS machines are now capable of analyzing a droplet containing a single cell for a variety of parameters, including size, refractility (granularity), and multiple antigens. The new generation of instruments can analyze up to five different antigens simultaneously by using antibodies labeled with different fluors and a combination of excitation and emission wavelengths to detect each. This capability allows the cell-surface phenotyping of cell populations and the discrimination of significant subpopulations. In Figure 12–27 the $CD4^+$ subpopulation of $CD3^+$ T cells has been identified in unseparated peripheral blood lymphocytes from a healthy adult by two-color analysis; the density profiles can be analyzed by the machine's computer to quantitate the number of cells in each sector and thus the distribution of cells within the entire lymphocyte population.

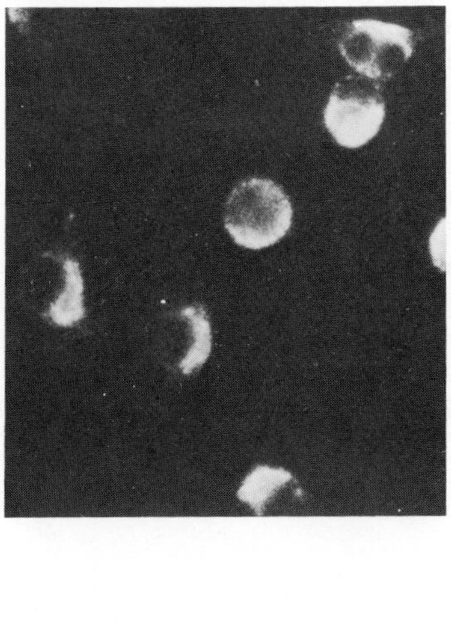

Fig. 12–26. Cytoplasmic staining of a tumor-associated embryonic antigen in acetone-fixed mouse L cells, using indirect immunofluorescence. The specific antibody is a rabbit antiserum to a mouse teratoma, and the developing serum is a goat antiserum to rabbit IgG conjugated with fluorescein. *(Courtesy of Dr. Linda R. Gooding.)*

Radioactive Binding Assays

Immunofluorescent detection of antibodies bound to cell surfaces is not a quantitative method. Enumeration of particular antigenic determinants on cells can be achieved by binding assays using anti-immunoglobulin reagents labeled with iodine 125 (^{125}I) or ^{125}I-protein A. Protein A, a molecule isolated from the cell wall of *Staphylococcus aureus,* can bind to the Fc region of most subclasses of the IgG of many mammals. Either protein A or an anti-immunoglobulin (frequently an affinity-purified $F[ab']_2$ preparation of, for example, rabbit anti-mouse [IgG]) can be labeled with ^{125}I without losing its binding capacity and then can be used in a manner analogous to indirect immunofluorescence. Cells are first incubated with specific antibody, washed, and then incubated with the ^{125}I-reagent. After further washes the amount of ^{125}I bound to the cells is determined. Using known numbers of cells and ^{125}I-reagents of known specific activity, estimates of the number of antigenic determinants per cell can be obtained. $F(ab')_2$ of rabbit anti-mouse IgG is particularly useful in binding assays using murine monoclonal antibodies.

Immunoferritin Techniques

The use of specific antibodies to detect cellullar antigens by electron microscopy is of increasing value. The principle is similar to that of immunofluorescence except that the antibody is conjugated to an electron-dense molecule such as the iron-containing molecule, ferritin. Cells are incubated with ferritin-conjugated antibody, and sections are examined by electron microscopy. Ferritin molecules can be observed on the cell surface where antibodies are bound. Other markers such as viruses have been used in place of ferritin and can be distinguished from ferritin morphologically, allowing the detection of two antigens on the same cell using antisera conjugated to ferritin and, for example, to tobacco mosaic virus.

Monoclonal, Hybridoma Antibodies

As mentioned earlier in the section describing serum paraproteins, techniques have been developed that allow the production by cell lines of monoclonal antibodies to virtually any designated antigens. The basic technique involves the polyethylene glycol–induced fusion of splenic B lymphocytes from an immunized mouse or rat with cells from a mutant myeloma lacking the gene for hypoxanthine-guanine-phosphoribosyl-transferase (HGPRT). The myeloma cell line is unable to grow in medium containing hypoxanthine, aminopterin, and thymidine (HAT medium) as a result of its enzyme deficiency, whereas hybrid cells containing the HGPRT gene donated by the splenocyte grow continuously, and unfused splenocytes die in this culture system. In addition to the expression of the HGPRT gene, the fused cells express the products of the immunoglobulin genes of the B lymphocytes, giving rise to "hybridoma" cell lines that produce antibodies

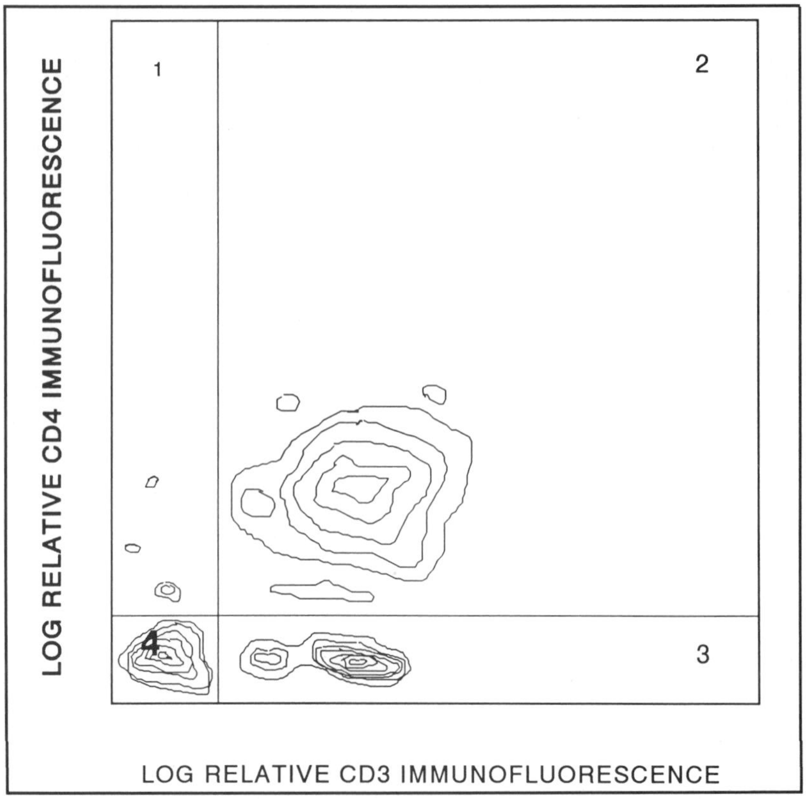

Fig. 12–27. Cell-surface phenotyping of human peripheral blood T lymphocytes by flow cytofluorimetry. Peripheral blood lymphocytes were stained with two different monoclonal antibodies, anti-CD3 and anti-CD4, each labeled with a distinctive fluorescent label (e.g., rhodamine and fluorescein). The stained population was analyzed by flow cytometry to detect cells that did not stain with either reagent (quadrant 4), cells that stained with only one of the reagents (quadrants 1 and 3), and cells that stained for both reagents—double positive cells (quadrant 2). The actual data consist of single points for each cell analyzed; a computer translates these data into contour maps indicating relative density of single data points. This representative figure shows approximately 60% of the $CD3^+$ cells are also $CD4^+$. The $CD3^+$, $CD4^-$ cells (quadrant 3) most likely consist of $CD8^+$ cells.

to the immunizing antigen. The use of a nonimmunoglobulin-secreting mutant myeloma in the fusion simplifies the pattern of immunoglobulin production by eliminating the light and heavy paraprotein chains. Cloning the hybrid cells after fusion results in cell lines producing monoclonal antibodies. Such cell lines can be grown in vitro or adapted to growth in animals for the production of large amounts of antibody of extremely high titer and with great specificity.

Many monoclonal antibodies of diagnostic and clinical relevance have been produced and are available commercially. They include blood group–specific reagents, antibodies that discriminate between subsets of human lymphocytes, and antibodies showing specificity for certain differentiated human tumors. Monoclonal antibodies are increasingly used as therapeutic tools in bone marrow transplantation and treatment of various tumors.

Methods for Enumerating and Classifying B Cells and T Cells and Assessing Their Function

B Lymphocytes

Enumeration and Cell-Surface Phenotyping

The technique of flow cytofluorimetry discussed previously can be used to identify the absolute number (and percentage) of B cells in peripheral blood. Cell-surface immunoglobulin is used as the unique marker to identify these cells. Fluorescently labeled antibodies to all classes of immunoglobulin usually are used, but subpopulations of B cells expressing a certain class of light chain, a distinct heavy chain class, or a particular allotype could be detected in the same way.

The stage of B cell differentiation might be assessed by quantifying the number of B cells that are membrane IgM^+ alone vs those that are IgM^+ and IgD^+, for example. Pre-B cells can be identified by detecting cells expressing cytoplasmic μ H chains but no cell-surface immunoglobulin. The state of B cell activation (in response to antigen) can be assessed by quantifying the level of expression of selected cell-surface markers such as increased expression of the receptor for transferrin (CD71) with B cell activation. An ever-increasing number of monoclonal antibodies have been described (many of which are commercially available) that identify B cells and distinct subpopulations based on the expression (or change in expression) of selected cell-surface markers.

Hemolytic Plaque Assays

In the plaque assays, cells producing hemolytic antibodies (B cells and plasma cells) are most readily detected. Antibody-secreting lymphoid cells (e.g., spleen cells from a mouse immunized against sheep red cells) are mixed with target erythrocytes in a warm (46C) isotonic 0.6% w/v agarose solution. This cell-laden agarose then is overlayered on a preformed 1.2% w/v agarose layer in a Petri dish. The plates are incubated at 37C in a humid atmosphere for 2 hours, during which time IgM and IgG secreted by the antibody-producing cells diffuse and bind to the target erythrocytes. With the addition of complement and further incubation, erythrocytes that have bound IgM antibody will lyse, causing visible, clear plaques in the otherwise red agarose, with a plasma cell or B lymphocyte at the center of each plaque (direct plaques). IgG antibodies do not cause lysis because of their lower lytic and complement-fixing activity, but including an anti-immunoglobulin serum in the top agarose layer enhances complement binding and hemolysis (indirect plaques).

The flexibility of the hemolytic plaque assay can be increased to include antigens other than erythrocytes by modification of erythrocytes with haptens or protein antigens as described previously for passive hemagglutination.

Stimulation of Immunoglobulin Synthesis and Secretion

The number of antigen-specific B cells in an unstimulated individual is too small to detect the in vitro response to a unique antigen. To assess the functional capabilities of the B cell population as a whole, polyclonal activators, or mitogens, are used to stimulate B cells, irrespective of their individual specifities. A combination of anti-immunoglobulin (anti-μ chain) and protein A from the Cowan strain of *S. aureus* can be used to stimulate B cells in vitro. Alternatively, the plant mitogen from pokeweed can be used as a polyclonal activator of B cells. Normal B cells should respond to these stimuli by synthesizing and secreting immunoglobulin at an enhanced rate and level. The response to these polyclonal activators can be quantitated at the mRNA level by Northern blot analysis (using labeled, specific oligonucleotide probes for heavy and light chain messages) or at the level of secreted immunoglobulin by radioimmunoassay (RIA) or ELISA techniques.

T Lymphocytes

Enumeration and Cell-Surface Phenotyping

Quantitation of human T cells from peripheral blood can be done in several ways. One of the simplest and least expensive methods is to take advantage of the observation that sheep erythrocytes spontaneously form a rosette around human T cells. Slight modification of the sheep erythrocytes by pretreatment with 2-aminoethylisothiouronium bromide hydrobromide (AET) renders them more avid for human T cells. The test is performed by mixing peripheral blood mononuclear cells with AET-treated sheep erythrocytes, incubating the mixture, and enumerating T cell rosettes (E-rosettes) microscopically. The T cell surface molecule responsible for the erythrocyte binding is the CD2 molecule.

Flow cytofluorimetry can be used to enumerate T cells and their subpopulations accurately, using the appropriate monclonal antibody-typing reagents. Fluorescently labeled antibodies specific for CD2, CD3 (the signal-transducing complex of the TCR), the αβ TCR, the δ TCR polypeptide chain, and a number of other T cell–associated cell-surface markers are available. In addition, monoclonal antibodies can identify immature thymocytes (such as anti-CD1), the MHC class II–restricted subset of T cells (anti-CD4), the MHC class I–restricted subset of T cells (anti-CD8), and memory (or activated) T cells vs virgin T cells. A number of T cell activation markers also have been identified that are useful in quantitating the T cell response to antigens or polyclonal activators in vitro.

T Cell Activation and Assessment of Response

A primary T cell immune response to a given antigen cannot be detected in vitro because of the limited number of specific T cells in unprimed populations. In primed populations, antigen can stimulate a proliferative T cell response in vitro. The proliferative response can be quantitated by measuring the incorporation of ^{3}[H]-thymidine into newly synthesized DNA. This assay is a rough in vitro correlate of the cutaneous delayed hypersensitivity response (Chap. 19).

The competence of T cells, in general, can be assessed by challenging unprimed peripheral blood mononuclear cells with polyclonal activators such as the plant mitogens pokeweed, Concanavalin A (Con A), and phytohemagglutinin (PHA) or with allogeneic lymphocytes in mixed lymphocyte reactions (Chap. 14). The ability of T cells to proliferate and to synthesize and secrete certain cytokines can be determined.

The secretion of cytokines such as IL-2, IL-4, and interferon-γ by antigen- or mitogen-stimulated T cells can be quantitated by RIA or ELISA; increased transcription of mRNA for each of these cytokines also can be detected by Northern analysis. Thus the functional capability of T cells can be determined through their synthesis of effector molecules in response to a stimulus.

Cytotoxic T Cell Assays

The interaction of virus-specific cytotoxic T lymphocytes (T_C cells) with infected target cells can be quantitated by modifying the ^{51}Cr-release assay described previously for antibody and complement. Infected target cells are prelabeled with $Na_2^{51}CrO_4$ and mixed with graded numbers of effector T_C cells. After incubation at 37C for 4 to 6 hours, the supernatant is counted to determine the amount of ^{51}Cr released by lysed target cells. T_C cells are virus (antigen) specific and are MHC restricted to killing virus-infected target cells expressing the appropriate MHC class I allele (Chap. 14). Thus very fine specificity involving the correct ternary complex of TCR, viral peptide, and MHC class I allele can be demonstrated in these assays.

FURTHER READING

General

Nisonoff A: Introduction to Molecular Immunology, ed 2. Sunderland, Mass, Sinauer, 1984

Roitt IM: Essential Immunology, ed 6. Oxford, Blackwell Scientific Publications, 1988

Antigens and Antigenic Determinants

Benjamin DC, Berzofsky JA, East IJ, et al: The antigenic structure of proteins: A reappraisal. Ann Rev Immunol 2:67, 1984

Davies DR, Padlan EA, Sheriff S: Antibody-antigen complexes. Ann Rev Biochem 59:439, 1990

Landsteiner K: The Specificity of Serological Reactions. New York, Dover Publications, 1962

Livingstone AM, Fathman CG: The structure of T-cell epitopes. Ann Rev Immunol 5:477, 1987

Senyk G, Williams GB, Nitecki, et al: The functional dissection of an antigen molecule: Specificity of humoral and cellular responses to glucagon. J Exp Med 133:1294, 1971

van Bleek GM, Natheson SG: Isolation of an endogenously processed immunodominant viral peptide from the class I H-$2K^b$ molecule. Nature 348:213, 1990

Immunogenicity

Sela M: Anigenicity: Some molecular aspects. Science 166:1365, 1969

Immunoglobulin Structure and Function

Burton DR: Immunoglobulin G: Functional sites. Mol Immunol 22:161, 1985

Childers NK, Bruce MG, McGhee JR: Molecular mechanisms of immunoglobulin A defense. Ann Rev Microbiol 43:503, 1989

Davies DR, Metzger H: Structural basis of antibody function. Ann Rev Immunol 1:87, 1983

Koshland ME: The coming of age of the immunoglobulin j chain. Ann Rev Immunol 3:415, 1985

Justement LB, Wienands J, Hombach J, et al: Membrane IgM and IgD molecules fail to transduce Ca^{2+} mobilizing signals when expressed on differentiated B lineage cells. J Immunol 144:3272, 1990

Moller G (ed): Immunoglobulin D. Immunol Rev 37, 1977

Moller G (ed): Immunoglobulin E. Immunol Rev 41, 1978

Antibody-combining Site

Capra JD, Kehoe JM: Hypervariable regions, idiotype, and the regions of Bence-Jones proteins and myeloma light chains and antibody combining site. Adv Immunol 20:1, 1975

Wu TT, Kabat EA: An analysis of the sequences of the variable regions of Bence Jones proteins and myeloma light chains and their implications for antibody complementarity. J Exp Med 132:211, 1970

Antigen-Antibody Interactions

Bhat TN, Bentley GA, Fischmann TO, et al: Small rearrangements in structures of Fv and Fab fragments of antibody D1.3 on antigen binding. Nature 347:483, 1990

Stanfield RL, Fieser TM, Lerner RA, Wilson IA: Crystal structure of an antibody to a peptide and its complex with peptide antigen at 2.8 Å. Science 248:712, 1990

Origin of Antibody Diversity

Black C, Hirama M, Lenhard-Schuller R, Tonegawa S: A complete immunoglobulin gene is created by somatic recombination. Cell 15:1, 1978

Blomberg B, Traunecker A, Eisen H, Tonegawa S: Organization of four mouse light chain immunoglobulin genes. Proc Natl Acad Sci U S A 78:3765, 1981

Early P, Huang H, Davis M, et al: An immunoglobulin heavy chain variable region gene is generated from three segments of DNA: V, D and J. Cell 19:981, 1980

Honjo T: The molecular mechanisms of the immunoglobulin class switch. Immunol Today 3:214, 1982

Rogers J, Early P, Carter C, et al: Two mRNAs with different 3′ ends encode membrane-bound and secreted forms of immunoglobulin chain. Cell 20:303, 1980

Seidman JG, Leder P: The arrangement and re-arrangement of antibody genes. Nature 276:790, 1978

Valbuena O, Marcu KB, Weigert M, Perry RP: Multiplicity of germline genes specifying a group of related mouse kappa chains with implications for the generation of immunoglobulin diversity. Nature 276:780, 1978

Antigen-specific T Cell Receptor

Brenner MB, McLean J, Scheft H, et al: Two forms of the T-cell receptor γ protein found on peripheral blood cytotoxic T-lymphocytes. Nature 325:689, 1987

Davis MM: T cell receptor gene diversity and selection. Ann Rev Biochem 59:475, 1990

Marrack P, Kappler J: The antigen specific major histocompatibility complex–restricted receptor on T-cells. Adv Immunol 38:1, 1986

Oettgen HC, Terhorst C: The T-cell receptor–T3 complex and T-lymphocyte activation. Hum Immunol 18:187, 1987

Raulet DH: The structure, function, and molecular genetics of the γ/δ T cell receptor. Ann Rev Immunol 7:175, 1989

Immunologic Assays and Techniques

Harlow E, Lane D: Antibodies: A Laboratory Manual. New York, Cold Spring Harbor Laboratory, 1988

Stites DP: Clinical laboratory methods for detection of cellular immune function. In Stites DP, Stobo JD, Wells JV (eds): Basic and Clinical Immunology, ed 6. Norwalk, Conn, Appleton & Lange, 1987

CHAPTER 13

Organization and Cellular Aspects of Immune Response and Immune Regulation

The immune system is primarily concerned with distinguishing between nonself- (usually microbial organisms) and self-components and eliminating undesirable invaders. Different classes of lymphocytes play a central recognition role in providing the specificity that initiates this process. Three major points are emphasized in this chapter. First, lymphoid organs are designed not only to produce lymphocytes but also to filter out and respond to foreign invaders (antigens). Second, lymphocytes possess specificity for these antigens, and specificity is clonally distributed (i.e., each lymphocyte has a slightly different specificity). Finally, lymphocytes recirculate throughout the body until they encounter trapped antigens, at which time they localize in the lymphoid tissue and respond to ultimately remove that antigen. In this chapter the organization, properties, and regulation of the various components of this immune system are considered.

Physical Components of Immune System

Barriers, Drainage, and Immune Response

All vertebrates possess primary barriers, such as the skin and mucosal surfaces, that prevent the invasion of most foreign organisms (Chap. 11). Thus the immune system per se is really a second line of defense that has evolved in multicellular, differentiated organisms. Once past these "walls," invaders drain into a web of lymphatics. The lymphatic system, schematically shown in Figure 13–1, extensively underlies the skin and permeates the body. Thin-walled lymphatic vessels carry lymphoid cells and foreign matter leaving the tissue spaces into larger lymphatics and ultimately, through the thoracic

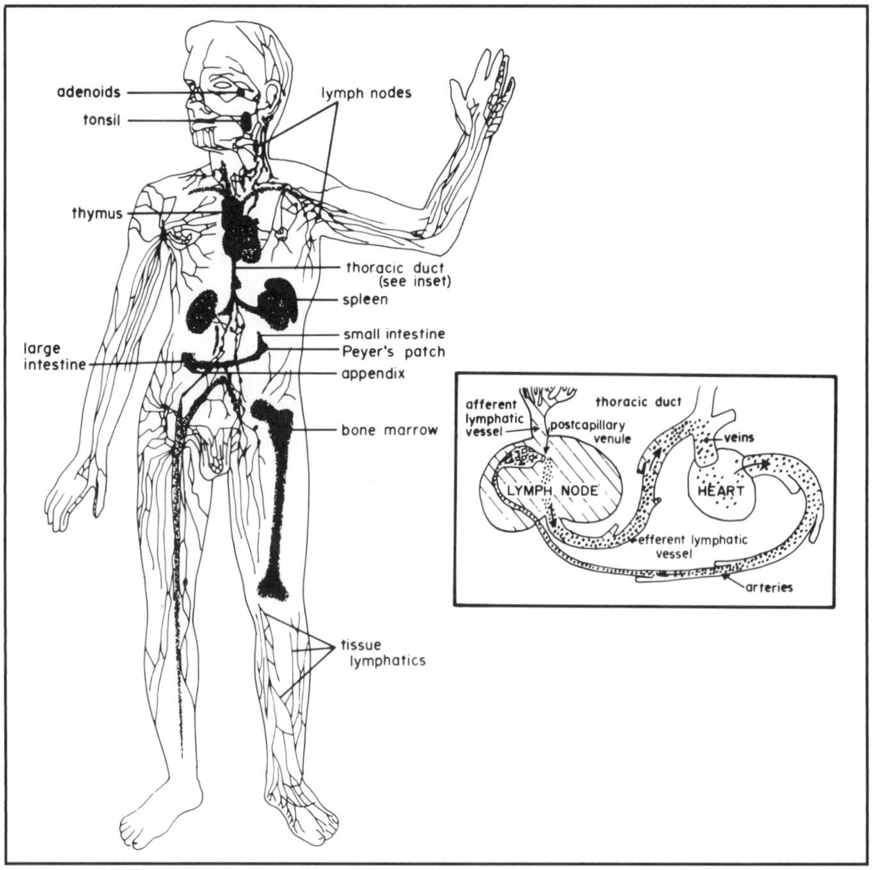

Fig. 13–1. The human lymphoid system, which includes a network of lymphatic vessels (thin lines) along which are lymph nodes (larger black dots). The spleen, blood lymphocytes, adenoids, tonsils, appendix, and Peyer's patches comprise the remainder of this system. The bone marrow (e.g., in the femur shown here) and the thymus are primary sites of lymphocyte production. The tissue lymphatics carry antigen, antibodies, and lymphocytes around the body. **Inset:** The lymphocyte recirculation pathway involves lymphocytes entering the nodes through the postcapillary venules (see Fig. 13–5C) and percolating through the node before exiting in the efferent lymphatics. They drain into larger vessels (e.g., the thoracic duct) and eventually enter the neck veins to join the blood circulation, and the process is repeated until antigen is detected in the nodes. Thereafter, recruitment of specific lymphocytes and immune response ensue. *(Adapted from Jerne: Sci Am 229:52, 1973; inset adapted from Gowans: Hosp Pract 3:34, 1968.)*

duct, into the bloodstream. Lymphocytes circulate through the lymphatics and into the lymph nodes so that antigens appearing in the node are exposed to a variety of circulating antigen-specific lymphocytes in a relatively brief time. Interposed along this network of lymphatics are the lymph nodes, into which foreign materials flow and are filtered out. In these nodes the immune responses are initiated.

The efficacy of filtration by this web of lymph nodes can be demonstrated by injecting an innocuous blue dye into a human foot. Within minutes the popliteal lymph node (behind the knee) becomes colored; later, any dye particles that escape the popliteal node pass through efferent lymphatics to the next node, the inguinal, and ultimately may transit to other nodes in the body. Such dyes normally do not immunize the

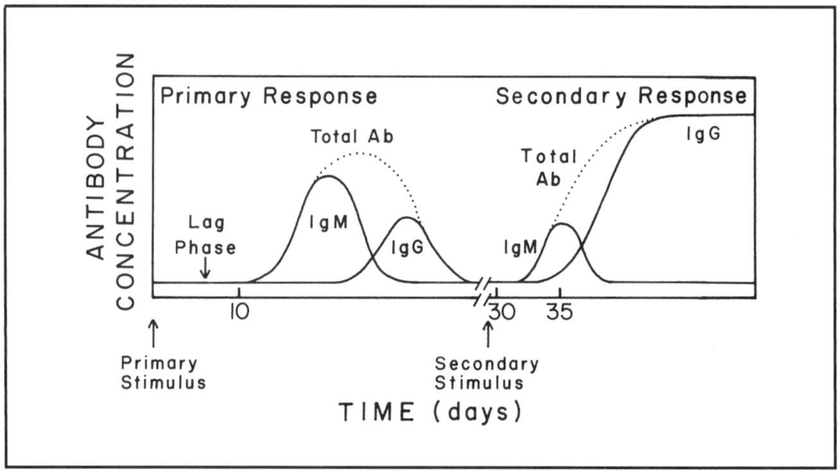

Fig. 13–2. Kinetics of a primary and secondary humoral immune response to a foreign antigen. After an initial lag period, IgM (and later, IgG) antibody is made. After a second exposure to antigen, a more rapid response occurs with a shorter lag period. This secondary or anamnestic response is characterized by a greatly increased production of IgG antibody.

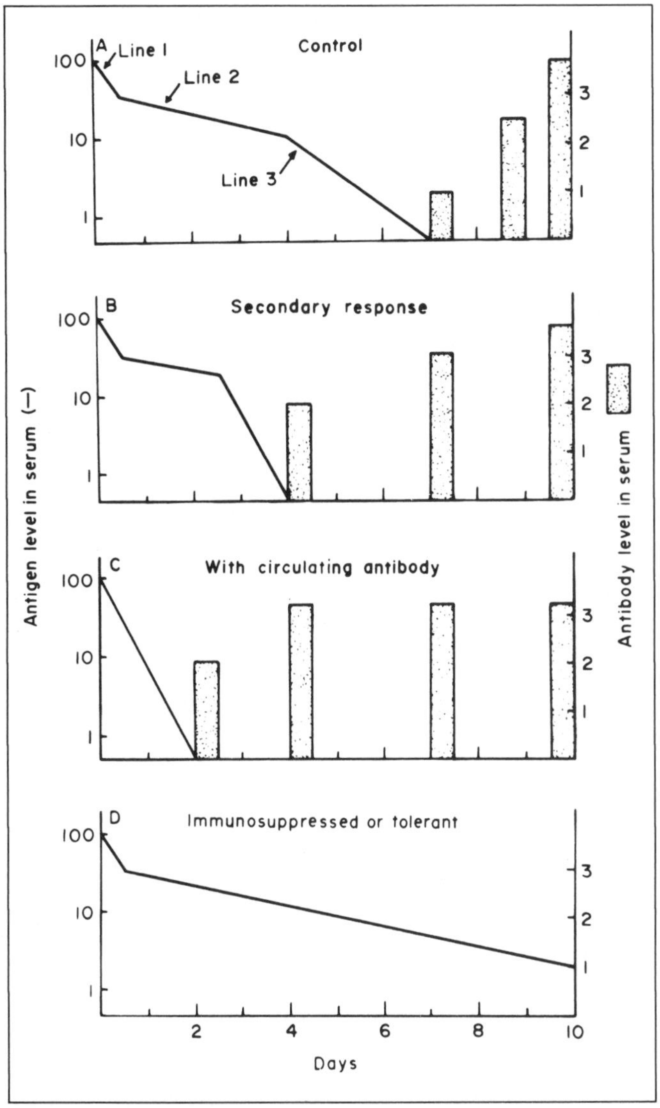

Fig. 13–3. Nonimmune and immune elimination of antigen. Radioactively labeled antigen is injected intravenously on day 0, and samples of blood serum are measured for remaining radioactivity (solid lines) or are titrated for free antibody activity (lightly shaded bars, arbitrary scale). Immune complexes are often detectable before free antibody. **A.** Normal animals not previously exposed to antigen. **B.** Previously immunized animals but with no antibody detectable on day 0 (secondary stimulus); note shorter lag period. **C.** Immunized animals with circulating antibody still present, showing accelerated (immune) elimination. **D.** Immunosuppressed animals or hosts tolerant to the antigen used; note extended nonimmune elimination (catabolism) and no antibody formation. *(Adapted from Talmage et al: J Immunol 67:243, 1951.)*

animal. If, instead, the host were injected with a killed virus vaccine through the same route, an antibody response would ensue over the course of the next 1 or 2 weeks as depicted in Figures 13–2 and 13–3.

Figure 13–2 depicts a typical humoral (antibody) response quantitated by the measurement of serum IgM, typical of the primary response to an antigen, and IgG, the predominant isotype observed after a secondary injection. After a lag period, which varies with the immunizing potential of the antigen (its immunogenicity), first IgM antibody and later IgG antibody appear in the serum. During a second exposure to the same antigen, a more rapid and greater response ensues, which is predominantly composed of IgG as the major class of antibody.

Figure 13–3 shows the same response from another perspective, that is, a typical immune elimination curve that further illustrates both the nonspecific and specific aspects of the entire immune system. An antigen such as bovine albumin, labeled with a radioactive tracer molecule, is introduced intravenously. The first phase is a brief period of equilibration between intravascular and extravascular spaces (line 1), occurring primarily through diffusion. Nonimmune catabolism of this foreign albumin antigen, during which time the albumin may be degraded, follows (line 2). This occurs with both self- and nonself-antigens. After a lag period, which usually lasts several days and is dependent on the half-life of the antigen, immune or rapid elimination of residual antigen begins (line 3). Immune elimination occurs after the immune system has started to produce antibodies that complex with the antigen. Complexes are taken up rapidly by phagocytic cells and are destroyed. Figure 13–3B shows the pattern in an animal that has seen this antigen previously. Line 1 is identical to that seen in a normal animal. However, line 2 is of shorter duration before the secondary immune response occurs, typifying the difference between a primary immune response and an anamnestic (meaning: not to forget) memory response (Fig. 13–2). Figure 13–3C depicts the situation in which antigen is introduced into an organism that still has circulating antibody present. No lag period is observed, and the antigen is eliminated in an immune fashion. Figure 13–3D exemplifies the "elimination" of an antigen to which the host is tolerant; the fall in antigen level is due only to catabolism. A similar pattern would occur in an irradiated or otherwise immunologically compromised host.

Phagocytic (Reticuloendothelial) System: Nonspecific Cellular Filters

An important adjunct of the immune response is provided by macrophages and other cells of the reticuloendothelial system. When any particle penetrates beyond the first line of defense, it usually is engulfed and removed by highly phagocytic (and some nonphagocytic) cells. The accessory cells include monocytes and polymorphonuclear neutrophils (PMNs) in the blood; macrophages in the lymphoid tissues; Kupffer's cells in the liver; Langerhans cells in the skin; and alveolar macrophages in the lungs. Many of these cells primarily function as scavenger cells, ingesting foreign or effete autologous materials; they also participate in inflammatory reactions. Some cells, such as medullary and dendritic macrophages in the lymph nodes, also process and present antigens to lymphocytes (see below), initiating the immune response.

Macrophages are derived ultimately from a hemopoietic stem cell in the bone marrow. The blood monocyte is the intermediate cell in this maturation process. Elegant studies have demonstrated the differentiation of rapidly dividing marrow stem cells to blood monocytes to tissue macrophages. During this process the cells change morphologically and biochemically, notably in the accumulation of lysosomal enzymes that ultimately destroy ingested particulate matter through a process of endocytosis, phagolysosomic localization, and enzyme release.

Specificity

The cells that carry out a specific immune response belong to the two major classes of lymphocytes—the T and B lymphocytes (or T and B cells)—named because of their origin and site of differentiation. T cells develop in the thymus, whereas B cells are derived from the bone marrow, or the so-called "bursal equivalent" in mammals. These small lymphocytes (which are 6 to 8 μm in diameter) comprise more than 95% of all cells traversing the lymphatics and 20% of the nucleated cells in the blood.

Although the involvement of antibody in immune responsiveness has been known since the last century, the source of antibody was unknown until its production by plasma cells—the end stage of differentiation of the B lymphocytes—was demonstrated just 35 years ago. The importance of small lymphocytes as the central defenders in this process was then elegantly demonstrated by Sir James Gowans. He inserted a cannula into the major lymphatic vessel (thoracic duct) of a rat and noted that the thoracic duct lymphocytes (TDL), those that flowed from this duct, could transfer the entire immune potential of the donor animal to an x-irradiated, immunologically incompetent recipient rat. Moreover, appropriately marked donor lymphocytes could be followed in their reemergence from the blood to the lymph and back again (Fig. 13–1 insert). Recently, it has been found that during this process lymphocytes in the blood attach to special ubiquitin-linked receptors on endothelial cells in the postcapillary venules (PCV) of the lymph nodes. The attached lymphocytes then migrate between the endothelial cells lining the PCV and begin to percolate through the node. If they do not meet their appropriate antigen, they are carried by the lymphatics back to the bloodstream and continue their shuttling through the system until they meet their specific antigen and are recruited into the immune response.

T and B cells also bear specific antigen-recognition units or receptors on their membranes. For B cells the receptor is an IgM heavy and light chain (H2L2) structure, whereas T cells possess a heterodimeric receptor (usually) comprised of α and β chains and the CD3 complex of proteins (i.e., αβ plus CD3 comprise the T cell receptor [TCR]). Indeed, these receptors give the B cells and T cells their specificity in recognizing different antigens. When lymphocytes pass through a lymph node in which antigen is trapped (see below), they bind to the antigen via these receptors. Antigen-specific lymphocytes are thus held out of the circulation, remain in the node, and are stimulated to join an immune response pattern. This process is called recruitment and is discussed further below. Before explaining the nature of the immune response, it is necessary to review the development of B and T cell repertoires and their differentiation before exposure to antigen.

Embryonic Development: Origins of Lymphoid Organs and Hematopoietic Cells

The Thymus: A T Cell Factory

Not all lymphoid organs are built for filtration; some are factories for making more lymphocytes. These so-called central, or primary, lymphoid organs are exemplified by the thymus, where the vast majority of T cells are produced and differentiate. Figure 13–4A shows a cross-section of the mammalian thymus, a bilobed organ in the anterior mediastinum. The thymus, the first lymphoid organ to appear in ontogeny, is derived from the third and fourth pharyngeal pouches and begins to develop at 4 to 5 weeks of gestation in humans. Although thymic lymphocytes (thymocytes) were originally believed to be formed directly from epithelial cells, cell transfer and parabiosis experiments established that stem cells migrate into the thymus through the bloodstream. Stem cells for the thymus are first identifiable in the yolk sac, then in the fetal liver, and still later in the bone marrow. Migration continues from the bone marrow even into adult life. Shortly after their arrival in the thymus, precursor (pre-T) cells organize into a thin layer in the outer cortex and begin producing progeny by dividing. Gradually, these cells migrate into the medulla, where they become smaller, acquire new cell-surface antigenic markers, and, most importantly, develop immunocompetence, and some then leave the thymus (still other thymic cells may leave directly from the cortical regions). Although the exact differentiation scheme(s) is still being investigated, evidence to date indicates that differentiation and maturation are under the influence of hormones such as thymopoietin and thymosin, produced by the epithelial elements in the thymus.

Thymic differentiation can be delineated by the presence of surface markers. The earliest of these to appear is the common leukocyte antigen, or T200, which is present on human T cells by 7 weeks gestation. T200 currently is called CD45 for "cluster of differentiation" antigen number 45. Because of its presence throughout the life of a T cell, CD45 is considered a "pan–T cell" marker.

The cortex contains mostly rapidly dividing immature thymocytes. These earliest cells lack the two major T cell markers (CD4 and CD8) and are termed *double-negative cells.* Soon they express the CD3 complex, which is an integral part of the TCR complex and contains critical transmembrane signaling molecules. The second group of T cells bears both CD4 and CD8 (double-positive cells), comprises about 80% of all cortical thymocytes, and is rarely seen in the peripheral circulation. Soon, two new populations, $CD4^+$,$CD8^-$ and $CD4^-$,$CD8^+$ thymocytes, the so-called single-positive T cells, appear, primarily in the medulla. These cells constitute most of the functionally mature thymic cells (10% to 15% of total thymocytes), are positive for the αβ TCR-CD3 complex, and are phenotypically similar to the majority of circulating T cells. $CD4^-$, $CD8^+$ cells, which comprise 20% to 30% of mature T cells in the circulation, recognize (or "are restricted to") class I major histocompatibility complex (MHC) molecules (Chap. 14) and have predominately cytotoxic or suppressor function, whereas $CD4^+$,$CD8^-$ cells (60% of circulating mature T cells) recognize class II MHC products and largely are involved in mediating B cell help and inflammatory responses.

A final minor population includes double-negative cells that express the γδ TCR-CD3 complex and are phenotypically similar to a subpopulation of peripheral cells found predominately in the skin and gut. Perhaps these $\gamma\delta^+$ thymocytes represent the thymic progenitors of the peripheral γδ T lymphocyte subpopulation. Although a proportion of the medullary and some cortical thymocytes exit from the thymus and are replaced continuously through cell division, there is also a great deal of intrathymic cell death. It is believed that the diversity of the immune system is generated in the thymus by rearrangements of the TCR; that is, V-J-C rearrangements

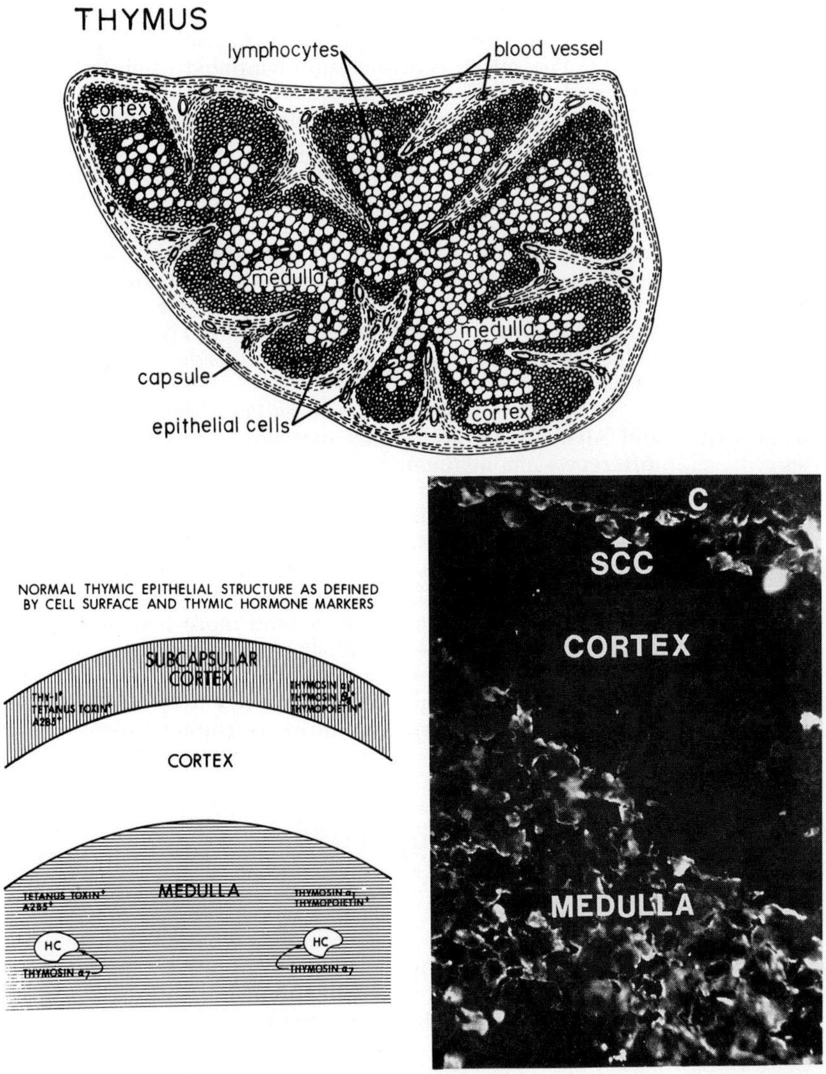

Fig. 13–4. Thymic architecture. Dense accumulation of thymic lymphocytes (thymocytes) in the cortex, surrounding a lighter medullary area composed primarily of epithelial cells and more mature thymocytes. Lower right: reactivity pattern of normal human thymus labeled with monoclonal antibody A2B5, which detects thymic hormones. Scheme at lower left depicts this pattern, which matches the staining observed with several thymic hormones. *(Courtesy of Dr. B. F. Haynes; from J Immunol 130:1182, 1983.)*

occur, and the maturing T cells are varied somatically. It is postulated that many of the cells, especially in the embryo, randomly express anti-self specificities and that these potentially autoreactive thymocytes are treated as lethal mutants and destroyed. Thus one way the immune system can become tolerant to self-antigens is by this negative selection in the thymus (see below).

B Cell Development

The thymus processes only T cells; there is no comparable organ regulating B cell development in mammals, although B cells also go through a series of maturational and developmental processes (Chap. 12). In birds the bursa of Fabricius (a lymphoid organ in communication with the cloaca) controls B cell development. In mammals, B cells probably develop in the microenvironment of the bone marrow or fetal liver. B cell maturation may also occur in other lymphoid organs, including the spleen, tonsils, and possibly in Peyer's patches of the gut. The first identifiable poststem cell stage is called the *pre-B cell.* Pre-B cells have rearranged immunoglobulin μ heavy chain genes. They possess heavy chains in their cytoplasm but not on their surface. Once light chains are rearranged, the cells assemble complete IgM dimers ($\mu 2$:L2), some of which are inserted into the membrane. Such a cell is surface IgM positive and is then, by definition, a B cell. It is believed that different V gene families are used in a preset pattern to be rearranged and somatically varied, thus giving rise to a programmed development of the B cell repertoire.

Subsequently the membrane IgM is joined by membrane IgD in most B cells (by appropriate V-C splicing; see Chap. 12). Although other surface markers have also been identified on developing B cells, surface IgM (with or without IgD) is the hallmark of B cells. B and T cell markers are discussed in more detail below.

Programmed Development of Repertoire

Immune competence develops gradually and not to all antigens simultaneously. This is called the programmed development of the repertoire. As T and B cells mature (e.g., in the thymus), reactivity to different antigens appears, as was shown by Silverstein and Klinman and their colleagues. For example, it was shown that fetal sheep make antibody to a bacterial virus by midgestation yet cannot respond to *Salmonella typhosa* until after birth. Klinman found that precursor frequencies to different haptens in mice occurred in a programmed pattern of repertoire development that could be mapped and predicted in a given mouse strain. Although such a program has not been delineated for responsiveness in humans, it probably could occur because of the evidence that the rearrangements necessary to make a complete Ig heavy (and light) chain or TCR may occur in a predetermined order, with the initial rearrangements involving V_H gene segments most proximal to the constant region. This process occurs in pre-B cells and cortical thymocytes in a totally antigen-independent manner, is genetically programmed, and, not surprisingly, shows marked differences between species.

Structure and Function of Peripheral Lymphoid Organs

The lymph nodes (and to a certain extent, the spleen) are intricate filters where immune recognition of foreign materials occurs. Figure 13–5, a lymph node, can be contrasted with the thymus shown in Figure 13–4. Lymph nodes have two main areas: a central medulla and a peripheral cortex without discrete borders. Lymph fluid enters through afferent lymphatics carrying cells, debris, and foreign particles from the extracellular spaces. It then passes through a series of sinusoids lined with phagocytic macrophages and B cells, both of which can bind and present antigens.

Within the superficial cortex, which is composed predominantly of B cells (Fig. 13–5A), are structures called primary follicles. These oval-shaped areas include a dense accumulation of lymphocytes in a mesh of macrophage-like cells called dendritic reticulum cells. During an immune response there is a burst of cell division augmented by recruitment from the blood. New germinal centers called *secondary follicles,* in which the developing germinal center is partially covered by a cap of phagocytic cells, are formed. The germinal center contains many lymphocytes, large, actively metabolizing lymphoblastoid cells, antigen-retaining dendritic reticulum cells, and some macrophages. The germinal center is the site of T:B cellular interactions and memory development.

Surrounding the follicles is the paracortical region, which is also called the deep cortex. It consists of further accumulations of lymphocytes, primarily T cells. Interspersed in the deep cortex are the PCV. Lymphocytes enter the node from the blood by traversing between the endothelial walls of the PCV. The role of the PCV in the recirculation of lymphocytes can be seen when radioactively labeled lymphocytes (obtained from the thoracic duct lymph) are injected intravenously. Within minutes, labeled cells cross the PCV into the deep cortex T cell area and later into the superficial cortex (B cell area). After percolating through the rest of the lymph node, most of these cells exit through efferent lymphatics and recirculate (Fig. 13–1 inset).

Like the lymph nodes, the spleen acts not only as a filter but also as a site of the immune response. The spleen has no lymphatic vessels and is supplied exclusively by the bloodstream. The spleen is divided into lymphoid white pulp and erythroid red pulp. The latter area removes old and damaged red cells. It also serves as a site of hematopoiesis and, in some species with a contractile spleen (e.g., dog), as a reservoir of red cells. The white pulp, surrounding the splenic arterioles, is analogous to the lymph node cortex (the so-called periarteriolar lymphocyte sheath) and contains numerous follicles and accumulations of less densely packed lymphocytes. Interposed between the sheath and the red pulp is the marginal zone, which is analogous to the lymph node medulla. In addition, mature plasma cells can be found in parts of the red pulp. Plasma cells are rarely found outside the organized lymphoid tissues.

Other lymphoid tissues such as Peyer's patches, tonsils, and adenoids are also highly specialized. The most obvious differences among them are the varying proportions of T and B cells and the class of antibody produced in different types of lymphoid tissue. (Peyer's patches, for example, contain many IgA-secreting cells.) Interestingly, the ratio of T and B cells within an organ is determined by interaction of lymphocyte homing receptors with ligands on endothelial cells in the PCV. That is, Peyer's patch PCV bind more B than T cells. Hence, this organ possesses nearly twice as many B as T cells, in contrast with the peripheral nodes. This allows more B cells to migrate through Peyer's patches to generate more antibody (e.g., IgA) responses during recruitment (see above).

Functional Properties of T and B Cells

The most notable property of the lymphocytes, aside from their ability to recirculate, is their specificity, which is endowed by surface receptors that bind specific antigen. The receptor on B cells is immunoglobulin. Although all B cells are surface Ig-positive, only a small proportion ($<0.1\%$) can interact with any given antigen. For example, one small fraction binds to tetanus toxoid, another fraction to poliovirus, and so on. Thus lymphocytes belong to many small clones, together representing every possible specificity in the repertoire of the host animal. Its surface antigen–specific receptors enable a given lymphocyte to respond to an antigen encountered in a lymph node during recirculation. During interaction with an antigen, the B lymphocyte's (Ig) receptors are cross-linked, and within seconds to minutes certain early metabolic signals are elicited that involve calcium ion changes, inositol phospholipid metabolism, and protein kinase activation. After several hours such cells exit G_0 and enter the G_1 phase of the cell cycle. During this process, antigen bound to B cell Ig receptors is internalized and later is presented to T cells along with class II MHC region–encoded antigens (D region in humans, Ia in mice).

In an analogous manner the T cell recognizes the complex of MHC class I or II molecules plus antigen with a receptor that is a heterodimer of disulfide-linked α and β chains of 45,000 Da. These chains contain rearranged regions such as immunoglobulins and are therefore called V, J, and C (Chap. 12). The T cell receptor is noncovalently associated with

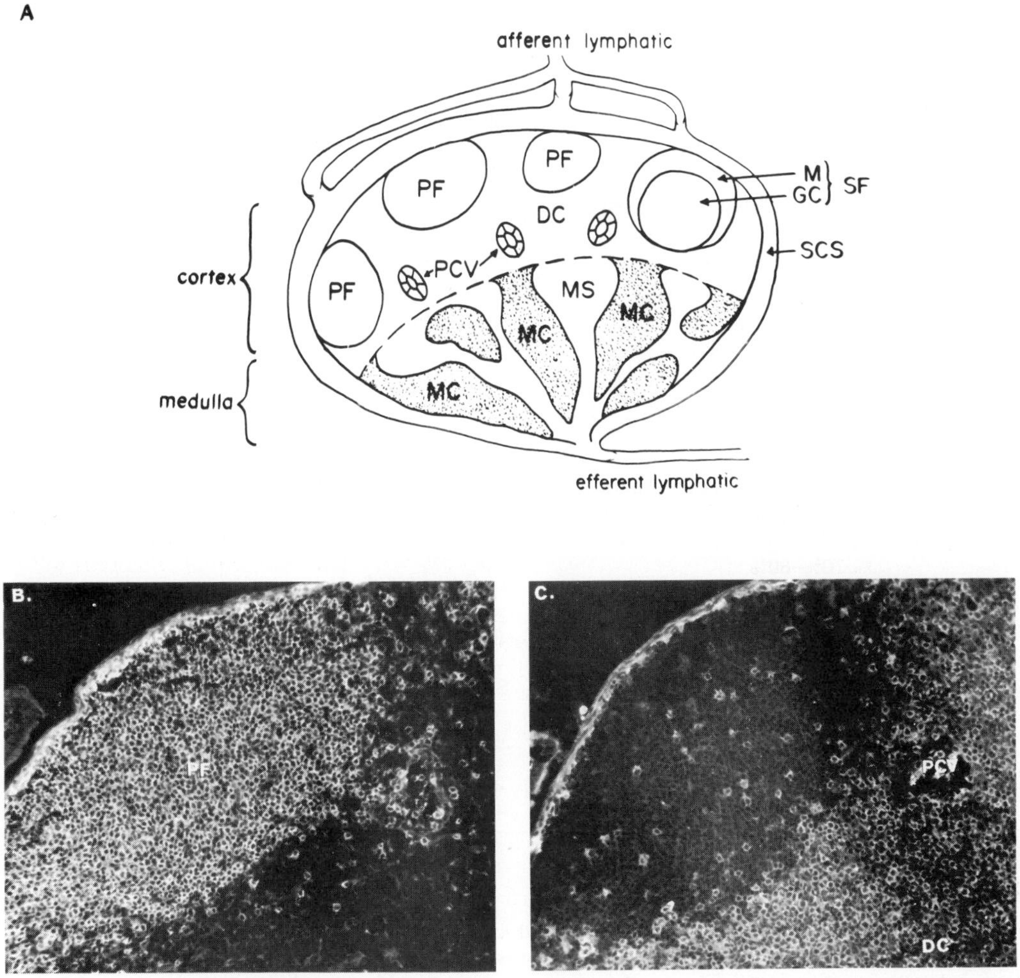

Fig. 13–5. Lymph node structure. **A.** Schematic drawing of a lymph node. PF, primary follicle; SF, secondary follicle containing a germinal center (GC) and mantle (M); DC, diffuse cortex containing the postcapillary venules (PCV); MS, medullary sinus; MC, medullary cords. **B.** and **C.** T and B cell localization. Frozen sections of a mouse lymph node were stained with fluorescein-labeled antibodies to mouse immunoglobulin (**B**), or with fluorescein-tagged anti-T-cell reagent (**C**). The anti-immunoglobulin stains B cells because of their surface immunoglobulin; they are localized in and around the primary follicle (light area in **B**). T cells in the diffuse cortex and a few in the PCV are labeled in **C.** There is little overlap of the two cell types. *(Photomicrographs courtesy of Dr. G. Gutman.)*

several other proteins called the CD3 complex. During interaction of this receptor complex with antigen (plus MHC) a cascade of changes occurs that is similar to that described previously for B cells, except that as T cells exit G_0 into G_1, receptors for interleukin-2 (IL-2) are expressed. Further changes and interactions are discussed below.

Numerous other markers help distinguish subsets of T and B lymphocytes (Table 13–1). Some markers are shared by both T and B cells (MHC class I), whereas others (e.g., Thy-1 in the mouse) are restricted to T cells. Other markers define B cells (e.g., membrane Ig), and a final group, the Fc receptors, are found on many cell types. The function of certain markers is apparent: for example, the membrane immunoglobulins bind antigen; the receptors for the constant domain of immunoglobulin (Fc receptors) on B cells interact with Fc to transmit positive or negative signals. Markers such as the histocompatibility antigens (Chap. 17) are critically essential for T:B or T:macrophage collaboration and communication between cells. T cells also carry many other markers related to adhesins that aid in cellular interactions with antigen-presenting cells. Many of these markers appear or disappear from the cell surface as a function of cell maturation. Such surface antigens were first observed in leukemic cells "frozen" in a given state of differentiation. They are exemplified by the murine TIa markers and the CD4 and CD8 markers referred to previously and by CD5, which is found on all T cells and subset of B cells (see above). The CD4 and CD8 antigens also reflect functionally different T cell subsets: CD4 generally function as helper cells, whereas CD8 cells are active as cytotoxic and suppressor cells. However, CD4 and CD8 reflect a most definitive T cell property: MHC restriction. Thus CD4 T cells only recognize antigens (or their fragment) in association with class II MHC, whereas CD8 T cells are restricted to recognizing MHC class I–associated antigens (Chap. 17). CD4 and CD8 markers actually aid in the interaction of the TCR with specific antigen and bind weakly to the MHC antigens. CD4 cells can be divided further in terms of their ability to secrete different lymphokines, some of which are cited in Table 13–2.

CD5 is expressed by a minority of B cells in the adult circulation and spleen (2% to 4%) but is the phenotype of 50% of the B cells in the murine peritoneal cavity. Such CD5+ B cells preferentially use V genes that differ from those used by the majority of CD5− (conventional) B cells in assembling

TABLE 13–1. T AND B LYMPHOCYTE AND MACROPHAGE PROPERTIES

	T Cells	B Cells	Macrophages
Differentiation site	Thymus	Marrow (bursa equivalent)	Marrow
Recirculation	Fast	Slower	
Life span	Long-lived	Short- to long-lived	
Specificity	Antigen and MHC	Antigen (hapten)	
Memory	+	+	—
Antigen receptor	α- and β-heterodimer (90 kDa)	Immunoglobulin heavy and light (150 kDa)	
Fc receptors	Some (Tγ, Tμ)	+	+
C3b receptors	—	+	+
SRBC receptor (CD2)	+ (human)	—	—
Major histocompatibility complex antigens (K/D-like)	+	+	+
Ia antigens	Minority	+	Some
Thy-1, brain-associated antigen	+	—	—
CD4 marker	Helpers	—	—
CD8 marker	Cytotoxic + suppressors	—	—
CD5 marker	All T cells	>5%	
Localization			
Peripheral blood	70%–80%	15%	+
Thoracic duct	90%	10%	—
Lymph node	75% (deep cortex)	25% (follicles)	+
Spleen	40%–50%	40%–50%	+
Thymus	100% (90% immature)	—	Few
Bone marrow	Few mature	Some mature B	+
Sensitivity to			
Corticosteroids	+	+	—
Irradiation	+	+ +	—
Antilymphocyte serum	+	+	±
Immunosuppressive drugs	+	+	—

their IgM receptors. It is thought that $CD5^+$ B cells play a role in immunoregulation and produce antibodies reactive with self-antigens (autoantibodies). Interestingly, humans with certain autoimmune diseases such as lupus possess an increased number of $CD5^+$ B cells in the circulation.

Results of Antigenic Encounter: Immune Response in Lymph Node

Role of Macrophages

Within minutes after an antigen enters a lymph node, it is taken up (phagocytized) by macrophages in the subcapsular sinus, the cortex, and the medulla. Similar events occur in the spleen if the antigen is blood-borne or in the tonsils and adenoidal lymphoid tissues if the portal of entry is nasal or oral. These sessile or tissue-bound macrophages comprise part of the reticuloendothelial system.

After uptake by macrophages, antigen enters cytoplasmic vacuoles called phagosomes, which fuse with lysosomes, organelles laden with hydrolytic enzymes. The number of lysosomes can increase during phagocytosis or after antigenic stimulation, the latter mediated by products of T cells. Such a cell is called an activated macrophage. Lysosomal enzymes degrade most of the antigen into peptides. Some antigenic material is preserved in a recognizable (or processed) form and is presented as peptides on the macrophage surface in association with class II MHC molecules. Processed antigen has been shown to be highly immunogenic for T lymphocytes. Indeed, T cells cannot recognize free antigen (unlike B cells) but only see peptides presented in association with MHC antigens. Some antigen, presumably in a highly immunogenic form, is also maintained on the surface of the nonphagocytic follicular dendritic reticulum cells of the lymph nodes. Antigen processing also occurs in B cells that have bound antigen via IgM receptors and may be as important as antigen processing by macrophages.

Studies in vitro have shown that macrophages are important in triggering the activation of specific lymphocytes. For example, spleen cells can be separated by exposure to a glass surface into an adherent, macrophage-rich fraction and a nonadherent lymphocytic fraction. Insoluble or cellular foreign antigens incubated with either fraction do not generally stimulate an immune response. However, antigen added to the adherent macrophages and followed by the addition of nonadherent (T and B) cells will stimulate the latter to produce antibody in vitro. This macrophage accessory function is relatively resistant to gamma- or x-irradiation, whereas B cell antigen processing is more radiosensitive.

The detailed knowledge of the localization of antigen in the lymph nodes is based largely on studies in Australia by Nossal and Ada involving radioiodinated flagellar proteins

TABLE 13–2. T LYMPHOCYTE–PRODUCED CYTOKINES (LYMPHOKINES)

Lymphokines	Biologic Activity
IL-2	T cell growth factor: Stimulates growth of activated T cells as well as natural killer and lymphokine-activated killer cells; can promote B cell growth and differentiation
IL-3	Stimulates growth of pluripotent hematopoietic stem cells
IL-4	Enhances class II gene expression; stimulates B cell proliferation; promotes switching to IgG1 and IgE production; stimulates subsets of T cells and mast cells to proliferate
IL-5	Enhances IgA switching, eosinophil growth factor, B cell growth factor
IL-6	Induces Ig secretion; also promotes hybridoma and hepatocyte growth
IL-7	Induces immature B and T stem cell growth
IL-9	Increases proliferation of long-term T cell lines, thymocytes, and mast cells
IL-10	Inhibits cytokine synthesis by other T cells; enhances survival of lymphoid cells; synergizes with IL-2 and IL-4 as a T cell growth factor
GM-CSF	Stimulates growth and differentiation of neutrophils and macrophages; activates macrophages
IFNγ	Inhibits viral proliferation; enhances macrophage activating factor; increases MHC expression of many somatic cells
TNF	Tumor necrosis factors α and β: cytotoxic for virally infected cells and induces cachexia and fever; activates osteoclasts

from *Salmonella* organisms. Their findings have been confirmed with other antigens. Classic studies visualized the localization of these antigens during the primary response in medullary macrophages and in the marginal sinus around the primary follicles, close to many B cells. In contrast, during a secondary response antigen was localized predominantly on the dendritic cells within the follicles. Follicular localization could be mimicked in unimmunized animals by the administration of preformed antigen-antibody complexes. This suggests that antigen combines with circulating antibody in already immune animals and is trapped quickly in the follicles where it can interact with T and B memory cells.

Morphologic Changes in Lymphoid Tissues During Immune Responses

Antigen processed by macrophages and B cells stimulates specific T lymphocytes. This results in the trapping of antigen-specific circulating small T and B cells in the responding lymph node and their transformation into large blast cells, which stain intensively with the RNA-stain pyronine (pyroninophilic cells) (Fig. 13–6). Blastogenesis is first seen in the diffuse cortex, the T cell area, and shortly thereafter in the superficial cortical region of B cells. The blast cells continue asymmetric division to yield clones of daughter cells, differentiated T and B effector cells, whereas some daughter cells persist as memory cells. Within days some of the stimulated T and B cells migrate to form secondary follicles and germinal centers; later plasma cells may be seen along the medullary cords.

The extent of the changes in the various lymphoid tissue regions depends on the nature of the antigen and on the route of injection. The picture described above is typical for the great majority of protein antigens, the so-called T-dependent antigens, which elicit both antibody formation and delayed hypersensitivity (see below).

Some antigens such as dinitrochlorobenzene or the urushiols of poison ivy stimulate a contact sensitivity (T cell) reaction. This form of stimulation is sharply localized to the paracortical region where activated T cells proliferate. Other antigens, primarily polysaccharides, elicit a pure antibody

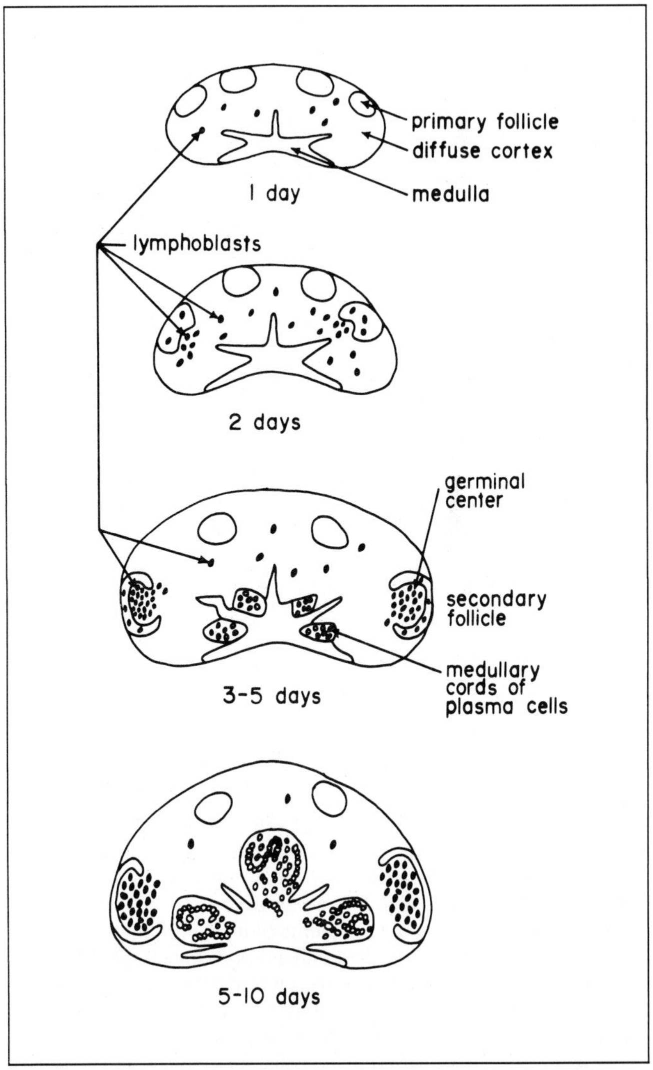

Fig. 13–6. Morphologic changes in a lymph node after stimulation with a thymus-dependent antigen. Lymphoblastoid cells (dark dots) increase with time after immunization to form the germinal center (by 3 to 5 days). *(Adapted from Hood et al (eds): Immunology. Benjamin/Cummings, 1978.)*

response in the absence of significant T cell reaction. The response to these antigens is largely in the superficial cortex and follicles.

Clonal Nature of Immune System

Each of the B and T lymphocytes in the immune system has specificity for a single antigen. That is, a given B cell, once stimulated, will produce antibody of the same specificity as its IgM receptor and of no other specificity. The frequency of lymphocytes with a specificity for a given foreign antigen is less than 1 in 1000. Once a lymphocyte encounters its antigen in the lymph node, it is recruited out of the circulation. Therefore, shortly after local antigenic stimulation, the lymphatics are relatively depleted of lymphocytes specifically reactive with that particular antigen, whereas the total numbers of circulating lymphocytes appear unchanged because the number responding to a single antigen is relatively small. This process is called *clonal selection* or *recruitment.* After the initial stage of activation is over, antigen-specific T and B cells reenter the circulation pool and disseminate throughout the body. The entire scenario of lymphocyte recruitment, stimulation, and release results in the temporary enlargement of lymph nodes. Part of the enlargement is from nonspecific vascular effects secondary to the release of lymphokines, monokines, and prostaglandins after the activation of T cells and macrophages. Enlargement lasts until the antigenic response (e.g., to a bacterial invader) wanes.

T and B Cell Collaboration

B cells generally require the presence of T cells for stimulation by antigen toward antibody formation. This process of T cell help was discovered in the late 1960s but only recently was the molecular basis of this process better understood (see below). Animals depleted of T cells (e.g., by neonatal thymectomy) fail to produce antibody to most antigens tested. When thymus cells are injected into these mice, the capacity to form antibody is restored (Fig. 13–7). Studies using labeled lymphocytes demonstrated that the antibody was produced by the B cells, not the added T cells. The capacity for T cell help is mediated by a subpopulation of T cells, which bear distinct markers such as CD4 or Lyt-1 (Table 13–1).

The mechanism by which helper T (T_H) cells and B cells collaborate is based on the fact that B cells bear class II MHC antigens on their surfaces and can process exogenous hapten (e.g., captured through Ig receptors) like macrophages. Originally, an absolute requirement for direct contact via an antigen bridge between T_H and B cells was considered unlikely because a response to antigen can occur when T and B cells were separated by a cell-impermeable membrane in vitro. However, more recent experiments demonstrating that B cells can bind, process, and present antigen to T cells suggest that a direct interaction may be physiologically relevant. It already has been mentioned that T cells can be stimulated by antigen presented on accessory cells such as macrophages (or the dendritic reticulum cells), which produce a factor called interleukin 1 (IL-1). Once activated, T cells produce a large number of growth and differentiation factors that promote their own continued proliferation as well as that of B cells (see Table 13–2). For example, T cells produce IL-2 (formerly called *T cell growth factor*) and use it by synthesizing the IL-2 receptor. A B cell–stimulating factor (IL-4) can activate B cells for increased class II MHC antigen expression, stimulate entry into S phase, and also cause isotype switching from IgM to IgG. In addition, at least two human B cell growth and differentiation factors (promoting division or antibody secre-

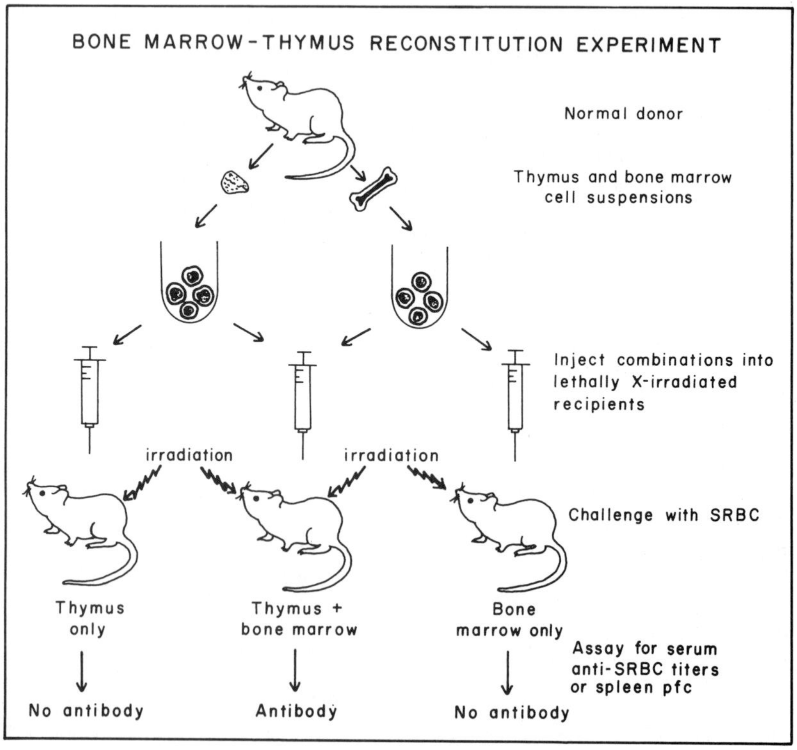

Fig. 13–7. Protocol to demonstrate that both T and B cells are needed to collaborate in antibody formation to certain antigens. Lethally irradiated mice received thymocytes, bone marrow cells, or mixtures of both types of cells. After immunization with a T-dependent antigen, only recipients of both thymus and marrow cells responded with antibody production. Subsequent experiments demonstrated that the antibody was made by the marrow-derived (B) cells, whereas the thymocytes provided carrier or helper cell recognition to those B cells. As shown in Figure 13–8, B and T cells may recognize different epitopes of the antigen, with B cells serving as antigen-presenting cells to some T cells. *(Adapted from Golub: The Cellular Basis of the Immune Response. Sinauer Associates, 1977.)*

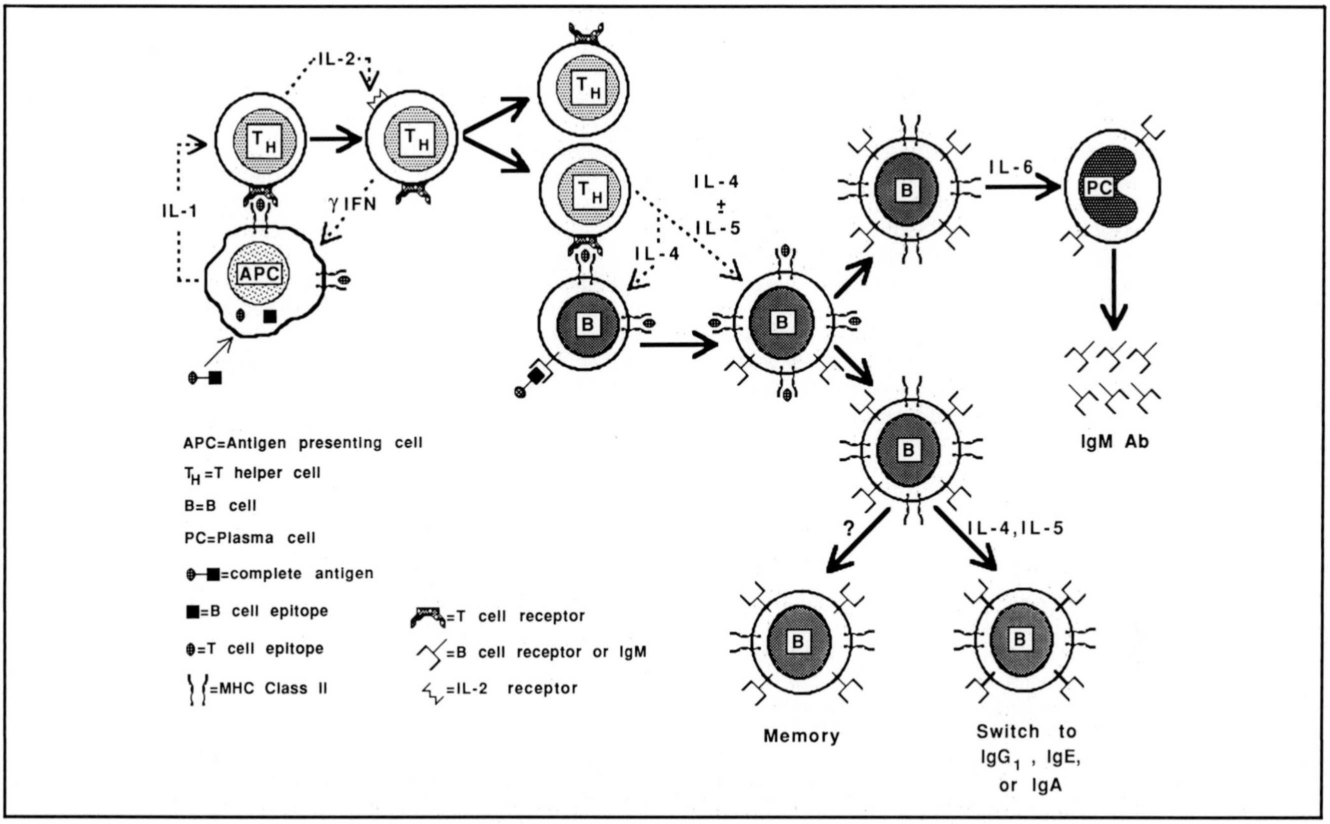

Fig. 13–8. Schematic of T:B collaboration and the role of cytokines. T cells bind to antigens processed and presented by so-called antigen-presenting cells (APC) such as macrophages or B cells, which produce IL-1 to promote T cell activation. The antigen actually is a peptide derived from the original antigenic protein and sits in a groove of the MHC class II antigen (e.g., DR). T cells recognizing this MHC class II–peptide complex are induced to express IL-2 receptors, make IL-2, and proliferate, yielding clones of T helper cells. These T cells also produce interferon γ (IFNγ), a cytokine that also causes macrophage activation, including increased MHC expression. Other stimulated T cells make IL-4, which stimulates B cells to enter the cycle and later proliferate. IL-4 promotes class II expression, which fosters further B:T interaction (since B cells can bind the antigen via their IgM receptors, process it, and present its peptides in their class II groove). In addition, other cytokines such as IL-5 and IL-6 enhance B cell proliferation and differentiation of immunoglobulin secretion, respectively. IL-4 and IL-5 are required in mouse systems for B cell isotype switching to IgE, IgG1, and IgA. Memory is poorly understood, but it may involve asymmetric division of B cells or the expansion of a different subset, as well as commitment to isotype switching. T cell memory is expressed by the clonal expansion shown across the top row and commitment to cytokine secretion.

tion or both) have been isolated from continuous T cell lines. Terminal differentiation of B cells to plasma cells is mediated by IL-6, formerly called interferon β. Another important lymphokine appears to be gamma interferon (IFNγ), which not only has important antiviral activity (Chap. 19) but also stimulates macrophages and can modulate B cell responses. A schematic showing interaction of B and T cells (and macrophages) is shown in Figure 13–8. Recent evidence suggests that distinct T cells secrete different lymphokines, and this leads to a different ability to provide help to B cells.

Some antigens, notably polysaccharides and lipopolysaccharides from bacteria, can stimulate without T cell help. These so-called T-independent antigens possess one or more of the following characteristics that enable them to trigger B cells directly: (1) They are usually large polymers with repeating antigenic determinants; (2) they are often mitogens that can cause B cell proliferation; and (3) many can activate the alternative pathway of the complement cascade (Chap. 15). Each of these properties has independently led to hypotheses of B cell activation. For example, repeating determinants can simultaneously interact with several immunoglobulin receptors on B cells, thus increasing the avidity of binding and receptor cross-linking, leading to "capping." Capping is also observed after B cells are incubated with bivalent $F(ab')_2$ but not with univalent Fab fragments of anti-immunoglobulin reagents. Most importantly, only the former can induce B lymphocyte proliferation. Movement of receptors into a "cap" is followed by their loss from the cell surface. They are soon resynthesized, often with an increased number of expressed receptors. Hence capping is considered an event that is necessary, but certainly not sufficient, for triggering B cells. Since many B cells possess receptors for activated complement components (Table 13–1), the ability of T-independent antigens to activate the complement sequence may play a role in their immunogenicity. Indeed, some complement components are involved in the generation of B cell memory in germinal centers.

Polysaccharide antigens discussed previously primarily stimulate an IgM response and little B cell memory, whereas T-dependent antigens (most proteins) elicit IgM and IgG responses and memory. Thus the IgG response is highly T cell dependent. In fact, it is clear that "switching" of murine B cells from the production of IgM to the IgG1 subclass can be facilitated by the cell lymphokine, IL-4. Hence any minimal hypothesis still requires B cell triggering to occur through the focusing of antigens on membrane Ig receptors and their internalization and eventual presentation to T cells that then elicits lymphokine production.

Memory and Affinity

The typical immune response illustrated by Figure 13–2 reflects one property that is the hallmark of immunity and the basis of prophylactic immunization: immunologic memory. Once an individual has been exposed to an antigen, the subsequent response to that antigen occurs more quickly and is usually of a different class—IgG rather than IgM. Memory for an anamnestic (secondary) response may persist in humans for decades. Memory is a property of both B and T cells and takes some time to develop adequately. For example, if a second antigen injection is given too soon after the first, a poor secondary response will be observed. In addition, although memory for some antigens (e.g., tetanus toxoid) can last for years, memory to other antigens can wane unless booster immunizations are given periodically. Thus there are empirically determined critical time course and booster immunization protocols for prophylactic vaccination with certain antigens. It is unwise for the clinician to deviate far from these protocols.

Memory still is poorly understood. Presumably it results from an expansion of specific T and B cell clones in a lymph node follicle during initial stimulation by a given antigen, X. Some of these progeny differentiate into effector cells such as T helper cells and plasma cells, whereas others remain as memory cells. When antigen is seen a second time, memory cells divide rapidly and presumably differentiate to yield the expanded clones of specific effector T and B cells that typify the anamnestic response.

Another feature of the secondary antibody response is a change in the affinity of the antibodies produced because cells vary in the affinity of their surface immunoglobulin receptors for antigen (e.g., poliovirus). During stimulation with a sufficient quantity of this virus, many B cells respond, and antipoliovirus antibodies of heterogeneous affinity are produced. The average affinity in this primary response is relatively low. By a combination of normal catabolic decay, immune elimination (Fig. 13–3), and the ability of antipoliovirus clones of higher affinity to react competitively with and be stimulated by decreasing amounts of virus, there is an increase in the average affinity with time after immunization. This is called the *maturation of the immune response*. Subsequent administration of antigen (poliovirus) leads to the immediate stimulation of these higher affinity clones of memory cells, which may have survived longer because of their better ability to compete for and be stimulated by small amounts of remaining antigen, and the typical high-affinity secondary response occurs, thus giving better protection against subsequent infection.

Immunologic tolerance, the process that prevents individuals from responding to their own antigens, may be considered the opposite of memory. Consistent with the above clonal observation of antibody affinity in secondary antibody responses, in experimental tolerance the highest affinity B cells would be the ones most likely to interact with antigen and therefore the most likely to be rendered tolerant. This would lead to a relatively low-affinity response (if any) to immunization of tolerant animals. This is indeed observed experimentally. It is also possible to show low-affinity autoantibodies in clinically normal individuals (see below and Chap. 17). This implies that self-tolerance reflects the elimination of high-affinity antiself-clones.

Effector Mechanisms in Cellular Immunity

Although this chapter so far has dealt with antibody production through B cells and T cell helpers, other types of T cells are needed for effective immunity. That is, the immune system must be able to cope with a variety of invaders, some producing harmful products (toxins) that must be neutralized quickly by antibodies but others growing intracellularly where antibodies cannot attack. Thus the need for the T cell limb of the immune system. Other cell types that are activated in these cases include delayed hypersensitivity T cells, cytotoxic or killer T cells, and regulatory or suppressor T cells. The reactions of these subpopulations are collectively termed *cellular immunity* because some forms of immunity historically could not be transferred with serum (humoral immunity) and could only be transferred in animals by lymph node or spleen cells from an immune donor. Since T cells active in cellular immunity must be able to recognize intracellular pathogens, they must also be able to see antigenic peptides derived from those pathogens associated with MHC antigens on the surface of cells harboring these invaders. This characteristic is called MHC restriction (see below) and is a unique property of T cells.

Delayed Hypersensitivity

Delayed hypersensitivity originally was described in the late nineteenth century in studies on immunity to tuberculosis (Chap. 19). The inflammatory response observed when guinea pigs exposed to tubercle bacilli were later inoculated with boiled bacterial culture filtrate (so-called old tuberculin, or OT) was the classic manifestation of a delayed hypersensitivity reaction. To this day skin testing with purified protein derivative (PPD) of OT from these organisms is used as a standard assay for prior exposure to tubercle bacilli. Delayed reactions, described below, are also used as a diagnostic aid with a variety of bacterial, fungal (e.g., coccidiomycosis), plant (e.g., poison ivy), and protozoan (e.g., leishmaniasis) antigens. Delayed reactions can also be elicited by hapten-carrier conjugates or even by haptens that spontaneously bind to tissue cells or products. Thus a patient's T cell competence can be tested by the ability to be sensitized against such simple compounds as dinitrochlorobenzene, which couples to self-MHC molecules on dermal cells.

Delayed hypersensitivity, by definition, differs from immediate-type hypersensitivity, not only in the time of appearance of the inflammatory response but also in its histologic character and specificity. In a tuberculin skin test little change is noted at the site of delayed hypersensitivity skin reaction during the first 12 hours after intradermal injection. Erythema and induration gradually progress during the next 24 to 48 hours. The induration is due to the influx of large numbers of mononuclear cells, notably macrophages, as well as a few lymphocytes. The macrophages are of hematogenous origin from monocytes originally derived from the marrow.

Mechanistically, delayed reactions depend on the release of lymphokines from a minority population of activated T cells (of the CD4 class) that both attract and hold inflammatory mononuclear cells at the skin test site. One lymphokine is a macrophage-monocyte chemotactic factor that is measured in the laboratory by the migration of mononuclear cells through the pores of a membrane. IFNγ is also produced; as stated previously, it activates these macrophages for more effective intracellular killing and also upregulates their MHC expression, thus making them more "visible" to T cells. Another important lymphokine is macrophage migration inhibitory factor (MIF). This designation is based on the fact that, when packed into a capillary tube by centrifugation, macrophages will begin to migrate out after a few hours. Migration is inhibited (hence the term *MIF*) if specific antigen and lymphocytes to which the donor is immune are present in the cell suspension. In cell-mixing experiments, reactions are positive if the suspension contains as few as 1% to 2% of T lymphocytes from a sensitized individual. Since other products of activated T cells and macrophages such as tumor necrosis factor (TNF) and prostaglandins affect vascular dilation and vascular permeability, one can envisage how this scenario leads to accumulation of leukocytes at the reaction sites. However, such "pure" delayed reactions are rare. That is, with many complex antigens, antibody is also present, and many reactions are intermediate between pure delayed-type and Arthus-type immediate reactions.

T Cell Cytotoxicity

Cell-mediated reactions of a substantially different nature are manifested by another subpopulation of T lymphocytes, the CD8 cells. They are called cytotoxic effector T cells because of their ability to destroy target cells bearing specific antigens. They are typified by the cytotoxic cells generated during allograft rejection (Chaps. 12 and 14). In the latter case cytotoxic cells can be generated in what is called a *mixed lymphocyte culture* (the MLC reaction), in which leukocytes from two unrelated (allogeneic) individuals are mixed in vitro. After 5 to 7 days, substantial proliferation can be measured because of the recognition of foreign major histocompatibility antigens on the leukocytes. The majority of the proliferating cells may be T helper, but many are cytotoxic. The latter are quantitated as follows. Target cells (e.g., mitogen-stimulated lymphocytes from the allogeneic donor) are labeled with chromium in the form of chromate, which remains inside viable cells. Putative cytotoxic cells are added, and damage is measured by determining the amount of radioactive chromium released from the labeled targets.

Cytotoxic reactions against targets carrying tumor or viral antigens also can be detected by this method. In this case of viral antigen the cytotoxic cells are often generated in vivo by first immunizing the animal with virally infected cells and restimulating immune lymphocytes in vitro. The $CD8^+$ effector cells generated destroy those target cells that simultaneously display viral antigens along with self-histocompatibility-antigens. Indeed, viral peptides are present in a groove or pocket of the MHC antigen like a hot dog in its bun! Cytotoxic T cells fail to react to the same virus presented on cells from a different (allogeneic) individual. This is called MHC restriction of cell-mediated cytotoxicity (Chaps. 12 and 14); it is also involved in T-B cell collaboration and in the transfer of delayed hypersensitivity reactions. In the first case, restriction requires a class I match, whereas in the last two examples a class II homology is needed for efficient interaction. The manner in which T cell receptors recognize self-MHC appears to depend on both α and β chains of the receptor. Once cytotoxic T cells encounter a virally infected target (with newly formed viral peptides associated with MHC class I), they physically conjugate briefly and release cytotoxic granules that soon destroy their target and eliminate the source of production of infectious virus.

Suppressor T Cells

A final category of cell-mediated reactions is manifested by suppressor T cells. These cells resemble cytotoxic T cells in some, but not all, surface markers (e.g., in humans suppressor and cytotoxic cells are $CD8^+$, but the suppressor cells may also carry other markers). The involvement of suppressor cells in the regulation of antibody responses is described later in this chapter. They also play a role in modulating other cell-mediated reactions. Gershon, the discoverer of suppressor cells, suggested that these T cells are the true "conductors of the immunologic orchestra," damping down or preventing unnecessary immunologic activity, including anti-self reactivity. However, the exact role and identity of suppressor cells remains unclear.

Immunoregulation

Specific self-nonself discrimination characterizes the immune system. Not only must subsets of interacting cells be organized in such a manner as to deal with pathogens (and other environmental agents), but they must do so in an optimal fashion. Once the hazards of infection are dealt with, this system must shut itself off. Moreover, to prevent autoimmunity, there must be methods of ensuring that serious anti-self reactions are not induced. Several levels of regulation therefore are necessary in the immune response; these are described in the following sections.

Regulation by Antigen: Immunologic Tolerance

Ehrlich realized the importance of lack of responsiveness to self when he coined the phrase *horror autotoxicus* to connote the possible consequences of anti-self reactivity. Self-tolerance is of critical importance to the well-being of the individual. Thus there must be a process by which anti-self B and T cells are functionally or physically eliminated to prevent autoantibody production.

An experimental basis for the development of self-tolerance is provided by observations on twin cattle of different sexes. These fraternal twins, unique in that they share hematopoietic stem cells in utero, fail to reject a skin graft from their twin after attaining immunologic competence. These animals maintain a stable chimeric state (mixture) of both their own and their twin's blood cells. Most importantly, they do not reject each other's skin grafts, although they can reject grafts from unrelated cattle. These observations were seized on by Sir MacFarlane Burnet and led to the suggestion that during prenatal exposure to their twin's cells (and therefore their allogeneic antigens), these dizygotic animals learn to accept the alloantigens as self. Burnet then proposed that during this prenatal period, tolerance would develop to any antigens to which the immature immune system was exposed. A corollary to this hypothesis was that tolerance represented the elimination (or repression) of the specific reactive lymphocyte clones; this was called *clonal deletion.* Experimental induction of unresponsiveness to foreign alloantigens in mice and chickens, respectively, by prenatal or perinatal injection of allogeneic cells verified this hypothesis. Since that time numerous systems have been developed to experimentally trick the immune system of even adult animals into specifically accepting foreign antigens as self. The factors affecting this process include the dose, form, and chemistry of the antigen and the age of the recipient.

In the 1960s it was reported that mice treated repeatedly with either very high (milligram) or very low (nanogram or lower) doses of antigen failed to make an immune response to an optimal immunizing challenge with the same antigen. These mice responded normally to unrelated antigens. Thus pretreatment led to specific unresponsiveness to subsequent antigenic challenge, which is the minimal definition of tolerance. It was later shown that high-dose tolerance somehow inactivated both T and B cells, whereas low-dose tolerance affected only T cells.

The importance of antigen form is exemplified by the fact that gamma globulin and other serum protein antigens, which normally are weakly immunogenic, become tolerogenic (i.e., would induce tolerance) after high-speed centrifugation to remove aggregates. The soluble supernatant preparations were tolerogens, whereas the aggregated proteins in the pellets were immunogens. This difference is probably due to the manner in which aggregates are taken up and presented (processed) by phagocytic cells in the immune system; it may also reflect uptake and presentation by cells other than the professional antigen-presenting cells (APC), e.g., macrophages and B cells.

Haptens coupled to self-serum-proteins (again notably gamma globulins) or even self-lymphocytes are tolerogenic. This property may reflect the ability of isologous gamma globulins and cells to pass unchecked through or even to localize in certain areas of lymphoid organs or react with Fc receptors on lymphocytes. Hence tolerance to the penicilloyl (the sensitizing portion of penicillin) group has been induced in mice by coupling it to self-IgG carriers (mouse IgG) to prevent or even reverse hypersensitivity to penicillin. Similarly, the anti-DNA autoimmunity syndrome of New Zealand black mice, which resembles lupus erythematosus (Chap. 17), has been prevented or ameliorated by coupling nucleosides to isologous gamma globulins.

As stated above, experimental tolerance as originally described is induced in the perinatal period when the immune system is immature. The manipulations reviewed above permit tolerance induction in adults, which is more clinically desirable. Compared to adults, however, neonatal animals are often much more susceptible to tolerance induction. This is particularly true in rats and mice, which are relatively immunoincompetent at birth; in contrast, the human neonate is fairly immunologically mature. Notable exceptions in humans include the failure to respond to certain polysaccharides such as the capsule of *Haemophilus influenzae.* The susceptibility of young animals to tolerance induction can be attributed to a combination of at least two factors: (1) a poor antigen-trapping network in lymphoid organs, which may enable antigens to contact many T lymphocytes via nonprofessional APC rather than be processed by macrophages, and (2) the presence of larger proportions of immature lymphocytes. Thus Waksman and colleagues demonstrated that tolerance was facilitated by injecting antigen directly into the thymus, which has an abundance of immature T cells. Also, the earliest B cells possess only surface IgM receptors; these cells may be more sensitive to in vitro tolerance induction than the more mature IgM^+ or IgD^+-bearing B cells, which appear later in ontogeny, although IgD per se does not delineate this difference. It has been suggested that adult B cells that have had their IgD removed revert to an immature B cell behavior, especially in terms of tolerance induction. Although this is clearly an oversimplification, it is possible that these receptors (IgM vs IgD) provide different (negative and positive) signals to the B cell bearing them. The results of possible tolerogenic signals are discussed later in this chapter.

Kinetics of Tolerance Induction and Waning

The immune response to a T-dependent antigen requires collaboration between both T and B cells. Hence tolerance to such antigens could be apparent if either T or B cells or both are unresponsive. T and B cells differ in terms of the kinetics of tolerance induction, the doses required, and the waning of tolerance. Unresponsiveness is seen in the recipients of T cells taken from donors 1 day after injection of tolerogen mixed with normal B cells, whereas B cells do not become unresponsive for at least 1 week after exposure to antigen. As shown in Figure 13–9, tolerance in T cells lasts longer than tolerance in B cells. *Tolerant donors remain unresponsive as long as their T cells are tolerant.* In addition, the dose of tolerogen required to induce unresponsiveness in B cells was at least 100-fold that required for T cell tolerance.

The waning of tolerance presumably is due to the gradual elimination of the tolerogen (below a tolerogenic threshold) and the generation of new antigen-reactive cells in the thymus and marrow. If tolerogen is reinjected before this waning occurs, tolerance can be induced in the newly generated cells, and unresponsiveness persists. The implications of this sequence of events for understanding self-tolerance and autoimmunity are obvious. Some self-antigens present in high concentrations may produce tolerance in both T and B cells. Other antigens, which may occur only at lower concentrations in the body, only produce T cell unresponsiveness. In the steady state, both kinds of self-antigens are tolerated by the host. Moreover, the presence of minimal amounts of self-

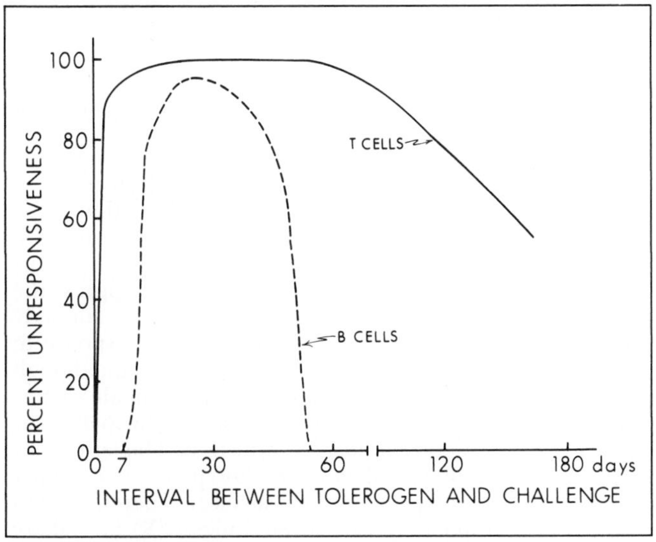

Fig. 13–9. Kinetics and waning of tolerance in T and B cells. Tolerance in helper T cells (solid line) was measured by the decrease in response to a hapten coupled to a carrier protein to which the donor was tolerant. This pattern was identical in kinetics to tolerance observed in thymocytes (not shown) and contrasts with bone marrow or B cell tolerance (dotted line). *(T cell data from Scott: Immunologic Tolerance: Mechanisms and Potential Therapeutic Applications. Academic Press, 1974. B cell data redrawn from Weigle et al: Prog Immunol 1:312, 1971.)*

antigen is sufficient to prevent loss of tolerance and autoimmunity. Under some circumstances the host can be tricked by altered self-antigens (e.g., tissue antigens altered during viral infection). Helper T cells recognizing virally modified self-antigens can cooperate with nontolerant B cells if present. This could circumvent self-tolerance and lead to an autoimmune response.

Pathways of Unresponsiveness

There is no single unifying mechanism of tolerance. Rather, it is likely that several mechanisms occur concurrently to maintain self-tolerance in T cells, B cells, or both. It was assumed from Burnet's hypothesis that self-tolerance is due to the absence (i.e., elimination) of autoreactive clones as they develop in the maturing immune system. Clear evidence for clonal deletion has been obtained in several antigenic systems for B and T cells. However, other data indicate the presence of some degree of autoreactivity, especially low-affinity antibody to certain self-antigens, including even those of the thymus. Low-avidity autoantibody-producing cells (to DNA) have been revealed in vitro in normal mouse strains, and low-avidity autoantibodies can be detected in clinically normal human sera. Interestingly, many autoantibody-producing cells can be derived from a separate lineage of B cells (CD5).

Because of these observations, three mechanisms for tolerance other than clonal deletion have received support and are discussed separately below: B and T cell anergy, control by antibody feedback, and active suppression by suppressor cells. Anergic B and T lymphocytes may actually persist for a brief period of time in the host. They cannot be triggered by antigen but sometimes can be triggered by mitogens. Evidence for B cell anergy has been obtained in transgenic mice, and T cell anergy has been induced in T cell clones in vitro.

Functional self-tolerance also could be due to the presence of so-called blocking antibodies (see below). Since blocking or enhancing antibodies can exert their effect in minute quantities, it sometimes is impossible to distinguish between antibody blockade, tolerance, and suppressor cells specific for certain (self) antigens.

Finally, a lack of responsiveness exists to many antigens that are physically sequestered from the immune system. Thus the immune system is essentially ignorant but not tolerant of their existence. They never induce tolerance while the immune system is developing. Thus sperm antigens, if exposed to the immune system (e.g., after vasectomy), can stimulate vigorous autoantibody production.

Tolerance to certain viruses can be beneficial to the host. For example, lymphocytic choriomeningitis virus (LCM) induces a vigorous inflammatory response in adult mice, leading to brain lesions and death. Mice exposed to LCM in utero become tolerant to the virus and survive when reinoculated as adults.

In summary, self-tolerance can be maintained at many levels. No single mechanism is sufficient to prevent autoreactivity to self-antigens, which differ greatly in concentration and chemistry.

Regulation by Antibody

As early as 1909, immunologists realized that specific antibody could influence the response to antigen. Preformed antigen-antibody complexes (especially in antibody excess) induced poor antibody responses, whereas free antigen or complexes in antigen excess were often potent immunogens. Thus the presence of antibody could modulate immune responsiveness. This has enormous practical consequences because the placental transfer of maternal antibodies against the poliovirus, for example, could possibly prevent adequate immunization of human infants. Hence vaccination is delayed until the infants are 3 to 9 months old, at a time when maternal antibody is no longer present in appreciable concentrations in the baby's circulation.

When passively administered, antibodies of the IgG class were more efficient at inhibiting the immune response than was IgM to the same antigen. However, not all IgG antibodies are effective. Thus murine IgG1 is quite effective at suppressing immunity, whereas IgG2 antibodies have little effect and may actually augment responsiveness. Intact IgG apparently is better than $F(ab')_2$ fragments, which are still superior to univalent Fab antibody fragments. This suggests that bivalency and the Fc portion of the antibody play important roles in antibody feedback (perhaps acting through Fc receptors on B cells, follicular dendritic cells, and macrophages) and that feedback is not simply due to masking antigenic determinants.

Passive IgG antibody can suppress immunity even when administered 24 hours after antigen. This observation has important clinical applications because an immune response might be aborted after antigen has already entered the body. In the case of hemolytic disease of the newborn (erythroblastosis fetalis), an Rh-negative mother delivering an Rh-positive infant can be treated with anti-Rh antibodies soon after parturition (i.e., after the mother has received a transfusion of the infant's cells during placental separation). This is thought to prevent sensitization to the infant's erythrocytes and has virtually eliminated the occurrence of this disease with subsequent Rh-positive pregnancies (Chap. 14).

Primary immune responses are the most readily inhibited by passive antibody, although the secondary response can be partially affected if enough high-affinity antibody is given with antigen. Inhibition of helper T cell priming is not generally affected greatly by antibody under conditions that would ablate primary B cell response to antigen. This may reflect the greater sensitivity of T cells to priming by low doses of antigen.

The affinity of passively administered antibody plays a critical role in the effectiveness of antibody-mediated regulation. High-affinity antibody, typified by the IgG antibody found late in the immune response, is more suppressive. Unlike tolerance, in antibody feedback the only antibody precursors that seem to escape regulation are those of *high* affinity (i.e., higher than the passive antibody administered).

Because the systems described above are artificial, it was important to show that antibody might in fact regulate its own formation homeostatically in vivo. Cyclical antibody formation, in which antibody levels fall after a single injection of antigen and then abruptly rise again, has been repeatedly reported as possibly due to antibody feedback acting on a reservoir of remaining antigen. In fact, when rabbits immunized to a given antigen were plasmapherized and their plasma replaced by normal plasma, the antibody titers, after an initial sharp drop, began to rise and plateaued at control values. This effect is due to de novo protein synthesis initiated by the drop in antibody titer leading to stimulation by retained antigen. Thus the antibody made in response to antigen X was regulating its own synthesis and level.

Regulation of Cell-mediated Immunity by Antibody: Enhancement

Antibodies to cell-surface antigens (e.g., histocompatibility antigens or tumor antigens) can suppress the immune response to an allograft or tumor, respectively. This phenomenon, called *immunologic enhancement,* is also discussed in Chapter 20 and can be demonstrated in two forms: active and passive. Active enhancement results from deliberate immunization with killed tumor cells and presumably is due to an ongoing antibody response to the tumor cells because killed cells are poor immunogens for a cellular immune response. The antibodies made actively by the host thus can prevent T cell sensitization to a subsequent viable tumor cell challenge immunization. These antibodies can be transferred to a normal recipient to suppress tumor graft rejection; this is called passive enhancement.

Several mechanisms of antibody-mediated suppression of cellular (and humoral) immunity are possible. Antibody can bind to and block cell surface antigens to prevent sensitization. Also, modulation (loss through capping) of cellular antigens can occur. Finally, immune elimination of the injected cells can prevent sensitization. These are all afferent mechanisms of regulation. Antibodies can allow tumor or graft survival by efferent suppression of induced immune effector function (e.g., by blocking target tumor antigens so killer T cells cannot destroy tumor cells [high-dose enhancement]). Finally, antibody, especially immune complexes, can directly inactivate immunocompetent cells, a "central mechanism."

Regulation by Antibodies to Idiotypes

Idiotypes (i.e., antigenic determinants of the antibody-combining site; Chap. 12) play an important role in immune regulation. Niels Jerne proposed that the immune system is a network of antibody idiotypes that is perturbed by antigenic exposure. That is, an idiotype (anti-X or Ab1) formed in response to antigen X could activate anti–anti-X (anti-idiotype or Ab2) formation and so on. Such anti-idiotypes can both suppress and augment the immune response. Heterologous IgG1 anti-idiotype under certain conditions will suppress the formation of a given idiotype but not reduce total antibody against antigen X. This is because the immune response to most antigens is idiotypically heterogeneous so that, although one idiotype is suppressed, other idiotypes can be made against a given antigen X. Heterologous anti-idiotype (in particular IgG2) augments idiotype (anti-X) production. The latter may occur as a result of stimulation of idiotype-positive helper cells (expressing idiotype X on their surface). Therefore both T and B cells responding to a given antigen (X) may share idiotypic determinants. Taking advantage of shared idiotypes, some investigators have used anti-idiotypes against an anti-MHC idiotype to successfully prolong allograft (MHC different) survival in rodents, thus regulating T cell responses by antibody, a potentially exciting clinical application derived from a basic research tool.

More recently, anti-idiotypes (some Ab2 may theoretically *look like* antigen X in that they combine with antibody to X [the idiotype]) have been used successfully as safe vaccines for both hepatitis and certain tumor antigens. This method can be useful in cases in which antigen supplies for vaccines are limited, the antigens are not readily purified, or the antigens are potentially hazardous.

Regulation by Suppressor T Cells

Subclasses of T cells (primarily of the $Ly2^+$ and $Ly1^+, 2^+$ phenotype in the mouse and bearing CD8 markers in humans) can actively suppress the immune response to an antigen specifically or nonspecifically. These cells produce factors (see below) that can interfere with a variety of immunologic activities such as T cell helper activity, IgE responses, delayed hypersensitivity, or even T-independent triggering of B cells. Their action can be direct or indirect (i.e., interference with helper factor activity or macrophage function). Suppressor T cell activity is itself regulated in a feedback loop in such a way that a homeostatic control of responsiveness can be maintained. Recently, this loop has been suggested to involve subsets of T suppressor cells that recognize antigen and others that recognize idiotypes. They communicate with each other through soluble factors presumably containing an antigen- or idiotype-specific binding site and other elements that restrict or focus their activity on appropriate acceptor or target cells. Unfortunately, so far these cells have resisted cloning, and the genes for these factors have not been isolated.

Non-antigen-specific suppressor T cells may also be involved in at least two clinical situations: immunodeficiency and autoimmunity. Patients with an acquired hypogammaglobulinemia may have normal B cell levels, but their T cells suppress the differentiation of these cells to plasma cells. A loss of suppressor activity in New Zealand black mice before the onset of autoimmune symptoms reminiscent of lupus also has been described. Understanding of immune reactivity by the induction of specific suppressor T cell clones has become an important goal for the future.

Summary

In summary, the immune system is built of tissues that make and educate lymphocytes to provide a network for antigen capture, T and B cell recirculation, and their interaction with antigen to generate an immune response. T and B cells interact with each other to produce antibody, whereas T cells are responsible for different forms of cell-mediated immunity. Antibody is important in eliminating bacterial invaders, whereas cell-mediated immunity is critical for the response to intracellular infectious agents such as viruses.

Just as each cell in the immune system has a specific function, these functions are regulated at many different levels. Both the quantity and quality of antigen control the nature of immune response and can induce unresponsiveness, thus avoiding autoimmunity. The antibody produced can provide feedback to regulate its own formation. Suppressor T cells, induced by antigen or even idiotype, also control the level of the immune response. All these control mechanisms ensure an appropriate immune response to foreign pathogens or autochthonous tumor cells and prevent overproduction or autoimmunity.

FURTHER READING

Books, Reviews, and Selected Papers

Allison JP, Lanier LL: The structure, function and serology of the T-cell antigen receptor complex. Ann Rev Immunol 5:503, 1987

Blackman M, Kappler J, Marrack P: The role of the T cell receptor in positive and negative selection of developing T cells. Science 248:1335, 1990

Ford WF: Lymphocyte migration and the immune response. Prog Allergy 19:1, 1975

Hanahan D: Transgenic mice as probes into complex systems. Science 246:1265, 1989

Kupfer A, Singer SJ: Cell biology of cytotoxic and helper T cell functions: Immunofluorescence microscopic studies of single cells and cell couples. Ann Rev Immunol 7:309, 1989

Lo D, Burkly LC, Flavell RA, et al: Antigen presentation in MHC class II transgenic mice: Stimulation versus tolerization. Immunol Rev 117:121, 1990

Miller JFAP, Morahan G, Allison J: Immunological tolerance: New approaches using transgenic mice. Immunol Today 10:53, 1989

Schwartz RH: Acquisition of immunologic self-tolerance. Cell 57:1073, 1989

Scott DW, Barth RK: Lymphocyte development, differentiation and function. In Hoffman R, Benz E, Jr, Shattil S, et al (eds): Hematology, Basic Principles and Practice. New York, Churchill Livingstone, 1990

Scott DW, Dawson JR: Key Facts in Immunology, New York, Churchill Livingstone, 1985

Sinha AA, Lopez MT, McDevitt HO: Autoimmune diseases: The failure of self tolerance. Science 248:1380, 1990

CHAPTER 14

The Major Histocompatibility Complex: Genes, Proteins, and Genetic Control of Immune Response

The major histocompatibility complex (MHC) is a remarkable cluster of genes that control T cell recognition of self and nonself. The complex was named *histocompatibility* because it was first detected through the rejection of tissue grafts exchanged between different strains of mice. It was a *major* system because rejection was rapid and difficult to control, and it was *complex* because many genes of differing function were clustered together. If the MHC were discovered today, it would undoubtedly be called something like the "major self-recognition complex," for example. However, MHC is still an appropriate name in the sense that MHC gene products are intricately involved in the recognition of foreignness.

Because of the importance and complexity of the MHC, many scientists from different disciplines—biochemists, geneticists, pharmacologists, anthropologists, virologists, physicians, surgeons, and even reproductive physiologists and behavioral psychologists—have collaborated with immunologists to unravel the molecular organization and functions of MHC genes. Their overwhelming importance in biology and medicine has been attested to by the Nobel Prize Committee. No less than eight Nobel prizes have been awarded to pioneers in transplantation and immunologic tolerance: Landsteiner received the prize in 1930 for study of human blood groups; Burnet and Medawar in 1960 for acquired immunologic tolerance; Benacerraf, Dausset, and Snell in 1980 for histocompatibility antigens and immune response genes; and Thomas and Murray in 1990 for bone marrow transplantation.

This chapter begins with the historical development of the MHC and is followed by the biochemistry of the gene products, the molecular organization of the genes, the antigen-presenting functions, and then the relevance of the human MHC (HLA) to transplantation and disease susceptibility. Some examples of other leukocyte and red cell histocompatibility antigens also are discussed briefly.

History of the Major Histocompatibility Complex

When skin or other tissue is transplanted from one place to another on the same individual (an autograft) or to an identical twin (an isograft), the graft survives for the life of the individual. Skin or kidney transplanted to another individual (allograft), even to a fraternal twin in the absence of immunosuppressive treatment, is almost certain to be rejected. Rejection, a complex process, was first studied systematically in rabbits by Medawar in England, in rabbits and humans by Shinoi in Japan, and later in humans by Rapaport. These investigators noted that skin allografts at first healed in as if they were autografts and became vascularized by day 6. By day 9, small blood vessels became dilated and tortuous and blood flow became sluggish. The allografts then died and were sloughed. Autografts continued healing in and became indistinguishable from nontransplanted skin. Gorer observed similar changes with transplanted tumors (sarcomas) in mice and noted that graft infiltration by macrophages was a prominent feature. The importance of lymphoid cells in graft rejection was shown by Mitchison. T cell deficient, athymic nude mice or mice thymectomized at birth could not reject skin grafts. In immunocompetent mice, immunity could be transferred by lymph node cells from an animal rejecting a graft (an adoptive transfer) but not by serum transferred passively. Rejection could be rapid or slow. Rapid rejection occurred when donor and recipient had major histocompatibility differences. Slow rejection was more typical of differences of so-called minor antigens.

Tumor Transplantation in Mice

The groundwork for all studies of the genetics of transplantation was laid by Tyzzer and Little. These biologists observed a tumor that grew in a stock of special mice called Japanese waltzing mice because they made slow circling movements. To keep the waltzing trait, it was necessary to inbreed them. One of these mice developed a tumor that was peculiar in that it could be easily transplanted to other waltzing mice but would not grow in ordinary white mice. To find out why this was so, Tyzzer and Little bred white mice to Japanese waltzers. The tumor could be transplanted to the hybrid (F_1 hybrid) between them. It would grow in all the progeny of F_1 hybrids bred back to Japanese waltzers (susceptible backcross), but only in a tiny fraction of the progeny of F_1 hybrids bred with white mice (resistant backcross). Little proposed that growth or rejection was genetically controlled. Another geneticist, Snell, later decided to determine the location of the relevant (histocompatibility) genes within the genome. Using many types of hybrids into which he had introduced marker genes, Snell tested for their ability to grow or reject tumors. One of his histocompatibility factors was linked to a series of genes for tail abnormalities. At about the same time, the English pathologist Gorer investigated some antigens of different mouse strains. Using alloantisera derived from mice that had rejected tumors from another inbred strain, he identified four distinctive antigens. In collaboration with Snell and Lyman, Gorer tested hybrids that accepted or rejected tumors with his antisera, and a consistent association was found with antigen 2. Animals with antigen 2 would accept tumors; mice lacking antigen 2 rejected them. Gorer, Lyman, and Snell designated the antigen as H-2, which later referred to the antigenic complex as well.

Extensive testing of other strains of mice revealed the existence of many H-2 alleles, two of which (D and K) occurred together on the chromosome. Although D and K were usually inherited as a unit, they could occasionally be separated by recombination, proving the existence of the two closely linked loci, H-2D and H-2K. From the original recombinants, recombinant inbred strains were created by crossing brothers and sisters. The gene products of these loci were called antigens H-2.4 and H-2.11 and could be identified by serologic reactions against red cells (by hemagglutination) or against lymphocytes, macrophages, and tumor cells (by leukoagglutination or cytotoxicity). Additional strains of mice were then immunized against each other. Antibodies produced after graft rejection permitted the identification of many new alleles of D or K. Although some antisera produced failed to react with red cells, they did react with a minority of splenic lymphocytes soon identified as B cells. A new locus, I, was postulated and mapped between H-2D and H-2K, and the map order was established as H-2K, H-2I, H-2D, respectively (see Fig. 14–1). Yet another locus, S, coded for the serum protein C4 and mapped between I and D. The I locus was later shown to be not one but two loci, I-A and I-E, and a suppressor "gene" I-J also appeared to map between I and S. I-J is an anomaly. No gene for H-2J has been identified, yet the functions ascribed to I-J map to this region, suggesting that I-J may be an epistatic interaction between an unknown structural gene and I-A or I-E.

Development of Inbred, Recombinant, and Congenic Mouse Strains

Genetic studies of the MHC were easier to perform in mice because numerous mouse strains had been inbred to homogeneity. Members of an inbred strain carry two copies of the same chromosome. Outbred species, human and dog, for example, do not; they are heterogeneous, as is the F1 hybrid between two inbred strains of mice. In addition, some special strains of mice were created that were identical to a parent strain except for a single locus or for one short segment of chromosome, usually the H-2 complex and its flanking genes. These were known as congenic strains and, along with recombinant mouse strains, have been used to pinpoint the functions of genes on that segment of chromosome.

Identification of Human Histocompatibility Antigens

The first human histocompatibility antigens were identified by Dausset in 1958 and then by Payne, van Rood, and others in the early 1960s. These investigators analyzed the reactions of antilymphocyte antibodies produced after blood transfusion or pregnancy and, in doing so, discovered the first of many human leukocyte antigens. Unlike H-2, there was no information about the chromosomal location of the leukocyte antigens. In fact, there was considerable disagreement even about their relationship to each other. The leading investigators met in 1964 and again in 1965 to test their antisera on cells from the same group of individuals in what was to become an increasingly comprehensive series of International Histocompatibility Testing Workshops. The 1964 Workshop

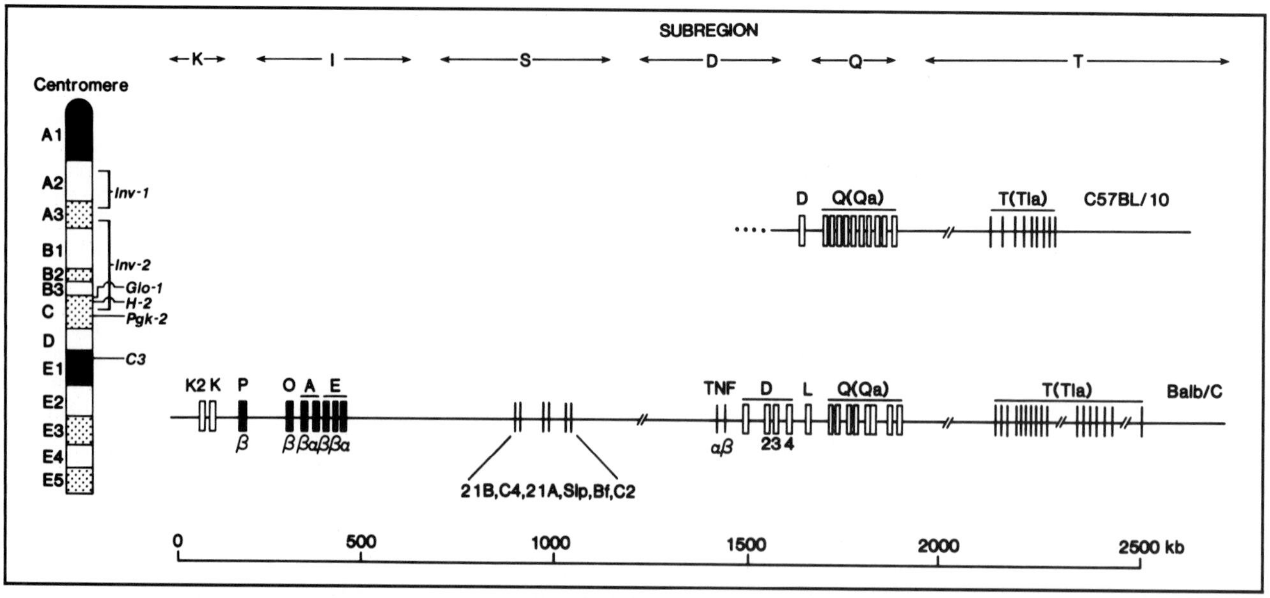

Fig. 14–1. Schematic of the murine major histocompatibility complex, H-2, illustrating subregions and encoded gene products for the BALB/c haplotype. The number of class I genes in the H-2 D, Qa, and T regions varies with the haplotype. For comparison, part of the C57BL/10 haplotype is shown. *(Adapted from Paul WE: Fundamentals of Immunology, Raven Press, 1990.)*

established the feasibility of such a collaborative endeavor. The 1965 Workshop proved that different laboratories were able to identify several antigens correctly, and Dausset and his colleagues predicted that each of the 10 antigens then detected belonged to the same system.

Amos and his colleagues soon established the truth of this in family studies. When tested against the available antisera, leukocytes from a father and some of his children reacted with distinct sets of sera (segregation); leukocytes from the mother were positive with other sera that also gave a segregating pattern in the children. From these patterns, it was deduced that the reactions revealed the inheritance of the father's gametes (usually designated as a and b) and the mother's (designated as c and d). Only four combinations (genotypes) were found in the children: ac, ad, bc, and bd (Fig. 14–2). If there were five children, the fifth gave the same pattern as one of the other siblings (e.g., two were ac). The gametic patterns were designated as *haplotypes,* a term now used for groups of closely linked genes that are inherited together as a unit. This inheritance pattern was confirmed extensively in the 1967 workshop. The two children inheriting the same haplotypes (e.g., ac and ac) were thereafter called an identical pair, and subsequent skin graft exchanges established that they were highly compatible. Identical pair skin grafts often persisted for more than 3 weeks. The pair sharing one haplotype (e.g., ac and ad; or bc and bd) were considered haploidentical and showed great variation in rejection times, from 8 to 30 days. Pairs sharing neither haplotype (ac and bd) were haplodistinct and always rejected skin grafts in less than 14 days. Dausset called the relevant genes Hu-1, a name later objected to because of a red cell antigen with a similar designation. In 1967, at the first of many convocations devoted to nomenclature, Hu-1 was officially changed to HL-A. In later years, the hyphen was dropped and the complex referred to simply as HLA.

An entirely different series of investigations led to a cellular technique that proved exceedingly sensitive in measuring histocompatibility differences between two individuals in vitro, and it ultimately led to the recognition of other loci in the HLA complex. The in vitro functional assay called the mixed lymphocyte culture response (MLC or MLR) was first introduced by Bach and Hirschhorn and by Bain and Lowenstein. Lymphocytes from two unrelated individuals almost invariably stimulated strong proliferative responses in each other when mixed together in culture for 5 to 7 days. Mixtures of cells from some pairs of siblings did not stimulate in MLR; cells from parents and children and from other sibling pairs stimulated to varying degrees. The MLR results correlated with the inheritance patterns shown by serology and also with skin graft rejection times; namely, HLA identical sibs did not stimulate while all other combinations did. Thus, HLA was assumed to be a single polymorphic locus that coded for major histocompatibility antigens, antigens that could be defined by serologic reactions or by functional tests in vitro or in vivo.

This oversimplified view was abandoned when exceptional families were encountered. These were of two types. In the first, segregation patterns of sera suggested that some haplotypes carried more than one antigen. This led to the realization that there were two closely linked loci, HLA-A and HLA-B. A third locus, HLA-C, was later evident. In the second, exceptional pairs of siblings that were HLA-A and -B identical by serology stimulated each other quite strongly in MLR. Often, one of these sibs would fail to stimulate one of his or her haploidentical family members (either parent or sib). This suggested the existence of another locus, initially called MLR stimulatory (MLR-S) and then later HLA-D. HLA-D was closely linked to HLA-A, -B, and -C (Fig. 14–3), but it was separable from them by recombination and was identified only by reactions in MLR.

A novel approach was introduced for the identification

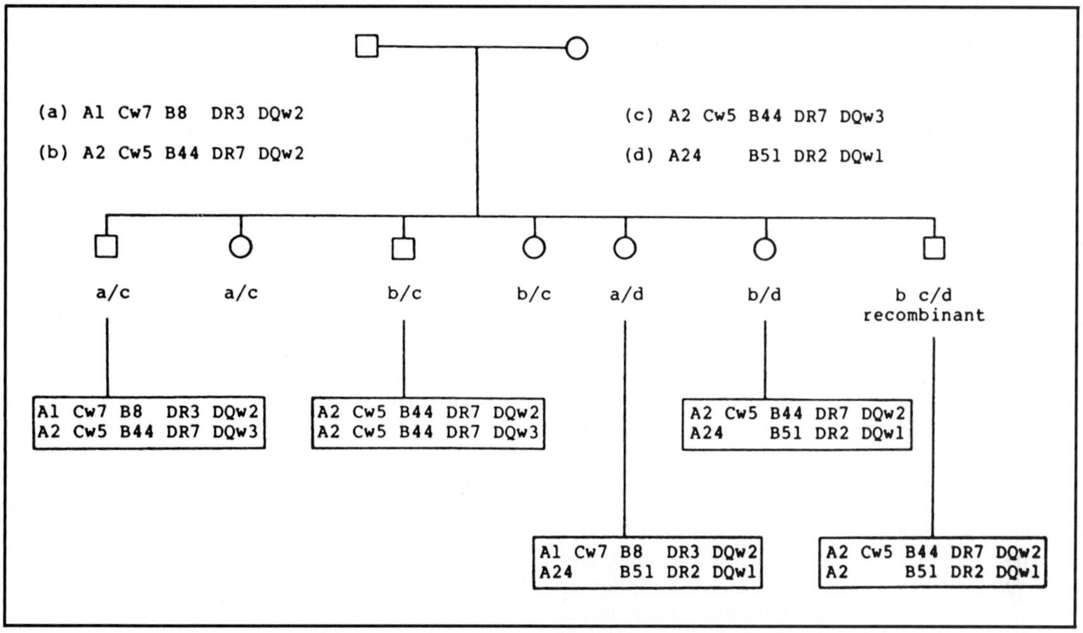

Fig. 14–2. Inheritance of HLA in a family. The paternal haplotypes are designated as a and b, while the maternal haplotypes are designated as c and d. One individual is an HLA-A–HLA-B recombinant.

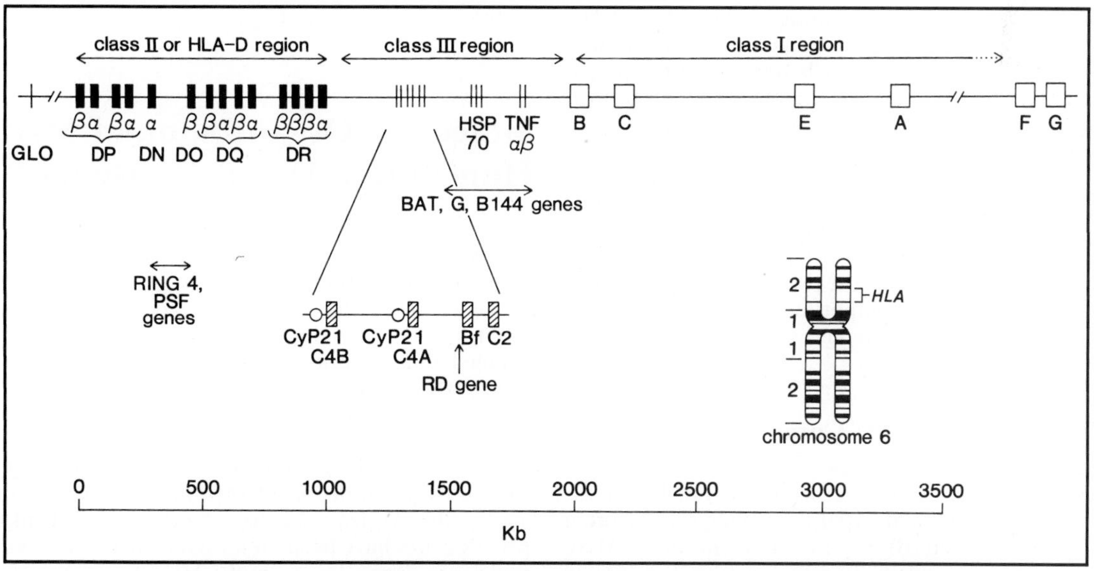

Fig. 14–3. Schematic of the human major histocompatibility complex, HLA. Class I genes are designated by open squares, class II genes by solid rectangles, and class III genes by vertical lines, circles, and striped rectangles. Newly defined but still uncharacterized genes include BAT, G, B144, RD, and Ring 4 and PSF (as described in the text).

of the 14 or so alleles of HLA-D. Children of consanguineous marriages sometimes inherited the same pair of haplotypes. A haplotype, c, would be passed from the grandmother to her two children and then to some of their offspring. Children of first cousins in such a family might inherit two copies of the c haplotype and would be homozygous for HLA. Their lymphocytes were designated as homozygous typing cells and became valuable reagents for typing for HLA-D. Within the family, these cells would not stimulate a response from the parents or the grandmother. They also would not stimulate occasional unrelated subjects who by chance had the same HLA-D allele.

Although there was great interest initially in determining if HLA-A, -B, -C, or -D was responsible for graft rejection, this became somewhat academic when van Leeuwen and van Rood discovered even further complexity. Certain antisera would block a mixed lymphocyte reaction. These sera recognized antigens present on B cells but not on T cells. The new antigens seemed to correlate closely (but not exactly) with HLA-D alleles and were subsequently designated as HLA-DR (for *D* related). As with other loci, HLA-DR was soon found to be not one locus but several; in addition new loci, HLA-DQ and HLA-DP, were identified through combined serologic, biochemical, and molecular studies. HLA-DR, -DQ, and -DP were each capable of stimulating in the mixed lymphocyte culture, although DP was relatively inefficient. Each locus, DR, DQ, and DP, as well as HLA-A, -B, and -C, was found to function as a target in graft rejection.

It was often remarked that the MHC could not have evolved simply to frustrate transplant surgeons; therefore, the true function of the MHC was still unknown. It is perhaps ironic that the essential physiologic role of the HLA molecules turned out to be the distinction between self and nonself. It was a very sensitive marker system for self-histocompatibility. How this occurs has come from sophisticated studies demonstrating that most, if not all, T cell functions are integrally associated with the recognition of antigens bound to MHC antigens. Studies in mice, later confirmed in humans, showed that cytotoxic and proliferative T cells responded to antigen only in the context of an MHC allele, a phenomenon termed *MHC restriction.* Speculation as to how a T cell receptor could see both antigen and MHC, and as to whether there was one receptor or two for MHC and antigen, ended for the most part in 1987 with the remarkable x-ray crystallographic study of the HLA-A2 molecule and the demonstration of a peptide-binding groove. The ramifications of this discovery are still being felt. Thus, the view of the MHC changed from a complex of genes functionally important in transplantation to a complex of genes that facilitate and control T cell recognition.

The MHC as a Supergene: Common Characteristics of All MHCs

Similar MHCs have now been identified in the rat (RT-1), the rhesus monkey (RhL-A), the dog (DLA), the pig (SL-A), other mammals, and the chicken (B). Some components of the MHC may also be present in the fish. In each instance, the content and molecular organization are surprisingly preserved. All MHCs examined have three basic families or "classes" of genes, each consisting of related genes with similar structure, tissue distribution, and function.

Class I genes code for a 44-kDa glycoprotein that is noncovalently bound to a small, non-MHC encoded β_2-microglobulin. The heterodimer is typically expressed on the plasma membrane of cells in nearly every tissue (except perhaps in brain, human red cells, and trophoblast) and functions in the binding of endogenous peptides and in the presentation of these to CD8+ T lymphocytes. Class I–like genes (sometimes called nonclassical class I genes) have been defined in the human, mouse, and chicken. These have a similar structure but different tissue distribution and unknown function (see discussion of H-2 below).

Class II genes code for the 33-kDa α chains and 27-kDa β chains that form transmembranous $\alpha\beta$ heterodimers expressed only on certain immunologically active cells. In humans, these cells include B lymphocytes, macrophages, vascular endothelial cells, activated T cells, precursors of myeloid cells of bone marrow, some cells of the thymic epithelium, and Langerhans cells of the skin. They have been found to be transiently expressed on activated cells of the thyroid and other organs. They are often called B cell antigens, because they were first discovered on B cells and are either absent from, or present in very low concentration, on resting T cells and resting somatic cells. The term "Ia," first used to designate the immune-associated genes of H-2, is also sometimes used to denote the multiple class II genes in humans and other species.

Class III is often used to denote the region between class I and class II that contains genes for several complement components, for heat shock proteins, for cytokine tumor necrosis factors (TNF) α and β and duplicated genes for a p450 cytochrome.

Other genes are scattered throughout the MHC. These include new genes in the class II region that appear to code for ATP-dependent proteins involved in intracellular transport of peptides, a low-molecular-weight protein (LMP) that is suspected of being a protease also involved in antigen processing, and still other genes in the HLA-B, class II, and class III regions that code for products unlike any current MHC product. Whether these have an immune function in addition is currently not known.

Molecular Organization of MHC in Human (HLA) and Mouse (H-2)

HLA

A schematic of human MHC is provided in Figure 14–3. Chromosome walking with cosmid clones, pulsed-field gel electrophoresis, and long-range genomic restriction maps have enabled definitive mapping and ordering of the genes. Although the boundaries are not precise, the HLA gene complex appears to span >3500 kb and includes an area sufficient for more than 50 genes.

The HLA-A, -B, and -C genes are class I genes coding for highly polymorphic glycoproteins expressed on all nucleated cells. At least 20 to 30 other class I–like genes or pseudogenes have been identified near HLA-A. Some of these nonclassic genes, for example, HLA-E, -F, and -G, appear to code for intact glycoproteins associated with β_2-microglobulin, but they are much less polymorphic, or nonpolymorphic, and have a limited tissue distribution. Expression of HLA-G is restricted to embryonic extravillous membranes. HLA-E and -F mRNA transcripts have been identified in a variety of human cells and tissues similar to that observed for the classic HLA-A, -B, and -C genes. Their function is unknown. It is

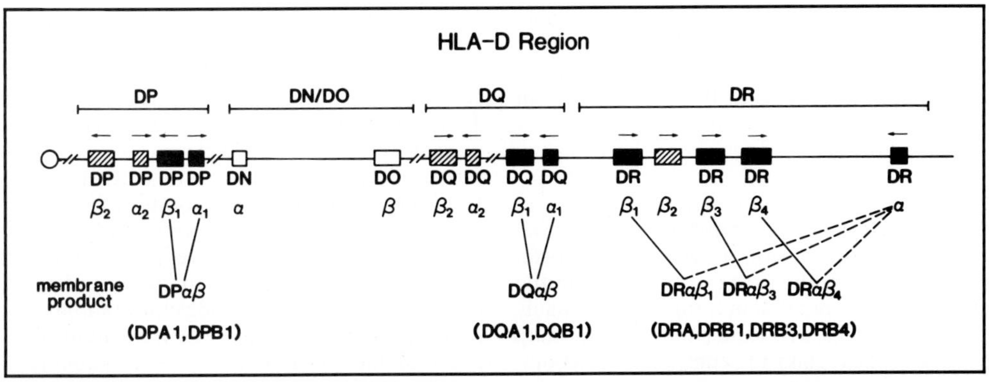

Fig. 14–4. Schematic of the HLA-D region. Filled squares represent expressed genes. Striped squares represent pseudogenes. Expression of some genes (empty squares) is still uncertain. The DR region contains a cluster of β chain genes, although the number of β genes present varies from person to person (see Fig. 14–5).

not clear if the many class I–like genes and pseudogenes are remnants of decaying genes that are no longer utilized, or if some have evolved unique functions other than antigen presentation.

Class II genes include the structural genes for the α and β chains that are tightly, but noncovalently bound to form functional DR, DQ, and DP molecules. In the DR subregion, a single nonpolymorphic DR α chain can join with any of several highly polymorphic DR β chains, the products of the DRA and DRB1, DRB3, DRB4, and DRB5 genes, respectively (see Fig. 14–4). The number of DRβ genes present varies from person to person. Some individuals possess only the DRβ1 gene and thus express only a single DR molecule. Others may possess DRB1, DRB3, DRB4, or DRB5 genes and thus express multiple DR molecules (Fig. 14–5). (The DRβ2 gene is a nonexpressed pseudogene.) The HLA-DQ subregion includes the DQA1 and DQB1 genes, which code for the DQ αβ chain heterodimer, as well as a set of duplicated αβ genes designated as DQA2 and DQB2, which are pseudogenes. In contrast to DR, both the DQ α and β chains are polymorphic. The HLA-DP subregion includes the DPA1 and DPB1 genes, which code for the DP αβ heterodimer, and the pseudogenes DPA2 and DPB2. The DP β chain is polymorphic, the DP α chain is less so. Other class II genes coding for a single α chain (the gene DNA) or β chain (DOB) have been identified at the molecular level, but it is not known if they are expressed, and if so, with what chain they pair.

Genes for ATP-dependent transport proteins (designated as PSF or peptide supply factor gene, probably identical to the RING 4 gene) map to the class II region between DOB and DNA. These are similar in size, sequence, and secondary structure to a superfamily of transporter genes that shuttle sugars, inorganic ions, amino acids, peptides, and proteins across cellular membranes. The localization of two of these genes to the MHC of humans, and the definition of similar genes in the MHC of mice and rats, suggests that they may operate as peptide pumps, ferrying peptides from the cytosol to the endoplasmic reticulum (ER), where peptides can bind to class I MHC molecules.

Class III genes include the four complement components: C2, C4A, C4B, and Bf. Also within this region are genes (CYP21 and CYP21P) for 21-hydroxylase (cytochrome p450) and a new gene designated as RD, which lies close to Bf. RD has an unusual repeated dipeptide structure unlike other MHC products; its function is unknown. Near HLA-B are genes for the two cytokines, α and β TNF. These lymphokines are secreted by activated macrophages and activated lymphocytes, respectively. Also near HLA-B are three genes for heat shock proteins (HSP-70-1, HSP70-2, and HSP70-Hom), a series of novel genes designated as BAT1-BAT9 (BAT stands

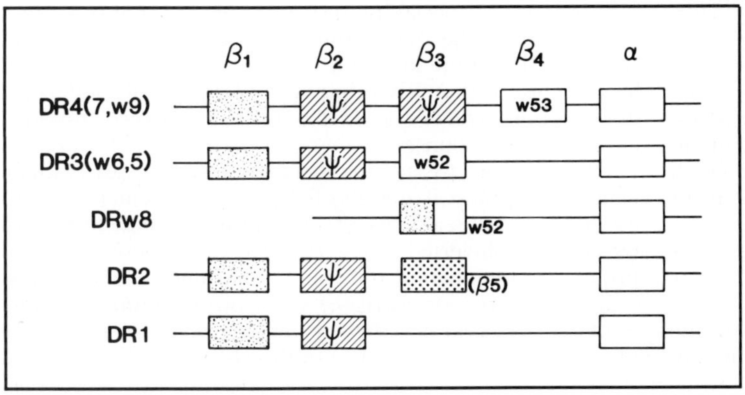

Fig. 14–5. Schematic of the HLA-DR region and variable number of β chains per haplotype. The DRβ1 gene codes for the commonly defined DR alleles. The β3 chain codes for the DRw52 antigen, while the DR β4 chain codes for the DRw53 antigen. DRw8 is believed to be a hybrid molecule, the result of a deletion from the 3′ end of the DRβ1 gene to the 5′ end of the DRβ3 gene. DR2 positive individuals express a DRβ1 and a DRβ5 molecule. *(Adapted from Arnett et al: J Autoimmunity 2:403, 1989.)*

for HLA-B associated transcripts, and these genes are probably identical to those designated as G1-G10), and a gene B144 that appears to be transcribed in B cells and macrophages. The structure and function of B144 and BAT genes are still unknown.

H-2

The murine MHC maps to an area on chromosome 17 (Fig. 14–1). The same three basic classes of genes have been identified as for HLA, although the order of the genes in the haplotype is slightly different from that in humans presumably because one of the class I genes, H-2K, has moved. The map order of the haplotype is H-K, class II genes, class III genes, and then H-2D and H-2L.

H-2D, H-2K, and H-2L are class I genes homologous to HLA-A, -B, and -C. In certain strains of mice, however, these genes have duplicated so that several H-2D-like or H-2K-like genes are present. Other, nonclassic class I genes were detected by using thymocytes as immunogens and thymocytes and leukemic cells as targets. These include genes distal to H-2D, known variously as Tl, Tla, and T. The products of Tl resemble the H-2 antigens structurally, but expression is restricted to the thymus and a very few leukemias (*t*hymus-*l*eukemia antigens). Some Tl-positive leukemias arise in Tl-negative strains. The Tl antigens also differ from H-2D, H-2K, and H-2L in that they rapidly modulate (or undergo endocytosis) when thymic or tumor cells are incubated with anti-Tl antibody. Possibly for this reason, the Tl alleles are not transplantation antigens. However, when certain pairs of mice congenic for Tl were tested in transplantation studies, their grafts were unexpectedly rejected. Further investigation revealed an additional family of class I–like genes designated as Q (Qa), which mapped between H-2D and Tl. The actual number of Q genes present varies with the mouse strain. The Q (Qa) antigens are found on splenic and other lymphocytes. Like Tl, Qa antigens are sometimes present in tumors from animals in which the antigen is not normally expressed (see Chap. 20 for other examples of anomalous expression of normal tissue antigens in tumors).

Like the human class II antigens, a mouse class II molecule also consists of two chains designated as α and β. The genes for these are H-2 Aa, Ab, Ea, Eb, Eb2, Ob, and Pb, where the A, E, O, and P refer to the gene and the a or b, to the α or β chain for which it codes. The Aa and Ab genes (in older forms of nomenclature, these were termed Aα and Aβ) code for the H-2 A αβ heterodimer, a molecule homologous to HLA-DQ. The Ea and Eb genes (previously Eα and Eβ) code for the H-2 E αβ heterodimer, a molecule homologous to HLA-DR. The Ob gene (previously Aβ2) and Pb gene (previously Aβ3) are homologous to the human DOB and DPB loci, respectively.

Immune response (Ir) genes involved in the genetic control of immune responses were originally mapped to the H-2I region by McDevitt and Benacerraf and colleagues. These genes were believed to determine specific recognition of foreign antigens, and they could be identified through functional assays. "Responders" could produce antibody or cellular responses to a limiting dose of branched-chain synthetic amino acids; "nonresponders" could not. In most cases responsiveness was dominant, although instances of recessivity and of transcomplementation between two nonresponders were occasionally observed. How the MHC could control the immune response to particular antigens was not readily apparent at the time Ir genes were identified, but now they would probably be considered to reflect the successful binding of a peptide to a particular MHC molecule and the presentation of the MHC-peptide complex to an immunocompetent T cell. In this sense, class I and class II genes, as well as transporter genes in the class II region that are responsible for translocating peptides to the ER, are all potential Ir genes. In humans, sporadic associations of HLA alleles with immune responsiveness (e.g., to streptococcal antigens or to ragweed antigen Ra5) have been noted, although Ir gene control has been difficult to identify in most studies. This is probably because the many MHC molecules can bind to the appropriate peptides, and most antigens have multiple and diverse epitopes. Deliberate immunization of humans with foreign antigens is rarely possible, and many studies have failed to use individuals sharing an HLA-restricting antigen or large families; therefore, it is not surprising that a simple pattern of responsiveness has not emerged.

H-2 also includes genes for class III complement genes; TNF α and β; an adjoining gene B144; the proposed transport genes HAM-1 and HAM-2; and a gene (Neu-1) that controls sialylation in some liver enzymes. A hematopoietic histocompatibility locus, Hh-1, that controls NK-mediated resistance to allografts, a gene (*Csp*-1) that determines susceptibility to cortisone-induced cleft palate, and genes involved in fertility and body size that are homologous to the *grc* (growth and reproduction complex) genes in the rat have also mapped to H-2. The gene for red cell glyoxalase is found centromeric to H-2. Recombinational hot spots have been identified in areas.

Although this chapter is devoted to the more well-characterized MHC genes with known immunologic function, it is important to know that genes centromeric to H-2 and designated as *t* are part of a complex series of recessive genes that function during differentiation and development of the embryo. Included among these are two distinct, but closely related gene families. One allele, *T*, found in laboratory stocks of mice, was mentioned earlier as giving a chromosomal location for H-2. *T*-region mutants (*t*) have been detected in all demes of wild mice so far tested. They are identified in crosses of wild mice to stocks carrying *T*, since *T*/*t* hybrids are viable tailless mice. *T* itself behaves as a multiallelic series of recessive lethals, as do most *t* mutants. The cross $T/t^x \times T/t^x$ yields only T/t^x offspring because T/T and t^xt^x are nonviable. Five separate genetic loci or complementation groups are clustered in the *T* region. The hybrid T^x/t^y is viable if t^x and t^y are from different complementation groups, but the embryo dies at a specific point in development if t^x and t^y are different members of the same complementation group. Male sterility and abnormal male transmission ratio are but two of many other features associated with this system. These studies, still in progress, are of special interest since they opened the way to an analysis of the extraordinary number of genes briefly activated during the different stages of embryogenesis. It has been suggested that *T* is as important for cell-cell cooperation during embryogenesis as H-2 is for cell-cell cooperation in immunologic responses.

In addition, *t* is notable because it suppresses recombination along most if not all of the mouse seventeenth chromosome. Short segments of an affected seventeenth chromosome are inverted when *t* is present. These inversions prohibit recombination with normal chromosomes. Paradoxically, recombination increases when two different *t* chromosomes are brought together in the heterozygote; at least two *t* loci are close to or even within the H-2 complex.

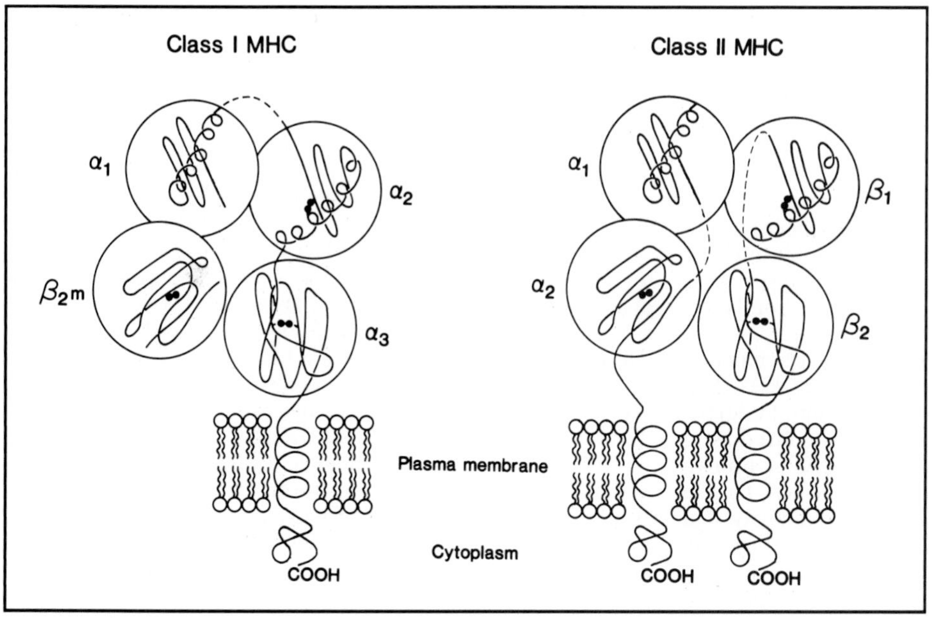

Fig. 14–6. Similar structure of class I and class II molecules. Despite different organization of genes at the molecular level, both molecules consist of four-domain structures with probably identical three-dimensional configuration (see Fig. 14–9 for more details).

Class I and Class II Genes and Products

Biochemistry

Class I molecules of all MHCs are heterodimers of a heavy chain of about 44 kDa molecular weight and a light chain (β_2-microglobulin) of 12 kDa (Fig. 14–6). The precise molecular weight of the heavy chain varies among species because of small differences in the length of the polypeptide chain and in the degree of glycosylation. Class I heavy chains are coded for by genes of the MHC, but the β_2m gene is on a different chromosome in both mouse and human.

Regardless of the number of class I genes expressed, there appears to be only one β_2m gene. The β_2m may be invariant as it is in humans, or it may have a rare second allele as it does in mice. β_2m does not contribute to the variability (polymorphism) of class I molecules, although it appears necessary for the intracellular processing of the molecule and for its antigenicity, possibly because it contributes to the conformation of the heavy chain. β_2m is noncovalently bound to the heavy chains and is in dynamic equilibrium. It can frequently be displaced by β_2m from another species.

Class I molecules are two-chain, four-domain globular structures. The heavy chain contributes the α1, α2, and α3 domains, β_2m contributes the fourth. The α1 and α2 domains are highly polymorphic, with amino acid substitutions concentrated in several hypervariable regions. The positions of these regions differ for each class I gene (Fig. 14–7). The α3 domain shows little variability, although the polymorphism that is present can be important. This is because the human α3 domain contains an interaction site for the CD8 α chain.

Each class I molecule has generally been assumed to carry a single antigenic site, and the official nomenclature reflects this. However, at least two separate epitopes have long been recognized on HLA-B, and there is growing evidence that each molecule expresses several polymorphic antigens. It is important to understand the nature of these epitopes. From x-ray crystallographic studies of class I molecules, discussed

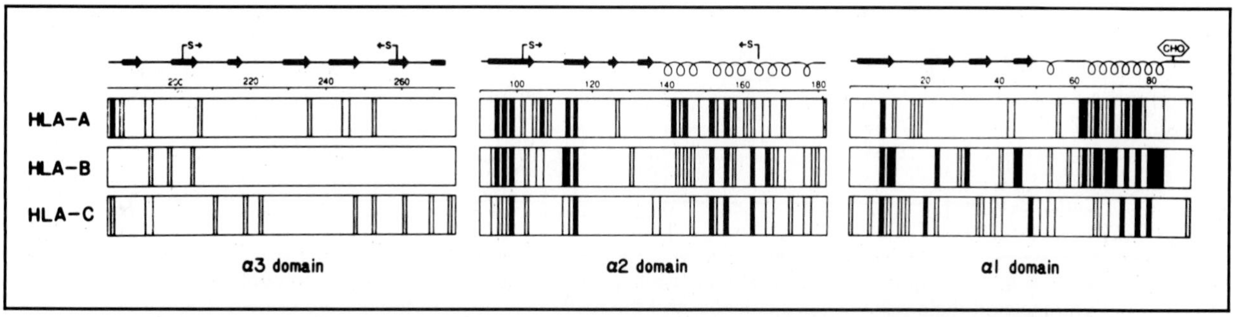

Fig. 14–7. Regions of amino acid polymorphism for class I α1, α2, and α3 domains. The parts of the molecule determined by each domain (e.g., β-pleated sheet denoted by arrows, α helix by coils) are noted above. *(Adapted from Bjorkman and Parham: Annu Rev Biochem 59:253, 1990.)*

in more detail below, it has been deduced that the hypervariable regions are located on the floor and sides of a peptide-binding groove formed by the α1 and α2 domains. Amino acid sequence differences contribute to the binding of a peptide. There is strong evidence that these hypervariable regions are also the sites recognized by antibodies and by T cells in allograft rejection.

A papain cleavage site lies external to the transmembranous hydrophobic segment. The existence of this cleavage site has facilitated purification and analysis. The cytoplasmic tail differs in length among different class I molecules and among different species; it has a half cysteine and a phosphorylation site.

Class II molecules are heterodimers of a heavy chain (α) of about 33 kDa and a light chain (β) of about 27 kDa (Fig. 14–6), both coded for by closely linked genes within the MHC. The α and β chains can be separated under nonreducing conditions, but only with difficulty. Finite analysis of human class II genes and products has been complicated by the multiplicity of HLA-DR β chains, by the cross-reactivity that is presumably due to amino acid sequences shared among genes, and by the fact that not all individuals carry all DRβ genes. Fortunately, the DR α chain is not polymorphic, although like β_2-microglobulin, it contributes to conformation; at least one HLA-DR molecule loses its ability to bind antibody when the chains are separated. For the DQ αβ heterodimer, both chains are polymorphic and the products of the α gene and β genes from the homologous chromosomes can interact in *cis* and *trans* manner to form hybrid DQ molecules. Thus, an individual can theoretically form four different DQ molecules on the cellular membrane.

Gene Structure and Regulatory Elements

The organization of class I and class II genes is shown in Fig. 14–8. For class I, a signal sequence is followed by the α1, α2, and α3 exons, each coding for the corresponding domain. One exon codes for the transmembranous domain, and three exons code for the cytoplasmic tail, followed by the 3′ untranslated sequence. For class II, the signal sequence of the α chain is followed by the α1 and α2 exons coding for the α1 and α2 protein domains, respectively. The cytoplasmic, transmembranous, and cytoplasmic tail peptides are coded for by a single exon followed by the 3′ untranslated sequence. The β chain gene similarly has two exons for the β1 and β2 domains, but part of the cytoplasmic tail is coded for by an exon adjacent to the 3′ untranslated sequence. All these exons are separated by introns.

Expression of the MHC class I and class II molecules is under complex regulatory control. Transcriptional regulation of class II genes occurs in the 5′ flanking and intronic regions, as illustrated for the DRα gene in Fig. 14–9. In B lymphocytes and cells constitutively producing high levels of DR, both the promoter (TATA and CAAT boxes) and enhancer regions are active. In macrophages, the promoter and enhancer elements are nonfunctional, but DR expression can be induced by IFN-gamma. In noninducible cells, the promoter and enhancer are inactive and interferon-induction sites are nonresponsive. Concentrations of CpG dinucleotides in the promoter, exon 1, and intron 1 regions of class II (and class I) genes form CpG-rich islands that are usually rare in eucaryotic genes. Demethylated cytosine residues in these regions may correlate with chromatin conformation and transcriptional activity. The DRα gene also contains three DNase I hypersensitivity sites to which *trans*-acting factors can bind. One site is present in all cells, the other two only in cells constitutively producing high levels of DR. In class I genes, regulatory elements flanking exon 1 include a promoter region of CAAT and TATA boxes, enhancers, and interferon responsive elements (Fig. 14–9). A negative regulatory element has been identified in a swine class I gene. Additional mechanisms may be responsible for the tissue specificity of nonclassic class I genes (e.g., HLA-G in extravillous membranes or H-2 Q10 in the liver).

Posttranscriptional regulation depends on splicing of primary transcripts, stability of mRNA, translational controls, sorting in the ER, glycosylation, or association with β_2m and peptide. Alternative splicing has been described for both class I and class II. Binding of peptide is required for cell surface

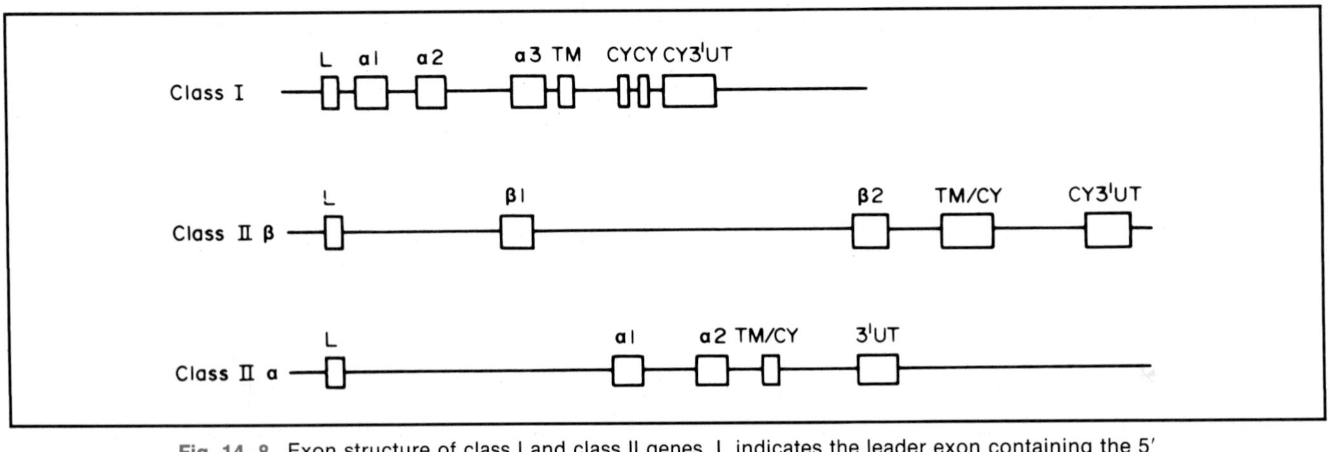

Fig. 14–8. Exon structure of class I and class II genes. L indicates the leader exon containing the 5′ untranslated region, the signal sequence, and the first amino acids of the mature protein. The α and β exons encode protein domains. TM and CY refer to the transmembranous region and cytoplasmic domain.

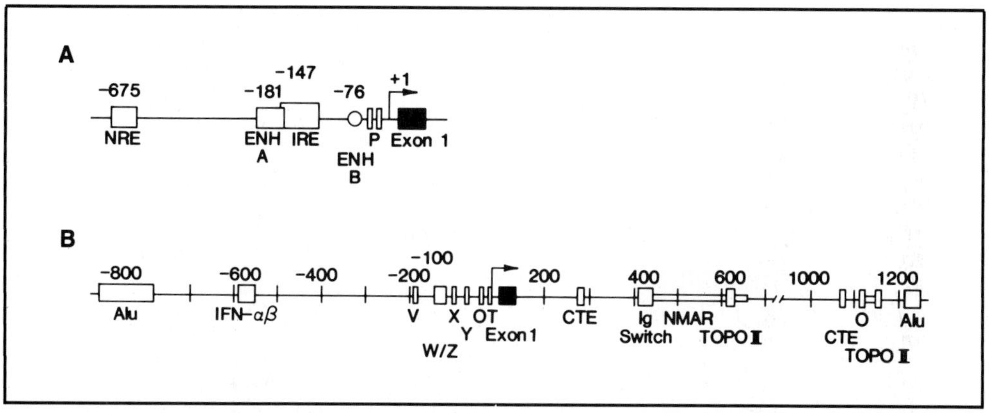

Fig. 14–9. **A.** Regulatory elements for the swine class I gene PD1. All elements except NRE are common to all class I genes analyzed and are similarly situated. NRE has so far only been identified in the PD1 gene. *P,* promoter, consisting of CAAT and TATA boxes (from −26 to −57). *ENH B,* enhancer B: in vivo function is unknown. *IRE,* interferon response element: homologous to the consensus sequences found in all IFN responsive genes. *ENH A,* enhancer A: usually a positive regulatory element that enhances transcription from downstream promoters (homologous to the Ig K gene enhancer NFKB), but also can exert negative regulatory effects; multiple binding factors have been identified. *NRE,* negative regulatory element. **B.** Regulatory elements of the HLA-DRα gene. Some are homologous to *cis*-acting elements that regulate expression of other gene families. The numbers indicate nucleotide position. *TOPO II,* sequences that represent potential binding sites for the enzyme topoisomerase II (involved in changing the geometric configuration of chromatin fibers during activation). *O,* octamer (GTTTGCAT): similar to O in the promoter region. *CTE,* three core transcriptional enhancer elements (TTGTGGTTTGG; TTGGTTTG; GTGTGTTTG): homologous to critical sequences for transcription of sv40 and polyoma viral enhancers. *NMAR,* nuclear matrix-associated region: may represent sequences involved in interaction of chromatin fibers and scaffolding of nuclear matrix. *Ig switch* $(TGGGGG)_4$: sequences within exon 1 that are implicated in immunoglobulin isotype switching; their function in the MHC is unknown. *T,* TATA box: important for initiation of transcription in a variety of genes. *O,* octamer (ATTTGCAT): positive transcriptional regulatory element also found in promoters of Ig H and L chains and in the transcriptional enhancer of the Ig H chain gene. *Y box* (CTGATTGGCCAAAG): positive transcriptional regulatory element that contains an inverted sequence of GGTTA to which the ubiquitous transcriptional activator CCAAT may bind. *X box* (CCTAGCAACAGATG): positive transcriptional regulatory element that may be responsible for tissue-specific class II expression and IFN-gamma inducibility. *WZ,* regulatory elements: W may also be responsible for tissue-specific class II expression and IFN-gamma inducibility. *V:* negative regulatory element. *IFNαβ consensus sequence* (GTGTTGAACCTCAGAGTTTCTCCTCTCAT): also involved in transcriptional regulation of class I genes by IFN-α and IFN-β. (**A** adapted from Singer and Maguire: CRC Crit Rev Immunol 10:235, 1990. **B** adapted from Sullivan et al: Immunol Today 8:289, 1987.)

expression of class I, since mutagenized B lymphoblastoid cell lines with depressed or absent class I expression were found to have a regulatory defect that mapped to the class II region, probably to genes that code for intracellular transport proteins. The failure to transport peptides from the cytoplasm to the ER appeared to result in peptide-deficient MHC class I molecules that were unstable and rapidly lost. Class I expression can also be modulated by viruses such as adenovirus, by tumor necrosis factors α and β, and by exogenous, nonviral agents such as ethanol and cycloheximide. Supragenic regulatory mechanisms such as chromatin organization, DNA sequence organization, and methylation are also likely to be important.

Congenital deficiencies in MHC expression result in what have been termed *bare lymphocyte syndromes.* Individuals with bare lymphocyte syndromes have variable deficits in immune response, including loss of lymphocyte function, depressed antibody production, delayed hypersensitivity, and increased susceptibility to infection. The syndromes can affect class I or class II genes or both and probably arise from defects in a variety of regulatory genes. In at least one instance, the regulatory gene is unlinked to the MHC.

Three-Dimensional Structure of HLA-A2

As mentioned earlier, the remarkable configuration of an HLA molecule was recognized in 1987 when the x-ray crystallographic structure of HLA-A2 was published. Up to that time, it was generally assumed that HLA would be immunoglobulin like. This assumption was based on the sequence homology of β_2-microglobulin and the α3 domain to immunoglobulin as well as on the molecule's appearance, which seemed to be organized into four Ig-like domains. This prediction was only partially correct. The HLA-A2 molecule has a unique structure (Fig. 14–10). The α1 and α2 domains

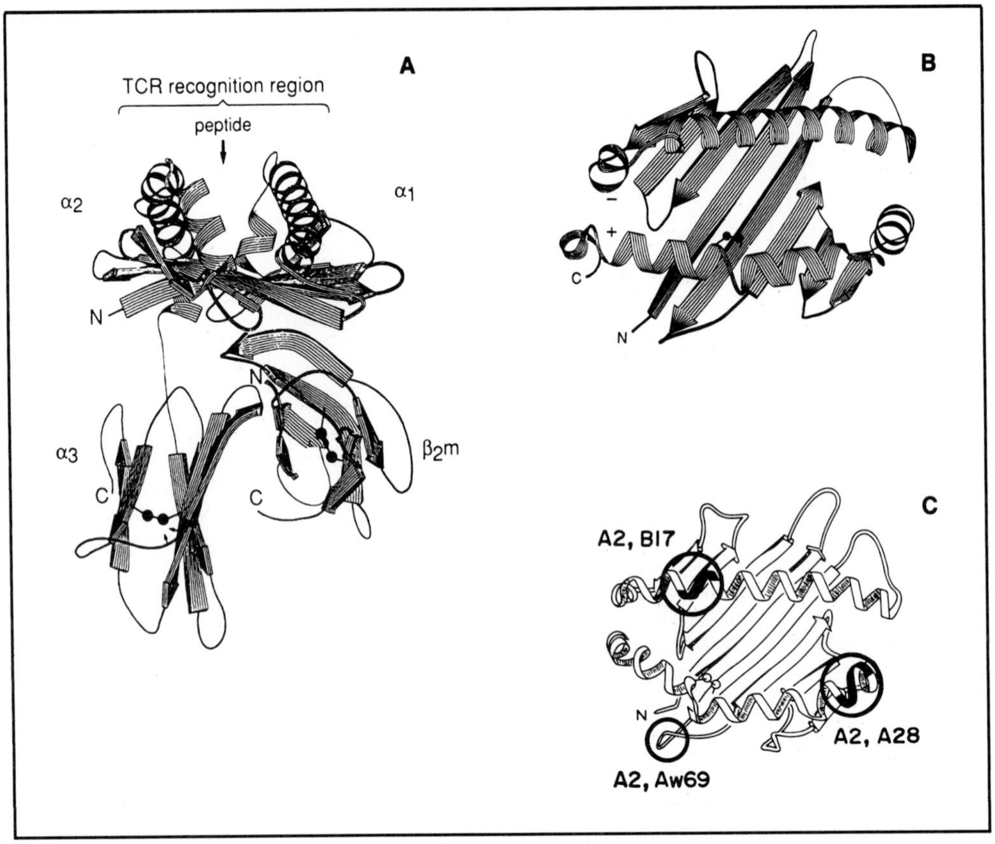

Fig. 14–10. Three-dimensional view of the HLA-A2 molecule from the side, **A**, and from the top, **B**. **C**. Location of three serologically defined epitopes on the HLA-A2 molecule. (**A** and **B** from Bjorkman and Parham: Annu Rev Biochem 59:253, 1990, with permission.)

each produce four antiparallel β strands followed by a long helical region. Together they form a structure similar to a set of "jaws," an eight-stranded β-pleated sheet platform topped with two long α helices and a long groove approximately 2.5 nm (25 Å) long and 1nm (10 Å) wide. This groove or cleft is lined with polar and nonpolar side chains capable of binding either processed exogenous or endogenous (self) peptides. The groove is large enough to accommodate an α helical peptide of 12 to 20 residues or a linear peptide of approximately 8 residues, although longer peptides, or native intact proteins such as fibrinogen, may be partially inserted into the groove. How and where a peptide binds to a class I or class II molecule is discussed in the following section. Most variable amino acids on the α helices or floor of the groove point into the groove, although a few on the α helices point directly upward and may interact directly with the T cell receptor (TCR). Beneath the platform of β-pleated sheet, the membrane-proximal α3 and β_2m domains consist of two antiparallel β-pleated sheets connected by an internal disulfide bond. Both resemble constant domains of immunoglobulins and are conserved in sequence. The α3 domain contains a site recognized by the CD8 α chain, suggesting that the membrane-proximal domains are more than structural supports.

The conformation of a class II molecule has not yet been fully defined because of difficulties in crystallization, but all available evidence suggests that it too has the same four-domain structure and antigen-binding groove. The membrane-distal platform is formed by the α1 domain of an α chain and the β1 domain of the β chain. The α2 and β2 domains form the membrane-proximal supporting structure. Class II molecules contain a binding site for CD4, but its location is not yet known.

Function

Helper T Cells Restricted for Class II Antigens. The importance of MHC determinants in controlling T cell function came from several sources. The first involved the reconstitution of congenitally athymic and immunoincompetent nude mice. These animals could be efficiently reconstituted only by thymocytes from mice of the same H-2 type. Then, T cell or B cell depleted mice that bore intra-H-2 recombinant haplotypes were reconstituted. It was found that antibody responses to a variety of antigens required the cooperation of T and B cells; the T and B cells had to be compatible in the H-2A (I-A) subregion. No other class I or class II region product was involved in restricting helper T cell function.

Immunogenetic analysis of T cell-macrophage interaction provided similar results. B cells and macrophages play essential roles in antigen presentation to T cells (Chap. 12). Only H-2 compatible, antigen-pulsed macrophages can efficiently present antigen to T cells. The response can be measured through the proliferation of T cells to homologous antigen in culture and through the helper cell activity of the sensitized T cells. B cells also present antigen in a highly specific manner. This ability was not observable when B cells in splenic or peripheral blood were tested (because of the heterogeneity of the B cells) but became apparent when cloned B cell lines became available.

Two other important features of these two systems are worth noting. First, T cells from F1 hybrids between two inbred strains (P1 × P2) that have been sensitized on antigen-pulsed macrophages from one parent (P1) will proliferate in response to a second challenge of the antigen only if F1 macrophages or P1 macrophages are present. These T cells will provide helper cell function only for B cells from the F1 hybrids or the parent that served as a source of antigen-presenting cells. Thus, T cell specificity is not for antigen per se, *but for antigen and the appropriate H-2 allele.* Whether the T cell recognition structure is composed of one receptor for an antigen-modified histocompatibility determinant or of two separate receptors—one for antigen and the other for the appropriate H-2 molecule—has been strongly debated. However, these studies and those in which cytotoxic T lymphocyte specificity was examined (see below) have demonstrated that the receptor specificity of T cells, in contrast to B cells, involves a self-MHC recognition unit. How this occurs became clear when the peptide-binding groove was identified. Implicit in this statement is a belief in the individuality (specificity) of the binding to a given MHC molecule only of those peptides with the correct conformation and charge.

The second important point from these studies is derived from experiments measuring responses to antigens under Ir gene control using F1 hybrids between responder and non-responder strains of mice. T lymphocytes from F1 mice primed to appropriate antigens are often restricted in their ability to interact with antigen-pulsed parental macrophages or parental B cells. Primed F1 T cells may interact with antigen-pulsed macrophages from high-responder macrophages but not from low-responder macrophages; or alternatively, they can be found to interact only with high-responder B cells to produce antigen. Such selectivity is not observed using antigens that are not demonstrably under Ir gene control.

Cytotoxic T Cells Restricted for Class I Antigens. Analyses of cytotoxic T cell responses against the lymphocytic choriomeningitis and influenza viruses demonstrated that CD4+ cytotoxic T cells recognize a viral antigen only in association with an MHC antigen. Surprisingly, the restricting molecules were not class II antigens, but class I. Similar results were obtained in cytotoxic responses against hapten-modified MHC molecules and later in studies of normal cellular components, such as the male H-Y antigen and minor histocompatibility antigens; class I restricted cytotoxic T lymphocytes (CTLs) could be elicited in genetically disparate individuals. These studies are notable because they identified a second type of restriction, this time involving class I MHC and CTLs. The specificity of the cytotoxic T cell response was paradoxically directed at internal viral products that are not expressed on the cell surface, leading to the conclusion that viral peptides associate with MHC molecules within the cell and are subsequently transported to the cell surface for presentation to CD8+ T cells.

Model of Antigen Presentation. The MHC class I and class II molecules constitute two separate but similar peptide-binding and transport systems. Class I antigens bring intracellular, endogenously synthesized peptides to the cell surface, whereas class II antigens bind extracellular, exogenous peptides from endocytosed and degraded antigens (Fig. 14–11). Each class of MHC molecules presents its peptides to different immunosurveillant T cells. The details of how class I and class II MHC molecules interact with antigen, and in what cellular compartments these interactions take place, are only now becoming clear. The following is a current interpretation of the sequence of events.

The class I heavy chain is synthesized, associates with β_2m, and then passes through the endoplasmic reticulum as a functional two-chain, four-domain structure with an accessible cleft. While in the endoplasmic reticulum, small peptides, including self-peptides or fragments of viral components, are bound in the groove. The peptides appear to be actively transported from the cytoplasm to the endoplasmic reticulum by intracellular transport proteins. Genes for two of these transport proteins (designated as HAM-1 and HAM-2 in mice; as mtp 1, mtp 2, and cim in rats; and as RING 4 or PSF in humans) map to the class II region of the MHC. The peptide/class I MHC complex is then transported through the Golgi complex to the surface, where it is "scanned" by T cells (Fig. 14–12) that have been educated in the thymus to discriminate self from nonself. Recognition of an aberrant MHC/peptide configuration triggers the series of interactions involving CD3, TCR, MHC class I, and CD8 (as described in Chaps. 12 and 13) and culminates in the triggering and activation of CD8+ cytotoxic T cells.

The trafficking of class II molecules is different. Class II α and β chains interact to form a two-chain, four-domain heterodimer in the endoplasmic reticulum. However, the cleft is thought to be inaccessible at this point, and a third chain, designated as the invariant or I chain, binds the $\alpha\beta$ heterodimer. The function of the I chain, which is the product of a gene unlinked to HLA, is not specifically known, although current thought is that it acts to obstruct or prevent peptide binding. The class II–invariant chain complex is routed through the Golgi and then to an endosomal compartment in which the I chain is degraded and the groove filled with one of the peptides generated by the degradation of endocytosed foreign proteins. The class II–peptide complex is then transported to the surface, where a set of interactions involving CD3, TCR, peptide, MHC, and CD4 trigger the activation of CD4+ T helper cells.

The development of a cytotoxic or T helper cell response thus depends on (1) whether a peptide interacts with a class I molecule in the endoplasmic reticulum or with a class II molecule in an endosomal compartment, (2) with the MHC allele involved (since each class I and class II molecule may bind nonoverlapping sets of peptides), and on (3) whether an appropriate T cell receptor recognizes and interacts with the MHC-peptide complex.

The antigen-presenting properties of the MHC and the discrimination of self and nonself become ingenious parts of an immune system designed to provide defense against infectious organisms and also to avoid destructive autoaggression. The large number of bacteria, viruses, fungi, protozoa, metazoa, and other organisms that challenge humans and higher animals has resulted in strong evolutionary pressures to develop diverse means of countering these infectious agents. Extracellular organisms are usually eliminated by antibody, complement, and phagocytes. Parasites, such as fungi and

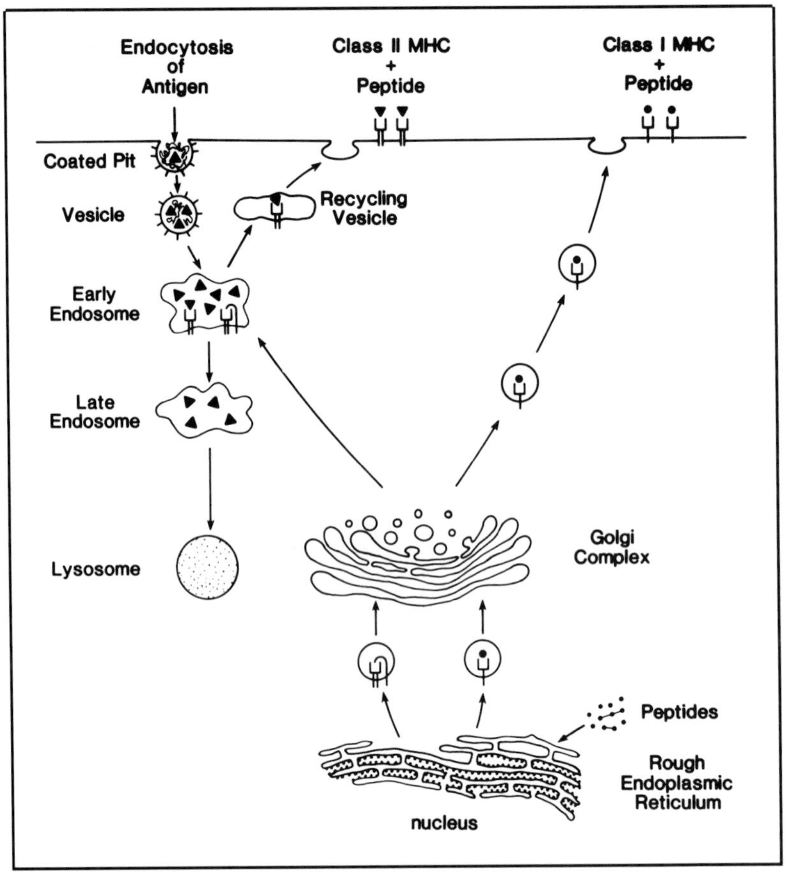

Fig. 14–11. Model of antigen presentation. Class I MHC molecules bind endogenous peptides in the endoplasmic reticulum and progress to the cell surface. Class II MHC molecules associate with an invariant chain in the endoplasmic reticulum and are then routed to an endosomal compartment, where the invariant chain is degraded and exogenous peptides bind.

tubercle bacilli, are controlled by macrophages activated by T cell lymphokines in the context of granulomatous inflammation. The first line of immune defense against viruses is usually antibody at the level of epithelial or endothelial cell contact. However, in the absence of sensitization or with the establishment of viral infection, host defenses are primarily cellular and often involve destruction of virally infected cells by cytotoxic T cells (Chap. 19).

The interaction of cytotoxic T cells with virus-MHC complexes establishes a means for recognizing virally infected cells while, at the same time, preventing effector cell neutralization or distraction by circulating virus or viral antigens. It also discourages cytotoxic responses against uninfected cells. Since class I molecules are present on nearly all body cells, protection extends to all tissues and organs. Class II MHC molecules are restricted in tissue distribution to those cells that can endocytose and degrade exogenous antigens. Again, the interaction of T cells with MHC class II-peptide complexes guards against unwarranted or uncontrolled T cell activation. It is not hard then to understand a selective advantage for an individual or species to maintain a high degree of polymorphism in the peptide-binding regions of class I and class II molecules.

Thymic Selection. The ability to discriminate between self and nonself is learned in the thymus. As described in Chapter 13, this is dependent on the elimination of T cells in which TCR gene rearrangements are unproductive, as well as on the elimination of T cells with productive rearrangements that recognize self MHC or self MHC–peptide complexes. How the selection process occurs is not well understood, but interaction of differentiating T cells with thymic epithelium appears to be essential. MHC molecules are expressed on the thymic epithelium, and it has been proposed that high-affinity TCR-MHC interactions lead to clonal deletion of autoreactive T cells, while low-affinity interactions select cells to be released to peripheral circulation. Numerous questions remain. We do not know, for example, how an individual becomes unresponsive to peptides not present in the thymus. The priming of the $CD4^-CD8^-$ gamma double-negative T cells that are MHC unrestricted is not yet understood, nor is it clear if the many autoimmune diseases associated with particular HLA alleles result from aberrant TCR-peptide-MHC interactions or from autoreactive T cells that have escaped from the thymus.

Polymorphism and Definition of Alleles. The MHC occupies only a relatively short segment of the sixth chromosome. As a result, crossing over within the MHC is infrequent and the whole complex is usually inherited as a single unit, the HLA haplotype. Because many linked HLA loci are polymorphic and because gene expression is codominant, the two HLA haplotypes carried by an individual can easily be distinguished by analyzing segregation patterns of HLA antigens in families (Fig. 14–2).

Testing for HLA within a family is relatively straightforward, even though there are very many HLA antigens. Highly

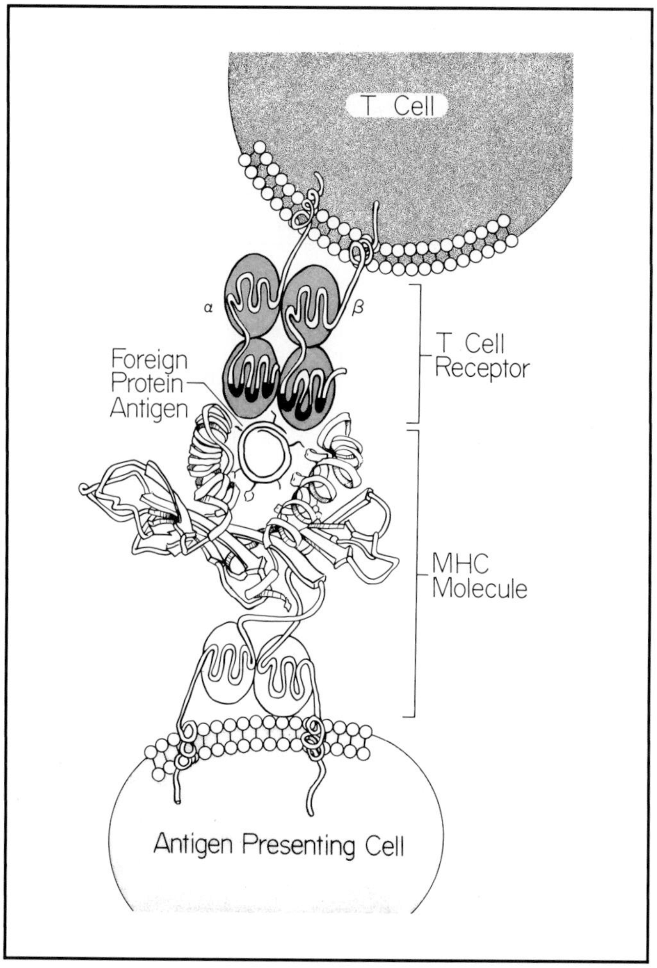

Fig. 14–12. Ternary MHC-peptide-TCR complex. (Adapted from Sinha et al: Science 248:1381, 1990.)

specific antibodies to most HLA antigens, and monoclonal antibodies to some, are available, and the test, a measurement of cell damage produced by complement after sensitization of lymphocytes with antibody (Chap. 12), is in theory simple. Serotyping for HLA-A, -B, and -C alleles requires relatively few peripheral blood lymphocytes. Typing for HLA-DR or -DQ alleles is more complex, as HLA-DR and -DQ molecules are found on B lymphocytes but not on resting T lymphocytes in the peripheral blood. Because B lymphocytes comprise only about 5% to 15% of human peripheral blood lymphocytes, modifications of the typing assay may entail larger volumes of blood, removal of T lymphocytes, selective enrichment of B lymphocytes, or use of two-color immunofluorescence to define B cell–specific reactions.

Typing for HLA-D is quite different and depends on results of stimulation in the MLR. The stimulator cells used for HLA-D typing are reference cells selected to carry two identical copies of the same HLA-D specificity and are called homozygous typing cells (HTCs). An HTC will stimulate cells from responders having a different HLA-D allele, but it will not stimulate cells having a copy of the same HLA-D allele. As an example, an HTC homozygous for the HLA-Dw1 allele will stimulate a positive mixed-lymphocyte response in HLA-Dw2-Dw3 subjects, but it will not stimulate Dw1-Dw1, Dw1-Dw2, or Dw1-Dw3 cells. HLA-D typing is slow, utilizes HTCs that are difficult to find, and requires large numbers of cells. A more efficient procedure, primed lymphocyte typing (PLT), uses HTCs that have been primed to a given specificity, but even this procedure is limited to specialty laboratories. HTC typing is therefore being replaced by serologic and molecular definition of individual class II loci, including HLA-DP alleles that have previously been defined by PLT.

There are numerous other methods of defining HLA alleles, including the use of cytotoxic T cells, isoelectric focusing, restriction fragment length polymorphisms, and sequencing. Most are performed only in more sophisticated laboratories usually when the goal is to identify precise differences in alleles that may be important in T cell restriction, in anthropologic studies, or in disease associations or to gain new insights retrospectively into the specificity of graft rejection.

A molecular typing method for class II alleles that has recently emerged promises to revolutionize HLA typing. The technique known as oligotyping is based on the amplification of α1 or β1 exons of class II genes (the exons that code for the more polymorphic domains) using the polymerase chain reaction. The amplified product is then hybridized with specific oligonucleotide probes in order to determine the presence or absence of allele-specific sequences. The method is extremely sensitive, allows for identification of alleles that are difficult if not impossible to identify with antibodies, and avoids some problems of cross-reactivity between class II loci that can cause ambiguity in serotyping or cellular typing. Oligotyping can be performed on minute amounts of blood or even on dead cells. This method is now being used in some clinical and forensic laboratories when there are insufficient cells for routine HLA-DR and -DQ typing, in place of MLR and HLA-D typing, and in many research laboratories. It should be noted that no procedure for HLA typing is unambiguous. Antisera, even monoclonal, can cross-react and oligomeric probes can hybridize to more than one sequence. Unambiguous typing requires skilled interpretation and controlled testing conditions.

Currently, >25 HLA-A alleles, >50 HLA-B alleles, >20 HLA-DR alleles, >15 HLA-DQ alleles, and >15 HLA-DP alleles have been recognized (Table 14–1). These numbers continue to grow as more sensitive typing techniques are used and as more ethnically diverse populations are tested. Revision of the nomenclature every 2 to 3 years affirms new antigens, identifies variants of old antigens, and discriminates between alleles defined at the protein level and those defined by DNA typing.

According to current nomenclature rules, alleles are prefixed with the letter of the locus and then by the number of the antigen, for example, A1, B8, DR3, and DQw2. The lower case "w" included in some designations identifies alleles that have been more difficult to recognize as they were defined during periodic workshops. For HLA-C, the "w" has been retained to prevent confusion with complement genes. As variants of alleles have been defined, they have been given new numbers; for example, two subtypes of A9 were designated as A23 and A24, two subtypes of B5 were designated as B51 and Bw52. It is interesting to note that Bw52 retains the "w" prefix although Bw52 and B51 were split from B5 many years ago. This is because there are few sera defining Bw52. It is a rather uncommon antigen in Caucasians, and few service laboratories type for it.

TABLE 14–1. PROTEIN-DEFINED AND DNA-DEFINED ALLELES AT HLA-A, -B, -C, -DR, -DQ, AND -DP

HLA-A		HLA-B		HLA-C		HLA-DR		HLA-DQ		HLA-DP	
Protein Defined[a]	DNA Defined[b]	Protein Defined	DNA Defined	Protein Defined	DNA Defined	Protein Defined	DNA Defined	Protein Defined	DNA Defined	Protein Defined	DNA Defined
A1	A*0101	B5		Cw1	Cw*0101	DR1	DRB1*0101–0103	DQw1		DPw1	DPB1*0101
A2	A*0201–0210	B7	B*0701, 0702	Cw2	Cw*0201, 0202	DR2		DQw2	DQB1*0201	DPw2	DPB1*0201, 0202
A3	A*0301, 0302	B8	B*0801	Cw3	Cw*0301	DR3	DRB1*0301, 0302	DQw3	DQB1*0301–0303	DPw3	DPB1*0301
A9		B12		Cw4		DR4	DRB1*0401–0411	DQw4	DQB1*0401, 0402	DPw4	DPB1*0401, 0402
A10		B13	B*1301, 1302	Cw5	Cw*0501	DR5		DQw5 (1)	DQB1*0501–0504	DPw5	DPB1*0501
A11	A*1101, 1102	B14	B*1401, 1402	Cw6	Cw*0601	DRw6		DQw6 (1)	DQB1*0601–0605	DPw6	DPB1*0601
Aw19		B15	B*1501	Cw7	Cw*0701, 0702	DR7	DRB1*0701, 0702	DQw7 (3)			DPB1*0801
A23 (9)		B16		Cw8		DRw8	DRB1*0801–0804	DQw8 (3)			DPB1*0901
A24 (9)	A*2401	B17		Cw9 (w3)		DR9	DRB1*0901	DQw9 (3)			DPB1*1001
A25 (10)	A*2501	B18	B*1801	Cw10 (w3)		DRw10	DRB1*1001				DPB1*1101
A26 (10)	A*2601	B21		Cw11	Cw*1101	DRw11 (5)	DRB1*1101–1104				DPB1*1301
A28		Bw22			Cw*1201, 1202	DRw12 (5)	DRB1*1201, 1202		DQA1*0101–0103		DPB1*1401
A29 (w19)	A*2901	B27	B*2701–2706		Cw*1301	DRw13 (6)	DRB1*1301–1305		DQA1*0201		DPB1*1501
A30 (w19)	A*3001	B35	B*3501, 3502		Cw*1401	DRw14 (6)	DRB1*1401–1405		DQA1*0301, 0302		DPB1*1601
A31 (w19)	A*3101	B37	B*3701			DRw15 (2)	DRB1*1501, 1502		DQA1*0401		DPB1*1701
A32 (w19)	A*3201	B38 (16)	B*3801			DRw16 (2)	DRB1*1601, 1602		DQA1*0501		DPB1*1801
A33 (w19)	A*3301	B39 (16)	B*3901			DRw17 (3)			DQA1*0601		DPB1*1901
Aw34 (10)		B40	B*4001, 4002			DRw18 (3)					
Aw36		Bw41	B*4101								DPA1*0101–0103
Aw43		Bw42	B*4201			DRw52a	DRB3*0101				DPA1*0201
Aw66 (10)		B44 (12)	B*4401, 4402			DRw52b	DRB3*0201, 0202				
Aw68 (28)	A*6801, 6802	B45 (12)				DRw52c	DRB3*0301				
Aw69 (28)	A*6901	Bw46	B*4601								
Aw74		Bw47	B*4701			DRw53	DRB4*0101				
(w19)											
		Bw48									
		B49 (21)	B*4901				DRB5*0101, 0102				
		Bw50 (21)					DRB5*0201, 0202				
		B51 (5)	B*5101								
		Bw52 (5)	B*5201								
		Bw53	B*5301								
		Bw54 (22)									
		Bw55 (22)									
		Bw56 (22)									
		Bw57 (17)	B*5701								
		Bw58 (17)	B*5801								
		Bw59									
		Bw60 (40)									
		Bw61 (40)									
		Bw62 (15)									
		Bw63 (15)									
		Bw64 (14)									
		Bw65 (14)									
		Bw67									
		Bw71 (70)									
		Bw72 (70)									
		Bw73									
		Bw75 (15)									
		Bw76 (15)									
		Bw77 (15)									
			B*7801								
		Bw4									
		Bw6									

[a] Protein-defined alleles are those that are recognized and defined primarily by reactions of alloantibodies, monoclonal antibodies, or T cells.
[b] DNA-defined alleles are those that are defined on the basis of nucleotide sequence. Note that there is much greater polymorphism at the DNA level; for example, the serologically defined HLA-DR4 allele can be subdivided into at least 8 variants (DRB1*0401–0408) when nucleotide sequences are examined.

TABLE 14–2. EXAMPLES OF H-2 HAPLOTYPES

		Composition of Haplotype					
Inbred Strains	**MHC Haplotype**	**K**	**Ab**	**Aa**	**Eb**	**Ea**	**D**
C57BL/6, C57BL/10	H-2^b	b	b	b	b	b	b
BALB/c, DBA/2	H-2^d	d	d	d	d	d	d
CBA, C3H, AKR	H-2^k	k	k	k	k	k	k
A*	H-2^a	k	k	k	k	k	d

* The H-2^a haplotype is the result of recombination between H-2^k and H-2^d.

For the class II region, serologically defined alleles are designated by the region and antigen number, for example, DR1, DQw1, DPw1, etc. Alleles defined functionally by MLC are designated with a capital "D" (e.g., Dw1, Dw2, etc.). Terminology for alleles defined on the basis of nucleotide sequence includes designation of region (DR, DQ, DP); gene (whether they code for an alpha (a) or beta (β) chain); number, if there is more than one α or β chain; and then an asterisk and a unique four-digit number. The first two numbers reflect the most closely related serologically defined antigen; the last two numbers are unique sequences. For example, the two variants of DR3 defined by sequence analysis of the DRB1 gene have been designated DRB1*0301 and DRB1*0302. Similar nomenclature applies to class I; for example, the DNA-defined alleles of B27 are designated as HLA-B*2701, B*2702, etc.

A full listing of the HLA types of an individual could therefore include serologic definitions as well as functionally or molecularly defined equivalents. An individual might therefore type as HLA-A1, A2, B27, B8, Cw3, Cw5, DR1, DR3, DRw52, DQw1, DQw2 (by antibody); Dw1, Dw3 (by MLC); DPw1, DPw2 (by PLT); and HLA-A*0204, B*2701, DRB1*0103, DRB1*0301, DRB3*0101, DQA1*0101, DQA1*0102, DQB1*0101, DQB1*0201, DPA1*0101, DPB1*0101, and DPB1*0102 (by oligotyping). The listing grows if one includes the polymorphic complement genes, especially when describing the haplotype in studies of the association of HLA and disease.

It can be noted that nomenclature is slightly different for the murine H-2 complex, where the H-2 type of each strain of mouse is considered in terms of a haplotype, not individual antigens (Table 14–2). For example, C57BL/10 mice are homozygous for the H-2^b haplotype and BALB/c mice for the H-2^d haplotype. Alleles of each locus are usually designated by the haplotype; for example, C57BL/10 mice have alleles designated as K^k, D^k, Aa^k, etc.

HLA and Population Genetics

As the first HLA population studies were carried out in Europe and North America, most of the initial information were from Caucasians. It was soon realized that different ethnic groups differ greatly in the HLA alleles represented. African and American blacks, American Indians, and Mongoloids have extreme differences in the frequencies of many class I and class II alleles; some alleles are found only in a particular ethnic group (Table 14–3). For example, HLA-A1 and B8 are both common in Caucasians but rare in Mongoloids. The allele Aw36 (a variant of HLA-A1) is almost exclusively confined to blacks, a Cw11 allele is exclusively confined to Asians, and a B21 variant called BN21 has been found only in North American Indians. Some differences between ethnic groups are believed to be due to founder effects, including distant mutations, and some to gene drift. These are common phenomena in small populations, especially when there is a degree of inbreeding. They may also reflect the evolutionary pressures of different environments.

The nonrandom association of alleles of closely linked genes on the haplotype is called linkage disequilibrium. The haplotypes HLA-A1, B8 and A3, B7 offer convenient examples. The alleles A1 and A3 and B7 and B8 have approximately the same frequencies in northern Europeans; therefore, either A1 or A3 would be expected to be found equally with B7 or B8. In practice, however, A1 is usually linked to B8 and A3 to B7 on the haplotype at frequencies much greater than expected. Linkage disequilibrium can extend from HLA-A to HLA-DR and -DQ, and occasionally to Glo, several centimorgans away. Several explanations have been advanced. One is that linkage disequilibrium is a consequence of the population explosion that began in former centuries; therefore, haplotypes in the founder populations became very frequent. One is that certain combinations of genes on a haplotype interact to confer a selective advantage. Another is that the MHC is riddled with deletions and insertions that make recombination between some haplotypes rare. From a practical point, it is noteworthy that many haplotypes showing pronounced linkage disequilibrium are frequently associated with disease, possibly favoring the selective hypothesis.

HLA and Disease

Because mice of certain H-2 type were found to be more susceptible to leukemogenesis or oncogenesis by specific tumor viruses, it seemed logical to search for a similar association in humans. Associations were indeed found between HLA-A2 and acute lymphocyte leukemia and between HLA-B5-related alleles and Hodgkin's disease, but these associations were not very strong. Studies of HLA and disease might have been discontinued had not extraordinarily strong associations been found in 1972. Two independent studies reported that over 90% of patients with ankylosing spondylitis, an inflammatory disease of the spine, were positive for HLA-B27 (an allele normally found in approximately 6% of the population). These findings immediately spurred a host of studies of other diseases. These searches were productive—many endocrine diseases, rheumatoid syndromes, and autoaggressive diseases were found to be associated with HLA antigens (Table 14–4)—and enigmatic because, in most instances, the reasons for the HLA associations could not be explained.

Two different types of disease studies have commonly been performed, one in populations and the other in multicase families. Population studies reveal associations between the HLA allele and the disease. The proportion of diseased individuals having the particular antigen is compared with the proportion of disease-free individuals in a comparable but disease-free control population with the same antigen. From this, an index called the relative risk (RR) is calculated, that is, by dividing the product of the proportion of patients with

TABLE 14–3. ETHNIC DISTRIBUTION OF HLA ANTIGENS

	European Whites	North American Whites	American Blacks	African Blacks	Japanese	American Indians
HLA-A	(228)[a]	(290)	(128)	(102)	(195)	(89)
A1	15.8	16.1	8.1	3.9	1.2	2.5
A2	27.0	28.0	16.3	9.4	25.3	45.3
A3	12.6	14.1	7.0	6.4	0.7	0.6
A23 } A9	2.4	1.9	10.6	10.8		
A24 } A9	8.8	7.3	5.1	2.4	37.2	23.2
A25 } A10	2.0	2.6	0.4	3.5		0.6
A26 } A10	3.9	3.4	2.3	4.5	12.7	—
A11	5.1	5.1	2.8	—	6.7	
A28	4.4	4.2	5.8	8.9	—	2.8
A29	5.8	3.6	2.3	6.4	0.2	0.6
A30	3.9	2.9	13.0	22.1	0.5	1.1
A31	2.3	4.5	2.8	4.2	8.7	19.9
A32	2.9	3.7	1.9	1.5	0.5	1.1
A33	0.7	1.2	5.1	1.0	2.0	0.6
Aw43	—	—	—	4.0	—	—
Blank	2.2	1.3	16.5	11.0	4.2	1.8
HLA-B	(228)	(290)	(128)	(102)	(195)	(89)
B5	5.9	5.9	4.9	3.0	20.9	14.0
B7	10.4	10.5	12.6	7.3	7.1	0.6
B8	9.2	10.4	5.5	7.1	0.2	1.7
B12	16.6	13.8	14.0	12.7	6.5	1.7
B13	3.2	2.6	0.4	1.5	0.8	—
B14	2.4	5.1	4.6	3.6	0.5	—
B18	6.2	3.1	3.6	2.0	—	0.6
B27	4.6	5.6	0.8	—	0.3	6.2
B15	4.8	5.9	4.7	3.0	9.3	13.7
B38 } Bw16	2.0	2.5	0.4		1.8	
B39 } Bw16	3.5	1.4	0.4	1.5	4.7	14.5
B17	5.7	4.9	11.2	16.1	0.6	—
B21	2.2	3.8	4.4	1.5	1.5	—
Bw22	3.6	2.3	3.9	—	6.5	0.6
B35	9.9	8.6	12.5	7.2	9.4	22.1
B37	1.1	1.7	1.2	—	0.8	—
B40	8.1	9.2	3.9	2.0	21.8	16.6
Bw41	—	—	—	1.5	—	—
Bw42	—	—	—	12.3	—	—
Blank	3.6	2.8	11.0	17.9	7.6	7.8

Adapted from Amos and Kostyu: Adv Human Genet 10:137, 1980.
[a] Number tested.

B27 (P+) and the population of B27− controls (C−) by the product of the proportion of patients without B27 (P−) and the proportion of controls with B27 (C+). For northern Caucasians and ankylosing spondylitis, P+ is approximately 90%, P− is 10%, C+ is 6%, and C− is 94%; therefore, the RR = (90 × 94)/(10 × 6) = 8460/60 = 141.

An absolute risk is calculated by multiplying P+ by the disease frequency F and dividing by C+. Because the frequency of ankylosing spondylitis is about 0.4%, the absolute risk is (90 × 0.4)/6 = 6; thus, only approximately 6% of HLA-B27$^+$ subjects are likely to develop ankylosing spondylitis. The actual incidence is likely to be higher than 6% in men and less in women because the disease phenotype is most common in men. Relative risks are considerably lower for most HLA-associated diseases, values of between 5 and 10 being reported for many of them (Table 14–4). However, for the sleep disorder narcolepsy, the association with DR2 is particularly strong, and 100% of Japanese patients with narcolepsy were found to have this allele.

Information of a different kind can be gained from family studies, especially when large kindreds having more than one affected member are available. The methods most widely used are linkage, or segregation, analysis and sib pair testing. In segregation analysis, a multigeneration family is HLA typed and the haplotypes assigned to each family member. Members are then assessed for the presence or absence of the gene predisposing them to the disease or trait, and a score called the lod (log odds) is calculated. The lod score links the disease-susceptibility gene to HLA and also estimates the frequency of recombination between HLA and the disease gene. Sib pair analysis is simple to perform; concordance for disease between sibs sharing a haplotype is compared to the frequency for sibs not sharing the haplotype. It is necessary to test a null hypothesis, namely, that there is no disease gene.

Population and family studies provide different information. Linkage analysis defines the distance of the disease gene from an HLA locus. Population associations can be suggestive for two genes that are linked, but the location of

TABLE 14–4. SOME SIGNIFICANT HLA AND DISEASE ASSOCIATIONS

Disease	Associated Allele	Frequency in		Relative Risk
		Patients	Controls	
Idiopathic hemochromatosis	A3	76	28	8.2
Behcet's disease	B5	41	10	6.3
Congenital adrenal hyperplasia	Bw47	9	1	15.4
Ankylosing spondylitis	B27	90	9	87.4
Reiter's disease	B27	79	9	37.0
Acute anterior uveitis	B27	52	9	10.4
Psoriasis vulgaris	Cw6	87	33	13.3
Dermatitis herpetiformis	DR3	85	26	15.4
Celiac disease	DR3	79	26	10.8
IgA deficiency	DR3	64	26	5.0
Idiopathic Addison's disease	DR3	69	26	6.3
Graves' disease	DR3	56	26	3.7
Insulin-dependent diabetes mellitus	DR3/4	91	57	7.9
Myasthenia gravis	DR3	50	28	2.5
Systemic lupus erythematosus	DR3	70	28	5.8
Narcolepsy	DR2	100	22	
Multiple sclerosis	DR2	59	26	4.1
Rheumatoid arthritis	DR4	50	19	4.2

Adapted from Svejgaard A et al: Immunol Rev 70, 1983.

the disease gene is not ascertained. HLA disease correlations defined by one method may not be demonstrable by the other. For instance, a disease may follow the HLA haplotype in several multicase families, but the haplotype involved in each family may be different and no single allele will be associated in population studies. This may be because the gene is at some distance from HLA or because more than one gene can cause the same disease phenotype. An example has been reported for some forms of the developmental abnormality spina bifida occulta. Loose linkage was reported in two studies but was not confirmed in others. Linkage rather than association may also be expected in cases in which other unlinked genes modify the disease phenotype. In contrast, the association of some diseases with HLA was first noticed in population surveys and later confirmed in linkage studies. Genes for 21-hydroxylase deficiency, C4 deficiency, and hemochromatosis are examples. Still other diseases show population associations but cannot be traced in families, either because of multigene effects, incomplete penetrance, or absence of enough informative families. The relationship between B27 and ankylosing spondylitis illustrates this. The population association is very strong, but multicase families are rare and linkage has not been established. Nevertheless, that HLA-B27 itself may be the disease-susceptibility gene has been suggested by experiments in transgenic rats, where introduction of B27 and β_2m genes into animals known to be susceptible to experimentally induced inflammatory disease led to the development of a disease reported to have a striking resemblance to the B27-associated human disorders. The human disease, however, may be multifactorial (see below).

Although there are more than a hundred diseases associated with particular HLA alleles, the reasons for such associations are rarely known. For example, hemochromatosis, an iron storage disease, is associated with HLA-A3. The fact that not all individuals with the disease are HLA-A3, and that the disease segregates in families with HLA haplotypes bearing an HLA-A allele other than A3, suggests the presence of a disease gene some distance from HLA-A. Further localization or identification of the involved gene has not yet been possible. The diseases most strongly associated with HLA-B are the inflammatory arthropathies (ankylosing spondylitis, Reiter's disease, anterior uveitis), all associated with HLA-B27 or one of its subtypes. Because many individuals with these diseases have a history of infection with gram-negative organisms, it has been postulated that infection of the intestine or urogenital tract serves as a trigger for an autoimmune or cross-reactive immune response. Whether HLA-B27 is modified by or cross-reacts with a bacterial product is not known.

The majority of HLA and disease associations have involved class II alleles. These include insulin-dependent diabetes mellitus (IDDM), chronic active hepatitis, gluten-sensitive enteropathy, dermatitis herpetiformis, Graves' disease (all associated with DR3 and DQw2), multiple sclerosis (associated with DR2), rheumatoid arthritis (DR4), and narcolepsy (DR2). All but narcolepsy are autoimmune diseases or have a component of autoimmunity, a fact perhaps reflecting the immune functions of class II molecules. For IDDM it has been suggested that susceptibility to disease correlates with the presence of a neutral residue (ala, val, ser) at amino acid position 57 on the DQ β chain, while resistance correlates with the presence of an asp at this position. It is possible that position 57 marks a region that presents an autoantigen, determines the selection of a particular T cell receptor during thymus maturation, or in some other way influences the conformation of the DQ β chain. Because of *cis/trans* pairing of DQ chains and the strong linkage disequilibrium between DR and DQ, however, it is possible that some diseases often associated with DR are really associated with DQ and that both DQα and DQβ genes play a role.

Suggested reasons for HLA disease associations have

included linked metabolic genes (e.g., hemochromatosis); molecular mimicry or cross-reactivity between viruses, bacteria, or environmental agents and HLA molecules (e.g., ankylosing spondylitis); complement deficiencies that may lead to aberrant immune responses; inappropriate expression of HLA class II genes on cells normally class II negative; ineffective blocking of class II in the endoplasmic reticulum (ER) so that self-peptides not normally bound and presented by class II are; or perhaps inappropriate transport of particular peptides into the ER. An early hypothesis that MHC genes themselves may be abnormal has been ruled out in studies of ankylosing spondylitis and IDDM where the amino acid sequence of the B27 or DQw2 molecules is the same in both affected and unaffected individuals. It is tempting to speculate that diseases associated with HLA-A will have different causes and etiologies from those associated with HLA-B, HLA-DR, or HLA-DQ. Undoubtedly, there is room for many additional genes in the HLA region, and some of these may be important in disease susceptibility. It is also possible that HLA genes have functions not yet realized, and it has been suggested that the haplotype rather than a specific allele at one locus is responsible.

MHC and Transplantation

Laws of Transplantion

The laws of transplantation could be readily formulated in mice because inbred strains of different H-2 types were available for testing the requisite genetic crosses. Tissue from one inbred strain was freely transplantable to another member of the same inbred strain, whereas it was usually promptly rejected by a mouse of a different strain. As mentioned briefly in the introduction, the F1 hybrid would accept a graft from either parent but could not donate to either. Either parent could donate tissue to a proportion of the progeny of a mating between two F1 hybrids (the F2), the proportion of successful "takes" being inversely proportional to the number of genes expressed on the tissue. After much investigation, it was proved that, although there were other antigens, the H-2 system was uniquely immunogenic in graft rejection and that a graft was accepted only if there were no H-2 antigens on the donor tissue that were not also present in the recipient. If the donor had H-2 antigens lacking from the recipient, antibodies and cytotoxic lymphocytes against H-2 were generated.

Gene-dose effects, in which the reaction against a donor sharing one antigen or haplotype is often less strong than that against a donor of a completely different type, have been observed for both H-2 and HLA. Skin grafts between HLA-different sibs (ad vs bc) are rapidly rejected (mean 11 days, range 6 to 14 days), whereas grafts between haploidentical sibs show a wide variation in rejection time, (mean 13 days, range 6 to 40 days). This is in contrast to HLA identical grafts that persist for several weeks (mean 24 days, range 14 to 40 days), and the delayed rejection observed is attributable to minor histocompatibility differences. A similar immunogenetic relationship holds true for kidney grafts. HLA-identical kidney grafts are readily accepted and require only moderate amounts of immunosuppressive drugs to prevent rejection. The immune response to haploidentical kidney grafts has been somewhat unpredictable; some have been very well accepted and some, irreversibly rejected. HLA-different sibling grafts are rarely performed because they offer few if any advantages over cadaveric grafts, and there is little ethical justification for using a live donor as it offers no clear advantage to the recipient. This is becoming increasingly true because the clear distinctions between compatible and incompatible grafts observed when azathioprine and steroids were used for immunosuppression have become blurred when cyclosporin A is used.

For various reasons, only a minority of kidney recipients receive an HLA-identical transplant, and most donor-recipient combinations are mismatched at one or more antigens or at one or both haplotypes. Because the majority of organs, including many kidneys and all hearts, lungs, and livers, are from cadaveric donors, there have been numerous attempts at reducing the antigenic disparity by selecting the most HLA-compatible recipient from a pool awaiting transplantation, by avoiding transplantion of a crossmatch positive graft into an already sensitized recipient (as these can reject a graft in hyperacute fashion), and by treating acute and chronic rejection with various immunosuppressive regimens. Many centers aim at a "6 antigen match," namely, HLA-A, -B, and -DR on donor and recipient should be the same. In the previous sections on polymorphism and structure and below, we point out how difficult this may be.

Avoiding Graft Rejection

The reasons why HLA or H-2 molecules are so immunogenic include the direct recognition of donor MHC molecules by the recipient and the high frequency of T cells that can react or cross-react with allo-MHC antigens. Disparity in HLA alleles between donor and recipient may be recognized at the level of class II positive endothelial, passenger leukocytes, or antigen-presenting cells within the graft through antigen-presenting cells of the recipient that have ingested small peptides of donor MHC class I or class II antigens. There may also be recognition of non-HLA peptides or organ- or tissue-specific antigens, either by themselves or in association with HLA. T cells that have been primed to respond to nominal antigen presented by self-MHC can, in a large proportion of cases, also respond to allo-MHC in the absence of nominal antigen (as, for example, in the MHC). Thus, the frequency of T cells in an individual capable of responding to allo-MHC is much greater than the number of T cells responding to more conventional antigens.

Antigenicity of a graft is also dependent on other factors. These include the physiology and architecture of the grafted organ or tissue; the degree of vascularization (skin, lung, and bowel, for example, are much more vascularized, are rich in lymphatics, and are more immunogenic than the less vascular cornea); the amount of MHC class I and class II expressed on cells of the graft (e.g., the high expression of class I on renal vascular endothelium vs the low expression on cardiac myocytes or liver hepatocytes); the number and location of antigen-presenting cells or passenger lymphocytes that may be highly antigenic in a graft; the possibility of damage to the organ or tissue during the procurement and waiting time, which can induce nonspecific inflammatory reactions; and in bone marrow transplantation, the grafting of immunocompetent cells and the probability of graft-versus-host disease.

Numerous measures are taken to prevent graft rejection. The relative importance of HLA matching, for example, depends on the type of graft. Bone marrow transplantation, because it involves the reconstitution of an immune system and carries the risk of graft-versus-host disease, has usually required full HLA matching. Only recently has a limited degree of mismatch been permissible because better immunosuppression is available. Indeed, a degree of mismatch can be beneficial in leukemic recipients, since donor cells preferentially attack the more immunogenic, residual leukemic cells. For kidneys, partially matched grafts are acceptable, although the benefits of a graft well matched for HLA are observed to have better long-term graft survival in most transplant centers.

Nationwide organ procurement and sharing organizations have evolved to produce the most equitable distribution of organs and the most well-matched donor-recipient pairs. National and international bone marrow registries are being used to build a large pool of donors that are necessary to meet the demands of a growing number of potential recipients. For heart, lung, and liver, little HLA matching is done because of insufficient time, because of graft physiology, and because of cyclosporin A, the immunosuppressive drug that can overcome any short-term effects against unmatched grafts involving these organs. Corneal grafts are another example. Primary corneal grafts are usually performed without HLA matching or immunosuppression. This is not because the cornea lacks antigens, but rather because the anterior chamber of the eye is one of a limited number of what are known as immunologically privileged sites. Privileged sites lack lymphatic drainage, and the small amount of antigen released into the bloodstream from grafts in these sites is not sufficient to trigger a cellular response. HLA matching is, however, indicated in corneal transplants when the recipient cornea is moderately vascularized or inflamed or when a previous cornea has been rejected. Class II expression increases rapidly when cells are exposed to IL2 and other cytokines present in inflammation.

There are other ways to avoid rejection or to reduce the severity of the immune response against a graft. In all cases, it is essential to crossmatch donor and recipient using donor lymphocytes as targets and serum from the recipient; recipients with preformed antibodies to HLA may reject a kidney from a donor giving a positive crossmatch within minutes (hyperacute rejection). A second and somewhat controversial measure for reducing rejection episodes has been to transfuse recipients with whole blood several weeks before a transplant. Although this procedure increases the risk of sensitization and formation of cytotoxic antibodies, a large proportion of transfused recipients do not form antibodies and therefore accept a graft more freely. Why improved graft survival is seen after transfusion is not clear, although it is probably due in part to the elimination of the most immunoreactive recipients and in part to the triggering of an as yet unknown state of immunosuppression. Finally, mention must be made of more powerful immunosuppressive drugs and anti–T cell monoclonal antibodies used to control acute and chronic rejection. Traditionally, corticosteroids and azathioprine were the drugs found empirically to be most effective. Cyclosporin A is more effective than older immunosuppressive agents but can be nephrotoxic and hepatotoxic in high doses. A new agent, FK506, originally isolated from a fungus found in Japanese soil, has shown exciting results. Antithymocyte serum has often been given in conjunction with other agents, especially with azathioprine. Unfortunately there is no reliable in vitro test for its potency, and different lots may vary. Monoclonal antibodies to T cell subsets have been used to reduce the severity of immune reactions against the transplant, but most patients quickly develop antibodies to these mouse proteins, so their use is limited. It should be noted that all current immunosuppressive agents act to dampen the entire (T cell) immune system, necessitating a careful balance between sufficient immunosuppression and overimmunosuppression, which can lead to opportunistic infections, drug toxicity, or neoplasia.

Other Histocompatibility Antigens: Platelet, Red Cell, and Granulocyte Antigens

Although a major component of immunogenetics is the study of HLA antigens, another branch involves the study of alloantigens of red blood cells, platelets, and neutrophils. Many antigens unique to red cells are of special importance in transfusion, in hemolytic disease of the newborn, and in autoimmune hemolytic anemias. Platelet and neutrophil antigens may also generate allo- or autoreactivity.

Recognition of red cell antigens preceded recognition of HLA antigens. Attempts at blood transfusion were first undertaken in the middle of the seventeenth century, but they were not successful. Several recipients died, and the practice was outlawed in both France and England. It was revived early in the nineteenth century by Blundell, a Scottish obstetrician, for saving patients with postpartum bleeding. Transfusion was sometimes successful, but often the patient died as a complication of the transfusion. The reason for these adverse reactions remained mysterious until 1904, when Landsteiner discovered that the serum of some normal human donors agglutinated the red cells of other donors. From an analysis of the pattern of reactions, he defined the major blood groups A, B, and O. Blood could usually be transfused safely when the groups of the donor and recipient were the same, but serious reactions occurred when the serum of the recipient agglutinated the donated cells. Since that time, more than 300 red cell alloantigens and many other blood groups have been described.

Examples of some of the clinically important antigens present on red blood cells, platelets, and granulocytes are given in Table 14–5. The ABO(H) antigens account for many

TABLE 14–5. EXAMPLES OF CLINICALLY RELEVANT ANTIGENS PRESENT ON RED BLOOD CELLS, PLATELETS, AND NEUTROPHILS

Red Blood Cell Antigens	Platelet Antigens	Granulocyte Antigens
ABO	ABO	ABO
Lewis	Lewis	Ii
Secretor systems	Ii	HLA
P	HLA	NA-NF (granulocyte specific)
MNSs	HPA (platelet specific)	
Rh		
Kell		
Duffy		
Kidd (JK)		
Ii		

of the serious hemolytic reactions that have occurred during blood transfusion. The Lewis antigens, P, MNSs, and others are also responsible for eliciting transfusion reactions. Rh incompatibility between mother and child can lead to hemolytic disease of the newborn (erythroblastosis fetalis). This occurs when an Rh negative mother is sensitized to Rh positive cells of the fetus and maternal antibodies cross the placenta to destroy fetal red blood cells. Fortunately, treatment of the mother with Rho-GAM, an anti-Rh immune serum, will block further sensitization.

Platelets carry some of the same antigens as leukocytes, either as integral membrane components or, in the case of HLA, as adsorbed from serum. They also carry antigens of several platelet-specific systems. Best known is human platelet antigen (HPA-1; previously designated as Pl^{A1} or Zw^{a}). Immunization of an HPA-1a negative mother by a positive child can lead to destruction of the child's platelets (neonatal purpura). Granulocytes also carry tissue-specific antigens called neutrophil antigens (NA), which are sometimes implicated in neonatal neutropenia.

In certain instances, immunologic tolerance is broken and an individual begins to make antibodies to antigens present on his or her own (autologous) blood cells. Classically, this process has involved red cells in the form of autoimmune hematolytic anemia, but the occurrence of thrombocytopenia (lack of platelets), leukopenia (lack of white cells), and neutropenia (lack of neutrophils) may be due to the same process. In most cases, the reason for the loss of tolerance is not known.

Transfusion reactions against HLA antigens can follow the administration of whole blood to a sensitized individual, most frequently a parous female, a subject who has been transfused, or an individual who has rejected a transplant. Often accompanied by severe chills, these reactions are rarely, if ever, fatal and can be readily avoided by substituting red cells or buffy-coat-free blood for the whole blood formerly used. Reactions against HLA antigens on platelets are a serious concern in aplastic anemia and thrombocytopenia, but they can be avoided by selecting donors lacking the antigen. Crossmatching is a necessity for any blood transfusion.

FURTHER READING

Evolution of the MHC

Goetz D (ed): The Major Histocompatibility System in Man and Animals. New York, Springer-Verlag, 1977

Guillemot F, Kaufman JF, Skjoedt K, Auffray C: The major histocompatibility complex in the chicken. Trends Genet 5:300, 1989

Hughes AL, Nei M: Pattern of nucleotide substitution at major histocompatibility complex class I loci reveals overdominant selection. Nature 335:167, 1988

Klein J, Figueroa F: Evolution of the major histocompatibility complex. CRC Crit Rev Immunol 6:295, 1986

H-2 Genes and Products

Artzt K, Shin H-S, Bennett D: Gene mapping within the T/t complex of the mouse. II. Cell 28:471, 1982

Flaherty L, Elliott E, Tine JA et al: Immunogenetics of the Q and TL regions of the mouse. CRC Crit Rev Immunol 10:131, 1990

Klein J: Biology of the Mouse Histocompatibility-2 Complex. New York, Springer-Verlag, 1975

Klein J, Benoist C, David CS et al: Revised nomenclature of mouse H-2 genes. Immunogenetics 32:147, 1990

Vincek V, Figueroa F, Gill TJ III et al: Mapping in the mouse of the region homologous to the rat growth and reproduction complex (grc). Immunogenetics 32:293, 1990

HLA Genes and Products

Awdeh ZL, Raum D, Yunis EJ, Alper A: Extended HLA complement allele haplotypes evidence for T/t like complex in man. Proc Nat Acad Sci USA 80:259, 1983

Bjorkman PJ, Parham P: Structure, function and diversity of class I major histocompatibility complex molecules. Annu Rev Biochem 59:253, 1990

Bjorkman PJ, Saper MA, Samraoui B et al: Structure of the human class I histocompatibility antigen, HLA-A2. Nature 329:506, 1987

Bjorkman PJ, Saper MA, Samraoui B et al: The foreign antigen binding site and T cell recognition regions of class I histocompatibility antigens. Nature 329:512, 1987

Dunham I, Sargent CA, Kendall E, Campbell RD: Characterization of the class III region in different MHC haplotypes by pulsed-field gel electrophoresis. Immunogenetics 32:175, 1990

Dupont B (ed): Immunobiology of HLA, vol 1 and 2. New York, Springer-Verlag, 1989

Hume CR, Shookster LA, Collins N et al: Bare lymphocyte syndrome: Altered HLA class II expression in B cell lines derived from two patients. Hum Immunol 25:1, 1989

Milner CM, Campbell RD: Structure and expression of the three MHC-linked HSP70 genes. Immunogenetics 32:242, 1990

Singer DS, Maguire JE: Regulation of the expression of class I MHC genes. CRC Crit Rev Immunol 10:235, 1990

Spies T, Blanck G, Bresnaham M et al: A new cluster of genes within the human major histocompatibility complex. Science 243:214, 1989

Strominger JL, Auffray C: Molecular genetics of the human major histocompatibility complex. Adv Hum Genet 15:197, 1986

Sullivan KE, Calman AF, Nakanishi M et al: A model for the transcriptional regulation of MHC class II genes. Immunol Today 8:289, 1987

Trowsdale J: Genetics and polymorphism: Class II antigens. Br Med Bull 43:15, 1987

Wei X, Orr HT: Differential expression of HLA-E, HLA-F, and HLA-G transcripts in human tissue. Hum Immunol 29:131, 1990

MHC and T Lymphocyte Function

Carreno BM, Anderson RW, Coligan JE, Biddison WE: HLA-B37 and HLA-A2.1 molecules bind largely nonoverlapping sets of peptides. Proc Nat Acad Sci USA 87:3420, 1990

Cresswell P, Blume JS: Intracellular transport of class II HLA antigens. In Pernis B, Silverstein SC, Vogel HJ (eds): Processing and Presentation of Antigens. New York, Academic Press, 1988, p 43

Grey HM, Sette A, Buus S: How T cells see antigen. Sci Am, Nov 1989, p 56

Salter RD, Benjamin RJ, Wesley PK et al: A binding site for the T-cell co-receptor CD8 on the α3 domain of HLA-A2. Nature 345:41, 1990

Spies T, Bresnahan M, Bahram et al: A gene in the human major histocompatibility complex class II region controlling the class I antigen presentation pathway. Nature 348:744–747, 1990

Teyton L, O'Sullivan D, Dickson PW et al: Invariant chain distinguishes between the exogenous and endogenous antigen presentation pathways. Nature 348:39, 1990

Trowsdale J, Hanson I, Mockridge I et al: Sequences encoded in the class II region of the MHC related to the "ABC" superfamily of transporters. Nature 348:741, 1990

Zinkernagel RM, Doherty PC: MHC restricted cytotoxic T cells: Studies on the biological role of polymorphic major transplantation antigens determining T-cell restriction specificity. Adv Immunol 27:51, 1979

HLA and Disease

French MAH, Dawkins RL: Central MHC genes, IgA deficiency and autoimmune disease. Immunol Today 11:271, 1990

Hammer RE, Maika SD, Richardson JA et al: Spontaneous inflammatory disease in transgenic rats expressing HLA-B27 and human β_2m: An animal model of HLA-B27-associated human disorders. Cell 63:1099, 1990

Khalil I, d'Auriol L, Gobet M et al: A combination of HLA-DQβ Asp-57-negative and HLA-DQα Arg-52 confers susceptibility to insulin-dependent diabetes mellitus. J Clin Invest 85:1315, 1990

Kostyu DD, Amos DB: The HLA complex: Genetic polymorphism and disease susceptibility. In Scriver CR, Beaudet AL, Sly WS et al (eds): Metabolic Basis of Inherited Disease. New York, McGraw-Hill, 1989

Sinha AA, Lopez T, McDevitt HO: Autoimmune diseases: The failure of self tolerance. Science 248:1380, 1990

Zielasek J, Jackson RA, Eisenbarth GS: The potentially simple mathematics of type I diabetes. Clin Immunol Immunopathol 52:347, 1989

Transplantation

Amos DB: Tissue transplantation immunity. In Smith DT, Conant NF, Willett HP (eds): Zinsser Microbiology, ed 14. New York, Appleton-Century-Crofts, 1968

Cramer DV: Cardiac transplantation: Immune mechanisms and alloantigens involved in graft rejection. CRC Crit Rev Immunol 7:1, 1987

Rolstad B: The popliteal lymph node graft-versus-host (GvH) reaction in the rat: A useful model for studying cell interactions in the immune response. Immunol Rev 88:153, 1985

Termijtelen A: T cell allorecognition of HLA class II. Hum Immunol 28:1, 1990

Platelet, Red Cell, and Granulocyte Antigens

Burns TR, Saleem A: Idiopathic thrombocytopenic purpura. Am J Med 75:1001, 1983

Court WS, Bozeman JM, Soong S-J et al: Platelet surface-bound IgG in patients with immune and nonimmune thrombocytopenia. Blood 69:278, 1987

Issitt PD: Applied Blood Group Serology, ed 3. Miami, Montgomery, 1985

Race RR, Sanger R: Blood Groups in Man, ed 6. Oxford, Blackwell, 1975

Salmon C, Cartron J-P, Rouget P: The Human Blood Groups. New York, Masson, 1984

Watkins WM: Blood group substances in the ABO system: The genes control the arrangement of sugar residues that determine blood group specificity. Science 152:172, 1966

CHAPTER 15

The Complement System

During the latter part of the nineteenth century, it became apparent that microbial invasion produced a number of human diseases and that specific immunization could provide an effective means of preventing many of them. Studies of immunologic mechanisms of host defense against bacteria demonstrated that microorganisms injected into the peritoneal cavity of immune animals underwent rapid dissolution. Bacteria were similarly lysed in vitro when added to the cell-free serum of immunized animals. Serum that had been aged for a few weeks or had been heated at 56C no longer supported a bactericidal reaction despite the fact that it still contained antibacterial antibody. The bactericidal reaction, therefore, required antibody and a heat-labile serum factor initially termed *alexin* (Greek, to ward off) and now called *complement.*

Complement consists of a series of interacting proteins that function as an immune effector of the acute inflammatory response. Activation of the complement system on the surface of cells results in the production of structural and functional membrane alterations that lead to cell death. During sequential activation of complement (C), a number of biologic events are initiated that facilitate the localization and destruction of foreign material by immune effector cells.

Biochemistry of Complement System

The realization that complement involved a number of components came about when it was found that different activities of complement could be inactivated by various physical or chemical means. Later, when the biochemical means became available, these components were more clearly defined, and it is now known that at least 16 proteins are engaged in the activation and regulation of complement (Table 15–1).

In general, these proteins circulate in the plasma in inactive form and are sequentially activated as a series of complexes with the following characteristics.

1. The complexes are localized by a stable interaction with the membrane of the cell under attack.
2. The complexes usually contain proenzymes that are converted to enzymes that act on subsequent components of the system. This allows amplification of the activation process.
3. The activity of the complex is modulated by inhibitory reactions. This modulation may be mediated by proteins of the plasma or of the cell surface.

The sum of the activation of complement is the localized generation of biologic mediators of immune reactions. The activation of the complement system may be initiated by either of two pathways.

1. The antibody-dependent or classic pathway. The reaction of antibody with antigens on the cell surface provides the localization of the reactions to specific cells.
2. The antibody-independent or alternative pathway. Antibody is not used for specific localization. Rather, the localization is provided by the reactions of specific components of complement.

The components and reactions of these pathways are analogous, and both result, through the production of ampli-

TABLE 15–1. THE COMPONENTS OF COMPLEMENT

	Function	Mol Wt (kDa)	Serum Concentration (g/mL)	Chain Structure
Classic Pathway				
C1q	Collagenlike	410	70	6 chains of 3 each
C1r	Serine protease	190	34	2 × 1 chain
C1s	Serine protease	85	31	2 × 1 chain
C4	Localizing	206	600	α, β, γ; anaphylotoxin, thioester
C2	Serine protease	117	25	1, 2 SCRs[a]
C3	Localizing	195	1,200	α, β; anaphylotoxin, thioester
Alternative Pathway				
C3b	Localizing	185		Generated from C3
B	Serine protease	95	225	1, 2 SCRs
D	Serine protease	25	1	1
Membrane Attack Complex				
C5	Localizing	180	85	α, β; anaphylotoxin
C6	Amphipathic	128	60	1
C7	Amphipathic	120	55	1 (like C6)
C8	Amphipathic	150	55	α, β, γ
C9	Amphipathic	79	60	1
Modulating Proteins				
Properdin	Stabilizes C3bBb	190	25	4 identical
C1 Inhibitor	Serpin	105	180	1
C4 Binding protein	Binding	560		8 identical, many SCRs
H	Binding	150	500	1, many SCRs
I	Serine protease	90	34	γ, β
S	Binding	80	600	1

[a] SCR (short consensus repeats) = tandem repeats or complement control repeats (CCR).

fication complexes, in the initiation of the final common pathway, the membrane attack complex.

Biochemical Characteristic of Complement Components

The proteins of the complement system can be divided into several families (Table 15–1, Fig. 15–1).

1. Serine proteases: C1r, C1s, C2, factor B, factor D, factor I.
   Each of these proteins includes a portion of about 25,000 Da that is constructed like the classic serine proteases, which, when activated, cleave peptide bonds having the general structure X-lys-X-arg. In addition, all except factor D have a portion that binds to other proteins and a portion that inhibits the enzymatic activity of the protease portion. Activation occurs when this inhibitor portion is cleaved away.
2. Localizing proteins: C3, C4, C5
   These three proteins have a number of similarities. Each consists of an α chain and either a β chain (C3 and C5) or a β and a γ chain (C4). In each, the amino terminal 77 amino acids of the α chain has a complex, cysteine-rich structure that, when cleaved from the native protein, can act as an anaphylotoxin. The remainder of all three proteins has considerable homology. In C3 and C4 there is a thioester bridge in the α chain that, when opened, forms a reactive group that can form covalent bonds with moieties on the membrane of the cell under attack. All three proteins are able to take part in protein-protein interactions with other components of the system.
3. Amphipathic proteins: C6, C7, C8, C9
   These proteins of the membrane attack complex (MAC) expose hydrophobic sequences when activated. These sequences interact with the lipid bilayer, allowing insertion of the proteins into the membrane.
4. C3–C4 binding proteins: factor H, C4 binding protein, decay accelerating factor, complement receptors.
   These proteins bind to C3, C4, or both and regulate interactions between them and other proteins of the complement system or other cells. All contain multiple copies (4 to 30) of a 60-amino-acid repeating sequence, and the genes for all are located in a limited area on chromosome 1. In some cases the binding with C3 or C4 results in immune adherence. In other cases the binding is part of the downregulation of the function of the protein.
5. C8 binding proteins: C8 binding protein (homologous

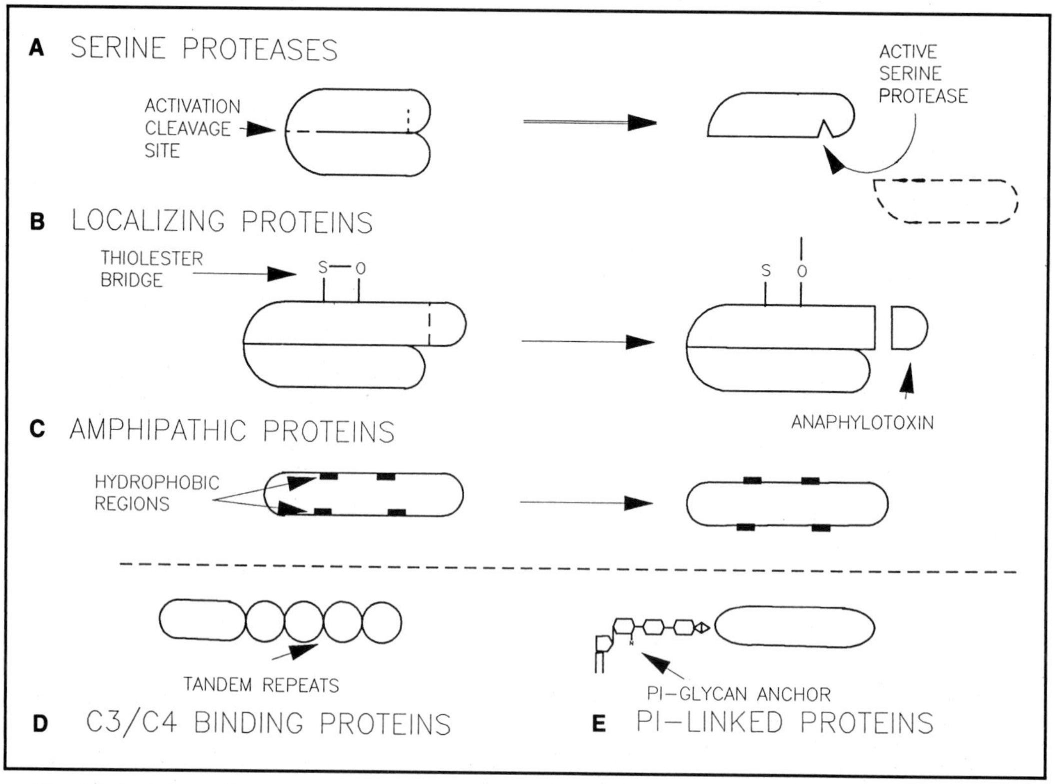

Fig. 15–1. Schematic representation of the classes of proteins of the complement components. **A.** Serine proteases are proenzymes that are activated by the cleavage of a portion of the molecule so that the active site is active. **B.** Localizing proteins (C3, C4, C5) are multichain molecules that are activated by proteolytic cleavage. In C3 and C4, this activates a covalent binding site by breaking a thiolester bridge. **C.** Amphipathic proteins (C6, C7, C9) expose hydrophobic areas when activated that permit them to interact with the lipid bilayer of cellular membranes. **D.** Complement-regulating proteins possess repeated elements that permit them to react with C3 and C4. **E.** Phosphatidylinositolglycan-linked proteins (decay accelerating factor, membrane inhibitor of reactive lysis [protectin, CD59]) are fixed in the membrane by a specific lipid–glycan anchor.

restriction factor), protectin (membrane inhibitor of reactive lysis [MIRL], CD59)
These regulatory proteins interact with C8 and prevent the formation of the polymeric C9 complex that is responsible for dissolution of the membrane and lysis of the cell by the MAC.

Activation of Complement

Classic Pathway

The initiation complex in the classic pathway of complement activation consists of antibody and the first component of complement. The fixation of antibody to antigen provides specific localization of the subsequent reactions. The activation step begins with the fixation of C1, which is in itself a complex of three molecules, C1q, C1r, and C1s (Fig. 15–2). C1q is a very complex molecule consisting of 18 peptide chains, each of which contains a portion closely resembling collagen and a portion resembling more conventional globular protein. These interact in groups of three to form six chains with collagenlike structure at one end and globular structure at the other. These six complex chains adhere to one another by the collagenlike portions. The six globular portions project from this structure and are capable of binding to the Fc portion of antibodies of particular isotypes (IgG3, IgG1, and IgM). To be fixed effectively, C1q must be affixed simultaneously to immunoglobulins by at least two of its binding areas. Thus, two subunits of one IgM molecule or two IgG molecules are capable of binding C1q, provided they are affixed to antigens that are sufficiently close together to allow the C1q molecule to span the doublet.

C1r and C1s are serine proteases and are arranged in a linear form as follows.

C1s····C1r····C1r····C1s

The binding of C1q activates (probably autoactivates) one of the C1r molecules, converting it from a proenzyme to an enzyme. This enzyme in turn cleaves the other C1r to activate it, and each C1r cleaves the adjacent C1s to activate a serine protease (Fig. 15–3A).

The activity of the initiation complex of the classic pathway is downregulated by several means.

1. The necessity for a specific geometric arrangement of antibody molecules limits the conditions for activation.

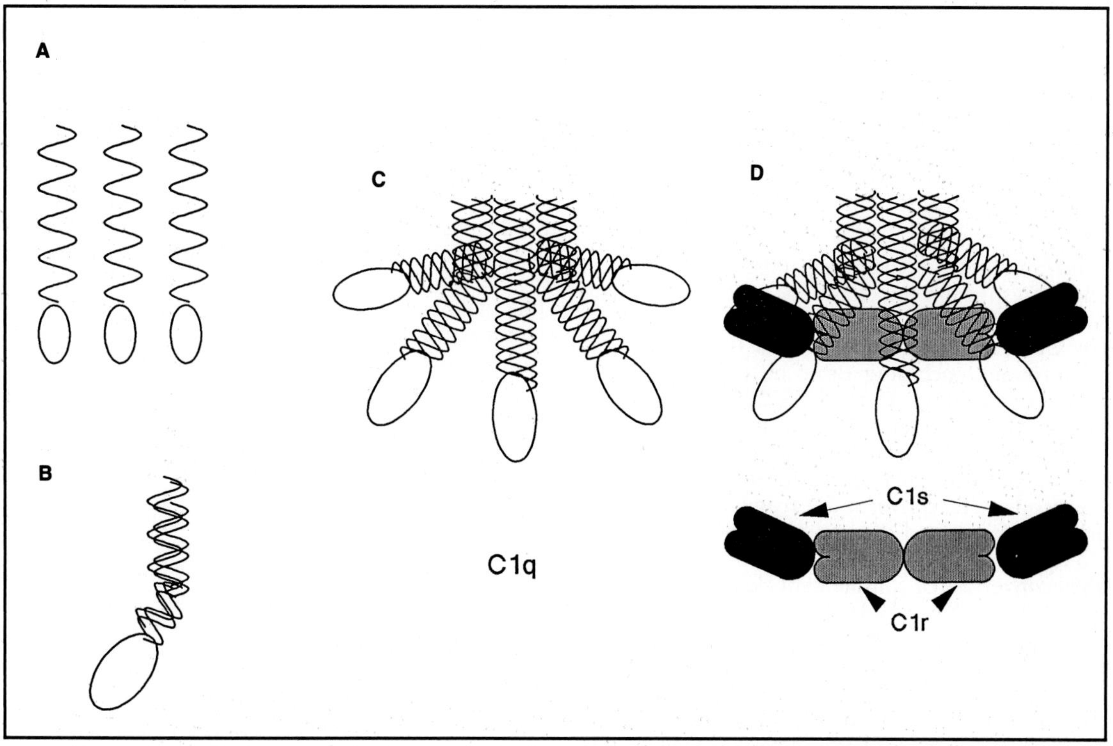

Fig. 15–2. Structure of C1. **A.** The basic molecules of C1q contains a collagenlike portion and a globular portion. There are three types of these molecules. **B.** Three of these molecules (one of each kind) form a collagenlike helical structure with a globular end. **C.** Six of these complexes combine by their collagenlike structures into a hexameric structure consisting of a core of collagenlike structures and an array of peripheral globular structures. The complete structure is called C1q. **D.** The tetrameric structure of two serine proteases, C1r and C1s, in the fomr C1s–C1r–C1r–C1s is noncovalently combined with the C1q complex.

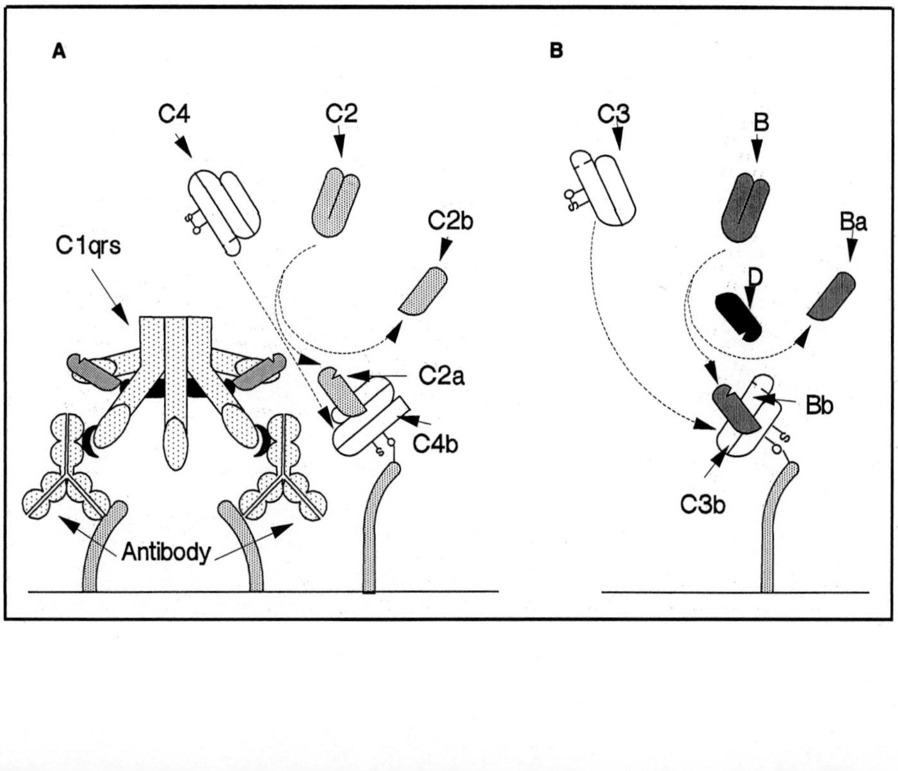

Fig. 15–3. Formation of the convertase complexes of complement. **A.** The amplification or convertase complex of the classic pathway is formed by C4b, the product of cleavage of the native protein by C1, which binds covalently to the membrane and which binds C2 using Mg^{2+} as the ligand. C2 is also cleaved by C1s to the active form, C2a, a serine protease. **B.** The convertase complex of the alternative pathway is formed on membrane-bound C3b derived from either the cleavage of C3 or the spontaneous activation of the native molecule. Factor B is bound by Mg^{2+} and cleaved to an active serine protease, Bb, by factor D.

2. Interactions between antibody and antigen and between antibody and C1q are unstable and, hence, reversible.
3. The enzymatic activity of C1r and C1s is inhibited by a plasma serpin (a suicide inhibitor of serine proteases) called C1 (esterase) inhibitor. The deficiency of this molecule results in the excessive activation of complement and the syndrome of hereditary angioedema (see below).

The second (amplification) complex of the classic pathway, C4b2a, is generated through the enzymatic action of C1s (Fig. 15–3A). C4a, the anaphylotoxin portion of native C4, is cleaved off by C1s, and the larger fragment (C4b) can covalently bind to proteins, including those on cell surfaces, by the opened thioester bridge. As many as 20 C4b molecules are scattered randomly about the activating antibody–C1 complex, providing a significant degree of amplification. Native C2, in the presence of magnesium ions, binds to C4 and is also cleaved by C1s, converting it from a proenzyme to an active serine protease, and the combination C4b2a forms an enzyme complex called a *convertase.*

The C4b2a convertase of complement cleaves two natural substrates, C3 and C5 (Fig. 15–4). In its first reaction, the C4b of the classic pathway convertase binds native C3 from plasma, and the C2a cleaves it into two fragments. C3a, the anaphylotoxin portion of the C3 molecule, is released into the fluid phase, and C3b is bound by the opened thioester linkage to polysaccharide structures on the cell surface. C3b molecules that bind near the enzyme complex serve as the attachment site of C5, the second substrate for classic pathway convertase. C5 is enzymatically cleaved by C2a into C5a and C5b. C5a is a potent chemotactic factor and anaphylatoxin. C5b is the first component taking part in the terminal attack complex.

Alternative (Properdin) Pathway

Early in the 1950s, Pillemer described a factor in serum that combined with zymosan, a yeast cell wall polysaccharide, and selectively consumed C3 in the absence of C1, C4, and C2. Pillemer termed the required new factor *properdin* (Latin, *perdere:* to destroy). Other workers subsequently demonstrated a similar activation of the late components in the absence of the early components when serum was incubated with a factor derived from cobra venom or with bacterial lipopolysaccharides (endotoxins).

In recent years the six protein components of this properdin system (now called *the alternative pathway of activation*) have been isolated and purified and found to be distinct from the early acting proteins of the classic-complement sequence. The biologic significance of the alternative pathway is that it allows activation of complement by microbial products before the development or in the absence of specific antibodies.

The biochemistry of the alternative pathway is entirely analogous to that of the classic pathway. The pathway is initiated with the formation of the convertase or amplification complex consisting of C3b and factor Bb (C3bBb) (Fig. 15–3B). In this, the role of C3b is analogous to that of C4b of the classic pathway in localizing the complex on the membrane and providing a binding site for an enzyme, factor B. C3 and C4 are closely related biochemically and genetically. The C3b on which the complex is built may be derived from activation of the classic pathway with cleavage of the C3a (anaphylotoxin portion) of the molecule. On the other hand, C3 may be affixed to the membrane as the result of spontaneous rupture of the thioester bond at residue 277. This affixes C3 to the membrane as though C3a had been cleaved away. This spontaneous fixation of C3 is more likely to occur on some bacterial cell walls than on host cells.

Once C3(b) is fixed to the membrane, factor B (a serine protease analogous to C2) is fixed to it by Mg^{2+} ions. Factor B is activated by the removal of a portion of the molecule, Ba, by another serine proteinase, factor D, which circulates in the plasma in the active form. The activated form of factor B, Bb, remains combined with C3b. The combination of C3b and factor Bb (C3bBb) constitutes the convertase complex of the alternative pathway. This complex acts exactly as does the

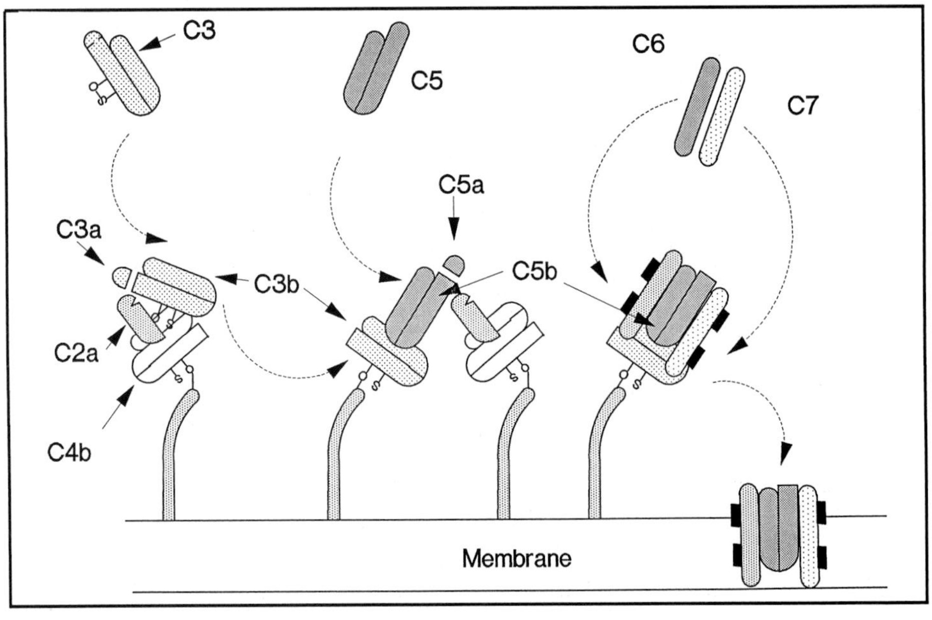

Fig. 15–4. Activation of C3 and C5 by the convertase convertase complex. The complex of the classic pathway is illustrated, but the reactions are the same with the alternative pathway complex, C3bBb, the binding protein of the complex [C4b or C3b binds C3, which is then cleaved by the enzyme of the complex (C2a or Bb)]. C3b is then attached to nearby membrane components. C3b thus bound binds native C5, which is cleaved by the convertase complex. C6 and C7 are bound to the activated C5b. The C5b-7 complex is then partially inserted into the membrane to initiate the membrane attack complex.

convertase complex of the classic pathway. C3b binds native C3, which is then cleaved (and activated) by factor Bb.

The activation of C5 by this enzyme system is also entirely analogous to that described previously (Fig. 15–4). Native C5 is held in place by a neighboring C3b molecule and cleaved by factor Bb. Thus, by the use of related molecules, the alternative pathway is activated without the limiting requirement for antibody.

Stabilization and Inactivation of Amplification Complexes

The amplification complexes of the alternative (C3bBb) and classic (C4b2a) pathways are very highly regulated. They are intrinsically unstable, since the two molecules of which they are comprised are held together only by Mg^{2+}. At 37C, the complexes remain intact, with a half-life measured in only a few minutes, and if the two molecules separate, the enzyme activity of the complex is lost. C4b2a may be stabilized artificially by altering the proteins or the ligand, but there is no known natural mechanism for doing this. On the other hand, C3bBb is stabilized by properdin, which appears to bind to both proteins. This complex also is stabilized by an antibody to neoantigens formed by the complex, the so-called C3 nephritic factor (C3NeF) found in some patients with hypocomplementemic glomerulonephritis.

The amplification complexes of complement are destabilized by a number of different proteins, all of which contain several tandem repeats described above. The blood cells and endothelial cells all possess a glycoprotein, decay accelerating factor, which is able to displace the enzymatic molecule (C2a or Bb) from the anchoring molecule (C4b or C3b). This reduces the length of time the enzyme is effective. Decay accelerating factor is missing on the blood cells of patients with paroxysmal nocturnal hemoglobinuria.

The complexes are also destabilized by two serum proteins, factor H and C4 binding protein (C4BP). These proteins likewise displace the enzymatic protein from the complex. Factor H does so by combining with C3b of the alternative pathway complex, C4 BP by combining with C4b. In addition to destabilizing the complex, these proteins serve as the binding site for yet another serine protease, factor I, which cleaves the α chain of both C3b and C4b. After the cleavage, the products (iC3b and iC4b) are no longer able to bind to the enzymatic proteins of the complex. A further cleavage in each case removes the major portion of the protein (C3c or C4c), leaving only a small remnant bound to the membrane [C3d(g) or C4d]. These steps tightly modulate the effectiveness of the amplification complexes.

Membrane Attack Complex

The C4b2a3b complex of the classic pathway and the C3bBbC3b complex of the alternative pathway are able to activate native C5 by enzymatic cleavage. The C5b that results rapidly combines with the next two components, C6 and its homologue, C7 (Fig. 15–4). This C5b67 complex is capable of binding to the membrane. C5b–7 complexes generated on one surface may land on an adjacent surface. This is called *reactive lysis.* The membrane-bound C5b–7 complex forms the nidus for the formation of the terminal complex or the MAC, which evolves when the final components, C8 and C9, are assembled (Fig. 15–5).

These protein are potentially amphipathic, bearing both hydrophobic and hydrophilic regions. During their activation, the hydrophobic regions are exposed to the lipids of the membrane, localizing the complex within the lipid bilayer. The complex contains one molecule each of C5b, C6, C7, and C8 combined with several (3 to 6) molecules of C9. The assembled complexes can be seen in electron microscopy as tubular structures of approximately 9 to 11 nm (Fig. 15–6). It is clear that the mere presence of such a complex is not a sufficient condition for penetration of the lipid bilayer and that some, perhaps two or more, MACs must be assembled together for penetration to occur. This process is relatively inefficient, particularly when the source of the complement

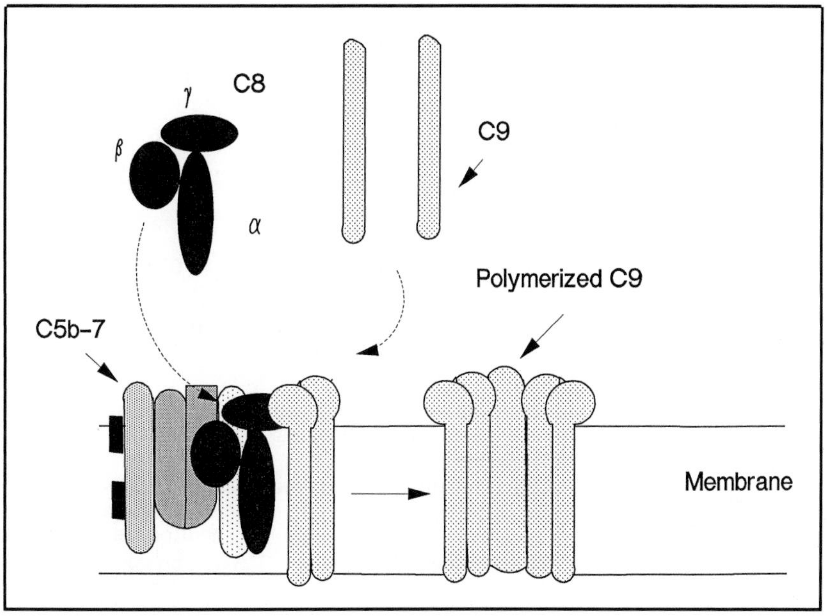

Fig. 15–5. The membrane attack complex of complement is assembled by the complex C5b–7. C8 is affixed from the serum, and it directs the polymerization of C9 into a lipid-penetrating array. If this complex goes through the membrane, the cell is lysed.

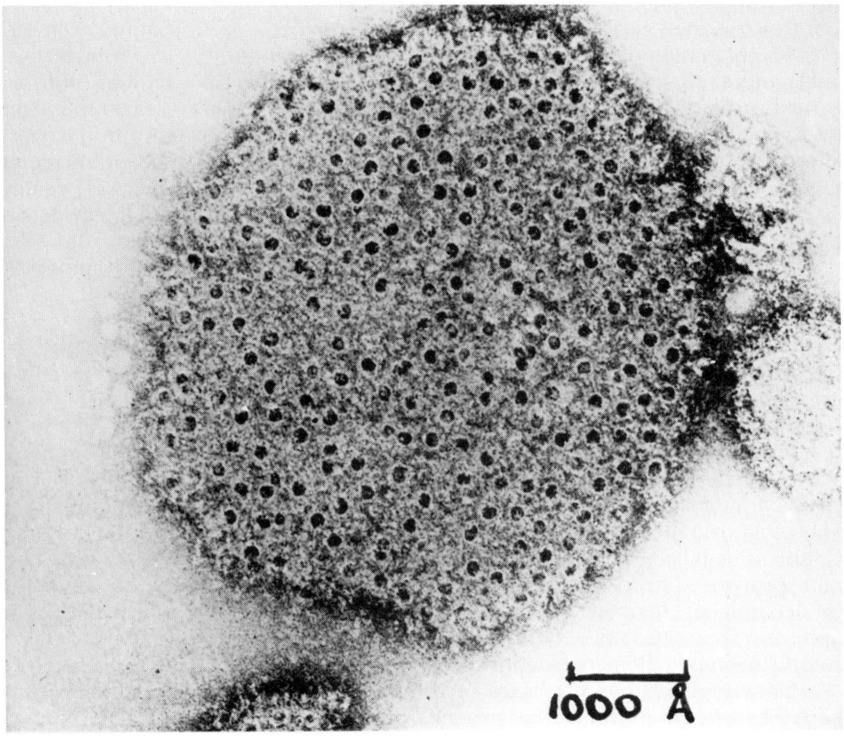

Fig. 15–6. Electron microscopic evidence of the action of complement. The small, dark ovoid structures are seen only after the addition of C9 to the membrane attack complex.

is from the same species as the cells under attack, since the membrane often has surface proteins that disrupt the formation of the final lytic complex. Two of these, protectin (CD59 [membrane inhibitor of reactive lysis]) and the C8 binding protein, have been identified on human cells. Further, in some bacteria that have capsules, this mechanism of membrane attack is totally ineffective, since the attack complex is assembled at some distance from the cell wall. Nevertheless, when membrane attack is effective, as typified by the reaction against red cells and lysable bacteria, a water-soluble passage is made in the lipid bilayer, and the cell is destroyed.

Biologic Activities Mediated by Complement System

Immune Adherence

Immune complexes that contain C3b or C4b (or their metabolites iC3b and iC4b) adhere to cells that possess specific receptors, which originally were called immune adherence (IA) receptors but now are called complement receptors (CR). Four different receptors are present on a variety of cells: phagocytes (macrophages, monocytes, neutrophils), lymphocytes (subsets of both B and T cells), other blood cells (erythrocytes, nonprimate platelets, endothelium), and perhaps other tissue cells (glomerular cells, and so on) (Table 15–2). These proteins bind to C3b and C4b and their inactivated derivatives (iC3b and iC4b, in particular). Two of these receptors belong to the family of complement regulatory proteins that includes factor H, DAF, and others. They contain the characteristic tandem repeats seen in this family of proteins. The other two (CR1 and CR4) belong to a large group of adherence mediating proteins called the *integrins* (Chap. 16). These proteins are characteristically heterodimers that have specific binding sites for groups on a number of proteins.

The binding of a target cell on which C3 or C4 is bound to a cell bearing a receptor for those components constitutes immune adherence that may lead to phagocytosis. The stimulus to phagocytosis of immune adherence mediated by complement components alone is less strong than that which follows the reaction of the Fc receptor with IgG molecules.

TABLE 15–2. BIOCHEMISTRY AND DISTRIBUTION OF THE COMPLEMENT RECEPTORS

	Preferred Substrate	Biochemistry	Distribution
CR1	C3b	Family of complement regulatory proteins, numerous tandem repeats	Neutrophils, monocytes, RBCs, lymphocytes
CR2	C3d	Family of complement regulatory proteins, few repeats	Lymphocytes (B cells)
CR3	iC3b	Integrins (heterodimer)	Monocytes, macrophages, neutrophils
CR4	iC3b	Integrin	Macrophages

However, the combination of immune adherence mediated by antibody acting in concert with that mediated by complement components is far more effective than either alone.

Immune adherence mediated by complement may also provide a mechanism for rapid clearance of immune complexes from the circulation by fixed phagocytic cells (macrophages) in the liver and spleen, and it may permit localization of nonphagocytized complexes at B lymphocyte–rich areas of the spleen and lymph nodes, facilitating additional antibody production.

Virus Neutralization

The binding of antibodies to certain viruses results in the formation of infectious virus-antibody complexes (VA). The addition of C1 and C4 to VA produces virus neutralization. Sequential addition of the later acting complement components produces additional virus neutralization. One mechanism of virus neutralization by complement may be to prevent the attachment of the virus to cells by steric hindrance produced by virus-bound complement.

Another mechanism by which complement may neutralize particular types of viruses does not require antibody. RNA tumor viruses (Chap. 62) are lysed by human serum but not by serum from many nonprimates. Although complement-mediated lysis of oncornaviruses does not require antibody to the virus, it does require an intact classic complement pathway. The complement sequence is activated by the direct interaction of C1q with the P15E component of the viral envelope. This leads to formation of C1 and subsequently to lysis of the viral envelope by the membrane attack complex. The ability of human serum to lyse oncornaviruses may provide a natural defense against RNA tumor viruses.

Anaphylatoxin Activity

Guinea pigs develop severe anaphylaxis when injected intravenously with serum that has been incubated with immune precipitates. Removal of the immune precipitates before injection does not prevent anaphylaxis, and a toxic factor, anaphylatoxin, produced by the interaction of serum with immune complexes, was proposed. It is now realized that anaphylaxis can be produced by IgE-mediated reactions (Chap. 17) as well as by complement activation. The term *anaphylatoxin* has persisted and is now restricted to activity of the complement system. It is used to describe a pharmacologically active substance derived from serum that (1) causes hypotension when injected intravenously, (2) causes abrupt contraction of guinea pig ileum, with subsequent tachyphylaxis, (3) is blocked from producing ileum contraction by antihistamines, (4) fails to contract estrous rat uterus, (5) increases vascular permeability in guinea pig skin, and (6) degranulates mast cells from guinea pigs but not from rat mesenteric preparations.

The cleavage products of complement activation, C3a and C5a, have activity of classic anaphylatoxin, that is, anaphylatoxin purified from complement-activated serum. C5a is 100 to 1000 times more potent than is C3a in contracting guinea pig ileum, whereas C3a produces degranulation of rat mesenteric mast cells, a property not shared by classic anaphylatoxin. C5a, therefore, appears to be anaphylatoxin as originally described, and C3a, although less potent, produces similar biologic effects. C4a, peptide cleaved from C4, also has anaphylatoxin activity but is less potent even than C3a. The primary amino acid structures of C5a, C3a, and C4a share considerable homology, and all react with a single receptor to mediate their biologic functions. The biologic function of anaphylatoxins in vivo may be to induce vascular permeability and stasis, thus allowing the efflux of serum proteins, including antibodies, into surrounding tissues and permitting establishment of stable chemotactic gradients necessary for recruitment of phagocytic cells.

A naturally occurring carboxypeptidase termed *anaphylatoxin inactivator* removes the C-terminus arginine from the anaphylatoxins and diminishes their biologic activities considerably.

Chemotactic Activity

Chemotaxis is the unidirectional migration of cells toward an increasing concentration of a chemical attractant (Chaps. 17 and 19). Leukocytes (including polymorphonuclear leukocytes, monocytes, macrophages, and even small lymphocytes) are capable of chemotactic migration. Activation of complement in serum by inflammatory agents, such as immune complexes or endotoxins, produces molecules, primarily C5a, capable of inducing chemotaxis for these cells. Loss of the terminal arginine by a plasma carboxypeptidase reduces but does not abrogate the chemotactic potency of C5a. Although C3a has amino acid sequence similarities to C5a, it lacks a methionyl residue present in C5a at the fifth position from the carboxy terminus. Purified C3a is not chemotactic, and it is noteworthy that human polymorphonuclear leukocytes contain a specific receptor for C5a but not for C3a. Serum from genetically C5-deficient individuals develops only low levels of activity when C is activated.

Injection of C5a into the skin produces vasodilatation, vascular stasis, and local accumulation of polymorphonuclear leukocytes and macrophages. The histologic picture looks quite similar to an Arthus reaction, and indeed C5a is an important mediator of the acute inflammatory response initiated by immune complexes. At concentrations higher than that required for chemotaxis, C5a initiates a respiratory burst and secretion of lysosomal enzymes by neutrophils and mononuclear phagocytes (Chap. 17).

Deficiencies of Complement System and Their Relationship to Human Diseases

Complete or partial deficiencies of most of the classic complement components, with the exception of some complement inhibitors, have been described in humans or animals (Table 15–3). Some of these complement deficiencies are associated with severe diseases, whereas in others, clinical manifestations are sporadic. Defects in the complement system could result in impaired elimination of microbial antigens or circulating immune complexes. Indeed, complement deficiencies have been associated with recurrent bacterial and fungal infections as well as with collagen-vascular inflammatory diseases.

TABLE 15–3. CONGENITAL DEFICIENCIES OF COMPLEMENT COMPONENTS

Component	Frequency of Symptomatic Disease[a]	Percent with Lupuslike Syndrome	Infections
Classic Pathway			
C1q	Rare (15)	90	Pyogenic
C1r or C1s	Rare (8)	75	Pyogenic
C4	Rare (14)	90	Pyogenic
C2	Not rare (66)	60	Pyogenic
Alternative Pathway			
B or D	None		
C3	Rare (11)	75	Severe pyogenic
Membrane Attack Complex			
C5	Rare (12)	8	*Neisseria*
C6	Rare (17)	15	*Neisseria*
C7	Rare (14)	7	*Neisseria*
C8	Rare (14)	7	*Neisseria*
C9	Common	No disease association	
Control Proteins			
C1 inhibitor	Common	2	Angioedema
I	Rare (5)	20	Severe pyogenic
H	Rare (2)	Hemolytic-uremic syndrome	

Adapted from Lachmann and Rosen: Springer Semin Immunopathol 1:399, 1978

[a] Numbers in parentheses indicate approximate number of reported cases as of 1983.

A deficiency or dysfunction of C1 esterase inhibitor results in hereditary angioedema, an autosomal dominant heritable disease. It is characterized by acute and transitory local accumulations of edema fluid, which, when localized in the larynx, can become life-threatening by obstructing the tracheal airways. During attacks, hemolytic complement activity in these individuals is markedly depressed due to consumption of C4 and C2 by unregulated C1s activity. The edema may be produced by a kinin cleaved from C2 by the action of C1s. Attacks appear to be triggered by activation of Hageman factor (factor XII, the plasma protein that initiates clotting), which leads to the formation of plasmin and kallikrein. These proteases cleave and activate C1s, resulting in activation of the complement system. The most promising approach to treating hereditary angioedema has been the use of androgen therapy with the attenuated sex hormones, such as fluoxymesterone and, particularly, danazol. These agents are quite effective in preventing attacks and appear to do so by increasing the synthesis of C1 esterase inhibitor.

Partial C1q deficiencies have been found in several patients with combined immunodeficiency disease. Normal levels of C1q were restored on bone marrow transplantation. Selective deficiency of C1r has been found in a few patients with glomerulonephritis and polyarthritis. C2 deficiency is the most common of the heritable complement deficiencies. Approximately half of the individuals with C2 deficiency enjoy normal health, while the remainder may have lupuslike diseases. Deficiencies of the fourth and second component of complement have been found in a number of patients with collagen-vascular diseases, particularly systemic and discoid lupus erythematosus. Genes, both regulatory or structural for C2 and C4, as well as for factor B, are closely linked to the major histocompatibility complex (HLA) of humans, and HLA-linked genes are involved in many diseases. Therefore, the lupuslike diseases may not have been directly due to lack of C2 or C4 but may be due to some other gene of this complex (Chap. 14).

Individuals with defects of C3 suffer from severe recurrent bacterial infections. Sera from these patients generate less chemotactic activity and support less phagocytic activity than do normal sera. It should be noted that an almost complete deficiency of these components is required to produce clinically apparent disease. A patient with a deficiency of factor H had very low levels of C3 because of hypercatabolism of C3, presumably because of constant activation of the alternative pathway by C3b. This patient suffered from bacterial infections, and serum from this individual was not able to generate chemotactic activity, probably because C3 is required for the activation of C5. The depression of C3 could be reversed in vivo by the administration of factor H.

Isolated deficiencies of each of the terminal complement components have been discovered in humans. Several families with heritable C5 deficiency have been found. In one, the proband had systemic lupus erythematosus. A sister with very low but detectable levels of C5 had several bouts of pneumococcal pneumonia. In another family, the proband had low but measurable levels of C5 (about 0.5% of normal hemolytic activity). She suffered from repeated episodes of disseminated gonococcal infections. Although two other family members with similar levels of C5 were healthy, their risk factor may have differed from that of the proband. However, individuals with isolated deficiencies of C5, C6, C7, or C8 do appear to be generally more susceptible to recurrent infection with neisserial organisms. Of 31 individuals found to be deficient in either C5, C6, C7, or C8, 15 have had infections with *Neisseria gonorrhoeae* or *Neisseria meningitidis*. Thus, the bactericidal activity of complement may be important for protection against neisserial infection.

The association of complement defects with infectious diseases could certainly be anticipated, but the high frequency of collagen-vascular inflammatory diseases with deficiencies of complement, particularly C1r, C4, and C2, was less predictable. Some individuals with terminal complement deficiencies have had rheumatic disorders. This latter association suggests that patients with isolated deficiencies of the early acting classic complement components are more susceptible to subtle infections that cause systemic inflammatory diseases, or that elimination of antigens and immune complexes in general by these individuals is suboptimal, thus producing chronic stimulation of the immune response. In any case, understanding the intriguing relationship of complement defects with inflammatory diseases will lead to a better understanding of the pathophysiology of these diseases, as well as of the biologic role of the complement system.

FURTHER READING

Bentley DR: Structural superfamilies of the complement system. Exp Clin Immunogenet 5:69, 1988

Complement. Springer Semin Immunopathol 7:117, 1983

Congenital deficiencies of complement. Immunodeficiency Rev 1:3, 1988
Lampris JD: The third component of complement: Chemistry and biology. Curr Topics Microbiol Immunol 153:1, 1990
Porter RR, Lachmann PJ, Reid KBM (eds): Biochemistry and genetics of complement. Phil Trans R Soc Lond [B] 306:277, 1984
Reid KBM, Day AJ: Structure–function relationships of the complement components. Immunol Today 10:177, 1989
Ross GD: The Immunobiology of the Complement System. Orlando, Fla., Academic Press, 1986
Ross GD, Medof ME: Membrane complement receptor specific for bound fragments of C3. Adv Immunol 37:217, 1985

CHAPTER 16

The Lymphocyte Surface: Molecules That Mediate Adhesion and Signaling

Cell-cell and cell-matrix interactions are critical for many aspects of the immune response. Included among these are the recirculation of lymphocytes and the interaction of developing lymphoid cells with their microenvironment (i.e., thymus, bursa, bone marrow). Cell adhesion processes also facilitate antigen presentation to T cells by macrophages or dendritic cells, interaction of regulatory and effector T cells, T cell interactions with B cells, tissue inflammation, and lysis by cytotoxic T cells of virally infected cells or tumor cells. Several examples of cell-cell adhesion are shown in Figure 16–1. Cell-cell and cell-matrix interactions are mediated by cell surface glycoproteins. This chapter focuses on the discovery and characterization of those cell surface molecules that mediate cell-cell and cell-matrix interactions in the immune system. An interesting aspect of the study of adhesion receptors in the immune response has been its convergence with studies on cell-cell and cell-matrix adhesion in other disciplines, such as developmental biology and neurobiology.

Historical Perspective

Our knowledge of cell-cell and cell-matrix interactions in the immune response has its historical basis in the study of two major areas of lymphocyte biology and function. The first of these is recirculation of lymphocytes. In the 1960s, Sir James Gowans performed elegant studies in rats showing that small lymphocytes recirculate in the body. Gowans and colleagues removed lymphocytes from rats, radioactively labeled them, and reinfused them (Chap. 13). The reinfused lymphocytes followed a defined pattern of recirculation from the blood into the lymph nodes and spleen and back into the lymph. To enter the peripheral lymphoid tissue, small lymphocytes migrated across the endothelium of a specialized group of blood vessels in lymph nodes called the *postcapillary venules* (PCV). Since pretreatment of lymphocytes with glycosidases

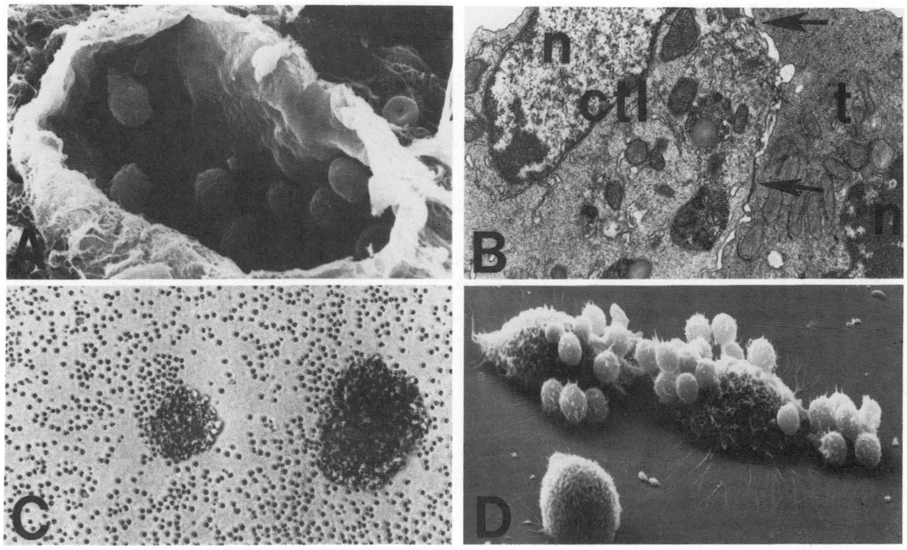

Fig. 16–1. Cell–cell adhesion is important in many aspects of leukocyte function and development. **A.** Leukocytes bind to vessel walls before extravasation into tissues during an inflammatory response. × 25,000. Scanning EM photomicrograph. **B.** Cytotoxic T lymphocytes (CTL) bind to their target cells. × 17,000. Transmission EM photomicrograph. **C.** Dendritic cells cluster with T lymphocytes during a primary MLR. **D.** Thymocytes bind to thymic epithelial cells. × 1500. *(**A** courtesy of Dr. M. J. Karnovsky. **B** courtesy of Dr. Janice Burkhardt and Susan Hester. **C** reproduced from Inaba and Steinman in the Journal of Experimental Medicine, 1987, 165:1403, by copyright permission of the Rockefeller University Press.)*

and proteinases inhibited migration, it was suggested that this process depended on glycoproteins expressed on the lymphocyte surface. An important step in lymphocyte recirculation is binding to vascular endothelial cells. This mechanism plays an important role in recirculation of lymphocytes (homing) as well as migration of lymphocytes and other leukocytes into infected tissues (inflammation) (Fig. 16–1A) (Chap. 19). Many of the molecules that mediate these important cell-cell and cell-matrix interactions have now been identified and are described here.

Another major lymphocyte function that was an early focus of cell-cell interaction studies was T cell–mediated cytotoxicity (Chap. 13). T cell–mediated cytolysis of target cells can be divided into stages based on temperature and anion requirements. The first stage is binding, or conjugation, of the effector cytotoxic T cell (CTL) with its target cell (Fig. 16–1B). Since T cell–mediated cytotoxicity is antigen-specific, it was assumed originally that interaction between a CTL and its target was mediated solely by the antigen-specific T cell receptor binding to a surface antigen on the target cell. This minimal model of CTL-target binding mediated solely by the T cell receptor is not correct. CTL-target cell binding is a complex interaction to which several other molecules contribute. This has been shown by inhibiting CTL with monoclonal antibodies and then using the antibodies to characterize the molecules to which they bind. Once these molecules were identified in CTL function, it was possible to show that they, along with related molecules, also participate in cell-cell and cell-matrix interactions important to other aspects of the immune response.

The molecules that participate in adhesive interactions in the immune response belong to at least three identified families of molecules. The integrin family includes the three leukocyte cell adhesion molecules (Leu-CAM)—LFA-1, Mac-1, and p150,95—and a series of receptors for extracellular matrix proteins. The immunoglobulin superfamily, in addition to immunoglobulin and the antigen-specific T cell receptor, includes the T cell coreceptor molecules CD4 and CD8, the T cell–activation antigen CD2 and its ligand LFA-3, and the T cell–activation molecules CD28 and Thy-1. In addition, the ligands ICAM-1, ICAM-2, and VCAM-1 are also members of the Ig family. Finally, the selectin family includes the MEL-14/LAM-1 and ELAM-1 molecules involved in leukocyte migration and homing, as well as the platelet adhesion molecule GMP-140. In addition to these recognized families, several other molecules not yet grouped into families play accessory roles and are discussed here, including the CD44 molecule and the leukocyte common antigen, CD45. Adhesion mediated by many of these molecules is under tight regulation, since it is advantageous to cells to make a rapid transition from a nonadherent to adherent state and vice versa.

Integrin Family of Adhesion Molecules

The identification of integrins as a family of proteins involved in cell-cell and cell-matrix adhesion followed a convergence of studies of adhesion receptors on platelets, receptors for cell matrix proteins, adhesion in embryonic development, and adhesion of leukocytes. The integrin family contains a group of related $\alpha\beta$ heterodimers (subunits of 95,000 to 200,000 Da) widely distributed in tissues and extending throughout most of the phylogenetic tree (Fig. 16–2). Integrins interact with cell matrix glycoproteins, complement components, and ligands expressed on cell surfaces. They link, or integrate, the cell and the cytoskeleton with the external microenvironment. Integrins also are involved in development, hemostasis, thrombosis, wound healing, and oncogenic transformation.

Subfamilies of integrins are recognized based on their usage of particular β subunits. Table 16–1 depicts in grid form the known possible combinations of α and β subunits and their ligands. Members of the β_1 subfamily, termed the VLA antigens, contain one β_1 subunit (CD29) in association with one of at least seven different α subunits. Additional molecules have been identified that use alternative β subunits in association with VLA α subunits (Table 16–2). Members of

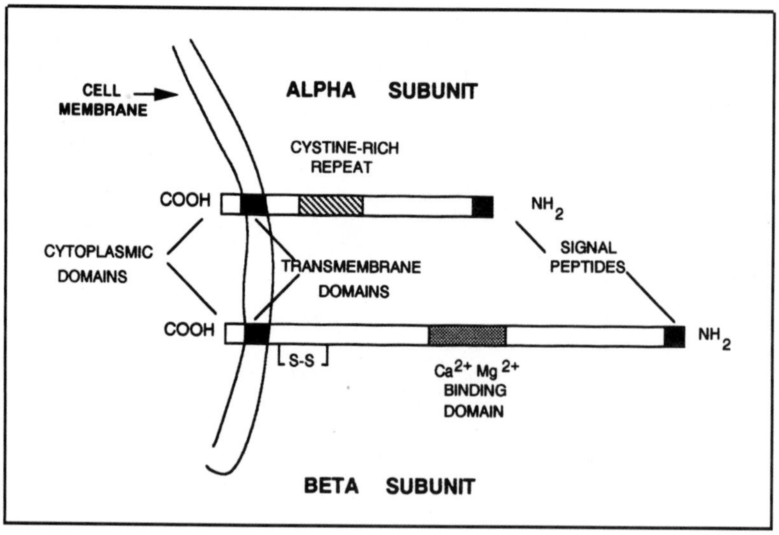

Fig. 16–2. The general structure of an integrin molecule anchored in a cell membrane. α and β subunits are noncovalently associated, transmembrane molecules with the COOH termini located in the cytoplasm. *(Adapted from Ruoslahti and Pierschbacher: Science 238:491, 1987.)*

the β_2 subfamily, termed *leukocyte cell adhesion molecules* or LeuCAMs, contain one β_2 (CD18) subunit in association with one of three different α subunits (CD11 a, b, or c). Members of the β_3 subfamily, termed the *vitronectin receptors,* contain one β_3 (CD61) subunit in association with one of two different α subunits. An additional member of this family has now been identified that uses an alternative β chain.

β_1 and β_3 Subfamilies

Interaction of Cells with Extracellular Matrix Proteins. In vivo cells of many types adhere to the extracellular matrix, an intricate network of macromolecules including polysaccharides and proteins that fill the extracellular space. In addition to serving as a scaffolding to stabilize the physical structure of tissues, the extracellular matrix also regulates the behavior of cells that come in contact with it by influencing development, migration, proliferation, shape, and function.

The extracellular matrix is made up of primarily two types of macromolecules, (1) polysaccharide glycosaminoglycans (GAGs), usually covalently linked to protein to form proteoglycans, and (2) fibrous proteins. The fibrous proteins include collagen, elastin, fibronectin, and laminin. Interaction of cells with the extracellular matrix can be demonstrated readily in vitro. Cells will adhere to surfaces coated with extracellular matrix (ECM) proteins. This type of study formed the early basis for the discovery of the β_1 and β_3 integrins. ECM proteins not only promote adhesion but also stimulate cell migration and differentiation.

Identification of ECM Protein Receptors. Fibronectin contains a cell-attachment domain. The amino acid sequence of the fibronectin binding domain has been determined, and

TABLE 16–1. INTEGRIN SUBUNIT COMBINATIONS AND LIGANDS

	β_1	β_2	β_3	β_4	β_5	β_6	β_7
α^1	Coll, Lm[a]						
α^2	Coll, Lm						
α^3	Fn, Lm, Coll						
α^4	Fn, VCAM-1						PP HEV
α^5	Fn						
α^6	Lm			?			
α^V	Fn, Vn?		Vn, Fb, Opn vWF, BSP, (Fn)		Vn, (Fn)	?	
α^{IIb}			Fb, Vn Fn, vWF				
α^L		ICAM-1,2					
α^M		C3bi, FX, Fb ICAM-1					
α^X		(C3bi)					

[a] Coll, collagen; Lm, laminin; Fn, fibronectin; Vn, vitronectin; FX, blood factor X; Fb, fibrinogen; Opn, osteopontin; PP HEV, Peyer's patch high endothelial venules; BSP, bone sialoprotein. (Courtesy of Dr. Martin E. Hemler.)

TABLE 16–2. TISSUE DISTRIBUTION OF MEMBERS OF THE INTEGRIN FAMILY OF ADHESION MOLECULES

Molecule	Other Names	Tissue Distribution
$\alpha^1\beta_1$	CD49a, VLA-1	Widespread, activated T cells, skin fibroblasts, mesangial cells, liver sinusoids
$\alpha^2\beta_1$	CD49b, VLA-2, ECMR-I	Widespread, activated T cells, platelets, most nonhematopoietic adherent cell lines
$\alpha^3\beta_1$	CD49c, VLA-3, ECMR-II	Widespread, kidney glomerulus, thyroid, most nonhematopoietic adherent cell lines
$\alpha^4\beta_1$	VLA-4, CD49d, LPAM-2	Lymphocytes, monocytes, most hematopoietic cell lines
$\alpha^4\beta_7$	VLA-4alt, LPAM-1	Lymphocytes, monocytes
$\alpha^5\beta_1$	VLA-5, CD49e, FNR	Widespread, variable on lymphocytes, monocytes, most cell lines
$\alpha^6\beta_1$	VLA-6, CD49f	Widespread
$\alpha^6\beta_4$	—	Epithelial cells
$\alpha^V\beta_1$	—	?
$\alpha^V\beta_3$	CD51	Endothelium, some tumor cells
$\alpha^V\beta_5$	$\alpha^V\beta_x$	Carcinomas
$\alpha^{IIb}\beta_3$	CD41a	Platelets
$\alpha^L\beta_2$	CD11a, LFA-1	Lymphoid cells, myeloid cells
$\alpha^M\beta_2$	CD11b, Mac-1, Mo-1 CR-3	Myeloid cells, NK[a]
$\alpha^X\beta_2$	p150,95, CD11c, CR-4	Myeloid cells, some B and T cell lines

[a] NK, natural killer cells.

the specific sequence of amino acids that is recognized by cells has been identified as Arg-Gly-Asp (RGD in the single letter code for amino acids). When RGD-containing peptides (usually the hexapeptide GRGDSP) are immobilized onto a surface, the peptides promote cell attachment in a manner similar to that promoted by the complete fibronectin molecule. A solution of RGD peptides inhibits attachment of cells to a surface coated with fibronectin, although this inhibition requires a substantial molar excess of peptide. Conservative changes in the peptides, such as an exchange of alanine for the glycine or glutamic acid for the aspartic acid, eliminate inhibitory properties. An RGD sequence also is found in a number of other matrix proteins and is important for binding of cells to many ECM proteins.

RGD-containing peptides have been used to identify the ECM protein receptors. ECM proteins (i.e., fibronectin, collagen) were covalently bound to Sepharose, and cell extracts were passed over a column of ECM protein–Sepharose. The material that bound to the ECM protein–Sepharose was eluted with an RGD-containing peptide (i.e., GRGDSP). Using this method, ECM protein receptors were isolated and characterized that bind to fibronectin, collagen, vitronectin, and von Willebrand factor. These receptors belong to the β_1 and β_3 integrin subfamilies.

Although several of the ECM protein receptors bind RGD sequences, their specificity apparently is dependent on other factors as well. For example, the fibronectin receptor $\alpha^5\beta_1$ binds to fibronectin and binding is inhibited by RGD-containing peptides. However, $\alpha^5\beta_1$ does not bind to vitronectin, which also contains an RGD sequence (Table 16–1). These data indicate that the specificity of $\alpha^5\beta_1$ receptors is not determined solely by RGD. It may be that the surrounding sequences are important for achieving the appropriate conformation of the RGD site. Alternatively, there may be a second binding site that contributes to specificity.

Biochemistry of β_1 Integrins. The members of the β_1 integrin subfamily frequently are called the *very late antigens,* or VLA, because two members, VLA-1 and VLA-2, originally were identified using monoclonal antibodies that detected protein heterodimers appearing on the surface of T cells 2 to 4 weeks after in vitro activation with mitogen or antigen. Four additional heterodimers and two alternative forms belonging to the same family have been described (Tables 16–1 and 16–2). The six VLA heterodimers are each composed of a distinct α subunit (α^1, α^2, ... α^6) noncovalently associated with a common β subunit (β_1). The alternative forms are VLA-4alt ($\alpha^4\beta_7$) and VLA-6alt ($\alpha^6\beta_4$). The VLA nomenclature has been retained to clarify the relationship between the molecules.

Expression of β_1 Integrins on Leukocytes. Although this discussion focuses on VLA proteins on leukocytes, it is important to note that VLAs are not restricted to leukocytes, and most cell types, except erythrocytes and granulocytes, express at least one of the VLA heterodimers. The distribution of VLA proteins on cells and tissues is shown in Table 16–2.

Although VLA-1 and VLA-2 are not expressed on resting T cells, the level of VLA-1 and VLA-2 on T cell slowly increases with time after activation with antigen or mitogen. The remaining VLAs are basally expressed on resting T cells, although expression can be variable and their expression may be altered by activation. VLA-3 increases with activation but to a lesser extent than VLA-1 and VLA-2. VLA-4 is variably expressed on activated T cells. VLA-5 expression increases, and VLA-6 expression decreases. Leukocytes express a diversity of β_1 integrins that may mediate adhesion to a variety of ligands.

Function of β_1 Integrins on Leukocytes. In vivo peripheral blood lymphocytes can be subdivided into populations expressing high or low levels of the β_1 subunit (CD29) using the monoclonal antibody 4B4. The subpopulation with higher CD29 levels also expresses increased levels of other adhesion molecules, such as LFA-3, CD2, LFA-1, CD44, and CD45RO. This phenotype is consistent with a memory cell phenotype, and such cells show an enhanced responsiveness to antigen. There is some evidence that suggests that ECM proteins modulate lymphocyte behavior, such as proliferation, lymphokine production, and motility. In addition to mediating interaction between cells and ECM proteins, some VLA proteins mediate cell–cell interactions. VLA-4alt ($\alpha^4\beta_7$) mediates binding of lymphocytes to Peyer's patch high endothelial venules (HEV) and thus plays a role in lymphocyte homing. VLA-4 ($\alpha^4\beta_1$) mediates binding of lymphocytes to endothelial cells. Its ligand, VCAM-1 (INCAM-110), is upregulated on endothelial cells by inflammatory cytokines. VLA-4/VCAM-1 interaction is probably critical for lymphocyte migration into tissues.

Regarding the role of β_1 integrins on monocytes and macrophages, it has been shown that fibronectin and laminin enhance phagocytosis and production of inflammatory mediators such as tumor necrosis factor α, colony stimulating factors, prostaglandins, and IL-1. Collagen has been reported to induce differentiation of monocytes to macrophages, and collagen and fibronectin are chemotactic for monocytes. It is likely that the basally expressed integrins, such as VLA-4, -5, and -6 on T cells and monocytes and VLA-4 on B cells, facilitate the initial extravasation and migration into tissues and that after activation, VLA-1 and VLA-2 are critically important.

β_2 Subfamily (Leu-CAM)

Biochemistry and Tissue Distribution. The β_2 subfamily of integrins consists of the three surface membrane heterodimeric glycoproteins: LFA-1 (CD11a/CD18), Mac-1 (CD11b/CD18), and p150,95 (CD11c/CD18). The 95 kDa β subunit (CD18) is shared among all three members and is noncovalently associated with a distinct α chain of 180 kDa (CD11a) in LFA-1, 155 kDa (CD11b) in Mac-1, or 150 kDa (CD11c) in p150,95. These three molecules also have been called *leukocyte integrins, leukocyte adhesion proteins* (LAP), and *Leu-CAM* because their distribution is limited to leukocytes. The leukocyte adhesion molecules have been characterized on human and mouse leukocytes. Although all three β_2 integrins are restricted to leukocytes, their expression varies among the three (Table 16–2). LFA-1 is expressed on all leukocytes with the exception of some peritoneal macrophages. Mac-1 is expressed on monocytes, macrophages, granulocytes, and natural killer (NK) cells. p150,95 is present on monocytes, macrophages, granulocytes, and some B cell lines and T cell lines in culture. In each case, the complex on the cell surface consists of one α chain and one β chain. The α and β subunits are synthesized as separate precursors containing N-glycoside high-mannose carbohydrate groups linked to polypeptides. The α and β precursors associate intracellularly before conversion of the high-mannose carbohydrates to a complex carbohydrate form in the Golgi. Only after this step can the αβ complex be expressed on the cell surface. In mouse-human hybrid cells, the α and β subunits of LFA-1 are capable of associating to form an interspecies complex, attesting to the degree of conservation in the LFA-1 molecules.

Function of LFA-1. As mentioned previously, the discovery of several of the adhesion molecules was linked to the demonstration that cell surface molecules other than the antigen-specific T cell receptor play a role in the binding of CTL to their targets. This was accomplished by demonstrating that the function of CTL could be inhibited by antibodies to cell surface molecules. Originally, antibodies to known cell surface molecules were used to show that antibody to the mouse Lyt-2 (CD8) antigen inhibited CTL function. This is discussed later. Afterward, strategies were developed to make monoclonal antibodies that inhibited CTL function. Using this approach, Springer and colleagues identified the lymphocyte function–associated antigen-1 (LFA-1) on both mouse and human cells and the lymphocyte-associated antigens 2 (LFA-2, CD2) and 3 (LFA-3) on human cells. CD2 and LFA-3 are discussed on pp 305–306.

Monoclonal antibodies to LFA-1 inhibit a wide variety of adhesion-dependent leukocyte functions, including CTL-mediated lysis, NK cell–mediated lysis, and antibody-dependent cytotoxicity by granulocytes and peripheral blood mononuclear cells. LFA-1 antibodies block CTL function at the Mg^{2+}-dependent binding stage rather than the Ca^{2+}-dependent lethal hit phase (Fig. 16–3) (Chap. 13). Interestingly, antibodies to the antigen-specific T cell receptor inhibit at the lethal hit phase, not the binding phase. Early studies on CTL primarily used in vivo–generated mouse CTL that recognized alloantigens on the sensitizing targets. In these studies, the specificity of binding was quite tight; that is, CTL bound only to their sensitizing targets, not to irrelevant targets. However, with increasing use of human CTL that were generated in vitro or of cloned lines of CTL, it became apparent that binding and killing did not always correlate tightly. Some cloned CTL lines bound to irrelevant target cells but did not kill them. This was termed *antigen-independent conjugation.* Antibodies to LFA-1 inhibit this antigen-independent conjugation.

Antibodies to LFA-1 also inhibit the proliferation of T cells in response to soluble antigens, viruses, alloantigens, and mitogens. To inhibit these functions, the antibody must be added within the first few hours of the assay, suggesting that the antibody blocks the induction of proliferation rather than proliferation itself. Antibody responses to T cell–dependent

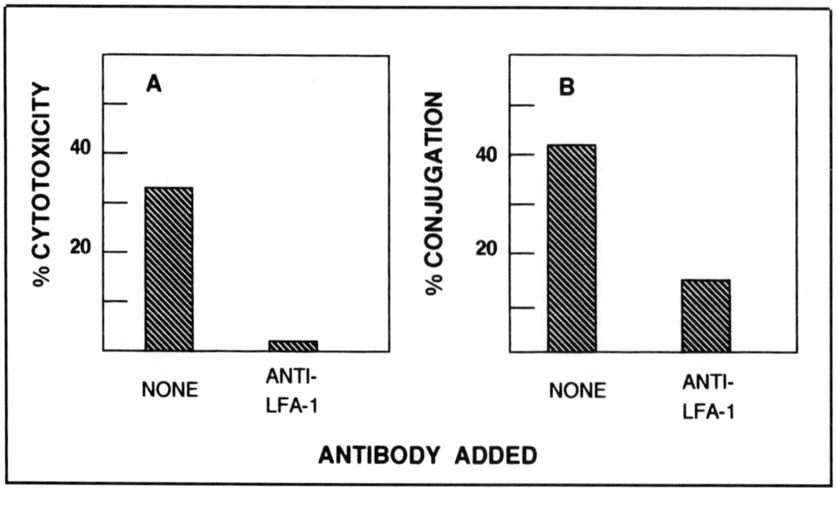

Fig. 16–3. **A.** Antibody to LFA-1 inhibits CTL-mediated lysis of ^{51}Cr-labeled tumor target cells. CTL were pretreated without antibody or with purified anti-LFA-1 antibody before relevant target cells were added. Percent cytotoxicity was determined by release of ^{51}Cr. **B.** Antibody to LFA-1 inhibits CTL-target conjugate formation. CTL were pretreated without antibody or with anti-LFA-1 antibody. Target cells were added, and cells were centrifuged and incubated at 37C for 21 minutes. After resuspension, cells were scored microscopically for the percentage of target cells conjugated to effector cells (% conjugation). *(Data from Davignon et al: J Immunol 127:590, 1981.)*

antigens also are inhibited by antibody to LFA-1, apparently by interfering with interactions of T cells and antigen-presenting cells.

LFA-1 is also a critical ligand for leukocyte binding to other nonhematopoietic cell types, including endothelial cells, fibroblasts, and epithelial cells. In addition to serving as an adhesion molecule, LFA-1 can convey an activation signal to T cells. Crosslinking of LFA-1 alone on the surface of T cells does not activate T cells to produce IL-2 and proliferate. However, when both LFA-1 and CD3 are crosslinked on the surface of T cells, IL-2 production and T cell proliferation are enhanced to a much greater extent than when CD3 is crosslinked alone. These data suggest that the interaction of LFA-1 on a T cell with its ligand facilitates adhesion but also may amplify T cell activation by delivering costimulatory signals.

Function of Mac-1 and p150,95. Mac-1 and p150,95 are similar in their expression and function. Mac-1 can function as a receptor for the C3bi component of complement as well as the clotting components fibrinogen and factor X. C3bi may also serve as a ligand for p150,95. Antibody to Mac-1 has been reported to enhance secretion of H_2O_2 by macrophages and decrease phagocytosis. Thus, like LFA-1, Mac-1 may be able to transduce signals.

Blocking studies using α chain–specific antibodies have shown that p150,95 is the most important of the leukocyte integrins in monocyte adhesion and chemotaxis, whereas Mac-1 is most important in the function of neutrophils. Mac-1 and p150,95 are stored in intracellular pools in circulating monocytes and granulocytes. Binding of chemoattractants to specific receptors results in translocation of Mac-1 and p150,95 to the cell surface. Through this mechanism, adhesion is increased, and the result is enhanced binding to endothelial cells and localization in inflammatory sites.

Leukocyte Adhesion Deficiency. From 1979 to 1982, several infants with widespread bacterial infections, defective neutrophil mobility, and delayed separation of the umbilical cord were described. Other patients with similar infections, accompanied by defects in neutrophil chemotaxis and function, also were reported. The neutrophil defects were secondary to an abnormality in adhesion, since patients' neutrophils only weakly adhered and failed to spread on Petri dishes. The patients' neutrophils lacked the common β subunit of the β_2 integrins. This defect, leukocyte adhesion deficiency (LAD), has been reported in a small number of individuals worldwide (<40). Patients are characterized by recurrent, life-threatening bacterial and fungal infections, progressive periodontitis, lack of pus formation, and leukocytosis. All leukocytes are affected, and there are two forms of the disease. In the severe form, patients' leukocytes express <1% of normal levels of LFA-1, Mac-1, and p150,95. In the moderate form, patients' leukocytes express 5% to 10% of normal levels. Life expectancy and the severity of clinical symptoms correlate with the level of expression.

The deficiency of expression of LFA-1, Mac-1, and p150,95 in LAD patients is due to a defect in the common β chain. Five distinct mutations have been described that affect either the amount of β chain precursor synthesized or the ability of the β chain to associate with the α chain in the endoplasmic reticulum after synthesis. B lymphoblastoid cell lines from LAD patients have been transfected with a vector containing the gene for the β subunit. Stably transfected patient cells expressed near normal levels of the LFA-1 complex on the cell surface. The LFA-1$^+$ transfected cells bound to a purified ligand for LFA-1, ICAM-1 (see below).

Identification of the Ligand for LFA-1. On activation, lymphocytes become more motile and sticky. Activated, antigen-specific lymphocytes show increased adhesion not only to cells expressing the relevant antigen but also to cells lacking the relevant antigen. Activated lymphocytes frequently form clusters (homotypic adhesion) (Fig. 16–4A). Homotypic adhe-

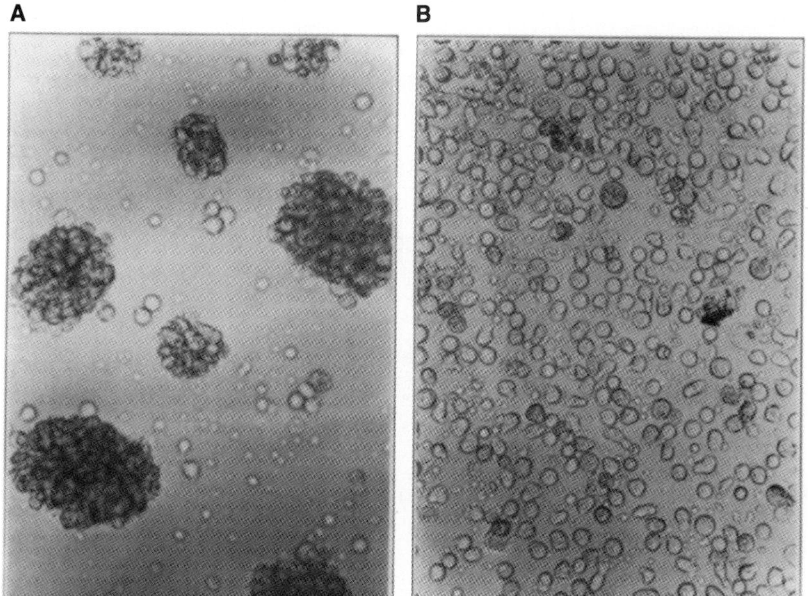

Fig. 16–4. Inhibition of homotypic adhesion of lymphoblastoid cells by antibody to LFA-1. JY cells were treated with PMA (**A**) or with PMA and anti-LFA-1 Ab (**B**) for 30 minutes. *(Reproduced from Rothlein and Springer in the Journal of Experimental Medicine, 1986, 163:1132, by copyright permission of the Rockefeller University Press.)*

sion can also be induced by phorbol myristate acetate (PMA), which directly stimulates protein kinase C. Similar aggregation is seen in lymphoblastoid cell lines, including Epstein-Barr virus-transformed B cell lines, and cloned cytotoxic T cell lines. Antibodies to LFA-1 inhibit homotypic adhesion (Fig. 16–4B), and homotypic adhesion of cell lines has been used as a model system for studying LFA-1-dependent adhesion. Along with the CTL system, this model has been used to show that LFA-1-mediated interactions are temperature and energy dependent and require an intact cytoskeleton and the presence of Mg^{2+}. The homotypic adhesion model system also was exploited to identify a ligand for LFA-1. PMA-activated lymphocytes from LAD patients (LFA-1$^-$) do not form homotypic clusters. However, PMA-activated LFA-1$^-$ cells do form clusters with LFA-1$^+$ activated cells from normal people. Clustering is LFA-1 dependent, since it is inhibited by antibodies to LFA-1. These data suggested that although the LAD patients' cells did not express LFA-1, they did express a ligand for LFA-1. Monoclonal antibodies were raised against activated cells from LAD patients and selected for inhibition of LFA-1-dependent homotypic adhesion. A ligand for LFA-1 was identified and called *intercellular adhesion molecule-1* (ICAM-1).

ICAM-1 (CD54) is a member of the immunoglobulin supergene family (Table 16–3). Unlike LFA-1 and its family members, ICAM-1 is not restricted to hematopoietic cells but can be expressed on a variety of cells. In the absence of an inflammatory response, ICAM-1 is expressed on only a few cells types, but the expression of ICAM-1 can be upregulated by inflammatory mediators, including interferon-γ, lipopolysaccharide, IL-1, and tumor necrosis factor. The increase in ICAM-1 expression by endothelial cells, epithelial cells, and fibroblasts is accompanied by an increase in the ability of these cells to bind activated LFA-1$^+$ lymphocytes. This is critically important, since binding of lymphocytes to endothelium is an early step in localizing circulating cells at an inflammatory site.

Like antibodies to LFA-1, antibodies to ICAM-1 inhibit CTL-mediated cytotoxicity. Fibroblasts transfected with the genes for ICAM-1 and major histocompatibility complex (MHC) class II molecules activate T helper cells more efficiently than those transfected with MHC class II alone. ICAM-1 is expressed on follicular dendritic cells and on activated B cells in germinal centers of lymph nodes and has been postulated to contribute to formation of germinal centers. In addition, ICAM-1 serves as a receptor for rhinoviruses.

Since some LFA-1-mediated binding was not inhibited by antibodies to ICAM-1, it was apparent that at least one other ligand for LFA-1 existed. A cDNA for a molecule called ICAM-2 was isolated from an expression library by screening for binding of transfected cells to Petri dishes coated with purified LFA-1. By screening in the presence of antibody to ICAM-1, it was possible to identify an alternative ligand for LFA-1. ICAM-2 is also a member of the immunoglobulin supergene family and is structurally similar to ICAM-1. Unlike ICAM-1, ICAM-2 is well expressed basally on endothelial cells and is not increased by inflammatory mediators (Table 16–3).

Regulation of LFA-1-mediated Adhesion. Binding mediated by LFA-1 is highly regulated over short periods of time. CTL adhere to their target cells, deliver a lethal hit, detach, and adhere to another target cell in just a few minutes. Treatment of T cells with PMA or with antibodies to the cell surface molecules CD2, CD3, and T cell receptor (TCR) (under conditions of crosslinking) stimulates LFA-1-dependent cell aggregation without increasing surface expression of LFA-1. These observations suggest that LFA-1 exists in at least two different forms, an inactive, low-avidity state and an active, high-avidity state. If LFA-1 were always in a high-avidity state and able to form high-avidity conjugates with ICAM-1$^+$ cells, spontaneous aggregation of peripheral blood leukocytes would cause clogging of blood vessels. A model has been proposed in which a number of stimuli, including PMA and activation through either the CD3-TCR or CD2 surface molecules, shift LFA-1 from an inactive to an active form. The model postulates that this shift involves phosphorylation of the β chain of LFA-1.

TABLE 16–3. TISSUE DISTRIBUTION AND FUNCTION OF SELECTED MEMBERS OF THE IMMUNOGLOBULIN SUPERGENE FAMILY

Molecule	Tissue Distribution	Ligand	Function
ICAM-1 (CD54)	Activated lymphoid cells, thymic epithelium, not basally expressed on most tissues but can be induced by mediators (IFN_α, TNF, IL-1)	LFA-1 (CD11a/CD18)	Adhesion, signaling(?), receptor for rhinoviruses
ICAM-2	Basally expressed on endothelium	LFA-1 (CD11a/CD18)	Adhesion
CD4	>95% thymocytes, 60% PBT,[a] monocytes/macrophages, Langerhans cells	MHC C1 II	Adhesion, signaling, receptor for HIV-1
CD8	>90% thymocytes, 40% PBT	MHC C1 I	Adhesion, signaling
CD2	>95% T cells, NK,[b] thymocytes	LFA-3, H19 others(?)	Adhesion, signaling
LFA-3 (CD58)	Widespread, hematopoietic and nonhematopoietic	CD2	Adhesion, signaling, regulates cytokine production
CD28	>90% CD4+ T cells, 50% CD8+ T cells, mature thymocytes	B7/BB1	Adhesion, signaling, regulates cytokine production
Thy-1	Mouse: PBT, thymocytes, fibroblasts, neural tissue Human: tissue, fibroblasts, neural tissue, not on PBT	?	Adhesion(?), signaling
VCAM-1 (INCAM-110)	Induced on endothelial cells by mediators (TNF_α, IL1)	VLA-4 ($\alpha^4\beta_1$)	Adhesion

[a] PBT, peripheral blood T cells.
[b] NK, natural killer cells.

CD4 and CD8 Accessory/Coreceptor Molecules

As is discussed in Chapter 12, early studies suggested that T lymphocytes could be divided into functional subclasses based on their expression of the cell surface molecules CD4 and CD8 (Table 16–3). On peripheral blood T cells, CD4 and CD8 are expressed on mutually exclusive populations of cells. It subsequently became apparent that assignment of function based on these molecules did not always hold but that the stronger association was that $CD4^+$ T cells recognize antigen in association with MHC class II molecules, and their function can be inhibited by CD4 antibodies, whereas $CD8^+$ T cells recognize antigen in association with MHC class I molecules, and their function can be inhibited by CD8 antibodies.

Biochemistry and Tissue Distribution of CD4 and CD8

CD4 is a 55 kDa glycoprotein expressed as a monomer on the surface of 60% of peripheral blood T (PBT) cells and on 95% of thymocytes (Table 16–2). CD4 also is expressed on human monocyte/macrophages and on Langerhans cells in the skin. In addition to its function in the immune response, CD4 serves as a receptor for the human immunodeficiency virus, HIV-1 (Chap. 19).

The gene encoding CD4 is a member of the immunoglobulin supergene family. The CD4 molecule has four external domains, a hydrophobic transmembrane stretch of amino acids, and a cytoplasmic tail of 40 residues. The most membrane distal external domain has striking homology to immunoglobulin light chain variable regions. Sequence comparison of cloned human and mouse CD4 cDNAs shows 55% amino acid homology overall, with the most extensive homology found in the cytoplasmic tail. The cytoplasmic domain contains three serine residues that may serve as substrates for phosphorylation by protein kinase C. The fact that the cytoplasmic tail is highly conserved across species suggests that it is involved in the function of the molecule and that CD4 can function as a signal-transmitting molecule.

CD8 is expressed on 40% of PBT cells and over 90% of thymocytes. Thus a large number of thymocytes are both $CD4^+$ and $CD8^+$ (Chap. 12). In mice, CD8 is expressed as disulfide-linked heterodimers of a 38 kDa α chain (Lyt-2) or a 34 kDa α' chain complexed with a 30 kDa β chain (Lyt-3). The α chain consists of an external domain with homology to the variable region of immunoglobulin light chains, a short extracellular hinge region, a hydrophobic transmembrane segment, and a highly charged cytoplasmic domain. The rat and mouse β chains are predicted to have a similar overall structure to the α chains, but there is little actual sequence homology between rat α and β chains. Human CD8 also consists of a 32 to 34 kDa α chain and a more recently discovered 32 to 34 kDa β chain. However, only 90% of human $CD8^+$ cells express CD8β chains. On the remaining cells, CD8α chains usually are found in dimers or multimers. Structural variants of the CD8β chain have been isolated that probably arise from alternative splicing of mRNA and differ in the sequencing encoding the cytoplasmic tail and may affect signal transduction.

Role of CD4 and CD8 as Adhesion Molecules

The first clues to the fact that CD4 and CD8 play a role in T cell function came from early studies showing that antibodies to these molecules inhibited CTL activity, lymphokine production, proliferation of T cells, and T cell help for B cell responses. Due to the association between expression of CD4 or CD8 and the recognition of antigen in the context of particular MHC elements, it was postulated that CD4 interacted with MHC class II molecules and CD8 interacted with MHC class I molecules. Several investigators demonstrated that $CD8^+$ CTL of low avidity were susceptible to inhibition by CD8 antibodies, whereas those of high avidity were not susceptible to inhibition by CD8 antibodies. This led to the suggestion that CD8 interacted with MHC class I molecules to stabilize antigen binding of CTL with low-affinity TCR but were not necessary to high-affinity CTL. Studies using CD4 antibodies to inhibit the recognition of antigen by $CD4^+$ cells gave similar results, suggesting that CD4 molecules stabilize low affinity TCR interactions by binding to class II molecules on antigen presenting cells.

Gene transfer studies have provided direct evidence that CD4 and CD8 can bind to MHC molecules. The gene for CD4 was transferred to fibroblasts that normally do not express CD4. This was accomplished by infecting the fibroblasts with a recombinant virus containing the gene for CD4 driven by the SV40 late promoter. The fibroblasts expressed high levels of CD4 on their surface. B cells bearing MHC class II molecules were added to a culture dish containing the $CD4^+$ fibroblasts. MHC class II^+ B cells bound to the $CD4^+$ fibroblasts, and binding was inhibited by antibodies to MHC class II and CD4. Likewise, the gene encoding human CD8 was transfected into chinese hamster ovary (CHO) cells, and a line of cells expressing CD8 was obtained. Human B cell lines expressing MHC class I bound to CHO cells expressing high levels of CD8. Studies using mutant HLA-A2 molecules mapped the binding site of CD8 to the α^3 domain of MHC class I.

Role of CD4 and CD8 as Signaling Molecules

In addition to their role in binding MHC molecules, CD4 and CD8 can serve as signal transducing molecules. Binding of CD4 antibodies to CD4 molecules inhibits T cell activation driven by non-MHC class II ligands, such as mitogenic lectins or antibody to CD3. In these experiments, inhibition by CD4 antibodies cannot be explained by inhibition of binding of CD4 to MHC class II. The fact that this is actually a negative signaling event is suggested from studies showing that bivalent CD4 antibodies inhibit T cell activation by mitogens, whereas the monovalent Fab fragment does not. Since both monovalent and bivalent antibody inhibited activation by antigen in association with MHC class II, it was concluded that the effect of bivalent antibody on mitogen activation was due to negative signaling. There is also evidence, however, that CD4 and CD8 can mediate positive signaling. Simultaneous stimulation of T cells with CD3 antibodies along with either CD4 or CD8 antibodies leads to the induction of IL-2 receptor expression and T cell proliferation.

CD4 and CD8 molecules are associated with a T cell–specific tyrosine kinase, $p56^{lck}$. The *lck* gene is a member of the *src* family of tyrosine protein kinase genes. The *lck* gene is expressed at relatively high levels in T cells and some B cells but only rarely in nonlymphoid cells. It encodes an internal plasma membrane–bound 56 kDa tyrosine kinase called $p56^{lck}$, which is associated with the cytoplasmic tail of CD4 and CD8 molecules. The $p56^{lck}$ is thought to be involved in normal T cell activation. $p56^{lck}$ can be activated by crosslinking CD4, and crosslinking CD4 can lead to tyrosine phosphorylation of the TCR zeta chain.

Role of CD4 and CD8 as Coreceptors

If CD4 and CD8 merely serve to strengthen adhesion between $CD4^+$ or $CD8^+$ cells and MHC class I or II cells, why is the expression of CD4 so tightly linked with recognition of class II molecules, whereas the expression of CD8 is linked with recognition of class I molecules? In order to explain this relationship, it has been suggested that rather than simply functioning as accessory molecules, CD4 or CD8 molecules actually are coreceptors and form a complex with the TCR on the surface of T cells. The result is that a CD4-TCR complex or CD8-TCR complex interacts with the same MHC class II–Ag complex on the antigen presenting cell surface (Fig. 16–5). Colocalization of CD4 and CD8 and the TCR to the same ligand might generate a more potent activating signal, allowing fewer ligands to activate a T cell. In addition, this model would explain the fact that $CD4^+$ cells recognize MHC class II and $CD8^+$ cells recognize MHC class I.

Several types of indirect evidence have been obtained to suggest that CD4 and TCR are associated on the cell surface. First, CD4 antibody inhibits responses induced by some anti-TCR antibodies directed at different TCR epitopes but not others. These data could be explained if the association between CD4 and TCR on the cell surface prevented binding of CD3 antibodies to TCR epitopes closely associated with or covered up by CD4 molecules. Second, some anti-TCR antibodies induce cocapping and comodulation of CD4. However, to date, attempts to coprecipitate CD4 or CD8 complexed to

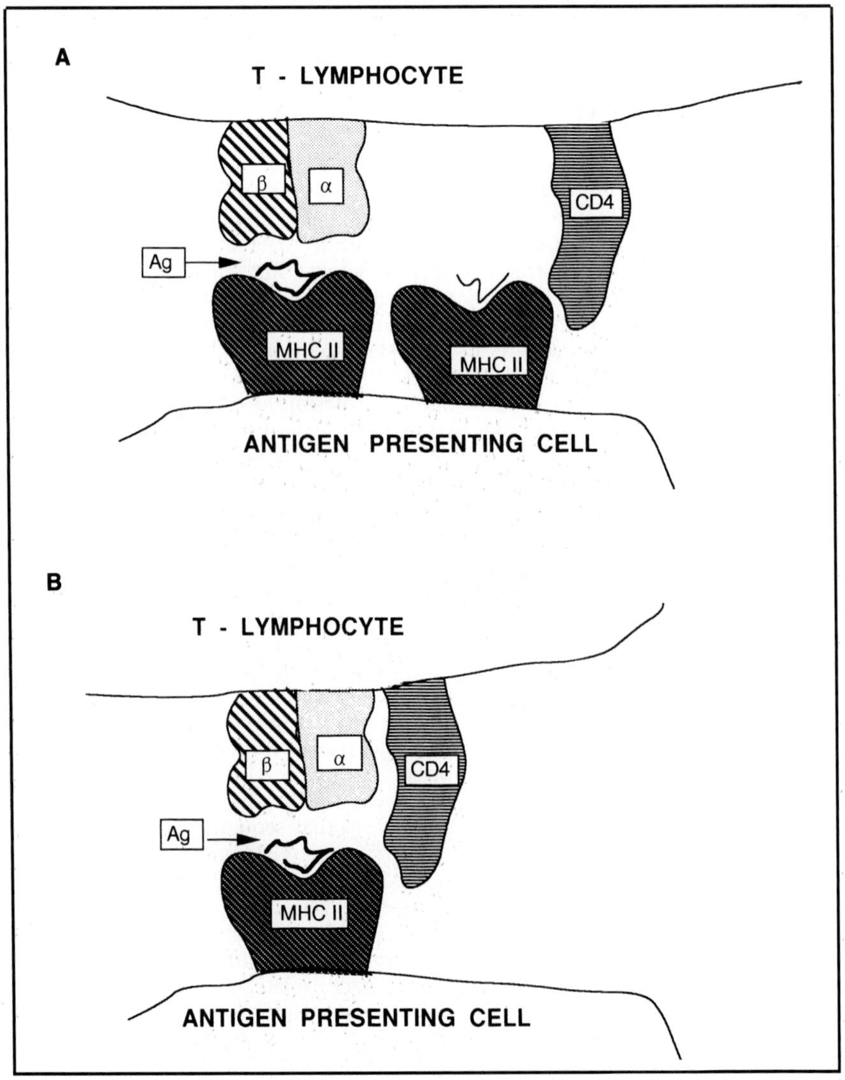

Fig. 16–5. Models contrasting the accessory molecule hypothesis and the coreceptor hypothesis of CD4 function. **A.** In the accessory molecule hypothesis, CD4 and the TCR bind to different MHC class II molecules on an antigen presenting cell (APC). CD4 increases the adhesion of the T cell to the APC, but no signal transduction is mediated by CD4. **B.** In the coreceptor hypothesis, CD4 physically associates with the TCR during antigen–MHC class II ligand recognition. Optimal signaling for T cell activation results from the interaction of CD4 and the TCR with the same Ag–MHC class II complex. *(Adapted from Janeway: Immunol Today 9:234, 1989.)*

TCR on the T cell surface have not been successful. Finally, studies using mutant MHC class I molecules support the model of CD8 function as a coreceptor by associating with the TCR on the T cell surface and forming a complex that binds to MHC class I.

Molecules that Induce T Lymphocyte Activation

Binding of monoclonal antibodies to a number of proteins on the surface of T lymphocytes induces activation of T lymphocytes. Frequently, an antibody must be used in combination with other antibodies or with agents, such as PMA or mitogens, to achieve activation. It is presumed that in these alternative pathways of T cell activation (non-TCR-mediated), the antibody mimics binding of an endogenous physiologic ligand. In some cases, a physiologic ligand has been identified, in some cases not.

CD2

As early as 1972, it was noted that T lymphocytes bind to sheep erythrocytes (sRBC). This phenomenon was used extensively to purify T lymphocytes and study their function. However, the ability to bind sRBC was not simply an epiphenomenon. By the early 1980s, several groups had shown that the same receptor on the surface of T cells that mediated binding to sRBC mediated binding to other cells as well, including targets of CTL. The receptor was originally called the E-rosette receptor. Subsequently, monoclonal antibodies were used to identify the receptor, and it was named T11. Now it is designated CD2, and a large number of antibodies to different epitopes on the molecule are available.

Biochemistry and Tissue Distribution. CD2 is a 50 kDa glycoprotein expressed by T lymphocytes, NK cells, and thymocytes (Table 16–3). The gene for CD2 has been cloned from humans, rats, and mice and has been shown to be a member of the immunoglobulin supergene family. The human gene encodes a polypeptide of 360 amino acids, including three potential N-glycosylation sites and a proline-rich cytoplasmic domain. There is significant homology between the human and rat, especially in the cytoplasmic domain, suggesting a relationship to the function of the molecule. In addition to their ability to block E-rosette formation, CD2 antibodies block binding of T cells to other nucleated cells, binding of cytotoxic T cells to their targets, binding of thymocytes to thymic epithelial cells, and T lymphocyte proliferation to antigens and mitogens. Thus, CD2 is considered an adhesion molecule that mediates T cell interaction with other cells.

Although antibodies to CD2 were first found to inhibit T cell function, primarily by inhibiting T cell interaction with other cells, later studies showed that under certain circumstances, CD2 antibodies can stimulate T cells to proliferate. CD2 expresses at least three different epitopes defined by specific CD2 antibodies ($T11_1$, $T11_2$, $T11_3$). When T cells are incubated with pairs of antibodies that bind to separate epitopes on CD2, T cell proliferation is enhanced (Fig. 16–6). It was postulated that natural ligands for each epitope exist, and through binding of the natural ligands, T cells could be activated by this alternative pathway, exclusive of the CD3-TCR pathway.

LFA-3: A Ligand for CD2. The search to identify the natural ligand for CD2 focused on both sRBC and nucleated cells to which T cells were known to bind using the CD2 molecule. Hunig and colleagues identified an sRBC structure called T11 target structure (T11TS), and Springer and colleagues raised monoclonal antibodies that identified a structure on target cells for CTL. This was called LFA-3 (CD58). CD58 is a highly glycosylated, broadly distributed, 55 to 70 kDa molecule expressed on endothelial, epithelial, and con-

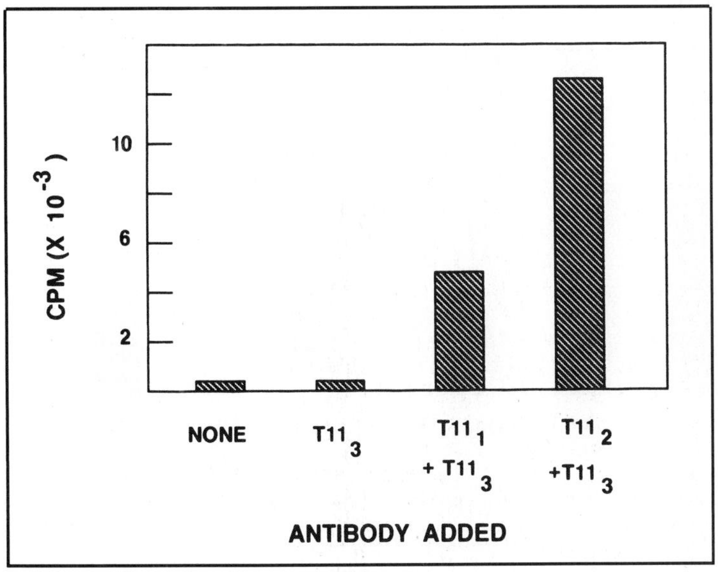

Fig. 16–6. Induction of T cell proliferation by combinations of monoclonal antibodies against distinct epitopes of CD2. Peripheral blood T cells were treated with medium alone or with antibodies as shown for 2 days. Proliferation was measured as cpm ^{3}H-thymidine incorporation after a 15-hour pulse. $T11_1$, $T11_2$, and $T11_3$ refer to antibodies that detect 3 different epitopes of the CD2 (T11) molecule. *(Adapted from Meuer et al: Cell 36:897, 1984.)*

nective tissue cells of most organs and on most blood cells, including erythrocytes (Table 16–3). T11TS is the sheep homologue of CD58.

CD58 antibodies inhibit a number of T cell–dependent functions, including conjugate formation between CTL and target cells. The gene for CD58 has been cloned and encodes a polypeptide backbone of 222 amino acids with a predicted molecular weight of 24 kDa. This is consistent with studies showing that the deglycosylated protein is around 25 kDa. However, deglycosylation studies also revealed two precursor forms of LFA-3, one of 25.5 kDa, the other of 29 kDa. These two precursors have been shown to correlate with two forms of mature LFA-3 expressed on the cells surface. The larger 29 kDa form is a typical membrane-bound form with a transmembrane hydrophobic segment. The smaller 25.5 kDa form can be released from the cell membrane with a phosphatidylinositol-specific phospholipase C (PI-PLC). Thus, the lower molecular weight form is attached to the cell membrane via a glycolipid membrane anchor. Other molecules, especially adhesion molecules and activation molecules, have been found to be attached to the membrane using this mechanism.

The relationship of LFA-3 and CD2 as a ligand pair was supported by studies on CTL binding to targets using antibodies to the three molecules LFA-1, CD2, and LFA-3. LFA-1 and CD2 antibodies inhibited binding by blocking the effector CTL, whereas LFA-3 antibodies blocked the target cell. It thus appeared that LFA-3 might be a ligand for either LFA-1 or CD2. Experiments using combinations of antibodies showed that the combination of CD2 and LFA-3 antibodies was not more inhibitory than either antibody alone (Fig. 16–7). By contrast, combining LFA-3 or CD2 antibodies with LFA-1 antibodies resulted in greater inhibition than using LFA-1 antibodies alone. These data suggested that there were at least two pathways of inhibition, one involving LFA-1 and the other perhaps involving LFA-3 and CD2. Direct confirmation was obtained by the demonstration that purified, ^{125}I-CD2 binds to LFA-3$^+$ cells, and binding is inhibited by antibody to LFA-3. Similarly, CD2$^+$ cells bind to LFA-3-containing planar membranes, and binding is inhibited by CD2 antibodies.

The CD2/LFA-3 ligand pair functions in cell-cell adhesion, and LFA-3 may serve as a naturally occurring ligand to bind T cells through one epitope of the activation antigen CD2. Ligands for other CD2 epitopes include H19, a 19 kDa molecule expressed on monocytes, erythrocytes, and T cells. Together, naturally occurring ligands for CD2 may function to provide activation signals to T cells. Molecular studies have used mutational analyses to identify regions of the CD2 molecule that are detected by different CD2 antibodies. Interestingly, after the cloning of the genes for CD2 and LFA-3, computer-generated comparisons indicated that the two molecules are in fact very similar and both members of the immunoglobulin supergene family. This suggested that the LFA-3/CD2 ligand system may have some similarities to neural cell adhesion molecules (N-CAMs). N-CAMs can exist in both transmembrane and PI-linked forms and are involved in cell-cell interactions mediated by like-like (N-CAM binding to N-CAM) interactions. LFA-3 and CD2 may have diverged from a common ancestral protein.

In addition to CD2-mediated signaling of T cells through CD2, signals can be delivered in the opposite direction; i.e., binding of CD2 to LFA-3 or other ligands can deliver signals to the LFA-3$^+$ cell. Ligand binding to LFA-3 molecules on the surface of epithelial cells of thymus and skin as well as monocytes results in enhanced production of the important immunoregulatory cytokine IL-1 by epithelial cells and monocytes (Table 16–4). LFA-3/CD2-mediated interactions thus provide a regulatory mechanism at the cell surface by which communication between CD2$^+$ T cells and LFA-3$^+$ epithelial cells, monocytes, or other cells can regulate local cytokine production. In the case of thymocyte–thymic epithelial (TE) interactions, this is highly relevant, since thymocytes proliferate in response to IL-1.

Other T Cell–activating Molecules

CD28. The cell surface antigen identified by CD28 antibodies is a disulfide-linked homodimer of heavily glycosylated 44 kDa subunits with a polypeptide backbone of 23 kDa. CD28

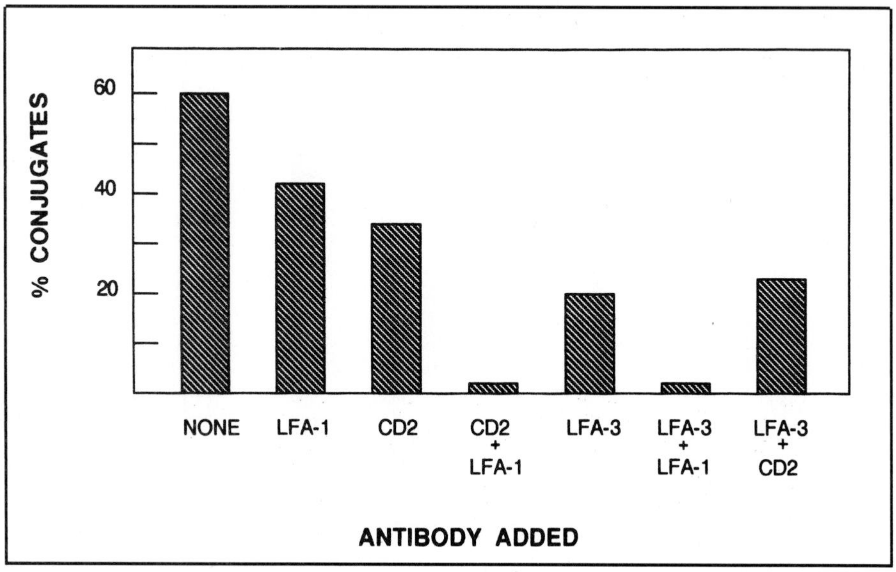

Fig. 16–7. Antibody inhibition of antigen-independent conjugate formation of CTL clones (anti-DPw2 specific) with target U266 (DPw2$^-$). CTL were pretreated with MAb directed against the antigens indicated along the abscissa before addition of target cells. Both cell types were labeled with fluorochromes, and conjugation was determined by flow cytometry. *(Adapted from Shaw et al: Nature 323:262, 1986.)*

TABLE 16–4. Anti-LFA-3 Monoclonal Antibody Augments IL-1 Release by Thymic Epithelial Cells

	Thymocyte Comitogenic Activity (Δcpm)[a]		
Experiment	No Ab	Control Ab	Anti-LFA-3 Ab
1	10,200	10,859	53,893
2	11,470	19,011	35,011
3	25,580	20,580	42,161

Adapted from Le et al: *J Immunol* 144:4541, 1990.

[a] Cultured human thymic epithelial (TE) cells were incubated without antibody or with control antibody or anti-LFA-3 Ab for 40 hours. Supernatants were harvested and assayed for IL-1 activity. The assay for IL-1 activity measures uptake of ^{3}H-thymidine by mouse thymocytes in the presence of submitogenic concentrations of phytohemagglutinin (PHA). Data are expressed as Δcpm (i.e., cpm ^{3}H-thymidine incorporation by thymocytes in the presence of TE supernatants plus PHA − cpm incorporated by thymocytes in the presence of PHA alone).

is a member of the Ig superfamily and is expressed on 95% of peripheral CD4$^+$ cells, 50% of peripheral CD8$^+$ cells, and a variable number of resting thymocytes, including most mature thymocytes (Table 16–3). The B cell activation antigen B7/BB1 has been identified as a natural ligand for CD28. CD28 antibody induces proliferation of peripheral blood T lymphocytes if PMA is present as a costimulator. Mature thymocytes that do not proliferate in response to combinations of CD2 antibodies do proliferate to CD2 antibodies in combination with an antibody to CD28. Activation through CD28 results in stabilization of lymphokine mRNA. Thus, interaction between CD28 and B7/BB1 may serve to regulate T cell cytokine levels at sites of B cell activation. CD28 antibodies also can partially block autologous and allogeneic mixed lymphocyte reactions.

CD45 (LCA,T200). CD45 is a family of membrane glycoproteins ranging from 180 to 240 kDa found in some form on all hematopoietic cells except erythrocytes and their progenitors. CD45 is complex with 6 to 8 isoforms differentially expressed on subpopulations of cells. The isoforms differ in primary structure as a result of alternative splicing of mRNA. They also differ in their pattern of glycosylation. There are several phosphorylation sites on the cytoplasmic domain of CD45. The cytoplasmic portion of CD45 is highly homologous to the protein tyrosine phosphatase 1B from human placenta, and CD45 can function as a protein tyrosine phosphatase. CD45 inhibits signal transduction, and this may occur via dephosphorylation of tyrosyl residues, such as those on the zeta chain of CD3. CD45 can also enhance CD4-mediated signaling.

Thy-1. Thy-1 has been used for many years as a marker for murine peripheral T cells and thymocytes. In the mouse, Thy-1 is also expressed on fibroblasts, epithelial cells, and neurons (Table 16–3). Mouse Thy-1 is a glycoprotein of 25 to 30 kDa and is expressed as two alleles Thy-1.1 and Thy-1.2, which differ by a single amino acid substitution. Thy-1 is a member of the Ig supergene family and is anchored to the cell membrane via a phosphatidylinositol linkage rather than by the conventional transmembrane linkage. Polyclonal antibodies to Thy-1 stimulate production of IL-2 and proliferation of murine T cells. Some monoclonal antibodies to Thy-1 also induce murine T cell production of IL-2 and proliferation. Expression of Thy-1 varies greatly between species, and Thy-1 is not found on rat and human peripheral T cells. In the rat, thymocytes express Thy-1, but in the human they do not. Since human T cells do not express the equivalent of mouse Thy-1, Thy-1 is probably not a T cell accessory molecule in humans. However, this does not exclude the possibility that in humans another molecule subserves the same function that Thy-1 does in mice.

Ly-6 or T Cell–activating Protein (TAP). Another surface molecule that may serve an accessory function is Ly-6 or TAP/TAPa. This complex set of molecules was identified originally in mice, and more recently a probable human homologue has been identified. It has been proposed that the mouse Ly-6 locus may control as many as seven distinct alloantigens. The ability of antibodies to Ly-6 to induce T cell activation has been demonstrated and requires both crosslinking of the antibodies on the cell surface and the addition of PMA as a costimulator.

Adhesion Molecules that Mediate Lymphocyte Migration

Recirculation and Inflammation

The ability of lymphocytes to recirculate is essential to the functioning of the immune system. Recirculation enhances immune surveillance by maximizing the potential for interaction between an antigen and the rare lymphocytes that recognize it. During an inflammatory response, lymphocytes along with other leukocytes, i.e., monocytes and neutrophils, migrate into lymphoid and nonlymphoid tissues, where they participate in the host response to infectious agents and, in some cases, are responsible for tissue damage as seen in hypersensitivity reactions (Chap. 19).

Leukocyte entry into tissues (extravasation) is mediated by cell-cell interactions with the vascular endothelium and involves binding of molecules on the surface of leukocytes to molecules on the surface of endothelial cells. Recirculation of lymphocytes into lymphoid organs (homing) is mediated by adhesion molecules on the surface of lymphocytes (homing receptors). These homing receptors bind to tissue-specific ligands called *vascular addressins* that are expressed on the surface of cells lining a specialized postcapillary venule, the high endothelial venule (HEV).

Cell Surface Molecules that Mediate Homing and Migration into Tissues

An in vitro assay developed by Woodruff and colleagues has been used to demonstrate organ-specific interactions between lymphocytes and vascular endothelial cells. In this assay, viable lymphocytes bind to HEV on tissue sections of lymphoid organs (Fig. 16–8). With the use of antibodies to inhibit this binding, several different lymphocyte–endothelial cell recognition systems have been described. Several molecules that participate in these interactions have been grouped in the

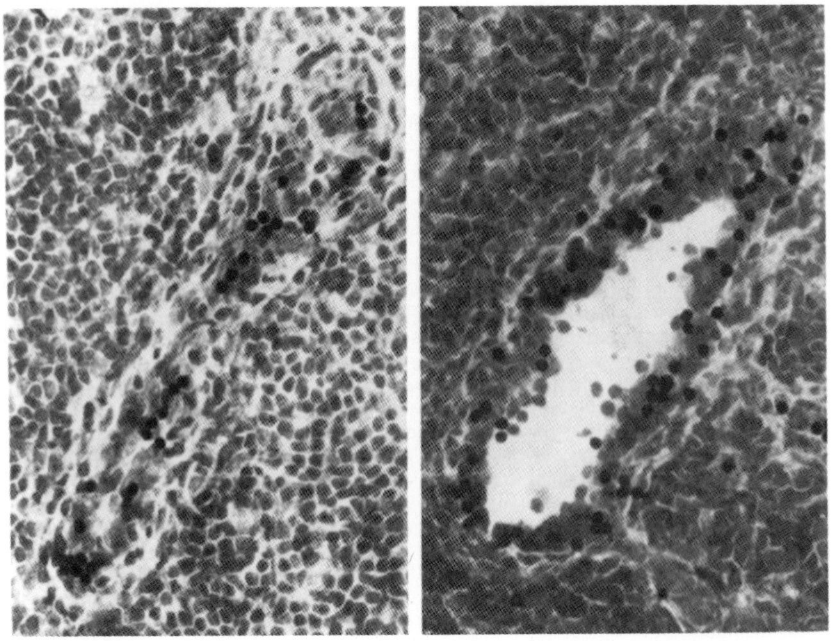

Fig. 16–8. Thoracic duct lymphocytes bind to HEV in sections of rat lymph nodes. The darkly stained cells above the plane of the tissue section are adherent overlaid lymphocytes. Most of the lymphoid cells bind at the endothelium of HEV. × 400. *(From Stamper and Woodruff: J Immunol 119:772, 1977.)*

selectin (LEC-CAM) family of adhesion molecules (Table 16–5).

The Selectin (LEC-CAM) Family of Adhesion Molecules. The first LEC-CAM described was the MEL-14 antigen. The monoclonal antibody MEL-14 was shown to inhibit mouse lymphocyte binding to HEV of peripheral lymph nodes. Expression of the MEL-14 epitope correlates with binding and recirculatory efficiency in lymphocytes; that is, high MEL-14 expression is associated with efficient binding to lymph node HEV in vitro and recirculation in vivo. MEL-14 antibody recognizes a highly glycosylated 85–95 kDa glycoprotein with an unusually low isoelectric point of 4.0 to 4.5.

The human homologue of the mouse lymphocyte homing receptor identified by the MEL-14 antibody is LAM-1 ($gp90^{MEL}$, TQ1, Leu-8). Other members of the LEC-CAM family are the human endothelial leukocyte adhesion molecule-1 (ELAM-1), which is expressed on activated endothelial cells, and the human granule-membrane protein (GMP-140, PADGEM, CD62), which is expressed on activated platelets and endothelial cells and mediates binding of platelets and endothelial cells to neutrophils. These proteins have an interesting structure. They contain an amino terminal lectinlike domain followed by an epidermal growth factor–like domain and a variable number of short consensus repeat sequences homologous to those found in complement-binding proteins. Members of the LEC-CAM family are involved in selective cell trafficking, mediated through binding of specific carbohydrate ligands to their lectinlike domains. The genes encoding LAM-1 and GMP-140 are on the same region of chromosome 1, suggesting that they arose from a common evolutionary precursor.

LAM-1 and MEL-14 share considerable amino acid sequence homology. LAM-1 is expressed only on lymphocytes, neutrophils, and monocytes and previously was detected using antibodies Leu-8 and TQ1. LAM-1 and MEL-14 are rapidly modulated from the cell surface after activation of neutrophils and lymphocytes.

ELAM-1 is expressed on the surface of endothelial cells treated with cytokines. ELAM-1 is important for the accumulation of lymphocytes at sites of inflammation by mediating adhesion of cells to the vascular lining. Thus, not only do the LEC-CAMs play a role in normal recirculation of lymphocytes, but some members also are likely to play a role in migration of leukocytes into tissues as part of the inflammatory response.

To mediate binding of leukocytes to vascular endothelial

TABLE 16–5. TISSUE DISTRIBUTION AND FUNCTION OF MEMBERS OF THE SELECTION FAMILY OF ADHESION MOLECULES

Molecule	Other Names	Tissue Distribution	Function
LAM-1/MEL-14	$gp90^{MEL}$, TQ1/Leu-8, LECAM1, Ly22	Leukocytes	Adhesion, lymphocyte homing
ELAM-1	LECAM2	Transiently expressed on vascular endothelium induced by IL-1, TNF	Adhesion
GMP-140	PADGEM, LECAM3, CD62	Platelet α granules, endothelial cell Weibel-Palade bodies, surface of activated platelets and endothelial cells	Adhesion

cells, homing receptors must recognize specific structures on the surface of the vascular endothelial cells. Several candidates for such target structures have been described. Monoclonal antibodies have been raised that selectively recognize molecules expressed on HEV in mucosal lymphoid tissue and HEV in peripheral lymph nodes. These molecules have been called *addressins.* It is likely that the selectins bind to the addressins by virtue of their lectin binding domains, and research in this area is focusing on the sugar specificity of the selectins.

CD44. Another molecule, CD44, has been implicated in the binding of lymphocytes to HEVs in a variety of tissues. The CD44 molecule was described in several different systems, and after the cloning of the CD44 gene, it became apparent that it encoded molecules that had been named Pgp-1, In(Lu)-related p80, Hermes, ECMR-III, and HUTCH-1. CD44 antibodies inhibit the binding of lymphocytes to HEV, suggesting that lymphocyte CD44 is involved in organ-specific lymphocyte homing. CD44 antibodies also augment T cell proliferation to other stimuli, and CD44 regulates other adhesion molecule-mediated interactions, most specifically CD2/LFA-3. Antibodies to CD44 enhance production of the immunoregulatory cytokine IL-1 by epithelial cells and monocytes. CD44 is the primary receptor for hyaluronate.

Summary

Adhesion of leukocytes to other cells and to the extracellular matrix is critically important for many aspects of the immune response, and adhesion is mediated by cell surface molecules. In addition to their adhesive function, many of these molecules also can play a role in either positive or negative signaling of leukocytes. The majority of the accessory/coreceptor molecules are members of the integrin, immunoglobulin, and selectin families. The integrin family includes the three leukocyte cell adhesion molecules (Leu-CAM)—LFA-1, Mac-1, and p150,95—and a series of receptors for extracellular matrix proteins. The immunoglobulin superfamily, in addition to immunoglobulin and the antigen-specific T cell receptor, includes the T cell coreceptor molecules CD4 and CD8, the T cell–activation antigen CD2 and its ligand LFA-3, and the T cell–activation molecules CD28 and Thy-1. In addition, the ligands ICAM-1, ICAM-2, and VCAM-1 also are members of the Ig family. Finally, the selectin family includes the MEL-14/LAM-1 and ELAM-1 molecules involved in leukocyte migration and homing, as well as the platelet adhesion molecule GMP-140. In addition to these recognized families, several other molecules not yet grouped into families play accessory roles, including the CD44 molecule and the leukocyte common antigen, CD45. Adhesion mediated by many of these molecules is under tight regulation, since it is advantageous to cells to make a rapid transition from a nonadherent to an adherent state and vice versa.

FURTHER READING

Books and Review Articles

Anderson DC, Springer TA: Leukocyte adhesion deficiency: An inherited defect in the Mac-1, LFA-1, and p150,95 glycoproteins. Annu Rev Med 38:175, 1987

Berke G: Functions and mechanisms of lysis induced by cytotoxic T lymphocytes and natural killer cells. In Paul WE (ed): Fundamental Immunology. New York, Raven Press, 1989, p. 735

Bierer BE, Burakoff SJ: T-lymphocyte activation: The biology and function of CD2 and CD4. Immunol Rev 111:267, 1989

Edelman GM: CAMs and Igs: Cell adhesion and the evolutionary origins of immunity. Immunol Rev 100:11, 1987

Ford WL, Gowans JL: The traffic of lymphocytes. Semin Hematol 6:67, 1969

Haynes BF, Telen MJ, Hale LP, Denning SM: CD44—A molecule involved in leukocyte adherence and T-cell activation. Immunol Today 10:423, 1989

Hemler M: VLA proteins in the integrin family: Structure, function and their role on leukocytes. Annu Rev Immunol 8:365, 1990

Hynes R: Integrins. A family of cell surface receptors. Cell 48:549, 1987

Janeway C: The role of CD4 in T cell activation: Accessory molecule or coreceptor? Immunol Today 10:234, 1989

Rudd CD, Anderson P, Morimoto C, et al: Molecular interactions, T-cell subsets and a role of the CD4/CD8:p56^{lck} complex in human T-cell activation. Immunol Rev 111:225, 1989

Ruoslahti E, Pierschbacher MD: New perspectives in cell adhesion: RGD and integrins. Science 238:491, 1987

Singer KH: Interactions between epithelial cells and T lymphocytes: Role of adhesion molecules. J Leukocyte Biol 48:367, 1990

Springer TA: Adhesion receptors of the immune system. Nature 346:425, 1990

Springer TA, Dustin ML, Kishimoto TK, Marlin SD: The lymphocyte function-associated LFA-1, CD2 and LFA-3 molecules: Cell adhesion receptors of the immune system. Annu Rev Immunol 5:223, 1987

Thomas ML, Lefrancois L: Differential expression of the leukocyte-common antigen family. Immunol Today 8:320, 1988

Yednock TA, Rosen SD: Lymphocyte homing. Adv Immunol 44:313, 1989

Articles

Bevilacqua M, Stengelin S, Gimbrone M, Seed B: Endothelial leukocyte adhesion molecule 1: An inducible receptor for neutrophils related to complement regulatory proteins and lectins. Science 243:1160, 1989

Davignon D, Martz E, Reynolds T, et al: Monoclonal antibody to a novel lymphocyte function–associated antigen (LFA-1): Mechanism of blockade of T lymphocyte-mediated killing and effects on other T and B lymphocyte functions. J Immunol 127:590, 1981

Doyle C, Strominger JL: Interaction between CD4 and class II MHC molecules mediates cell adhesion. Nature 330:256, 1987

Dustin ML, Springer TA: T-cell receptor cross-linking transiently stimulates adhesiveness through LFA-1. Nature 341:619, 1989

Greve JM, Davis G, Mayer AM, et al: The major human rhinovirus receptor is ICAM-1. Cell 56:839, 1989

Haskard D, Cavender D, Beatty P, et al: T lymphocyte adhesion to endothelial cells: Mechanisms demonstrated by anti-LFA-1 monoclonal antibody. J Immunol 137:2901, 1986

Hemler ME, Sanchez-Madrid F, Flotte TJ, et al: Glycoproteins of 210,000 and 130,000 MW on activated T cells: Cell distribution and antigenic relation to components on resting cells and T cell lines. J Immunol 132:3011, 1984

Keizer GD, Visser W, Vliem M, Figdor CG: A monoclonal antibody (NKI-L16) directed against a unique epitope on the α-chain of human leukocyte function-associated antigen 1 induces homotypic cell-cell interactions. J Immunol 140:1393, 1988

Meuer S, Hussey R, Fabbi M, et al: An alternative pathway of T-cell activation: A functional role for the 50 Kd T11 sheep erythrocyte receptor protein. Cell 36:897, 1984

Salter RD, Benjamin RJ, Wesley PK, et al: A binding site for the T cell co-receptor CD8 on the α_3 domain of HLA-A2. Nature 345:41, 1990

Stamper HB, Woodruff JJ: An in vitro model of lymphocyte homing. I. Characterization of the interaction between thoracic duct lymphocytes and specialized high endothelial venules of lymph nodes. J Immunol 119:772, 1977

Yang SY, Denning SM, Mizuno S, et al: A novel activation pathway for mature thymocytes. Costimulation of CD2 (T,p50) and CD28 (T,p44) induces autocrine interleukin 2/interleukin 2 receptor-mediated cell proliferation. J Exp Med 168:1457, 1988

CHAPTER 17

Immunopathology

Immunopathology is the study of diseases caused by host immunologic processes. Immunologically mediated diseases may exhibit a spectrum of systemic or organ-specific clinical manifestations. It is interesting to note how many diseases formerly considered idiopathic are now known to be immunopathologic in nature. Many other common diseases, such as type I diabetes, are also being found to have important immunologic components.

The immune system plays a protective role for the host against infection, tumors, and other toxic agents. This chapter deals with inflammatory and immune responses that cause injury to the host. The sequence of events leading to an immunologically mediated inflammatory reaction generally involves (1) binding of a recognition component (e.g., antibody, cell receptor) to an antigen, resulting in (2) the activation or release of immune effector molecules, which act to (3) produce a local inflammatory reaction by altering vascular permeability, increasing vascular stasis, and chemotactically attracting and activating immune effector cells. Because these processes have evolved primarily to provide for host defense against infectious organisms and the elimination of dead, injured, or neoplastic cells (as well as toxins), they are of necessity highly destructive and may affect normal tissues as innocent bystanders. Not infrequently, these reactions are directed at host components that harbor infectious agents or express determinants that resemble foreign antigens. Moreover, inflammatory responses are influenced and regulated by a large number of complex cellular and molecular mechanisms, and alterations or perturbations affecting any of these factors can lead to inappropriate reactions. Thus, immune mechanisms can injure or destroy host tissues for a variety of reasons and cause a number of important and diverse types of inflammatory and autoimmune diseases.

Understanding how inflammation is initiated and regulated is thus essential for understanding immunopathologic processes as well as immunologically mediated host defense. This chapter reviews the mechanisms of inflammation and conditions related to abnormal (pathologic) immune responses, with specific emphasis on several important hypersensitivity and autoimmune diseases.

Mechanisms of Inflammation

Inflammatory Cells

A wide range of cells participate in inflammatory responses, with macrophages, lymphocytes, and granulocytes playing the dominant role. Other cells, such as vascular endothelial cells, platelets, basophils, and mast cells, also are involved, especially in the production of inflammatory molecules. The major inflammatory cell types differ to some extent in several characteristics: antigen recognition, trafficking, activation, and effector function.

Antigen Recognition

Although antigen specificity is a hallmark of the immune response, all of the cells in the immune system express antigen-nonspecific receptors that are capable of initiating or modifying immune responses (Table 17–1). These include receptors for monokines, lymphokines, the constant region of immunoglobulins, and complement breakdown products. Immune responses usually are initiated by antigen presenting cells (APC), which typically are macrophages or dendritic cells of the mononuclear-phagocyte system that constitutively express class II major histocompatibility complex (MHC) antigens (Chap. 13). These cells can recognize a wide range of antigens using a variety of surface proteins and receptors, with the MHC antigens themselves playing an important direct role in antigen binding. Different APCs can express different levels of class II (as well as class I) MHC antigens, which affect their ability to bind antigen or present it in an immunogenic fashion.

The type of APC that reacts with a given antigen depends on the portal of entry and the chemical characteristics of the antigen. For example, antigens that enter through the skin usually attach to the surface of Langerhans cells. These cells cannot phagocytize large molecules but instead are specialized for transporting small molecules to regional draining lymph nodes to initiate immune reactions. In contrast, antigens that enter the respiratory or gastrointestinal tracts initially are exposed to the substantial macrophage-phagocyte systems of the lung (alveolar macrophages) and liver (Kupffer cells). Antigens that escape these defenses or enter the systemic circulation directly are likely to be phagocytized by splenic macrophages. Several specialized macrophages are located in different compartments of the spleen, and the distribution of antigen among these macrophages is determined by certain characteristics of the antigen (e.g., charge, size).

Lymphocyte recognition of antigen is mediated by a variety of surface receptors, including some that are on other leukocytes. However, in contrast to all other cells involved in inflammation, lymphocytes alone express receptors that have antigen specificity (Chaps. 12 and 13). For T lymphocytes, the clonotypic αβ T cell receptor (TCR) is associated with the CD3 complex and recognizes antigen plus autologous MHC proteins, that is, MHC restricted or associative recognition of antigen. Helper T cells generally recognize foreign antigen together with self–class II MHC antigens and express the CD4 receptor, which itself binds to a common class II MHC antigenic determinant. Cytotoxic or suppressor T lymphocytes usually are class I MHC restricted and express the CD8 receptor, which binds to a common class I MHC determinant. Thus, the recognition system of T lymphocytes selects the antigenic specificity and, to some extent, the function and cell binding properties of the responding T cell population. In contrast, B cells recognize antigenic determinants alone by means of surface immunoglobulin as a receptor.

Although T and B lymphocytes synthesize their own antigen-specific receptor molecules, they can be activated by antigen-nonspecific stimuli, such as various viral and bacterial products. Moreover, antigen-specific immune responses usually result in the release of lymphokines, immunoglobulins, and complement breakdown products, which themselves may act locally to expand the inflammatory response in an antigen-nonspecific manner. The recruitment and expansion of antigen-nonspecific cells can be so efficient that antigen-specific cells sometimes constitute only a small percentage of cells at the site of inflammation.

Granulocytes and mast cells are other leukocytes that often are involved in inflammatory reactions but do not express antigen-specific receptors (as do lymphocytes) or class II MHC molecules (as do macrophages and APC). However, like macrophages and lymphocytes, they can recognize antigen indirectly via receptors for immunoglobulin or complement products that may be bound to antigens.

Trafficking and Activation

The accumulation and activation of inflammatory cells at sites of antigen deposition are central to the inflammatory process. To accumulate at sites of inflammation, leukocytes emigrate from the blood (diapedesis), a process that requires their binding to vascular endothelium and subsequent migration through gaps between endothelial cells. The binding of leukocytes to endothelial cells is mediated by adhesion molecules present on both cell types, a process that can be upregulated by inflammatory stimuli (see below and Chap. 16). Lymphocytes, while motile, do not respond to the same chemotactic factors as do polymorphonuclear leukocytes (PMN) and macrophages. The migration of lymphocytes is stimulated primarily by cytokines produced by other lymphocytes.

Macrophages and PMN are motile phagocytic cells that can perceive gradients of molecules with chemotactic activity

TABLE 17–1. RECEPTORS OF IMMUNOCOMPETENT HUMAN LEUKOCYTES

Cell Type	Antigen-Specific	Fc Receptors	Complement Receptors	Cytokine Receptors
Macrophages/APC		FcγRI, FcγRII, FcγRIII, FcεRII	CR1, CR3, C1q, C5a	IL-2, IL-3, IL-4, IFN-γ, TNF_{α}
Lymphocytes				
T helper cells	TCR	(Fcμ)[a]	(C5a)[a]	IL-1, IL-2, IL-10
T cytotoxic/suppressor cells	TCR	(FcγRIII)[a]	(CR1)[a]	IL-1, IL-2
B cells	sIg	FcμR, FcγRII, FcαR	CR1, CR2, C1q	IL-1, IL-2, IL-4, IL-5, IL-6, IFN-γ
Granulocytes				
Neutrophils		FcγRII, FcγRIII, FcαR	CR1, CR3, C1q, C3a/4a, C5a	IL-1, IL-8
Eosinophils		FcγRII, FcγRIII, FcεRII FcμR	CR1, C3a/4a, C5a	IL-1, IL-5
Basophils		FcεRI	CR1, C5a	IL-1, IL-8
Mast cells		FcεRI	CR1, C5a, C3a/4a	IL-3, IL-4

[a] Not an absolute correlation.

by means of specific surface receptors. Proinflammatory chemoattractants include formylpeptides, which are analogous to bacterial products, a cleavage component of the fifth component of complement (C5a), leukotriene B_4 (LTB_4), platelet activity factor (PAF), interleukin 8 (IL-8), and other cytokines. Interaction with chemoattractants can result in activation and directional migration of leukocytes, as well as the upregulation of adhesion molecules and enhanced binding to endothelial cells. The binding of chemoattractants to the surface of phagocytes results in their loss of a normally round configuration. They become triangular, with the base of the triangle facing toward the chemoattractant gradient. This change in cell shape requires rearrangement of intracellular cytoskeletal elements. Microtubules provide a front-to-back polarization, and actin filaments accumulate at the front and back of the cells to provide the contractile forces required for movement.

Following the binding of chemotactic factors to their receptors on phagocytic cells, a series of biochemical events is initiated that lead to either chemotaxis (and associated shape changes) or the activation of the respiratory burst, production of superoxide anions, and secretion of lysosomal enzymes. Chemoattractant receptors initiate these events by interacting with a membrane-associated guanine nucleotide regulatory protein termed $G_{i\alpha2}$. G proteins couple membrane-associated receptors to their effector enzymes (e.g., adenylate cyclase for β-adrenergic receptors). The binding of chemoattractants to their receptors activates $G_{i\alpha2}$, which then complexes with a membrane-associated phospholipase C and hydrolyzes the membrane phospholipid termed phosphatidylinositol 4,5-bisphosphate (PIP_2). This process leads to the production of two second messengers, 1,2-diacylglycerol (DAG) and inositol 1,4,5-trisphosphate (IP_3). The former activates protein kinase C, and the second mobilizes intracellular calcium. These events are critical for leukocyte activation by chemoattractants, since their blockage (e.g., by *Bordetella pertussis* toxin, which inactivates $G_{i\alpha2}$) inhibits all leukocyte responses to chemoattractants. The activation of phospholipase C by chemoattractants occurs rapidly and is associated with motility-related cellular events.

Activation of the respiratory burst and secretion of lysosomal enzymes requires additional biochemical events that can be initiated by sustained activation of the receptor in the presence of higher concentrations of chemoattractant. These events appear to result in the enhanced permeability of the leukocyte to calcium, allowing a more prolonged intracellular calcium mobilization. Sustained production of phosphatydic acid and DAG through activation of phospholipase D and hydrolysis of phosphotidylcholine promotes initiation of the respiratory burst (Fig. 17–1).

As mentioned, chemotactic factors can, in addition to stimulating direct migration, initiate cytotoxic responses by PMN. Cytotoxic activity includes the production of superoxide anions and other toxic oxygen metabolites and secretion of lysosomal constituents. The concentration of chemotactic factors required to initiate cytotoxicity is approximately 20-fold higher than that required for the induction of chemotaxis. This threshold may be important in preventing the release of potentially toxic products from the cells until they arrive at an inflammatory site.

The migration of leukocytes through vessel walls first requires their binding to the vascular endothelium, which is mediated by a variety of adhesion molecules that currently are grouped into families (Chap. 16). The integrin family of adhesion molecules is expressed on leukocytes and consists of heterodimers of α and β chains. One subfamily using the β_1 chain is termed the *very late antigens* (VLA); another uses the β_2 chain (CD18), and a third, the β_3 chain. Whereas some integrins, such as LFA-1 (CD11a/CD18), are expressed on all leukocytes, others show more restricted expression. For example, the heterodimers of CR3 (C11b/CD18), and gp150/95 (CD11c/CD18) normally are expressed on only phagocytes and large granular lymphocytes. T cells express several adhesion molecules, including CD2, CD4, CD8, LFA-1, VLA-1, VLA-2, LAM-1, and CD44.

Vascular endothelial cells also express a variety of adhesion molecules and receptors. These include intercellular adhesion molecule (ICAM)-1, which is inducible on a variety of other cells, inducible cell adhesion molecule (INCAM)-110, vascular cell adhesion molecule (VCAM)-1, and at least two members of the LEC-CAM family of adhesion molecules: endothelial-leukocyte adhesion molecule (ELAM)-1, and

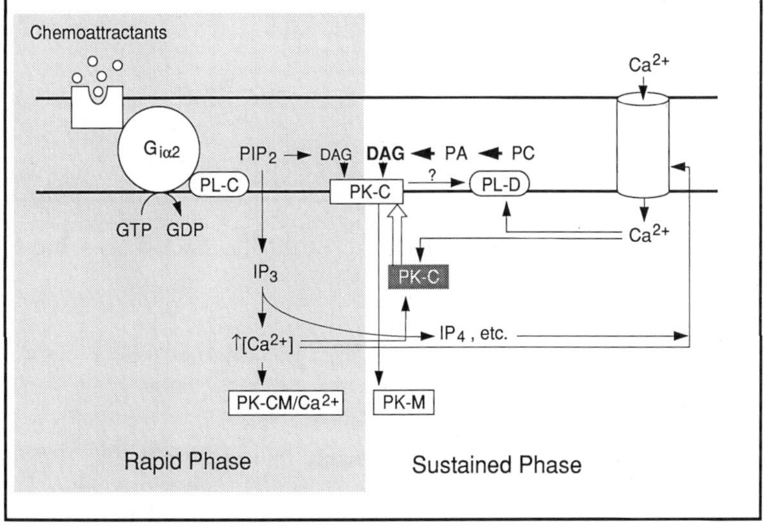

Fig. 17–1. Model for regulation of phagocyte activation. As determined from the data presented, products from the rapid phase initiate activation of the sustained phase pathway. Solid arrows indicate activation; stippled area indicates inhibition. PL-C, phospholipase C; PK-C, protein kinase C; PK-CM/CA^{2+}, calcium-calmodulin-dependent protein kinase; PK-M, phospholipid-independent form of protein kinase C; PA, phosphatidic acid; PC, phosphatidylcholine; PL-D, phospholipase D. *(From Snyderman et al. In Moss (ed): ADP Ribosylating Toxins and G Proteins: Insights into Signal Transduction. American Society for Microbiology, 1990, pp 295–323.)*

GMP-140, which is expressed on activated endothelial cells and platelets. These molecules also exhibit differential specificity: ICAM-1 binds LFA-1 and, therefore, all leukocytes, whereas ELAM-1 binds neutrophils and INCAM-110 binds lymphocytes. LHR (also termed LAM-1/MEL-14 in the mouse, and Leu-8/TQ1 in humans) serves as a leukocyte homing receptor for high endothelial venules (HEV) and is important for T cell recirculation from the blood to lymph. GMP-140 (CD62) is expressed primarily on platelets, venules, and small veins and is important in platelet aggregation.

The expression of various adhesion receptors and ligands can be regulated by different inflammatory reactions and soluble mediators. In particular, activated T cells express CD11b, CD11c, and HLA-DR. Interferon-gamma (IFN-γ) can upregulate HLA-DR and ICAM-1 expression on endothelial cells, and IL-1, tumor necrosis factor $(TNF)_\alpha$ and lymphotoxin (also termed TNF_β) can stimulate ELAM-1 and ICAM-1 expression on vascular endothelial cells. The importance of these molecules is best demonstrated by physiologic and pathologic consequences after their altered expression. Numerous reports have demonstrated that normal leukocyte responses can be inhibited significantly in vitro by blocking these molecules. Various clinical immunodeficiency syndromes are associated with their absence in vivo.

As discussed in detail in Chapter 13, activation of lymphocytes generally involves an antigen-specific as well as a second signal, usually provided by a cytokine. For T cells, the antigen-specific signal is provided by ligand binding to the clonotypic receptor complex, whereas surface immunoglobulin serves as the antigen-specific receptor for B lymphocyte stimulation. An additional cytokine signal generally is needed for lymphocyte activation: IL-1 (from APCs) for T helper cells, IL-2 (from T helper cells) for T cytotoxic cells, and IL-4 (from T helper cells) for B cells. Under some circumstances, activation of these lymphocyte populations may occur by extensive crosslinking of antigen-specific receptors with complex antigens having many similar determinants (e.g., B cells with lipopolysaccharide).

Effector Function

Macrophages provide an important constitutive defense against infection (Chap. 19) and can act as inflammatory effector cells in addition to serving as APC to initiate specific immune responses. Nonimmunologic inflammatory stimuli can increase many macrophage functions, but complete activation of macrophages occurs as a result of their interaction with lymphokines, products of complement activation, or IFN-γ. Activated macrophages become larger, spread more quickly, and adhere more firmly to surfaces, whereas phagocytosis of particulate matter coated with immunoglobulin and complement fragments increases (Fig. 17–2), as does pinocytosis. In addition, macrophages secrete an array of biologically and immunologically active products (Table 17–2), including cellular growth and differentiation factors, cytokines that stimulate acute phase reactions, arachidonic acid metabolites that have local and systemic inflammatory effects, and numerous toxic compounds that cause direct tissue injury. Feedback stimulation by lymphokines produced by T cells also causes an increase in microbicidal and tumoricidal activity of macrophages.

Lymphocytes, on activation, exhibit a variety of functions that contribute to inflammatory responses. T lymphocytes, in particular, produce a variety of inflammatory mediators (Table 17–3). Helper T lymphocytes produce multiple lymphokines that promote proliferation, activation, or both, of other T cells (e.g., IL-2), B cells (e.g., IL-4, IL-5, IL-6), macrophages (e.g., IFN-γ), and granulocytes and mast cells (e.g., IL-3, IL-5). Some of these stimulatory lymphokines are counterbalanced by suppressive factors produced by T cells (e.g., TGF_β and IL-10). In addition, cytotoxic T cells can attach directly to target cells and lyse them by the release of serine esterases, lymphotoxin (TNF_β), and pore-forming protein (perforin), which is similar to the membrane attack complex of complement. In humoral immune responses, B lymphocytes differentiate into plasma cells and produce large quantities of antibodies, which can initiate a variety of inflammatory reactions (Chap. 12).

Granulocytes are activated via their Fc and complement receptors. All of the members of the granulocyte family have receptors for C3a, C5a, C3b (CR1), iC3b (CR3), and the Fc portion of IgG (FcγRIII). Mast cells, basophils, and eosinophils also have Fc receptors for IgE (FcϵRI). When two surface bound IgE antibodies on mast cells are crosslinked by binding to antigen, a spectrum of preformed and newly synthesized mediators is released (see below). C3a and C5a, the anaphylatoxic products of complement activation, also can cause degranulation. Neutrophils are more versatile in that they are also capable of phagocytosis and internal microbicidal activity. As with macrophages, neutrophil phagocytosis is greatly augmented by the presence of IgG and complement components on the microbial surface.

Platelets are another pharmacologically potent cell with Fc receptors for IgG and IgE. Platelets can release chemotactic factors as well as vasoconstrictors. Moreover, early complement components (C1q, C4, C2, and C3) are present on the platelet surface and, on activation, cause the release of C3a and C3b. Thus, antibody-directed platelet binding can secondarily activate the complement cascade as well as initiate thrombosis.

Inflammatory Molecules

Inflammatory reactions result from the local release of a number of mediators derived from humoral or cellular sources (Tables 17–2 and 17–3). A complex interplay of stimulatory and suppressive mechanisms modulates the type and magnitude of the inflammatory response that develops.

Lipid Mediators

Phospholipids are major constituents of cell membranes (including those of leukocytes and platelets) and are subject to degradation by cellular phospholipases under certain conditions, such as exposure of cells to inflammatory or toxic stimuli. Cleavage of phospholipids results in the release of arachidonic acid, which can be further metabolized into a number of biologically potent mediators and modulators of inflammation. The enzymes cyclooxygenase and lipoxygenase initiate the two major pathways of arachidonic acid metabolism. Prostaglandins (PG) are synthesized from arachidonic acid after the action of cyclooxygenase, forming PGG_2, which is then reduced to PGH_2. Depending on the isomerase enzymes present in the particular tissue, prostaglandins (PGE_2, PGF_{2a}), thromboxanes, or prostacyclins will be formed. Leukocytes and explants of rheumatoid synovia produce predominantly PGE_2, platelets produce thromboxane A_2 (TxA_2), macro-

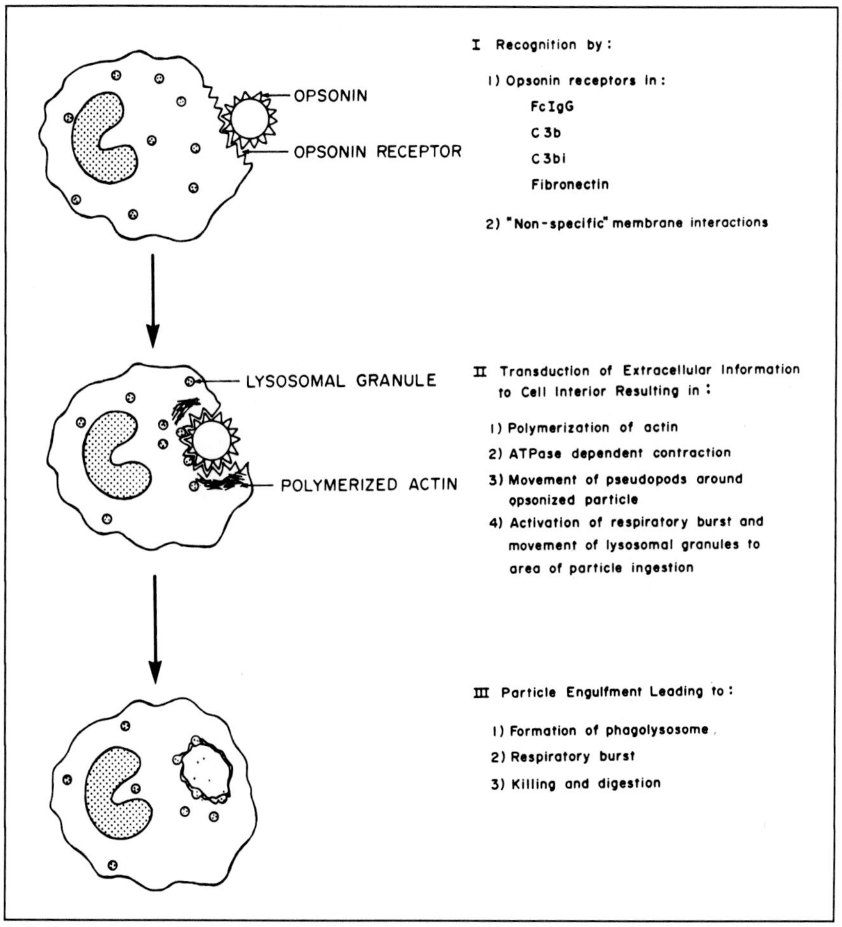

Fig. 17–2. Mechanisms of phagocytosis. *(From Snyderman. In McCarthy (ed): Arthritis and Allied Conditions. Lea & Febiger, p 287.)*

phages produce PGE_2, PGI_2, and TxA_2, and endothelial cells can produce prostacyclin and TxB_2. Thromboxanes are vasoconstrictors, whereas prostacyclins are potent vasodilators.

PGE_2 modulates a number of inflammatory events. It enhances vascular permeability, is pyrogenic, and increases sensitivity to pain. PGE_2 also stimulates the formation of cAMP in many types of inflammatory cells and thereby suppresses a number of immunologic responses, including lymphocyte blastogenesis, lymphocyte-mediated cytotoxicity, and the release of mediators from mast cells. An important source of PGE_2 in immunologic reactions is the macrophage. Supernatant fluids from explants of rheumatoid synovium stimulate bone resorption by enhancing osteoclast activity and the release of bone calcium. This phenomenon probably is mediated in large part by PG, since it is inhibitable by indomethacin (which blocks PG formation). PGE_2 also may play an important role in inhibiting IL-2 production by helper T cells.

Arachidonic acid can be metabolized into another class of biologically active products by the lipoxygenase pathway. The hydroxyeicosatetraenoic acids (HETEs) and the derivatives of 5-hydroperoxyeicosatetraenoic acid (termed *leukotrienes*) are examples of these arachidonic acid metabolites and are synthesized by granulocytes, macrophages, and basophils. 5,12-HETE, also termed leukotriene B_4 (LTB_4), is a potent chemotactic factor, whereas LTC_4 and D_4 stimulate smooth muscle constriction. LTB_4 has been identified in the synovial effusions of patients with rheumatoid arthritis and ankylosing spondylitis. Large amounts of LTB_4 are produced when granulocytes phagocytize monosodium urate crystals, and production of LTB_4 is inhibited by colchicine, which is an effective therapeutic agent for gout. Platelet-activating factors (PAF) are a group of 1-acetyl-2-alkyl-*o*-glyerol-ether analogues of alkylphosphatidylcholine. PAF causes platelet aggregation and is a potent leukocyte activator and chemoattractant. It is produced by leukocytes after their stimulation by inflammatory mediators.

Biologically Active Amines

Histamine is derived from the decarboxylation of histidine by the enzyme L-histidine decarboxylase. It is stored in mast cells and basophils and is complexed with mucopolysaccharides such as heparin. Stimulation of mast cells and basophils by a number of mechanisms can cause secretion of histamine. This agent has diverse biologic activities that include constriction of smooth muscle, enhancement of vascular permeability, depression of leukocyte chemotaxis, T lymphocyte inhibition, and reduction of further histamine release from mast cells and basophils. Histamine thus modulates both acute and chronic inflammatory responses. Serotonin (5-hydroxytryptamine) is produced by the decarboxylation of 5-hydroxytryp-

TABLE 17–2. EFFECTOR MOLECULES RELEASED BY MACROPHAGES

Mediator	Activity
Cellular Differentiation Factors	
M-CSF	Differentiation of macrophages
GM-CSF	Differentiation of macrophages, granulocytes, eosinophils
G-CSF	Differentiation of granulocytes
IL-3	Differentiation and growth of granulocytes, mast cells, erythrocytes, macrophages
Cellular Growth Factors	
Platelet-derived growth factor (PDGF)	Induces platelet growth
IL-1	T and B lymphocyte growth
IL-6	Plasma cell growth
Epidermal growth factor (EGF)	Promotes granulation tissue formation
Fibroblast growth factor (FGF)	Angiogenesis
Transforming growth factor-β (TGF-β)	Inhibits lymphocyte growth/activity; promotes wound repair
Acute Phase Stimulants	
IL-1	Pyrogenic; activation of lymphocytes, endothelial, dendritic, osteoclast, and synovial cells; increased adhesion molecule expression
TNF_{α}	Similar to IL-1; neutrophil activation
IL-6	Pyrogenic; lymphocyte, NK cell activation
Arachidonic Acid Metabolites	
Leukotrienes	Chemotaxis, vasoconstriction
Thromboxanes	Vasoconstriction
Prostaglandins	Pain, pyrogenic increased vascular permeability, bone resorption immunomodulation
Platelet activating factor (PAF)	Chemotaxis, thrombosis, stimulates granule release by neutrophils, eosinophils
Others	
IL-8	Neutrophil chemotaxis and degranulation
Complement components	Opsonization, chemotaxis, anaphylatoxins
Lysosomal enzymes	Tissue injury
Interferon (IFN)-α, β	Immunomodulation, promotes myeloid differentiation

TABLE 17–3. EFFECTOR MOLECULES RELEASED BY T CELLS

Mediator	Activity
IL-2	Promotes proliferation and differentiation of T (and B) cells; induction of adhesion molecules
IL-3	Promotes growth and differentiation of granulocytes, mast cells, eosinophils, macrophages
IL-4	Promotes B cell growth, proliferation and production of IgG1 and IgE; induction of MHC class II and IgE-FcR; activation of T cells, macrophages
IL-5	Stimulates eosinophil activity; B cell proliferation and IgA production; IL-2R induction
IL-6	Promotes macrophage, neural cell differentiation; B cell/plasma cell growth and Ig production; T cell activation, growth, and differentiation (cytotoxic T cells)
IL-7	Stimulates T and B cell maturation and differentiation
IL-8	Promotes neutrophil degranulation and chemotaxis
IFN-γ	Activation of macrophages and endothelial cells; induction of MHC class I and II, adhesion molecules
TNF_{β} (lymphotoxin)	Cytolysis; MHC class I induction; stimulates B cell growth and differentiation; inhibits T cell activity; stimulates osteoclasts and endothelial cells
Perforin	Cytolysis
Serine esterases	Cytolysis
IL-10	Inhibition of helper T cells

tophan. More than 90% of body stores of serotonin is found in the gastrointestinal tract and the central nervous system. The remainder is present in the dense granules of platelets. The biologic role of serotonin in inflammation is not well understood, but it enhances the chemotactic responses of leukocytes, increases fibroblast growth in vitro, and stimulates collagen formation.

Complement Cleavage Products

The complement system is an important amplifier of inflammatory reactions that are initiated by immunoglobulins and the release of hydrolytic enzymes from traumatized cells or leukocytes. The biology and biochemistry of this complex series of proteins are described in Chapter 15. Two complement cleavage products, C3a and C5a, which are derived from the third and fifth complement components, respectively, are important mediators of inflammation in host defense as well as immunopathologic reactions.

Enzymatic cleavage of the α chain of C3 by the earlier acting complement components or by other proteases releases C3a, a peptide consisting of 77 amino acids. C3a mediates a number of biologic responses, including smooth muscle contraction, vasodilatation, enhanced vascular permeability, the degranulation of mast cells and basophils, and the secretion of lysosomal enzymes by leukocytes. C3a also has immunoregulatory effects and suppresses humoral immune responses in vitro by affecting T lymphocytes. C3a is the most abundant of the complement activation peptides released in serum. The COOH-terminal arginine of C3a is required for its biologic activity, and cleavage of this amino acid by a carboxypeptidase-B-like enzyme in serum renders the peptide inactive.

C5a has a number of structural and biologic similarities to C3a. C5a consists of 74 amino acids, with the COOH-terminal constituent also being arginine. C5a is derived from cleavage of the α chain of C5. In addition to having all the biologic activities of C3a, C5a is an extremely potent chemoattractant for PMN, monocytes, and macrophages. C5a is the major source of chemotactic and anaphylatoxic activity generated in serum treated with immune complexes or endotoxin and also is an important source of chemotactic activity in rheumatoid synovial fluids. In contrast to C3a, C5a potentiates humoral immune responses in vitro. Cleavage of the terminal arginine of C5a by a serum carboxypeptidase-B markedly diminishes its biologic activity.

Cytokines

Cytokines are low-molecular-weight (<80 kDa) immunoregulatory proteins produced predominantly by T cells and macrophages. They bind to specific receptors on target cells (primarily leukocytes and endothelial cells), are effective at very low concentration, and have a wide range of overlapping effects. Major activities of cytokines involve regulation of cellular growth, proliferation, differentiation, activation, and expression of various molecules, including receptors, accessory molecules, and MHC molecules.

Cytokines characterized to date include the interleukins (IL-1 through 8), the interferons (IFN-α, β, and γ), tumor necrosis factors (TNF_{α} and $_{\beta}$), growth factors (TGF, PDGF, EGF, and FGF), and colony-stimulating factors (G-, M-, and GM-CSF). A summary of some of their activities is provided in Tables 17–2 and 17–3.

Lysosomal Enzymes

Lysosomal enzymes are contained in subcellular organelles termed *lysosomal granules.* Leukocytes contain several types of lysosomal granules, some of which contain antimicrobial constituents, such as myeloperoxidase and lactoferrin. Lysosomal enzymes degrade complex macromolecules and digest antigens following phagocytosis. However, since these enzymes also may be released during phagocytosis or on cell death, they can cause host tissue destruction that sometimes accompanies inflammatory reactions.

Lysosomal proteases found in leukocytes include collagenase, elastase, cathepsin D, cathepsin G, and gelatinase. These enzymes are capable of destroying extracellular structures and may thus participate in mediating tissue injury in various inflammatory reactions. Cathepsin D cleaves cartilage proteoglycan, whereas granulocyte collagenase is active in cleaving type I and, to a lesser degree, type III collagen substrates found in bone, cartilage, and tendon. The substrates of granulocyte elastase include collagen crosslinkages and proteoglycans, as well as the elastin components of blood vessels, ligaments, and cartilage. Lysosomal hydrolyases also produce mediators of inflammation through their direct action on complement components, such as C5. Leukocytic hydrolyases can liberate kinin from kininogen. Plasminogen activator, an enzyme that converts plasminogen to plasmin (which stimulates fibrinolysis) is found in both granulocyte and macrophage lysosomes. Rheumatoid synovial collagenase usually is present as an inactive lysosomal proenzyme that requires plasminogen activator for conversion to its active form.

Regulation of the tissue-destructive potential of the lysosomal proteases is mediated by protease inhibitors, such as α_2-macroglobulin and α_1-antiprotease. These antiproteases are present in serum and in synovial fluids and inhibit protease enzymes by binding to them and blocking their active sites. In addition, α_2-macroglobulin binds numerous cytokines and inhibits their activity by direct inactivation (e.g., IL-2) or by inhibition of their release (e.g., TNF).

Oxygen Metabolites

The production of various toxic oxygen metabolites by neutrophils undergoing respiratory burst plays an important role in the killing of ingested microbes (Chap. 19). These intermediates include the superoxide anion radical, hydrogen peroxide, hydroxyl radicals, and halide radicals, all of which can lead to local cell injury when released during an inflammatory response.

Heat Shock Proteins

Heat shock proteins (HSP), also termed *stress proteins,* are highly conserved proteins produced in response to stress by virtually all procaryotic and eucaryotic cells. They have been divided into four major families based on molecular weight and have been described as *molecular chaperones* because of their physiologic capacity to associate and interact with other proteins. They also have been implicated as important targets in autoimmune responses. The smallest family (10–30 kDa) of HSP, termed *ubiquitin,* may function to assist in the degradation of endogenous (cytoplasmic) proteins and the association of their products with MHC class I molecules. They also show sequence homology with fragments of the LAM-1 selectin molecule, which acts as a homing receptor for leukocytes to high endothelial venules. Two other families (HSP60, HSP70) appear to promote protein folding and unfolding, as well as assembly of multichained proteins. HSP70 molecules are involved in immunoglobulin molecule assembly and possibly the processing and association of exogenous peptide fragments with MHC class II in endosomes. Interestingly, the genes encoding at least some of these HSP have been linked to the MHC in several species examined. Members of the largest family (HSP90) may be preferentially expressed on transformed cells and thus function as tumor-specific antigens.

The HSPs represent major antigens of many pathogens and have been identified as targets of host immune responses in numerous autoimmune diseases. Antibodies to specific HSP are seen in patients with rheumatoid arthritis, systemic lupus erythematosus, ankylosing spondylitis, and other rheumatic diseases. In addition, T cells expressing the less polymorphic γδ TCR antigen receptor appear to recognize HSP, which because of their highly conserved nature may require a less diverse T cell repertoire for recognition.

Others

Kinin-Forming System. An intimate association exists between the activation and regulation of the intrinsic clotting, fibrinolytic, and kinin-forming systems. Hageman factor (HF), or factor XII of the clotting system, is central to the activation of all three systems. HF is activated by a number of agents, including crude preparations of collagen, vascular basement membranes, monosodium urate crystals, calcium pyrophosphate crystals, and endotoxin. Negatively charged surfaces also activate HF. On activation, HF (an 80 kDaβ globulin) is cleaved, and its active form HF_a initiates the conversion of factor XI of the clotting pathway to XIa and the conversion of prekallikrein to kallikrein. Kallikrein activates plasminogen, a key enzyme involved in promoting fibrinolysis. Kallikrein also cleaves a high molecular weight serum protein to form bradykinin, a nonapeptide with potent biologic activities. C1 esterase inhibitor (C1INH), a protein that inhibits activated C1, is also an important inhibitor of HF_a and kallikrein. Bradykinin and two other kinins produced by tissue kallikreins from kininogen induce smooth muscle contraction, increased vascular permeability, and pain. Cleavage of fibrinogen by plasmin results in the production of a number of products, including fibrinopeptide B, an agent that potentiates the action of bradykinin and itself has chemotactic activity.

Substance P. Substance P is an oligopeptide released by nerve endings that has numerous immunmodulatory effects, including the ability to enhance the response of leukocytes to other inflammatory stimuli. This inflammatory mediator also is present in rheumatoid synovial fluid and is capable of causing synovial cell proliferation.

Regulatory Mechanisms

Regulatory mechanisms are involved in the initiation, expansion, focusing, and termination of diverse immune responses that are necessary to protect the body from infections. If an antigen-specific immune response is not initiated and expanded rapidly, an invading organism may overcome immune defenses. However, it is also important that specific immune responses remain focused so as to avoid unnecessary damage to adjacent tissues as innocent bystanders. Many of the molecules that can modulate the magnitude and type of ongoing immune responses have been discussed previously, including the monokines and lymphokines listed in Tables 17–2 and 17–3.

Regulation also occurs on an antigen-specific level. First, genetic information determines the capacity to respond to any given antigen by defining the repertoire of possible antigen-specific receptors on B cells (i.e., surface immunoglobulin) and T cells (i.e., TCR). If the genetic capacity to produce certain receptors is lacking, an immune response to the corresponding antigen will not be generated. On the other hand, if a given receptor is preferentially expressed by certain cells or molecules, a selected immune response may occur. For example, the binding site for some antigens preferentially is associated with antibodies of the IgG4 immunoglobulin subclass, which are not bound by the Fc receptor of macrophages and do not fix complement. As a result, most of the antibodies produced against such antigens will not activate complement or macrophages, critically affecting the type of inflammatory reactions evoked. Complement-fixing antibodies have been shown to be important in focusing the uptake of antigen by follicular dendritic cells, which bear complement receptors and are the APC in the B lymphocyte–rich compartments of the spleen and lymph nodes. Complement-mediated attachment of opsonized antigens to follicular dendritic cells is a major factor in the intense activity observed in germinal centers during memory immune responses.

B lymphocyte function can be regulated directly by antibody. Circulating antibody titers that are temporarily decreased by plasmapheresis (without supplementary immunosuppression) will subsequently overshoot the original levels. This type of antibody feedback operates at two levels. First, circulating antibody competes with B lymphocyte surface Ig receptor for antigen. Second, antigen-antibody complexes bound by B lymphocyte Fc receptors (or T suppressor cells) may directly or indirectly inhibit antibody production by B lymphocytes. Thus, physical removal of antibody or immune complexes from the circulation may, in effect, stimulate increased antibody production.

Another mechanism of antibody-mediated regulation of immune responses is through anti-idiotypic antibodies, which bind to the antigen receptor site of antibodies (paratope) or T lymphocyte receptors. These antibodies can have multiple effects. Anti-idiotypic antibodies that have a mirror image of the internal portion of the antigen receptor can block the interaction of antigen with antibodies, surface Ig receptors on B lymphocytes, or T lymphocyte receptors. Alternatively, the same antibodies may act like antigen and directly trigger T or B lymphocyte function. This type of internal image anti-idiotypic antibody can have special applications as vaccines to immunize individuals to certain viral and bacterial antigens without exposing the individual to the hazards of an attenuated live virus (Chap. 19). Anti-idiotypic antibodies that bind to the external components of the antigen recognition structure (idiotope) do not necessarily interfere with antigen binding but can still stimulate specific B or T lymphocytes by interacting with their antigen receptors. Such anti-idiotypic antibodies may be effective in modulating ongoing immune responses without interfering with effector functions. An analogous situation may exist for regulatory suppressor T cells that may be directed at other T cell receptors.

The MHC phenotype and T cell repertoire of an individual also may affect the level and type of responses evoked. Since T cells recognize foreign antigen in association with self-MHC antigens, the immunogenicity of particular antigens can be strongly influenced by the class I or II MHC antigen profile of the host. This has been demonstrated by the clinical association between certain HLA phenotypes and the level of host responsiveness to particular microbial and other antigens and by the in vitro finding that the repertoire of T cells (identified by specific variable region sequences expressed on the β-chain [Vβ] of the TCR) that is responsive to an antigen can be affected by the host MHC haplotype.

T lymphocytes can produce antigen-specific and antigen-nonspecific suppressor factors that can inhibit helper T lymphocytes and B lymphocytes (Table 17–3). Suppressor factors act to terminate completed or inappropriate antigen-specific immune responses and may help to focus immune responses by regulating polyclonal responses to mitogenic products of viruses and bacteria. Although the mechanisms of suppressor T cells remain unresolved, it has been proposed that they may recognize antigen and suppress effector cells or act directly on helper T cells.

Immunopathologic Processes

The most practical system for classifying immunopathologic reactions was first described in the early 1960s by Gell and Coombs and still remains useful. This classification is based on the general mechanism of immune reactivity and also provides some information about the pathologic manifestation of tissue damage. These four categories (and their associated diseases) are listed in Table 17–4.

Type I Immediate hypersensitivity: anaphylactic, allergic or atopic diseases
Type II Humorally mediated cytotoxic reactions: autoimmune diseases, cytotoxic diseases, antibody diseases
Type III Immune complex reactions: serum sickness diseases
Type IV Delayed-type hypersensitivity: cell-mediated cytotoxic diseases, granulomatous diseases

Type I Reactions (Immediate Hypersensitivity)

Type I or immediate hypersensitivity reactions are typically mediated by IgE antibodies, which bind via characteristic Fc domains with very high affinity to specific Fc receptors (FcεRI) on the surface of mast cells and basophils. Such binding is independent of the antigen specificity of the IgE antibodies. However, on crosslinking of such antibodies by multivalent antigen, the effector cell is stimulated to release preformed and newly formed soluble mediators (Table 17–5). Preformed mediators are released almost immediately (within 1 minute in vitro) and include histamine, eosinophil chemotactic factors (ECF), various proteolytic enzymes, and heparin. The release of histamine results in almost immediate increased vascular permeability and smooth muscle contraction, whereas heparin inhibits coagulation, and ECFs, which include two tetrapeptides, attract eosinophils. The release of proteolytic enzymes (such as trypsin from mast cells) may result in the activation of complement or other pathways.

The stimulation of mast cells and basophils also leads to the rapid synthesis (within minutes) of several soluble mediators, including PAF and products of arachidonic acid metabolism, such as leukotrienes and prostaglandins. The release of leukotrienes C_4, D_4, and E_4, also termed *slow-reacting substance of anaphylaxis* (SRS-A), causes increased vascular permeability and smooth muscle contraction. LTB_4 is chemotactic for eosinophils and neutrophils, and PAF stimulates platelet aggregation and leukocyte chemotaxis. The synthesis and release of cytokines, including IL-3, IL-4, IL-5, and IL-6, promote further IgE production and mast cell and granulocyte growth and differentiation. These late or newly formed mediators act to enhance and potentate the major effects of immediate mediators, i.e., smooth muscle contraction, increased vascular permeability, and chemotaxis. Eosinophils attracted and activated by these mediators, however, may be involved in feedback regulation. Their release of histaminase, phospholipase D, and oxygen metabolites can neutralize histamine, PAF, and LTB_4, respectively.

Since mast cells and basophils remain viable after initial stimulation, the immunopathologic manifestations of type I reactions depend not only on the initial number of cells sensitized by surface-bound IgE but also on the level of specific IgE antibody present and the amount of antigen to which the host is exposed. Both genetic and environmental factors can influence the magnitude of type I responses.

The typical histopathologic features of these responses include congestion and edema (secondary to vasodilatation) as well as the presence of eosinophils. The clinical manifestations of type I reactions may vary in intensity from life-threatening systemic anaphylaxis to localized reactions, such as urticaria, allergic rhinitis, sinusitis, and certain types of bronchial asthma. Common allergens include pollens, drugs (especially penicillin), and microbial products (especially from parasites and helminths) (Chap. 19).

Type II Reactions (Antibody-mediated)

The development of antibodies against components of an individual's own cells and tissues normally is downregulated but, in some cases, can be stimulated and lead to a variety of disease states. Production of antihost antibody responses may result from abnormal antigenic challenge, abnormal immune regulation, or both. The effects of antibody directed against, or crossreactive with, host components may result in several types of reactions, including localized tissue inflammation, complement-mediated toxicity, and altered host regulation due to antibody-mediated stimulation or damage.

Tissue-specific Inflammation

The development of autoantibody to various cellular and structural host components most typically results in a localized organ-specific inflammatory disease. In general, the binding of antibody to a fixed tissue antigen will lead to an inflammatory response as a result of complement activation, release of chemotactic factors, and the localization of inflammatory cells and soluble mediators as described in the preceding

TABLE 17–4. IMMUNOPATHOLOGIC REACTIONS

Type of Inflammation	Immune Recognition	Soluble Component	Inflammatory Response	Disease Example
I. Immediate hypersensitivity	IgE	Basophil, mast cell products	Immediate flare and wheal, smooth muscle constriction, eosinophil, neutrophil infiltrates	Atopy, anaphylaxis, urticaria, asthma
II. Cytotoxic antibody	IgG, IgM	Complement	Lysis or phagocytosis of circulating antigens, acute inflammation in tissues	Autoimmune hemolytic anemia, Goodpasture's syndrome
III. Immune complex	IgG, IgM, IgA	Complement	Accumulation of neutrophils, eosinophils, and macrophages	Rheumatoid arthritis, systemic lupus erythematosus
IV. Delayed-type hypersensitivity	T cells	Lymphokines, monokines	Mononuclear cell infiltrate	Tuberculosis, sarcoidosis, polymyositis, contact dermatitis

TABLE 17–5. MEDIATORS OF IMMEDIATE HYPERSENSITIVITY

Mediator	Source	Activity
Histamine	Preformed: Mast cell, basophil	Smooth muscle contraction, increased vascular permeability, increased mucus secretion
ECF-A	Preformed: Mast cell, basophil	Eosinophil chemoattractant
Heparin	Preformed: Mast cell, basophil	Anticoagulant
Proteases	Preformed: Basophils, lung	Complement, kinin activation
Serotonin	Preformed: Platelets, mast cells	Enhances vasoactive and chemotactic factors
Cytokines (IL-3,4,5,6)	Stimulated	Eosinophil, neutrophil activation, growth, differentiation
LTC_4, D_4, E_4 (SRS-A)	Stimulated: Mast cell, PMNs	Smooth muscle contraction, increased vascular permeability
LTB_4	Stimulated: PMNs, mast cells	PMN chemoattractant
PGD_2	Stimulated: Mast cells	Vasodilatation
PGE_1, E_2	Stimulated: Neutrophils, macrophages	Bronchodilation, vasodilatation
Platelet activating factor (PAF)	Stimulated: Basophils, alveolar macrophages	Platelet aggregation, chemotaxis, bronchoconstriction

discussions. Although the mechanisms by which particular autoantibodies are produced vary (see below), the early inflammatory tissue changes are similar, with the appearance of granulocytes, congestion, and edema.

A wide range of autoantibodies has been identified in association with various organ-specific and systemic inflammatory diseases. Many of these involve antibodies directed against endocrine cells and their hormone receptors, whereas others have specificity against cytoplasmic, nuclear, or circulating antigens that in some instances can lead to type III (immune complex) reactions. Several of the most classic examples of type II inflammatory diseases involve antibodies against structural determinants, such as basement membrane glycoproteins (e.g., Goodpasture's syndrome, bullous pemphigoid) and the intercellular matrix of skin and mucosa (e.g., pemphigus). In Goodpasture's syndrome, host IgG autoantibodies bind in situ to collagen antigens expressed on glomerular and alveolar basement membranes (Fig. 17–3), leading to localized complement activation and inflammation. This results in a characteristic acute exudative glomerulonephritis and hemorrhagic alveolitis. In an analogous manner, subepidermal exudative bullae are seen in patients with pemphigoid, and intraepidermal inflammation is seen in patients with pemphigus.

Complement-mediated Toxicity

The ability of the membrane attack complex (MAC) of complement to mediate direct cytotoxicity in vivo is limited primarily to the lysis of erythrocytes. A wide range of immune hemolytic anemias has been identified and is associated with host antibodies to various blood group and red cell–bound antigens. Alloimmune antibodies directed against ABO and Rh blood group antigens are seen most commonly in transfusion reactions, where mismatched blood is given to the host, and in hemolytic disease of the newborn, where maternal anti-Rh antibodies are transmitted into the fetal circulation. Responses to Rh and most other blood group antigens require prior stimulation, in contrast to reactions involving antibodies against ABO blood group antigens, where naturally occurring isohemagglutinins are present and prior exposure to mismatched blood is not necessary.

Autoimmune antibodies to blood group antigens often are elicited by secondary diseases. The most common autoimmune hemolytic anemias are caused by IgG (and occasionally by IgA or IgM) antibodies directed against Rh antigens, which react in vitro at 20C or 37C (warm reactive). These autoantibodies often are associated with prior viral infection, leukemia, systemic lupus erythematosus (SLE), or other systemic autoimmune diseases. Antibodies that have activity at less than 20C (cold reactive) are less common and usually are associated with specific target reactions. Cold agglutinin diseases are seen in patients with *Mycoplasma pneumoniae* infections, who develop IgM anti-I blood group antibodies, and in patients with infectious mononucleosis, who develop IgM anti-i antibodies. In contrast, paroxysmal cold hemoglobinuria involves an IgG anti-P antibody that binds in the cold but leads to full complement activation at 37C.

Certain drugs can react with antibody and red cells, leading to hemolysis. In some cases (e.g., with quinidine or phenacetin), antibodies to the drug will form complexes that bind to red cells, fix complement, and result in hemolysis. In other cases (e.g., with penicillins and cephalosporins), the drug is first absorbed onto red cell membranes and antidrug antibody is subsequently bound, leading to complement activation and hemolysis.

Although direct complement-mediated lysis can play a major role in hemolytic anemia, phagocytes and effector lymphocytes often contribute to the destruction of antibody and complement-coated targets via Fc and complement receptor interactions. Antibody-mediated reactions against platelet and leukocyte antigens also can lead to thrombocytopenia and leukopenia by mechanisms involving complement deposition, causing direct toxicity or secondary destruction by phagocytosis and antibody-dependent cell-mediated cytotoxicity (ADCC)-type reactions.

Altered Host Regulation

Autoantibody reactions often can be directed against molecules that are involved in homeostatic pathways, such as soluble mediators or cell surface receptors. Patients with autoimmune diseases (e.g., SLE) may exhibit antibodies that interfere directly with coagulation pathways (e.g., anticoagulant antibodies against factor VIII) or indirectly with complement pathways (e.g., depressed complement levels due to increased complement-fixing immune complexes). In some cases, patients actually may develop antibodies to components of the

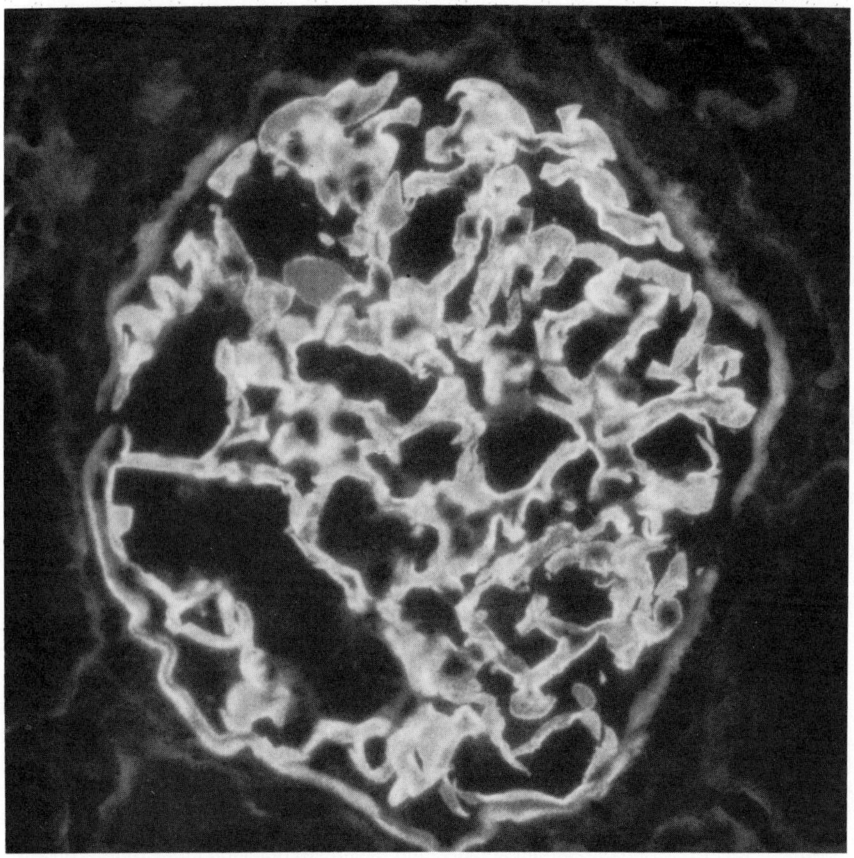

Fig. 17–3. Antibody deposition along glomerular basement membranes in a patient with Goodpasture's syndrome. Staining with fluoresceinated antihuman IgG shows uniform linear deposits.

immune system, as, for example, with anti-immunoglobulin antibodies (rheumatoid factors) in patients with rheumatoid arthritis and anti–T cell antibodies in patients with SLE.

The most dramatic effects of altered regulation due to type II reactions involve antibodies directed against cell-specific receptors or their natural ligands. These reactions can lead to specific organ failure, often with the presence of a tissue-specific inflammatory response. Several well-characterized diseases (and their associated autoantibody) include Graves' disease (anti-TSH receptor), Hashimoto's thyroiditis (antithyroglobulin), myasthenia gravis (antiacetylcholine receptor), pernicious anemia (anti-intrinsic factor), and insulin-resistant diabetes (anti-insulin receptor, anti-insulin). Other diseases are associated with antibodies to adrenal cells (Addison's disease), oxyphil cells (primary hypoparathyroidism), theca interna cells (ovarian failure), and spermatozoa (infertility). The effect of such autoantibodies is usually to depress endocrine function by receptor blockade or secondary inflammation. However, in some cases, an antireceptor antibody may actually mimic the hormone, resulting in overstimulation. This is the case, for example, in Graves' disease, where an anti-TSH receptor autoantibody (termed *long-acting thyroid stimulator,* or LATS) results in hyperthyroidism.

Type III Reactions (Immune Complex)

Antigen-antibody complexes commonly are formed in response to a wide range of microbial and other foreign antigens and usually are cleared by phagocytic cells without any host damage. Under certain conditions, however, antigen-antibody or antibody-antibody (e.g., rheumatoid factor, cryoglobulin) complexes may lead to localized tissue inflammation. In general, this depends on the ability of an immune complex to form or deposit at a fixed tissue site and then activate the complement system. These characteristics, in turn, are dependent on a variety of physical, chemical, and biologic properties of the immune complex, including its size, charge, solubility, antibody-binding affinity, and immunoglobulin class and subclass.

The development of disease after immune complex deposition and complement activation usually involves the same inflammatory mechanisms and pathologic changes discussed for complement-fixing autoantibody deposition. A number of important clinical diseases are associated with inflammatory immune complex deposition, including many types of vasculitis, glomerulonephritis, as well as rheumatoid arthritis and SLE. In some cases, however, immune complexes may not efficiently activate complement or may deposit in sites that are less accessible to mediators of inflammation, so that disease results from structural damage caused by the complexes. For example, in idiopathic-type membranous glomerulonephritis, immune complexes appear to form in situ along glomerular basement membranes, without inducing significant inflammation. However, they can alter membrane permeability, resulting in proteinuria that often leads to the nephrotic syndrome.

Two basic models of immune complex-mediated disease

have been well characterized: the Arthus reaction and serum sickness. These differ somewhat in both their mode of development and their clinical manifestations.

Arthus Reaction

In 1903, N. M. Arthus described the localized inflammatory effects of intradermal injection of antigen into previously sensitized animals. In this model, a host receives primary immune stimulation to a particular antigen, leading to systemic antibody production. On local (not systemic) secondary challenge with the same antigen, antigen-antibody complexes form within adjacent vessels or tissue. Complement activation by these localized immune complexes results in the release of chemotactic factors (C5a) and anaphylatoxins (C5a, C3a), causing infiltration of inflammatory cells (predominantly neutrophils and macrophages), which release other inflammatory mediators (see above), leading to local tissue injury. Particularly damaging is the destruction of endothelial cell basement membrane due to the exocytosis of phagocytic cells that have been stimulated by immune complexes embedded in the basement membrane itself. As the immune complexes are cleared, the picture of acute inflammation may change to one with a predominantly chronic mononuclear inflammatory cell infiltrate.

Serum Sickness Models

In contrast to the localized formation of immune complexes seen in the Arthus reaction, serum sickness represents a model of systemic challenge with formation of circulating immune complexes. Although the mode of immune complex formation differs, once circulating complexes are deposited in various tissue sites, they lead to the same local picture of inflammation as in the Arthus reaction.

Two models of serum sickness have been described, which differ in terms of sensitization but are similar in their resulting disease. The acute or one-shot serum sickness model is demonstrated by a single systemic challenge with a large amount of antigen (Fig. 17–4). In this case, systemic antibody production occurs before the loss of circulating antigen, resulting in the formation of antigen-antibody complexes in circulation. Initially, circulating antigen is in excess, leading to small, nonpathogenic complexes. However, as antigen decreases and antibody increases, intermediate-sized complexes are formed that are potentially able to deposit within vessel walls or basement membranes and provoke inflammatory reactions similar to that of the Arthus reaction. Certain tissues are more likely to have immune complex deposition due to their anatomic structure. Renal glomeruli, dermal papillae, joints, and small vessels are particularly common targets of immune complex reactions (Fig. 17–5). A characteristic feature of this model is the temporal similarity of inflammation in tissues affected, since complexes are formed and deposited in various sites at the same time.

The model of chronic serum sickness involves the same type of primary systemic sensitization with antigen resulting in circulating antibody but, in contrast, is followed by a second (or repeated) systemic exposure to antigen, leading to antigen-antibody complex formation in the circulation. The repeated exposure to the antigen results in the continuous formation of complexes that sequentially deposit in different tissues, thus yielding a more heterogeneous pattern of local tissue inflammatory reactions than is seen in the one-shot model.

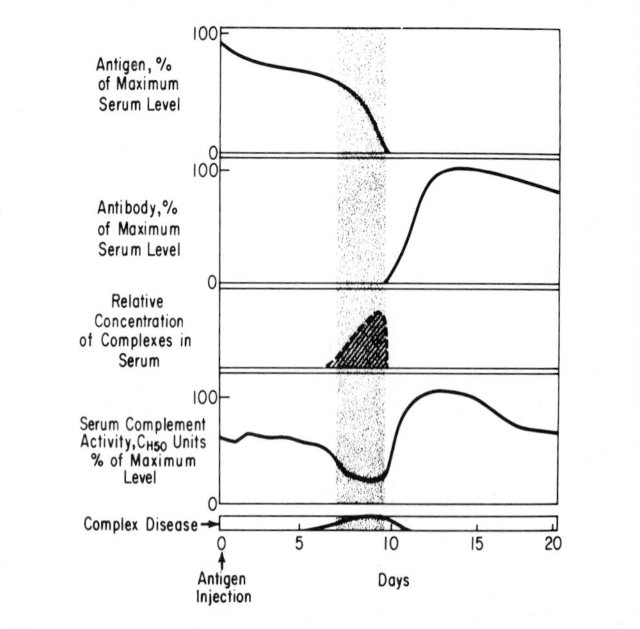

Fig. 17–4. Relationships between the serologic events and experimental immune complex disease. Injected antigen is equilibrated with body fluid and undergoes gradual catabolic attrition until day 6, when antibody production begins. Rapid attrition of antigen characteristic of immune elimination occurs between day 7 and day 10. During this interval, antibody production results in the presence of identifiable antigen-antibody complexes in the serum, depression of complement activity, and tissue changes in kidney glomeruli and blood vessel walls characteristic of immune complex disease. Free antibody appears after antigen elimination and is followed by a rebound in serum complement activity.

Circulating immune complexes also may have direct effects on leukocytes, platelets, and other cells having Fc or complement receptors. The binding of complexes by such cells may lead to activation (via surface receptor interactions) or destruction (due to clearance by other phagocytes) or suppression (due to crosslinking of Fc and C receptors). The development of fever and rashes in patients with serum sickness is largely due to release of pyrogens (e.g., IL-1, TNF_{α}, IL-6) from affected leukocytes and platelets.

Type IV Reactions (Delayed-type Hypersensitivity)

Unlike the other three types of immunopathologic reactions, which are all induced by antibody, type IV responses are initiated by antigen-specific T cells. The typical delayed-type hypersensitivity (DTH) reaction is perhaps best demonstrated by the tuberculin test, in which an intradermal injection of purified protein derivative (PPD) of tuberculin is given to a presensitized individual, resulting in a local area of induration that appears 24 to 72 hours later. The histologic picture of this reaction shows an intense mononuclear cell (granulomatous) inflammatory infiltrate comprised of lymphocytes and macrophages, without the edema or significant numbers of

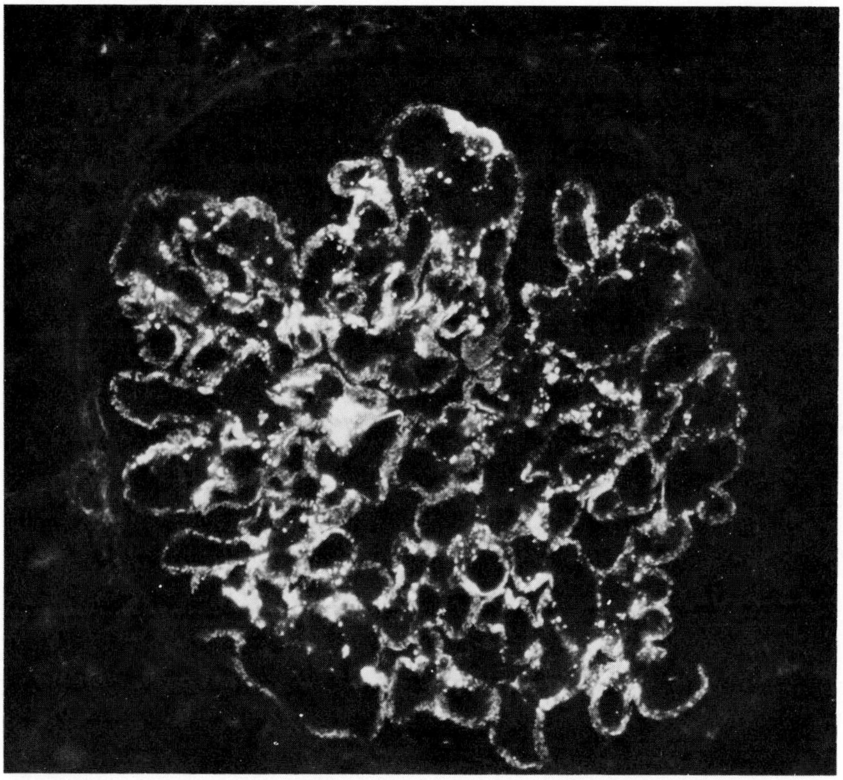

Fig. 17–5. Immune complex glomerulonephritis from a patient with serum sickness after treatment with horse antithymocyte globulin. Staining with fluoresceinated antihorse IgG shows immune complex deposits along glomerular basement membranes.

granulocytes that are hallmarks of antibody and complement-mediated reactions. DTH responses usually can be elicited by injection of antigen with dead tubercle bacilli in an oil emulsion (Freund's adjuvant). The damage seen in type IV reactions is largely the result of inflammatory mediators released from activated macrophages (Table 17–2), lymphocytes (Table 17–3), and sometimes basophils (Table 17–5). However, the reaction can be transferred in vivo with sensitized T cells alone.

As discussed above and in Chapter 13, both humoral and cellular immune responses are initiated after antigen processing and presentation by macrophages (or other APCs) to helper T lymphocytes, which in turn provide necessary signals (via lymphokines) to those B cell and T effector cell clones that have received an antigen-specific signal (via their antigen-specific receptors). The factors promoting cell-mediated (T effector) rather than humoral-mediated (B cell) responses are directed primarily by T helper cell subpopulations and are affected by the mode of antigen presentation, the physicochemical characteristics of the antigen, the antigenic specificities involved, and the state of host presensitization. In the mouse, two subpopulations of T helper cells (T_{h1} and T_{h2}) have been identified. They produce (and respond to) different cytokines. T_{h1} cells preferentially activate macrophages (e.g., IFN-γ) and effector T cells (e.g., IL-2), whereas T_{h2} cells preferentially stimulate B cells (e.g., IL-4, -5, -6). Thus, preferential stimulation of T_{h1} is more likely to promote a cellular immune response. In some cases, type IV reactions occur with an inflammatory infiltrate of mostly lymphocytes and basophils, termed a *Jones-Mote reaction*. The factors leading to this type of response also involve the nature of antigen, route of challenge, and regulatory T cell activity.

The most common clinical examples of type IV reactions are seen in infections with intracellular parasites or microbes that can resist phagocytosis (e.g., viruses, mycobacteria, and fungi). A second major category of type IV reactions is seen with contact sensitivity to various substances, such as plant catechols (e.g., poison ivy, poison oak), drugs (e.g., sulfonamides), and metals (e.g., nickel). In contact sensitivity reactions, Langerhans cells of the skin are able to present unprocessed antigen to stimulate host responses. Although many of the substances that cause contact sensitivity are of low molecular weight and would normally be nonantigenic haptens, they often bind to endogenous epithelial proteins, which act as carrier moieties to provide an immunogenic stimulus.

A third major clinical example of type IV reactions is seen in response to transplanted organs and tissues, which express allogeneic MHC molecules that can be recognized by host T cells directly as intact antigens or as processed peptides associated with self-MHC determinants. Autoimmunity is responsible for or contributes to a wide range of diseases that can be of rapid or insidious onset, mild or severe in intensity, localized to particular tissues or multisystemic in nature, and of transient duration or prolonged and progressive.

Mechanisms of Autoimmunity

No single pathogenic mechanism can account for the diversity of disease states associated with autoimmunity. In fact, several different pathogenic processes may underlie disorders that

TABLE 17–6. POTENTIAL CONTRIBUTING FACTORS TO AUTOIMMUNE DISEASES

Variations in Genetic Programming of Immunocompetent Cells

Defects in thymic selection against forbidden clones
Abnormal T lymphocyte receptor genes
High responder immune response genes
Abnormal immunoglobulin genes
Defective clearance of antigen by macrophages
Somatic mutation of lymphocyte receptors

Defects in Immune Regulation

Increased helper T cell function
Decreased suppressor T cell function
Refractory responses to suppressor signals
Idiotype–antiidiotype network defects

Alternations in the Normal Antigenic Environment

Release or exposure of sequestered antigens
Ectopic expression of class II antigens
Virally or chemically altered self-antigens

Secondary Influences on Immune Response Hormones

Viral, bacterial, fungal infections
Environmental factors

are clinically indistinguishable and categorized as single disease entities.

As discussed in Chapters 12 and 13, autoreactive T cells normally undergo negative selection in the thymus, whereas autoreactive antibodies are downregulated to low levels compatible with health. Although escape from these controls can lead to autoimmune reactivity, the majority of autoimmune diseases probably reflect a genetic predisposition toward hyperresponsiveness to certain antigens. This can be exacerbated by intrinsic and extrinsic factors, such as hormone levels, anatomic peculiarities or injury, and exposure to infectious agents. Some of the factors that may contribute to autoimmune diseases are categorized in Table 17–6.

Numerous observations indicate that genetic factors have an influence on the incidence, onset, type, and severity of autoimmune diseases. The most compelling evidence for this comes from animal models of autoimmune diseases in which crossbreeding experiments have led to the identification of genes that control both the occurrence of disease and the organ systems involved. Often, two or three genes on different chromosomes must act in concert to result in disease with these animal models. In humans, many autoimmune diseases also have been correlated with certain genes, but as with the animal models, the inheritance of any single gene is rarely sufficient to cause autoimmunity. Rather, certain genes are associated with increased relative risks for given autoimmune diseases, which are triggered by a precipitating stimulus. Autoimmune diseases have been associated with certain MHC antigens (particularly class II) and immunoglobulin allotypes. The association of MHC antigens with autoimmunity may rest at the level of antigen presentation or recognition. Certain foreign antigens may associate most easily with given MHC antigens, resulting in pathologically increased responses. Other foreign antigens may actually resemble host MHC antigens, leading to crossreactive immune responses. The major HSPs expressed by microbial organisms are highly conserved across species and closely resemble autologous HSP in the infected host, potentially leading to autoimmune responses (see above).

The intensity of some immune responses may be controlled by MHC genes (high responder immune response genes), whereas other genes control the type of response that is generated. Studies of allergic patients, for instance, have revealed that the ability to respond to particular ragweed pollen antigens is governed by two HLA-linked genes, whereas the level of IgE production is associated with a non-HLA-linked gene. Thus, for this reaction, at least three genes are involved in determining exactly which antigens elicit an allergic response and the intensity of the response.

Because some HLA gene associations differ among ethnic groups, the primary association of some diseases may not be with known MHC antigens but rather with some closely linked, as yet unidentified gene on the HLA haplotype (Chap. 14). For example, Graves' disease initially was associated with HLA-B8/DR3 in Caucasians but with DR5 and 8 in Japanese. More recent studies show that a stronger association is with DQw2. The initial correlation in type I diabetics with the HLA-DR3, 4 heterozyous phenotype has been replaced with homozygosity of HLA-DQβ3.2, with an amino acid substitution for Asp at position 57.

Some autoimmune diseases associated with the HLA-B8/DR3 haplotype may be related to decreased function of the mononuclear phagocyte system due to defects in Fc receptors for IgG on Kupffer cells. This defect leads to a decreased capacity to clear IgG-antigen immune complexes and an increased possibility of their deposition causing tissue injury. Genetic deficiencies in individual complement components are another cause of decreased efficiency in clearance of immune complexes and are associated with autoimmune diseases.

Several different mechanisms may account for autoantibody production. This has been demonstrated in a spontaneous disorder of different inbred strains of mice that resembles SLE in humans. Genetically determined defects of B lymphocytes underlie the excessive polyclonal antibody production in BXSB and NZB/W mice, whereas in the MRL/l mouse, increased levels of IgG autoantibody production are related to a chronic hypersecretion of lymphokines by T cells. Similarly, humans with SLE have been demonstrated to have abnormal IL-2 production, increased amounts of IFN-γ, and depressed T suppressor cells. The incomplete deletion of autoreactive T cells in the thymus during development also may lead to the development of autoimmune reactivity.

Although the predisposition toward autoimmune disorders is genetically influenced, various secondary factors may initiate or exacerbate the abnormality into a clinically apparent disease. Infectious agents, particularly viruses and bacteria, have been associated with several autoimmune diseases. Viral infections produce alterations in tissue antigens by the insertion of viral antigens on cell surfaces. This may alter the conformation of adjacent self-antigens or provide determinants that may on their own resemble self-antigens. Either of these two phenomena—altered self-antigens or antigenic mimicry—may stimulate immune responses that crossreact with self-antigens. Antigenic mimicry is responsible for immune reactions to heart muscle and nervous tissues after infections with certain streptococci. Likewise, there are structural similarities between measles virus antigens and myelin basic protein, between various bacterial antigens and acetylcholine receptors, and between coxsackie B virus and heart muscle.

Viruses also have the potential to alter indirectly the normal antigenic composition of host cells by stimulation of class II MHC expression as a result of IFN-γ production. Such cells may then stimulate helper T lymphocytes to respond to host cells. Thyroid cells isolated from patients with Graves' disease have been found to express such ectopic class II HLA antigens, as have beta cells in the pancreatic islets of patients with type I diabetes. The observation for diabetics is particularly interesting in the light of the correlation between viral illness and inflammatory cell reactions in the pancreatic islets of patients who develop the disease.

The regulation of T and B lymphocytes can be directly modified by virus infection or by secondary interactions with viral or bacterial products. Epstein-Barr virus infects B lymphocytes through binding to their C3d receptors (CR2) and can transform these cells, resulting in continuous antibody secretion. Cytomegalovirus infections increase suppressor T lymphocyte numbers and immunosuppressive functions of macrophages, possibly through direct infection. Likewise, HIV preferentially infects T helper cells, decreasing their regulatory function. In addition, various viral and bacterial products (most notably lipopolysaccharide) stimulate lymphocyte mitosis and polyclonal antibody production, and HSP released by microorganisms may result in immune responses directed at analogous host antigens.

FURTHER READING

Books and Reviews

Albelda SM, Buck CA: Integrins and other cell adhesion molecules. FASEB J 4:2868, 1990

Balkwill FR, Burke F: The cytokine network. Immunol Today 10:299, 1989

Basten A: The Florey Lecture, 1989. Self-tolerance: The key to autoimmunity. Proc R Soc Lond [B] 328:1, 1989

Colvin RB, Bhan AK, McCluskey RT: Diagnostic Immunopathology. New York, Raven Press, 1988

Galli SJ: New insights into "The riddle of the mast cells": Microenvironmental regulation of mast cell development and phenotypic heterogeneity. Lab Invest 62:5, 1990

Goodacre J, Dick WC: Immunopathogenetic Mechanisms of Arthritis. Lancaster, MTP Press, 1988

Klein J: Immunology. Boston, Blackwell, 1990

Lydyard PM, vanEden W: Heat shock proteins: Immunity and immunopathology. Immunol Today 11:228, 1990

Möller G (ed): Autoreactive T cells and clones. Immunol Rev vol 116, 1990

Paul WE (ed): Fundamental Immunology, 2nd ed. New York, Raven Press, 1989

Pober JS, Cotran RZ: The role of endothelial cells in inflammation. Transplantation 50:537, 1990

Prud'homme GJ, Parfrey NA: Role of T helper lymphocytes in autoimmune disease. Lab Invest 59:158, 1988

Rodnan GP, Schumacher HR, Zvaifler NJ (eds): Primer on the Rheumatic Diseases, 8th ed. Atlanta, Arthritis Foundation, 1983

Rose NR, Friedman H, Fahey JL (eds): Manual of Clinical Laboratory Immunology, 3rd ed. Washington, DC, American Society for Microbiology, 1986

Salyer JL, Bohnsack JF, Knape WA, et al: Mechanisms of tumor necrosis factor-α alteration of PMN adhesion and migration. Am J Pathol 136:831, 1990

Swanborg RH: Horror autotoxicus and homing: Implications for autoimmunity. Lab Invest 63:141, 1990

Tan EM: Antinuclear antibodies: Diagnostic markers for autoimmune diseases and probes for cell biology. Adv Immunol 44:93, 1989

Todd JA: Genetic control of autoimmunity in type I diabetes. Immunol Today 11:122, 1990

Walsh LJ, Lavker RM, Murphy GF: Determinants of immune cell trafficking in the skin. Lab Invest 63:592, 1990

Wilson K, Eisenbarth GS: Immunopathogenesis and immunotherapy of type I diabetes. Annu Rev Med 41:497, 1990

Winchester R (ed): Immunopathology of SLE and Related Diseases. New York, Springer, Semin Immunopathol 9, 1986

Selected Articles

Beekhuizen H, Corsèl-van Tilburg AJ, vanFurth R: Characterization of monocyte adherence to human macrovascular and microvascular endothelial cells. J Immunol 145:510, 1990

Benichou G, Takizawa PA, Ho PT, et al: Immunogenicity and tolerogenicity of self-major histocompatibility complex peptides. J Exp Med 172:1341, 1990

Chin Y-H, Cai J-P, Johnson K: Lymphocyte adhesion to cultured Peyer's patch high endothelial venule cells is mediated by organ-specific homing receptors and can be regulated by cytokines. J Immunol 145:3669, 1990

Christie MR, Vohra G, Champagne P, et al: Distinct antibody specificities to a 64-kd islet cell antigen in type I diabetes as revealed by trypsin treatment. J Exp Med 172:789, 1990

de Graeff-Meeder ER, Voorhorst M, van Eden W, et al: Antibodies to the mycobacterial 65-kd heat-shock protein are reactive with synovial tissue of adjuvant arthritic rats and patients with rheumatoid arthritis and osteoarthritis. Am J Pathol 137:1013, 1990

Groggel GC, Terreros DA: Role of the terminal complement pathway in accelerated autologous anti-glomerular basement membrane nephritis. Am J Pathol 136:533, 1990

Guidos CJ, Danska JS, Fathman CG, Weissman IL: T cell receptor-mediated negative selection of autoreactive T lymphocyte precursors occurs after commitment to the CD4 or CD8 lineages. J Exp Med 172:835, 1990

Hammer RE, Maika SD, Richardson JA, et al: Spontaneous inflammatory disease in transgenic rats expressing HLA-B27 and human β_2m: An animal model of HLA-B27-associated human disorders. Cell 63:1099, 1990

Kalish RS, Johnson KL: Enrichment and function of urushiol (poison ivy)-specific T lymphocytes in lesions of allergic contact dermatitis to urushiol. J Immunol 145:3706, 1990

Klinman DM, Eisenberg RA, Steinberg AD: Development of the autoimmune B cell repertoire in MRL-1pr/1pr mice. J Immunol 144:506, 1990

Leeuwenberg JFM, Von Asmuth EJU, Jeunhomme TMAA, Buurman WA: IFN-γ regulates the expression of the adhesion molecule ELAM-1 and IL-6 production by human endothelial cells in vitro. J Immunol 145:2110, 1990

Mosman TR, Cherwinski H, Bond MW, et al: Two types of murine helper T cell clones. I. Delineation according to profiles of lymphokine activity and secreted proteins. J Immunol 136:2348, 1986

Nepom GT: HLA and type I diabetes. Immunol Today 11:314, 1990

Patarca R, Wei F-Y, Singh P, et al: Dysregulated expression of the T cell cytokine Eta-1 in $CD4^-8^-$ lymphocytes during the development of murine autoimmune disease. J Exp Med 172:1177, 1990

Picker LJ, Terstappen LWMM, Rott LS, et al: Differential expression of homing-associated adhesion molecules by T cell subsets in man. J Immunol 145:3247, 1990

Pullen AM, Marrack P, Kappler JW: The T cell repertoire is heavily influenced by tolerance to polymorphic self-antigens. Nature 335:976, 1988

Rico MJ, Korman NJ, Stanley JR, et al: IgG antibodies from patients with bullous pemphigoid bind to localized epitopes on synthetic peptides encoded by bullous pemphigoid antigen cDNA. J Immunol 145:3728, 1990

Sakaguchi S, Sakaguchi N: Thymus and autoimmunity: Capacity of the normal thymus to produce pathogenic self-reactive T cells and conditions required for their induction of autoimmune disease. J Exp Med 172:537, 1990

Strominger JL: Biology of the human histocompatibility leukocyte antigen (HLA) system and a hypothesis regarding the generation of autoimmune diseases. J Clin Invest 77:1411, 1986

Wuthrich RP, Jevnikar AM, Takei F, et al: Intercellular adhesion molecule-1 (ICAM-1) expression is upregulated in autoimmune murine lupus nephritis. Am J Pathol 136:441, 1990

CHAPTER 18

Abnormal Development of the Immune System

Since the first example of a human host deficit was described in 1952, more than 40 genetically determined immunodeficiency syndromes have been reported in the world's literature. This growing list of diseases includes defects in all components of the immune system, including T, B, and natural killer (NK) lymphocytes, phagocytic cells, and complement proteins. Extensive information has accrued about inheritance patterns, clinical features, and cellular abnormalities in each of these conditions, and there is now information about the primary biologic errors in a number of them. Examples include an-adhesion protein deficiency, which is due to genetic abnormalities in a 95 kDa β chain (CD18, encoded by a gene on chromosome 21q22.3) common to three different leukocyte surface glycoprotein heterodimers; and combined immune defects caused by deficiencies of one of the purine salvage pathway enzymes, adenosine deaminase (ADA, encoded by a

TABLE 18–1. PROBABLE CHROMOSOMAL MAP LOCATIONS FOR FAULTY GENES IN PRIMARY IMMUNODEFICIENCY DISEASES

Chromosome	Disease
1q25	Chronic granulomatous disease (NCF2[a])
2p11	κ chain deficiency
6p21.3	(?)Common variable immunodeficiency and selective IgA deficiency
7q11.23	Chronic granulomatous disease (NCF1[b])
11q22.3	Ataxia telangiectasia
14q13.1	Purine nucleoside phosphorylase deficiency[c]
14q32.3	Immunoglobulin heavy chain deletion
20q13-ter	Adenosine deaminase deficiency[c]
21q22.3	Leukocyte adhesion deficiency (CD11:CD18 deficiency)[c]
Xp21.1	Chronic granulomatous disease[c]
Xp11-11.3	Wiskott-Aldrich syndrome
Xq13-21.1	Severe combined immunodeficiency
Xq21.3-22	X-linked agammaglobulinemia
Xq24-27	Immunodeficiency with hyper-IgM
Xq24-26	X-linked lymphoproliferative syndrome

[a] Neutrophil cytoplasmic factor 2.
[b] Neutrophil cytoplasmic factor 1.
[c] Gene cloned and sequenced, gene product known.

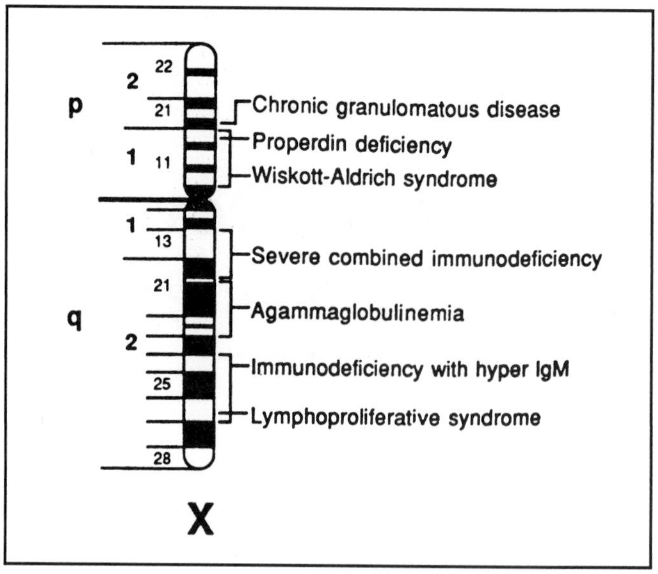

Fig. 18–1. The human X chromosome and the locations of the X-linked primary immunodeficiency diseases. *(From Winkelstein and Fearon: Carrier detection of the X-linked primary immunodeficiency diseases using X-chromosome inactivation analysis. J Allerg Clin Immunol 85:1091, 1990.)*

gene on chromosome 20q13-ter) or purine nucleoside phosphorylase (PNP, encoded by a gene on chromosome 14q13.1) (Table 18–1).

The faulty genes in many other immunodeficiencies are known to be on the X chromosome. They have been localized to specific sites in the case of X-linked agammaglobulinemia, X-linked severe combined immunodeficiency, the Wiskott-Aldrich syndrome, X-linked lymphoproliferative disease, properdin deficiency, and X-linked chronic granulomatous disease (CGD), but only in the last case has the abnormal gene been identified (Fig. 18–1). In addition, the genes for two autosomal recessive forms of CGD have been assigned to specific locations on chromosomes 1 and 7. Lethal immunodeficiency can also be due to broad deficiencies of HLA class I and II antigens, and these have been shown to be due to different mutations in *trans*-acting factors governing the surface expression of these molecules.

Since trace amounts of immunoglobulins of all five isotypes usually can be found in the sera of most agammaglobulinemics, it is unlikely that most immunoglobulin deficiency states are attributable to deletions of immunoglobulin genes. Exceptions include rare patients with deletions of genes encoding the κ light chain or the heavy chains of immunoglobulin G subclasses (Table 18–1). Monoclonal antibody studies have shown that cells having surface markers characteristic of mature B or T cells or their subsets are rarely completely lacking in any of these conditions.

Genetically determined immunodeficiency is considered rare. Although general population statistics are not available, it has been estimated that agammaglobulinemia occurs with a frequency of 1:50,000 and severe combined immunodeficiency with a frequency of 1:100,000 to 1:500,000 live births. Selective absence of serum and secretory IgA is the most common defect, with reported incidences ranging from 1:333 to 1:700. However, racial differences have been noted, as selective IgA deficiency is much less common in Japanese and genetic defects in immunity have been noted most often among Caucasians. An exception appears to be an unusually high incidence of one form of severe combined immunodeficiency among Navajo Indians. In contrast to the rarity of genetic defects in immunity, the acquired immunodeficiency syndrome (AIDS) has a new case acquisition rate of more than 350 per week.

Classification of Genetically Determined Immunodeficiency Syndromes Involving Lymphocytes

Various attempts have been made by World Health Organization (WHO) committees over the past 20 years to classify the known primary immunodeficiency disorders. Table 18–2 lists the current state of knowledge about 20 of the better-known primary immunodeficiency syndromes involving lymphocytes, giving the most prominent functional deficits and the presumed cellular or molecular levels of the defects.

Antibody Deficiency Disorders

Antibody deficiency may occur clinically either as a congenital or as an acquired abnormality, although in both situations it appears to be genetically determined. There may be deficiencies in all immunoglobulin classes (agammaglobulinemia or hypogammaglobulinemia) or in one or more but not all classes (selective immunoglobulin deficiencies). In addition, antibody

TABLE 18–2. CLASSIFICATION OF PRIMARY IMMUNODEFICIENCY DISORDERS

Disorder	Functional Deficiencies	Presumed Cellular Level of Defect
X-linked agammaglobulinemia	Antibody	Pre-B cell
Common variable immunodeficiency (CVID; "acquired" hypogammaglobulinemia)	Antibody	B lymphocyte
IgG subclass deficiencies; κ chain deficiency	Antibody	B lymphocyte; immunoglobulin heavy or light chain gene deletions
Selective IgA deficiency	IgA antibody	IgA B lymphocyte
Secretory component deficiency	Secretory IgA	Mucosal epithelium
Selective IgM deficiency	IgM antibody	T helper cells
Immunodeficiency with elevated IgM	IgG and IgA antibodies	B lymphocytes; "switch" T cells
Transient hypogammaglobulinemia of infancy	None; immunoglobulins low but antibodies present	Unknown
Antibody deficiency with near-normal immunoglobulins	Antibody	Unknown; (?)B cell
X-linked lymphoproliferative disease	Anti-EBNA antibody	B cell; (?)also T cell
DiGeorge syndrome	T cellular; some antibody	Dysmorphogenesis of 3rd and 4th branchial pouches
Nezelof syndrome (including PNP deficiency)	T cellular; some antibody	Unknown; (?)thymus; (?)T cell; metabolic defects
Severe combined immunodeficiency syndromes (autosomal recessive; ADA deficiency; X-linked recessive; defective expression of HLA antigens; reticular dysgenesis)	Antibody and T cellular phagocytic in reticular dysgenesis	Unknown; metabolic defect(s); (?)T cell; (?)stem cell; (?)thymus; regulatory gene defects
Wiskott-Aldrich syndrome	Antibody, T cellular	Unknown; (?)CD43 expression
Ataxia telangiectasia	Antibody; T cellular	B lymphocyte; helper T lymphocyte
Cartilage hair hypoplasia	T cellular	G1 cycle of many cells
Immunodeficiency with thymoma	Antibody; some T cellular	B lymphocyte; excessive T suppressor cells
Hyperimmunoglobulinemia E	Specific immune responses; excessive IgE	Unknown; (?)deficient CD43RO+ TH1 memory cells
Leukocyte adhesion deficiency (LAD, CD11/18 deficiency)	Cytotoxic lymphocytes, phagocytic cells	95 kDa β chain (CD18) of LFA-1, CR3, and p150,95
Lymphocyte activation defects	T cellular; some antibody	Decreased CD3/Ti expression; defective signal transduction; defective IL-2 and other cytokine production

deficiency may occur in the presence of normal or near normal serum immunoglobulin or immunoglobulin subclass concentrations. Most patients with these disorders are recognized because they have recurrent infections with high-grade bacterial pathogens, but some with selective IgA deficiency or infants with transient hypogammaglobulinemia may have few or no infections. Table 18–3 lists some of the general features of these disorders.

X-linked (Bruton's) Agammaglobulinemia. This rare disorder, which appears to selectively involve very early B lineage cells, was the first recognized of all of the primary immunodeficiencies and was discovered in 1952 by Colonel Ogden Bruton. The abnormal gene in X-linked agammaglobulinemia was mapped recently to a region on the proximal part of the long arm of the X chromosome. This was accomplished by restriction fragment length polymorphism (RFLP) studies, using DNA probes for the loci DXS17 and DXS3 that mapped the abnormal gene to the q21.3-q22 region (Fig. 18–1). Carriers can be detected by the finding of nonrandom X-chromosome inactivation in B cells in RFLP studies of hamster–human B cell hybrids or of differences in methylation patterns.

Most boys afflicted with this malady remain well during the first 6 to 9 months of life, presumably by virtue of maternally transmitted IgG antibodies. Thereafter, they repeatedly acquire infections with extracellular pyogenic organisms, such as pneumococci, streptococci, and *Haemophilus*, unless given prophylactic antibiotics or gammaglobulin therapy. Infections with other organisms, such as meningococci, staphylococci, and *Pseudomonas*, occur less frequently. These

TABLE 18–3. CLINICAL CHARACTERISTICS OF ANTIBODY DEFICIENCY DISORDERS

1. Recurrent infections with high-grade extracellular encapsulated pathogens
2. Few problems with fungal or viral (except enteroviral) infections
3. Chronic sinopulmonary disease
4. Growth retardation not striking
5. Antibody deficiency in serum and secretions
6. May or may not lack B lymphocytes with surface immunoglobulins or complement receptors
7. Absence of cortical follicles in lymph node and spleen in X-linked agammaglobulinemia
8. Paucity of palpable lymphoid and nasopharyngeal tissue in X-linked agammaglobulinemia
9. Compatible with survival to adulthood or for several years after onset except for those with persistent enteroviral infections, autoimmune disorders, or malignancy

include not only mucous membrane infections (sinusitis, pneumonia, otitis, and conjunctivitis) but also life-threatening systemic infections (septic arthritis, meningitis, and septicemia). Despite these chronic or recurrent infections, patients with this disorder usually grow normally unless they develop bronchiectasis or persistent enteroviral infections. Chronic fungal infections are not usually present, and *Pneumocystis carinii* pneumonia rarely occurs unless there is an associated neutropenia. Viral infections are usually handled normally, with the notable exceptions of hepatitis and enteroviruses. There have been several instances of meningoencephalitis or paralysis after live polio (an enterovirus) vaccine administration because of failure of immune elimination by secretory IgA antibodies, subsequent viremia, and then central nervous system (CNS) infection because of a lack of circulating IgG antibody. In addition, chronic progressive, eventually fatal CNS infections with various echoviruses have occurred in more than 40 such patients. These observations suggest a primary role for antibody, particularly secretory IgA, in host defense against this group of viruses, since normal T cell function has been present in all X-linked agammaglobulinemics with persistent enteroviral infections reported thus far.

The diagnosis of X-linked agammaglobulinemia is suspected if serum concentrations of IgG, IgA, and IgM are far below the 95% confidence limits for appropriate age- and race-matched controls (i.e., usually <100 mg/dL total immunoglobulin). Tests for natural antibodies to blood group substances, for antibodies to antigens given during standard courses of immunization (e.g., diphtheria, tetanus, *Haemophilus influenzae,* and pneumococci), and for antibodies to bacteriophage ϕX 174 are useful in distinguishing this disorder from transient hypogammaglobulinemia of infancy. Polymorphonuclear functions usually are normal if heat-stable opsonins (e.g., IgG antibodies) are provided, but some patients with this condition have had transient, persistent, or cyclic neutropenia.

The number of T cells usually is increased, and the percentages of T cell subsets have been found to be normal in most of these patients. By contrast, blood lymphocytes bearing surface immunoglobulin, Ia-like antigens, the EBV receptor or reacting with monoclonal antibodies specific for B cell antigens are absent or are present in very low numbers. Nevertheless, normal numbers of pre-B cells are found in the bone marrow. Hypoplasia of adenoids, tonsils, and peripheral lymph nodes is the rule. Germinal centers are not found in these tissues, and plasma cells rarely are found. Mixed lymphocyte responsiveness, cell-mediated lympholysis, and lymphocyte proliferative responses to antigens and mitogens are normal. Cell-mediated immune responses can be detected in vivo, and the capacity to reject allografts is intact. NK cell function is normal. The thymus is morphologically normal. Hassall's corpuscles are present, and lymphoid cells are abundant in thymus-dependent areas of peripheral lymphoid tissues.

Except in those unfortunate patients who develop polio, persistent enteroviral infection, rheumatoid arthritis, or lymphoreticular malignancy (an incidence as high as 6% has been reported), the overall prognosis is reasonably good if IgG replacement therapy is instituted early. Systemic infection can be prevented by administration of intravenous immune serum globulin (IVIG) at a dose of 400 mg/kg every 3 to 4 weeks. Such preparations are known to be free of hepatitis viruses and the HIV viruses. Many patients go on to develop crippling sinopulmonary disease despite IVIG therapy, since no effective means exists for replacing secretory IgA at the mucosal surface. Chronic antibiotic therapy usually is necessary for the management of such patients.

Common Variable Immunodeficiency. Common variable immunodeficiency (CVID), also known as acquired hypogammaglobulinemia or idiopathic late-onset immunoglobulin deficiency, may appear similar clinically in many respects to X-linked agammaglobulinemia. The principal differences are the generally later age of onset, the somewhat less severe infections, an almost equal sex distribution, and a tendency to autoantibody formation. In addition, patients with CVID may have normal-sized or enlarged tonsils and lymph nodes, and splenomegaly occurs in approximately 25%. The serum immunoglobulin and antibody deficiency are usually just as profound as in the X-linked disorder, and the kinds of infections experienced and bacterial etiologic agents involved generally are the same for the two defects. Fortunately, however, echovirus meningoencephalitis is rare in patients with CVID. Autoimmune diseases are not, however, and there are now several cases of lupus erythematosus converting to CVID.

CVID has been variably associated with a spruelike syndrome with or without nodular follicular lymphoid hyperplasia of the intestine, thymoma, alopecia areata, hemolytic anemia, gastric atrophy, achlorhydria, and pernicious anemia. Frequent complications include giardiasis (seen far more often than in X-linked agammaglobulinemia), bronchiectasis, gastric carcinoma, lymphoreticular malignancy (an 8- to 13-fold increase over normal), and cholelithiasis. Lymphoid interstitial pneumonia, pseudolymphoma, amyloidosis, and noncaseating granulomas of the lungs, spleen, skin, and liver have been seen. There is a 438-fold increase in lymphomas in affected women in the fifth and sixth decades.

Despite the normal numbers of circulating immunoglobulin-bearing B lymphocytes and the presence of lymphoid cortical follicles, blood lymphocytes from CVID patients do not differentiate into immunoglobulin-producing cells when stimulated with pokeweed mitogen in vitro, even when cocultured with normal T cells. Thus, in most patients, the defect appears to be intrinsic to the B cell, resulting in abnormal terminal differentiation. T cells and subsets usually are present in normal percentages, although T cell function may be depressed in some patients. Because this disorder occurs in first-degree relatives of patients with selective IgA deficiency (A def) and some patients with A def later become panhypogammaglobulinemic, it is possible that these diseases have a common genetic basis. The high incidences of abnormal immunoglobulin concentrations, autoantibodies, autoimmune disease, and malignancy in families of both types of patients also suggest a shared hereditary influence. This concept is supported by the recent finding of rare alleles or deletions of class III major histocompatibility complex (MHC) genes in individuals with either A def or CVID, suggesting that the susceptibility gene(s) are in this region on chromosome 6.

The treatment of patients with CVID is essentially the same as for the X-linked disorder.

IgG Subclass Deficiency. A number of patients have been reported to have deficiencies of one or more subclasses of IgG, despite normal total IgG serum concentrations. Most of those with absent or very low concentrations of IgG2 have been patients with selective IgA deficiency (see below). It is difficult to know the biologic significance of the multiple moderate deficiencies of IgG subclasses that have been reported, particularly when completely asymptomatic individuals have been described who totally lack IgG1, IgG2, IgG4, and IgA1 due to gene deletion. The more relevant question to ask is "What is the capacity of the patient to make specific antibodies to protein and polysaccharide antigens?" since profound deficiencies of antipolysaccharide antibodies have been noted even in the presence of normal concentrations of IgG2. IVIG should not be given to IgG subclass-deficient patients unless they are shown to have a deficiency of antibodies to a broad array of antigens.

Selective IgA Deficiency. An isolated absence or near-absence (i.e., <10 mg/dL) of serum and secretory IgA is thought to be the most common well-defined immunodeficiency disorder, a frequency of 1:333 being reported among some blood donors. Although this disorder has been observed in apparently healthy individuals, it commonly is associated with ill health.

As would be expected when there is a deficiency of the major immunoglobulin of external secretions, infections occur predominantly in the respiratory, gastrointestinal, and urogenital tracts. Bacterial agents responsible are essentially the same as in other types of antibody deficiency syndromes. There is no clear evidence that patients with this disorder have an undue susceptibility to viral agents. Children with IgA deficiency (A def) vaccinated with killed poliovirus intranasally produced local IgM and IgG antibodies. Several children later contracted rubella, and IgM and IgG antirubella antibodies were found in their secretions during convalescence. Serum concentrations of other immunoglobulins usually are normal in patients with selective A def, although an IgG2 subclass deficiency has been reported, and IgM (usually elevated) may be monomeric.

Patients with A def frequently have IgG antibodies against cow milk and ruminant serum proteins. These antiruminant antibodies often falsely detect IgA in immunoassays that employ goat (but not rabbit) antisera. A high incidence of autoantibodies has been noted. This may have bearing on the frequent association of A def with collagen-vascular and autoimmune diseases. A spruelike syndrome has occurred in adults with A def, which may or may not respond to a gluten-free diet. As in patients with CVID, there is an increased incidence of malignancy.

The basic defect leading to selective IgA deficiency is unknown. In 10 of 11 IgA-deficient individuals studied, more than 80% of the IgA bearing B cells also coexpressed surface IgM and IgD (similar to cord blood B cells), as compared with less than 10% triple isotype-bearing IgA B cells in healthy persons, suggesting a B cell maturation arrest. In others, treatment with phenytoin, sulfasalazine, D-penicillamine, or gold has been suspected as being the cause of the IgA deficiency. In some A def patients the defect may disappear spontaneously with time, whereas in others it may evolve into CVID. The occurrence of IgA deficiency in both males and females and in families is consistent with autosomal inheritance. In some families this appears to be dominant with variable expressivity.

Of possible etiologic and great clinical significance is the presence of antibodies to IgA in the sera of as high as 44% of patients with selective IgA deficiency. Anti-IgA antibodies can fix complement and remove IgA from the circulation 4 to 20 times faster than the normal catabolic rate for IgA. A number of IgA-deficient patients have had severe or fatal anaphylactic reactions after intravenous administration of blood products containing IgA, and anti-IgA antibodies (particularly IgE anti-IgA antibodies) have been implicated. For this reason, only five times–washed (in 200 mL volumes) normal donor erythrocytes or blood products from other IgA-absent individuals should be administered to these patients. IVIG (which is >99% IgG) is not indicated, because most A def patients make IgG antibodies normally. Moreover, many IVIG preparations contain sufficient IgA to cause anaphylactic reactions.

Currently there is no treatment for A def beyond the vigorous treatment of specific infections with appropriate antimicrobial agents. Even if serum IgA could be replaced (a dangerous thing to attempt), it could not be transported into the external secretions, since such transport is an active process involving only locally and endogenously produced IgA.

Secretory Component Deficiency. A patient with chronic intestinal candidiasis and diarrhea was found to lack IgA in his external secretions, despite having a normal serum IgA concentration. This ultimately was traced to a lack of secretory piece, which prevented the normal secretion of locally produced IgA onto his mucous membrane surfaces. This case further illustrates the importance of secretory IgA in protecting the mucous membrane surfaces.

Selective IgM Deficiency. Selective IgM deficiency (<10 mg/dL IgM) is a rare condition. Septicemia due to meningococci and other gram-negative organisms, pneumococcal meningitis, tuberculosis, recurrent staphylococcal pyoderma, periorbital cellulitis, bronchiectasis, recurrent otitis, and other respiratory infections have been reported in this disorder.

Immunodeficiency with Elevated IgM. Immunodeficiency with elevated IgM (hyper M) is characterized by very low serum IgG and IgA but either a normal or, more frequently, a markedly elevated concentration of polyclonal IgM. Some of these patients have low-molecular-weight IgM molecules that give falsely high IgM values in radial immunodiffusion assays. High titers of IgM antibodies to blood group substances and to *Salmonella* O antigen have been found in some patients, but very low titers or no IgM antibody has been noted in others.

Patients with hyper M may become symptomatic during the first or second year of life with recurrent pyogenic infections, including otitis media, sinusitis, pneumonia, and tonsillitis. In contrast to patients with X-linked agammaglobulinemia, however, the frequent presence of lymphoid hyperplasia in hyper M patients often is misleading. Even more than with some of the other antibody-deficiency syndromes, there is an increased frequency of autoimmune disorders in the hyper IgM syndrome. Hemolytic anemia and thrombocytopenia have been seen in several patients, and transient, persistent, or cyclic neutropenia is a common feature. The neutropenia is considered a possible explanation for the occurrence of *P. carinii* pneumonia and extensive verruca vulgaris lesions in some such patients. Thymic-dependent lymphoid tissues and T cell functions usually are normal, but several hyper M patients have had partial T cell deficiencies. A sex-linked mode of inheritance has been noted in some pedigrees. The abnormal gene in the X-linked type has been localized to Xq24-Xq27. Several examples in females suggest that this phenotype has more than one genetic cause.

Normal or only slightly reduced numbers of IgM or IgD

B lymphocytes or both have been found in the blood of these patients. However, cultured B cell lines from such patients have shown the capacity to synthesize only IgM and a defect of switch recombination. B cells from a few such patients have shown the capacity to synthesize IgM, IgA, and IgG when cocultured with a switch T cell line, suggesting that in those patients the defect lay in T lineage cells. Because these patients have an inability to make IgG antibodies, the treatment for this condition is the same as for agammaglobulinemia, i.e., monthly IVIG infusions.

Transient Hypogammaglobulinemia of Infancy. Unlike patients with X-linked agammaglobulinemia or CVID, patients with transient hypogammaglobulinemia of infancy (THI) can synthesize antibodies to human type A and B erythrocytes and to diphtheria and tetanus toxoids, usually by 6 to 11 months of age, and well before immunoglobulin concentrations become normal. Lymphocyte studies in vitro show no abnormalities in the percentages of cells in the different subpopulations or in their responses to mitogens. THI has been found in pedigrees of patients with other immune defects, including CVID and severe combined immunodeficiency (SCID).

IVIG therapy is not indicated in this condition. In addition to the known risk of inducing antiallotype antibodies, passively administered IgG antibodies could suppress endogenous antibody formation to infectious agents in the same manner that RhoGAM suppresses anti-D antibodies in Rh-negative mothers delivering Rh-positive infants. IVIG may also suppress immune responses by Fc receptor interaction and by the presence or induction of anti-idiotypic antibodies.

Antibody Deficiency with Near-Normal Immunoglobulins. Only scattered reports have appeared in the literature describing patients with apparently normal T cell function and normal or near-normal immunoglobulin concentrations but with deficient antibody responses. Such individuals have recurrent pyogenic infections similar to those with agammaglobulinemia. Indeed, with time, serum immunoglobulin concentrations may decline to levels seen in CVID patients. This has led to speculation that this condition may be an early stage of CVID. Blood group antibody titers frequently are absent. Diphtheria, tetanus, *H. influenzae,* and pneumococcal antibody titers are significantly lower than normal, and primary immune responses to bacteriophage ϕX 174 are far below the normal range. Because these patients do not have the ability to produce antibodies normally, they are candidates for monthly IVIG infusions.

X-linked Lymphoproliferative Disease. X-linked lymphoproliferative disease, also referred to as Duncan's disease (after the original kindred in which it was described), is a recessive trait characterized by an inadequate immune response to infection with Epstein-Barr virus (EBV). The defective gene has been localized to the distal long arm of the X-chromosome (q.26). A few apparent examples in women suggest that non-X-linked inheritance of this susceptibility also may exist. The affected patients are apparently healthy until they experience infectious mononucleosis. Two thirds of the more than 100 patients studied thus far died of overwhelming EBV-induced B cell proliferation during mononucleosis. Most patients surviving the primary infection developed hypogammaglobulinemia or B cell lymphomas. There is a marked impairment in production of antibodies to the EBV nuclear antigen (EBNA), and titers of antibodies to the viral capsid antigen have ranged from zero to markedly elevated. Antibody-dependent cell-mediated cytotoxicity (ADCC) against EBV-infected cells has been low in many, and NK function also is depressed. There is a deficiency in long-lived T cell immunity to EBV. These patients frequently have elevated percentages of $CD8^+$ T cells. Immunoglobulin synthesis in response to pokeweed mitogen stimulation in vitro is markedly depressed. Thus, both EBV-specific and nonspecific immunologic abnormalities occur in these patients.

Cellular and Combined Immunodeficiency Disorders

In general, patients with partial or absolute defects in T cell function have infections or other clinical problems that are of a more severe nature than those with antibody deficiency disorders (Table 18–4). It is rare that such individuals survive beyond infancy or childhood.

Thymic Hypoplasia (DiGeorge Syndrome). Thymic hypoplasia results from dysmorphogenesis of the third and fourth pharyngeal pouches during early embryogenesis, leading to hypoplasia or aplasia of the thymus and parathyroid glands. Other structures forming at the same age also are frequently affected, resulting in anomalies of the great vessels (right-sided aortic arch), esophageal atresia, bifid uvula, congenital heart disease (atrial and ventricular septal defects), a short philtrum of the upper lip, hypertelorism, an anti-Mongoloid slant to the eyes, mandibular hypoplasia, and low-set, often notched ears. The diagnosis usually is first suggested by the presence of hypocalcemic seizures during the neonatal period. DiGeorge syndrome has occurred in both males and females, and chromosomal abnormalities (monosomy 22q11 and 10p13) have been noted in approximately 10% to 15%. It has been hypothesized that deletion of contiguous genes on chromosome 22 results in DiGeorge syndrome and that the critical region may be in proximity to the BCRL2 locus. Familial occurrence is rare but has been reported. Because the characteristic facies and conotruncal heart lesions seen in DiGeorge patients also have been noted in the fetal alcohol syndrome, it has been proposed that the DiGeorge anomaly may be a polytypic field defect of diverse etiology involving cephalic neural crest cells.

Since the original description of the syndrome, it has become apparent that a variable degree of hypoplasia is more frequent than total aplasia of the thymus and parathyroid glands. Some children have little trouble with life-threatening infections and grow normally. Such patients often are referred

TABLE 18–4. CLINICAL CHARACTERISTICS OF CELLULAR IMMUNODEFICIENCY DISORDERS

1. Recurrent infections with low-grade or opportunistic infectious agents, such as fungi, viruses, and *Pneumocystis carinii*
2. Delayed cutaneous anergy
3. Accompanied by growth retardation, short life span, wasting, and diarrhea
4. Susceptible to graft-versus-host disease (GVHD) if given nonirradiated blood products or unmatched allogeneic bone marrow
5. Fatal reactions from live virus or BCG vaccination
6. High incidence of malignancy

to as having partial DiGeorge syndrome. Those with complete DiGeorge syndrome may resemble patients with SCID in their susceptibility to infections with opportunistic pathogens (i.e., fungi, viruses, and *P. carinii*). They also may develop graft-versus-host disease (GVHD) from nonirradiated blood transfusions.

Concentrations of serum immunoglobulins usually are near normal for age, but IgA may be diminished and IgE may be elevated. T cell numbers are decreased, and, as a result, there is a relative increase in the percentage of B cells. Despite decreased numbers of $CD3^+$ T cells, there are usually normal proportions of $CD4^+$ and $CD8^+$ cells. Lymphocyte responses to mitogen stimulation, like the intradermal delayed hypersensitivity response, have been absent, reduced, or normal, depending on the degree of thymic deficiency. Thymic tissue, when found, does contain Hassall's corpuscles and a normal density of thymocytes. Corticomedullary distinction is present. Lymphoid follicles usually are present, but lymph node paracortical areas and thymus-dependent regions of the spleen show variable degrees of depletion. Because of variability in the severity of the immunodeficiency, it is difficult to evaluate claimed benefits of fetal thymus transplantation. Some patients have experienced immunologic reconstitution after unfractionated HLA-identical bone marrow transplantation.

Cellular Immunodeficiency with Immunoglobulins (Nezelof Syndrome). Nezelof syndrome is characterized by lymphopenia, diminished lymphoid tissue, abnormal thymus architecture, and the presence of normal or increased levels of most of the five immunoglobulin classes. Nezelof syndrome is the primary immunodeficiency disorder most likely to be confused with AIDS in the pediatric age group because of its features. During infancy, patients may experience recurrent or chronic pulmonary infections, failure to thrive, oral or cutaneous candidiasis, chronic diarrhea, recurrent skin infections, gram-negative sepsis, urinary tract infections, and severe varicella. Other findings include neutropenia and eosinophilia. Serum immunoglobulins may be normal or elevated for all classes, but selective IgA deficiency, marked elevation of IgE, and elevated IgD levels have been found in some cases. Although antibody-forming capacity has been impaired in a majority, it has not been absent and has been apparently normal in roughly one third of the reported cases. Moreover, plasma cells usually are abundant in the lamina propria and lymph nodes.

Studies of cellular immune function have shown delayed cutaneous anergy to ubiquitous antigens in all such patients and extremely low lymphocyte proliferative responses to mitogens, antigens, and allogeneic cells in vitro. Such patients have profound deficiencies of $CD3^+$ T cells but usually normal proportions of $CD4^+$ and $CD8^+$ cells, in contrast to patients with AIDS, who characteristically have a selective deficiency of $CD4^+$ cells. Peripheral lymphoid tissues demonstrate paracortical lymphocyte depletion. The thymuses are very small and have a paucity of thymocytes and usually no Hassall's corpuscles. However, again in contrast to AIDS, thymic epithelium is intact. Despite the profound cellular immunodeficiency, however, Nezelof patients usually survive longer than do infants with SCID. An autosomal recessive pattern of inheritance often is seen. Although patients with this disorder have been reconstituted successfully by matched sibling bone marrow transplants, most other forms of therapy have been unsuccessful.

NEZELOF SYNDROME WITH PURINE NUCLEOSIDE PHOSPHORYLASE DEFICIENCY. More than 33 patients with Nezelof syndrome have been found to have PNP (encoded by a gene on chromosome 14q13.1) deficiency. In contrast to patients with ADA deficiency, serum and urinary uric acid are markedly deficient, and no characteristic physical or skeletal abnormalities have been noted. Deaths have occurred from generalized vaccinia, varicella, lymphosarcoma, and GVHD following blood transfusions or allogeneic bone marrow transplantation. Unlike most Nezelof patients, the thymuses of PNP-deficient patients have had occasional Hassall's corpuscles at postmortem examination, reminiscent of some patients with ADA deficiency. Analyses of lymphocyte subpopulations with monoclonal antibodies have demonstrated a marked deficiency of T cells and T cell subsets but increased numbers of cells with NK phenotype and function. Attempts to correct the immunologic and enzymatic deficiencies of PNP-deficient patients by enzyme replacement or deoxycytidine therapy have not been successful.

Severe Combined Immunodeficiency Disorders

The syndromes of SCID are characterized by (1) absence of all adaptive immune function from birth and (2) great cellular, molecular, and genetic diversity. Patients with this group of disorders have the most severe of all of the recognized immunodeficiencies. Unless immunologic reconstitution can be achieved through immunocompetent tissue transplants or enzyme replacement therapy or gnotobiotic isolation can be carried out, death usually occurs before the patient's first birthday and almost invariably before the second.

Autosomal Recessive Severe Combined Immunodeficiency Disease. This was the first described of the SCID syndromes, reported initially by Swiss workers in 1958. Affected infants, within the first few months of life, have frequent episodes of diarrhea, pneumonia, otitis, sepsis, and cutaneous infections. Growth may appear normal initially, but extreme wasting usually develops after infections and diarrhea begin. Persistent infections with opportunistic organisms, such as *Candida albicans*, *P. carinii*, varicella (Fig. 18–2), measles, parainfluenzae 3, cytomegalovirus, Epstein-Barr virus, and BCG lead to death. These infants also lack the ability to reject foreign tissue and are, therefore, at risk for GVHD. GVHD reactions can result from maternal immunocompetent cells crossing the placenta or from the administration of nonirradiated blood products or allogeneic bone marrow containing T lymphocytes.

Infants with SCID have profound lymphopenia, an absence of lymphocyte proliferative responses to mitogens, antigens, and allogeneic cells in vitro, and delayed cutaneous anergy. Serum immunoglobulin concentrations are diminished to absent, and no antibody formation occurs after immunization. Analyses of lymphocyte populations and subpopulations have demonstrated marked heterogeneity among SCID patients, even among those with similar inheritance patterns or with ADA deficiency. Despite the uniformly profound lack of T or B cell function, many patients have elevated percentages of B cells. Monoclonal antibody studies generally have shown extremely low percentages of T cells and subsets. There is no increase in circulating lymphocytes bearing CD1,

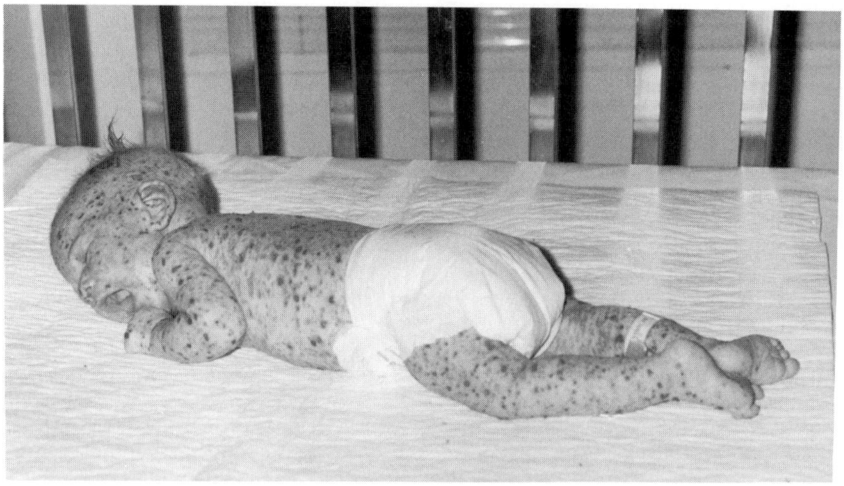

Fig. 18–2. Progressive varicella in an infant with severe combined immunodeficiency. *(From Buckley: JAMA 258:2845, 1987.)*

an antigen present on immature cortical thymocytes. Thus, the few T lymphocytes present appear to have acquired surface markers characteristic of mature T cells. Recently, a new phenotype of SCID was characterized by the author in which all or most of the lymphocytes present in some SCID infants were large granular lymphocytes with NK cell phenotype and function. NK function has been totally lacking in other SCID patients, again illustrating the striking heterogeneity at a cellular level. Typically, SCID patients have very small thymuses (less than 1 g), which usually fail to descend from the neck, contain few thymic lymphocytes, lack corticomedullary distinction, lack epithelial GD and GT gangliosides, and usually lack Hassall's corpuscles. It should be noted that despite the profound thymocyte depletion in SCID patients, thymic epithelium appears histologically normal, in contrast to the situation in AIDS, where there is marked epithelial atrophy. Both the follicular and paracortical areas of the peripheral lymph nodes are depleted of lymphocytes in SCID patients. Tonsils, adenoids, and Peyer's patches are absent or extremely underdeveloped.

Replacement therapy with IVIG fails to halt the progressively downhill course of SCID. Conversely, transplantation of bone marrow cells from HLA-identical or haploidentical donors has resulted in correction of the immunologic defect in a number of these patients, with over 200 known long-term survivors.

AUTOSOMAL RECESSIVE SCID WITH ADENOSINE DEAMINASE DEFICIENCY. An absence of the enzyme ADA (encoded by a gene mapped to chromosome 20q.13-ter) has been observed in approximately 40% of patients with autosomal recessively inherited SCID. Marked accumulations of adenosine, 2′-deoxyadenosine and 2′-O-methyladenosine directly or indirectly lead to lymphocyte toxicity, which causes the immunodeficiency. Adenosine and deoxyadenosine are apparent suicide inactivators of the enzyme, S-adenosylhomocysteine (SAH) hydrolase, resulting in the accumulation of SAH. SAH is a potent inhibitor of virtually all cellular methylation reactions. Such patients usually have more profound lymphopenia than other SCID infants and rarely have elevated percentages of B cells. In further contrast to infants with other types of SCID, a few ADA-deficient patients have been found to have rare Hassall's corpuscles in their thymuses and changes suggestive of early thymic differentiation.

Other distinguishing features of ADA-deficient SCIDs have included the presence of ribcage abnormalities similar to a rachitic rosary and multiple skeletal abnormalities of chondroosseous dysplasia on radiographic examination. These occur predominantly at the costochondral junctions, at the apophyses of the iliac bones, and in the vertebral bodies. As with other types, ADA-deficient SCID can be cured by HLA-identical or haploidentical T cell–depleted bone marrow transplantation, which remains the treatment of choice. Enzyme replacement therapy with polyethylene glycol–modified bovine ADA (PEG-ADA) administered subcutaneously once weekly has resulted in both clinical and immunologic improvement in more than 15 ADA-deficient patients. However, this therapy should not be initiated if bone marrow transplantation is contemplated, since it will confer graft-rejection capability. ADA-deficient SCID recently became the first genetic defect in which gene therapy was attempted. However, that particular effort is not likely to be successful in the long term, since mature T cells rather than stem cells were transfected with a vector carrying the normal ADA gene.

X-linked Recessive Severe Combined Immunodeficiency Diseases. This is thought to be the most common form of SCID in this country. The abnormal gene has been mapped by RFLP analysis to the Xq13-21.1 region. Carriers can be detected by demonstration of the presence of nonrandom X chromosome inactivation in T lymphocytes. Clinically, immunologically, and histopathologically, patients with the X-linked form usually appear similar to those with the autosomal recessive form, except that they generally tend to have higher percentages of B cells. However, results of X chromosome inactivation studies suggest that the genetic defect affects their B lineage cells as well as those of T lineage.

Defective Expression of Major Histocompatibility Complex Antigens. There are two main forms: (1) class I MHC antigen deficiency (bare lymphocyte syndrome) and (2) class I MHC antigen deficiency plus absence of class II MHC antigens. These conditions are inherited in an autosomal recessive pattern. The defect is not linked to genes encoding

MHC antigens on chromosome 6 (6p21.3). In some patients lacking class II MHC antigens, the defect appears to be due to a defective X-box binding protein that binds to the HLA-DR promoter. Sera from affected infants contain normal quantities of class I MHC antigens and β_2-microglobulin. Patients (usually of North African descent) have persistent diarrhea in early infancy and have oral candidiasis, bacterial pneumonia, *Pneumocystis* pneumonia, septicemia, and undue susceptibility to enteroviruses, herpes, and other viral agents. Those with both class I and class II antigen deficiencies also have malabsorption. There is variable hypogammaglobulinemia, with decreased serum IgM and IgA and poor to absent antibody production. B cell percentages usually are normal, but plasma cells are absent in tissues. Lymphopenia is only moderate. T cell functions are decreased in vivo and in vitro but are not absent. The thymus and other lymphoid organs are severely hypoplastic. Most of those affected die in the first 3 years of life. The associated defects of both B and T cell immunity and of HLA expression reinforce the important biologic role for HLA determinants in effective immune cell cooperation (Chap. 17).

Severe Combined Immunodeficiency with Leukopenia (Reticular Dysgenesis). In 1959 identical twin male infants were described who exhibited a total lack of both lymphocytes and granulocytes in their peripheral blood and bone marrow. Seven of the eight infants thus far reported with this defect died between 3 and 119 days of age from overwhelming infections. The eighth underwent complete immunologic reconstitution from a bone marrow transplant. Mature normal-appearing granulocytes (although markedly reduced in number) were noted in three patients, and a normal percentage of E rosetting T cells was found in the cord blood of a fourth patient, arguing against a total failure of stem cell differentiation in this defect. However, despite the normal percentage of T cells in the fourth patient's cord blood, the cells failed to give an in vitro proliferative response to mitogens. The thymus glands have all weighed less than 1 g, no Hassall's corpuscles have been present, and few or no thymocytes have been seen. An autosomal-recessive mode of inheritance seems most likely.

Partial Combined Immunodeficiency Disorders

Immunodeficiency with Thrombocytopenia and Eczema (Wiskott-Aldrich Syndrome). Wiskott-Aldrich syndrome is an X-linked recessive syndrome that is characterized clinically by the triad of eczema, thrombocytopenic purpura with normal-appearing megakaryocytes but small defective platelets, and undue susceptibility to infection. The abnormal gene responsible for this defect was shown by deSaint Basile et al to be closely linked to the novel hypervariable locus DXS255 on the proximal arm of the X chromosome between DXS7 (Xp11.3) and DXS14 (Xp11). Carriers can be detected by nonrandom X chromosome inactivation in several hematopoietic cell lineages. Often there is prolonged bleeding from the circumcision site or bloody diarrhea during infancy. The thrombocytopenia appears to be caused by an intrinsic platelet abnormality. Survival times of allogeneic but not autologous ^{51}Cr-platelets have been normal in these patients.

Atopic dermatitis and recurrent infections also usually develop during the first year of life. In younger patients, infections are commonly those produced by pneumococci and other bacteria having polysaccharide capsules, resulting in episodes of otitis media, pneumonia, meningitis, and sepsis. Later, infections with such agents as *P. carinii* and the herpesviruses become more frequent. Survival beyond the teens is rare. Infections and bleeding are major causes of death, but there is also a 12% incidence of fatal malignancy in this condition.

Patients with this defect uniformly have an impaired humoral immune response to polysaccharide antigens, as evidenced by absent or markedly diminished isohemagglutinins and poor or absent antibody responses after immunization with polysaccharide antigens. Antibody titers to proteins also fall with time, and anamnestic responses are often poor or absent. Studies of immunoglobulin metabolism have shown an accelerated rate of synthesis as well as hypercatabolism of albumin, IgG, IgA, and IgM, resulting in highly variable concentrations of different immunoglobulins, even within the same patient. The predominant pattern is a low serum IgM, elevated IgA and IgE, and a normal or slightly low IgG concentration. Lymphocyte responses to mitogens are moderately depressed, and cutaneous anergy is a frequent finding. Analyses of blood lymphocytes have shown moderately reduced percentages of T cells reacting with monoclonal antibodies to CD3, CD4, and CD8. In addition, there is defective expression of the sialoglycoprotein CD43 on all circulating leukocytes and platelets of Wiskott-Aldrich patients due to instability of this molecule on the cell surfaces. Sialophorin is encoded by a gene on the short arm of chromosome 16, whereas the susceptibility gene for this immunodeficiency disease is on the short arm of the X chromosome. The interrelationship of the two genes or their products (if any) in causing this disorder is unknown.

Several patients who required splenectomy for uncontrollable bleeding had impressive rises in their platelet counts and have done well clinically while on chronic antibiotic and antibody replacement therapy with IVIG. A number of patients with this disorder have had complete corrections of both the platelet and immunologic abnormalities by HLA-identical sibling bone marrow transplants.

Ataxia Telangiectasia. Ataxia telangiectasia is a complex syndrome with neurologic, immunologic, endocrinologic, hepatic, and cutaneous abnormalities. Inheritance follows an autosomal-recessive pattern. The abnormal gene has been mapped to the long arm of chromosome 11 (11q22-23). The most prominent clinical features are progressive cerebellar ataxia, oculocutaneous telangiectasias (Fig. 18–3), chronic sinopulmonary disease, a high incidence of malignancy, and variable humoral and cellular immunodeficiency. Ataxia typically becomes evident soon after the child begins to walk and progresses until he or she is confined to a wheelchair, usually by the age of 10 to 12 years. The telangiectasias develop between 3 and 6 years of age. Recurrent, usually bacterial, sinopulmonary infections occur in roughly 80% of these patients, but common viral exanthems have not usually resulted in untoward sequelae. However, fatal varicella occurred in one of the author's patients.

Cells from patients as well as those of heterozygous carriers have increased sensitivity to ionizing radiation, defective DNA repair, and frequent chromosomal abnormalities.

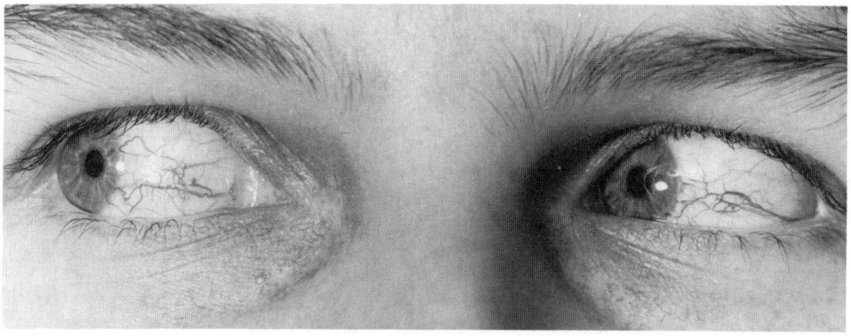

Fig. 18–3. Ocular telangiectasias in a patient with ataxia telangiectasia. *(From Buckley: JAMA 258:2847, 1987.)*

The sites of chromosomal breakage involve chromosomes 7 and 14 in more than 50% of patients. The breakpoints involve the genes that code for the T cell receptor and immunoglobulin heavy chains, most likely accounting for the combined T and B cell abnormalities seen. Inversion of chromosome 7-inv (7)(p14q35) is the most frequent rearrangement seen, although others involve chromosome 14 and the X chromosome. These rearrangements may be clonal and either may be stable or may undergo malignant transformation. The malignancies reported in this condition have usually been of the lymphoreticular type, but adenocarcinoma and other forms also have been seen. There is also an increased incidence of malignancy in unaffected relatives. The most frequent humoral immunologic abnormality is the selective absence of IgA, found in from 50% to 80% of these patients. Hypercatabolism of IgA also is known to occur. IgE concentrations are usually low, and the IgM may be of the low molecular weight variety. IgG2 or total IgG may be decreased. Specific antibody titers may be decreased or normal. In vivo there is impaired (but not absent) cell-mediated immunity, as evidenced by delayed cutaneous anergy and prolonged allograft survival. In vitro tests of lymphocyte function generally have shown moderately depressed proliferative responses to T and B cell mitogens. There are moderately reduced percentages of $CD3^+$ and $CD4^+$ T cells, with normal or increased percentages of $CD8^+$ and elevated numbers of Ti γ/δ^+ T cells. Studies of immunoglobulin synthesis have shown both helper T cell and intrinsic B cell defects. The thymus is hypoplastic, exhibits poor organization, and lacks Hassall's corpuscles. No satisfactory treatment has been found.

Cartilage Hair Hypoplasia. In 1965 an unusual form of short-limbed dwarfism with frequent and severe infections was reported among the Pennsylvania Amish. Severe and often fatal varicella infections, progressive vaccinia, and vaccine-associated poliomyelitis have been observed.

The severity of the immunodeficiency varies. In one series, 11 of 77 patients died before age 20. Three patterns of immune dysfunction have emerged: defective antibody-mediated immunity, defective cellular immunity (most common form), and severe combined immunodeficiency. In vitro studies have shown decreased numbers of T cells and defective T cell proliferation due to an intrinsic defect related to the G1 phase, resulting in a longer cell cycle for individual cells. This abnormality also occurs in fibroblasts from these patients. However, NK cells are increased in number and function. Cartilage hair hypoplasia appears to be autosomal recessive with variable penetrance. Bone marrow transplantation has resulted in immunologic reconstitution in some cartilage hair hypoplasia patients with the SCID phenotype.

Immunodeficiency with Thymoma. Patients with immunodeficiency with thymoma are adults who almost simultaneously develop recurrent infections, panhypogammaglobulinemia, deficits in cell-mediated immunity, and benign thymoma. They may also have eosinophilia or eosinopenia, aregenerative or hemolytic anemia, agranulocytosis, thrombocytopenia, or pancytopenia. Antibody formation is poor, and progressive lymphopenia develops, although percentages of Ig-bearing B lymphocytes usually are normal. Several patients with this disorder have been shown to have excessive suppressor T cell activity. The thymomas are predominantly of the spindle cell variety, although other types of benign and malignant thymic tumors also have been seen.

Hyperimmunoglobulinemia E Syndrome. The hyper-IgE syndrome is a relatively rare primary immunodeficiency syndrome characterized by recurrent severe staphylococcal abscesses and markedly elevated levels of serum IgE. The disorder was first reported by the author and coworkers in two young boys in 1972. Since then, the author has evaluated a total of 25 patients with the condition, and many other examples have been reported. These patients all have histories of staphylococcal abscesses involving the skin, lungs, joints, and other sites from infancy. Persistent pneumatocoeles develop as a result of their recurrent pneumonias. The pruritic dermatitis that occurs is not typical atopic eczema, and it does not always persist. Respiratory allergic symptoms usually are absent.

Laboratory features include exceptionally high serum IgE, elevated serum IgD, usually normal concentrations of IgG, IgA, and IgM, pronounced blood and sputum eosinophilia, abnormally low anamnestic antibody responses to booster immunizations, and poor antibody and cell-mediated responses to neoantigens. In vitro studies have shown normal percentages of $CD2^+$, $CD3^+$, $CD4^+$, and $CD8^+$ lymphocytes, and there is no increase in the percentage of IgE-bearing B lymphocytes. Most have normal lymphocyte proliferative responses to mitogens but very low or absent responses to antigens or allogeneic cells from family members. Possibly related to this is the recent observation by the author of a decreased percentage of T cells with the memory (CD45RO) phenotype in the blood of these patients. Blood, sputum, and histologic sections of lymph nodes, spleen, and lung cysts show striking eosinophilia. Hassall's corpuscles and normal thymic architecture were observed at postmortem examination of one patient.

Phagocytic cell ingestion, metabolism, killing, and total hemolytic complement activity have been normal in all patients. Defects of mononuclear or polymorphonuclear chemotaxis have been present in some but not all patients and, hence, are not the basic problem in these patients.

The fact that both males and females have been affected, as have members of succeeding generations, suggests an autosomal dominant form of inheritance with incomplete penetrance. The most effective management for this condition consists of chronic administration of therapeutic dosages of a penicillinase-resistant penicillin, with the addition of other antibiotics or antifungal agents as required for specific infections and appropriate thoracic surgery for superinfected pneumatoceles or those persisting beyond 6 months.

Leukocyte Adhesion Deficiency. Leukocyte adhesion deficiency (LAD or CD11/CD18 deficiency) is due to mutations in the gene on chromosome 21q22.3 encoding the 95 kDa β subunit (CD18) shared by three adhesive heterodimers: LFA-1 on B, T, and NK lymphocytes, complement receptor type 3 (CR3) on neutrophils, monocytes, macrophages, eosinophils, and NK cells, and p150,95 (function unknown but thought to be another complement receptor, Chap. 16). The α chains of these three molecules (encoded by genes on chromosome 16) are not expressed because of the abnormal β chain. Those so affected have histories of delayed separation of the umbilical cord, omphalitis, gingivitis, recurrent skin infections, repeated otitis media, pneumonia, peritonitis, perianal abscesses, and impaired wound healing. Severe, widespread, and life-threatening bacterial and fungal infections account for the high mortality. They do not have increased susceptibility to viral infections or malignancy. All cytotoxic lymphocyte functions are markedly impaired because of a lack of the adhesion protein LFA-1. Deficiency of LFA-1 also interferes with immune cell interaction and immune recognition. CR3 binds fixed iC3b fragments of C3 and β glucans. Its absence causes abnormal phagocytic cell adherence and chemotaxis and a reduced respiratory burst with phagocytosis. Blood neutrophil counts usually are significantly elevated even when no infection is present. Deficiencies of these glycoproteins can be screened for by cytofluorography of blood leukocytes with any of the following monoclonal antibodies: anti-Mac-1, OKM1, Leu-15, or anti-Mo1, which react with the α chain of CR3, or with Leu-M5, specific for the α chain of p150,95. This disease can be corrected by bone marrow transplantation. Since the CD18 gene has been cloned and sequenced, this disorder is considered a leading candidate for gene therapy.

T Cell–Activation Defects. These conditions are characterized by the presence of T cells that appear phenotypically normal by many criteria but that fail to proliferate or produce cytokines in response to stimulation with mitogens, antigens, or other signals delivered to the T cell antigen receptor (TCR). Recently a number of these defects have been characterized at the molecular level, including those in patients who had either (1) defective surface expression of the CD3/TCR complex because of failure of the CD3 ζ chain to associate with the rest of the components, (2) defective signal transduction from the TCR to intracellular metabolic pathways, or (3) pretranslational defects in IL-2 (T cell growth factor) or in other cytokine production or in both. These patients have clinical problems similar to those of other T cell–deficient individuals, although they are somewhat less severe than in SCID patients.

Acquired Immunodeficiency Syndrome

First recognized in late 1980, the acquired immunodeficiency syndrome (AIDS) is now known to be due to highly lethal, progressively epidemic viral infections that destroy the immune system. The causative agents are the human immunodeficiency viruses, HIV-1 (the cause of almost all cases in the United States) and HIV-2, both of which have affinity for the CD4 antigen on T lymphocytes, macrophages, and other cells. It is estimated that nearly 1.5 million Americans are infected with HIV-1. More than 100,000 cases of advanced infection (AIDS) have been reported to the U.S. Communicable Diseases Center, and over half of these people are dead. Predictions are that most HIV-infected individuals ultimately will die from the disease.

Patients with this syndrome have life-threatening opportunistic infections, Kaposi's sarcoma, or both. The opportunistic infectious agents have now included most of the bacterial, fungal, and parasitic agents customarily associated with cellular immunodeficiency, with *P. carinii, C. albicans, Mycobacterium avium-intracellulare,* herpes simplex, *Toxoplasma gondii,* hepatitis B, cytomegalovirus, and *Cryptococcus* leading the list. Until 1979, Kaposi's sarcoma was a tumor rarely seen in North America or Europe, occurring only in persons aged 50 years or older and responding well to chemotherapy or irradiation. A rapidly fatal form of it has been reported to be endemic in equatorical Africa, predominantly in black boys and young men, and several hundred cases of this type of Kaposi's sarcoma have been reported in the United States in young homosexual males over the past 10 years. In addition to the classic presentation with either severe opportunistic infections or Kaposi's sarcoma, a prodromal phase characterized by generalized adenopathy, recurrent fever, weight loss, and leukopenia occurs with high frequency in HIV-infected individuals (AIDS-related complex, or ARC). The fact that the prodromal phase can last for many months, together with other epidemiologic data, indicates a prolonged incubation period for the causative agent (i.e., 6 months to more than 8 years).

HIV infection is not acquired by casual contact, possibly because these are fragile enveloped viruses. Infection occurs primarily through intimate contact with blood or blood products or through sexual activity. There is no evidence for spread by insects or other routes. Although a majority of persons infected with HIV are homosexual or bisexual men, there is a rapidly increasing percentage of patients who are intravenous drug users, their sexual partners, and their children. The development of highly sensitive and specific tests for HIV infection, including the polymerase chain reaction (PCR), has permitted remarkable protection of the blood supply for those dependent on blood products for surgery or survival.

The immunologic abnormalities found in AIDS are those of a severe and profound cellular immunodeficiency. These include an absence of delayed hypersensitivity, lymphopenia caused by an absolute deficiency of $CD4^+$ T cells, reversal of the usual 2:1 ratio of $CD4^+/CD8^+$ blood lymphocytes, depressed lymphocyte responses to mitogens, and impaired NK cell function in vitro. The profound level of immunodeficiency occurs because 1 in every 100 $CD4^+$ T cells is infected and their helper function is lost, the gp120 coat protein is able to disrupt antigen presentation by macrophages to T cells, and viral materials from infected cells have immunosuppressive properties or can induce normal immune system cells to inhibit the hosts' immune responses. Paradoxically, marked hypergammaglobulinemia is present in most cases due to polyclonal B cell activation, and antibody titers to a wide range of antigens often are very high. Nevertheless, there is clear evidence for defective B cell responses to neoantigens. For this reason, AIDS patients are highly susceptible to high-grade bacterial infections.

Even though infected individuals have high titers of antibodies to HIV, these antibodies fail to prevent HIV from infecting new cells and, under conditions of limited amounts of virus, may even facilitate increased viral uptake by cells. Thymus glands from patients dying from this disorder show marked epithelial atrophy despite variable persistence of lymphoid elements. This picture is the opposite of that seen in thymuses of SCID patients, where epithelium is preserved but thymocytes are markedly depleted.

For the present there is no known effective treatment, although there is some evidence that therapy with zidovudine (AZT) may prolong survival in persons with AIDS, as well as in those with less advanced HIV infection. Other antivirals, such as 2′3′-dideoxyinosine (ddI), are promising, but both efficacy and toxicities need to be fully defined. An enormous effort is underway to develop an effective vaccine, and clinical trials are now beginning in the United States. Prevention based on the known epidemiologic features and treatment of those opportunistic infections for which therapies are available are still the principal approaches to management. Interferon-α has been effective in treating some patients with Kaposi's sarcoma. Bone marrow transplantation was successful in transiently correcting the immunodeficiency in one patient with AIDS who had a normal identical twin donor but was ultimately unsuccessful in this and in 14 other patients who also had identical twin donors because of infection of the transplanted cells with HIV.

Phagocytic Cell Disorders

The essential role of phagocytic cells in host defense is seen in those patients who, although fully endowed with all the necessary components and functions needed for specific immune responsiveness, have either an insufficient number or inadequate function of polymorphonuclear cells or macrophages or both. Infections experienced by such individuals are similar in many respects to those of patients with antibody and complement deficiencies (e.g., primarily with high-grade encapsulated pathogens). Unlike patients with the latter defects, however, those with phagocytic cell dysfunction rarely have meningitis or septicemia but are more likely to experience subcutaneous abscesses or abscesses of lymph nodes, lungs, liver, and bones. Staphylococcal and gram-negative enteric organisms predominate, but infections with certain fungi, such as *Aspergillus* or *Nocardia* species, can be particularly problematic. Phagocytic cell deficiencies or dysfunctions can be a result of iatrogenic or genetic causes.

Disorders of Production

Polymorphonuclear neutrophils are the first cells of the immune system to arrive at sites of injury, and they are soon joined by mononuclear phagocytes from the circulation. Patients with insufficient numbers or reserves of phagocytic cells are likely to be susceptible to serious bacterial or fungal infections and to respond poorly to antimicrobial therapy.

Hereditary Neutropenias. These are autosomal traits that occur in both recessive and dominant forms. The recessive (Kostmann) form is characterized by $<500/mm^3$ granulocytes in the peripheral blood from birth. Arrested myeloid differentiation is the apparent cause of this condition, for the bone marrows of these patients contain an increased number of granulocyte precursors. Until recently, Kostmann's syndrome was invariably fatal in the first year of life. Patients with this disorder can now be treated effectively with injections of recombinant human granulocyte colony-stimulating factor (G-CSF) (Chap. 17) or by bone marrow transplantation. The dominant form of hereditary neutropenia is a benign condition in which the life span is normal and the abnormality is detected only as an incidental finding. A compensatory monocytosis is thought to be the explanation for the latter.

Cyclic Neutropenia or Periodic Myelodysplasia. Cyclic neutropenia is characterized by a periodic diminution in the number of peripheral blood polymorphonuclear neutrophils. Serial bone marrow studies have shown an intermittent failure of bone marrow neutrophil maturation at the promyelocyte stage. The rhythmicity of the disorder is remarkably uniform, the neutropenia occurring every 21 days in most instances. The condition occurs in both sexes with approximately equal frequency. In women the rhythmicity ordinarily has no relationship to menstruation. Fever, malaise, and ulcers on the oral mucous membranes and, occasionally, arthritis, abdominal pain, sore throat, lymphadenitis, and cutaneous ulceration accompany the neutropenia. All other aspects of immunity usually are normal. Interestingly, splenectomy has relieved the clinical symptoms of some patients, even though it did not alter the neutropenic episodes. A few instances of familial cyclic neutropenia are known, but there is no clear evidence for a genetic mechanism.

Neutropenia with Immunodeficiency. As noted earlier in this chapter, neutropenia may occur in association with several of the primary immunodeficiency disorders, most often in reticular dysgenesis, infantile X-linked agammaglobulinemia, and X-linked immunodeficiency with hyper IgM. When neutropenia occurs, it may be transient, persistent, or cyclic in nature, with the transient variety being most common. In the transient type, neutropenia may occur at the onset of a severe infection and give way to leukocytosis later in the course of the illness. The cyclic variety is different from the periodic myelodysplasia described previously in that the periodicity usually is not uniform.

Acquired Neutropenia. This may occur secondary to toxic effects of drugs, pollutants, or irradiation or as a consequence of autoimmune reactions involving leukocytes. The latter may be seen as a transient phenomenon in the newborn as a consequence of maternal isoimmunization by NA series antigens (Chap. 14) on fetal neutrophils during pregnancy. Neutropenia has been noted also in patients with neoplasms, overwhelming infections, or endotoxemia. Neutropenia is frequent in hypersplenism, in aplastic anemia (the most common cause of persistent neutropenia), and in certain forms or stages of leukemia.

Disorders of Function

In disorders of function, the number of peripheral blood leukocytes usually is normal, but their function is impaired in one or more of the following properties: adherence, locomotion, directional response to chemotactic stimulation, deformability, recognition, attachment, engulfment, phagosome formation, metabolic response during phagocytosis, degranulation, microbial killing, or digestion of engulfed material. Most of these disorders have been described within the past 25 years. Currently there are approximately 15 primary disorders of phagocytic cell function, and at least 35 other conditions have been reported in which there is a secondary decrease in phagocytic cell function.

Disorders of Deformability. The normal newborn's polymorphonuclear cells are characterized by abnormal deformability, which results in defective locomotion and chemotactic responsiveness, both of which are thought to require glycolysis. In neonates stressed by immaturity, hypoxia, or an overwhelming bacterial infection, intracellular killing of bacteria also may be abnormal. Moreover, the granulocyte reserves in neonatal bone marrow are extremely limited, so that granulocytopenia is the usual response to bacterial as well as viral infections.

Disorders of Adherence. Granulocytes must adhere to vascular endothelium before they can leave the circulation to enter the tissues. For this they must have a normal capacity for cell-cell adherence. Certain drugs, namely, corticosteroids and salicylates, interfere with adherence by preventing changes in plasma membrane surface charge. Neutrophils from patients with myotonic dystrophy also exhibit defective adherence and locomotion.

The best-known disorder of granulocyte adherence is seen in the LAD or CD11/18 syndrome caused by the profound deficiency or absence of complement receptor type 3 (CR3), which normally binds iC3b fragments. This deficiency results in abnormal phagocytic cell adherence and chemotaxis and a reduced respiratory burst on phagocytosis of iC3b-coated particles. The clinical and immunologic features of these patients are discussed under LAD (see above).

Disorders of Locomotion. For phagocytic cells to localize effectively an infectious process, they must be capable of rapid locomotion in response to chemotactic stimulation. A delay in this process results in an inflammatory lesion, as opposed to an abortive infection. Phagocytic cell locomotion depends on a contractile system that includes actin, myosin, actin-binding protein, and gelsolin and that is regulated by methylation of proteins and a calcium shift. Abnormal neutrophil locomotion had earlier been detected in children with the lazy leukocyte syndrome, who had recurrent gingivitis, stomatitis, otitis, and low-grade fever associated with severe neutropenia. Their granulocytes fail to respond normally to chemotactic stimuli and mobilize poorly from the bone marrow, which contains normal numbers of myeloid precursors and mature neutrophils. The cells also have reduced random mobility. Their serum does not contain inhibitors of chemotaxis, and the phagocytic and killing capacities of their polymorphonuclear cells are normal. Patients with thalassemia are susceptible to serious bacterial infection, even before splenectomy, because of depressed locomotive response of their granulocytes to chemotactic stimuli and defective neutrophil adherence.

Occasional instances of recurrent severe bacterial infections are thought to be due to the absence of specific granule antimicrobial peptides, termed *defensins.* Azurophilic granule constituents myeloperoxidase and lysozyme are present in normal quantity. Margination in response to endotoxin, aggregation, adherence, and ingestion of bacteria is normal. Findings in such patients support the concept that specific granules and their contents are important for oxidative metabolism and other neutrophil functions.

Chemotactic Defects. These occur in two forms: (1) those in which the blood chemotactic activity is diminished and (2) those in which the cellular response is impaired. In the first instance, diminished chemotactic activity has been attributed to the presence of plasma or serum inhibitors of chemotaxis in patients with Hodgkin's disease, with hepatic cirrhosis, with chronic mucocutaneous moniliasis (CMC), and with Wiskott-Aldrich syndrome. Controversy exists as to whether the inhibitors are abnormal constituents or a normal factor that is unopposed by an absence of a normal antagonist to the inhibitor, since the inhibitor could be neutralized by normal plasma in some instances. Polymeric IgA is a prime candidate for the serum inhibitor in patients with CMC. Bacterial products such as lipopolysaccharide and aspirates from staphylococcal abscesses also can be inhibitory. Such drugs as colchicine and steroids can act as inhibitors of chemotaxis. Chemotactic factors can be diminished in conditions in which C3 or C5 is diminished or dysfunctional (Chap. 13). Other examples of such deficiencies are seen in the normal newborn, in whom both components are low, and in acute glomerulonephritis and in Klinefelter's syndrome, where C3 is markedly reduced.

Intrinsic polymorphonuclear unresponsiveness to chemotactic stimuli has been noted in all disorders of deformability, adherence, and locomotion referred to previously and also in patients with diabetes mellitus or in terminal shock, in alcoholics, in patients with the Schwachman-Diamond syndrome, in two kindreds with ichthyosis, and in the immotile cilia syndrome. Decreased numbers of microtubules have been found in the pericentriolar region of granulocytes from patients with immotile cilia disorders, as well as in their respiratory ciliary cells.

Abnormal granulocyte chemotactic responsiveness was found in two children congenitally deficient in α-mannosidase. In such patients, large quantities of mannose-rich material accumulated within body cells, including granulocytes. The affected patients had severe recurrent infections. Their leukocytes also evidenced delayed phagocytosis of *Staphylococcus aureus* and *Escherichia coli.* The abnormal metabolites are suspected of interfering either with neutrophil membrane function or with cell locomotion.

Chediak-Higashi-Steinbrink syndrome is a rare but important disorder characterized by gigantism of cytoplasmic lysosomes in white cells, melanocytes, Schwann cells, and possibly other tissues. Clinically, affected individuals have partial (oculocutaneous) albinism with resultant photophobia, undue susceptibility to viral and enteric bacterial infections, hepatosplenomegaly, lymphadenopathy, anemia, and leukopenia, cutaneous ulcers, and neurologic changes, including cerebral atrophy. Peripheral blood smears show abnormally large peroxidase-positive granules in the neutrophils and eosinophils. Depressed responsiveness of polymorphonuclear cells to normal chemotactic stimuli has been noted, as well as an intracellular microbicidal defect. The latter appears to be due to a marked deficiency of the granule proteases cathepsin G and elastase. All aspects of adaptive immunity are normal, but there is a marked deficiency of NK cell function. Death from infection generally occurs before the fifth year of life. Heterozygous carriers of this autosomal recessive trait have been identified by the presence of the granulation anomaly in leukocytes.

Opsonic Defects. Opsonic defects may be due to deficiencies of the heat-labile (complement-derived C3b) or heat-stable (IgM and IgG antibodies) opsonins that alter the surfaces of bacteria to facilitate phagocytosis. As pointed out earlier, newborn serum is deficient in C3 and C5. Thus, it not only is incapable of generating normal quantities of C3a and C5a chemotactic factors but also cannot provide adequate quantities of the opsonin, C3b. In addition to a deficiency of heat-labile opsonins, cord serum is virtually devoid of IgM antibodies to gram-negative bacteria. Patients with congenital deficiencies of C3 or C3b inactivator or with dysfunction of C5 (Chap. 13) produce inadequate quantities of heat-labile opsonins and may have recurrent, often severe, infections. Heat-stable opsonins (antibodies) are severely lacking in patients with B cell functional deficiencies, accounting to a large extent for their special tendency to develop pyogenic infections.

Ingestion Defects. The capacity of the phagocytic cell to ingest bacteria is determined by the maturity of the cell, the presence of specific membrane receptors, and the energy potential of the cell. In acute myelocytic leukemia, the ingestion capacity of the cells is severely limited. Phagocytic cell membrane receptors for C3b and the Fc portion of IgG often are saturated in such conditions as systemic lupus erythematosus, rheumatoid arthritis, multiple myeloma, and macroglobulinemia, where circulating immune complexes or immunoglobulin aggregates interact continuously with the cells. A deficiency of a phagocytosis-promoting tetrapeptide, threonyl-L-lysyl-L-arginine or tuftsin, was reported to result in diminished ingestion of staphylococcal organisms by polymorphonulear cells in nine patients from four families. The affected patients had recurrent lower respiratory infections, enlarged fluctuant lymph nodes, and documented infections with *S. aureus, Candida,* and pneumococci. Tuftsin is synthesized in the spleen in the form of a cytophilic gammaglobulin termed *leukokinin,* which binds to granulocytes and is cleaved by the enzyme leukokinase to form tuftsin, which in turn enhances the phagocytic capacity of granulocytes. The negative surface charge of the phagocyte membrane can be altered by such drugs as levorphanol, a morphine analogue, or by viruses, such as influenza, that bind to the membrane. Any condition in which there is an associated inhibition of glycolysis, such as that due to hypophosphatemia of malnutrition, can produce a phagocytic defect on the basis of diminished cellular energy potential.

Killing Defects. A variety of disorders can alter the phagocytic cell's ability to kill bacteria, even though the cells may have responded normally to chemotactic stimuli and the bacteria have been well opsonized and ingested normally. Among the best known of these conditions is chronic granulomatous disease (CGD). This syndrome is characterized by chronic suppurative infections, draining adenopathy, pneumonia, hepatomegaly with liver abscesses, osteomyelitis, splenomegaly, hypergammaglobulinemia, and dermatitis, with onset of symptoms usually before 1 year of age.

In the syndrome of CGD, three different molecular defects have been delineated, one of which involves a gene on the X-chromosome (62% of cases) and two more that affect genes on chromosomes 1 (5% of cases) and 7 (33% of cases). When normal granulocyte membranes are stimulated during phagocytosis, there is activation of the membrane-bound electron-transport chain, NADPH-oxidase, which acts on NADPH to reduce molecular oxygen to the superoxide anion. The NADPH-oxidase system is known to consist of at least two components, a flavoprotein and cytochrome *b* 245. The gene that is abnormal in X-linked CGD (X-CGD) was mapped to Xp21.1 by deletion and formal linkage analysis. Using this information, it was possible to clone the gene and demonstrate that its transcripts were absent or structurally abnormal in four patients with X-CGD. The nucleotide sequence of the complementary DNA (cDNA) clones led to the prediction that the gene product is a polypeptide of at least 468 amino acids. Further characterization of the protein showed it to be the 90 kDa transmembrane β chain of the cytochrome *b* 245 heterodimer. Since the gene for this polypeptide has been cloned and sequenced, CGD is another candidate disease for gene therapy. Two other autosomal recessively inherited molecular defects have been described that affect cytosolic factors important in the electron transport complex. These include a 47 kDa factor (neutrophil cytoplasmic factor 1 or NCF1) encoded by a gene on chromosome 7q11.23 and (less commonly) a 67 kDa factor (NCF2) encoded by a gene on chromosome 1q25.

Leukocytes from these patients have normal increments of glucose consumption, lactate production, Krebs or tricarboxylic acid (TCA) cycle activity, and lipid turnover during phagocytosis of latex particles. In contrast, their leukocytes fail to show normal oxygen consumption, direct oxidation of glucose, and hydrogen peroxide formation. The inability of leukocytes from patients with chronic granulomatous disease to lyse bacteria is related to their inability to stimulate the direct pathway of glucose metabolism to form hydrogen peroxide during phagocytosis. The myeloperoxidase, iodide (or other halide), hydrogen peroxide system is an important bactericidal system of human polymorphonuclear cells. Thus, the failure of CGD cells to generate peroxide, the superoxide anion radical, or singlet oxygen provides an explanation for their impaired microbicidal activity.

Because of defective triggering of oxidative metabolism, neutrophils from such patients are unable to kill catalase-positive bacteria (e.g., *S. aureus, Klebsiella aerobacter, Proteus,* and *Serratia marcesens*) and fungi despite normal chemotactic responsiveness and a normal ability to phagocytize these organisms. Moreover, these intracellular bacteria or fungi enjoy protection from antibiotics and can later seed out into the body fluids. These intracellular organisms evoke granulomatous reactions in the liver, the spleen, and other organs they invade. Pigmented histiocytes are found in such reactions. Granulomatous reactions (usually to gram-negative organisms) in the gastrointestinal and urinary tracts cause frequent problems with obstruction, and smaller granulomas in the lungs account for persistent reticulonodular densities on x-ray. Catalase-negative organisms, such as group A streptococci, *H. influenzae,* and pneumococci, which generate peroxide, are killed normally by their phagocytic cells. Patients with CGD have a particular susceptibility to resistant and recurrent pulmonary and bone infections with *Aspergillus* sp. Other fungi, such as *Nocardia, Candida,* and *Torulopsis,* also have caused such infections.

Failure of phorbol myristate acetate (PMA)–stimulated polymorphonuclear cells from affected individuals to reduce the colorless redox dye, nitroblue tetrazolium (NBT), to purple formazan during phagocytosis serves as a simple screening diagnostic test for this disorder. The slide test version of this can be used also to detect carriers. During phagocytosis, free oxygen radicals normally are generated. When they react with oxydizable substrates, they form unstable intermediates. As these intermediates return to their ground state, light energy measurable as chemiluminescence is released. A direct correlation has been shown between defective bacterial killing and failure to generate chemiluminescence in the neutrophils and monocytes of CGD patients. Because chemiluminescence is easily measured with a β-scintillation spectrometer, this assay has become another valuable diagnostic test, one that is also useful in determining CGD carriers in family studies. Unlike many of the other X-linked immunodeficiencies, however, X-chromosome inactivation is random in all cell lineages examined from obligate carriers of X-linked CGD.

In vitro fungicidal and bactericidal activity is markedly diminished in the neutrophils and monocytes of patients with congenital absence of myeloperoxidase. This is now believed to be the most common granulocyte defect, with an incidence of 28 in 60,000 subjects. There is increased susceptibility to infections with *C. albicans,* particularly if the patient also has diabetes mellitus, but resistance to bacterial infection appears normal. Myeloperoxidase levels are often lower than normal in patients with myeloblastic leukemia or in those with severe or overwhelming infections. Bactericidal capacity may be depressed in patients with severe (e.g., <1% of normal) deficiencies of glucose-6-phosphate dehydrogenase (G6PD), but most individuals with this hereditary defect (that involves both erythrocytes and leukocytes) have 20% to 50% of the normal amount of G6PD and no problems with infections. Finally, healthy newborns, despite their (1) abnormal granulocyte deformability and lack of responsiveness to chemotactic factors and (2) inadequate heat-labile and heat-stable opsonins, usually have no intrinsic phagocytic cell microbicidal defects. They do, however, have increased resting rates of oxygen consumption, HMP activity, and NBT dye reduction.

Intrauterine Diagnosis and Carrier Detection

Intrauterine diagnosis of ADA and PNP deficiencies can be made by enzyme analyses on amnion cells (fresh or cultured) obtained before 20 weeks' gestation and of several X-linked defects by RFLP studies of the X chromosome in amnion cells from male infants whose mothers have been identified as carriers and who are heterozygous for informative DNA polymorphisms. Diagnosis of enzyme-normal SCID or other severe T cell deficiencies, MHC class I or class II antigen deficiencies, CGD, or Wiskott-Aldrich syndrome (by platelet size) can be made by appropriate tests of phenotype or function on small samples of blood obtained by fetoscopy at 18 to 22 weeks of gestation. In the case of those disorders in which the defective gene has been cloned and cDNA probes are available (CGD, ADA, PNP, and LAD), the diagnosis can be made by deletional or RFLP analyses of chorionic villus samples obtained during the first trimester.

Carriers of X-linked CGD can be detected by NBT or chemiluminescence studies of their blood neutrophils. Carriers of ADA and PNP deficiency can be detected by quantitative enzyme analyses of blood samples. Carriers of X-linked agammaglobulinemia, X-linked SCID, or the Wiskott-Aldrich syndrome can be identified by one of two techniques designed to detect nonrandom X chromosome inactivation in one or more blood cell lineages. One method employs somatic cell hybrids that selectively retain the active X chromosome, and the other depends on methylation differences between the active and inactive X chromosomes. Either method can be used successfully even when only one member of a family (or no previous members) has been affected, since neither of these methods depends on linkage analysis.

Treatment

The principal modes of therapy for the primary immunodeficiency disorders include protective isolation, use of antibiotics for the eradication or prevention of bacterial and fungal infections, and attempted replacement of missing humoral or cellular immunologic functions. The complexities of both the immune deficiency diseases and their treatment emphasize the need for all such patients to be evaluated in centers where detailed studies of immune function can be conducted before therapy is selected or begun.

Antibody Deficiency Disorders

Judicious use of antibiotics and regular administration of antibodies are the only treatments that have proved effective for this group of disorders. Patients with agammaglobulinemia, X-linked immunodeficiency with hyper IgM, antibody deficiency with near-normal immunoglobulins, Wiskott-Aldrich syndrome, and all forms of SCID are candidates for immunoglobulin replacement therapy. The most common form of replacement therapy currently is with immune serum globulin modified for safe intravenous use (IVIG). All six FDA-approved IVIG preparations in the United States consist primarily of IgG antibodies, with small amounts of antibodies of the other classes. Recent experience suggests that 400 mg/kg per month of IVIG permits achievement of trough IgG levels close to the normal range. HIV is inactivated by the ethanol used in preparation of ISG and IVIG, and such preparations are also free of hepatitis antigen. Systemic reactions to IVIG may occur, but rarely are these true anaphylactic reactions. Anaphylactic reactions caused by IgE antibodies (in the patient) to IgA (in the IVIG preparation) may, however, occur in patients with common variable immunodeficiency who have absent serum IgA. All newly diagnosed patients with CVID should be screened for anti-IgA antibodies through the American Red Cross before undergoing IVIG therapy. If such antibodies are detected, IVIG therapy may still be possible by use of the one available IVIG preparation containing almost no IgA (Gammagard, Baxter-Hyland).

Immunoglobulin replacement therapy is contraindicated in patients with selective absence of serum and secretory IgA because of the high frequency of anti-IgA antibodies and because these patients usually have normal quantities of IgG antibodies. IVIG should not be given to infants with transient hypogammaglobulinemia of infancy because it could suppress their innate capacity to form antibodies. There is no indication for the use of gammaglobulin therapy in patients with IgG subclass deficiencies unless they have been shown to have a broad defect in antibody-forming capacity.

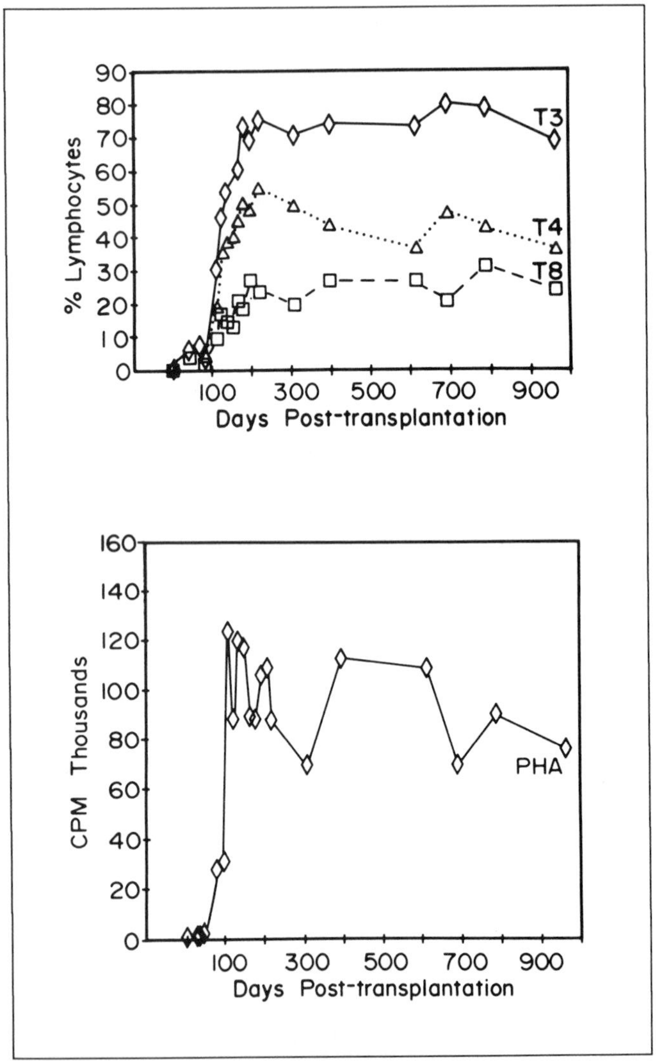

Fig. 18–4. Development of lymphocytes with mature T cell phenotypes (**top**) and function (**bottom**) in a male infant with severe combined immune deficiency after a maternal bone marrow stem cell transplant. All cells dividing in response to phytohemagglutinin had a female karyotype. The 90- to 100-day lag before the maternal stem cells have been matured completely by the infant's thymus is reminiscent of the time it takes for mature T cells to appear in the human embryo.

Cellular Immunodeficiency

The only adequate therapy for patients with severe forms of cellular immunodeficiency is immunologic reconstitution by means of an immunocompetent tissue transplant. Mature bone marrow that is MHC compatible or haploidentical (Chap. 17) with the recipient is the tissue of choice, except in the case of the complete DiGeorge syndrome, in which fetal thymic tissue has been recommended. However, there is no convincing evidence that thymic transplants cause immunologic reconstitution in that syndrome, whereas unfractionated HLA-identical bone marrow transplantation has been effective in all three DiGeorge syndrome patients in whom this was attempted. The major risk to the recipient from transplants of bone marrow or fetal tissues is that of GVHD. The recent development of techniques to deplete all postthymic T cells from donor marrow have, however, permitted the safe and successful use of haploidentical (half-matched) bone marrow cells for the correction of SCID. These techniques have employed (1) initial incubation with soybean lectin, followed by two rosette-depletion steps with sheep erythrocytes (the most successful approach) or (2) incubation with monoclonal antibodies to T cells plus complement. Both methods enrich the final cell suspension for stem cells. To date, more than 150 infants with SCID who lacked an HLA-identical donor have been treated with T cell-depleted haploidentical parental bone marrow, with usually little or no GVHD. Approximately 60% survive with successful immune reconstitution (Fig. 18–4).

Patients with less severe forms of cellular immunodeficiency reject such grafts unless they are treated with immunosuppressive agents before transplantation, and even then, there has been a high incidence of resistance to engraftment. Several patients with Wiskott-Aldrich syndrome and other forms of partial cellular immunodeficiency have been treated successfully with (usually HLA-identical) bone marrow transplants after immunosuppression. It is entirely possible that a number of genetic defects, including ADA and PNP deficiencies, LAD, and CGD, will be correctable in the future by gene therapy.

FURTHER READING

Books and Reviews

Bortin MM, Rimm AA: Severe combined immunodeficiency disease. Characterization of the disease and results of transplantation. JAMA 238:591, 1977

Buckley RH: Advances in the diagnosis and treatment of immunodeficiency diseases. Arch Intern Med 146:377, 1986

Buckley RH: Immunodeficiency diseases. JAMA 258:2841, 1987

Buckley RH: Primary immunodeficiency diseases. In Wyngaarden JB, Smith LG (eds): Cecil Textbook of Medicine, 19th ed. Philadelphia, WB Saunders Co, 1991

Buckley RH, Sampson HA: The hyperimmunoglobulinemia E syndrome. In Franklin EC (ed): Clinical Immunology Update. New York, Elsevier North-Holland, 1981, p 147

Buckley RH, Schiff RI: The use of intravenous immune globulin in immunodeficiency diseases. N Engl J Med 325:110, 1991

Buckley RH, Schiff SE, Sampson HA, et al: Development of immunity in human severe primary T cell deficiency following haploidentical bone marrow stem cell transplantation. J Immunol 136:2398, 1986
Calvelli TA, Rubinstein A: Pediatric HIV infection: A review. Immunodef Rev 2:83, 1990
Clark EA, Lanier LL: Report from Vienna: In search of all surface molecules expressed on human leukocytes. J Clin Immunol 9:265, 1989
Cunningham-Rundles C: Clinical and immunologic analysis of 103 patients with common variable immunodeficiency. J Clin Immunol 9:22, 1989
Eibl MM, Wedgwood RJ: Intravenous immunoglobulin: A review. Immunodef Rev 1:1, 1989
Fauci AS: The human immunodeficiency virus: Infectivity and mechanisms of pathogenesis. Science 239:617, 1988
Fischer A, Landais P, Friedrich W, et al: European experience of bone marrow transplantation for severe combined immunodeficiency. Lancet 336:850, 1990
Fischer A, Lisowska-Grospierre B, Anderson DC, Springer TA: Leukocyte adhesion deficiency: Molecular basis and functional consequences. Immunodef Rev 1:39, 1988
Frank MM: Complement in the pathophysiology of human disease. N Engl J Med 316:1525, 1987
Griscelli C, Lisowska-Grospierre B, Mach B: Combined immunodeficiency with defective expression in MHC class II genes. Immunodef Rev 1:135, 1989
Hirschhorn R: Inherited enzyme deficiencies and immunodeficiency: Adenosine deaminase (ADA) and purine nucleoside phosphorylase (PNP) deficiencies. Clin Immunol Immunopathol 40:157, 1986
Hong R: Update on the immunodeficiency diseases. Am J Dis Child 114:983, 1990
Johnston RB: Monocytes and macrophages. N Engl J Med 318:747, 1988
Lawton AR: Ontogeny of B cells and pathogenesis of humoral immunodeficiencies. Clin Immunol Immunopathol 40:5, 1986
Lehrer RI: Neutrophils and host defense. Ann Intern Med 109:127, 1988
Lobach DF, Haynes BF: Ontogeny of the human thymus during fetal development. J Clin Immunol 7:81, 1987
McAlpine PJ, Shows TB, Boucheix C, et al: Report of the nomenclature committee and the 1989 catalog of mapped genes. Cytogenet Cell Genet 51:13, 1989
Orkin SH: Reverse genetics and human disease. Cell 47:845, 1986
Polmar SH, Pierce GF: Cartilage hair hypoplasia: Immunological aspects and their clinical implications. Clin Immunol Immunopathol 40:87, 1986
Preud'Homme J-L, Hanson LA: IgG subclass deficiency. Immunodef Rev 2:129, 1990
Primary immunodeficiency diseases. Report of a WHO sponsored meeting. Immunodef Rev 1:173, 1989
Ratech H, Hirschhorn R, Greco MA: Pathologic findings in adenosine deaminase deficiency severe combined immunodeficiency. II. Thymus, spleen, lymph node, and gastrointestinal tract lymphoid tissue alterations. Am J Pathol 135:1145, 1989
Remold-O'Donnell E, Rosen FS: Sialophorin (CD43) and the Wiskott-Aldrich syndrome. Immunodef Rev 2151, 1990
Ross SC, Densen P: Complement deficiency states and infection: Epidemiology, pathogenesis and consequences of neisserial and other infections in an immune deficiency. Medicine 63:243, 1984
Stiehm ER: Human gamma globulin as therapeutic agent. Adv Pediatr 35:1, 1988
Swift M: Genetic aspects of ataxia telangiectasia. Immunodef Rev 2:67, 1990
Tiller TL, Buckley RH: Transient hypogammaglobulinemia of infancy: Review of the literature, clinical and immunologic features of 11 new cases and long-term follow-up. J Pediatr 92:347, 1978
Winkelstein JA, Fearon E: Carrier detection of the X-linked primary immunodeficiency diseases using X-chromosome inactivation analysis. J Allergy Clin Immunol 85:1090, 1990

Selected Articles

Akahori Y, Kurosawa Y, Kamachi Y, et al: Presence of immunoglobulin (Ig) M and IgG double isotype-bearing cells and defect of switch recombination in hyper IgM immunodeficiency. J Clin Invest 85:1722, 1990
Akeson AL, Wiginton DA, Hutton JJ: Normal and mutant human adenosine deaminase genes. J Cell Biochem 39:217, 1989
Alarcon B, Regueiro JR, Arnaiz-Villena A, Terhorst C: Familial defect in the surface expression of the T cell receptor CD3 complex. N Engl J Med 319:1203, 1988
Ambrosino DM, Umetsu DT, Siber GR, et al: Selective defect in the antibody response to *Haemophilus influenzae* type B in children with recurrent infections and normal serum IgG subclass levels. J Allergy Clin Immunol 81:1175, 1988
Barrett MJ, Buckley RH, Schiff SE, et al: Accelerated development of immunity following transplantation of maternal marrow stem cells into infants with severe combined immunodeficiency and transplacentally acquired lymphoid chimerism. Clin Exp Immunol 72:118, 1988
Biron CA, Byron KS, Sullivan JL: Severe herpesvirus infections in an adolescent without natural killer cells. N Engl J Med 320:1731, 1989
Bonilla MA, Gillio AP, Ruggeiro M, et al: Effects of recombinant human granulocyte colony-stimulating factor on neutropenia in patients with congenital agranulocytosis. N Engl J Med 320:1574, 1989
Carbonari M, Cherchi M, Paganelli R, et al: Relative increase of T cells expressing the gamma/delta rather than the alpha/beta receptor in ataxia telangiectasia. N Engl J Med 322:73, 1990
Chatila T, Wong R, Young M, et al: An immunodeficiency characterized by defective signal transduction in T lymphocytes. N Engl J Med 320:696, 1989
Clark RA, Malech HL, Gallin JI, et al: Genetic variants of chronic granulomatous disease: Prevalence of deficiencies of two cytosolic components of the NADPH oxidase system. N Engl J Med 321:647, 1989
Clement LT, Plaeger-Marshall S, Haas A, et al: Bare lymphocyte syndrome: Consequences of absent class II major histocompatibility antigen expression for B lymphocyte differentiation and function. J Clin Invest 81:669, 1988
Conley ME, Brown P, Pickard AR, et al: Expression of the gene defect in X-linked agammaglobulinemia. N Engl J Med 315:1418, 1986
Conley ME, Lavoie A, Briggs C, et al: Non-random X chromosome inactivation in B cells from carriers of X-linked severe combined immunodeficiency. Proc Natl Acad Sci USA 85:3090, 1988
Cunningham-Rundles C: Clinical and immunologic analyses of 103 patients with common variable immunodeficiency. J Clin Immunol 9:22, 1989
Cunningham-Rundles C, Siegal FP, Cunningham-Rundles S, Lieberman P: Incidence of cancer in 98 patients with common varied immunodeficiency. J Clin Immunol 7:294, 1987
deSaint Basil G, Arveiler B, Oberle I, et al: Close linkage of the locus for X chromosome-linked severe combined immunodeficiency to polymorphic DNA markers in Xq11-q13. Proc Natl Acad Sci USA 84:7576, 1987
deSaint Basil G, Fraser NJ, Craig IW, et al: Close linkage of hypervariable marker DXS255 to disease locus of Wiskott-Aldrich syndrome. Lancet 1:1319, 1989

deWolf F, Lange JM, Houweling JT, et al: Numbers of $CD4^+$ cells and the levels of core antigens of and antibodies to the human immunodeficiency virus as predictors of AIDS among seropositive homosexual men. J Infect Dis 158:615, 1988

Dinauer MC, Orkin SH, Brown R, et al: The glycoprotein encoded by the X-linked chronic granulomatous disease locus is a component of the neutrophil cytochrome b complex. Nature 327:717, 1987

Ezekowitz RAB, Dinauer MC, Jaffe HS, et al: Partial correction of the phagocyte defect in patients with X-linked chronic granulomatous disease by subcutaneous interferon gamma. N Engl J Med 319:146, 1988

Fibison WJ, Budarf M, McDermid H, et al: Molecular studies of DiGeorge syndrome. Am J Hum Genet 46:888, 1990

Francke U, Hsieh CL, Foellmer BE, et al: Genes for two autosomal recessive forms of chronic granulomatous disease assigned to 1q25 (NCF2) and 7q11.23 (NCF1). Am J Hum Genet 47:483, 1990

Ganz T, Metcalf JA, Gallin JI, et al: Microbicidal/cytotoxic proteins of neutrophils are deficient in two disorders: Chediak-Higashi syndrome and "specific" granule deficiency. J Clin Invest 82:552, 1988

Geisler C, Pallesen G, Platz P, et al: Novel primary thymic defect with T lymphocytes expressing gamma/delta T cell receptor. J Clin Pathol 43:705, 1989

Goldsobel AB, Haas A, Stiehm ER: Bone marrow transplantation in DiGeorge syndrome. J Pediatr 111:40, 1987

Gougeon M-L, Drean G, le Deist F, et al: Human severe combined immunodeficiency disease. Phenotypic and functional characteristics of peripheral B lymphocytes. J Immunol 145:2873, 1990

Greer WL, Kwong PC, Peacocke M, et al: X-chromosome inactivation in the Wiskott-Aldrich syndrome: A marker for detection of the carrier state and identification of cell lineages expressing the gene defect. Genomics 4:60, 1989

Hershfield MS, Buckley RH, Greenberg ML, et al: Treatment of adenosine deaminase deficiency with polyethylene glycol-modified adenosine deaminase (PEG-ADA). N Engl J Med 316:589, 1987

Hume CR, Lee JS: Congenital immunodeficiencies associated with absence of HLA class II antigens on lymphocytes result from distinct mutations in *trans*-acting factors. Hum Immunol 26:288, 1989

Jackson GG, Paul DA, Falk LA, et al: Human immunodeficiency virus (HIV) antigenemia (p24) in the acquired immunodeficiency syndrome (AIDS) and the effect of treatment with zidovudine (AZT). Ann Intern Med 108:175, 1988

Kwan S-P, Sandkuyl LA, Blaese M, et al: Genetic mapping of the Wiskott-Aldrich syndrome in two highly linked polymorphic DNA markers. Genomics 3:39, 1988

Lammer EJ, Opitz JM: The DiGeorge anomaly as a developmental field defect. Am J Med Genet 2:113, 1986

Lau YL, Levinsky RJ: Prenatal diagnosis and carrier detection in primary immunodeficiency disorders. Arch Dis Child 63:758, 1988

Lefranc G, Chaabani H, Van Loghem E et al: Simultaneous absence of the human IgG1, IgG2, IgG4 and IgA1 subclasses: Immunological and immunogenetic considerations. Eur J Immunol 13:240, 1983

Malech HL, Gallin JI: Neutrophils in human diseases. N Engl J Med 317:687, 1987

Markert ML, Norby-Slycord C, Ward FE: A high proportion of ADA point mutations associated with a specific alanine to valine substitution. Am J Hum Genet 45:354, 1989

Markert ML, Hershfield MS, Wiginton DA, et al: Identification of a deletion in the adenosine deaminase gene in a child with severe combined immunodeficiency. J Immunol 138:3203, 1987

Moss AR, Bacchetti P, Osmond D, et al: Seropositivity for HIV and the development of AIDS or AIDS-related condition: Three year follow-up of the San Francisco General Hospital cohort. Br Med J 296:745, 1988

Nunoi H, Rotrosen D, Gallin JI, Malech HL: Two forms of autosomal chronic granulomatous disease lack distinct neutrophil cytosol factors. Science 242:1298, 1988

Pahwa R, Chatila T, Pahwa S, et al: Recombinant interleukin 2 therapy in severe combined immunodeficiency disease. Proc Natl Acad Sci USA 86:5069, 1989

Peterson RDA, Funkhouser JD: Ataxia telangiectasia: An important clue. N Engl J Med 322:124, 1990

Reith W, Barras E, Satola S, et al: Cloning of the major histocompatibility complex class II promoter binding protein affected in a hereditary defect in class II gene regulation. Proc Natl Acad Sci USA 86:4200, 1989

Roberts JL, Volkman DJ, Buckley RH: Modified MHC restriction of donor-origin T cells in humans with severe combined immunodeficiency transplanted with haploidentical bone marrow stem cells. J Immunol 143:1575, 1989

Schaffer FM, Palermos J, Zhu ZB, et al: Individuals with IgA deficiency and common variable immunodeficiency share complex polymorphisms of major histocompatibility complex class III genes. Proc Natl Acad Sci USA 86:8015, 1989

Stern MH, Lipkowitz S, Aurias A, et al: Inversion of chromosome 7 in ataxia telangiectasia is generated by a rearrangement between T cell receptor beta and T cell receptor gamma genes. Blood 74:2076, 1989

Teahan C, Rowe P, Parker P, et al: The X-linked chronic granulomatous disease gene codes for the beta chain of cytochrome b-245. Nature 327:720, 1987

Weinberg K, Parkman R: Severe combined immunodeficiency due to a specific defect in the production of interleukin 2. N Engl J Med 322:1718, 1990

CHAPTER 19

Immune Responses to Infection

The study of immune reactions to pathogenic organisms has provided much of the framework for the current understanding of basic immunology. Indeed, many of the fundamental concepts of immunology were developed by microbiologists studying natural host reactions to infectious organisms (Table 19–1). Although much of the recent progress in understanding basic immune responsiveness has involved studies using unusual or artificial antigens, cloned cells, manipulated hosts, and purely in vitro models, the concepts and mechanisms derived from such data ultimately must be considered in terms

TABLE 19–1. EARLY MICROBIOLOGISTS-IMMUNOLOGISTS AND THEIR CONTRIBUTIONS

Scientist	Discovery (Year)	Organism or Model
Jenner	Vaccination, cross-reactivity (1796)	Cowpox, smallpox
Pasteur	Attenuated vaccine (1878)	Cholera
Metchnikoff	Phagocytosis (1882–1884)	Bacteria, fungi
Richet and Hericourt	Serologic immunity (1888)	*Staphylococcus*
Charrin and Roger	Serum agglutinins (1889)	*Pseudomonas aeruginosa*
Pfeiffer	Serologic specificity (1889)	Cholera
Behring and Kitasato	Serologic antitoxins, neutralization (1890)	*Clostridium tetani*
Pfeiffer and Isaeff	Bacteriolysis (1894)	Cholera
Bordet	Complement (1895)	Cholera
Kraus	Serum precipitins (1897)	Culture supernates
Neufeld	Quellung reaction (1902)	*Streptococcus pneumoniae*
Richet and Portier	Anaphylaxis (1902)	Actinaria
Wright and Douglas	Opsonization (1903)	Bacteria

of their relevance to natural biologic phenomena. Even today, the interface between immunology and microbiology becomes most evident with the infected patient. For example, a major component of clinical immunology involves serologic and other immunologic measures of the host response to infection. Defense against infectious agents is clearly the major function of host immunity, and this chapter examines immune reactions to infection, considering the influence of both the host and the offending organism.

Infectious Organisms: Basis for Host Immune Diversity

The complexity of the mammalian immune system largely reflects the variety of infectious organisms encountered. In turn, the emergence of new pathogenic organisms reflects (to some extent) changes in host defense mechanisms that ensure their evolutionary survival. Thus it is not surprising that humans, as one of the most mobile and ubiquitous species, have developed a highly sophisticated means of immunologic defense for protection against the wide range of pathogens to which they are exposed. The diversity of immunologic protection is reflected at several distinct levels: (1) mechanistic variety, (2) the broad range of specific antigens recognized by antibody and T cell receptors (TCR), and (3) polymorphism of the major histocompatibility complex (MHC).

Mechanistic Variety

The human host has developed a variety of immunologic defenses for coping with the many different characteristics of infectious organisms. Some of the major factors that influence the effectiveness of specific immune mechanisms include the mode of microbial invasion, methods of intrahost spread, and structural features that protect the organism from certain types of immune-mediated damage. Therefore, depending on the organism, the most effective type of immune response might be local or systemic and involve cellular or humoral mechanisms. Moreover, the most useful mechanism might involve physical inhibition (e.g., by antibody-mediated neutralization), opsonization and phagocytosis (mediated by antibody, complement, and phagocytes), direct lysis (mediated by antibody and complement or cytotoxic T lymphocyte responses), or other more complex responses (regulated by cytokines produced by lymphocytes and macrophages).

Range of Specificity

The human host has the capacity to recognize 10^6 to 10^8 different antigenic determinants (epitopes) by both humoral (through antibodies) and cellular (through TCR) responses. This high degree of diversity is essential considering the tremendous number of microbes that may be encountered and the variety of antigens and toxins they express. The diversity of immunoglobulin specificities is based on the recombination of genes coding for the hypervariable, joining, diversity, and constant regions of heavy and light chains (Chap. 12). This mechanism provides the host with the potential ability to produce antibody that will recognize virtually any immunogenic combination of epitopes expressed by an organism. An analogous mechanism accounts for the diversity of T cell receptor (TCR) specificities, yielding a T cell repertoire capable of recognizing most antigens in association with polymorphic class I and class II self-MHC determinants.

Polymorphism of Major Histocompatibility Complex

The discovery of MHC-encoded transplantation antigens in mice and man during the 1940s and 1950s raised fundamental questions about their true function in biologic processes, as tissue transplantation cannot be considered a naturally occurring event. Moreover, the biologic basis for the high degree of MHC polymorphism was difficult to explain until it was shown in the 1970s that T cell–mediated lysis of virus-infected cells involves dual recognition of both viral and MHC antigens expressed by the target cell. Since then the critical role of class I and class II MHC gene products in regulating immune responses at the level of antigen recognition by effector and regulatory T cells has been more clearly elucidated (Chap. 13).

In general, regulatory *helper* T (T_h) cells have receptors that recognize antigen plus polymorphic class II MHC products, whereas *effector* or *cytotoxic* T (T_c) cells express receptors that generally recognize antigen plus polymorphic class I MHC products. T cells also express other receptors (i.e., CD8 and CD4), which bind to monomorphic (common) determinants of class I and class II MHC molecules, respectively, to promote cell-cell interaction (Chap. 16). Both of these characteristics presumably evolved to ensure the close physical contact of T cells with other cells expressing host MHC molecules and microbial or other antigens. Important physical interactions between T cells and other cells include helper T cells with stimulator macrophages expressing class II MHC and processed microbial antigens; cytotoxic T cells with infected target epithelial cells expressing class I MHC and virus surface antigens; and in some cases helper T cells with B cells expressing class II MHC and antigen bound to surface immunoglobulin. Moreover, MHC polymorphism may have evolved to provide a selective advantage for host responses against specific endemic organisms based on differences in the immunogenicity of particular microbial and polymorphic MHC antigen combinations (see below).

Constitutive Defenses

Components

In general, constitutive defenses provide the first line of protection against infections until antigen-specific immune defenses can be fully activated. Constitutive and immunologic defenses differ in several important ways. First, constitutive mechanisms are normally in place or are activated within minutes to hours after exposure. In contrast, activation and differentiation of lymphocytes to produce significant effector T cell or antibody responses (particularly with the initial exposure) usually require several days or more. Second, many different organisms may activate or be damaged by the same constitutive mechanism, whereas immune defenses are generally targeted for specific agents. Consequently, the immune response to one agent can, within some limits, be regulated independently of the responses to other agents. Third, whereas immune responses are usually enhanced (or, in some cases, depressed) by previous exposure to an agent, constitutive defenses generally remain unchanged. Finally, immune (but not constitutive) responses to pathogens depend on the activity of antigen-activated lymphocytes. Major components of constitutive defenses are listed in Table 19–2 and include physical and biologic barriers, the inflammatory responses, and the reticuloendothelial system.

Physical and Biologic Barriers

The most basic defense against microorganisms is provided by preventing their attachment, surface colonization, or penetration of the host. The skin and epithelial linings of the respiratory, urogenital, and gastrointestinal tracts form the major physical points of contact with infectious agents, and the constant turnover and sloughing of epithelia act to eliminate attached or colonizing microorganisms, and the action of epithelial cilia also restricts attachment. Since the outer layer of intact skin is composed of dead and decaying cells, it is not a useful substrate for viral replication, which is dependent on host cell metabolism. A virus on the skin surface is also susceptible to inactivation by dehydration; with loss of viral capsid integrity, nucleases from the skin can rapidly degrade free nucleic acids.

Another physical defense mechanism is temperature. For example, the relatively cool environment of the nasal passages (33C to 35C) is not ideal for many temperature-sensitive species of virus. However, the rhinoviruses, which are a chief cause of the common cold, have adapted to the cool environ-

TABLE 19–2. COMPONENTS OF CONSTITUTIVE DEFENSES

Component	Examples	Immune Regulation
Physical barriers	Skin, epithelia, hair	Minimal or none
Chemical barriers	Mucus, enzymes, fatty acids in sweat, tears, secretions	Minimal or none
Phagocytic or exocytic cells		
Fixed in tissues	Reticuloendothelial system, splenic macrophage, Kupffer's cells, dendritic cells, Langerhans' cells, mast cells	Activated by lymphokines; receptors for Ig, complement
Inflammatory cells	Neutrophils, granulocytes, monocytes, natural killer cells	Receptors for Ig, complement chemotaxins; some activation by lymphokines
Vasoactive agents	C3a, C5a, histamine, serotonin, kinins	Antibody, complement, and clotting cascades
Coagulation	Clotting cascade	Antibody effects on C; acute phase reactions
Complement	Opsonic and chemotactic activity of C3a and C5a; lytic activity of C5–C9 complex	Antibody activation; acute phase reactions
Other acute phase reactants	Protease inhibitors, transport proteins, adherence, agglutinating proteins, pyrogens	Cytokines
Interferons	Alpha and beta forms made by nonimmune cells	IFNγ made by T cells

ment of the nasal passages and grow preferentially in that environment. Fever, especially with temperatures greater than 38.5C, can inhibit replication of some viruses to the extent that the use of antipyretics (aspirin, acetaminophen) is really of questionable therapeutic benefit with these infections.

Chemical and biologic defenses can augment these physical barriers by directly neutralizing microorganisms or mechanically blocking their further dissemination into the body. The skin, for example, provides habitats for a variety of bacterial species that comprise the normal (usually harmless) commensal microbial flora. Some of these species produce substances that can inhibit the growth of pathogenic organisms; inhibition of *Staphylococcus aureus* growth by products of *Propionibacterium acnes* is an example. Substances that inhibit bacterial growth, block attachment to or penetration of surface layers, or directly kill microbes are present in the fluids and secretions that bathe the body surface and epithelia. For example, lysozyme in tears, saliva, and nasal secretions can digest the muramic acid in bacterial cell walls, and lactic acid in sweat, lactoperoxidase in saliva, unsaturated fatty acids in sebum, and gastric acids in the digestive tract also can directly inhibit bacterial growth. Although the nonenveloped enteroviruses and rotaviruses are stable in gastric acids, the more labile enveloped viruses are not as well adapted to gastric conditions; therefore their entry must occur either through breaks in the skin or through other mucosal surfaces.

When these various constitutive barriers are altered, the ability to resist infection becomes severely impaired. For example, overwhelming infection is a major, life-threatening risk to burn victims who have lost the protection of their skin; chronic damage to the respiratory epithelium from smoking or other causes increases the risk of pulmonary infections; urinary retention as a result of obstructive urologic disorders frequently is associated with urinary tract infections; and decreased gastric acidity can increase the risk of enteric infections. Diseases that perturb normal protective secretions can increase the risk of infections, for example, patients with Sjögren's syndrome (a condition with decreased tear and saliva production) have more frequent ocular and gingival infections, and those with cystic fibrosis (in which mucus becomes markedly thickened) are more susceptible to pulmonary infections.

Inflammatory Response

The activation of local inflammatory responses after microbial penetration of skin or another epithelial barrier provides a constitutive defense mechanism that inhibits microbes from spreading locally or systemically through the circulation. These inflammatory responses have two interacting components involving cells and soluble mediators as discussed in detail in Chapter 17.

Inflammatory Cells. Leukocytes are motile cells that respond chemotactically to a variety of stimuli. These stimuli include products released by microorganisms and damaged tissue or that are formed during the activation of various antimicrobial defense mechanisms. Consequently, leukocytes tend to accumulate at sites of infection or tissue damage. Changes in blood flow and vascular permeability at these sites potentiate migration of inflammatory cells into the tissue space.

The types of cells that dominate an inflammatory population depend strongly on the chemotactic signals that are produced, which change as inflammation progresses. Neutrophils normally predominate early in inflammation because they are the most numerous in the leukocyte population and respond to a wide variety of common signals. Basophils and eosinophils are more scarce in the blood but can become important inflammatory cells in special cases such as helminth infections. Monocytes usually are recruited into inflammatory sites later than granulocytes and often in response to lymphokines released by antigen-activated T cells. The presence of monocyte and lymphocyte infiltrates is often characteristic of an ongoing, chronic immune response at the inflammatory site. Detailed discussions of phagocytic cell migration, activity, and interaction with immune defenses are given below and in Chapter 17.

Various lymphocyte populations also provide constitutive defenses, the most prominent of which involves natural killer (NK) cells. These cells are predominantly large granular lymphocytes (LGLs), which can be identified with monoclonal antibodies to surface markers and by the presence of receptors for the Fc fragment of IgG. NK cells can be stimulated by interferon produced by virally infected cells or proliferating lymphocytes, but they exhibit limited specificity in vitro by lysing both infected and uninfected targets. Stimulated NK cells may also produce interferon, which up-regulates their own activity, protects uninfected cells from NK lysis, and causes NK cells to lyse other NK cells as a type of negative-feedback control. Although NK cells do not appear to recognize fine epitope differences, they do tend to respond to certain broad classes of target antigens. For example, a given NK cell clone might be very efficient at lysing a particular tumor cell line or one type of virus-infected cell but not others. NK cells are also probably involved in antibody-dependent cellular cytotoxicity (ADCC) reactions against viruses.

T cells expressing the $\gamma\delta$ TCR recognize a more limited range of antigenic determinants than those with the $\alpha\beta$ TCR but nevertheless are highly reactive with certain microorganisms such as mycobacteria and, in particular, the heat shock proteins (HSP) they produce. Moreover, such HSP-reactive $\gamma\delta$ T cells are present at birth (in the mouse) and thus may represent a form of constitutive defense.

Inflammatory Plasma Proteins. Inflammatory plasma proteins (Chap. 17) are produced in the acute-phase host response to infection or trauma and include complement and coagulation proteins; transport proteins (e.g., hemopexin, ceruloplasmin, ferritin, and haptoglobin) that compete for nutrients, making them unavailable to pathogens; protease inhibitors that limit tissue damage and regulate enzyme cascades; and adherence proteins (e.g., C-reactive protein, serum amyloid, and fibronectin), which may cause microbial agglutination, potentiate phagocytosis, or block adherence to host target cells. Synthesis of acute-phase proteins can be induced by the macrophage cytokines interleukin-1 (IL-1) and tumor necrosis factor-α (TNF-α) which also potentiate the release of inflammatory neutrophils into the blood and help restrict microbial growth by inducing fever. Macrophage synthesis of IL-1 and TNF-α is increased by bacterial products such as endotoxin or by lymphocyte products such as gamma interferon (IFNγ). Although most plasma proteins are synthesized in hepatocytes, many of the early-acting components of the complement and coagulation systems are also synthesized by resident and inflammatory macrophages. Thus these components are replaced to some degree at the sites of inflammation where they are consumed.

The coagulation and kinin systems, which control the flow of blood and lymph to and from sites of infection, can be activated directly by a variety of mediators such as bacterial components or products, enzymes released from damaged tissues or inflammatory host cells, endothelial cell products from damaged blood vessels, and other inflammatory plasma proteins. Factors generated during complement activation can directly affect vasodilation, coagulation, and kinin activities. Platelets can release vasoactive substances and complement components, as well as coagulation factors, at inflammatory sites. Fibrin deposition and blood clotting can trap microorganisms mechanically, and vasodilation increases lymph flow and can sweep microbes into the reticular fibers of lymph nodes where they can be killed by resident macrophages (see below). Vasodilation can also accelerate the infiltration of blood-borne inflammatory cells at the site of infection.

Components of the alternative complement pathway can be activated directly by the surface of many microorganisms without participation of antibody. As discussed in more detail in Chapter 15, complement activation involves formation of a covalent bond between complement component C3 and a suitable substrate on the microbial surface. Fixation of C3 can lead to formation of multienzyme complexes that cleave more C3 and C5. Surface-bound fragments of C3 and C5 and their soluble cleavage products C3a and C5a have important effects on microorganisms and inflammation: C3a and C5a are chemotactic and can mobilize cellular mediators of defense (see below) and also are vasodilators and smooth muscle contractants that can control hemodynamics locally; C3b and C3bi fragments on the microbial surface can potentiate receptor-mediated phagocytosis; and C3 and C5 membrane-bound fragments ultimately can activate the membrane attack complex of complement, leading to lysis of some microbes.

Although many microbes induce complement activation, some can actually escape the harmful effects of complement by using surface characteristics that destabilize complement complexes or facilitate complement inactivation. The pathogenicity of certain encapsulated strains of *Escherichia coli* has been ascribed to their ability to resist lysis by the membrane attack complex of complement. Blood parasites in particular (e.g., trypanosomes) have developed ways of inactivating or evading effects of the alternative complement pathway.

Reticuloendothelial System

The reticuloendothelial system (RES) includes phagocytes that line endothelial sinuses, especially in the liver (Kupffer's cells) and spleen, as well as phagocytes in tissue spaces attached to connective tissue (reticular) fibers. These resident "tissue" or "fixed" macrophages remove invading microbes from the blood and the lymph. Unlike inflammatory phagocytes, the cells in this system are derived primarily from the monocyte rather than the granulocyte lineage. Although not classically included in the RES, Langerhans' cells in the skin and dendritic cells in the lymph nodes are functionally similar to other RES phagocytes in that they can present antigens to and stimulate T cells. The RES is a last line of constitutive defense; organisms that penetrate physical and biologic barriers and resist local inflammatory responses then meet tissue macrophages of the RES. If the invading microbes are still not destroyed, they can enter the lymph nodes or the blood where they again must deal with constitutive phagocytic cell defenses and are likely to stimulate an immune response.

Phagocytic Cell Activity

Two distinct cell types are recognized as "professional phagocytes": the polymorphonuclear phagocytes (neutrophils) and the mononuclear phagocytes (monocytes or macrophages). These phagocytes can engulf particles at a high rate as opposed to the low-level phagocytosis that occurs with other cell types such as fibroblasts.

The proper functioning of phagocytes is critical for host defenses against microorganisms. Phagocytes are phylogenetically the most primitive host defense cells and likely have provided the foundation on which the extraordinarily complex cellular and humoral elements of the mammalian immune system have evolved. Despite the presence of complex regulatory and effector T lymphocyte populations, immunoglobulin classes and subclasses, and protein cascades yielding opsonins, chemotaxins, and bacteriolysins, phagocytic cell defenses have not been replaced in higher species. On the contrary, evolutionary refinements have brought about changes that amplify and increase the efficiency of phagocytic function. Phagocytes appear to be absolutely essential for the survival of both vertebrates and invertebrates. This is indicated by the following observations: animals with a congenital absence of phagocytes have not been described (suggesting that such a mutation would be lethal); humans with a genetic defect in one of the phagocyte-killing pathways (Chap. 18) have recurrent severe infections and a markedly shortened lifespan; and cancer chemotherapy, which impairs production of phagocytes, is associated with lethal opportunistic infections.

Production

Neutrophils are short-lived cells having a life span of approximately 4 days. Their production is a tightly regulated hematopoietic process centered in the bone marrow. A variety of cells, including macrophages, T cells, vascular endothelial cells, and fibroblasts, produce neutrophil growth factors such as colony-stimulating factor-G (CSF-G) and IL-3, which regulate the division and differentiation of neutrophil progenitor cells (called myeloblasts). The myeloblasts differentiate into mature neutrophils, which then leave the bone marrow and enter the circulation. There are about 3 to 7 million neutrophils per milliliter of blood in the normal state. During bacterial infections this circulating cell concentration may rise to 20 to 30 million neutrophils per milliliter of blood. Estimates of the number of neutrophils emigrating from the circulation into a tissue abscess are approximately 10^{10} to 10^{11} neutrophils per milliliter of abscess fluid.

Mononuclear phagocytes (monocytes) are also produced in the bone marrow and emigrate into the tissues where they can differentiate further into macrophages. Macrophages live longer than neutrophils and are prominent in tissues infected with facultative or obligate intracellular microbes. Tissue macrophages are present in all organs, especially along the sinusoids of the liver, spleen, and lymph nodes, and are a key component of the RES (see above). Tissue macrophages are produced in both the bone marrow and by in situ cell division in various organs. However, most tissue macrophages that respond to microbial infection are newly produced in the bone marrow.

Adherence

Neutrophils circulating in the blood adhere to capillary endothelial cells adjacent to infected tissue as a result of the interaction of adhesion molecule receptors and ligands on both cell types (Chaps. 16 and 17). This is a critical step in mobilizing phagocytes into an infected area. Phagocytes possess several types of surface receptors that facilitate adherence to other cells and targets. These include complement receptors, immunoglobulin Fc fragment receptors, and the integrin family of receptors, which bind to such ligands as fibronectin, collagen, and laminin. The importance of these receptors in immunologic defense is illustrated by newborns with leukocytes that lack the complement receptor (CR2) for the inactivated large proteolytic fragment of the third complement component (C3bi). These infants develop serious bacterial infections despite high circulating neutrophil counts. Their neutrophils tend not to accumulate in infected foci and fail to spread on plastic or glass surfaces when tested in vitro. Congenital absence of integrins has also been associated with increased rates of infection with pyogenic bacteria.

Chemotaxis

Leukocytes adhering to capillary endothelial cells crawl between the endothelial cells, a process called diapedesis. They traverse the capillary basement membrane to enter the interstitial space and then the parenchyma of various organs. This motility may exhibit a directional preference relative to a chemical gradient (i.e., chemotaxis; Chap. 17). Phagocyte receptor–ligand binding of chemotaxins leads to generation of an intracellular second messenger involving guanine nucleotides and phospholipid-derived inositol phosphates. Cytoplasmic calcium increases in response to the chemotactic stimulus.

Although many chemotaxins are produced by the host, some are direct microbial products. An important microbial chemotaxin is the formyl tripeptide characteristic of the initiation of protein synthesis in prokaryotes: formyl-methionine-leucine-phenylalanine. The small proteolytic fragment of the fifth component of complement (C5a) is an important endogenous chemotaxin, and the lipoxygenase pathway of arachidonic acid oxidation yields another important chemotaxin, leukotriene B_4 (LTB_4). Endogenously produced chemotaxins arise under conditions of inflammation. They are generated in plasma or extracellular fluid (i.e., complement activation) or are secreted from inflammatory cells (i.e., platelets and leukocytes in the case of LTB_4). Genetic defects in phagocytic chemotaxis have been described in humans (Chap. 18), and the propensity for pyogenic infections in these individuals demonstrates the importance of this physiologic process in maintaining host defense.

Phagocytosis

There are two key steps in phagocytosis: attachment of the object particle to the phagocyte, followed by ingestion of the particle into an internalized phagocytic vacuole called the primary phagosome. Phagocytes possess plasma membrane receptors for the Fc portion of IgG molecules and separate receptors for C3b (CR1), C3d (CR2), and C3bi (CR3) (Chaps. 15 and 17). After attachment the phagocyte membrane moves around the microorganism sequentially and circumferentially, engaging the protein ligands in a stepwise fashion. This movement requires that the receptors for these ligands have mobility in the plane of the membrane and has been termed the *zipper mechanism* of phagocytosis (Fig. 19–1). Ingestion is highly energy and temperature dependent. Plasma membrane

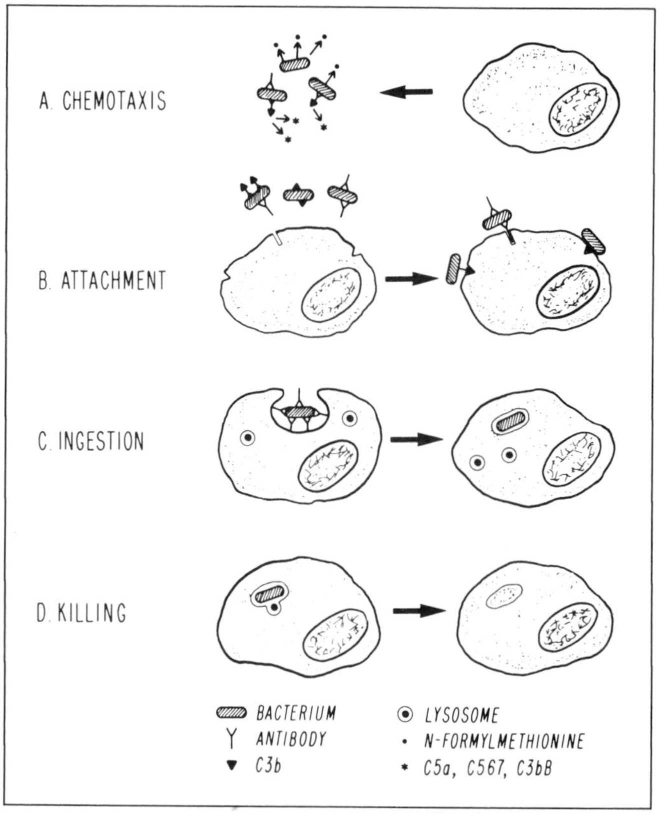

Fig. 19–1. Phagocytosis. Chemotaxis of phagocytes is mediated by bacterial products and complement activation. Attachment of phagocytes is enhanced by opsonins bound to the microorganism, such as the Fc portion of immunoglobulin and C3b. Engulfment of the microorganism results in the formation of a phagosome, which then fuses with cytoplasmic lysosomes, destroying the microbe by oxygen-dependent or oxygen-independent reactions (see text).

movement requires actin, myosin, actin-binding protein, and a cofactor protein that stimulates Mg^{2+}-dependent ATPase activity. Gelsolin controls the cross-linking of actin filaments by actin-binding protein. Contraction occurs when myosin contracts the actin gel into an aggregate, a process accelerated by the cofactor protein.

Many microorganisms have evolved antiphagocytic surface structures. Examples are the polysaccharide capsules of *Streptococcus pneumoniae* and *Cryptococcus neoformans*, the M-protein of *Streptococcus pyogenes*, and the pili of *Neisseria gonorrhoeae*. Mutant clones lacking these factors are avirulent. Phagocytosis of encapsulated microorganisms requires that specific antibodies or C3 or both be deposited on the surfaces of these microorganisms. Of the several classes of immunoglobulins, only IgG promotes phagocytosis, and C3b on the surface of microorganisms is probably the most important plasma ligand for phagocytosis. IgG enhances complement-mediated ingestion by localizing C3b on the most external parts of the microbial antiphagocytic structures. Individuals born with IgG agammaglobulinemia develop more frequent and more serious infections with encapsulated microorganisms, but animals or humans incapable of generating C3b (i.e., absence of both the classic and alternative complement pathways) have not been described. Both neutrophils and macrophages phagocytize microorganisms by using receptors for IgG and the products of C3, although the particle ingestion rate of neutrophils exceeds that of monocytes by tenfold.

Killing Mechanisms

Both neutrophils and macrophages have evolved multiple mechanisms to eliminate microbes. It was observed more than 50 years ago that neutrophils actively phagocytizing bacteria consumed oxygen at a high rate. It was presumed that this was due to increased electron transport activity in response to a demand for chemical energy to power phagocytosis. Later experiments showed that cyanide, which blocks mitochondrial oxygen uptake, did not block O_2 consumption of phagocytizing neutrophils, and a new oxygen-consuming pathway was discovered for neutrophils and monocytes. This pathway has been called the *respiratory burst* because the oxygen consumption occurs suddenly and wanes within approximately 30 minutes. Phagocytes contain an oxidase system that produces the superoxide radical during reduction of O_2 with one electron. This is a complex collection of proteins, including a membrane flavoprotein, a *b*-type cytochrome, and two cytosolic regulatory proteins. When the neutrophil is triggered by contacting a microorganism, the *b*-cytochrome is transported to the developing phagocytic vacuolar membrane. This process leads to NADPH oxidase activation and hence superoxide production. The initiation of this process involves perturbation of the neutrophil plasma membrane, for example, by receptor-ligand interactions with IgG or C3b bound to a microorganism.

The reducing equivalents that drive the respiratory burst are supplied by NADPH, which is oxidized to NADP by NADPH oxidase. NADPH is regenerated by the two redox reactions occurring in the hexose monophosphate shunt pathway. Thus glucose is the ultimate substrate for this process. Once superoxide is produced, additional enzymatic and nonenzymatic reactions occur. These reactions lead to highly reactive intermediates that kill bacteria and to reactions that detoxify these intermediates so that the host's own tissues are not destroyed. These reactions include the following:

$$NADPH + O_2 \xrightarrow{E1} NADP + O_2^-\cdot + H^+ \quad (1)$$

$$2O_2^-\cdot + 2H^+ \xrightarrow{E2} H_2O_2 + O_2 \quad (2)$$

$$2H_2O_2 \xrightarrow{E3} 2H_2O + O_2 \quad (3)$$

$$H_2O_2 + O_2^-\cdot \xrightarrow[\text{or } Cu^{2+}]{Fe^{3+}} OH\cdot + OH^- + O_2 \quad (4)$$

$$H_2O_2 + X^- \xrightarrow{E4} XO^- + H_2O \quad (5)$$

where E1 = NADPH oxidase, E2 = superoxide dismutase, E3 = catalase, and E4 = myeloperoxidase.

Overall, O_2 is ultimately reduced to H_2O. But in this reduction, superoxide (reaction 1), hydrogen peroxide (reaction 2), and the hydroxyl radical, OH^- (reaction 4), are produced. These oxygen species are toxic for microorganisms, with the hydroxyl radical in particular being one of the most highly reactive compounds known. It can damage membranes, cross-link proteins, and cause nucleic acid scissions. Neutrophils also contain myeloperoxidase, which utilizes H_2O_2 and halide ions to produce hypohalite ions (reaction 5) such as hypochlorite (ClO^-), which is highly microbicidal. Inherited enzyme defects in these systems have been described and include chronic granulomatous disease (NADPH oxidase), enzyme defects of certain hexose monophosphate shunt reactions, and myeloperoxidase deficiency.

These reactions occur within the enclosed phagolysosome or secondary phagosome of the phagocyte, although some of these products can also be detected extracellularly. Neutrophils and other host cells contain superoxide dismutase, catalase, and glutathione peroxidase, which help detoxify the oxygen intermediates that leak back into the neutrophil cytoplasm and extracellular fluid.

The NADPH oxidase system requires a continued supply of both glucose and oxygen. In bacterial infections that progress to abscess formation the steady-state concentrations of glucose and oxygen in abscess fluid are low or undetectable. There is a long-standing medical tenet that abscesses must be drained to produce cure. The most beneficial effect of abscess drainage may actually be to "let O_2 in" rather than to "let the pus out."

Other oxygen-independent mechanisms for phagocytic toxicity exist. For example, neutrophil granules contain proteins called *defensins* that are highly cationic at neutral pH and bind to the negatively charged bacterial surface, forming channels analogous to the membrane-attack complex of the complement system. Other phagocyte products such as lysozyme, cathepsins, serine esterases, acid phosphatase, lipases, phospholipase, histones, and lactoferrin are also microbicidal.

It is likely that additional phagocyte antimicrobial mechanisms exist. For example, macrophages normally arrest the replication of intracellular bacteria, fungi, and protozoans. These organisms, which may persist in the host for decades as static but living commensals, can suddenly begin to replicate, producing reactivation infections such as seen in pulmonary tuberculosis, cerebral toxoplasmosis, and disseminated histoplasmosis. Although the mechanisms normally preventing such reactivation infections are unclear, their development often is associated with an acquired immunodeficiency.

Microbial Digestion

Phagocyte function does not end with the death of the invading microbe. The cell walls of bacteria and fungi are composed of complex carbohydrate and glycolipid polymers that must be eliminated. Were this not the case, host tissues eventually would become repositories of dead microorganisms, leading to a type of "bacterial storage disease." The lysosomes of neutrophils and macrophages contain enzymes that degrade carbohydrates, proteins, and lipids but do not necessarily kill or degrade living bacteria. However, after bacterial cell death, changes occur that allow the enzymatic dissolution of complex cell wall polymers. In this way phagocytes are able to digest the bacteria that they kill by other means.

Interactions Between Constitutive and Immune Defenses

Antibody

Antimicrobial antibody augments several constitutive defense mechanisms. Perhaps the most important involves antibody enhancement of phagocytosis caused by physical aggregation and opsonization of pathogens. Because of their high valency, IgM and IgA antibodies are efficient at aggregating microbes. Besides helping to retard microbial spread, such aggregation increases the ability of macrophages to take up many bacteria simultaneously. This can be of considerable importance in early primary immune responses or in T cell–independent responses to bacterial cell-wall antigens, which both tend to involve IgM production predominately. Antibody also augments constitutive defenses by activating complement on microbial surfaces that alone might not directly activate the alternative pathway. IgM antibodies activate the classic pathway more efficiently than IgG since one molecule of IgM carries several of the sites necessary for binding C1q, whereas at least two adjacent IgG molecules are required for complement activation. Thus the chemotactic and hemodynamic effects of complement-cleavage peptides C3a and C5a are heightened at sites where antibody binds to antigen and activates complement.

In addition to enhancing constitutive defense mechanisms, antibody is a major component of specific host immune defense mechanisms, which include the following.

Complement-dependent Cytotoxicity. Complement-mediated lysis of certain organisms has been demonstrated in vitro and probably plays some role in host defense. For example, the pathogenicity of some gram-negative bacteria has been attributed to a relative resistance of their outer cell wall to lysis by complement. Likewise, patients with deficiencies in only late complement components, which are necessary for lysis but not immune adherence, handle most infections normally but have an increased susceptibility to *Neisseria* species, especially gonococci and meningococci.

Neutralization. Binding of antibody to functionally important sites can directly inhibit the spread or growth of pathogens and inactivate their *toxic* products. No additional cells or molecular mediators are required for this neutralizing activity, although in some cases complement components may add additional conformational or steric effects that help inactivate critical functions. Neutralizing antibodies (primarily secretory IgA dimers) constitute the first line of immunologic defense against intestinal and respiratory pathogens by preventing colonization of epithelial cells (Chap. 18). This is critical for protection against intracellular parasites of epithelia such as viruses. Neutralization is virtually the only immune reaction that can be mounted on the external side of an epithelium where plasma proteins, phagocytic cells, and other accessory factors of immune effector mechanisms are absent or only present in low concentrations.

IgE-mediated Reactions. IgE responses often are considered in the sense of allergic or immunopathologic (Chap. 17) host reactions, but they may also play an important role in the immune defense at epithelial surfaces. In particular, IgE responses can mediate the secretion of factors into and smooth muscle contraction of the gastrointestinal and respiratory tracts to assist in the defense against protozoa and helminths. This effect is dependent on the interaction between microbial antigens and antigen-specific IgE antibodies that are cytotropically bound to mast cells in or near the epithelium.

Antibody-dependent Cellular Cytotoxicity. Many circulating cells have receptors for the Fc portion of specific immunoglobulin isotypes (Chap. 17). Whereas Fc receptors of neutrophils and macrophages potentiate phagocytosis, other cells use receptor-bound immunoglobulin to mediate additional defense reactions. Usually, these involve binding of the effector cells to a pathogen through the antibody molecule, with subsequent release of factors that kill the pathogen. Neutrophils, for example, can adhere to the cuticle of schistosome cercaria and release the content of granules on the worm surface in the presence of certain IgG antibodies. ADCC involving eosinophil degranulation and release of major basic protein may be particularly important in resistance to helminths; IgE and IgG antibodies both can mediate this response. Monocytes and certain lymphoid cells can also mediate ADCC reactions with IgG antibodies.

T Cells

T cells regulate (directly or indirectly) virtually all aspects of immune host resistance to infection, which include macrophage activity, antibody synthesis, synthesis of other inflammatory proteins, generation of inflammatory cells in the bone marrow and their recruitment into the circulation, and differentiation of other effector and regulatory lymphocytes (Chaps. 13 and 17).

T cells primarily enhance constitutive defense mechanisms by promoting the growth, differentiation, and activation of macrophages. Lymphokines from activated T cells that are involved in this process include IFNγ, IL-3, IL-4, and IL-6. Some characteristics of macrophage activation include increased chemotaxic behavior, adherence properties, phagocytic activity, microbicidal activity, and release of inflammatory mediators. Macrophage activation is important in providing host resistance to many pathogens and is essential for resistance to organisms that multiply as intracellular parasites of macrophages. T cells can induce macrophages to synthesize IL-1, and TNF-α, thereby activating the acute phase reaction. T cells also produce IFN-γ, which can supplement the antiviral activities of nonimmune interferons produced by other cell types. T cells and their products also can be directly involved in stimulating antigen nonspecific, lymphokine-activated killer (LAK) lymphocytes in local inflammatory reactions.

Immune Defenses

Immune Defenses Against Viruses

The wide variety of viruses and their ability to spread by different mechanisms require that the immune system be capable of responding with an equally diverse repertoire (Fig. 19–2). This requirement is perhaps best demonstrated by the susceptibility to viral infections associated with virtually all human immunodeficiency diseases. However, even in the immunocompetent host, defenses against viral infection are less than perfect. The symptoms of viral infections are often more a result of the immune response to the virus than of cellular injury produced by the viral infection itself.

Some viruses (e.g., most picornaviruses) are intrinsically cytolytic. They release themselves from the intracellular environment by destroying the integrity of the cell in which they are replicating. These viruses have a mandatory extracellular phase during which the virus potentially is exposed to neutralizing antibodies that can block the virus from infecting other susceptible cells. However, many viruses have developed means for avoiding destruction during the extracellular phase.

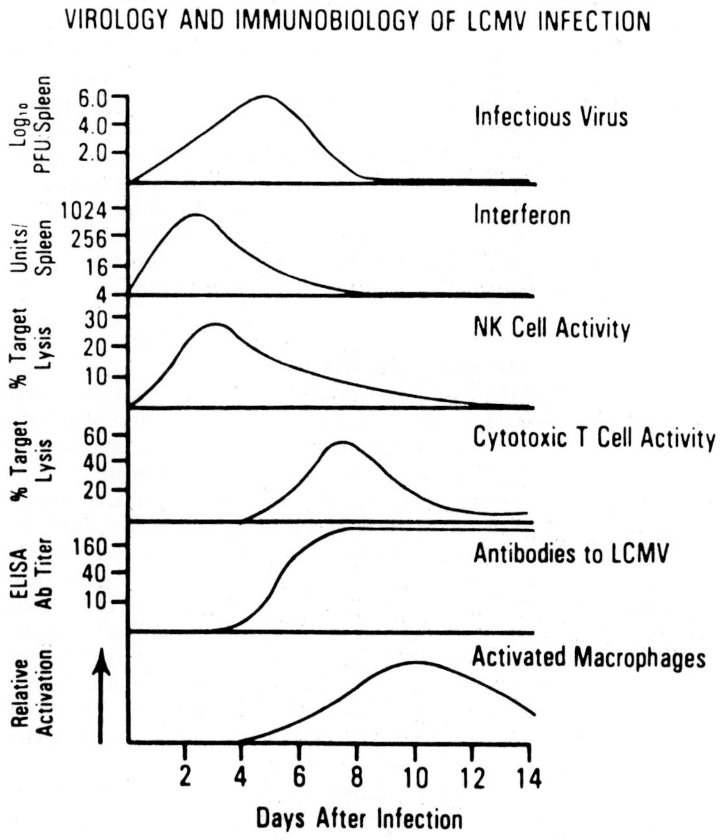

Fig. 19–2. Virus titer, nonspecific, and specific host response after inoculation of lymphocyte choriomeningitis virus (LMCV) in adult mice. *(Adapted from Buchmeier et al: Adv Immunol 30:275, 1980.)*

Some of the viral and host strategies for defense are discussed below.

Patterns of Viral Infection

Many viruses disseminate from cell to cell through intercellular bridges. This technique allows the virus to spread without exposure to the extracellular environment and the effects of neutralizing antibodies. Most viruses that use intercellular bridges are also shed through the outer cell membrane of infected cells via a process called *budding*. As the viral capsid exits the cell, it acquires a coat or envelope composed of virally encoded proteins and lipids from the plasma membrane. Antibodies can be directed at the virally encoded proteins, both on the virus and intercalated on the cell surface. In contrast, specific cytotoxic T cells only recognize viral proteins on the cell surface in association with host MHC antigens (Chaps. 13 and 17).

Viruses can also cause cells to fuse, forming multinucleated cells known as syncytia. This mechanism again allows the virus to move from cell to cell without being exposed to antibodies. To facilitate the process of cell fusion, some viruses (e.g., the myxoviruses) have "fusion proteins" that allow the membrane of one infected cell to mesh with adjacent uninfected cell membranes. An effective neutralizing antibody response against viruses of this type includes antibodies directed against such fusion proteins.

Not all viruses are engaged in a constant process of transmission from cell to cell. Some viruses are capable of "latency." Latent viruses have infected a cell but either are not multiplying or are replicating at a slow rate. In many cases the nucleic acids of a latent virus will be integrated into the host-cell genome, moving from the integrated, latent state into a replicating phase under the correct conditions such as when the infected cell is activated to replicate. One advantage to latency is that the virus can remain hidden, since there is no means for the immune system to recognize cells that are infected when the virus is not expressing antigens.

Humoral Mechanisms

The primary humoral immune defense mechanism against viruses is antibody-mediated neutralization. Virus-specific immunoglobulins, mostly of the IgA class, are present in virtually all body secretions (e.g., mucus, tears, saliva, urine). If sufficient preexisting antibody is present at the time the virus arrives at the mucosal surface, the virus will be neutralized before it has a chance to bind or penetrate the superficial cells. These specific antibodies are generated during the first infection with a virus and are maintained by reexposure to the same or cross-reactive antigens. The process of neutralization can occur with antibodies that (1) bind to the virus and hinder the absorption of the virus to a cell surface; (2) stabilize the virus capsid so that the nucleic acids within the capsid cannot be released; or (3) fix complement on the protein and lipid coat of an enveloped virus, causing structural or toxic damage. A virus that has been neutralized by antibodies is no longer infectious, at least while the antibody remains attached.

One important function of neutralizing antibodies is to block attachment of the virus to the cell surface. Theoretically, this can occur through steric hindrance of the interaction between the viral attachment protein and cell-surface receptor. In some cases complement may enhance this type of neutralization. Experimentally, antibodies have been developed against cell-surface receptors of picornaviruses (rhinovirus 14, Coxsackie B viruses). These antibodies prevent the in vitro binding of the virus to the cell surface and can completely terminate an infection in tissue culture. However, such antibodies have not been demonstrated as active in vivo, and the therapeutic utility of heterologous antireceptor antibody therapy has not been determined.

Altering certain characteristics of the viral capsid is a second means by which neutralization occurs. Neutralizing antibodies may simply increase the stability of the capsid (e.g., by cross-linking proteins) and thus prevent release of the viral genome (uncoating) after virus entry into the cell. They can also change in the capsid conformation so that the viral attachment protein no longer identifies the receptor for which it should be specific, or they can alter the isoelectric point (pI) of the virus and diminish the attraction of the virus to the cell. Antibodies can also neutralize viruses by initiating complement fixation directly on the viral surface, which can then lead to viral lysis. However, this mechanism is probably significant only for large enveloped viruses.

Immunoglobulin binding to virus can enhance constitutive defense mechanisms. Some antibodies aggregate virus particles into clumps that are more easily engulfed by phagocytes in the reticuloendothelial system. Similarly, bound antibody and complement may act as opsonins to promote phagocytosis. Enveloped viruses express virally encoded proteins on the surface of infected host cells, which provide potential targets for antibody binding. In this setting immunoglobulins can promote lysis of infected host cells via ADCC mechanisms. If the viral antigen is one for which preformed antibody exists, this type of cytolytic response may develop more quickly than the expansion of appropriate cytotoxic T cell clones.

The antibody responses in viral infections are fairly typical of those made against most new antigens, with initial IgM production followed by higher titer and longer lasting IgG responses. Neutralizing antibodies rise quickly in the serum, whereas complement-fixing antibodies, which tend to be directed to a greater degree at internal capsid proteins (nucleoproteins), rise more slowly. After an early antibody peak, titers generally decline in the months and years after infection. An exception is the case of latent viruses, particularly the herpesviruses, in which there are periodic brief escapes from latency that serve to restimulate the immune system. During these viral reactivations there may be a new elevation in IgM antibodies and an increase in the total IgG antibody titers. Because of this recurrent antigenic stimulation, antibody titers against the herpesvirus family tend to stay high long after the primary infection.

Respiratory viruses such as influenza, parainfluenza, and respiratory syncytial virus (RSV) also are associated with high antibody titers because of their repeated circulation in the community. These agents spread each winter in the temperate climate zones, reexposing the population on a regular basis and boosting antibody titers. If a new strain of virus (particularly influenza) is of enough genetic distance, the preexisting antibodies developed during the last infection may be only partially protective. In contrast, some viruses are genetically very stable and have only one major serotype (e.g., measles), and as a result a single infection can offer lifelong protection. This type of antigenic uniformity was true of smallpox (variola) and contributed greatly to its eradication as a wild-type infection by worldwide vaccination programs.

Cellular Mechanisms

One of the major functions of the cellular immune system is to eliminate intracellular viruses, largely by destroying infected cells. This is a particularly important step in eradicating those viruses that can spread from cell to cell without having to move through the extracellular environment. Cytotoxic T cells are able to recognize infected cells specifically and lyse them under certain conditions. The antigen receptors of cytotoxic T cells recognize polymorphic (host) MHC gene products together with proteins encoded by the viral genome. In general, T lymphocytes bearing the CD8 surface antigen have receptors that recognize viral proteins plus HLA class I antigens and comprise the predominant cytotoxic effector T cell population. T cells that recognize viral antigens in the context of HLA class II antigens generally express the CD4 surface antigen and predominantly provide helper T cell activity, although a subset of such cells may also be cytotoxic against targets expressing viral antigen and MHC class II determinants.

The generation of cytotoxic T cells (Tc) is a complex and multistep process involving antigen-presenting cells (APC), amplification by $CD4^+$ helper lymphocytes, and the cytotoxic T lymphocytes themselves (Fig. 19–3; Chaps. 13 and 17). MHC class I or II molecules on an APC act to bind the viral protein in position for the T cell to recognize specific antigenic determinants. The association of antigen and MHC class I molecules occurs in the endoplasmic reticulum of the cell, with the complex then carried to the cell surface; MHC class I bound peptides are derived from endogenous (intracellular) proteins. Thus viral antigens, which are produced by infected cells, are typically associated with MHC class I, allowing for responsiveness by MHC class I restricted T cells, generally $CD8^+$ cytotoxic T cells. The association of antigens with MHC class II for presentation to MHC class II restricted T cells is blocked within the cell by the invarient (I) chain. Thus peptides bound to MHC class II are generally derived from exogenous antigens and involve interactions on the surface of the APC.

Once $CD8^+$ cells are primed by seeing the antigen for which they are specific in the context of an MHC molecule, they are ready for clonal expansion. $CD4^+$ T cells facilitate this multiplication through the release of various lymphokines, especially IL-2. For a primary infection this clonal expansion takes several days before it becomes detectable. The expanded pool of activated cytolytic T cells remains in circulation for weeks but then begins to decline and may not be detectable within months. Nevertheless, after clonal expansion more antigen-specific memory T cells are present than before the primary infection. As a result, when the host is reinfected with the same virus, the presence of a larger number of

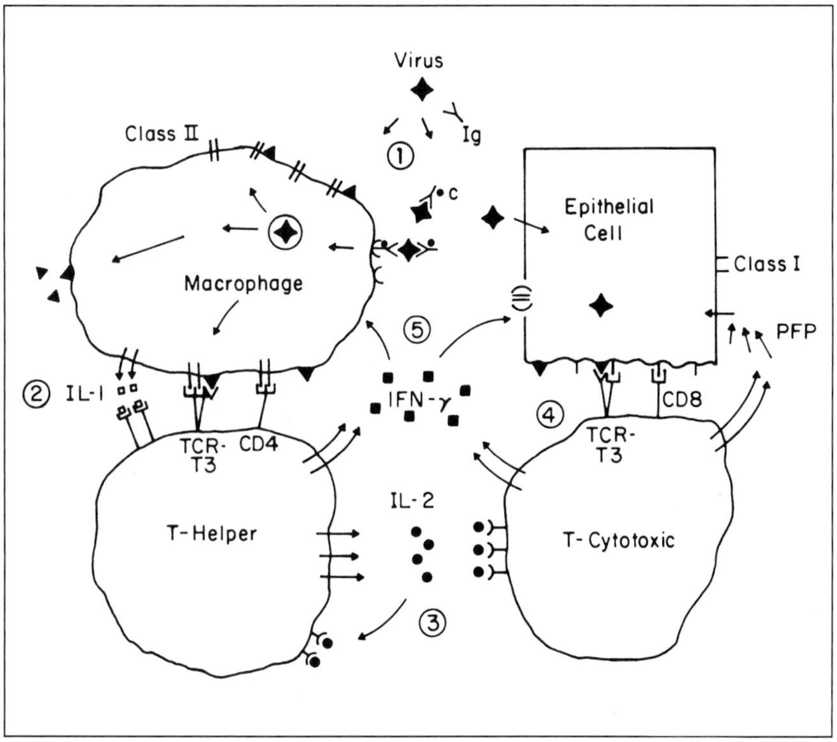

Fig. 19–3. Host interactions with virus leading to cellular immune responses. **1.** Virus is processed by a phagocyte (e.g., macrophage), and viral antigens are presented on antigen-presenting cells (APC; e.g., macrophage, dendritic cell). This process is enhanced by macrophage Fc and complement receptor binding of immunoglobulin (Ig) and complement (C) components bound to the virus. **2.** The antigen receptors (TCR-T3 complex) of T helper (T_h) cells recognize antigen and self-class II MHC, whereas CD4 molecules enhance the binding interactions of T_h with common class II MHC determinants. Interleukin-1 (IL-1) from the APC promotes T_h cell stimulation by antigen. **3.** Interleukin-2 (IL-2) from activated T_h enhances effector T cytotoxic (T_c) and T_h activity. **4.** Activated T_c cells recognize viral antigen and self-class I MHC, whereas CD8 molecules enhance the binding interactions with common class I determinants. **5.** Activated T cells produce IFNγ, which stimulates macrophages and induces increased class II MHC expression on APC and target cells. Activated T_c cells also produce pore-forming protein (PFP, perforin), which can lyse infected targets. Additional inflammatory mediators are also produced by activated T cells and macrophages.

antigen-specific precursor cells means the generation of an adequate cytolytic T cell response will occur within 1 or 2 days. Because of their ability to become latent and to recur endogenously, some viruses such as the herpes group produce a cytotoxic T cell response that is both strong and persistent.

Constitutive cellular responses augment several stages of the immune response to viral infection. Macrophages act as APCs and after activation are rich in HLA class II antigens. Both macrophages and polymorphonuclear leukocytes are capable of phagocytosing virus particles that have been opsonized with antibody or complement or both and can engage in ADCC reactions. However, some viruses such as the dengue virus use nonneutralizing but opsonizing antibodies as a means to gain entry to the macrophage's cytoplasm, an environment it seems to prefer. In cases like that of dengue, nonneutralizing antibodies actually make the clinical syndrome worse.

The infrequency of unusually serious viral infections in purely neutropenic hosts suggests that the effective role of granulocytes in the immune response to viral infection is small. NK cells also play a role in constitutive defense against viral infection, directly by lytic activity or indirectly through the production of lymphokines, especially interferon.

Interferons

The interferons are proteins with antiviral activity elaborated by infected cells and stimulated lymphocytes in response to certain intracellular stimuli. Some of the interferons also act as intercellular messengers. Because interferons are species specific, this discussion is limited to human interferons.

There are three basic subtypes of human interferon: alpha, beta, and gamma. The first two of these, alpha and beta, are type I interferons, which can be made by cells other than those of the immune system. Type I interferons can protect cells that have not yet been infected and additionally can stimulate NK cells into lytic and replicative states. Alpha-interferons originally were isolated from leukocyte suspensions, hence their old name *leukocyte interferon*. These proteins are encoded by 13 to 18 human alpha genes, each producing a slightly different molecule with some minor variations in function. These genes are clustered on chromosome 9 and are notable for their lack of introns. Because the alpha-interferons are not glycosylated by the cell in which they are produced, the genes can be cloned into prokaryotes and the proteins produced in large quantity. The alpha-interferons are 166 amino acids long, with the first 23 being a hydrophobic signal that is cleaved off by the cell as the protein is released.

Beta-interferon is similar to alpha-interferon in that it also is a type I interferon, is coded on chromosome 9, and has a gene devoid of introns. However, there are several important differences between alpha- and beta-interferons. Beta-interferon was originally produced from infected fibroblast cultures and is 166 amino acids long, with a 21 amino acid hydrophobic signal tail. There is probably only one beta-interferon gene, and the proteins translated from that gene are glycosylated before the protein is released. Human alpha- and beta-interferon gene sequences show approximately 30% homology.

The most distinct of the human interferons is gamma-interferon (IFNγ), a type II, or immune, interferon. This designation refers to the production of IFNγ by lymphocytes during blastogenesis. IFNγ is an acid-labile glycoprotein coded by a single gene on chromosome 12. The gene has three introns and encodes a protein 166 amino acids long, with a signal peptide chain of 20 amino acids. IFNγ is a major cytokine involved in macrophage activation. Its activities include increasing the expression of HLA class II antigens on macrophages (and other cells) and thus enhancing their ability to present antigens for helper T cell stimulation; promoting the cytolytic activity of macrophages; increasing the expression of adhesion molecules and thus promoting cell-to-cell interactions; and increasing the elaboration of other cytokines such as IL-1.

Several steps in the production and function of interferon are still not clearly understood. Viral infection of the host cell triggers transcription and translation of the interferon genes. These proteins are transported to the cell surface; glycosylation occurs in the case of the beta- and gamma-interferons, and the signal peptides are cleaved off as the protein is released from the cell. The free interferon molecules bind to surface receptors on uninfected cells (infected cells may also have interferon binding, but the effects are not very clear), and eventually an intracellular messenger protein is produced. This protein has several effects, but the most important seems to be an inhibition of RNA translation, an effect that is greater on viral metabolism than on host cellular protein synthesis.

Viruses provoke a variable amount of interferon production. One of the most powerful interferon generators is influenza virus. The myalgias, fever, and headache of influenza are probably the result of the host immune response and interferon synthesis, since the influenza virus itself typically replicates in the surface epithelial cells of the respiratory tract. Different viruses also have varying sensitivity to the effects of interferons, one of several factors that makes the standardization of interferon bioassays difficult.

Immunodeficiency Patients

Patients with serious defects in their immune system, particularly patients with congenital immunodeficiencies (Chap. 18) are uncommon, but much of what is known currently about the human immune response to viral infections is a result of examining the pathogenesis of infections in these "experiments of nature."

Patients with a congenital deficiency in B cells can have a virtual absence of immunoglobulins. These patients do not have problems with the enveloped viruses (which primarily operate by budding), such as herpesviruses, measles, influenza, or other orthomyxoviruses and paramyxoviruses. Instead, the worst problems for agammaglobulinemic patients and those who have a selective IgA deficiency are with small, cytolytic viruses such as poliomyelitis, in which even attenuated strains used in vaccines can lead to severe disease. This increased risk is at least partially due to the patients' inability to eradicate the virus from the gastrointestinal tract. During their prolonged gastrointestinal excretion the polioviruses are able to mutate away from their attenuated vaccine genotype to a more virulent, wild-type character. In addition to poliomyelitis, agammaglobulinemic patients are also at high risk for a unique form of chronic meningoencephalitis, usually caused by an echovirus serotype. In patients with this disease the virus can remain in the central nervous system for years, slowly causing a loss in neurologic function and occasionally disseminating from its central nervous system reservoir to cause myositis and a cutaneous disease much like dermatomyositis. The fact that this syndrome only occurs in patients severely lacking in the ability to make antibodies emphasizes the importance of humoral immunity in enteroviral infections.

Children with pure T cell defects have much more trouble with enveloped, budding viruses. They are unable to eradicate infected cells, so that free virus still is released even if there is antibody available to neutralize those particles. Cell-to-cell spread can progress largely unhindered, so diseases such as varicella, measles, and primary herpes simplex become potentially lethal. Children with combined T and B cell defects have by far the most problems. After maternally transferred antibodies wane, these children are immunologically defenseless and as a result are susceptible to both the enveloped and nonenveloped viruses. In a similar manner, patients treated with immunosuppressive drugs and patients with human immunodeficiency virus infection are most susceptible to the enveloped viruses, particularly to the herpes group (e.g., cytomegalovirus, herpes simplex).

Immunosuppressive Effects of Viral Infections

The interaction of viruses and the immune system is made particularly complex by the ability of viruses to affect the immune system directly. There are several well-known examples of virus-induced immunosuppression, with the most well-known being the action of human immunodeficiency virus (HIV) on $CD4^+$ (T helper cell) lymphocytes (Chap. 18). However, long before HIV became widely known, other immunologic effects of viral infection were recognized.

One of the first viral diseases to be associated with immunosuppression was measles. In 1908 vonPirquet noted that a recent measles infection could impair tuberculin skin test responsiveness. Since then, researchers have recognized that even the attenuated measles vaccine is capable of producing anergy in purified protein derivative (PPD) skin tests. The mechanism for this immunosuppression is not entirely clear, but there is evidence that the measles virus can infect all lymphocyte types. The infection does not kill the lymphocytes but does depress the ability of an uncommitted cell to begin replication and differentiation. There may also be generation of suppressor T cell populations that actively restrict lymphocyte proliferation. Other viruses exert their immunosuppressive effect by lysis of immune cells. HIV, which lyses $CD4^+$ cells and may cause dysfunction of macrophages and reticuloendothelial cells, is an excellent example of this mode of immunosuppression.

The ability of some respiratory viruses to change the oxidative metabolic capabilities of polymorphonuclear leukocytes has been proposed as another mechanism for immune system suppression. With animal models, influenza virus and RSV have been shown to decrease the oxidative burst in stimulated neutrophils. As a result of these studies, researchers have been investigating whether this change in the oxidative pathway might contribute to the long-recognized role of viral infections as predisposing factors in the acute bacterial middle ear infections of childhood.

The ability of many viruses to multiply in macrophages, which play a key role in initiating an immune response, makes virus-macrophage interactions another possible mechanism for immunosuppression. Although viruses can effect macrophage functions in vitro, the in vivo significance of these phenomena is still under investigation.

Slow and Persistent Viruses

There are several mechanisms by which viruses establish long-term relationships with a host organism. The first of these patterns is latency. A latent virus is associated with a cell but cannot be detected unless genetic probes are used. In the proper environment the latent virus begins to replicate, and complete viral particles are constructed. Some latent viruses will integrate into the host genome, whereas others can exist independently in the cell.

The slow viruses are agents with very long incubation times. They are often referred to as "unconventional viruses" because of the atypical features in their pathogenesis, and many aspects of slow viral disease are still not well understood. The best-known human examples are kuru (a disease found in certain New Guinea tribes that performed ritualistic cannibalism) and Creutzfeldt-Jakob disease. These agents have very limited contagiousness, with the only known examples of transmission coming after direct contact with infected central nervous system tissues.

Conventional viruses can also cause persistent infections. Hepatitis B virus (HBV), adenoviruses, rubella virus (in congenital infection), and echoviruses (in the central nervous system of agammaglobulinemic patients) can all cause persistent infections without latency. The mechanisms used by the virus to escape host defenses are not known, although the variability in the occurrence of persistent infections implies that there are important contributions made to the viral pathogenesis by host factors.

Some viruses use the immune system to establish persistence. For example, antiviral antibodies can lead to modulation of the viral proteins from the surface of infected cells, leaving the cell infected but immunologically unrecognizable. In other instances the cells of the immune system themselves become infected. The effects of infecting the immune system vary with the cell type involved. The most striking example is with HIV. Another example is the Epstein-Barr virus (EBV), which infects B cells and epithelial cells. Once a person has been infected with EBV, a certain small percentage of B cells will continue to be infected with the virus. In general, the virus will remain latent and undetectable, but a few B cells will be "transformed," with the ability to proliferate in an unregulated manner. To control such transformed B cells, cytotoxic and suppressor T cell responses are stimulated. If these effector and regulatory T cells are themselves hindered, for example, by the immunosuppression needed for organ transplantation or by an HIV infection, EBV-associated B cell lymphomas can develop.

Immune Defenses Against Bacteria

Bacterial Clearance

Phagocytes kill bacteria by oxygen-dependent and oxygen-independent mechanisms as described previously. These bactericidal mechanisms require that the phagocyte physically engage the microorganism. However, some bacteria (especially those that are encapsulated) are able to resist attachment to phagocytes. When encapsulated bacteria such as *S. pneumoniae* or *Haemophilus influenzae* gain access to the circulation, host defenses must operate to remove them from the blood. When this clearance function fails, the host is at jeopardy for seeding sequestered sites such as the subarachnoid, pleural, and pericardial spaces, the peritoneal cavity, joint spaces, and at the site of an implant or prosthesis. Infections at these sites are dangerous and often lethal.

Fixed macrophages of the liver and spleen are of primary importance for clearance of bacteria from the circulation. When radiolabeled encapsulated pneumococci are injected intravenously in experimental animals, they initially are filtered in the pulmonary capillaries. However, within 30 minutes almost all of the label is redistributed to the liver and spleen, with the organisms sequestered within hepatic Kupffer's cells and splenic macrophages. This clearance is complement dependent. If the animals are treated with cobra venom factor to deplete critical complement components, bacterial clearance does not occur, and the animals die. Passively administered anticapsular IgG enhances the efficiency of bacterial clearance in the normal animal but does not repair the clearance defect in cobra venom factor–treated animals. The importance of specific IgG appears to be its targeting of C3b deposition onto the bacterium and perhaps protecting against C3b inactivation. With alternative pathway activation, C3b is deposited on the surface of the pneumococcal cell wall, deep within the matrix of the polysaccharide capsule. The capsular material blocks the binding of C3b to its receptors on phagocytes. In contrast, specific IgG localizes C3b deposition throughout the capsule matrix, making C3b molecules more accessible to macrophage and neutrophil receptors.

Less virulent strains of pneumococci are cleared predominantly by Kupffer's cells of the liver, whereas highly virulent strains of encapsulated bacteria escape hepatic clearance but are cleared by splenic macrophages. This difference may relate to the unique anatomy of the spleen in which the fenestrated reticular membrane is found partitioning the white from the red pulp. Here blood flow is extremely slow and provides splenic macrophages with a greater potential for phagocytosis. Asplenic humans are susceptible to overwhelming bacteremia because of encapsulated bacteria, especially *S. pneumoniae.*

Bacterial Killing

There are two ways in which host immune defenses kill bacteria: by complement-mediated lysis and by phagocytes. Lymphocytes do not usually function as effector cytotoxic cells in the killing of bacteria but contribute in host defense by producing opsonic immunoglobulins and lymphokines (e.g., IFNγ), which facilitate phagocyte binding (through increased adhesion molecule expression), engulfment, and activation.

Fluid-phase killing requires assembly of the membrane attack complex, C5 to C9, by either the classic or alternative complement pathways. Membrane-attack complexes insert into the outer membranes of gram-negative bacteria and lead to bacteriolysis. However, many bacteria, especially gram-positive bacteria, are resistant to complement-mediated lysis. Their thick peptidoglycan cell walls prevent access of C5–C9 complexes to the vulnerable cytoplasmic membrane. Some species of gram-negative bacteria are complement sensitive but readily yield clones that are resistant to bacteriolysis. The basis for this change involves alterations of the bacterial outer membrane, with the result that C5–C9 complexes are deposited superficially and are shed into the surrounding medium. The polysaccharide chains of endotoxin and a specific outer-membrane protein cause this effect in *Salmonella* and *Neisseria* species, respectively. Species of the genus *Neisseria* can be killed by the complement cascade in concert with bactericidal antibody. Patients with inherited deficiencies in the terminal complement proteins are at increased risk for developing disseminated *Neisseria* infections.

Site of Infection

Certain anatomic locations present unique problems for host defense, and infections at these sites tend to be particularly severe. Obligate anaerobic bacteria such as *Clostridia* species and *Bacteroides fragilis* almost never cause disease in healthy oxygenated tissue. However, serious gas-forming infections can occur in traumatized anoxic muscle, subcutaneous tissue, or intestine. Bone has a limited blood supply within a solid-phase matrix so that phagocytic cells and humoral factors may not gain easy access to foci of infection. Consequently, bone infections (osteomyelitis) may become chronic and difficult (if not impossible) to cure and often result in skeletal destruction. The cornea is an avascular structure, and since emigration of leukocytes requires proximity to a capillary, bacterial keratitis may progress to produce corneal opacity (and neovascularization) before the infection can be contained. Heart valves are also avascular so that microorganisms growing in fibrinous vegetations on the valve leaflets are sometimes inaccessible to phagocytes. Before the use of antibiotic drugs, bacterial endocarditis was always fatal. Serous cavities of the body (e.g., subarachnoid, peritoneal, synovial, pleural spaces) present a different problem when infected with bacteria. These fluid-filled spaces present a circulating growth medium for bacteria, and since phagocytes commonly migrate toward a characteristic stimulus by crawling (not swimming), phagocyte-microbe interaction in the fluid phase of the meningeal space depends on chance collisions. The host counters this disadvantage by mounting a phagocyte influx that may be so massive that the entire fluid phase is replaced by a thick exudate composed primarily of leukocytes.

The presence of foreign bodies is important in the genesis of bacterial infections as illustrated by the following observations. When *S. aureus* is injected into normal skin or into skin surrounding a suture, both sites form abscesses and drain spontaneously. However, the lesion in normal skin heals promptly, whereas a chronic, nonhealing infection occurs around the suture site. The difficulties in healing bacterial infections adjacent to foreign bodies are well recognized; examples include patients with prosthetic heart valves, bone hardware, artificial joints, and ventricular catheters within the brain. Although reasons for this phenomenon are unclear, neutrophils harvested from foreign body sites have reduced respiratory burst activity and hence may be incapable of generating sufficient oxygen metabolites to kill bacteria. It is known that if the respiratory burst is triggered prematurely by one stimulus (e.g., a foreign body), a much-reduced respiratory burst occurs with a second stimulus (e.g., a microorganism).

Virulence Factors

Pathogenic bacteria have evolved mechanisms that facilitate their survival as successful parasites. These mechanisms circumvent host resistance factors or increase transmissibility of the parasite. The adaptations required may be complex, especially if the parasite exists in markedly different environments during its life cycle.

The typhoid bacillus, *Salmonella typhi,* exists in water and sewage during intervals between parasitization of the human host. After ingestion by the host, the organism is exposed to acid pH in the stomach and then must invade the intestinal epithelium, survive within phagocytes, and ultimately establish a carrier state for further transmission by a fecal-freeliving-oral route. Hence it may not be surprising that a highly adapted parasite such as this one has evolved a complex genetic program that is switched on and off in certain environments.

Intestinal pathogens, including salmonellae, possess virulence genes that regulate a battery of other structural genes located at different sites on the bacterial chromosome. Mutations in these virulence-regulatory genes yield organisms with a marked reduction in virulence. In *Salmonella* a virulence regulatory gene may be activated after engulfment by a macrophage. The regulator gene induces expression or repression of more than 30 structural genes. Some of these gene products promote survival in the macrophage. They have been correlated with bacterial resistance to leukocyte-derived defensin molecules. Other bacterial genes may be turned on by contact with gut epithelial cells. These genes promote invasion of the intestinal pathogen into the host epithelial cell.

Environmental factors that activate virulence regulatory genes are "stress related" and include, for example, increased osmolarity or very low phosphate concentration of culture medium. Genes encoding major heat shock proteins are transcribed in response to activation of virulence regulatory genes. A great challenge in microbial virulence involves unraveling the complex networks that regulate the proteins responsible for the many virulence phenotypes that have been observed in infections in experimental animals and in natural populations.

Other bacteria thwart host immunity by avoiding detection. They may express nonimmunogenic determinants; may shed, modify, or alter their antigens; may interfere with antigen processing; or may even mimic or assume host antigens. *Borrelia recurrentis,* the spirochete that produces epidemic relapsing fever, is sequestered within internal organs during afebrile periods but reemerges into the circulation with modified antigenicity. This cyclical process of antigenic variation followed by specific antibody production is responsible for the relapsing course of the disease.

Some bacteria produce inhibitory products that help them survive as successful parasites. *S. aureus* secretes leukocidin, a toxin lethal for neutrophils. *Pseudomonas aeruginosa* exoprotease may cleave and hence inactivate immunoglobulins. Some *Shigella* species kill phagocytes after their ingestion. However, the best known of the inhibitory products are the antiphagocytic devices or capsules. Numerous bacteria elaborate polysaccharide or glycoprotein structures external to the cell wall that profoundly inhibit non-opsonin-mediated phagocytosis. This has been demonstrated in experiments comparing wild-type and acapsular mutants of particular bacterial species.

Immune Defenses Against Fungi

As with bacteria, the fungi are found ubiquitously in nature. However, certain fungi have evolved a dual life-style. They may live as saprophytes (usually in decaying organic material in the soil), or they may parasitize animal tissues as potential pathogens. Such pathogenic fungi present a unique and difficult problem for the host. Compared to bacteria, they are highly evolved eukaryotes that undergo morphogenetic changes coupled with sexual reproduction. This genetic versatility accounts for the expression of virulence in pathogenic fungi. A prime example is the infection caused by *Coccidioides immitis,* one of the pathogenic fungi found in soil in the southwestern United States. Freeliving fungal cells growing as filaments (mycelia) transform into single-cell arthrospores during nutrient deprivation and desiccation. Arthrospores are very light, becoming easily airborne and thus inhaled. At 37C in the lung the inhaled cells change into a new vegetative state (the yeast form) in which they replicate by budding, and a second tissue stage called the spherule may form. This cystlike structure, harboring hundreds of daughter yeast cells, has a thick impenetrable wall and may render the fungus highly resistant to host killing mechanisms.

In *Cryptococcus neoformans* the heteropolysaccharide capsule is an important virulence factor. The rate of synthesis of this structure is in part regulated by the environment. Increasing the carbon dioxide concentration induces a marked stimulation of capsular polysaccharide biosynthesis. The maximal rate of synthesis occurs at approximately the carbon dioxide concentration of the tissues. Thus when the fungus is inhaled into the lungs, the sudden increase in the partial pressure of carbon dioxide maximally stimulates capsule synthesis, and within a few hours exuberant capsular polysaccharide surrounds each microorganism.

Phagocytic Defenses

Ubiquitous fungi pass through the alimentary tract or are inhaled from the air (e.g., *Candida albicans* and *Aspergillus fumigatus*, respectively) but provide little risk to the immunocompetent host. For the compromised host, however, infections with such fungi often become systemic and lethal. Gastrointestinal candidiasis and pulmonary aspergillosis are not uncommon in patients who are neutropenic, and these infections often become invasive. When neutrophils phagocytize yeast cells or conidiospores, they undergo the respiratory burst, and fungicidal oxygen metabolites are produced. Neutrophils and macrophages also synthesize cationic proteins, the defensins, which bind to the negatively charged fungal cell surface and are highly perturbing to cell membranes. However, aspergillus hyphae and *C. albicans* pseudohyphal forms are relatively resistant to killing by this mechanism so that a quantitative deficiency of neutrophils allows these opportunistic fungi to undergo morphogenic transformation to their more resistant forms.

Cell-mediated Immunity

Several fungi (e.g., *C. immitis, Histoplasma capsulatum, C. neoformans, Blastomyces dermatitidis, Paracoccidioides braziliensis, Sporothrix schenckii*) have evolved virulence factors enabiling them to cause a spectrum of disease in man. They are facultative intracellular parasites and generally are capable of undergoing asexual reproduction in a yeast phase within macrophages: first within the phagocytic vacuole and then, after rupture of the vacuole, within the cytoplasm of the phagocyte. In addition, some of these species (especially *Histoplasma*) can establish dormant states within host phagocytes, leading to latent foci of living organisms in the lung, liver, or spleen. The severity of disease caused by these fungi is highly dependent on cell-mediated immune competence. Macrophages (from experimental animals) that are activated by exposure to IFNγ produced by NK and T cells become fungistatic for *Histoplasma, Blastomyces* and *Cryptococcus*. After engaging the fungus, the macrophage message is induced for TNF-α. This important cytokine activates the macrophage in an autocrine loop but only for macrophage populations previously primed by IFNγ. Thus macrophage activation is a two-step process in which the chemical signals, acting sequentially, first prime (IFNγ) and then trigger (TNF-α) the phagocyte. The second signal (TNF-α) is induced by the microbe itself, and the two signals have a synergistic effect. Activation of mouse macrophages leads to synthesis of a cytosolic nitric oxide synthetase. This enzyme utilizes arginine as substrate, oxidizing one of its nitrogen atoms to nitric oxide gas. This dissolved gas or possibly other nitrogen oxides diffuse into the microorganism and react with iron-containing enzymes such as those necessary for electron transport in oxidative phosphorylation and for ribonucleotide reduction. Reaction with such iron prosthetic groups leads to inhibition of critical metabolic processes in the microorganism, thereby blocking its replication and possibly killing it. Certain fungi, protozoa, and bacteria are directly sensitive to inhibition by nitric oxide.

Resistance to Dermatophytes

The pathogenic fungi that cause systemic or deep mycotic infections may disseminate to the skin, producing hyperkeratotic, fungating lesions, whereas a select group of fungi called *dermatophytes* preferentially infects skin, hair, and nails. Dermatophytes have essentially no propensity to invade beyond the superficial dermis and almost never cause deep infections. Fungi invading the most superficial layers of the epidermis and the nail matrix may be inaccessible to secondary constitutive and primary immune defenses, resulting in characteristic chronic and indolent infections.

Immune Defenses Against Protozoa

Just as bacteria and fungi have evolved particular strategies for evading host defenses, the parasites, which represent a more formidable pathogen in terms of size and complexity, have also developed their means of protection. Some parasitic protozoa have simple life cycles in which only one or two developmental stages come into contact with humans. These cycles involve contaminative transmission through the gut (*Entamoeba, Toxoplasma, Giardia*) or the vagina (*Trichomonas*). In these cases the immune response is truly focused on a single stage of the organism. Agents of the more serious protozoal diseases, however, tend to have more complex life cycles so that humans are exposed to at least two, and sometimes several, developmental forms that differ considerably in antigenicity and sensitivity to immune mediators. Thus the basis for host defense and potential approaches to vaccination or immunodiagnosis must be considered separately for each stage of these diseases. For a general description of these organisms and their life cycles see Chapter 19.

Stage-specific Immune Responses

In most cases the parasite is at an extracellular stage at the time of infection and therefore is accessible to the full range of immunologic responses of the host. Immunity to reinfection, if established, often is expressed against this stage. During or after penetration of epithelial barriers, most protozoan parasites differentiate into at least one other life-cycle stage that multiplies in the host, resulting in a new immune response against these subsequent stages. The only major exceptions, the amebae, remain as trophozoites after invasion of the tissues.

The location in the host where protozoa develop and multiply usually determines which immune responses are generated against the later life-cycle stages. Most pathogenic protozoa have at least one (e.g., *Leishmania, Toxoplasma*) and sometimes several (e.g., *Plasmodium, Trypanosoma cruzi*) intracellular life-cycle stages in the mammal. Intracellular parasites are not directly exposed to antibody, although antibody to parasite antigens expressed on the surface of infected cells may help control infections. Intracellular stage forms that are released from ruptured host cells and parasites that live extracellularly in the blood or the tissue space (e.g., *T. cruzi, T. rhodesiense,* and *T. gambiense*) can be inactivated by antibody. Antibody also controls infections with *Giardia, Entamoeba,* and *Trichomonas* species by neutralization, opsonization for phagocytes (especially neutrophils), and complement activaton. Protective immune responses to organisms at intracellular stages often involve other effector mechanisms. Phagocytosis by normal macrophages does not contribute to resistance against some parasites (e.g., *Leishmania, Toxoplasma, T. cruzi*) that can actually live in these cells; macrophage activation is necessary to kill these intracellular parasites. Control of parasites that infect host cell types that do not have intrinsic antimicrobial activity such as muscle cells (*Toxoplasma, T. cruzi*), erythrocytes (*Plasmodium*), and hepatocytes (*Plasmodium*) may involve T cell–mediated responses such as cell-mediated cytotoxicity or delayed-type hypersensitivity reactions.

Transmission-blocking antibodies in patients with malaria illustrate another type of stage-specific immunity. A low percentage of intraerythrocytic malarial parasites differentiate into gametocytes. Gametocyte antigens stimulate antibody production. Feeding mosquitoes ingest both gametocytes and antigametocyte antibodies. Some of these antibodies can stop transmission of malaria by mosquitoes by blocking development of gametes or fusion of gametes to produce oocysts in the mosquito gut. Humans in endemic areas make transmission-blocking antibodies, and available evidence suggests that they help control seasonal malaria outbreaks. Transmission-blocking antibodies do not help limit disease in an infected individual but probably reduce the risk of disease spread to other people in the same population.

Immune Evasion and Host Counterattack

Most protozoan parasites persist even in immunocompetent hosts. Some parasites (e.g., *T. cruzi*) can cause chronic disease for years. Others (e.g., *Plasmodium*) can persist as cryptic infections for as long as decades before a change in the health of the infected individual results in a disease expression. African trypanosome infections may be acute or chronic but are inevitably fatal if untreated. The actual course of infection with a particular parasite varies considerably among different strains and, at least in animal models, depends strongly on genetic factors of the host. *Leishmania* strains give disease patterns that range from immunologically controlled local lesions that eventually heal to widely disseminated mucocutaneous or lethal visceral infections. In virtually all protozoan infections, immune host defenses are activated but often fail to eliminate infections because of special evasion mechanisms of the parasite.

The most spectacular mechanism of immune evasion is antigenic variation, and it is best demonstrated by African trypanosomes. Both the invasive metacyclic form and the bloodstream form are covered with a dense surface coat of the variant-specific glycoprotein (VSG). This coat restricts the interaction of macromolecules such as antibody and complement with components of the parasite membrane. It also is the major antigen exposed on the surface of intact parasites and consequently is the dominant target of host responses to these parasites. Trypanosomes carry several hundred to a thousand different genes for VSG, but only one of these VSG genes is expressed at a time. New VSG genes are activated spontaneously at a rather high frequency in individual cells of bloodstream populations. Thus although the host mounts a strong (usually IgM) antibody response to the dominant VSG, which usually clears this variant from the body, new clones of variants expressing different VSG genes are always present in the blood and escape immune destruction (Fig. 19–4). The infection can thus persist in the bloodstream despite a strong immune response, and successive cycles of antibody synthesis and antigenic variation account for the relapsing nature of trypanosome infections. Antigens expressed on the surface of erythrocytes infected with malarial parasites also undergo some degree of variation during infection.

The different ways protozoa escape death after phagocytosis can also be viewed as mechanisms of immune evasion. *Leishmania* amastigotes are adapted for life in the phagolysosome. Amastigotes have enzymes that enable them to detoxify mediators of phagocytic oxygen metabolism, to neutralize the acidity of the phagolysosome (thereby controlling phagocytic enzyme activity), and to use protons in the phagolysosome as cosubstrates in transport processes. When the defensive ac-

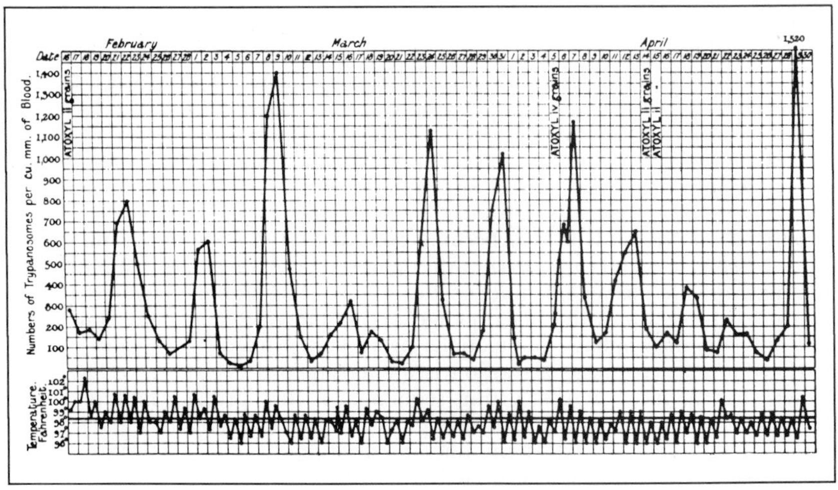

Fig. 19–4. Cyclical reappearance of trypanosomes in the peripheral blood of a patient with African sleeping sickness. Each peak corresponds to the appearance of a new antigenic variant. A number of variants are present in the infecting inoculum, but many more are generated by activation of different variant-specific glycoprotein (VSG) genes as the infection progresses. Antibody plays a passive selective role in the appearance of new variants. *(From Ross and Thomas: Proc R Soc Lond (Biol) 82:411, 1910.)*

tivities of macrophages are enhanced during immune-mediated activation, however, *Leishmania* are killed.

In animal models, activation of type 1 helper T cells (T_h1) that produce gamma-interferon and IL-2 in response to *Leishmania* antigens leads to protective immunity. Activation of type 2 helper cells that generate IL-3 and IL-4 can exacerbate leishmaniasis. Activation of suppressor T cells that restrict mediator production of T_h1 cells leads to rapidly fatal, disseminated leishmaniasis. IFNγ is probably the major lymphokine responsible for activation of macrophages during the resolution of human cutaneous leishmaniasis.

Other protozoans avoid destruction after phagocytosis in different ways. Trypomastigotes of *T. cruzi* produce a protein that disorganizes the macrophage phagolysosome membrane, allowing the parasite to escape from microbicidal mediators and to develop in the cytoplasm. Activated macrophages are more able to kill or at least stop reproduction of intracellular *T. cruzi. Toxoplasma* infects cells that are not normally phagocytic or defensive (e.g., fibroblasts, muscle cells), and the membrane surrounding the intracellular parasite does not fuse with phagolysosomes. Host defense mechanisms against the tissue stages of this parasite are not known. However, antibody is produced, and phagosome-lysosome fusion does occur when fibroblasts take up antibody-coated or killed trophozoites. T cells are known to activate macrophages that destroy trophozoites and may also play a role in clearing the tissue stages of the parasite; large granulomas often form at sites of persistent *Toxoplasma* infections.

One final example of the balance between immune responses and immune evasion occurs with *Plasmodium falciparum* infections. The erythrocytic stages are protected from direct phagocytosis and antibody-mediated damage by the erythrocyte membrane. However, infected erythrocytes express parasite antigens and exhibit other surface alterations. These infected blood cells may be removed by splenic macrophages. At certain stages of development *P. falciparum* synthesizes a glycoprotein that causes infected erythrocytes to adhere to the endothelial lining of small blood vessels. This adherence sequesters the developing parasites in small capillary beds, especially those in the brain, which may cause many of the symptoms of cerebral malaria. For protection, antibody produced to the glycoprotein can prevent or reverse endothelial attachment and in effect flushes infected erythrocytes into the circulation where they are cleared by the reticuloendothelial system.

Immune Defenses Against Helminths

Worms, like protozoa, have complex life cycles in which a variety of immunologically distinct forms confront the immune system. These include infectious stages, various migratory or larval forms, adult worms of both sexes, and eggs or other transmission forms. Each life-cycle form is metabolically active and releases antigenic products. The immune system usually responds actively to worms and their products, but because of some specialized immune evasion strategies, worms frequently establish chronic infections.

Several aspects of antihelmintic immune responses are unique. Helminths are large, metazoan organisms that cannot be readily taken up by phagocytic host cells. Thus phagocytosis, a major defense mechanism used to control other types of infections, is not effective against worms. Instead, ADCC reactions, including those mediated by IgE antibodies that involve secretion of mediators from a variety of cell types, play a more important role in the immunologic control of helminths.

Cellular Mechanisms

Eosinophils, neutrophils, monocyte-derived macrophages, platelets, and other cell types can all damage helminths under appropriate conditions in vitro. Which of these reactions is most important in controlling helminth infections and which contribute to immune pathology in humans are matters of controversy. Different types of cells and antibody isotypes probably will prove dominant in different types of infection. However, most immune reactions involve IgE and IgG or complement receptor–mediated adherence of the effector cell to the surface of the worm or both. Subsequently, toxic molecules are deposited on the parasite. Different mediators appear to be important with each cell type. Cationic proteins are released during eosinophil degranulation, but oxygen metabolites may mediate damage after neutrophil and monocyte adherence. Cytotoxic T cells do not appear to damage worms directly, regulatory T cells, however, play a major role in controlling helminth infections as described below. The cell-mediated reaction of most importance varies with the species and life-cycle stage of the parasite and host used in experimental studies. Eosinophils and IgE play a significant role in immune defense, and it is believed that IgE-eosinophil mechanisms may have evolved primarily in response to the selective pressure of helminth infections.

IgE-eosinophil defenses involve a highly regulated immune response. Tissue mast cells and inflammatory basophils bearing cytophilic IgE release a variety of mediators (Chap. 17), which preferentially attract eosinophils in response to parasitic antigens. Eosinophils can adhere to worms by receptor-linked IgE to mediate killing. Some worms activate complement directly; in other cases complement can be activated by antibodies to surface antigens. In either case C3 fragments on worms also can cause receptor-mediated adherence of effector cells (including eosinophils). T cells stimulated by helminth antigens produce chemoattractants, and IgE production is highly dependent on helper T cell activation of B cells. Other T cell lymphokines (e.g., IL-3) alter hematopoiesis and promote the development of eosinophilia that is characteristic of helminth infections. T cell–induced macrophage activation can increase IL-1 and TNF production, leading to synthesis of other acute phase reactants that also can damage worms. Schistosome killing by platelets, for example, may involve C-reactive protein. Mast cells play an additional role in resistance to intestinal parasites: IgE-mediated release of histamine and other substances that stimulate contraction of smooth muscles in the gut may enhance expulsion of nematodes. All of these reactions are controlled by regulatory T cells, and as already noted in connection with leishmaniasis, different subclasses of helper T cells produce different mediators in response to helminth antigens.

Immune Evasion

In spite of this assortment of defense mechanisms, worms persist in immunocompetent hosts. Adult schistosomes, for example, may resist immunologic attack for years. This is particularly noteworthy since these parasites such as microfilaria live in the bloodstream where they are exposed to the full spectrum of immunologic mediators. The basis of this resistance is unknown, although several phenomena have been described that may play a role in immune evasion by helminths. For example, the glycoproteins rapidly shed from the cuticular surface of schistosomules appear to prevent deposition of complement on the parasite surface and probably interfere with antibody-mediated adherence of effector cells. Cestodes also shed antigenic material, and depletion of complement in the fluid phase by shed immune complexes may help worms survive antibody-mediated damage. The cuticle of schistosomules may fuse with the plasma membrane of neutrophils under some conditions, thus blocking degranulation and the release of mediators. Schistosomes also have proteolytic enzymes that can cleave surface-bound immunoglobulin molecules and thereby inhibit their effector functions. Individuals who are chronically infected with schistosomes, filarial worms, or cestodes often show significant suppression in their ability to react to antigens in general.

Host tissue damage from antihelminth responses is also common, for example, with the formation of granulomas around schistosome eggs deposited in the liver or bladder. In mouse models the intensity of granuloma formation also reflects the strength of resistance to superinfection by schistosomules. Maintenance of such resistance to superinfection (sometimes referred to as concomitant immunity) seems to depend on continued stimulation of the immune system by adult worms. Concomitant immunity has also been reported in patients with cestode infections.

Host Characteristics That Influence Susceptibility to Infection

Age

Changes that occur in the immune system during fetal, neonatal, and adult development greatly affect the host response to different types of infection. Placental transfer of maternal IgG plays an important role in providing passive fetal immunity, but some synthesis of IgM and IgG can be elicited by the second and third trimesters. During fetal development, susceptibility is generally limited to those organisms that are blood borne and can be transmitted by the maternal circulation (e.g., cytomegalovirus, rubella, *Toxoplasma,* and syphilis). At birth, neonatal levels of maternally transferred IgG are relatively high and slowly begin to decrease, whereas IgM levels are low but slowly rise. Milk and colostrum provide immunoglobulins (especially IgA) and leukocytes; indeed, the number of leukocytes in a daily feeding of milk is roughly equivalent to those already in the neonate. Epidemiologic studies suggest that this transferred immunity is important because breastfed infants appear to be less susceptible to viral and bacterial infections.

Cell-mediated immunity is relatively well developed in the neonate, although natural killing activity directed against some virus-infected cells (e.g., herpes simplex) appears to be low. A major deficit in children less than 2 years old is their inability to make antibodies against polysaccharide antigens. As a result, young children are susceptible to infections with encapsulated bacteria such as *H. influenzae, S. pneumoniae,* and *Neisseria meningitidis.* There is a period of 2 to 3 months after birth when the transferred maternal antibodies are protective, followed by 2 years of relatively high danger from infection as passively transferred antibody declines. When exposed to a polysaccharide antigen, children in this age range can transiently make IgM antibodies (often in a delayed manner), but IgG antibodies do not develop, and no memory B cells are established. The reason for this inability to make antipolysaccharide IgG antibodies is not clearly understood, but methods for stimulating the production of anticapsular antibodies are being studied. The most successful approach to date has been in conjugating the polysaccharide onto a protein carrier. Children respond both to the carrier protein and to the polysaccharide antigen, giving protective antibody levels against the encapsulated organisms.

Genetic Factors

The inheritance of genes that control the type and magnitude of immune responses to specific antigens appears to influence host responsiveness to infection. For example, the level of host immunity appears related to the clinical course of hepatitis B virus infection. Vaccinated hosts are generally protected, but nonvaccinated hosts develop different types of disease, depending in part on their ability to respond immunologically; strong responders generally experience acute (transient) hepatitis, whereas weak responders have a mild, indolent infection with little liver damage. Intermediate responders, unable to eliminate infection, develop persistent and often severe cellular immune-mediated hepatic damage (chronic active hepatitis). Similarly, weak responders to *Mycobacterium leprae* develop lepromatous leprosy, as opposed to the tuberculoid leprosy seen in strong responders. Particular HLA phenotypes have been associated with these and other infection-related, autoaggressive diseases such as type 1 diabetes mellitus, ankylosing spondylitis, and anterior uveitis, suggesting a genetic influence at the level of immune recognition or responsiveness (Chaps. 13 and 17).

Other genetic factors may also indirectly affect host susceptibility to certain organisms. Individuals who do not have the Duffy a and b erythrocyte antigens (Fy a^-b^-) are resistant to *Plasmodium vivax* infection, correlating with the inability of the organism to bind and penetrate these red blood cells. Likewise, individuals who have sickle cell trait (HbS) have increased resistance to *P. falciparum.* In the homozygous condition (S-S) this is probably due to a decreased survival rate of infected red blood cells that become sickled by oxygen metabolism of the organism within the red blood cell. In the heterozygous condition (S-A), growth of the organism is arrested at the large ring stage.

Nutritional Factors

Dietary requirements in humans include the need for vitamins, minerals, and trace elements, essential fats, carbohydrates and fats (to provide calories), and sufficient protein to provide the essential amino acids for synthesis of proteins and nucleic acids. Malnutrition affects host susceptibility to certain microorganisms, especially bacteria. The complexity of the human nutritional requirements makes it difficult to associate the deficiency of a particular nutrient with an increased propensity for certain infections. The malnutrition that occurs in developing countries is often present with other multiple dietary deficiencies. Protein-calorie malnutrition produces striking effects on various facets of immunocompetence, especially those involving complement, secretory IgA, and cell-mediated immunity. Complement proteins are synthesized primarily by hepatocytes, although macrophages can synthesize complement components as well. The plasma concentrations of C3, C5, and factor B are decreased in malnourished humans. This decrease may be a consequence of reduced synthesis in the liver or increased consumption due to intercurrent infections and the increased formation of immune complexes.

Secretory IgA levels in nasopharyngeal and other external secretions are low in individuals with protein-calorie malnutrition. Furthermore, the production of specific IgA in response to immunization with viral vaccines is reduced. This may be the result of reduced production of secretory component due to atrophic mucosal epithelium. Secretory IgA deficiency has been associated with an increased incidence and severity of diarrheal and pneumonic infections, especially in undernourished children.

Resistance to tuberculosis in a population with a high prevalence of dormant infection is a clinical index of cell-mediated immune competence. Historical examples provide provocative evidence for the role of cell-mediated immunocompetence in controlling the activity of this (and other) facultative intracellular microbial infections relative to nutrition. During World War I most people living in western Europe had acquired tubercle bacilli at a young age, resolved the primary infection, and therefore harbored dormant but living bacilli in their lungs. The tuberculosis death rate, largely due to reactivation of dormant lesions, could be directly correlated with the food supply and was independent of military campaigns, poor living conditions, or other stress factors of wartime.

Acquired immunity to tubercle bacilli or *Pneumocystis carinii* is a complex process involving the coordinated interaction of T lymphocyte subsets and macrophages. The effect of protein-calorie deprivation on this process is undoubtedly multifactorial. In malnutrition the number of circulating T-helper lymphocytes is significantly decreased, and there is loss of cutaneous delayed hypersensitivity. Likewise, in vitro T cell responses to mitogens and alloantigens are depressed. Under these conditions the amplification and activation processes and their effects in activating macrophages are depressed. The consequence is that microorganisms such as *Mycobacterium tuberculosis* replicate freely within host macrophages.

Immunopathologic Reactions to Infection

An infection can have three different pathologic effects: no host damage, damage caused by the organism, or damage caused by the host response to the organism or infected cells. Normally, an inflammatory response benefits the host by resolving the infection. In some cases, however, host damage from inflammation exceeds damage caused by the organism, as, for example, with chronic active hepatitis, cavitating tuberculosis, and tuberculoid leprosy. In these diseases the organism itself causes minimal damage, whereas damage from the host response can lead to significant morbidity and death.

All four major types of immunopathologic reactions (Chap. 17) may take place in response to infection. Type I (IgE-mediated) reactions, which occur in response to many metazoan infections, type IV (cell-mediated) reactions, which occur with intracellular microbes, and some aspects of type II (cytotoxic-antibody) reactions have been discussed earlier in this chapter. However, infections may also induce other types of immunopathologic responses such as type III (immune-complex) reactions and various autoimmune diseases.

Immune Complex Diseases

Immune complexes commonly form during infections but infrequently cause significant host injury. Nevertheless, certain organisms can induce severe immune complex diseases such as the acute glomerulonephritis associated with streptococcal infection. Typically, 1 to 2 weeks after pharyngeal or skin infection with a nephritogenic strain of *S. pyogenes,* hematuria and proteinuria develop concomitantly with large immune complexes that bind complement along glomerular basement membranes (Fig. 19–5). These lesions usually heal with minimal impairment, although acute complications may occur. Other organisms associated with immune complex glomerulonephritis include bacteria (e.g., staphylococci, enterococci), fungi (e.g., *Candida*), protozoa (e.g., malaria), and viruses (e.g., HBV). Other clinical manifestations of immune complex diseases associated with infection include vasculitis (e.g., polyarteritis nodosa with hepatitis B virus), dermatitis (e.g., erythema nodosa with leprosy), and pneumonitis (e.g., allergic alveolitis with actinomyces). Although identification of specific microbial antigens within the immune complexes is often difficult, the characteristic temporal, clinical, and morphologic features associated with the formation of these complexes provide presumptive evidence of their etiology.

Autoimmune Diseases

Infectious organisms often are involved in the pathogenesis of autoimmune diseases. Some microbes or their products may induce nonspecific immune reactions; B cells, for example, can undergo polyclonal (nonspecific) activation in response to certain organisms (e.g., mycoplasma, trypanosoma, plasmodia, measles, EBV) and bacterial products (e.g., lipopolysaccharide, *S. aureus* protein A, PPD of tuberculin). Such stimulation may actually detract from the specific response required for protection and thus potentiate the infection. Animal models have implicated infectious organisms in autoimmune diseases such as systemic lupus erythematosus and rheumatoid arthritis. Several rheumatic, endocrinologic, and neurologic diseases with autoimmune features have been associated with particular microorganisms, especially in individuals with certain HLA phenotypes. As mentioned previously, some infections cause secondary disease as a result of autodestructive immune mechanisms (e.g., hepatitis, leprosy). Other organisms appear to stimulate host responses to cross-reactive self-antigens (e.g., rheumatic fever with streptococcal antigens). Some autoimmune hemolytic anemias are also associated with specific infectious organisms; a cold agglutinin to the I blood group can be seen in patients infected with *M. pneumoniae.* Interestingly, some microbial enzymes can convert the A_1 blood group to B, which results in a hemolytic anemia from the normal circulating anti-B isohemagglutinins in patients with the A blood type.

Immune-mediated host tissue damage accompanies many

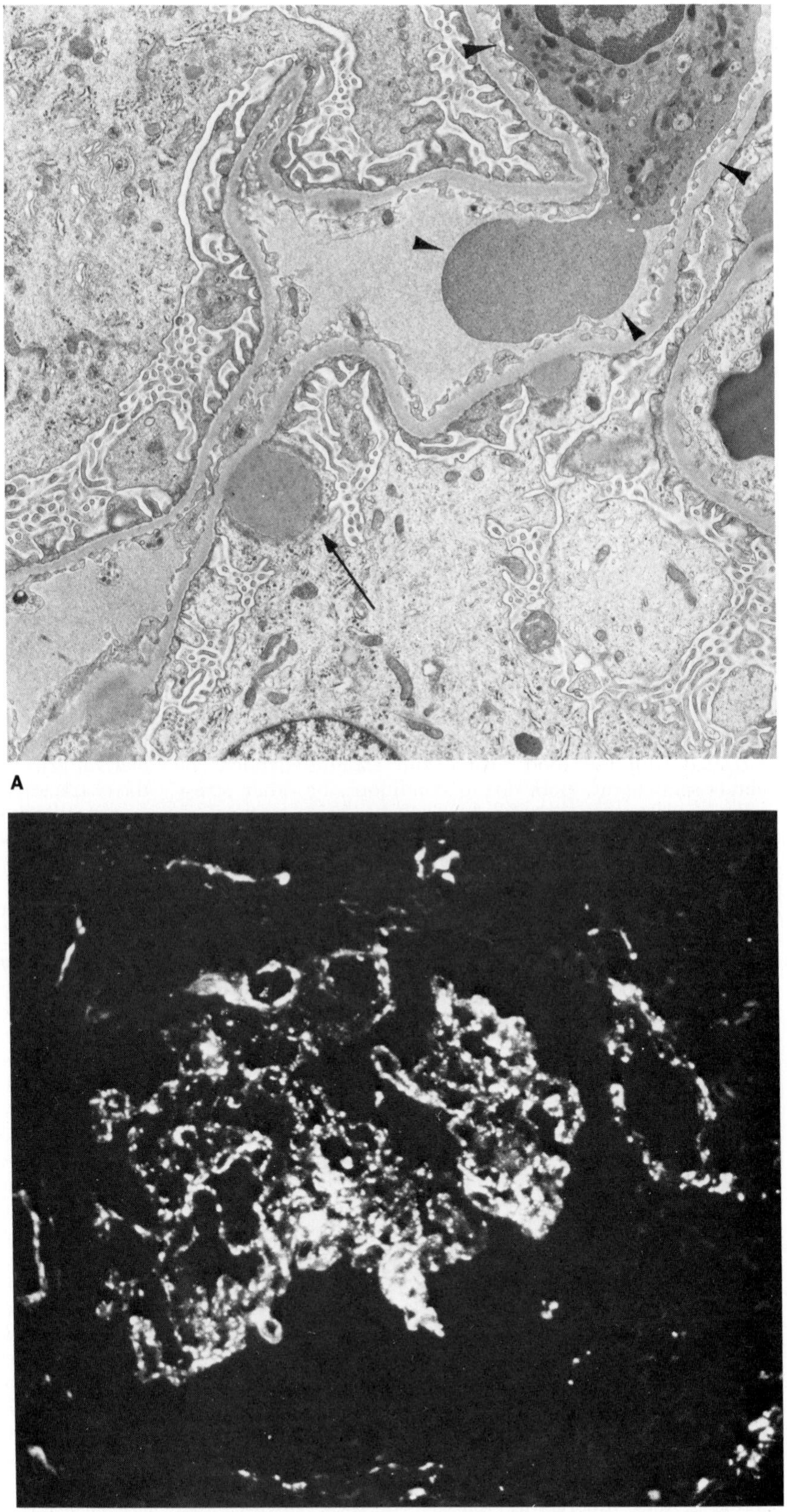

A

B

Fig. 19–5. Postinfectious glomerulonephritis. **A.** The typical appearance of electron-dense, subepithelial immune complex deposit (arrow) associated with postinfectious glomerulonephritis. An attracted neutrophil (arrowhead) is seen nearby in the glomerular capillary loop. × 5000. **B.** Immunofluorescent staining shows abundant C3 deposits in these complexes. × 250.

chronic protozoan infections. Much of the symptomatology of African trypanosomiasis, for example, results from immune complex formation. The immunopathologic effects of induced IgG antibodies are primarily responsible for damage to tissue and blood cells in this disease. In trypanosomiasis and malaria, alterations of host immune regulation are evident; for example, polyclonal B cell activation is common. Thus serum IgM antibodies are usually elevated in human trypanosomiasis but are not specific for trypanosomes and express activity against a wide variety of unrelated antigens, including autoantigens. Autoantibody has been postulated to play a role in the pathogenesis of several protozoal diseases. Paradoxically, individuals with chronic parasitic infections often show depressed immunologic responsiveness to other organisms. This anergic state can be clinically significant because concurrent bacterial infections may be lethal in patients infected with these parasitic diseases.

Immunization

The two basic categories of immunization are (1) passive immunization, in which an already created specific immune effector is transferred to a new host (generally antibodies in humans, but immune cells can be transferred in infants or in genetically identical animal strains), and (2) active immunization, or vaccination, in which an antigenic material is inoculated so the host organism will actively create its own immune response.

Passive Immunization

Most passive immunization in humans involves the injection of antibody or antiserum preparations. The most widely used antibody preparations are "immune-specific globulin" (ISG) and intravenous immune globulin, which are both made by pooling serum from hundreds of donors, then separating out the immunoglobulin fraction of the serum. For many years injections of ISG ("gamma globulin shots") were given to patients exposed to measles to attenuate their infection. ISG shots are still used as prophylaxis against hepatitis A virus in people traveling to endemic areas. Intravenous immune globulin is given as replacement therapy for patients who are antibody or immunoglobulin deficient and for its immunomodulating properties. Products with high antibody titers against specific pathogens such as varicella zoster immune globulin or rabies immune globulin are used to protect nonimmune or immunocompromised individuals after a known exposure to an infected person or animal. One shortcoming with the use of passive immunization is that the antibodies must be given before or within a short time after exposure to have maximal efficacy. In addition, the transferred antibodies have a fairly short half-life so that the protection offered by passive immunization is more transient than that offered by vaccination.

Passive transfer of specific cellular immune effectors is not technically feasible in humans because of the need for complete HLA matching to avoid rejection of (or graft-vs-host reaction from) the transfused cells. Another limitation is the low number of specific T cell effectors in a donor's blood or bone marrow at any time other than immediately after an acute infection. The primary use of cellular passive immunization has been in studying the immune response to infections, using inbred animal strains.

Active Immunization

Live Attenuated and Inactivated Vaccines

Most of the attenuated viral vaccines currently in use (measles, mumps, rubella, oral poliomyelitis, and many others) have been created by sequentially growing the viruses on several different cell types in vitro. Serial tissue culture passages seem to decrease the virulence of the virus, probably as a result of point mutations. In some cases an opposite mutational pattern occurs when the attenuated virus from tissue culture is introduced back into the human host. As an example, there is a tendency for the attenuated poliovirus vaccine strains to evolve back toward a more virulent form while they are replicating in the gastrointestinal tract. This more virulent strain has the potential to spread to new hosts from the infected child, although, fortunately, this is an uncommon event.

There are several advantages of live attenuated vaccines over killed vaccines. Both categories of vaccine generally produce high levels of serum IgG neutralizing antibodies. However, the process of inactivating a virus can modify its antigens so that the same antibody specificities generated against a wild-type virus are not produced. For example, the inactivated measles and RSV vaccines both failed to generate effective antibodies against the fusion proteins in the envelope of the virus. Exposure to wild-type virus resulted in infection in many of the vaccinated patients, and symptomatic illness was not prevented. The inactivated RSV vaccine altered the immune response in such a way that children infected with RSV after the vaccine actually had more serious respiratory disease than children who had never been vaccinated. In the case of measles, children who had been vaccinated with the inactivated vaccine developed a form of serious but modified measles when they were subsequently infected with wild-type virus.

Another advantage of live attenuated viruses is that most replicate in the parts of the body where immunity is needed. In the case of poliovirus, oral administration causes secretory IgA synthesis against viral replication in the oral and gastrointestinal mucosa. These secretory antibodies protect against subsequent viral infection of mucosal cells. In contrast, secretory IgA antibodies are not made against inactivated virus vaccine administered by intramuscular injection. As a result, when a person who has been immunized with the killed poliomyelitis vaccine swallows a wild-type poliovirus, the gastrointestinal tract replication and fecal excretion of the virus will be greater than that of a person who received the live attenuated vaccine. Since gastrointestinal replication is a major community reservoir for the virus, the use of attenuated oral poliomyelitis vaccine has the potential to decrease the circulation of wild-type poliovirus.

The major advantage of inactivated vaccines is their safety. Live attenuated poliovirus vaccine has the potential to cause paralytic poliomyelitis in a few cases each year. In addition, the live attenuated vaccines can mutate toward the wild type from which they were derived. If the preparation of the inactivated vaccines is monitored carefully so that no contaminating live virus is contained in the vaccine, the inactivated vaccines have little or no risk. An occasional individual may have an allergic reaction to a component of the vaccine, and, rarely, unusual immunologically mediated reactions can occur (e.g., Guillain Barré syndrome after the swine flu vaccine in 1976), but in general their safety is excellent.

Toxoids

The use of toxoids is quite similar to the use of inactivated vaccines in that a potentially virulent material (i.e., toxin) is modified to render it nonpathogenic but antigenically intact. A classic example of a toxoid is the tetanus vaccine. *Clostridium tetani,* an anaerobic bacteria that lives in dead tissues, produces an extremely powerful neurotoxin. Disease can result from so little neurotoxin that most patients who have clinical tetanus never develop an antibody response against the toxin. Tetanus toxoid is produced by inactivating toxin with formalin, and it can be injected in large enough quantities for the host to develop antibodies that neutralize the toxin before it binds to peripheral nerves.

Anti-Idiotype Antibodies

Anti-idiotype antibodies can be directed against the binding site (paratope) of other antibodies specific for a given antigenic determinant (epitope). This mechanism might be compared to a lock and key. The target epitope from the pathogen (usually a factor related to virulence) is the lock, and the idiotype (paratope) of the antibody is the key. The anti-idiotype is a model of the lock, created to fit the key. The hope in immunizing with anti-idiotypes is that the host will respond to this nontoxic version of the lock (virulent pathogen factor) by forming antibodies identical to the original key (which was directed against the real virulent host factor). To date, anti-idiotypes have not been used as human vaccines, but their potential remains of research interest.

Vector Vaccines

A relatively new area in vaccine development is the use of vectors as immunizing agents. A "vector" is an organism that is modified to include genes from another organism or source (some genes might be artificially created). As a result, the vaccine recipient is able to generate an immune response without risking the dangers of the pathogen, although the side effects of the vector itself must be considered.

Using a virus as a vector has several advantages. Once the virus is internalized into the cell, translation of the genes inserted into the vector can begin. These proteins can associate with the MHC molecules in such a way that both class I and class II antigen presentation occurs. The vector enables the antigens to be processed in a manner essentially identical to that for the wild-type infection, but by selecting which antigens are translated, an immune cellular and antibody response can occur without the virulence of the wild-type virus.

Another advantage of vector vaccines is in the ability to choose which antigens to include. This control can be useful both in research and in designing a vaccine that maximizes protection while minimizing side effects. The vector virus that has been studied most intensively is vaccinia. Vaccinia is a large and complex poxvirus that previously was used as the smallpox vaccine. It has several advantages making it well suited for vector use. The virus has a large double-stranded DNA genome that can be easily manipulated to include genes in addition to those of the vaccinia itself. Promoters are inserted along with the desired genes to get expression of the inserted genomic material. Another advantage of vaccinia is the large number of genes that can be inserted—enough so that one vaccinia vector vaccine may be able to protect against several diseases simultaneously. Unfortunately, vaccinia virus strains used in the past as vaccines against smallpox caused many complications, including disseminated vaccinia and an allergic encephalitis. The strains currently being used as vectors have been attenuated beyond the previously used vaccinia strains, but it is still unknown whether complications will be reduced.

Bacterial vaccine vectors have also been created. These agents include gram-negative enteric bacteria modified so that their replication in the gastrointestinal tract is severely limited. The most studied example is a galactose epimerase deficient (gal E) mutant of *S. typhi.* This organism cannot grow in the presence of galactose and has itself been used as an attenuated typhoid vaccine. When used as a vector, genes can be added to the basic bacterial gene complement, usually as plasmids. The resulting proteins can include virulence factors from other organisms for which neutralizing antibodies (particularly secretory IgA) would be advantageous. Because the epimerase gene is deleted in the *S. typhi* vaccine strain, the attenuation is stable. Removing a gene from an organism makes restoring virulence much more difficult than the changing of point mutation back to the wild-type pattern.

Vaccines Produced from Cloned Genes

Another area in which contemporary molecular biology has had an enormous impact on vaccine development is in the ability to produce huge quantities of pure proteins from isolated genes. Once the gene encoding a protein has been isolated, it can be cloned in bacteria to obtain large quantities of genomic material. These cloned nucleic acids can then be translated into proteins using many different systems. Bacteria, yeast, viruses, and even a combination of an insect virus (baculoviruses) and the fall army worm (*Spodoptera fugiperda*) have been used to synthesize relatively pure proteins in large amounts. The first human vaccine commercially produced from a cloned gene is a hepatitis B vaccine synthesized in yeast and approved for use in 1986. However, having purified proteins available is not always sufficient to make an effective vaccine. Many proteins in isolation do not achieve the same conformation they have in situ on the organism. In addition, there are advantages to having several different antigenic sites so that antibodies can attach to more places on the target organism.

Parasite Immunoprophylaxis

Attempts to develop a vaccine against *P. falciparum* malaria illustrate important factors that influence the effectiveness of human vaccines. Studies with monoclonal antibodies identified circumsporozoal proteins that cover the surface of *Plasmodium* sporozoites. These proteins have highly repeated amino acid sequences that form immunodominant epitopes, and monoclonal antibodies to these repeated epitopes neutralize sporozoites and protect animals from infection by mosquito bite. This immunodominant epitope is conserved in *P. falciparum.* Immunizing humans with a synthetic peptide corresponding to the conserved, immunodominant epitope coupled to protein carriers elicited antibody production in human volunteers who had not been exposed to malaria; unfortunately, this method was not highly effective in protecting humans against malaria in field trials in an endemic area. Subsequent work has shown that portions of the circumsporozoal protein outside the peptide strongly influence the ability of animals and people to mount an effective antibody response to the peptide. These other epitopes are recognized by helper T cells that potentiate antibody synthesis by B cells. Consequently, further work on synthetic subunit vaccines will involve incorporating into the immunogen epitopes that activate both B and T cell responses.

The circumsporozoite vaccine that was field tested was a monovalent vaccine: the immunogen was a single antigen derived from only one life-cycle stage of malaria. Vaccines that incorporate antigens expressed on erythrocytic stages of malaria have also been tested in humans, and more extensive field trials are forthcoming. Epidemiologic evidence suggesting that transmission of blocking antibodies can protect human populations against the spread of malaria has encouraged efforts to develop an antigametocyte vaccine. Ultimately, multivalent vaccines that include antigens derived from several life-cycle stages may prove most effective.

Genetic factors strongly influence the intensity of the T cell response of mice and people to a given epitope on circumsporozoal and other malaria antigens. In some cases, responsiveness to an antigen may reflect the ability of the antigen to be presented to T cells in association with class II MHC molecules. Responses to other malaria antigens do not show MHC restriction. What types of T cells respond to a given antigenic epitope is also an important concern in vaccine development. As already noted, only some types of helper T cells potentiate protective immune responses in schistosome and *Leishmania* infections. Other T helper or suppressor cells may actually exacerbate disease.

Thus the work on malaria vaccines has shown that identifying antigens that can elicit strong protective antibody responses in animal model systems is only the first stage in vaccine development. Subunit vaccines must be engineered so antigens can be effectively presented to T cells that will potentiate beneficial and long-lasting immune responses, including antibody production, in genetically heterogeneous populations. This will require detailed analysis of the human immune response to future vaccine candidates.

Summary

Infectious organisms are largely responsible for the development of the complex nature of host immunity, and over the years they have provided practical models for studying immunologic mechanisms. Despite tremendous advances in our understanding of host-microbial interactions and in the development of new and varied antimicrobial drugs and therapies, infection still remains the greatest cause of human morbidity and mortality. The ability to intervene and amplify host immunity, especially by immunization, has already had a dramatic effect in reducing (and even eradicating) previously widespread diseases such as smallpox, but such developments are only a beginning. Continued progress over the next few years in prevention and therapy, based on an increased understanding of immunologic mechanisms, should provide the basis for greater success in the defense against infectious organisms.

FURTHER READING

Books and Reviews

Blackwell JM: Immunology of leishmania. In Lachmann PJ, Black DK, Rosen FS, Walport MJ (eds): Clinical Aspects of Immunology. Oxford, Blackwell Scientific Publications, 1990

Butterworth AE: Control of schistosomiasis in man. In Englund PT, Sher A (eds): The Biology of Parasitism. New York, Alan R Liss, 1988

Cross GAM: Cellular and genetic aspects of antigenic variation in trypanosomes. Ann Rev Immunol 8:83, 1990

Devreotes PN, Zigmond SH: Chemotaxis in eukaryotic cells: A focus on leukocytes and diclyostelium. Ann Rev Cell Biol 4:649, 1988

Gordon AH, Koj A: The Acute Phase Response to Injury and Infection: The Roles of Interleukin 1 and Other Mediators. Amsterdam, Elsevier, 1985

Grau GE, Piguet PF, Vassalli P, Lambert PH: Tumor necrosis factor and other cytokines in cereberal malaria: Experimental and clinical data. Immunol Rev 112:49, 1989

Hynes RO: Integrins: A family of cell surface receptors. Cell 48:549, 1987

Kaufmann SHE: T cell paradigms in parasitic and bacterial infections. Curr Top Microbiol Immunol 155:1–160, 1990

Kraus R (ed): Immunopathology of parasitic diseases. Springer Semin Immunopathol 2:355, 1980

Lachmann PJ, Ivanyi J (eds): Immunology of mycobacterial disease. Springer Semin Immunopathol 10:279–391, 1988

Miller JF, Makalanos JJ, Falkow S: Coordinate regulation and sensory transduction in the control of bacterial virulence. Science 243:916, 1989

Mims CA: The Pathogenesis of Infectious Disease. New York, Academic, 1982

Mims CA: Virus immunity and pathogenesis. Brit Med Bull 41:1, 1985

Mitchell GH: An update on candidate malaria vaccines. Parasitology 98:S21 1989

Modabber F: Experience with vaccines against cutaneous leishmaniasis of mice and men. Parasitology 98:S49, 1990

Moeller G (ed): MHC restriction of anti-viral immunity. Immunol Rev 58:1, 1981

Moulder J: Intracellular parasites. Microbiol Rev 49:298, 1986

Perlmann P, Wigzell H: Malaria Immunology, Progress Allergy. Karger, Basel, 1988

Rouse BT, Norley S, Martin S: Antiviral cytotoxic T lymphocyte induction and vaccination. Rev Infect Dis 10:16, 1988

Segal AW: The electron transport chain of the microbicidal oxidase of phagocytic cells and its involvement in the molecular pathology of chronic granulomatous disease. J Clin Invest 83:1785, 1989

Sher A, James SL, Correa-Oliviera R, et al: Schistosome vaccines: Current progress and future prospects. Parasitology 98:561, 1989

Stiehm ER, Kronenberg LH, Rosenblatt HM, et al: Interferon: Immunobiology and clinical significance. Ann Intern Med 96:80, 1982

Welsh RM: Natural cell-mediated immunity during viral infections. Curr Top Microbiol Immunol 92:83, 1982

Selected Papers

Andrews NW, Abrams CK, Slatin SL, Griffiths G: A *Trypanosoma cruzi*–secreted protein immunologically related to complement component C9: Evidence for membrane pore forming activity at acid pH. Cell 61:1277, 1990

Babior BM: The respiratory burst of phagocytes. J Clin Invest 73:599, 1984

Brown EJ, Hosea JW, Frank MM: The role of antibody and complement in the reticuloendothelial clearance of pneumococci from the bloodstream. Rev Infect Dis 5:797, 1983

Buchmeier NA, Heffron F: Induction of *Salmonella* stress proteins upon infection of macrophages. Science 248:730, 1990

Bukowski JF, Warner JF, Dennert G, Welsh RM: Adoptive transfer studies demonstrating the antiviral effect of natural killer cells *in vivo.* J Exp Med 161:40, 1985

Bukowski SF, Welch RM: Interferon enhances the susceptibility of virus-infected fibroblasts to cytotoxic T cells. J Exp Med 161:257, 1985

Capron A, Dessaint JP, Capron M, et al: Immunity to schistosomes: Progress toward vaccine. Science 238:1065, 1987

Casali P, Rice GPA, Oldstone MBA: Viruses disrupt functions of human lymphocytes: Effects of measles virus and influenza virus on lymphocyte-mediated killing and antibody production. J Exp Med 159:1322, 1984

Chandra RK, Tejpar S: Diet and immunocompetence. Int J Immunopharmacol 5:175, 1983

Cox JH, Yewdell JW, Eisenlohr LC, et al: Antigen presentation requires transport of MHC class I molecules from the endoplasmic reticulum. Science 247:715, 1990

Densen P, Mandrell GL: Phagocyte strategy vs microbial tactics. Rev Infect Dis 2:817, 1981

De Vries RRP, Mehra NK, Vaidya MC, et al: HLA-linked control of susceptibility to tuberculoid leprosy and association with HLA-DR types. Tissue Antigens 16:294, 1980

Ding AH, Nalhan CT, Steuhr DJ: Release of reactive nitrogen intermediates and reactive oxygen intermediates from mouse peritoneal macrophages: Comparison of activating cytokines and evidence for independent production. J Immunol 141:2407, 1988

Fujinami RS, Oldstone MBS: Antiviral antibody reacting on the plasma membrane alters measles virus expression inside the cell. Nature 279:579, 1979

Ganz T, Selsted ME, Harwig SL, et al: Defensins. Natural peptide antibiotics of human neutrophils. J Clin Invest 76:1427, 1985

Gao X-M, Liew FY, Tite JP: Identification and characterization of T helper epitopes in the nucleoprotein of influenza A virus. J Immunol 143:3007, 1989

Good MF, Miller LH: Involvement of T cells in malaria immunity: Implications for vaccine development. Vaccine 7:3, 1989

Griffin DE, Ward BJ, Jauregui E, et al: Immune activation during measles: Interferon-γ and neopterin in plasma and cerebrospinal fluid in complicated and uncomplicated disease. J Infect Dis 161:449, 1990

Gustafson TL, Lievens AW, Brunell PA, et al: Measles outbreak in a fully immunized secondary-school population, N Engl J Med 316:771, 1987

Horowitz MA: Phagocytosis of microorganisms. Rev Infect Dis 4:104, 1982

Johnston JM, Harmon SA, Binn LN, et al: Antigenic and immunogenic properties of a Hepatitis A virus capsid protein expressed in *Escherichia coli.* J Infect Dis 157:1203, 1988

Joyner KA, Brown EJ, Frank MM: Complement and bacteria. Ann Rev Immunol 2:461, 1984

Kierszenbaum F: Autoimmunity in Chagas disease. J Parasitol 72:201, 1986

Klavinskis LS, Tishon A, Oldstone MBA: Efficiency and effectiveness of cloned virus-specific cytotoxic T lymphocytes in vivo. J Immunol 143:2013, 1989

Kornfeld SJ, Plaut AG: Secretory immunity and the bacterial IgA proteases. Rev Infect Dis 3:521, 1981

Leclerc C, Martineau P, van der Werf S, et al: Induction of virus-neutralizing antibodies by bacteria expressing the C3 poliovirus epitope in the periplasm: The route of immunization influences the isotypic distribution and the biologic activity of the antipoliovirus antibodies. J Immunol 144:3174, 1990

Lightowlers MW, Rickard MD: Excretory-secretory products of helminth parasites: Effects on host immune responses. Parasitology 96:S123, 1988

Masson SJ, Miller LH, Shiraishi T, et al: The Duffy blood group determinants: Their role in the susceptibility of human and animal erythrocytes to *P. knowlesi* malaria. Br J Haematol 36:327, 1977

Nutman TB: Protective immunity in lymphatic filariasis. Exp Parasitol 68:248, 1989

Parkhouse RM, Harrison LJ: Antigens of parasitic helminths in diagnosis, protection, and pathology. Parasitology 99:55, 1989

Petersen BH, Lee TJ, Snyderman R, et al: *Neisseria meningitidis* and *Neisseria gonorrhoeae* bacteremia associated with C6, C7, or C8 deficiency. Ann Intern Med 90:917, 1979

Premawansa S, Peiris JS, Perera KL, et al: Target antigens of transmission blocking immunity of *Plasmodium vivax* malaria. Characterization and polymorphism in natural parasite populations. J Immunol 144:4376, 1990

Ross, R, Thomas D: A case of sleeping sickness studied by precise enumerative methods: Regular, periodical increase of the parasites disclosed. Proc R Soc Lond (Biol) 82:411, 1910

Scott P: The role of TH1 and TH2 cells in experimental cutaneous leishmaniasis. Exp Parasitol 68:369, 1989

Sher A, Hall BF, Vadas MA, et al: Acquisition of murine major histocompatibility complex gene products by schistosomula of *Schistosoma mansoni.* J Exp Med 148:46, 1978

Sissons JGP, Oldstone MBS: The antibody-mediated destruction of virus-infected cells. Adv Immunol 29:209, 1980

Thomas DB, Hodgson J, Riska PF, Graham CM: The role of the endoplasmic reticulum in antigen processing. *N*-glycosylation of influenza hemagglutinin abrogates $CD4^+$ cytotoxic T cell recognition of endogenously processed antigen. J Immunol 144:2789, 1990

Zhaori G, Sun M, Ogra PL: Characteristics of the immune response to poliovirus virion polypeptides after immunization with live or inactivated polio vaccines. J Infect Dis 158:160, 1988

Zinkernagel RM, Doherty PC: H-2 compatibility requirement for T cell–mediated lysis of target cells infected with lymphocytic choriomeningitis virus. Different cytotoxic T cell specificities are associated with structures coded for in H-2K or H-2D. J Exp Med 141:1427, 1975

CHAPTER 20

Immunity to Tumors and Pregnancy

Tumor Antigens

Historical Perspective

Tumors occasionally regress spontaneously. This is a rare event and, paradoxically, is confined largely to such highly malignant tumors as melanoma, to some rare childhood tumors such as neuroblastoma and retinoblastoma, and to choriocarcinomas. Spontaneous regressions always have attracted attention in the press and in the medical literature, and they provided the basis for believing that tumors can be regulated immunologically. Other observations that supported the concept of immunologic control included the sudden loss of delayed hypersensitivity that often accompanied the appearance of metastatic spread and the explosive growth of some tumors after surgery or after years of remission. This has been reinforced by the occasional success associated with immunostimulation by endotoxin and other potentiators.

The first experiments to determine if the immune system responded to tumors relied on transplantable murine tumors. These usually were transferred to allogeneic hosts, where they regressed; thus cellular and humoral responses could be demonstrated. These experiments allowed steady progress in the understanding of antigens (especially class I) of the major histocompatibility complex (MHC) but afforded little understanding of any tumor-specific antigen (TSA).

The first definitive experiments showing immunity to autochthonous (meaning in the same place) tumors were performed in the 1950s with chemically induced rodent tumors. Ligation or surgical removal rendered the animal resistant to reimplantation with a fragment of the original tumor whereas a fragment of another similarly induced tumor would grow progressively (Table 20–1). The antigens, known as tumor-specific transplantation antigens (TSTA) could not be biochemically characterized because no specific antisera were available and each chemically induced tumor had its own unique TSTA. In contrast, rodent tumors induced with viruses such as Friend, Rauscher, or Maloney virus often could be placed in cross-reactive groups. Serum from regressors could be protective against murine tumors induced by the same, or a cross-reactive, murine leukemia virus (MuLV) such as Maloney virus. Tumors induced with the Bittner mammary tumor virus (MTV) did not confer cross-reactive immunity with MuLV-induced tumors, thus demonstrating some virus specificity as well. These animal experiments all pointed toward the existence of families of tumor antigens.

Early findings in humans were highly contradictory. Patients with cancer frequently showed seemingly positive skin test reactions (delayed hypersensitivity) against extracts of their own or other patients' tumors, and many apparently

TABLE 20–1. IMMUNITY TO METHYLCHOLANTHRENE-INDUCED TUMORS—LIVE TUMOR CELL CHALLENGE OF EITHER NONIMMUNE MICE SYNGENEIC TO THE TUMOR CELL DONOR OR SYNGENEIC MICE PREIMMUNIZED WITH IRRADIATED TUMOR CELL VACCINES

Tumor Used for Immunization[a]	Lethal Dose in Nonimmune Animals (Cell No.)	Consecutive Doses Given Preimmunized Animals Resulting in No Tumor Growth (Cell No.)	Lethal Dose in Preimmunized Animals (Cell No.)	Comments
MDAD	10^3	10^3, 10^4, 10^5, 10^6, 10^7	NT	Mice preimmunized with irradiated MDAD resist a challenge of 10^7 live MDAD tumor cells, but succumb to 10^5 live MDAQ tumor cells.
MDAQ	10^4	10^4, 10^5, 10^6	10^7	

Adapted from Klein et al: Cancer Res 20:1561, 1960.
[a] Tumors were induced on the right hind leg of mice with methylcholanthrene. The mice were cured by amputation at 3 months. A tumor cell suspension was used either live for challenge of x-irradiated for immunization.

interesting leads developed. Unfortunately, all too often the immunity that could be demonstrated would later prove to be against microorganisms colonizing the tumors and present in the sample used to prepare the skin test extract.

In vitro reactions against cultured tumor cell lines appeared, at one time, to avoid some of the difficulties of in vivo experiments. T cell–mediated cytotoxicity and growth inhibition of these tumor cell lines by lymphocytes from cancer patients were two of the procedures used. These tests showed patterns of reactivity that appeared to be tumor-type specific, for example, carcinoma of breast. Subsequently, some of these results were attributed to the reactivity of natural killer (NK) cells. Conducting the tests in vitro did not automatically avoid artifacts. Immunity to the serum supplement used to grow tumor cells in vitro or the trypsin used in the preparation of the cell suspension was responsible for much of the reactivity reported. After much study it was acknowledged that there was little direct evidence in humans for a tumor-specific cellular immunity to TSAs or, more important, for the TSTA required for T cell recognition and activation leading to tumor rejection. This was too pessimistic a view.

Recent findings in animals and humans have provided evidence for the existence of true TSA and, more important, for TSTA. TSAs do not necessarily provoke a cytotoxic response, but by definition TSTAs do, although the immunity may not be easy to demonstrate for several reasons. First, it has been known for some time that animals neonatally infected with MTV are difficult to immunize against their own tumors. In contrast, virus-free syngeneic animals are easily immunized; specific tolerance to MTV and tumors induced by it had been inadvertently effected in the neonatally infected mice. Because of the possibility of neonatal tolerance to viral and oncofetal antigens, it is not surprising that most tumors are feebly immunogenic in the original host. Second, there is more than a slight resemblance between immunity to tumors and immunity to parasites (Chap. 19), wherein the invader (tumor or parasite) escapes detection or destruction by any of several processes. Third, changes in the tumor cell–surface expression of MHC antigens required for T cell recognition of TSA have now been documented with the use of monoclonal antibodies. Finally, much of the preceding work focused on antigens expressed at the tumor cell surface, and these were predominantly glycoproteins and glycolipids. There is now a growing awareness of protein and nucleoprotein antigens found only inside the cell. Many of these have been analyzed by virologists, but they have been less intensively studied by tumor immunologists because they were thought to be inaccessible to defense mechanisms confined largely to the surface of the tumor cell. Although this was true for antibodies, more recent work suggests that fragments of intracellular protein and nucleoprotein antigens are accessible to T cells and can be recognized in the context of self-MHC antigens. Thus the search for TSA, whether intracellular or cell surface, is now in progress again. The following sections review tumor development (or oncogenesis) and its consequences with respect to expression of TSA, TSTA, and tumor-associated antigen (TAA) and the immunity that can be developed against them.

Oncogenesis and Oncogenes

The initiation of a tumor and its subsequent development ultimately depend on fundamental, stable changes in the cellular genome. These changes occur as a result of the introduction of exogenous oncogenes (viral transforming elements, *v-onc*) or the aberrant activation of silent cellular oncogenes (*c-onc*). Cellular oncogenes normally serve important roles at different stages of somatic cell differentiation and activation. Both cellular and viral oncogenes encode a number of growth-related and regulatory proteins that include protein kinases, nuclear regulatory proteins, cytoplasmic regulators of second messages, and plasma membrane receptors for a number of growth-regulating factors. The consequences of oncogene activation are manifested outwardly as a transformed cellular phenotype, characterized by altered cellular properties, including growth patterns, responses to tissue-specific chalones (growth regulatory molecules), state of differentiation, cell metabolism, and possible changes in the level and molecular composition of certain cell-surface components. Several lines of investigation have led to the formulation of the oncogene hypothesis; that is, oncogenesis occurs through sequential activation of two or more key oncogenes.

Cell transformation may result from infection with an acute transforming virus such as a double-stranded DNA virus (SV40) or an RNA retrovirus (Harvey sarcoma virus). Acute transforming viruses contain a linked transforming element or a gene (e.g., *Ha-v-ras* from Harvey sarcoma virus). The transforming properties of these genes can be assayed biologically by transfection of fibroblast cell lines (previously selected for long-term, in vitro growth patterns). The presence of the transfected gene results in transformation of the fibroblasts and loss of contact inhibition. The transformed cells overlay each other in a haphazard fashion, whereas the original fibroblast cell line grows to a confluent monolayer and cells stop dividing when they come into contact. When this same experiment is attempted with freshly explanted fibroblasts, tranfection with a single oncogene fails to induce the transformed phenotype.

Transformation of fresh fibroblasts, and perhaps most normal cells, requires the synergistic action of at least two distinct types of oncogenes. One type is typified by oncogenes like *myc, N-myc, fos,* and *jun* that encode nuclear proteins that regulate transcription (*trans*-acting factors). The second type of oncogene encodes cytoplasmic proteins that relate either to growth factor receptors like *erb*B or to regulators of second messengers such as the products of the *ras* gene family. Thus oncogenesis is thought to occur through a series of sequential steps leading to the transformed phenotype—the oncogene hypothesis. (The indicator, long-term cultured fibroblasts used in the initial biologic assays above are thought to be partially transformed variants that survived the selection process for long-term growth in vitro.)

Transgenic mice that carry a single exogenous oncogene have now been created and are being used to determine the biologic effects of a single oncogene; the oncogene can be expressed either in all tissues of the transgenic mouse or in selected tissues, depending on the use of particular 5′ regulatory sequences. Further, isolated cells from the transgenic mouse can be used to examine the effects of a second, transfected oncogene. Thus the steps in oncogenesis may be delineated through the use of this important animal model.

Oncogenesis also may result from the activation or alteration of one of several normal cellular oncogenes. These cellular genes may normally function at different stages of cell differentiation, and their expression is strictly regulated. For example, the different stages of B lymphocyte differentiation may represent the phenotypic expression of distinct cellular oncogene subsets. B cell lymphomas arrested at an early, a middle, or a late stage of B cell differentiation may represent aberrant function of one of the subsets. Activation or alteration of a cellular oncogene (*c-onc*) may occur after (1) viral activation, (2) chromosome breaks and translocation, (3) deletion or single point mutations, or (4) loss of a critical tumor suppressor gene, as has been described for certain retinoblastomas. Viruses implicated in causing human cancer, such as the DNA-containing Epstein-Barr virus in Burkitt's lymphoma and human T cell leukemia virus (HTLV), an RNA retrovirus, may facilitate activation or alteration, or both, of normal cell oncogenes. This may occur through proximal effects (insertion close to a cellular oncogene) or induction of chromosome breaks and translocation of a cellular oncogene. For Burkitt's lymphoma, translocations involving chromosomes 8 and 14, 8 and 2, and 8 and 22 have been characterized.

Altered cellular oncogenes have been reported. The data for T24 bladder carcinoma indicate that a single base change (thymidine for guanine) results in coding for a valine residue (vs. a glycine residue) at position 12 of the first exon (Fig. 20–1), encoding a protein, p21. Protein p21 in the bladder tumor cells differs from the p21 product of the normal cell oncogene by a single amino acid. This change, which has a dramatic effect on the structure of p21, is associated with cell transformation. DNA restriction fragments of the T24 altered oncogene (encoding the altered p21) transform suitable target fibroblasts; corresponding fragments from normal cells do not. Tumors from human colon and lung appear to carry altered cellular oncogens that are comparable to those of bladder. Whereas some bladder cancers show activation or alteration of the oncogene cHa-*ras* (with sequence homology to the transforming element of Harvey sarcoma virus), others do not; the implication is that different cellular oncogenes may be activated in other bladder tumors.

Activation of normal cellular oncogenes also may occur if tumor suppressor genes are inactivated. Recently, several tumor suppressor genes have been described (e.g., Rb, a retinoblastoma suppressor gene, and *p53*, a suppressor gene found in many different types of cancer). The protein products of these normal genes suppress, in as yet an unidentified manner, the activity of a number of normal cellular oncogenes. Inactivation (or deletion) of one copy of the *Rb* gene predisposes individuals to retinoblastoma; inactivation of both copies of the Rb gene causes eye tumors. The *p53* suppressor gene product can have two different activities. In its normal form, it functions as a regulator of proliferation; in a mutated form, it can function as a oncogene itself. These exciting new developments have encouraged other investigators to look for tumor suppressor genes in other types of cancer. There are preliminary reports of candidate suppressor genes in colon carcinoma, Wilms' tumor, neurofibromatosis, breast cancer, and bladder cancer.

The oncogene hypothesis and the role of tumor suppressor genes provide a basis for understanding the antigenic changes that accompany cell transformation. It may be possible to predict what types of antigens (and, more important, what peptide fragments thereof) might be detected, and, one hopes, whether these abnormally expressed cellular oncogene products or altered gene products might function as TSTA.

Changes in Expression of Cellular Antigens

Neoantigens

TSA and TSTA (Table 20–2) most likely represent neoantigens encoded by altered genes (not necessarily restricted to oncogenes) and are due to single point mutations and deletions, or translocations of the cellular genes, or inserted viral genes. The encoded antigens frequently are specific for a particular tumor; that is, two methylcholanthrene tumors induced in the same inbred strain or even at different sites on the same animal express unique TSTA. Despite histologic and other similarities, the tumors are antigenically disparate and reflect distinct genetic alterations.

Oncogenic viruses may induce the expression of several neoantigens. Some of these are attributed to viral-encoded components used either in packaging the virus or in its synthesis. Viral-encoded neoantigens may be group specific (common to all viruses of a group, e.g., herpes viruses) or type specific. Group-specific neoantigens are common to all tumors induced by viruses in the same group (e.g. the MuTV discussed earlier). Retroviruses (oncogenic RNA viruses) possessing acute transforming elements (viral oncogenes) also may express neoantigens encoded by these genes. These neoantigens are common to all tumors induced by retroviruses carrying the same oncogene (e.g., the *ras* gene). Finally, retroviruses lacking an oncogene (therefore they are less oncogenic) may insert next to or within a cellular oncogene and modify it. If the viral promoters and transcriptional elements influence only the level of cellular oncogene expression, no new antigen should be expressed, but if the cellular oncogene affected is genetically altered, a new antigen also may be expressed. Because the particular cellular oncogene affected and the mode of alteration may vary from one viral-

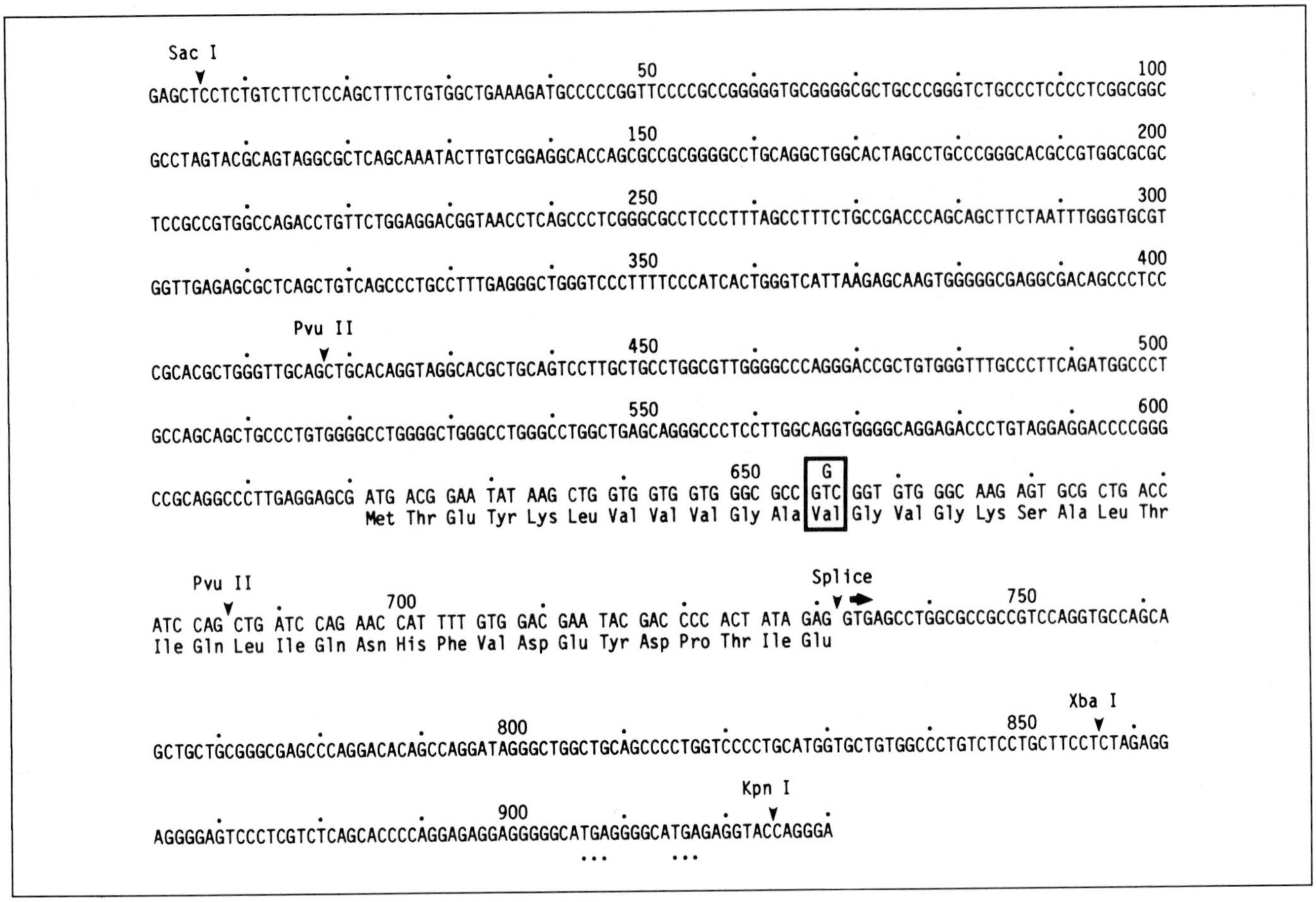
Sac I
50
100
GAGCTCCTCTGTCTTCTCCAGCTTTCTGTGGCTGAAAGATGCCCCCGGTTCCCCGCCGGGGGTGCGGGGCGCTGCCCGGGTCTGCCCTCCCCTCGGCGGC
150
200
GCCTAGTACGCAGTAGGCGCTCAGCAAATACTTGTCGGAGGCACCAGCGCCGCGGGGCCTGCAGGCTGGCACTAGCCTGCCCGGGCACGCCGTGGCGCGC
250
300
TCCGCCGTGGCCAGACCTGTTCTGGAGGACGGTAACCTCAGCCCTCGGGCGCCTCCCTTTAGCCTTTCTGCCGACCCAGCAGCTTCTAATTTGGGTGCGT
350
400
GGTTGAGAGCGCTCAGCTGTCAGCCCTGCCTTTGAGGGCTGGGTCCCTTTTCCCATCACTGGGTCATTAAGAGCAAGTGGGGGCGAGGCGACAGCCCTCC
Pvu II
450
500
CGCACGCTGGGTTGCAGCTGCACAGGTAGGCACGCTGCAGTCCTTGCTGCCTGGCGTTGGGGCCCAGGGACCGCTGTGGGTTTGCCCTTCAGATGGCCCT
550
600
GCCAGCAGCTGCCCTGTGGGGCCTGGGGCTGGGCCTGGGCCTGGCTGAGCAGGGCCCTCCTTGGCAGGTGGGGCAGGAGACCCTGTAGGAGGACCCCGGG
650
G
CCGCAGGCCCTTGAGGAGCG ATG ACG GAA TAT AAG CTG GTG GTG GTG GGC GCC GTC GGT GTG GGC AAG AGT GCG CTG ACC
Met Thr Glu Tyr Lys Leu Val Val Val Gly Ala Val Gly Val Gly Lys Ser Ala Leu Thr
Pvu II
Splice
700
750
ATC CAG CTG ATC CAG AAC CAT TTT GTG GAC GAA TAC GAC CCC ACT ATA GAG GTGAGCCTGGCGCCGCCGTCCAGGTGCCAGCA
Ile Gln Leu Ile Gln Asn His Phe Val Asp Glu Tyr Asp Pro Thr Ile Glu
Xba I
800
850
GCTGCTGCGGGCGAGCCCAGGACACAGCCAGGATAGGGCTGGCTGCAGCCCCTGGTCCCCTGCATGGTGCTGTGGCCCTGTCTCCTGCTTCCTCTAGAGG
Kpn I
900
AGGGGAGTCCCTCGTCTCAGCACCCCAGGAGAGGAGGGGGCATGAGGGGCATGAGAGGTACCAGGGA

Fig. 20–1. A comparison between the DNA fragment encoding the T24 bladder carcinoma oncogene (the first exon of the p21 protein) and the normal human oncogene homologue. The DNA sequence reads 5′ to 3′ from left to right. *Sac I, Pva II, Xba I,* and *Kpa I* indicate restriction enzyme cleavage sites (arrow). *Splice* indicates where the first exon terminates. The sequences are identical save a single base change in the codon originally coding for glycine (*GGC*) in the normal cell oncogene homologue to a codon coding for valine (*GTC*) (broad arrow). *(Adapted from Reddy et al: Nature 300:149, 1982).*

TABLE 20–2. ANTIGENIC CHANGES ASSOCIATED WITH ONCOGENESIS[a]

Change Detected	Virally Induced Tumors	Chemically Induced Tumors	Spontaneous Tumors
Expression of neoantigens			
Tumor-specific transplantation antigens	+	+ +	±
Individually specific	±	+ +	?
Common neoantigens	+	±	?
Oncofetal/developmental antigens reexpressed	+	+	+
Decreased expression of normal surface components (e.g., histocompatibility antigens, blood group antigens)	+	+	+

+, occasionally detected; + +, frequently detected; ±, seldom; ?, unknown.

[a] Tumor-specific transplantation antigens detected by tumor transplantation; others detected serologically.

induced tumor to another, the neoantigens are likely to be different.

Oncofetal and Developmental Antigens

In addition to the tumor- (or virus-) specific antigens described above, tumors, whether chemically induced, virally induced, or spontaneous, sometimes express tumor-associated antigens (TAA). These antigens, for example, may be components also found on fetal tissue or tissues in intermediate stages of differentiation, or both. Cellular oncogenes usually active during normal embryogenesis and early development may be directly affected by the transforming event or indirectly through alteration of a regulatory element. Few of the oncofetal antigens encoded by these genes are very immunogenic; none appear to act as TSTA. Many are designated antigens because they can be detected and characterized with xenogeneic antibodies raised against either tumor or fetal tissues. Some oncofetal antigens are cell-associated but sometimes can be shed (e.g., carcinoembryonic antigen, or CEA), whereas others are actively secreted (e.g., alpha-fetoprotein and human chorionic gonadotropin, or HCG). Some oncofetal antigens such as HCG are common to tumors of a given histologic type; others such as CEA are expressed by a variety of tumors of distinct histologic type. Oncofetal antigens such as CEA often are expressed at low levels on normal tissue, and thus their increased expression in tumor tissue appears to reflect enhanced synthesis or decreased catabolism.

Altered Expression of Normal Surface Components (Antigens)

Cell surface histocompatibility antigens (MHC) (Chap. 17) or blood group antigens, or both, sometimes are absent from tumor tissue, although they are expressed in adjacent normal tissue. In the case of blood group antigens (notably ABH), the terminal carbohydrates determining blood group specificity are missing; the core oligosaccharide structure may still be present. If present, the core structure may be modified by changes in fucose or sialic acid residues. Sometimes it is possible to detect a host response associated with these antigenic changes. For example, serum anti-I/i blood group immunoglobulins may be detected in cancer patients, and their appearance correlates with the loss of blood group ABH activity.

As mentioned earlier, the first experiments that attempted to demonstrate cancer-specific antigens were disappointing. Even as late as 1951, Hauschka in an extensive update of earlier reviews, concluded there was little substantial evidence for the existence of TSA, but he and other investigators did find that aneuploid tumors could be less strain specific and express lower levels of MHC class I antigens than more nearly diploid tumors. Thus, quantitative differences in the expression of MHC antigens could correlate with malignancy. In some recent studies, loss of HLA class I molecules correlated with dedifferentiation in colorectal cancer; other malignant tumors also may express lower concentrations of these antigens.

The importance of MHC antigens on tumor surfaces is believed to lie in their role in the normal processes of T cell recognition and regulation of tissues and in the discrimination of self from nonself. After much uncertainty, it is becoming clear that there are surveillance mechanisms for the control of tumor growth and that these operate, in part, through the MHC. Thus there is interest in the mechanisms that regulate the level of MHC antigens expressed at the tumor cell surface, as well as in the processes that can lead to qualitative changes in the MHC antigens expressed (see later discussion).

The expression of MHC antigens at the cell surface is controlled at the level of transcription through the activity of various *cis*-acting DNA regulatory sequences (promoters and enhancers) 5′ to the transcription initiation site. *Trans*-acting DNA-binding (and protein-binding) factors interact with these regulatory sequences (and other regulatory factors) to control the rate of transcription. The activity of these *trans*-acting factors is developmentally controlled, relating to the tissue type and its stage of differentiation. Thus dedifferentiated tumors may down-regulate the expression of MHC class I (and class II) molecules and reexpress special class I genes normally silent in differentiated cells, such as certain Qa-like or Tla-like genes in the mouse.

Hypomethylation of these 5′ regulatory DNA sequences is associated with increased expression of class I and class II MHC antigens in T cell lines. On the other hand, hypermethylation of DNA has been associated with reduced expression of HLA-D region antigens in acute lymphocytic T cell leukemia but not in adult T cell leukemia. Hormones (e.g., glucocorticoids) and lymphokines (e.g., interferons [IFN] α, β, and γ, and tumor necrosis factor–alpha [TNF-α]) that interact with *trans*-acting regulatory factors have been shown to affect the expression of the MHC gene product. For example, the interferons induce increased expression of either class I antigens or class II antigens, or both. IFNγ also may affect MHC class I expression in a posttranscriptional stage. Prostaglandins, in general, down-regulate the expression of MHC antigens, and pharmacologic reagents that counteract the effect of prostaglandins, such as indomethacin, increase the expression of MHC antigens. More recently, 1,23-dihydroxy vitamin D_3 (calcitriol) and sodium butyrate have been added to the growing list of biologic regulators affecting the cell-surface expression of MHC antigens.

Cell-surface expression of MHC also is regulated at the translational and posttranslational levels. The synthesis, assembly, and transport to the cell surface of functional class I and class II MHC molecules are regulated by other, as yet largely uncharacterized, proteins, one example of which is the invariant chain (I chain) associated with MHC class II molecules (Chap. 14).

The effect of MHC class I expression is illustrated in the growth potentials of tumor cell clones that express different levels of H-2 class I antigens from the same chemically induced murine sarcoma (GR9) and that have been compared in syngeneic hosts. Clone A7 expressed high levels of H-2 class I antigens but was of low malignancy; clone B9 had no detectable H-2 and was highly malignant. Both expressed comparable levels of TAA. Although the direct involvement of MHC in this and other comparable studies is inferential, more compelling are the growing numbers of transfection experiments. H-2^k fibroblasts were transfected with the H-$2K^b$ or H-$2D^d$ gene and with AKR MuLV. Cytotoxic T (T_c) cells raised against the transfectants showed the effectiveness of H-$2K^b$ in presenting *gag* and *env* MuLV antigens, although a small but significant H-$2D^b$ restricted killing also was demonstrated. Killing of double transfectants expressing both H-2^b and MuLV was 10 times as effective as killing of single transfectants. Induced murine fibrosarcomas that have lost H-2 also can be transfected. Hammerling and coworkers reported that approximately half the sarcomas studied by them lost H-2 antigens. Of these, about half lost only H-2K^b (or H-2K^k), whereas none lost H-2D^b (or H-2K^b) alone. Some recently derived hypermethylated H-2K loss variants were inducible with 5-azacytidine (and INFγ), whereas long transplanted tumors were not inducible. Thus, in different experimental approaches, immune recognition (and subsequent killing) of syngeneic tumors depended on the level of H-2 class I expression. These findings are consistent with the important role of MHC class I in presentation of tumor antigens to T cells.

MHC class II antigens expressed at the cell surface of normal cells are involved in the stimulation of regulatory T cells (i.e., CD4$^+$ helper/inducer or suppressor/inducer cells). When these antigens are expressed on the surface of certain tumor cells, including cells from tissues that do not normally express class II molecules, they can have a paradoxical role, namely, immune stimulation. Immunostimulation has been proposed as one factor that promotes rapid tumor cell growth. Murine reticulum cell sarcomas (RCSs), which can be transplanted to normal SJL mice, will not grow in immunodeficient animals. The class II antigens on these tumors, like the HLA-DR antigens of some human melanomas, appear to be abnormally glycosylated and induce T cell responses (presumably T_h) that facilitate tumor growth. In contrast, increased class II expression can also be associated with the antitumor effect of IFNα. One of the most interesting of the alpha interferons is the A species, which has significant antitumor effects in the treatment of hairy cell leukemia and large cell B lymphomas. It also increases HLA-DR expression in hairy cell leukemia. IFNγ may also increase or induce HLA-DR expression, but studies of colorectal cancer indicate that for this tumor, IFN alone is insufficient to alter class II antigen levels. HLA-DR antigens were expressed on the epithelium of 23/32 colorectal cancers, HLA-DP on 13/23, and HLA-DQ on 7/23. None of these antigens were expressed on normal colonic epithelium nor on epithelium from benign or inflammatory tissues; however, epithelial cells adjacent to the tumor sometimes showed positive reactions. Noncoordinate expression of DR, DP, and DQ antigens, as seen in the colorectal tumors, also occurs in activated T cell clones from normal subjects and is believed to reflect stages in differentiation. Levels of both class I and class II antigen can thus be influenced either by the normal processes of differentiation or by the effect of biologic modifiers, including the interferons and prostaglandins.

The number of T cells and NK cells and the extent of macrophage infiltration vary from location to location within a tumor. Focal necrosis and microbial infection also can be expected to alter host responses locally. Processes such as these affect the local production of interferons and other inducers that can modify antigen expression. Local production of inducers complicates the fluctuating balance between differentiation and regulation of growth and may result in the stimulation of new growth and the emergence of more malignant variant clones. The influence of MHC antigens in these processes is becoming more and more clear. Macrophage-lymphocyte and T-B interactions, which are class II dependent, modify lymphocyte proliferation and function. Lymphocyte-tumor interactions may induce both class I and class II antigens on the tumor cell surface.

In animal studies qualitative changes in the MHC antigens expressed at the tumor cell surface also have been documented. For example, "alien" H-2 antigens appear at the surface of certain UV-induced tumors or in the induced fusion of different lines of cultured mouse L cells. Although these manipulations do not allow a particular change in antigen expression to be predetermined and thus are not as precise as transfection, they provide additional insights into the phenotype modifications that can be developed by physical agents. A UV radiation–induced fibrosarcoma of C3H inbred mice (1591) expressed its own H-2K^k and D^k molecules; however, it also expressed unique H2-L^d molecules, as determined serologically. This and other lines of evidence suggest that sister chromatid exchange, unequal crossing over, or some other method of gene conversion can affect the expression of MHC antigens in somatic cells. Mutations of this type might be missed if tumors are screened with antibodies to normal HLA antigens. They might be detected with monoclonal antibodies, but the generation of new, specific monoclonals is time-consuming. Mutations would be more likely to be revealed after endonuclease digestion of DNA. DNA changes would show up as new restriction fragment length polymorphisms (RFLP).

Tumor Immunity

Evidence for Tumor Immune Responses In Vivo

Tumor-specific immunity frequently can be transferred from an immune animal to a nonimmune, syngeneic animal by the transfer of lymphocytes (adoptive transfer of immunity). The strongest protection is given by lymphocytes from the node draining the site of the original tumor (Mitchison assay), especially if the node cells are mixed with the tumor cell inoculum (Winn assay). If these procedures are repeated by draining lymph node B cells alone or T cell subsets (Chap. 14), the optimum protection is afforded either by T cells of the subset conferring delayed hypersensitivity or by cytotoxic T cells, depending on the model system used.

Evidence for tumor-specific immunity in humans is much more inferential. The primary evidence consists of three different types of observation: infiltration of human tumors with lymphocytes and macrophage in vivo, in vitro evidence of tumor-reactive lymphocytes, and the production of tumor-reactive antibodies. The infiltration of breast tumors with T lymphocytes has been associated with a favorable prognosis. In patients with melanoma who respond to interleukin [IL]-2 therapy (see later discussion), the regressing lesions were permeated with macrophage and CD4$^+$ and CD8$^+$ T cells; before therapy the majority of the biopsy specimens showed no infiltrating cells.

There also is evidence that tumors can be immunosuppressive in humans. Many manifestations of cellular immunity are lost as the tumor becomes enlarged and especially when it becomes metastatic. This is clearly reflected in skin tests with antigen and in the normal lymphocyte transfer (NLT) test of Brent and Medawar. This test, which is in many ways an in vivo correlate of the mixed lymphocyte response (MLR) (Chap. 14), is performed by injecting lymphocytes into the dermis of a second individual. An inflammatory reaction develops at the injection site in 24 to 48 hours, which is accompanied by the release of angiotensin. As mentioned earlier, patients with advanced disease not only fail to react to many environmental antigens, including tuberculin, *Candida, Tricophyton,* or mumps, but also frequently give markedly impaired responses to allogeneic lymphocytes in the NLT, especially if the cells transferred were from another patient with advanced malignancy, for example, Hodgkin's disease. Rather disquietingly, skin transplanted from patients with advanced tumors (or mice with some, but not all, transplanted tumors) underwent very delayed rejection. Lack of availability of highly purified tumor-associated antigen for skin testing, immunosuppression related to chemotherapy, dietary deficiencies, and many other variables also interfere with many of the clinical tests that have been tried; therefore, tests of tumor-associated cell-mediated responses often are determined in vitro in a more controlled but less informative environment.

In Vitro Evidence for Tumor Immunity

The early attempts to detect in vitro proliferative responses to tumor cells (or tumor cell extracts) also were clouded by extraneous influences, among them failure to account for MHC restiction. Thus, although there have been reports of in vitro tumor-specific response, these findings are difficult to interpret as evidence for significant tumor immunity. With better technique and an understanding of MHC restriction, it has been possible to show $CD4^+$ T cell responses to autochthonous tumor with apparent specificity. However, the controls for these experiments involve, at a minimum, the response of the patients' lymphocytes to their own Epstein-Barr virus (EBV)–transformed B cell lines. These are not always readily available, nor are they entirely satisfactory.

Attempts to characterize tumor-infiltrating lymphocytes (TIL)—lymphocytes infiltrating the solid tumor mass or found in the ascites associated with the malignancy—have met with some success. A majority of $CD8^+$ and some $CD4^+$ T cells have been recovered from tumor (or ascites). When assayed for cytotoxic function shortly after isolation, TIL generally are unreactive to specific tumor cells or cell extracts, but if they are cultured in vitro with IL-2 (or a mixture of IL-2 with either IL-4 or TNF-α) and regularly stimulated with irradiated autologous tumor cells, their cytotoxic or proliferative potential can be demonstrated. Both tumor-reactive, MHC-restricted T_c cell lines and tumor-reactive, MHC-unrestricted T_c cell lines have been established from TIL. In the latter studies the MHC-unrestricted T_c cell line was found to react with a tumor-associated mucin in which the T cell epitope is repeated many times in the polypeptide backbone of the mucin molecule.

Humoral responses to tumors have often been reported, but the interpretation is difficult. Tumor-reactive antibodies in serum and malignant effusions have been detected by immunofluorescence, immunohistochemical, and radioisotopic assays. The serum level of these tumor-reactive antibodies may change with tumor reduction or growth, that is, increasing after cytoreductive therapy and decreasing with increased tumor growth. Sometimes the antibody may form a complex with antigen, and there may be a reciprocal relationship between the serum level of free, tumor-reactive antibody and the level of immune complex detected. The significance of malignancy-associated immune complexes is unknown; they are not necessarily protective, and a deleterious consequence of antitumor antibody production is the high incidence of complex-induced glomerular nephritis (about 10% of all patients with cancer).

Controversy concerns the specificity of these antibodies. Early claims of tumor specificity were supported by the apparent specificity of (1) inhibition of cell-mediated cytotoxicity in vitro (blocking antibodies) or (2) enhancement of animal tumor growth in vivo (enhancing antibodies). Extensive, subsequent analyses have demonstrated that although the antibodies are tumor reactive, the initial hopes that they would be tumor specific have not been realized. They may detect autoantigens, including antigens in necrotic areas and oncofetal antigens and, not infrequently, histocompatibility antigens of the tumor. The lack of absolute tumor specificity for the majority of tumor-reactive antibodies does not rule out a significant role in control of neoplastic growth in vivo, but the clinician is rightly concerned that any induced antibody might enhance, rather than suppress, tumor growth (see later sections).

In a few cases, notably murine leukemias, it is possible to induce a tumor-reactive antibody of exquisite specificity and significant protective activity. In this case, the antibody is specific for an idiotypic determinant (Chap. 12) expressed by the characteristic surface immunoglobulin of the malignant B cell. The idiotypic antibody has been used therapeutically. Attempts to use this approach in human leukemia have not been promising.

Evidence for Natural Resistance to Tumor Growth and Metastasis

There is excellent evidence for natural cytotoxic (NC) cells and natural killer (NK) cells during the very early stages of tumor growth. They also may prevent, to a limited extent, the metastatic spread of tumor cells. The available evidence in human and animal studies also suggests potent activity against certain lymphosarcomas. Few freshly isolated primary carcinomas, however, are susceptible to natural killing.

Up to 5% of all blood mononuclear cells in humans and rodents function as NK cells. These MHC-unrestricted cells bind to and kill a variety of transformed cell types, as well as a subpopulation of immature, normal cells in the thymus and bone marrow. An additional set of target cells is recognized by NK cells but is resistant to cell lysis (e.g., preplasma cells in the B cell differentiation pathway). In this case, binding promotes synthesis and secretion of several cytokines, including IFNγ and TNF by NK cells that then function as regulatory cells.

NK activity is strongly associated with large granular lymphocytes (LGLs) that can be readily isolated because of their low buoyant density and their distinct cytoplasmic granules (Fig. 20–2). LGLs have a greater cytoplasmic to nuclear ratio than do most peripheral blood lymphocytes and contain cytoplasmic, azurophilic granules. These cytoplasmic granules, which are specialized lysosomes, are important in the NK cell's cytolytic activity.

Although several cell types exhibit NK activity, the most significant population has the $CD16^+$, $CD56^+$, $CD3^-$, $CD4^-$, $CD8^{\pm}$, TCR $\alpha\beta^-$, and TCR $\gamma\delta^-$ cell-surface phenotype. Human NK cells weakly bind to sheep erythrocytes and can be readily separated from strong E-rosetting cells (T cells)

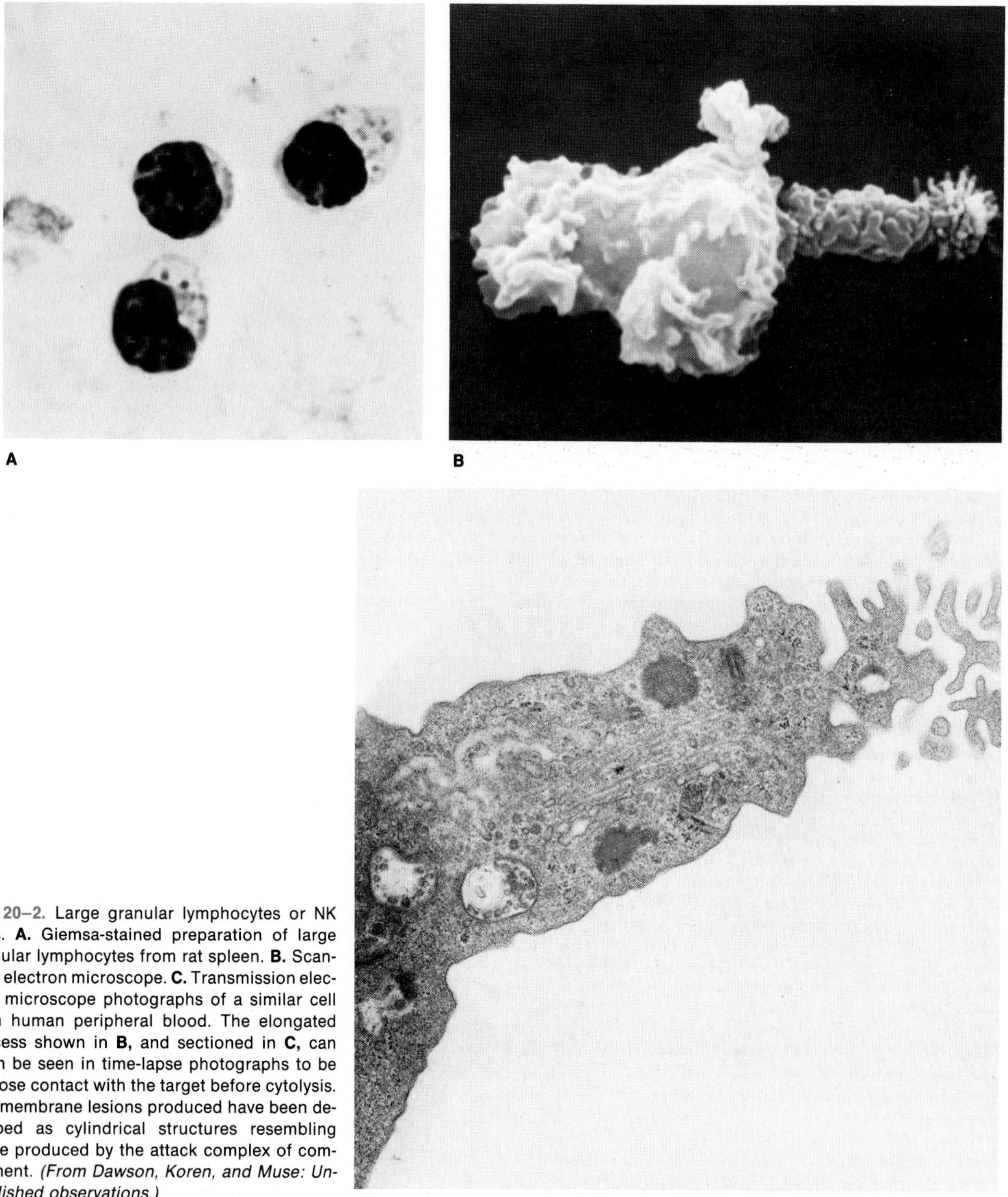

A B C

Fig. 20–2. Large granular lymphocytes or NK cells. **A.** Giemsa-stained preparation of large granular lymphocytes from rat spleen. **B.** Scanning electron microscope. **C.** Transmission electron microscope photographs of a similar cell from human peripheral blood. The elongated process shown in **B,** and sectioned in **C,** can often be seen in time-lapse photographs to be in close contact with the target before cytolysis. The membrane lesions produced have been described as cylindrical structures resembling those produced by the attack complex of complement. *(From Dawson, Koren, and Muse: Unpublished observations.)*

because they are low expressers of CD2, the sheep cell receptor. Activated T cells may exhibit NK-like MHC-unrestricted killing; however, cytokine stimulation usually is required to demonstrate this kind of killing. The NK cells express the low affinity Fc(γ) receptor (CD16), but the ability to bind tumor cells (targets) does not depend on the presence of Fc receptors or, therefore, on natural or specific antibodies.

NK cells also may function as killer cells in conjunction with specific antibody (antibody-dependent cell-mediated cytotoxicity, or ADCC). Their activity in this case does depend on expression and utilization of the CD16, Fc receptor for IgG. Additional cell types, including activated macrophages, polymorphonuclear leukocytes, eosinophils, and platelets, may function as ADCC effector cells against antibody-coated targets.

The in vivo relevance of NK cells to control of malignancy has been demonstrated by animal experiments in which a cell suspension has been depleted or enriched of NK activity in vitro and transferred to NK cell–deficient mice that are subsequently challenged with a murine leukemia or melanoma. Cloned NK cells also have been reported to afford NK cell–deficient mice protection against NK-sensitive tumors. Beige mutant mice (*bg/bg*) are NK cell deficient and succumb to murine leukemias and melanomas, whereas heterozygous littermates (*bg*/+) are resistant. Like the beige mouse, the Chédiak-Higashi syndrome in humans (Chap. 18) is characterized by a cellular deficiency with large, aberrant cytoplasmic granules. These patients are susceptible to many infections despite their ability to mount normal delayed hypersensitivity and antibody responses. Little NK-cell activity can be demonstrated in vitro with their lymphocytes, and 85% of the young patients enter a lymphoma-like phase before they die. Patients deficient in cell-surface expression of the cellular adhesion molecule LFA-1 and a single known female patient with a complete absence of $CD16^+$ cells are also NK deficient. Although these young patients show decreased ability to handle certain herpes viral infections, as yet they have not evidenced any malignancies.

Specific and Nonspecific Antitumor Reactions

The T cell subpopulation responsible for delayed hypersensitivity may be as or more important than cytotoxic T cells in the rejection of syngeneic tumors in Winn assays and the adoptive transfer of immunity. In contrast to tumor-specific elimination by cytotoxic T cells, the specific recognition of tumor cells by delayed hypersensitivity T cells leads to the indirect, nonspecific elimination of tumor by activated macrophages and, perhaps, NK cells. Activation of these effector cells occurs upon antigen stimulation of the delayed hypersensitivity T cells and their elaboration of cytokines, including macrophage activating factor (MAF), IL-2, IFN, and TNF. Activated macrophages, in contrast to resting macrophages, show greatly enhanced tumoricidal activity and secrete significant levels of potent proteases and reactive oxygen intermediates. The tumoricidal activity of NK cells also can be increased in vitro twofold to fivefold by pretreatment with IL-2, IL-4, or the interferons.

In clinical trials IFNα or IFNγ therapy has been reported to result in transient increases of NK cell activity in the peripheral blood of cancer patients. Few objective tumor-specific responses, however, have been reported from these trials, with two notable exceptions. Patients with hairy cell leukemia or large-cell B lymphomas have shown dramatic, objective responses to IFN immunotherapy. Tumor regression most likely is due to a direct effect of the IFN on the tumor and not the activation of natural effector cells. Similarly, IL-2 (or a combination of IL-2 with IL-4 or TNF-α) therapy for patients with cancer appears to stimulate increased NK activity and lymphokine-activated killing (LAK) (see below) in the peripheral blood compartment. However, the levels of IL-2 required to achieve objective responses border on toxic levels and frequently are associated with a plethora of undesirable side effects.

TABLE 20–3. MECHANISMS BY WHICH TUMORS MIGHT ESCAPE IMMUNE ELIMINATION

1. The host develops tolerance to his or her tumor
2. Tumors may be selected (by interaction with the immune system) that are weakly immunogenic or that have developed mechanisms for resisting immune-specified lysis
3. Immunogenic components may be modulated in the presence of an immune response
4. Suppression of the immune response:
   a. Nonspecific factors elaborated by the tumor cells
   b. Nonspecific suppressor macrophage induced by either the tumor or the immune response
   c. Nonspecific, T suppressor cells induced by the immune response
   d. Specific, T suppressor cells
   e. Therapy-related immunosuppression
5. Immune stimulation or enhancement of tumor growth by products of the immune response
6. An imbalance between the mass of tumor cells and specific and nonspecific components of the immune system

Interrelationship Between Tumor and Immune System

The vast majority of tumors progress despite the immunity discussed above. There are several reasons why some tumors escape immune elimination (Table 20–3). First, the tumor immunity that can be demonstrated early in tumor growth gradually declines with time, which suggests the induction of tolerance. Second, tumors that become clinically apparent are weakly immunogenic, implying that immunogenic tumor cells may be eliminated at early stages. In addition, tumors may adapt to an immune response by developing mechanisms to repair damage or to circumvent immune lysis. Thus drugs that inhibit protein synthesis may increase the sensitivity to lysis of some tumors. Third, tumor cell surface components may be modulated, or down-regulated, in the presence of an immune effector cell or molecule. This has been most clearly documented with thymic leukemias in the presence of antibody. In addition, loss of histocompatibility antigens would, of necessity, interrupt reactivity against viral tumors in which major histocompatibility complex restriction operates (Chap. 14).

The immune response may be suppressed through one of several mechanisms:

1. Tumor cells themselves may suppress immunity by synthesis and release of nonspecific immunoregulatory proteins and polypeptides, prostaglandins, and corticosteroids.
2. Macrophages recovered from tumor infiltrates may also nonspecifically suppress NK and T cell proliferative responses, both specific and nonspecific.
3. T suppressor cells detected in some animal tumor inflammatory cell infiltrates may suppress an antitumor response.
4. Antineoplastic chemotherapy and radiation therapy are themselves strongly suppressive of the immune system.

Antibodies or blocking factors may result in increased growth of the tumor. Blocking factors may combine with antigen and interfere with effector function; under certain conditions they also may down-regulate the immune response. In animals, enhancing antibodies may directly stimulate tumor growth or inhibit the immune system. As with ADCC, very small (as little as 0.5 μL in animal experiments) amounts of antibody are required. Finally, just as a patient may succumb to overwhelming infection in the face of demonstrable immunity to a pathogen, the mass of a tumor also may exceed the capacity of the immune system to bring about its rejection.

Immunotherapy

Active Specific Immunotherapy

Active immunization with tumor cell vaccines is a very attractive ideal that has had no conspicuous success in humans. Experimentation is limited because clinicians are concerned that the use of crude tumor cell extracts or irradiated tumor cells as vaccines could result in active enhancement of tumor growth rather than in immunoprophylaxis. If purified tumor antigens are to be used in future studies, suitable immunogenic components must be identified and purified and incorporated in suitable vectors, yeast or vaccinia virus, and this is not yet possible in humans. For ethical reasons, experimental active immunotherapy of humans has been attempted only in the late stages of disease, that is, at a stage when the patient is already anergic.

Passive Antibody Immunotherapy

Tumor-reactive antibodies have been effective in preventing the growth of feline and murine leukemias if given simultaneously with or shortly after challenging the animal with live tumor cells. With few exceptions, however, this technique is unsuccessful against established leukemias and lymphomas; it has failed against carcinomas. Tumor-reactive antibodies cannot easily be delivered to the center of a large tumor mass, and much of the antibody is trapped or eliminated nonspecifically in liver, lungs, and kidney. In addition, the role of antibody- and complement-mediated cytolysis of tumor cells in vivo is minimal despite its effectiveness in vitro, perhaps because of the inefficiency of homologous complement (Chap. 15). The contribution of ADCC in vivo is unknown.

Early in this century, Paul Ehrlich thought that antibody could be used to deliver a "magic bullet" in the form of a cytotoxic drug conjugated to an antibody. Later it was believed that if the antibody could be made radioactive (e.g., with ^{125}I or ^{131}I), it would home to the tumor, and the radioactivity would be tumoricidal. Unfortunately, conjugates are rapidly eliminated from the circulation and highly radioactive antibodies lose appreciable binding capacity. The recipient also may become sensitized to the foreign antibody and develop anaphylaxis. Also, those conjugates that require not only specific homing and binding to the tumor cell, but also endocytosis and release inside the appropriate subcellular compartment for maximum biologic activity, have additional limitations. Nevertheless this approach continues to be actively pursued.

Recent attempts at immunotoxin therapy have concentrated on the use of monoclonal, tumor-reactive antibodies. Their homogeneity reduces some of the problems associated with administration of complex, polyclonal reagents, but it does not eliminate them. More recently, mouse monoclonal antibodies have been "humanized" by genetically engineering the construction of mouse Fab regions with human Fc regions. Immunotoxins under investigation include monoclonal antibodies coupled to ricin, to diphtheria toxin, to potent chemotherapeutic drugs, or to cytokines such as the interferons (see below). In addition, new techniques for labeling antibodies, including chelation of indium 111 (^{111}In) and technetium 99m (^{99m}Tc) labeling, are promising in terms of preserving antibody-binding capacity and in vivo localization. It is hoped that monoclonal reagents and new methods of labeling will allow the radiologist to detect the location of otherwise unsuspected metastases through the use of antibody sufficiently radioactive, and with a half-life long enough, to be detected even though the conjugate might not in itself be therapeutic.

Two recent variations of immunoconjugates involving bifunctional immunoglobulins include heteroconjugates and immunoglobulins produced by "quadromas." Heteroconjugates are produced by chemically linking two different monoclonal antibodies to one another. One of the monoclonal antibodies is tumor-reactive and the other may be reactive with an activation determinant expressed on an effector cell such as CD16 on an NK cell and CD3 or the TCR on a cytotoxic T cell. Heteroconjugates thus may focus a cytotoxic cell to the tumor cell regardless of the intrinsic antigenic specificity of the effector cell. Quadromas are produced by fusing two hybridoma cell lines, each producing a distinct monoclonal antibody, and selecting hybrid immunoglobulin molecules secreted by the quadromas that express two distinct binding activities, for example, reactivity with a specific tumor and an effector cell or molecule. Unfortunately, the immune system is capable of recognizing and eliminating molecules that differ by as little as one amino acid or by slight changes in conformation, so that until this property is circumvented, these approaches have limited usefulness.

Biologic Response Modifiers

Bacteria and bacterial cell wall products increase the activity of nonspecific effector cells such as macrophages and NK cells. One of the first of these microbial vaccines was Coley's toxins. This was a form of endotoxin treatment that probably increased cytokine production (see below). Attenuated *Mycobacterium tuberculosis* (bacille Calmette-Guérin [BCG]) therapy has been used in the management of melanoma. The organism is used live and is given intralesionally. *Corynebacterium parvum* therapy has been used in conjunction with chemotherapy; its advantage is that a formalin-fixed vaccine is used. In many of the *C. parvum* trials the reagent was administered intravenously and the results were equivocal. In those cases where intratumor inoculation with the formalin-fixed vaccine was used, significant activation of macrophage and NK cells that correlated with a partial clinical response was observed. A lyophilized vaccine of heat- and penicillin-treated *Streptococcus pyogenes* A3, Su strain (OK432), also augments NK activity in vivo and in vitro and has significant antitumor activity.

Synthetic muramyl dipeptides and tripeptides activate macrophage in vivo when incorporated in liposomes. A corresponding reduction in the ability of B16 murine melanoma to metastasize to the lung was obtained by this therapy. The list of natural cell wall components and synthetic compounds under investigation is impressive. Most result in macrophage activation and augmentation of NK cells; some may achieve this through stimulation of IL-1, interferons, or TNF.

Cytokine therapy has been under active consideration since interferons were shown to augment NK activity in vitro. The major limiting factor has been the amount of cytokine available for therapeutic use. With the advent of recombinant sources of lymphokines it has been possible to show, for example, that the major types of interferon (α, β, and γ) and their subtypes differ in their ability to augment NK activity. Unfortunately, some can paradoxically protect tumor cells from immune lysis, but, as discussed earlier, interferon therapy has proved particularly useful in the treatment of hairy cell leukemia and large-cell, B cell lymphomas.

IL-2 also has been given considerable prominence as a potential therapeutic agent. IL-2 (T cell growth factor) has been used to culture and expand tumor-reactive, cytotoxic T lymphocytes, to augment NK activity after short-term incubation of NK effector cells, and to promote the development of LAK cells over a 3 to 5-day incubation of lymphocytes in vitro. Recombinant IL-2 (rIL-2) has made it possible to follow up these in vitro findings with clinical trials. In particular, the characterization of LAK cells and their effect on tumor cells have received considerable interest in the last few years. These cells show significant activity against a variety of freshly isolated tumor cells, in contrast to NK cells. LAK effectors also are relatively specific for tumor cells compared with normal somatic cells. Several cell types are capable of demonstrating LAK activity after activation with rIL-2; thus LAK is defined by a cellular activity and not a particular cell type. One of the major LAK precursors is the $CD16^+$, $CD56^+$ NK cell, but $CD3^+$ T cells also can be stimulated to show considerable LAK activity. Attempts to treat cancer patients with rIL-2 have led to mixed results; an objective, therapeutic result may be noted but only at concentrations close to or exceeding toxic levels. IL-2 therapy has been combined with passive cellular immunotherapy (see below) with considerable success.

TNF originally was described as a powerful cytokine that destroyed certain types of tumor cell. Two types of TNF are released by leukocytes activated by various agents, including endotoxin. TNF-α is produced by many different cells, including lymphocytes and cells of the monocyte-macrophage lineage; TNF-β (lymphotoxin) is synthesized by T lymphocytes. Therapeutic applications of TNF initially were limited by the amount of cytokine that could be produced in vitro from activated macrophages and the relative impurity of the preparations. With the advent of recombinant forms of TNF, extensive evaluation of TNF as a therapeutic agent has begun. TNF has additional biologic activities that can be demonstrated on cells resistant to its cytotoxic effects. For example, monocytes themselves express receptors for TNF; its binding induces the synthesis of IL-1. Indeed, this recent observation explains why both TNF and IL-1 share many common biologic activities such as the induction of prostaglandin E_2, collagenase, fibroblast proliferation, and colony-stimulating factor (CSF) and the inhibition of lipoprotein lipase. Inhibition of lipase activity is associated with cachexia, or a wasting syndrome, and has identified TNF as identical to the factor cachetin. The cloning of TNF genes also resulted in two interesting facts. First, the TNF genes map to the MHC in mouse and humans, and second, one of the TNF gene products (TNF-β) is identical to classic lymphotoxin, an earlier described cytotoxic factor produced by activated T lymphocytes.

Based on the supposition that an ineffective antitumor response reflects an immunodeficiency (which might be imposed by either the tumor itself or an early immune suppressor cell response), attempts to reconstitute the immune system with hormones known to stimulate T cell differentiation have been contemplated. Thymosin 1, thymopoietin fraction 5, thymic hormone factor (THF), and factor thymique sérique (FTS) have been isolated and shown to exhibit thymic hormone–like activity. Patients with immunosuppressive malignancies, such as Hodgkin's lymphoma, treated with THF have shown increases in T cell number, proliferative responses to mitogens, and cutaneous delayed hypersensitivity to recall antigens.

Passive Cellular Immunotherapy

Cloned cytotoxic T lymphocytes specific for murine tumors have been expanded in vitro and adoptively transferred to nonimmune, syngeneic animals before challenge with live tumor cells. The results of these experiments have been disappointing; it is now thought that the transferred cells require additional IL-2 to maintain significant activity in vivo (see below). In contrast, transfer of cloned NK effector cells to NK cell–deficient mice, such as bg/bg mice, does protect the recipients from challenge with live, NK-sensitive tumor cell lines. The transfer of cloned NK effector cells also protects C57 Bl/6 mice from developing x-irradiation-induced leukemia, if given soon after the final x-irradiation. Transfer at later stages fails to suppress development of leukemia.

LAK effectors, like cytotoxic T lymphocytes, when transferred to tumor-bearing hosts, show little or no effect on tumor growth. In contrast, if the tumor-bearing animal is treated with syngeneic, LAK effector cells and IL-2, variable—although sometimes striking—tumor rejection has been reported. In clinical trials a combination of IL-2 treatment with transfer of the patient's own cells (activated in vitro) as LAK effectors has resulted in objective tumor regressions, notably for melanoma and renal cell carcinomas. It has been proposed that LAK effector cells (and perhaps the tumor-specific, cytotoxic T cells noted above) require an elevated level of IL-2 for maintaining their cytolytic potential in vivo. This combination therapy can be used with concentrations of rIL-2 below toxic levels, but not without a number of side effects of variable seriousness. Questions remain about why some patients respond while others do not, how long an objective response can be maintained, and the side effects of this therapy.

Variability in response is now attributed to the relative concentration of tumor-specific T cells in the general LAK cell population. If instead of patient peripheral blood lymphocytes, tumor-infiltrating cells are restimulated with antigen and IL-2, it is possible to develop highly efficacious cell lines. Moreover, it has been found that a mixture of IL-2 and Il-4 promotes the stimulation of tumor-reactive T cells and suppresses the development of nonspecific LAK cells. Combinations of IL-2 and TNF-α also have been used to promote the growth of tumor-reactive T cell lines.

Other Therapeutic Procedures

Considerable interest was aroused by reports that the filtration of tumor-bearer plasma through a column containing formalin-fixed Cowan strain staphylococci (or protein A derived from this strain and conjugated to an inert matrix) removed immune complexes (blocking factors). Reinfusion of the column-treated plasma correlated with rapid necrosis of mammary and other tumors. Unfortunately, this treatment often resulted in extreme toxicity, presumably by leaching of toxins from staphylococci.

Lawrence and co-workers discovered in the 1960s that cell-free extracts of human peripheral blood leukocytes from tuberculin-positive patients could transfer tuberculin-specific reactivity to unreactive patients. The authors named the active moiety *transfer factor*. Transfer factor subsequently was found to be heat-stable, dialyzable, and of low molecular weight. Transfer factor has been used to achieve conversions of bacterial and fungal reactivities. Patients with severe fungal infections such as candidiasis have benefited from this treatment. Transfer factor therapy has been used in malignant melanoma, and prolonged remissions have sometimes been noted. Although not harmful to the patient (as some other potentializing agents have been), transfer factor was not standardized and therapy often was ineffective. A recent suggestion that transfer factor consists of processed antigen plus a fragment of the T cell receptor may allow a more objective evaluation.

Human Tumor Markers

The ectopic production of certain enzymes and hormones has been used to confirm the presence of certain tumors and has an important use in monitoring the response of these tumors to therapy. The classic example of ectopic production of a hormone by a tumor is the synthesis of HCG by choriocarcinoma and trophoblastic tumors. HCG can be detected in serum by radioimmunoassay or enzyme immunoassay (Chap. 12), and monoclonal anti-HCG antibodies have been developed for this purpose. Serum levels provide an excellent assessment of tumor response to therapy. Antibodies to alphafetoprotein (AFP) can be used in a similar way to monitor the response of patients with hepatomas and germinal yolk sac tumors to therapy. The association between a rising serum AFP level and the growth of AFP-producing tumors is excellent. Pregnancy must be excluded, because AFP levels rise in pregnancy and AFP is concentrated in amniotic fluid.

Antibodies to β_2-microglobulin, a polypeptide associated with certain products of major histocompatibility gene complex (Chap. 14), have been used in radioimmunoassays and enzyme-linked immunoassays to determine serum concentrations. Changes in the serum level of β_2-microglobulin are useful in determining the prognosis of Hodgkin's disease, non-Hodgkin's lymphoma, chronic lymphocytic leukemia, and multiple myeloma. β_2-microglobulin levels also are raised in AIDS (Chap. 17).

Antibodies to carcinoembryonic antigen (CEA) were at first thought to be specific for colon carcinoma and fetal tissue. With the advent of sensitive radioimmunoassays, this strong association failed. Several other tumors express and shed CEA, and normal tissues express a low level of CEA. Serum detection of CEA is subject to a number of variables; for example, smokers and noncancer patients with liver disease also may show elevated levels of serum CEA. Nonetheless, for some patients with CEA-producing tumors, serum CEA monitoring has been used as a valuable adjunctive assay. Furthermore, xenogeneic anti-CEA and, recently, monoclonal anti-CEA have been labeled with ^{131}I, ^{111}In, or ^{99m}Tc and administered intravenously to detect small primary and metastatic CEA-producing tumors by radiographic imaging techniques.

Figure 20–3 illustrates the radioimmunodetection of a human cancer with a radiolabeled antitumor monoclonal antibody. The monoclonal antibody, 791T/36, was produced against an osteosarcoma cell line (791T) but cross-reacts with some malignant lung, cervix, and bladder cell lines. It may identify an antigen of the oncofetal or developmental type but, nevertheless, has been used effectively in applications of this type.

Similar tumor-reactive antibodies have been developed for a variety of cancers, including those of the lung, ovary, breast, and brain. None has proved to be absolutely specific; they either react at low levels with normal tissue or they cross-react with other histologic type of tumor. For example, antibodies to a high molecular weight secreted mucin associated with pancreatic cancer have been developed and characterized. One of these antibodies, DUPAN-2, also reacts with normal tissues, albeit at a much reduced level. Nevertheless the DUPAN-2 monoclonal antibody has been very useful in monitoring the response to therapy of patients with pancreatic cancer. Thus the available polyclonal antibodies and monoclonal reagents can be used in assays to monitor the serum level of a variety of tumor-associated molecules and, therefore, the response of the tumor to therapy. They can be used to detect the metastatic spread of tumor cells in lymph node biopsy specimens by immunohistochemical techniques. They have found use in the in vivo detection of occult metastases and small primary tumors by radiographic techniques. They might be used in the form of reagent conjugates for passive immunotoxin therapy if tumor localization can be improved and if expression of the tumor-reactive epitope on normal tissues is limited.

Maternofetal Relationship

Without an efficient defense system, the individual would die; the immune system provides for specific defense and to do so it must monitor self and nonself. The embryo and fetus are nonself, but if the immune system destroyed the fetus, the species would die. Not only the fetus but the male gamete and the fertilized ovum also must avoid immunologic attack. This section examines some of the ways in which avoidance is accomplished.

The Fetus As Allograft

A provocative consideration of the relationship between mother and fetus was presented by Medawar, who correctly considered the fetus to be a form of allograft and advanced several possibilities to explain why it was not rejected by the mother. These factors have been added to and tested by many others—by Beer and Billingham and by Faulk and MacIntosh. One possibility was that the embryo and fetus might fail to express any antigens that could be recognized as foreign or that the uterus might provide an especially privileged site where immune reactions did not occur. The mother's immune system might be paralyzed for the period of gestation, either specifically by development of tolerance or nonspecifically by

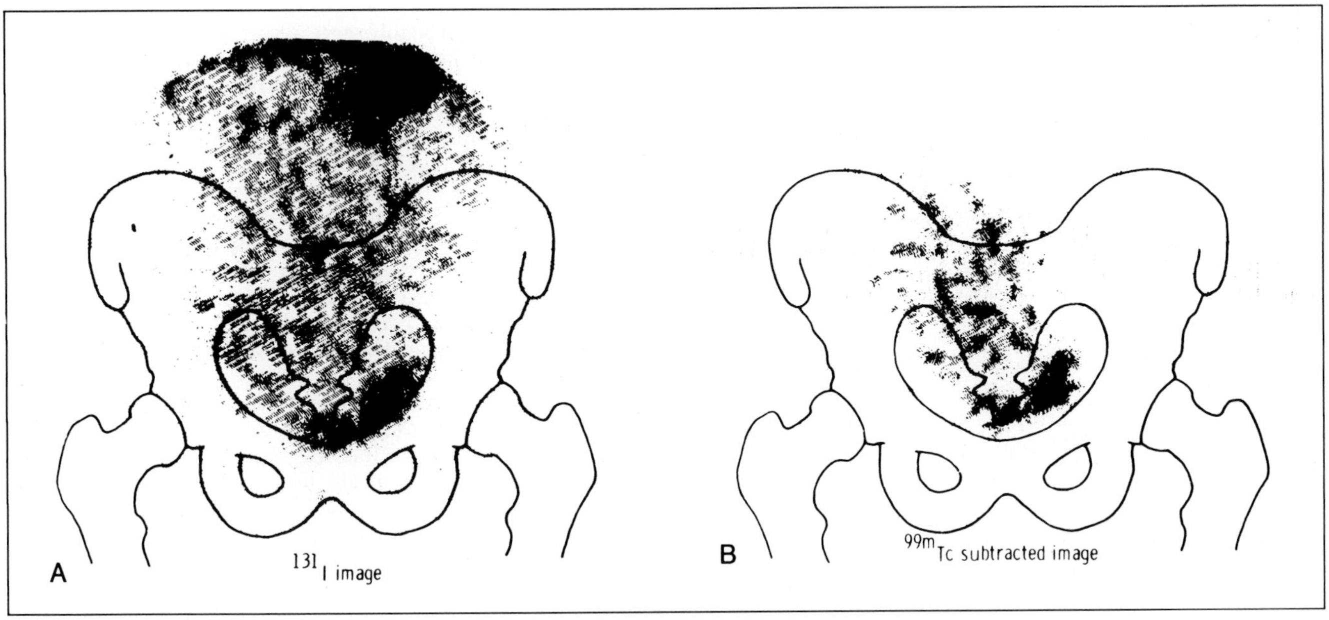

Fig. 20–3. An anterior radionuclide image of the pelvis of a colorectal cancer patient showing localization of the monoclonal, ^{135}I-labeled 791T/36 antibody. ^{99m}Tc was used to label red blood cells, and ^{113m}In was used to label blood transferrin. **A.** Radiographic analysis before image enhancement. **B.** Analysis after image enhancement by subtraction of ^{99m}Tc and ^{113m}In backgrounds. *(From Farrands et al: Lancet 21:399, 1982).*

suppressor factors. The mother could subvert the immune attack by providing blocking antibodies. The placenta might provide a barrier between the mother and the fetus. An analysis of these points follows.

Lack of Antigenicity

It is possible to examine embryonic antigens in early cleavage embryos in vitro and later during fetal development. By direct cytotoxicity or binding assays it has been established that the early embryo expresses at least some of the paternal antigens. The amount of tissue available for testing is extremely small, and these studies are difficult to carry out. An ingenious innovation by Simmons and Russel was to implant the developing embryo of a mouse under the kidney capsule of an allogenic recipient. The investigators then observed the growth of the transplant. Extraembryonic tissue—the ectoplacental cone—survived. The embryo itself did not; thus it was inferred that the very early embryo did carry immunogenic forms of transplantation antigens, although the trophoblast apparently did not. There subsequently have been numerous transplant studies with fetal skin and other tissues (including hearts). Although there may be some prolongation of survival, the eventual outcome is rejection, confirming that the fetus is immunogenic. In humans, the HLA antigens are well expressed by week 12 of gestation, and in the mouse, H-2 can be detected beginning at about day 12. These findings are inconsistent with the hypothesis that the fetus lacks antigens, although the tissues of the early embryo probably are less immunogenic than those of the mature fetus, and some early skin transplantation studies reported that neonatal skin was more slowly rejected than was adult skin.

In humans, certain cases of repeated spontaneous abortions have been attributed to an immune response to paternal antigens expressed by the fetus. The nature of the immune response intitiating abortion is not yet clear, but on the basis of animal model studies, cytokine-activated NK cells with LAK activity are thought to play an important role in the effector phase. Animal models have been used in which there is a high rate of embryo resorption, for example, CBA/J × DBA/2 matings versus CBA/J × BALB/c matings. In these studies, administered high levels of TNF-α and IFNγ, in particular, reproduce the resorption findings, suggesting that an immune response giving rise to these cytokines may be harmful to embryo survival.

The Uterus as Privileged Site

A privileged site can be defined as one in which a transplant can grow without being destroyed by an immunologic reaction. From studies with allografts and xenografts—for example, human tumors transferred to the cheek pouch of the Syrian hamster or to a raised skin pedicle—it has been learned that a tissue often will not immunize the recipient unless it can establish connections with lymphatic vessels. The anterior chamber of the eye and the surface of the brain, like the cheek pouch, also are privileged sites. Because the decidua of the uterus was, for a long time, believed to be devoid of lymphatic vessels, it was logical to examine the possibility that the uterine cavity was a privileged site; however, fragments of tumor placed on the decidua were rejected normally. Because tumor might be more immunogenic than were normal tissues, other cell types also were grafted to the uterus. The most ingenious experiments were those of Billingham, who cut a longitudinal slit in one horn of the bifid uterus of a rat and inserted a graft made by everting a cylinder of rat tail skin. Not only was the tube of skin rejected; the draining lymph nodes also became hypertrophic. In addition, other studies have shown hyperplasia of the regional nodes in pregnancy. Thus the fetus is recognized, and the uterine cavity is not a privileged site.

Hormonal Modification of Maternal Immune Responses

Hormonal modification during pregnancy remains one of the more complex aspects of the immune response to the fetus. Subtle changes in immune responsiveness occur. Some parameters appear to be unchanged, isoagglutinin levels are unchanged in the human, and humans and mice both can produce antibodies to paternal antigens. Grafts of tumor or of skin, however, may persist longer than they would on the nonpregnant animal, and secondary antibody responses may be reduced. Infections are more frequent during pregnancy, especially those with opportunistic organisms, including *Candida albicans* and cytomegalovirus, suggesting an impairment of the effector cells of cellular immunity. It has been mentioned above that the lymph nodes draining the uterus may become enlarged in pregnancy as they are in graft rejection. In pregnancy, T cells from the nodes can produce migration inhibitory factor, but they do not generate cytotoxic effectors, again supporting the concept of selective immunologic unresponsiveness. Pharmacologic doses of steroid hormones have been reported to depress T cell responses, but this is disputed and neither estrogen nor progesterone appear to prolong skin graft survival. The protein hormones, especially HCG, can decrease spleen and lymph node weights and depress immune responses. The mixed lymphocyte response (MLR) in humans and the graft-versus-host response in experimental animals is depressed by HCG, and phytohemagglutin (PHA) responses are impaired in a dose-related manner. HCG is placentally derived; thus the most profound effects on the immune system may be caused by placental metabolites. Much attention is now being focused on prolactin, AFP, estradiol, calcitriol, and certain cytokines (see above) in addition to HCG, especially as factors in spontaneous abortion and in early pregnancy.

The Placenta as Immunologic Barrier

Although there has been widespread support for the idea that the placenta, by separating maternal and fetal circulations, acts as a barrier, there was for many years a controversy as to how the barrier functioned. It was believed that an inert fibrinoid substance constituted a barrier. In fact, the barrier is a dynamic one. When surgically transplanted to ectopic sites, trophoblasts are as invasive as certain types of malignant cells, if not more so. Yet under the influence of the decidua, their invasiveness is allowed to progress to a certain point and is then tightly regulated. The leading edge of these cells is composed of syncytiotrophoblasts, which are multinucleated cells with ill-defined cell borders. Falk has shown these cells, which communicate directly with the maternal circulation, to be negative for expression of MHC class I and II antigen.

Just beneath the syncytiotrophoblasts lie the villous cytotrophoblasts that probably serve as stem cells for the syncytia. The cytotrophoblasts are also cell-surface negative for MHC class I and II antigens, but, in contrast, these cells contain cytoplasmic messenger RNA (mRNA) for class I molecules. A third type of trophoblast, the extravillous cytotrophoblast, makes contact with maternal stromal cells and vessel endothelial cells at a later time in pregnancy. The cytoplasm of extravillous cytotrophoblasts contains significant mRNA for fully translated class I molecules; weak but significant cell-surface expression of class I molecules has been reported. The class I molecule expressed by these cells has been characterized as HLA-G, a unique class I species of limited polymorphism and tissue distribution (Chap. 14). The function of HLA-G, that is, whether it acts as a class I restricting element for a trophoblast antigen(s), is not known. Thus the placenta does function as a dynamic barrier with trophoblasts that interact with the underlying maternal decidua, and it may or may not be antigenically inert. The barrier also is not absolute; trophoblasts occasionally escape into maternal circulation, and the passage of Rh-positive red cells to the Rh-negative mother can lead to *erythroblastosis fetalis*. Lymphocytes and granulocytes also may enter the maternal circulation during parturition and may contribute to the development of anti-HLA, anti-Lewis, and other antibodies by the mother.

There is still some uncertainty about the antigenicity of nontrophoblastic cells in the placenta. Immunoglobulins, including antibodies to HLA, are recovered commercially from human placentas. Palm proposed that graft-versus-host reactions occurring in the placentas of rats were protective. The maternal cells that might otherwise pass into the fetus and cause injury were by this hypothesis immobilized by the graft-versus-host reaction. In support of this suggestion are the observations (1) that the placentas of hybrid rodents are heavier and more densely cellular than are the placentas of inbred strains and (2) that male rats died from a runting syndrome when the parents were compatible for Rt-1, the major histocompatibility complex of the rat, which is incompatible for minor antigens. The mother would of course lack the male-associated antigen of the male offspring and could respond to it, thus producing male runting.

Protective Antibodies

Antibodies can depress cellular responses. This is called *immunologic enhancement* in tumor-host relationships and *blocking* in most other situations. Female mice mated to a male of another strain form enhancing antibodies, as well as antibodies to H-2, the amount of antibody formed being a function of the number of pregnancies. Rocklyn demonstrated the formation of blocking antibodies by healthy gravid humans and found these antibodies to be absent from the serum of women with a history of repeated abortion. Buckley and colleagues used the MLR-blocking antibodies present in a multiparous woman to suppress graft-versus-host reactions that otherwise might have developed when her bone marrow was transplanted to her immunodeficient child. Unfortunately, not all pregnancy sera have this effect on the MLR or on graft-versus-host reactions.

Immunization and Abortion

Spontaneous abortion is quite frequent in first pregnancies. Some women, however, repeatedly abort (see above) and may lack the protection to the fetus afforded by blocking antibodies. Skin grafts from the father or a third-party donor have been reported to reduce this tendency. Beer, Faulk, and others have immunized women with histories of repeated abortion with skin grafts or injections of lymphocytes and have reported the subsequent delivery of healthy infants at term. Although it might appear that immunization could lead to adverse reactions against the fetus, these have not been reported. Care is taken of course to avoid sensitization against ABH or Rh antigens. Anti-HLA antibodies reactive with the infant probably do not cross the placenta, and there are no known adverse effects to the fetus from maternal immunity to HLA. McIntyre and Faulk have reported on two glycoproteins from the placenta that appear at the blastocyst stage. Immunization against the trophoblast-lymphocyte cross-reactivity (TLX) of one of these antigens is regarded as protective of the fetus. Recent findings have shown one of the TLX antigens is identical to a complement regulatory protein MCP, also designated CD46. Restriction fragment length polymorphisms (RFLPs) in CD46 have been reported; in patients with recurrent spontaneous abortion, some of these RFLPs occurred less frequently than in the normal control population. Thus the CD46 allelic system may have an important function in protecting the fetus from complement-mediated attack.

Conclusion

Tumor host relationships and the immune response to pregnancy are two of the most challenging and important topics in immunobiology. In each condition there are subtle variations in the display of antigens presented to the host and also in host reactivity. Neoantigens in the tumor may be shared by different tumors of the same type or may be uniquely specific to the individual tumor. The array of antigens present on the embryo and fetus may change from day to day as different genes are activated during development. In both conditions, too, the extraneous tissue modifies the ability of the host to mount a response. The abrupt loss of cellular reactivity, often coincident with metastatic spread, and the more elusive alterations that occur in pregnancy have not, so far, been adequately explained. This chapter has drawn attention to some of the false leads that have been explored. Other misconceptions undoubtedly will arise because of the numerous pitfalls, but in learning about these complex relationships, the immunologist will learn much about immunoregulation. The knowledge gained will be used in addressing other complex diseases, including AIDS, parasite infections, and autoimmunity.

FURTHER READING

General

Beer AE, Billingham RE: Immunobiology of mammalian reproduction. Adv Immunol 14:1, 1971

Mettler L, Billington WD (eds): Reproductive Immunology 1989. Amsterdam, Elsevier Science Publishers, 1990

Risk JM, Flanagan BF, Johnson PM: Polymorphism of the human CD46 gene in normal individuals and in recurrent spontaneous abortion. Hum Immunol 30:162, 1991

Sell S: Immunology, Immunopathology and Immunity, ed 4. New York, Elsevier Science Publishing Co, 1987

Tumor Antigens/Oncogenes and Human Tumor Markers

Carney W: Human tumor antigens and specific tumor therapy. Immunol Today 9:363, 1988

Cooper GM: Cellular transforming genes. Science 218:801, 1982

Cory S, Adams JM: Transgenic mice and oncogenesis. Annu Rev Immunol 6:25, 1988

Hellstrom KE, Hellstrom I, Brown JP: Human tumor associated antigens identified by monoclonal antibodies. In Baldwin RW, Miescher PA, Muller-Eberhard HJ (eds): Springer Seminars in Immunopathology, vol 5. New York, Springer-Verlag, 1982, p 127

Muschel RJ, Khoury G, Lebowitz P, et al: The human *c-ras*, oncogene: A mutation in normal and neoplastic tissue from the same patient. Science 219:853, 1983

Premkumar Reddy E, Reynolds RK, Santos E, et al: A point mutation is responsible for the acquisition of transforming properties by the T24 human bladder carcinoma oncogene. Nature 300:149, 1982

Schreiber H, Ward PL, Rowley DA, Stauss HJ: Unique tumor-specific antigens. Annu Rev Immunol 6:465, 1988

Tabin CJ, Bradley SM, Bargmann CI, et al: Mechanism of activation of a human oncogene. Nature 300:143, 1982

Touchette N: Tumor suppressors: A new arena in the war against cancer. J NIH Res 2:62, 1990

Weinberg RA: The retinoblastoma gene and cell growth control. Trends Biochem Sci 15:199, 1990

Tumor Immunity

David-Watine B, Israël A, Kourilsky P: The regulation and expression of MHC class I genes. Immunol Today 11:286, 1990

Foley EJ: Antigenic properties of methylcholanthrene-induced tumors in mice of strain of origin. Cancer Res 13:853, 1953

Kaliss N: Immunological enhancement of tumor homografts in mice: A review. Cancer Res 18:992, 1958

Kawase I, Urdal DL, Brooks CG, et al: Selective depletion of NK cell activity in vivo and its effect on the growth of NK-sensitive and NK-resistant tumor cell variants. Int J Cancer 29:567, 1982

Klein G, Sjogren HO, Klein E, et al: Demonstration of resistance against methylcholanthrene-induced sarcomas in the primary autochthonous host. Cancer Res 20:1561, 1960

Lawrence HS, Valentine FT: Transfer factor and other mediators of cellular immunity. Am J Pathol 60:437, 1970

Mitchison MA: Passive transfer of transplantation immunity. Proc R Soc Lond [Biol]: 143:72, 1954

Moller, G (ed): Experiments and the concept of immunological surveillance. Transplant Rev 28:1, 1976

Prehn RT, Main JM: Immunity to methylcholanthrene induced sarcomas. J Natl Cancer Inst 18:769, 1957

Rubin JT, Elwood LJ, Rosenberg SA, Lotze MT: Immunohistochemical correlates of response to recombinant interleukin-2-based immunotherapy in humans. Cancer Res 49:7086, 1989

Storkus WJ, Dawson JR: Target structures involved in natural killing (NK): Characteristics, distribution, and candidate molecules. CRC Rev Immunol 10:393, 1990

Tanaka K, Yoshioka T, Bieberich C, Gilbert J: Role of the major histocompatibility complex class I antigens in tumor growth and metastases. Annu Rev Immunol 6:359, 1988

Winn HJ: Immune mechanisms in homotransplantation. II. Quantitative assay of the immunologic activity of lymphoid cells stimulated by tumor homografts. J Immunol 86:228, 1961

Immunotherapy

Goldenberg DM: Targeted cancer treatment. Immunol Today 10:286, 1989

Jung G, Muller-Eberhard HJ: An in vitro model for tumor immunotherapy with antibody heteroconjugates. Immunol Today 9:257, 1988

Lotze MT, Custer MC, Bolton ES, et al: Mechanisms of immunologic antitumor therapy: Lessons from the laboratory and clinical applications. Hum Immunol 28:198, 1990

Parmiani G: An explanation of the variable clinical response to interleukin-2 and LAK cells. Immunol Today 11:113, 1990

Rosenberg SA, Lotze MT: Cancer immunotherapy using interleukin-2 and interleukin-2-activated lymphocytes. Annu Rev Immunol 4:681, 1986

SECTION III

MEDICAL BACTERIOLOGY

CHAPTER 21

Host-Parasite Relationships

Infectious disease is the result of an unsuccessful relationship between parasite and host. It is the summation of the vectors of both agents and ranges in severity from human rabies, which is almost invariably fatal, to the common cold, which is almost invariably nonfatal. In between lie the common infectious diseases, the etiologic agents of which are described in this book. Although new agents of infectious disease continue to be described—for example, human immunodeficiency virus (AIDS)—the rate of new discovery has slowed remarkably. Increasing attention is being paid to perturbations in the host defense mechanisms that open the doors to infections with our own microbial flora, a subject that is only now beginning to be understood. The advances in public health services, vaccines, antibiotics, and improved nutrition have tremendously reduced infection as one of the common causes of death in advanced societies. It has been the advances in therapeutics and consequent alteration of host defense mechanisms that have tremendously increased the incidence of infectious diseases resulting from medical progress. Although there are many general principles regarding host defense mechanisms and determinants of microbial pathogenicity, each individual patient and each specific pathogen must be carefully studied for clues as to why that particular combination produced a particular illness. In many instances, however, the specific reasons why a particular combination results in a given clinical picture are not clearly discernible. This chapter discusses a few of the host factors that may modify infection, the problem of the compromised host, clinical manifestations of infectious diseases, and a few of the microbial attributes that are cited as the explanations for what is seen clinically. For a more detailed discussion of the immune responses to infection and virulence determinants, the reader is referred to Chapter 19 and to the chapters dealing with specific organisms.

The Host

To a considerable extent, chance plays a role in any infectious disease. An individual must be in the wrong place at the wrong time: historically, using a blanket previously used by a patient with smallpox, being in the center of a typhoid epidemic, living with someone who has active tuberculosis, or being a member of a family in which there is a case of meningococcal meningitis. What then ensues depends on a number of host factors. All infectious diseases begin at the surface of the host, with the exception of certain intrauterine-transmitted infections. The first barrier, therefore, is the gross surface area, which usually is skin, respiratory tract, gastrointestinal tract, or genitourinary tract. The specific surface involved relates to how the pathogenic microorganism reaches the host, for example, puncture of the skin by a needle, inhalation of an aerosolized droplet, swallowing of an infected substance, or sexual transmission of a microbe. Starting with the skin, there is an obvious physical barrier aided by frequent desquamation. The spraying of a suspension of bacteria on the skin usually produces no untoward effect. Simple drying is sufficient to eliminate most bacteria, and the fatty acids on the surface layers, as well as the skin pH, exert an antibacterial effect. Direct intradermal inoculation of volunteers with virulent bacteria may require as many as 5 to 10 million viable organisms to produce infection. There are exceptions, however, such as in the case of *Francisella tularensis,* which in human volunteers may require a very small number of viable organisms to produce serious tularemia infection. Any break in the integrity of the skin will, of course, remove the physical barrier. This could range from a simple abrasion to a severe burn or drug-related exfoliative dermatitis. More commonly, a puncture wound with a foreign body, such as a splinter, a suture, or an indwelling intravenous needle and/or plastic catheter, can provide a nidus for initiating infection.

In addition to the integrity of the mucosal lining, the gastrointestinal tract is protected to a great extent by the acid secreted in the stomach, which is inimical to most microbial forms of life. The stomach's acidity, however, can be modified by the ingestion of food or other substances that neutralize the acid, by certain diseases, and by surgery of the stomach. This barrier also can be overcome by the ingestion of large numbers of bacteria; for example, the ingestion of a million *Salmonella* organisms, a common cause of food poisoning, will provoke disease in volunteers. Another property that protects the gastrointestinal tract is its fairly rapid motility, resulting in a rapid transit time for microbes that survive the stomach acid. In addition, the lower parts of the gastrointestinal tract have an enormous indigenous bacterial flora that play a competitive role in the establishment of an exogenous pathogenic organism; these flora, however, also can be altered by the use of antibiotics, thereby allowing new pathogens to flourish.

The respiratory surface has as its physical protection a mucous coating that can entrap most microbial forms of life. This mucous coating is swept up from the respiratory tree by cilia, where it is coughed up and swallowed reflexively, thereby depositing the potentially infectious material into the sterilizing environment of the stomach. Finally, the surface of the urinary tract—the ureter, bladder, urethra—has as its protective barrier the simple flow of urine. Instillation into the bladder of organisms capable of causing urinary tract infections is followed by their prompt excretion in the urine, with no untoward effects. Many of these cellular surfaces, however, which provide the first barrier to infection, have receptors to which pathogenic organisms can attach and thereby lessen the effectiveness of the simple physical means of eliminating these agents. Obstruction in any of these areas—the gastrointestinal tract, the respiratory tract, the genitourinary tract—either from a physical agent or from disease can alter these bacteria-removing barriers in such a way that either resident microbial flora or invasive organisms can replicate and produce disease.

Once these gross physical barriers have been breached, microorganisms encounter an extremely hostile environment. At this particular point, they encounter a very complex cellular response called *inflammation.* This response is as old as recorded history: *rubror et tumor cum calore et dolore.* The type of cellular response varies with both time and the specific type of microorganism. In very general terms, the polymorphonuclear leukocyte is primarily effective against extracellular bacteria. This effectiveness is greatly enhanced by the presence of complement, which possesses a wide range of antimicrobial properties such as chemotaxis, opsonization, and lysis. The later appearance of specific antibody tremendously improves the efficiency of these cells. If there is preexisting antibody in the serum, disease usually does not occur. The macrophage and subsequently the multinucleated giant cell and epithelioid cell are most effective against mycobacterial and mycotic infections. Interferon, lymphocytes, and specific antibody globulin are the most effective deterrents to progressive viral infection. Last, the eosinophil plays a role in certain parasitic infections.

It should be pointed out, however, that in addition to microbial invasion, the inflammatory response may be triggered by many other events—physical, chemical, or immunologic—resulting in a clinical picture that at times is difficult to differentiate from infection. In bacterial infections the first 20 minutes of the host response usually determines whether a given invading organism will produce disease. At the cellular level, one of the earliest responses is that of polymorphonuclear leukocyte migration. Chemotaxis, the attraction of phagocytic cells to the site of infection or tissue injury, is an early event in response to infection. When the polymorphonuclear leukocyte arrives at the site of the invading microorganism, a change occurs in the plasma membrane of the phagocytic cell, resulting in invagination around the bacterial cell with subsequent fusion to produce a phagocytic vacuole. Biochemical changes within the leukocyte at the time of phagocytosis may kill the ingested organism. In addition, fusion of lysosomes with the phagocytic vacuole to produce a phagolysosome may result in digestion of the organism by the enzymatic contents of the lysosome.

In general, the antimicrobial systems of the polymorphonuclear leukocyte are of two types, the oxygen-dependent and the oxygen-independent systems. The oxygen-dependent system can be further subdivided into myeloperoxidase (MPO)-mediated systems, which when combined with hydrogen peroxide and appropriate oxidizable cofactor (iodide, bromide, or chloride) have marked antimicrobial activity. MPO-independent systems include the production of hydrogen peroxide, superoxide anion, hydroxyl radicals, and singlet oxygen. Oxygen-independent microbial systems include the acid pH within the phagocytic vacuole and the release of lysozyme, lactoferrin, and granular cationic proteins. Antimicrobial systems similar to these also have been described in macrophage cell cultures.

Complement possesses a dual role in the phagocytic process. Fission of fragments C3 and C5a generates chemotactic factors, whereas bound C3b has primarily the function of opsonization. This opsonic function is based on the ability of these fragments to bind bacteria or other microbial forms to sites that can specifically interact with receptors on the surface of phagocytic cells. The presence of preformed antibody to the invading agent tremendously improves the efficiency of phagocytosis. This preformed antibody may be from previous infection or from stimulation by a related but not necessarily microbiologic source of antigen. Any event that interferes with this classic inflammatory response obviously will allow microbes to become established. Interfering effects may range from simple foreign bodies and impaired blood supply that prevents adequate polymorphonuclear leukocyte response to blatant leukopenia due either to natural disease or the effects of drug therapy. More subtle changes in chemotaxis, phagocytosis, complement, and intracellular killing are also now recognized as being responsible for certain infectious diseases.

In addition to the classic defense mechanisms of the polymorphonuclear leukocyte, specific antibody globulin, and complement, many microbial pathogens, upon invasion of the host, generate a cell-mediated immunity. This type of immunity is mediated by the action of specifically sensitized T lymphocytes and is effected by an interaction of lymphocytes and macrophages, with the result that both cellular types play a role in resistance to certain types of infection. Cell-mediated immunity is most important in defense against facultative intracellular pathogens, including representatives of the bacterial, mycotic, viral, and parasitic groups. Unfortunately, a number of diseases, as well as certain therapeutic agents, can interfere with cell-mediated immunity, thereby permitting replication of the aforementioned group of agents and resulting in disease.

Should the invading organism survive the immediate localizing effect of inflammation, there exist simple gross physical barriers, such as fascial planes, muscles, serosal cavities, and bone. More effective is the extensive barrier of the lymphatic system, with its filtering lymph nodes and phagocytic potential. It is possible, however, for microorganisms to overcome this barrier either through gross numbers or through a remarkable ability to resist phagocytosis, with the result that the bloodstream is invaded. Bacteremia (also fungemia, viremia, parasitemia) signals a failure of these local barriers and usually portends more significant illness. Even here, however, there is an incredibly effective clearance mechanism scattered throughout the body, characterized as the reticuloendothelial system but concentrated in the liver, spleen, bone marrow, and lung. This system, which comprises a remarkably efficient phagocytic macrophage process, is capable of clearing the blood of a wide range of foreign agents. Despite this effective clearance mechanism, however, some organisms can survive to set up sites of infection distal to the site of primary invasion, with the result that patients may present with metastatic disease involving the brain, heart, joints, and other organ sites.

The Compromised Host

Every patient with an infectious disease is to some extent a compromised host. In some instances, we know enough about the defense mechanisms to pinpoint the area compromised. In many instances, however, we are unable to define the defect. With continued observations of infectious diseases, however, it has been possible to define certain settings in which increased infection can be predicted. Among the most common compromised hosts are the very young and the very old. Certain prevalent basic diseases, such as alcoholism and diabetes, often are associated with infection. Less commonly, the patient with uremia is a source of host-parasite problems. Nutritional deficiency is recognized as a contributor to infection. Natural diseases involving the hematopoietic system, Hodgkin's disease, and other lymphomas, leukemias, and multiple myeloma are notoriously associated with high attack rates of infection. Various solid tumors, such as carcinomas and sarcomas, also present problems with increased infection attack rates. Infection with the human immunodeficiency virus (HIV) that results in AIDS has become an increasingly important setting for secondary microbial invasion. Inherited and acquired primary immunodeficiency diseases also present problems.

In addition to these basic illnesses, there exist superimposed conditions, which in some respects are the diseases of medical progress. For this reason, they are commonly encountered in hospitals and are associated with hospital-acquired infection or nosocomial infection. The normally effective physical barriers to infection may be altered by the use of indwelling intravenous and urethral catheters. One can change the normal indigenous flora by the use of broad-spectrum antibiotics, thereby leaving a void to be filled by drug-resistant microorganisms, which in themselves have a low degree of pathogenicity but which in the compromised host are capable of producing significant illness. A decrease in the total circulating pool of phagocytic cells can be caused by cytotoxic chemotherapy of cancers and by irradiation. Patients with altered leukocyte responses, such as decreased migration, diminished phagocytosis, and decreased bactericidal capacity, have presented problems. Finally, interference with the classic immunoglobulin production or impairment of cell-mediated immunity by therapy with steroids or cytotoxic drugs, irradiation, or antilymphocytic globulins can lead to infection. In the compromised host, one does not necessarily have problems with the usual pyogenic cocci. Instead, one may see organisms usually selected by prior chemotherapy, such as *Pseudomonas* species, Enterobacteriaceae, anaerobic bacteria, *Mycobacterium,* fungi, herpes viruses, and such parasites as nematodes, protozoa, and *Pneumocystis.*

Clinical Manifestations of Infectious Diseases

Most infectious diseases start with exposure to the infectious agent, followed by an incubation period and then manifestations of the disease. Patients ill enough to enter the health care system are usually evaluated by obtaining a history from the patient, doing a complete physical examination, and then using selected laboratory procedures. Fever is almost always an accompaniment of clinical infectious diseases, although it also may accompany a wide variety of illnesses totally unrelated to infection. The fever may be subtle or abrupt in its onset, and it may move with great speed or at a very slow tempo. It usually is the inflammatory response that brings a patient to a physician because of the attendant pain and loss of function. It generally is possible by history or physical examination, or both, to localize the site of the infection. By virtue of the tempo and clinical appearance of the infection, differentiation among the usual subdivisions of microbiology is made, that is, bacterial, virus, fungal or mycobacterial, or parasitic. The specific cause of any given infectious disease, however, can be proved only by demonstrating the infectious agent in smears or cultures or by an appropriate antibody response. Because the number of antimicrobial drugs is so great and the spectrum so varied, it is necessary that some attempt be made to identify specifically the etiologic agent of any infectious disease. Additional laboratory procedures, such as x-ray studies, sometimes are helpful in defining infectious illnesses more precisely. The more recent advent of computed tomography (CT) scans has revolutionized the localization of abscesses. In addition, the host response to the infectious agent may be roughly gauged by measuring the number and types of peripheral white blood cells. Classically, an excessive production of polymorphonuclear leukocytes with the appearance of early forms suggests bacterial infection. Normal or low white blood cell counts with prevalent lymphocytes suggest viral infection. Eosinophilia has been associated with some types of parasitic infections. Nonspecific parameters of inflammation, such as the sedimentation rate and C-reactive protein, can be measured, and the lack of an increase in such measurements may suggest a viral infection. The least reliable, but nonetheless commonly used parameter, is the response of the patient to antimicrobial therapy.

Most infectious diseases run a reasonably predictable course, with spontaneous resolution. How antimicrobial therapy changes this clinical course is an extremely important element of infectious diseases. Finally, it should be stressed that certain infections, although they may resolve either spontaneously or with therapy, can persist in a latent form to reappear at a later date. This problem has become of increasing significance, since immunosuppression due to therapy or disease may allow these diseases to change from a latent host-parasite relationship to an overt disease-producing relationship.

The Parasite

Of the many thousands of known microorganisms, fewer than 300 have acquired the ability to produce disease in humans and animals. Organisms capable of producing disease usually are referred to as *pathogens.* One of the most fundamental properties of such a microorganism is its ability to multiply within the human host. Even here, however, there are a few exceptions wherein organisms multiply on the surface of the host and produce disease. In addition, there are not uncommon intoxications as opposed to infections resulting from products produced outside the host but coming in contact with the host. *Virulence* is a quantitative measure of the degree of pathogenicity of a particular microorganism or of a specific strain. Virulence usually is measured by the numbers of microorganisms necessary to kill or alter a particular animal species or test system under standardized conditions. The importance of genetic variability in both pathogenicity and virulence has been repeatedly demonstrated. *Communicability* may be defined as the ability of the organism to spread under natural conditions from human to human, from animal to human, or from human to animal. The mechanisms of such communicability cover a remarkable range, such as simple respiratory droplet nuclei, anal or oral ingestion, contact, and insect or animal bite.

Surface Factors

Most infectious diseases require that the parasitic agent initiate infection on the body surfaces—the skin or the mucous membranes of the respiratory, gastrointestinal, or genitourinary tract. The initial contact resulting in adherence of the microorganism to the underlying cell is an important determinant of pathogenicity. The presence of receptor sites on both bacteria and host surface cells allows the microorganism to attach to host tissue and thereby gain pathogenic advantage over organisms that do not possess these receptors. This has been abundantly documented, especially in the area of virology. A number of bacteria and protozoa also have been shown to take advantage of this mechanism of pathogenicity. In *Chlamydia* a cell surface lectin is produced with binding affinity for *N*-acetyl-D-glucosamine in the host cell receptors. *Mycoplasma* has a protein adhesin localized in a specialized tip structure for adherence to sialic acid–containing cell receptors. Enterobacteriaceae utilize specific adhesive organelles, pili (or fimbriae), for adherence to host cell surfaces. The archetypical pilus of this family is type I or common pili, which are expressed under a wide variety of cultural conditions. These pili attach to uroepithelial cells and play a role in the pathogenesis of urinary tract infections. In *Escherichia coli,* a different class of pili (K88) is associated with the enterotoxigenic strains that colonize the intestinal tract. *Vibrio cholerae* and *Shigella dysenteriae* also adhere to gastrointestinal epithelium, and *Plasmodium* species, the cause of malaria, use this mechanism for initial attachment to the susceptible erythrocyte.

In addition to attachment to a susceptible host cell, the microbial surface can play a significant role in resisting phagocytosis, thereby adding another dimension of pathogenicity. These surface properties usually are in the form of a slime layer or capsule of either polysaccharide or polypeptide. Examples of such surface structures are the polysaccharide capsules of *Streptococcus pneumoniae, Neisseria meningitidis,* and *Haemophilus influenzae.* Patients with defective reticuloendothelial systems (e.g., as a result of splenectomy) are particularly susceptible to bacteremic infections with these pathogens. In addition, *Bacillus anthracis* presents an example of a surface capsule of polypeptide composition. Although the presence of a surface capsule can explain why a particular organism can multiply within the human host, it does not explain why disease is produced. Antibodies directed specifically against these surface antigens dramatically eliminate the organism's resistance to phagocytosis. Such antibodies are called *opsonins* and, in the presence of complement and an intact polymorphonuclear leukocyte, present the most fundamental mechanism of resistance against bacteria that have crossed the surface barriers of the host. A small number of microorganisms, however, have developed an ability to survive within phagocytic cells, a property contributing to their pathogenicity.

Toxins

A large number of substances have been described in association with bacteria that can either damage host cells or interfere with defense mechanisms. In only a relatively few instances, however, do these substances explain what is seen clinically or provide a rationale for treatment or prevention. These examples are limited to toxins, the mechanisms of action of some of which have been clearly described at the biochemical level. The exotoxins of diphtheria and tetanus are thought to act as single determinants to produce disease. Other diseases in which toxins play a major role are cholera, bacillary dysentery, botulism, anthrax, scarlet fever, and pertussis.

Toxins are of two major types: the exotoxins, which are easily separated from the bacterial cell, and the endotoxins, which are intimately associated with the bacterial cell wall.

Extracellular Toxins

Exotoxins are released from the cell during exponential growth. They are protein in nature, possess enzymatic activity, and are toxic for target cells. A number of the exotoxins are two-component toxins and conform to a general structural model. The others are broadly referred to as bacterial cytolysins.

Two-component Toxins. The isolation, purification, and chemical characterization of the two-component toxins have revealed a fascinating thread of similarity despite the startling diversity of the organisms and the diseases from which they were isolated. Usually one component is composed of a binding (B) domain associated with absorption to the surface of a susceptible cell (implying specificity) and is necessary for the transfer of the enzymatic component (A) across the cell membrane. Once inside the cell, the toxic A component exerts an enzymelike effect that alters the normal function of the susceptible cell. Isolated A subunits are enzymatically active but lack binding and cell entry capability. Isolated B subunits bind to target cells, but they are nontoxic and biologically inactive.

Diphtheria toxin is the prototype two-component adenosine diphosphate (ADP)–ribosylating toxin that inhibits cellular protein synthesis by catalyzing the transfer of ADP-ribose from nicotinamide-adenine dinucleotide (NAD) to elongation factor–2 (EF2). Although many types of cells can be damaged by this toxin, the major clinical manifestations, in addition to the pharyngitis, are carditis and peripheral neuropathy. A similar toxin is produced by *Pseudomonas aeruginosa,* a gram-negative rod commonly associated with nosocomial infections because of its extensive antibiotic-resistance spectrum. However, the role of this toxin in the pathogenesis of disease caused by this organism is less clear.

The enzymatic A–subunit of cholera toxin catalyzes the ADP ribosylation of the B-subunit of the stimulatory guanine nucleotide protein G_s. This results in a profuse outpouring of fluid and electrolytes, resulting in a profound life-threatening diarrhea. Interestingly, some strains of *E. coli* capable of producing enteritis have been found to produce a similar heat-labile toxin.

Tetanus and botulinum toxins are less well understood because their molecular site of action is not known. The B component of both toxins binds to a neuroreceptor ganglioside. Determination of whether the A chain is responsible for the toxicity must await the discovery of the molecular site of toxin activity. Clinically, the tetanus toxin releases inhibitory impulses, with the production of trismus (lockjaw) and tetanic convulsions. Botulinum toxin is among the most potent of all biologic toxins. It inhibits the release of acetylcholine at the myoneural junction, resulting clinically in the development of profound paralysis that frequently is fatal.

A few of the aforementioned toxins can be altered by exposure to dilute concentrations of formaldehyde, with the production of toxoids—substances that have retained antitoxic antigenicity but have lost physiologic toxicity. These have provided powerful tools for the prevention of disease (e.g., tetanus and diphtheria).

Bacterial Cytolysins. These substances initially were discovered because their damage to erythrocyte membranes produces a readily observable effect—hemolysis. Much of the earlier work thus refers to these toxins as *hemolysins.* Some of these toxins, however, have a much broader range of target cell membranes, and some that are quite toxic to certain intact cells have no effect on red blood cells. Although hemolysis occasionally is seen as a clinical complication of infectious diseases, the fact that these toxins can produce tissue necrosis and are lethal when administered intravenously to experimental animals has resulted in their receiving a great deal of attention as a possible explanation for certain clinical syndromes. Although some of these cytolysins probably explain what is seen clinically, there are as yet few therapeutic or preventive applications. The three major types of cytolysins are (1) those that hydrolyze membrane phospholipids (phospholipases), as seen in pathogenic *Clostridium* and *Staphylococcus* species, (2) thiol-activated cytolysins (also referred to as *oxygen-labile*) that alter membrane permeability by binding to cholesterol and that are found in pathogenic *Streptococcus* and *Clostridium* species, and (3) the cytolysins in pathogenic staphylococci that exert a detergentlike activity on cell membranes and that have a rapid rate of lysis and a remarkable range of activity in membrane systems. In addition, there also are bacterial cytolysins for which at present there is no explanation of their mechanism of action.

Endotoxins

The second large category of toxins, the endotoxins, are a major component of the outer membrane of gram-negative bacteria. They are lipopolysaccharide in composition and are heat stable. Unlike exotoxins, they do not form toxoids, are less specific in their action, and are considerably less toxic on a weight basis. Although the intact lipopolysaccharide molecule is of considerable immunologic significance, the toxic activity resides in the lipid moiety. Endotoxins are potent pharmacologic agents. A large number of toxic effects have been described after the administration of endotoxins to experimental animals. However, the relationships of these effects to the clinical manifestations of disease are not clear. The most obvious effects, such as pyrogenicity, the ability to produce shock mediated through cachectin, and their effect on nonspecific immunity, are among the most important.

Host Response

There are a number of microbial agents for which no toxic substance has been implicated in the pathogenesis of the disease. In many infections the response of the host may constitute a substantial portion of the disease process. This may range from the sudden outpouring of polymorphonuclear leukocytes producing the consolidation of the lung seen in *S. pneumoniae* infections to the cell-mediated immunity resulting in the activated macrophages, granuloma reaction, and caseous tissue necrosis seen with *Mycobacterium* infections.

FURTHER READING

Books and Reviews

Atkins E: Fever: The old and the new. J Infect Dis 149:339, 1984

Beutler B, Cerami A: Cachectin: More than a tumor necrosis factor. N Engl J Med 316:386, 1987

Brown MRW, Williams P: The influence of environment on envelope properties affecting survival of bacteria in infections. Annu Rev Microbiol 39:527, 1985

Brubaker RR: Mechanisms of bacterial virulence. Annu Rev Microbiol 39:21, 1985

Ciba Foundation Symposium 80: Adhesion and Microorganism Pathogenicity. London, Pitman Medical, 1981

Ciba Foundation Symposium 112. Microbial Toxins and Diarrheal Disease. London, Pitman Medical, 1985

Cohen P, van Heyningen S (eds): Molecular Action of Toxins and Viruses. New York, Elsevier Biomed Press, 1982

Costerton JW, Irvin RT, Cheng KJ: The role of bacterial surface structures in pathogenesis. CRC Crit Rev Microbiol 8:303, 1981

Dixon RE (ed): Nosocomial Infections. New York, Yorke Medical Books, 1981

Eidels L, Proia RL, Hart DA: Membrane receptors for bacterial toxins. Microbiol Rev 47:596, 1983

Finlay BB, Falkow S: Common themes in microbial pathogenicity. Microbiol Rev 53:210, 1989
Foster JW, Kinney DM: ADP-ribosylating microbial toxins. CRC Crit Rev Microbiol 11:273, 1984–85
Gallin JI, Fauci AS (eds): Advances in Host Defense Mechanisms, vol 1: Phagocytic Cells. New York, Raven Press, 1982
Gallin JI, Fauci AS (eds): Advances in Host Defense Mechanisms, vol 2: Lymphoid Cells. New York, Raven Press, 1983
Gallin JI, Fauci AS (eds): Advances in Host Defense Mechanisms, vol 4: Mucosal Immunity. New York, Raven Press, 1985
Gallin JI, Fauci AS (eds): Advances in Host Defense Mechanisms, vol 6: Davis JM, Shires GI (guest eds): Host Defenses in Trauma and Surgery. New York, Raven Press, 1986
Gill DM: Bacterial toxins: A table of lethal amounts. Microbiol Rev 46:86, 1982
Grieco MH (ed): Infections in the abnormal host. New York, Yorke Medical Books, 1980
Hahn H: The role of cell-mediated immunity in bacterial infections. Rev Infect Dis 3:1221, 1981
Hanson JM, Rumjanek VM, Morley J: Mediators of cellular immune reactions. Pharmacol Ther 17:165, 1982
Hirsch RL: The complement system: Its importance in the host response to viral infections. Microbiol Rev 46:71, 1982
Horwitz MA: Phagocytosis of microorganisms. Rev Infect Dis 4:104, 1982
Iglewski BH, Clark VL: Molecular Basis of Bacterial Pathogenesis. New York, Academic Press, 1990
Jeljaszewicz J, Wadstrom T (eds): Bacterial Toxins and Cell Membranes. New York, Academic Press, 1978
Kilian M, Mestecky J, Russell MW: Defense mechanisms involving Fc-dependent functions of immunoglobulin A and their subversion by bacterial immunoglobulin A proteases. Microbiol Rev 52:296, 1988
Mackowiak PA: Microbial latency. Rev Infect Dis 6:649, 1984
Middlebrook JL, Dorland RB: Bacterial toxins: Cellular mechanisms of action. Microbiol Rev 48:199, 1984
Mims CA: The Pathogenesis of Infectious Disease. New York, Academic Press, 1982
Mizuro D, Cohn ZA, Takeya K, et al (eds): Self-defense Mechanisms—Role of Macrophages. Tokyo, University of Tokyo Press/Elsevier Biomed Press, 1982
Moulder JW: Comparative biology of intracellular parasitism. Microbiol Rev 49:298, 1985
Neville DM, Hudson TH: Transmembrane transport of diphtheria toxin, related toxins and colicins. Annu Rev Biochem 55:195, 1986
O'Grady F, Smith H (eds): Microbial Perturbation of Host Defenses. New York, Academic Press, 1981
Powanda MC, Canonico PG (eds): Infection—The Physiologic and Metabolic Responses of the Host. New York, Elsevier Biomedical Press, 1981
Proctor RA: Handbook of Endotoxin, vol 4: Clinical Aspects of Endotoxin Shock. New York, Elsevier, 1986
Root RK, Cohen MS: The microbiocidal mechanisms of human neutrophiles and eosinophiles. Rev Infect Dis 3:565, 1981
Rosenstreich DL, Weinblatt AC, O'Brien AD: Genetic control of resistance to infection in mice. CRC Crit Rev Immunol 3:263, 1982
Smith H, Skehel JJ, Turner MJ: The Molecular Basis of Microbial Pathogenicity. Deerfield Beach, Fla, Verlag Chemie, 1980
Swanson J, Sparling PF, Puziss M (eds): Bacterial virulence and pathogenicity. Rev Infect Dis 5:633, 1983
Taylor PW: Bactericidal and bacteriolytic activity against gram-negative bacteria. Microbiol Rev 47:46, 1983
Wolbach B, Baehner RL, Boxer LA: Review: Clinical and laboratory approach to the management of neutrophil dysfunction. Isr J Med Sci 18:897, 1982
Zabriskie JB, Gibofsky A: Genetic control of the susceptibility to infection with pathogenic bacteria. Curr Top Microbiol Immunol 124:1, 1986

Selected Papers

Densen P, Weiler JM, Griffiss JM: Familial properdin deficiency and fatal meningococcemia. N Engl J Med 316:922, 1987
Devita VT Jr, Broder S, Fauci AS: Developmental therapeutics and the acquired immunodeficiency syndrome. Ann Intern Med 106:568, 1987
Edén CS, Hausson S, Jodal U, et al: Host-parasite interaction in the urinary tract. J Infect Dis 157:421, 1988
Franzon VL, Arondel J, Sansonetti PJ: Contribution of superoxide dismutase and catalase activities to *Shigella flexneri* pathogenesis. Infect Immun 58:529, 1990
Miles AA, Miles EM, Burke J: The value and duration of defense reactions of the skin to the primary lodgement of bacteria. Br J Exp Pathol 38:79, 1957
Quie PG: Perturbations of the normal mechanisms of intraleukocytic killing of bacteria. J Infect Dis 148:189, 1983
Reinholdt J, Tomana M, Mortensen SB, Kilian M: Molecular aspects of immunoglobulin Al degradation by oral streptococci. Infect Immun 58:1186, 1990
Stibitz S, Weiss AA, Falkow S: Genetic analysis of a region of the *Bordetella pertussis* chromosome encoding filamentous hemagglutinin and the pleiotropic regulatory locus *vir*. J Bacteriol 170:2904, 1988

CHAPTER 22

Normal Flora and Opportunistic Infections

Ecologic Relationships

Ecology is the study of the interactions between organisms and their environment. The environment of an organism is as much a product of the presence and activities of the organisms that inhabit it as it is of nonliving chemical and physical forces. This is especially so in the case of microorganisms, which in nature occur almost always in association with other microorganisms and with animals and plants. Microorganisms are ubiquitous and are present under all conditions that permit the existence of any form of life. Because these conditions are diverse, organisms tend to segregate and to become adapted to a particular habitat or environmental niche. In this ecologic niche they are constantly engaged in the synthesis of new organic compounds and in the degradation of complex animal and plant tissues. Here, as among the higher forms of life, there is a constant struggle for survival between individuals and various species.

Microbial Interactions. The complex relationships among the different microbial species may be classified as neutral, antagonistic, or synergistic. Few species are strictly neutral in their reactions because they interfere in a passive manner by using the available food supply or by excreting toxic metabolites. The majority of microbial species exhibit positive antagonism, which arises from alterations in the physical environment or the elaboration of antibiotics and bacteriocins that are specifically inhibitory for certain organisms. These factors are important both in soil and water ecology and in animal ecology. Antagonism between the gram-positive cocci and gram-negative bacilli of the respiratory tract and their independent and mutual antagonism to fungi were not suspected until the clinical introduction of antibiotics. After a patient is treated with penicillin, for example, the normal flora (predominantly streptococci, and *Neisseria* and *Haemophilus* species) are replaced by gram-negative enteric bacilli, or *Pseudomonas*. On the other hand, broader-spectrum antibiosis (as achieved by chloramphenicol and tetracyclines or combinations of penicillins, cephalosporins, and aminoglycosides) may result in the emergence of resistant bacteria or overgrowth by *Candida* species.

Synergism may be described as a cooperative effort by two or more microbial species that produces a result that could not be achieved individually. This phenomenon may be relatively frequent in nature but is uncommon in disease states. Examples of the latter are the synergistic gangrene described by Meleney and some forms of anaerobic lung abscess caused by organisms that are ordinarily normal mouth flora (Chap. 43).

Host-Parasite Interactions. The various ecologic relationships that exist between microorganisms and the human host are of three types: commensalism, symbiosis, and parasitism. *Commensalism* refers to the mutual but almost inconsequential association between bacteria and higher organisms. *Symbiosis* refers to a mutually beneficial relationship between two species. *Parasitism* is that complex spectrum of relationships whereby one organism derives benefits at the expense of another. These interactions were analyzed in a classic monograph by Theobald Smith in 1934. Smith emphasized the concept that the phenomenon of disease caused by infectious agents is largely a by-product of evolving parasitism; that is, violent reactions between host and parasite tend to lessen as parasitism approaches a biologic equilibrium. The rapid and destructive actions of some microorganisms are expressions of bungling parasitism. The skillful or well-adapted parasite enters its host with ease and may produce lesions only as a means of securing exit to infect a new host. In a sense, commensalism represents an ideal form of parasitism.

The terms *pathogen* and *opportunist* require definition. In general, a pathogen is a microorganism that is capable of infecting or parasitizing "normal" individuals. As the field of immunology becomes more sophisticated, we may find that no one is normal and that this terminology is artificial. At the present time, however, the terms are useful. Certain organisms appear to represent bona fide pathogens in that their hosts comprise sufficiently large numbers of the general population who lack demonstrable underlying disease. Among these are the bacterial species *Staphylococcus aureus, Streptococcus pyogenes,* and *Streptococcus pneumoniae; Histoplasma capsulatum* and *Coccidioides immitis* among the fungi; and the plethora of common cold viruses and viruses that cause childhood diseases (measles, mumps, varicella, rubella). On the other hand, such organisms as *Pseudomonas aeruginosa, Serratia marcescens, Candida albicans, Pneumocystis carinii,* and *Nocardia asteroides,* which are referred to as *opportunists,* uncommonly cause de novo disease but almost always are encountered under unusual circumstances, either in abnormal hosts or in situations in which the normal flora have been supplanted. The factors responsible for the pathogenic potential of various microorganisms are discussed in the chapters that follow.

Natural Habitats

The diversity of physical and chemical conditions present in different environments results in the segregation of microorganisms into different physical niches, depending on available nutrients, temperature, moisture, and other conditions. Knowledge of the flora of various natural habitats is important in understanding human acquisition of disease.

Soil

The soil is a great reservoir of microorganisms, the majority of which are nonpathogenic. Some microorganisms reach the soil in the excreta or cadavers of animals; others, such as the autotrophic bacteria, actinomycetes, and fungi, are indigenous. Among the pathogens that may be present in soil are *Clostridium tetani* and *Clostridium perfringens,* the etiologic agents of tetanus and gas gangrene. These organisms can be cultured from uncontaminated soil and thus are able to grow in this environment, as well as from soil contaminated by animal and human feces. Another species, *Clostridium botulinum,* whose toxin is responsible for the symptoms of botulism, also is present in soil and from this source may find its way into improperly processed foods or contaminated wounds. *Bacillus anthracis,* the causative agent of anthrax, is deposited in the soil when animals die of the disease. It infects herbivorous animals and occasionally humans by entering the body through the skin or mucous membranes. *Clostridium* and *Bacillus* species produce endospores that are of survival advantage to the bacterial cell in that they confer resistance to adverse environmental conditions. Certain of the pathogenic fungi, *C. immitis, H. capsulatum, Cryptococcus neoformans,* and *Blastomyces dermatitidis,* also have been grown from the soil. Inhalation of spores aerosolized from soil results in entry of the organism into the respiratory tract of humans and other animals.

Water

Most bodies of saltwater and freshwater contain microorganisms, many of which are adapted to extremely adverse conditions (e.g., psychrophilic, halophilic, and thermophilic bacteria). Pathogenic bacteria, however, usually are not present except in water that is directly contaminated by human or animal urine and feces. Among the pathogenic organisms that often reach water used for drinking or recreational purposes are the enteric pathogens *Salmonella* and *Shigella* species, *Vibrio cholerae,* hepatitis A virus, polio viruses, and other enteroviruses. These organisms, however, are infrequently isolated directly from water. Therefore the isolation of *Escherichia coli,* which is a hardier organism and persists in water for longer periods, serves as an index of fecal contamination. *Legionella pneumophila,* the agent of Legionnaires' disease, also has been isolated from water. Aerosolization of water contaminated with this organism has resulted in epidemics of this disease.

Air

Although microorganisms frequently are found in air, they do not multiply in this medium. The outdoor air rarely contains pathogens, probably because of the bactericidal effects of desiccation, ozone, and ultraviolet radiation. Indoor air, however, may contain pathogenic viruses and bacteria that are shed by humans from the skin, hands, clothing, and especially the upper respiratory tract.

Talking, coughing, and sneezing produce progressively larger numbers of respiratory droplets, many of which contain bacteria and viruses. A sneeze (Fig. 22–1) may produce as many as 10^6 particles from 10 μm to 2 mm in diameter. The larger droplets may travel a distance of 1 to 3 m before reaching the ground. These larger droplets rapidly settle to the floor and dry, leaving organisms attached to dust particles. The smaller droplets remain suspended in air and evaporate rapidly, leaving behind droplet nuclei a few micrometers in diameter, which may or may not contain organisms. These droplet nuclei settle very slowly and, in an ordinary room filled with people, are wafted about in air currents and remain suspended almost indefinitely. Under such conditions great accumulations of potentially infective particles may occur.

Animals and Animal Products

Animals are hosts for many of the microorganisms that produce disease in humans (e.g., tularemia, brucellosis, psittacosis, salmonellosis, plague, anthrax, insect-borne viral and

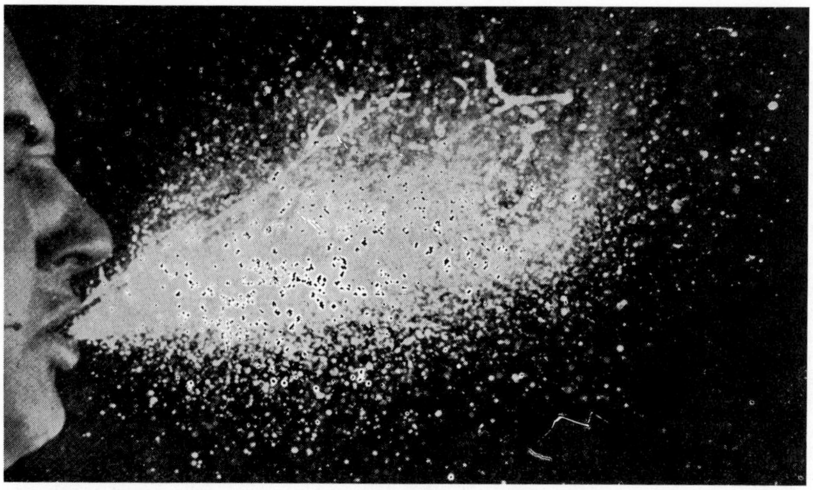

Fig. 22–1. Droplet dispersal after a sneeze by a patient with a cold. Note strings of mucus. *(From Jennison: Aerobiology 17:106, 1947.)*

rickettsial diseases, and parasitic diseases). These diseases may be transmitted directly; by vectors; by contamination of soil, water, or other materials; or by ingestion of meat or dairy products.

Milk from healthy cows, even when drawn under aseptic conditions, usually contains from 100 to 1000 nonpathogenic organisms per milliliter. Other organisms may be present when cows are diseased or may be added during collection. Diseases that may be transmitted by diseased cows or milk handlers include tuberculosis, salmonellosis, streptococcal infection, diphtheria, shigellosis, brucellosis, and staphylococcal food poisoning. Pasteurization processes and the destruction of diseased cattle have decreased the incidence of milk-borne infections.

Microbial Flora of Normal Human Body

Humans are consistently bombarded by the myriads of microorganisms that occupy the environment. Fortunately, however, humans do not provide a favorable habitat for most of these saprophytes because they must compete with the commensal flora that is already adapted to the human environment. Those organisms that constitute the normal flora must overcome barriers to colonization produced by the flow of body juices, mucociliary clearance, and local immune mechanisms (Table 22–1). In addition, the persistence of various organisms in their specific niches may depend on attachment to host cells in these areas (Chap. 21).

Skin

Human skin normally contains a varied microbial population. The predominant organisms are *Staphylococcus epidermidis*, aerobic and anaerobic diphtheroids (*Corynebacterium* spp and *Propionibacterium acnes*), and *Micrococcus* species. *Staphylococcus aureus* regularly inhabits only the nose and perhaps the perineum, but transient colonization by this and other bacteria, such as alpha and nonhemolytic streptococci, may occur at any site. Saprophytic mycobacteria occasionally are found on the skin of the external auditory canal and the genital and axillary regions. Two lipophilic yeasts (*Pityrosporum ovale* and *Pityrosporum orbiculare*) frequently are present on the scalp or chest and on the back, respectively. Nonlipophilic yeasts are also variably present.

Most of these organisms inhabit the stratum corneum and the upper parts of hair follicles. A small number, however, are present deeper within follicles and serve as a reservoir for replenishing the flora after washing. Washing may decrease skin counts by 90%, but normal numbers are found again within 8 hours. Abstinence from washing does not lead to an increase in numbers of bacteria on the skin. Normally 10^3 to 10^4 organisms are found per square centimeter. However, counts may increase to $10^6/cm^2$ in more humid body areas such as the groin and axilla. Small numbers of bacteria are dispersed from the skin to the environment, but certain individuals may shed up to 10^6 organisms in 30 minutes of exercise. Many of the fatty acids found on the skin may be bacterial products that inhibit colonization by other species. The flora of hair is similar to that of the skin.

Conjunctivae. The relative freedom of the normal conjunctivae from infections may be explained by the mechanical action of the eyelids, the washing effect of the normal secretions that contain the bacteriolytic enzyme lysozyme, and the production of inhibitors by the normal flora of the eye. *S. epidermidis* and various aerobic and anaerobic diphtheroids frequently are isolated from the conjunctival sac, presumably arising from the flora of the eyelids.

Nose and Nasopharynx

Innumerable bacteria are filtered from the air as it passes through the nasopharynx, trachea, and bronchi. The majority of these organisms are trapped in mucous secretions and are swallowed. Thus the sinuses, trachea, bronchi, and lungs usually are sterile. The nasopharynx is the natural habitat of the common pathogenic bacteria and viruses that cause infections in the nose, throat, bronchi, and lungs. Humans are the primary host for these organisms. Thus individuals with active infection, or convalescent and symptom-free carriers, maintain the reservoir from which others become infected. Certain

TABLE 22–1. PREDOMINANT NORMAL FLORA AT VARIOUS BODY SITES

Body Site	Microbial Flora
Skin	*Staphylococcus epidermidis, Corynebacterium, Propionibacterium, Micrococcus*, yeasts
Conjunctivae	*Staphylococcus epidermidis*
Nose and nasopharynx	*Staphylococcus epidermidis, Staphylococcus aureus, Streptococcus* spp
Mouth and oropharynx	*S. epidermidis*, non–group A streptococci, *Streptococcus pneumoniae, Streptococcus mitis, Streptococcus salivarius, Neisseria, Haemophilus, Veillonella, Bacteroides, Fusobacterium, Treponema, Lactobacillus*, yeasts
Intestinal tract	
Small intestine	*Lactobacillus, Streptococcus* spp, *Enterococcus, Veillonella*, actinomycetes, yeasts
Large intestine	*Bacteroides, Clostridium, Fusobacterium, Eubacterium, Bifidobacterium, Lactobacillus, Peptostreptococcus, Enterococcus*, Enterobacteriaceae
Genitourinary tract	*Corynebacterium*, alpha and nonhemolytic streptococci, *Staphylococcus epidermidis, Enterococcus, Lactobacillus, Mycobacterium smegmatis*, Enterobacteriaceae, *Bacteroides, Fusobacterium*
Blood and cerebrospinal fluid	Sterile
Tissues, bladder, uterus and fallopian tubes, middle ear, paranasal sinuses	Sterile

individuals become nasal carriers for streptococci and staphylococci and discharge these organisms in enormous numbers from the nose into the air. These staphylococci frequently produce skin infections that tend to recur. Efforts to eradicate *S. aureus* from the nares of such individuals by the use of antibiotics have met with limited success.

The nasopharynx of the newborn infant is sterile, but within 2 to 3 days the infant acquires the common commensal flora and the pathogenic flora carried by the mother and nursing staff. The carrier rate of pathogens (such as group A streptococci, *Haemophilus influenzae*, and pneumococci) may be almost 100% in infants and is higher in children than in adults.

Mouth and Oropharynx

The pharynx usually contains a mixture of viridans (alpha and nonhemolytic) streptococci, nonpathogenic *Neisseria* species, *Branhamella catarrhalis*, and *S. epidermidis*. The streptococci and staphylococci are inhibitory to *S. aureus* and *Neisseria meningitidis*. Many strains of viridans streptococci also are inhibitory to *S. pyogenes*. Children infected with *S. pyogenes* may have fewer inhibitory strains than those who are not infected. Also, colonization with inhibitory flora increases with age. The normal flora of the pharynx may be eradicated by high doses of penicillin, thereby resulting in colonization and overgrowth with gram-negative organisms such as *E. coli, Klebsiella, Proteus*, and *Pseudomonas*. If the viridans streptococci, however, are made resistant to penicillin by stepwise increases in dosage, no abnormal colonization occurs.

Streptococcal species constitute 30% to 60% of the bacterial flora of the surfaces within the mouth. These are primarily viridans streptococci: *Streptococcus salivarius, Streptococcus mitis, Streptococcus mutans*, and *Streptococcus sanguis*. *S. mitis* is found primarily on the buccal mucosa, *S. salivarius* on the tongue, and *S. mutans* and *S. sanguis* on the teeth and dental plaque. Specific binding to mucosal cells or to tooth enamel has been demonstrated with these organisms. Bacterial plaque developing on teeth may contain as many as 10^{11} streptococci per gram in addition to actinomycetes, *Veillonella* bacteria, and *Bacteroides* species. Anaerobic flora, such as *Bacteroides melaninogenicus, Treponema, Fusobacterium, Clostridium, Propionibacterium*, and *Peptostreptococcus*, are present in gingival crevices where the oxygen concentration is less than 0.5%. Many of these organisms are obligate anaerobes and do not survive in higher oxygen concentrations. These organisms, when aspirated into the tracheobronchial tree, may play a role in the pathogenesis of anaerobic pneumonia and lung abscess. The natural habitat of the pathogenic species *Actinomyces israelii* is the gingival crevice. Among the fungi, species of *Candida* and *Geotrichum* are found in 10% to 15% of individuals.

The newborn infant's mouth is not sterile but, in general, contains the same types of organisms present in the mother's vagina, which usually consists of a mixture of *Lactobacillus, Corynebacterium, Staphylococcus, Micrococcus, Streptococcus*, coliforms, and yeasts. Among the streptococci are enterococci—microaerophilic and anaerobic species—and of specific importance in neonatal sepsis and meningitis, group B streptococci. These organisms diminish in number during the first 2 to 5 days after birth and are replaced by the types of bacteria present in the mouth of the mother or nurse. Anaerobic flora appear after the eruption of teeth and the production of gingival crevices.

Intestinal Tract

Stomach and Small Intestine. In normal fasting individuals the stomach and upper portion of the small intestine usually are sterile or contain fewer than 10^3 organisms per milliliter. Organisms swallowed from the mouth are either killed by the hydrochloric acid and enzymes in gastric secretions or passed quickly into the small intestine where forward peristalsis, bile, and pancreatic enzymes are responsible for maintaining sterility or keeping the number of organisms fewer than 10^3/mL. When the gastric pH is greater than 5, salivary, nasopharyngeal, and fecal-type flora may colonize the stomach. When organisms are present in the duodenum or jejunum, they usually consist of small numbers of *Streptococcus, Lactobacillus, Haemophilus, Veillonella*, actinomycetes, and yeasts, especially *C. albicans*. Larger numbers of bacteria normally are found in the terminal ileum. Under abnormal conditions, such as gastric achlorhydria, abnormal peristalsis (scleroderma and diabetes), or blind loops after gastric surgery, bacterial overgrowth may occur. This may result in megaloblastic anemia due to bacterial depletion of vitamin B_{12} or in fat malabsorption and diarrhea secondary to deconjugation of bile salts and release of free deoxycholic acid, which may be toxic to small bowel mucosa.

Large Intestine. In contrast to the small numbers of organisms found in the small intestine, the microflora of the colon represents a rich ecosystem composed of metabolically active microorganisms in close proximity to an absorptive mucosal surface. Approximately 20% of the fecal mass consists of bacteria (10^{11} organisms per gram wet weight). It is estimated that 400 different species of bacteria comprise the intestinal flora of any given person. Most of these are obligate anaerobes that predominate over facultative organisms by a factor of 1000:1. Major species of organisms in the colon are *Bacteroides, Bifidobacterium, Fusobacterium, Eubacterium, Lactobacillus,* coliforms, aerobic and anaerobic streptococci, *Clostridium,* and variable numbers of yeasts. More than 90% of the fecal flora consist of *Bacteroides* and *Bifidobacterium,* both of which are obligate anaerobes. The relative numbers of the bacteria may vary from population to population. Factors that determine the balance of these bacterial species are poorly understood. The production of colicins by enterobacteria perhaps accounts for the predominance of a few serotypes of these species. In addition, the normal flora of the large intestine is more resistant to bile and pancreatic enzymes (enterococci, enterobacteria, *Bacteroides*).

INTESTINAL TRACT OF NEWBORN. The intestinal tract of the newborn child usually is sterile, although a few organisms may be acquired during delivery. Under normal circumstances, intestinal flora are established within the first 24 hours after delivery, primarily from the aforementioned organisms. The stool of the breast-fed infant is soft and light yellowish brown, and it has a faintly acid odor. *Lactobacillus bifidus* is the prominent organism in these stools, others being enterococci, coliforms, and staphylococci. In contrast, artificially fed infants have hard, dark brown, foul-smelling stools that contain *Lactobacillus acidophilus,* coliforms, enterococci, and anaerobic bacilli, including clostridial species. *L. bifidus* may return after the addition of 12% lactose to cow's milk or other formulas.

ANTIBIOTIC ALTERATION OF FLORA. The flora may be altered by the administration of antibiotics; for example, cephalosporins decrease aerobic and anaerobic streptococci and *Lactobacillus,* whereas clindamycin may totally eradicate most of the anaerobic species (*Bacteroides, Bifidobacterium,* and *Lactobacillus*). Eradication of normal flora and overgrowth by enterotoxin-producing *Clostridium difficile* are responsible for some forms of antibiotic-induced colitis. Colonic flora also may play a role in disease when the integrity of the gut is compromised, as in appendicitis, diverticulitis, intestinal perforation, and postoperative infections, and may supply the flora (coliforms) that are the major cause of urinary tract infection and gram-negative bacteremia.

SIGNIFICANCE OF INTESTINAL FLORA. Since the time of Pasteur, the significance of the intestinal flora has been a controversial issue. Are the microorganisms essential for life, a natural but inevitable handicap, or a nonessential asset? Pasteur's studies on microbial fermentations suggested that the intestinal organisms might play an essential role in the metabolism of foodstuffs, analogous to that of the protozoa in the gut of termites, but subsequent studies in germ-free animals have shown that these flora are not essential. Intestinal flora do, however, have complex effects on the rate of maturation of intestinal epithelial cells, as well as on the levels of various cytoplasmic enzymes in these cells.

The bacteria of the intestinal tract possess an impressive array of enzymes that can convert endogenous and exogenous substrates into a wide spectrum of metabolites. Among the most active of these are the glycosidases that break down dietary sugars or glucuronide metabolites excreted by the liver. In individuals with a lactase deficiency (which occurs in up to 80% of some populations), lactose is metabolized by intestinal bacteria, which results in abdominal discomfort, flatulence, and diarrhea due to increased water retention and lowered pH. Many bacteria attack nitrogen-containing compounds. Urease-producing organisms hydrolyze urea to CO_2 and NH_3; amino acids are deamidated; and diazo compounds are esterified, dealkylated, hydrolyzed, or reduced. Bile acids (cholanic acids conjugated with taurine or glycine) are dehydroxylated or hydrolyzed to free bile acids. Bilirubin is metabolized by intestinal microorganisms to urobilinogen, which is reabsorbed and excreted in the urine or bile.

Considerable interest recently has focused on the possible role of intestinal bacteria as a metabolic intermediary in colon cancer. A number of bacterial enzymes in the intestinal microflora have been implicated in the generation of mutagens and carcinogens. Among the most active of these are β-glucuronidase, β-glucosidase, β-galactosidases, azoreductase, and nitroreductase. Bacterial β-glucuronidase appears to play an especially important role in the metabolism of colon carcinogens. It has wide substrate specificity and can alter or amplify the biologic activity of exogenous and endogenous compounds. Among the intestinal bacteria that produce high levels of this enzyme are *Bacteroides, Eubacterium, Peptostreptococcus* and *E. coli.* These organisms have been shown to hydrolyze glucuronides secreted into the bile to potent mutagenic aglycones. Intestinal bacteria have been incriminated in the generation of mutagens from a number of azo dyes used as color additives in food and textile industries. Bacterial azoreductases reductively hydrolyze the azo bond, which results in the formation of aromatic amines, some of which are highly carcinogenic. The reduction of nitro groups by intestinal microflora is another source of aromatic amines.

The role of bacteria in the metabolism of drugs is poorly understood. An interesting phenomenon, however, is known to occur with salicylazosulfapyridine, a drug used in the treatment of inflammatory bowel diseases. This compound is metabolized to sulfapyridine and 5-aminosalicylate by the intestinal microflora; this does not occur in germ-free animals. It is possible that the antiinflammatory effects of the drug are related to its intraluminal cleavage and high local levels of 5-aminosalicylate. Chemical modification, however, may alter drug activity; for example, *Eubacterium lentum* has been shown to reduce digoxin to dihydrodigoxin, which leads to increased dosage requirements in some patients. Many antibiotics are inactivated by the intestinal flora. Clinical evidence indicates that the intestinal bacteria also serve as the major reservoir for antibiotic-resistance plasmids. If individuals carrying these drug-resistant saprophytic species in their gut become infected with pathogenic organisms, the drug-resistance plasmids may be transmitted to the drug-susceptible pathogen.

A beneficial role for intestinal bacteria also can be demonstrated. They produce a number of the vitamins, especially those of the B complex. The treatment of patients with broad-spectrum or poorly absorbable oral antibiotics may greatly reduce or alter the normal flora, thereby inducing vitamin deficiencies in individuals with poor nutrition.

The normal flora have an immense but still incompletely understood effect on the immune system. Some of the organisms that colonize the gut share cross-reactive antigens with many bacterial species. The natural antibodies that arise in response to these antigens of the normal gut flora are of great importance in immunity to a number of pathogenic species, especially encapsulated organisms such as *Haemophilus influenzae* type b and *Neisseria meningitidis*. Blood group antibodies are a consequence of constant immunization against intestinal flora that possess cross-reactive antigens.

Genitourinary Tract

The genitourinary tract and its unique microflora form a finely balanced ecosystem. The genitourinary environment controls the types of organisms present, and the microflora exert their effects and controls on the environment of the ecosystem. The microflora are not a static population but fluctuate in response to environmental changes.

External Genitalia and Anterior Urethra. In addition to the normal "skin flora" (diphtheroids, alpha and nonhemolytic streptococci, *S. epidermidis*), the anterior urethra of both males and females may contain *Mycobacterium smegmatis* and species of Enterobacteriaceae, *Bacteroides*, and *Fusobacterium*. The female flora also contain many *Lactobacillus* species, including both facultative and obligate anaerobes. Sexually active individuals may harbor such organisms as mycoplasmas and ureaplasmas. The sterility of the internal urethra is maintained primarily by the normal flow of urine and evacuation of the bladder. Urine aspirated from the bladder with a needle normally is sterile.

Vagina. The vulva of the newborn child is sterile, but after the first 24 hours of life it gradually acquires a rich and varied flora of nonpathogenic organisms such as diphtheroids, micrococci, and nonhemolytic streptococci. After 2 to 3 days, estrogen from the maternal circulation induces the deposition of glycogen in the vaginal epithelium, which facilitates the growth of *Lactobacillus* (Döderlein's bacillus). These organisms produce acid from glycogen, and a flora develops that resembles that of the adult female. After the passively transferred estrogen is excreted, the glycogen disappears, the lactobacilli are lost, and the pH again becomes alkaline. At puberty the glycogen reappears, and an adult flora again returns. On both aerobic and anaerobic cultures, these flora usually consist of diphtheroids, lactobacilli, micrococci, *S. epidermidis, Enterococcus faecalis,* microaerophilic and anaerobic streptococci, ureaplasmas, and yeasts. The presence of *Gardnerella vaginalis, Mobiluncus,* or *Chlamydia* is usually associated with symptomatic vaginitis.

Despite the close proximity of the anus, the vaginal flora of healthy women only rarely shows even small numbers of coliforms. It has been shown, however, that women who are prone to recurrent urinary tract infection generally demonstrate vaginal and urethral colonization with coliforms before the invasion of the bladder by these organisms. Normal flora probably play an important role in inhibiting the attachment of pathogens. During pregnancy, 15% to 20% of women are colonized with group B streptococci (*Streptococcus agalactiae*), an agent that has assumed increased importance in the etiology of neonatal sepsis and meningitis. After menopause the flora resembles that found before puberty.

Blood and Tissues

Occasionally commensals from the normal flora of the mouth, nasopharynx, and intestinal tract are carried into the blood and to tissues. Under normal circumstances, they are eliminated by normal defense mechanisms, particularly phagocytosis by reticuloendothelial cells. A few organisms may remain viable for a time in lymph nodes and may be cultured from biopsy specimens of such tissues. Any unusual organisms of questionable pathogenicity that appear in only one of a series of blood cultures should be regarded as a contaminant from the skin or a stray transient. Simple manipulations, such as chewing, tooth brushing, dental work, genitourinary catheterization or instrumentation, and proctosigmoidoscopy, also may be associated with transient bacteremia. This phenomenon generally is of little consequence in the normal host. In the presence of abnormal heart valves, prosthetic heart valves, or other prosthetic devices made of foreign materials, however, these bacteremias may lead to colonization and infection by pathogenic organisms or saprophytes of low pathogenicity.

Nosocomial Infections

Nosocomial or hospital-acquired infections are of particular concern to the medical and nursing professions. These infections are transmitted to patients by hospital personnel and other patients, or they may arise from the patient's own endogenous flora. Modes of acquisition include surgical procedures, indwelling intravenous or bladder catheters, endotracheal tubes, intravenous fluids, and equipment used for respiratory support. Of particular importance is the seemingly innocuous acquisition of pathogenic or opportunistic organisms into the pool of normal flora that predispose compromised individuals to subsequent invasion by their own indigenous organisms. This is particularly true of postoperative patients and individuals treated with antibiotics, immunosuppressants, or antineoplastic agents. These organisms include the usual pathogens such as *S. aureus* and invasive strains of *E. coli,* as well as other enterobacteria, *Pseudomonas,* opportunistic fungi, and viruses (Table 22–2).

Nosocomial infections occur in approximately 5% of all patients admitted. These rates vary depending on the type of hospital (e.g., acute versus extended care facilities). More than 80% of these infections involve the urinary and respiratory tracts and surgical wounds. The use of antibiotics in hospitals predisposes to the selection of resistant organisms that may inadvertently be passed from patient to patient by the mechanisms described above. In addition, the duration of hospitalization plays a significant role in the development of pharyngeal colonization by gram-negative bacteria. Thus physicians and nursing personnel should be constantly aware of the role of antibiotics and person-to-person transmission in the genesis of hospital-acquired infections. Infection committees with surveillance programs must be an integral part of the modern hospital.

TABLE 22–2. NOSOCOMIAL INFECTIONS IN ACUTE CARE INSTITUTIONS

Infection Site	Percentage of All Nosocomial Infection	Most Common Agents
Urinary tract	40%	*Escherichia coli, Enterococcus, Proteus, Klebsiella, Pseudomonas aeruginosa*
Surgical wound	20%	*Staphylococcus aureus, Staphylococcus epidermidis, Escherichia coli*
Pulmonary	10%	*Klebsiella, Pseudomonas, Escherichia coli, Staphylococcus aureus*
Primary bacteremia	5%–10%	*Staphylococcus aureus, Staphylococcus epidermidis,* gram-negative rods
Others	20%–25%	*Staphylococcus aureus, Escherichia coli*

TABLE 22–3. MISCELLANEOUS CONDITIONS PREDISPOSING TO COMPROMISED HOST DEFENSES

Drugs: immunosuppressive, antibiotics, anesthetics
Alcoholism
Malnutrition
Viral infections, e.g., influenza, measles, human immunodeficiency virus
Alterations in normal mucosal-cutaneous barriers
Iatrogenic procedures
Prosthetic devices
- Intravenous catheters, bladder catheters
- Respiratory assist devices, i.e., inhalation therapy, nebulizers, respirators
- Whirlpools

Opportunistic Infections

Infections that occur as a result of abnormalities in host defenses generally are referred to as *opportunistic.* These infections may be caused by bona fide pathogens or by organisms of low virulence such as those that constitute the normal body flora or are a part of the nonpathogenic transient flora. Opportunistic infection may occur either as a complication of abnormal defense mechanisms or as a result of various iatrogenic or nosocomial factors. For example, diabetics and alcoholics, two groups of individuals at increased risk for gram-negative rod pneumonias, have twice the normal incidence of gram-negative rods as part of their resident pharyngeal flora. Similar increases in pharyngeal colonization may be observed after the administration of broad-spectrum antibiotics such as ampicillin, cephalosporins, clindamycin, and tetracyclines. Tetracyclines frequently are associated with *Candida* vaginitis or thrush. Many of these drugs may result in pseudomembranous colitis, which is caused by an overgrowth of the colonic flora by *C. difficile.*

Other infections, such as measles or influenza, may lead to superinfections through depression of phagocytosis and chemotaxis, decreased cell-mediated immunity, or damage to the respiratory epithelium. Infection with the human immunodeficiency virus produces destruction of T4 lymphocytes and markedly impaired cell-mediated immunity.

Hospital admission results in the acquisition of new flora, many of which may be potential pathogens. Many of the procedures performed on hospitalized patients lead to colonization and potential superinfection. These are outlined in the section on nosocomial infections and in Table 22–3.

Inherited or acquired disorders of immune function may result in abnormal antibody synthesis, absence of cell-mediated immunity, or impaired neutrophil killing or chemotaxis. In addition, iatrogenic factors such as immunosuppression in cancer patients or transplant recipients produce broad disorders of normal defenses. Neutropenia induced by antitumor

TABLE 22–4. INFECTIONS MOST COMMONLY ASSOCIATED WITH IMMUNE DEFICIENCIES

Defect	Predisposing Condition	Infection
Phagocytic abnormalities	Acute leukemia, cytotoxic drugs, radiation therapy, corticosteroid therapy, diabetes	Localized and systemic infection with *Staphylococcus aureus, Staphylococcus epidermidis, Pseudomonas aeruginosa,* Enterobacteriaceae, *Candida, Aspergillus,* Zygomycetes
	Splenectomy	Bacteremias with *Streptococcus pneumoniae, Haemophilus influenzae*
Complement abnormalities	Genetic disorders	
	C3 deficiency	Bacteremias and pneumonias with encapsulated organisms
	C5–C9 deficiency	Disseminated *Neisseria* infections
Antibody deficiency	Hypogammaglobulinemia, multiple myeloma, lymphocytic leukemias, lymphomas, nephrotic syndrome, steroids or cytotoxic drug therapy	Systemic infections with encapsulated and extracellular bacteria, enteroviruses, *Giardia*
Cell-mediated immunity dysfunction	Hodgkin's disease, steroid therapy, cytotoxic drug therapy, uremia, malnutrition, AIDS	Systemic infection with *Mycobacterium* and other intracellular bacteria, *Candida* and systemic fungi, DNA viruses, protozoa, *Pneumocystis, Strongyloides*

drugs may turn such commensals as *S. epidermidis*, *Propionibacterium acnes*, *Candida* species, bacilli, and micrococci into virulent pathogens. Examples of associations between various host defects and infecting organisms are presented in Table 22–4. With these patients great care must be taken to prevent introduction of organisms from the environment; for example, patients with neutropenia should not be given raw fruits or vegetables, which frequently are contaminated with *P. aeruginosa*. An outbreak of aspergillosis in patients with leukemia has been associated with the intake of air from a construction site into the ventilation system of a hospital.

Control of the resident flora has been attempted in some of these instances. Gut *sterilization* by orally administered antibiotics and placement of patients in isolation laminar flow rooms may decrease the incidence of infection. Infants with severe combined immunodeficiency (total absence of cell-mediated and humoral immunity) have been kept alive in a sterile environment while awaiting bone marrow transplantation. These procedures, however, are extraordinarily expensive. More recently, antibiotics, such as co-trimoxazole, aztreonam, and the quinolones, which preferentially inhibit gram-negative aerobic pathogens, have been used to *selectively* decontaminate the intestinal tract.

Ultimately, the successful treatment of such inherited disorders and neoplastic diseases will rest on the ability of medical science to control and prevent infections from the body's resident flora.

FURTHER READING

Books and Reviews

Britton G, Marshall KC: Adsorption of Microorganisms to Surfaces. New York, Wiley, 1980

Hentges DJ: Human Intestinal Microflora in Health and Disease. New York, Academic Press, 1983

McDermott W: Conference on air borne infections. Bacteriol Rev 25:173, 1961

Noble WC: Microbiology of Human Skin. London, Lloyd-Luke, 1981

Rosebury T: Microorganisms Indigenous to Man. New York, McGraw-Hill, 1962

Skinner FA, Carr JG: The Normal Microbial Flora of Man. New York, Academic Press, 1974

Smith T: Parasitism and Disease. Princeton, NJ, Princeton University Press, 1934

Selected Papers

Beachey EH: Bacterial adherence: Adhesion-receptor interactions mediating the attachment of bacteria to mucosal surfaces. J Infect Dis 143:325, 1981

Brun-Buisson C, Philippon, Ansquer M, et al: Transferable enzymatic resistance to third-generation cephalosporins during nosocomial outbreak of multiresistant *Klebsiella pneumoniae*. Lancet 2:302, 1987

Cohen R, Roth FJ, Delgado E, et al: Fungal flora of the normal human small and large intestine. N Engl J Med 280:638, 1969

Craven DE, Kunches LM, Kilinsky V, et al: Risk factors for pneumonia and fatality in patients receiving continuous mechanical ventilation. Am Rev Respir Dis 133:792, 1986

Daifuku R, Stamm W: Bacterial adherence to bladder uroepithelial cells in catheter-associated urinary tract infection. N Engl J Med 314:1208, 1986

Drasar BS, Shiner M, McLeod GM: Studies on the intestinal flora. I. The bacterial flora of the gastrointestinal tract in healthy and achlorhydric persons. Gastroenterology 56:71, 1969

Edens CS, Eriksson B, Hanson LA: Adhesion of *Escherichia coli* to human uroepithelial cells in vitro. Infect Immun 18:767, 1977

Evaldson G, Heimdahl A, Kager L, et al: The normal human anaerobic microflora. Scand J Infect Dis [suppl] 35:9, 1982

Goldacre MF, Watt B, Loudon N, et al: Vaginal microbial flora in normal young women. Br Med J 1:1450, 1979

Gossling J, Slack JM: Predominant gram-positive bacteria in human feces: Numbers, variety, and persistence. Infect Immun 9:719, 1974

Jennison MW: Atomizing of mouth and nose secretions into the air as revealed by high-speed photography. Aerobiology 17:106, 1947

Mackowiak PA: The normal microbial flora. N Engl J Med 307:83, 1982

Mobley HLT, Chipendale GR, Tenney JH, et al: MR/K hemagglutination of *Providencia stuartii* correlates with catheter adherence and with persistence in catheter-associated bacteriuria. J Infect Dis 157:264, 1988

Nord CE, Heimdahl A, Kager L, et al: The impact of different antimicrobial agents on the normal gastrointestinal microflora of humans. Rev Infect Dis 6 [suppl 1]:270, 1984

Patterson TF, Patterson JE, Masecar BL, et al: A nosocomial outbreak of *Branhamella catarrhalis* confirmed by restriction endonuclease analysis. J Infect Dis 157:996, 1988

Platt R, Polk BF, Murdock B, et al: Risk factors for nosocomial urinary tract infection. Am J Epidemiol 124:977, 1986

Saigh JH, Sanders CC, Sanders WE Jr: Inhibition of *Neisseria gonorrhoeae* by aerobic and facultatively anaerobic components of the endocervical flora: Evidence for a protective effect against infection. Infect Immun 19:704, 1978

Schimpff SC: Surveillance cultures. J Infect Dis 144:81, 1981

Schimpff SC, Green WH, Young VM, et al: Infection prevention in acute nonlymphocytic leukemia. Laminar air flow room reverse isolation with oral, nonabsorbable antibiotic prophylaxis. Ann Intern Med 73:351, 1975

Sen P, Kapila R, Chmel H, et al: Superinfection: Another look. Am J Med 73:707, 1982

Warren JW, Damron D, Tenney JH, et al: Fever, bacteremia, and death as complications of bacteriuria in women with long-term urethral catheters. J Infect Dis 155:1151, 1987

CHAPTER 23

Staphylococcus

Staphylococci are ubiquitous organisms and among the most commonly encountered in medical practice. In spite of the introduction of antimicrobial agents and improvements in hygiene, which have been pivotal in reducing the frequency and morbidity of staphylococcal diseases in the twentieth century, staphylococci have persisted as an important hospital and community pathogen. They are responsible for more than 80% of the suppurative diseases encountered in medical practice and are second only to *Escherichia coli* as a cause of hospital-acquired infections.

The primary natural habitat of staphylococci is mammalian body surfaces, where the organisms are found in large numbers. In their adaptation to parasitism, staphylococci have been among the most versatile and successful of the pathogenic bacteria. Their latent aggressivity is manifested, however, only if the surface barrier is breached because of trauma or surgery and organisms gain access to the underlying tissue. Once the bloodstream is invaded, staphylococci can produce acute endocarditis and widespread metastatic lesions. A major factor in the persistence of the organism in spite of the introduction of many effective antistaphylococcal antibiotics during the past 40 years is the ability of the staphylococcus to develop resistance to these agents. Of primary concern has been the development of strains resistant to penicillin and its derivatives and the association of these strains with epidemic outbreaks of severe nosocomial infections.

The Genus *Staphylococcus*

Staphylococcus is the only genus of medical importance in the family Micrococcaceae. It contains gram-positive cocci that are

TABLE 23–1. CHARACTERISTICS DISTINGUISHING MEMBERS OF THE GENERA *STAPHYLOCOCCUS* AND *MICROCOCCUS*

	Staphylococcus	*Micrococcus*
Anaerobic growth, fermentation of glucose	+	–
Cell wall:		
Glycine-containing penta- or hexapeptide cross-bridges	+	–
Ribitol or glycerol teichoic acids	+	–
DNA: G + C content (mol%)	30–40	66–75

From Baird-Parker: Ann NY Acad Sci 236:8, 1974.
+, 90% or more strains positive; –, 90% or more strains negative.

facultatively anaerobic and grow in irregular clusters. Properties that distinguish staphylococci from members of the genus *Micrococcus,* which are also often present in soil, water, and on the skin of humans, are shown in Table 23–1. The name *staphylococcus,* derived from the Greek noun *staphyle* (a bunch of grapes) and *coccus* (a grain or berry), was introduced by early investigators to describe the organisms seen in pus from surgical infections. Since most strains freshly isolated from staphylococcal infections produced a golden yellow pigment, the organism was named *Staphylococcus aureus* to distinguish these strains from the less pathogenic staphylococci that usually produce white colonies. Pigment production, however, is a variable trait of staphylococci, and its correlation with pathogenicity is unreliable. Its use has been superseded by coagulase production, which is the most useful single criterion for the recognition of *S. aureus.* A staphylococcus that produces coagulase is *S. aureus,* irrespective of colony pigmentation.

Of the more than 20 species of *Staphylococcus,* only three are clinically significant: *S. aureus, S. epidermidis,* and *S. saprophyticus.* Properties useful for distinguishing the three species are shown in Table 23–2. Although *S. aureus* is the most significant pathogen for man, coagulase-negative staphylococci have emerged as pathogens causing nosocomial bacteremias. *S. epidermidis,* although relatively avirulent, is associated with hospital-acquired infections, especially in patients whose susceptibility is increased and in whom there is a nidus of foreign material, such as a prosthesis or plastic catheter. *S. saprophyticus* can cause urinary tract infections in women.

Staphylococcus aureus

Morphology

S. aureus is a nonmotile coccus, 0.8 to 1.0 μm in diameter, that divides in three planes to form irregular grapelike clusters of cells (Fig. 23–1). In smears from pus, the cocci appear singly, in pairs, in clusters, or in short chains. The irregular clusters are found characteristically in smears from cultures grown on solid media, whereas in broth cultures, short chains and diplococcal forms are common. A few strains produce a capsule or slime layer that enhances the virulence of the organisms. *S. aureus* is a gram-positive organism, but old cells and phagocytized organisms stain gram-negative.

Ultrastructure and Cell Composition. The architecture of a staphylococcus is similar to that of other gram-positive organisms. Thin sections of log phase cells reveal nucleoids, mesosomes, and a trilaminar cytoplasmic membrane that is separated from the cell wall by a periplasmic region. In encapsulated strains, a loose fimbriate or capsular layer also may be seen.

The cell wall of *S. aureus* consists of three major components: peptidoglycan, teichoic acids, and protein A. The composition of these materials has been useful in distinguishing *Staphylococcus* from *Micrococcus* and *S. aureus* from *S. epidermidis* (Tables 23–1 and 23–2). The peptidoglycan comprises 40% to 60% of the weight of the cell wall; the amounts of the other major components vary.

PEPTIDOGLYCAN. The primary structure of the staphylococcal peptidoglycan is distinctive for the species (see Fig. 6–2B). As

TABLE 23–2. CHARACTERISTICS DISTINGUISHING MAJOR SPECIES OF THE GENUS *STAPHYLOCOCCUS*

	S. aureus	*S. epidermidis*	*S. saprophyticus*
Coagulase	+	–	–
Anaerobic growth and fermentation of glucose	+	+	–
Mannitol			
Acid aerobically	+	v	v
Acid anaerobically	+	–	–
α-Toxin	+	–	–
Heat-resistant endonucleases	+	–	–
Biotin required for growth	–	+	NT
Cell wall			
Ribitol	+	–	+
Glycerol	–	+	v
Protein A	+	–	–
Novobiocin sensitivity[a]	S	S	R

From Baird-Parker: Ann NY Acad Sci 236:9, 1974.
+, 90% or more strains positive; –, 90% or more strains negative; v, some strains positive, some negative; NT, not tested.
[a] R, MIC > 2.0 μg/mL; S, MIC < 0.6 μg/mL.

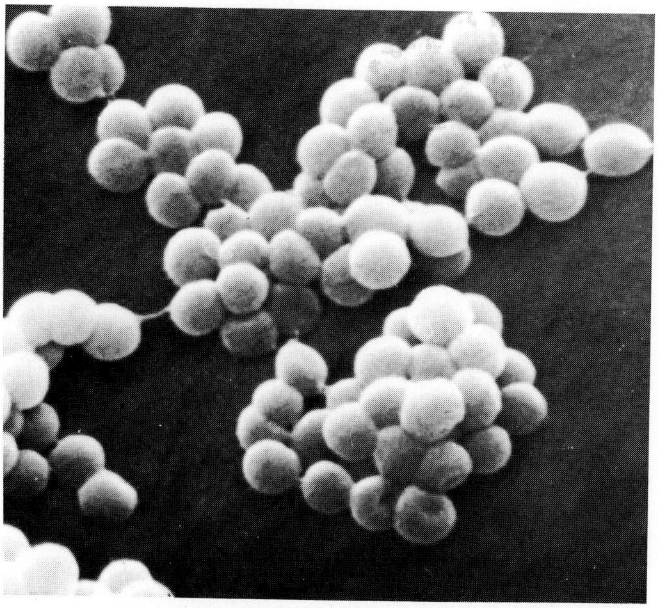

Fig. 23–1. Scanning electron photomicrograph of *S. aureus* in serum-salts broth. *(From Watanakunakorn: Infect Immun 4:73, 1971.)*

in most bacteria, the glycan portion of the molecule consists of alternating *N*-acetylglucosamine and *N*-acetylmuramic acid residues joined through β-1,4 glycosidic linkages. In staphylococci, however, all of the *N*-acetylmuramic acid residues carry tetrapeptide chains that are cross-linked by pentaglycine bridges. The extensive cross-linking of the peptide moiety gives the staphylococcal wall a tight structure that aids the cell in its quest for survival in the host tissues. Antibodies to the peptidoglycan are produced.

TEICHOIC ACID. In *S. aureus* the wall teichoic acid is of the ribitol phosphate type (see Fig. 6–4). The walls of *S. epidermidis* contain a glycerol teichoic acid, whereas in micrococci there is another type of teichoic acid or, usually, no teichoic acid at all. Teichoic acid is an essential component of the phage receptor of *S. aureus.* It also plays an important role in the maintenance of normal physiologic functions. By regulating the cationic environment of the bacterial cell, it controls the activity of autolytic enzymes that function in growth of the cell wall and separation of daughter cells. Although mutants completely lacking teichoic acid do exist, showing that the polymer is not essential for viability, such mutants are phage-resistant, grow more slowly than wild-type organisms, and produce large, bizarre, nonseparating cells with an abnormal crosswall structure (p. 405).

PROTEIN A. The major protein component of the cell wall of *S. aureus* is protein A, about one third of which is released into the medium during cell growth. This is a group antigen specific for most strains of *S. aureus;* it is not found in other staphylococci or in the micrococci. In the cell it is covalently linked to the peptidoglycan structure and uniformly distributed in the whole cell wall. Considerable interest has focused on protein A because of its unique property of interacting nonspecifically with immunoglobulins. The immunologic importance of protein A is discussed on page 405.

Physiology

Cultural Characteristics. The staphylococcus is a facultative anaerobe but growth is more abundant under aerobic conditions. Some strains also require an increased CO_2 tension. Growth occurs over a wide temperature range, from 6.5C to 46C, with an optimum for *S. aureus* of 30C to 37C. The pH optimum is 7.0 to 7.5, with growth occurring over a range of pH 4.2 to 9.3. Staphylococci have complex nutritional requirements but grow well on most routine laboratory media, such as nutrient agar or trypticase soy agar. For primary isolation from clinical materials, sheep blood agar is recommended. Human blood should not be used in the preparation of blood agar because it contains nonspecific inhibitors or antibodies.

On agar plates, colonies are smooth, opaque, round, low-convex, 1 to 4 mm in diameter. Most strains of *S. aureus* produce golden yellow colonies on primary isolation. The color can be attributed to carotenoid pigments and is extremely variable, ranging from deep orange to pale yellow. Because of this variability and the dependency of pigment production on growth conditions, colony pigmentation is not a valid criterion for the separation of *S. aureus* and *S. epidermidis.* Pigment production is best observed by growth on agar plates at 37C for 24 hours, followed by incubation at room temperature for an additional 24 to 48 hours. No pigment is produced under anaerobic conditions or in liquid media.

On blood agar, a zone of β hemolysis surrounds colonies of organisms that produce soluble hemolysins. Although primarily associated with *S. aureus,* β hemolysis also may be produced by strains of *S. epidermidis* and, as with pigmentation, is a variable property of the staphylococcus.

Metabolism. Energy is obtained via both respiratory and fermentative pathways. Intact pathways for glycolysis, the pentose phosphate pathway and the citric acid cycle are operative under appropriate growth conditions. The ability of the staphylococcus to exist under conditions of both high and low oxidation-reduction potential is an obvious advantage to the organism in its battle for survival in its natural habitat on mucosal surfaces and in competition with other bacterial species in the mixed microflora at the site of infection.

Catalase is produced by aerobically grown cells. In testing for this enzyme in blood agar cultures, precaution must be taken to avoid carryover of blood cells with the organisms. Catalase is present in red blood cells, which, if present in the bacterial mixture, may lead to a false-positive reaction.

A wide range of sugars and other carbohydrates are used by staphylococci. Under aerobic conditions the major product of glucose dissimilation is acetic acid with small amounts of carbon dioxide. Under anaerobic conditions, lactic acid is the principal product; acetoin also is usually produced. The fermentation of mannitol by most strains of *S. aureus* is helpful in its differentiation from *S. epidermidis.*

Identification. Major characteristics for distinguishing *S. aureus* from other staphylococci are shown in Table 23–2. Of these, the most convenient and reliable property for diagnostic purposes is the production of coagulases, enzymes that cause the coagulation of plasma. Approximately 97% of staphylococci isolated from pathologic processes elaborate these enzymes. In testing for coagulase, the test tube method should be employed. The slide test, although useful for screening purposes and usually correlating well with test tube results, detects a clumping factor on the surface of the organism that is distinct from the free coagulase. It is less reliable than the test tube method.

Classification

BACTERIOPHAGE TYPING. Most strains of *S. aureus* are lysogenic: they carry phages to which they themselves are immune but which will lyse some of the other members of the species. Susceptibility of *S. aureus* strains to the various temperate bacteriophages provides the basis for a phage-typing system that has been useful in epidemiologic studies. The system is based on patterns of sensitivity shown by each strain to various phages. The phage patterns of different strains fall essentially into three broad groups, phage groups I to III. The term *group* refers to strains of *S. aureus* with related phage patterns as well as to corresponding groups of phages with host range for these strains. The phages within a group are unrelated and possess different morphologic and serologic properties (groups A–L). The grouping of strains appears to be less fortuitous; that is, group II strains of staphylococci are often associated with skin infections, such as impetigo and pemphigus of the newborn, and the production of enterotoxin is confined primarily to phage group III. Group III phage types and strains within the 80/81 complex are most often incriminated in outbreaks of infection among newborn infants, older surgical and medical patients, and hospital personnel. Strains that cause exfoliative diseases usually belong to phage group II, and most of them are lysed only by phage 71. Strains untypable by the typing scheme currently in use are now being isolated with increasing frequency. The basis of phage patterns appears to lie in the strain-dependent restriction-modification systems on which lysogenic immunity and phage-dependent restriction are superimposed (Chap. 8).

The 23 phages that now constitute the basic set of typing phages are shown in Table 23–3. Only coagulase-positive staphylococci may be typed with the basic set of phages. For typing, each specific phage of the basic set is grown on its homologous propagating strain of *Staphylococcus*, separated from the bacterial cells by centrifugation and filtration, and after proper dilution a single drop is placed on separate squares of an agar plate previously seeded with a young broth culture of the organism to be typed. The plate is air-dried and incubated overnight at 30C. Phage typing results are recorded by listing only the phages that exhibit strong lysis (i.e., a 2^+ reaction indicating more than 50 plaques).

SPECIATION. In animals, variants of *S. aureus* have arisen as a result of adaptation to a particular host. Schemes that recognize such biotypes or ecotypes have been useful for epidemiologic and ecologic studies (Table 23–4). They have provided the basis for an emerging new classification of the *Staphylococcus* in which new species are recognized.

TABLE 23–3. LYTIC GROUPS OF *STAPHYLOCOCCUS* TYPING PHAGES IN THE BASIC SET OF TYPING PHAGES

Lytic Group	Phages in Group				
I	29	52	52A	79	80
II	3A	3C	55	71	
III	6	42E	47	53	54 75 77 83A 84 85
Unassigned	81	94	95	96	

TABLE 23–4. MAJOR NATURAL HOSTS OF *STAPHYLOCOCCUS* SPECIES

Species	Host(s)
S. hominis, S. epidermidis, S. capitus	Humans
S. haemolyticus, S. warneri, S. aureus, S. saprophyticus, S. simulans	Humans and nonhuman primates
S. cohnii	Humans, nonhuman primates, tree shrews
S. simians	Nonhuman primates
S. xylosus	Primates, carnivores, artiodactyls, perissodactyls, rodents, marsupials
S. intermedius	Carnivores
S. hyicus	Artiodactyls
S. sciuri	Mammals
S. lentus	Artiodactyls

Data from Kloos and Schleifer: In Starr et al. (eds): The Prokaryotes, vol. 2. New York, Springer-Verlag, 1981.

Genetics. The extreme flexibility of the staphylococcus has always made difficult the characterization of a typical *S. aureus*. The medical implications of this variability were not fully realized, however, until the spectacular emergence of antibiotic-resistant strains, first to penicillin and then successively to each antibiotic included in the therapeutic regimen. The serious epidemiologic and therapeutic problems created by these drug-resistant strains prompted genetic studies on the staphylococcus similar to those carried out with the enteric organisms. It has been shown that in *S. aureus*, as in the Enterobacteriaceae, most antibiotic resistance is plasmid mediated and that the genetics of the staphylococcus is basically analogous to the genetics of *E. coli*.

About 10% of the total cell DNA in naturally occurring organisms is plasmid DNA. Since these genetic elements have the capacity to evolve rapidly, they impart to the population of cells carrying them a better ability to survive under changing environmental conditions than cells containing a uniform DNA content.

Two distinct classes of staphylococcal plasmid have been demonstrated. One class comprises relatively large plasmids that often carry a variety of recognizable resistance markers and are present in the cell in a small number of copies. These large plasmids are either non-self-transmissible or can mediate a conjugation-like process. The second class comprises small plasmids that encode only one resistance determinant each and are present in a large number of copies (Table 23–5). The best example of plasmid-determined resistance in *S. aureus* is the production of penicillinase. Many strains carry this trait on 18- to 21-megadalton plasmids. In addition, these plasmids often carry resistance determinants to certain heavy metals and can also carry determinants for resistance to erythromycin, fusidic acid, or the aminoglycosides.

Some of the R-determinants in *S. aureus* are part of transposable DNA sequences that can undergo *rec*-independent translocation to multiple chromosomal and plasmid sites. Whole plasmids can also be stably integrated into the chromosome. A number of transposition elements have been described in *S. aureus:* Tn 551 is similar to many of the transposons from *E. coli* in that it is capable of insertion into

TABLE 23–5. TYPICAL *STAPHYLOCOCCUS AUREUS* PLASMIDS

Plasmid	Incompatibility Type	Incompatibility MW	Copies per Cell	Genotype[a]
pI258	Inc 1	18×10^6	2.7	*pen*$^+$ *asa*$^+$ *asi*$^+$ *ant*$^+$ *ero*$^+$ *inc 1*$^+$ *mer*$^+$ *bis*$^+$ *cad*$^+$ *lea*$^+$
pII147	Inc 2	21×10^6	2.7	*pen*$^+$ *asa*$^+$ *inc 2*$^+$ *cad B*$^+$ *bis*$^+$ *lea*$^+$ *mer*$^+$ *cad A*$^+$
pT169	Inc 3	2.7×10^6	~30	*tet*
pC221	Inc 4	3.0×10^6	>20	*cml*

Adapted from Novick et al: In Schlessinger (ed): Microbiology—1974. Washington DC, American Society for Microbiology, 1975.
[a] The following genotype abbreviations are used for loci: *asa, asi, ant, bis, lea, cad, mer, pen, ero, tet, cml* for response to arsenate, arsenite, antimony, bismuth, lead, cadmium, and mercuric ions and to penicillin, erythromycin, tetracycline, and chloramphenicol; *inc* is for incompatibility specificity.

various chromosomal and plasmid sites. Transposons encoding gentamicin resistance (Tn 4001, Tn 3851) also encode resistance to tobramycin and kanamycin.

In staphylococci, bacteriophages are closely associated with the expression and spread of antibiotic-resistance determinants. Bacteriophages mediate transfer of antibiotic resistance by transduction or by phage-mediated conjugation. Most clinical isolates of *S. aureus* harbor one or more prophages that presumably are integrated into the bacterial chromosome. Of the large number of staphylococcal phages, however, only those of serogroup B are transducing and thus potentially capable of the transfer of plasmids. In nature, transduction is of the generalized type. Almost any character can be transduced at a frequency of about 10^{-4} to 10^{-10} per plaque-forming unit of phage.

A conjugative mechanism of transfer independent of bacteriophage has also been documented for the transfer of aminoglycoside-resistance plasmids among staphylococci. These conjugative gentamicin R plasmids are capable of mobilizing nonconjugative coresident plasmids as a part of the conjugation process. This conjugative mechanism of exchange thus provides a mechanism for the "stacking" of multiple resistance traits within staphylococci as a result of a one-transfer event.

Some strains of *S. aureus* carry plasmid genes for bacteriocin production. These genes are analogous in many ways to the colicinogenic factors of the enteric bacteria. The production of the bacteriocin, staphylococcin, is limited to phage group II strains of *S. aureus*. Staphylococcin is a heat-stable protein distinct from other extracellular products of *S. aureus*, and is a specific phage product. Its spectrum is wide and includes β-hemolytic streptococci, pneumococci, other staphylococci, corynebacteria, and *Bacillus* species. Gram-negative bacteria and producer strains are resistant to its action.

Although plasmids have been implicated in the synthesis of a number of virulence factors of the staphylococcus, their precise role as structural or regulatory genes has not been defined. In the case of α-toxin, the gene for toxin production appears to be associated with a transposon. There are both chromosomal and plasmid genes for the synthesis of exfoliative toxin, each producing a distinct species of toxin.

Resistance. Staphylococci are more resistant to adverse environmental conditions than are most nonsporulating bacteria. They survive for weeks in dried pus and sputum and, on sealed agar slants, remain viable for several months. Most strains are relatively heat resistant, and killing them requires a temperature of 60C for 1 hour. Staphylococci are also more resistant than most bacteria to the common chemical disinfectants, such as the phenols and mercuric chloride, but like other gram-positive organisms they are sensitive to concentrations of unsaturated fatty acids and basic dyes that do not inhibit most gram-negative organisms.

Antigenic Structure

The phagocytic response of the host is a crucial factor in determining the initiation and the outcome of staphylococcal infections. In this process of host recognition and immunity, the cellular antigens of the staphylococcal cell, especially the surface ones, are major determinants. The antigenic structure of *S. aureus* is complex; of the more than 30 antigens observed, the biologic and chemical properties of only a few have been well characterized.

Teichoic Acid. A major antigenic determinant of all strains of *S. aureus* is the group-specific ribitol teichoic acid of the cell wall. The serologic determinant of this polysaccharide is *N*-acetylglucosamine. In the cell wall, teichoic acid is associated with the peptidoglycan in an insoluble state and requires lytic enzymes for release. Ribitol teichoic acid is not found in *S. epidermidis*, which contains, instead, glycerol teichoic acid.

Most adults have a cutaneous hypersensitivity reaction of the immediate type to teichoic acid, and low levels of precipitating antibodies are found in their sera. Elevated levels of teichoic acid antibodies result from recent staphylococcal disease, such as endocarditis or bacteremia, with metastatic foci of abscesses in which drainage or antibiotic therapy is delayed. Increases in teichoic acid antibodies are infrequent, however, in transient staphylococcal bacteremia.

Extracellular teichoic acid is responsible for the rapid consumption of early-reacting complement components up to and including C5 in human serum. Complement activation occurs as a consequence of immune complex formation between the antigen and specific human IgG antibodies. By induction of abortive, complement-consuming reactions, teichoic acid protects staphylococci from complement-dependent opsonization.

Protein A. Protein A is a group-specific antigen unique to *S. aureus* strains. Ninety percent of protein A is found in the cell wall covalently linked to the peptidoglycan. During cell growth, protein A is also released into the culture medium, where it comprises about one third of the total protein A produced by the organism.

Protein A consists of a single polypeptide chain with a molecular weight of 42 kDa. Four tyrosine residues fully exposed on the surface are responsible for biologic activity. The uniqueness of protein A is centered on its ability to interact with normal IgG of most mammalian species. Within a species the interaction may be restricted to certain subgroups of IgG. Unlike a specific antigen-antibody reaction, binding involves not the Fab fragment but the Fc portion of the immunoglobulin. Protein A consists of five regions: four highly homologous domains, which are Fc-binding, and a fifth, C-terminal domain, which is bound to the cell wall and does not bind Fc (Fig. 23–2).

Protein A provokes a variety of biologic effects. It is chemotactic, anticomplementary, and antiphagocytic and elicits hypersensitivity reactions and platelet injury. It is mitogenic and potentiates natural killer activity of human lymphocytes. Although there is good correlation between protein A production and coagulase activity, there is no correlation between the absence or presence of protein A and any pathogenic property. Its ability to bind to the Fc region of IgG has led to numerous applications in immunochemical and cell-surface structural studies.

Peptidoglycan. Staphylococcal peptidoglycan elicits both humoral and cellular immune responses. Virtually all healthy donors have antibodies to the peptidoglycan in their serum. They are primarily of the IgG class and can cross the placenta. The antipeptidoglycan IgG level is increased by *S. aureus* infections, especially when accompanied by a bacteremic phase. Whereas these antibodies are potentially beneficial because of their opsonizing capacity, increased levels may predispose some patients to immune complex disorders.

Clumping Factor. The component on the cell wall of *S. aureus* that results in the clumping of whole staphylococci in the presence of plasma is referred to as the clumping factor. This component binds human fibrinogen and differs from free coagulase in both its mechanism of action and its antigenic properties. The cellular fibrinogen-binding component is found almost exclusively in strains that produce the extracellular coagulase; however, capsulated strains give a negative clumping reaction, presumably because the clumping factor is covered by extracellular polysaccharide.

Capsular Polysaccharide. The presence of a capsule in *S. aureus* is a variable trait. Although only a few strains possess a morphologically distinct capsule, it is probable that encapsulation in vivo is not a rare phenomenon. When tested with monospecific antisera, most strains isolated from clinical material are found to carry immunologically significant polysaccharide surface antigens. These antigens are antiphagocytic. They interfere with the interaction between the underlying teichoic acid–peptidoglycan complex and complement, which is activated primarily through the alternative pathway.

Determinants of Pathogenicity

One of the essential attributes of a successful parasite is the ability to survive in the animal host. In this respect the staphylococcus has exhibited exceptional adaptive potential. Of special importance is its ability to bind specifically to a variety of mammalian proteins in the extracellular matrix and thereby breach the normal barriers between host tissues. A number of hydrolytic enzymes for a wide range of substrates, including native animal proteins, are elaborated and undoubtedly contribute to the organism's versatility. Proteases, lipases, esterases, and lyases are among the more important enzymes facilitating establishment of the organism on the skin and mucous membranes of the host. To survive in a hostile environment, however, the successful parasite must also counteract host defenses. For more than half a century, a wide array of extracellular enzymes, toxins, and cellular components of the more virulent strains of *Staphylococcus* have been examined, but unfortunately, at present no single factor can be equated with virulence. It is probable that virulence is multifactorial in the staphylococci and that many factors are involved, each constituting an important link in a complex chain of interactions culminating in overt staphylococcal infection.

Surface Antigens

Polysaccharides. Surface components that possess antiphagocytic activity are of obvious advantage to the staphylococcus in its initial establishment in the host. By protecting the organisms from the complement-mediated attack of polymorphonuclear leukocytes, encapsulated staphylococci are able to spread rapidly through tissue. For colonization to occur, however, and the infectious process to be sustained, adhesion of the organisms to a biosurface is the essential initiating event. The production of an exopolysaccharide by some strains of *Staphylococcus* may be the critical factor in the organism's successful colonization of implanted prosthetic devices such as cardiac valves and intravascular catheters. In

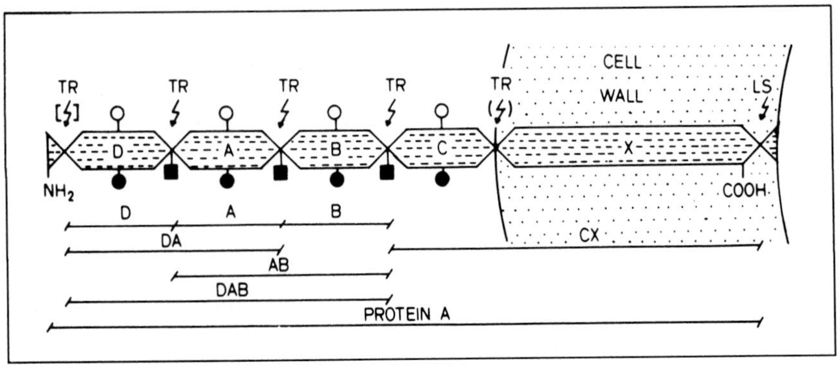

Fig. 23–2. Proposed structure of protein A. Arrows indicate points of enzymic cleavage. TR, trypsin; LS, lysostaphin. Arrow in round brackets indicates no cleavage of cell wall–bound protein; arrow in square brackets indicates that site may constitute the *N*-terminus of the protein. Fc receptor (○), structures evoking precipitation against rabbit antiprotein-A serum; (●), present in all Fc-binding regions; (■), demonstrated only in the polyvalent fragments. These structures are not necessarily true antigenic determinants but may be related to the Fc receptors. *(From Sjodahl: Eur J Biochem 73:343, 1977.)*

the competitive natural environment, bacterial glycocalyx production results in the formation of adherent microcolonies surrounded by a biofilm that enmeshes the organisms. This biofilm not only stabilizes their adhesion to prosthetic surfaces but also protects the organism from antibiotics and natural host defenses.

Protein Receptors. A number of specific binding sites for mammalian proteins have been identified on the staphylococcal cell surface. These receptors provide the organism with an adhesion mechanism by which infective foci become established. Among the plasma proteins that bind specifically to *S. aureus* are fibronectin, fibrinogen, immunoglobulin G, and C1q. Staphylococci also bind to components of the extracellular matrix (e.g., laminin, collagen, and fibronectin). The most extensively studied of these is fibronectin, a glycoprotein ubiquitous in wounds. Fibronectin mediates the adherence of vital cells such as fibroblasts, epithelial cells, and monocytes to an injured site. By specifically binding *S. aureus,* fibronectin may serve as a bridge between the organism and the host wound tissue. Laminin, another mammalian protein for which *S. aureus* has receptors, is the major glycoprotein in human basement membranes. The metastasis-like potential of staphylococci to breach the normal barriers between host tissues may be related to its ability to bind specifically to basement membranes.

The variety of mammalian proteins capable of binding specifically to *S. aureus* strongly suggests the existence of more than one adhesion gene. At least one of these genes is located on a plasmid. If adhesion genes are located on plasmids and can be readily mobilized, they provide a mechanism for the distribution of virulence traits between staphylococcal strains and an explanation for the wide diversity in pathogenic potential among isolates.

Extracellular Enzymes

Coagulases. Although the correlation between coagulase production and pathogenicity provides a convenient virulence marker, there is no definite evidence that coagulase is directly involved in pathogenicity.

The action of coagulase in the clotting of plasma is similar to the thrombin-catalyzed conversion of fibrinogen to fibrin. For full enzymatic activity, coagulase requires a plasma component, either prothrombin or a prothrombin derivative, referred to as coagulase reacting factor (CRF). The coagulase-thrombin product (CT) not only causes fibrinogen clotting but also possesses proteolytic and esterolytic activity similar to that of thrombin. The fibrinopeptides released are indistinguishable from thrombin-induced fibrinopeptides, some of which possess pharmacologic activity comparable to that of bradykinin on smooth muscle.

Lipases. Staphylococci produce several lipid hydrolyzing enzymes collectively referred to as lipases. The lipases are active on a variety of substrates, including plasma and the fats and oils that accumulate on the surface areas of the body. The utilization of these materials has survival value for the organism and explains the intense colonization of staphylococci in the sebaceous areas of greatest activity. The production of lipase apparently is essential in the invasion of healthy cutaneous and subcutaneous tissues. In primary human isolates, there is a close correlation between in vitro production of lipase and the ability to produce boils. The decreased virulence of hospital staphylococci observed during the last 20 to 30 years parallels a decrease in staphylococcal isolates that produce large amounts of the enzyme. The decrease apparently is due to the presence of a prophage that blocks lipase production by insertional inactivation.

Hyaluronidase. More than 90% of *S. aureus* strains produce hyaluronidase. This enzyme hydrolyzes the hyaluronic acid present in the intracellular ground substance of connective tissue, thereby facilitating spread of the infection. Since inflammation antagonizes the spreading action by hyaluronidase, its importance in staphylococcal infections is limited to the very early stages of infection.

Staphylokinase (Fibrinolysin). One of the proteolytic enzymes of staphylococci has fibrinolytic activity but is antigenically and enzymatically distinct from the streptokinase of the streptococci. The determinant for staphylokinase production is dependent on a phage genome and is expressed during lysogeny. In the dissolution of clots by the staphylococcal enzyme, the proenzyme plasminogen is converted to the fibrinolytic enzyme plasmin. Although produced by most strains of *S. aureus,* there is little evidence that it is a major factor in pathogenicity.

Nuclease. The elaboration of a heat-resistant nuclease appears to be uniquely associated with *S. aureus.* The enzyme, which is present in, at, or near the cell surface, is a compact globular protein consisting of a single polypeptide chain. Heating at 65C causes structural disruptions, but the changes are rapidly and completely reversible. The nuclease is a phosphodiesterase with both endonucleolytic and exonucleolytic properties and can cleave either DNA or RNA.

Toxins

Cytolytic Toxins. A number of bacteria produce toxins that cause physical dissolution of mammalian or other cells in vitro. Most of these are proteins, are extracellular, and induce the formation of neutralizing antibodies. There is considerable diversity, however, in the manner in which the various cytolytic toxins interact with the cell surface. The hemolysins and leukocidin elaborated by *S. aureus* are among the best defined of the cytolytic toxins, a group of toxins that also includes streptolysin O and S and various toxins of *Clostridium.* Four distinct hemolytic toxins (α-, β-, δ-, and γ-hemolysins) are produced by *S. aureus,* although different strains may vary in the levels that they express.

ALPHA TOXIN (α-HEMOLYSIN). α-Toxin exhibits a wide range of biologic activities, including the hemolytic, lethal, and dermonecrotic effects observed after the injection of broth culture filtrates. α-Toxin disrupts lysosomes and is cytotoxic for a variety of tissue culture cells. Human macrophages and platelets are damaged, but monocytes are resistant. There is injury to the circulatory system, muscle tissue, and tissue of the renal cortex. Although not the sole virulence factor for the staphylococci, the α-toxin contributes significantly to pathogenicity by producing tissue damage after the establishment of a focus of infection.

The gene for α-toxin production appears to be associated with a transposon. The pure toxin has a molecular weight of

34 kDa and is secreted by most strains as a water-soluble monomer. It consists of four different conformational forms, separable by electrophoresis. Rapid interconversion of these forms occurs on storage. The pure 3S α-toxin monomer polymerizes and aggregates reversibly to form both soluble and insoluble 12S products. These forms, which are biologically inactive, are referred to as toxoids.

The precise mechanism of membrane damage has not been established, but it is currently believed to involve the following sequence of events: (1) binding of toxin monomers to the cell surface, (2) hexamer formation to form transmembrane channels 2 to 3 nm in diameter, (3) leakage of small ions through the channels, and (4) colloid osmotic lysis of the cell. Triggering of the hexamerization process is not dependent on the presence of a specific receptor molecule on the membrane, but certain cells do possess high-affinity binders that render them more highly sensitive to toxin-binding and subsequent secondary pathophysiologic events.

BETA TOXIN (STAPHYLOCOCCAL SPHINGOMYELINASE). The most striking activity of β-toxin is its ability to produce a "hot-cold" lysis (i.e., an enhanced hemolytic activity if incubation room temperature). The toxin is an enzyme with substrate specificity for sphingomyelin (and lysophosphatides). Sphingomyelin degradation is the membrane lesion that leads to hemolysis when the cells are chilled.

$$\text{Sphingomyelin} + H_2O \xrightarrow[Mg^{2+}]{\beta\text{-toxin}} N\text{-Acylsphingosine} + \text{Phosphorylcholine}$$

Erythrocytes from different animal species exhibit impressive differences in their sensitivity to β-toxin. A correlation exists between toxin sensitivity and content of sphingomyelin, most of which is located in the outer leaflet of the lipid bilayer of the erythrocyte membrane and thus is accessible to exogenous toxin.

DELTA TOXIN. δ-Toxin is a relatively thermostable surface-active toxin whose strong detergent-like properties are responsible for its damaging effects on membranes. It exhibits a high degree of aggregation and is electrophoretically heterogeneous. The toxin has a high content of hydrophobic amino acids, which, if localized in one area, could make the molecule amphipathic and strongly surface active. The membrane receptor site is thought to be a straight-chain fatty acid with 13 to 19 carbons. δ-Toxin exhibits a broad spectrum of biologic activity and displays no pronounced specificity for cells of a particular species; erythrocytes, macrophages, lymphocytes, neutrophils, and platelets are all damaged.

In addition to the gross cytolytic effects of the toxin, a number of more subtle responses can be induced at very low concentrations. δ-Toxin inhibits water absorption by the ileum, stimulates accumulation of adenosine monophosphate, and alters ion permeability in the guinea pig ileum. Other effects of δ-toxin include its influence on human polymorphonuclear leukocyte functions and platelet-activating factor metabolism. These proinflammatory effects may be the result of its capacity to increase (1) Ca^{2+} influx, (2) generation of oxygen radicals, and (3) activation of acetyltransferase, leading to formation of the potent lipid mediator, platelet-activating factor.

GAMMA TOXIN. γ-Toxin has pronounced hemolytic activity, but its precise mode of action is not known. It consists of two protein components that act synergistically, both being essential for hemolysis and toxicity. The finding of elevated levels of specific neutralizing antibodies in human staphylococcal bone disease suggests a possible role of this toxin in the disease state.

LEUKOCIDIN. The Panton-Valentine leukocidin produced by most strains of *S. aureus* attacks polymorphonuclear leukocytes and macrophages but no other cell type. The toxin is composed of two protein components (S and F) that act synergistically to induce cytolysis. The S and F components are bound preferentially by Gm_1-ganglioside and phosphatidylcholine. The primary step in leukocytolysis is the activation of methyltransferases subsequent to the binding of the S component. This leads to the activation of phospholipase and an increase in membrane phosphatidylcholine binding sites for the F component. The unique response of leukocytes to leukocidin is an altered permeability to cations. Other changes that occur are secondary to this initial event. In the presence of calcium, large amounts of protein derived from the cytoplasmic granules are secreted. This degranulation may be observed microscopically. Both components of leukocidin are highly antigenic and have been toxoided.

Enterotoxins. Approximately one third of all clinical isolates of *S. aureus* produce exotoxins. These exotoxins are members of a large group of pyrogenic protein toxins that mediate a spectrum of diseases with similar clinical manifestations and organ involvements. Included in this family of toxins in addition to the staphylococcal enterotoxins are the toxic shock syndrome toxin 1 (TSST-1) and the streptococcal pyrogenic exotoxins A through C. All of these toxins are pyrogenic and immunosuppressive as a result of their ability to induce nonspecific T lymphocyte mitogenicity and enhance host susceptibility to lethal endotoxin shock. A unique feature of the staphylococcal enterotoxins is their ability to provoke vomiting and diarrhea in humans after oral administration.

The staphylococcal enterotoxins have been serologically classified into six groups: A, B, C, C_2, D, and E. At present enterotoxin A is most frequently associated with staphylococcal food poisoning in the United States. Although these toxin groups are antigenically distinct when evaluated by immunodiffusion assays, shared antigenic determinants between some of the toxins can be demonstrated in neutralization and other more sensitive immunoassays. The genetic control of staphylococcal enterotoxins has not been clearly defined. However, analyses of the chromosomal DNA of enterotoxin-producing strains have shown that the enterotoxin B gene (ent B) is a part of a discrete element, 26.8 kb in size. It is possible that the ent B gene is part of a bacteriophage or a large integrated plasmid.

The mechanism of action of staphylococcal enterotoxins has not been well defined. The major hindrance to an understanding of their pathogenesis and mode of action has been the lack of a practical and sensitive assay system. Except for man, the only reliable experimental animal for testing enterotoxin activity is the monkey. The emetic receptor site for staphylococcal enterotoxin is the abdominal viscera, from which site the sensory stimulus reaches the vomiting center via the vagus and sympathetic nerves. Enterotoxin-induced diarrhea has been attributed to inhibition of water absorption from the lumen of the intestine and to increased transmucosal fluid flux into the lumen. More recent studies on the enterotoxins have focused on their function as biologic response modifiers which affect host immune defense mechanisms. Because of this activity, they have been referred to as "superantigens." They are powerful T cell mitogens whose activity leads to the activation of T lymphocytes, a process that requires the involvement of major histocompatibility complex (MHC) class II molecules. Investigations are also under way to find an explanation for the clinical symptoms and pathologic lesions indicative of shock. Enterotoxin directly stimulates macrophages to produce tumor necrosis factor, and it is also associated with endotoxin-induced shock. The accumulated data show that prostaglandin E and other arachidonic acid cascade metabolites may play a crucial role in illness induced by this toxin. These mediators have been implicated as chemotactic factors for neutrophil accumulation and as agents that increase vascular permeability and inflammation.

Exfoliative Toxins. The staphylococcal scalded-skin syndrome is caused by toxins produced predominantly by bacteriophage group II strains. Two serologically and biochemically distinct forms of exfoliative toxin—ETA and ETB—have been identified. The gene for ETA is chromosomal, whereas the gene for ETB resides on a family of plasmids. For isolation and characterization of exfoliative toxin, a newborn mouse model is used. In mice the toxin produces a severe form of the disease that is indistinguishable histologically and clinically from the human disease. The purified toxins are proteins with molecular weights of approximately 30 and 29.5 kDa. They cause lysis of the intracellular attachment between cells of the granular layer of the epidermis but do not elicit an inflammatory response and do not primarily cause cell death. There is evidence that exfoliative toxin is a sphingomyelinase but that it is different from the staphylococcal β-toxin. Exfoliative toxin is a potent mitogen, primarily of T cells.

Toxic Shock Syndrome Toxin-1. *S. aureus* is associated with toxic shock syndrome (TSS), a severe and often fatal disorder characterized by multiple organ dysfunction (p. 412). In most cases of TSS associated with menstruation and in approximately 50% of nonmenstrual cases, TSS toxin-1 (TSST-1)–producing strains of *S. aureus* are involved. TSST-1 is a 22 kDa exotoxin with pronounced and diverse immunologic effects. These include the induction of interleukin-2 receptor expression, interleukin synthesis, proliferation of human T lymphocytes, and stimulation of interleukin-1 synthesis by human monocytes. The major binding site for TSST-1 on human mononuclear cells has been identified as major histocompatibility complex (MHC) class II molecules.

Clinical Infection

Epidemiology. The staphylococcus is a normal component of man's indigenous microflora and is carried asymptomatically in a number of body sites. Its transmission from these sites causes both endemic and epidemic disease. The acquisition and carriage of *S. aureus* is a complex problem that is incompletely understood. Colonization of the infant with staphylococci occurs within a few days after birth, but because of antibodies passively received through the placenta the carrier rate drops during the first 2 years of life. By the age of 6 the child has acquired an adult carrier rate of approximately 30%. Some persons who harbor staphylococci are chronic or persistent carriers, but most are intermittent carriers who harbor the organism for only a few weeks. *S. aureus* is found in the symptom-free carrier in a number of body sites, but the anterior nares is the major reservoir of infection and source of disease. The perineum is also an important carriage site.

The carrier problem is an especially serious one in the newborn nursery. The umbilicus and the groin are usually the sites of primary colonization. By maintaining sterility of the umbilical stump, the nasal carrier rate can be markedly reduced. The carriage rate is determined by the presence or absence in the nursery of an epidemic strain. If such a strain is present, most of the infants will be colonized, but if a number of different strains are present, less than 20% will be colonized. Many of the staphylococcal lesions that develop during early infancy are thus due to nursery-acquired strains. Staphylococci are disseminated from these newborn infants with lesions to other infants and nursery personnel and to their families. Also, since lesions may not develop until after hospital discharge, newborn infants and patients with postoperative wound infections may transmit hospital strains of *Staphylococcus* into the community.

The source of staphylococcal infection is a patient or a member of the hospital staff with a staphylococcal lesion. Patients with lesions draining pus externally are dangerous to others because of their ability to disseminate the organisms by contamination of the environment. Direct contact via the hands is the single most important route of transmission. There are documented cases of hospital personnel with mild staphylococcal lesions, such as furuncles, paronychia, or styes, who have initiated epidemics. An infected surgeon is a common source of infection in surgical patients.

The carrier state is a potentially serious problem in chronic users of parenteral drugs, in whom an increased carrier rate of *S. aureus* has been found. It is probable that the high frequency of staphylococcal endocarditis in the narcotic addict is attributable to the increased opportunity for the introduction of staphylococci into the circulation as the skin barrier is penetrated by injections of narcotic.

ANTIBIOTIC RESISTANCE. A better understanding of the origin and epidemiology of staphylococcal disease was provided during the 1950s after the appearance of epidemics caused by antibiotic-resistant strains of the 80/81 complex. The appearance of epidemics at that particular time apparently resulted from a set of new circumstances that had evolved as a result of medical progress. When first introduced, penicillin was dramatically effective in the treatment of staphylococcal infections. By 1946, however, an increasing number of penicillin-resistant strains were isolated from hospital infections. As penicillin became less useful clinically and as other antibiotics were introduced, resistance to these agents also rapidly appeared. Resistance to the new antibiotics was associated almost exclusively with penicillinase production and the development of multiple resistance in a few strains, which then became established endemically in the hospitals. The increasing number of highly susceptible persons congregated in hospitals contributed to the epidemic appearance of staphylococcal disease. Resistance to penicillin and methicillin first appeared in group III before it developed in other strains. Hospital epidemics started with strains of a few phage patterns (phages 75, 77) in group III and group I (phage 80) but soon shifted to resistant strains of the 52/52A/80/81 complex (group I), to be followed by strains lysed by phage 83A (group III) and strains of the 83A/84/85 complex.

Pathogenesis. In the typical staphylococcal skin infection, the organisms penetrate a sebaceous gland or hair shaft, where they find an environment nutritionally suitable for growth. The defense mechanisms of the host and the size and virulence of the infective dose determine the likelihood of development of a staphylococcal infection. Although benign skin infections are common, serious staphylococcal disease is infrequent, emphasizing the excellent protective barrier provided by the skin and mucous membranes. Any condition that destroys the integrity of these surface areas predisposes the person to infection. Third-degree burns, traumatic wounds, surgical incisions, decubitus or trophic ulcers, and certain viral infections are among the many precipitating causes of staphylococcal disease.

Phagocytosis of Staphylococci. The granulocyte is primarily responsible for resistance to staphylococcal infections. Once the organisms have penetrated the skin or mucous membranes, mobile phagocytes migrate into the area in response to the stimulus of chemotactic factors. Chemotactic activity is generated by a number of different mechanisms, each of which is significant at a different stage of the infection. Early in the infection, staphylococcal proteases generate their own chemotactically active fragments of complement components. Later in the course of infection, or with repeated antigenic challenge, specific antibody may generate chemotactic activity through the classic complement pathway (Chap. 13). By virtue of their ability to activate complement, all major cell wall components of *S. aureus* contribute to the generation of chemotactic factors.

The inflammatory reaction induced after the accumulation of phagocytes at the site of the invading bacteria facilitates contact between organisms and phagocytic cells. This interaction of staphylococci with phagocytic cells plays a central role in the critical early stages of infection. Phagocytosis of nonencapsulated strains is promoted by either complement or antibody. For efficient phagocytosis of the more resistant encapsulated strains, however, both antibody and complement are required. In most healthy persons, as well as in many persons with staphylococcal infections, complement is the primary source of opsonic factors. Although specific IgG antibodies are present in the serum of most persons as the result of subclinical infection with staphylococci, the titer of these antibodies is relatively low. In the absence of antibody or a functional classic complement pathway, staphylococcal opsonization may proceed by activation of the alternate complement pathway, which is mediated by peptidoglycan. Activation of complement by either the classic or the alternative complement pathway leads to the deposition of opsonic C3b on the bacterial surface and engulfment of the organism by means of C3b receptors of the leukocyte.

Once they are phagocytized, most staphylococci are rapidly killed and degraded within the phagocytic vacuoles. The intracellular killing is mediated primarily by oxygen-dependent bactericidal mechanisms (p. 351). In patients with chronic granulomatous disease, the phagocytic cells are deficient in their bactericidal capacity against staphylococci. Leukocytes of these patients do not exhibit the normal metabolic response to phagocytosis that results in hydrogen peroxide accumulation. As a result, engulfed staphylococci remain viable within phagocytic vacuoles. Catalase-negative organisms, however, such as the streptococci, are unable to break down the hydrogen peroxide produced by their own metabolism and accumulate it. They are, therefore, readily killed by chronic granulomatous disease leukocytes (p. 340).

Oxygen-independent staphylocidal systems that are also operative in the phagocytes include the low pH within the vacuole, lysozyme, lactoferrin, and granular cationic proteins.

Immunity. Humans are highly resistant to infection by staphylococci. Billions of organisms must be introduced to elicit an observable response. How much of this resistance is of a natural (inherited) type and how much is acquired in response to repeated natural exposure to organisms that constitute part of the natural flora has not been clearly defined. Most adults possess serum antibodies to a number of cell wall antigens and toxins of the organism, but none of these gives full protection against *S. aureus* infection. Antibody levels (IgM and IgG) to both peptidoglycan and teichoic acid are usually elevated in the more serious staphylococcal infections of deep tissue sites.

DELAYED HYPERSENSITIVITY. A small number of organisms may survive for prolonged periods within the phagocytic cell. These survivors may outlive the phagocyte cell, which could explain the occurrence of chronic, latent, or smoldering infections. An important aspect of this intimate host-parasite relationship is the development of delayed hypersensitivity to staphylococcal antigens, which has been demonstrated both experimentally and in patients with various types of recurrent *S. aureus* infections. The exaggerated hypersensitivity response may impair local resistance and increase tissue destruction. Both cell wall peptidoglycan and membrane proteins are thought to contain the major determinants of delayed hypersensitivity.

Clinical Manifestations. The characteristic feature of staphylococcal infection is abscess formation. This can occur in any part of the body, but in each area the basic lesion consists of inflammation, leukocyte infiltration, and tissue necrosis. In a fully developed lesion there is a central necrotic core filled with dead leukocytes and bacteria separated from the surrounding tissue by a relatively avascular fibroblastic wall.

CUTANEOUS INFECTIONS

Furuncles and Carbuncles. Staphylococcal infection of the skin is the most common bacterial infection in man. The most superficial of these is folliculitis, in which there is infection of the hair follicle. An extension into the subcutaneous tissue results in the formation of a focal suppurative lesion, the boil or furuncle. A carbuncle is similar to a furuncle but has multiple foci and extends into the deeper layers of fibrous tissue. Carbuncles are limited to the neck and upper back, where the skin is thick and elastic. In children, cutaneous lesions are less well localized than they are in adults.

Little or no pain is associated with folliculitis, but as the infection penetrates into the subcutaneous tissues and inflammation progresses, exquisite tenderness appears. Most furuncles evolve in 3 to 5 days and are followed by spontaneous drainage, relief of pain, and onset of healing. Satellite lesions and secondary lesions at new sites as a consequence of autoinoculation are frequent, and a small number of patients develop chronic recurrent furunculosis extending over months or years. Dissemination from cutaneous lesions occurs by contiguous extension or hematogenous spread.

Impetigo. In the newborn infant, pustules or impetiginous lesions are the most frequent staphylococcal skin manifestations. Staphylococcal impetigo also is common in young children, often occurring around the nose. It is characterized by the formation of encrusted pustules on the superficial layers of the skin. When crusts are removed, a red weeping denuded surface is exposed. The disease is highly contagious and, when introduced into a nursery or school, spreads in an epidemic manner. In the United States, staphylococci appear to participate with streptococci in most common impetiginous lesions.

Scalded Skin Syndrome. The scalded skin syndrome comprises a spectrum of dermatologic diseases with a common etiology, the staphylococcal exfoliative toxin. All of the clinically recognizable features of this syndrome are attributable to this toxin, the effects of which are separable from the effects of the staphylococcal infection itself (Fig. 23–3). The scalded skin syndrome comprises three distinct but related clinical entities:

1. Generalized exfoliative dermatitis (Ritter's disease, staphylococcal toxic epidermal necrolysis) is the most severe form. It is characterized by generalized painful erythema and dramatic bullous desquamation of large areas of skin. The focus of infection may be at a distant site.
2. Bullous impetigo is a localized form of the syndrome in which the infection occurs at the site of the lesion.
3. Staphylococcal scarlet fever is a mild generalized form of the scalded skin syndrome, clinically similar to streptococcal scarlet fever. A localized infection from which staphylococci may be isolated is the usual focus.

The scalded skin syndrome primarily afflicts neonates and children under 4 years of age. Its relatively rare occurrence in adults, except in immunologically compromised patients, suggests the presence of neutralizing antibodies in the majority of the population.

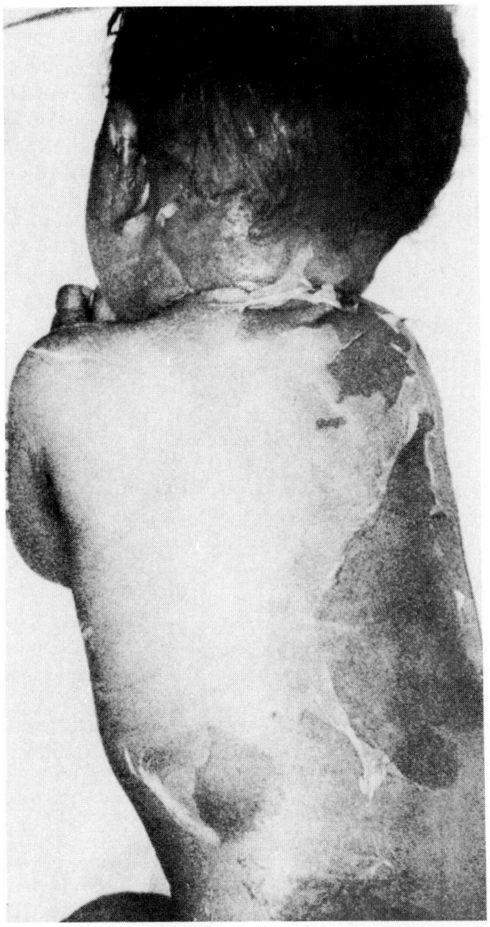

Fig. 23–3. Scalded-skin syndrome produced by the exfoliative toxin of *S. aureus*. In the generalized exfoliative form the epidermis separates and peels off, leaving rolled skin at the margins and revealing a moist, red glistening area. *(From Melish et al: Zentralbl Bakteriol 1 Abt. 5(suppl):473, 1976.)*

PNEUMONIA. Staphylococcal pneumonia is an important disease because of its high mortality rate (up to 50%). It may be a fulminant process in all age groups, but it is relatively rare except during epidemic periods of influenza. Infants less than 1 year of age appear to be the most susceptible and account for about 75% of the cases. Primary staphylococcal pneumonia is most often seen in patients with impaired host defense: children with cystic fibrosis or measles, influenza patients, or debilitated, hospitalized persons being treated with antimicrobials, steroids, cancer chemotherapy, or immunosuppressants. Necrosis, with formation of multiple abscesses, is characteristic of the infection. The pneumonia usually is patchy and focal in nature.

Staphylococcal bacteremia from a focus elsewhere may result in hematogenous or secondary pneumonia. In recent years this has been seen most often among heroin addicts with endocarditis, predominantly in the adolescent–young adult age group.

OSTEOMYELITIS. *S. aureus* is the cause of the majority of cases of primary osteomyelitis. This disease occurs primarily in male children under the age of 12 years, and in most cases it follows hematogenous spread from a primary focus, usually a wound or furuncle. The organisms localize at the diaphysis of long bones, probably because the arterial circulation in this area consists primarily of terminal capillary loops. As the infection progresses, pus accumulates and emerges to the surface of the bone, raising the periosteum and producing a subperiosteal abscess. Clinical symptoms of acute osteomyelitis include fever, chills, pain over the bone, and muscle spasm around the area of involvement. When the infection occurs near a joint, staphylococcal pyoarthrosis is a common complication.

Secondary staphylococcal osteomyelitis is associated with a penetrating trauma or surgery and is frequent in patients with diabetes mellitus or peripheral vascular disease. Two increasingly common forms of osteomyelitis are vertebral osteomyelitis, seen in adults (especially intravenous drug users), and clavicular osteomyelitis, a complication of subclavian catheter use.

PYOARTHROSIS. Approximately 50% of all cases of bacterial

arthritis are caused by *S. aureus*. Staphylococcal pyoarthrosis may occur after orthopedic surgery, in conjunction with osteomyelitis or local skin infections, or as a result of direct inoculation of staphylococci into the joint during intraarticular injections, especially in patients with rheumatoid arthritis who are receiving corticosteroids. Staphylococcal joint infection destroys the articular cartilage and may result in permanent joint deformity.

BACTEREMIA AND ENDOCARDITIS. Bacteremia may occur with any localized staphylococcal infection, but infections of the skin, the respiratory tract, or the genitourinary tract provide the primary focus for most of these lesions. Approximately 50% of staphylococcal septicemias are acquired in the hospital. It is uncommon to observe staphylococcal bacteremia in persons who do not have an associated disease that predisposes to infection. It is most commonly seen in persons with diabetes mellitus, cardiovascular disease, granulocyte disorders, and immunologic deficiency. Also, foreign bodies such as intravascular prostheses and intravenous plastic catheters provide a medium for vascular infection and bacteremia. An increasing number of community-acquired cases of *S. aureus* bacteremia are found among drug addicts.

Fever, shaking chills, and systemic toxicity are usually associated with staphylococcal bacteremia. A frequent complication is endocarditis, which is usually acute and malignant, with heart valve destruction within a few days. In spite of appropriate antibiotic treatment, *S. aureus* endocarditis has a high mortality, varying from 40% to 80%, depending on the underlying medical problem, the age of the patient, and resistance of the infecting strain to penicillin.

METASTATIC STAPHYLOCOCCAL INFECTIONS. One of the characteristic features of *S. aureus* bacteremia is the production of metastatic abscesses. The most frequent sites of the metastatic abscesses are the skin, the subcutaneous tissues, and the lungs. Internal abscesses of the kidneys, the brain, and the spinal cord are not uncommon.

FOOD POISONING. In the United States, staphylococcal food poisoning is the most common form of bacterial food poisoning. It is caused by the ingestion of food that contains the preformed toxin elaborated by enterotoxin-producing strains (p. 408). The food is usually contaminated by food handlers who have the organisms on their hands. The foods most commonly involved are improperly refrigerated custard or cream-filled bakery products. Ham, processed meats, ice cream, cottage cheese, hollandaise sauce, and chicken salad are foods that are often implicated. Foods containing the enterotoxin are normal in odor, appearance, and taste. Sufficient toxin is produced in 4 to 6 hours at 86F, but not at refrigerator temperatures, to produce symptoms of food poisoning.

Symptoms, which appear abruptly 2 to 6 hours after ingestion of the food, consist of severe cramping, abdominal pain, nausea, vomiting, and diarrhea. Sweating and headache are seen, but fever is not a common feature. Recovery is usually rapid, within 6 to 8 hours.

TOXIC SHOCK SYNDROME (TSS). Toxin-producing strains of *S. aureus* have been implicated in most cases of TSS, a multisystem disease that primarily afflicts young women. Most cases occur in menstruating women who use tampons; however, nonmenstruating women, children, and men with boils or staphylococcal infections of wounds can also have TSS. Clinical features include fever, marked hypotension, diarrhea, conjunctivitis, myalgias, and a scarlatiniform rash followed by fine desquamation. There appears to be no significant correlation between outcome of the acute illness and type of antimicrobial therapy. However, the use of β-lactamase-resistant drugs does reduce the rate of recurrence, probably by reducing or oblating colonization with toxin-producing *S. aureus* strains (p. 409). Levels of antibody to the TSS toxin in the sera of women with TSS or a history of TSS are lower than levels in sera of women with no prior evidence of TSS. This suggests that the absence of antibodies to the TSS toxin may be a predisposing factor in the development of clinical disease.

Laboratory Diagnosis. Because of the widespread distribution of staphylococci, meticulous care must be taken in the collection of specimens. If the material for culture requires aspiration, the skin in the area must be properly sterilized. The finding of typical irregular clusters of gram-positive cocci on direct microscopic examination of purulent material is presumptive evidence of the presence of staphylococci, but definitive identification requires laboratory isolation.

Pus, purulent fluids, sputum, and urine specimens should be streaked directly on a blood agar plate and inoculated into a tube of thioglycollate broth. For blood cultures, 10 ml of venous blood should be inoculated into 50 ml of tryptose-phosphate broth. Identification of staphylococci and differentiation of *S. aureus* from *S. epidermidis* is based on colonial and microscopic morphology, catalase and coagulase production, and acid production from certain carbohydrates (Table 23–2). Staphylococci and micrococci are catalase-positive; pneumococci and streptococci are catalase-negative. By definition, all strains of *S. aureus* are coagulase-positive.

Treatment. In the management of localized staphylococcal infections, the basic principle of therapy is adequate drainage. Foreign bodies at the site of infection should be removed. Although antibacterial agents may control spread of the organisms from the abscess, they are less effective on bacteria within the abscess and do not facilitate its resolution.

Antibiotic sensitivity testing is important in the selection of the appropriate antibiotic and in evaluation of its effectiveness during the course of infection. Although many antibiotics are now available for the treatment of staphylococcal infections, the unpredictable sensitivity of a particular isolate narrows the initial choice. Unless the patient is allergic, bactericidal penicillin analogues are recommended. The initial choice should be limited to penicillinase-resistant drugs, since most isolates from both hospital and community infections are resistant to penicillin G, penicillin V, and ampicillin. If, however, sensitivity testing proves the staphylococcal isolate to be sensitive to penicillin, this is the drug of choice for continued treatment because it is more active and less expensive.

For cutaneous infections, oral therapy with a semisynthetic penicillin, such as cloxacillin or dicloxacillin, is usually efficacious. Oxacillin and nafcillin are not recommended for oral therapy because their absorption is too unpredictable. If the patient is allergic to penicillin, erythromycin may be used.

For serious systemic staphylococcal disease, parenteral administration of nafcillin or oxacillin is recommended. Vancomycin or cephalosporins are suitable parenteral substitutes in the allergic patient. Staphylococcal infections often respond slowly and relapses often occur if therapy is terminated too early. The development of resistance to penicillin during the course of treatment is unusual, but with erythromycin it is not uncommon. Treatment of most serious staphylococcal infections should be continued for 4 to 6 weeks to prevent the later emergence of metastatic abscesses.

Staphylococci that are resistant to the β-lactam antibiotics are usually referred to as "methicillin-resistant staphylococci." Methicillin, however, is simply the drug used in testing the resistance of these organisms in the laboratory. When any staphylococcus isolated is identified as being resistant to methicillin, this implies that it is also resistant to nafcillin and oxacillin and to all β-lactam antibiotics, including the cephalosporins. Although methicillin-resistant strains of *S. aureus* have not been a common problem in the United States, they are now being seen with increased frequency. Most significant outbreaks have occurred in hospitals, but methicillin-resistant infection may also arise in the community and has the potential to disseminate in both settings. Drug abusers and debilitated patients represent major sources of methicillin-resistant *S. aureus*. These organisms may also be resistant to gentamicin, tobramycin, and clindamycin. Vancomycin, alone or in combination with rifampin, is the recommended treatment of infections caused by methicillin-resistant strains. Rifampin should be used only in combination with another antibiotic to prevent the emergence of rifampin resistance.

Prevention. Staphylococcal infection will never be completely controlled because of the carrier state in humans. In the home as well as in the hospital, spread of infection can be limited only by proper hygienic care and disposal of contaminated materials. In the hospital setting, one is more likely to encounter a more virulent organism as well as a very susceptible patient population. Persons with staphylococcal lesions should be segregated from newborn infants and from highly susceptible adults. Indiscriminate use of antibiotics should be avoided to prevent establishment and spread of resistant strains throughout the hospital. All surgical procedures and instrumentation should be performed with maximal attention to aseptic techniques. In the newborn infant, proper care should be given the umbilical stump, and personnel in the nursery should be screened for staphylococcal carriers. Infection committees that have been set up in hospitals to control nosocomial infections should provide effective surveillance and follow-through of problems that are uncovered.

Other Medically Significant Staphylococci

With advances in medical knowledge, staphylococci other than *S. aureus* have become increasingly important as true pathogens. Previously regarded as contaminants or harmless commensals on the skin, coagulase-negative staphylococci are now recognized as a major cause of infections associated with the use of prosthetic devices and of urinary tract infections. At least 11 human coagulase-negative species of staphylococci have been recognized, of which *S. epidermidis* and *S. saprophyticus* are the most important.

Staphylococcus epidermidis

Identification. *S. epidermidis* characteristically produces white colonies on blood agar. It may be distinguished from *S. aureus* and from other coagulase-negative species by a number of biochemical properties, the most useful of which are listed in Table 23–2.

Epidemiology. *S. epidermidis* appears to be host-specific for humans. All human beings carry the organisms as part of their normal skin flora. Most frequent sites include the axillae, head, arms, nares, and legs. Humans thus serve both as an exogenous source of contamination for infection to others and as an endogenous source. Virtually all *S. epidermidis* infections are hospital acquired and result from contamination of a surgical site by organisms from the patient's skin or nasopharynx or from hospital personnel. Hospital-associated *S. epidermidis* isolates are usually resistant to multiple antibiotics, including methicillin and penicillin G. Biotyping and phage-typing techniques have been devised for *S. epidermidis* to trace specific isolates from the environment to the patient, but as a general epidemiologic tool these have proved inadequate. Plasmid pattern analysis, currently being evaluated, shows promise as an epidemiologic marker for clinically important isolates.

Pathogenesis. In the normal host, *S. epidermidis* is an organism with low virulence, but when host defenses are breached, it may cause serious and often life-threatening infections. *S. epidermidis* has a distinct predilection for foreign bodies, such as artificial heart valves, indwelling intravascular catheters, central nervous system shunts, and hip prostheses. These foreign bodies are susceptible to bacterial contamination during implantation and seeding from bacteremias postoperatively. The adhesion of organisms to the surface of the prosthetic device is the initiating step in the pathogenesis of infection. Some strains of *S. epidermidis* produce a viscous extracellular substance that appears to facilitate colonization on smooth surfaces, such as plastic or metal. Scanning electron microscopy of intravascular catheters removed from patients with *S. epidermidis* infections has demonstrated bacteria embedded in deposits of an amorphous material. The glycocalyx that enmeshes the organisms not only facilitates adhesion to the smooth prosthetic surfaces but also contributes to their pathogenesis by protecting them from antibiotics and natural host defenses. The adherence of *S. epidermidis* also causes erosive changes in the inert surface of polyethylene catheters and may in this way contribute further to the adherence potential of the organism.

Clinical Infection. The association of *S. epidermidis* with infections involving prosthetic devices is unique and accounts for a high morbidity. *S. epidermidis* is the single most common isolate from infections associated with cardiac valve or total hip replacement and central nervous system shunt insertion. It causes infections of pacemakers, vascular grafts, and prosthetic joints as well as peritonitis in patients undergoing peritoneal dialysis. It is the single most common organism infecting intravenous catheters, and in the last few years it has accounted for an increasing number of documented cases of true *S. epidermidis* bacteremias. These infections are often occult in nature and difficult to manage. In addition, *S. epidermidis* can cause urinary tract infections, especially in elderly hospitalized men, and occasionally natural valve endocarditis in intravenous drug abusers. Coagulase-negative species have recently been shown to produce one or more of the toxins involved in TSS and to be clinically important in this syndrome.

Treatment. Multiple antibiotic resistance, including resistance to methicillin, is a common feature of disease-producing strains of *S. epidermidis*. There is no single recurring pattern of antibiotic resistance. Multiple antibiotic resistance not only complicates therapy but also provides a reservoir of genetic antibiotic resistance for the more virulent *S. aureus*. The choice of appropriate therapy should be based on the local antibiogram to *S. epidermidis*. In the absence of this, an initial regimen should include an aminoglycoside (gentamicin or tobramycin) with cephalothin or rifampin or vancomycin alone.

Staphylococcus saprophyticus

This coagulase-negative staphylococcus can be distinguished from *S. epidermidis* by its resistance to novobiocin and by its failure to ferment glucose anaerobically. It is nonhemolytic and does not contain protein A. In contrast to other staphylococci, most strains have the ability to agglutinate sheep erythrocytes.

S. saprophyticus occurs on the normal skin and in the periurethral and urethral flora, but transiently and in small numbers. Only recently has its pathogenic potential been fully appreciated. *S. saprophyticus* is a common cause of urinary tract infections in sexually active young women and is second only to *Escherichia coli* as the most frequent causative agent of such infections. Urinary tract infections caused by this organism are less frequent in men than in women. They can occur at any age but are more common in patients over 50 years of age. Urinary tract infection by *S. saprophyticus* is usually symptomatic, and in approximately one half of all cases the upper urinary tract is involved.

S. saprophyticus shows a tropism for the epithelial lining of the urinary tract, the only organ system in which it causes disease. The organism selectively adheres to urothelial cells via specific oligosaccharide receptors on the cell membrane. Certain strains of *S. saprophyticus* are able to suppress growth of other bacteria, such as *Neisseria gonorrhoeae* and *S. aureus*. An extracellular enzyme complex is responsible for this inhibitory activity.

FURTHER READING

Books and Reviews

Arbuthnott JP: Staphylococcal toxins. In Schlessinger D (ed): Microbiology—1975. Washington, DC, American Society for Microbiology, 1975, p 267

Archer GL: *Staphylococcus epidermidis* and other coagulase-negative staphylococci. In Mandell GL, Douglas RG Jr, Bennett JE (eds): Principles and Practice of Infectious Diseases, ed 3, vol 2. New York, Churchill Livingstone, 1990, p 1489

Bhakdi S, Tranum-Jensen J: Membrane damage by pore-forming bacterial cytolysins. Microbial Pathogen 1:5, 1986

Chesney PJ, Bergdoll MS, Davis JB, Vergeront JM: The disease spectrum, epidemiology, and etiology of toxic-shock syndrome. Annu Rev Microbiol 38:315, 1984

Cohen JO (ed): The Staphylococci. New York, Wiley, 1972

Forsgren A: Immunological aspects of protein A. In Schlessinger D (ed): Microbiology—1977. Washington, DC, American Society for Microbiology, 1977, p 353

Freer JH, Arbuthnott JP: Biochemical and morphologic alterations of membranes by bacterial toxins. In Bernheimer AW (ed): Mechanisms in Bacterial Toxinology. New York, Wiley, 1976, p 169

Hirsch ML, Kass EH: An annotated bibliography of toxic shock syndrome. Rev Infect Dis 8(Suppl 1):1, 1986

Hovelius B, Mardh P-A: *Staphylococcus saprophyticus* as a common cause of urinary tract infections. Rev Infect Dis 6:328, 1984

Kloos WE, Jorgensen JH: Staphylococci. In Lennette EH, Balows A, Hausler WJ Jr, Shadomy HJ (eds): Manual of Clinical Microbiology, ed 4. Washington, DC, American Society for Microbiology, 1985, p 143

Kloos WE, Schleifer K-H. The genus *Staphylococcus*. In Starr MP, Stolp H, Trüper HG, et al (eds): The Prokaryotes, vol 2. New York, Springer-Verlag, 1981, p 1548

Lacey RW: Antibiotic resistance plasmids of *Staphylococcus aureus* and their clinical importance. Bacteriol Rev 39:1, 1975

Misfeldt ML: Microbial "superantigens." Infect Immun 58:2409, 1990

Novick R, Wyman L, Bouanchaud D, et al: Plasmid life cycles in *Staphylococcus aureus*. In Schlessinger D (ed): Microbiology—1974. Washington, DC, American Society for Microbiology, 1975, p 115

Rogolsky M: Nonenteric toxins. Microbiol Rev 43:320, 1979

Schaberg DR, Zervos M: Plasmid analysis in the study of the epidemiology of nosocomial gram-positive cocci. Rev Infect Dis 8:705, 1986

Sheagren JN: Staphylococcal infections. In Wyngaarden JB, Smith LH Jr (eds): Textbook of Medicine, ed 18, vol 2. Philadelphia, WB Saunders, 1988, p 1596

Sheehy RJ, Novick RP: Penicillinase plasmid replication in *Staphylococcus aureus*. In Schlessinger D (ed): Microbiology—1974. Washington, DC, American Society for Microbiology, 1975, p 130

Sneath PHA, Mair NS, Sharpe ME, Holt JG (eds): Bergey's Manual of Systematic Bacteriology, vol 2. Baltimore, Williams & Wilkins, 1986, p 999

Waldvogel FA: *Staphylococcus aureus* (including toxic shock syndrome). In Mandell GL, Douglas RG Jr, Bennett JE (eds): Principles and Practice of Infectious Diseases, ed 3, vol 2. New York, Churchill Livingstone, 1990, p 1489

Wiseman GM: The hemolysins of *Staphylococcus aureus*. Bacteriol Rev 39:317, 1975

Selected Papers

Altboum Z, Hertman I, Sarid S: Penicillinase plasmid-linked genetic determinants for enterotoxins B and C, production in *Staphylococcus aureus*. Infect Immun 47:514, 1985

Archer GL, Dietrick DR, Johnston JL. Molecular epidemiology of transmissible gentamicin resistance among coagulase-negative staphylococci in a cardiac surgery unit. J Infect Dis 151:243, 1985

Baughn RE, Bonventre PF: Acquired cellular resistance following transfer of lymphocytes from mice infected repeatedly with *Staphylococcus aureus*. Cell Immunol 27:287, 1976

Betley MJ, Löfdahl S, Kreiswirth BN, et al: Staphylococcal enterotoxin A gene is associated with a variable genetic element. Proc Natl Acad Sci USA 81:5179, 1984

Bodén MK, Flock J-I: Fibrinogen-binding protein/clumping factor from *Staphylococcus aureus*. Infect Immun 57:2358, 1989

Carney DN, Fossieck BE Jr, Parker RH, et al: Bacteremia due to *Staphylococcus aureus* in patients with cancer: report on 45 cases in adults and review of the literature. Rev Infect Dis 4:1, 1982

Chesney PJ, Davis JP, Purdy WK, et al.: Clinical manifestations of toxic shock syndrome. JAMA 246:741, 1981

Choi Y, Kotzin B, Herron L, et al: Interaction of *Staphylococcus aureus* toxin "superantigens" with human T cells. Proc Natl Acad Sci USA 86:8941, 1989

Clewell DB, An FY, White BA, Gawron-Burke C: *Streptococcus faecalis* sex pheromone (cAM373) also produced by *Staphylococcus aureus* and identification of a conjugative transposon (Tn918). J Bacteriol 162:1212, 1985

Crass BA, Bergdoll MS: Toxin involvement in toxic shock syndrome. J Infect Dis 153:918, 1986

Craven DE, Rixinger AI, Goularte TA, et al: Methicillin-resistant *Staphylococcus aureus* bacteremia linked to intravenous drug abusers using a "shooting gallery." Am J Med 80:772, 1986

Crossley K, Landesman B, Zaske D: An outbreak of infections caused by strains of *Staphylococcus aureus* resistant to methicillin and aminoglycosides. II. Epidemiologic studies. J Infect Dis 139:280, 1979

Davis JP, Osterholm MT, Helms CM, et al: Tri-state toxic-shock syndrome study. II. Clinical and laboratory findings. J Infect Dis 145:441, 1982

de Azavedo JCS, Foster TJ, Hartigan PJ, et al: Expression of the cloned toxic shock syndrome toxin 1 gene (tst) in vivo with a rabbit uterine model. Infect Immun 50:304, 1985

Dunkle LM, Blair LL, Fortune KP: Transformation of a plasmid encoding an adhesin of *Staphylococcus aureus* into a nonadherent staphylococcal strain. J Infect Dis 153:670, 1986

Edwin C, Parsonnet J, Kass EH: Structure-activity relationship of toxic-shock-syndrome toxin-1: Derivation and characterization of immunologically and biologically active fragments. J Infect Dis 158:1287, 1988

Elias PM, Fritsch P, Tappeiner G, et al: Experimental staphylococcal toxic epidermal necrolysis (TEN) in adult humans and mice. J Lab Clin Med 84:414, 1974

Espersen F, Clemmensen I: Isolation of a fibronectin-binding protein from *Staphylococcus aureus*. Infect Immun 37:526, 1982

Espersen F, Clemmensen I, Barkholt V: Isolation of *Staphylococcus aureus* clumping factor. Infect Immun 49:700, 1985

Espersen F, Frimodt-Møller N: *Staphylococcus aureus* endocarditis: A review of 119 cases. Arch Intern Med 146:1118, 1986

Fast DJ, Schlievert PM, Nelson RD: Toxic shock syndrome-associated staphylococcal and streptococcal pyrogenic toxins are potent inducers of tumor necrosis factor production. Infect Immun 57:291, 1989

Garbe PL, Arko RJ, Reingold AL, et al: *Staphylococcus aureus* isolates from patients with nonmenstrual toxic shock syndrome. JAMA 253:2538, 1985

Gatermann S, Marre R: Cloning and expression of *Staphylococcus saprophyticus* urease gene sequences in *Staphylococcus carnosus* and contribution of the enzyme to virulence. Infect Immun 57:2998, 1989

Herrmann M, Vaudaux PE, Pittet D, et al: Fibronectin, fibrinogen, and laminin act as mediators of adherence of clinical staphylococcal isolates to foreign material. J Infect Dis 158:693, 1988

Hill HR, Williams PB, Krueger GG, et al: Recurrent staphylococcal abscesses associated with defective neutrophil chemotaxis and allergic rhinitis. Ann Intern Med 85:39, 1976

Holderbaum D, Hall GS, Ehrhart LA: Collagen binding to *Staphylococcus aureus*. Infect Immun 54:359, 1986

Holmberg SD, Blake PA: Staphylococcal food poisoning in the United States. JAMA 251:487, 1984

Ishak MA, Gröschel DHM, Mandell GL, et al: Association of slime with pathogenicity of coagulase-negative staphylococci causing nosocomial septicemia. J Clin Microbiol 22:1025, 1985

Jackson MP, Iandolo JJ: Cloning and expression of the exfoliative toxin B gene from *Staphylococcus aureus*. J Bacteriol 166:574, 1986

Jett M, Brinkley W, Neill R, et al: *Staphylococcus aureus* enterotoxin B challenge of monkeys: Correlation of plasma levels of arachidonic acid cascade products with occurrence of illness. Infect Immun 58:3494, 1990

Johnson GM, Lee DA, Regelmann WE, et al: Interference with granulocyte function by *Staphylococcus epidermidis* slime. Infect Immun 54:13, 1986

Johns MB Jr, Khan SA: Staphylococcal enterotoxin B gene is associated with a discrete genetic element. J Bacteriol 170:4033, 1988

Kaplan MH, Chmel H, Hsieh HC, et al: Importance of exfoliative toxin A production by *Staphylococcus aureus* strains isolated from clustered epidemics of neonatal pustulosis. J Clin Microbiol 23:83, 1986

Kasimir S, Schönfeld W, Alouf JE, König W: Effect of *Staphylococcus aureus* delta-toxin on human granulocyte functions and platelet-activating-factor metabolism. Infect Immun 58:1653, 1990

Kohashi O, Pearson CM, Watanabe Y, et al: Structural requirements for arthritogenicity of peptidoglycans from *Staphylococcus aureus* and *Lactobacillus plantarum* and analogous synthetic compounds. J Immunol 16:1635, 1976

Kondo I, Fujise K: Serotype B staphylococcal bacteriophage singly converting staphylokinase. Infect Immun 18:266, 1977

Kuusela P, Vartio T, Vuento M, Myhre EB: Attachment of staphylococci and streptococci on fibronectin, fibronectin fragments, and fibrinogen bound to a solid phase. Infect Immun 50:77, 1985

Lee CY, Iandolo JJ: Lysogenic conversion of staphylococcal lipase is caused by insertion of the bacteriophage L54a genome into the lipase structural gene. J Bacteriol 166:385, 1986

Leijh PCJ, van den Barselaar MTh, Daha MR, et al: Stimulation of the intracellular killing of *Staphylococcus aureus* by monocytes: Regulation by immunoglobulin G and complement components C3/C3b and B/Bb. J Immunol 129:332, 1982

Lillibridge CB, Melish ME, Glasgow LA: Site of action of exfoliative toxin in the staphylococcal scalded-skin syndrome. Pediatrics 50:728, 1972

Lowy FD, Hammer SM: *Staphylococcus epidermidis* infections. Ann Intern Med 99:834, 1983

Maxe I, Rydén C, Wadström T, Rubin K: Specific attachment of *Staphylococcus aureus* to immobilized fibronectin. Infect Immun 54:695, 1986

Melish ME, Glasgow LA: The staphylococcal scalded-skin syndrome: Development of an experimental model. N Engl J Med 282:1114, 1970

Morgan NG, Montague W: Studies on the interaction of staphylococcal δ-haemolysin with isolated islets of Langerhans. Biochem J 204:111, 1982

O'Reilly M, de Azavedo JCS, Kennedy S, Foster TJ: Inactivation of the alpha-haemolysin gene of *Staphylococcus aureus* 8325-4 by site-directed mutagenesis and studies on the expression of its haemolysins. Microbial Pathog 1:125, 1986

Osterholm MT, Davis JP, Gibson RW, et al: Tri-state toxic-shock syndrome study. I. Epidemiologic findings. J Infect Dis 145:431, 1982

Parsonnet J, Gillis ZA, Pier GB: Induction of interleukin-1 by strains of *Staphylococcus aureus* from patients with nonmenstrual toxic shock syndrome. J Infect Dis 154:55, 1986

Peacock JE, Moorman DR, Wenzel RP, et al: Methicillin-resistant *Staphylococcus aureus:* Microbiologic characteristics, antimicrobial susceptibilities, and assessment of virulence of an epidemic strain. J Infect Dis 144:575, 1981

Pead L, Maskell R, Morris J: *Staphylococcus saprophyticus* as a urinary pathogen: a six year prospective survey. Br Med J 291:1157, 1985

Peterson PK, Wilkinson BJ, Kim Y, et al: Influence of encapsulation on staphylococcal opsonization and phagocytosis by human polymorphonuclear leukocytes. Infect Immun 19:943, 1978

Poindexter NJ, Schlievert PM: Suppression of immunoglobulin-secreting cells from human peripheral blood by toxic-shock-syndrome toxin-1. J Infect Dis 4:772, 1986

Ponce de Leon S, Guenthner SH, Wenzel RP: Microbiologic studies of coagulase-negative staphylococci isolated from patients with nosocomial bacteremias. J Hosp Infect 7:121, 1986

Ruby C, Novick RP: Plasmid interactions in *Staphylococcus aureus:* Nonadditivity of compatible plasmid DNA pools. Proc Natl Acad Sci USA 72:5031, 1975

Saravolatz LD, Markowitz N, Arking L, et al: Methicillin-resistant *Staphylococcus aureus:* Epidemiologic observations during a community-acquired outbreak. Ann Intern Med 96:11, 1982

Schlievert PM, Shands KN, Dan BB, et al: Identification and characterization of an exotoxin from *Staphylococcus aureus* associated with toxic-shock syndrome. J Infect Dis 143:509, 1981

Schmeling DJ, Gemmell CG, Craddock PR, et al: Effect of staphylococcal α-toxin on neutrophil migration and adhesiveness. Inflammation 5:313, 1981

Schmitt D, Bandyk DF, Pequet AJ: Mucin production by *Staphylococcus epidermidis.* Arch Surg 121:89, 1986

Scholl P, Diez A, Mourad W, et al: Toxic shock syndrome toxin 1 binds to major histocompatibility complex class II molecules. Proc Natl Acad Sci USA 86:4210, 1989

Speziale P, Raucci G, Visai L, et al: Binding of collagen to *Staphylococcus aureus* Cowan 1. J Bacteriol 167:77, 1986

Stewart PR, Waldron HG, Lee JS, Matthews PR: Molecular relationships among serogroup B bacteriophages of *Staphylococcus aureus.* J Virol 55:111, 1985

Stolz SJ, Davis JP, Vergeront JM: Development of serum antibody to toxic shock toxin among individuals with toxic shock syndrome in Wisconsin. J Infect Dis 151:883, 1985

Tuazon CU, Sheagren JN, Choa MS, et al: *Staphylococcus aureus* bacteremia: Relationship between formation of antibodies to teichoic acid and development of metastatic abscesses. J Infect Dis 137:57, 1978

Vaudaux P, Pittet D, Haeberli A, et al: Host factors selectively increase staphylococcal adherence on inserted catheters: A role for fibronectin and fibrinogen or fibrin. J Infect Dis 160:865, 1989

Vaudaux P, Suzuki R, Waldvogel FA, et al: Foreign body infection: Role of fibronectin as a ligand for the adherence of *Staphylococcus aureus.* J Infect Dis 150:546, 1984

Verbrugh HA, Peters R, Rozenberg-Arska M, et al: Antibodies to cell wall peptidoglycan of *Staphylococcus aureus* in patients with serious staphylococcal infections. J Infect Dis 144:1, 1981

Weinstein RA, Kabins SA, Nathan C, et al: Gentamicin-resistant staphylococci as hospital flora: Epidemiology and resistance plasmids. J Infect Dis 145:374, 1982

Wheat LJ, Kohler RB, Tabbarah ZA, et al: IgM antibody response to staphylococcal infection. J Infect Dis 144:307, 1981

Wilkinson BJ, Kim Y, Peterson PK, et al: Activation of complement by cell surface components of *Staphylococcus aureus.* Infect Immun 20:388, 1978

CHAPTER 24

Streptococcus

The genus *Streptococcus* comprises a large and biologically diverse group of gram-positive cocci that grow in pairs or chains. A number of species within the genus cause major human diseases, such as streptococcal pharyngitis, scarlet fever, impetigo, urinary tract infections, and bacterial endocarditis. In addition, infection caused by group A streptococci may lead to the postinfectious syndromes of acute rheumatic fever, rheumatic heart disease, and acute glomerulonephritis.

Streptococci were first described by Billroth in 1874 in exudates from erysipelas and wound infections, and in 1879 Pasteur found similar organisms in the blood of a patient with puerperal sepsis. Subsequently, organisms with similar characteristics were obtained from a variety of different types of material, but it was many years before the diverse nature of the various species within this genus was fully understood. A major turning point in our understanding of the epidemiology of streptococcal infections came in 1933 with the introduction by Lancefield of a useful serologic system for the classification of β-hemolytic streptococci. The system was based on the antigenic composition of cell wall carbohydrates and provided a mechanism for the unraveling of the spectrum of streptococcal infections and their nonsuppurative complications. To date, serogroups A to H and K to V have been designated. Groups A, B, C, D, and G are those most commonly found associated with human infections.

Twenty-seven recognized species are currently included in the genus *Streptococcus*, a phylogenetically loosely related group of gram-positive cocci. Many of the species exist as commensals or parasites on man or animals. Some are highly pathogenic. Others are saprophytes present in the natural

TABLE 24–1. STREPTOCOCCAL SEROGROUPS ASSOCIATED WITH HUMAN INFECTIONS

Lancefield Serogroup	Hemolysis on Blood Agar	Representative Species	Major Clinical Syndromes
A	β	*S. pyogenes*	Pharyngitis, scarlet fever, septicemia, erysipelas, impetigo, rheumatic fever, acute glomerulonephritis
B	β	*S. agalactiae*	Neonatal sepsis and meningitis, urinary tract infection, puerperal sepsis
C	β	—[b]	Pharyngitis
D	V[a]	*Enterococcus faecalis*	Genitourinary tract infections, endocarditis
		Nonenterococci (*S. bovis*)	Endocarditis
G	β	—	Pharyngitis

[a] Variable, usually nonhemolytic.
[b] *Streptococcus equisimilis* has the group C antigen but is not at present an approved *Streptococcus* species.

environment. The most important of the human pathogens are *Streptococcus pyogenes* (group A), *Streptococcus agalactiae* (group B), *Enterococcus faecalis* (*Streptococcus faecalis*) (group D), *Streptococcus pneumoniae* (Chap. 25), and some of the oral streptococci (Table 24–1). Although *Bergey's Manual of Systematic Bacteriology* has retained the enterococci as a subgroup within the genus *Streptococcus*, current schemes of classification now recognize a new genus, *Enterococcus*. In the discussion that follows, this designation will be employed for currently recognized species of enterococci that were previously included among the group D species.

Properties of the Genus

Streptococci are gram-positive organisms, spherical to ovoid in shape and less than 2 μm in diameter. When grown in liquid media, they occur in pairs or chains, the chain length varying according to the species and the composition of the culture medium. Growth of streptococci occurs by elongation on the axis parallel to the chain. Cross walls form at right angles to the chain, and after cell division an appearance of pairing may remain. Streptococci are facultative anaerobes with a fermentative metabolism. Fermentation is primarily homolactic, and no gas is produced. They are catalase-negative, an important and convenient property for the initial separation of streptococci from staphylococci.

One of the most useful schemes for the preliminary classification of streptococci is based on the type of hemolysis produced on blood agar plates. Some streptococci produce a clear zone of hemolysis (β-hemolysis) around the colony as a result of the complete lysis of the red blood cells. Other streptococci produce a zone of partial hemolysis with a greenish discoloration (α-hemolysis) of the medium, whereas some species are nonhemolytic and produce no hemolysis (γ-hemolysis) on blood agar. Because of the lack of a recognizable group antigen in most α-hemolytic and nonhemolytic streptococci and the variability of their hemolytic activity, there is at present no satisfactory method for their classification.

Group A Streptococci: *Streptococcus pyogenes*

Streptococcus pyogenes constitutes Lancefield's group A streptococci. It is one of the most important human pathogens. It can produce an exceptionally wide variety of systemic and cutaneous infections and is the most common cause of acute pharyngitis.

Morphology

S. pyogenes are spherical to ovoid organisms, 0.5 to 1.0 μm in diameter. The organism grows in short or moderately long chains, the chain length being dependent on the strain and culture medium. When grown in liquid medium, some strains produce very long chains (Fig. 24–1).

The ultrastructure of the group A streptococcus is typical of other gram-positive bacteria in that there is a rigid cell wall, an inner plasma membrane with mesosomal vesicles, cytoplasmic ribosomes, and nucleoid. In addition, external to the cell wall are surface, fimbriae-like appendages that contain the type-specific M protein (Fig. 24–2). Some strains produce a capsule of hyaluronic acid, which may be demonstrable during the first 2 to 4 hours of growth. Since many strains also produce the enzyme hyaluronidase later during the growth cycle, capsules may not be seen in older cultures.

Physiology

S. pyogenes, like all members of the genus *Streptococcus*, is a facultative anaerobe. It is catalase-negative and oxidase-negative, and it does not contain any heme compounds. The

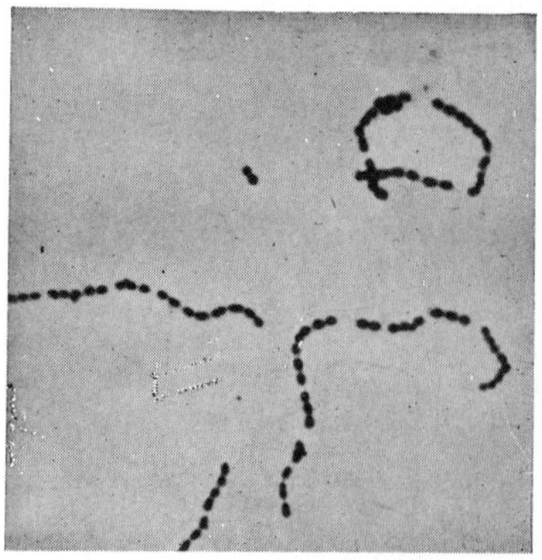

Fig. 24–1. *Streptococcus pyogenes.* Gram stain. × 1200.

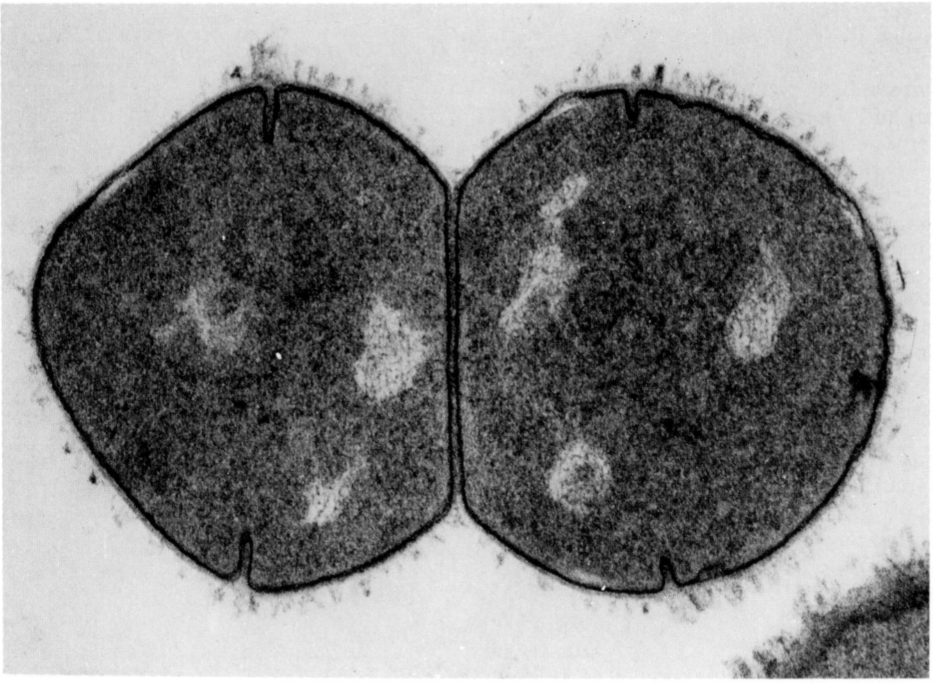

Fig. 24–2. Electron micrograph of group A streptococcus, M type 23, showing external fuzz with M protein and cell wall with electron-dense inner layer and closely adherent plasma membrane. The cytosol shows numerous homogeneous ribosomes and lighter nucleoid areas. This pair of organisms demonstrates one complete crosswall and the beginning of secondary septations. Glutaraldehyde-osmium fixation. × 84,000. *(Courtesy of Dr. Roger M. Cole.)*

minimal nutritional requirements of the streptococcus are complex because of the organism's inability to synthesize many of its required amino acids, purines, pyrimidines, and vitamins. Group A streptococci are killed in 30 minutes at 60C, a property that is useful in their differentiation from certain other streptococci, for example, group D, that are more heat resistant.

Cultural Characteristics. For primary isolation of group A streptococci from clinical materials, media containing blood or blood products are preferred. The optimal pH for growth is 7.4 to 7.6 at 37C. An enhancement of growth of many strains can be obtained by culture at a reduced oxygen tension or an increased level of CO_2. Most group A streptococci are β-hemolytic on sheep blood agar, although the presence of small amounts of fermentable carbohydrate (0.05% glucose) may decrease the reaction around surface colonies (Fig. 24–3). Since hemolysis is enhanced under anaerobic conditions, it is recommended that the agar be slashed by the loop at the primary site of inoculation to ensure subsurface growth. Sheep blood is preferred for primary isolation because it is inhibitory to the growth of *Haemophilus haemolyticus,* an organism whose colonial morphology and β-hemolytic reaction may cause it to be confused with the hemolytic streptococci. Human blood should not be used unless it is known to be free of inhibitory substances.

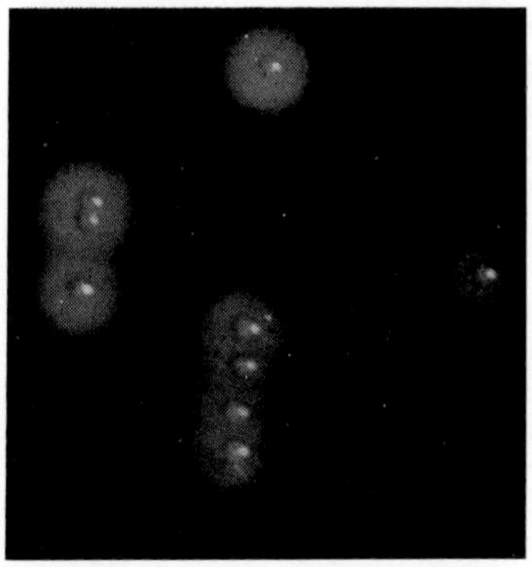

Fig. 24–3. Hemolytic streptococcus. Yeast blood agar. × 3. Note β-type hemolysis. *(From Li and Koibong: J Bacteriol 69:326, 1955.)*

Laboratory Identification. For primary culture, clinical specimens may be processed by both pour and streak plate techniques. Characteristically, after 18 to 24 hours of growth on blood agar, *S. pyogenes* colonies are 0.5 mm in diameter, domed, grayish to opalescent, and surrounded by a zone of β-hemolysis several times greater than the diameter of the colony. β-Hemolysis serves as the marker for primary isolation. Group A streptococci vary considerably in their colonial morphology. Strains that synthesize large amounts of hyaluronic acid produce mucoid colonies that, on continued incubation, collapse as a result of drying or hyaluronidase activity.

Group A streptococci must be distinguished from other β-hemolytic streptococci (primarily groups B, C, and G) that are often present in the pharynx and other tissue sites. The serologic group may be determined by a variety of techniques, such as Lancefield extraction and precipitation, fluorescent antibody, or coagglutination. The bacitracin test, used primarily for pharyngeal cultures, may be useful for presumptively distinguishing between β-hemolytic streptococci. This test is based on the sensitivity of group A streptococci to bacitracin and predicts with 95% accuracy the presumptive identification of pharyngeal isolates. Various rapid identification tests based on extraction of group A carbohydate directly from throat swabs have been devised. These tests are rapid (less than 1 hour) and highly specific. Negative tests, however, should be followed up with culture of the throat swab since the rapid tests lack the sensitivity of culture techniques.

Streptococci are differentiated from staphylococci on the basis of cellular and colonial morphology and the catalase test. Streptococci are catalase-negative, whereas staphylococci are catalase-positive.

Lysogeny. Lysogeny is very common among all groups of streptococci. In group A, estimates of lysogeny range as high as 90% to 100%. Some of the bacteriophages associated with the lysogenized state may play an important role in directing the synthesis of various group A streptococcal enzymes and toxins. This relationship has been especially well established with the pyrogenic exotoxin (erythrogenic toxin). Phage-associated muralysins are produced by virulent phages of both groups A and C during infection of streptococcal cultures. The group C lysin has been particularly useful in studies on the cell wall structure of group A streptococci. The enzyme is an *N*-acetylmuramyl-L-alanine amidase that is capable of lysing streptococci of many groups. This enzyme has also been useful in the production of L forms and in the preparation of purified membranes and M protein.

Antigenic Structure

C-Polysaccharide. The work of Rebecca Lancefield in 1933 laid the groundwork for the serologic classification of β-hemolytic streptococci based on their cell wall polysaccharide antigen. A variety of techniques have been used for the extraction of the group antigens, including the use of dilute hydrochloric or nitrous acid, formamide, or cell wall lytic enzymes. The extracts thus obtained are then tested against group-specific antisera by capillary tube precipitation reactions. This is the most accurate method employed for defining the various serologic groups. A variety of agglutination techniques using extracts or whole cells may also be used.

The C polysaccharide, which is specific to the species, is composed of a branched polymer of L-rhamnose and *N*-acetyl-D-glucosamine in a 2:1 ratio, the latter being the antigenic determinant. The polysaccharide is linked by phosphate-containing bridges to the peptidoglycan, which consists of *N*-acetyl-D-glucosamine, *N*-acetyl-D-muramic acid, D-glutamic acid, L-lysine, and D- and L-alanine.

Proteins

TYPING. Group A streptococci produce two major classes of protein antigens, the M and T antigens, that are responsible for type specificity in the group. Both antigens are sufficiently stable and immunologically distinct to provide useful serologic methods of typing. More than 90% of all group A strains may be typed by use of these antigens. The M antigens are resistant to heat and acid but are destroyed by trypsin; the T antigens are heat and acid stable but are resistant to trypsin. Routine M typing is performed by capillary tube precipitin tests using a hydrochloric acid extract of harvested cells as antigen against absorbed rabbit type-specific hyperimmune sera. For expression of the M protein, organisms should be grown on media containing peptides, and to avoid destruction of the M protein by proteinase activity, the pH should not be allowed to fall below 6.5.

T typing is an effective adjunct to M typing and a useful epidemiologic marker for routine surveillance of isolates. It has also been useful for typing group A streptococcal strains that cannot be serotyped with anti-M sera. Many of these strains are associated with cases of pyoderma for which antisera are not available.

TABLE 24–2. RELATION OF T PATTERNS TO M TYPES

T Complex	M Types Bearing T Complex
1	1
2	2
3/13/B3264	3, 13, 33, 39, 41, 43, 52, 53, 56
8/25/Imp. 19	2, 8, 25, 55, 57, 58
5/11/12/27/44	5, 11, 12, 27, 44, 59, 61
14/49	14, 49
15/17/19/23/47	15, 17, 19, 23, 30, 47, 54

T typing is performed by a slide agglutination test that uses trypsin-treated whole streptococci. Some T antigens are restricted to a single M type, whereas others may be shared by several M types (Table 24–2). T antigens are not associated with surface fuzz or with virulence; antibodies to T antigens are not protective.

Another antigen, M-associated protein (MAP), is found in all M protein-containing group A streptococci and some strains of groups C and G but not in M-negative strains. It is antigenically related to sarcolemmal components of the myocardium. Antibody responses to MAPs are usually highest in patients with acute rheumatic fever.

The serum opacity factor (SOF) is a trypsin-sensitive protein antigen with the ability to opacify horse serum. It is produced by 16 of the currently recognized M serotypes but is absent from all of the other strains. It is type-specific and antigenic and has proved useful for the typing of group A streptococci that are nontypable with M antigen.

M PROTEIN. Streptococcal M protein is an antiphagocytic fibrillar molecule located on the surface of group A organisms. It is an alpha helical coiled-coil dimer, which may extend 60 nm (600 Å) or more from the cell surface and which appears in thin-section electron micrographs as hairlike projections on the cell wall (Fig. 24–4). More than 70 antigenically distinct serotypes have been described. The amino-terminal portion of the M protein contains the antigenically variable determinants of type specificity. Homology among the various M protein serotypes progressively increases at sites that are closer to the carboxyterminus and more proximal to the cell wall. A major portion of the M protein gene consists of three large regions of tandem repeats that, through homologous recombination, generate M protein size variants. It is likely that intragenic homologous recombination events contribute to the antigenic diversity between serotypes.

The M protein is the major virulence factor of group A streptococci and renders the organisms resistant to phagocytosis. In the absence of type-specific antibody, streptococci producing M protein persist in infected tissues until antibodies appear. The antiphagocytic activity of the M protein is attributed to an interference with the deposition of the complement component C3b onto the streptococcal cell surface. Activation of the alternate complement pathway and opsonization of the streptococcus is thus inhibited. With the appearance of type-specific antibodies, M protein activity is nullified. The immunity that develops is type-specific and long-lasting.

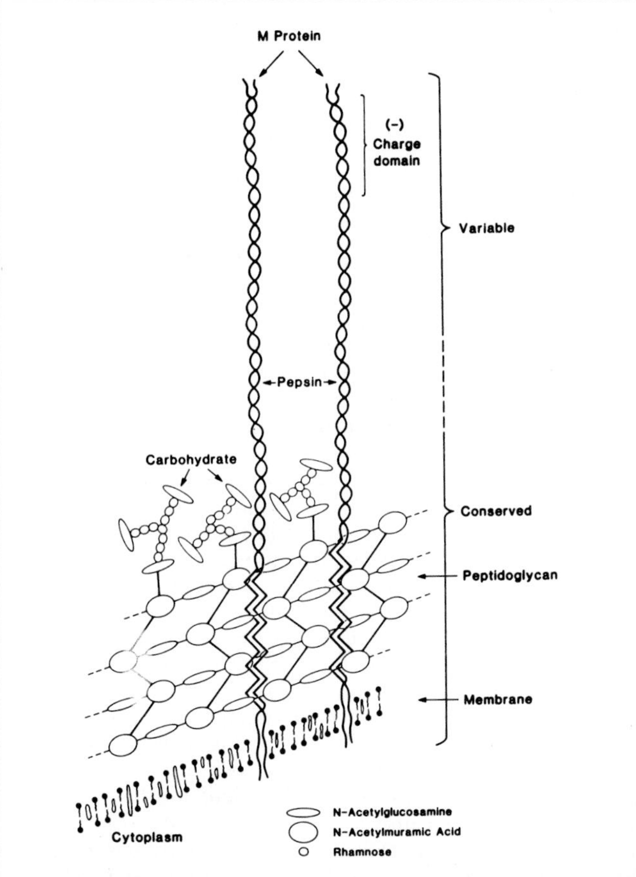

Fig. 24–4. Schematic representation of the coiled-coil M protein molecule on the streptococcal cell wall. Pepsin represents the region of the molecule cleaved by pepsin at pH 5.8. A negative charge domain is located at the *N*-terminal region. Variable and conserved regions are defined on the basis of DNA hybridization studies between other M serotypes and reactivity with monoclonal antibodies. The molecule is held in the cell by both a membrane anchor at the C-terminus and a stabilization domain embedded in the peptidoglycan. Carbohydrate represents the group A–specific carbohydrate. *(From Fischetti et al: In Horwitz (ed): Bacteria-Host Cell Interaction. Alan R Liss, 1988.)*

Determinants of Pathogenicity

The pathogenicity of *S. pyogenes* is multifactorial. A number of virulence factors are produced, which are of survival value and permit the organism to interact with tissue receptors, resist host defenses, and multiply within the host. Some of these have recently been shown to belong to a common operon that is globally controlled in response to environmental changes and the general physiologic state of the cell.

Cellular Components

Lipoteichoic Acid (LTA). For an organism to infect its intended host, it must be able to gain a foothold on the surface of cells at the portal of entry. It has been shown that adherence to buccal epithelial cells is mediated by the lipoteichoic acid that is present in the cell wall of group A streptococci. LTA is an amphipathic and amphoteric molecule. It is highly cytotoxic for a variety of host cells and is capable of a wide array of biologic activities. LTA has been identified as the streptococcal colonization ligand that forms a complex network with M protein and binds via its lipid moiety to fibronectin on epithelial cells.

M Protein. Once adherence has taken place, those strains that are able to resist phagocytosis and killing by leukocytes (i.e., those organisms rich in M protein) proliferate and begin to invade local tissues. Local pharyngeal or cutaneous infection may ensue, or the organism may invade contiguous tissues or distant tissues via the bloodstream. Once an antibody response is induced, organisms may be rapidly engulfed and killed by phagocytes. The cell walls of group A streptococci have been shown to react with immunoglobulin (IgG) in a nonimmune manner similar to that of staphylococcal protein A. The cell walls are also potent activators of the alternative complement pathway. The presence of M protein on the surface of the cell wall prevents these reactions from occurring and hence may explain the rapid recognition and phagocytosis of M-negative strains. The antiphagocytic activity of streptococcal M protein has been attributed to the inhibition of complement, mediated by the binding of factor H, the serum control protein of the alternative complement pathway.

In addition to M protein, which has long been thought to be the key determinant of virulence for *S. pyogenes,* the organism possesses additional virulence factors, at least some of which appear to be under the control of a virulence regulon. One of these, a C5a peptidase, which is located on the cell surface, destroys chemotactic signals by removing a six-amino-acid peptide from the carboxyterminus of the complement component C5a. The biosynthesis of M protein and C5a peptidase is coordinately regulated and subject to simultaneous phase regulation. Phase switching of both proteins is at the transcriptional level. The serum opacity factor, which is very closely associated with the M protein, is a distinct gene product subject to phase variation and is also coregulated with the M protein by a genetic switch that controls colony morphology and M protein expression.

A unique surface protein that binds to the Fc region of mammalian IgG is also expressed by *S. pyogenes.* The importance of these receptors to the virulence of the organism is at present unknown; however, studies suggest that they may possess an internal image of certain rheumatoid factors. An analysis of the cloned receptor protein has shown a high degree of similarity between the M protein and the Fc receptor protein in their secondary structure and in the organization of functional domains. There is extensive amino acid sequence similarity between the two proteins in their signal peptides. On the basis of these similarities, it has been postulated that the M protein and Fc receptor genes of group A streptococci are the products of gene duplication from a common ancestral gene and that the DNA sequence similarity between these two genes may permit homologous recombination as a potential means for the streptococci to develop antigenic diversity.

The etiologic role of *S. pyogenes* in acute rheumatic fever and poststreptococcal glomerulonephritis is well established, but the mechanisms of pathogenicity in these poststreptococcal sequelae are poorly understood. The development of these diseases is thought to be due in part to an abnormal immune response to streptococcal antigens. Elevated levels of heart-reactive antibodies have been found in the sera of patients with acute rheumatic fever; myosin-cross-reactive epitopes of streptococcal M protein have been identified. Monoclonal antibodies recognizing both heart and streptococcal M protein have identified myosin, actin, and DNA as autoantigens involved in cross-reactions between the heart and streptococci. There is evidence, however, that antigens other than M protein may also be involved in immunologic cross-reactivity with the heart and other tissues.

Capsular Polysaccharide. Many group A streptococci produce a diffuse hyaluronic acid capsule, which mimics the ground substance of animal tissues. Although less important as a virulence factor than M protein, it assists the organism in avoiding the phagocytic defenses of the host.

Extracellular Products

Hemolysins. Two hemolytic and cytolytic toxins—streptolysin O (SLO) and streptolysin S (SLS)—are produced by most strains of group A streptococci and many strains of groups C and G. They are responsible for the clear zones of β-hemolysis around the colonies in blood agar media.

STREPTOLYSIN O. SLO is an immunogenic single-chain protein (ca 60 kDa) released into the culture medium during growth. It is the prototype of a group of oxygen-labile or thiol-activated bacterial cytolytic protein toxins produced by diverse species of *Streptococcus, Bacillus, Clostridium,* and *Listeria.* The toxins produced by these gram-positive organisms are immunologically cross-reactive and share a number of common biochemical and physical properties. Their biologic and lethal effects are rapidly lost by oxidation but are completely restored by thiols or other reducing agents. The toxins are inactivated irreversibly by cholesterol and structurally related sterols. Their cytolytic activity, which is attributed to their damage of cholesterol-containing membranes, extends to a wide range of eucaryotic cells, including red blood cells, polymorphonuclear leukocytes, and platelets. The toxins bind to the membrane and oligomerize in the membrane to form large arc- and ring-shaped structures composed of 25 to 100 toxin monomers. The role of the toxin oligomers has not been clearly established, but they appear to span the membrane, and concomitant with their formation, high-molecular-weight cytoplasmic components leak from the cell, resulting in cell death.

Following pharyngeal or systemic infections, SLO induces a brisk antibody response, usually within 10 to 14 days. A more rapid anamnestic response occurs after repeated infection. Because of this good antibody response, the measurement of antistreptolysin O (ASO) antibodies in human sera has proved exceedingly useful as an indicator of recent streptococcal infection. In pediatric populations, where these organisms are frequently encountered, antibody titers of 300 to 500 may be seen normally, but titers are considerably lower in adults. Immune responses to SLO after skin infection are considerably lower, possibly because of local inactivation of SLO by skin lipids. It has also been postulated that SLO may reach the circulation and be involved in immune complexes in patients with rheumatic fever.

STREPTOLYSIN S. SLS is an oxygen-stable, nonantigenic toxin that is extractable from streptococcal cells only when a carrier or inducer is added to the culture or to resting cell suspensions. Serum, albumin, and a RNase-resistant fraction of RNA are among the most potent inducers and have permitted the successful separation of a hemolytically active peptide of about 1.8 kDa. Although detailed information on the chemical and biologic properties of SLS is lacking, the available evidence suggests that the hemolysin consists of a polypeptide attached to an oligonucleotide. It is lytic for red and white blood cells and also for wall-less forms (protoplasts and L forms) from various species. The lytic effects are inhibited by phospholipids, which suggests their involvement in the cytolytic activity of the toxin. Most strains of group A streptococci produce SLS, which is responsible for the surface hemolysis seen on blood agar plates. Those occasional strains that lack SLS may appear nonhemolytic on surface growth.

Pyrogenic Exotoxins (Erythrogenic Toxins). More than 90% of all group A streptococci isolates produce pyrogenic exotoxins. There are at least three different serotypes (A, B, and C), which have molecular weights of 8, 17.5, and 13.2 kDa, respectively. They are heat labile but are stable to acid, alkali, and pepsin. The structural gene for these toxins, as is the case with diphtheria toxin, is carried by a temperate bacteriophage. Historically, much attention has been paid to the scarlet fever rash produced by the toxins. Fever instead of rash, however, appears to be the primary effect of the toxins. Dermal reactivity is, at least in part, secondary to hypersensitivity. In addition to pyrogenicity, these exotoxins also increase the susceptibility of rabbits to lethal endotoxic shock, cause reticuloendothelial blockade, act as specific and nonspecific mitogens, produce myocardial and hepatic necrosis in rabbits, and cause a decrease in antibody synthesis. Because of these properties, streptococcal pyrogenic toxins (SPEs) are members of a larger family of pyrogenic toxins that have a number of biologic and biochemical properties in common. Other members include the staphylococcal enterotoxins, the staphylococcal pyrogenic exotoxins, and the toxic shock syndrome toxin. These toxins serve as immunomodulators of the host defense system; because of their ability at very low concentrations to stimulate T cells to proliferate, they are referred to as "superantigens."

The type C toxin causes increased permeability of the blood-brain barrier to endotoxin and bacteria and exerts its pyretic effect by direct action on the hypothalamus. Traditionally, it has been thought that these toxins cause an erythematous reaction in the skin of nonimmune persons (positive Dick test) and no reaction in persons with immunity (negative Dick test). Antitoxin injected into the skin of a patient with scarlet fever causes localized blanching as a result of neutralization of erythrogenic toxin (Schultz-Charlton reaction). Recently it has been proposed, however, that the rash in some persons may be related more to hypersensitivity than to lack of immunity and that the occurrence of the rash may depend on an interplay between cellular and humoral factors.

Nucleases. There are four antigenically distinct nucleases (A, B, C, and D) in *S. pyogenes* that assist in the liquefaction of pus and presumably help to generate substrates for growth. All strains of *S. pyogenes* produce at least one nuclease, usually the B enzyme. Nucleases A and C have only DNase activity, whereas B and D also possess RNase activity. All have molecular weights of 25 to 30 kDa and require calcium and magnesium for optimal activity. Antibody titers to DNase B are of great value in the serodiagnosis of pharyngeal or skin infection, especially the latter, where the SLO response may be blunted.

Other Enzymes. During growth the group A streptococcus releases a large number of proteins into its external environment. The role of these enzymes and toxins in pathogenicity versus the generation of amino acids or nucleic acid substrates for growth is unclear. Two different streptokinases are produced by group A streptococci. These enzymes are antigenically distinct from the streptokinase of the group C streptococcus (which is the source for the commercial production of streptokinase for use as a thrombolytic agent in humans). Streptokinase forms a complex with plasminogen activator and catalyzes the conversion of plasminogen to plasmin, thus leading to the digestion of fibrin. This reaction also leads to the cleavage of the third component of complement into the chemotactic factor C3a. Streptococcal hyaluronidase hydrolyzes hyaluronic acid, both that present in the streptococcal capsule and that found in animal tissues. Both streptokinase and hyaluronidase are antigenic and may thus be of value in serodiagnosis. Many strains of streptococci also produce a proteinase (especially as the environmental pH falls during growth), NADase, ATPase, phosphatase, esterases, amylase, *N*-acetylglucosaminidase, neuraminidase, lipoproteinase, and a cardiohepatic toxin, possibly distinct from pyogenic exotoxin.

Clinical Infection

Historically, the streptococcus has been a major human pathogen. In the preantibiotic era, streptococci were among the most frequent pathogens and produced significant mortality. Since the introduction of antibiotics, streptococcal diseases have been well controlled, and deaths are uncommon. The major pathogen for humans is the group A streptococcus (*S. pyogenes*), which is also responsible for the nonsuppurative postinfectious sequelae of rheumatic fever and glomerulonephritis.

Acute Streptococcal Infection

Epidemiology. Pharyngitis and impetigo are the most common streptococcal infections. The true incidence is not known, but it is unlikely that a child would reach the age of 10 years without having encountered such an infection. Surveys of schoolchildren for antibodies to SLO or other streptococcal exoproducts have shown that the majority have significant titers, indicating infection within the preceding 3 to 6 months.

Upper respiratory infections occur most frequently during the winter months, when asymptomatic nasal and pharyngeal carriage is also increased and there is a greater tendency for crowding. Group A streptococci are primarily transmitted by droplets from respiratory secretions. Transmission in milk and milk products has been largely controlled by pasteurization. However, explosive common-source epidemics may result from the contamination of foods by carriers or by infected persons. Hospital-acquired infections are occasionally caused by medical personnel with minimal infections.

Streptococcal pyoderma (impetigo) is predominantly a disease of temperate climates, and it occurs with highest frequency in late summer and early fall. Organisms first colonize normal skin and appear secondarily in the pharynx. Although the exact mode of transmission is unknown, insects such as mosquitoes and flies have long been suspected.

Pathogenesis. Group A streptococci possess numerous factors that enhance virulence and allow establishment of infection in the host. Many strains have a predilection for the upper respiratory tract as opposed to the skin, but the mechanisms responsible for tissue specificity are unclear. Recently, however, it has been shown that pharyngeal or cutaneous strains may bind selectively to epithelial cells at these sites. These phenomena have been discussed above in the section on Determinants of Pathogenicity.

Streptococci are rapidly killed after ingestion, and disintegration of most organisms occurs within 1 to 4 hours. The cell wall, however, is resistant to lysozyme and lysosomal enzymes and may persist indefinitely in cells or tissues. The cell walls and peptidoglycan of group A streptococci may produce chronic inflammatory lesions in animal tissues and induce cutaneous nodules and myocarditis in rabbits. In addition, cell walls and peptidoglycan activate complement in vitro, with generation of chemotactic factors capable of inducing inflammation. The role of these phenomena in the induction of poststreptococcal diseases has been postulated but unproved.

Clinical Manifestations

PHARYNGITIS AND SCARLET FEVER. Streptococcal pharyngitis is usually associated with group A organisms, although sporadic cases and epidemics have been reported with groups C and G. When infection is caused by a lysogenized strain, scarlet fever may ensue. In the preantibiotic era, streptococcal pharyngitis was frequently associated with suppurative (tonsillar abscess, otitis, mastoiditis, septicemia, osteomyelitis) as well as nonsuppurative (acute rheumatic fever or glomerulonephritis) complications. Whether associated with the earlier administration of antibiotics or with changes in virulence, the incidence of serious sequelae has progressively declined in the United States and many European countries. Rheumatic fever and glomerulonephritis remain important problems in developing countries, and reports of multifocal resurgence in the United States in the mid-1980s are especially alarming.

Pharyngeal infection may be asymptomatic or may be associated with all gradations of the syndrome of sore throat, fever, chills, headache, malaise, nausea, and vomiting. Occasionally abdominal pain is seen in children and may be confused with appendicitis. The pharynx may be mildly erythematous or beefy red with grayish yellow exudates and may bleed when swabbed for culture. Anterior cervical adenopathy and leukocytosis are usually present. Clinical syndromes indistinguishable from streptococcal pharyngitis may be seen with diphtheria, infectious mononucleosis, gonorrhea, and infections with many respiratory viruses, such as adenoviruses, coxsackie virus, rhinoviruses, and herpes simplex virus.

The association of a scarlatinal rash is almost diagnostic of streptococcal infection. This rash characteristically blanches on pressure and begins on the trunk and neck, with spread to the extremities. Desquamation may occur during convalescence. This may be very similar to the rash of toxic shock syndrome caused by a similar toxin of *Staphylococcus aureus.*

Immunity. Pharyngeal infection probably confers lifelong type-specific immunity. Early treatment, however, may prevent or modify the immune response.

TABLE 24–3. ASSOCIATION OF CERTAIN SEROTYPES WITH ACUTE NEPHRITIS

M Type	Pharyngitis-associated	Pyoderma-associated
1	+ + +	
2	0	+ + +
3	+ +	±
4	+ + +	±
12	+ + + +	±
25	+ +	±
49	+ +	+ + + +
55	0	+ + +
57	0	+ +

From Wannamaker: N Engl J Med 282:78, 1970.
+ + + +, strong evidence of association; ± or 0, questionable or no evidence.

SKIN INFECTION. Group A streptococci produce the syndromes of impetigo, cellulitis, erysipelas, wound infection, and gangrene.

Impetigo is a superficial infection that usually begins as small vesicles, progressing to weeping lesions with amber crust and slightly cloudy purulent exudate. The early lesions usually contain only streptococci but may be superinfected with staphylococci later in the course. Many serotypes have been associated primarily with impetigo and occasionally with outbreaks of nephritis (e.g., M types 2, 49, 55, and 57) (Table 24–3). Most of the "skin strains" tend to comprise the higher number M types. In addition, many isolates either lack detectable M protein or, more likely, represent as yet undescribed M types. T agglutination patterns have been especially useful in defining the epidemiology of non-M typable strains (Table 24–2).

Cellulitis with lymphangitis and lymphadenitis may occur after deeper invasion by streptococci. Systemic symptoms, such as fever, chills, and malaise, occasionally complicated by bloodstream invasion, may be seen. Erysipelas is an infection of the skin and subcutaneous tissues that usually occurs on the face or the lower extremities. This lesion is characterized by erythema, edema, and induration, which usually has a distinct advancing border. Streptococci may be isolated from the subcutaneous tissues and occasionally from the blood. Some persons are prone to recurrences, usually at the same site. Superficial cellulitis may spread to cause gangrene, especially in patients with peripheral vascular disease or diabetes. In addition to group A, groups B, C, and D and anaerobic streptococci may be involved. Sporadic outbreaks of omphalitis occasionally are seen in newborn infants. When caused by a group A streptococcus, acute glomerulonephritis may follow any of these infections. Rheumatic fever, however, occurs only after respiratory infection.

Immunity. The development of type-specific immunity is not well documented in streptococcal impetigo. Antibody to M protein has been demonstrated in fewer than 10% of the infections.

PUERPERAL SEPSIS. In the preantibiotic era, puerperal sepsis or childbed fever was a common cause of maternal death. In recent years, however, with better obstetric techniques, puerperal infections are uncommon. Streptococci causing the infection may be part of the normal vaginal flora or may be introduced by the attending physician or nurse during delivery. Some of the outbreaks that still occur occasionally, even in hospitals, may be traced to respiratory or anal carriers of streptococci. The usual syndrome is characterized by chills, fever, facial flushing, abdominal distention with pelvic tenderness, and serosanguineous vaginal discharge.

Group A streptococci are frequently isolated from the uterus or blood. Mortality has been significantly reduced with antibiotics, but even with therapy, recovery may be complicated and prolonged.

Laboratory Diagnosis. The definitive diagnosis of streptococcal pharyngitis can be made only by direct culture of the posterior pharynx and tonsils. Swabs may be inoculated into broth and examined by fluorescent antibody techniques or onto blood agar, with subsequent grouping by bacitracin disk sensitivity or commercial techniques. Commercial kits are now available for serologic grouping. The bacitracin sensitivity is an inexpensive screening procedure for the identification of group A streptococcal isolates; the fluorescent antibody techniques are also excellent for specifically identifying group A organisms. More recently, rapid detection commercial kits for the identification of group A carbohydrate extracted directly from throat swabs have also been introduced. The results obtained with these kits are highly specific, but they are less sensitive than throat cultures. Whereas a positive reaction obviates the need for a throat culture, negative test results should be confirmed by a routine throat culture.

Streptococci can be best recovered from impetigo lesions early in the infection. Vesicular or pustular fluid inoculated onto blood agar may reveal a pure culture of streptococci. As lesions become older, streptococci and staphylococci may be isolated concomitantly. For culture of cellulitis and erysipelas, material from tissue fluids can be best obtained by needle aspiration, especially from the advancing border in erysipelas, or by subcutaneous injection of a small amount of sterile saline solution followed by reaspiration. Streptococci may also be isolated from the blood in patients with septicemia and deeper infections.

Treatment. Streptococcal pharyngitis is frequently a self-limited disease that may resolve without complication or antibiotics. Therapy is directed primarily at the prevention of suppurative complications and the late sequelae of rheumatic fever and at decreasing the incidence of glomerulonephritis. The treatments of choice are intramuscular benzathine penicillin given in a single dose or oral penicillin V given for 10 days. Alternatives in the penicillin-allergic patient include erythromycin, clindamycin, and cephalexin (Table 24–4). Tetracyclines and sulfonamides are contraindicated because of increased resistance of streptococci and lack of prevention of rheumatic fever. Recurrences of streptococcal infection in patients with previous rheumatic fever may be prevented by

TABLE 24–4. TREATMENT OF STREPTOCOCCAL PHARYNGITIS OR IMPETIGO

Parenteral benzathine penicillin	Children: 600,000 to 900,000 units Adults: 1,200,000 units
Oral penicillin V, erythromycin, cephalexin, or clindamycin	15mg/kg/d in 4 divided doses

TABLE 24–5. PROPHYLACTIC REGIMENS AND RECURRENCE RATES OF RHEUMATIC FEVER

	Parenteral Benzathine Penicillin	Oral Penicillin	Oral Sulfadiazine
Number of patient years	560	545	576
Rate of recurrence[a]	0.4	5.5	2.8

From Wood et al.: Ann Intern Med 60:31, 1964.
[a] Rate per 100 patient years (patient year = number of patients × number of years followed).

monthly injections of benzathine penicillin, by oral penicillin V, or by sulfonamides (Table 24–5). Sulfonamides are effective in prevention but not in therapy.

Impetigo is best treated with parenteral benzathine penicillin or with oral penicillin V, erythromycin, clindamycin, or cephalexin (Table 24–4). However, parenteral high-dose therapy may be required for deeper, more invasive infections. Surgical debridement and even amputation may be required in severe infections, especially when complicated by peripheral vascular disease.

Prevention. Infection may be prevented by prompt therapeutic intervention during epidemics or prophylactic therapy given to persons at high risk, such as military recruits or patients with rheumatic heart disease. Although immunization with M protein vaccines has been shown to be effective, the use of such vaccines in selected populations remains to be explored.

Impetigo is commonly observed in hot, humid climates, especially where crowded living conditions exist. A majority of these infections could be prevented by improved skin hygiene. Epidemics are best halted by improving hygiene and treatment of all cases with effective antibiotic regimens.

Puerperal sepsis may be prevented, for the most part, by strict attention to aseptic techniques during deliveries.

Sequelae of Acute Streptococcal Infection

Acute Rheumatic Fever (ARF). Rheumatic fever is a nonsuppurative inflammatory reaction that is epidemiologically and serologically related to antecedent group A streptococcal infection. It is manifested by arthritis, carditis, chorea, erythema marginatum, or subcutaneous nodules. This constellation of symptoms usually occurs within 2 to 3 weeks of the onset of streptococcal infection, although chorea and erythema marginatum may be seen as much as 6 months later. The clinical experience of T. Duckett Jones led to the establishment of the Jones criteria for diagnosis of acute rheumatic fever (Table 24–6).

In addition to the clinical criteria, the documentation of recent streptococcal infection by culture or serology is of utmost importance. Since the causative streptococcal infection may have resolved or may have been asymptomatic, it is necessary to detect an increase in antibody titer to at least one of several streptococcal antigens (streptolysin O, DNase B, hyaluronidase, or streptokinase). The ability to document a change in titer depends on the length of the latent period, since many patients will have a maximal response at the time of acute illness. Rheumatic fever most commonly occurs after infection by serotypes 1, 3, 5, 6, 14, 18, 19, 24, 27, or 29.

During epidemics of pharyngitis, rheumatic fever may occur in as many as 3% of affected persons. In contrast, in the nonepidemic situation, rheumatic fever will occur in as few as 1 per 1000 episodes of streptococcal pharyngitis. Milder poststreptococcal inflammatory states, characterized by fever, arthralgia without arthritis, and erythema nodosum, may also be seen but are not classified as acute rheumatic fever unless associated with major manifestations (Table 24–6). The major causes of morbidity and mortality associated with rheumatic fever are linked to the subsequent development of rheumatic valvular heart disease. With the decline that has occurred in the incidence of rheumatic fever, rheumatic heart disease probably accounts for fewer than 15,000 deaths per year in the United States.

PATHOGENESIS. The pathogenesis of rheumatic fever is poorly understood. Various theories have been proposed, including antigenic cross-reactivity between streptococcal antigens and heart tissue, direct toxicity due to streptococcal exotoxins, actual invasion of the heart by streptococci, or localization of antigens within damaged muscle or valvular tissues. Circulating immune complexes have been found in the serum of patients with acute rheumatic fever. There is considerable controversy over the relationship of host factors such as the human HLA system and other immune response genes in the susceptibility to poststreptococcal syndromes. Experimental models for streptococcal cell wall–induced arthritis have also indicated a requirement for thymic tissue. The true pathogenesis of ARF, however, may not be elucidated until there is a suitable experimental model.

TREATMENT. The treatment of rheumatic fever depends on the severity of the illness. Prolonged bed rest is no longer recommended unless it is necessary to control congestive heart failure. Salicylates and corticosteroids are of equal benefit in the reduction of acute symptoms and control of long-term sequelae. Corticosteroids are usually administered to patients with moderate to severe heart failure. Although penicillin does not alter the course of ARF, it is usually administered once the diagnosis is definitive or when group A streptococci are cultured from the pharynx.

TABLE 24–6. MODIFIED JONES CRITERIA FOR THE DIAGNOSIS OF RHEUMATIC FEVER

Major Manifestations[a]	Minor Manifestations
Carditis	Fever
Arthritis	Arthralgia
Chorea	Elevated sedimentation rate or C-reactive protein
Erythema marginatum	Electrocardiographic changes
Subcutaneous nodules	History of previous rheumatic fever or rheumatic heart disease

Plus evidence of preceding streptococcal infection (scarlet fever, culture-proven group A streptococcal pharyngitis, or elevated streptococcal antibody test)

[a] Two major or one major and two minor manifestations with evidence of previous streptococcal infection indicate a high probability of rheumatic fever.

PREVENTION. The prevention of streptococcal infections will prevent the development of rheumatic fever. In addition, the prompt treatment of patients with streptococcal pharyngitis within 10 days of onset greatly reduces the incidence of rheumatic fever. Patients who have had previous episodes of rheumatic fever should be placed on a regimen of continuous antibiotic prophylaxis. The therapy of streptococcal pharyngitis and the prophylaxis of streptococcal infection are outlined in Tables 24–4 and 24–5.

Acute Poststreptococcal Glomerulonephritis (AGN). AGN is another postinfectious complication of group A streptococcal infection. In contrast to rheumatic fever, which occurs only after pharyngitis, AGN may be seen after either a pharyngeal or a cutaneous infection. It is primarily associated with a well-defined group of serotypes (1, 2, 3, 4, 12, 15, 49, 55, 57, 59, 60, and 61). Type 12 has been most frequently associated with AGN after pharyngeal infection, with the majority of the other strains being associated with pyoderma. The incidence of AGN in epidemics or in sporadic streptococcal infections may vary from less than 1% to as high as 10% to 15%.

AGN is most often seen in children and may be associated with the acute onset of edema, oliguria, hypertension, congestive heart failure, or seizures. Laboratory findings include dark or smoky urine with red blood cells, red blood cell casts, white blood cells, proteinuria, depressed serum complement, decreased glomerular filtration rate, and serologic evidence of recent streptococcal infection. In addition, less severe cases frequently occur and may be associated with minimal urinary sediment changes or depressed serum complement without symptoms. These changes are frequently seen in the siblings of patients with AGN.

The latent period between streptococcal infection and the development of nephritis is 1 to 2 weeks after pharyngitis and 2 to 3 weeks after skin infection. Hematuria may occur during the latent period both in patients in whom clinical AGN develops and in those in whom it does not. To establish a streptococcal etiology, it is necessary to document previous or concurrent streptococcal infection or an immune response to streptococcal products. Most patients will show a serologic response either to SLO or to DNase B. Since the SLO response is poor after skin infection, it is important to look for antibodies to the latter in patients with impetigo.

Renal biopsy in the typical patient with AGN shows edema and hypercellularity of the glomerular tuft, with red blood cells in Bowman's space or in the tubular lumina. Immunofluorescent examination may show a granular pattern of complement components with or without immunoglobulins, and in electron microscopic preparations subepithelial deposits on the glomerular basement membrane may be seen.

PATHOGENESIS. Granular accumulations of immunoglobulin, commonly seen by immunofluorescent staining, correspond to the subepithelial deposits seen with the electron microscope. The inflammatory response is probably due to deposition of immune complexes within the kidney, although the localization of streptococcal cellular components or exotoxins may also play a role. Circulating immune complexes have been found in the serum of patients with acute poststreptococcal glomerulonephritis. Streptococcal components are almost certainly present within the glomerulus, although controversy exists over the exact nature of these materials.

TREATMENT. Therapy is directed at the secondary phenomena of volume excess, hypertension, and seizures. This consists primarily of sodium restriction, diuretics, and anticonvulsants. Recovery is usually complete in children, although fatalities may occur during the acute phase. AGN in adults may be associated with a poorer prognosis and a higher incidence of chronic renal failure.

PREVENTION. Treatment of streptococcal pharyngitis probably lowers the subsequent incidence of AGN. Therapy, therefore, is directed toward the prevention of transmission of infection, especially when known nephritogenic strains are involved. Effective regimens are presented in Table 24–3.

Other Streptococci Pathogenic for Humans

Group B Streptococci: *Streptococcus agalactiae*

Morphology and Physiology. These organisms cannot be distinguished on a morphologic basis from other β-hemolytic streptococci. In liquid media, however, they tend to grow as diplococci or in short chains in contrast to the longer chains usually seen with groups A, C, and G. Colonies on blood agar are usually large and mucoid (1 to 2 mm) with a relatively small zone of β-hemolysis. A double zone of hemolysis on rabbit blood agar may be observed when the blood is refrigerated after initial incubation. As many as 5% to 15% of isolates may be nonhemolytic. Ninety-seven percent of the strains produce yellow, red, or orange pigment when incubated anaerobically on appropriate media. These pigments (carotenoids) are associated with the cell membrane fraction; pigment production is suppressed by the addition of glucose to the medium. The β-hemolysis is attributed to a hemolysin distinct from those of the group A streptococcus. Its properties are more similar to those of streptolysin S than to those of streptolysin O in that it is not excreted into the medium but is extracted by serum or detergents.

S. agalactiae may be presumptively identified by its ability to hydrolyze sodium hippurate and by a positive CAMP test. The latter phenomenon is characterized by an accentuated zone of complete hemolysis when the group B streptococcus is inoculated perpendicular to the streak of colonies of *Staphylococcus aureus*. The CAMP factor has a molecular weight of 23.5 kDa, is thermostable and antigenic, and acts in conjunction with staphylococcal β-lysin (sphingomyelinase C) to complete the lysis of erythrocyte membranes. A majority of strains can also grow in 6.5% sodium chloride, and a few grow in the presence of 50% bile. Esculin is not hydrolyzed, a feature that distinguishes group B streptococci from group D streptococci. A small percentage are sensitive to bacitracin and thus may be falsely identified as belonging to group A. Group B organisms also produce DNases, hippuricase, neuraminidase, and hyaluronidase.

Antigenic Structure. The group-specific carbohydrate of *S. agalactiae* is composed of D-glucosamine, D-galactose, glucitol, and L-rhamnose, with rhamnose being the major antigenic determinant. There are at least six capsular serotypes

(Ia, Ib/c, Ia/c, II, III, and IV). In some of these serotypes, surface proteins serve as antigenic markers in addition to the capsular type-specific polysaccharide. The frequency of isolations of various serotypes varies from locale to locale, with types II and III usually being most common.

Clinical Infection

EPIDEMIOLOGY. Group B streptococci are commonly found among the flora of the pharynx, gastrointestinal tract, and vagina. Approximately 15% to 20% of pregnant women may be vaginal carriers. The exact rates of transmission of group B streptococci to the newborn infant are variable but may be as high as 50% to 60% in infants born of maternal carriers. The incidence of disease in colonized infants is low but may have disastrous consequences.

CLINICAL MANIFESTATIONS. Group B streptococci cause skin infection, endocarditis, puerperal infection, neonatal septicemia, and meningitis. Skin infections are most common on the lower extremities in patients with diabetes mellitus and peripheral vascular disease. In the last 20 years, group B streptococci have been noted with increasing frequency as causes of neonatal septicemia and meningitis (see Table 25–2). The organism is acquired from the mother during delivery, and clinical disease may be higher after obstetric complications, such as prolonged labor, premature rupture of the membranes, or obstetric manipulation. Mortality rates in neonates may be as high as 50% and are higher when the onset of infection is within 10 days of delivery. Transmission to the infant may be prevented by administration of ampicillin to the mother before delivery, but this is not standard practice.

TREATMENT. Penicillin G is the antibiotic of choice for group B streptococcal infections. A majority of strains are also sensitive to erythromycin, chloramphenicol, cephalosporins, vancomycin, imipenem, and clindamycin. The prevention of neonatal disease by the prophylactic administration of penicillin or by immunization has been considered but is as yet controversial.

Group C Streptococci

In addition to *Streptococcus equi,* which causes disease in horses, a single taxon designated "group C" currently contains those streptococci previously classified as *Streptococcus equisimilis, Streptococcus zooepidemicus,* and *Streptococcus dysgalactiae.* Because of the importance of these species as pathogens for humans and animals, the older designations have been retained for discussion purposes. The group C antigen is also found in some of the minute colony forms of *Streptococcus anginosus* (*Streptococcus milleri*).

Morphology and Physiology. The morphology of the large-colony group C streptococci is similar to that of group A organisms. All species of group C are β-hemolytic, with the exception of *S. dysgalactiae,* which may be α-hemolytic or nonhemolytic. *S. equisimilis* produces streptolysin O, streptokinase (antigenically distinct from that of the group A streptococci), and other extracellular products. Increases in antibody titers may thus be seen following infection with this organism. *S. equisimilis* serves as the source of streptokinase used in thrombolytic therapy in humans.

Antigenic Structure. The group-specific carbohydrate is a polymer of L-rhamnose and *N*-acetyl-D-galactosamine, the latter being the major antigenic determinant. Serotypes within species may be conferred by surface protein antigens that are similar to M protein. Group C streptococci differ from group A streptococci primarily in the substitution of *N*-acetyl-D-galactosamine for *N*-acetyl-D-glucosamine, but group C organisms are not associated with rheumatic fever, perhaps because they lack virulence factors of equal importance to the proteins of the group A streptococcus.

Clinical Infection. Streptococci of group C are important causes of disease in a wide variety of animal species and are not infrequently associated with human infections. The species of major interest in human infections is *S. equisimilis,* which has been isolated from the upper respiratory tracts of normal and diseased swine, cows, horses, and humans. It has been implicated as a cause of pharyngitis, puerperal sepsis, endocarditis, bacteremia, osteomyelitis, brain abscess, postoperative wound infection, and pneumonia. With the exception of an isolated epidemic of pharyngitis that was associated with acute glomerulonephritis, poststreptococcal sequelae do not occur. Treatment is similar to that used for group A streptococcal infections.

Enterococcus species and Group D Streptococci

The group D streptococci have traditionally been divided into two groups, the enterococcal species (*Enterococcus faecalis, Enterococcus faecium, Enterococcus durans*) and the nonenterococci (*Streptococcus equinus* and *Streptococcus bovis*). The previous distinction was based on the ability of the enterococci to grow in the presence of 6.5% sodium chloride. In a recent major reclassification of the streptococci based on DNA/DNA and DNA/rRNA hybridization studies, the enterococci were elevated to genus status.

Morphology and Physiology. Group D streptococci commonly grow as diplococci or short chains. Rare motile strains are sometimes encountered. Organisms in the group differ from most other streptococci in their capacity to grow at 45C and to withstand temperatures above 60C. In addition, they grow in the presence of 40% bile and hydrolyze esculin. All give the alpha or gamma reaction on blood agar, with the exception of a subgroup of *E. faecalis* formerly known as the subspecies var. *zymogenes,* which is β-hemolytic. The species with the group D antigen may be separated on the basis of their biochemical reactions, which are listed in Table 24–7.

Antigenic Structure. In contrast to most of the other groups of streptococci, the group D antigen is not a cell wall carbohydrate but a lipoteichoic acid associated with the cytoplasmic membrane. It is a polyglycerol phosphate in which some of the glycerol is substituted with D-alanine and glucose. The cell wall polysaccharides in the species serve as type-specific antigens. They are acid-labile and do not contain rhamnose. Variations in peptidoglycan structure exist between the species of group D, specifically as additions to the peptide portion: *E. faecalis* contains only glutamic acid, lysine, and alanine, while *E. faecium* and *E. durans* also contain aspartic acid, and

TABLE 24–7. BIOCHEMICAL AND GROWTH CHARACTERISTICS OF GROUP D STREPTOCOCCI

	E. faecalis	*E. faecium*	*E. durans*	*S. bovis*	*S. equinus*
Bile esculin	+	+	+	+	+
6.5% NaCl	+	+	+	−	−
Sorbitol	+	−	−	±	−
Mannitol	+	+	−	±	−
Lactose	+	+	+	+	−
Starch	−	−	−	+	+

±, variable within species.
S. faecalis var *zymogenes* is β-hemolytic and *S. faecalis* var *liquefaciens* liquefies gelatin.

S. bovis and *S. equinus* contain threonine. This group of organisms exhibits a taxonomic problem common to groups C and G and viridans streptococci (i.e., biochemical and antigenic heterogeneity within the Lancefield serogroup).

Clinical Infection. Group D streptococci commonly inhabit the skin and upper respiratory, gastrointestinal, and genitourinary tracts. A majority of infections apparently result from invasion by these normal flora. Person-to-person transmission is not of documented importance.

Group D organisms, most commonly *E. faecalis*, are frequently associated with urinary and biliary tract infections, septicemia, endocarditis, wound infection, and intra-abdominal abscesses complicating diverticulitis, appendicitis, and other diseases that alter the integrity of the gastrointestinal tract. These bacteria are a frequent cause of bacterial endocarditis, especially in the elderly or in patients with underlying valvular heart disease who undergo manipulation of the genitourinary or gastrointestinal tracts. A recent association has been made between endocarditis or bacteremias due to *S. bovis* and underlying gastrointestinal tumors. It has been suggested that isolation of this organism from the blood should alert the clinician to a possible occult malignancy.

TREATMENT. The proper identification of group D streptococci is of practical importance in that the enterococcal strains are generally resistant to penicillin G, ampicillin, and the penicillinase-resistant penicillins. However, many infections may show a synergistic response when treated with penicillin and an aminoglycoside, such as gentamicin or streptomycin. Other antibiotics useful in patients who are allergic to penicillin are vancomycin and erythromycin. The nonenterococcal strains (*S. bovis* and *S. equinus*) are generally sensitive to penicillin G.

Group G Streptococci: *Streptococcus* sp

The strains containing the group G antigen, for the most part, do not have species designations. The large-colony form of group G streptococcus gives a wide zone of β-hemolysis on blood agar and resembles *S. pyogenes* in a number of respects. It produces streptolysin O, streptokinase, NADase, DNase, and hyaluronidase and after infection may elicit increases in antibody levels, especially to streptolysin O, after infection. In addition to these organisms, a small number of the minute-colony and small-cell variants of *Streptococcus anginosus* (*S. milleri*) contain the group G polysaccharide.

The group G carbohydrate is composed of galactose, galactosamine, and rhamnose, with the last being the major antigenic determinant. There are several serotypes within the group, but the antigens have been poorly studied. Strains have been isolated that contain an antigen similar to, or identical with, group A type 12 M protein.

These organisms occasionally cause cellulitis and bone or joint infections, which are frequently resistant to therapy with penicillin alone and often require the addition of an aminoglycoside, such as gentamicin.

Streptococcus anginosus-milleri Group

The *S. anginosus-milleri* group of streptococci includes a biochemically, serologically, and genetically heterogeneous collection of strains referred to variously as *Streptococcus milleri, Streptococcus anginosus, Streptococcus* MG, *Streptococcus intermedius, Streptococcus constellatus,* and minute β-hemolytic colony-forming streptococci of Lancefield groups F and G. Controversy continues regarding the classification of this clinically important group of organisms and will be resolved only when the DNA/DNA homology studies have been expanded to include a greater number of strains. However, as with organisms in group D and the viridans strains discussed below, serologic identification and type of hemolysis of these organisms have less meaning than with the β-hemolytic Lancefield groups A and B. The species name *S. anginosus* has priority taxonomically, but the species name *S. milleri* is preferred by many workers in laboratories throughout the world. The species *milleri* has yet to be officially accepted as a valid species, but, because of its inclusive nature, it is a clinically useful term for a group of organisms with a propensity for causing invasive pyogenic disease.

Growth of many strains on solid media either requires or is enhanced by an increased level of carbon dioxide in the atmosphere. Hemolysis on blood agar is a variable property. Since some strains are α-hemolytic, they are often listed with the viridans or oral streptococci. The *S. anginosus-milleri* group of organisms are found as part of the normal oral flora, principally in the gingival crevice and in dental plaque. They have been isolated from abscesses in many body sites, which, although uncommon, are dramatic and frequently life threatening. Their most common associations are with dental abscesses, brain abscesses, intra-abdominal abscesses, lung abscesses, and empyema.

Viridans Streptococci

Morphology and Physiology. The designation "viridans group" has been assigned to a large number of alpha-reacting streptococci that resist classification by group-specific carbohydrates. This heterogeneous collection of streptococci, generally found in the mouth or upper respiratory tract, includes the following species: *S. sanguis, Streptococcus salivarius, S. mutans, S. mitis* (*mitior*), *S. anginosus* (*S. milleri, S. intermedius,* and *S. constellatus*). They are usually classified by fermentation patterns, cell wall sugar composition, and production of dextrans (glucose 1-6 polymers) or levans (fructose 2-6 polymers) from sucrose. Strict criteria for speciation have yet to be evolved; however, physiologic schemes, such as that presented in Table 24–8, are useful in characterizing species. *S. mutans*, an organism important in the formation of dental plaque, possesses a cellular and extracellular dextran sucrase that produces an insoluble dextran polymer from sucrose. This polymer is an important component of dental plaque, which, in addition, may contain up to 10^{11} streptococci per gram wet weight.

Antigenic Structure. This group of organisms has been notoriously resistant to serologic characterization. Although many strains may possess antigens characteristic of groups F or K (and others), physiologic heterogeneity within these groups makes this phenomenon seem of less importance. Physiologic schemes, such as the one described in Table 24–8, would therefore seem to better characterize a species.

Clinical Infection. The viridans streptococci are frequently found in the nasopharynx, mouth, gingival crevices, gastrointestinal tract, female genital tract, and occasionally on the skin. From these sites the organisms may invade the bloodstream after chewing, dental manipulation, or gastrointestinal or genitourinary instrumentation. In addition, cellulitis or wound infection, meningitis, sinusitis, biliary or intra-abdominal infection, or endocarditis may occur. It has recently been noted that *S. anginosa* has an unusual predilection to produce abscesses in tissues such as those of the brain or the liver. *S. sanguis*, on the other hand, is the most frequent single species causing bacterial endocarditis (see below).

DENTAL CARIES. The role of the viridans streptococci, especially of *S. mutans*, in the production of dental plaque and dental diseases is a complex phenomenon and will be discussed in detail in Chapter 45.

Other Streptococcal Infections

Infective Endocarditis. Infective endocarditis may be defined as implantation of bacteria or fungi on the endocardial surface of the heart. Endocarditis is most frequently encountered on damaged heart valves, in congenital heart disease, or on prosthetic valves. The majority of cases are caused by streptococci (viridans, pneumococci, group D) and staphylococci. Endocarditis may follow a fulminant course (acute) or be a prolonged insidious illness (subacute). Streptococci are most commonly associated with the latter presentation. Endocarditis may complicate infection at other sites, such as pneumonia, abscesses, or urinary tract infection, or it may be a result of transient bacteremia, such as that associated with dental manipulation.

The symptoms and signs of endocarditis are fever, weight loss, anemia, heart murmur, splenomegaly, and peripheral embolization. The diagnosis is confirmed by repeated blood culture. In most cases, more than 90% of blood cultures are positive. Endocarditis may be caused occasionally by nutritionally deficient (vitamin B_6-dependent) streptococci, which require supplemented media for isolation.

The duration of therapy and the choice of antibiotic are determined by the sensitivity of the isolated organism to various antimicrobial agents. Parenteral therapy is given for 2 to 6 weeks. Many cases of endocarditis may be prevented by prophylactic administration of antibiotics to patients with underlying heart disease who undergo procedures associated with transient bactermia (dental work or genitourinary manipulation).

Miscellaneous Infections. Streptococci of all groups and those that are not identified by species or group may cause

TABLE 24–8. SCHEMA FOR BIOCHEMICAL SPECIATION OF VIRIDANS STREPTOCOCCI[a]

	Mannitol[b]	Lactose[b]	Sucrose[b]	Raffinose[b]	Inulin[b]	Esculin[c]	Hippurate[c]	Arginine[c]	Litmus[d]	40%[e] Bile	Glucan[f] Agar	Glucan[f] Broth
S. mutans	+	+	+	+	+	+	−	−	+	v[e]	+	+
S. uberis	+	+	+	+	v	+	v	v	+	+	−	−
S. sanguis 1	−	+	+	v	+	v	−	v	+	v	+	v
S. sanguis 2	−	+	+	+	−	−	−	v	+	v	v	v
S. salivarius	−	+	+	+	+	+	−	−	+	v	v	−
S. mitis (*mitior*)	−	+	+	−	−	−	−	v	+	v	v	−
S. intermedius (*milleri*-MG)	−	+	+	v	−	+	−	v	+	v	v	−
S. anginosus	−	−	+	−	−	v	−	v	+	v	−	−
S. morbillorum	−	−	v	−	−	−	−	−	−	−	−	−
S. acidominimus	−	−	v	−	−	+	+	v	v	+	−	−

From Facklam: J Clin Microbiol 5:184, 1977.

+, ≧80%; −, ≦10%, v, 11%–79%.

[a] Species designations in this group of organisms remain controversial. This schema is given because analysis of cell wall carbohydrates is not required. Lancefield antisera for groups A through G should be used only for β-hemolytic isolates. All bile-esculin-positive strains should be tested serologically for presence of group D antigen (see Table 26–7). Growth in 6.5% sodium chloride or at 10C is rarely observed. All strains were bile-insoluble and optochin-resistant.

[b] Production of acid.

[c] Hydrolysis.

[d] Reduction of litmus milk.

[e] Tolerance.

[f] Production of gel or partial gel in 5% sucrose broth.

pneumonia, septic arthritis, biliary or intra-abdominal infection, urinary tract infection, cellulitis or wound infection, meningitis, osteomyelitis, or sinusitis. Today, with improved techniques of anaerobic bacteriology, microaerophilic and anaerobic streptococci are frequently isolated from patients with lung abscess, septic abortion or puerperal infection, endocarditis, empyema, and intra-abdominal infection. The anaerobic streptococci are discussed in Chapter 43.

FURTHER READING

Books and Reviews

Bisno AL: Treatment of Infective Endocarditis. New York, Grune & Stratton, 1981

Breese BB, Hall CB (eds): Beta Hemolytic Streptococcal Disease. Boston, Houghton Mifflin, 1978

Brennan RO, Durack, DT: The viridans streptococci in perspective. In Remington JS, Schwartz MN (eds): Current Clinical Topics in Infectious Disease, vol 5. New York, McGraw-Hill, 1984

Christensen KK, Christensen P, Ferrieri P (eds): Neonatal Group B Streptococcal Infections. Antibiotics and Chemotherapy, vol 35. New York, Karger, 1985

Cimolai N, Elford RW, Bryan L, Anand C: Do the β-hemolytic non-group A streptococci cause pharyngitis? Rev Infect Dis 10:587, 1988

Gullberg RM, Homann SR, Phair JP: Enterococcal bacteremia: Analysis of 75 episodes. Rev Infect Dis 11:74, 1989

Kimura Y, Kotami S, Shiokawa Y (eds): Recent Advances in Streptococci and Streptococcal Diseases. Bracknell, Berkshire, Reedbooks, 1985

Mandell GL, Douglas RG, Bennett JE (eds): Principles and Practice of Infectious Diseases, ed 3. New York, Churchill Livingstone, 1990, p 1518

Markowitz M, Gordis L: Rheumatic Fever. Philadelphia, WB Saunders, 1972

Ortel TL, Kallianos J, Gallis HA: Group C streptococcal arthritis: Case report and review. Rev Infect Dis 12:829, 1990

Quinn RW: Comprehensive review of morbidity and mortality trends for rheumatic fever, streptococcal disease, and scarlet fever: The decline of rheumatic fever. Rev Infect Dis 11:928, 1989

Tuazon CU, Gill V, Gill F: Streptococcal endocarditis: Single vs. combination antibiotic therapy and role of various species. Rev Infect Dis 8:54, 1986

Uhr JW: The Streptococcus, Rheumatic Fever, and Glomerulonephritis. Baltimore, Williams & Williams, 1964

Wannamaker LW, Matsen JM: Streptococci and Streptococcal Diseases. New York, Academic Press, 1972

Selected Papers

Barnett LA, Cunningham MW: A new heart-cross-reactive antigen in *Streptococcus pyogenes* is not M protein. J Infect Dis 162:875, 1990

Bergey EJ, Stinson MW: Heparin-inhibitable basement membrane-binding protein of *Streptococcus pyogenes*. Infect Immun 56:1715, 1988

Bisno AL, Dismukes WE, Durack DT, et al: Antimicrobial treatment of infective endocarditis due to viridans streptococci, enterococci, and staphylococci. JAMA 261:1471, 1989

Caparon MG, Scott JR: Identification of a gene that regulates expression of M protein, the major virulence determinant of group A streptococci. Proc Natl Acad Sci USA 84:8677, 1987

Chhatwal GS, Valentin-Weigand P, Timmis KN: Bacterial infection of wounds: Fibronectin-mediated adherence of group A and C streptococci to fibrin thrombi in vitro. Infect Immun 58:3015, 1990

Chun CSY, Brady LJ, Boyle MDP, et al: Group B streptococcal C protein-associated antigens: association with neonatal sepsis. J Infect Dis 163:786, 1991

Cleary PP, Kaplan EL, Livdahl C, Skjold S: DNA fingerprints of *Streptococcus pyogenes* are M type specific. J Infect Dis 158:1317, 1988

Craven DE, Rixinger AI, Bisno AL, et al: Bacteremia caused by group G streptococci in parenteral drug abusers: Epidemiological and clinical aspects. J Infect Dis 153:988, 1986

Duma RJ, Weinber AN, Medrek JR, et al: Streptococcal infections: Bacteriologic and clinical study of streptococcal bacteremia. Medicine 48:87, 1969

Facklam RR: Physiological differentiation of viridans streptococci. J Clin Microbiol 5:184, 1977

Facklam RR: The major differences in the American and British *Streptococcus* taxonomy schemes with special reference to *Streptococcus milleri*. Eur J Clin Microbiol 3:91, 1984

Facklam RR, Washington JA III: *Streptococcus* and related catalase-negative gram-positive cocci. In Balows A, Hausler WJ Jr, Herrmann KL (eds): Manual of Clinical Microbiology, ed 5. Washington DC, American Society for Microbiology, 1991, p 154

Fischetti VA, Jones KF, Hollingshead SK, Scott JR: Molecular approaches to understanding the structure and function of streptococcal M protein: A unique virulence molecule. In Horwitz MA (ed): Bacteria-Host Cell Interaction. New York, Alan R Liss, 1988, p 99

Freedman P, Meisler HR, Lee JH, et al: The renal response to streptococcal infection. Medicine 49:433, 1970

Ginsburg I: Mechanisms of cell and tissue injury induced by group A streptococci: Relation to poststreptococcal sequelae. J Infect Dis 126:294, 419, 1972

Goshorn SC, Schlievert PM: Bacteriophage association of streptococcal pyrogenic exotoxin type C. J Bacteriol 171:3068, 1989

Gupta RC, Badhwar AK, Bisno AL, et al: Detection of C-reactive protein, streptolysin O, and anti-streptolysin O antibodies in immune complexes isolated from the sera of patients with acute rheumatic fever. J Immunol 137:2173, 1986

Hafez M, Chakravarti A, El-Shennawy F, et al: HLA antigens and rheumatic fever. Genet Epidemiol 2:273, 1985

Hardie JM: Streptococci; oral streptococci. In Sneath PHA, Mair NS, Sharpe ME, Holt JG (eds): Bergey's Manual of Systematic Bacteriology, vol 2. Baltimore, Williams & Wilkins, 1986, p 1043

Heath DG, Cleary PP: Fc-receptor and M-protein genes of group A streptococci are products of gene duplication. Proc Natl Acad Sci USA 86:4741, 1989

Herzberg MC, Gong K, MacFarlane GD, et al: Phenotypic characterization of *Streptococcus sanguis* virulence factors associated with bacterial endocarditis. Infect Immun 58:515, 1990

Horstmann RD, Sievertsen HJ, Knoblach J, Fischetti VA: Antiphagocytic activity of streptococcal M protein: Selective binding of complement control protein factor H. Proc Natl Acad Sci USA 85:1657, 1988

Johnson LP, Tomai MA, Schlievert PM: Bacteriophage involvement in group A streptococcal pyrogenic exotoxin A production. J Bacteriol 166:623, 1986

Kellogg JA, Manzella JP: Detection of group A streptococci in the laboratory or physician's office. JAMA 255:2638, 1986

Leon O, Panos C: *Streptococcus pyogenes* clinical isolates and lipoteichoic acid. Infect Immun 58:3779, 1990

Ludwig W, Seewaldt E, Kilpper-Balz R, et al: The phylogenetic position of *Streptococcus* and *Enterococcus*. J Gen Microbiol 131:543, 1985

McCarty M: An adventure in the pathogenetic maze of rheumatic fever. J Infect Dis 143:375, 1981

Morrison AJ, Wenzel RP: Nosocomial urinary tract infections due to enterococcus. Arch Intern Med 146:1549, 1986

Mosquera JA, Katiyar VN, Coello J, Rodriguez-Iturbe B: Neuraminidase production by streptococci from patients with glomerulonephritis. J Infect Dis 151:259, 1985

Mundt JO: Enterococci. In Sneath PHA, Mair NS, Sharpe ME, Holt JG (eds): Bergey's Manual of Systematic Bacteriology, vol 2. Baltimore, Williams & Wilkins, 1986, p 1063

Murray BE, Singh KV, Markowitz SM, et al: Evidence for clonal spread of a single strain of β-lactamase-producing *Enterococcus (Streptococcus) faecalis* in six hospitals in five states. J Infect Dis 163:780, 1991

Nealon TJ, Beachey EH, Courtney HS, Simpson WA: Release of fibronectin-lipoteichoic acid complexes from group A streptococci with penicillin. Infect Immun 51:529, 1986

Nealon TJ, Mattingly SJ: Role of cellular lipoteichoic acids in mediating adherence of serotype III strains of group B streptococci to human embryonic, fetal, and adult epithelial cells. Infect Immun 43:523, 1984

O'Connor SP, Darip D, Fraley K, et al: The human antibody response to streptococcal C5a peptidase. J Infect Dis 163:109, 1991

Pancholi V, Fischetti VA: Isolation and characterization of the cell-associated region of group A streptococcal M6 protein. J Bacteriol 170:2618, 1988

Pulliam L, Dall L, Inokuchi S, et al: Effects of exopolysaccharide production by viridans streptococci on penicillin therapy of experimental endocarditis. J Infect Dis 151:153, 1985

Reinholdt J, Tomana M, Mortensen SB, Kilian M: Molecular aspects of immunoglobulin A1 degradation by oral streptococci. Infect Immun 58:1186, 1990

Rýc M, Beachey EH, Whitnack E: Ultrastructural localization of the fibrinogen-binding domain of streptococcal M protein. Infect Immun 57:2397, 1989

Shigeoka AO, Rote NS, Santos JI, Hill HR: Assessment of the virulence factors of group B streptococci: Correlation with sialic acid content. J Infect Dis 147:857, 1983

Simpson WJ, Cleary PP: Expression of M type 12 protein by a group A streptococcus exhibits phaselike variation: Evidence for coregulation of colony opacity determinants and M protein. Infect Immun 55:2448, 1987

Simpson WJ, LaPenta D, Chen C, Cleary PP: Coregulation of type 12 M protein and streptococcal C5a peptidase genes in group A streptococci: Evidence for a virulence regulon controlled by the *vir R* locus. J Bacteriol 172:696, 1990

Spanier JG, Cleary PP: Integration of bacteriophage SP24 into the chromosome of group A streptococci. J Bacteriol 164:600, 1985

Speziale P, Hook M, Switalski LM, Wadstrom T: Fibronectin binding to a *Streptococcus pyogenes* strain. J Bacteriol 157:420, 1984

Stevens DL, Tanner MH, Winship J, et al: Severe group A streptococcal infections associated with a toxic shock-like syndrome and scarlet fever toxin A. N Engl J Med 321:1, 1989

Stimpson SA, Esser RE, Cromartie WJ, Schwab JH: Comparison of in vivo degradation of ^{125}I-labeled peptidoglycan-polysaccharide fragments from group A and group D streptococci. Infect Immun 52:390, 1986

Stollerman GH: Rheumatogenic and nephritogenic streptococci. Circulation 43:915, 1971

Switalski LM, Murchison H, Timpl R, et al: Binding of laminin to oral and endocarditis strains of viridans streptococci. J Bacteriol 169:1095, 1987

Wannamaker LW: Differences between streptococcal infections of the throat and of the skin. N Engl J Med 282:23, 78, 1970

Weeks CR, Ferretti JJ: The gene for type A streptococcal exotoxin (erythrogenic toxin) is located in bacteriophage T12. Infect Immun 46:531, 1984

Weinstein L, Schlesinger JJ: Pathoanatomic, pathophysiologic and clinical correlations in endocarditis. N Engl J Med 291:832, 1122, 1974

Zabriskie J: The role of streptococci in human glomerulonephritis. J Exp Med 130:180s, 1971

CHAPTER 25

Streptococcus pneumoniae

In spite of modern antimicrobial agents, *Streptococcus pneumoniae,* or the *pneumococcus* as it is commonly referred to, remains a leading cause of morbidity and mortality in persons of all ages. It is the most common cause of community-acquired pneumonia and an important cause of otitis media, meningitis, and septicemia. Pneumococcal pneumonia is the classic prototype from which our present concepts of the pathogenesis of pneumonia have evolved.

S. pneumoniae has a long and fascinating history. It was isolated from human saliva in 1881 in independent studies by Sternberg and Pasteur. The following year Friedlander demonstrated its association with acute lobar pneumonia, and within the next 10 years the range of pneumococcal infection was elucidated with remarkable speed.

Some of the most important achievements in biology and medicine have resulted from studies on the pneumococcus. The recognition of different types of pneumococci on the basis of serologic differences in capsular material provided the foundation for specific serum therapy and for the classic studies at the Rockefeller Institute by Avery and his collaborators on the immunologic and chemical properties of the capsular polysaccharides. These studies also formed the basis for the development of the polyvalent polysaccharide vaccine that currently is used in high-risk patients for the prevention of bacteremic pneumococcal pneumonia. The most revolutionary, however, of the many contributions originating from the study of the pneumococcus was the elucidation of the mechanism of transformation of pneumococcal types. The discovery that DNA is the transforming material provided the cornerstone of the modern discipline of molecular genetics.

Pneumococcal pneumonia is no longer the "captain of the men of death" described by Sir William Osler in his famous textbook before the advent of the sulfonamides and introduction of penicillin. Although many factors, such as antimicrobial therapy, increasing age of our hospitalized population, and modern immunosuppressive and tumor chemotherapy, have altered its clinical and epidemiologic manifestations, pneumococcal pneumonia remains an important cause of morbidity and mortality. There are an estimated 150,000 to 570,000 cases per year, with 40,000 deaths. Pneumonia is the only infectious disease among the 10 most common causes of death in the United States today. This continued frequency and severity of pneumococcal infections, coupled with the emergence of strains resistant to most antimicrobial agents, underscores the need for a better understanding of the pathogenesis of these infections.

Morphology

S. pneumoniae is an encapsulated gram-positive coccus, oval or spherical in shape and 0.5 to 1.25 μm in diameter. Characteristically, the organism is lancet-shaped, and as observed in direct smears of sputum and body fluids, it occurs singly, in pairs, and short chains (Figs. 25–1 and 25–2). Continued laboratory cultivation, especially on unfavorable media, leads to the formation of longer chains. Pneumococci are highly sensitive to the products of their fermentative metabolism, resulting in a gram-negative staining reaction as the culture ages. Capsules may be readily demonstrated by examination of wet mounts of virulent organisms in India ink or by use of homologous type-specific antibody in the quellung reaction

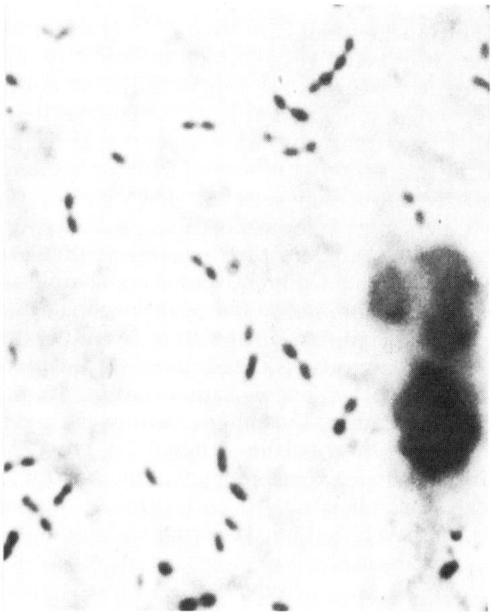

Fig. 25–1. *Streptococcus pneumoniae* in sputum smear. Gram stain. *(Courtesy of Dr. Leon J. LeBeau, University of Illinois Medical Center.)*

(p. 434). The size of the capsule varies considerably with the pneumococcal type and is especially large in types 3, 8, and 37.

Ultrastructure and Cell Composition. The outermost boundary of the pneumococcus is a typical gram-positive cell wall composed of peptidoglycan and teichoic acid. The cell wall teichoic acid contains the determinant for C polysaccharide antigenic activity. At least some of the teichoic acid units are located on the outer surface of the cell wall inasmuch as live pneumococci can be agglutinated with antisera against the C polysaccharide. An important structural component of teichoic acid is the amino alcohol choline, which is unique to the pneumococcal wall and is thought to function as a regulatory ligand.

Essentially all the lipid that is extractable from pneumococci is present in the plasma membrane. Also found in the membrane is a choline-containing teichoic acid, similar to that present in the wall but covalently bound to fatty acids. This membrane lipoteichoic acid is the carrier of the F antigen, an immunologic determinant that cross-reacts with the Forssman series of mammalian surface antigens. Lipoteichoic acid is also a potent inhibitor of the homologous autolytic enzyme, an *N*-acetylmuramyl-L-alanine amidase, and thereby regulates peptidoglycan hydrolase activity.

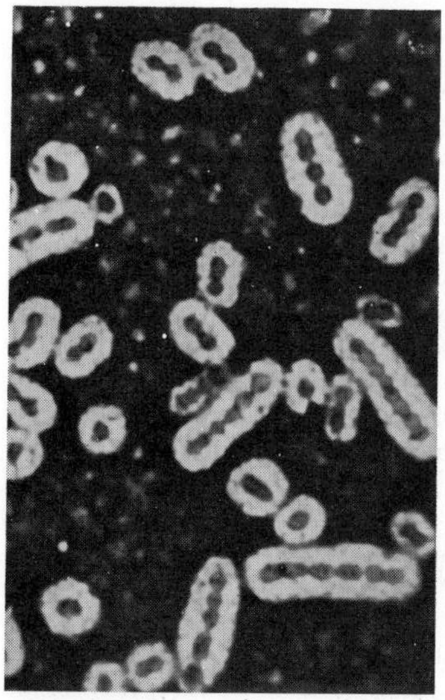

Fig. 25–2. Pneumococcus from spinal fluid. Preparation stained by P. Bruce White method to show capsules. × 1800. *(Courtesy of Dr. Josephine Bittner and Dr. C. F. Robinow.)*

Physiology

S. pneumoniae is a facultative anaerobe that can use a wide variety of fermentable carbohydrates. Its energy-yielding metabolism is primarily of the lactic acid type, but the amount of acid accumulating is small unless the culture is periodically neutralized. Under aerobic conditions a significant amount of hydrogen peroxide is formed, along with acetic and formic acids. Because *S. pneumoniae* does not produce catalase or peroxidase, the accumulation of hydrogen peroxide kills the organism unless catalase is provided by the addition of red blood cells to the culture medium.

Cultural Characteristics. The pneumococcus has complex nutritional requirements. It can be grown on chemically defined synthetic media, but for primary isolation and routine culture, enriched infusion agar and broth such as tryptic soy or brain heart infusion enriched with 5% defibrinated blood, is recommended. The optimum pH for growth is 7.4 to 7.8. Inasmuch as 5% to 10% of all pneumococcal strains require an increased CO_2 concentration for primary isolation on solid media, a candle jar or CO_2 incubator should be used.

On blood agar plates, young cultures of encapsulated pneumococci produce circular, glistening, dome-shaped colonies about 1 mm in diameter. Colonies produced by type 3 organisms usually are larger and more mucoid than those produced by the other types, a reflection of the greater size of its capsule. As pneumococcus colonies on blood agar become older, autolytic changes result in a collapse of the center of the colony, giving it an umbilicate appearance. Unencapsulated strains produce small rough colonies. Colonies incubated aerobically are surrounded by a zone of alpha hemolysis similar to the greenish discoloration observed with the viridans streptococci. Under anaerobic conditions, however, a zone of beta hemolysis is produced around the colony by an oxygen-labile pneumolysin 0 (p. 436).

CHOLINE REQUIREMENT. Unlike other streptococci, *S. pneumoniae* has an absolute nutritional requirement for choline. If ethanolamine is substituted for choline during growth, a number of physiologic defects are observed. Among these are resistance to autolysin, aberrant cell division, incompetence in transformation, and phage resistance. Most of these defects can be directly attributed to changes in the choline-containing teichoic acid of the cell surface. About 85% of the cell's choline is found in the teichoic acid of the cell wall. The remaining 25% is localized in the membrane lipoteichoic acid.

Laboratory Identification

OPTOCHIN SENSITIVITY. The procedures used in the laboratory for the identification of *S. pneumoniae* are designed primarily to distinguish it from the viridans streptococci, both of which produce alpha hemolysis on blood agar. The test most widely used for the presumptive identification of the pneumococcus is the optochin disk sensitivity test. Optochin (ethylhydrocupreine hydrochloride) is a quinine derivative that inhibits the growth of pneumococci but not of viridans streptococci. For testing, a filter paper disk impregnated with drug is applied to the surface of a blood agar plate that has been streaked with a pure culture of the organism.

BILE SOLUBILITY. Another useful test for identifying pneumococci is based on the presence in pneumococci, but not in the viridans streptococci, of an autolytic amidase that cleaves the bond between alanine and muramic acid in the peptidoglycan. The amidase is activated by surface-active agents such as bile or bile salts, resulting in lysis of the organisms. For testing, a neutral pH, 10% deoxycholate, and viable young organisms should be used.

QUELLUNG REACTION. The most useful and rapid method for the identification of *S. pneumoniae* is the Neufeld quellung or capsular precipitation reaction. The test not only identifies an organism as a pneumococcus but also specifies its type. It can be used directly for the identification of pneumococci in sputum, spinal fluid, exudates, or culture. The test is performed by mixing on a slide a loopful of emulsified sputum (or other clinical material) with a loopful of antipneumococcal serum and methylene blue and examining the mixture under the oil-immersion lens. In a positive reaction, which occurs when pneumococci are brought into contact with homologous capsular antiserum, the capsule becomes more refractile and greatly swollen in appearance.

At the present time, the only source of pneumococcal antisera is the Statens Seruminstitut in Copenhagen. Because the prevalence of different types varies with time and geographic area, typing surveillance is necessary to ensure the optimal composition of pneumococcal polysaccharide vaccines for use in different areas. The typing of isolates from vaccines also must be continued to determine whether vaccine use leads to a predominance of different types.

ANIMAL INOCULATION. The mouse is exquisitely sensitive to most types of pneumococci. When injected intraperitoneally with sputum containing pneumococci, the mouse succumbs to fatal infection within 16 to 48 hours. Other organisms that may be present in the sputum usually are eliminated, and pneumococci may be isolated in pure culture from the heart blood. Several types of pneumococci, such as the commonly encountered type 14, however, are essentially avirulent for mice and do not produce fatal infections within 4 days. Although the mouse virulence test rarely is used for diagnostic purposes at the present time because it is expensive and time-consuming, it remains an excellent experimental model in the research laboratory in testing the virulence of a particular isolate or type.

Genetic Variation. The possession of a capsule by the pneumococcus provides an easily recognized marker for genetic studies. When cultured on the surface of solid media, encapsulated organisms form characteristic glistening colonies composed of mucoid or smooth (S) cells. If such organisms are cultured in the presence of homologous antiserum, they produce rough, granular colonies composed of nonencapsulated, rough (R) cells. In such a culture the antiserum selects for R mutants present in any pneumococcal culture. Conversely, when broth cultures of R pneumococci are inoculated into mice, the R organisms are replaced by S pneumococci of the same serologic type as that from which the R strain was derived. In the animal, the less virulent organisms are destroyed by the host, and the more virulent encapsulated forms survive and are specifically selected. The exquisite sensitivity of the mouse to most pneumococcal capsular types permits detection of small numbers of S organisms that arise from back mutations and that would be undetectable unless cultured in a selective environment. The conventional method of maintaining the maximum virulence of a culture by several passages through a mouse is based on this principle.

Another type of genetic variation that occurs in *S. pneumoniae* is transformation. This phenomenon was first observed in 1928 by Griffith and further studied by Avery, MacLeod, and McCarty in classic experiments that demonstrated conclusively the genetic role of DNA. In Griffith's original experiment, it was observed that mice injected with nonencapsulated avirulent type 2 *S. pneumoniae*, together with heat-killed cells from a virulent encapsulated type 3 strain, frequently succumbed to the infection. From these infected animals living organisms of the virulent encapsulated type 3 could be isolated. The active principle in the heat-killed organisms responsible for transforming the avirulent organisms to virulent ones was later identified by Avery's group as DNA. The transformation in pneumococci of a number of additional characteristics other than capsular type also has been demonstrated, as has been the transformation of genetic markers between pneumococci and other species of streptococci. The discovery of plasmids in *S. pneumoniae* and the designing of successful plasmid transformation systems also have provided an accessible model for the cloning of recombinant DNA in this species.

Pneumococcal bacteriophages provide an additional genetic tool for study of the organism. Both lytic and temperate phages have been isolated from a variety of geographic areas and thus are thought to be of widespread occurrence (Fig. 25–3). These phages vary in their morphology, serology, and ability of their DNA to transfect pneumococci. The presence of capsular polysaccharide appears to protect pneumococci from infection by all lytic phages isolated to date. A high frequency of lysogeny, however, has been demonstrated among the capsular types of pathogenic strains that most frequently cause infections.

Antigenic Structure

Capsular Antigens. Pneumococcal capsules consist of complex polysaccharides that form hydrophilic gels on the surface of the organism. These polysaccharides are antigenic and form the basis for the separation of pneumococci into 84 different serotypes. Some of the serotypes form serogroups—types carrying the same number but different capital letters—such as serogroup 7, which consists of serotypes 7F, 7A, 7B, and 7C. The pneumococcal polysaccharides vary in their monosaccharide and disaccharide components, but at present the chemical structure of the polysaccharide of only a few types is completely known.

Some pneumococcal types exhibit no or very few cross-reactions, whereas other types have antigens in common with several pneumococcal types. Also, antisera to some of the types cross-react with polysaccharides from a number of other bacteria, including *Klebsiella, Rhizobium, Salmonella, Escherichia*

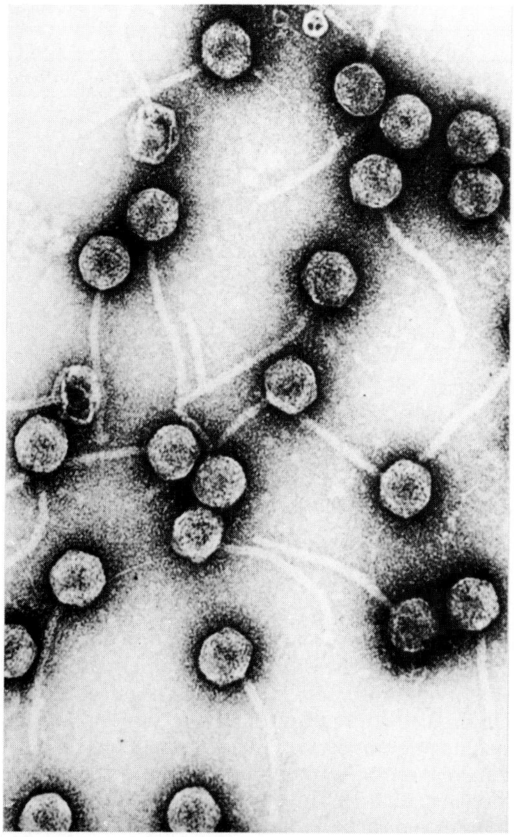

Fig. 25–3. Electron micrograph of purified phage 2, a pneumococcal bacteriophage isolated from a throat swab of an adult in the infirmary at the Massachusetts Institute of Technology. From 62 different throat swabs collected during a single week, 43 gave plaques on the standard laboratory pneumococcus strain 662. The hexagonal heads of two are one third the size of coliphage T4. *(From Tiraby: Virology 68:566, 1975.)*

coli, Haemophilus influenzae type b, and viridans streptococci. In addition, type 14 polysaccharide cross-reacts with human ABO blood group isoantigens. This cross-reaction probably is attributable to *N*-acetyl D-glucosamine, which is the common terminal end group shared by these polysaccharides. The polysaccharide capsule is essential for the pathogenicity of the pneumococcus and stimulates the production of antibodies that are protective against subsequent infection with pneumococci of the homologous type.

Somatic Antigens

C POLYSACCHARIDE. This species-specific carbohydrate, which is a major structural component of the cell wall of all pneumococci, is uniformly distributed on both the inside and the outside of the wall. It is a teichoic acid polymer containing phosphocholine as a major antigenic determinant. Phosphocholine is responsible for the agglutination of pneumococci by certain myeloma proteins and for the interaction of the C polysaccharide with a serum beta globulin in the presence of calcium. This beta globulin, referred to as *C-reactive protein* (CRP), is not an antibody but a protein that is present in low concentrations in normal blood but that is elevated in patients with acute inflammatory diseases. The binding of CRP to C polysaccharide can activate complement and mediate phagocytosis.

In addition to phosphocholine, C polysaccharide contains galactosamine, glucose, phosphate, ribitol, and a trideoxydiaminohexose. The complete structure of the repeating unit has been elucidated and has been shown to be identical in C polysaccharide derived from a number of pneumococcal types (Fig. 25–4).

F ANTIGEN. Another major antigenic component of the pneumococcus is the F or Forssmann antigen, a determinant that cross-reacts with the Forssmann series of mammalian cell surface antigens. The F antigen is a lipoteichoic acid. It consists of the C polysaccharide covalently linked to a lipid moiety. Unlike the C antigen, however, it is distributed uniformly on the outer surface of the cell membrane. The F antigen is a powerful inhibitor of the *N*-acetylmuramyl-L-alanine amidase, which suggests a specific physiologic role for lipoteichoic acids in the in vivo regulation of peptidoglycan hydrolase activity in the organism.

M PROTEIN. Type-specific protein antigens, analogous to the M protein of *Streptococcus pyogenes* but immunologically distinct, are present in pneumococci. No correlation has been shown between the presence of a specific type of M protein and type of organism based on capsular polysaccharide. Antibodies to the pneumococcal M protein are not protective.

Determinants of Pathogenicity

Polysaccharide Capsule. The pneumococcus is an excellent example of an extracellular parasite that damages the tissues of the host only as long as it remains outside the phagocytic cell. Protection against phagocytosis is provided by the capsule, which exerts an antiphagocytic effect. This can be readily demonstrated by comparing the behavior in mice of an encapsulated S strain with that of a nonencapsulated R strain. The S organism is highly virulent for the mouse, whereas the R strain is avirulent and is rapidly phagocytized. Removal of the capsule by treatment with an enzyme specific for the polysaccharide renders the organism nonpathogenic and readily susceptible to phagocytosis. Antibodies against the capsular polysaccharide combine specifically with it, rendering the organism susceptible to phagocytosis.

Many aspects of the pathogenesis of pneumococcal infection remain ill defined. The capsular polysaccharide is present in a soluble form in the body fluids of infected individuals. It is relatively nontoxic, but high levels in the serum or urine are associated with severe infections accompanied by bacteremia, empyema, and a high mortality rate. The excessive amounts of free polysaccharide neutralize anticapsular antibody, making it inaccessible to the invading organisms.

Adherence. Attachment to the mucosal surface is an initial event in colonization and infection. *S. pneumoniae* attaches by interacting with the *N*-acetylglucosamine-galactose moiety of cell surface glycolipids. The capacity to adhere to epithelial cells is important for pneumococci colonizing the nasopharynx or inducing otitis media. In studies on the adherence of *S. pneumoniae* to human pharyngeal cells, differences observed between the adhesive capacity of the various strains could be

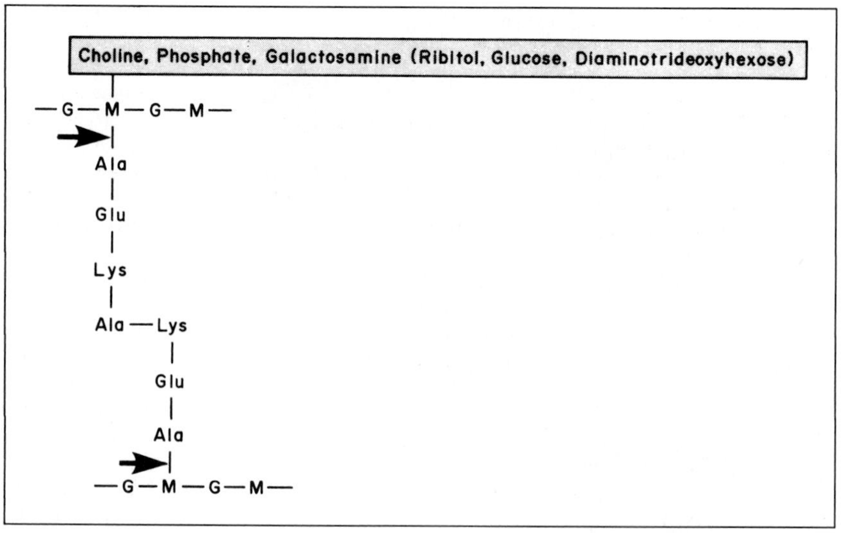

Fig. 25–4. Schematic diagram of proposed cell wall structure of *S. pneumoniae*. The basic element is the *N*-acetylglucosamine *N*-acetylmuramic acid backbone of a typical peptidoglycan, which has two kinds of substituents attached to it: (1) the usual tetrapeptides (two alanine, one glutamic acid, one lysine), which are further cross-linked, and (2) chains of a teichoic acid polymer. The arrows indicate site of action of autolysin. *(Adapted from Mosser and Tomasz: J Biol Chem 245:287, 1970.)*

correlated with the clinical origin of the strain. Otitis strains belonging to the capsular types most often associated with otitis media adhered in high numbers. The capsular polysaccharide, however, appears not to determine the adhesive capacity.

Enzymes

NEURAMINIDASE. A number of organisms that colonize the respiratory tract produce the glycosidic enzyme neuraminidase. The production of this enzyme by log-phase cells from fresh clinical isolates of *S. pneumoniae* has been detected. In its attack on the glycoprotein and glycolipid components of the cell membrane, neuraminidase cleaves a terminal *N*-acetylneuraminic acid from an adjacent sugar. Although a specific role for the pneumococcal enzyme in disease has not been demonstrated, the organism's ability to grow in the human nasopharynx and in the mucous secretions within the bronchial tree requires special metabolic capacities. Neuraminidase is only one of the factors contributing to the invasiveness of the organism.

PROTEASES. Pneumococci produce immunoglobulin-degrading extracellular proteases. Proteases that degrade secretory IgA (S-IgA), IgA, IgG, and IgM have been found in a large number of isolates from acutely ill patients, as well as in symptomless carriers. By eliminating immunoglobulins, these enzymes are thought to play an important role in facilitating bacterial colonization on mucosal surfaces.

Toxins

PNEUMOLYSIN O. Pneumococci produce a hemolysin, pneumolysin O, with properties similar to those of streptolysin O, the oxygen-labile hemolysin of *S. pyogenes*. Pneumolysin is a thiol-activated toxin that is cytolytic for eucaryotic cells that have cholesterol as a component of their cell membranes. Its specific role in the pathogenesis of human pneumococcal infections is unknown, but there is increasing evidence that it is involved in pneumococcal pathogenesis. At very low doses pneumolysin inhibits the respiratory burst and chemotaxis of polymorphonuclear leukocytes; at higher concentrations it activates the classic pathway of complement in an antibody-independent manner. Immunization of mice with purified pneumolysin also confers partial protection against challenge with virulent pneumococci. Pneumolysin exerts a toxic effect on human respiratory epithelium in organ cultures. It causes ciliary slowing, changes in epithelial cell ultrastructure, and disruption of epithelial integrity. Additional proof of the importance of pneumolysin as a virulence factor also has come from a molecular genetic assessment. The pneumolysin gene has been cloned in *E. coli*, and a defined pneumolysin-negative mutant of an encapsulated pneumococcus has been constructed by insertion-duplication mutagenesis. The pneumolysin-negative mutant showed reduced virulence for mice when compared with the parent strain. When pneumolysin production was reinstated by transformation with the cloned pneumolysin gene, virulence of the organism was fully restored.

PURPURA-PRODUCING PRINCIPLE. This substance produces purpura and dermal hemorrhage in experimental animals. Purpurogenic activity resides in the peptidoglycan of the cell wall, which is solubilized by the organism's own autolysin. Intact β-1,4-glycosidic linkages of the peptidoglycan molecule are required for expression of toxicity. There is as yet, however, no conclusive evidence for a role of this toxic principle in the pathogenesis of human infections.

Autolysin. The role of pneumococcal cell wall autolysin in cell division is well recognized, as is its role in causing lysis of pneumococci in the presence of surface-active agents and antimicrobial agents that inhibit cell wall synthesis. Evidence is accumulating, however, that it also contributes to the organism's virulence. Its involvement may not be limited to facilitating the release of pneumolysin, which is located in the cytoplasm of *S. pneumoniae*, but also may include release of other toxic proteins or inflammatory substances from the cells. Autolysin-negative mutants show a markedly reduced virulence for mice; reinstatement of autolysin production by back transformation with the cloned autolysin gene results in a concomitant increase in virulence. These findings, as well as immunization studies in mice which show that purified autolysin significantly increases the survival time, suggest that it is a potential vaccine antigen.

Cell Wall Components. The pneumococcal cell wall is accessible to and reactive with the host environment in spite of its location beneath the capsular polysaccharide. It appears to be a potent activator of meningeal inflammation, with both major cell wall components—teichoic acid and peptidoglycan—contributing to the inflammatory activity. Extensive degrading of either component markedly reduces activity. This inflammatory activity of the cell wall and its components has biologic significance in that these components could be released in the cerebrospinal fluid during the course of meningitis and contribute to further injury of host tissues.

Clinical Infection

Epidemiology

INCIDENCE. Pneumococcal pneumonia is the most common form of bacterial pneumonia. Although it is not a reportable disease in the United States, the estimated attack rate is 68 to 260 cases per 100,000 population, or between 150,000 and 300,000 cases annually. The incidence is three to four times greater in patients older than 40 years of age in whom occurrence often is conditioned by underlying chronic obstructive pulmonary disease. It is increased in closed population groups such as schools, the military, and the institutionalized chronically ill. Pneumococcal infections usually are more numerous during the winter months when frequent viral infections of the upper respiratory tract predispose to infection and spread of the organisms.

THE CARRIER STATE. Pneumococci are carried in the nasopharynx of healthy contact carriers who constitute the major reservoir for pneumococcal infections. Multiple infections within family units, however, indicate that infections also may result from contact with another case. The carrier rate varies with age, environment, and the presence of upper respiratory infections. Carriage rates are highest in children of preschool age (25% to 50%) and with increasing age tend to decrease to about 18% in the adult. The carriage rate for adults who have no contact with children is only 5%. In military installations where the incidence of pneumococcal infections also is very high, rates may be as high as 60%.

PNEUMOCOCCAL TYPES. Although 84 pneumococcal capsular serotypes have been identified, all pneumococcal types are not equally invasive. Well-known differences exist in pathogenicity, resistance to phagocytosis, and stimulation of antibody response. In a surveillance study of more than 4000 isolates from municipal hospitals in several geographic areas throughout the United States, epidemiologic data have shown that 12 types account for about 80% of the infections. Types or groups 8, 4, 3, 14, 7, 12, 9, 1, 18, 19, 6, and 23, in the order given, are the 12 most frequent isolates. In the pediatric age-group, the same types are associated with most bacteremic infections, except for the rare occurrence of type 12 in this age-group. Approximately 65% of the isolates from infants and children are of types or groups 6, 14, 18, 19, and 23.

Although there is remarkable similarity and constancy in the types responsible for infections, the rank order of frequency of different types does tend to shift slowly, and an invasive type may with time assume lesser clinical importance in a particular area. During the past 40 years a shift has been observed away from the predominance of types 1, 2, and 3 infections previously observed to a more balanced distribution. Except for type 3, which is a common inhabitant of the normal pharynx, pneumococci of the higher-numbered types usually are associated with the carrier state, rather than the more virulent lower-numbered types.

Pathogenesis. Pneumococcal pneumonia rarely is a primary infection and results only when the normal defense barriers of the respiratory tract are disturbed. Chilling, anesthesia, morphine, and alcoholic intoxication commonly predispose to pneumococcal disease. By slowing epiglottal reflex, these factors facilitate aspiration of infected secretions from the upper respiratory tract. Viral infections of the upper respiratory tract are a major contributory cause of pneumococcal pneumonia and often precede its abrupt onset. Pneumococci present in the nasopharynx proliferate in the viral-modified environment and are carried down into the alveoli by the thin bronchial secretions. A number of additional clinical conditions also predispose to acute pneumococcal pneumonia: congestive heart failure, noxious gases, and pulmonary stasis resulting from prolonged bed rest. In all these cases, fluid accumulates in the alveoli, providing an excellent culture medium for the organism.

THE PNEUMOCOCCAL LESION. Invasion of alveolar tissue by pneumococci results in an outpouring of edema fluid that facilitates rapid multiplication and spread of the organisms to other alveoli. Polymorphonuclear leukocytes and red blood cells accumulate in the infected alveoli, leading to complete consolidation of the lobe or segment. Crowding of leukocytes in the alveoli promotes phagocytosis and destruction of the invading organisms. Macrophages participate in the final stages of resolution, and in less serious cases recovery is complete and the lung parenchyma is restored to its normal state. Effective antibiotic therapy, however, frequently alters or halts the classic inflammatory response so that the distinguishing histologic features of the spreading pneumonic lesion are obscured.

In the adult, pneumococcal pneumonia characteristically involves one or more complete lobes. In infants, young children, and elderly persons, however, the lesions may be more patchy in their distribution and are localized around the bronchi. From the primary lesion in the lung, pneumococci may invade the pleural cavity and pericardium with the formation of extensive purulent foci (empyema). In fulminating infections, bacteremia also is common and may lead to infections of the meninges, heart valves, or joints.

PHAGOCYTIC DEFENSE. The phagocytic cells in the lungs provide the major line of defense against pneumococcal infections. Before phagocytosis can proceed, the encapsulated pneumococcus must be opsonized by serum components. In human serum, clearance of bacteria by polymorphonuclear neutrophils (PMNs) depends primarily on complement deposition on the surface of the organism. The third component of complement, C3, is of central importance, both as the site of convergence of the classic and alternative pathways and as the source of the opsonically active fragments C3b and iC3b. Virulent serotypes of *S. pneumoniae* differ in the amount, localization, and degradation of covalently bound C3b. In the nonimmune individual, opsonization occurs mainly through the alternative complement (properidin) pathway. In the immune individual, however, the full effect of type-specific antibody requires both an intact alternative and classic pathway of complement activation. The unusually high frequency of severe pneumococcal infections in children with sickle cell disease is attributed to an impairment of serum opsonization of the organism. There is a defect in alternative complement function, as well as in the formation of antibodies to the capsular polysaccharide.

A single specific mechanism for the killing of intracellular pneumococci by phagocytes has not been defined. There is, however, strong evidence that bacterial killing at least partially depends on an intact peroxide-generating system. During aerobic phagocytosis peroxidation of pneumococcal lipids is associated with the generation of peroxide and probably contributes significantly to effective phagocytic killing. Killing by human blood leukocytes proceeds independently of the bacterial autolytic system. An evaluation of the microbicidal capacity of the serum can be made by measuring the chemoluminescent response generated subsequent to the oxidation of the ingested organism by singlet molecular oxygen.

Clinical Manifestations

PNEUMONIA. Classic pneumonia strikes suddenly with a single violent shaking chill and fever that ranges between 102F and 106F (38.8C and 41.1C). The patient usually reports a history of a mild upper respiratory infection preceding the acute onset by a few days. Severe pleuritic pain often is present, and a cough developing during the course of the disease is productive of "rusty" mucopurulent sputum. In untreated cases recovery may be as dramatic as the onset, with fever terminating abruptly by "crisis" 5 to 10 days after onset. In other cases, fever subsides more gradually by lysis. A dramatic crisis often occurs within 24 hours in patients receiving effective antibiotic therapy.

The classic presentation of acute pneumococcal pneumonia is unmistakable. Atypical cases often occur, however, in which a diagnosis is less obvious. This is especially true in the case of the alcoholic, elderly, or debilitated patient in whom symptoms may be less dramatic or overshadowed by symptoms of severe prostration, confusion, or delirium.

Complications. The most common complication of pneumococcal pneumonia is pleural effusion, which results from inflammation of the pleura overlying the parenchymal lesion of the lung. If bacteria gain access to the effusion, the leukocyte response is greatly increased and empyema results. Empyema, meningitis, pericarditis, and endocarditis are serious complications associated with an increased risk of death. Bacteremia occurs in approximately 25% to 30% of the patients with pneumococcal pneumonia and carries with it a twofold increase in mortality. An especially fulminant clinical course is seen in asplenic patients with pneumococcal bacteremia. Patients infected with human immunodeficiency virus (HIV) also are at increased risk for invasive pneumococcal disease.

Prognosis. The case fatality rate of untreated pneumococcal pneumonia is about 30%. With specific therapy the overall fatality rate is about 5%. In adults with bacteremic pneumococcal disease, however, there remains a high case fatality rate (approximately 25%) despite antibiotic treatment, improved intensive care facilities, and shift in prevalent capsular types (Table 25–1). Prognosis is influenced adversely by increasing age, an extrapulmonary site of infection, the presence of cirrhosis or diabetes mellitus, immunodeficiency disease, and infection with certain capsular types, especially type 3. The case fatality rate in type 3 bacteremic pneumococcal pneumonia is more than 50% even with antibiotic therapy.

TABLE 25–1. CASE FATALITY RATE BY AGE FROM PNEUMOCOCCAL BACTEREMIA AMONG ADULTS WITH PNEUMONIA OR EXTRAPULMONARY DISEASE

Category	Age (y)	No. in Group	Deaths No.	Deaths %
Bacteremic pneumococcal pneumonia	14–29	30	1	3
	30–49	130	20	15
	50–69	87	33	38
	70+	15	8	53
TOTAL		262	62	24
Extrapulmonary disease with or without pneumonia	14–29	9	1	20
	30–49	26	9	35
	50–69	24	12	50
	70+	8	6	75
TOTAL		63	28	44

From Mufson et al: Arch Intern Med 134:505, 1974.

UPPER RESPIRATORY TRACT INFECTIONS. *S. pneumoniae* is a leading bacterial pathogen in infants and young children, accounting for a large number of infections of the respiratory tract and adjacent structures, such as the middle ear. By the age of 3 years more than two thirds of children have had at least one attack of otitis media. Many children have recurrent attacks with persistent middle ear effusions and hearing loss. *S. pneumoniae* is the most frequent cause, accounting for 35% to 50% of all cases.

Prevention of pneumococcal otitis media by use of a polyvalent pneumococcal polysaccharide vaccine has been attempted, but its efficacy appears to be limited by the impaired immune response in young children to polysaccharide antigens.

EXTRAPULMONARY INFECTIONS

Meningitis. The pneumococcus is the most common cause of bacterial meningitis in adults and of recurrent meningitis in all age groups (Table 25–2). It is the most serious pneumococcal infection, with a case fatality rate of 40%. Half the cases are in young children aged 1 month to 4 years. Pneumococcal meningitis usually is preceded by pulmonary infection or by symptomatic primary infection of the upper respiratory tract and continguous structures, that is, sinusitis, mastoiditis, or otitis media. Alcoholism, head trauma, sickle cell disease, multiple myeloma, and general debility predispose to pneumococcal meningitis.

Immunity

NATURALLY ACQUIRED IMMUNITY. In the normal adult, natural host resistance is high, and even without treatment, seven of every ten patients with pneumococcal pneumonia will recover. Spontaneous recovery depends on the production of type-specific antibodies to the capsular polysaccharide.

TABLE 25–2. BACTERIAL CAUSES OF MENINGITIS

	Neonates (<1 mo) (%)	Children (1 mo–15 y) (%)	Adults (>15 y) (%)
Streptococcus pneumoniae	0–5	10–20	30–50
Neisseria meningitidis	0–1	25–40	10–35
Haemophilus influenzae	0–3	40–60	1–3
Streptococcus, groups A, B	20–40 [a]	2–4	5
Staphylococcus aureus	5	1–2	5–15
Listeria monocytogenes	2–10	1–2	5
Gram-negative bacilli	50–60 [b]	1–2	1–10

From Swartz: In Wyngaarden and Smith (eds); Cecil Textbook of Medicine, ed 18. Saunders, 1988, vol 2.
[a] Almost all isolates from neonatal meningitis are group B streptococci.
[b] Of all cases of neonatal meningitis. *E. coli* accounts for about 40% and *Klebsiella-Enterobacter* for about 8%.

These are first demonstrable in the serum 5 to 6 days after onset of the disease. In vivo the primary role of protective antibody is opsonic, but the precise mode of clearance in most naturally occurring pneumococcal infections is unknown. The development of measurable type-specific antibody is delayed in patients with capsular polysaccharide antigenemia, but it is not known whether this delay is due to decreased antibody production or to the neutralization of antibody by circulating antigen.

The bactericidal power of the blood of normal individuals varies with the type of pneumococcus and with the age of the individual. Blood of newborn babies has the same killing power as that of their mothers, but this is lost within 3 to 5 weeks. After that, it is observed in an increasing number of persons as they become older until the age of 55 years, when the bactericidal capacity decreases.

Type-specific immunity to pneumococcal infections is long-lasting. Recurrent attacks of pneumococcal infection usually are caused by pneumococci of a different serologic type. Also, the persistence of pneumococci in sputum and throat cultures from patients with pneumococcal pneumonia may be attributed to new types of pneumococci acquired during the course of infection. Multiple types are more frequently encountered in patients with chronic respiratory tract infections in whom pneumococci persist longer than in uncomplicated cases. Persistence is not related to the patient's inability to develop antibodies to specific pneumococcal types.

ARTIFICIALLY ACQUIRED IMMUNITY. Immunity to specific pneumococcal types may be induced by immunization with a polyvalent vaccine consisting of capsular polysaccharides obtained from several of the most prevalent or invasive pneumococcal types. The vaccine currently employed is composed of 23 capsular polysaccharides and provides protection against 90% of the pneumococcal infections acquired in the United States and in Europe at the present time (p. 440). The preventive efficacy of the vaccine in healthy young men in epidemic conditions is 80% to 95% (Table 25–3). Similar responsiveness has been demonstrated for elderly persons and for patients with sickle cell disease and diabetes.

Protection against pneumococcal infection, however, is complex. Such protection depends on the host's ability to produce both opsonizing antibody and complement, the presence of a functioning spleen, and leukocytes able to phagocytize the opsonized pneumococci. Any disease state, therapy, or condition that seriously impairs the host's defense mechanisms may reduce vaccine effectiveness in that patient. These same patients are those at greatest risk of significant morbidity and mortality from pneumococcal infection. The vaccine has yet to be fully assessed in all high-risk groups, but studies to date have shown that even in patients with serious chronic diseases its use is indicated. For maximum antibody response, however, adults should be immunized at about 55 years of age.

TABLE 25–3. BACTEREMIC INFECTION CAUSED BY TYPES OF *STREPTOCOCCUS PNEUMONIAE* WHOSE CAPSULAR POLYSACCHARIDES WERE INCLUDED IN VACCINES

Group	No. at Risk	No. with Bacteremia[a]
Vaccinees	3,975	10
Controls	8,035	113
TOTAL	11,992	123

From Austrian: J Infect Dis 136[suppl]:S38, 1977.
[a] Infection occurred in vaccinees and in controls later than 2 weeks after inoculation.
Note: These data show a protection rate of 82.3% (x^2 = 34.759; $P < 0.0001$).

Laboratory Diagnosis. The collection of appropriate clinical specimens is the physician's responsibility. Sputum specimens must be mucus expectorated from the lungs rather than samples of saliva. The pneumococcus does not survive for long periods on dry swabs or in physiologic saline. For culture, swabs should be placed immediately in nutrient broth for transport to the laboratory. When pneumococcal pneumonia is suspected in a hospitalized patient, blood should be drawn for culture before the administration of antibiotics.

DIRECT EXAMINATION OF SPUTUM. A direct examination of gram-stained smears should be made to determine the probable cause of infection. If the smears are positive for gram-positive lancet-shaped diplococci, a presumptive diagnosis of pneumococcal pneumonia may be made. Cultural identification, however, is required to distinguish the pneumococcus definitively from certain other gram-positive cocci. If typing sera are available, the most simple, rapid, and accurate method for the identification of pneumococci by direct examination is the quellung reaction (p. 434).

CULTURE. Specimens for culture should be planted immediately (1) on an enriched medium such as brain-heart infusion or trypticase soy agar and broth containing 5% blood and (2) in thioglycolate broth. For blood culture, 5 to 15 mL of blood should be inoculated into trypticase soy broth and thioglycolate broth, maintaining a ratio of approximately 1:10 between blood and culture medium. Subcultures should be made by streaking the surface of a blood agar plate. Pour plates with samples of blood provide valuable information on the magnitude of the bacteremia and prognosis of the infection. For culture of body fluids, blood agar plates should be streaked, and 0.5 to 1 mL of the specimen should be inoculated into blood broth. Presumptive identification of pneumococci is based on the appearance of α-hemolytic colonies containing organisms that are bile soluble and optochin sensitive, that ferment inulin, and that have a positive quellung reaction (p. 434).

SEROLOGIC DIAGNOSIS

Detection of Pneumococcal Antibodies. A number of techniques have been employed for the demonstration of an immunologic response to pneumococcal infection. Among the most useful is the radioimmunoassay technique. This test, employing as antigen pneumococcal polysaccharide labeled intrinsically with carbon 14, has been widely used in the detection not only of an immunologic response to infection but also of a response after the administration of pneumococcal vaccines. The method is exquisitely sensitive, is capable of detecting specific capsular antibody in nanogram amounts, and requires very small amounts of serum for the assay procedure.

Detection of Capsular Polysaccharide. Capsular polysaccharide appears in the serum and body fluids of patients with pneumococcal infection. The presence of large quantities of the soluble polysaccharide is associated with severe infection accompanied by bacteremia, empyema, and a high mortality rate. In some patients, especially those with slowly resolving infection, capsular polysaccharide may be detected in the urine for several months. Counterimmunoelectrophoresis has been used to demonstrate pneumococcal polysaccharide in the blood, urine, and spinal fluid of patients and to establish a diagnosis of pneumococcal infection. The pneumococcal capsular antigen present in serum or in pleural or cerebrospinal fluids is similar physically and immunologically to purified pneumococcal polysaccharide (PPP). The polysaccharide in urine, however, is a smaller molecule and has only partial immunologic identity with the PPP. The precise role played by this polysaccharide in the overall disease process is unknown. Also unknown is the mechanism by which polysaccharide is ultimately eliminated from the body, because there is no evidence that mammalian cells can degrade pneumococcal polysaccharides.

Treatment. Penicillin is the drug of choice for all types of pneumococcal infection. Antimicrobial therapy should be started immediately after specimens are obtained for culture and should not be withheld until culture results are available. The choice of drug in the treatment of bacterial pneumonia is based on the results of gram-stained smears of sputum and usually is directed against the pneumococcus. Delay in the administration of specific antipneumococcal therapy probably accounts for the high death rate that is still observed in patients with bacteremic pneumococcal pneumonia.

Penicillin G, given intramuscularly, is the drug of choice in the treatment of uncomplicated pneumococcal pneumonia. Oral penicillin also may be used effectively for outpatients with mild symptoms, but its absorption from the gastrointestinal tract is less predictable, especially in acutely ill patients. For patients in shock, or with pneumonia plus meningitis, endocarditis, or arthritis, aqueous crystalline penicillin should be given intravenously. Patients allergic to penicillin can be given a cephalosporin or erythromycin for pneumonia, and chloramphenicol for meningitis. Response to penicillin therapy usually is dramatic, and bacteremia, if present, will clear in a few hours.

Penicillin-resistant organisms, although still unusual, have been recovered from patients in many parts of the world. Most of these strains are of intermediate resistance with minimal inhibitory concentrations (MICs) for penicillin of 0.1 to 1.0 μg/mL, a MIC that is 10 to 100 times greater than those for susceptible strains. Persons with pneumonia caused by these organisms usually respond to conventional penicillin therapy, but the response in patients with meningitis is more irregular. In 1977, however, strains were isolated from patients with MICs of penicillin 100 to 10,000 times greater than those for susceptible strains. Particularly alarming was the emergence in South Africa of multiple resistant pneumococci with decreased susceptibility to all penicillins and cephalosporins, aminoglycosides, chloramphenicol, clindamycin, erythromycin, sulfonamides, tetracycline, and rifampin. Most of these highly resistant clinical isolates are of type 19A (United States type 57) and have been found associated with both nosocomial and community-acquired infections. Except for a small focus of multiple antibiotic–resistant serotype 19A in Brooklyn, New York, pneumococci highly resistant to penicillin have been isolated only rarely in the United States.

Epidemiologic evidence suggests that the overall susceptibility to penicillin of clinical isolates has changed significantly during the past 40 years of penicillin use. In some areas the incidence of isolates of intermediate resistance is as high as 20%. In the pneumococcus, penicillin resistance is a multigenic property acquired in a stepwise fashion, and it is associated with the development of altered penicillin-binding proteins (PBPs) that have greatly decreased affinity for the antibiotic (p. 185). Selection by penicillin during treatment may play a major role in the upward shift of MICs of penicillin for clinical isolates. There is strong evidence that at least some of the penicillin-resistant clinical isolates are of clonal origin.

Prevention. In the United States the case fatality rate of 25% in bacteremic pneumococcal pneumonia has remained unacceptably high and essentially unchanged by 4 decades of antibiotic therapy (Table 25–1). Attempts to reduce this rate have focused on the development of a pneumococcal vaccine for use in certain high-risk groups. The composition of the vaccine is based on epidemiologic evidence collected during the past 4 decades. The vaccine is composed of capsular polysaccharide antigens of 23 different serotypes of *S. pneumoniae* that cause 90% of the documented pneumococcal disease in this country. The present vaccine consists of types 1, 2, 3, 4, 5, 8, 9, 12, 14, 17, 19, 20, 22, 23, 26, 34, 43, 51, 54, 56, 57, 68, and 70. The antigen content of the vaccine is 25 μg of each serotype of polysaccharide per 0.5 mL dose. Adverse reactions usually are mild and consist principally of local erythema and induration at the injection site. Immunity lasts for at least 5 years after vaccination.

Clinical indications for the administration of the vaccine include all patients who are at increased risk for pneumococcal pneumonia and who possess the immunologic ability to respond to polysaccharide antigen challenge with the production of adequate homotypic antibody. It is probable that the greatest number of reported vaccine failures among high-risk patients is attributable to an inadequate immune response to the pneumococcal polysaccharide antigens. The vaccine should not be given to children younger than 2 years of age. Currently it is recommended for patients with chronic cardiac or respiratory disease, sickle cell disease, splenic hypofunction or asplenia, cirrhosis, diabetes mellitus, and chronic renal disease. The vaccine also should be offered to elderly persons, especially those in chronic care facilities. Although antibody responses in immunosuppressed patients such as those with multiple myeloma, Hodgkin's disease, and asymptomatic or symptomatic HIV infection are likely to be impaired, most patients do respond to the pneumococcal vaccine. Whether the response is sufficient to protect against invasive disease is unknown, but because of its potential benefit in this population group at increased risk from pneumococcal bacteremia, its use is recommended.

FURTHER READING

Books and Reviews

Briles DE, Horowitz J, McDaniel LS, et al: Genetic control of the susceptibility to pneumococcal infection. Curr Top Microbiol Immunol 124:103, 1986

Burman LA, Norrby R, Trollfors B: Invasive pneumococcal infections: Incidence, predisposing factors, and prognosis. Rev Infect Dis 7:133, 1985

Finland M: Excursions into epidemiology: Selected studies during the past four decades at Boston City Hospital. J Infect Dis 128:76, 1973

Geiseler PJ, Nelson KE, Levin S, et al: Community-acquired purulent meningitis: A review of 1,316 cases during the antibiotic era, 1954–1976. Rev Infect Dis 2:725, 1980

Kass EH (ed): Assessment of the pneumococcal polysaccharide vaccine. Rev Infect Dis 3 [suppl]:S1, 1981

Kass EH, Green, GM, Goldstein E: Mechanisms of antibacterial action in the respiratory tract. Bacteriol Rev 30:488, 1966

Quie PG, Giebink GS, Winkelstein JA (eds): The pneumococcus. A symposium. Rev Infect Dis 3:183, 1981

Schwartz JS: Pneumococcal vaccine: Clinical efficacy and effectiveness. Ann Intern Med 96:208, 1982

Swartz MN: Bacterial meningitis. In Wyngaarden JB, Smith LH Jr (eds): Cecil Textbook of Medicine, 18th ed. Philadelphia, Saunders, 1988, vol 2, p 1604

Tomasz A: New and complex strategies of β-lactam antibiotic resistance in pneumococci and staphylococci. In Ayoub EM, Cassell GH, Branche WC Jr, Henry TJ (eds): Microbial Determinants of Virulence and Host Response. Washington, DC, American Society for Microbiology, 1990, p 345

Ward J, Koornhof: Antibiotic-resistant pneumococci. In Remington JS, Swartz MN (eds): Current Clinical Topics in Infectious Diseases. New York, McGraw-Hill, 1980, vol 1, pp 265–287

Selected Papers

Alvarez S, Guarderas J, Shell CG, et al: Nosocomial pneumococcal bacteremia. Arch Intern Med 146:1509, 1986

Avery OT, MacLeod CM, McCarty M: Transformation of pneumococcal types induced by a deoxyribonucleic acid fraction isolated from *Pneumococcus* type III. J Exp Med 79:137, 1944

Bernheimer HP: Lysogeny in pneumococci freshly isolated from man. Science 195:66, 1977

Berry AM, Lock RA, Hansman D, Paton JC: Contribution of autolysin to virulence of *Streptococcus pneumoniae.* Infect Immun 57:2324, 1989

Bolan G, Broome CV, Facklam RR, et al: Pneumococcal vaccine efficacy in selected populations in the United States. Ann Intern Med 104:1, 1986

Briles DE, Forman C, Horowitz JC, et al: Antipneumococcal effects of C-reactive protein and monoclonal antibodies to pneumococcal cell wall and capsular antigens. Infect Immun 57:1457, 1989

Brunell PA, Bass JW, Daum RS, et al (Committee on Infectious Diseases, American Academy of Pediatrics): Recommendations for using pneumococcal vaccine in children. Pediatrics 75:1153, 1985

Centers for Disease Control: Pneumococcal polysaccharide vaccine. MMWR 38:64, 1989

Claverys JP, Lefevre JC, Sicard AM: Transformation of *Streptococcus pneumoniae* with *S. pneumoniae*–phage hybrid DNA: Induction of deletions. Proc Natl Acad Sci USA 77:3534, 1980

Cohn DA, Schiffman G: Immunoregulatory role of the spleen in antibody responses to pneumococcal polysaccharide antigens. Infect Immun 55:1375, 1987

Crain MJ, Waltman WD II, Turner JS, et al: Pneumococcal surface protein A (Psp A) is serologically highly variable and is expressed by all clinically important capsular serotypes of *Streptococcus pneumoniae.* Infect Immun 58:3293, 1990

Dowson CG, Hutchison A, Brannigan JA: Horizontal transfer of penicillin-binding protein genes in penicillin-resistant clinical isolates of *Streptococcus pneumoniae.* Proc Natl Acad Sci USA 86:8842, 1989

Finland M, Barnes MW: Changes in occurrence of capsular serotypes of *Streptococcus pneumoniae* at Boston City Hospital during selected years between 1935 and 1974. J Clin Microbiol 5:154, 1977

Gordon DL, Johnson GM, Hostetter MK: Ligand-receptor interactions in the phagocytosis of virulent *Streptococcus pneumoniae* by polymorphonuclear leukocytes. J Infect Dis 154:619, 1986

Gray BM, Dillon HC Jr: Epidemiological studies of *Streptococcus pneumoniae* in infants: Antibody to types 3, 6, 14, and 23 in the first two years of life. J Infect Dis 158:948, 1988

Griffith F: The significance of pneumococcal types. J Hyg 27:113, 1928

Guckian JC, Christensen GD, Fine DP: The role of opsonins in recovery from experimental pneumococcal pneumonia. J Infect Dis 142:175, 1980

Handwerger S, Tomasz A: Alterations in penicillin-binding proteins of clinical and laboratory isolates of pathogenic *Streptococcus pneumoniae* with low levels of penicillin resistance. J Infect Dis 153:83, 1986

Heidelberger M, Nimmich W: Additional immunochemical relationships of capsular polysaccharides of *Klebsiella* and pneumococci. J Immunol 109:1337, 1972

Henderson FW, Gilligan PH, Wait K, Goff DA: Nasopharyngeal carriage of antibiotic-resistant pneumococci by children in group day care. J Infect Dis 157:256, 1988

Holtze JV, Tomasz A: Lipoteichoic acid: A specific inhibitor of autolysin activity in pneumococcus. Proc Natl Acad Sci USA 72:1690, 1975

Horne D, Tomasz A: Pneumococcal Forssman antigen: Enrichment in mesosomal membranes and specific binding to the autolytic enzyme of *Streptococcus pneumoniae.* J Bacteriol 161:18, 1985

Hostetter MK: Serotype variations among virulent pneumococci in deposition and degradation of covalently bound C3b: Implications for phagocytosis and antibody production. J Infect Dis 153:682, 1986

Istre GR, Tarpay M, Anderson M, et al: Invasive disease due to *Streptococcus pneumoniae* in an area with a high rate of relative penicillin resistance. J Infect Dis 156:732, 1987

Jabes D, Nachman S, Tomasz A: Penicillin-binding protein families: Evidence for the clonal nature of penicillin resistance in clinical isolates of pneumococci. J Infect Dis 159:16, 1989

Kasper, DL: Bacterial capsule—old dogmas and new tricks. J Infect Dis 153:407, 1986

Klein RS, Selwyn PA, Maude D, et al: Response to pneumococcal vaccine among asymptomatic heterosexual partners of persons with AIDS and intravenous drug users infected with human immunodeficiency virus. J Infect Dis 160:826, 1989

Klugman KP, Koornhof HJ: Drug resistance patterns and serogroups

of pneumococcal isolates from cerebrospinal fluid or blood, 1979–1986. J Infect Dis 158:956, 1988
LaForce FM, Eickhoff TC: Pneumococcal vaccine: An emerging consensus. Ann Intern Med 108:757, 1988
MacLeod CM, Hodges RG, Heidelberger M, et al: Prevention of pneumococcal pneumonia by immunization with specific capsular polysaccharides. J Exp Med 82:445, 1945
McDonnell M, Ronda-Lain C, Tomasz A: "Diplophage": A bacteriophage of *Diplococcus pneumoniae.* Virology 63:577, 1975
Mosser JL, Tomasz A: Choline-containing teichoic acid as a structural component of pneumococcal wall and its role in sensitivity to lysis by an autolytic enzyme. J Biol Chem 245:287, 1970
Mufson MA, Kruss DM, Wasil RE, Metzgar WI: Capsular types and outcome of bacteremic pneumococcal disease in the antibiotic era. Arch Intern Med 134:505, 1974
Prober CG, Frayha H, Klein M, Schiffman G: Immunologic responses of children to serious infections with *Streptococcus pneumoniae.* J Infect Dis 148:427, 1983
Redd SC, Rutherford GW III, Sande MA: The role of human immunodeficiency virus infection in pneumococcal bacteremia in San Francisco residents. J Infect Dis 162:1012, 1990
Ripley-Petzoldt ML, Giebink GS, Juhn SK, et al: The contribution of pneumococcal cell wall to the pathogenesis of experimental otitis media. J Infect Dis 157:245, 1988
Robbins JB, Austrian R, Lee C-J, et al: Considerations for formulating the second-generation pneumococcal capsular polysaccharide vaccine with emphasis on cross-reactive types within groups. J Infect Dis 148:1136, 1983
Ronda C, Lopez R, Garcia E: Isolation and characterization of a new bacteriophage, Cp-1, infecting *Streptococcus pneumoniae.* J Virol 40:551, 1981
Ronda-Lain C, Lopez R, Tapia A, Tomasz A: Role of the pneumococcal autolysin (murein hydrolase) in the release of progeny bacteriophage and in the bacteriophage-induced lysis of the host cells. J Virol 21:366, 1977
Ronda C, Lopez R, Tomasz A, Portoles A: Transfection of *Streptococcus pneumoniae* with bacteriophage DNA. J Virol 26:221, 1978
Ruben FL, Uhrin M: Specific immunoglobulin-class antibody responses in the elderly before and after 14-valent pneumococcal vaccine. J Infect Dis 151:845, 1985
Seto H, Tomasz A: Early stages in DNA binding and uptake during genetic transformation of pneumococci. Proc Natl Acad Sci USA 71:1493, 1974
Shohet SB, Pitt J, Baehner RL, Poplack DG: Lipid peroxidation in the killing of phagocytized pneumococci. Infect Immun 10:1321, 1974
Simberkoff MS, Cross AP, Al-Ibrahim M, et al: Efficacy of pneumococcal vaccine in high-risk patients. Results of a Veterans Administration Cooperative Study. N Engl J Med 315:1313, 1986
Simberkoff MS, Lukaszewski M, Cross A, et al: Antibiotic-resistant isolates of *Streptococcus pneumoniae* from clinical specimens: A cluster of serotype 19A organisms in Brooklyn, New York. J Infect Dis 153:78, 1986
Simberkoff MS, Sadr WE, Schiffman G, Rahal JJ Jr: *Streptococcus pneumoniae* infections and bacteremia in patients with acquired immune deficiency syndrome, with report of a pneumococcal vaccine failure. Am Rev Respir Dis 130:1174, 1984
Sims RV, Steinmann WC, McConville JH, et al: The clinical effectiveness of pneumococcal vaccine in the elderly. Ann Intern Med 108:653, 1988
Stassi DL, Lopez P, Espinosa M, Lacks SA: Cloning of chromosomal genes in *Streptococcus pneumoniae.* Proc Natl Acad Sci USA 78:7028, 1981
Steinfort C, Wilson R, Mitchell T, et al: Effect of *Streptococcus pneumoniae* on human respiratory epithelium in vitro. Infect Immun 57:2006, 1989
Thore M, Löfgren S, Tärnvik A, et al: Anaerobic phagocytosis, killing, and degradation of *Streptococcus pneumoniae* by human peripheral blood leukocytes. Infect Immun 47:277, 1985
Tiraby JG, Tiraby E, Fox MS: Pneumococcal bacteriophages. Virology 68:566, 1975
Tuomanen E, Hengstler B, Zak O, Tomasz A: The role of complement in inflammation during experimental pneumococcal meningitis. Microbial Pathogen 1:15, 1986
Tuomanen E, Liu H, Hengstler B, et al: The induction of meningeal inflammation by components of the pneumococcal cell wall. J Infect Dis 151:859, 1985
Wikström MB, Dahlen G, Kayser B, Nygren H: Degradation of human immunoglobulins by proteases from *Streptococcus pneumoniae* obtained from various human sources. Infect Immun 44:33, 1984
Williams WW, Hickson MA, Kane MA, et al: Immunization policies and vaccine coverage among adults: The risk for missed opportunities. Ann Intern Med 108:616, 1988
Wilson D, Braley-Mullen H: Antigen requirements for priming of type III pneumococcal polysaccharide-specific IgG memory responses: Suppression of memory with the T-independent form of antigen. Cell Immunol 64:177, 1981
Winkelstein JA, Abramovitz AS, Tomasz A: Activation of C3 via the alternative complement pathway results in fixation of C3b to the pneumococcal cell wall. J Immunol 124:2502, 1980
Winkelstein JA, Shin HS: The role of immunoglobulin in the interaction of pneumococci and the properdin pathway: Evidence for its specificity and lack of requirement for the Fc portion of the molecule. J Immunol 112:1635, 1974

CHAPTER 26

Neisseria

Neisseria

Two species of the genus *Neisseria* are of major medical importance, *Neisseria meningitidis* and *Neisseria gonorrhoeae*. The organisms are genetically very closely related, but the clinical manifestations of the diseases they produce are quite different. Discovered in 1885 by Neisser, for whom the genus is named, *N. gonorrhoeae* is the etiologic agent of gonorrhea, the most prevalent of the classic venereal diseases. The last decade of the twentieth century finds a worldwide epidemic of gonorrhea in progress.

N. meningitidis is the causative agent of meningococcal meningitis, a disease that has the potential for occurring in epidemic form. Because of the tendency of this illness to occur in clusters, there is a great deal of concern when a patient with meningococcal infection is identified. Within the last decade, the identification and purification of capsular antigens of several types of *N. meningitidis* have resulted in the preparation and commercial availability of vaccines for use in epidemic situations.

Humans are the only known reservoir of the members of the genus *Neisseria,* which includes, in addition to *N. meningitidis* and *N. gonorrhoeae,* organisms that inhabit the upper respiratory tract and other mucosal surfaces of the body. In these positions as resident flora, the other *Neisseria* can be confused with *N. gonorrhoeae* and *N. meningitidis.* Unusual situations occur in which certain of the other species may be responsible for invasive disease in the human host. Species within the genus are shown in Table 26–1.

The genus *Neisseria* is one of four genera included in the family Neisseriaceae. Other genera in the family include *Moraxella* (*Branhamella*), *Acinetobacter,* and *Kingella.* The taxonomic classification and an outline of the distinguishing characteristics of the four genera of the family Neisseriaceae are

TABLE 26–1. CHARACTERISTICS DIFFERENTIATING THE SPECIES OF GENUS *NEISSERIA* ASSOCIATED WITH HUMAN INFECTION

	N. gonorrhoeae	*N. meningitidis*	*N. sicca*	*N. subflava*	*N. flavescens*	*N. mucosa*	*N. lactamica*
Acid from							
Glucose	+	+	+	+	−	+	+
Maltose	−	+	+	+	−	+	+
Sucrose	−	−	+	±	−	+	−
Lactose	−	−	−	−	−	−	+
Polysaccharide produced from 5% sucrose	−	−	+	±	+	+	−
Reduction of							
Nitrate	−	−	−	−	−	+	−
Nitrite	±[a]	±[a]	+	+	+	+	−
Pigment	−	−	±	+	+	±	+
Extra CO_2 for growth	+	+	−	−	−	−	−

[a] Nitrite in low concentrations can be reduced by *N. gonorrhoeae* and by serogroups A, D, and Y of *N. meningitidis*.

given in Table 26–2. *Moraxella* organisms have come to be appreciated as significant pathogens in otitis media of childhood and in respiratory infection in adults. Persons with chronic obstructive pulmonary disease are predisposed to bronchitis and pneumonia with these bacteria alone or in conjunction with other organisms. Unusual disease, including bacteremia, has been reported in children and adults. These bacteria are nosocomial pathogens and cause disease in hospitalized patients. The other genera cause occasional invasive disease and are opportunistic agents.

Morphology

Neisseria are gram-negative cocci, 0.6 to 1.0 μm in diameter. The organisms usually are seen in pairs with adjacent sides flattened. Fresh isolates of most *N. meningitidis* serogroups are encapsulated. Other *Neisseria* species produce surface polysaccharides as loosely associated envelopes or intact capsules. Fimbriae or pili are present on virulent *N. gonorrhoeae,* and although they frequently are present on *N. meningitidis* isolates, there is no correlation with virulence. *Neisseria* are not motile.

The *Neisseria* are structurally like other gram-negative bacteria. The ultrastructure of the cytoplasm and the cell wall of the meningococcus and the gonococcus are similar. The cell envelope is composed of three major elements: the cytoplasmic membrane; the rigid peptidoglycan layer; and the outer membrane, which contains lipopolysaccharide, phospholipid, and proteins that are immunologically significant.

Physiology

Neisseria are aerobic or facultatively anaerobic organisms. Most strains of *N. meningitidis* and *N. gonorrhoeae* utilize glucose, but the acid produced arises primarily from an oxidative pathway rather than by fermentation, which explains the weak reaction that usually is observed. All *Neisseria* produce catalase and cytochrome oxidase.

Members of the genus are highly susceptible to adverse environmental conditions, such as drying, chilling, and exposure to unfavorable pH or to sunlight. They should be handled in the laboratory with minimal delay.

Cultural Characteristics

N. meningitidis and *N. gonorrhoeae* are fastidious organisms with complex nutritional growth requirements. Iron is required for growth, and the ability of the organism to compete for transferrin-bound iron is discussed below under Determinants of Pathogenicity. Starch, cholesterol, or albumin should be added to the media to neutralize the inhibitory effect of fatty acids.

Laboratory Identification

Cultures derived from normally sterile sites, such as cerebrospinal fluid, blood, or synovial fluid, can be inoculated on nonselective media, such as chocolate agar. Growth of primary

TABLE 26–2. DIFFERENTIAL PROPERTIES OF THE GENERA OF THE FAMILY NEISSERIACIAE

Genus	Morphology	Dissimilation of Glucose	Oxidase	Catalase	G + C (moles %)
Neisseria[a]	Gram-negative cocci	+	+	+	46.5–53.5
Moraxella					
Subgenus *Moraxella*	Gram-negative rods	−	+	+	40–47.5
Subgenus *Branhamella*	Gram-negative cocci	−	+	+	40–47.5
Acinetobacter	Gram-negative rods	±	−	+	38–47
Kingella	Gram-negative rods	+	+	−	47–55

[a] Species: *N. gonorrhoeae, N. meningitidis, N. lactamica, N. sicca, N. subflava, N. flavescens, N. mucosa, N. cinerea, N. dentrificans, N. elongata, N. canis.*

isolates is enhanced by incubation in the presence of 3% to 10% CO_2. Some of the apparently beneficial effects of the CO_2 atmosphere may be a result of the increased moisture present in the incubator.

Thayer-Martin or Martin-Lewis selective media permit recognition of *N. meningitidis* and *N. gonorrhoeae* from materials contaminated with other bacterial flora. The media contain chocolate agar modified by the addition of vancomycin to inhibit gram-positive bacteria; colistin for the inhibition of gram-negative enteric flora; and nystatin for the inhibition of yeast. Most nonpathogenic *Neisseria* species also fail to grow on these media. Recently, *N. gonorrhoeae* organisms sensitive to vancomycin have been recognized, but using a low concentration of vancomycin will solve this problem. Only rarely are meningococci inhibited. A number of biochemical reactions are useful in the differentiation of *N. meningitidis* and *N. gonorrhoeae* from other species that are present in clinical material (Table 26–1). Colonies of *Neisseria* species may be recognized by use of the oxidase test that employs the indicator dye tetramethyl-*p*-phenylenediamine dihydrochloride. When exposed to this dye, colonies turn dark purple within seconds. Because all *Neisseria* are oxidase positive, however, the finding of oxidase-positive, gram-negative diplococci in a clinical specimen requires additional tests for confirmation and identification of species. Organisms are rapidly killed by the oxidase reagent; therefore subculture to chocolate agar of the unused portion of the colony should be made immediately.

The distinction between *N. gonorrhoeae* and *N. meningitidis* usually is based on the metabolism of carbohydrates. *N. meningitidis* produces acid from both glucose and maltose, whereas *N. gonorrhoeae* produces acid from glucose only. These differential tests of pure cultures can be complicated by some of the growth characteristics of these organisms. For example, the production of acid from carbohydrate sources may be masked by the alkaline products of enzymatic peptone degradation. Supplementary methods of identification may thus be required. Isoenzyme electrophoresis has been used to analyze the hexokinase from Neisseriaceae. Gonococci and meningococci each have a characteristic hexokinase isoenzyme that is species specific and that distinguishes these two organisms from each other and from other species of Neisseriaceae. The isoenzyme remains constant after transformation that alters carbohydrate utilization by the transformant. The carbohydrate utilization pattern may be an imperfect means of distinguishing species; thus the electrophoresis of hexokinase enzymes may be important because it is more precise.

A valuable but not fully appreciated differential diagnostic test is based on the synthesis from 5% sucrose of an iodine-reacting polysaccharide by *Neisseria* species other than *N. gonorrhoeae, N. meningitidis,* and *Neisseria lactamica.* The test is done simply by incubating a streaked culture on 5% sucrose agar for 48 hours and then treating the culture with modified Gram's iodine. A positive test shows a darkening of the colonies to red-blue or blue-black.

Other techniques that are not generally available in service laboratories may become practical as the methodology is standardized. DNA hybridization using the 2.6 MDa gonococcal cryptic plasmid as a radiolabeled probe detects as few as 100 colony-forming units of *N. gonorrhoeae.* The technique provides a means of detecting nonviable organisms, and the specimens placed on nitrocellulose filter paper can be mailed. Evaluation of the method has been in symptomatic males with urethritis, but additional data are needed. At present it is not as sensitive in female infections as culture is and is not generally available. In summary, the identification of isolates as *Neisseria* species is based on the growth of gram-negative, oxidase-positive, catalase-positive diplococci that produce characteristic colonies on blood and chocolate agar plates. The differential utilization of carbohydrates forms the basis of initial speciation. Immunoserologic diagnosis of *N. meningitidis* or recognition of antigen in specimens can be accomplished by means of specific antisera as discussed on page 449.

Neisseria meningitidis

Antigenic Structure

Nine serotypes of *N. meningitidis,* designated A, B, C, D, X, Y, Z, W-135, and 29-E, have been identified on the basis of immunologic specificity of capsular polysaccharides. Organisms in groups A, B, and C are most often responsible for clinically recognized disease. The structural repeating unit of the capsular polysaccharides of all serotypes except D is known and listed in Table 26–3. Identification and purification of the groups A, C, Y, and W-135 polysaccharide antigens have resulted in the production and licensure of effective vaccines. The type B polysaccharide has been purified but is nonimmunogenic.

Antigenic similarities to meningococci have been found in unrelated bacteria. Thus *Escherichia coli* isolated from cerebrospinal fluids of newborn infants with meningitis have a K_1 capsular polysaccharide antigen that is immunologically identical to that of group B meningococcus and correlates with the apparent invasiveness of the organism in the neonate. This K_1 antigen is easily degraded in the host and also is a very poor immunogen in humans. Organisms with K_1 capsule are opsonized poorly by activation of the alternate complement pathway and are phagocytosed poorly in the absence of antibody. Two polysialosylglycopeptides (GM_3 and GD_3) of human fetal brain have been shown to react with antibodies raised to group B meningococcus capsule. The inability of the host to produce antibody may contribute to the virulence.

Surface antigens other than the group polysaccharides may stimulate bactericidal antibodies. Physicochemical characterization of the four to five major outer membrane proteins designates classes 1 to 5 on the basis of peptide mapping. Originally, 18 reported protein serotypes of group B and C were established and are now known to be associated with proteins of classes 1, 2, 3, or 5 (Table 26–4). Either class 2 or class 3 major outer membrane protein is present in all meningococcal strains and is analogous to protein I in the gonococcus. Variable hydrophilic regions are probably surface exposed and responsible for serotype specificity. The class 5 proteins are comparable to protein II in the gonococcus and are highly immunogenic. Their antigenic specificities are identifiable in the currently used protein serotypes. The class 2 and 3 proteins are proposed as the basis for a new and uniform protein serotyping system. One or the other protein class is present in all meningococci. They are the predominant outer membrane protein. There is a useful degree of antigenic variability between strains but sufficient stability to be useful epidemiologically. An association of specific serotype either with asymptomatic carriage or with disease can be shown by using these two proteins.

The scheme proposed for standardization of strain des-

TABLE 26–3. POLYSACCHARIDE CAPSULES OF MENINGOCOCCI

Serogroup	Structure of Repeating Unit	Repeating Unit
A (homopolymer)	ManNAc-(1-P$\xrightarrow{\alpha}$6)--- 3 ⋮ OAc	2-acetamido-2-deoxy-D-mannopyranosyl-phosphate
B (homopolymer)	NeuNAc-(2$\xrightarrow{\alpha}$8)---	α-2,8 *N*-acetyl neuraminic acid
C (homopolymer)	NeuNAc-(2$\xrightarrow{\alpha}$9)--- 7 8 ⋮ ⋱ OAc OAc	α-2,9 *O*-acetyl neuraminic acid
W-135 (disaccharide repeating unit)	6-D-Gal(1$\xrightarrow{\alpha}$4)-NeuNAc(2$\xrightarrow{\alpha}$6)---	4-O-α-D-galactopyranosyl-*N*-acetylneuraminic acid
X	DOGlcNAc(1-P$\xrightarrow{\alpha}$4)---	2 acetamido-2-deoxy-D-glucopyranosyl-phosphate
Y(Bo) (disaccharide repeating unit)	6-D-Glc(1$\xrightarrow{\alpha}$4)-NeuNAc(2$\xrightarrow{\alpha}$6)--- ⋮ OAc	4-O-α-D-glucopyranosyl-*N*-acetylneuraminic acid
Z (monosaccharide-glycerol repeating unit)	D-GalNAc (1$\xrightarrow{\alpha}$1′)-glycerol-(3′-P→4)---	
29-e (disaccharide repeating unit)	D-GalNAc(1$\xrightarrow{\beta}$7)-KDO(2$\xrightarrow{\alpha}$3)--- 4,5 ⋮ OAc	1′-O-2-acetamido-2-deoxy-α-D-galactopyranosylglycerol 3-deoxy-D-manno-oculosonic acid

Data from DeVoe: Microbiol Rev 46:162, 1982; Jennings et al: J Infect Dis 136:S78, 1977; Jennings et al: Can J. Biochem 57:2902, 1979.
Gal, galactose; Glc, glucose; GlcNAc, *N*-acetylglucosamine (2-acetamido-2-deoxy-D-glucose); KDO, 3-deoxy-D-manno-octulosonic acid; ManNAc, *N*-acetylmannosamine (2-acetamido-2-deoxy-D-mannose); NeuNAc, *N*-acetyl neuraminic acid (sialic acid); OAc, *O*-acetylated; NAc, *N*-acetylated; phosphate, phosphodiester linkage.

ignation would indicate serogroup, protein serotype (classes 2 and 3) with subtyping based on differences in class 1 and 5 proteins and lipopolysaccharide (LPS). For example, B:2a:L3,7 is group B, major outer membrane protein 2a; and 3 and 7 are the LPS determinants. Further typing of the outer membrane proteins 1 and 5 could be done for epidemiology and indicated as P1.1:P5.2. The entire designation becomes B:2a:P1.1:P5.2:L3,7.

TABLE 26–4. CHARACTERISTICS OF THE MAJOR CELL-SURFACE OUTER MEMBRANE PROTEIN CLASSES IN *NEISSERIA MENINGITIDIS*

Class of Protein	Molecular Weight (kDa)	Properties
1	44–47	Quantitatively variable, absent in few strains, trypsin-sensitive, and deoxycholate-insoluble
2	40–42	Quantitatively predominant, trypsin-resistant, and deoxycholate-insoluble; exists as a trimer and functions as a porin
3	37–39	Similar to class 2; classes 2 and 3 mutually exclusive
4	33–34	Present in all strains, trypsin-resistant, 2-mercaptoethanol-modifiable
5	26–30	Highly variable in expression and molecular weight; more than one class-5 protein may be expressed simultaneously; very sensitive to proteolytic enzymes, deoxycholate-soluble, and heat-modifiable

Adapted from Frasch et al: Rev Infect Dis 7:504, 1985.

Humans produce antibodies to the serotype proteins of groups B and C meningococci in response to both nasopharyngeal carriage and to systemic infection. These antibodies may be specific for the serotype proteins or LPS antigens, or both. Fortunately, a few serotypes seem to be responsible for the majority of illnesses, and others more often are found in symptom-free carriers. For example, serotype 2 (old classification) has been reported to account for 65% of group B and 78% of group C disease in Canada and Belgium. Thus persons may lack anticapsular antibody and yet have demonstrable bactericidal antibody against a specific protein serotype. It therefore may be possible to utilize selected outer membrane protein antigens to induce a protective response against the strains of both the B and C groups having this particular antigen. As already noted, the group B polysaccharide is nonimmunogenic in humans, and natural infection with these organisms does not seem to result in a strong antibody response to the group B polysaccharides. Membrane protein that has been detergent treated to remove LPS is a highly soluble immunogen in combination with high molecular weight group B polysaccharide.

In addition to the surface capsular polysaccharide antigens and outer membrane protein antigens, there are somatic antigens, which include a nucleoprotein fraction and a carbohydrate antigen. These have not been chemically defined but appear to be common to the *Neisseria* within a specific serogroup.

Determinants of Pathogenicity

The capsular polysaccharides contribute to the invasive properties of the meningococci by inhibiting phagocytosis. In the presence of specific antibody, organisms are readily destroyed by the phagocytic leukocytes. Organisms visualized on Gram stain may appear to be in an intracellular location, but these are likely to be organisms that adhere to the surface of the neutrophil. There is no evidence that these organisms survive within phagocytes.

The endotoxins of the meningococci are basically similar to those of other gram-negative bacteria. These organisms produce large amounts of LPS-containing outer membrane, and during division, vesicles of this material are released extracellularly. The LPS from meningococci is a more potent inducer of the dermal Shwartzman phenomenon than that from *E. coli* or *Salmonella typhimurium.* It is thought that as organisms invade and multiply, they release large quantities of LPS, as do the neutrophil-ingesting organisms. These materials released in cells of the vascular endothelium cause vascular necrosis and induce an inflammatory response. Thus endotoxin is implicated in the vascular damage, especially that visualized in the characteristic skin lesions that are a varying component of the disease that is produced. Antibody produced to a mutant strain of *E. coli* (J5 mutant of 0111) deficient in uridine 5′-diphosphate (UDP)–galactose epimerase protects animals against endotoxemia due to *N. meningitidis, Klebsiella, E. coli,* and *Pseudomonas.* The antibodies are directed against the core glycolipid because of the absence of complete O side chains in the mutant. This suggests a similarity among the endotoxins from diverse bacteria.

In patients with meningitis, circulating antigen-antibody complexes have been demonstrated in the weeks after initiation of therapy. A decreased serum complement also has been seen, and the late manifestations of infection such as arthritis may be attributable to these immune complexes. Pathology of the synovium is consistent with this hypothesis inasmuch as mononuclear cells are present that contain IgM, C3, and meningococcal antigen.

All strains of every *N. meningitidis* serogroup produce an IgA1 protease that is excreted into the extracellular environment. All pathogenic *Neisseria* species have this capacity. These enzymes are neutral endopeptidases with a substrate specificity for human IgA1. The proteases cleave the heavy chain of IgA1 in the hinge region. Two enzymes, types 1 and 2 from *N. meningitidis,* have been shown to cleave a proline-serine or prolyl-threonyl bond, producing intact Fc and Fab fragments, respectively. The role of these enzymes in the pathogenesis of human infection remains to be characterized, but the limitation of these enzymes to pathogenic *Neisseria* species suggests that they may contribute to the ability of the organism to produce disease.

N. meningitidis is exclusively a human pathogen and therefore must be able to multiply in a host in whom iron sequesters either intracellularly or in association with high-affinity iron-binding proteins. Iron is essential for growth of the organism, and in vitro experiments have demonstrated conclusively that *N. meningitidis* can utilize transferrin-bound iron as the sole iron source. Organisms in an iron-depleted environment for a few hours acquire the ability to obtain iron from transferrin by a saturable nonenergy-requiring cell surface mechanism. There is no evidence that *N. meningitidis* has a siderophore. Uptake of iron from the bacterial cell surface and its subsequent metabolism are accomplished by an unknown energy-dependent mechanism. Nonpathogenic *Neisseria* species lack the ability to use iron from transferrin.

Clinical Infection

The first recognition of disease caused by *N. meningitidis* occurred in 1805 with the description of an epidemic of meningitis in Geneva, Switzerland. One year later, an outbreak in Medfield, Massachusetts, marked the first recognized outbreak in North America. The causative organism, however, was not identified until 1887, when Weichselbaum described the gram-negative diplococci in the spinal fluid of patients.

Epidemiology

Meningococcal disease is worldwide in distribution and varies from sporadic cases observed in a community to epidemics of infection. *N. meningitidis* causes 20% of meningitis and therefore is the second commonest cause of this illness. The reported number of cases of meningitis is about 3000 to 4000 per year in the United States. Serogroup B accounts for 50% to 55% of all cases, serogroup C for 20% to 25%, and serogroup W135 for 15%. Serogroups Y (10%) and A (1% to 2%) cause almost all remaining cases. In 1946 an outbreak of group A meningococcal disease occurred with a reported case rate of 14/100,000 population (Fig. 26–1). There has been no major epidemic in the United States since then. The potential for a meningococcal epidemic is illustrated by the urban epidemic that began in São Paulo, Brazil, in June 1971. The disease outbreak continued for 3 years, with an attack rate of 65/100,000 population per month. In February and March of 1974 the predominant strain of *N. meningitidis* changed from serotype C to serotype A.

Starch gel electrophoresis of seven cytoplasmic enzymes and SDS polyacrylamide gel electrophoresis (PAGE) of two outer membrane proteins have been used to resolve the clonal population structures of serogroup A meningococci. Almost 500 strains from 23 epidemics over the past two decades were

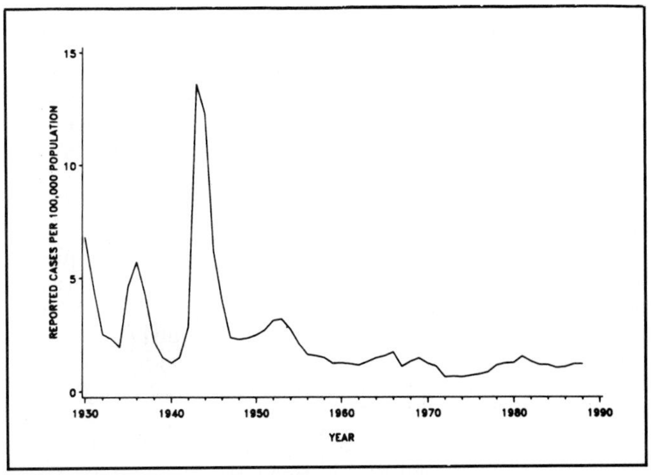

Fig. 26–1. Meningococcal infections—rates, by year, United States, 1930 to 1989. *(From Centers for Disease Control: MMWR 38(54):32, 1989.)*

available for study. Most outbreaks had a predominant clone, and seven clones that had caused outbreaks since 1915 were recognizable. These data and analysis of isolates from the outbreak in Gambia suggest that a major epidemic is related to emergence of an antigenically distinct virulent strain in a susceptible population. The adult nasopharyngeal carrier is important in the transmission of meningococci and provides a reservoir of infection from which the organisms are introduced into a household. The median duration of carriage in a nonepidemic setting is 10 months. The carrier rate is higher in members of the household of a patient with meningococcal disease. In community epidemic situations, carriage rates of 15% have been observed in households with identified disease as compared with 3.6% in households without disease. An investigation of an extended family with several infected children revealed a 44% carriage rate, whereas a rate of 3% was found in samples of unrelated population in the same geographic area.

The peak occurrence of disease is in children from 6 to 24 months of age. A similar peak in incidence occurs in the 10- to 20-year-old age-group and is related primarily to outbreaks of disease in the military population. Meningococcal disease in military populations is associated with nasopharyngeal carriage rates as high as 90%. The intimate contact provided by army barracks increases exposure of susceptible recruits from a variety of geographic areas to carriers harboring the organism.

It is of practical importance to emphasize that susceptible intimate contacts, primarily those within a household and potentially those in a day-care setting, have the greatest risk of acquiring meningococcal disease. Attention should be focused on young children within the intimate setting of recognized cases, and the fear of acquisition of disease, placed in the proper perspective.

Immunity

Purification and use of the A, B, C, Y, and W-135 polysaccharides have extended our information concerning immunity to meningococci. The A, C, Y, and W-135 polysaccharides in humans induce group-specific antibodies measured by a passive hemagglutination test, bactericidal assay, opsoninization (chemoluminescence assay), and a radioactive antigen-binding assay. The radioactive antigen-binding assay measures total anticapsular antibody, whereas the bactericidal antibody assay measures the ability of antibody to initiate immune lysis. The antibodies that induce lysis are thought to be protective, and opsonization also is a functional assessment of antibodies. Therefore, bactericidal antibody induction and potentially opsonization are used as the means to assess efficacy of the meningococcal polysaccharides. The bactericidal activity is complement dependent. The terminal complement sequence is essential for this antibody-associated serum bactericidal activity but does not enhance either phagocytosis of these organisms or intracellular killing. Clinical evidence for these observations is provided by the severe, chronic, or recurrent *Neisseria* infections that have been documented in persons naturally deficient in C5, C6, C7, C8, or C9. The serum from these persons lacks complement-dependent bactericidal activity; however, it does support phagocytosis.

Antibody-dependent, complement-mediated immune lysis or bactericidal antibodies restrict the meningococcus to mucosal surfaces. Antibodies as measured by the bactericidal assay are present in the blood of very young infants. These antibodies, detectable at birth and for the subsequent few months of life, presumably are transplacentally acquired. The lowest antibody titer is present in infants between 6 and 24 months of age, which correlates well with the peak incidence of sporadic meningococcal disease. Thus there is an inverse correlation between age-related incidence of disease and age-specific prevalence of serum bactericidal activity. Prospective longitudinal studies of army recruits also confirms that the absence of bactericidal titers correlates with susceptibility to infection.

Antibodies to the meningococcus may be of any of the three major classes (IgG, IgM, and IgA) of immunoglobulin. However, their ability to induce immune lysis is variable. IgM is always bactericidal, whereas IgG at best is only one half as effective because doublet formation is necessary for activation of complement. In fact, IgG2 and IgG4 poorly activate complement. IgA does not induce immune lysis, and probably of even greater relevance is the observation that IgA can block initiation of lysis by either IgM or IgG. This blocking effect is antigen specific; that is, IgA must compete for the same antigenic sites as the lytic antibody. Clinically, this observation has been linked to disseminated disease by the demonstration of the absence of bactericidal activity for the infecting strain of *N. meningitidis,* which can be restored if IgA is absorbed from the patient's serum. The uncovered bactericidal antibody is IgM. On the other hand, IgA antibody to the meningococcal capsule has been demonstrated to be necessary for complement-independent opsonophagocytosis of organisms by circulating monocytes. It has been postulated that this is a mechanism capable of destroying small numbers of invading organisms.

Phagocytic killing is also of importance in the host's ability to control infection. Antibody-dependent, complement-mediated phagocytic killing of meningococci deposits C3b on the surface of the organism, promoting the ingestion and killing by phagocytes. Persons lacking specific antibody do not activate the classic complement pathway and fail to eradicate organisms by opsonophagocytosis. The alternate complement pathway and serum bactericidal activity are then operative to contain infection.

The phagocytosis and killing of meningococci also vary with the serogroup. Group B organisms are susceptible to phagocytosis and resistant to complement-mediated serum bactericidal activity, whereas those in groups A, C, Y, and W-135 are killed by serum bactericidal activity. Persons with complement deficiency have proportionally more infections with group Y organisms, perhaps because these organisms are less susceptible to phagocytosis and the host lacks serum bactericidal activity. Disease caused by group B organisms predominates in the general population. Susceptible persons lack specific antibody, thereby becoming dependent on the serum bactericidal activity to which group B organisms are more resistant.

In the United States and several other developed nations, there has not been a nationwide epidemic of meningococcal infection since the 1940s. Recently, a hypothetic immunoepidemiologic model was proposed to explain the epidemic occurrence of meningococcal infection. Enteric bacteria with surface antigens that are immunologically cross-reactive with *N. meningitidis* capsular polysaccharides have been identified, for example, group C *N. meningitidis* with *E. coli* K92 and *Streptococcus faecalis* with group A *N. meningitidis.* These colonizing organisms would not cause recognizable infection, are fecally to orally transmissible, and could stimulate the gastrointestinal tract–associated lymphoid tissue to produce IgA. Ultimately, serum IgA would be detectable. Variations in the IgA could be anticipated, depending on the stimulus and the ability of the liver to transport circulating IgA to bile. If an individual had high circulating IgA levels to *N. meningitidis* at the time this organism colonized the respiratory tract, any IgM antibodies might be blocked by the circulating IgA. Immune lysis thus would be transiently blocked and the person would be susceptible to invasive disease. The basic premise of this hypothesis is that an epidemic of invasive disease is realized when the *N. meningitidis* cocirculates with a nonpathogenic enteric organism, elaborating a cross-reactive surface antigen. It is consistent with observed features such as the slow contiguous spread of epidemics and involvement that frequently is limited to socioeconomically deprived persons. As with many other infections, poor sanitation enhances fecal to oral spread.

Respiratory infection has been suggested as a predisposing factor in meningococcal infection. In a case-controlled study of patients with meningitis in Chad, coincident upper respiratory tract infection with viruses or *Mycoplasma* species was more common. The mechanism of interaction of these agents colonizing the respiratory tract and increasing the risk of meningitis is unknown. However, this link of meningococcal disease with other agents is another approach that has been taken to explain the seasonal and age-related epidemiology of meningococcal disease. There are no studies to suggest that these organisms have cross-reacting antigens or stimulate blocking antibodies to the meningococcus.

Pathogenesis and Clinical Manifestations

Meningococci enter the body via the upper respiratory tract, including the conjunctiva and establish themselves on the mucous membrane of the nasopharynx. Systemic but not topical antimicrobial treatment of conjunctivitis will prevent invasive disease. Nasopharyngeal acquisition of the organism precedes hematogenous dissemination by an indeterminate length of time. The incubation period is a matter of days and usually is less than 1 week. Dissemination of meningococci via the bloodstream results in metastatic lesions in various areas of the body, such as the skin, meninges, joints, eyes, and lungs. The clinical manifestations vary, depending on the site of localization.

The spectrum of illness includes a mild febrile disease, which may be accompanied by pharyngitis but is without other specific manifestations of meningococcal infection. Systemic disease characterized by fever and prostration is more readily identified. Infrequently an erythematous macular rash is observed, which usually is superseded by the appearance of a petechial eruption rapidly developing into large areas of ecchymosis. This vasculitic purpura is initiated by emboli of meningococci and is considered the hallmark of meningococcal disease. It is characteristic of the more severe fulminant disease. Meningococcemia may be accompanied by meningitis, arthritis, pericarditis, and involvement of virtually any organ system. Disseminated intravascular coagulation and gram-negative shock may be present. Hemorrhage into adrenal tissue with the resultant hypoadrenergic state is referred to as the *Waterhouse-Friderichsen syndrome*. The patient may survive meningococcal disease with no detectable sequelae or with direct residua of the infection that are evident for the remainder of his or her life. Such sequelae include eighth nerve deafness and central nervous system damage and may include necrosis of large areas of the skin or tissue secondary to vascular thrombosis. These lesions may require skin grafting or amputation of necrotic digits or of an even larger portion of an extremity. The characteristic petechial eruption present in the majority of patients permits an accurate presumptive diagnosis and allows appropriate initial therapy of the illness.

In children, presentation with hypothermia, seizures, shock, white blood cell count less than 5000/mm^3, platelet count less than 100,000/mm^3, or purpura fulminans has a poor prognosis. Overall mortality of approximately 10% is reported in developed nations and has been unchanged for three decades.

Laboratory Diagnosis

Meningococcal infection is specifically diagnosed by the identification of *N. meningitidis* in materials obtained from the patient. If inflammatory exudates, such as spinal fluid, are available, a rapid presumptive diagnosis may be made by finding the characteristic gram-negative diplococci in stained smears. The organisms also may be occasionally demonstrated in Gram stains of petechial lesions. In cases of overwhelming septicemia, the meningococci have been demonstrated in buffy coat smears from peripheral blood or, rarely, in a drop of blood obtained from an earlobe or even a fingertip for routine differential white cell count.

The materials submitted to the laboratory for culture vary with the illness of the patient. Blood, cerebrospinal fluid, material from petechial skin lesions, synovial fluid, and a nasopharyngeal or throat swab may yield positive culture results. Thayer-Martin selective medium is used for the culture of materials expected to yield a mixture of organisms. Specimens of blood, spinal fluid, or other normally sterile materials are inoculated into blood culture bottles of trypticase soy broth with increased CO_2, and on the surface of a chocolate agar plate.

Detection of meningococcal polysaccharide in the cerebrospinal fluid, synovial fluid, and urine is possible by such techniques as countercurrent immunoelectrophoresis (CIE), latex agglutination, or coagglutination employing staphylococci with protein A. The antibody molecule will bind to the meningococcal antigen if present, resulting in visible coagglutination of the staphylococci or agglutination of latex particles. These antigen-detection systems are more widely used and reproducible than immunofluorescence is.

The research methods for demonstrating the serologic response of a patient with meningococcal infection are discussed on page 445. The radioactive antigen-binding assay is the most sensitive method, but antibodies cannot be detected until several days after symptoms of disease have appeared.

Treatment

Penicillin remains the drug of choice for therapy of meningococcal infections. *N. meningitidis* is exquisitely sensitive to penicillin, with minimal inhibitory concentrations usually in the range of 0.05 μg/mL. Therapy consists of high-dosage aqueous penicillin G administered intravenously. In penicillin-sensitive individuals, chloramphenicol is an effective alternative form of therapy. Ceftriaxone also has been used successfully and may provide logistic advantages when frequent intravenous administration of drug is a problem. In addition to the essential specific antimicrobial therapy, supportive measures for possible complications, such as gram-negative shock or disseminated intravascular coagulation, are important aspects of the care of such patients.

Prevention

Prophylaxis. Antimicrobial prophylaxis of exposed persons remains a controversial issue. Before the emergence of resistance to sulfonamide therapy, this drug was used efficiently to eradicate the organisms from the nasopharynx of affected individuals. It has been an interesting puzzle to microbiologists and clinicians that similar use of penicillin, to which the organism is sensitive, fails to eradicate the carrier state. Currently, when prophylaxis seems advisable, a choice may be made between rifampin and minocycline. Treatment with rifampin for a short period eliminates *N. meningitidis* from the nasopharynx, but during subsequent weeks, rifampin-resistant strains may recolonize the nasopharynx. Minocycline also eradicates the carrier state, but a recognized side effect of the drug—vestibular dysfunction with resultant disturbance of equilibrium—has limited its use. The combined use of two drugs probably has the greatest efficacy but is a practical impossibility because of the high incidence of side effects in patients receiving the combination. Ciprofloxin also can eradicate carriage.

Decisions concerning the use of such prophylaxis should be made with a complete awareness of the persons at greatest risk. These usually include (1) children, primarily those younger than 6 years of age who have household-type intimate contact with the index case and (2) recruits in the setting of an army camp. If prophylaxis is given, this does not obviate the need for close observation of contact persons. Meningococcal meningitis has been reported in a patient who received rifampin prophylaxis. Similarly, penicillin at the prophylactic dosage employed does not appear to prevent meningococcal disease.

Within the hospital setting, it usually is unnecessary to use prophylactic therapy for personnel exposed to meningococcal disease. The occurrence of secondary disease among this group is exceedingly rare. In this setting, recognition of disease and prompt therapy of the patient with appropriate antimicrobial agents tend to decrease the spread of illness. Personnel who have intimate contact with an untreated patient may take prophylaxis, depending on the specific situation.

Immunization. Group A, C, Y, and W-135 meningococcal vaccines are licensed and available. The vaccines consist of purified group-specific meningococcal polysaccharide and are administered as a single dose of 50 μg to adults and children older than 2 years. Large-scale field trials in the United States Army with group C vaccine demonstrated 90% efficacy in the prevention of group C disease and a decrease in the number of meningococcal carriers. Subsequent field trials of groups A and C polysaccharides in Brazil, Egypt, the Sudan, and Finland have established the safety and efficacy of these vaccines in persons older than 2 years. These trials suggest that a measurable concentration of antibody protein of approximately 2 μg/mL is necessary for protection.

The immunogenicity of these polysaccharides is age dependent. Infants can respond to the group A polysaccharide as early as 3 months of age and will show an anamnestic rise in serum antibody when given a second dose of the vaccine 3 to 4 months later. The level of antibody achieved is 2 to 3 μg/mL. A large field trial in Finland demonstrated complete protection against meningococcal group A disease in 130,000 children from 3 months to 5 years of age. Two 25-μg doses of vaccine were administered at 3-month intervals to children 3 to 18 months of age, and a single 50-μg dose was administered to children 1.5 to 5 years of age.

In contrast, group C, W-135, and Y polysaccharides are more age dependent. Vaccine will induce antibodies in infants older than 6 months in 40% to 100% infants, depending on age and specific polysaccharide. A second dose should be given after 3 months to infants younger than 24 months. The group C vaccine did not protect infants from 6 to 24 months of age during the epidemic in São Paulo, Brazil, and efficacy of the other polysaccharides in young infants remains to be established.

In summary, group A vaccine offers effective protection for patients of all ages, and control of group A epidemics is feasible. Group C, Y, and W-135 vaccine will induce antibodies to varying degree in infants younger than 2 years and will protect persons older than 2 years of age. Therefore these vaccines offer significant control of epidemics because they are effective for 60% to 80% of expected cases. These vaccines are available for use in military populations, in which epidemic disease is likely, and by specific request for control of an outbreak of infection. At the present time these vaccines are not recommended for routine use in childhood.

The development of type-specific vaccines for group A and C meningococci constitutes a significant contribution to preventive medicine. The group B organisms continue to pose a problem because the polysaccharide is a very poor immunogen. Successful stimulation of IgG antibodies to individual serotype outer membrane proteins of group B meningococci has been accomplished. Protection against group B disease is being approached by use of these protein antigens and by use of the core oligosaccharide of the LPS. Theoretically it is possible that immunization with the group A and a group C, Y, or W-135 polysaccharide will prevent disease from the organisms within these serogroups but will allow other serogroups of organisms to emerge as epidemiologically significant, but confirmation awaits the test of experience with the present vaccines. The persistence of antibody and duration of protection are being assessed longitudinally. Some data suggest that children immunized with one dose of type A vaccine at an age younger than 4 years have decreased protection in the second and third years after vaccination. In developing nations, the logistics of multiple immunizations may be difficult to overcome.

Neisseria gonorrhoeae

Physiology

Cultural Characteristics. *N. gonorrhoeae* is more fastidious in its growth requirements than is *N. meningitidis*. Approximately 20% of strains require glutamine for primary isolation, and most freshly isolated strains also have a requirement for CO_2 or HCO_3^-.

When gonococci are grown on a solid transparent medium, they exhibit several colonial forms that have been useful in our understanding of certain biochemical and virulence properties of the organism. Four major colony types can be distinguished: T1, T2, T3, and T4. The T1 and T2 colonies

TABLE 26–5. SYSTEMS FOR TYPING *NEISSERIA GONORRHOEAE*

System	Types	Comment
Coagglutination using monoclonal antibodies to OMPIA and OMPIB	50	This system may be used in conjunction with auxotyping
Coagglutination after cross-absorption using *Staphylococcus aureus* protein A	WI–WIII	Results correlate with monoclonal methods
Auxotyping based on nutritional requirements	1–30	DGI strains[a] are $A^-H^-U^-$
Pilus typing	>8	Pilus variation occurs in vivo

OMPIA and OMPIB, outer membrane proteins A and B; DGI, disseminated gonococcal infections; $A^-H^-U^-$, arginine, hypoxanthine, and uracil.
[a] Most strains from persons with DGI are type WI and correspond to OMPIA types.

are produced on primary culture and are small and dome-shaped, whereas after subsequent in vitro unselected passage, gonococci grow as larger, flatter colonies (T3 or T4). Pili are present on the small colony variants but are absent from the large colonies. In addition, colonies of both piliated and nonpiliated organisms exhibit variation in their color and opacity characteristics.

Metabolism. The gonococcus is an aerobic organism. Glucose, which is the preferred carbon and energy source, is dissimilated via the Entner-Doudoroff and pentose phosphate pathways and a heme-containing respiratory chain. Acetic acid is the principal nongaseous end product of glucose dissimilation by growing organisms. Although *N. gonorrhoeae* is considered to be an obligate aerobe, some features of its metabolism differ from those of other *Neisseria* species and from aerotolerant organisms. Some strains of *N. gonorrhoeae* lack detectable levels of the O_2^--scavenging enzyme superoxide dismutase (SOD), and those strains that do possess the enzyme have very low levels of activity. The high tolerance of the organism for extracellular O_2^- and H_2O_2 generated by vigorously metabolizing polymorphonuclear neutrophils (PMNs) in purulent exudates appears to be due to very high constitutive levels of peroxidase and catalase activity together with a cell envelope impervious to O_2^-. It has been shown, however, that *N. gonorrhoeae* can grow in the absence of oxygen by using anaerobic respiration with nitrite as a terminal electron acceptor. This provides a possible mechanism for the survival and proliferation of the organism in the genitourinary tract, along with obligate anaerobes, provided an alternative electron acceptor is present.

Typing. Several methods for distinguishing strains of *N. gonorrhoeae* are currently available (Table 26–5). These methods have been especially useful in epidemiologic studies of the transmission of infection and in studies of virulence determinants. The most useful of these employ serologic techniques and auxotyping. Auxotyping is based on the nutritional requirement of a strain for one or more metabolites, primarily amino acids and nitrogenous bases. More than 30 different auxotypes have been defined by this method. It is significant that the majority of strains that are derived from patients with disseminated gonococcal infection are auxotrophic for arginine, hypoxanthine, and uracil ($A^-H^-U^-$). It also has been found that organisms cultured from sexual partners are of a similar auxotype.

Several systems for the serologic classification of strains of *N. gonorrhoeae* have been proposed. Among the most refined of these is a coagglutination test that uses monoclonal antibodies to the gonococcal protein I molecule of the outer membrane. All strains can be separated into two serogroups, IA and IB. By the use of 12 monoclonal antibodies to protein I, more than 1400 isolates in a worldwide collection could be assigned to one of 46 different serovars. Furthermore, a combination of auxotyping and serotyping provides an even more detailed classification scheme for populations of *N. gonorrhoeae* strains and is especially useful in epidemiologic studies. The dual system can be used to analyze patterns of antibiotic resistance, the movement of gonococcal strains between different geographic areas, and temporal changes that occur in gonococcal populations.

Antigenic Structure

The antigenic composition of *N. gonorrhoeae* is complex. Associated with the surface layers are at least three major classes of antigens: (1) pilus antigen; (2) lipooligosaccharide (LOS), and (3) the outer membrane protein constituents. The presence of antigenically distinct forms of these components results in considerable variation in the antigenic structure of the cell surface of the various gonococcal strains.

Pilus Antigen. Pili are nonflagellar surface appendages constructed from identical protein subunits (pilin) linked in tandem to form long thin polymers (Fig. 26–2). Gonococcal pili are serologically heterogeneous. The molecular weight of each pilin subunit ranges from 17 to 22 kDa, depending on the *N. gonorrhoeae* strain. Piliated organisms predominate in colony types T1 and T2 of fresh isolates from genitourinary tract infections, whereas colony types T3 and T4 appear on

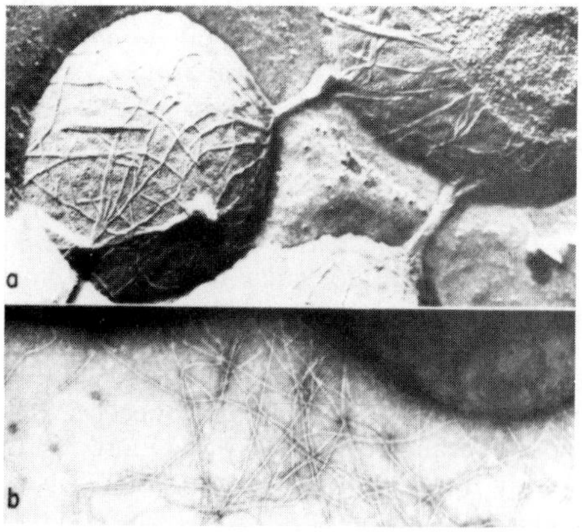

Fig. 26–2. Gonococci and gonococcal pili. **a.** Freeze-fracture, freeze-etch preparation of gonococci with pili on surface. × 80,000. **b.** Negatively stained gonococcus with pili radiating from surface. Uranyl acetate. × 70,000. *(From Buchanan et al: J Clin Invest 52:2896, 1973.)*

subculture and consist of nonpiliated organisms. Many strains from extragenital sites also are found to be nonpiliated even in fresh isolates.

The pili of *N. gonorrhoeae* undergo both phase and antigenic variations. Phase variation, which refers to a reversible switch between alternative states, such as pilus expressing (P^+) or pilus nonexpressing (P^-), occurs at high frequencies (about 10^3 or 10^4) and is easily recognized by attendant changes in colony morphology on solid clear medium. Pilus antigenic variation also occurs at high frequencies as determined both by in vitro observations and by comparing pilus antigens from different clinical isolates. A single gonococcal cell has the genetic capacity to produce at least eight antigenically variant pili. The gonococcal pilin molecule can be divided into three regions: a constant (C) region in which the amino acids always are conserved, a semivariable (SV) region in which many amino acid substitutions are found, and a highly variable (HV) region at the carboxyterminal that, in addition to amino acid substitutions, contains insertions and deletions of one to four codons. This part is immunodominant over the conserved portion of the molecule.

A genetic analysis of pilus production in the gonococcus has shown that pilus expression is regulated at two expression loci on the chromosome, although many other regions contain silent pilin information. When the cell is in the P^+ state, either one or both expression sites contain an intact pilin gene. In most cases, a P^+ to P^- switch results in the deletion of pilin information from either one or both of the expression sites. The generation of a complete pilin gene within the expression loci is the result of multiple recombination events. At the DNA level, the mixing and matching of individual SV and HV gene segments by recombination increases the number of new pilin epitopes any one cell is capable of producing. An understanding of pilus antigenic variation and genetics is important for the development of a clinically successful vaccine against all strains of *N. gonorrhoeae.*

Antipilus antibody appears to be responsible for immune-enhanced phagocytosis in vitro. After the use of parenteral pilus vaccine in humans, mucosal IgA immunoglobulin is produced and is capable of blocking attachment to epithelial cells of homologous types of gonococci. There also is some protection against mucosal cell attachment by heterologous strains. Because of the organism's potential to readily change its pili or lose the ability to produce pili, gonococci may quite successfully evade the effects of local antibody production.

Outer Membrane Proteins. The cell envelope contains a number of proteins, one of which is protein I (PI), which accounts for about 60% of the total weight of the outer membrane. It has a molecular weight of 32 to 36 kDa and is present in the same submolecular weight in gonococci from each of the different colony types from any one strain. PI is, however, antigenically variable and has been used as the basis for the enzyme-linked immunosorbent assay (ELISA) and the coagglutination assay for serotyping gonococci. PI is located in the outer membrane in such a way that most of the molecule, including both the N- and C-terminal ends, is within the membrane and only a small part of the central portion of the molecule is exposed on the surface. In the membrane, PI is complexed with protein III to form porins. A correlation has been found between the molecular weight of PI and the type of gonococcal infection. *N. gonorrhoeae* strains with a low molecular weight PI are found in patients with disseminated infection whereas *N. gonorrhoeae* strains with a high molecular weight PI usually are found in symptomatic genital infections. Also, organisms with the low molecular weight PI usually are resistant to killing by serum, but organisms with the high molecular weight PI usually are highly sensitive. PI of a given strain is invariable. Epidemiologic evidence indicates that this protein is a target of protecting antibody so that repeat invasive infections with the identical type are very unusual. PI also may serve to trigger a phagocytic response from nonprofessional phagocytes, such as mucosal cells.

The protein IIs (PIIs) are a series of heat-modifiable proteins that are subject to phase variation. They have subunit molecular weights ranging from 24 to 30 kDa. Because they were initially described as proteins present in the outer membrane of opaque colony variants and generally absent in transparent variants of the same strain, they also have been referred to as *opacity-associated protein.* At least six to eight antigenically distinct PII proteins have been described, and a single cell may express from zero to as many as three PII species at one time. PII^+ cells are characterized by clumping (autoagglutination) and by adherence to mucosal cells and neutrophils. Organisms expressing these proteins usually are isolated from localized infections, whereas organisms that lack PIIs are recovered from disseminated infections. The PIIs are structurally related but contain variable hydrophilic regions, which appear to be located on surface-exposed portions of the protein. The presence of monoclonal antibodies specific for unique epitopes in individual proteins emphasizes the extensive intrastrain and interstrain variability in their antigenic structure. The gonococcus is capable of rapid, reversible changes in the expression of the PIIs. This variation is believed to contribute to the evasion of host immune responses and may account in part for recurrent gonococcal infections.

Protein III (PIII) occurs in the outer membrane complexed with PI to form porins. PIII appears to be the major binding site for IgG blocking antibody, which interferes with complement-mediated killing of serum-resistant *N. gonorrhoeae* by immune serum.

Protein H8 is a recently detected antigen found in all strains of *N. gonorrhoeae* and *N. meningitidis* tested, but not in saprophytic *Neisseria* species. Within a given strain the H8 antigen appears to be antigenically homogeneous irrespective of piliation or opacity colony type, and all strains have in common one or more surface-exposed epitopes of this antigen. Monoclonal antibodies to the H8 protein are bactericidal for gonococcal strains that are susceptible to killing by normal human serum. Because of its surface location and widespread distribution among all pathogenic *Neisseria,* the H8 antigen has been suggested as a possible candidate for a vaccine against both gonococcal and meningococcal infection.

Lipooligosaccharide. The lipooligosaccharide (LOS) of the gonococcal outer membrane plays an important role in immunity to infection. It is the primary surface antigen involved in the serum bactericidal reaction. Although basically similar in structure to the lipopolysaccharides of other gram-negative organisms, individual LOS units have a lower molecular weight and do not contain repeating O-antigenic side chains. Gonococcal LOS has, however, a complex antigenic structure. It has at least six antigenically distinct serotype determinants, as well as two additional antigens that are shared by all (the common determinant) or by some (the variable) strains.

Some LOS epitopes are similar to precursors of the human

erythrocyte i antigen. This ability to mimic host cell antigens may be central to the capacity of *N. gonorrhoeae* to survive in and to infect human mucosal surfaces.

Determinants of Pathogenicity

Gonorrhea is a disease essentially confined to the mucus-secreting epithelial surface of humans. For expression of their pathogenic potential, gonococci must possess the ability not only to multiply on and invade through these mucosal surfaces but also to resist attack by host defenses. This often induces conflicting requirements and necessitates a response by the organism to a wide variety of environmental conditions. Major changes in the surface properties of the gonococcus result from the selective pressures encountered in its in vivo environment.

Pili. Organisms from T1 and T2 colonies are piliated and are associated with virulence for humans even after many in vitro selected passages. Gonococci from the T3 and T4 colony types are nonpiliated, and although they have selective advantage in vitro, they are unable to cause infection in human volunteers. Piliated gonococci adhere to a variety of epithelial cells of human origin much more avidly than do nonpiliated cells and thus are thought to act as virulence factors by anchoring the organisms to mucosal infection sites. The mechanisms responsible for pilus-mediated adherence are not known. Attachment occurs at the tips of microvilli on nonciliated cells, followed by phagocytosis and transport of gonococci in vacuoles to the base of the cell and into the subepithelial tissues.

Outer Membrane Components. Another gonococcal surface constituent that promotes adherence is PII. The presence of this protein is reflected in the colony form and usually is associated with opaque colonies that exhibit extensive intergonococcal aggregation. Like pili, PII functions as an adhesin and is one of the most variable constituents of the organism's surface. Each specific PII arises from a family of genetically and antigenically related proteins that exhibit phase variation (see above). Modulation of the adhesion properties of the cell surface by rapid gain or loss of a particular PII, as well as changes in the structure of the pilus subunit, would enable the organism to cope with the different anatomic and environmental niches that are encountered in the human host. Different PII variants behave differently in respect to their adherence capabilities for certain types of cells. Consistent differences have been observed in the opacity or PII phenotypes of clinical isolates from men and women, from women at different times in their menstrual cycles, and from different anatomic sites in the same woman. Different PIIs in a given strain thus may contribute to the organism's ability to survive in a particular anatomic site that may be undergoing cyclic changes.

The mechanisms by which gonococci damage host cells are poorly understood. Studies designed to provide a better understanding of the complex mechanisms involved have led to the separation of all strains of *N. gonorrhoeae* into two phenotypes on the basis of their sensitivity to killing by normal human serum—serum sensitive and serum-resistant strains. Strains isolated from uncomplicated genital infections are serum sensitive, whereas those from patients with a functionally intact complement pathway who have disseminated infections are serum resistant. Because of this relationship, resistance to the bactericidal effect of normal human serum is considered to be a virulence factor. Antigenic determinants on LOS have been implicated as the target of bactericidal antibodies in normal serum. It is assumed that these antibodies are induced by commensal and enteric gram-negative organisms that colonize a variety of mucosal surfaces. Indeed it has been shown that these antibodies are directed against a site on the LPS moiety that shares antigenicity with gonococcal LOS. LOS also has been implicated as a major contributor to the damage of host cells. In a fallopian tube organ culture, LOS damages the mucosa, resulting in loss of ciliary activity and sloughing of ciliated epithelial cells in a manner similar to that observed during active gonococcal infection. Toxicity is due to the lipid A portion of the molecule, whereas the oligosaccharide side chain is important in antibody- and complement-mediated killing. Patients develop increased levels of IgG and IgM antibodies against the oligosaccharide and provide some protection against gonococcal bacteremia caused by serum-sensitive strains.

Peptidoglycan. Soluble monomers of gonococcal peptidoglycan represent a second class of heat-stable components of the gonococcus that are thought to contribute to the pathogenesis of gonococcal infection. These monomers are biologically active with properties that include activation of human complement and modulation of mononuclear cell proliferation. During exponential growth, gonococci have the unique ability to shed large amounts of a mixture of unusual nonreducing disaccharide peptide monomers and the corresponding disaccharide tetrapeptide. These monomers result from the action of a gonococcal transglycosylase and differ from the analogous reducing monomeric fragments derived from the action of muramidase of host origin. Both monomers are thought to be released during infection. In addition to their diverse biologic activities, both nonreducing and reducing peptidoglycan monomers possess intrinsic toxicity for human fallopian tube mucosa. The resultant damage consists of a sloughing of ciliated cells from the mucosa and closely resembles the damage observed in active gonococcal infection.

IgA Protease. IgA is the predominant immunoglobulin involved in mucosal defense. All gonococci produce a protease that specifically cleaves the subclass IgA1 molecule and inactivates it. This enzyme presumably permits gonococci to adhere to mucosal surfaces even in the presence of a secretory antibody response. The finding of IgA1 protease only in pathogenic *Neisseria* but not in commensal species of this genus suggests an association of the production of this enzyme with the virulence of *N. gonorrhoeae*.

Strains of *N. gonorrhoeae* produce one of two types of IgA1 protease, each of which cleaves the IgA1 molecule at a distinct peptide bond in the hinge region. The production of type 1 IgA1 protease is characteristic of strains that require arginine, hypoxanthine, and uracil for growth and that are serovar 1A. Other serovars and auxotypes usually produce type 2 IgA1 protease.

Clinical Infection

The term *gonorrhea,* meaning *flow of seed,* was introduced by Galen in AD 130. Although ancient writings refer to medical

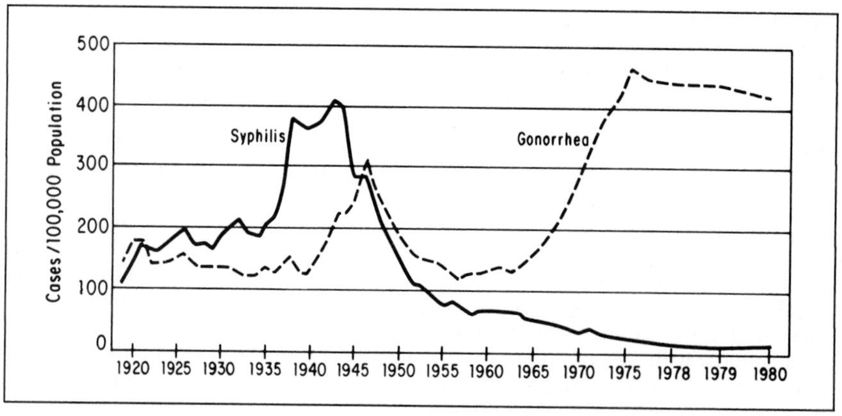

Fig. 26–3. Reported cases of gonorrhea and syphilis in the United States per 100,000 population, 1919 to 1981. Since 1975 there has been an arrest of the annual increase in gonorrhea that occurred through the middle 1970s. From 1975 to 1984, rates of gonorrhea declined by 20% for the United States and declined by 17% for combined metropolitan areas. *(Data from the Centers for Disease Control, Atlanta.)*

conditions characterized by a urethral discharge, it was not until the thirteenth century that physicians were definitely applying the term to a sexually transmitted disease similar to gonorrhea as we know it. Syphilis and gonorrhea often were acquired simultaneously, and descriptions of the two diseases were intermingled. In 1767, the widely known physician John Hunter acquired both syphilis and gonorrhea during an autoinoculation experiment in which he used urethral exudate from a patient erroneously thought to have only gonorrhea. Hunter ascribed his subsequent syphilitic symptoms to gonorrhea, and the confusion of the two diseases became complete. They were not effectively differentiated until the middle of the nineteenth century.

Epidemiology

Gonorrhea is the most common of the classic sexually transmitted diseases. Most areas of the world are now affected by the current pandemic. Since the beginning of the twentieth century, when rates of gonorrhea were first recorded, increases and decreases in incidence have been associated with major social changes and with disruptions caused by wars. Before the present period, the highest rates in the United States occurred during and just after World War II (Fig. 26–3). The current pandemic began in the early 1960s when the number of gonorrhea cases reported to the Centers for Disease Control increased from about 300,000 in 1964 to more than 1 million reported cases per year during the peak years from 1975 to 1980. Since 1980 there has been a slow but steady decline in incidence of reported cases, with approximately 700,000 reported cases in 1990 with a rate of 282/100,000 population.

Seasonal peaks of incidence of gonorrhea occur from July through September in both the southern and the northern areas of the United States. The prevalence of gonorrhea in the United States is markedly affected by age. More than 80% of the documented gonorrhea cases in the United States occur in persons between the ages of 15 and 29 years. In both men and women, the disease is most common in persons 20 to 24 years of age (1546/100,000) and is second highest among teenagers 15 to 19 years old. Most cases of gonorrhea are casually acquired, but prostitution presently is responsible for the spread of antibiotic-resistant disease in the United States. There is a general trend toward increased prevalence in nonwhite individuals, persons of low socioeconomic groups, and urban dwellers (Fig. 26–4).

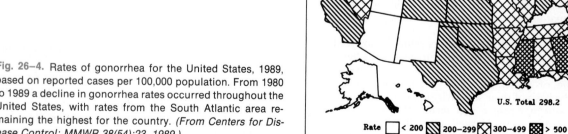

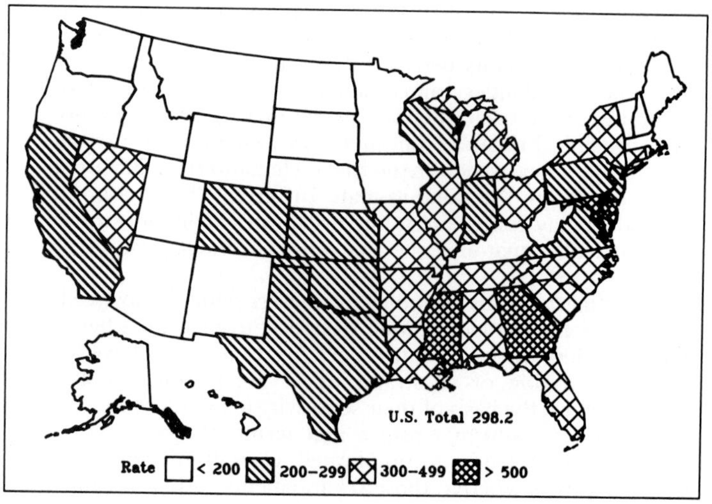

Fig. 26–4. Rates of gonorrhea for the United States, 1989, based on reported cases per 100,000 population. From 1980 to 1989 a decline in gonorrhea rates occurred throughout the United States, with rates from the South Atlantic area remaining the highest for the country. *(From Centers for Disease Control: MMWR 38(54):23, 1989.)*

Pathogenesis

Autopsy material from persons who have died of intercurrent disease during the acute phase of gonorrhea has provided some information on the histopathology of acute infection. The primary infection usually begins at the columnar epithelium of the urethra and periurethral ducts and glands of either sex. Cervical, conjunctival, and rectal mucosa also can serve as the portal of entry. Within less than 1 hour after contact with the mucosal surface, the infection is established and gonococci are anchored by pili to surface urethral cells. Penetration occurs through intercellular spaces, and organisms reach the subepithelial connective tissue by the third day. The resulting inflammatory response consists of a dense infiltration of PMNs. Obstruction of ducts and glands by this exudate results in retention cysts and abscesses. Spread to other areas often occurs by direct extension through lymphatic vessels and, less commonly, by blood vessels.

In vitro perfusion of human fallopian tubes has provided a suitable model for electron microscopic study of the disease process. Initial contact between the organism and the host is with cell receptors of the microvilli. Gonococcal pili extend over the membrane of the epithelial cells as the attached cocci penetrate the mucosal lining of the fallopian tube. Foci of infection develop in the subepithelial connective tissue, resulting in disorganization of collagen connective tissue and local extension of disease. Destruction of ciliated epithelial cells by gonococci depletes the mucosal lining, thereby permitting more rapid penetration by other gonococci, as well as the mixed flora that characterizes pelvic inflammatory disease (PID).

Resistance to Gonococcal Infection

Both specific and nonspecific factors play an important role in host defense against gonococcal infection. Among the nonspecific mechanisms in women that have been implicated are cyclic changes in hormone levels and genital pH that are associated with the menstrual cycle. Disseminated gonococcal infection occurs most frequently during the perimenstrual period. Variations in the pH, osmolarity, and urea concentrations of the urine also appear to be important and may explain why some men fail to acquire infection upon exposure. As previously indicated, the presence of "natural antibodies" derived from gram-negative bacteria with antigens cross-reactive with gonococcal antigens undoubtedly are very important in the natural resistance to infection for some persons.

The specific host defenses that are most important in gonococcal infection are those of the humoral immune system. Antibodies on the mucosal surfaces constitute the primary line of defense and consist primarily of IgA and IgG. Vaginal secretion antibodies that are reactive with pili, outer membrane proteins, and LOS have been demonstrated, but the relative importance in infection of antibodies to any specific antigen has been difficult to assess. Because of the importance of pili as attachment effectors and virulence factors, most of the efforts directed toward the development of a vaccine have utilized the pilus antigen. Mucosal antibody production does follow immunization of human volunteers with pilus vaccine, but data supporting the protective effect of antipili antibodies in naturally acquired infection are not clear, probably because of the antigenic heterogeneity of different pilins.

Systemic immunity constitutes an important secondary line of defense against gonococcal infection. Complement activation by the classic pathway appears to be more important than activation by the alternative pathway. In the presence of antibody and complement, serum-sensitive gonococci are killed. Naturally occurring, nonimmune antibodies may participate in the bactericidal reaction, but immune antibodies usually are active in higher titer. IgM is much more active than IgG in the in vitro bactericidal reaction, and IgA is not bactericidal. There is some evidence that IgA and IgG antibody actually may block the bactericidal effects of IgM antibody. Outer membrane PIII appears to be the target of this blocking effect. Bacteremia with serum-sensitive gonococci does not occur in persons with normal antibody and complement systems because of the antibody-complement-mediated killing of the organisms. Disseminated infections, however, commonly occur in patients infected with gonococci that are resistant to the bactericidal action of antibody and complement. LOS is the primary surface antigen of the gonococcus that is involved in the bactericidal effect of antibody. It is significant that the presence of bactericidal activity in the serum does not protect an individual from acquiring a genital infection. The central role of complement in protection against bacteremia caused by serum-sensitive *N. gonorrhoeae* is emphasized by the finding that patients with deficiencies of one of the terminal complement components, C5 to C9, have deficient bactericidal systems and are at risk for bacteremia caused by the gonococcus but not by other kinds of organisms.

Antibody-complement-mediated opsonization, phagocytosis, and PMN killing is an important component of the host response to gonococcal infection, especially in mucosal or other localized gonococcal infections. Large numbers of PMNs are found in urethral or endocervical exudates of patients, attracted to the site of infection by chemotactic agents such as gonococcal LOS and complement cleavage products. Some of the PMNs contain large numbers of organisms presumably as a consequence of opsonization and phagocytosis. PII, also known as *leukocyte association factor,* is one of the surface components of the gonococcus that mediates attachment to the PMNs. Once ingested, the bactericidal systems of the PMNs are activated. It is unlikely that the organisms multiply within the PMNs or that these cells serve as a reservoir of infection.

Clinical Manifestations

Disease in Men. When compared with many other infectious diseases, gonorrhea is not highly contagious. An unprotected man has an approximately 22% chance of acquiring gonorrhea from intercourse with an infected woman, and the risk is considerably reduced by use of a condom. Acute gonorrhea in a man has an incubation period of 2 to 8 days, with most cases occurring within 4 days of infection. The patient presents with burning on urination and a yellow purulent urethral discharge that signifies acute anterior urethritis. The patient may be febrile and have a leukocytosis, but systemic signs generally are lacking. The infection is asymptomatic in approximately 10% of cases, but the patient retains the capacity to transmit infection. In the preantibiotic era the disease resolved in most men within a month; however, complications develop in approximately 1% of men, the most common being urethral strictures, epididymitis, and prostatitis. Less common are septicemia, peritonitis, and meningitis. Another frequent sequela of gonorrhea in men is the subsequent development of nongonococcal urethritis (postgonococcal urethritis, often caused by *Chlamydia trachomatis* and *Ureaplasma* species: Chaps. 52 and 53).

Disease in Women. Screening of some groups of symptom-free women has shown prevalence rates of gonorrhea between 1% and 8%. Lower rates of infection are observed for such groups as private obstetric practices and higher rates for groups such as manpower training programs, neighborhood clinics, and venereal disease clinics. The risk to a woman from intercourse with an infected man is not definitely known but probably is higher than for the man.

Between 20% and 80% of women with gonorrhea have no symptoms, depending on the population studied. Signs of disease in those with symptoms include burning or frequency of urination, vaginal discharge, fever, and abdominal pain. The major complication of gonorrhea in women is the development of PID by gonococcal infection of the fallopian tubes. This disease affects approximately 15% of women with gonorrhea and has two important consequences: (1) Gonococcal PID is a major cause of sterility and ectopic pregnancies because the scars from the infection may block the passage of ova through the fallopian tubes. (2) Scar formation also blocks the normal flow of fluid through the fallopian tubes. In areas with fluid accumulation, infection by other bacteria, especially anaerobic organisms, may develop. This leads to chronic PID, a debilitating and painful disease without satisfactory forms of therapy. Other complications occasionally encountered are infectious perihepatitis and generalized peritonitis.

Approximately 50% of women with gonorrhea have concomitant rectal colonization, and proctitis occasionally develops. In 10% of women the rectal site is the only area colonized. Few heterosexual men have rectal colonization, but in male homosexuals, it is common.

The other major site of extragenital colonization in both men and women is the pharynx. In about 5% of persons who practice fellatio, it is the only site of infection. Although pharyngeal gonococcal infection most often produces no symptoms, in some instances it is associated with clinically apparent pharyngitis.

Disseminated Gonococcal Disease. The gonococcal arthritis-dermatitis syndrome, which is the most common manifestation of disseminated gonococcal disease, is the result of gonococcal bacteremia. Male and female patients in whom this syndrome occurs usually have had asymptomatic genitourinary infection. Although more cases have been reported in women, men with asymptomatic gonorrhea also are at risk. The incidence of gonococcal bacteremia is approximately 1% of all persons with gonorrhea.

The acute form of the gonococcal dermatitis syndrome is heralded by fever, chills, malaise, intermittent bacteremia, polyarticular arthritis or tenosynovitis, and the development of typical skin lesions. The small distal joints are the predominant sites of involvement, and there usually is a paucity of synovial effusion. Joint fluid, if obtained, most often is sterile. The characteristic skin lesions are few in number; occur on the distal dorsal surfaces of the wrists, elbows, and ankles; and usually begin as small petechial or papular lesions. Suppuration, bullous formation, and central necrosis also are common.

If therapy is not received during this stage, which usually lasts about 3 days, the disease may progress to the septic joint stage. With this form of the disease, blood cultures rarely yield *N. gonorrhoeae.* Symptoms of septicemia such as fever and chills cease, and the disease becomes prominent in a single joint as overt arthritis. The synovial fluid is characteristic of pyarthrosis, with decreased sugar, poor mucin clot formation, and a pronounced granulocytic response.

Other rare forms of gonococcal disease that may follow bacteremic spread include subacute bacterial endocarditis and meningitis. The organisms responsible for disseminated gonococcal infection usually are highly sensitive to penicillin.

Disease in Children. Although gonorrhea most commonly is acquired during sexual contact between adults, a significant number of cases each year occur in infants and children. Gonorrhea in this age-group may be a result of sexual abuse, but in infancy it usually results from contamination during passage through an infected birth canal.

In the perinatal period, infection of the eye is the most common manifestation of gonorrhea. Before the use of silver nitrate for ophthalmic prophylaxis, gonococcal ophthalmia was the cause of blindness in approximately half the children admitted to schools for the blind. Although gonococcal ophthalmia neonatorum continues to occur, the disease is now a rare cause of blindness. Prevention of disease is based on diagnosis and treatment of the mother before delivery or on prophylactic treatment of the eyes of the newborn after birth. After birth, all states require prophylactic care of the eyes of the newborn; 1% silver nitrate remains the most satisfactory agent. Failure of silver nitrate prophylaxis does occur, however, and is more common in premature infants or after prolonged rupture of membranes. Because silver nitrate instillation is inadequate treatment for established infection, some of the failures may be due to the presence of active disease by the time of birth.

Relatively little is known of the hazard to the fetus of maternal gonorrhea, but there are indications of increased rates of premature birth and of perinatal morbidity. In addition, the mother may suffer complications of delivery. For these reasons, good obstetric care now includes repeated gonococcal screening during pregnancy. Table 26–6 summarizes four separate studies on the outcome of pregnancy in women who had gonococcal disease during gestation.

Neonatal gonococcal arthritis is a highly destructive form of infectious arthritis. The organism usually is acquired from the infected mother at the time of birth. Infection of any mucous membrane may enable dissemination to occur. In

TABLE 26–6. OUTCOME OF PREGNANCY IN MOTHERS WHO WERE INFECTED WITH *NEISSERIA GONORRHOEAE* AT DELIVERY

	No. of Cases (%)			
Outcome	Sarrell	Israel	Amstey	Edwards
Total No. in study	37	39	222	19
Normal or term infant	13(35)	30(77)	142(64)	7(37)
Aborted	13(35)	1	24(11)	—
Perinatal death	3(8)	1	15(7)	2(11)
Premature	6(17)	5(13)	49(22)	8(42)

Data from Sarrell and Pruett: Obstet Gynecol 32:670, 1968; Israel et al: Clin Obstet Gynecol 18:143, 1975; Amstey and Steadman: J Am Vener Dis Assoc 3:14, 1976; Edwards et al: Am J Obstet Gynecol 132:637, 1978.

several instances in which neonatal gonococcal arthritis has occurred, the mother also has had disseminated disease, a finding consistent with the observations that certain strains have increased invasive capacity.

Gonorrheal vulvovaginitis usually occurs in girls 2 to 8 years of age. The alkaline pH of the prepubescent vagina is cited as one factor favoring the establishment of gonococcal disease in this age-group. The disease usually is self-limited but occasionally progresses to invasion of the fallopian tubes or to peritonitis.

An area of rapidly increasing interest and understanding concerns the role of sexual abuse of children in the acquisition of childhood gonococcal infections, as well as other sexually transmitted infections. Pediatricians now recognize sexual abuse as one aspect of the larger spectrum of child abuse and neglect.

Laboratory Diagnosis

The laboratory diagnosis of gonococcal infection is based primarily on the identification of *N. gonorrhoeae* in infected sites by (1) microscopic examination and (2) culture.

Microscopic Examination. In urethral smears from men with symptoms of urethritis, the Gram stain is considered positive for gonorrhea when gram-negative diplococci of typical morphology are found within or closely associated with PMNs. It is equivocal if only extracellular organisms or atypical intracellular gram-negative diplococci are seen. Nonpathogenic *Neisseria* species usually are not cell associated. In symptomatic cases, the Gram stain is both sensitive and specific. Approximately 90% to 98% of culture-positive men with a purulent discharge have a positive smear. This contrasts with a sensitivity of only 60% in men with symptom-free gonococcal urethritis. Smears from the endocervix are less sensitive (50% to 60%) than those for the urethra but are highly specific when examined by experienced personnel. Extreme care must be taken to avoid mistaking morphologically similar saprophytic organisms of the normal flora for *N. gonorrhoeae,* and only smears containing several PMNs with multiple intracellular gram-negative diplococci with typical morphology should be labeled presumptively positive for gonorrhea. Endocervical smears have a higher predictive value in women suspected of having gonorrhea than in symptom-free persons with normal physical findings.

Culture. A definitive diagnosis is established by isolating the gonococcus in the laboratory. The materials submitted include urethral exudate and endocervical secretions. The pharynx and rectum also may be colonized in infected persons, and cultures may provide evidence of infection. In disseminated disease, blood cultures often are positive, and synovial fluid from patients with pyarthrosis usually yields the gonococcus. In the neonate, cultures of gastric aspirate and the conjunctivae also are helpful. The laboratory processing and identification of materials are discussed on page 444.

Isolates from patients suspected of having either meningococcal or gonococcal infection should be completely identified inasmuch as *N. meningitidis* has been recovered from all the sites in which *N. gonorrhoeae* commonly is found.

Serologic Tests. Because of the difficulty in obtaining an adequate endocervical specimen for culture from women and because a single endocervical culture from women with symptom-free gonorrhea fails to provide a diagnosis in at least 20% of cases, a serologic method for the diagnosis of gonorrhea would be useful. A number of these have been developed to detect antibody in a patient's serum to *N. gonorrhoeae* or its components, but none of these has been sufficiently reliable for serodiagnostic purposes. Newer techniques, some using monoclonal antibodies, currently are being evaluated.

Other Diagnostic Tests. Isolation of *N. gonorrhoeae* is the diagnostic standard, in part because of the importance of having an isolate whose antimicrobial sensitivity pattern can be determined. Other, and more rapid, diagnostic methods are in common use but do not allow susceptibility testing. Those other tests include the detection of gonococcal antigens by enzyme immunoassay. It is sensitive and specific for men patients but less so for women. Nonculture methods should not be used for diagnosis of gonorrhea in children or for testing for cure.

Treatment

Standards for the treatment of all forms of gonorrhea are regularly revised and published by the Centers for Disease Control. As modifications of these recommendations are needed, they are published in the weekly issue of *Morbidity and Mortality Report* and should be consulted by physicians who treat any patient with gonorrhea. Treatment recommendations of gonococcal disease are determined by age, sex, type of clinical disease, site of disease, and local prevalence of penicillinase-producing *N. gonorrhoeae* (PPNG) or chromosomally mediated resistant *N. gonorrhoeae* (CMRNG). Until recently, standard courses of therapy were based on the assumption that the patient had a penicillin-sensitive strain unless there was epidemiologic reason to expect a resistant strain. More recently, the emergence of multiple foci of isolates of *N. gonorrhoeae* that are resistant to a variety of antimicrobial agents has led to the use of regimens to which resistant strains have been rare or unreported.

For uncomplicated infections of mucosal surfaces, ceftriaxone is now most commonly recommended. For persons older than 8 years of age, doxycycline should be added, and for younger patients with gonorrhea, erythromycin in a base may be added. Alternatives to ceftriaxone include spectinomycin, trimethoprim-sulfamethoxazole, ciprofloxacin, and cefuroxime.

Although there had been a gradual increase in minimal inhibitory concentrations (MIC) of penicillin and other agents for gonococcal isolates as a result of chromosomally mediated resistance, until the last 15 years the level of resistance was low and could be overcome with increased dosage regimens. Beginning in the middle 1970s, however, strains of gonococci were isolated in the Far East that were resistant to levels of penicillin greater than could be achieved in the serum. Since that time PPNG strains have become widespread in some geographic areas and, in parts of Africa and the Far East, now outnumber penicillinase-negative strains. PPNG strains were first recognized in the United States in 1976, and although the number of reported PPNG cases has increased, it continues to remain low (Fig. 26–5). Most cases can no longer be linked to persons who have traveled overseas but are attributed to sustained domestic transmission. In some areas, PPNG now represents as much as 2% of all cases of

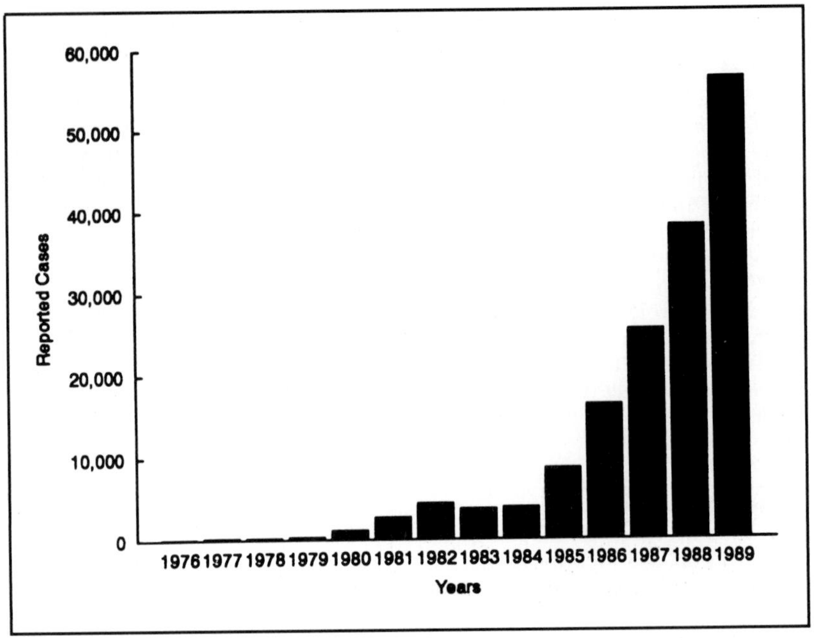

Fig. 26–5. Total resistant strains of *Neisseria gonorrhoeae* in the United States, 1976 to 1989. First case was reported in March 1976. Greater than 95% of resistant strains represents penicillinase-producing *N. gonorrhoeae* (PPNG). *(From Centers for Disease Control: MMWR 38(54):25, 1989.)*

gonorrhea. In 1986, approximately 17,000 cases of PPNG were reported to the Centers for Disease Control. Because local epidemiologic conditions vary in different parts of the country, the selection of a particular regimen should take into account the local incidence of penicillin-resistant strains.

Resistance in PPNG strains from the Far East, and in most but not all U.S. strains, is due to the presence of a plasmid-borne gene for the production of a TEM-1 type of β-lactamase (penicillinase). These plasmids are either 3.4 or 4.7 MDa in size, and they are closely related to each other and to penicillinase plasmids from some *Haemophilus* species.

Since 1980 strains of *N. gonorrhoeae* have been identified that are intrinsically resistant to penicillins. In these strains, resistance is caused by altered penicillin-binding proteins and is chromosomally mediated. An outbreak involving 199 cases occurred in 1983 in North Carolina. The prevalence of resistant strains of this type is increasing nationally.

Control

Each case of gonorrhea should be reported to the local public health department. In some instances, contact tracing by the private physician may supplement public health efforts to control disease. A number of factors contribute to the difficulties encountered in the control of gonorrhea: (1) Gonococcal infection has a very short incubation period, making it possible for secondary and tertiary cases to transmit disease before recognition and treatment of the primary case. (2) The disease frequently is symptom free, and the diagnosis is made only with appropriate cultures. (3) Social acceptance of sexual activity with multiple partners provides the opportunity for wide and rapid dissemination of gonorrhea and other sexually transmitted diseases. (4) During the past decade, gonococcal isolates have undergone a progressive increase in the mean MICs for penicillin. This has made the use of single injection therapy of disease increasingly difficult.

FURTHER READING

Books and Reviews

BRANHAMELLA CATARRHALIS

Hager H, Verghese A, Alvarez S, Berk S: *Branhamella catarrhalis* respiratory infections. Rev Infect Dis 9:1140, 1987

NEISSERIA MENINGITIDIS

Devoe IW: The meningococcus and mechanisms of pathogenesis. Microbiol Rev 46:162, 1982

Frasch CE, Zollinger WD, Poolman JT: Serotype antigens of *Neisseria meningitidis* and a proposed scheme for designation of serotypes. Rev Infect Dis 4:504, 1985

Griffiss JM: Epidemic meningococcal disease: Synthesis of a hypothetical immunoepidemiologic model. Rev Infect Dis 4:159, 1982

Olyhoek T, Crowe BA, Achtman M: Clonal population structure of *Neisseria meningitidis* serogroup A isolated from epidemics and pandemics between 1915 and 1983. Rev Infect Dis 9:665, 1987

NEISSERIA GONORRHOEAE

Braude AI: Resistance to infection with the gonococcus. J Infect Dis 145:623, 1982

Brooks GF, Donegan EA: Gonococcal Infection. London, Edward Arnold, 1985

Brunton J, Clare D, Meier MA: Molecular epidemiology of antibiotic resistance plasmids to *Haemophilus* species and *Neisseria gonorrhoeae.* Rev Infect Dis 8:713, 1986

Holmes KK, Mardh P-A, Sparling PF, Wiesner PJ: Sexually Transmitted Diseases. New York, McGraw-Hill, 1984

Lossick JG: Epidemiology of sexually transmitted diseases. In Spagna VA, Prior RB: Sexually Transmitted Diseases. A Clinical Syndrome Approach. New York, Marcel Dekker, 1985

Selected Papers

NEISSERIA MENINGITIDIS

Archibald FS, Devoe IW: Iron acquisition by *Neisseria meningitidis* in vitro. Infect Immun 27:322, 1980

Brandtzaeg P, Mollnes TE, Kierulf P: Complement activation and endotoxin levels in systemic meningococcal disease. J Infect Dis 160:58, 1989

Braude AJ, McCutchan JA, Ison C, and Sargeaunt PR: Differentiation of Neisseriaceae by isoenzyme analysis. J Infect Dis 147:247, 1983

Caugant DA, Mocca LF, Frasch CE, et al: Genetic structure of *Neisseria meningitidis* populations in relation to serogroup, serotype, and outer membrane protein pattern. J Bacteriol 169:2781, 1987

Centers for Disease Control: Meningococcal vaccines. MMWR 34(18):255, 1985

Crowe BA, Wall RA, Kusecek B, et al: Clonal and variable properties of *Neisseria meningitidis* isolated from cases and carriers during and after an epidemic in the Gambia, West Africa. J Infect Dis 159:686, 1989

Frasch CE, Zahradnik JM, Wang LY, et al: Antibody response of adults to an aluminum hydroxide-adsorbed *Neisseria meningitidis* serotype 2b protein-group B polysaccharide vaccine. J Infect Dis 158:710, 1988

Gotschlich EC, Liu TY, Artenstein MS: Human immunity to the meningococcus. III. Preparation and immunochemical properties of the group A, group B, and group C meningococcal polysaccharides. J Exp Med 129:1349, 1969

Halstensen A, Haneberg B, Froholm LO, et al: Human opsonins to meningococci after vaccination. Infect Immun 46:673, 1984

Havens PL, Garland JS, Brook MM, et al: Trends in mortality in children hospitalized with meningococcal infections, 1957 to 1987. Pediatr Infect Dis 8:8, 1989

Jarvis GA, Vedros NA: Sialic acid of group B *Neisseria meningitidis* regulates alternative complement pathway activation. Infect Immun 55:174, 1987

Lowell GH, Smith LF, Griffiss JM, et al: IgA-dependent, monocyte-mediated, antibacterial activity. J Exp Med 152:452, 1980

Moore PS, Hierholzer J, DeWitt W, et al: Respiratory viruses and mycoplasma as cofactors for epidemic group A meningococcal meningitis. JAMA 264:1271, 1990

Nicholson A, Lepow IH: Host defense against *Neisseria meningitidis* requires a complement-dependent bactericidal activity. Science 25:298, 1979

Peltola H, Safary A, Kayhty H, et al: Evaluation of two tetravalent ($ACYW_{135}$) meningococcal vaccines in infants and small children. A clinical study comparing immunogenicity of O-acetyl-negative and O-acetyl-positive group C polysaccharides. Pediatrics 76:91, 1985

Ross SC, Rosenthal PJ, Berberich HM, Densen P: Killing of *Neisseria meningitidis* by human neutrophils: Implications for normal and complement-deficient individuals. J Infect Dis 155:1266, 1987

Soderstrom C, Braconier JH, Danielsson D, Sjoholm AG: Bactericidal activity for *Neisseria meningitidis* in properdin-deficient sera. J Infect Dis 156:107, 1987

Stephens DS, Hoffman LH, McGee ZA. Interaction of *Neisseria meningitidis* with human nasopharyngeal mucosa: Attachment and entry into columnar epithelial cells. J Infect Dis 148:369, 1983

Stephens DS, Whitney AM, Melly MA, et al: Analysis of damage to human ciliated nasopharyngeal epithelium by *Neisseria meningitidis.* Infect Immun 51:579, 1986

Weidmer CE, Dunkel TB, Pettyjohn FS, et al: Effectiveness of rifampin in eradicating the meningococcal carrier state in relatively closed populations. Emergence of resistant strains. J Infect Dis 124:172, 1971

NEISSERIA GONORRHOEAE

Apicella MA, Mandrell RE, Shero M, et al: Modification by sialic acid of *Neisseria gonorrhoeae* lipooligosaccharide epitope expression in human urethral exudates: An immunoelectron microscropic analysis. J Infect Dis 162:506, 1990

Apicella MA, Shero M, Jarvis GA, et al: Phenotype variation in epitope expression of the *Neisseria gonorrhoeae* lipooligosaccharide. Infect Immun 55:1755, 1987

Archibald FS, Duong M-N: Superoxide dismutase and oxygen toxicity defenses in the genus *Neisseria.* Infect Immun 51:631, 1986

Bergstrom S, Robbins K, Koomey JM, Swanson J: Piliation control mechanisms in *Neisseria gonorrhoeae.* Proc Natl Acad Sci USA 83:3890, 1986

Bessen D, Gotschlich EC: Interactions of gonococci with HeLa cells: Attachment, detachment, replication, penetration, and the role of protein II. Infect Immun 54:154, 1986

Bessen D, Gotschlich EC: Chemical characterization of binding properties of opacity-associated protein II from *Neisseria gonorrhoeae.* Infect Immun 55:141, 1987

Bohnhoff M, Morello JA, Lerner SA: Auxotypes, penicillin susceptibility, and serogroups of *Neisseria gonorrhoeae* from disseminated and uncomplicated infections. J Infect Dis 154:225, 1986

Britigan BE, Cohen MS, Sparling PF: Gonococcal infection: A model of molecular pathogenesis. N Engl J Med 312:1683, 1985

Brunham RC, Plummer F, Slaney L, et al: Correlation of auxotype and protein I type with expression of disease due to *Neisseria gonorrhoeae.* J Infect Dis 152:339, 1985

Clark VL, Campbell LA, Palermo DA, et al: Induction and repression of outer membrane proteins by anaerobic growth of *Neisseria gonorrhoeae.* Infect Immun 55:1359, 1987

Handsfield HH, Lipman JO, Harnisch JP, et al: Asymptomatic gonorrhea in men. Diagnosis, natural course, prevalence and significance. N Engl J Med 290:117, 1974

Handsfield HH, Sandstrom EG, Knapp JS, et al: Epidemiology of penicillinase-producing *Neisseria gonorrhoeae* infections. N Engl J Med 306:950, 1982

Hoehn GT, Clark VL: Distribution of a protein antigenically related to the major anaerobically induced gonococcal outer membrane protein among other *Neisseria* species. Infect Immun 58:3929, 1990

Holmes KK, Counts GW, Beaty HN: Disseminated gonococcal infection. Ann Intern Med 79:979, 1971

Ingram DL, White ST, Durfee MF, Pearson AW: Sexual contact in children with gonorrhea. Am J Dis Child 136:994, 1982

Johnson SC, Chung R CY, Deal CD, et al: Human immunization with Pgh 3-2 gonococcal pilus results in cross-reactive antibody to the cyanogen bromide fragment-2 of pilin. J Infect Dis 163:128, 1991

Knapp JS, Tam MR, Nowinski RC, et al: Serological classification of *Neisseria gonorrhoeae* with use of monoclonal antibodies to gonococcal outer membrane protein I. J Infect Dis 150:44, 1984

McKenna WR, Mickelsen PA, Sparling PF, Dyer DW: Iron uptake from lactoferrin and transferrin by *Neisseria gonorrhoeae.* Infect Immun 56:785, 1988

Meitzner TA, Bolan G, Schoolnik GK, et al: Purification and characterization of the major iron-regulated protein expressed by pathogenic *Neisseriae.* J Exp Med 165:1041, 1987

Melly MA, McGee ZA, Rosenthal RS: Ability of monomeric peptidoglycan fragments from *Neisseria gonorrhoeae* to damage human fallopian-tube mucosa. J Infect Dis 149:378, 1984

Miettinen A, Hakkarainen K, Gronroos P, et al: Class-specific antibody response to gonococcal infection. J Clin Pathol 42:72, 1989

Moran JS, Zenilman JM: Therapy for gonococcal infections. Options in 1989. Rev Infect Dis 12:S633, 1990

Mulks MH, Knapp JS: Immunoglobulin AI protease types of *Neisseria gonorrhoeae* and their relationship to auxotype and serovar. Infect Immun 55:931, 1987

Newhall WJ, Mail LB, Wilde CE III, Jones RB: Purification and

antigenic relatedness of proteins II of *Neisseria gonorrhoeae.* Infect Immun 49:576, 1985
Rice PA, Kasper DL: Characterization of gonococcal antigens responsible for induction of bactericidal antibody in disseminated infection. The role of gonococcal endotoxins. J Clin Invest 60:1149, 1977
Rice PA, Kasper DL: Characterization of serum resistance of *Neisseria gonorrhoeae* that disseminate. Roles of blocking antibody and gonococcal outer membrane proteins. J Clin Invest 70:157, 1982
Sandstrom EG, Knapp JS, Buchanan TB: Serology of *Neisseria gonorrhoeae:* W-antigen serogrouping by coagglutination and protein I antigens. Infect Immun 35:229, 1982
Schoolnik GK, Buchanan TM, Holmes KK: Gonococci causing disseminated gonococcal infections are resistant to the bactericidal action of normal human sera. J Clin Invest 58:1163, 1976
Segal E, Hagblom P, Seifert HS, So M: Antigenic variation of gonococcal pilus involves assembly of separated silent gene segments. Proc Natl Acad Sci USA 83:2177, 1986
Sparling PF, Cannon JG, So M: Phase and antigenic variation of pili and outer membrane protein II of *Neisseria gonorrhoeae.* J Infect Dis 153:196, 1986
Weber RD, Britigan BE, Svendsen T, Cohen MS: Energy is required for maximal adherence of *Neisseria gonorrhoeae* to phagocytic and nonphagocytic cells. Infect Immun 57:785, 1989
Woods ML, Bonfiglioli R, McGee ZA, Georgopoulos C: Synthesis of a select group of proteins by *Neisseria gonorrhoeae* in response to thermal stress. Infect Immun 58:719, 1990

CHAPTER 27

Haemophilus

The genus *Haemophilus* comprises a group of small, pleomorphic, gram-negative rods with fastidious growth requirements. The name of the genus comes from the requirement by these organisms for accessory growth factors found in blood, that is, *haemo* (Greek for blood) and *philos* (Greek for loving).

Members of the genus are obligate parasites for humans and other vertebrates. They exhibit a pronounced host specificity, and with few exceptions, each species is exclusively associated with one specific host. In humans, most *Haemophilus* species are members of the indigenous flora of the upper respiratory tract.

Historical and Clinical Perspective. As a cause of human infection, *Haemophilus influenzae* is the most important species in the group. Although it is not the cause of epidemic influenza as its name suggests, it is responsible for a number of severe infections. In infants and young children, it causes acute bacterial meningitis and several other serious pediatric diseases. In adults, it is primarily associated with chronic pulmonary disease.

The organism was first isolated by Pfeiffer during the 1892 influenza pandemic. The frequency of its presence in the nasopharynx of patients with influenza and in postmortem lung cultures led to the erroneous assumption that it was the etiologic agent of influenza—thus the designation *the influenza bacillus*. As was later shown, influenza is caused by a virus. The role of *H. influenzae* during the pandemics of 1890 and 1918 was apparently that of a secondary invader. This type of synergistic interaction was subsequently demonstrated for the influenza virus of swine and a closely related organism, *Haemophilus suis*. However, because *H. influenzae* has not played a similar role in more recent influenza pandemics, the importance of viral-bacterial synergism in human disease is unknown.

The strains of *H. influenzae* that cause meningitis and other acute infections differ from those found in the respiratory tract of healthy persons in that these strains possess capsules. This important observation by Pittman has provided the basis for our current understanding of *H. influenzae* disease. The experience of the last 50 years has shown that of the six capsular serotypes demonstrated by Pittman, serotype b organisms are responsible for virtually all acute infec-

TABLE 27–1. PERCENTAGE DISTRIBUTION OF *HAEMOPHILUS* ISOLATES FROM HUMAN INFECTIONS AND NORMAL FLORA

Source (No.)	*H. influenzae* (%)	*H. parainfluenzae*[a] (%)	*H. haemolyticus* (%)	*H. segnis* (%)	*H. paraphrophilus* (%)	*H. aphrophilus* (%)
Meningitis and epiglottitis (157)	100	0	0	0	0	0
Ear infections (53)	100	0	0	0	0	0
Conjunctivitis (104)	96[b]	4	0	0	0	0
Lower respiratory tract (patients with CF) (56)	89	11	0	0	0	0
Healthy upper respiratory tract (496)	11	73	1	11	5	0
Oral cavity (649)	0	74	0	19	2	5

Adapted from Kilian and Biberstein: In Krieg and Holt (eds): Bergey's Manual of Systematic Bacteriology, vol 1. Williams & Wilkins, 1986, p 561.
CF, cystic fibrosis.
[a] Includes hemolytic strains.
[b] Includes strains with the characteristics of *Haemophilus aegyptius*.

tions caused by *H. influenzae*. *H. influenzae* type b is the most common cause of acute bacterial meningitis in infancy and early childhood, being responsible in the United States for approximately 8000 cases annually in children younger than 5 years of age. It also is the cause of such invasive diseases as pyarthrosis, cellulitis, pneumonia, and acute epiglottitis. Species other than *H. influenzae* that may be encountered in clinical material are listed in Table 27–1.

Haemophilus influenzae

Morphology

H. influenzae, as all members of the genus, is pleomorphic. In spinal fluid, joint fluid, or primary cultures of these materials on an enriched medium, the organisms are predominantly coccobacillary and uniform in shape, 0.2 to 0.3 by 0.5 to 0.8 μm (Fig. 27–1). Faint refractile capsules, demonstrable by quellung reactions with type-specific antisera, may be present. *H. influenzae* is gram-negative but may appear gram-variable unless the staining procedure is very carefully carried out. Unencapsulated organisms from sputum or ear aspirates often are more elongated than the encapsulated organisms and may exhibit bipolar staining with Gram stain, leading to an erroneous diagnosis of *Streptococcus pneumoniae*. Organisms from rough colonies are very pleomorphic, often appearing as long threads and filaments (Fig. 27–2). The ultrastructure of *H. influenzae* is similar to that of other gram-negative organisms.

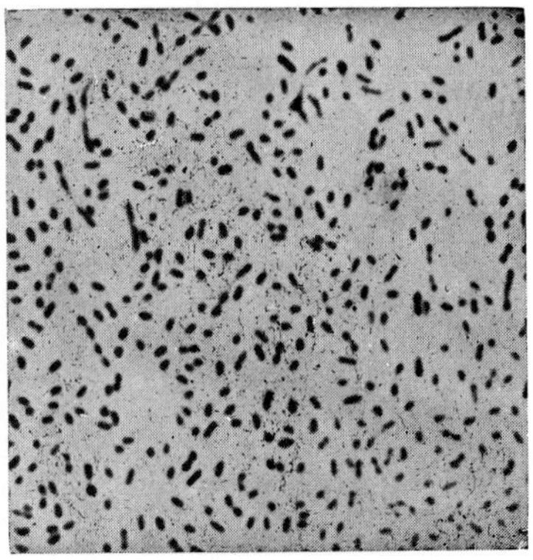

Fig. 27–1. Primary growth of *Haemophilus influenzae* on chocolate agar.

Physiology

Cultural Characteristics. Chocolate agar is the most generally used culture medium for the isolation of *Haemophilus* species. In its preparation, blood is added to an agar base and heated at 80C until a brown color appears. The mild heat releases the X and V factors from the blood cells and also inactivates V factor splitting enzymes without destroying the V factor itself. Also useful for the culture of clinical specimens are Levinthal and Fildes enriched agar media. Because it is colorless and transparent, Levinthal agar is especially useful for differentiating between encapsulated and nonencapsulated strains. Ordinary blood agar permits growth of *H. influenzae* only when the agar plate is cross-inoculated with a *Staphylococcus* or other V factor–excreting microorganism. Sizable colonies appear as satellite colonies in the vicinity of the feeder

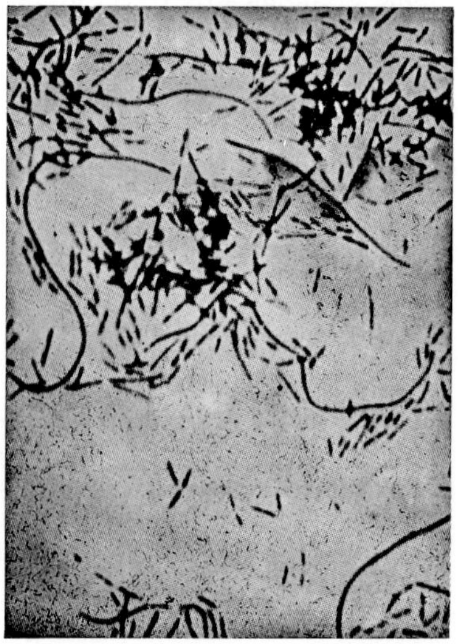

Fig. 27–2. Pleomorphic growth of *Haemophilus influenzae* from rough colony.

strain. Fresh human or sheep blood agar plates should not be used, however, because they contain heat-labile V factor inhibitors. Maximum growth occurs at 37C and pH 7.4 to 7.8 under aerobic conditions. For primary isolation, incubation in the presence of 10% CO_2 is recommended because of its enhancing effect on the growth of some strains.

Growth on semisolid agar is apparent 18 to 24 hours after inoculation. Since most clinical isolates are from respiratory specimens and are nonencapsulated, colonies usually are very small and dewlike and develop a coarse or rough appearance. These colonies usually are 0.5 to 1.5 mm in diameter. Encapsulated *H. influenzae* from invasive disease (usually type b from blood or cerebrospinal fluid) produces mucoid, glistening colonies that are characteristically iridescent on Levinthal agar. These may reach 3 or 4 mm in diameter on enriched medium. During the second 24 hours of incubation, a central umbilication develops because of the excretion of capsular polymer. Mucoid colonies often spontaneously convert to rough colonies because of loss of encapsulation (p. 464). Cultures of *H. influenzae* are difficult to maintain in the laboratory because of their tendency to autolyze. Proper maintenance of viable virulent organisms requires frequent transfers on chocolate agar or other enriched media.

Nutritional Requirements. All species of *Haemophilus* require either one or both of the two growth factors present in blood designated as X and V (Table 27–2). The heat-stable X factor is protoporphyrin IX, the precursor of hemin that is the prosthetic group in the cytochromes and in heme enzymes such as catalase and peroxidase. Hemin-independent species such as *H. parainfluenzae* synthesize hemin by the common tetrapyrrole pathway, but hemin-dependent organisms have lost the ability to convert δ-aminolevulinic acid to protoporphyrin. Hemin-dependent species appear to lack all the enzymes in tetrapyrrole synthesis except the ferrochelatase or heme synthase, which is variably present and catalyzes the final insertion of Fe^{2+} or Fe^{3+} into the protoporphyrin ring:

$$\text{Succinyl CoA} + \text{Glycine} \longrightarrow \delta\text{-Aminolevulinate}$$
$$\longrightarrow \text{Porphobilinogen}$$
$$\text{Uroporphyrinogen} \longrightarrow \text{Coproporphyrinogen}$$
$$\text{Protoporphyrin IX} \xrightarrow{Fe^{2+} \text{ or } Fe^{3+}} \text{Heme or hemin}$$

When grown anaerobically, *H. influenzae* shifts to an anaerobic metabolism and does not produce cytochromes. The hemin requirement is therefore greatly reduced if not completely absent. Since *H. parainfluenzae* has no requirement for an exogenous source of iron and thus is metabolically less flexible, under anaerobic conditions it continues to produce and utilize the cytochrome system (p. 43).

The heat-labile V factor is minimally nicotinamide mononucleoside, but usually is described as nicotinamide adenine dinucleotide (NAD) or NAD phosphate (NADP), which function as coenzymes for pyridine-linked dehydrogenases. Species of *Haemophilus* designated *para-* have a requirement only for the V factor, a differential property used in the laboratory identification of species by the use of disks impregnated with the X and V factors.

Metabolism. *Haemophilus* is aerobic but facultatively anaerobic. In an oxygen-free environment, nitrate is used as the final electron acceptor. The sole quinone produced by *H. influenzae* is demethylmenaquinone (DMK), but some species also produce ubiquinone. Whereas ubiquinone is used in electron transport systems leading only to high-potential acceptors such as oxygen or nitrate, DMK may be used for both aerobic and anaerobic electron transport. The possession of DMK thus enables *H. influenzae* to produce energy both by substrate-level phosphorylation and oxidative phosphorylation.

BIOTYPING. A separation of strains of *H. influenzae* into subgroups or biotypes may be accomplished by a battery of biochemical tests based on phenotypic properties of the organism (Table 27–3). The data that have accumulated from biotyping studies suggest that *H. influenzae* is biochemically heterogeneous and that noncapsular factors, frequently predictable by biovar, are associated with virulence. In a study of 157 isolates from *H. influenzae* meningitis, 94% belonged to biovar I, a biovar that is uncommon in the respiratory tract. The nonencapsulated strains that often are implicated in conjunctivitis, chronic bronchitis, sinusitis, and otitis media usually belong to biovars II and III, the same biovars that colonize the nasopharynx of most healthy persons (Table 27–1).

Genetics. In *H. influenzae,* a striking correlation exists between the colony type, antigenic structure, and virulence of

TABLE 27–2. DIFFERENTIAL PROPERTIES OF *HAEMOPHILUS* SPECIES THAT COLONIZE HUMANS

Species	V Factor Requirement	X Factor Requirement	Increased CO_2 Requirement	Hemolysis	Acid from D-Xylose
H. influenzae	+	+	−	−	+
H. aegyptius	+	+	−	−	−
H. haemolyticus	+	+	−	+	±
H. ducreyi	−	+	−	(±)	−
H. parainfluenzae	+	−	−	−	−
H. parahaemolyticus	+	−	−	+	−
H. paraphrohaemolyticus	+	−	+	+	−
H. aphrophilus	−	+	+	−	−
H. paraphrophilus	+	−	+	−	−
H. segnis	+	−	−	−	−

Adapted from Kilian and Biberstein. In Krieg and Holt (eds): Bergey's Manual of Systematic Bacteriology, vol 1. Williams & Wilkins, 1986, p 564.
( ), delayed.

TABLE 27–3. BIOCHEMICAL PROPERTIES OF *HAEMOPHILUS INFLUENZAE*

Biovar	Indole	Urease	Ornithine Decarboxylase	D-Glucose (Acid Only)	Nitrate Reduction	Catalase	Oxidase
I	+	+	+	+	+	+	+
II	+	+	−	+	+	+	+
III	−	+	−	+	+	+	+
IV	−	+	+	+	+	+	±
V	+	−	+	+	+	+	+
VI	−	−	+	+	+	+	+

Adapted from Kilian and Biberstein. In Krieg and Holt (eds): Bergey's Manual of Systematic Bacteriology, vol 1. Williams & Wilkins, 1986, p 564.

the organism. Mucoid to rough transitions in colony morphology, as observed when clinical isolates from invasive disease are subcultured on artificial media, reflect loss of specific capsular polysaccharide synthesis by mutation. The spontaneous mutation rate for this property is relatively high and may be increased by suboptimal culture conditions or by the presence of type-specific antisera.

The elaboration of a type-specific polysaccharide capsule by *H. influenzae* provides a convenient marker for genetic studies dealing with the transfer of DNA from one organism to another. Transformation and transfection mediated by DNA from the different serovars and other species of *Haemophilus* have been extensively studied, and the enzymology and genetics of these restriction and modification systems have been characterized. In *H. influenzae,* strain-specific restriction endonucleases recognize DNA from other strains as foreign. Protection against restriction is provided by a modification methylase that methylates a limited number of adenine or cytosine residues in the recognized nucleotide sequence. Each serovar of *H. influenzae* carries different DNA restriction and modification systems. These systems are powerful tools for the molecular biologist who has successfully used *Haemophilus*-derived enzymes to analyze the structure and function of specific genome fragments.

In *H. influenzae,* plasmids have been implicated in the transfer of antibiotic resistance, significantly affecting the clinical treatment of acute *Haemophilus* infections. Two types of plasmids are present: (1) a large conjugative 30 to 38 MDa plasmid and (2) a small nonconjugative plasmid with a 2.5 to 4.4 MDa molecular weight. Both plasmids contain a transposon (TnA) that codes for β-lactamase. This transposon resembles that of the transposable element Tn3 originally found in the Enterobacteriaceae. The cores of the conjugative *H. influenzae* R plasmids isolated in different parts of the world have similar base sequences but are not identical. Although the small 3 MDa plasmids are unable to mediate their own conjugal transfer, nonconjugative plasmids may be conjugally transferred if a self-transmissible plasmid also is present in the cell. Such an indigenous *H. influenzae* plasmid has been found, supporting the hypothesis that the *H. influenzae* R plasmids could have arisen simultaneously, as a result of the integration of the β-lactamase transposon, into different but closely related indigenous *H. influenzae* plasmids in various parts of the world. In *Haemophilus ducreyi* a similar plasmid transfer system that will cross species and generic lines also has been demonstrated.

Resistance to chloramphenicol and tetracycline also is plasmid-mediated in *H. influenzae.* Conjugative R plasmids for these drugs are closely related to the ampicillin plasmids and have most of their base sequences in common, as would be expected from the hypothesized origin of *H. influenzae* plasmids.

Antigenic Structure

H. influenzae contains three major classes of surface antigens: the capsular polysaccharide, lipopolysaccharide, and outer membrane proteins. A number of typing and subtyping schemes based on the diversity of these antigens have been introduced. Such schemes have revealed the extreme genetic variability of *H. influenzae* strains.

Capsular Antigens. The major antigenic determinant of encapsulated *H. influenzae* is the capsular polysaccharide. This polysaccharide confers type specificity on the organism and is the basis for the grouping of the organism into six serovars, designated a through f. Virtually all the strains associated with invasive disease belong to serovar b.

The capsular antigens produced by serovars a, b, c, and f are of the teichoic acid type, whereas those from serovars d and e are polysaccharides. The distinct chemical specificity of each type is shown in Table 27–4. The serovar b capsular polymer is unique in that it contains the pentose sugars, ribose and ribitol phosphate, instead of hexoses or hexosamines as found in the other serovars. Antibody to this polyribosylribose phosphate capsular antigen plays a key role in protection from *H. influenzae* type b (Hib) infection. It is bactericidal in the presence of complement and is opsonic and protective. The human response to antigenic challenge with the Hib capsule results in the production of antibodies of the IgG, IgM, and IgA classes. IgG antibody is bactericidal and opsonic for human polymorphonuclear neutrophils (PMNs) in the presence of complement and is protective in an animal model. Although IgM is bactericidal and protective, it is poorly

TABLE 27–4. CAPSULAR POLYSACCHARIDES OF *HAEMOPHILUS INFLUENZAE*

Type	Sugar	PO_4	Acetyl
a	Glucose	+	−
b	Ribose and ribitol	+	−
c	Galactose	+	−
d	Hexose	−	−
e	Hexosamine	−	+
f	Galactosamine	+	+

opsonic for bacteria; IgA is not bactericidal, nor is it opsonic or protective. A number of organisms in other genera have been shown to have antigens cross-reactive with the serovar b polysaccharide of *H. influenzae.* Cross-reactions are known to occur between Hib and a diverse group of gram-negative and gram-positive organisms. Cross-reactivity between *Escherichia coli* and Hib has been attributed to shared specificities of acidic polysaccharides or K antigens, whereas in gram-positive species the cross-reacting antigens are cell wall polyribitol phosphate teichoic acids.

SEROLOGIC CAPSULAR REACTIONS. Encapsulated *H. influenzae* may be typed by the quellung (capsular swelling) reaction using serovar-specific antisera. Typing may be done directly on fresh clinical specimens or on primary isolates. Slide agglutination is a simple, rapid, and accurate technique for routine laboratory use but must be interpreted carefully and confirmed with another procedure such as counterimmunoelectrophoresis or coagglutination.

The serovar of free capsular polysaccharide antigen that is found in culture filtrates and body fluids may be identified serologically by counter immunoelectrophoresis or latex particle agglutination (p. 467). Since type b organisms cause more than 95% of invasive disease, detection of the type b capsular antigen is especially important.

Somatic Antigens. The cell envelope of *H. influenzae* consists of an outer and an inner membrane containing protein and lipooligosaccharide (LOS) antigens. The major antigenic component of LOS is its nontoxic oligosaccharide fraction. Antibodies to this somatic antigen are age-independent in contrast to the age-dependent responses to the capsular polysaccharide. Hib LOS consists of only lipid A and a structure analogous to the core oligosaccharide of the lipopolysaccharide (LPS) of enteric bacteria. There is cross-reactivity between the core glycolipid of *H. influenzae* LOS and the LPS of *E. coli. H. influenzae* LOS lacks an O-antigen repeat unit and exhibits little antigenic heterogeneity among the different strains. It contains at least three O-antigenic determinants. The antigenic determinants of Hib LOS have been highly conserved over time in that strains isolated from cases of systemic disease more than 40 years ago react with the same set of monoclonal antibodies that recognize recent Hib isolates. The lipid A component of the LOS is highly specific for *H. influenzae* but is antigenically heterogeneous among *Haemophilus* strains and species.

Of the two to three dozen proteins detected in the outer membrane of *H. influenzae,* a small number account for most of the protein content of the cell surface. Some are consistently present in all strains of *Haemophilus,* whereas others vary with the serovar of capsulated and noncapsulated strains. Substantial antigenic variation in some of the major outer membrane antigens also occurs among the various Hib strains. By using a system for subtyping isolates based on their outer membrane protein profiles, 13 different antigenic groups have been defined. Subtyping schemes have proved especially useful in comparing epidemiologically related isolates.

Interest in the outer membrane protein antigens has been intensified by the failure of the vaccine prepared from Hib capsular polysaccharide to confer on infants younger than 2 years of age protective immunity against systemic disease. Since both animals and humans develop antibody to outer membrane antigens during Hib infection, the outer membrane proteins currently are being characterized and assessed for their vaccine potential. Especially promising are the type b polysaccharide-protein conjugates, which apparently are thymic-dependent and induce an enhanced anti–type b antibody response.

Determinants of Pathogenicity

Capsule

The phosphoribosylribitol phosphate (PRRP) capsule of Hib plays a critical role in the pathogenesis of invasive disease caused by this organism. Systemic infections always are caused by encapsulated strains and virtually always by those elaborating the type b capsular polysaccharide. In humans, susceptibility to systemic infections is highly correlated with the absence of serum antibodies to the type b capsule. Antibodies to the type b capsule also effectively promote phagocytosis of Hib in vitro. The reason for the proclivity of type b for bacteremic infections is unknown, but it is believed to be attributable to the unique structure of its capsular polysaccharide, which in the absence of specific antibody imparts to the organism an effective resistance to complement (p. 467).

Other Virulence Factors

Outer Membrane Components. Although the type b capsular polysaccharide is the critical determinant of virulence, it is likely that in *Haemophilus,* virulence is multifactorial and that, at present, other ill-defined factors contribute to virulence in different time-site sequences. Among the components most likely to influence the disease process are outer membrane proteins and LOS. Each of a number of different surface molecules may be responsible for a specific function associated with virulence, such as attachment, invasiveness, and resistance to phagocytosis. The differences that have been found in the outer membrane proteins of type b organisms may reflect a modulation of some of these functions. The importance of noncapsular somatic antigens in the pathogenesis of *H. influenzae* is emphasized by a number of studies in both human and experimental animal systems, which show that antibody directed against these antigens also may be important in immunity to *H. influenzae* disease.

Surface somatic antigens of nonencapsulated *H. influenzae* also contribute to the pathogenesis of chronic nonspecific lung diseases such as asthmatic bronchitis. *H. influenzae* LOS exerts a paralyzing action on the ciliated respiratory epithelium and promotes proliferation of the organism in the bronchial tree. The chemical composition of the lipid A component of *H. influenzae* LOS is similar to that of enterobacterial LPS, but free lipid A does not exhibit all the classic biologic activities of other lipid A preparations.

Adherence. Little is known about the role of adherence of *H. influenzae* to epithelial surfaces in the pathogenesis of infection. Studies indicate, however, that most (more than 90%) nontypeable strains are adherent to human buccal epithelial cells, whereas only a few (5%) of type b strains are adherent. These differences may contribute to the variations in colonization observed between type b and nontypeable strains and may explain the tendency for nontypeable strains to cause localized infection whereas type b strains are associated with invasive disease.

IgA Proteases. *H. influenzae* is one of five bacterial species known to produce IgA proteases, enzymes that have the unique ability to hydrolyze the human IgA1 heavy chain as their only known substrate. The IgA proteases are neutral endopeptidases, distinguishable from other microbial enzymes in that their cleavage fragments, Fab-α and Fc-α, do not undergo a secondary degradation. Because *H. influenzae* primarily infects human mucosal surfaces where host defense is mediated by secretory IgA, cleavage of IgA may contribute to the organism's virulence potential. *H. influenzae* is the only member of the genus that produces this enzyme. Strains of *H. influenzae* produce three distinct types of IgA proteases that cleave different peptide bonds within the IgA1 hinge region. The type of protease produced correlates with the serotype of the isolate. Each nontypeable strain also produces one of the three protease types.

Clinical Infection

Epidemiology

Unencapsulated *H. influenzae* organisms are commonly carried in the nasopharynx of symptom-free persons. Rates of carriage are about 60% to 90% in healthy young children and 35% in adults. Of the isolates from children, about 5% are encapsulated, one half of which are type b. In the adult, only 0.4% of the isolates are type b.

The frequency of invasive infections is inversely related to age; only a small percentage occurs in adults and older children. Infections in the first 2 months of life are rare, probably because of transplacental transfer of maternal antibody (p. 467). Most cases of meningitis, pyarthrosis, and cellulitis occur in children younger than 2 years of age, and the mean age of children with epiglottitis is 3 to 5 years. Systemic *H. influenzae* in the adult, previously thought to be uncommon, now is being recognized with increasing frequency. Also, the overall incidence of invasive *Haemophilus* disease has increased fourfold over the last two decades, possibly because of improved laboratory techniques for identification.

H. influenzae diseases are worldwide in their occurrence and are for the most part endemic in nature. An increased incidence of secondary cases, however, occurs among susceptible persons in families and day-care centers who are exposed to an index case. Systemic infections occur more commonly among the poor and the black population. Host factors that appear to contribute to increased susceptibility include immunoglobulin deficiencies, sickle cell disease, splenectomized state, and chronic pulmonary infections. In the adult, alcoholism increases the risk of *H. influenzae* pneumonia.

Pathogenesis

Respiratory Portal of Entry. Infection with *H. influenzae* occurs after the inhalation of infected droplets from clinically active cases, convalescent patients, and carriers. Nonhuman reservoirs of *H. influenzae* are unknown. The natural history of infections in children is poorly understood, but clinical experience suggests that the organisms initially colonize the nasopharynx. Both rough and smooth variants of *H. influenzae* are carried at this site. These relatively common asymptomatic infections occasionally develop into symptomatic disease that may spread contiguously to the sinuses, middle ear, or bronchi. The organisms are established in the tracheobronchial tree, perhaps in synergy with a virus, or by paralysis of normal cilia clearance functions. The relevance, however, of viral synergy, toxic bacterial products, and local immunity in producing clinical disease remains to be proved. The strains usually associated with chronic respiratory disease are nonencapsulated and probably do not invade tissues. The presence of Hib in sputum or ear aspirates may indicate tissue invasion. Respiratory infections are important sources for the seeding of the blood to produce metastatic disease in the meninges or joints and for the invasion of local tissues to cause epiglottitis, pneumonia, or cellulitis.

Bloodstream Invasion. The critical pathogenic event for most serious diseases caused by type b organisms is invasion of the organisms from the respiratory mucous membranes and their survival in the blood. Although the precise mechanisms mediating this invasion are ill-defined at present, both bacterial virulence determinants and host resistance factors are involved. The type b capsule is essential for invasiveness. The presence of a type b capsular polysaccharide enables the organism to resist the action of complement, permitting longer survival and eventual multiplication in the blood. The increased incidence of invasive disease in nonimmune and genetically susceptible individuals emphasizes the critical role of host factors in *H. influenzae* infections. Viral synergy also may play an important role in the host-parasite interaction.

After implantation within the tissues, *H. influenzae* characteristically evokes a nonspecific acute neutrophilic exudation that is rich in fibrin. The heavy plastic nature of the exudate may be important in protecting the organisms against the host defenses.

Clinical Manifestations

In one survey of hospitalized children, Hib was the most common cause of bacteremic disease. Of those with *H. influenzae* disease, meningitis was the most common manifestation (54%), followed by pneumonia (14%), bacteremia without focus (11%), cellulitis (11%), epiglottitis (10%), and pericarditis (4%).

Meningitis. The most serious of the diseases produced by *H. influenzae* is an acute bacterial meningitis. *H. influenzae* meningitis occurs rarely in infants younger than the age of 3 months and is uncommon in children older than 6 years of age. Cases have been reported, however, both in neonates and in adults. The distribution of disease is equal in males and females and in races, except for the increased susceptibility in association with sickle cell anemia. Patients with humoral immunodeficiency are especially susceptible. The incidence of disease is approximately 5/100,000 population and is reported to be increasing in recent years. Overt symptoms, cerebrospinal fluid pleocytosis, and positive culture reactions often are preceded by several days of respiratory symptoms, during which invasion presumably occurs. Clinical and laboratory findings are typical of a pyogenic infection. Therapy can prevent mortality in 90% to 97% of cases, but residual central nervous system deficits are demonstrable in one third of patients.

Acute Bacterial Epiglottitis. This disease, rarely caused by organisms other than Hib, has an acute onset and a dramatically rapid course. It occurs in children who are older than patients with meningitis and even occasionally in adults. The genetic makeup of children with epiglottitis appears to be different from those with *H. influenzae* meningitis. There is a striking predominance of occurrence in white children. The infected epiglottis has microabscesses, and the marked edema may cause complete airway obstruction, requiring emergency tracheotomy within 12 hours of onset. Severe septicemia frequently occurs in this too often fatal illness.

Cellulitis. *H. influenzae* causes cellulitis in children younger than 2 years of age and, rarely, in older adults. The most commonly involved site is the cheek, but cellulitis may occur in the periorbital area and other locations, especially the upper extremities. Classically, *H. influenzae* cellulitis of the cheek has an acute onset, develops rapidly within a few hours, and is accompanied by pain and edema. A distinctive bluish-purple occurs late in the infection. Inasmuch as cellulitis due to *H. influenzae* usually is a bacteremic disease, metastatic infection may result.

Bacteremia Without Local Disease. *H. influenzae* is responsible for about 20% of the bacteremias that occur in febrile children without any evidence of local disease. Children 6 to 36 months of age who have sickle cell disease or who have undergone splenectomy are particularly susceptible. Unsuspected *H. influenzae* bacteremia also occurs in adults with neoplastic disease who are undergoing chemotherapy. The clinical course may progress to septic shock and often death within hours of the initial medical evaluation.

Other Infections. Hib is a common cause of childhood pyarthrosis and is associated with pericarditis, usually as a part of a pneumonic episode. Most cases of *H. influenzae* pneumonia are due to type b and occur in very young children. In adults, pneumonia occurs more frequently in elderly persons with chronic lung disease, alcoholism, or immunologic deficiency, but it also may develop in previously healthy individuals.

H. influenzae is second in frequency to *Streptococcus pneumoniae* as the cause of otitis media. The strains isolated usually are nontypeable, but in 10% of the cases, type b organisms are associated with the infection. Nontypeable strains often cause acute sinusitis in adults and frequently are associated with purulent sputum and clinical exacerbations of chronic bronchitis.

Immunity

One of the most striking features of *H. influenzae* disease is the relationship between age and susceptibility. The frequency of meningitis is inversely related to the bactericidal activity of the blood, whether passively acquired from the mother or actively formed. Invasive disease occurs during the age of relative humoral immunodeficiency—3 months to 3 years. Although it is now apparent that immunity to Hib is mediated by antibody of multiple specificities, anticapsular antibody is the factor in serum that correlates with protection. The anticapsular antibody titer of serum varies with age in the same manner as the bactericidal activity. Anticapsular antibody is bactericidal in the presence of complement, promotes phagocytosis, and is protective in animal models and in humans.

Antibodies to the type b capsular polysaccharide can be generated by infection with bacteria that possess cross-reacting surface antigens (p. 465). These antibodies are bactericidal in vitro and protective in experimental disease. It has been suggested that the incidence of Hib carriage or disease is too low to account for the rapid and extensive age-related acquisition of anticapsular antibodies and that cross-reacting organisms may serve as the primary immunogen. Antibodies to *H. influenzae* outer membrane antigens also appear to play a role in immunity. They are bactericidal, promote complement-mediated phagocytosis, and are protective in animal model systems. In certain adults and older children, resistance to clinical infection has correlated with antibody titers to somatic antigens in the absence of anticapsular type b activity. Therefore, natural resistance to *H. influenzae* is based on a multifactorial antibody response to *H. influenzae* itself, as well as heterologous antigens cross-reactive with the type b capsular polysaccharide.

The antibody response of patients recovering from systemic Hib disease is age related. Infants respond infrequently and with low antibody levels. High titers develop in older children and adults. This same type of response is observed after immunization with capsular type b polysaccharide, severely limiting the effectiveness of this antigen for the vaccination of children younger than 18 months of age. Failure to develop a consistent antibody response to natural Hib exposure or to vaccination with type b capsular polysaccharide probably is related to the young child's immunologic immaturity in processing carbohydrate antigen.

Laboratory Diagnosis

Accurate identification of the causative agent is a prerequisite for the proper management of *H. influenzae* disease.

Direct Examination. Gram-stained smears of clinical specimens are useful in providing a rapid presumptive identification. Specimens suitable for direct examination include those from cerebrospinal fluid; arthrocentesis, thoracentesis, or middle ear aspirates; and sputum samples. However, because of the organism's tendency to retain the Gram stain, unless extreme care is taken during the staining procedure to decolorize sufficiently, the organism's coccobacillary forms may be erroneously interpreted as pneumococci. The use of carbolfuchsin as a counterstain in the Gram stain is recommended.

Culture. Because *H. influenzae* is fastidious and dies quickly in clinical materials at room temperature, specimens should be planted immediately. They should be streaked directly on the surface of a chocolate agar or other suitable media, then incubated aerobically in an atmosphere of 10% CO_2 (p. 462). In addition, blood cultures should be performed for every patient thought to have meningitis or other invasive disease.

Antigen Detection. The detection of specific polysaccharide antigen in body fluids also is a valuable diagnostic aid and provides a presumptive diagnosis of *H. influenzae* infection even in the absence of a positive culture reaction. The techniques that have proved most useful are counter immunoelectrophoresis (CIE), latex particle agglutination, and enzyme-linked immunosorbent assay (ELISA), all of which provide rapid and semiquantitative results. With use of CIE, rapid diagnosis can be made in 90% of confirmed cases of Hib meningitis and in a majority of other infections caused by this organism. CIE may be especially helpful in establishing a diagnosis for patients who have received antibiotic therapy before lumbar puncture and who often pose a more complicated diagnostic challenge because of negative results on Gram stain and culture.

Treatment

The treatment of invasive *H. influenzae* disease, especially meningitis and epiglottitis, is a medical emergency. Any unnecessary delay in starting treatment may make the difference between life and death or, in the case of meningitis, between a normal and a brain-damaged child or adult.

About 24% of all strains of *H. influenzae* isolated in this country from systemic infections are now resistant to ampicillin. Because of this prevalence of resistant strains, until the etiologic agent is proved to be sensitive to ampicillin, all systemic illnesses suspected of having an *H. influenzae* etiology should be treated with chloramphenicol alone or in combination with ampicillin.

Ampicillin or amoxicillin, each of which is active against *S. pneumoniae* and most strains of *H. influenzae,* is the drug of choice for initial treatment of otitis media in children. Alternatives include trimethoprim-sulfamethoxazole, the combination of penicillin (or erythromycin) with a sulfonamide, or cefaclor. Because ampicillin-resistant strains rarely cause *H. influenzae* pneumonia in the adult, initial treatment of these infections should be with ampicillin. Cephalosporins also are often used. Ampicillin is a suitable initial antibiotic choice for acute sinusitis.

Passive Immunotherapy. As an adjunct to antibiotics in the treatment of severe infections, passive immunization with hyperimmunoglobulin has been shown to be effective. More recently, monoclonal antibody to the capsular polysaccharide has been produced, and although still in the experimental stage, results in animal models suggest that passive immunotherapy with monoclonal antibody will have a future role in the treatment of *H. influenzae* disease.

Prevention

Active Immunization. In 1985, after two decades of intensive investigation and development of a vaccine against Hib, a vaccine consisting of purified capsular polysaccharide was licensed in the United States. This vaccine, although safe and moderately effective in lowering the incidence of Hib infections in children 24 months of age or older, was ineffective in children younger than 18 months of age, when the incidence of infection is greatest. Ambitious and creative programs led to the development of polysaccharide-protein conjugate vaccines, a new class of vaccines designed to immunize infants against diseases caused by encapsulated bacteria such as Hib. Type b capsular polysaccharide is coupled to protein carriers, such as a variant of diphtheria toxin, diphtheria toxoid, or outer membrane proteins. These conjugate vaccines stimulate higher concentrations of preponderantly IgG immunoglobulin, are more immunogenic in young infants, and elicit booster response with subsequent doses, all of which characterize thymic-dependent antigens. Of the conjugate vaccines currently licensed for use, two have been approved for use in infants at 2 months of age. In one of these an oligosaccharide derivative of Hib capsular polysaccharide is coupled to a nontoxic mutant diphtheria toxin. In the second and most recently approved vaccine, Hib polysaccharide is linked to the outer membrane protein of *Neisseria meningitidis* group B. The latter vaccine is approved for use in a two-dose primary immunization schedule for infants at 2 and 4 months of age, with a booster dose at the age of 12 months (Table 27–5). Clinical evaluation of the various conjugate vaccines in diverse locations throughout the United States shows that they are highly immunogenic and that they are compatible with other pediatric vaccines. Their inclusion among the routine childhood immunizations would have a definite impact on pediatric morbidity.

TABLE 27–5. ACIP-RECOMMENDED *HAEMOPHILUS INFLUENZAE* TYPE B (Hib) ROUTINE VACCINATION SCHEDULE

	Vaccine	
Month	HbOC[a]	PRP-OMP[b]
2	dose 1	dose 1
4	dose 2	dose 2
6	dose 3	
12		booster
15	booster	

From Centers for Disease Control: MMWR 40(RR-1):1, 1991.
ACIP, Immunization Practices Advisory Committee; PRP-OMP, polyribosylribitolphosphate–outer membrane protein.
[a] CRM_{197} mutant *C. diphtheriae* toxin used as protein carrier.
[b] *N. meningitidis* outer membrane protein complex used as protein carrier.

Passive Immunization. Children with congenital or acquired deficiencies of immunoglobulin synthesis probably will not benefit from vaccination and should receive periodic doses of immunoglobulin. A single 0.5 ml/kg intramuscular dose of human hyperimmunoglobulin will protect children for 4 months. Immunoglobulin also may be indicated in other high-risk groups of children, such as those with sickle cell disease or asplenia, socioeconomic or racial predisposing factors, or exposure to another individual with Hib. The significantly increased rate of secondary cases of invasive *H. influenzae* diseases among young children who have intimate contacts with primary cases indicates the need for an effective prophylactic program. No specific antibiotic regimen tested has proved reliably effective, and the issue of chemoprophylaxis of contacts of patients with invasive *H. influenzae* infection remains controversial, especially in day-care settings.

Other *Haemophilus* Species

Human disease caused by species of *Haemophilus* other than *H. influenzae* has been considered rare. Because of recent interest in these organisms and improved techniques for their isolation and identification, it is apparent that they are more frequent causes of infection than previously thought.

Sixteen species of *Haemophilus* currently are recognized and included in the genus in *Bergey's Manual of Systematic Bacteriology*. Ten of the species are found in humans either as part of the normal flora or associated with infection. The species *H. parainfluenzae, H. parahaemolyticus, H. paraphrohae-*

molyticus, H. segnis, H. aphrophilus, and *H. paraphrophilus* are opportunistic pathogens present in the mouth and nasopharynx of healthy persons. Clinical infection caused by these species is the result of local or bloodstream invasion from sites of colonization. Infections that have been attributed to these organisms include endocarditis, brain abscesses, dental abscesses, jaw infections, and infections after human bites or finger sucking.

Haemophilus aegyptius (Koch-Weeks Bacillus)

H. aegyptius is associated with a communicable purulent conjunctivitis, especially in children in hot climates. *H. aegyptius* is indistinguishable from *H. influenzae* biovar III, and because of difficulties in differentiating *H. aegyptius* from *H. influenzae,* which also may cause conjunctivitis, the natural history of *H. aegyptius* infections is poorly understood. *H. aegyptius,* however, appears to be associated with a more acute form of conjunctivitis and, in contrast to *H. influenzae,* can colonize eyes in the absence of any predisposing condition. Outbreaks of seasonal conjunctivitis occur during the summer and early fall. A mechanical vector transmission by gnats is believed to play an important role, especially in many areas of the southern United States.

H. aegyptius has been differentiated from *H. influenzae* on the basis of its hemagglutinating ability, but this property is not universally characteristic of all strains causing acute conjunctivitis. Also, authentic and freshly isolated *H. aegyptius* strains are notably more fastidious than *H. influenzae* and differ from it in a number of additional properties such as the failure to produce indole and ferment xylose. It can be differentiated serologically. The conjunctivitis usually responds to topically applied sulfonamides.

Haemophilus parainfluenzae

This species is part of the normal flora of the mouth and nasopharynx. Clinical infection is the result of local or bloodstream invasion from these sites, usually after dental disease, dental procedures, or other oral trauma. Additional predisposing factors include respiratory tract infections, alcoholism, and other conditions that compromise host defense mechanisms. The most common *H. parainfluenzae* infection is endocarditis. Approximately 5% of all infective endocarditis is caused by this organism. Known preexisting cardiac disease such as congenital or rheumatic heart disease is present in about 50% of the cases. Most cases occur in young or middle-aged adults. The recommended treatment is ampicillin alone or in combination with gentamicin. *H. parainfluenzae* also is a rare cause of meningitis, epiglottitis, otitis media, bacteremia, brain abscess, and pneumonia in the adult. Ampicillin is the drug of choice unless resistance requires the use of an alternate regimen employing chloramphenicol.

Haemophilus ducreyi

H. ducreyi is the cause of chancroid, a sexually transmitted disease worldwide in distribution. In temperate climates, *H. ducreyi* may be responsible for up to 10% of venereal disease in civilian populations, but during periods of war chancroid may be nearly as great a problem as gonorrhea. In civilian populations it is most common among nonwhite men and usually is associated with poor socioeconomic and hygienic conditions.

After exposure, there is a 2- to 14-day incubation period before the appearance of a single lesion or multiple lesions that develop into sharply circumscribed, nonindurated, painful ulcers. These usually are confined to the genitalia and perianal areas and rarely are accompanied by systemic symptoms. Suppurative inguinal buboes are characteristic and develop in about one half of the patients. Oral erythromycin is the treatment of choice. An alternative effective regimen is oral trimethoprim-sulfamethoxazole.

A laboratory diagnosis is made by finding *H. ducreyi* in gram-stained smears of ulcer exudate or bubo aspirate. The organisms are pleomorphic and may occur both extracellularly and intracellularly. The classic microscopic appearance is that of a school of red fish, but interpretation of smears may be difficult because organisms in fresh smears may appear to be gram-positive or other organisms may be mistaken for *H. ducreyi.* Culture of material from the ulcer or bubo should be attempted. Although primary isolation may be difficult, a positive culture provides a definitive diagnosis. The best culture results have been obtained with a chocolate agar medium containing vancomycin.

FURTHER READING

Books and Reviews

Albritton WL: Biology of *Haemophilus ducreyi.* Microbiol Rev 53:377, 1989

Centers for Disease Control: *Haemophilus* b conjugate vaccines for prevention of *Haemophilus influenzae* type b disease among infants and children two months of age and older: Recommendations of the Immunization Practices Advisory Committee (ACIP). MMWR 40(RR-1):1, 1991

Daum RS, Granoff DM, Gilsdorf J, et al: *Haemophilus influenzae* type b infections in day care attendees: Implications for management. Rev Infect Dis 8:558, 1986

Geiseler PJ, Nelson KE, Levin S, et al: Community-acquired purulent meningitis: A review of 1,316 cases during the antibiotic era, 1954–1976. Rev Infect Dis 2:725, 1980

Hammond GW, Slutchuk M, Scatliff J, et al: Epidemiologic, clinical, laboratory, and therapeutic features of an urban outbreak of chancroid in North America. Rev Infect Dis 2:867, 1980

Kilian M, Biberstein EL: Genus II. *Haemophilus.* In Krieg NR, Holt JG (eds): Bergey's Manual of Systematic Bacteriology, vol 1. Baltimore, Williams & Wilkins, 1986, p 558

Klein JO, Gerety RJ: Current status of *Haemophilus influenzae* type b vaccines. Pediatrics 85(suppl):631, 1990

Murphy TF, Apicella MA: Nontypable *Haemophilus influenzae:* A review of clinical aspects, surface antigens, and the human immune response to infection. Rev Infect Dis 9:1, 1987

Musser JM, Kroll JS, Granoff DM, et al: Global genetic structure and molecular epidemiology of encapsulated *Haemophilus influenzae.* Rev Infect Dis 12:75, 1990

Smith AL: Antibiotic resistance in *Haemophilus influenzae.* In Ayoub EM, Cassell GH, Branche WC Jr, Henry TJ (eds): Microbial Determinants of Virulence and Host Response. Washington, DC, American Society for Microbiology, 1990, p 321

Turk DC, May RF: *Haemophilus influenzae:* Its Clinical Importance. London, English Universities Press, 1967

Wallace RJ Jr, Baker CJ, Quinones FJ, et al: Nontypable *Haemophilus influenzae* (biotype 4) as a neonatal, maternal, and genital pathogen. Rev Infect Dis 5:123, 1983

Selected Papers

Alexander HE, Ellis C, Leidy G: Treatment of type-specific *Haemophilus influenzae* infections in infancy and childhood. J Pediatr 20:673, 1942

Ambrosino DM, Landesman SH, Gorham CC, Siber GR: Passive immunization against disease due to *H. influenzae* type b: Concentration of antibody to capsular polysaccharide in high-risk children. J Infect Dis 153:1, 1986

Amir J, Liang X, Granoff DM: Variability in the functional activity of vaccine-induced antibody to *Haemophilus influenzae* type B. Pediatr Res 27:358, 1990

Anderson P: Antibody responses to *Haemophilus influenzae* type b and diphtheria toxin induced by conjugates of oligosaccharides of the type b capsule with the nontoxic protein CRM_{197}. Infect Immun 39:233, 1983

Apicella MA, Dudas KC, Campagnari A, et al: Antigenic heterogeneity of lipid A of *Haemophilus influenzae.* Infect Immun 50:9, 1985

Arditi M, Ables L, Yogev R: Cerebrospinal fluid endotoxin levels in children with *H. influenzae* meningitis before and after administration of intravenous ceftriaxone. J Infect Dis 160:1005, 1989

Bakaletz LO, Tallan BM, Hoepf T, et al: Frequency of fimbriation of nontypable *Haemophilus influenzae* and its ability to adhere to chinchilla and human respiratory epithelium. Infect Immun 56:331, 1988

Barenkamp SJ, Munson RS Jr, Granoff DM: Subtyping isolates of *Haemophilus influenzae* type b by outer membrane protein profiles. J Infect Dis 143:668, 1981

Berk SL, Holtsclaw SA, Wiener SL, Smith JK: Nontypable *Haemophilus influenzae* in the elderly. Arch Intern Med 142:537, 1982

Bradshaw M, Schneerson R, Parke JC, Robbins JB: Bacterial antigens cross reactive with the capsular polysaccharide of *Haemophilus influenzae* type b. Lancet 1:1095, 1971

Cope LD, Yogev R, Mertsola J, et al: Effect of mutations in lipooligosaccharide biosynthesis genes on virulence of *Haemophilus influenzae* type b. Infect Immun 58:2343, 1990

Crisel RM, Baker RS, Dorman DE: Capsular polymer of *Haemophilus influenzae,* type b. I. Structural characterization of capsular polymer of strain Eagan. J Biol Chem 250:4926, 1975

Degré M, Solber LA: Synergistic effect in viral-bacterial infection. Acta Pathol Microbiol Scand [B] 79:129, 1971

Deneer HG, Slaney L, MacLean IW, Albritton WL: Mobilization of nonconjugative antibiotic resistance plasmids in *Haemophilus ducreyi.* J Bacteriol 149:726, 1982

Denny F: Effect of a toxin produced by *Haemophilus influenzae* on ciliated epithelium. J Infect Dis 219:93, 1974

Elwell LP, Roberts M, Falkow S: Common β-lactamase–specifying R plasmid isolated from the genera *Haemophilus* and *Neisseria.* In Schlessinger D (ed): Microbiology 1978. Washington, DC, American Society for Microbiology, 1978, p 255

Eskola J, Kayhty H, Takala AK, et al: A randomized, prospective field trial of a conjugate vaccine in the protection of infants and young children against invasive *Haemophilus influenzae* type b disease. N Engl J Med 323:1381, 1990

Eskola J, Peltola H, Takala AK, et al: Efficacy of *Haemophilus influenzae* type b polysaccharide-diphtheria toxoid conjugate vaccine in infancy. N Engl J Med 317:717, 1987

Fothergill LD, Wright J: Influenzal meningitis: The relationship of age incidence to the bactericidal power of blood against the causal organism. J Immunol 24:273, 1933

Gigliotti F, Insel RA: Protection from infection with *Haemophilus influenzae* type b by monoclonal antibody to the capsule. J Infect Dis 146:249, 1982

Glode MP, Daum RS, Boies EG, et al: Effect of rifampin chemoprophylaxis on carriage eradication and new acquisition of *Haemophilus influenzae* type b in contacts. Pediatrics 76:537, 1985

Granoff DM, Sheetz K, Pandey JP, et al: Host and bacterial factors associated with *Haemophilus influenzae* type b disease in Minnesota children vaccinated with type b polysaccharide vaccine. J Infect Dis 159:908, 1989

Green BA, Metcalf BJ, Quinn-Dey T, et al: A recombinant non-fatty acylated form of the Hi-PAL (P6) protein of *Haemophilus influenzae* elicits biologically active antibody against both nontypable and type b *H. influenzae.* Infect Immun 58:3272, 1990

Grundy FJ, Plaut AG, Wright A: Localization of the cleavage site specificity determinant of *Haemophilus influenzae* immunoglobulin A1 protease genes. Infect Immun 58:320, 1990

Hansen EJ: Noncapsular surface antigens and their association with virulence of *Haemophilus influenzae* type b. In Ayoub EM, Cassell GH, Branche WC Jr, Henry TJ (eds): Microbial Determinants of Virulence and Host Response. Washington, DC, American Society for Microbiology, 1990, p 45

Hansen EJ, Pelzel SE, Orth K, et al: Structural and antigenic conservation of the P2 porin protein among strains of *Haemophilus influenzae* type b. Infect Immun 57:3270, 1989

Herrington DA, Sparling PF: *Haemophilus influenzae* can use human transferrin as a sole source for required iron. Infect Immun 48:248, 1985

Hill MR, McKinney KL, Marks MI, Hyde RM: Comparative analysis of *Haemophilus influenzae* type b and *Escherichia coli* J5 lipopolysaccharides. J Med Microbiol 21:25, 1986

Hoiseth SK, Connelly CJ, Moxon ER: Genetics of spontaneous, high-frequency loss of b capsule expression in *Haemophilus influenzae.* Infect Immun 49:389, 1985

Hunter KW Jr, Hemming VG, Fischer GW, et al: Antibacterial activity of a human monoclonal antibody to *Haemophilus influenzae* type b capsular polysaccharide. Lancet 2:798, 1982

Insel RA, Anderson PW Jr: Cross-reactivity with *Escherichia coli* K100 in the human serum anticapsular antibody response to *Haemophilus influenzae* type b. J Immunol 128:1267, 1982

Insel RA, Anderson PW Jr: Oligosaccharide-protein conjugate vaccines induce and prime for oligoclonal IgG antibody responses to the *Haemophilus influenzae* b capsular polysaccharide in human infants. J Exp Med 163:262, 1986

Käyhty H, Eskola J, Peltola H, et al: Immunogenicity in infants of a vaccine composed of *Haemophilus influenzae* type b capsular polysaccharide mixed with DPT or conjugated to diphtheria toxoid. J Infect Dis 155:100, 1987

Kimura A, Gulig PA, McCracken GH, et al: A minor high-molecular-weight outer membrane protein of *Haemophilus influenzae* type b is a protective antigen. Infect Immun 47:253, 1985

Kimura A, Hansen EJ: Antigenic and phenotypic variations of *Haemophilus influenzae* type b lipopolysaccharide and their relationship to virulence. Infect Immun 51:69, 1986

Klein JO, Feigin RD, McCracken GH: Report of the task force on diagnosis and management of meningitis. Pediatrics 78:501, 1986

Lampe RM, Mason EO Jr, Kaplan CL, et al: Adherence of *Haemophilus influenzae* to buccal epithelial cells. Infect Immun 35:166, 1982

Laufs R, Riess F-C, Jahn G, et al: Origin of *Haemophilus influenzae* R factors. J Bacteriol 147:563, 1981

Lepow ML, Barkin RM, Berkowitz CD, et al: Safety and immunogenicity of *Haemophilus influenzae* type b polysaccharide-diphtheriae toxoid conjugate vaccine (PRP-D) in infants. J Infect Dis 156:591, 1987

Levy SB, Buu-Hoi A, Marshall B: Transposon Tn10–like tetracycline resistance determinants in *Haemophilus parainfluenzae.* J Bacteriol 160:87, 1984

Loeb MR, Connor E, Penney D: A comparison of the adherence of fimbriated and nonfimbriated *Haemophilus influenzae* type b to human adenoids in organ culture. Infect Immun 56:484, 1988

Loeb MR, Smith DH: Outer membrane protein composition in disease isolates of *Haemophilus influenzae:* Pathogenic and epidemiological implications. Infect Immun 30:709, 1980

Loeb MR, Smith DH: Human antibody response to individual outer membrane proteins of *Haemophilus influenzae* type b. Infect Immun 37:1032, 1982

Long SS, Teter MJ, Gilligan PH: Biotype of *Haemophilus influenzae:* Correlation with virulence and ampicillin resistance. J Infect Dis 147:800, 1983

MayoSmith MF, Hirsch PJ, Wodzinski SF, Schiffman FJ: Acute epiglottitis in adults. An eight-year experience in the state of Rhode Island. N Engl J Med 314:1133, 1986

Michaels RH, Myerowitz RL, Klaw R: Potentiation of experimental meningitis due to *Haemophilus influenzae* by influenza A virus. J Infect Dis 135:641, 1977

Moxon ER, Murphy PA: *Haemophilus influenzae* bacteremia and meningitis resulting from survival of a single organism. Proc Natl Acad Sci USA 75:1534, 1978

Mulks MH, Kornfeld SJ, Frangione B, Plaut AG: Relationship between the specificity of IgA proteases and serotypes in *Haemophilus influenzae.* J Infect Dis 146:266, 1982

Munson RS Jr, Granoff DM: Purification and partial characterization of outer membrane proteins P5 and P6 from *Haemophilus influenzae* type b. Infect Immun 49:544, 1985

Murphy TF, Apicella MA: Antigenic heterogeneity of outer membrane proteins of nontypable *Haemophilus influenzae* is a basis for a serotyping system. Infect Immun 50:15, 1985

Murphy TF, Bartos LC: Human bactericidal antibody response to outer membrane protein P2 of nontypable *Haemophilus influenzae.* Infect Immun 56:2673, 1988

Musser JM, Barenkamp SJ, Granoff DM, Selander RK: Genetic relationships of serologically nontypable and serotype b strains of *Haemophilus influenzae.* Infect Immun 52:183, 1986

Musser JM, Granoff DM, Pattison PE, et al: A population genetic framework for the study of invasive diseases caused by serotype b strains of *Haemophilus influenzae.* Proc Natl Acad Sci USA 82:5078, 1985

Mustafa MM, Ramilo O, Sáez-Llorens X, et al: Role of tumor necrosis factor alpha (cachectin) in experimental and clinical bacterial meningitis. Pediatr Infect Dis J 8:907, 1989

Osterholm MT, Pierson LM, White KE, et al: The risk of subsequent transmission of *Hemophilus influenzae* type b disease among children in day care. Results of a two-year statewide prospective surveillance and contact survey. N Engl J Med 316:1, 1987

Peter G, Smith DH: *Haemophilus influenzae* meningitis at the Children's Hospital Center in Boston, 1958–1973. Pediatrics 55:523, 1975

Pifer ML: Plasmid establishment in competent *Haemophilus influenzae* occurs by illegitimate transformation. J Bacteriol 168:683, 1986

Pittman M: Variation and type specificity in the bacterial species *Haemophilus influenzae.* J Bacteriol 59:413, 1950

Porras O, Caugant DA, Gray B, et al: Difference in structure between type b and nontypable *Haemophilus influenzae* populations. Infect Immun 53:79, 1986

Quinn PH, Crosson FJ, Winkelstein JA, et al: Activation of the alternative complement pathway by *Haemophilus influenzae* type b. Infect Immun 16:400, 1977

Ramadas K, Petersen GM, Heiner DC, Ward JI: Class and subclass antibodies to *Haemophilus influenzae* type b capsule: comparison of invasive disease and natural exposure. Infect Immun 53:486, 1986

Robbins JB, Schneerson R, Argaman M, et al: *Haemophilus influenzae* type b: Disease and immunity in humans. Ann Intern Med 78:259, 1973

Schneerson R, Barrera O, Sutton A, Robbins JB. Preparation, characterization, and immunogenicity of *Haemophilus influenzae* type b polysaccharide-protein conjugates. J Exp Med 152:361, 1980

Schreiber JR, Barrus V, Cates KL, Siber GR: Functional characterization of human IgG, IgM, and IgA antibody directed to the capsule of *Haemophilus influenzae* type b. J Infect Dis 153:8, 1986

Sell SH, Merrill RE, Doyne EO, et al: Long-term sequelae of *Haemophilus influenzae* meningitis. Pediatrics 49:206, 1972

Setlow JK, Notani NK, McCarthy D, Clayton N-L. Transformation of *Haemophilus influenzae* by plasmid RSF0885 containing a cloned segment of chromosomal deoxyribonucleic acid. J Bacteriol 148:804, 1981

Shenep JL, Munson RS Jr, Granoff DM: Human antibody responses to lipopolysaccharide after meningitis due to *Haemophilus influenzae* type b. J Infect Dis 145:181, 1982

Shope RE: The influenza of swine and man. Harvey Lect 36:183, 1935

Siber GR, Santosham M, Reid GR, et al: Impaired antibody response to *Haemophilus influenzae* type b polysaccharide and low IgG2 and IgG4 concentrations in Apache children. N Engl J Med 323:1387, 1990

Spagnuolo PJ, Ellner JJ, Lerner PI, et al: *Haemophilus influenzae* meningitis: The spectrum of disease in adults. Medicine 61:74, 1982

Spinola SM, Peacock J, Denny FW, et al: Epidemiology of colonization by nontypable *Haemophilus influenzae* in children: A longitudinal study. J Infect Dis 154:100, 1986

St. Geme JW III, Falkow S: *Haemophilus influenzae* adheres to and enters cultured human epithelial cells. Infect Immun 58:4036, 1990

Stuy JH: Transfer of genetic information within a colony of *Haemophilus influenzae.* J Bacteriol 1:162, 1985

Sutter VL, Finegold SM: *Haemophilus aphrophilus* infections: Clinical and bacteriological studies. Ann NY Acad Sci 174:468, 1970

Sutton A, Schneerson R, Kendall-Morris S, Robbins JB: Differential complement resistance mediates virulence of *Haemophilus influenzae* type b. Infect Immun 35:95, 1982

Syrogiannopoulos GA, Hansen EJ, Erwin AL, et al: *Haemophilus influenzae* type b lipooligosaccharide induces meningeal inflammation. J Infect Dis 157:237, 1988

Tarr PI, Hosea SW, Brown EJ, et al: The requirement of specific anticapsular IgG for killing of *Haemophilus influenzae* by the alternative pathway of complement activation. J Immunol 128:1772, 1982

Umetsu DT, Ambrosino DM, Quinti I, et al: Recurrent sinopulmonary infection and impaired antibody response to bacterial capsular polysaccharide antigen in children with selective IgG-subclass deficiency. N Engl J Med 313:1247, 1985

van Alphen L, van den Berghe N, van den Broek LG: Interaction of *Haemophilus influenzae* with human erythrocytes and oropharyngeal epithelial cells is mediated by a common fimbrial epitope. Infect Immun 56:1800, 1988

Ward J, Brenneman G, Letson GW, et al: Limited efficacy of a *Haemophilus influenzae* type b conjugate vaccine in Alaska native infants. N Engl J Med 323:1393, 1990

Ward JI, Margolis H, Lum M, et al: *Haemophilus influenzae* disease in Alaskan Eskimos: Characteristics of a population with an unusual incidence of invasive disease. Lancet 1:1281, 1981

Weiser JN, Love JM, Moxon ER: The molecular mechanism of phase variation of *H. influenzae* lipopolysaccharide. Cell 59:657, 1989

Weiser JN, Williams A, Moxon ER: Phase-variable lipopolysaccharide structures enhance the invasive capacity of *Haemophilus influenzae.* Infect Immun 58:3455, 1990

Wenger JD, Hightower AW, Facklam RR, et al: Bacterial meningitis in the United States, 1986: Report of a multistate surveillance study. J Infect Dis 162:1316, 1990

Winkelstein JA, Moxon ER: Role of complement in the host's defense against *Haemophilus influenzae*. In Sell SH, Wright PF (eds): *Haemophilus influenzae*. Epidemiology, Immunity and Prevention of Disease. New York, Elsevier Biomedical, 1982, p 135

Zamenhof S, Leidy G, Fitzgerald PL, et al: Polyribosephosphate, the type-specific substance of *Haemophilus influenzae* type b. J Biol Chem 203:695, 1953

Zwahlen A, Rubin LG, Connelly CJ, et al: Alteration of the cell wall of *Haemophilus influenzae* type b by transformation with cloned DNA; association with attenuated virulence. J Infect Dis 152:485, 1985

CHAPTER 28

Bordetella

The clinical syndrome of whooping cough or pertussis has been traced to a classic description given in the latter part of the sixteenth century. Paroxysmal coughing has been the hallmark of this acute bacterial infection of the respiratory tract. The severity of the illness prompted early investigative work, and the causative organism, *Bordetella pertussis,* was first isolated in 1906 by Bordet and Gengou. Subsequently, occasional instances of similar illness were attributed to *Bordetella parapertussis* and rarely to *Bordetella bronchiseptica.* In the United States, widespread use of standardized vaccine has resulted in a dramatic decline in the incidence of the disease and its attendant morbidity and mortality. As pertussis became rare, investigative interest in the organism and in the pathogenesis of clinical disease declined concomitantly. A resurgence of laboratory research and renewed interest in the development of less reactogenic vaccine for immunization has occurred with the technologic advances of the past decade.

Morphology

The three species of the genus *Bordetella* are *B. pertussis, B. parapertussis,* and *B. bronchiseptica.* The close genetic relationship, similar physiology, and comparable antigenic and isozyme properties place these organisms in one genus. The bacteria are small, gram-negative coccobacilli measuring 0.2 to 0.3 μm by 0.5 to 1.0 μm; they appear singly, in pairs, and in small clusters. On primary isolation, cells are uniform in size, but in subcultures they become quite pleomorphic and filamentous, and thick bacillary forms are common. Bipolar metachromatic staining may be demonstrated with toluidine blue. The only motile species of the genus is *B. bronchiseptica,* which possesses lateral flagella. Capsules are produced but can be demonstrated only by special stains and not by capsular swelling.

Physiology

Bordetellae are highly communicable, obligatory parasites of man and animals. They multiply among cilia of epithelial cells. Man is the only natural host of *B. pertussis* and *B. parapertussis,* whereas *B. bronchiseptica* is mainly a pathogen of animals. *Bordetella* organisms are strict aerobes with a respiratory metabolism. They do not produce hydrogen sulfide, indole, or acetylmethylcarbinol. *Bordetella* organisms have no specific growth requirement for hemin (X factor) and coenzyme I (V factor).

Cultural Characteristics. Modified Bordet-Gengou medium (potato-glycerol-blood agar) and charcoal oxoid medium with horse blood (Regan-Lowe) have been recommended for primary isolation of phase I *B. pertussis* to neutralize the growth-inhibiting and toxin-suppression effects of such substances as peptone, unsaturated fatty acids, colloidal sulfur, sulfides, or peroxides. A synthetic medium, modified Stainer-Scholte agar supplemented with cyclodextrin and cephalexin, has been used as a selective medium and has the advantage of a longer shelf-life, which facilitates the direct plating of organisms. Colonies of *B. pertussis* are pinpoint in size, smooth, convex, glistening, almost transparent, and pearl-like in appearance. All three species produce a zone of hemolysis that varies with cultural conditions.

Variation. *B. pertussis* freshly isolated from patients in the catarrhal stage of pertussis are smooth colony–forming organisms (phase I or X mode) and fully virulent. Serial mutational changes occur with passage on culture media, such as blood or chocolate agar. These mutations result in irreversible transition through intermediate forms (phases II and III) to the avirulent rough colony–producing form (phase IV). In the avirulent phase IV mutant, there is a loss of the production of pertussis toxin, adenylate cyclase, hemolysin, dermonecrotic toxin, filamentous hemagglutinin, agglutinogens, cytochrome d-G29 and changes in cell envelope profile.

A second type of variation, antigenic modulation, is phenotypic and involves a change in phenotype of the organism that occurs in almost all members of a population of *B. pertussis* as a result of environmental conditions. Media containing a high level of magnesium sulfate or culture at 25C can induce this reversible modulation. Phenotypically, these organisms are similar to the avirulent phase IV organisms and lack the properties enumerated above that are correlated with virulence for animals. The mechanism is unknown.

Antigenic Structure

The single heat-stable surface O antigen common to smooth strains of *B. pertussis, B. parapertussis,* and *B. bronchiseptica* and to rough strains of *B. pertussis* and *B. bronchiseptica* is a protein easily extracted from cells. It is found in the supernatant fluids of cell cultures but does not confer protection against infection.

Surface antigens called agglutinogens have been classified according to the heat-labile (120C) or capsular antigens of Kauffmann. The serotype is often indicated by numbers (e.g., *B. pertussis* 1.2.4). The existence of 14 K antigens, designated as factors, has been demonstrated on the basis of agglutinin adsorption tests. This scheme explains most of the observed serologic relationships. Factors 1 through 6 are found only in strains of *B. pertussis.* Factor 7 is common to all strains of the three species of *Bordetella* organisms. Factor 14 is specific for *B. parapertussis* and factor 12 is specific for *B. bronchiseptica.* The serotypes per se of *B. pertussis* are not significant determinants of the severity of disease or of protection against infection. Factor 1 antigen is present in all strains of *B. pertussis* and is probably the agglutinating antigen (agglutinogen) of the organism. Isolated agglutinogen is nontoxic but does not protect animals against *B. pertussis* infection. Agglutinins or antibodies to agglutinogen are a measurable response in persons immunized with whole-cell vaccine or some of the acellular vaccines and in those sustaining natural infection. These antibodies are not themselves completely protective.

Other antigenic components of *Bordetella* organisms that are probably responsible for inducing the protective antibody response are discussed in the following section.

Determinants of Pathogenicity

B. pertussis is a pathogenic organism with unique properties. The antigenicity and multiple biologic activities of the bacterium have long been recognized, but only within the last decade has whooping cough been recognized as a toxin-mediated disease. Pertussis toxin (TOX) affects host cells by ADP-ribosylating the alpha subunits of susceptible G proteins. This uncouples the proteins from their receptors and blocks signal transduction. The G proteins are involved in a variety of regulatory pathways. Other antigens, including the fimbrial hemagglutinin, hemolysin, and extracellular adenylate cyclase, are probably also involved in disease production, or immunity, or both. Expression of the majority of the known virulence factors is regulated coordinately.

Pertussis Toxin: Histamine-sensitizing Factor, Lymphocytosis-promoting Factor, and Islet-activating Protein. The histamine-sensitizing factor (HSF) has been known for years, but only with the purification of a single protein from the *B. pertussis* envelope has it become clear that this one protein with a molecular weight of approximately 73 to 77 kDa is also the lymphocytosis-promoting factor (LPF) and the islet-activating protein (IAP). Other *Bordetella* species have toxin gene sequences, but they are not expressed. The protein diffuses into the culture medium and, when treated with formaldehyde, loses its biologic activity but not its antigenicity. The homogeneous protein is thermostable, and its molecular structure and mode of catalytic activity are compatible with the A-B model of toxins.

The protein is a hexamer with subunits 1 to 5 designated by molecular weight from largest to smallest. All five subunits are coded by closely linked cistrons in a region of the genome. The A or "active" protomer is the S-1 subunit. The B or "binding" oligomer contains two dimers (S-2 + S-4) and (S-3 + S-4) and a connecting subunit S-5. The toxin binds to cells, and the A protomer then reaches its enzymatic site of action inside the cell. This peptide is an ADP-ribosyl transferase and its substrate is G_i, a regulatory protein involved in GTP-dependent receptor-mediated inhibition of cellular adenylate cyclase in eucaryotic cells. Since the inhibitory control is removed, basilar cAMP is increased and the cell's response to stimulatory ligands is exaggerated with increased cAMP production and cAMP-dependent processes. For example, the production of insulin in response to glucose is increased; experimentally the effect has been shown to persist for more than 1 month.

The striking lymphocytosis observed in association with clinical pertussis has been duplicated in the mouse with pertussis toxin (HSF-LPF-IAP). It has been proposed that lymphocyte migration from small vessels is hindered by the adsorption of the protein onto lymphocyte surfaces. The adherence to postcapillary venules with entrapment of lymphocytes in the vascular and lymphatic compartments creates the lymphocytosis. Also, LPF is known to be a polyclonal activator of human T lymphocytes. It is a potent T cell mitogen in vitro at concentrations in excess of those that produce lymphocytosis in vivo. The significance in human infection of the mitogenicity of LPF is unknown.

Mice given *B. pertussis* develop lethal sensitivity to histamine. Such variables as dose, route of administration, and genetic strain of mice influence the response. This is associated with greatly increased vascular permeability. Specific antiserum can prevent or block all three of these biologic activities. Clinical and experimental data demonstrate that after toxin binds to the cell the biologic activities are no longer affected by antiserum. Antibody to toxin can protect mice against lethal challenge with *B. pertussis* intranasally, intraperitoneally, and intracerebrally. Because of the toxicity of this protein, its use as an immunogen requires conversion to toxoid. Many of the nonrespiratory tract symptoms of *B. pertussis* infection will undoubtedly be found to be attributable to this toxin, and it is reasonable to predict that circulating antibody will be shown to neutralize toxin or inhibit the attachment to cells in humans, as in the animal model.

Hemagglutinins. *B. pertussis* has two hemagglutinins that mediate adherence of these bacteria to mammalian respiratory cilia. One of these is a filamentous protein with an estimated molecular weight of 130,000. This hemagglutinin (FHA) is a surface-associated and secreted protein on the surface of the organism. The structural gene is adjacent to the *vir* locus. FHA is the dominant adhesin for the organisms' adherence to cilia of respiratory epithelial cells and, therefore, presumably to ependymal cells in the mouse and to erythrocytes. Either FHA or TOX is sufficient for binding to macrophages. The FHA has an RGD (arginine glycine aspartic acid) site, which interacts with CR3 of macrophages. Antibody to FHA protects mice against lethal aerosol challenge with *B. pertussis.* Antibody directed against FHA should help to provide protection against infection by altering the adherence of these bacteria to respiratory epithelial cells. Although local or respiratory tract antibody should be more important in providing this protection than humoral antibody, infant mice receiving only passive humoral antibody have been protected from subsequent intranasal challenge.

The second hemagglutinin, pertussis toxin-hemagglutinin (TOX-HA), is a round molecule with one twentieth of the hemagglutinating activity of the FHA. There is no recognized role in clinical disease for the hemagglutinating properties of this protein. This hemagglutinin adheres to sialic acid–containing receptors and is expressed only by phase I organisms. The hemagglutinin portion of the molecule may therefore be important in the adherence of toxin to cells. Antibody to TOX decreases colonization by the organism. Sialoproteins, including haptoglobin and ceruloplasmin, can compete for the toxin HA, thereby inhibiting attachment to cell receptors in the respiratory tract. Recent study has shown that these two hemagglutinins or adhesins can enhance the adherence of other respiratory pathogens such as *Haemophilus influenzae* or *Streptococcus pneumoniae.* This potential "piracy of adhesins" by other organisms may contribute to secondary bacterial invasion in pertussis.

Adenylate Cyclase. There are at least two adenylate cyclase (AC) complexes stimulated by intracellular calmodulin in *B. pertussis.* One is intracellular, heat stable at 100C, and found only in *B. pertussis.* The second is extracytoplasmic, soluble, labile at 56C, and produced by phase I *B. pertussis, B. parapertussis,* and *B. bronchiseptica.* The species-common adenylate cyclase may be involved in activation of heat-labile toxin (HLT). This enzyme is an exotoxin with a molecular weight of about 70.6 kDa. It gains entry into eucaryotic cells, where it is activated by calmodulin to produce cAMP from host cell ATP. AC is obligatory for virulence in animals. The AC toxin is a hemolysin that produces pores in red blood cell membranes. However, the hemolysis and the enzymatic activity of the molecule are independent functions. In vitro, AC can alter chemotaxis and inhibit the oxidative burst of polymorphonuclear neutrophils (PMNs). The role of this protein in disease has not been clearly defined.

Heat-labile Toxin or Dermonecrotic Toxin. The heat-labile toxin (HLT) produced by all species of *Bordetella* appears to be a cytoplasmic protein that occurs in bacteria in precursor form, requiring activation to induce toxicity. Released by lysis of phase I cells, HLT is destroyed when heated to 56C for 15 minutes. It is dermonecrotic and, when given intraperitoneally or intravenously, is lethal for mice. It is a poor antigen unless converted to toxoid by formaldehyde treatment of lysed cells but not intact cells. Toxoid-stimulated antibody does not protect mice against intracerebral challenge or children against infection. HLT is not known to stimulate antibody production in humans, and its role in the pathogenesis of human illness is unknown.

Lipopolysaccharide (Heat-stable Toxin). The lipopolysaccharide (LPS) or endotoxin of the cell wall is heat stable and basically similar to the endotoxins of Enterobacteriaceae except for differences in macromolecular structure and in a lower pyrogenic activity. It consists of two different polysaccharides, each terminated by a molecule of 3-deoxy-2-octulosonic acid. Two distinct lipid fragments, lipid A and lipid X, are present and contain glucosamine, fatty acids, and esterified phosphate in similar proportions. Lipid X, which is the minor lipid, has 2-methyl, 3-hydroxydecanoic, and tetradecanoic acids, which are absent from lipid A. Lipid X appears to be responsible for the acute toxicity of this endotoxin. The LPS does not induce the formation of antibodies with protective activity.

Antibody to LPS in the presence of complement determines the bactericidal activity of serum against *B. pertussis.* Bactericidal activity, however, is not correlated with protection against intracerebral challenge of mice with *B. pertussis* or with protection of children vaccinated against disease.

Tracheal Cytotoxin. The tracheal cytotoxin (TCT) molecule is a monomeric fragment of peptidoglycan with a molecular weight of 921 daltons. TCT is a specific product released into the culture supernatant by growing organisms. This toxic component damages ciliated cells and inhibits nonciliated cell differentiation, thus possibly hindering repair of the mucosa and prolonging the effects of destroyed mucociliary clearance. The sugars in the molecule are not important for the activity of this molecule, suggesting receptors that are different from those for other muramyl peptides. TCT competitively inhibits the binding of 5-hydroxytryptamine (5 HT) on respiratory epithelial cells. Interference with the effects of 5 HT is perhaps important for TCT toxicity.

69 kDa Outer Membrane Protein (Pertactin). Pertactin, which has been identified in some vaccines, may contribute to adherence of the organism. Measurable antibodies to this protein may be detected in patients convalescing from illness and in recipients of whole-cell vaccine. This protein provides protection against intranasal challenge with *B. pertussis* in mice, but in this model it is not additive with PT or with PT plus FHA. In this same model PT and FHA confer almost complete protection. In the intracerebral mouse model challenge, however, the 69 kDa protein increases the protection induced by PT and FHA to a level equal to that of the whole-cell vaccine.

Experimental In Vitro and In Vivo Models. Some of the most useful current data regarding the pathogenesis of *B. pertussis* infection comes from ultrastructural analysis of an in vitro model consisting of hamster tracheal organ culture. Phase I organisms, but not phase IV organisms, selectively

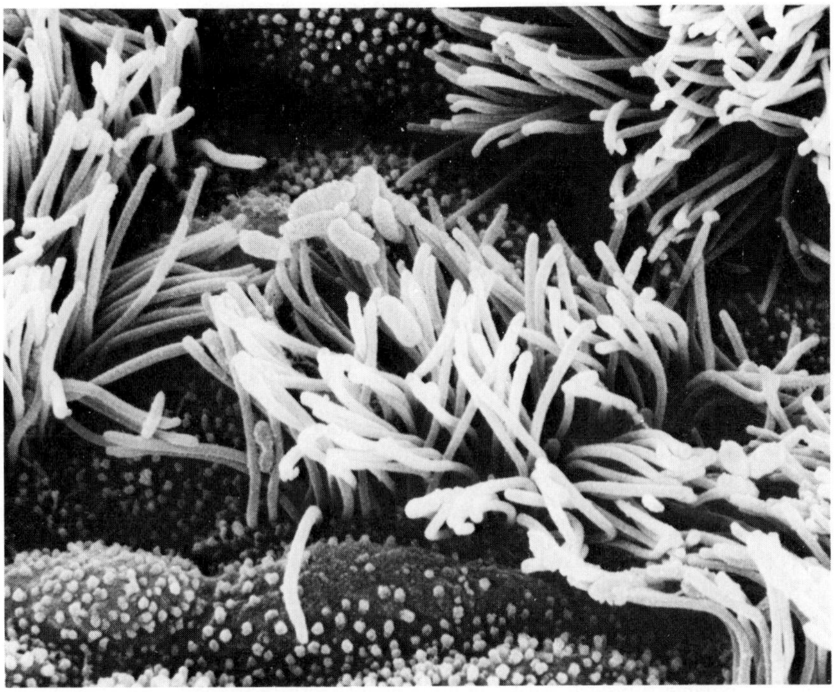

Fig. 28–1. Scanning electron micrograph of *Bordetella pertussis*–infected hamster tracheal organ culture. Unciliated cells covered with microvilli are adjacent to parasitized ciliated cells. Rod-shaped bacteria are attached to the cilia. × 6000. (*Courtesy of Dr. Kenneth E. Muse.*)

adhere to the ciliated epithelial cells (Fig. 28–1). Bacterial attachment is essential for production of diminished ciliary activity, which is the first demonstrable effect of *B. pertussis* infection. The ciliated cells are then extruded from the epithelial surface, with subsequent necrosis. The fimbrial hemagglutinin and pertussis toxin are implicated in the attachment of organisms to the ciliated cells. The subsequent cell damage is not a result of cell invasion by *B. pertussis* and may be attributed to exotoxin(s) release and adherence to cells.

Mice provide an in vivo model that allows study of the host response to infection. Pathologically, experimental *B. pertussis* respiratory infection in mice is similar to that of infants, as is the duration of excretion of bacteria, the lymphocytosis, and the higher mortality in infant mice. Moreover, the interval from infection to the onset of histamine sensitization and the persistence of sensitization parallel the catarrhal and paroxysmal stages in the child. Mice that recover from respiratory infection are then resistant to intracerebral challenge. Intracerebral challenge with *B. pertussis* induces a fatal infection. Organisms multiply among ciliated ependymal cells and not in parenchyma. Antibodies that protect against intracerebral challenge are induced by PT. This assay best correlates with protection induced by vaccine. Sera obtained from mice or infants more than 4 weeks after onset of illness can provide protection to the homologous species.

Clinical Infection

Epidemiology

Several features of the epidemiology of pertussis have intrigued students of this disease for a number of years. Pertussis usually has not been a disease with marked seasonal variation. The disease is worldwide in its distribution. The number of reported cases in the United States declined from approximately 120,000 in 1950 to 1730 in 1980 (Fig. 28–2), but it has been increasing, with 4157 cases reported in 1989. Reported deaths declined from approximately 1100 in 1950 to 12 in 1970. The case rate is highest and most deaths occur in infants under 1 year of age (Fig. 28–3). In 1984, 73% of infants less than 1 year of age with the disease were hospitalized; 3% had at least one seizure, and 1% died.

The illness is highly communicable, as evidenced by attack rates of 90% in unimmunized household contacts of persons with pertussis. Humans are the only known source of *B. pertussis*, and excretion of organisms is limited almost entirely to persons with active infection. However, immunization seems to have altered the epidemiologic pattern. In recent epidemics, persons with modification or absence of clinical illness have been shown to excrete *B. pertussis*. These persons are thought to be partially immune as a result of prior immunization. Adults and older children are infected and introduce the organism into a household. Prolonged presence of organisms during convalescence is extremely rare.

Pathogenesis

After inhalation of infected droplets, the organisms colonize the respiratory tract. The specificity of attachment of *B. pertussis* to ciliated respiratory epithelial cells is attributable to the F-HA, to PT, and to the 69 kDa protein. Such adherence is essential for production of disease, as specific antibody can prevent damage to ciliated cells in vitro or prevent disease in an animal model. Development of local antibody against the F-HA has been shown to occur after natural infection in children. Also, parenteral administration of F-HA induces systemic anti-F-HA antibodies that can protect mice against disease after lethal aerosol challenge. The organisms evade nonspecific host defenses. It is presumed that the incubation period and the initial mild symptoms of rhinitis, cough, sneezing, and sometimes conjunctivitis are caused by local

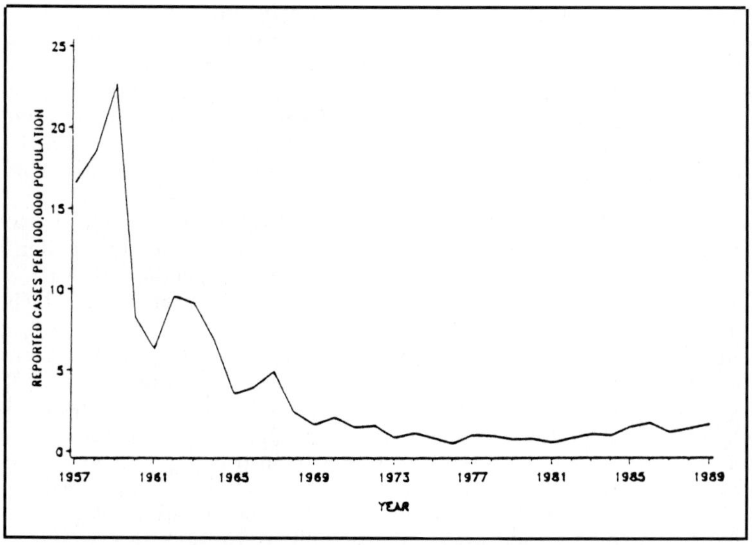

Fig. 28–2. Pertussis (whooping cough) rates by year. United States, 1957–1989. (*From the Centers for Disease Control: MMWR 38(54):33, 1990.*)

multiplication of the organisms in the respiratory tract. Diminished ciliary activity, as observed in vitro, would lead to poorer clearance of bacteria and secretions, resulting in their accumulation in the respiratory tract. Multiplication of organisms and local toxin production would be facilitated. The toxins would then contribute to necrosis and sloughing of ciliated cells. It is also tempting to speculate that the lack of bacteremia and invasion of other tissues by *B. pertussis* is related to the lack of receptors for the organism on other cell types. Bacterial multiplication in other tissues does not occur. The systemic manifestations of disease are probably due to severe respiratory compromise and to circulating pertussis toxin, with another contributing virulence factor being adenylate cyclase. The paroxysmal coughing, the central nervous system manifestations, and even the rarely observed hypoglycemia, as well as the leukocytosis and lymphocytosis, may be attributable to the effects of pertussis exotoxin. Bacteria are less readily detectable in the respiratory tract during the paroxysmal stage of the disease; the persistence of cough and lymphocytosis would thus result from the fixation of toxin to cells. Experimentally, the leukocytosis is clearly reproduced by purified toxin. It is conceptually easy to attribute the multiple systemic manifestations of disease to circulating exotoxin with an array of defined biologic activities. Antibody to the toxin prevents the lymphocytosis and also provides protection against disease in the mouse. It is thus highly likely that whooping cough results from local bacterial colonization of the respiratory tract and subsequent systemic circulation of bacterial exotoxin. The enzymatic mechanism(s) of the toxin has been delineated, but the specific target cells for induction of paroxysmal coughing are unknown.

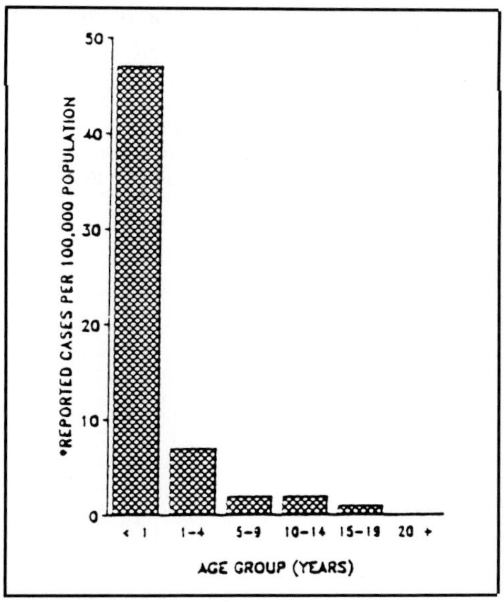

Fig. 28–3. Pertussis (whooping cough) rates by age group. United States, 1989. (*From the Centers for Disease Control: MMWR 38(54):33, 1990.*)

Clinical Manifestations

The clinical syndrome of pertussis is readily defined in the presence of the paroxysmal cough and associated whoop, but the illness is of variable severity, and the milder respiratory syndromes caused by *B. pertussis* are impossible to distinguish on clinical grounds alone. As many as 20% of pertussis infections have been estimated to be atypical illnesses, and those patients are infectious to others.

Following inhalation of infected droplets, the organisms colonize the respiratory tract. Symptoms almost always begin within 10 days after exposure to pertussis, although the incubation period can vary from 5 to 21 days. The clinical illness is divided into three separate stages for descriptive purposes. The catarrhal or prodromal stage lasts from 1 to 2 weeks. During this period, the child exhibits only mild symptoms of an uncomplicated upper respiratory infection. Physical examination does not reveal any serious objective findings.

The second stage usually lasts from 1 to 6 weeks and is characterized by progression to a paroxysmal cough. A characteristic paroxysm is one in which 5 to 20 forcible hacking coughs are produced in 15 to 20 seconds, often terminating with production of mucus or associated vomiting. There is no time for breathing between coughs, and the paroxysm may be sufficiently prolonged to induce anoxia. The final inspiratory breath takes place through the narrowed glottis and produces the characteristic whoop. These early stages of illness are frequently associated with leukocytosis of 12,000 to 200,000/mm^3 and a lymphocytosis of 60%.

The third stage of illness is that of convalescence. Coughing may persist for several months after the initial onset of illness. An understanding of the pathogenesis of the cough is of potential therapeutic importance, as the clinical course of the disease and the morbidity are not appreciably altered by administration of specific antimicrobial agents.

The morbidity and mortality associated with the disease have resulted primarily from compromise of the central nervous system during the acute illness and from secondary bacterial infection, usually involving the ears, sinuses, or lower respiratory tract. The neuropathology of infants dying of pertussis with central nervous system involvement is nonspecific and indistinguishable from changes produced by anoxia. Central nervous system compromise is clearly not a result of actual invasion by *B. pertussis.*

Laboratory Diagnosis

Culture. Definitive diagnosis depends on isolation of *B. pertussis* (or, less commonly, *B. parapertussis* or *B. bronchiseptica*) from the patient. The isolation rate of the organism from the respiratory tract is greatest during the catarrhal stage, as organisms are not usually detectable for longer than the first 4 weeks of illness. The appropriate specimen for cultivation from patients is a nasopharyngeal swab (calcium alginate).

Isolation of *B. pertussis* from clinical specimens is dependent on careful transport and efficient processing of the materials obtained for culture. If the specimen will not be cultured for 1 to 2 hours, the swab should be placed in 0.25 to 0.50 mL of casamino acid solution with a pH of 7.2 to prevent drying of the swab. When the specimen is shipped to another laboratory, or if the holding time exceeds 2 hours, other organisms may overgrow *B. pertussis.* Swabs should therefore be placed in a selective enrichment medium. Regan-Lowe, a half-strength charcoal agar medium with horse blood and cephalexin, is better able to maintain the viability of organisms and to support growth under conditions of transport. There is a decreased recovery rate of *B. pertussis* from transport media as compared with direct inoculation. Modified Stainer-Scholte agar supplemented with cyclodextrin and cephalexin is the preferred medium for primary isolation of organisms.

In addition to the biochemical reactions listed in Table 28–1, serologic identification of *B. pertussis* confirms its identity. A slide agglutination test can be performed with a standard inoculum of organisms and specific antiserum, which is available commercially.

New approaches are also being investigated for their diagnostic utility in the identification of *B. pertussis* in clinical specimens. Radionucleotide-labeled probes (single-stranded DNA or RNA sequences) for hybridization with complementary nucleic acid sequences are currently being evaluated. The sensitivity for detection of LPF is less than that for the detection of the organism by culture. The detection of adenylate cyclase by this method would be especially useful since this protein is a specific product of *B. pertussis.*

Direct Microscopic Examination. Fluorescent antibody (FA) staining has been used for the identification of *B. pertussis* in direct smears from nasopharyngeal swabs and for identification of organisms growing on plates. The FA examination of nasopharyngeal swab material, however, is less sensitive than culture, even in experienced hands. Although the FA procedure cannot substitute for the isolation of the organism by culture, it can offer the advantage of more rapid laboratory identification of organisms after isolation.

Serologic Tests. A specific and reliable assessment of the humoral response to *B. pertussis* infection or immunization has been developed but is not widely available. The agglutination test, which has been used by some laboratories in the past, is not adequate because agglutinin titers do not necessarily correlate with the immune status, and a rise in titer does not occur until too late in the infection to be of diagnostic value.

TABLE 28–1. DIFFERENTIAL CHARACTERISTICS OF SPECIES OF GENUS *BORDETELLA*

	B. pertussis	*B. parapertussis*	*B. bronchiseptica*
Motility	−	−	+
Growth on MacConkey agar	−	+	+
Growth on peptone agar			
Phase I	−	+	+
Phase IV	+	+	+
Browning	−	+	−
Growth on Bordet-Gengou agar			
1–2 days	−	+	+
3–6 days	+	−	−
Reduces nitrate	−	−	+[a]
Utilizes citrate	−	+	+
Produces urease	−	+	+[b]
Oxidase	+	−	+
Mol % G + C content of DNA (T_m)	67–70	66–70	68.9

From Krieg and Holt (eds): Bergey's Manual of Systematic Bacteriology, vol 1. 1984, p 392.

[a] Exceptions occur in conventional nitrate test medium, but test reactions are regularly positive when medium is supplemented with NAD and serum.

[b] Positive within 4 hours.

New assay techniques measure antibody to pertussis toxin (LPF) and the fimbrial hemagglutinin (FHA) that develop after immunization or natural disease. Appropriately timed paired sera are usually not available, and one serum is submitted. Enzyme-linked immunosorbent assays (ELISA) measuring IgG and IgA antibodies to FHA and LPF are standardized and can be used for diagnosis. More than 90% of infected persons produce IgG-LPF antibodies, and 80% to 90% produce IgG-FHA antibodies; 50% to 60% produce IgA-FHA, and 40% to 50% produce IgA-TOX antibodies. Infants may respond more slowly with IgA. A method for detection of specific IgA antibodies to FHA and LPF in respiratory secretions has demonstrated that IgA is formed in response to infection but only minimally in response to immunization. An assay for serum antibody neutralization of the cytopathic effects of pertussis toxin on Chinese hamster ovary cells also provides evidence of infection or immunization.

Treatment

Erythromycin is currently the drug of choice for treatment of pertussis infection. The organism is sensitive to this drug in vitro, and administration eliminates the organism from the nasopharynx in 3 to 4 days, thereby shortening the period of communicability. There is some evidence that if erythromycin is administered early during the catarrhal stage, the paroxysmal manifestations may be shortened. Tetracycline, chloramphenicol, or possibly trimethoprim-sulfamethoxazole are considered adequate alternative antimicrobial agents. Secondary bacterial infection may necessitate additional therapy directed at the responsible pathogen. Supportive measures, such as careful suction to remove tenacious secretions, hydration, nutrition, and electrolyte balance, are of great importance. Oxygen therapy with increased humidity appears to be beneficial.

Prevention

Children under 4 years of age who have been previously immunized against pertussis should receive a booster dose of vaccine after coming in contact with an infected person. They should also receive erythromycin, since immunity conferred by vaccine is not absolute. Treatment may also curtail spread of infection from immunized persons who may harbor organisms but have no symptoms. Unimmunized contacts should receive chemoprophylaxis with erythromycin for approximately 10 days after contact with the patient has ceased. The best protective measures in early infancy are adequate immunization and avoidance of contact with pertussis.

Active Immunization. Protection of the young infant against pertussis is important because the greatest number of severe complications and the highest morbidity occur in this age group. Passive protection is not afforded by the quantity of antibody that traverses the placenta. Routine primary immunization is begun at about 2 months of age unless pertussis is prevalent in the community, in which case immunization should begin earlier. A total of 12 protective units of whole-cell pertussis vaccine is recommended; this is divided into three equal doses given at 4- to 8-week intervals. The vaccine is usually given in a combined preparation containing absorbed diphtheria and tetanus toxoids and pertussis vaccine (DPT). These are depot antigens and appear to be more immunogenic and less reactive than a similar plain antigen product without adjuvant. A booster injection is given 12 to 18 months after primary immunization or before the child enters school.

Immunization has been successful in the prevention of disease, and widespread use of vaccine has been associated with the continued decline of reported cases of pertussis in countries in which immunization is mandatory.

Additional evidence of vaccine efficacy has unfortunately accrued as a result of diminished immunization in several countries, including Denmark, the United Kingdom, and Japan. In Denmark an upswing in the number of cases from a few hundred to thousands per year has occurred within several years after alterations in immunization requirements, including the use of smaller quantities of antigen. In the United Kingdom, diminished public acceptance of immunization since 1974 has resulted in pertussis reaching epidemic proportions, beginning in 1977. It is estimated that vaccine acceptance has declined from a rate of 70% to 80% before 1974 to less than 40% in 1982. The resulting epidemic occurred in younger children who had not received pertussis vaccine. The epidemic in 1982 was the largest since 1957, with 47,508 cases reported from January to September. Studies during these epidemics suggest that current vaccine is 90% effective in the prevention of pertussis.

The effectiveness of the vaccine in young children temporarily discouraged the development of purified immunogens. Increased concern with the reputed reactogenicity of the formalinized whole-organism vaccine revived studies of the organism and the pathogenesis of infection. The factors that produce toxicity or contribute to postvaccination encephalopathy have not been defined, and thus it is impossible to test vaccines for this activity. To date, the mouse weight-gain test has been employed in the United States as the most accurate animal assessment of potential toxicity of vaccine for humans. More important, the definition of FHA, pertussis toxin, and adenylate cyclase, the 69 kDa outer membrane protein, and agglutinins has greatly advanced understanding of the antigens of *B. pertussis* necessary to induce protection. Recent work has demonstrated that the formaldehyde treatment of LPF diminishes its antigenicity, and early studies of an LPF produced by genetic mutation show promise of improved antigenicity.

Studies conducted in Japan indicate that partially purified vaccines containing primarily FHA and pertussis toxin produce fewer local effects and less fever in children. Efficacy data on vaccinees who have had household contact with *B. pertussis* suggest that the more purified vaccine does provide protection. A randomized placebo-controlled trial of two acellular (FHA and LPF or LPF) vaccines was performed in Sweden. The vaccines were efficacious but without direct comparison to whole-cell vaccine. It is unclear whether the efficacy is as good as current whole-cell vaccine. These acellular vaccines will be available for administration as booster doses to children in the United States.

Persistent neurologic damage associated with vaccine administration was estimated to occur at a rate of one in 310,000 immunizations (95% confidence limits = 1 in 5,310,000 to 1 in 54,000) on the basis of a preliminary analysis of the national childhood encephalopathy study in the United Kingdom. A subsequent review with longer follow-up of the children has failed to show any permanent neurologic sequelae attributable to vaccine. The estimated incidence of central nervous system complications of natural disease has ranged from 1.5% to 14% in hospitalized patients. One third of these patients recover;

one third have varying neurologic sequelae; and one third die or have severe deficits. The morbidity of prolonged illness and the necessity for hospitalization with natural disease make it clear that the theoretical risks of immunization are far less than the documented risks associated with the natural disease.

FURTHER READING

Manclark CR (ed): Proceedings of the sixth international symposium on pertussis. DHHS Public No. (FDA) 90-1164,408. Bethesda, Md., Department of HHS, USPHS, 1990

Pittman M: Pertussis toxin: The cause of the harmful effects and prolonged immunity of whooping cough. A hypothesis. Rev Infect Dis 1:401, 1979

Pittman M: The concept of pertussis as a toxin mediated disease. Pediatr Infect Dis J 3:467, 1984

Wardlaw AC, Parton R: Bordetella pertussis toxins. Pharmacol Ther 19:1, 1983

Weiss AA, Hewlett EL: Virulence factors of *Bordetella pertussis.* Ann Rev Microbiol 40:661, 1986

REFERENCES

Bass JW: Erythromycin for treatment and prevention of pertussis. Pediatr Infect Dis J 5:154, 1986

Cowell JL, Urisu A, Zhang JM, et al: Filamentous hemagglutinin and fimbriae of *Bordetella pertussis:* Properties and roles in attachment. In Leive L (ed): Microbiology 1986. Washington, DC, American Society for Microbiology, p. 55

Goldman WE, Klapper DG, Baseman JB: Detection, isolation, and analysis of a released *Bordetella* product toxic to cultured tracheal cells. Infect Immun 36:782, 1982

Granstrom M, Granstrom G, Gulinius P, Askelof P: Neutralizing antibodies to pertussis toxin in whooping cough. J Infect Dis 151:646, 1985

Hewlett EC, Weiss AA: Pertussis toxin: Mechanism of action, biological effects and roles in clinical pertussis. In Leive L (ed): Microbiology, 1986. Washington, DC, American Society for Microbiology, p. 75

Masure HR, Shattuck RL, Storm DR: Mechanisms of bacterial pathogenicity that involve production of calmodulin-sensitive adenylate cyclases. Microbiol Rev 51:60, 1987

Pittman M: Neurotoxicity of *Bordetella pertussis.* Neurotoxicology 2:53, 1986

Sato H, Sato Y: *Bordetella pertussis* infection in mice: Correlation of specific antibodies against two antigens, pertussis toxin, and filamentous hemagglutinin with mouse protectivity in an intracerebral or aerosol challenge system. Infect Immun 46:415, 1984

Thomanen E: Adherence of *Bordetella pertussis* to human cilia: Implications for disease prevention and therapy. In Leive L (ed): Microbiology, 1986. Washington, DC, American Society for Microbiology, p. 59

Weiss AA, Myers GA, Crane JK, Hewlett EL. *Bordetella pertussis* adenylate cyclase toxin: Structure and possible function in whooping cough and the pertussis vaccine. In Leive L (ed): Microbiology, 1986, Washington DC, American Society for Microbiology, p. 70

CHAPTER 29

Listeria and Erysipelothrix

Medical Significance. *Listeria monocytogenes* is a facultative intracellular gram-positive bacillus that causes serious infections, mainly in immunocompromised patients and newborn infants. Meningitis and bacteremia are the most frequent manifestations of listeriosis, but the most unique of its many clinical forms is infection of the genital tract of the gravid female and infection of the offspring, either before birth or during delivery (Table 29–1). *Erysipelothrix rhusiopathiae* is the cause of erysipeloid in man, an acute self-limited infection of the skin that occurs primarily in occupational groups that handle animals and animal products.

Although morphologically resembling the corynebacteria, *Listeria* and *Erysipelothrix* are genetically more related to *Lactobacillus,* with which they are currently grouped.

Listeria monocytogenes

Morphology and Physiology

Morphology. *Listeria* are small gram-positive coccobacilli that have a tendency to occur in short chains of three to five organisms. In stained preparations they often assume a typical diphtheroid palisade arrangement, a property that was responsible for their previous incorrect classification with the corynebacteria. *L. monocytogenes* is 0.4 to 0.5 μm by 0.5 to 2.0 μm in size. In cultures incubated for 3 to 6 hours at 37C, the bacillary forms predominate, but thereafter the prevalent form is coccoid. In cultures 3 to 5 days old, long filamentous structures 6 to 20 μm or more in length often occur, especially in rough strains. At temperatures of 20C to 25C, *L. monocytogenes* is actively motile by means of four peritrichous flagella, but at 37C only one polar flagellum is formed. The motility of listeria is useful in their differentiation from *Erysipelothrix* and the corynebacteria.

Cultural Characteristics. The optimum temperature for growth is 37C, but growth occurs over a wide temperature range down to 2.5C. This ability to grow at low temperatures is the basis for the cold-enrichment technique used in the clinical laboratory for the isolation of *Listeria* from specimens containing a mixed flora (p. 484).

Listeria are not fastidious organisms, and they grow well on tryptose agar and sheep blood agar media. On the clear colorless tryptose agar, colonies are translucent and are easily recognized by their characteristic blue-green color when viewed with oblique light. On sheep blood agar, colonies resemble *Streptococcus* colonies and are 0.5 to 1.5 mm in diameter. Strains isolated from pathologic specimens of human or animal origin produce β-hemolysis on blood agar. *L. monocytogenes* produces a very distinct narrow band of hemolysis that distinguishes it from the animal pathogen *Listeria ivanovii,* which produces a much more pronounced zone of hemolysis. In contrast with the β-hemolytic pathogenic isolates of *L. monocytogenes* from clinical infections, isolates of *Listeria innocua* from the feces of healthy humans and animals are nonhemolytic and nonpathogenic.

Metabolism. *L. monocytogenes* is aerobic to microaerophilic, but growth is improved when cultures are incubated under reduced oxygen and a 5% to 10% concentration of CO_2. Catalase is produced, a property that is useful in differentia-

TABLE 29–1. PRIMARY CLINICAL MANIFESTATIONS OF HUMAN LISTERIOSIS

Manifestation[a]	Cases
Meningitis, meningoencephalitis, or encephalitis	496
Septicemia	
Neonates	51
Others	59
Pregnant women	
Prepartum flu-like symptoms	5
Abortion	12
Postpartum, or infected infant	17
Endocarditis	7
Abscess	5
Pneumonia	5
Conjunctivitis	2
Infectious mononucleosis	2
Pharyngitis	2
Cutaneous papules and pustules	1
Persistent headache	1
Fever	2
No disease, routine culture	1
Total cases	641

From Killinger and Schubert: Proceedings of the Third International Symposium on Listeriosis, Bilthoven, The Netherlands, July 13, 1966.
[a] One or more manifestations may be observed in each case.

tion of the organism from streptococci. *L. monocytogenes* ferments a number of sugars with the formation of acid only (Table 29–2). Most strains from clinical material do not ferment mannitol; this property is useful in separating *L. monocytogenes* from the morphologically similar but serologically distinct nonpathogenic species, *Murraya grayi* (*L. grayi* and *L. murrayi*), which do ferment mannitol.

Antigenic Structure

On the basis of their O (somatic) and H (flagellar) antigens, strains of *L. monocytogenes* have been separated into 13 serotypes (serovars). No correlation has been detected between the various serotypes and any particular clinical syndrome or specific host. There is, however, a striking difference in the geographic distribution of the various serotypes and a tendency for shifts in the prevalent serotype. In the United States and Canada, serotype 4b is the predominant strain. At the present time, three strains (1/2a, 1/2b, and 4b) cause at least 90% of all clinical *Listeria* infections throughout the world.

Significant antigenic differences exist between the pathogenic *L. monocytogenes* and the nonpathogenic species *L. grayi* and *L. murrayi,* supporting the proposal that a new genus, *Murraya,* be designated to encompass these nonpathogenic organisms. (Recommendation of the *Listeria* subcommittee of the International Committee on Systematic Bacteriology).

Determinants of Pathogenicity

L. monocytogenes is a facultative intracellular organism that invades and grows in a variety of mammalian cells, including macrophages, epithelial cells, and fibroblasts. The capacity of the organism to enter the cytoplasm of the cell, to grow, and to spread to adjacent cells is essential for the full expression of its pathogenic potential. The morphologic stages observed in the spread of *L. monocytogenes* from cell to cell have been described and are summarized in Fig. 29–1. Subsequent to internalization, the organism escapes from a host vacuole and undergoes rapid division in the cytoplasm of the host cell before becoming encapsulated by short actin filaments. These filaments reorganize into a long tail extending from only one end of the bacterium. The tail mediates movement of the organism through the cytoplasm to the surface of the host cell. At the periphery, protrusions are formed that can then penetrate neighboring cells and allow the bacterium to enter. This method of spread from cell to cell explains the requirement for a cell-mediated immunity. Since the organisms are never extracellular, host humoral antibody would not be effective.

Soluble Products. The virulence of *L. monocytogenes* is multifaceted and is apparently due both to antiphagocytic components that are present at the cell surface of the organism and to soluble products that are excreted during growth. The best characterized of the soluble products is a hemolysin, listeriolysin O, that plays an important role in the pathogenesis of infection. Listeriolysin O belongs to a family of cytolysins whose prototype is streptolysin O and which are produced by various gram-positive species. The hemolysin, which is secreted into the culture medium during growth, is a sulfhydryl-activated antigenic protein. It is sensitive to oxidative inactivation and can be reactivated by reducing agents. Among the cytolysins, however, listeriolysin O is the only one produced by an intracellular bacterium, and the only one active at the

TABLE 29–2. DISTINGUISHING PROPERTIES OF CERTAIN NONSPORING GRAM-POSITIVE RODS

	Listeria monocytogenes	*Erysipelothrix rhusiopathiae*	*Lactobacillus* sp.	*Corynebacterium* sp.
β-Hemolysis	+	–	–	±
Catalase	+	–	–	+
Motility	+	–	–	–
Acid from				
Glucose	+	+	+	±
Mannitol	–	–	±	±
H_2S Production	–	+	–	–
Mol%, G + C	37–39	36–40	32–53	51–60

G + C, Guanosine plus cytosine.

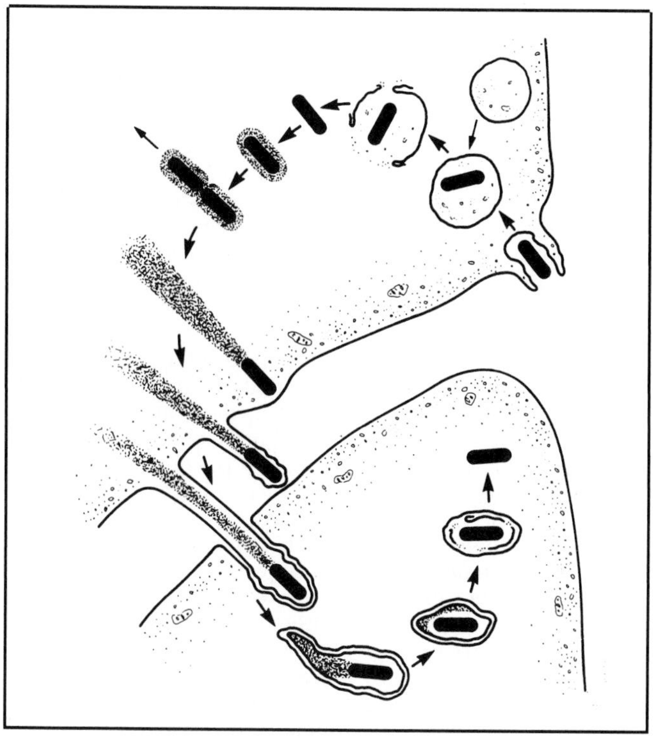

Fig. 29–1. Stages in the entry, growth, movement, and spread of *Listeria* from one macrophage to another. (*From Tilney and Portnoy: J Cell Biol 109:1597, 1989.*)

low pH found within the phagocyte. Listeriolysin O is efficiently produced by virulent strains under heat-shock conditions, and in this respect it resembles the heat-shock proteins produced by a number of other intracellular bacteria. These stress proteins are apparently produced by invasive intracellular bacteria to enable them to cope with the hostile environment within the phagocyte. During listeric infection, *Listeria* hemolysin disrupts membranes, especially those of the phagolysosome, leading to unrestricted growth of the organism within the cytoplasm of the phagocyte. Listeriolysin O has also been shown to contribute to the virulence of the organism by inhibiting macrophage-mediated antigen processing.

A soluble antigen(s) with lipolytic activity is also produced, but the precise nature and role of this substance is unclear. A correlation exists, however, between hemolysin production, lipolytic activity, and virulence.

Surface Components. Several antiphagocytic factors have been described, but only one—an endotoxin-like material—has been well characterized. The chemical, physical, and biologic properties of the purified cell wall component are strikingly similar to those of the classic lipopolysaccharide (LPS) endotoxins of gram-negative bacteria. The listerial LPS is believed to be responsible for the transient cold-agglutinin syndrome observed in some patients with septicemic listerial infections. Antibodies induced in these patients can, under appropriate conditions, react with the host's own erythrocytes, causing a complement-mediated in vivo lysis. The antibodies responsible are of the IgM class and appear to be directed against the blood group I system.

Clinical Infection

Epidemiology. *L. monocytogenes* typically is sporadic in occurrence and is worldwide in its distribution. It has been isolated from humans with disease, from healthy carriers, and from a wide range of other mammals, birds, fish, ticks, and crustacea. There also is a high incidence in plant and soil samples and in animal feces. The basic question of whether *L. monocytogenes* is primarily borne in soil or originates from animals excreting the organisms in their feces has not been resolved. It is currently believed, however, that *L. monocytogenes* is a saprophytic organism that lives in a plant-soil environment and can thus be contracted by humans and animals from many sources.

Although direct transmission has been reported in high-risk occupational groups, such as veterinarians and farm workers, most infections in the United States occur in urban dwellers with no history of direct contact with animals or potentially infected materials. Recent epidemiologic data now implicate food as the most common vehicle for transmission of human listeriosis in both adults and neonates. As many as 20% of cases in the United States are associated with food. Evidence of this has come from several large outbreaks in which several foods were directly implicated. In an outbreak in Canada in 1981 involving 41 cases, indirect transmission from an animal reservoir was documented when the contaminated product, coleslaw, was traced to its source—a cabbage farm with previously documented cases of listeriosis in its sheep herd. Raw vegetables, dairy products, and meats have been directly implicated in separate outbreaks of human infection. In the United States raw hot dogs and undercooked chicken account for most food-associated cases.

The significance of the symptom-free carrier, especially the fecal excretor, as a reservoir of infection is unknown. At least 1% of normal adults excrete *Listeria,* and the percentage is higher in household contacts of infected persons. The only proved example, however, of human-to-human transmission is infection of the fetus transplacentally through the umbilical vein with production of septicemia. Infection may also be acquired during delivery through contact with infective secretions.

The incidence of human listeriosis in the United States appears to be increasing. Some of this apparent increase may be due to greater awareness and improved methods for identification, but some is attributable to the increasing numbers of patients with immunosuppressive disorders that predispose to infectious complications. The age distribution of listeriosis is uneven, with most cases occurring among neonates and the elderly. Between these extremes, it occurs primarily in immunocompromised patients. Renal transplant recipients are now one of the largest groups infected by *Listeria,* approximating in frequency that of malignancy associated with *Listeria* infection.

Pathogenesis. The gastrointestinal tract is probably the major portal of entry for extrauterine *Listeria* infections. Studies in experimental animals demonstrate infection via this route and stress the role of the normal microbial flora in modulating *Listeria* colonization of the gut and subsequent penetration of the intestinal epithelial barrier. Determinants necessary to establish mucosal colonization or to explain the infectivity for humans of a limited number of serotypes have not been defined. Intraluminal bacteria are presumed to gain entrance to the circulatory system when the host's defense is altered, followed by seeding of various sites.

In humans, the usual histologic response is a polymorphonuclear leukocytosis with microabscess formation, although a monocytic reaction may occur. *L. monocytogenes* exhibits a striking tropism for the fetus and placenta of most animals and for the central nervous system of monkeys and humans. Listeriosis of the newborn, contracted intrapartum, usually is localized to the central nervous system. In prepartum infection, *Listeria* organisms from the infected placenta are widely disseminated, resulting in granulomatous foci in many organs, including the liver, spleen, lungs, and central nervous system.

Clinical Manifestations. A wide variety of clinical syndromes is caused by *L. monocytogenes,* ranging from a mild influenza-like illness to fulminant neonatal listeriosis associated with mortality rates of 54% to 90%. In the adult the major infections are meningitis (55%), primary bacteremia (25%), endocarditis (7%), and nonmeningitic central nervous system infection (6%). More than half of these patients have underlying disorders, such as malignancy, alcoholism, cirrhosis, diabetes, or vasculitis, or are receiving immunosuppressive drugs. Relatively few cases of listeriosis, however, have been reported in patients infected with human immunodeficiency virus (HIV) or in patients with acquired immunodeficiency syndrome (AIDS).

NEONATAL INFECTIONS. Genital tract infection in the gravid female with infection of the offspring is the most distinctive of infections caused by *L. monocytogenes.* Usually the mother has no symptomatic illness, or a history of only a benign and self-limited influenza-like illness during the last trimester of pregnancy. Infection in the infant may take one of two forms. The early type, granulomatosis infantiseptica, results from infection in utero and appears within 2 days of birth. Abortion, premature birth, stillbirth, or death within a short period after birth may occur. If the infant is born alive, symptoms of septicemia develop within a few hours, often followed by fetal distress, pneumonia, diarrhea, seizures, and maculopapular skin lesions on the legs and trunk. This form of the disease has a very high mortality rate, which is largely due to the failure to consider the diagnosis in the early stages.

The second or late form of neonatal listeriosis appears after the fifth day of life, with meningitis as the usual presentation. Infection is believed to be acquired either during or after birth rather than in utero. The mother is almost always free of symptoms. About 10% of all cases of neonatal meningitis are due to *L. monocytogenes.*

ADULT INFECTIONS. Meningitis is the most commonly recognized form of listeriosis in the adult, and it is a leading cause of bacterial meningitis in patients with cancer and in renal transplant recipients. About 30% of meningitis patients, however, have no preceding disease. Clinically, meningitis caused by *L. monocytogenes* cannot be distinguished from meningitis caused by other bacteria. The overall mortality rate among patients with meningitis is 30%, but among cancer patients with *Listeria* meningitis the mortality rate is 60%.

Primary *Listeria* bacteremia usually affects patients under 50 years of age. Pregnant persons and those with underlying diseases are particularly prone to this form of the disease. As with other listerial infections, diagnosis depends on laboratory identification of the organism, since there are no specific clinical features. Endocarditis and pneumonia are among the rare focal infections that may result from bloodstream invasion.

Immunity. *L. monocytogenes* is readily phagocytosed by normal macrophages after activation of the alternative complement pathway by cell wall components. In addition to the C3b generated, natural antibody is also believed to contribute to opsonization. Once within the cell, the organism can survive and multiply, their eventual elimination depending on a cell-mediated immune response. Immunity is dependent on macrophage-activating lymphokines produced by the $CD8^+$ T cell subset.

The genetics of resistance to *Listeria* infections has been examined in inbred strains of mice that exhibit differences in responsiveness to infection. The resistance trait is apparently controlled by a single autosomal, dominant non-H-2-linked gene termed *Lr.* The gene is expressed phenotypically in the enhanced response of the mononuclear phagocyte system to infection. In the *Listeria*-resistant host, the *Lr* gene product appears to promote the early arrival of immature macrophages that develop potent antibacterial activity.

As is the case with several other bacteria, *L. monocytogenes* has an array of cell surface components that are capable of interacting in a variety of ways with participants of the immune response. One of the most unique of these is a factor with monocytosis-producing activity. In some animals, monocytosis is a hallmark of listeria infection and the property for which the organism was named. Various cell wall fractions that have been obtained are mitogenic for bone marrow–derived cells, act as an adjuvant, and are immunosuppressive.

No second clinical infections with *Listeria* have been observed in patients or animals cured of proven listeriosis.

Laboratory Diagnosis. The diagnosis of listeriosis is based on the isolation of *L. monocytogenes* from the appropriate clinical materials, depending on the syndrome. The usual materials include blood, cerebrospinal fluid, amniotic fluid, and genital tract secretions. The key to the diagnosis of listeriosis is awareness. Laboratory personnel should be alerted when *Listeria* infection is suspected, as in a setting of diminished host defenses. A frequent error made by the clinical laboratory is to assume that all diphtheroid isolates are contaminants and thus are unimportant. Gram stains should be made of the infected material and examined for the presence of typical pleomorphic gram-positive bacilli. A positive finding is extremely useful, but in 60% of the patients with *Listeria* meningitis, organisms are not seen in a Gram stain of the spinal fluid. Also, the organisms may sometimes be mistaken for streptococci or, when poorly stained, may resemble *Haemophilus influenzae.*

When the organisms are numerous and are not mixed with other bacteria, *Listeria* is not difficult to grow from infected material unless the patient has received antibiotics. A 2% tryptose agar medium is excellent for cultivation and propagation. When the organisms are to be grown from tissues, successful isolation requires homogenization to release the organisms that are incarcerated, often intracellularly in the focal lesions.

If the primary culture fails to reveal *L. monocytogenes* from a suspected *Listeria* infection, the clinical specimen should be held at 4C for several weeks and replated after storage for 6 weeks and 3 months. The combination of the cold-enrichment technique and the use of oblique lighting for the examination of colonies is basic for the isolation of *Listeria* from specimens where the organisms are sparse or are mixed with other bacteria. Accurate identification of an isolate as *L. monocytogenes* is based on the demonstration of β-hemolysis, catalase production, and a tumbling motility at room temperature. Useful procedures for the differentiation of *L. monocytogenes* from diphtheroids and other gram-positive bacilli with which it may be confused are listed in Table 29–2. Cultures identified as *L. monocytogenes* should be sent to the Centers for Disease Control for complete serologic identification.

Although antibodies appear in the serum of patients during and after *Listeria* infections, serologic diagnosis of listeriosis is unreliable because *L. monocytogenes* cross-reacts with a number of other gram-positive organisms, including staphylococci.

Treatment. Penicillin G or ampicillin is the recommended treatment for *Listeria* infections. Erythromycin and the tetracyclines are also effective, but cephalosporins should not be used because of their variable activity and limited penetration of the meninges. For high-risk patients, such as neonates and immunosuppressed patients, administration of either penicillin or ampicillin and an aminoglycoside is recommended as initial therapy. Trimethoprim-sulfamethoxazole appears to be effective in the treatment of patients allergic to penicillin.

Prevention. There is no vaccine for the prevention of listeriosis. Effective control of *Listeria* infections is hampered by difficulties in recognition of human and animal infection. In the newborn infant, listeriosis is preventable by early recognition and prompt treatment of the mother. Prevention should center on elimination of animal reservoirs, and contact with infected animals or animal products should be avoided. Careful attention should be given to the handling of infected infants in a neonatal unit to prevent nosocomial transmission, and patients with immunosuppressive disorders and those receiving immunosuppressive drugs should be protected from contact with cases of listeriosis.

Erysipelothrix rhusiopathiae

Morphology and Physiology. *E. rhusiopathiae* is a nonsporogenous, nonmotile, nonencapsulated gram-positive rod. The organism has a strong tendency to dissociate from the S to the R form, resulting in changes in virulence and antigenic properties. In smears from acute forms of *Erysipelothrix* disease, organisms of the smooth colony form are seen, whereas in chronic cases the rough form occurs. In smooth colonies, the organisms are short, slender, straight, or slightly curved and measure 0.2 to 0.4 μm by 0.5 to 2.5 μm. In rough colonies, long filamentous structures and chains of up to 60 μm or more are present.

When first isolated, *E. rhusiopathiae* is microaerophilic and grows in a band a few millimeters below the surface of a semisolid tube of agar. Heart infusion agar containing rabbit blood and incubation at 37C in the presence of 5% CO_2 is suitable for primary isolation. On blood agar plates, colonies are small, round, and grayish white, somewhat similar to the colonies of *Streptococcus viridans*. They are α-hemolytic, although a slight but definite clearing occurs around the colonies on prolonged incubation. Black colonies are produced on tellurite media. Properties useful in the identification and differentiation of *Erysipelothrix* from *Listeria* and corynebacteria are listed in Table 29–2. The former's resistance to neomycin also provides a useful rapid means of differentiating *E. rhusiopathiae* from *L. monocytogenes.*

Most strains produce hyaluronidase. A correlation has been observed between hyaluronidase production, antigenic structure, and virulence. Several serovars have been described, but most of the virulent strains belong to serogroup A and are good hyaluronidase producers. Neuraminidase also appears to contribute to the pathogenic potential of some strains.

Clinical Infection. *Erysipelothrix* is widely distributed in nature in all parts of the world. Many wild and domestic animals, fish, and birds harbor the organism, usually as a commensal. It occurs in the surface slime of freshwater and saltwater fish and is found in sewage effluent from abbatoirs and in the feces of infected animals. The disease is most common in swine, sometimes occurring in epizootics and causing considerable economic loss. Infections also occur in horses, sheep, cows, and a number of other animals. Man acquires the infection by contact with animals or animal products. The disease is more prevalent in the male, especially abattoir employees, butchers, and those handling fish, animal hides, and bones. Most infections are related to skin injury.

The disease in humans, erysipeloid, is characterized by a nonsuppurative purplish erythematous lesion at the site of inoculation, which is usually on the hand or fingers. The lesions burn and itch, and there is usually pain which often extends to the adjacent joint. Lymphangitis occurs in about 20% of the cases and is sometimes accompanied by constitutional symptoms. Most localized disease runs a self-limited course of approximately 3 weeks. Rarely, *Erysipelothrix* infections may be disseminated, causing infective endocarditis and septic arthritis.

A laboratory diagnosis can be made by culture of the organism from aspirated material or biopsy specimens taken from the margin of the local lesion. Blood cultures are necessary for a diagnosis of endocarditis.

Penicillin is the drug of choice. In patients sensitive to penicillin, erythromycin may be used.

FURTHER READING

Books and Reviews

Armstrong D: *Listeria monocytogenes.* In Mandell GL, Douglas RG Jr, Bennett JE (eds): Principles and Practice of Infectious Diseases, ed 3. New York, Churchill Livingstone, 1990

Bortolussi R: Listeriosis: Systemic infection due to *Listeria monocytogenes.* Clin Invest Med 7:211, 1984

Bortolussi R, Schlech WF III, Albritton WL: In Lennette EH, Balows A, Hausler WJ Jr, Shadomy HJ (eds): Manual of Clinical Microbiology, ed 4. Washington DC, American Society for Microbiology, 1985, chap 19

Dee RR, Lorber B: Brain abscess due to *Listeria monocytogenes:* Case report and literature review. Rev Infect Dis 8:968, 1986

Ewald FW: The genus *Erysipelothrix.* In Starr MP, Stolp H, Truper HG, et al (eds): The Prokaryotes, vol II. New York, Springer-Verlag, 1981, chap 133

Gorby GL, Peacock JE: *Erysipelothrix rhusiopathiae* endocarditis: Microbiologic, epidemiologic and clinical features of an occupational disease. Rev Infect Dis 10:317, 1988

Gray ML, Killinger AH: *Listeria monocytogenes* and listeria infections. Bact Rev 30:309, 1966
Grieco MH, Sheldon C: *Erysipelothrix rhusiopathiae.* Ann NY Acad Sci 174:523, 1970
Hahn H, Kaufmann SHE: The role of cell-mediated immunity in bacterial infections. Rev Infect Dis 3:1221, 1981
Kongshavn PAL: Genetic control of resistance to *Listeria* infection. Curr Top Microbiol Immunol 124:67, 1986
Nieman RE, Lorber B: Listeriosis in adults: A changing pattern. Report of eight cases and review of the literature, 1968–1978. Rev Infect Dis 2:207, 1980
Proceedings of the Third International Symposium of Listeriosis, Bilthoven, The Netherlands. July 13–16, 1966
Seelinger HPR: Listeriosis. New York, Hafner, 1961
Seelinger HPR, Jones D: Genus Listeria. In Sneath PHA, Mair NS, Sharpe ME, Holt JG (eds): Bergey's Manual of Systematic Bacteriology, vol 2. Baltimore, Williams & Wilkins, 1986, pp 1235–1245
Stamm AM, Dismukes WE, Simmons BP, et al: Listeriosis in renal transplant recipients: report of an outbreak and review of 102 cases. Rev Infect Dis 4:665, 1982
Welshimer HJ: The genus *Listeria* and related organisms. In Starr MP, Stolp H, Truper HG, et al (eds): The Prokaryotes, vol II. New York, Springer-Verlag, 1981, chap 132

Selected Papers

Baker LA, Campbell PA: *Listeria monocytogenes* cell walls induce decreased resistance to infection. Infect Immun 20:99, 1978
Baldridge JR, Barry RA, Hinrichs DJ: Expression of systemic protection and delayed-type hypersensitivity to *Listeria monocytogenes* is mediated by different T-cell subsets. Infect Immun 58:654, 1990
Bortolussi R, Issekutz A, Faulkner G: Opsonization of *Listeria monocytogenes* type 4b by human adult and newborn sera. Infect Immun 52:493, 1986
Buchmeier NA, Schreiber RD: Requirement of endogenous interferon-γ production for resolution of *Listeria monocytogenes* infection. Proc Natl Acad Sci USA 82:7404, 1985
Cheers C, Ho M: Resistance and susceptibility of mice to bacterial infection. IV. Functional specificity in natural resistance to facultative intracellular bacteria. J Reticuloendothel Soc 34:299, 1983
Cheers C, McKenzie IFC, Mandel TE, Chan YY: A single gene (*Lr*) controlling natural resistance to murine listeriosis. In: Skamene E, Kongshavn PAL, Landy M (eds): Genetic Control of Natural Resistance to Infection and Malignancy. New York, Academic Press, 1980, p 141
Chen-Woan M, McGregor DD, Noonan SK: Isolation and characterization of protective T cells induced by *Listeria monocytogenes.* Infect Immun 52:401, 1986
Cluff CW, Garcia M, Ziegler HK: Intracellular hemolysin-producing *Listeria monocytogenes* strains inhibit macrophage-mediated antigen processing. Infect Immun 58:3601, 1990
Cossart P, Vicente MF, Mengaud J, et al: Listeriolysin O is essential for virulence of *Listeria monocytogenes:* direct evidence obtained by gene complementation. Infect Immun 57:3629, 1989
Filice GA, Cantrell HF, Smith AB, et al: *Listeria monocytogenes* infection in neonates: Investigation of an epidemic. J Infect Dis 138:17, 1978
Fleming DW, Cochi SL, MacDonald KL, et al: Pasteurized milk as a vehicle of infection in an outbreak of listeriosis. N Engl J Med 312:404, 1985
Galsworthy SB, Gurofsky SM, Murray RGE: Purification of a monocytosis-producing activity from *Listeria monocytogenes.* Infect Immun 15:500, 1977
Geoffroy C, Gaillard J-L, Alouf JE, Berche P: Purification, characterization, and toxicity of the sulfhydryl-activated hemolysin listeriolysin O from *Listeria monocytogenes.* Infect Immun 55:1641, 1987
Havell EA: Augmented induction of interferons during *Listeria monocytogenes* infection. J Infect Dis 153:960, 1986
Ho JL, Shands KN, Friedland G, et al: An outbreak of type 4b *Listeria monocytogenes* infection involving patients from eight Boston hospitals. Arch Intern Med 146:520, 1986
Kathariou S, Pine L, George V, et al: Nonhemolytic *Listeria monocytogenes* mutants that are also noninvasive for mammalian cells in culture: evidence for coordinate regulation of virulence. Infect Immun 58:3988, 1990
Kongshavn PAL, Sadarangani C, Skamene E: Cellular mechanisms of genetically determined resistance to *Listeria monocytogenes.* In Skamene E, Kongshavn PAL, Landy M (eds): Genetic Control of Natural Resistance to Infection and Malignancy. New York, Academic Press, 1980, p 149
Kuhn M, Goebel W: Identification of an extracellular protein of *Listeria monocytogenes* possibly involved in intracellular uptake by mammalian cells. Infect Immun 57:55, 1989
Kuhn M, Prévost M-C, Mounier J, Sansonetti PJ: A nonvirulent mutant of *Listeria monocytogenes* does not move intracellularly but still induces polymerization of actin. Infect Immun 58:3477, 1990
Paquet A Jr, Raines KM, Brownback PC: Immunopotentiating activities of cell walls, peptidoglycans, and teichoic acids from two strains of *Listeria monocytogenes.* Infect Immun 54:170, 1986
Petit J-C, Richard G, Burghoffer B, Daguet G-L: Suppression of cellular immunity to *Listeria monocytogenes* by activated macrophages: Mediation by prostaglandins. Infect Immun 49:383, 1985
Saiki I, Kamisango K, Tanio Y, et al: Adjuvant activity of purified peptidoglycan of *Listeria monocytogenes* in mice and guinea pigs. Infect Immun 38:58, 1982
Schlech WF III, Lavigne PM, Bortolussi RA, et al: Epidemic listeriosis—evidence for transmission by food. N Engl J Med 308:203, 1983
Schuffler C, Campbell PA: Listeria cell wall fraction. Characterization of *in vitro* adjuvant activity. Immunology 31:323, 1976
Schwartz B, Hexter D, Broome CV, et al: Investigation of an outbreak of listeriosis: New hypotheses for the etiology of epidemic *Listeria monocytogenes* infections. J Infect Dis 159:680, 1989
Sokolovic Z, Fuchs A, Goebel W: Synthesis of species-specific stress proteins by virulent strains of *Listeria monocytogenes.* Infect Immun 58:3582, 1990
Sun AN, Camilli A, Portnoy DA: Isolation of *Listeria monocytogenes* small-plaque mutants defective for intracellular growth and cell-to-cell spread. Infect Immun 58:3770, 1990
Tilney LG, Portnoy DA: Actin filaments and the growth, movement, and spread of the intracellular bacterial parasite, *Listeria monocytogenes.* J Cell Biol 109:1597, 1989
Virgin HW IV, Unanue ER: Suppression of the immune response to *Listeria monocytogenes.* I. Immune complexes inhibit resistance. J Immunol 133:104, 1984
Virgin HW IV, Wittenberg GF, Bancroft GJ, Unanue ER: Suppression of immune response to *Listeria monocytogenes:* Mechanism(s) of immune complex suppression. Infect Immun 50:343, 1985
Wexler H, Oppenheim JD: Isolation, characterization, and biological properties of an endotoxin-like material from the gram-positive organism *Listeria monocytogenes.* Infect Immun 23:845, 1979
Wexler H, Oppenheim JD: Listerial LPS: An endotoxin from a gram-positive bacterium. In Agarwal (ed): Bacterial Endotoxins and Host Response. New York, Elsevier/North-Holland Biomedical Press, 1980, p 27
Zinkernagel RM, Althage A, Adler B, et al: H-2 restriction of cell-mediated immunity to an intracellular bacterium: Effector T cells are specific for *Listeria* antigen in association with H-2I region-coded self-markers. J Exp Med 145:1353, 1977

CHAPTER 30

Corynebacterium

Corynebacterium diphtheriae

Diphtheria is an acute infection caused by *Corynebacterium diphtheriae*. The primary lesion usually occurs in the throat or nasopharynx and is characterized by the presence of a spreading grayish pseudomembranous growth. As the organisms multiply at this site, they elaborate a potent exotoxin that is transported by the blood to remote tissues of the body causing hemorrhagic and necrotic damage in various organs. Whereas both toxigenic and nontoxigenic strains of *C. diphtheriae* can cause disease, only strains that produce toxin cause the systemic manifestations more often associated with severe or fatal illness.

The history of diphtheria is a fascinating account of the successful application of basic research to the control of an infectious disease. Diphtheria was first established as a specific clinical entity in 1826 after publication of a classic monograph by Pierre Bretonneau, but its bacterial etiology was not fully established until 1888. Klebs had earlier described the characteristic bacilli in pseudomembranes from diphtheritic throats, and Löffler had isolated the organism in pure culture, but complete understanding of the pathogenesis of the infection was provided only with the discovery by Roux and Yersin of a soluble exotoxin in the filtrates of cultures. This finding opened the door to immunologic studies that resulted in the discovery of antitoxin and toxoid, the two biologicals that have been so successfully employed in passive and active immunization against the disease.

C. diphtheriae is the only major human pathogen of the corynebacteria group of organisms, a group that also contains a number of opportunistic species and harmless, poorly described saprophytes frequently found on the surfaces of mucous membranes. The corynebacteria are taxonomically related to the mycobacteria and nocardia. There are similarities in the composition of their cell walls, and they exhibit cross-reactivity. Peptidoglycans of the three genera contain *meso*-α, ϵ-diaminopimelic acid; the major sugars of their walls polysaccharide are arabinose and galactose. The lipids associated with the outer envelope of corynebacteria also contain considerable amounts of mycolic acids, which are similar to the large saturated, α-branched, β-hydroxy fatty acids of the mycobacteria but contain fewer carbon atoms (p. 82).

Morphology

C. diphtheriae is a slender, gram-positive, rod-shaped organism that is not acid-fast and does not form spores. Cells are 1.5 to 5 μm in length and 0.5 to 1.0 μm in width. In stained smears, they characteristically appear in palisades or as individual cells lying at sharp angles to each other in V and L formations. These Chinese character–like formations are caused by the "snapping" movement involved when two cells divide. When grown on nutritionally complete media, diphtheria bacilli are uniform in shape. However, when grown in suboptimal media, such as Löffler's coagulated serum or Pai's coagulated egg medium, the cells are pleomorphic and stain irregularly with methylene blue or toluidine blue. Club-shaped swellings and beaded and barred forms are common. The metachromatic (Babès-Ernst) granules that are responsible for the beaded appearance represent accumulations of polymerized polyphosphates.

Physiology

Cultural Characteristics. *C. diphtheriae* is an aerobic and facultatively anaerobic organism but grows best under aerobic conditions. Complex media are required for primary isolation and characterization. Most strains grow as a waxy pellicle on the surface of liquid media. On Löffler's coagulated serum medium, which is useful for the primary isolation of the organism, minute, grayish white glistening colonies appear after 12 to 24 hours' incubation at 37C. Löffler's medium is also useful because it does not support growth of streptococci and pneumococci that may be present in the clinical specimen.

The addition of tellurite salts to media used for primary isolation also reduces the number of contaminants. On tellurite media, colonies of *C. diphtheriae* assume a characteristic gray or black color and may be differentiated into three major colonial types: gravis, mitis, and intermedius. Colonies of gravis strains are large, flat, and gray to black with a dull surface; mitis organisms produce medium-sized colonies that are smaller, blacker, glossy, and more convex; and colonies of intermedius strains are very small and either smooth or rough. The tellurite ion passes through the cell membrane into the cytoplasm, where it is reduced to the metal tellurium and precipitated. There is no constant relationship between the severity of the disease and the three colony types.

Resistance. *C. diphtheriae* is more resistant to the action of light, desiccation, and freezing than are most non-spore-forming bacilli. On dried fragments of pseudomembranes, organisms survive for at least 14 weeks. They are readily killed, however, by a 1-minute exposure to 100C or a 10-minute exposure to 58C. They are susceptible to most of the routinely used disinfectants.

Antigenic Structure

C. diphtheriae is an antigenically heterogeneous species. Agglutination tests with whole-cell suspensions show a large number of serologic types. The three major colonial types—gravis, mitis, and intermedius—reflect differences in the cell surface and constitute the major biotypes of the organism. Within each of these biotypes is a more or less separate group of agglutinating serotypes. Additional differences in cell surface components have also been detected by bacteriophage typing and bacteriocin production. Regardless of type, however, all toxigenic strains produce a biologically and immunologically identical toxin.

K Antigen. The antigens responsible for the type specificity of *C. diphtheriae* strains are heat-labile proteins, the K antigens, localized in the superficial layers of the wall. These antigens play an important role in antibacterial immunity and hypersensitivity separate from antitoxic immunity. The occurrence of different antigenic types of *C. diphtheriae* probably explains the occurrence of diphtheria in immunized persons who show a detectable level of circulating antitoxin. The K antigens on the surface, together with the glycolipid cord factor (see below), are major determinants of invasiveness and virulence in diphtheria bacilli.

O Antigen. The heat-stable O antigen of *C. diphtheriae* is a group antigen common to the corynebacteria parasitic for humans and animals. It is a polysaccharide containing arabinogalactans and is the antigen responsible for the cross-reactivity with mycobacteria and nocardia. Corynebacterial cells and their subcellular components are excellent antigens. When administered to animals with immunizing agents, they also function as adjuvants (p. 220).

Determinants of Pathogenicity

Invasiveness. Since both toxigenic and nontoxigenic strains of *C. diphtheriae* are capable of colonizing mucous membranes, factors other than toxin production contribute to the organism's invasiveness and ability to establish and maintain itself in the human host. The precise relationship of these traits to the pathogenesis of the disease, however, is ill defined. In addition to the surface K antigens, the organisms contain a cord factor that is considered to be a necessary adjunct of virulence. The cord factor, a toxic glycolipid, is a 6-6′ diester of trehalose containing the mycolic acids characteristic of *C. diphtheriae*, corynemycolic acid ($C_{32}H_{62}O_3$), and corynemycolenic acid ($C_{32}H_{64}O_3$) (see p. 82). The pharmacologic activity of the cord factor of *C. diphtheriae* is similar to that of the cord factor from *Mycobacterium tuberculosis*. In the mouse, it causes a disruption of mitochondria, reduction of respiration and phosphorylation, and death.

Other factors that probably contribute to the invasive potential of *C. diphtheriae* are neuraminidase and *N*-acetylneuraminate lyase. By degrading the *N*-acetylneuraminic acid residues cleaved from its mucinous environment, these enzymes could provide a readily available source of energy for bacteria inhabiting the mucous membranes.

Exotoxin. Most naturally occurring diseases are too complex at the cellular level to dissect successfully and define definitively the primary biochemical lesion. In diphtheria, however, the exotoxin produced by *C. diphtheriae* is the major biochemical determinant in the pathogenesis of the infection and accounts for essentially all of the pathologic systemic effects.

LYSOGENY AND TOXIN PRODUCTION. Toxin is produced only by strains of *C. diphtheriae* infected with a temperate bacteriophage carrying the structural gene for toxin production. Nontoxigenic strains may be converted to the lysogenic, toxigenic state by infection with a suitable tox^+ corynephage. Conversion to toxigenicity, however, is not an obligatory property of corynephages. Although most of the studies on toxin production have been conducted with β corynephage, the *tox* gene occurs in a number of corynephages that differ both genetically and serologically.

The production of toxin by a lysogenic strain does not require lytic growth of the phage. The *tox* gene can be expressed when corynebacteriophage β is present in *C. diphtheriae* as a vegetatively replicating phage, as a prophage, or as a superinfecting, nonreplicating exogenote in immune lysogenic cells. Under laboratory conditions, the toxin appears to serve no essential viral function. Under natural conditions in

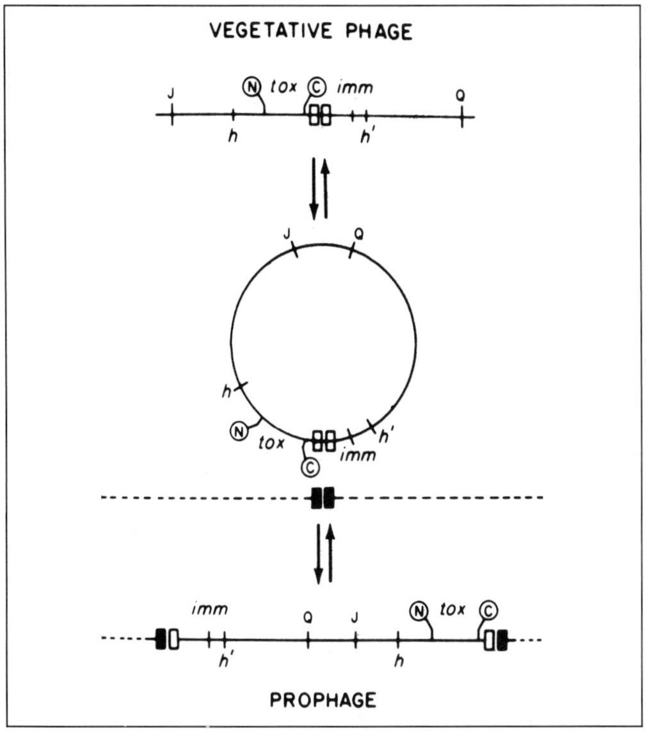

Fig. 30–1. Orientation of the *tox* gene in the β bacteriophage and prophage. The figure shows the interconversion of the prophage and vegetative phage states. The *tox* gene has been enlarged, and its boundaries are defined by N and C, the locations of the codons for the N-terminal and C-terminal amino acids. Phage chromosome (——); bacterial chromosome (- - -). The open and closed rectangles represent phage and bacterial attachment sites, respectively. (*From Laird and Groman: J Virol 19:228, 1976.*)

the nasopharynx of humans, however, the *tox* gene imparts survival value both to the phage and to *C. diphtheriae*, its lysogenized host.

The life cycle of corynebacteriophage β is similar to that of coliphage λ, growing productively in most infected cells but lysogenizing a small number. Phage mutants that produce antigenically similar but nontoxic proteins (crm proteins) have been used to construct a map of the vegetative and prophage genomes of the β phage. The prophage map appears to be a cyclic permutation of the vegetative map, with the *tox* gene at one end of the prophage map next to the attachment site on the host chromosome and the immunity gene at the other end of the map (Fig. 30–1). Insertion into the bacterial chromosome occurs by a mechanism similar to that found in coliphage λ. The position of the integrated *tox* gene suggests that it may have evolved from a bacterial gene.

REGULATION OF *TOX* GENE EXPRESSION. Regulation of the synthesis of diphtheria toxin encompasses both genetic and physiologic factors and involves both the bacterium and the bacteriophage. Different strains of *C. diphtheriae* vary greatly in their capacity for toxin production when infected by specific tox^+ corynebacteriophages. Also, some phages may be nontoxicogenic for some host strains but tox^+ for other *C. diphtheriae*. The λ corynephage, a nonconverting phage closely related to β-phage, carries the *tox* gene in an inactive form. In the λ phage, a complete phage genome is present plus an adjacent small loop of bacterial DNA. It is probable that this additional DNA represents an insertion element or a transposon and that the *tox* gene of λ phage has been inactivated by its insertion.

The yield of toxin is markedly influenced by growth conditions, especially the inorganic iron content of the medium. Diphtheria toxin is produced at maximal levels only during the decline phase of the bacterial growth cycle, when iron becomes the rate-limiting substrate. The addition of iron to iron-starved cultures of lysogenic *C. diphtheriae* inhibits the production of toxin almost immediately. The successful use for many years of the Park-Williams no. 8 strain for the commercial production of toxin is linked to its ability to grow in media containing very low levels of iron. Under such conditions, growth is slow, but toxin may account for approximately 5% of the total bacterial protein.

At the molecular level, regulation of diphtheria toxin production occurs independently of other phage functions and is directed at the level of transcription. According to the proposed model, *C. diphtheriae*, irrespective of its lysogenic state, carries a gene coding for the synthesis of the diphtheria *tox* aporepressor. In the presence of iron, a repressor-iron complex forms that binds specifically at the phage β *tox* operator locus. Under conditions of iron limitation, the repressor-iron complex dissociates and the diphtheria *tox* gene is derepressed (Fig. 30–2). Nothing is known at present concerning the identity and function in the bacterial host of the repressor protein.

PROPERTIES. Diphtheria toxin is synthesized in precursor form on membrane-bound polysomes in *C. diphtheriae* and is cotranslationally secreted as a single polypeptide chain with a molecular weight of approximately 58 kDa (Fig. 30–3). When released, the native toxin molecule is nontoxic until exposure of the active enzymatic site by mild trypsin treatment. The biologically active molecule consists of two functionally distinct polypeptide chains, fragments A and B, linked by a disulfide bridge. Both of these fragments are essential for cytotoxicity. The aminoterminal portion of the toxin, fragment A (ca 21 kDa), contains the enzymatically active site of the toxin. Fragment B (ca 37 kDa), from the carboxyterminal of the toxin, contains the eucaryotic cell receptor binding domain, as well as two lipid associating domains that appear to be essential in the membrane translocation of fragment A into the eucaryotic cell cytosol.

UPTAKE BY EUCARYOTIC CELLS. To express toxicity in living cells, diphtheria toxin must cross a membrane barrier and reach its target in the cytosol. In spite of intensive study on the mechanism of the entry of diphtheria toxin into cells, the process is still not completely understood. The specific membrane receptor has not been identified, although current data indicates that both the peptide backbone of a glycoprotein and membrane phospholipids are involved in the binding of the toxin. It is hypothesized that toxin is internalized by receptor-mediated endocytosis and finds its way into an acidified endocytic vesicle, where it is triggered by the low pH to escape into the cytoplasm. According to this model, anion transport appears to be necessary for entry of the A fragment into the cytosol, which occurs through ion-permeable channels formed by insertion of the hydrophobic domain of the B fragment into the membrane. At some point before or during the translocation, disulfide reduction and cleavage of one or

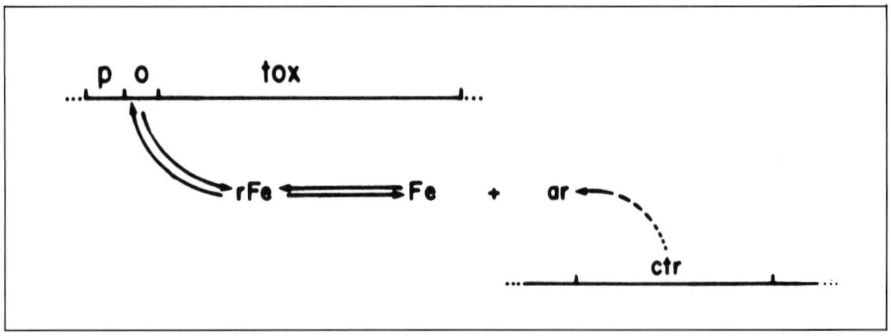

Fig. 30–2. Hypothetic model of the corynebacterial regulation of the corynephage β *tox* gene. *C. diphtheriae* carries the structural information (ctr) for the synthesis of the diphtheria tox aporepressor (ar). In the presence of iron, a repressor-iron complex would form and bind to the corynephage β *tox* operator locus. Under conditions of iron limitation, the equilibrium would shift to the right, and the diphtheria *tox* gene would become depressed. (*From Murphy and Bacha: Microbiology-1979. Washington, DC, American Society for Microbiology.*)

more peptide bonds are required to release fragment A from fragment B.

MODE OF ACTION. On reaching the cytoplasm, fragment A disrupts protein synthesis by catalyzing transfer of the adenosine-diphosphoribose (ADPR) moiety of nicotinamide adenine dinucleotide (NAD) to the eucaryotic peptidyl-tRNA translocase, elongation factor 2 (EF2). This adenosine diphosphate (ADP)-ribosylation of EF2 is the primary target of diphtheria toxin.

$$\text{NAD} + \text{EF2} \rightleftharpoons \text{ADPR-EF2} + \text{Nicotinamide} + \text{H}^+$$

Although the reaction is reversible, its equilibrium at physiologic pH lies far to the right. Only soluble EF2 can serve as substrate, and once it is fixed to ribosomes, it cannot be ADP-ribosylated.

The specific site in EF2 to which ADPR becomes covalently linked is diphthamide, a unique amino acid that results from a novel posttranslational modification of a histidine residue. Diphthamide has not been found in any other eucaryotic protein. Toxin has no effect on polypeptide chain elongation in procaryotic systems or in mitochondria, where a different protein, elongation factor G (EFG), replaces EF2.

Although it is widely accepted that the killing mechanism of diphtheria toxin is linked to its ability to inhibit protein synthesis, a second cytotoxic pathway may also be involved. On exposure to diphtheria toxin, human target cells show widespread membrane blebbing and extensive prelytic internucleosomal DNA cleavage. Discovery of this nuclease activity suggests that diphtheria toxin-induced cell lysis is not a simple consequence of protein inhibition but is also linked to chromosomal degradation.

HOST SUSCEPTIBILITY. Animals vary greatly in their susceptibility to diphtheria toxin. Doses as low as 160 ng/kg of body weight are lethal for humans, rabbits, guinea pigs, and birds. Rats and mice, however, are highly resistant unless the toxin is administered intracerebrally.

ANTITOXIN. Both A and B moieties of toxin contain a number of antigenic determinants. As a consequence, antitoxin consists of a heterogeneous mixture of antibodies specific for different domains of the toxin molecule. In native toxin or toxoid, most

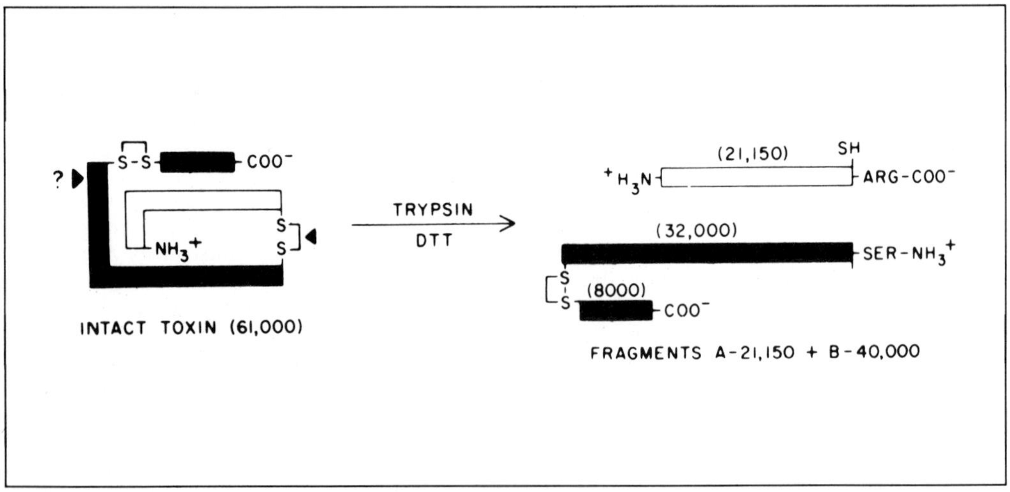

Fig. 30–3. Diagram of diphtheria toxin and its fragments. Toxin is released into the culture medium as a single polypeptide chain. The intact molecule contains two disulfide bridges. The peptide loop contained within the first disulfide bridge is extraordinarily sensitive to proteolytic cleavage and is opened after mild digestion by trypsin. Subsequent reduction of the disulfide results in splitting of the nicked toxin into two fragments, A and B. (*From Pappenheimer: Microbiology-1979. Washington, DC, American Society for Microbiology.*)

of the antigenic determinants in fragment A are deeply buried and are not available either to stimulate antibody production or to participate in the precipitation of antibody. Also, although anti-A antibody inhibits the enzymic activity of toxin, it does not protect animals or cells against the lethal action of toxin. Antibodies directed against fragment B, however, neutralize toxin with great efficiency, supporting the theory that antitoxin acts by competing with toxin for surface receptors on sensitive eucaryotic cells and that fragment B is required for the initial attachment.

Active antitoxic immunization against diphtheria toxin by use of a synthetic oligopeptide has been accomplished. The synthetic antigen is a tetradecapeptide consisting of the loop of 14 amino acids subtended by the disulfide bridge nearer the N-terminus of the molecule. This tetradecapeptide, when linked covalently with a carrier, will elicit in guinea pigs antibodies that not only bind specifically with the toxin but neutralize its dermonecrotic and lethal effects. This represents the first example of successful active immunization against a lethal bacterial toxin by use of a synthetic antigen.

TOXOID. The addition of low concentrations of formaldehyde to diphtheria toxin destroys its toxicity and converts it to toxoid. Detoxification by formaldehyde alters both the enzymatic activity of fragment A and the binding of fragment B to cells. The alteration may be due either to the chemical modification of essential residues in the toxin or to intramolecular cross-linking of lysine and tyrosine via methylene bonds. The increased stability and resistance to proteolysis of toxoid is attributed to the cross-linking effects. Toxoid cannot be cleaved into A and B fragments. It possesses no ADP-ribosylating activity and does not bind to cell membranes of sensitive cells.

Clinical Infection

Epidemiology. Diphtheria has a worldwide distribution but is now relatively uncommon in the United States and Western Europe. In many developing countries, however, where fewer than 10% of the infants are fully immunized, an estimated 1 million deaths a year are caused by diphtheria. The marked decrease in incidence in the United States from more than 200,000 cases in 1921 to only 27 cases of respiratory diphtheria in the 10-year period from 1981 through 1990 is attributable to successful programs for the active immunization of preschool children and to an apparent reduction in the circulation of toxigenic strains of *C. diphtheriae.* Even though the annual number of cases is small, the problem remains a serious one in certain population clusters. The immunization status of the adult population in the United States is low, and therefore diphtheria occurs in the older age groups at about the same low frequency as in the past. Diphtheria may occur and give rise to epidemics during any month of the year, but crowding and close interpersonal contact during the winter results in a higher frequency from September through March.

Humans are the only natural hosts of *C. diphtheriae* and thus the only significant reservoir of infection. Symptom-free carriers and persons in the incubation stage of the disease are the major sources of most infections. The primary habitat of *C. diphtheriae* is the upper respiratory tract, from which site the organisms are transmitted from person to person, either directly or indirectly. Transmission via droplet infection is the major mechanism of transfer in respiratory disease. Discharges from extrarespiratory sites, such as skin ulcers, also provide a source of pharyngeal as well as cutaneous disease. In tropical and subtropical areas, the skin provides a major reservoir of *C. diphtheriae* infection. Skin infections are more contagious than respiratory disease; as a result, a higher environmental carrier level is maintained. The precise role played by skin diphtheria in instituting respiratory tract diphtheria in both tropical and temperate climates remains to be clarified.

Immunity. In diphtheria, immunity against clinical disease depends on the presence in the blood of antitoxin produced in response to either clinical or subclinical infection or as a result of artificial active immunization with toxoid. Under the age of 6 months, infants are passively protected from diphtheria by the transplacental passage of antitoxin from immune mothers. The antibodies present in antitoxin are of the IgG and IgA classes.

The widespread immunization of infants and preschool children with toxoid has materially reduced the incidence of diphtheria in children and in doing so has decreased the carrier rate and opportunity for natural reinforcement of immunity by subclinical infection. As a result, an increasing number of adults are without protective antitoxic immunity. Also, a much lower percentage of newborn infants are immune during the first months of life. The immune status of a person may be assessed by the determination of serum antitoxin levels or by the Schick test.

SCHICK TEST. The Schick test is performed by injecting into the skin of the forearm 0.1 ml of highly purified toxin.* When the Schick test is administered, a control consisting of a similar amount of toxin heated to 60C for 30 minutes should be injected into the other arm. A positive reaction, indicating the absence of immunity to diphtheria, is characterized by a local inflammatory reaction that reaches a maximal intensity within 4 to 7 days and fades gradually. A negative Schick test reaction signifies that the antitoxin level is greater than 0.03 U/mL of blood and that the person is immune under ordinary conditions of exposure. Allergic reactions are sometimes observed in adults and older children, especially in endemic areas. These reactions probably result from previous infections with corynebacteria or from artificial immunization with toxoid. If such persons are immune, they will give a pseudoreaction characterized by erythema at both test and control sites. Such reactions reach maximum intensity within 24 to 36 hours but fade and disappear completely within the next 72 hours. If the persons are allergic but have no antitoxin or a low level of antitoxin, they will give a combined reaction—the reaction in the control arm subsides by the fifth or sixth day, whereas that in the test arm reaches its maximum on the fifth day and persists for several days.

Pathogenesis. After exposure to *C. diphtheriae,* there is an incubation period of 1 to 7 days during which the organism

* The Schick test dose (STD) was previously defined as 1/50 MLD (minimal lethal dose) for the guinea pig. Because of the difficulty of standardizing the lethal activity of the toxin for the guinea pig, a change was made to the use of the animal erythema potency test. The STD is now defined as that amount of standard toxin that, when mixed with 0.001 unit of the U.S. standard diphtheria antitoxin and injected intradermally into a guinea pig, will induce an erythematous reaction 10 mm in diameter.

establishes itself at the infected site. The initial lesion usually occurs on the tonsils and oropharynx and from this site may spread to the nasopharynx, larynx, and trachea. The organisms multiply rapidly on epithelial cells in the local lesion, producing an exotoxin that causes necrosis of cells in the area. An inflammatory reaction results, accompanied by the outpouring of a fibrinous exudate. At first patchy in appearance, as the local exudative lesions coalesce a very tough adherent pseudomembrane forms. This is grayish to black and is composed of fibrin, necrotic epithelial cells, lymphocytes, polymorphonuclear leukocytes, erythrocytes, and diphtheria bacilli. The pseudomembrane adheres very tenaciously to the underlying tissues, and if attempts are made to forcibly remove it, a raw bleeding surface is exposed. Edema of the soft tissues beneath the membrane may be pronounced.

Growth of *C. diphtheriae* is restricted to the mucosal epithelium and rarely, if ever, do the organisms invade the deeper tissues and produce lesions in other parts of the body. The reasons for this high degree of tissue specificity are not known. The absorption of the toxin into the general circulation, however, results in degenerative lesions in a number of organs. The most serious of these are usually associated with nasopharyngeal diphtheria and involve the heart, the nervous system, and the kidneys.

Clinical Manifestations

RESPIRATORY DISEASE. The clinical manifestations vary, depending on the virulence of the organism, host resistance, and anatomic location of the lesion. In tonsillar diphtheria, the most common clinical presentation, there is an abrupt onset characterized by low-grade fever, malaise, and a mild sore throat. The cervical lymph nodes become edematous and tender, especially when there is involvement of the nasopharynx. Swelling may be so pronounced that the classic bull neck appearance results. Extension from the nasopharynx to the larynx and trachea results in a very severe form of the disease in which mechanical obstruction of the airway by the membrane and accompanying edema introduce the risk of suffocation. Death ensues unless the airway is restored by tracheotomy or intubation.

EXTRARESPIRATORY DISEASE. Although diphtheria is usually a disease of the upper respiratory tract, primary or secondary lesions may occur in other parts of the body. The most common extrarespiratory site is the skin. In tropical areas, cutaneous diphtheria is relatively common, especially as a secondary infection of septic skin lesions. Although less common in temperate zones, there have been outbreaks of cutaneous diphtheria in the United States and Canada, primarily in indigent and derelict groups. In skin diphtheria, lesions usually appear at the site of minor abrasions as chronic, spreading, nonhealing ulcers covered with a grayish membrane. The etiology of cutaneous diphtheria is complex. In addition to *C. diphtheriae,* either *Streptococcus pyogenes* or *Staphylococcus aureus* is usually present in the lesion, which fails to heal until appropriate therapy for both organisms is instituted. Mitis strains are usually associated with such infections, which are usually milder with much less systemic illness.

Rarely, diphtherial infections of the conjunctiva, cornea, vagina, and ear occur. These are almost always secondary to pharyngeal or skin infection.

COMPLICATIONS. The most serious complications of diphtheria are those affecting the cardiovascular and nervous systems. Cardiac abnormalities that appear after the second week of the disease are seen in approximately 20% of patients with diphtheria and are responsible for more than half of the case fatalities. Diphtheria toxin causes fatty myocardial degeneration, resulting in cardiac dysfunction and circulatory collapse. The myocardial damage is reversible, and if the patient survives, recovery is usually complete.

When neurologic symptoms occur, they usually appear in the third to fifth week of the disease. Involvement of the cranial nerves characteristically leads to paralysis of the soft palate, with resultant difficulty in swallowing and nasal regurgitation of fluids. The most common manifestation of peripheral nerve involvement is a polyneuritis of the lower extremities, varying in severity from a mild weakness to paralysis of certain muscle groups. Recovery from both cranial and peripheral nerve dysfunction is usually complete.

Laboratory Diagnosis

CULTURE. Isolation of the organism is necessary for the microbiologic diagnosis of diphtheria. Because early administration of antitoxin is of paramount importance, the clinician should institute therapy immediately on the basis of clinical findings without waiting for laboratory confirmation. Streptococcal pharyngitis and Vincent's infection may be confused with diphtheria and should always be considered when a laboratory diagnosis is made. Swabs containing material from both the nasopharynx and the throat should be transported promptly to the laboratory, and personnel should be alerted to the presumptive diagnosis of diphtheria. A Löffler or Pai slant, a tellurite plate, and a blood agar plate should be inoculated immediately, and a smear stained with gentian violet should be examined to rule out infection with Vincent's fusospirochetal organisms. No attempt should be made to identify *C. diphtheriae* directly from smears of clinical material. Löffler's slants should be examined after 16 to 24 hours by staining with methylene blue and looking for the typical pleomorphic forms (p. 487). Blood agar plates should be examined for β-hemolytic streptococci, and any characteristic grayish or black colonies on tellurite media should be transferred to Löffler slants. Confirmatory biochemical characterization may be carried out, and the isolate on Löffler's medium may be tested for pathogenicity either with the in vivo virulence test or the in vitro immunodiffusion technique.

IN VIVO TEST. Animal inoculation is recommended for laboratories that seldom isolate *C. diphtheriae.* Either guinea pigs or rabbits may be used, and one animal is sufficient for both test and control inoculations. The test is performed by injecting intracutaneously into the shaved animal 0.2 mL of a 48-hour infusion broth culture of the test organism. Five hours later, 500 units of diphtheria antitoxin is injected intraperitoneally into the guinea pig (or into the ear vein of the rabbit), and after 30 minutes a second 0.2 mL broth sample is injected intracutaneously into the control area opposite the test site. Preliminary readings are made at 24 and 48 hours. If a toxigenic strain is present, a necrotic area appears at the site of the test injection after 48 to 72 hours. At the control site, only a pinkish nodule develops but does not proceed to ulceration because of the prior administration of antitoxin.

IN VITRO TEST. The gel diffusion test for determining

pathogenicity is more rapid than the in vivo method, but unless plates are carefully prepared, false-negative results may be obtained. In this test, antitoxin-soaked strips of filter paper are placed on the surface of a serum agar medium and the plate is inoculated heavily by streaking a line of inoculum perpendicular to the strip. The plates should be read daily for 3 days. If the organism is toxigenic, a white line of toxin-antitoxin precipitate appears, extending out at a 45-degree angle from the intersection of the line of inoculum and the front of antitoxin diffusing from the filter paper.

Treatment

ANTITOXIN. Administration of diphtheria antitoxin in adequate amounts is the only specific and effective treatment for diphtheria. The antitoxin should be administered as soon as a presumptive diagnosis of diphtheria is made clinically, without waiting for a laboratory confirmation. In severe cases the prognosis depends to a great extent on how early in the course of the infection antitoxin therapy is initiated. The toxin binds rapidly to susceptible tissue cells. The initial binding is reversible but is quickly followed by an irreversible phase as fragment A gains entrance into the cell. At this stage toxin cannot be displaced by antitoxin. The role of antitoxin is to prevent any further binding to undamaged cells of free toxin circulating in the blood. It does this by binding to determinants on the toxin molecule at the C-terminal (17 kDa) end, thereby preventing attachment of fragment B to the tissue cell (p. 30).

Diphtheria antitoxin should be administered intramuscularly or intravenously in a single dose. The amount of antitoxin given depends on the severity of the infection, but there is a general lack of agreement as to what constitutes adequate therapy. One conservative scheme specifies 20,000 to 50,000 units intramuscularly for mild or moderate cases and 80,000 to 100,000 units intravenously for severe cases.*

Because commercial diphtheria antitoxin is usually produced in horses, to avoid the possible occurrence of anaphylaxis, the patient should be tested for hypersensitivity to horse serum before therapy is started.

CHEMOTHERAPY. *C. diphtheriae* is susceptible to a number of antimicrobials that should be used as an adjunct to, not as a substitute for, antitoxin in the patient with diphtheria. Penicillin G is the drug of choice, and erythromycin is effective in the patient who is allergic to penicillin. Antibiotics are especially useful in the prevention of secondary infections and in treatment of chronic carriers. Without chemotherapy, from 1% to 15% of persons who recover from diphtheria become carriers, harboring *C. diphtheriae* for weeks or months after infection. Carriage of the organism is greater after nasal infection.

Prevention

ACTIVE IMMUNIZATION. Active immunization is the key to control and prevention of clinical diphtheria. For this purpose, toxoid is administered as an aluminum salt–adsorbed preparation. Toxoid is prepared by treating diphtheria toxin with 0.3% formalin at 37C until the product is completely nontoxic. The addition of alum to fluid toxoid yields a partially purified preparation with increased antigenic efficiency because of the local stimulatory effect of the alum.

The primary course of immunization should be started during the first 6 to 8 weeks of life. It consists of four 0.5 mL doses of toxoid combined with tetanus toxoid and pertussis vaccine (DPT) given intramuscularly on four occasions—the first three doses at 4- to 8-week intervals and the fourth dose approximately 6 to 12 months after the third. Children receiving all four primary immunizing doses before the age of 4 should receive a single booster dose of DPT before entering kindergarten.

Young children rarely exhibit either local or general hypersensitivity reactions to the toxoid, but in older children and adults one must be alert to the possibility of a hypersensitivity reaction. This may be detected by administration of a skin test in which 0.1 mL of a 1:10 dilution of fluid toxoid is given intracutaneously. A positive reaction indicates hypersensitivity to the proteins of *C. diphtheriae* or other corynebacteria or to the toxin itself. Approximately 50% of persons over the age of 15 years have positive reactions to the test. Such reactions present a problem in the immunization of adult population groups and require that the toxoid be administered cautiously in multiple small doses. For persons 7 years of age and older a combined preparation of tetanus and diphtheria toxoids (Td) is recommended. This product contains a smaller amount of diphtheria toxoid than is present in DPT. A booster dose of Td should be given every 10 years because immunity after the original immunization series wanes. Often diphtheria infection does not confer adequate immunity against subsequent infection. Therefore, active immunization should be initiated or the primary course should be completed during convalescence.

PROPHYLAXIS FOR CASE CONTACTS. All household contacts and persons with intimate exposure to a patient with respiratory diphtheria should be placed immediately under close surveillance. Contacts immunized within the previous 5 years should receive a booster dose of toxoid, and unimmunized or inadequately immunized persons should complete the immunization sequence and should also receive a chemoprophylactic course of penicillin or erythromycin.

Passive immunization with 5,000 to 10,000 units of antitoxin may be employed for the protection of nonimmunized persons who are heavily exposed to toxigenic organisms. Because such protection is of short duration and introduces the risk of inducing sensitization or of eliciting an anaphylactic reaction in a previously sensitized person, its use should be limited to high-risk situations.

Other Corynebacteria

Traditionally, with the exception of *C. diphtheriae*, corynebacteria have been considered unimportant as producers of disease in humans. Because of the presence of such organisms as common contaminants of clinical material, they have been recognized and accepted with reservation as the cause of infection. There has been, however, an increasing awareness that in the proper setting, especially in the immunocompro-

* Diphtheria antitoxin is standardized in units by comparing its ability to neutralize toxin with that of the official standard unit of antitoxin, maintained in vacuo at the State Serum Institute in Copenhagen. In terms of protective units the standard unit of antitoxin will neutralize 100 MLD of toxin.

mised host, diphtheroids may assume the role of opportunistic invaders. A number of cases of endocarditis after cardiac surgery, meningitis, and osteomyelitis have been attributed to a diphtheroid. Therapy with the penicillins or with erythromycin has usually proved effective for such infections, although there has been an increase in the prevalence of resistant strains.

The tendency in the past to classify many organisms as corynebacteria solely on the basis of morphology has resulted in the placing of a number of unrelated or distantly related organisms in the genus. The 1986 edition of *Bergey's Manual of Systematic Bacteriology* has clarified and limited the definition of the genus *Corynebacterium,* which is now well defined on the basis of chemical criteria. Only organisms with a directly cross-linked peptidoglycan based on *meso*-diaminopimelic acid, a wall arabinogalactan polymer, short-chain mycolic acids, and a mole percent guanosine-plus-cytosine (G + C) content in the range of 51 to 65 are included in the genus. As now constituted, 16 species are recognized in the genus, which includes human and animal pathogens and saprophytes. Species of selected corynebacteria and related organisms associated with nondiphtheria infections in humans are listed in Table 30–1. *Corynebacterium ulcerans* is no longer recognized as a distinct species but is considered a variant of *C. diphtheriae.*

Corynebacterium pseudotuberculosis. Except for *C. diphtheriae, Corynebacterium pseudotuberculosis* is the only species producing an exotoxin. This exotoxin, however, is antigenically distinct from that of *C. diphtheriae.* Closely related to *C. diphtheriae, C. pseudotuberculosis* is susceptible to some of the bacteriophages used in typing the diphtheria bacillus and, when lysogenized with a tox^+ phage, synthesizes diphtheria toxin. *C. pseudotuberculosis* causes ulcerative lymphangitis and abscesses in sheep, horses, cattle, and other warm-blooded animals. Human infections characteristically occur as a subacute or chronic lymphadenitis and appear to arise from contact with infected animals.

Corynebacterium pseudodiphtheriticum* and *Corynebacterium xerosis. *C. pseudodiphtheriticum* and *C. xerosis* are the two species most frequently cultured from clinical materials. *C. pseudodiphtheriticum* is found in the nasopharynx of humans. It is a short, rather uniform rod that stains evenly except for a transverse medial unstained septum. Metachromatic granules and club forms are usually absent. *C. xerosis* inhabits the skin and mucous membranes, especially the conjunctiva, of humans. Infections with these organisms occur particularly in immunocompromised patients or in those with mucocutaneous defects facilitating bacteremia. Prosthetic valve endocarditis is one of the most prevalent infections attributed to these species.

Corynebacterium bovis. The taxonomic position of *C. bovis* is uncertain, although for the present it remains affiliated with the genus *Corynebacterium.* It is a lipophilic organism that requires unsaturated long-chain fatty acids. *C. bovis* is a commensal in the bovine udder and can be a cause of bovine mastitis. A variety of different human infections caused by this organism have been reported, but their relationship to an animal source has not been documented. It is the most frequent *Corynebacterium* species associated with CNS "shunt nephritis."

Corynebacterium minutissimum. *C. minutissimum* is the organism that causes erythrasma, a disease that occurs in the intertriginous areas and is characterized by the presence of scaly plaques that fluoresce coral red under Wood's light at 365 nm. *C. minutissimum* is a nutritionally exacting organism. When grown aerobically on a solid medium containing tissue culture medium base and 20% bovine fetal serum, porphyrins are produced and give the colonies a coral red to orange fluorescence similar to that of the skin lesions. Colonies grown on blood agar do not produce this characteristic fluorescence.

Arcanobacterium haemolyticum (Corynebacterium haemolyticum). *Corynebacterium haemolyticum* is distinct from all *Corynebacterium* and *Actinomyces* species and has been reclassified as a new genus, *Arcanobacterium.* It is a short, irregular gram-positive rod, but after 18 hours of growth on a blood agar plate the organisms become granular and resemble small and irregular cocci. On Löffler's media they remain bacillary and are pleomorphic at 48 hours. *A. haemolyticum* is present on the skin and in the nasopharynx of healthy persons, but it can also cause acute pharyngitis similar to that resulting from group A streptococcal infection. In contrast to streptococcal pharyngitis, *A. haemolyticum* infection affects mostly teenagers and young adults, and in about half of the cases there is a scarlatiniform rash. The cause of the rash is not known, but

TABLE 30–1. CORYNEFORM ORGANISMS ASSOCIATED WITH NONDIPHTHERIA INFECTIONS

Organism	Major Animal Reservoir	Human Commensal	Predominant Human Infections
C. pseudotuberculosis	Sheep, cattle, horses	No	Subacute relapsing lymphadenitis
C. xerosis	None	Skin, pharynx, conjunctivae	Bacteremia, skin infections, pneumonia in immunocompromised hosts
C. pseudodiphtheriticum	None	Nasopharynx	Endocarditis
C. minutissimum	None	Skin	Erythrasma
C. matruchotii	Primates	Oral cavity	Dental plaque
C. bovis[a]	Cows	No	CNS, bloodstream
Arcanobacterium haemolyticus[b]	None	Skin, pharynx	Pharyngitis, skin infections, brain abscess
Rhodococcus equi[c]	Horses, cattle, swine	No	Pneumonia

[a] Not a member of genus *Corynebacterium* but not reassigned to new genus.
[b] Formerly *Corynebacterium haemolyticus.*
[c] Formerly *Corynebacterium equi.*

it is conceivable that the operative mechanism is similar to that in *C. diphtheriae*.

Actinomyces pyogenes (Corynebacterium pyogenes). *A. pyogenes* is an aerotolerant anaerobe and is biochemically similar to *Actinomyces bovis*, except that it is hemolytic and proteolytic. It produces a variety of pyogenic infections in a number of domestic animals, but the reports of human infections have not been well documented.

Rhodococcus equi (Corynebacterium equi). *Rhodococcus equi* is a gram-positive aerobic nocardioform organism that exhibits a rod-coccus morphogenetic cycle. It is found in soil and herbivore dung and causes several important zoonoses, including bronchopneumonia in horses. A number of human infections have been reported in young, immunocompromised adults with severely impaired cell-mediated immunity and with histories of animal exposure. The infection in these patients runs a subacute course, and the necrotizing pneumonia produced by *R. equi* resembles mycobacterial or nocardial infection.

Group JK. Unaccounted for in the present classification of the corynebacteria is a group of coryneform organisms, designated the JK group, which are highly resistant to multiple antibiotics. These organisms appear to be part of the normal flora of the skin, especially in the inguinal, axillary, and rectal areas. They rarely colonize healthy, nonhospitalized persons but can be found in 10% to 15% of hospitalized general patients and in 25% to 35% of hospitalized neutropenic patients. Most infections with JK organisms have occurred in patients with hematologic malignancies, where they have been most commonly associated with bacteremia, cutaneous infections at intravenous entry sites, and pneumonia. JK organisms are a well-established cause of prosthetic valve endocarditis. Patients at greatest risk of infection by JK strains are those with prolonged neutropenia and broad-spectrum antibiotic therapy. All isolates have been susceptible to vancomycin.

On gram stain, the JK organisms show gram-positive coccobacillary or coccal forms resembling streptococci. They are slow-growing and produce small, gray to white colonies on blood agar. The JK strains resemble aerobic lipophilic diphtheroids from human skin. They have a strict nutritional requirement for lipid and are similar in their composition of cellular fatty acid, mycolic acid, and peptidoglycan. These similarities have led to the suggestion that JK bacteria represent resident lipophilic diphtheroids that have acquired antibiotic resistance.

Group D2. *Corynebacterium* group D2 is a gram-positive rod whose biochemical and culture characteristics are similar to those of *Corynebacterium* group JK. Unlike group JK, however, these organisms are urease-positive, and they do not use glucose. They are highly resistant to most antibacterial agents. Most of the infections with which they have been associated have been in patients who are immunosuppressed, instrumented, or undergoing antibacterial therapy. Group D2 has been isolated from transtracheal aspirates of an elderly patient with pneumonia and has played an important role in the development of encrusted cystitis, a chronic inflammatory condition of the bladder characterized by deposits of ammonium magnesium phosphate on the surface and walls of the ulcer. Urologic manipulations, renal grafts, previous urinary infections, and intense antibiotic treatment predispose to colonization of the urinary tract by group D2. The organisms respond to treatment with vancomycin.

FURTHER READING

Books and Reviews

Barksdale L: *Corynebacterium diphtheriae* and its relatives. Bacteriol Rev 34:378, 1970

Barksdale L: Immunobiology of diphtheria. In Nahmias AJ, O'Reilly RJ (eds): Immunology of Human Infection. New York, Plenum Publishing Corporation, 1981, pp 171–199

Barksdale L, Arden SB: Persisting bacteriophage infections, lysogeny, and phage conversions. Annu Rev Microbiol 28:265, 1974

Collier RJ: Diphtheria toxin: Mode of action and structure. Bacteriol Rev 39:54, 1975

Hewlett EL: Selective primary health care: Strategies for control of disease in the developing world. XVIII. Pertussis and diphtheria. Rev Infect Dis 7:426, 1985

Jones D, Collins MD: Irregular, nonsporing gram-positive rods. In Sneath PHA, Mair NS, Sharpe ME, Holt JG (eds): Bergey's Manual of Systematic Bacteriology, vol 2. Baltimore, Williams & Wilkins, 1986, pp 1261–1288

Lipsky BA, Goldberger AC, Tompkins LS, et al: Infections caused by nondiphtheria corynebacteria. Rev Infect Dis 4:1220, 1982

Murphy JR: The diphtheria toxin structural gene. Curr Top Microbiol Immunol 118:235, 1985

Neville DM Jr, Hudson TH: Transmembrane transport of diphtheria toxin, related toxins, and colicins. Annu Rev Biochem 55:195, 1986

Pappenheimer AM Jr: Diphtheria toxin. Annu Rev Biochem 46:69, 1977

Singer RA: Lysogeny and toxinogeny in *Corynebacterium diphtheriae.* In Bernheimer AW (ed): Mechanisms in Bacterial Toxinology. New York, John Wiley & Sons, 1976, pp 1–30

Washington JA II: Bacteriology, clinical spectrum of disease, and therapeutic aspects in coryneform bacterial infection. In Remington JS, Swartz MN (eds): Current Clinical Topics in Infectious Diseases. New York, McGraw-Hill, 1981, vol 2, pp 68–88

Selected Papers

Aguado JM, Ponte C, Soriano F: Bacteriuria with a multiply resistant species of *Corynebacterium* (*Corynebacterium* group D2): An unnoticed cause of urinary tract infection. J Infect Dis 156:144, 1987

Barile MF, Kolb RW, Pittman M: United States standard diphtheria toxin for the Schick test and the erythema potency assay for the Schick test dose. Infect Immun 4:295, 1971

Bayston R, Higgins J: Biochemical and cultural characteristics of "JK" coryneforms. J Clin Pathol 39:654, 1986

Bezjak V, Farsey SJ: *Corynebacterium diphtheriae* in skin lesions in Ugandan children. Bull WHO 43:643, 1970

Buck GA, Cross RE, Wong TP, et al: DNA relationships among some *tox*-bearing corynebacteriophages. Infect Immun 49:679, 1985

Buck GA, Groman NB: Genetic elements novel for *Corynebacterium diphtheriae:* Specialized transducing elements and transposons. J Bacteriol 148:143, 1981

Centers for Disease Control: Diphtheria, tetanus, and pertussis: Guidelines for vaccine prophylaxis and other preventive measures. Recommendation of the Immunization Practices Advisory Committee. Ann Intern Med 103:896, 1985

Chang MP, Baldwin RL, Bruce C, Wisnieski BJ: Second cytotoxic pathway of diphtheria toxin suggested by nuclease activity. Science 246:1165, 1989

Chang T-m, Neville DM Jr: Demonstration of diphtheria toxin receptors on surface membranes from both toxin-sensitive and toxin-resistant species. J Biol Chem 253:6866, 1978

Chen RT, Broome CV, Weinstein RA, et al: Diphtheria in the United States, 1971–81. Am J Public Health 75:1393, 1985

Cianciotto N, Rappuoli R, Groman N: Detection of homology to the beta bacteriophage integration site in a wide variety of *Corynebacterium* spp. J Bacteriol 168:103, 1986

Collier RJ, Kandel J: Structure and activity of diphtheria toxin. I. Thiol-dependent dissociation of a fraction of toxin into enzymatically active and inactive fragments. J Biol Chem 246:1496, 1971

Colombatti M, Greenfield L, Youle RJ: Cloned fragment of diphtheria toxin linked to T cell-specific antibody identifies regions of B chain active in cell entry. J Biol Chem 261:3030, 1986

Creagan RP: Genetic analysis of the cell surface: Association of human chromosome 5 with sensitivity to diphtheria toxin in mouse-human somatic cell hybrids. Proc Natl Acad Sci USA 72:2237, 1975

Dan M, Somer I, Knobel B, Gutman R: Cutaneous manifestations of infection with *Corynebacterium* group JK. Rev Infect Dis 10:1204, 1988

Donovan JJ, Simon MI, Montal M: Requirements for the translocation of diphtheria toxin fragment A across lipid membranes. J Biol Chem 260:8817, 1985

Drazin R, Kandel J, Collier RJ: Structure and activity of diphtheria toxin. II. Attack by trypsin at a specific site within the intact toxin molecule. J Biol Chem 246:1504, 1971

Fourel G, Phalipon A, Kaczorek M: Evidence for direct regulation of diphtheria toxin gene transcription by an Fe^{2+}-dependent DNA-binding repressor, Dtox R, in *Corynebacterium diphtheriae*. Infect Immun 57:3221, 1989

Gerry JL, Greenough WB III: Diphtheroid endocarditis: Report of nine cases and review of the literature. Johns Hopkins Med J 139:61, 1976

Gibson LF, Colman G: Diphthericin types, bacteriophage types and serotypes of *Corynebacterium diphtheriae* strains isolated in Australia. J Hyg (Camb) 71:679, 1973

Halsey N, Galazka A: The efficacy of DPT and oral poliomyelitis immunization schedules initiated from birth to 12 weeks of age. Bull WHO 63:1151, 1985

Holmes RK: Characterization and genetic mapping of nontoxicogenic (*tox*) mutants of corynebacteriophage beta. J Virol 19:195, 1976

Honjo T, Nishizuka Y, Kato I, et al: Adenosine diphosphate ribosylation of aminoacyl transferase II and inhibition of protein synthesis by diphtheria toxin. J Biol Chem 246:4251, 1971

Hranitzky KW, Durham DL, Hart DA, Eidels L: Role of glycosylation in expression of functional diphtheria toxin receptors. Infect Immun 49:336, 1985

Hu VW, Holmes RK: Evidence for direct insertion of fragments A and B of diphtheria toxin into model membranes. J Biol Chem 259:12226, 1984

Kagan BL, Finkelstein A, Colombini M: Diphtheria toxin fragment forms large pores in phospholipid bilayer membranes. Proc Natl Acad Sci USA 78:4950, 1981

Kandel J, Collier J, Chung DW: Interaction of fragment A from diphtheria toxin with nicotinamide adenine dinucleotide. J Biol Chem 249:2088, 1974

Keen JH, Maxfield FR, Hardegree MC, et al: Receptor-mediated endocytosis of diphtheria toxin by cells in culture. Proc Natl Acad Sci USA 79:2912, 1982

Laird W, Groman N: Orientation of the *tox* gene in the prophage of corynebacteriophage beta. J Virol 19:228, 1976

Larson EL, McGinley KJ, Leyden JJ, et al: Skin colonization with antibiotic-resistant (JK group) and antibiotic-sensitive lipophilic diphtheroids in hospitalized and normal adults. J Infect Dis 153:701, 1986

McCloskey RV, Saragea A, Maximescu P: Phage typing in diphtheria outbreaks in the southwestern United States, 1968–1971. J Infect Dis 126:196, 1972

McCloskey RV, Eller JJ, Green M, et al: The 1970 epidemic of diphtheria in San Antonio. Ann Intern Med 75:495, 1971

Miller LW, Bickham S, Jones WL, et al: Diphtheria carriers and effect of erythromycin therapy. Antimicrob Agents Chemother 6:166, 1974

Miller RA, Brancato F, Holmes KK: *Corynebacterium hemolyticum* as a cause of pharyngitis and scarlatiniform rash in young adults. Ann Intern Med 105:867, 1986

Moynihan MR, Pappenheimer AM Jr: Kinetics of adenosinediphosphoribosylation of elongation factor 2 in cells exposed to diphtheria toxin. Infect Immun 32:575, 1981

Murphy JR, Bacha P: Regulation of diphtheria toxin production. In Schlessinger D (ed): Microbiology-1979. Washington, D.C., American Society for Microbiology, 1979, p 181

Murphy JR, Skiver J, McBride G: Isolation and partial characterization of a corynebacteriophage β *tox* operator constitutive-like mutant lysogen of *Corynebacterium diphtheriae*. J Virol 18:235, 1976

Pappenheimer AM Jr, Harper AA, Moynihan M, et al: Diphtheria toxin and related proteins: Effect of route of injection on toxicity and the determination of cytotoxicity for various cultured cells. J Infect Dis 145:94, 1982

Pappenheimer AM Jr, Moynihan MR: Diphtheria toxin: A model for translocation of polypeptides across the plasma membrane. In Middlebrook JL, Kohn LD (eds): Receptor-Mediated Binding and Internalization of Toxins and Hormones. New York, Academic Press, 1981, p 31

Platts-Mills TAE, Ishizaka K: IgG and IgA diphtheria antitoxin responses from human tonsil lymphocytes. J Immunol 114:1058, 1975

Riebel W, Frantz N, Adelstein D, Spagnuolo PJ: *Corynebacterium* JK: A cause of nosocomial device-related infection. Rev Infect Dis 8:42, 1986

Rittenberg MB, Pinney CT Jr, Iglewski BH: Antigenic relationships on the diphtheria toxin molecule: Antitoxin versus antitoxoid. Infect Immun 14:122, 1976

Roblas RF, Prieto S, Santamaria M, et al: Activity of nine antimicrobial agents against *Corynebacterium* group D2 strains isolated from clinical specimens and skin. Antimicrob Agents Chemother 31:821, 1987

Rolf JM, Gaudin HM, Tirrell SM, et al: Anti-idiotypic antibodies that protect cells against the action of diphtheria toxin. Proc Natl Acad Sci USA 86:2036, 1989

Russell LM, Holmes RK: Highly toxinogenic but avirulent Park-Williams 8 strain of *Corynebacterium diphtheriae* does not produce siderophore. Infect Immun 47:575, 1985

Sandvig K, Olsnes S: Interactions between diphtheria toxin entry and anion transport in Vero cells. IV. Evidence that entry of diphtheria toxin is dependent on efficient anion transport. J Biol Chem 261:1570, 1986

Soriano F, Aguado JM, Ponte C, et al: Urinary tract infection caused by *Corynebacterium* group D2: Report of 82 cases and review. Rev Infect Dis 12:1019, 1990

Soriano F, Ponte C, Santamaría M, et al: In vitro and in vivo study of stone formation by *Corynebacterium* group D2 (*Corynebacterium urealyticum*). J Clin Microbiol 23:691, 1986

Van Ness BG, Howard JB, Bodley JW: ADP-ribosylation of elongation factor 2 by diphtheria toxin. J Biol Chem 255:10710, 1980

Welkos SL, Holmes RK: Regulation of toxinogenesis in *Corynebacterium diphtheriae*. J Virol 37:936, 1981

CHAPTER 31

Mycobacterium

Mycobacterium

The most distinctive property of organisms within the genus *Mycobacterium* is their characteristic staining. They stain with difficulty, but once stained, they are resistant to decolorization with acid alcohol. For this reason, they are often referred to as acid-fast bacilli. The genus contains a wide range of nutritional types, including saprophytic species that are present in the soil as well as parasitic organisms that have not been cultured in vitro. Within the genus are species responsible for two of the most dreaded diseases in the history of mankind—tuberculosis and leprosy. Both remain major public health priorities of many of the developing countries. A number of species that usually exist as environmental saprophytes are also causes of human infections and are now being seen with increasing frequency.

The mycobacteria are aerobic, slightly curved or straight rods 0.2 to 0.6 μm wide and 1.0 to 10 μm long. The most distinctive structure of the mycobacterial cell is its cell wall, a multilayered structure containing an abundance of complex lipids, some of which are unique to the mycobacteria and exhibit profound biologic effects in the host.

Because of tradition and their unique properties, the 1986 edition of *Bergey's Manual of Systematic Bacteriology* places the mycobacteria in a separate section and treats them as a distinctive family. The mycobacteria, however, have a number of important properties in common with the genera *Corynebacterium* and *Nocardia,* and the three genera are sometimes referred to as the CNM group because of this relatedness. All produce mycolic acid and have a similar guanine-plus-cytosine (G + C) content.

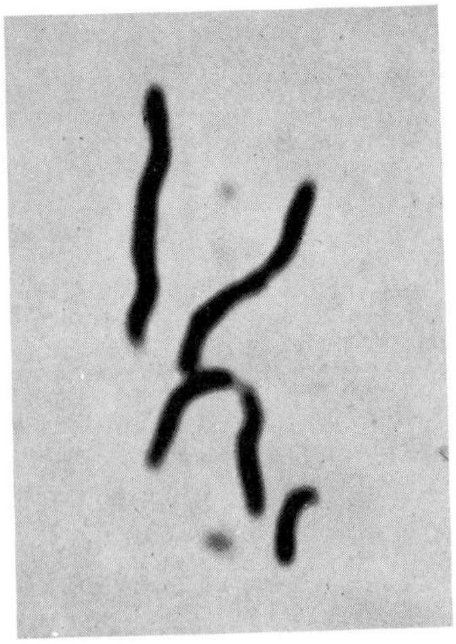

Fig. 31–1. Tubercle bacilli stained uniformly by the Ziehl-Neelsen method. × 3600, *(From Yegian and Kurung: Am Rev Tuberc 56:36, 1947.)*

Mycobacterium tuberculosis

Tuberculosis is an ancient disease, recognizable in skeletons from the Stone Age and in bones from some of the early Egyptian mummies. Although the infectious nature of tuberculosis was established by Villemin around 1865, the protean nature of its clinical manifestations delayed understanding of the disease until Koch's discovery of the causative agent in 1882. Koch always found the organism associated with the clinical disease, isolated it in pure culture, reproduced the disease in animals, and recovered the bacillus in pure culture from the experimentally infected animals. For the last century, these rigid requirements—referred to as Koch's postulates—have provided criteria considered essential for the complete acceptance of a particular microorganism as the cause of a specific infectious disease.

Morphology

M. tuberculosis is a slender, straight, or slightly curved rod with rounded ends. The organisms vary in width from 0.3 to 0.6 μm and in length from 1 to 4 μm. True branching, occasionally seen in old cultures and in smears from caseous lymph nodes, may also be produced in vitro under specific cultural conditions.

The bacilli are acid-fast, nonsporogenous, and nonencapsulated. The Ziehl-Neilsen acid-fast stain is useful in staining organisms either from cultures or from clinical material. With this stain, the bacilli appear as brilliantly staining red rods against a blue background (Fig. 31–1). Organisms in tissue and sputum smears often stain irregularly and have a beaded appearance, presumably because of their vacuoles and polyphosphate content (Fig. 31–2). Although the acid-fastness of mycobacteria is attributable to their lipid content, the physical integrity of the cell is also essential. The best explanation of the acid-fastness of mycobacteria is based on a lipid-barrier principle, according to which an increased hydrophobicity of the surface layers follows the complexing of dye with mycolic acid residues that are present in the cell wall. This prevents exit of carbolfuchsin that has become trapped in the interior of the cell.

Tubercle bacilli are difficult to stain with the Gram stain; although they are usually considered to be gram-positive, staining is poor and irregular because of failure of the dye to penetrate the cell wall. Gram stains of clinical material are thus invalid for the identification of mycobacteria.

Mycobacterial Cell Wall. Electron micrographs of thin sections show a thick wall composed of three layers enclosing a plasma membrane that is also a three-layered structure. Chemically, the wall is very complex and unlike that of either gram-positive or gram-negative organisms. It contains an abundance of complex lipophilic macromolecules, many of which are unique to the organism and are biologically very

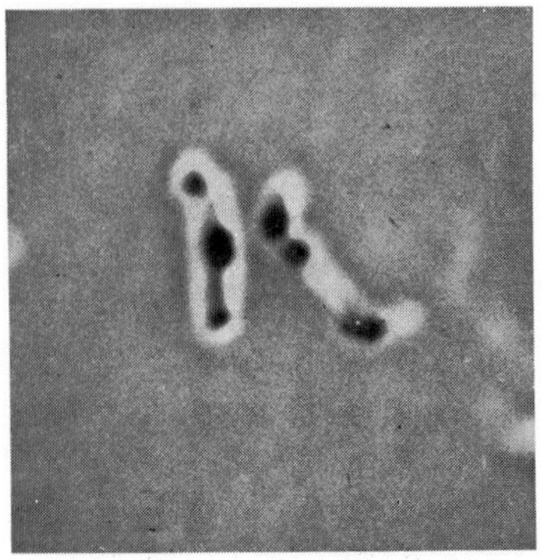

Fig. 31–2. Tubercle bacilli. The protoplasm of the bacillus has been stained by the Ziehl-Neelsen method and the unstained cell wall outlined by the addition of nigrosin. × 3600 *(From Yegian and Vanderlinde: J Bacteriol 54:777, 1947.)*

active. Lipids account for approximately 60% of the dry weight of the wall and confer properties that enable the organism to resist adverse environmental conditions.

The backbone of the mycobacterial cell wall is a covalent structure consisting of two polymers covalently linked by phosphodiester bonds, a peptidoglycan and an arabinogalactan. To this covalent structure are attached a large number of other complex materials (Chap. 6, p. 81). Three features distinguish the peptidoglycans of mycobacteria: (1) the presence of *N*-glycolylmuramic acid instead of the usual *N*-acetyl derivative, (2) the presence of two amide groups, on both glutamate and *meso*-diaminopimelic acid (DAP) in the peptides of the repeating subunit, and (3) the presence of two kinds of interpeptide linkage: D-ala—*meso*-DAP and *meso*-DAP—DAP. As much as 70% of the cross-linking in the peptidoglycan consists of interpeptide bridges between *meso*-DAP residues. Interpeptide bridges of this type appear to occur only in the mycobacteria. A unit of the mycobacterial peptidoglycan is shown in Fig. 31–3.

The peptidoglycan is linked to the arabinogalactan polymer by phosphodiester linkages between muramic acid residues and an arabinose of the arabinogalactan. About one in ten of the arabinose residues of the polymer is esterified by a molecule of mycolic acid. The terminal branches of the arabinogalactan are linear oligosaccharides, which constitute the main immunogenic determinant of the molecule. An oligomer of the cell wall, Wax D, is of special interest because of its immunoadjuvant activity (p. 502).

A large number of other materials are also associated with the mycolate-arabinogalactan-peptidoglycan complex. Crude cell walls contain large amounts of most protein amino acids, which are probably present in the wall as lipoproteins or glycolipoproteins. These peptide-containing constituents are essential for tuberculin activity of wall preparations. One of the most abundant polypeptides, a partly amidated poly-

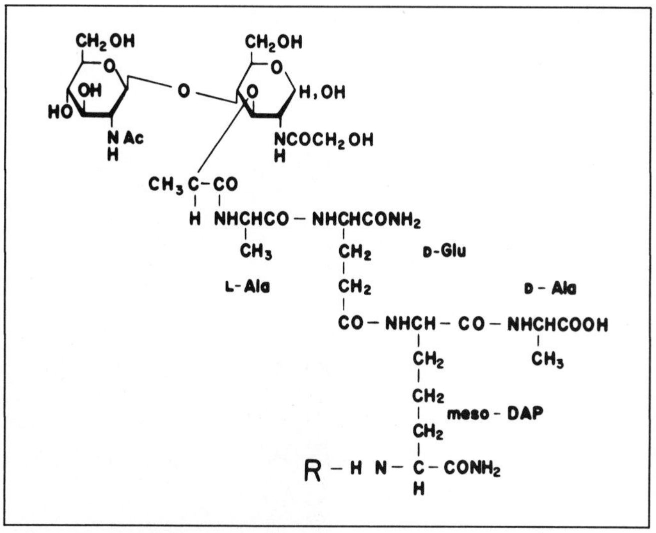

Fig. 31–3. Mycobacterial peptidoglycan unit consisting of *N*-acetylglucosamine, muramic acid, L-alanine, D-glutamic acid, *meso*-diaminopimelic acid, and D-alanine. R, Another unit beginning with an interpeptide bridge between the *meso*-DAP (shown) and a second *meso*-DAP linked in turn to D-Glu, L-Ala, and additional amino acids. *(From Barksdale and Kim: Bacteriol Rev 41:217, 1977.)*

α-L-glutamic acid, is of special interest because it is present in human and bovine tubercle bacilli but is lacking in saprophytic species. In some strains, it accounts for up to 8% of the total weight of the wall.

In addition to the glycolipids bound to the peptidoglycan, other important lipid substances are present on the cell surface. The three most important of these are cord factor (trehalose 6, 6′-dimycolate), sulfatides, and mycosides, all of which have specific biologic activity (p. 503).

Physiology

Cultural Characteristics. *M. tuberculosis* is an obligate aerobe and will not grow in the absence of oxygen. Even a small reduction in the oxygen tension results in an appreciable decrease in the rate of growth. Tubercle bacilli will grow on a very simple synthetic medium, but for primary isolation from clinical material, a more complex medium containing either an egg-potato base or a serum-agar base is required. The organisms are very slow growing even under optimal growth conditions, and 10 to 20 days of incubation at 37C is required before growth can be visualized. Colonies are small, dry, and scaly in appearance. In synthetic liquid media the hydrophobic properties of the organism's cell surface result in a pellicle growth that is confined to the surface of the medium. The addition to broth media of the nonionic detergent Tween 80 (polyoxyethylene derivative of sorbitan monooleate) deters aggregation of cells and permits them to grow diffusely and to be assayed turbidimetrically. Aeration of cultures by rotary shaking markedly increases the growth rate and shortens the lag phase of growth. Growth is also enhanced by an increased CO_2 tension. The optimal pH for growth is 7.0 but a pH range of 6.0 to 7.6 will permit growth. For *M. tuberculosis* the optimal temperature is 37C, but for a number of other mycobacteria species the optimal temperature corresponds to the body temperature of their specific natural host, a property that must be taken into account in their isolation from clinical material.

Metabolism. The mycobacteria are strictly aerobic organisms that fulfill their energy requirements by the complete oxidation of glucose or glycerol to carbon dioxide and water. Glycerol is the preferred carbon and energy source. Although both Embden-Meyerhof (EMP) and pentose phosphate pathways are present, the EMP pathway is used predominantly. The tricarboxylic acid (TCA) and glyoxylate cycles are operative, and three distinct respiratory chains using molecular oxygen as terminal electron acceptor have been described. Catalase and peroxidase are present in all mycobacteria for the disposal of hydrogen peroxide generated in the final reaction of the terminal respiratory chain. Catalases that are different with respect to their heat stability have been identified in various species of the mycobacteria (p. 511).

Under optimal culture conditions, the doubling time of tubercle bacilli is 14 to 15 hours. This is also the in vivo generation time calculated from experimentally infected animals.

OXYGEN REQUIREMENT. Oxygen is critical for the growth of *M. tuberculosis*, both in vitro and in vivo. This is demonstrated very clearly by a comparison of growth curves of Tween 80–grown organisms in aerated vs nonaerated cultures. In cultures well aerated by constant shaking, the growth pattern is exponential. In nonaerated cultures, an initial period of exponential growth is followed by an arithmetic linear growth period in which the bacilli replicate in the upper oxygen-rich portion of the medium at a rate that is just balanced by the rate at which the bacilli settle toward the bottom of the tube. During the settling process the organisms adapt to survival under anaerobic conditions; when resuspended in an oxygen-rich medium, they exhibit synchronous replication. The resting bacilli in this system may be analogous to the condition of tubercle bacilli lying quiescent in the host but retaining the potential of proliferating and producing overt disease after years of latency. In the in vitro system, adaptation to dormant survival under anaerobic conditions is accompanied by a marked shift to the anaplerotic glyoxylate bypass as oxygen becomes limiting. Also brought into play is a unique glycine dehydrogenase that catalyzes reductive deamination in *M. tuberculosis*. Diversion of glycine and TCA cycle intermediates to glyoxylate synthesis serves mainly to provide a substrate for the regeneration of NAD that may be required for the orderly shutdown before oxygen limitation stops growth completely.

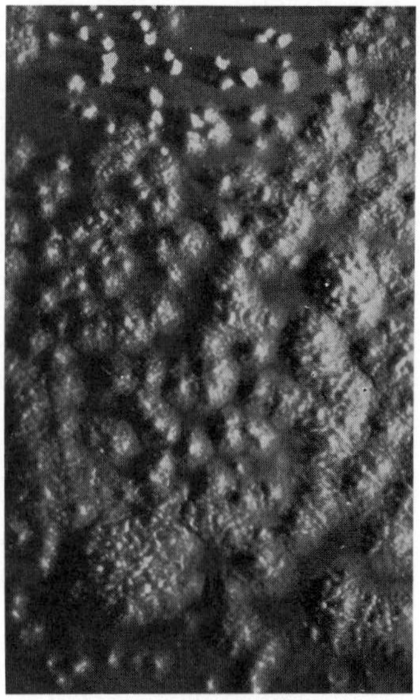

Fig. 31–4. Rough colonies of the human virulent strain H37 Rv. *(Grown by William Steenken, photographed by Joseph Kurung.)*

NUTRITIONAL REQUIREMENTS. Tubercle bacilli are prototrophic for all the amino acids, purine and pyrimidine bases, and B-complex vitamins. After primary isolation, they adapt readily to growth on simple salt solutions with ammonium ion as the nitrogen source and glucose as a source of carbon. The most important source of carbon is glycerol, and asparagine is the preferred nitrogen source.

IRON ASSIMILATION. Trace metal deficiencies have observable consequences on the structure and metabolism of the mycobacteria. Especially pronounced are those caused by a deficiency of iron. The insoluble nature of iron at physiologic pH values has resulted in the evolution of systems for its transport into the cell. Because of the thick lipid-rich cell wall of the mycobacteria, the system employs two iron-chelating components: (1) an extracellular water-soluble compound, exochelin, which can rob iron from ferritin (storage form of iron in the mammalian cell), and (2) mycobactin, a lipophilic molecule located in discrete regions of the cell envelope close to the cytoplasmic membrane. In the model proposed, ferric iron in the extracellular milieu is solubilized by exochelins, which then act in concert with mycobactin to transport the iron through the wall. Mycobactin, originally isolated from *Mycobacterium phlei* as a growth factor for *Mycobacterium paratuberculosis*, is present in all mycobacteria and appears to be confined to this genus (Chap. 5, p. 60). The basic mycobactin molecule varies only slightly from species to species.

Genetics. Genetic studies on the mycobacteria have been greatly hampered by the slow growth of the organism. Although the existence of genetic variation within members of the group is well recognized, only in the case of drug resistance have the observed phenomena been subjected to critical genetic analysis. With the use of fluctuation test analysis for the calculation of mutation rates, mutations are observed to occur in *M. tuberculosis* at very low frequencies comparable to those of other bacteria.

Another commonly observed class of spontaneous mutations is that causing alterations in colony morphology. Different colonial types are observable between strains as well as within a species. Smooth (S) and rough (R) variants of tubercle bacilli have been described. With few exceptions, virulent organisms produce R colonies (Fig. 31–4), but avirulent strains may also produce colonies of the R type (Fig. 31–5). The best example of this is the H37 strain of *M. tuberculosis* which, by manipulation of culture conditions, has been dissociated into the rough virulent (Rv) and rough avirulent (Ra) variants. Although both variants are rough, their colonial morphology on both egg and liquid media is different and characteristic. These classic strains have been extensively used in experimental studies for more than 50 years.

Mycobacteriophages. Numerous phages with activities on many mycobacterial species, including *M. tuberculosis*, have been isolated from both clinical and environmental sources. Soil, human excreta, polluted water, and biopsy specimens of patients with sarcoid and lung cancer are among the sources that have yielded phages on each of several occasions. Myco-

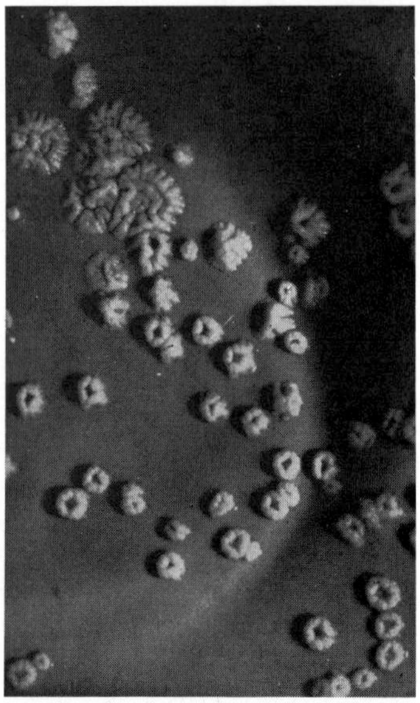

Fig. 31–5. Rough colonies of the human avirulent strain H37 Ra. Note the large, flatter, intermediate colonies. *(Grown by William Steenken, photographed by Joseph Kurung.)*

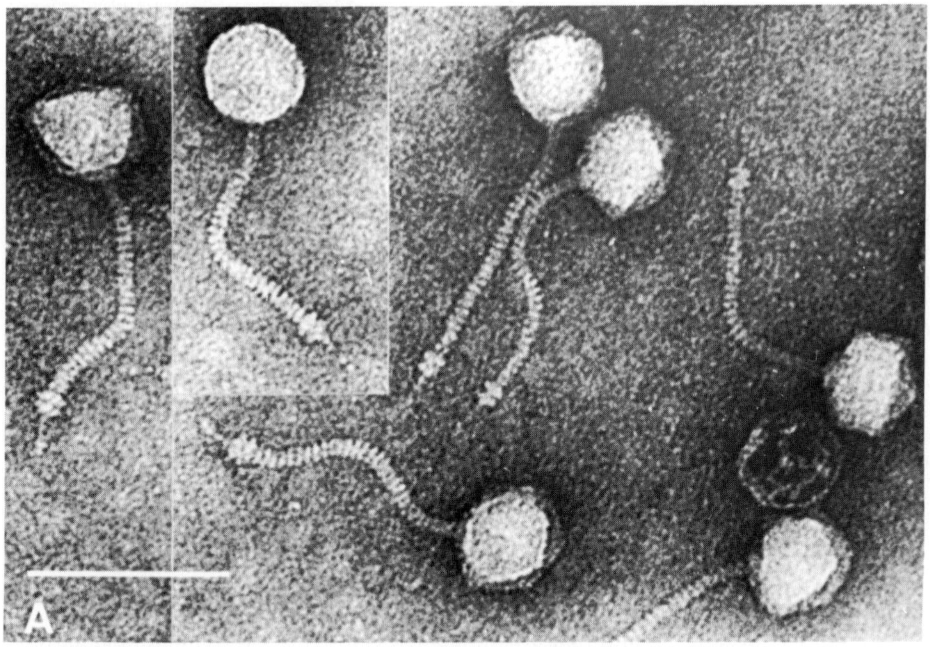

Fig. 31–6. Mycobacteriophage MC-1. As with most mycobacteriophages, the symmetrical hexagonal head suggests an icosahedron. The long, noncontractile tail exhibits distinct cross-striations and ends in a single fiber extending from the tail plates. × 270,000. Bar = 0.1 μm. *(From Barksdale and Kim: Bacteriol Rev 41:217, 1977.)*

bacteriophages are double-stranded DNA phages with a G + C content similar to that of the host bacterium. Most of them possess a hexagonal or oval head and a long noncontractile tail (Fig. 31–6).

In addition to protein, some mycobacteriophages, including a phage grown on the host strain *M. tuberculosis* H37 Rv, also contain lipid. A high percentage of the lipid in the H37 Rv phage is phospholipid and appears to be newly synthesized. The mycobacteriophage lipids appear to be present as a bilayer membranelike structure essential for maintaining the structural integrity and infectivity of the phage.

In *Mycobacterium smegmatis,* the peptidoglycolipid, mycoside C, serves as a phage receptor, but in *M. tuberculosis* the specific phage receptor has not been characterized. Although basic information on the mycobacterial host-virus relationship is still extremely limited, mycobacteriophages may either multiply within their hosts, thereby causing cell death by lysis, or establish a nonlytic lysogenic relationship with the host. Pseudolysogeny is also particularly common in the mycobacteria. The establishment of lysogeny induces changes in various biologic properties of mycobacteria: colony morphology, growth rate, enzymic activity, and antigenic composition. Virulence, however, does not appear to be conditioned by the lysogenic state.

BACTERIOPHAGE TYPING. Phage typing as a tool for the classification of mycobacteria is of limited value because the host range of many mycobacteriophages is not restricted to the species of the propagator strain. In the species *M. tuberculosis,* however, which comprises a single homogeneous serotype, bacteriophage typing offers a potentially valuable tool for genetic and epidemiologic studies. *M. tuberculosis* is divisible into several types on the basis of their susceptibility to lysis by bacteriophages. The original scheme separated all freshly isolated strains into three major and one intermediate phage types (A, B, C, I). The geographic distribution of the phage types varies considerably, suggesting that the major phage types form distinct groups within *M. tuberculosis* rather than minor mutational variants. Type A predominates in west and central Africa, Uganda, Japan, and Hong Kong. Types A and B are common in Europe and North America, and type C occurs predominantly in the United States. Type I, as well as type A, is common in India but is rare elsewhere. Strains of phage type I are of special interest because they differ from the other types in a number of properties, including virulence, lipid content, and susceptibility to various antibacterial agents. Phage types are very stable, the mutation rate to resistance to a single phage being less than 1.3×10^{-8}. Mutation to drug resistance in *M. tuberculosis* is not associated with a change in phage type.

Useful epidemiologic information on the spread of tubercle bacilli from person to person may be provided by phage typing. One of the most interesting findings is that a person may be concurrently infected with more than one phage type. An examination of sputum from a large number of Eskimo patients showed that 14% contained more than one phage type of organism. Although members of the *M. tuberculosis* complex (*M. tuberculosis, M. bovis, M. africanum, M. microti*) cannot be distinguished by phage typing, one phage, 33D, has the useful property of distinguishing the bovine strain bacillus Calmette-Guerin (BCG) from other strains of tubercle bacilli by its inability to lyse BCG. Since BCG is used as an immunostimulant in tumor therapy and in vaccination against tuberculosis, its rapid identification would be helpful to the clinician.

Resistance. Tubercle bacilli are highly resistant to drying. Cultures maintained at 37C have been found both viable and virulent after storage for 12 years. The environment in which bacilli are found is an important factor in their viability. When exposed to direct sunlight, organisms from cultures are killed in 2 hours, but bacilli contained in sputum require an exposure of 20 to 30 hours. Bacilli remain viable for as long as 6 to 8 months in dried sputum protected from direct sunlight. The tubercle bacillus is generally more resistant to chemical disinfection than other non-spore-formers, especially when present in sputum. However, they possess no greater resistance to moist heat than other bacteria and are killed by pasteurization temperatures.

Antigenic Structure

Mycobacteria contain many unique immunoreactive substances, most of which are components of the cell wall. In spite of intensive study for more than 50 years, however, the antigenic composition of *M. tuberculosis* is not clearly defined. Few antigens that compose this complex mosaic have been obtained in chemically pure form to permit full evaluation of their immunologic potential. Since protective immunity to mycobacterial infections is mediated primarily by the cellular arm of the immune system, proteins are regarded as the key immunogens.

Old Tuberculin. Old tuberculin (OT) is the original test reagent for the tuberculin test, a diagnostic skin test for tuberculosis infection. First described by Koch in 1881, tuberculin is an antigenically crude extract prepared from 6-week-old broth cultures by boiling the culture, filtering off the organisms, and concentrating the filtrate tenfold by steaming. The active component of this preparation is a heat-stable protein.

Purified Protein Derivative. Purified protein derivative (PPD) is a partially purified preparation of OT prepared by ammonium sulfate fractionation. The product consists primarily of a mixture of small tuberculoproteins (2 and 9 kDa, respectively) in contrast to the 32 kDa of the native immunogenic tuberculoprotein. One large batch of PPD, made by Seibert in 1939, has been designated PPD-S and adopted by the World Health Organization as the International PPD-Tuberculin. Currently, PPD is the test reagent used for tuberculin skin testing (p. 507).

Purified Antigens. Although tuberculin has been invaluable for immunodiagnostic purposes, its complex and ill-defined composition and lack of specificity for *M. tuberculosis* have considerably limited its usefulness. Numerous attempts have been made during the past several decades to isolate more species-specific protein antigens, but all efforts using classic methods of purification have been unsuccessful. Modern technology, however, has provided new approaches for the identification and purification of mycobacterial antigens. Among the most promising of these are (1) use of recombinant DNA techniques and antigen expression in *Escherichia coli* and (2) affinity purification of antigen preparations using monoclonal antibody immunoadsorbent columns. With these approaches a large number of monoclonal antibodies that react with *M. tuberculosis* antigens have been raised. Some of the reagents have been used to create new serodiagnostic assays for tuberculosis and to screen genomic DNA libraries of *M. tuberculosis* in a bacteriophage expression vector. The recombinant antigens isolated by genetic engineering have been used to define the reactivity of specific T cell clones derived from patients with tuberculosis.

One of the purified mycobacterial antigens of special interest is the 65 kDa antigen. This is a highly immunoreactive protein capable of eliciting a strong delayed-type hypersensitivity reaction in experimental animals. In humans, antibodies and T cells directed against the 65 kDa antigen can be isolated from persons infected with *M. tuberculosis* or *M. leprae*. The 65 kDa antigen is a member of an antigenically related family of proteins, the heat shock proteins (HSP), which are widely distributed in nature. There is also evidence that this protein has an etiologic role in autoimmune disease, a role based on the molecular mimicry between the 65 kDa mycobacterial HSP and a number of human proteins.

Polysaccharides. The protein-free polysaccharides (arabinogalactans and arabinomannans) are immunogenic and serologically active. They elicit immediate skin reactions in sensitized guinea pigs but do not elicit delayed-type hypersensitivity. Polysaccharides give precipitin reactions with antisera and are active in complement fixation and hemagglutination reactions. The significance of these humoral antibodies, however, has not been established.

Phosphatidyl Inositol Mannosides. The phosphatidyl inositol mannosides (PIMs) are a family of amphipathic polar lipids present in the plasma membrane of mycobacteria and related organisms. They serve an important structural role, providing a noncovalent link between the membrane and cell wall. Although purified PIMs are primarily haptenic, in the host they are undoubtedly presented in an immunogenic form and are serologically active. In the past, the major interest in this group of glycolipids has focused on their use as potential serodiagnostic agents. More recently, however, with the purification of an antigenic lipoarabinomannan from *M. tuberculosis* and a similar one from *Mycobacterium leprae,* there is renewed interest in these components and the belief that they are important lipoteichoic acidlike polymers with a role in macrophage recognition and perhaps in cross-protective immunity.

Other Immunoreactive Components

WAX D AND MURAMYLDIPEPTIDE (MDP). The waxes D are a heterogeneous group of peptidoglycolipids composed of all of the components of the cell wall (Chap. 6, p. 81). When extracted from *M. tuberculosis,* they have unique adjuvant activity in that they not only enhance antibody production against a protein antigen incorporated in a wax D water-in-oil emulsion but also induce a cell-mediated immune response against the protein. Wax D duplicates the adjuvant activity of Freund's complete adjuvant, a water-in-oil emulsion of dead mycobacterial cells widely used in immunologic studies. The immunotherapeutic effects of *M. bovis* BCG in producing regression of certain tumors are due to the adjuvant activity of their cell walls.

The least common denominator of adjuvant activity of wax D is muramyl dipeptide (MDP), *N*-acetyl-muramyl-L-alanyl-D-isoglutamine (p. 499). When MDP is combined with trehalose dimycolate, the combination possesses synergistic immunostimulatory activity and is highly effective against certain tumors and infections that do not respond to either compound alone.

TREHALOSE-6,6′-DIMYCOLATE. Often referred to as the cord factor because of its association with the cording tendency of virulent tubercle bacilli (Chap. 6, p. 82), trehalose-6,6′-dimycolate has a number of immunoreactive properties, including adjuvant activity. It elicits extensive pulmonary granulomas of the foreign body type, which are also associated with some level of protection against challenge with virulent *M. tuberculosis*. Cord factor activates the alternative complement pathway and is endowed with demonstrable antitumor properties. A further discussion of cord factor is found below.

SULFATIDES. Sulfatides, sulfur-containing glycolipids often referred to as sulfolipids, are trehalose 2′-sulfates esterified with long-chain fatty acids (Chap. 6, p. 82). Primarily of interest because of their association with neutral red reactivity of virulent *M. tuberculosis* strains, the sulfatides, although lacking adjuvant activity, can effectively replace cord factor as a component of an oil-BCG cell wall or endotoxin preparation causing tumor regression. Although intralesional injection of tumors with mutant *Salmonella* endotoxin admixed with sulfatide gives high cure rates, its specific role in immunostimulation may be a minor one attributable to its amphipathic properties. For further discussion of the sulfatides see below.

Determinants of Pathogenicity

M. tuberculosis produces neither exotoxins nor endotoxins. No single structure, antigen, or mechanism can explain the virulence of the organism. There is likewise no simple in vitro test based on colony morphology or serologic differences that can distinguish a virulent tubercle bacillus from its avirulent variant, a distinction that can be provided only by virulence testing in animals. A number of properties, however, are usually associated with the capacity of virulent strains of *M. tuberculosis* to produce progressive disease; although none of these, either singly or together, can account completely for virulence, each undoubtedly plays a crucial role in the pathogenesis of infection.

Cord Factor. There is a high correlation between the virulence of strains of tubercle bacilli and their morphologic appearance in culture in the form of serpentine cords consisting of bacilli in close parallel arrangements (Fig. 31–7). Attenuated and avirulent forms grow in a random brush-heap pattern without this characteristic orientation (Fig. 31–8).

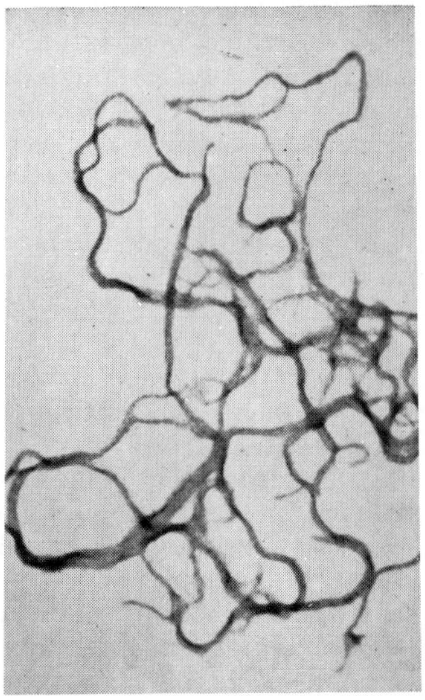

Fig. 31–7. Cord growth of virulent H37 Rv. *(From Yegian and Kurung: Am Rev Tuberc 65:181, 1952.)*

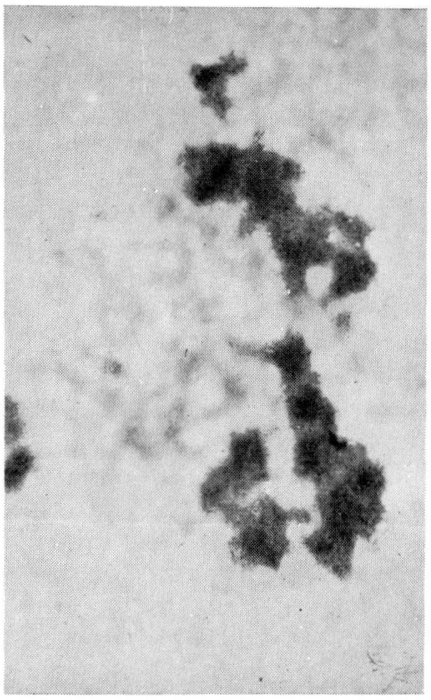

Fig. 31–8. Absence of cord growth with avirulent H37 Ra. *(From Yegian and Kurung: Am Rev Tuberc 65:181, 1952.)*

Growth in cords can be correlated with the presence of the glycolipid trehalose 6,6′-dimycolate peripherally located in the organism (p. 31 and Chap. 6, p. 81). A number of biologic responses to mycobacterial infection can be duplicated by treatment with this material. It has a peculiar and characteristic toxicity for mice, inhibits migration of polymorphonuclear leukocytes, elicits granuloma formation, and stimulates protection against virulent infection. Cord factor also attacks mitochondrial membranes, causing functional damage to respiration and oxidative phosphorylation. In spite of these varied activities of cord factor, its specific role in the pathogenesis of tuberculosis is unknown.

Sulfatides. Sulfatides are peripherally located glycolipids responsible for the neutral red reactivity associated with virulent strains of *M. tuberculosis*. A significant correlation has also been demonstrated between the elaboration of sulfatides in culture and the rank order of virulence for the guinea pig among a series of wild-type strains spanning a broad spectrum of virulence. Although sulfatides are not toxic themselves, when administered simultaneously with cord factor, they potentiate synergistically the toxicity of cord factor. Sulfatides are readily endocytosed by macrophages in culture and, from within secondary lysosomes, inhibit fusion of these organelles with phagosomes. Thus since *M. tuberculosis* is an intracellular parasite, it may promote its own survival within the host by acting from within phagosomes to prevent phagolysosome formation, thus avoiding exposure to the lysosomal hydrolases.

Clinical Infection

Epidemiology. Tuberculosis is a global problem. Although effective methods for its control are available and have been applied successfully for several decades, in some regions the prevalence of tuberculosis is still inordinately high, and a plateau in reduction of incidence is evident. Tuberculosis also remains the leading cause of death among notifiable infectious diseases.

At the present time, there are an estimated 8 to 10 million

new cases of tuberculosis each year throughout the world and about 3 million deaths. Whereas the annual case rate in the United States in 1989 was 9.5 per 100,000, the rates in many developing countries, especially in some areas of Africa, Asia, and Oceania, often exceed 300 per 100,000. The large numbers of immigrants entering the United States from the developing countries bring with them rates of tuberculosis similar to those seen in their native countries. These newcomers pose a serious public health problem.

Tuberculosis is not evenly distributed throughout the population. In the United States certain groups are known to have a high incidence: blacks, Asians and Pacific Islanders, American Indians and Alaskan natives, and Hispanics. Also at greater risk are current or former prison inmates, alcoholics, intravenous drug users, the elderly, and foreign-born persons from areas of the world with a high prevalence of the disease. The tuberculosis case rates are influenced by the race, sex, and age of the population group (Fig. 31–9). Nearly two thirds of all cases of tuberculosis occur in racial and ethnic minorities. Fifty years ago the death rate from tuberculosis in the United States was exceedingly high in infants, adolescents, and young adults and relatively low among persons in late middle and old age. With improved standards of living and the adoption of control measures, a high percentage of the open carriers of tubercle bacilli have been identified and treated. This has resulted in a sharp reduction of deaths in infancy, adolescence, and the early years of adult life. However, the influence of puberty on the activation of clinical disease is still apparent. Fifty years ago the death rate for females was always higher than that of males in all age groups and all races. This is no longer true. The highest death rates now occur in nonwhite and white men past the age of 30 and in nonwhite and white women past the age of 60.

Since 1984 there has not been the steady decline in case rate that had been witnessed annually for the past 100 years. In 1990, 23,720 new cases of tuberculosis were reported to the Centers for Disease Control. There is considerable variation in the new case rate by states. Before 1984 the highest case rates were concentrated in a broad band across the southeastern United States and in states with Indian reservations. These rates reflected the influence of low socioeconomic status on the activation of clinical disease. Poverty and tuberculosis have always been close allies. Since 1984 the largest increases have occurred among blacks and white Hispanics in the 25- to 44-year age group (Fig. 31–9). Nearly two thirds of all cases of tuberculosis occur in racial and ethnic minorities. The increase has been especially marked in areas where there is a high incidence of human immunodeficiency virus (HIV) infection, such as New York City, Florida, and California (Fig. 31–10). HIV infection is now the strongest known risk factor for the development of active, frequently disseminated tuberculosis. It is estimated that the rate of tuberculosis in patients with AIDS is 100 times that in the general population.

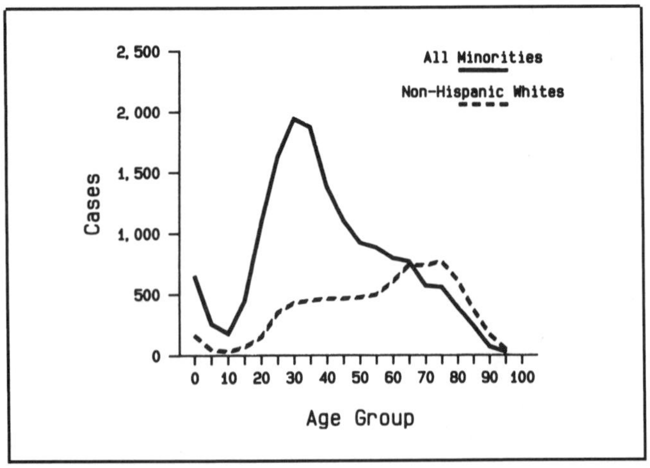

Fig. 31–9. Frequency distribution of tuberculosis cases by age, race, and ethnicity, United States, 1989. *(From Centers for Disease Control: MMWR 38(54):45, 1989.)*

Tuberculosis spreads in an epidemic wave similar to that seen with other infectious diseases, but with a time course measured in decades instead of weeks. Morbidity and mortality rates rise steeply, peak, and then show a more gradual decline. The present worldwide tuberculosis epidemic began in England in the sixteenth century. Since then, large epidemics have been precipitated when tubercle bacilli were introduced for the first time into groups or races that had never been exposed to the infection. The Alaskan Indians and Eskimos are only now emerging from a major epidemic that has persisted on a high level for about 100 years.

TRANSMISSION. Tuberculous infection is acquired primarily by the inhalation of dried residues of droplets containing tubercle bacilli that have been expelled in an aerosol created in coughing, sneezing, or talking. These droplet nuclei remain suspended in the air for prolonged periods, and those particles 1 to 10 μm in diameter are sufficiently small to reach the alveoli and initiate infection. The most important source is the infectious person with undiagnosed cavitary tuberculosis. Patients receiving effective chemotherapy rapidly lose their infectiousness for other persons.

Although still a problem in some parts of the world, bovine tuberculosis caused by *M. bovis* is an uncommon disease in the United States today. *M. bovis* infection results from the drinking of contaminated milk and can be prevented by milk pasteurization and the slaughter of all infected cattle. Tuberculous infection may also be acquired by direct inoculation of abraded skin by pathologists and laboratory personnel handling contaminated tissues.

RISK OF TUBERCULOUS INFECTION VERSUS TUBERCULOUS DISEASE. Humans are very susceptible to tuberculous infection but remarkably resistant to tuberculous disease. Although the prevalence of tuberculous infection as estimated by tuberculin testing of sample populations, has demonstrated that both geographic and socioeconomic characteristics affect the risk of infection, in all cases the risk factors appear to be related to the likelihood of coming into contact with an infectious case. The degree of infectiousness of the source case is the chief factor that determines whether or not a contact will become infected.

Tuberculosis is less infectious than the common communicable diseases of childhood. Frequent and fairly prolonged association with an infectious patient is usually required for infection. Recent reports indicate that at present only 22% of household associates of all ages are infected. Although the household contacts of an infected adult or adolescent patient are at greatest risk, small epidemics within certain closed environments have been attributed to schoolteachers, students, or bus drivers who were unusually good spreaders of infection. In one well-studied epidemic in Denmark, a schoolteacher

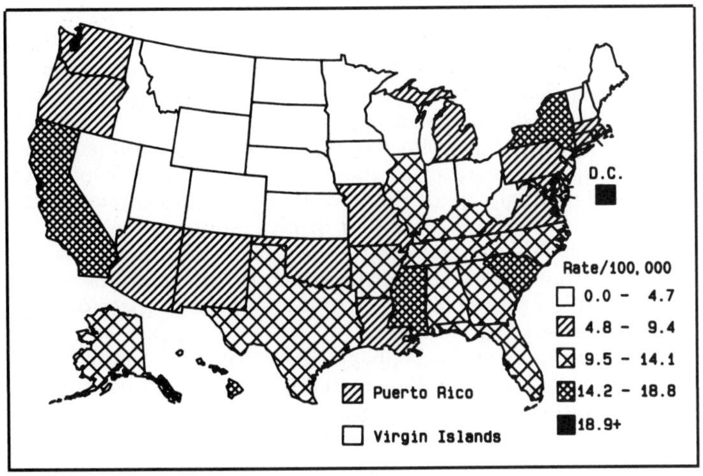

Fig. 31–10. Case rates of tuberculosis by state, United States, 1989. *(From Centers for Disease Control: MMWR 38(54):44, 1989.)*

infected 70 of 105 tuberculin-negative students. After infection, 41 of the 105 developed primary infections demonstrable by x-ray and cultures and 15 of the students developed postprimary progressive tuberculosis during the next 12 years. Tuberculosis has become an increasingly greater problem in correctional institutions where the environment is often conducive to airborne transmission of infection among inmates and staff. Nursing homes for the elderly and shelters for the homeless also provide a high-risk situation for the transmission of tuberculosis and the occurrence of microepidemics.

It has been estimated that for all persons newly infected with tubercle bacilli, about 5% will have clinical disease within a year of their infection. The remainder carry a lifelong risk of potential disease. Risk factors for development of tuberculous disease after infection are primarily intrinsic characteristics of the individual, such as age, sex, body build, and genetic susceptibility. In addition, the following special risk factors predispose to disease among infected persons: use of adrenocorticosteroids and other immunosuppressive agents, hematologic and reticuloendothelial diseases that suppress cellular immunity, diabetes mellitus, and silicosis. Patients with HIV infection or those at risk of HIV infection, particularly intravenous drug abusers, also have a higher than expected tuberculosis attack rate, especially extrapulmonary and disseminated forms.

Pathogenesis. The response of a person after exposure to virulent tubercle bacilli depends on an interplay of two major immunologic responses: acquired cellular immunity and delayed hypersensitivity. The emergence of hypersensitivity to the proteins of the tubercle bacillus is responsible for the tissue destruction characteristic of the disease. Sensitization appears about 3 to 4 weeks after infection and is detected by the tuberculin test. Once a person converts to a tuberculin-positive reaction, he or she usually remains sensitive as long as viable organisms remain in the body (p. 507).

Individual responses after exposure are thus determined by the previous immunologic experience with the tubercle bacillus. The initial infection with *M. tuberculosis* is referred to as a primary infection. Subsequent disease in a previously sensitized person, either from an exogenous source or by reactivation of a primary infection, is known as secondary or reinfection tuberculosis.

PRIMARY INFECTION. After inhalation of virulent tubercle bacilli in droplet nuclei, the organisms reach the alveolar spaces where they are phagocytosed by alveolar macrophages. Within the macrophages, bacterial multiplication proceeds with minimal reaction and spreads to the regional nodes in the hilum of the lung and thence into the bloodstream, with a seeding of bacteria in almost all parts of the body. Asymptomatic lymphohematogenous dissemination of the primary infection occurs before the acquisition of tuberculin hypersensitivity and sets the stage for later "reactivation" to present clinically as pulmonary or extrapulmonary disease. Circulating bacilli are efficiently cleared from the bloodstream by reticuloendothelial organs, but bacterial multiplication continues in the apices of the lungs and to a lesser extent in the kidneys, vascular skeletal areas, and lymph nodes. The high oxygen tension in the lung apices provides a favorable environment for the organisms and probably accounts for their predilection for these areas.

About 3 to 4 weeks after infection the development of cellular immunity and tuberculin hypersensitivity greatly alters the course of infection. Activated macrophages limit further bacterial growth and reduce the number of organisms in both primary and metastatic foci.

Tubercle Formation. The appearance of hypersensitivity to tuberculin provokes a dramatic change in the host's response to the organisms. The nonspecific inflammatory response evoked on first exposure to tubercle bacilli becomes granulomatous, evoking the formation of tubercles. The tubercle comprises an organized aggregation of enlarged macrophages that, because they resemble epithelial cells, are referred to as epithelioid cells. A peripheral collar of fibroblasts, macrophages, and lymphocytes surrounds the granuloma. Frequently the central region of epithelioid cells undergoes a characteristic caseous necrosis to produce a "soft" tubercle, the most characteristic hallmark of tuberculosis. When the antigen load at the initial infection site and regional lymph nodes is large, caseation necrosis may develop and lesions may later calcify. These calcified lesions of the primary site are referred to as the Ghon complex.

After the development of hypersensitivity, the infection becomes quiescent and asymptomatic in the majority of patients (about 90%). In some, however, especially the very young and adults who are immunocompromised or who have other predisposing illnesses, the primary infection may evolve into clinical disease. The progression may be local at the site of the primary lesion, or it may be at one or more distant sites where bacilli have arrived during the early hematogenous spread.

SECONDARY OR REINFECTION TUBERCULOSIS. In a small number of persons whose initial tuberculous infection subsides, secondary disease occurs in spite of acquired cellular immunity. Although the question of whether reinfection tuberculosis results from the breakdown of quiescent foci (endogenous) or from acquisition of new infection from an active case has long been a controversial issue, current opinion favors the endogenous source. In this phase of the disease, lesions are usually localized in the apices of the lungs. In about 5% of patients, apical pulmonary tuberculosis manifests itself within 2 years of the primary infection. In others, however, clinical disease may evolve many decades later whenever resistance is lowered. Quiescent foci that harbor viable organisms thus remain a potential hazard throughout a person's lifetime.

Because of the acquired cellular immunity, bacilli are more promptly phagocytized and destroyed by the activated macrophages. As a result, in secondary tuberculosis, lesions remain localized and dissemination of organisms via the lymphatic vessels is usually prevented. Hypersensitivity promotes a more rapid caseation and fibrotic walling-off of the focus. Histologically the reaction is characteristic of tubercle formation, manifested by a local accumulation of lymphocytes and macrophages. T lymphocytes and their chemotactic lymphokines play a major role in the development of tuberculous granulomas. The chronicity of these lesions appears to be due to the persistence within them of wax D components of tubercle bacilli.

Immunity. Infections caused by *M. tuberculosis* produce a range of immunologic reactions, but since its first demonstration by Koch immunity to tuberculosis has remained an elusive concept. Two immunologic responses—antituberculous immunity and tuberculin hypersensitivity—develop simultaneously in the naturally infected host. Koch made the initial observation of an accelerated inflammatory and healing response in guinea pigs superinfected with tubercle bacilli. In animals injected subcutaneously, the primary infection site was associated with a slowly progressive granulomatous ulcer with extensive lymph node involvement and fatal outcome. If during this infection an intradermal injection of organisms was given at a different site, an early localized indurative response occurred, followed by rapid healing and no lymph node involvement. This observation, referred to as the *Koch phenomenon*, demonstrates acquired increased resistance in the infected animal, but the level of immunity is inadequate to protect the animal against death from the initial infection. Koch subsequently demonstrated that a similar localized allergic response could be induced in the skin of tuberculous animals or persons by the injection of culture filtrates of the tubercle bacillus (*tuberculin reaction*). Since these early observations of Koch, it has become generally recognized that neither response can be transferred to naive recipients by means of hyperimmune serum but require an infusion of lymphoid cells from tuberculin-hypersensitive donors. Although humoral antibodies are produced in response to naturally occurring tuberculous infection, they appear to play no beneficial role in host defense.

Acquired antituberculous immunity is the prototype of cell-mediated immunity invoked by facultative intracellular bacteria. Its development requires the cooperation of two cell types: specific T-lymphocytes that act as specific inducers and mononuclear phagocytes that serve as nonspecific effector cells. The dual role of the T cells is to recruit mononuclear phagocytes for the formation of granulomatous lesions and to activate the phagocytes for enhanced bactericidal activity within the lesions. The expression of immunity ultimately depends on the performance of the nonspecific effector cells, the activated macrophages.

Activation of macrophages is mediated by lymphokines, biologically active substances released by immunocompetent T cells when they contact processed antigens of the tubercle bacillus. Within the developing tuberculous lesion lymphokines with chemotactic, migration-inhibitory, and mitogenic properties cause macrophage and lymphocyte infiltration, macrophage activation, and macrophage and lymphocyte division. Activated macrophages exhibit a number of morphologic and physiologic properties that endow them with enhanced phagocytosis and bactericidal potential. Once the enhanced microbicidal activity of activated macrophages is established, it is nonspecific and can be directed against a number of unrelated microbial species, viruses, and tumor cells. This activity is the basis for the use of BCG vaccine in tumor therapy.

Macrophage activation is most pronounced within granulomas, which provide a specific focusing mechanism. Within these lesions, cells are tightly packed, facilitating cell-to-cell interactions and effective containment of the infection. Macrophages near the center of granulomas appear to be the richest in lysosomal enzymes and the most capable of destroying tubercle bacilli. The alveolar macrophage is thus the key cell that determines the outcome for the host when virulent tubercle bacilli are implanted on the alveolar surface. The macrophage cytoplasm of some mammalian species is probably not favorable for growth of the organisms, especially after acquired resistance is superimposed on the basic native resistance.

The delayed hypersensitivity that develops concomitant with infection is a beneficial reaction when low amounts of bacillary antigens are involved. When large doses of antigen are present, however, the hypersensitivity reaction itself causes cell death and tissue destruction and almost all the tissue damage characteristic of the disease. Whether a causal relationship exists between delayed hypersensitivity and cell-mediated immunity to tubercle bacilli remains a controversial issue. A precise definition of the underlying pathologic mechanisms and specific antigens and T cell subsets involved is required for a clear understanding of these two immunologic phenomena.

Both experimental and clinical studies have demonstrated that quiescent tuberculosis shows a high incidence of recrudescence if there is little or no response to the tuberculin reaction, whereas moderate responders show a low incidence of relapse. A high incidence of relapse is also seen in patients with a very pronounced tuberculin reaction. The magnitude of the response is thus important in assessing protective and nonprotective sensitivity.

Failure of patients to react to tuberculin, a condition known as anergy, is considered an ominous sign in clinical medicine. It occurs in patients with miliary tuberculosis and may also be relatively common among patients with pulmonary tuberculosis if the patients are tested while acutely ill, before their disease has become chronic or has responded to therapy. Studies suggest that suppressor T cells and macrophages are responsible for the increasing degree of immunosuppression that develops in severe progressive disease in humans.

Clinical Manifestations. *M. tuberculosis* can cause disease in any organ of the body. In the United States, however, pulmonary tuberculosis accounts for 85% of the cases. Infection at other sites usually results from a dissemination of organisms from the primary lesion in the lungs. Most patients with tuberculosis experience nonspecific symptoms, such as malaise, fatigue, and low-grade fever. The development of more specific symptoms depends on the organs involved and the extent of the infection.

PULMONARY TUBERCULOSIS

Primary Infection. In approximately 50% of patients recently infected with tuberculosis some nonspecific clinical symptoms develop at the time of tuberculin conversion. Although undetectable clinically, the hallmark of initial tuberculosis infection is the prominence of hilar adenopathy compared with the relatively insignificant size of the initial focus in the lung.

In the majority of patients, the primary lesion heals completely, leaving no clinical evidence of prior infection other than hypersensitivity to tuberculin. In some patients, however, the primary infection progresses directly, evolving into a pneumonic caseous process as the organisms spread through the bronchi or when a tuberculous node ruptures into a bronchus. Contiguous spread can cause infection in the pleural and pericardial spaces. In fact, pleurisy and effusion are important and not uncommon complications occurring soon after infection. The onset of pleurisy is usually abrupt, resembling bacterial pneumonia, with fever, chest pain, and shortness of breath.

Chronic Pulmonary Tuberculosis. In adults, pulmonary tuberculosis is usually caused by organisms hematogenously seeded in the apices of the lungs during the preallergic stage of the primary infection. These metastatic foci may evolve fairly soon after seeding or after a long period of quiescence. Small patches of pneumonia develop around the foci, which become caseous as inflammation increases. The center then liquefies and empties into an adjacent bronchus, creating a cavity in open communication with inspired air from which organisms can be further disseminated to other parts of the lung and to the outside environment. As the disease progresses, there is an insidious onset and development of nonspecific constitutional symptoms, such as fever, fatigue, anorexia, night sweats, and wasting. Cough and sputum are variable in both degree and time of onset but denote more advanced disease. Hemoptysis and chest pain may also be pronounced in late chronic disease.

Extrapulmonary Tuberculosis. Miliary tuberculosis occurs when tubercle bacilli gain access to the lymphatics and bloodstream and seed distant organs. The term *miliary* is descriptive of the small, barely visible foci, which resemble millet seeds, in the sites of localization. Miliary lesions may develop in almost any organ of the body, but the most favored sites for progressive tuberculous infection that develops in the absence of an adequate immunologic response are bones and joints, the genitourinary tract, the meninges, the lymph nodes, and the peritoneum. The primary infection is especially likely to evolve into progressive miliary tuberculosis in very young children and, together with the associated meningitis, is responsible for most tuberculosis deaths in this age group. In AIDS patients with tuberculosis, there is an increased risk of the development of progressive tuberculosis with severe and unusual manifestations, predominantly extrapulmonary and disseminated.

Tuberculin Test. The tuberculin skin test plays an essential role in the control of tuberculosis. It identifies tuberculosis infection, recent or past, with or without disease. The test is based on the fact that persons infected with tubercle bacilli develop hypersensitivity to the proteins of the organism.

Purified protein derivative (PPD) is the skin test reagent that is primarily used to detect hypersensitivity in these persons. In order that comparable reactions may be obtained when different batches of PPD are used, each batch requires accurate standardization in humans against the standard PPD-S, which has been arbitrarily designated as containing 50,000 tuberculin units (TU) per milligram of protein. Table 31–1 gives the relationship between the various doses of OT and PPD.

ADMINISTRATION OF TEST. The standard dose for tuberculin testing is 0.1 mL of PPD biologically equivalent to 5 TU of PPD-S (p. 502). The test is performed by intracutaneous injection (Mantoux method) and, when properly performed, will produce a discrete pale elevation of the skin (wheal). To minimize reduction in potency caused by adsorption, skin tests should be given immediately after the syringe has been filled. In children or persons suspected of having ocular involvement, a 1 TU dose should be used. The 250 TU dose should be used only for assessing the immunologic status of patients who are negative to the 5 TU test dose.

Multiple puncture methods are also in general use for the administration of the tuberculin test. They are not recommended for diagnostic use. However, because they are cheaper and easier to apply than the Mantoux test, they are widely used for screening and survey purposes. The exact amount introduced in a test cannot be measured. Multiple puncture devices introduce concentrated tuberculin into the skin either by puncture with an applicator with points coated with dried tuberculin or by puncture of the skin through a film of concentrated liquid tuberculin. Although these methods may be the practical answer for the busy physician in office or clinic practice, doubtful reactions should be confirmed by the Mantoux test.

READING AND INTERPRETATION OF TEST. Tuberculin tests should be read 48 to 72 hours after injection. The reading is based on the presence or absence of induration, which may be determined visually and by palpation. The diameter of induration should be measured transversely to the long axis of the forearm and recorded in millimeters. A 5 TU dose that produces 10 mm or more of induration is considered virtually diagnostic of infection with *M. tuberculosis*. A reaction that is larger than 5 mm but less than 10 mm in diameter is of doubtful significance because it may be due to other mycobacterial infections. If there is erythema without induration, or induration of less than 5 mm, the reaction should be considered negative, and the patient should be retested with

TABLE 31–1. COMPARABLE DOSES OF OLD TUBERCULIN AND PURIFIED PROTEIN DERIVATIVE

Dilution of Old Tuberculin	Tuberculin Injected (mg)[a]	Purified Protein Derivative Injected (mg)[b]	Tuberculin Units[c]	Strength
1:100,000	0.001		0.1	
1:10,000	0.01	0.00002	1.0	First
1:2,000	0.05	0.0001	5.0	Intermediate
1:1,000	0.1		10.0	
1:100	1.0	0.005	250.0	Second

From Smith: Am Rev Resp Dis 99:820, 1969
[a] Based on 1 mL of concentrated old tuberculin equaling 1000 mg.
[b] Based on milligrams of protein.
[c] One milligram of purified protein derivative-S contains 50,000 TU.

250 TU. If a positive reaction to this second-strength dose is obtained, it is of doubtful significance and may reflect cross-reactions to other mycobacteria. A negative reaction, however, in nonfebrile persons who are in relatively good physical condition and in whom anergy can be ruled out is strong evidence against infection with *M. tuberculosis* or other mycobacteria species. For persons with HIV infection a reaction of ≥5 mm is considered positive.

The use of PPD in the recommended skin test doses does not induce delayed hypersensitivity in a person, even when administered over a period of months or years. Nor does tuberculin testing activate a quiescent infection. Occasionally, exquisitely hypersensitive persons respond to tuberculin testing with vesicular and ulcerating cutaneous reactions, but only rarely does a febrile or constitutional reaction follow.

False-Negative Reactions. There are a number of potential causes of false-negative reactions. Most of these are the result of injecting the tuberculin into the deeper layers of the skin, where it drains away from the local area through the lymphatics. Improper storage and handling of the tuberculin used also accounts for some errors.

About 10% or more of patients critically ill with tuberculosis may fail to react to the 5 TU dose of tuberculin or may react only to the 250 TU dose. In most of these patients the test response becomes positive after a few weeks of therapy. The intensity of a tuberculin reaction may also be diminished by a number of associated illnesses and conditions: acute viral exanthems or vaccinations with live virus vaccines; immunosuppression by disease, drugs, or steroid hormones; or a state of general anergy such as that associated with sarcoidosis or malignant disease, especially lymphoma. Persons with HIV infection are likely to have false-negative skin test reactions, especially in the more advanced stages of the disease.

Fifty years ago, when almost everyone over 20 years of age had a positive tuberculin test reaction, it was assumed that once acquired, tuberculin sensitivity would persist for the remainder of the person's life. This is true at present when tubercle bacilli persist in quiescent foci. If the organisms are completely eliminated, however, the tuberculin reaction is slowly diminished and finally disappears with advancing age or if the infection is treated in its earliest stages. This also occurs in persons who have been vaccinated with BCG but not superinfected with virulent tubercle bacilli.

False-Positive Reactions. The major cause of false-positive reactions is hypersensitivity to mycobacteria other than *M. tuberculosis*. Although these cross-reactions tend to be smaller than reactions caused by tuberculous infections, there is no definitive point of separation. The specificity of the tuberculin test varies geographically according to the prevalence of other mycobacterial infections. In geographic areas where nontuberculous mycobacteria are prevalent in the environment, false-positive reactions to 5 TU of PPD-S, particularly 4 to 12 mm reactions, are also common.

Booster Effect. The reaction to a tuberculin test that has waned with time below the level of positivity may be boosted by the stimulus of a retest, sometimes causing an apparent conversion or development of sensitivity. Although it may occur at any age, it is most frequently encountered among persons over 55 years of age. The booster effect can be seen after a second test done as early as 1 week after the initial stimulating test, and it can persist for a year or more. The booster effect is clinically important, especially in programs of yearly tuberculin testing of hospital personnel in whom a positive reaction on the second annual test actually caused by the booster effect may be interpreted as new infection and lead to inappropriate chemoprophylaxis. To avoid the booster phenomenon in serial tuberculin testing, it has been recommended that a repeat test be given to persons with negative reactions 1 week later and that those with positive reactions on the second test be classified as boosters rather than new infections.

Laboratory Diagnosis. Many species of mycobacteria, both saprophytes and potential pathogens, may be isolated from humans. For the individual patient, a clear-cut separation of pathogen from saprophyte is not always possible. If an isolate proves to be a mycobacterium other than *M. tuberculosis*, the diagnostic laboratory should be able to provide a precise species identification by the use of a few in vitro tests (p. 511).

COLLECTION OF SPECIMENS. Specimens submitted for culture should be collected before antituberculosis drug therapy is started. They should be collected in sterile containers, preferably 50 mL plastic tubes with screw caps, and sent immediately to the laboratory for processing. A series of three to five single early morning samples of sputum and a volume of 5 to 10 mL is recommended. Since tuberculosis and other mycobacterial diseases may affect almost any organ of the body, a wide variety of other specimens, such as pus, cerebrospinal fluid, urine, gastric lavage material, and fluids from inflamed serous cavities, are also suitable for culture.

MICROSCOPIC EXAMINATION. The detection of acid-fast bacilli in stained smears is the easiest and most rapid procedure for evaluating a clinical specimen. Since most patients with symptomatic tuberculosis will demonstrate acid-fast bacilli in the sputum, sputum examinations play an important role in tuberculosis-control programs.

For making the smear, small caseous areas of the sputum should be selected, spread in a thin layer on a new slide, and stained with the Ziehl-Neelsen or Kinyoun stain. Where facilities are available, fluorescent staining with auramine 0 or rhodamine facilitates more rapid scanning of a sputum smear. A recommended method for examining the smear microscopically is to make three longitudinal sweeps of the stained area, parallel to the length of the slide. A report from the laboratory should provide an estimate of the number of acid-fast bacilli detected. The following method is recommended by the American Lung Association:

Number of Bacilli	Report
0	No acid-fast bacilli seen
1–2 per slide	Report number found and request repeat specimen
3–9 per slide	Rare or +
10 or more per slide	Few or + +
1 or more per field	Numerous or + + + +

DIGESTION AND DECONTAMINATION OF SPECIMENS. Most clinical specimens contain an abundance of contaminants that grow much faster than the mycobacteria and must, therefore, be decontaminated before culture. Also, since organisms are usually trapped within cellular and organic debris, exudates must be liquefied before cultures are made. The usefulness of most of the digestion-decontamination procedures depends on the greater resistance of acid-fast bacilli to strong alkaline or acidic solutions. These solutions, however, are also toxic for the mycobacteria, and overdigestion causes a marked reduction in the numbers of survivors. The currently recommended technique used at the Centers for Disease Control employs a mixture of the mucolytic agent, *N*-acetyl-L-cysteine, and sodium hydroxide.

CULTURE. A number of very sensitive culture media are available that are capable of detecting as few as 10 organisms per milliliter of digested concentrated material. They are of two types: egg-potato-base media (e.g., Löwenstein-Jensen) and agar-base media (e.g., Middlebrook 7H-10). Both types should be inoculated and the culture incubated in an atmosphere of 5% to 10% CO_2. The time from the laboratory's receipt of the specimen to the clinician's receipt of the culture report is usually 3 to 6 weeks.

Treatment. The availability of effective antituberculosis drugs has radically changed the management of patients with active disease. Surgical therapy is rarely needed, and sanatoriums have almost vanished. At present the majority of patients with pulmonary tuberculosis in the United States are being treated in public health clinics, but the family physician and the internist have increased responsibilities in the diagnosis, treatment, and follow-up evaluation of tuberculous patients.

Five first-line antituberculosis drugs—isoniazid (INH), rifampin, pyrazinamide, streptomycin, and ethambutol—and a number of second-line agents—cycloserine, ethionamide, *p*-aminosalicylic acid, viomycin, capreomycin—are available for use in a variety of combinations.

Treatment of tuberculosis is based on the use of two or more drugs in concert to prevent the emergence of resistant mutants. There are several highly successful drug regimens that can achieve actual sterilization of the tuberculous lesion within a 9-month treatment period. The initial choice of regimen depends on the patient population. For patients with newly diagnosed tuberculosis, in whom the risk of initial isoniazid resistance is small, the treatment of choice consists of the combination of the two bactericidal drugs, isoniazid and rifampin, for a 9-month period. This two-drug bactericidal therapy for 9 months also appears adequate for the treatment of extrapulmonary tuberculosis. When there is reason, however, to suspect isoniazid resistance, pyrazinamide plus either streptomycin or ethambutol should be added to the two-drug regimen. Patients who may harbor INH-resistant bacilli include those who (1) have received previous chemotherapy, (2) have received INH preventive therapy, (3) have disease acquired through contact with an isoniazid-resistant patient, or (4) have infection probably acquired in countries with high prevalence of isoniazid resistance, such as Southeast Asia, Africa, and Latin America.

At present the role of bacteriostatic drugs (ethambutol, ethionamide, and cycloserine) is limited to their use in situations where drug toxicity or the presence of multiple drug resistance precludes the use of two effective bactericidal drugs. At present the principal use of the previously standard chemotherapeutic regimen of isoniazid and ethambutol for 18 to 24 months is in patients who have hepatitis or impending hepatic failure.

Prevention. The prevention of tuberculosis involves either prevention of infection or, if infection has already occurred, elimination of viable populations of organisms within the host. There are two relatively effective methods for preventing clinical tuberculosis—INH prophylaxis and BCG vaccination. These methods should be considered as complementary and not competitive. The BCG vaccination is useless after the patient has been infected with tubercle bacilli, and isoniazid prophylaxis affords no protection to the uninfected person after treatment is stopped.

ISONIAZID PROPHYLAXIS. Preventive therapy with isoniazid has become a frequently used and well-established procedure, especially in the treatment of the recent tuberculin converter. Chemotherapy with INH for 1 year has been shown to reduce the risk of the evolution of a dormant infection into tuberculous disease by approximately 75%. INH prophylaxis is recommended for all household contacts of persons with newly diagnosed active tuberculosis. Its greatest use is in a person whose tuberculin conversion has occurred within the previous 2 years. Treatment of children under 5 years of age who have a positive reaction to a 5 TU dose of tuberculin is recommended without exception. Persons under the age of 20 years with a positive tuberculin reaction of unknown duration or history are generally treated. However, for patients above the age of 20 years, and especially those beyond the age of 35 years, there is an increased risk of isoniazid-induced hepatitis. In addition, isoniazid is recommended for patients whose health and defenses may be compromised by diabetes, alcoholism, gastrectomy, silicosis, malignancy, or prolonged corticosteroid therapy.

BACILLUS OF CALMETTE AND GUERIN (BCG) PROPHYLAXIS. After years of investigation, Calmette and Guerin obtained a strain of the bovine tubercle bacillus, *M. bovis,* with a low and relatively fixed degree of virulence (see below). This attenuated organism, known as the bacillus of Calmette and Guerin or BCG, has been used to vaccinate approximately 10 million persons. Although some of the data are conflicting, most of the evidence indicates that BCG vaccination will result in a 60% to 80% decrease in the incidence of tuberculosis in a given population group. The vaccine is harmless when properly prepared and administered, but it gives a relative, rather than absolute, immunity. It does reduce the immediate complications of infection stemming from lymphatic or lymphohematogenous spread, especially miliary tuberculosis and tuberculous meningitis.

The value of BCG vaccination depends on the infection rate in the population to be vaccinated, and the proportion of the population that is uninfected. In the United States, where the general population is at low risk of acquiring tuberculous infection, BCG vaccination for the entire population is not indicated. The BCG vaccination can be recommended, however, for special groups in which the morbidity rates are high and the factors favoring rapid transmission of the organisms are temporarily uncontrollable. Such groups include American Indians residing on reservations and inhabitants of certain slum areas in large cities. It is also recommended for infants and children with negative tuberculin skin tests who have intimate and prolonged exposure to persons with active disease.

The vaccine should be administered only to those persons who have a negative tuberculin reaction to 100 TU of PPD. If a positive reaction to a 100 TU dose of PPD does not develop by the end of the third month after vaccination, the procedure may be repeated. Positive tuberculin reactions usually are obtained in 92% to 100% of persons who receive the vaccine, and the hypersensitivity persists for 3 to 4 years or longer. The accidental vaccination of a tuberculin-positive person results in the rapid development, at the site of inoculation, of a superficial ulceration that persists for a few weeks but does not injure the patient. Administration by the intracutaneous method is recommended, but in the United States a vaccine for transcutaneous administration is also available.

Mycobacterium bovis

Although most cases of tuberculosis are caused by *M. tuberculosis,* two additional species—*M. bovis* and *M. africanum*—also cause tuberculosis in humans. *M. africanum* has been isolated only in certain parts of Africa, but there remains a substantial residue of infection with *M. bovis* in many countries where raw milk is ingested.

Sixty years ago dairy herds in the United States were heavily infected with bovine tubercle bacilli, and the milk from these animals provided a common source of infection in humans. Tuberculin testing of cows and slaughter of all cows with positive reactions have dramatically reduced the incidence of infection in cows in the United States to less than 1%. Infection in humans has been almost eliminated in countries where pasteurized milk is consumed. However, until it is completely eradicated as a source of disease, *M. bovis* must be included in the differential diagnosis.

Morphologic and Cultural Characteristics. This species is often shorter and plumper than the human tubercle bacillus, and its primary isolation is usually more difficult. Because glycerol selectively inhibits growth of the bovine species, glycerol should not be included in the Löwenstein-Jensen or 7H10 culture media for primary isolation. The addition of 0.4% sodium pyruvate is stimulatory, especially for the growth of primary isolates. Strains of *M. bovis* grow more slowly, and the colonies are smaller than most clinical isolates of the human species.

In general, *M. bovis* is less aerotolerant than *M. tuberculosis,* but it is more pathogenic for experimental animals. In the laboratory, the most useful single test for differentiating *M. bovis* from *M. tuberculosis* is the niacin test, a test based on the difference between the amount of free nicotinic acid produced by the two species (Table 31–2).

Pathogenesis. *M. bovis* produces spontaneous tuberculosis in a wide range of animals, including cats, dogs, and primates. In man the portal of entry is usually the gastrointestinal tract. Extrapulmonary lesions are prevalent, especially in the cervical and mesenteric lymph nodes, bones, and joints. When inhaled, *M. bovis* can also cause pulmonary tuberculosis indistinguishable from that caused by *M. tuberculosis.*

Bacillus of Calmette and Guerin (BCG). BCG is an attenuated mutant of *M. bovis* isolated in 1908 by the French workers Calmette and Guerin by repeated subculture on a glycerol-potato-bile medium. Subcultures of the original isolate are maintained as *M. bovis* strain BCG and used as an immunizing agent against tuberculosis and in cancer immunotherapy. Since BCG organisms are often isolated from abscesses arising after BCG vaccination or from the lymph nodes draining the vaccination site, the laboratory must ensure proper identification of the isolate.

Mycobacteria Associated with Nontuberculous Infections

The existence of mycobacteria having culture characteristics different from *M. tuberculosis* had been recognized for many years, but their wide distribution in nature and their lack of virulence for the guinea pig led workers to conclude that they were strictly saprophytic species. Their occasional isolation from clinical material was assumed to be completely fortuitous. Only within the last 30 years has there been a full awareness of the clinical significance of a number of these organisms. Often referred to as "atypical" mycobacteria, these organisms can and do produce severe and even fatal disease in humans.

Identification. Organisms in this group grow well on Löwenstein-Jensen, 7H10, and other media commonly used for the culture of *M. tuberculosis.* A useful system for their classification is based on Runyon's scheme, in which organisms are subdivided into four groups on the basis of their rate of growth and pigment production. Groups I, II, and III are slow-growers, requiring 7 days or more to yield visible colonies, and Group IV includes the rapid growers that produce visible growth within less than 7 days. Group I organisms are photochromogenic, producing pigmented colonies only on

TABLE 31–2. DIFFERENTIAL PROPERTIES OF SELECTED PATHOGENIC AND OPPORTUNISTIC SPECIES OF *MYCOBACTERIUM*

Species	Rate of Growth	Pigment		Niacin Production	Nitrate Reduction	Catalase		Tween[b] Hydrolysis (10 Day)	Urease	Arylsulfatase (10 day)	Growth on		
		Dark	Light			>45 mm	Heat Stable[a]				5% NaCl	TCH, 1 μg/mL	THZ, 10 μg/mL
M. tuberculosis	S	–	–	+	+	–	–	±	+	–	–	+	–
M. africanum	S	–	–	±	±	–	–		+		–	–	
M. bovis	S	–	–	–	–	–	–	–	+	±	–	+	–
M. ulcerans	S	–	–	±	–		+	–	–	–		+	
Photochromogens													
M. kansasii	S	–	+	–	+	+	+	+	+	+	–	+	–
M. marinum	S	–	+	–	–	±	+	+	+	+	±	+	±
M. simiae	S	–	+	±	–	+	+	–		±	–	+	+
M. asiaticum	S	–	+	–	–	+	+	+	–	±	–	+	+
Scotochromogens													
M. scrofulaceum	S	+	+	–	–	+	+	–	+	–	–	+	±
M. szulgai	S	+[c]	+	–	+	+	+	±	±	±	–	+	+
M. xenopi	S	+	+	–	–	–	+	–	–	+	–	+	+
M. gordonae	S	+	+	–	–	+	+	+	–	±	–	+	+
M. flavescens	S	+	+	–	+								
Nonphotochromogens													
M. avium–M. intracellulare	S	–	–	–	–	–	±	–	–	±	–	+	+
M. gastri	S	–	–	–	–	–	–	+	+	+	–	+	–
M. malmoense	S	–	–	–	–	–		+	±	±	–	+	+
M. terrae	S	–	–	–	±	+	+	+	–	±	–	+	+
M. triviale	S	–	–	–	+	+	+	+	–	±	+	+	+
Rapid-growing species													
M. fortuitum	R	–	–	–	+	+	+	±	+	+	+	+	+
M. chelonei	R	–	–	–	–	+		±	+	+	±	+	+
M. flavescens	I	+	–	–	+	+	+	+	+	+	±	+	+
M. smegmatis	R	–	–	–	+	+	+	+			+	+	+

Data from Wayne and Kubica: In Sneath et al (eds): Bergey's Manual of Systematic Bacteriology, vol 2. Williams & Wilkins, 1986; Good: Annu Rev Microbiol 39:347, 1985.

S, slow grower, requires more than 7 days; R, rapid grower, requires less than 7 days; I, intermediate growth rate, 7 to 10 days; +, 85% or more of strains are positive; –, 15% or less of strains are positive; ±, high degree of variability.

[a] Resists 68C.

[b] Polysorbate.

[c] At 37C; may be photochromogenic at 25C.

exposure to light. Group II is scotochromogenic, being pigmented without light exposure, and Group III is nonphotochromogenic, either nonpigmented or having a very light yellow color that does not change with exposure to light. Within each group are numbers of species whose biochemical, epidemiologic, and clinical characteristics are well-defined (Table 31–2). Although the number of species that has been isolated from clinical specimens is somewhat bewildering to the clinician, only a relatively few of these are known human pathogens.

Epidemiology. The mycobacteria in these groups are ubiquitous and are found in all parts of the world. They are endemic in certain geographic areas, as has been impressively demonstrated by extensive skin testing and by culture from clinical specimens and the environment. The organisms have no known primary animal host but apparently exist in the soil. The species distribution depends on locale, type of soil, and other climatic and environmental factors. There is no evidence of direct transmission of organisms from man to man. Epidemiologic aspects of mycobacterial pulmonary disease point strongly to the probability that most disease of this type occurs only in persons whose lungs have already sustained damage. The current view is that mycobacterial disease caused by these organisms results from two coinciding events: (1) a colonization by large numbers of mycobacteria and (2) a localized or generalized impairment of the body's defense mechanisms.

Clinical Manifestations. The diseases produced by this group of mycobacteria have roentgenologic, pathologic, and, to some extent, clinical similarities to tuberculosis, but there are important differences in virulence, treatment, and prognosis. Species designation of a particular infection is important because of differences in treatment and prognosis. Clinically, these mycobacterioses may be grouped according to organ involvement as pulmonary disease, localized lymphadenitis, cutaneous disease, and rarely disseminated disease. The most common manifestation in the United States is pulmonary disease, which occurs mainly in older white men with chronic bronchitis and emphysema. *M. kansasii* and organisms of the *M. avium–M. intracellulare* and *M. fortuitum* complexes are usually associated with this form of the infection. Lymphadenitis, which occurs primarily in children, is usually caused by *M. scrofulaceum*, but any of the slowly growing species may occasionally be the causative agent. Superficial skin diseases are restricted to occupational or recreational activities involving fish. *Mycobacterium marinum* is responsible for most skin infections in the United States, whereas *M. ulcerans* is restricted to specific areas of Africa and the southeast Pacific. Other infections with which these mycobacteria have been associated include a large number of injection abscesses and cardiac surgery infections. Most of these have been caused by the saprophytes *M. fortuitum* and *M. chelonei.* Fatal cases of disseminated infection have been reported in young children and immunologically deficient adults. Many different mycobacteria have been implicated, including *M. kansasii* and organisms of the *M. avium–M. intracellulare* and *M. fortuitum* complexes. In patients with AIDS, however, in whom disseminated mycobacterial disease is very common, the *M. avium–M. intracellulare* complex is the predominant bacterial isolate (page 514).

Laboratory Diagnosis. Diagnosis of the specific organism is crucial in determining therapy. Simply grouping the organisms into one of Runyon's groups is inadequate. Diagnosis depends completely on bacteriologic identification of the organism and its repeated demonstration in patient secretions in the absence of other potential pathogens. Skin testing is generally not helpful in nontuberculous mycobacterial disease. A positive acid-fast smear with a negative skin test reaction to PPD-S, however, may lead one to suspect the diagnosis.

Treatment. Only *M. kansasii* shows significant susceptibility to the antituberculosis drugs. Organisms of the *M. avium–M. intracellulare* and *M. fortuitum* complexes and all other saprophytic species of mycobacteria are highly resistant in vitro. In spite of this, various combinations of three or more antituberculosis drugs are used by many physicians, some of whom report improvement.

Slowly Growing Mycobacteria

Mycobacterium kansasii. *M. kansasii* organisms are usually longer and wider than tubercle bacilli and, with the acid-fast stain, characteristically stain unevenly to give a barred or beaded appearance. The organisms are usually arranged in curving strands.

M. kansasii is photochromogenic. Colonies, which are demonstrable after 1 to 2 weeks of incubation in the dark on glycerol egg slants, are usually smooth and ivory in color. If grown in the light, the colonies are lemon-yellow, becoming orange or reddish orange with age.

In terms of common antigens, *M. kansasii* is closer to *M. tuberculosis* than any of the other mycobacteria species. Also, in a comparison of skin-test reactions to PPDs from *M. tuberculosis* and *M. kansasii* in patients with known disease, patients reacted with complete crossover. Experimentally, *M. kansasii* produces almost as much protection against a challenge with *M. tuberculosis* as does BCG, whereas other mycobacteria are less effective.

PATHOGENESIS. Pathogenicity for animals is extremely limited, and in most experimental animals only local lesions are produced. Of relevance to the pathogenesis of human disease, however, is the demonstration that guinea pigs exposed to a carbon aerosol or to a mixed carbon dust–silica dust aerosol contracted progressive pulmonary disease when they were exposed to *M. kansasii,* whereas control animals exposed only to *M. kansasii* contracted minimal or no disease. Preexisting lung disease is present in a large number of persons who develop clinically significant *M. kansasii* infections.

The pulmonary changes seen at surgery or autopsy are indistinguishable from those caused by *M. tuberculosis.* Skin lesions and lymph node lesions due to *M. kansasii* may be granulomatous or suppurative.

CLINICAL INFECTION

Epidemiology. Subclinical infection with *M. kansasii,* as shown by positive skin test reactions, indicates a definite geographic distribution. In the United States, *M. kansasii* infections are more frequent in the areas of Chicago, Louisiana, and Texas. There is also a high incidence of isolates in northeast London, where *M. kansasii* has been isolated from the water supply. It has also been cultured from milk and animals, but its natural habitat remains unclear. In contrast to *M. avium–M. intracellulare*, *M. kansasii* appears to occur most frequently in urban areas.

There is no evidence that the organism spreads directly from man to man or that children become infected when a sputum-positive member remains in a family for months to years. In Oklahoma, an area of high infectivity, children have positive skin test reactions to PPDs made from *M. kansasii* much earlier than to PPDs from *M. tuberculosis* or from other mycobacteria species. A positive skin test rate of 50% by the age of 17 does not increase much after that age.

Clinical Manifestations. Pulmonary disease is the most common clinical form of *M. kansasii* infection. It occurs primarily in middle-aged or elderly white men, most of whom have some preexisting form of lung disease. Clinically, it resembles tuberculosis except that symptoms, when present, tend to be mild. Usually there is a very gradual progression of the disease over a period of many years, with multiple thin-walled cavity formation.

M. kansasii may also occasionally cause infections of the cervical lymph nodes, penetrating wound infections, and granulomatous synovitis. Although uncommon, dissemination does occur especially in patients with conditions known to impair cell-mediated immunity. AIDS patients are at increased risk from disseminated *M. kansasii* infection.

Treatment. Isolates of *M. kansasii* vary in their susceptibility to the various antituberculosis agents and, in general, require higher doses than *M. tuberculosis.* Therapy should be begun with three agents. One recommended regimen that has resulted in healing in 90% to 95% of cases is an 18-month course of INH, ethambutol, and streptomycin. Rifampin should be included if disease is extensive or if the patient is severely immunocompromised.

Mycobacterium marinum

MORPHOLOGIC AND CULTURAL CHARACTERISTICS. *M. marinum* is a photochromogenic species implicated in a granulomatous skin disease commonly known as swimming pool granuloma. In tissues, the organisms may appear in clumps as short, thick, and uniformly staining rods or as long, thin, beaded, and barred bacilli scattered throughout the tissue. *M. marinum* grows readily at 30C to 32C on any medium commonly employed for mycobacteria. On Löwenstein-Jensen medium, colonies are grayish white with pale yellow streaks but, on exposure to light at room temperature, develop an intense orange-yellow pigmentation that eventually turns red.

CLINICAL INFECTION. Since the first isolation of *M. marinum* from granulomatous lesions of marine fish, it has been found widely distributed in nature, occurring in soil, water, and freshwater fish. Its association with human infection was first described during an epidemic in 1954, when it was isolated both from skin lesions of patients and from the rough cement of swimming pools. Since that time, epidemics of granulomatous skin disease have been traced to infected swimming pools, freshwater lakes, and beaches of several of the Hawaiian Islands. Sporadic cases have also been reported, a number of which were associated with the cleaning of tropical fish aquariums. Epidemic cases are readily recognized, but the sporadic single case is usually misdiagnosed.

Lesions occur at the site of minor abrasions, especially on the elbows, but also on the knees, toes, fingers, and dorsa of the feet. The infection usually begins 2 to 3 weeks after exposure as a small papule, which slowly increases in size, ulcerates, and discharges pus containing the acid-fast organisms.

In most cases, the lesions heal spontaneously after several months, but in some patients healing is prolonged, requiring 2 years or more. Tetracycline has been recommended for an initial conservative approach, to be replaced by rifampin and ethambutol if there is no response.

Mycobacterium simiae. *M. simiae* was first isolated in 1965 during a bacteriologic survey of a colony of *Macaca rhesus* monkeys in which disease was prevalent. Since then it has been found associated with human disease in Europe, Cuba, and the United States. It has also been isolated from an environmental water supply.

CULTURAL CHARACTERISTICS. The organism is photochromogenic, producing small dysgonic colonies, which are initially buff in color but which gradually turn yellow on exposure to light. Its most distinctive property is the production of niacin, a trait not seen in the other nontuberculous mycobacteria.

CLINICAL INFECTION. In humans disease due to *M. simiae* has not been well defined, and there is relatively little epidemiologic information. It is quite probable, however, that infected *Macaca* monkeys might transmit this mycobacterium to humans. Disease in some patients has been marked by rapid progression and extensive pulmonary cavitation, but in most patients the clinical picture has been confused by the simultaneous use of corticosteroids or by the presence of other underlying disease.

M. simiae is highly resistant to the antituberculosis drugs. An in vitro evaluation, however, should include pyrazinamide, cycloserine, capreomycin, and kanamycin, as well as the tetracyclines and erythromycin.

Mycobacterium scrofulaceum. As its name suggests, *M. scrofulaceum* is most frequently associated with a scrofula-like disease involving the cervical lymph nodes. It has been isolated from many environmental sources, from sputum, and lesions in pigs.

MORPHOLOGIC AND CULTURAL CHARACTERISTICS. Microscopically, *M. scrofulaceum* is longer, thicker, and more coarsely beaded than *M. tuberculosis.* In liquid media organisms are randomly distributed and display no evidence of cording. It is scotochromogenic, producing compact, domed colonies, which are yellow to orange when grown in the dark but which develop a reddish orange pigmentation on continuous exposure to light.

CLINICAL INFECTION. Cervical lymphadenitis in children is the major clinical manifestation of *M. scrofulaceum* infection. The organism is very widespread in its occurrence and has been isolated from cervical lymph nodes in various parts of the world. Reports from a number of countries indicate that 75% of granulomatous cervical adenitis suggestive histologically of tuberculosis is actually caused by mycobacteria other than *M. tuberculosis.* In some areas, especially the Great Lakes region, Canada, and Japan, *M. scrofulaceum* appears to be the predominant cause of mycobacterial lymphadenitis, but this is not true for all regions. The widespread incidence of infection with this organism is also emphasized by the demonstration of a reaction rate of 49% in 30,000 naval recruits skin-tested with PPD prepared from a scotochromogenic organism.

The portal of entry in children with mycobacteriosis of the cervical nodes appears to be the oropharynx. Throat swabs and tonsils of healthy children reveal a high incidence of mycobacteria of this type, but only a relatively few children in the same area have manifest disease. As a rule, children who contract mycobacterial scrofula have been healthy and have not exhibited any obvious abnormalities or undue susceptibility to other infections. In some reports, however, the disease may have been preceded by a bacterial or viral pharyngitis that permitted mycobacterial invasion.

In adults, chronic pulmonary disease in association with scotochromogenic organisms has been reported but is difficult to assess. In some of these cases, *M. scrofulaceum* has colonized old tuberculosis cavities of the lung and is thus suggestive of secondary invasion. Skin ulcers and abscesses, bone infections, and generalized dissemination also occur but are uncommon. Disseminated disease is almost invariably associated with some other serious disease.

The treatment of mycobacterial lymphadenitis consists of complete excision of the node. Strains of *M. scrofulaceum* vary in their susceptibility to antituberculous and other antibacterial agents. Initial treatment of severe and threatening disease should consist of a combination of isoniazid, streptomycin, cycloserine, and rifampin until sensitivity tests on the specific strain are available.

Mycobacterium szulgai. *M. szulgai* superficially resembles *M. scrofulaceum* and the nonpathogenic *M. gordonae,* but it differs from them both biochemically and serologically. *M. szulgai* is widespread in its distribution. Most clinical isolates to date have been from patients with pulmonary disease, rarely from patients with lymphadenitis and bursitis. The recommended treatment is a combination of rifampin, streptomycin, and either ethambutol or isoniazid. The organism must be differentiated from *M. gordonae,* a slow-growing scotochrome that is frequently isolated from the sputum of patients who do not have mycobacterial infections.

Mycobacterium xenopi. *M. xenopi* is probably the most easily recognized of potential mycobacterial pathogens. Although it was first isolated from a cold-blooded animal, the toad *Xenopus laevis,* it is unique among mycobacteria in that it grows poorly at 37C, preferring temperatures of 42C to 45C. For primary isolation, 3 to 4 weeks or longer is required. Colonies are characteristically very small and granular and microscopically show a peripheral network of hyphae. A yellow pigmentation gradually develops on prolonged incubation. In stained smears, the bacilli are unusually long and thin and are often arranged in typical arching patterns.

M. xenopi has been isolated from water, from both hot and cold taps, and from granulomatous lesions in swine. It is more limited in its geographic distribution than other opportunistic mycobacterial pathogens, with more reported clinical isolations coming from northwestern Europe than from America. Since most of these have been from areas near the coast or tidal estuaries, an ecologic association with the sea or with seabirds is suggested. *M. xenopi* produces a chronic slowly progressive pulmonary disease, which is clinically and radiologically similar to tuberculosis. Accurate identification of the organism is important since it is more amenable to drug therapy than *M. scrofulaceum* or *M. avium–M. intracellulare,* with which it may be confused. Initial treatment should consist of isoniazid, rifampin, and ethambutol. The organism is also generally sensitive to the other antituberculosis drugs.

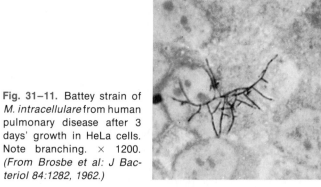

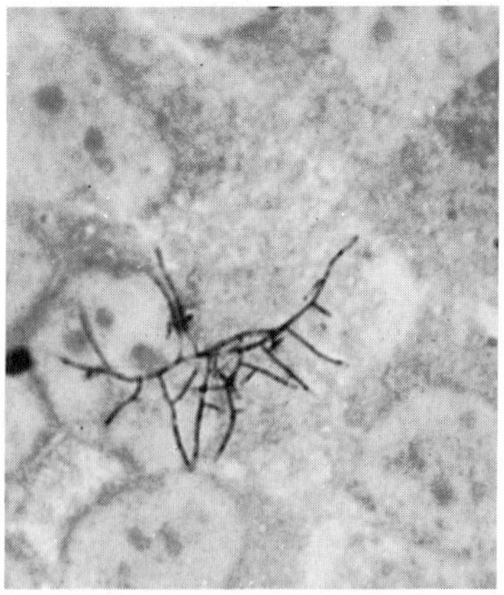

Fig. 31–11. Battey strain of *M. intracellulare* from human pulmonary disease after 3 days' growth in HeLa cells. Note branching. × 1200. *(From Brosbe et al: J Bacteriol 84:1282, 1962.)*

Mycobacterium avium–Mycobacterium intracellulare. There is considerable overlap between the properties of the two major nonphotochromogenic pathogens, *M. avium* and *M. intracellulare,* making speciation of strains extremely difficult. Because of what some mycobacteriologists consider needless concern over the separation of the two species, the term *M. avium–M. intracellulare* complex (MAC) is used for these mycobacteria.

Serotyping of strains by agglutination and agglutinin absorption is a useful tool for epidemiologic studies. The basis for the serologic specificity of the serotypes is a unique class of C-mycoside glycopeptidolipids, which are present in the organism as a superficial sheath. *M. avium* is composed of three distinct agglutination serotypes, whereas *M. intracellulare* contains 25 serotypes. Neither the temperature at which a serotype grows best nor pathogenicity for birds is adequate for distinguishing strains.

MORPHOLOGIC AND CULTURAL CHARACTERISTICS. In clinical materials, the organisms are pleomorphic, but on culture media they usually appear as short rods with bipolar acidfast granules (Fig. 31–11). Most virulent avian strains grow better at 44C than at 37C, whereas most strains of *M. intracellulare* prefer the lower temperature. On repeated subculture in the laboratory, however, avirulent variants of avian strains may adapt to good growth at 37C and are then indistinguishable by the usual tests from avirulent *M. intracellulare* strains. Colonies of primary isolates are predominantly thin, translucent, and smooth, but a few rough colonies are also often produced (Fig. 31–12). On subculture, colonies become more opaque and domed. Correlated with these colony variations are changes in virulence and other properties.

CLINICAL INFECTION

Epidemiology. Organisms of this group are worldwide in distribution. They are ubiquitous in the environment and have been isolated from water, soil, and dairy products as well as from the tissues of both birds and mammals. Avian serotypes produce spontaneous disease in domestic fowl and other birds and can spread from these sources to cows, swine, and man.

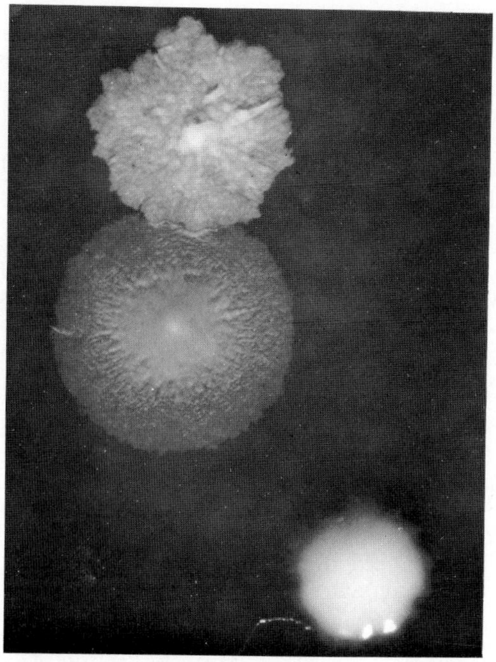

Fig. 31–12. Rough, transparent, and opaque colonies of *M. avium*, serotype 2, on oleic acid-albumin agar. Original magnification × 15. *(From Schaefer et al: Am Rev Respir Dis 102:499, 1970.)*

M. intracellulare serotypes are associated with insects, sawdust, soil, and environmental sources. There is no accurate estimate of the prevalence of *M. avium–M. intracellulare* infections, although skin test surveys indicate that inapparent infection is common, especially in the southeastern United States. It appears to be more frequent than infection with *M. tuberculosis* but less frequent than *M. scrofulaceum* infection.

Clinical Manifestations. Chronic pulmonary disease caused by *M. avium–M. intracellulare* is clinically and pathologically indistinguishable from tuberculosis, but symptoms are generally quite mild, and the disease usually follows an indolent course. The incidence is highest among middle-aged to elderly white men, most of whom have preexisting pulmonary disease. Before 1982 and the onset of the AIDS era, extrapulmonary involvement was rare except in some geographic areas where *M. avium–M. intracellulare* was associated with cervical adenitis. Only 14 documented cases of disseminated infection in adults had been described, all in immunosuppressed persons. Since that time, however, there has been an astonishingly high incidence of cases of disseminated *M. avium–M. intracellulare* infection. At present *M. avium–M. intracellulare* infection is recognized as one of the most common complications of AIDS. Symptoms of disseminated *M. avium–M. intracellulare* infection in patients with AIDS are nonspecific and include high fever, night sweats, progressive weakness, diarrhea, and overall deterioration. In patients with AIDS and other immunodeficiencies, blood is the specimen of choice for culture. Culture of stool specimens is also important since the most likely route of transmission is via the gastrointestinal tract.

Treatment. *M. avium–M. intracellulare* organisms are generally highly resistant to most antituberculous drugs. Clinically ill patients with progressive pulmonary disease or disseminated disease should be treated with four- to six-drug regimens including isoniazid, rifampin, ethambutol, streptomycin, cycloserine, and ethionamide. At present, there is no treatment regimen that is convincingly effective against *M. avium–M. intracellulare* infections in patients with AIDS.

***Mycobacterium malmoense* and *Mycobacterium haemophilum*.** *M. malmoense* and *M. haemophilum* are nonphotochromogenic species with biochemical properties similar to those of *M. avium. M. malmoense* appears to elicit a distinct agglutinating serotype and is associated with pulmonary disease. *M. haemophilum* is unique among slow-growing mycobacteria in its inability to grow in the absence of hemin. It also requires a temperature of 30C to 32C and will not grow at 37C. It is probable that this organism is sometimes not isolated from clinical material because of failure to use the appropriate media and conditions for culture. *M. haemophilum,* first isolated in Israel from granulomatous skin lesions of a patient with Hodgkin's disease, has subsequently been found in skin lesions from immunosuppressed patients in Australia and the United States.

Rapidly Growing Mycobacteria

***Mycobacterium fortuitum* and *Mycobacterium chelonei*.** The rapidly growing mycobacteria are widely distributed in both aquatic and terrestrial habitats. Most of these are purely environmental saprophytes, but two species, *M. fortuitum* and *M. chelonei,* are occasional pathogens of humans, birds, and poikilothermic animals.

MORPHOLOGIC AND CULTURAL CHARACTERISTICS. *M. fortuitum* and *M. chelonei* are now well-defined species, but because they share a number of similar metabolic characteristics and are not infrequently found in the same types of infection, they are sometimes referred to as the *M. fortuitum–M. chelonei* complex. Organisms of this group are pleomorphic and exhibit various degrees of acid-fastness. Long, filamentous forms are seen in pus, sometimes with definite branching. Colonies that appear after 72 hours' incubation at 37C on the 7H10 medium are unpigmented and are usually large and rough, but smooth, waxy, butyrous colonies may also be seen on some media. Many strains of *M. fortuitum* may be incorrectly identified as *M. tuberculosis* if the cultures are not inspected for 3 to 4 weeks after inoculation. At that time *M. fortuitum* presents an unpigmented, somewhat rough growth that may closely resemble that seen with the human tubercle bacillus. The key to the identification of *M. fortuitum* is the inspection of cultures at 4 to 14 days and selection of the colorless rapid growers for further study.

M. fortuitum is characterized by its rapid growth on routine media at room temperature as well as at 37C and by its uniform resistance to isoniazid, streptomycin, and *p*-aminosalicylic acid. Strains exhibit marked variability in their biochemical properties, especially on primary isolation, making speciation of strains extremely tedious and of questionable clinical importance. *M. fortuitum* and *M. chelonei* can be distinguished by their growth and physiologic properties and their antigenic structure.

CLINICAL INFECTION. Organisms of the *M. fortuitum–M.*

chelonei complex have been found in 30% to 78% of soil samples from various areas of the United States. They have been isolated from the sputum and saliva of healthy persons and from scrub sinks in operating rooms. In skin tests, *M. fortuitum* gives a specific reaction to PPD-F and exhibits very slight cross-reactivity with other tuberculins. In a large study of naval recruits, only 7.7% had skin reactions to 5 TU of PPD-F.

The most common clinical manifestation is an abscess appearing at the site of trauma, usually at the injection site of supposedly sterile products. Less frequent are corneal ulcers after some type of penetrating injury and pulmonary infection. Pulmonary *M. fortuitum* infection cannot be distinguished by x-ray from typical tuberculosis. In most of these infections, there has been evidence of preexisting disease, concomitant injury by other material, or suppression of immunity, which permitted invasion by an organism that is rarely pathogenic. Serious infections have developed in wounds after open heart surgery or venous stripping and in renal homograft recipients. A *M. chelonei*–like organism has also been responsible for outbreaks of peritonitis associated with the use of intermittent chronic peritoneal dialysis by patients with renal disease.

M. fortuitum–M. chelonei organisms are highly resistant in vitro to antituberculosis drugs. In spite of this, some success has been achieved with multiple-drug regimens that include four to six drugs. If drug therapy fails, surgical resection may be necessary.

Saprophytic Species. The widespread occurrence of saprophytic species of mycobacteria leads to their frequent isolation as contaminants in clinical material. *Mycobacterium gordonae* and *Mycobacterium terrae* are among the saprophytic species that have been associated with human disease on rare occasions. Both have been isolated from treated and natural water samples and are able to colonize respiratory and skin surfaces. In most cases, their isolation from clinical material represents contamination. However, *M. terrae* has been implicated in pulmonary disease and arthritis, whereas documented infections of the respiratory tract, bursa, and prosthetic aortic valve have been attributed to *M. gordonae*. *M. gordonae* has also been the cause of an increasing number of disseminated mycobacterial infections in patients with AIDS.

Two species, *Mycobacterium smegmatis* and *Mycobacterium phlei,* do not cause disease but have been used extensively in biochemical and genetic studies because they grow rapidly on simple media and constitute no health hazard in the laboratory. All studies on the structure and function of the mycobacterial genome and all successful attempts at genetic transfers have employed *M. smegmatis,* while *M. phlei* has been used in studies on mutagenesis. *M. smegmatis* is usually nonchromogenic, while the pigmentation of *M. phlei* varies with the medium on which it is grown. *M. phlei* can grow at temperatures up to 52C and, unlike *M. smegmatis,* can survive for 4 hours at 60C. Both organisms are present in the soil. *M. phlei* occurs only occasionally in the sputum of patients with pulmonary cavities or bronchiectasis, while *M. smegmatis* is often present in the smegma around the genitals.

Mycobacterium ulcerans

Mycobacterium ulcerans produces a destructive, primarily tropical skin disease that, if not treated early, produces chronic ulcers with necrotic centers. The disease was first described in a small group of patients in Victoria, Australia, but has since been reported from a number of tropical countries in Asia, Africa, and South America.

MORPHOLOGIC AND CULTURAL CHARACTERISTICS. In culture preparations the bacilli are 0.5 μm wide and 1.5 to 3.0 μm long, but in tissue sections they are usually larger and are beaded in appearance. The optimal temperature for growth is 30C to 33C, with no growth occurring at either 25C or 37C. It is very slow-growing, requiring 6 to 12 weeks for primary isolation. Rough domed, lemon yellow colonies are produced on Löwenstein-Jensen medium. *M. ulcerans* is biochemically unreactive.

PATHOGENESIS. Pathologic changes in the skin of patients infected with *M. ulcerans* do not resemble those of tuberculosis. No caseation and only rare granulomas are seen. The base of the ulcer usually displays a rapid, undermining necrosis. Most laboratory animals are resistant to infection, but mice may be infected by the injection of *M. ulcerans* into their footpads, a site with a low body temperature.

CLINICAL INFECTION. *M. ulcerans* infection is the third in importance of the mycobacterial diseases. It has been most frequently encountered in isolated pockets in Australia, Africa, and Mexico. Proximity to rivers or swampy areas appears to be an important factor, but no studies have demonstrated the existence of the organism outside the human body. Lesions usually occur on the legs or arms, beginning as a single subcutaneous nodular lesion that gradually breaks down to form a chronic necrotizing, undermining skin ulcer. The lesion is somewhat similar to leprosy but more superficial and without nerve involvement. Acid-fast bacilli may be demonstrated in the lesions. Treatment consists of wide surgical excision, and skin grafting may be necessary when lesions are extensive. In general, drug regimens have not proved effective.

Mycobacterium leprae

Leprosy is an ancient disease whose origin is shrouded in antiquity. As early as 1400 BC, reference to it as an old disease in India may be found in the sacred Hindu writings of the Veda. Many accounts of leprosy may also be found in the ancient Hebrew writings, and although some of the skin lesions considered to be leprosy in the Old Testament of the Bible were probably not leprosy, many undoubtedly were.

Hansen, in 1874, described the presence of myriads of bacilli in the lesions of leprosy patients. Although this was one of the first descriptions of a microorganism as the cause of human disease, the organism is still an enigma. All attempts to culture *Mycobacterium leprae* in vitro have failed. It is difficult to propagate and transmit to experimental animals, and its slow growth, both in animals and in patients, has drastically hampered investigative efforts.

Stimulated in large part by the World Health Organization, in recent years there has been renewed interest in leprosy, a disease that continues to threaten the quality of life of more than 12 million people in all parts of the world. The movement of the world's growing population and today's means of rapid transportation have resulted in increased contact between susceptible travelers and the millions of patients who have leprosy. The current concern with leprosy is thus of global importance.

Morphology and Physiology

When stained by the Ziehl-Neelsen method, the leprosy bacilli are seen as acid-fast rods predominantly in modified mononuclear or epithelioid structures called lepra cells. Organisms are found singly or in large masses called globi. Large numbers of bacilli may be packed in the cells in an arrangement that suggests packets of cigars. The individual rods vary in length from 1 to 8 μm and in width from 0.3 to 0.5 μm. The rods are usually straight or slightly curved and may stain uniformly or show granules and beads that are slightly larger than the average diameter of the cell. Bacilli that uniformly stain acid-fast are healthy viable cells, whereas bacilli that show beading are probably nonviable. Acid-fastness of *M. leprae* may be removed by preliminary extraction with pyridine, a useful property in distinguishing it from most other mycobacteria.

In thin sections of *M. leprae* in lepromatous nodules, the organism's structure resembles that of *M. tuberculosis* with a three-layered cell wall and a complex intracytoplasmic membrane system that connects with the plasma membrane.

All well-controlled attempts to culture *M. leprae* have met with failure, including attempts to grow the organism in tissue cultures of various types of human cells. Up to the present time, no published paper has produced proof of multiplication of *M. leprae* in either the presence or the absence of cultured cells. It can be grown experimentally only in animals.

The presence of a phenolase in *M. leprae* obtained from lepromatous skin nodules provides a simple test for separating *M. leprae* from other mycobacteria and from nocardias in which activity has never been detected. The phenolase converts 3,4-dihydroxyphenylalanine (dopa) to a colored product that has an absorption peak at 540 nm.

Experimental Disease in Animals

Since *M. leprae* cannot be grown in vitro, animal models have been extensively used for study of the organism and experimental leprosy. The most frequently used animals are the normal mouse injected in the footpad and the nine-banded armadillo. In the mouse, infections can be initiated with as few as 1 to 10 bacilli. Footpad temperatures of 30C, obtained by controlling air temperatures at 20C to 25C, are the secret of the footpad success. The intravenous injection of *M. leprae* into mice results in lesions in the nose and front feet. In humans, the bacilli that are shed from the nose have been growing at that site at a temperature of approximately 30C.

In the footpad of the mouse the multiplying *M. leprae* produce a growth curve and histologic pattern sufficiently distinctive to permit its differentiation from other mycobacteria. During its logarithmic phase of growth, it has a generation time of approximately 12 days. Multiplication at this rate continues for 150 to 180 days after inoculation until the number of bacilli in the footpad reaches a level of about 1×10^6 organisms. At this time, multiplication stops, apparently because of the triggering of cell-mediated immunity. Lymphocytes infiltrate the area, and macrophages in the center of the lesion enlarge. The infection in mice remains localized and self-healing, and dissemination does not occur unless the animals are subjected to thymectomy and irradiation. The mouse model has been especially useful for drug screening and vaccination experiments. The armadillo has also been used extensively as an experimental model. In this animal, the disease becomes disseminated to all organs, in contrast to the disease in man.

The armadillo has been especially useful in providing a system for the study of immunologic factors that control development of the disease. It is also useful in providing large numbers of *M. leprae* for laboratory investigation vaccination attempts. Approximately 200 g of *M. leprae* (1×10^{12} organisms) can be obtained from one animal 15 months after inoculation. The potential usefulness of the armadillo model, however, has been threatened by the finding of a naturally occurring leprosy-like disease among wild armadillos. Until the armadillo can be bred in captivity and pathogen-free animals are available, its full-scale use as an experimental model is hampered. Man is highly resistant to experimental infection. A number of attempts have been made to infect humans experimentally, but most have ended in failure.

Antigenic Structure

A number of highly immunogenic substances have been identified in *M. leprae*. Among these are a unique phenolic glycolipid, lipoarabinomannan, and proteins that are integral parts of the peptidoglycan layer. The phenolic glycolipid is serologically active, and has been biochemically characterized and synthesized. An enzyme-linked immunosorbent assay (ELISA) based on the use of this antigen is currently being evaluated for clinical use. The lipoarabinomannan is clearly a dominant antigen of the leprosy bacillus and is immunologically cross-reactive with a similar product from *M. tuberculosis*.

The most recent advances in the identification of major antigenic determinants have resulted from the use of monoclonal antibodies and the construction of genomic libraries for the characterization and expression of genes specifying *M. leprae* protein antigens. A number of these have now been characterized and are currently being studied for their potential use in immunodiagnosis and as a vaccine component for protection against leprosy.

Clinical Infection

Epidemiology. There are approximately 12 million persons with leprosy throughout the world at the present time. The disease is most prevalent in tropical areas, especially in Africa, South and Southeast Asia, and parts of Central and South America. In endemic areas of Africa, 20 to 50 persons in every 1000 may be infected. Within the United States, leprosy is endemic in Hawaii and in small areas of Texas, California, Louisiana, and Florida. In recent years there has been a continuous increase in the number of new cases reported each year, mostly in foreign-born immigrants from leprosy-endemic areas, especially Mexico, the Philippines, Southeast Asia, and Cuba.

Humans appear to be the only natural host for *M. leprae*. Infection is acquired by contact with patients with lepromatous leprosy who shed large numbers of organisms in their nasal secretions and ulcer exudates, but the precise modes of transmission have not been established. The major portal of entry is probably the respiratory tract. Biting insects and breast milk may also be potential sources of infection. Spread by the cutaneous route through excoriations in the skin can occur but is not believed to play a significant role.

Although humans have traditionally been considered the sole natural hosts of *M. leprae*, an organism indistinguishable from the leprosy bacillus has been recovered from wild armadillos captured for use in experimental research. Up to 10% of the animals in certain regions of Louisiana are infected with a disseminated disease resembling lepromatous leprosy. Also, in addition to their occurrence in wild armadillos, organisms indistinguishable from *M. leprae* have been recovered from lesions in a sooty mangabey monkey from Africa. The organisms are transmissible to monkeys of the same species, where they produce a disseminated disease similar to human leprosy. These findings, coupled with observations that show that certain arthropods may play a role in the transmission of infection, provide additional parameters in the currently ill-defined epidemiology of this disease.

Both environmental and host factors determine susceptibility to infection with *M. leprae*. Geographic, ethnic, and socioeconomic factors contribute to the spread of leprosy by affecting the number of untreated or ineffectively treated lepromatous cases and the opportunities for exposure. Persons in household contact with lepromatous leprosy have a five- to tenfold increase in risk compared with persons with no known household contact.

Genetic factors have been shown to contribute considerably to the striking individual differences in susceptibility and in type of response to infection with *M. leprae*. The most convincing evidence to date has been provided by studies designed to detect linkage by comparing HLA segregation patterns with the distribution of leprosy within sibships. There is evidence of the existence of a gene predisposing to tuberculoid leprosy that is linked to HLA. In the multiple-case families the HLA-linked susceptibility gene appears to be either DR2 itself or a gene associated with DR2. Genetic differences among hosts in response to infection with *M. leprae* reflect differences in specific immunologic competence among persons and are consistent with the variation in pathologic types that is manifested by patients with leprosy along the spectrum of the disease.

Pathogenesis. The spectrum of disease activity in leprosy is very broad, characterized by pronounced variations in clinical, histopathologic, and immunologic findings. On the basis of these properties, Ridley and Jopling have established a classification scheme consisting of five forms of leprosy: tuberculoid (TT), borderline tuberculoid (BT), borderline (BB), borderline lepromatous (BL), and lepromatous (LL). In this spectrum, which is summarized in Table 31–3, only two forms—TT and LL—are stable. The others are unstable, especially BT, which in the absence of treatment can regress to BB or BL.

TABLE 31–3. CLINICAL, HISTOLOGIC, BACTERIOLOGIC, AND IMMUNOLOGIC FEATURES OF THE DIFFERENT TYPES OF LEPROSY

	Types of Leprosy				
Feature	Tuberculoid	Borderline Tuberculoid	Borderline	Borderline Lepromatous	Lepromatous
Skin lesions					
Numbers	1 to 3	Few to moderate	Moderate	Many	Very many
Symmetry	Very asymmetrical	Asymmetrical	Asymmetrical	Slightly asymmetrical	Symmetrical
Anesthesia	Very marked	Marked	Moderate	Slight	None
Nerve enlargement[a]					
Cutaneous sensory	Common	May occur	0	0	0
Peripheral nerves	0 to 1	Common, asymmetrical	Common, asymmetrical	Moderately asymmetrical	Symmetrical
Skin histology					
Granuloma cell	Epithelioid	Epithelioid	Epithelioid	Histiocyte	Foamy histiocyte
Lymphocytes	+ + +	+ + +	+	± or + +	±[b]
Dermal nerves	Destroyed	Mostly destroyed	Some visible	Visible	Easily visible
Bacilli numbers (routine examination)	0	0, +, or + +	+, + +, or + + +	+ + + +	+ + + + +
Lymph nodes					
Paracortical infiltrate	Nil, immunoblasts	Sarcoid-like	Diffuse epithelioid	Diffuse histiocytes	Massive infiltrate with foamy histiocytes and Virchow cells
Germinal centers	Normal	Normal	Normal	Some hypertrophy	Gross hypertrophy
Lepromin test	+ + +	+ +	± or 0	0	0
Reactions					
ENL	0	0	0	Rare	Very common
Lepra	?	Common	Very common	Very common	(Rare)[c]

From Grove et al: J Infect Dis 134:205, 1976.

ENL, erythema nodosum leprosum. Mahmoud: J Infect Dis 134:205, 1976.

[a] Nerves of predilection: ulnar, median, lateral popliteal, facial, great auricular, and posterior tibial.

[b] In lepromatous leprosy the peripheral blood shows an absolute decrease in T lymphocytes and an absolute increase in B lymphocytes.

[c] Lepra reactions are occasionally seen in treated lepromatous patients whose leprosy developed from borderline forms that were not treated.

M. leprae is an obligate intracellular parasite that multiplies very slowly within the mononuclear phagocytes, especially the histiocytes of the skin and Schwann cells of the nerves. It has an especially strong predilection for nerves.

TUBERCULOID LEPROSY. In tuberculoid leprosy, skin biopsies show mature granuloma formation in the dermis consisting of epithelioid cells, giant cells, and rather extensive infiltration of lymphocytes. Acid-fast bacilli usually cannot be demonstrated. The organisms invade the nerves and selectively colonize the Schwann cells. The cutaneous nerve twigs are obliterated, and the larger nerves are swollen and destroyed by granulomas. The nerve damage is nonspecific and arises as a consequence of the cell-mediated immune response.

LEPROMATOUS LEPROSY. The histopathologic findings in lepromatous leprosy are strikingly different. Epithelioid and giant cells are absent, and lymphocytes are rare and diffusely distributed. The inflammatory infiltrate consists largely of histiocytes with a unique foamy appearance resulting from the accumulation of bacterial lipids. Massive numbers of acid-fast bacilli are found within the macrophages. Skin biopsy specimens may contain up to 10^9 bacilli per gram of tissue. *M. leprae* tends to invade vascular channels, resulting in a continuous bacteremia in lepromatous patients and consistent involvement of the reticuloendothelial system. The nerves are also infected, and numerous bacilli can be seen within the Schwann cells. Damage to the nerve structure, however, is less than in tuberculoid leprosy.

Immunity. Leprosy is a disease of low infectivity (Fig. 31–13). Most persons never have clinical manifestations of disease, while many others have a localized lesion that heals spontaneously. This implies that those who develop disease are immunologically defective with respect to *M. leprae*. Also, in leprosy there is a close correlation between the various clinical forms and the cell-mediated immune response of the host. This is shown in Figure 31–14, which illustrates the inverse relationship between the intensity of the delayed hypersensitivity response to *M. leprae* and the humoral response throughout the clinical spectrum of the disease. Patients with tuberculoid leprosy exhibit a strong delayed-type hypersensitivity to lepromin, and the histology of lesions is that of hypersensitivity granulomas. As the disease progresses across the leprosy spectrum, there is a progressive loss of hypersensitivity and development of an anergic state in the patient with lepromatous leprosy. A concomitant loss of cell-mediated immunity parallels the decline of delayed hypersensitivity to *M. leprae* antigens. Conversely, a high serologic response characterizes lepromatous leprosy, and polyclonal hypergammaglobulinemia is a characteristic feature. Antibodies to *M. leprae* that cross-react with other mycobacteria may be detected

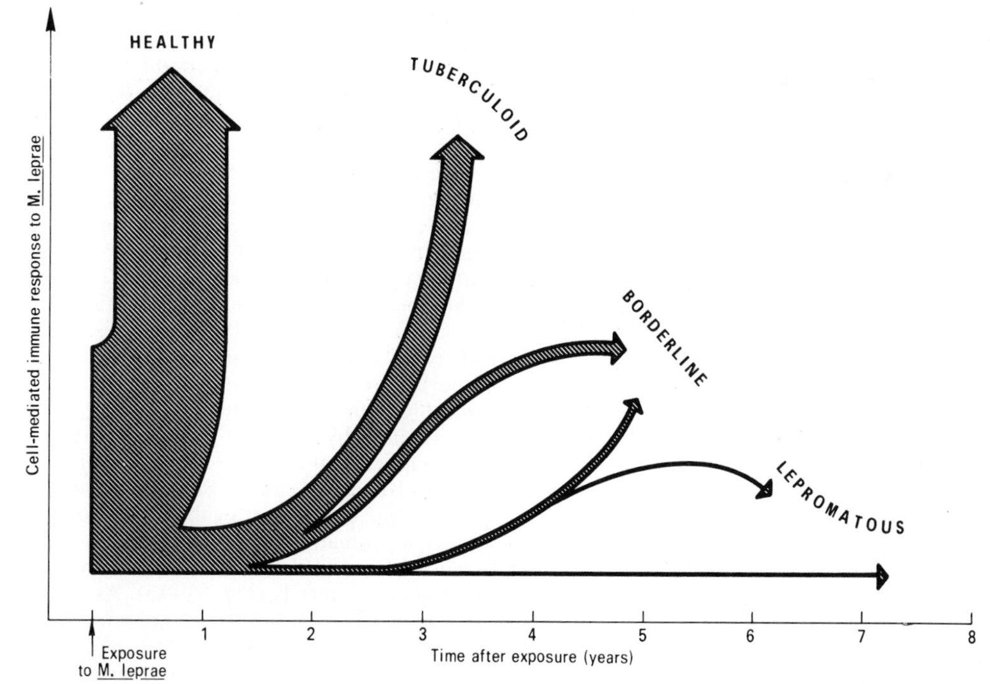

Fig. 31–13. A schematic representation of the hypothesis of how the development of subclinical infection and various types of leprosy is related to time of onset of cell-mediated immune response to *M. leprae* antigens after the initial exposure. The thickness of the lines indicates the proportion of individuals from the exposed population that is likely to fall into each category. The indicated incubation periods, 2 to 3 years in tuberculoid and 6 to 7 years in lepromatous leprosy, probably represent the shortest incubation periods. They are often considerably longer. *(From Godal et al: Bull Inst Pasteur 72:273, 1974.)*

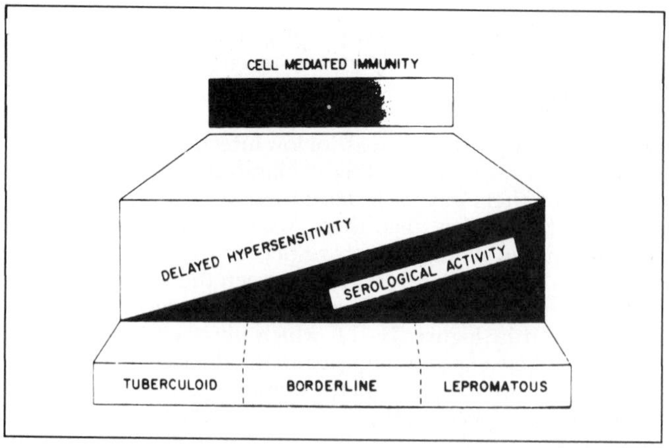

Fig. 31–14. A schematic representation of the relationship between antibody production, delayed hypersensitivity, and cell-mediated immunity as related to severity of intracellular infections. *(From Bullock: J Infect Dis 137:341, 1978, as modified from Adv Intern Med 21:149, 1976.)*

in the sera of 75% to 95% of the patients with the lepromatous form of the disease. Humoral antibodies play no protective role, however, in immune defense.

In patients with lepromatous leprosy, erythema nodosum sometimes occurs spontaneously or is precipitated by treatment. It results from immune-complex deposition in the tissues. A number of abnormal serologic activities are also associated with lepromatous leprosy, including a biologic false-positive reaction in routine serologic tests for syphilis (Table 31–4).

Lepromin Test. Skin testing is not diagnostically useful but is of value in determining the position of the patient on the immunologic spectrum. The skin test material, lepromin, consists of a heat-killed suspension of *M. leprae* prepared from lepromatous nodules. When injected intracutaneously, two types of reaction occur. The first, an early reaction (Fernandez reaction), resembles the tuberculin reaction and appears in 24 to 48 hours. In the late reaction (Mitsuda reaction) an indurated nodule develops after 3 to 4 weeks. This corresponds to the formation of an immunologic granuloma. If the intact organisms are removed or if more purified preparations of lepromin are employed, the late lepromin reaction can be reduced or eliminated and the 48-hour reaction intensified. The early reaction is an indication of a delayed hypersensitivity to soluble *M. leprae* antigens by a previously sensitized person. The late granulomatous reaction corresponds to the ability of the person, sensitized or nonsensitized, to produce an immunologic granuloma in the presence of whole bacteria. Patients with tuberculoid leprosy usually exhibit both early and late lepromin reactions, but lepromatous patients never show these reactions because of complete anergy to the antigens of *M. leprae*. This anergy is very persistent in spite of long-term therapy.

Lepromin lacks specificity. Positive lepromin tests are elicited in patients with tuberculosis in areas of the world where no leprosy exists. Also, a positive lepromin test can be induced in normal, healthy children by vaccination with BCG.

TABLE 31–4. ABNORMAL SEROLOGIC ACTIVITIES ASSOCIATED WITH LEPROMATOUS LEPROSY

Abnormality	Prevalence[a] (%)
False-positive VDRL test	>10
Autoantibodies	
To testicular germinal cells	b
To thyroglobulin	b
Antinuclear factors	0–30
Rheumatoid factor	0–50
Amyloid-related serum component protein	>50
Elevated level of C-reactive protein	b
Circulatory suppressor factor(s)	b
Elevated level of chemotactic factor inactivator	b
Cryoglobulinemia	>30
Elevated level of Clq reacting substances	b

From Bullock: J Infect Dis 137:341, 1978.
[a] Approximate prevalence based on published literature.
[b] Prevalence not established.

Clinical Manifestations. The incubation period is long, usually ranging from about 2 to 5 years, although periods as short as 3 months and up to 40 years have been reported. The presence of bacilli in the skin can often be demonstrated before the recognition of clinical symptoms. In one reported case, leprosy bacilli were seen in smears from an apparently normal earlobe 2 years before cutaneous and neural leprosy of the forearms and legs developed.

The earliest symptom of leprosy is usually an asymptomatic, slightly hypopigmented macule several centimeters in diameter, which usually occurs on the trunk or distal portion of the extremities. Approximately three fourths of all patients with an early solitary lesion heal spontaneously (Fig. 31–13). In some patients, however, the infection progresses to one of a wide spectrum of patterns, which vary markedly in histopathologic and clinical manifestations. The immunologic status of the patient determines the prognosis. At one end of the spectrum is tuberculoid leprosy, a relatively benign form characterized by skin lesions 3 to 30 cm in diameter and few in number. Intermediate in its position in the spectrum, as well as in its severity of infection, is borderline leprosy in which skin lesions are more numerous and nerve involvement is more severe. Patients with borderline leprosy may move toward either end of the spectrum. Such movements are accompanied by serious hypersensitivity reactions, especially as the clinical status of the patient improves, typically from a BL to a BB classification. Such reactions are regarded as an "upgrading" of the host's cellular immune response.

In lepromatous leprosy, which is the most severe and extensive form of the disease, the lesions are multiple and are distributed bilaterally (Fig. 31–15). As the disease progresses, the lesions coalesce and there is a marked folding of the skin, especially of the forehead, eyebrows, nose, and earlobes, resulting in the classic leonine facies. The eyebrows and eyelashes are often lost, and the gradual destruction of the small peripheral nerves leads to trauma and secondary infection. Erythema nodosum leprosum (ENL) is a serious reactional state that occurs in more than 50% of patients within the first year of effective antileprosy treatment. It is believed that ENL triggered by antimycobacterial therapy is precipitated by the release of antigenic material after the degradation of large numbers of leprosy bacilli. Antibodies to *M. leprae*

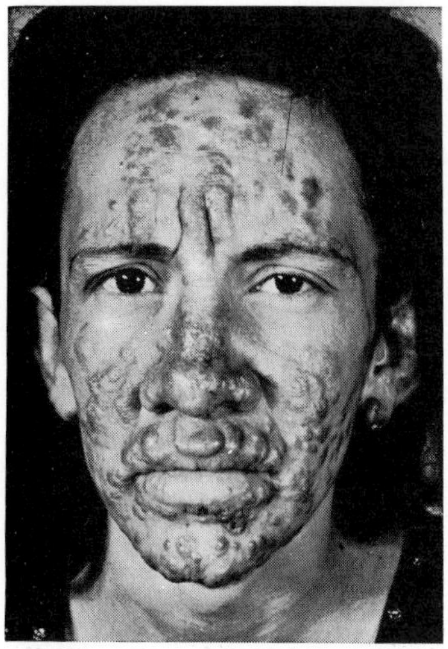

Fig. 31–15. Leprosy patient before treatment. *(From Johansen et al: Public Health Rep 65:204, 1950.)*

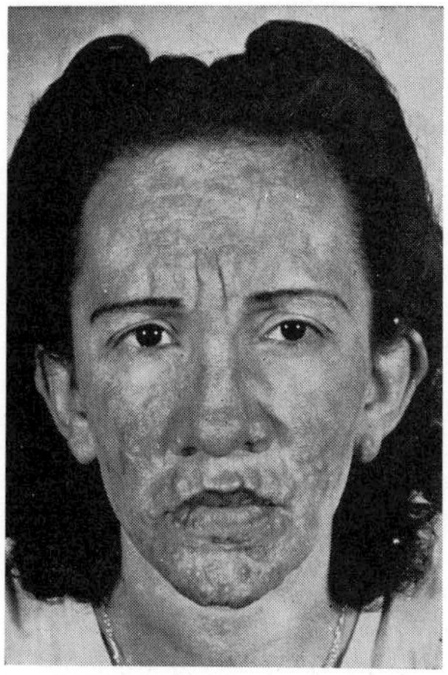

Fig. 31–16. Leprosy patient in Fig. 31–15 after 12-month treatment with the sulfone promacetin. *(From Johansen et al: Public Health Rep 65:204, 1950.)*

are presumed to complex with these antigens, thereby inducing severe constitutional reactions. In untreated cases, death results from respiratory obstruction, renal failure, or secondary infection.

Laboratory Diagnosis. A diagnosis of leprosy may be suspected from the symptoms, the type and distribution of the lesions, and a history of having lived in an endemic area. Diagnosis is made by the demonstration of acid-fast bacilli in smears of skin lesions, nasal scrapings, earlobes, and tissue secretions. The bacilli are numerous in lepromatous leprosy, but in tuberculoid leprosy they are very difficult and often impossible to detect. The characteristic histologic response in biopsy material is helpful in such cases and is essential for accurate classification of the disease within the disease spectrum. Since *M. leprae* in paraffinized tissues is frequently not acid-fast when stained by the Ziehl-Neelsen method, interpretation of tissue sections can be improved by use of the Wade-Fite technique, which restores acid-fastness.

Treatment. For many years the mainstay of treatment for leprosy has been 4,4′-diaminodiphenylsulfone (DDS or dapsone). Since its first use on a wide scale in 1950, almost all of the treatment has consisted of dapsone alone (Fig. 31–16). As a consequence of its long-term use as the single therapeutic agent for leprosy, a marked increase in the prevalence of both primary and secondary resistance to dapsone now threatens its future usefulness. Drug resistance has been reported from 25 countries where overall rates of secondary drug resistance range from 2% to 19%, depending on locale. Rates of resistance as high as 40% have been reported in some areas. In response to this threat, the World Health Organization has recommended a combined regimen of dapsone, rifampin, and clofazimine for all patients with lepromatous leprosy and a regimen of dapsone and rifampin for all those with tuberculoid disease. Treatment should be continued until skin smears are free of bacilli. This may permit treatment to be stopped after a minimum of 2 years, in contrast to the traditional dapsone regimen of lifelong chemotherapy.

Prevention. The control of leprosy, and perhaps its eventual elimination from the world, should be possible. Unfortunately, however, progress in this direction has been slow, primarily because of ignorance, superstition, poverty and overpopulation in endemic areas of the world that account for most of the cases.

Early detection and rigid isolation of all acute lepromatous and indeterminate types of leprosy are important. This should be followed by prophylactic chemotherapy for persons in close contact with the patient. For long-term effective control and eventual eradication of leprosy, however, a method of primary prevention is an urgent need. Largely under the auspices of the World Health Organization, a global effort is currently being made to develop an effective antileprosy vaccine. Three major trials using BCG for the active immunization of children in villages where lepromatous leprosy is highly endemic have yielded widely divergent results. A new WHO vaccine containing *M. leprae* derived from armadillos is currently being tested in large-scale clinical trials in India. The objectives are to evaluate the prophylactic efficacy of the vaccine and to assess its value with and without accompanying BCG.

Mycobacteria Associated with Animal Diseases

Mycobacterium lepraemurium. *M. lepraemurium,* the causative agent of rat leprosy, is a chronic disease that occurs spontaneously among house rats in many parts of the world. The disease is probably transmitted naturally from rat to rat by fleas. It is a disease characterized by subcutaneous indurations, swelling of lymph nodes, emaciation, and sometimes ulceration and loss of hair. Acid-fast bacilli resembling *M. leprae* are found in large numbers in the mononuclear cells of the subcutaneous tissues, lymph nodes, and nodules in the liver and lungs. Because of the similarity of the disease to human leprosy, it was thought at one time that rats could be a potential source of the human disease. The geographic distribution of rat leprosy, however, does not correspond with the distribution of human leprosy. At present it appears that *M. lepraemurium* and *M. leprae* are not related species but that there is a relatedness between *M. lepraemurium* and *M. avium.*

M. lepraemurium can be maintained for months in tissue cultures of monocytes, where it has a generation time of about 7 days. It has also been cultured in rat fibroblasts, and in vitro in a cysteine-containing medium. *M. lepraemurium* has provided a useful model system for the study of host-parasite relationships of an intracellular parasite.

Mycobacterium paratuberculosis. *M. paratuberculosis,* often referred to as Johne's bacillus, produces a chronic enteritis in ruminants. The disease is of major economic concern in cattle and sheep, as entire herds may become infected through contact with infected feces. The lesions, which are confined to the intestinal tract, are proliferative and granulomatous and contain enormous numbers of acid-fast bacilli within the monocytes. The disease is invariably fatal.

M. paratuberculosis can be grown in the laboratory only by supplementing the medium with killed mycobacteria or with mycobactin, an iron-chelating compound unique to the mycobacteria and required for iron transport (Chap. 5, p. 500). Taxonomically, *M. paratuberculosis* bears a strong resemblance to members of the *M. avium* complex. Strong skin test cross-reactivity has also been observed between *M. avium* and *M. paratuberculosis.*

Mycobacterium microti. *M. microti* causes generalized tuberculosis in the vole. Commonly referred to as the vole bacillus, it is somewhat longer and thinner in culture than other mammalian species. Irregular S-shaped, hook-shaped, semicircular, and circular forms have been seen in tissues of infected voles. Primary growth does not occur on media containing glycerol. The organism grows more slowly than the human and bovine species, requiring 4 to 8 weeks for the appearance of minute colonies.

Immunologically, *M. microti* is closely related to *M. tuberculosis* and *M. bovis.* For this reason, it was included in pilot studies with BCG to test its effectiveness when compared with BCG in the immunization of humans against tuberculosis. A level of protection was provided after 7.5 to 10 years, which was almost identical to that provided by BCG.

FURTHER READING

Books and Reviews

MYCOBACTERIUM

Asselineau C, Asselineau J: Lipides specifiques des mycobacteries. Ann Microbiol (Inst Pasteur) 129A:49, 1978

Barksdale L, Kim K-S: *Mycobacterium.* Bacteriol Rev 41:217, 1977

Casal M (ed): Mycobacteria of Clinical Interest. Proceedings of International Symposium, Cordoba, Spain, Sept. 27–28, 1985. New York, Excerpta Medica, Int Congress Series 697:3, 1986

Chaparas SD: The immunology of mycobacterial infections. CRC Crit Rev Microbiol 12:139, 1982

Daniel TM, Janicki BW: Mycobacterial antigens: A review of their isolation, and immunological properties. Microbiol Rev 42:84, 1978

Goren MB: Mycobacterial lipids. Bacteriol Rev 36:33, 1972

Grange, JM: Mycobacterial Disease. New York, Elsevier, 1980

Hahn H, Kaufmann SHE: The role of cell-mediated immunity in bacterial infections. Rev Infect Dis 3:1221, 1981

Høiby N, Döring G, Schiøtz PO: The role of immune complexes in the pathogenesis of bacterial infections. Ann Rev Microbiol 40:29, 1986

Ratledge C, Stanford J: The Biology of the Mycobacteria. Vol 1. Physiology, Identification and Classification. New York, Academic Press, 1982

Skamene E: Genetic control of resistance to mycobacterial infection. Curr Top Microbiol Immunol 124:49, 1986

Stewart-Tull DES: The immunological activities of bacterial peptidoglycans. Ann Rev Microbiol 34:311, 1980

United States-Japan Cooperative Medical Science Program: Immunology of Tuberculosis and Leprosy: A Symposium. In Leive L, Schlessinger D (eds): Microbiology—1984. Washington DC, American Society for Microbiology, 1984, p 335

Wayne LG, Kubica GP: Family Mycobacteriaceae. In Sneath PHA, Mair NS, Sharpe ME, Holt JG (eds): Bergey's Manual of Systematic Bacteriology, vol 2. Baltimore, Williams & Wilkins, 1986, p 1436

Young LS, Inderlied CB, Berlin OG, Gottlieb MS: Mycobacterial infections in AIDS patients, with an emphasis on the *Mycobacterium avium* complex. Rev Infect Dis 8:1024, 1986

MYCOBACTERIUM TUBERCULOSIS

Eickhoff TC: The current status of BCG immunization against tuberculosis. Annu Rev Med 28:411, 1977

Luri MB: Resistance to Tuberculosis: Experimental Studies in Native and Acquired Defensive Mechanisms. Cambridge, Harvard University Press, 1964

Redmond WB, Bates JH, Engel HWB: Methods for bacteriophage typing of mycobacteria. In Bergan T, Norris JR (eds): Methods in Microbiology, vol 13. New York, Academic Press, 1979, p 345

Snider D Jr, Bridbord K, Hui F (guest eds): Research towards global control and prevention of tuberculosis with an emphasis on vaccine development. Rev Infect Dis 11:S335, 1989

White RG: The adjuvant effect of microbial products on the immune response. Annu Rev Microbiol 30:579, 1976

Wiegeshaus E, Balasubramanian V, Smith DW: Immunity to tuberculosis from the perspective of pathogenesis. Infect Immun 57:3671, 1989

Wolinsky E: Tuberculosis. In Wyngaarden JB, Smith LH Jr (eds): Cecil Textbook of Medicine, ed 18. Philadelphia, WB Saunders, 1988, vol 2, p 1682

Youmans GP: Tuberculosis. Philadelphia, WB Saunders, 1979

NONTUBERCULOUS MYCOBACTERIA

Blaser MJ, Cohn DL: Opportunistic infections in patients with AIDS: Clues to the epidemiology of AIDS and the relative virulence of pathogens. Rev Infect Dis 8:21, 1986

Chapman JS: The Atypical Mycobacterial and Human Mycobacterioses. New York, Plenum, 1977

Davidson PT (ed): International Conference on Atypical Mycobacteria. Rev Infect Dis 3:813, 1981

Desforges JF: *Mycobacterium avium* complex infection in the acquired immunodeficiency syndrome. N Engl J Med 324:1332, 1991

Good RC: Opportunistic pathogens in the genus *Mycobacterium.* Annu Rev Microbiol 39:347, 1985

Tellis CJ, Putnam JS: Pulmonary disease caused by nontuberculosis mycobacteria. Med Clin North Am 64:433, 1980

Wayne LG: The "atypical" mycobacteria: Recognition and disease association. CRC Crit Rev Microbiol 12:185, 1982

MYCOBACTERIUM LEPRAE

Bloom BR, Godal T: Selective health care: Strategies for control of disease in a developing world. V. Leprosy. Rev Infect Dis 5:765, 1983

Bullock WE: Anergy and infection. Adv Intern Med 21:149, 1976

Bullock WE: Leprosy (Hansen's disease). In Wyngaarden JB, Smith LH Jr (eds): Cecil Textbook of Medicine, ed 18. Philadelphia, WB Saunders, 1988, vol 2, p 1696

Fine PEM: Leprosy: The epidemiology of a slow bacterium. Epidemiol Rev 4:161, 1982
Gaylord H, Brennan PJ: Leprosy and the leprosy bacillus: Recent developments in characterization of antigens and immunology of the disease. Annu Rev Microbiol 41:645, 1987
Godal T: Immunological aspects of leprosy—Present status. Prog Allergy 25:211, 1978
Hill GH: Leprosy in Five Young Men. Boulder, Colo, Colorado Associated University Press, 1970
Pan American Health Organization Proceedings: Leprosy: Cultivation of the Etiologic Agent, Immunology, Animal Models. Washington, DC, World Health Organization, 1977
Sansonetti P, Lagrange PH: The immunology of leprosy: Speculations on the leprosy spectrum. Rev Infect Dis 3:422, 1981

Selected Papers

MYCOBACTERIUM TUBERCULOSIS

Bass JB Jr, Serio RA: The use of repeat skin tests to eliminate the booster phenomenon in serial tuberculin testing. Am Rev Respir Dis 123:394, 1981
Bothamley GH, Beck JS, Schreuder GMT, et al: Association of tuberculosis and *M. tuberculosis*-specific antibody levels with HLA. J Infect Dis 159:549, 1989
Brennan PJ: Structure of mycobacteria: Recent developments in defining cell wall carbohydrates and proteins. Rev Infect Dis 11:S420, 1989
Britton WJ, Hellqvist L, Basten A, Inglis AS: Immunoreactivity of a 70 kd protein purified from *Mycobacterium bovis* bacillus Calmette-Guerin by monoclonal antibody affinity chromatography. J Exp Med 164:695, 1986
Catanzaro A: Nosocomial tuberculosis. Am Rev Respir Dis 125:559, 1982
Centers for Disease Control, US Dept Health and Human Services: Diagnosis and management of mycobacterial infection and disease in persons with human immunodeficiency virus infection. Ann Intern Med 106:254, 1987
Centers for Disease Control: Tuberculosis in minorities—United States. MMWR 36:6, 1987
Chaisson RE, Slutkin G: Tuberculosis and human immunodeficiency virus infection. J Infect Dis 159:96, 1989
Chaparas SD, Brown TM, Hyman IS: Antigenic relationships of various mycobacterial species with *Mycobacterium tuberculosis.* Am Rev Respir Dis 117:1091, 1978
Chase MW: The cellular transfer of cutaneous hypersensitivity to tuberculins. Proc Soc Exp Biol Med 59:134, 1945
Collins FM: The immunology of tuberculosis. Am Rev Respir Dis 125 (suppl 3):42, 1982
Comstock GW: Epidemiology of tuberculosis. Am Rev Resp Dis 125 (suppl 3):8, 1982
Comstock GW, Ferebee SH, Hammes LM: A control trial of community wide isoniazid prophylaxis in Alaska. Am Rev Respir Dis 95:935, 1967
Daniel TM, Oxtoby MJ, Pinto ME, Morano SE: The immune spectrum in patients with pulmonary tuberculosis. Am Rev Respir Dis 123:556, 1981
Dannenberg AM Jr: Pathogenesis of pulmonary tuberculosis. Am Rev Respir Dis 125(suppl 3):25, 1982
Dannenberg AM JR: Immune mechanisms in the pathogenesis of pulmonary tuberculosis. Rev Infect Dis 11:S369, 1989
de Bruyn J, Bosmans R, Turneer M, et al: Purification, partial characterization, and identification of a skin-reactive protein antigen of *Mycobacterium bovis* BCG. Infect Immun 55:245, 1987
Edwards LB, Livesay VT, Acquaviva FA, Palmer CE: Height, weight, tuberculous infection and tuberculous disease. Arch Environ Health 22:106, 1971
Eisenach KD, Crawford JT, Bates JH: Genetic relatedness among strains of the *Mycobacterium tuberculosis* complex. Analysis of restriction fragment heterogeneity using cloned DNA probes. Am Rev Respir Dis 133:1065, 1986
Farer LS: Chemoprophylaxis. Am Rev Respir Dis 125 (suppl 3):102, 1982
Goren MB: Immunoreactive substances of mycobacteria. Am Rev Respir Dis 125 (suppl 3):50, 1982
Goren MB, Cernich M, Blokl O: Some observations on mycobacterial acid-fastness. Am Rev Respir Dis 118:151, 1978
Goren MB, Hart PD, Young MR, Armstrong JA: Prevention of phagosome-lysosome fusion in cultured macrophages by sulfatides of *Mycobacterium tuberculosis.* Proc Natl Acad Sci USA 73:2510, 1976
Grange JM, Aber VR, Allen BW, et al: The correlation of bacteriophage types of *Mycobacterium tuberculosis* with guinea-pig virulence and in vitro-indicators of virulence. J Gen Microbiol 108:1, 1978
Hardy MA, Schmidek HH: Epidemiology of tuberculosis aboard a ship. JAMA 203:175, 1968
Higuchi S, Suga M, Dannenberg AM Jr, et al: Persistence of protein, carbohydrate and wax components of tubercle bacilli in dermal BCG lesions. Am Rev Respir Dis 123:397, 1981
Holoshitz J, Klajman A, Drucker I, et al: T lymphocytes of rheumatoid arthritis patients show augmented reactivity to a fraction of mycobacteria cross-reactive with cartilage. Lancet 2:305, 1986
Hyde L: Clinical significance of the tuberculin test. Am Rev Respir Dis 105:453, 1972
Jones WD Jr, Good RC, Thompson NJ, Kelly GD: Bacteriophage types of *Mycobacterium tuberculosis* in the United States. Am Rev Respir Dis 125:640, 1982
Kato K, Yamamoto K-I, Kimura T: Migration of natural suppressor cells from bone marrow to peritoneal cavity by live BCG. J Immunol 135:3661, 1985
Katz P, Goldstein RA, Fauci AS: Immunoregulation in infection caused by *Mycobacterium tuberculosis:* The presence of suppressor monocytes and the alteration of subpopulations of T lymphocytes. J Infect Dis 140:12, 1979
Kaufmann SHE, Flesch I: Function and antigen recognition pattern of L3T4$^+$ T-cell clones from *Mycobacterium tuberculosis*–immune mice. Infect Immun 54:291, 1986
Kent DC, Schwartz R: Active pulmonary tuberculosis with negative tuberculin skin tests. Am Rev Respir Dis 95:411, 1967
Lederer E: Structure de constituants mycobacteriéns: Relation avec l'activité immunologique. Annu Microbiol 129:91, 1978
Magnus K, Edwards LB: The effect of repeated tuberculin testing on postvaccination allergy. Lancet 2:643, 1955
Matthews R, Scoging A, Rees ADM: Mycobacterial antigen-specific human T-cell clones secreting macrophage activating factors. Immunology 54:17, 1985
Morse DL, Hansen RE, Swalbach WG, et al: High rate of tuberculin conversion in Indochinese refugees. JAMA 248:2983, 1982
Ottenhoff THM, Torres P, de las Aguas, et al: Evidence for an HLA-DR4-associated immune-response gene for *Mycobacterium tuberculosis.* Lancet 2:310, 1986
Palmer CE, Long MW: Effects of infection with atypical mycobacteria on vaccination and tuberculosis. Am Rev Respir Dis 94:553, 1966
Retzinger GS, Meredith SC, Takayama K, et al: The role of surface in the biological activities of trehalose 6,6′-dimycolate. J Biol Chem 256:8208, 1981
Rideout VK, Hiltz TE: Epidemic in a high school in Nova Scotia. Can J Public Health 60:22, 1969
Shinnick TM: The 65-kilodalton antigen of *Mycobacterium tuberculosis.* J Bacteriol 169:1080, 1987

Small PM, Schecter GF, Goodman PC: Treatment of tuberculosis in patients with advanced human immunodeficiency virus infection. N Engl J Med 324:289, 1991

Smith DT: The tuberculin unit. Am Rev Respir Dis 99:820, 1969

Smith DT: The diagnostic and prognostic value of the second strength dose of PPD (5 micrograms). Am Rev Respir Dis 101:317, 1970

Snider DE Jr: The tuberculin skin test. Am Rev Respir Dis 125 (suppl 3):108, 1982

Stead WW: Pathogenesis of first episode of chronic pulmonary tuberculosis in man: Recrudescence of residuals of primary infection on exogenous reinfection. Am Rev Respir Dis 95:729, 1967

Stead WW, Bates JH: Evidence of "silent" bacillemia in primary tuberculosis. Ann Intern Med 74:559, 1971

Sunderam G, McDonald RJ, Maniatis T: Tuberculosis as a manifestation of the acquired immunodeficiency syndrome (AIDS). JAMA 256:362, 1986

Suzuki Y, Yoshinaga K, Ono Y, et al: Organization of rRNA genes in *Mycobacterium bovis* BCG. J Bacteriol 169:839, 1987

Thole JER, Dauwerse HG, Das PK, et al: Cloning of *Mycobacterium bovis* BCG DNA and expression of antigens in *Escherichia coli*. Infect Immun 50:800, 1985

van Eden W, Holoshitz J, Nevo Z, et al: Arthritis induced by a T-lymphocyte clone that responds to *Mycobacterium tuberculosis* and to cartilage proteoglycans. Proc Natl Acad Sci USA 82:5117, 1985

Wayne LG: Microbiology of tubercle bacilli. Am Rev Respir Dis 125 (suppl 3):31, 1982

Wayne LG, Lin K-Y: Glyoxylate metabolism and adaptation of *Mycobacterium tuberculosis* to survival under anaerobic conditions. Infect Immun 37:1042, 1982

Young RA, Bloom BR, Grosskinsky CM, et al: Dissection of *Mycobacterium tuberculosis* antigens using recombinant DNA. Proc Natl Acad Sci USA 82:2583, 1985

NONTUBERCULOUS MYCOBACTERIA

Adams RM, Remington JS, Steinberg J, Seibert JS: Tropical fish aquariums: A source of *Mycobacterium marinum* infection resembling sporotrichosis. JAMA 211:457, 1970

Band JD, Ward JI, Fraser DW, et al: Peritonitis due to a *Mycobacterium chelonei*–like organism associated with intermittent chronic peritoneal dialysis. J Infect Dis 145:9, 1982

Barrow WW, Brennan PJ: Immunogenicity of type-specific C-mycoside glycopeptido-lipids of mycobacteria. Infect Immun 36:678, 1982

Brooks RW, Parker BC, Gruft H, Falkinham JO III: Epidemiology of infection by nontuberculous mycobacteria. V. Numbers in eastern United States soils and correlation with soil characteristics. Am Rev Respir Dis 130:630, 1984

Camphausen RT, Jones RL, Brennan PJ: Structure and relevance of the oligosaccharide hapten of *Mycobacterium avium* serotype 2. J Bacteriol 168:660, 1986

Conner DH, Lunn HF: Buruli ulceration: A clinicopathologic study of 38 Ugandans with *Mycobacterium ulcerans*. Arch Pathol 81:183, 1966

Donta ST, Smith PW, Levitz RE, Quintiliani R: Therapy of *Mycobacterium marinum* infections. Arch Intern Med 146:902, 1986

Edwards LB, Acguaviva FA, Livesay VT, et al: An atlas of sensitivity to tuberculin PPD-B and histoplasmin in the United States. Am Rev Respir Dis 99:1, 1969

Edwards LB, Palmer CE: Isolation of "atypical" mycobacteria from healthy persons. Am Rev Respir Dis 80:747, 1959

Feldman RA, Long MW, David HL: *Mycobacterium marinum:* A leisure time pathogen. J Infect Dis 129:618, 1974

Jacobs WR, Snapper SB, Tuckman M, Bloom BR: Mycobacteriophage vector systems. Rev Infect Dis 11:S404, 1989

Johnston WW, Smith DT, Vandiviere HM III: Simultaneous or sequential infection with different mycobacteria. Arch Environ Health 11:37, 1965

Morris SL, Rouse DA, Hussong D, Chaparas SD: Isolation and characterization of recombinant λgtll bacteriophages expressing four different *Mycobacterium intracellulare* antigens. Infect Immun 58:17, 1990

Orme IM, Collins FM: Crossprotection against nontuberculous mycobacterial infections by *Mycobacterium tuberculosis* memory immune T lymphocytes. J Exp Med 163:203, 1986

Palmer CE, Long MW: Effects of infection with atypical mycobacteria on BCG vaccination and tuberculosis. Am Rev Respir Dis 94:553, 1966

Rivoire B, Ranchoff BJ, Chatterjee D, et al: Generation of monoclonal antibodies to the specific sugar epitopes of *Mycobacterium avium* complex serovars. Infect Immun 57:3147, 1989

Yanagihara DL, Barr VL, Knisley CV, et al: Enzyme-linked immunosorbent assay of glycolipid antigens for identification of mycobacteria. J Clin Microbiol 21:569, 1985

MYCOBACTERIUM LEPRAE

Abou-Zeid C, Harboe M, Sundsten B, Cocito C: Cross-reactivity of antigens from the cytoplasm and cell walls of some corynebacteria and mycobacteria. J Infect Dis 151:170, 1985

Britton WJ, Hellqvist L, Basten A, Raison RL: *Mycobacterium leprae* antigens involved in human immune responses. I. Identification of four antigens by monoclonal antibodies. J Immunol 135:4171, 1985

Bullock WE: Leprosy: A model of immunological perturbation in chronic infection. J Infect Dis 137:341, 1978

Chiplunkar S, de Libero G, Kaufmann SHE: *Mycobacterium leprae*–specific Lyt-2^+ T lymphocytes with cytolytic activity. Infect Immun 54:793, 1986

Clark-Curtiss JE, Walsh GP: Conservation of genomic sequences among isolates of *Mycobacterium leprae*. J Bacteriol 171:4844, 1989

Emmrich F, Thole J, van Embden J, Kaufmann SHE: A recombinant 64 kilodalton protein of *Mycobacterium bovis* bacillus Calmette-Guerin specifically stimulates human T4 clones reactive to mycobacterial antigens. J Exp Med 163:1024, 1986

Garsia RJ, Hellqvist L, Booth RJ, et al: Homology of the 70-kilodalton antigens from *Mycobacterium leprae* and *Mycobacterium bovis* with the *Mycobacterium tuberculosis* 71-kilodalton antigen and with the conserved heat shock protein 70 of eucaryotes. Infect Immun 57:204, 1989

Gelber RH, Brennan PJ, Hunter SW, et al: Effective vaccination of mice against leprosy bacilli with subunits of *Mycobacterium leprae*. Infect Immun 58:711, 1990

Grosskinsky CM, Jacobs WR Jr, Clark-Curtiss JE, Bloom BR: Genetic relationships among *Mycobacterium leprae, Mycobacterium tuberculosis,* and candidate leprosy vaccine strains determined by DNA hybridization: identification of an *M. leprae*-specific repetitive sequence. Infect Immun 57:1535, 1989

Hunter SW, Fujiwara T, Brennan PJ: Structure and antigenicity of the major specific antigen of *Mycobacterium leprae*. J Biol Chem 257:15072, 1982

Hunter SW, Gaylord H, Brennan PJ: Structure and antigenicity of the phosphorylated lipopolysaccharide antigens from the leprosy and tubercle bacilli. J Biol Chem 261:12345, 1986

Hunter SW, McNeil M, Modlin RL, et al: Isolation and characterization of the highly immunogenic cell wall-associated proteins of *Mycobacterium leprae*. J Immunol 142:2864, 1989

Jacobs WR, Docherty MA, Curtiss R III, Clark-Curtiss JE: Expression of *Mycobacterium leprae* genes from a *Streptococcus mutans* promoter in *Escherichia coli* K-12. Proc Natl Acad Sci USA 83:1926, 1986

Mohagheghpour N, Munn MW, Gelber RH, Eagleman EG: Identification of an immunostimulating protein from *Mycobacterium leprae*. Infect Immun 58:703, 1990

Ridley DS: Histological classification and the immunological spectrum of leprosy. Bull WHO 51:451, 1974

Ridley DS, Jopling WH: Classification of leprosy according to immunity: A five-group system. Int J Lepr 34:255, 1966

Sathish M, Esser RE, Thole JER, Clark-Curtiss JE: Identification and characterization of antigenic determinants of *Mycobacterium leprae* that react with antibodies in sera of leprosy patients. Infect Immun 58:1327, 1990

Shankara MK, Narayanan E, Kasturi G, et al: Non-cultivable mycobacteria in some field collected arthropods. Lepr India 45:231, 1973

Shepard CC, McRae DH: *Mycobacterium leprae* in mice: Minimal infectious dose, relation between staining quality and infectivity, and effect of cortisone. J Bacteriol 80:365, 1965

Shinnick TM, Sweetser D, Thole J, et al: The etiologic agents of leprosy and tuberculosis share an immunoreactive protein antigen with the vaccine strain *Mycobacterium bovis* BCG. Infect Immun 55:1932, 1987

Van Eden W, deVries RRP, Mehra NK, et al: HLA segregation of tuberculoid leprosy: Confirmation of the DR2 marker. J Infect Dis 141:693, 1980

Van Voorhis WC, Kaplan G, Sarno EN, et al: The cutaneous infiltrates of leprosy. Cellular characteristics and the predominant T-cell phenotypes. N Engl J Med 26:1593, 1982

Williams DL, Gillis TP, Booth RJ, et al: The use of a specific DNA probe and polymerase chain reaction for the detection of *Mycobacterium leprae*. J Infect Dis 162:193, 1990

CHAPTER 32

Actinomycetes

Actinomycetous Bacteria

Comprising a large and diverse group of bacteria, the actinomycetes are gram-positive bacilli with a characteristic tendency to form chains or filaments. The actinomycetes include a number of higher taxa that vary in morphology, oxygen requirements, cell wall composition, and the ability to form spores. These bacteria are classified together because of morphologic similarities and related pathogenicities. Phylogenetic relationships are possible but largely unproven. Actinomycetes cause three major infections—actinomycosis, nocardiosis, and actinomycetoma—which are discussed in this chapter.

The common feature of all actinomycetes is their tendency, differing in degree, to form filaments. To a varying extent, as the bacilli grow, they may fail to separate after cell division, and consequently they form elongated chains of cells about 1 μm in width. In some taxa the filaments become quite long and branch extensively. Actinomycetous filaments are often termed *hyphae* or *mycelia* because of their resemblance to molds (Chap. 80). The initial filaments from which colonies develop are called *substrate* or *vegetative* filaments, and the extent to which substrate filaments develop and branch or fragment into cocci or bacilli after formation is an important characteristic. The higher actinomycetes produce filaments that project above the colony; these *aerial* filaments may branch, fragment into spores, or acquire a characteristic surface structure or pigmentation. Such variations in morphology produce distinct characteristics for the separation and identification of different taxa.

Some actinomycetes grow as rod-shaped cells and filaments that fragment soon after formation to yield individual cells. Nocardioforms produce branching filaments that fragment into cocci and rods. Higher actinomycetes develop extensive, branching filaments and spores. Another type of growth is exhibited by *Dermatophilus,* which produces filaments that divide lengthwise as well as transversely to produce coccoid cells or spores. Recent chemical studies have indicated that morphologic complexity does not necessarily reflect phylogenetic proximity. The corynebacteria are morphologically simple yet linked to the more complex mycobacteria and nocardiae. The highly filamentous *Thermoactinomyces* appears to be closely related to bacilli with simpler forms of growth.

Taxonomists have evaluated many characteristics of the members of this group, including such physiologic properties as enzymatic activity, temperature and oxygen requirements, and fermentation products. Detailed studies have compared DNA content (mole percent guanine plus cytosine [G + C] and homology studies), rRNA oligonucleotide catalogues, antigenic determinants, and analyses of fatty acids, phospholipids, menaquinones, and cell wall composition. Some of these features are compared in Table 32–1.

Cell Wall. Analysis of cell wall composition is one of the most useful taxonomic aids in the classification of the actinomycetous genera. As expected, all the cell walls possess the basic components of the peptidoglycan cell wall material—*N*-acetylglucosamine, muramic acid, alanine, and glutamic acid—but the genera can be characterized by the presence or absence of certain other amino acids and sugars. Chromatographic analysis of cell walls have defined eight chemotypes on the basis of the content of a few sugars and amino acids such as arabinose, galactose, glycine, DL- or LL-diaminopimelic (DAP) acid.

The basic morphology and a few stable distinguishing features of several genera of medically important actinomycetes are summarized in Table 32–1. For comparison, three genera of gram-positive bacilli are included: *Corynebacterium, Propionibacterium,* and *Mycobacterium.* Some genera such as *Mycobacterium* and *Nocardia* have the same chemotype. To further distinguish such genera, a subset of four additional chemotypes has been devised based on the presence or absence of arabinose, galactose, xylose, and madurose in whole cells.

Streptomycetes

The streptomycetes are represented by the genus *Streptomyces* and three related genera. The streptomycetes are the most abundant actinomycetes in nature, with more than 140 species of *Streptomyces.* The most distinctive morphologic feature of this group is the formation of extensively branching aerial and substrate filaments. Streptomycetes are found naturally a few inches below the surface in soil, in water, and on organic debris. Only a few species may, on rare occasions, be patho-

TABLE 32–1. GENERAL CHARACTERISTICS OF ACTINOMYCETES AND SIMILAR GENERA OF NONMOTILE, GRAM-POSITIVE RODS

		Filaments								
Genera	Morphology	Substrate	Aerial	Fragmentation	Spores	Oxygen Requirement	Cell Wall[a] Chemotype	Mol% G + C	Mycolic Acids (No. of Carbons)	Catalase
Corynebacterium	Pleomorphic rods, club-shaped cells	–	–		–	A, F	IV	51–59	+ (22–38)	+
Actinomyces	Rods, filaments, some branching	+	–	+	–	A, F, An	V, VI	57–69	–	–[b]
Arachnia	Rods, filaments, some branching	+	–	+	–	A, M	I	63–65	–	–
Bifidobacterium	Irregular rods with branching	–	–		–	An	VIII	55–67	–	–
Mycobacterium	Rods, some branched filaments	v	–	+	–	A	IV	62–70	+(60–90)	+
Dermatophilus	Large, irregular branched filaments and cocci	+	–	+	+[c]	A, M	III	57–59	–	+
Rhodococcus	Rods, fragmentation into cocci	v	+	+	–	A	IV	59–72	+ (34–64)	+
Propionibacterium	Pleomorphic rods, branched forms, cocci	–	–		–	F	I	53–68	–	+
Nocardia	Rods, filaments, fragmentation into rods and cocci	+	v	+	v	A	IV	64–72	+ (46–60)	+
Nocardiopsis	Branched filaments	+	+	+	+	A	III	64–69	–	+
Actinomadura	Rods, filaments, cocci	+	v	–	+	A	III	65–77	–	+
Streptomyces	Branched filaments	+	+	–	+	A	I	69–78	–	+
Faenia	Branched filaments	+	+	v	+	A	IV	66–68	–	+
Thermoactinomyces	Branched filaments	+	+	–	+	A	III	53–55	–	+

Data from Sneath et al (eds): Bergey's Manual of Systemic Bacteriology, vol 2, Williams & Wilkins, 1986; Williams et al (eds): Bergey's Manual of Systematic Bacteriology, vol 4, Williams & Wilkins, 1989; Goodfellow et al (eds): The Biology of the Actinomycetes. Academic Press, 1984.

+, 90% or more of species positive; –, 10% or less of species positive; v, 11% to 89% of species positive; A, aerobic; F, facultative; M, microaerophilic; An, anaerobic.

[a] I, LL-diaminopimelic acid (DAP) and glycine; III, DL-DAP; IV, DL-DAP, arabinose, and galactose; V, lysine and ornithine; VI, lysine, aspartic acid, and galactose; VIII, ornithine.

[b] *A. viscosus* is catalase-positive.

[c] Motile spores; multilocular sporangia.

genic. Most are ubiquitous, benign bacteria that provide an essential ecologic function in the soil.

Much of the pioneering and continuing knowledge of streptomycetes and other soil microorganisms has been obtained at the Rutgers University Institute of Microbiology, New Brunswick, New Jersey. The inspiration for the institute was Selman Waksman, in whose laboratory the antibiotic streptomycin was discovered in 1944.

Morphology and Physiology

The streptomycetes are aerobic, filamentous bacteria. They produce filaments (or mycelia) that are long, highly branched, and nonfragmenting. Aerial filaments may be rudimentary or extensive and may be embellished with spirals, coils, or multiple branching. The aerial filaments of many species produce spores, often in chains. The identification of a species of *Streptomyces* uses morphologic criteria. The spore chains may be straight to flexuous, looped or spiral. Other important characteristics include the spore surface (e.g., smooth, rugose, spiny); fragmentation or sporulation of substrate filaments; and pigments associated with the spores (blue, gray, green, red, violet, white, or yellow), substrate filaments, or diffusible pigments. Other useful phenotypic properties include the presence of various enzymes (e.g., proteinases, hydrolases), patterns of carbohydrate and nitrogen assimilation, the ability to degrade a variety of compounds (e.g., tyrosine, xanthine), susceptibility to antibiotics and chemicals, and growth temperature.

Cultural Characteristics. Colonies grow relatively slowly and require several days to become visible. The colonies are tenacious and adhere to the agar because the substrate filaments penetrate the medium and anchor the colony. After 7 to 10 days, aerial spore-bearing filaments proliferate, and colonies typically lose their luster. As indicated above, spore color and chain morphology are helpful in beginning to identify species of the genus *Streptomyces*. In stationary broth cultures the organisms grow on the surface as a mat until they sink under their own weight. In aerated, shaken liquid cultures, streptomycetes grow in spherical microcolonies and do not produce aerial filaments.

Ecologic and Medical Importance. In their natural habitat in the soil, streptomycetes decompose organic matter. As the filaments render clay more adherent, they may also affect the texture of soil. The presence of streptomycetes contributes to the odor of soil. Indeed, cultures often elaborate the familiar aroma of aged straw or freshly turned earth.

The major medical importance of the streptomycetes is the production of antibiotics. Collectively, the streptomycetes are responsible for about 85% of the known antibiotics, the remaining ones being derived from fungi and other bacteria. Among the most important antibiotics synthesized by streptomycetes are streptomycin, chloramphenicol, tetracycline, neomycin, erythromycin, kanamycin, cycloheximide, amphotericin B, and nystatin. In addition to these antibacterial and antifungal antibiotics, various species of *Streptomyces* produce antiviral, antiparasitic, and anticancer agents. Although the medical potential of this group of bacteria has long been exploited by pharmaceutical companies, the impact of antibiotic production in nature on maintenance of microbial balance or evolution is unknown.

Actinomycosis

Actinomyces israelii, Actinomyces naeslundii, and *Arachnia propionica*

A chronic, both suppurative and granulomatous infection, actinomycosis is characterized by pyogenic lesions with interconnecting sinus tracts that contain granules, which are composed of microcolonies of the bacterial pathogen embedded in tissue elements. The name *actinomycosis* derives from two Greek words that describe the appearance of the granules in tissue as being "ray like" (*actino*), because of the array of peripheral filaments, and similar to a "fungus" (*mykēs*). Actinomycosis can be caused by any of several closely related species of actinomycetes, all of which are members of the normal flora of the mouth and gastrointestinal tract, as are numerous species of similar bacteria that are benign commensals. Based on the site of involvement, three clinical forms of actinomycosis are recognized: cervicofacial, thoracic, and abdominal. A fourth entity, genital actinomycosis, has been described in women with intrauterine devices.

The etiologic agents of actinomycosis, in decreasing order of frequency, are *Actinomyces israelii, Arachnia propionica,* and *Actinomyces naeslundii.* Very rarely, the disease has been attributed to *Bifidobacterium dentium.* All of these bacteria colonize the healthy mucous membranes of the mouth and gastrointestinal tract of all humans. At least two additional *Actinomyces* species, *A. viscosus* and *A. odontolyticus,* are also found among the oral flora; these species have rarely been implicated as agents of actinomycosis but are important causes of or contributors to dental caries. *Actinomyces meyeri* has been reported to cause thoracic actinomycosis. In cattle the predominant agent of actinomycosis is *Actinomyces bovis.* Although the clinical disease in cattle called *lumpy jaw* is similar to human actinomycosis, *A. bovis* is not associated with humans either as a commensal or pathogen.

Morphology and Physiology

The three genera *Actinomyces, Arachnia,* and *Bifidobacterium* share similarities in morphology and physiology. On an enriched solid medium (e.g., brain-heart infusion agar) or thioglycollate broth at 37C, they produce initial microcolonies composed of branching substrate filaments that after 24 to 48 hours fragment into diphtheroids, short chains, and coccobacillary forms (Figs. 32–1 and 32–2). They develop neither aerial filaments nor spores. They are not acid-fast, and their cell walls do not contain arabinose or mycolic acids. They may resemble other diphtheroidal bacteria such as *Propionibacterium* and *Corynebacterium,* which also reside on the oral and intestinal mucosa.

Most strains of the five species of *Actinomyces* referred to above are facultative anaerobes that grow best in the presence of carbon dioxide. *A. propionica* is also a facultative anaerobe, but its growth is not affected by carbon dioxide. *B. dentium* is strictly anaerobic. Table 32–2 indicates the biochemical and physiologic characteristics that are most helpful in speciating these actinomycetes. *A. bovis* is included for comparison.

Species of *Actinomyces* and *Arachnia* resemble other diphtheroidal or filamentous bacteria in morphology and in many physiologic characteristics. Although quite similar to *Actinomyces israelii, Arachnia propionica* can be differentiated serol-

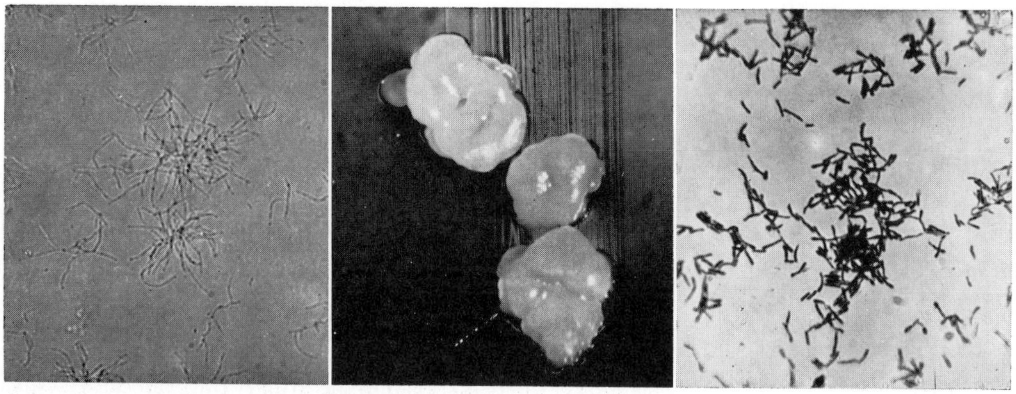

A B C

Fig. 32–1. **A.** *Actinomyces israelii.* Spidery colony on brain-heart infusion agar plate, 24 hours. × 500. **B.** *A. israelii.* Molar tooth colony on brain-heart infusion agar plate, 15 days. **C.** *A. israelii.* Gram stain of smear from rough colony, showing diphtheroid forms. × 1200. *(Courtesy of Mycology Unit, Centers for Disease Control, Atlanta, Ga.)*

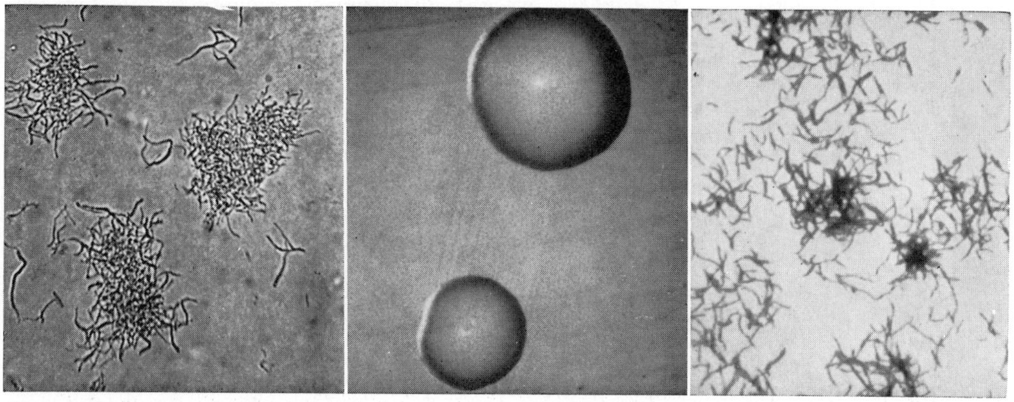

A B C

Fig. 32–2. **A.** *Actinomyces naeslundii.* Dense, tangled colony on brain-heart infusion agar plate, 24 hours. × 475. **B.** *A. naeslundii.* Smooth colony on brain-heart infusion agar plate, 7 days. **C.** *A. naeslundii.* Gram stain smear from smooth colony, showing branching diphtheroid forms. × 900. *(Courtesy of Mycology Unit, Centers for Disease Control, Atlanta, Ga.)*

TABLE 32–2. DIFFERENTIAL CHARACTERISTICS OF *ACTINOMYCES* SPECIES, *BIFIDOBACTERIUM DENTIUM*, AND *ARACHNIA PROPIONICA*

	A. bovis	*A. israelii*	*A. naeslundii*	*A. odontolyticus*	*A. viscosus*	*B. dentium*	*A. propionica*
Oxygen requirement	An	An	F	F	F	An	F
Catalase	−	−	−	−	+	−	−
Nitrate reduction	−	V	+	+	+	−	+
Gelatin hydrolysis	−	−	−	−	−	−	−
Esculin hydrolysis	+	+	+	V	+	V	−
Fermentation (acid production)							
Arabinose	−	V	−	V	−	+	−
Glucose	+	+	+	+	+	+	+
Lactose	+	+	V	V	V	+	+
Mannitol	−	V	−	−	−	+	+
Raffinose	−	V	+	V	+	+	+
Sucrose	V	+	+	+	+	+	+
Trehalose	V	+	V	V	V	+	+
Xylose	V	+	−	V	−	+	−

F, facultative anaerobe; An, anaerobe; +, 90% or more of strains tested positive; −, 90% or more strains tested negative; V, variable reactions, strains positive or negative.

ogically by the presence of LL-DAP in the cell wall and by the production of propionic acid during fermentation of glucose. *Arachnia* can be distinguished from *Propionibacterium* by its morphology, cell wall composition, and other (e.g., catalase activity) features (Table 32–1).

A. naeslundii, A. viscosus, and *A. odontolyticus* are more aerotolerant than *A. israelii* and *A. bovis.* Most strains of the latter two species grow better under anaerobic conditions, but all members of the genus *Actinomyces* are enhanced by carbon dioxide. Indeed, they vary in oxygen tolerance but require carbon dioxide.

Clinical Infection

Epidemiology. Actinomycosis has been observed in persons of all ages, but the disease is rare in children less than 10 years of age. Most cases occur between the ages of 15 and 35 years. The infection rate in males is approximately twice that in females. Most patients do not have compromised defenses or other diseases.

Pathogenesis. Two of the four etiologic agents listed in Table 32–3, *A. israelii* and *A. propionica,* cause most cases of actinomycosis. However, the pathology and pathogenesis are the same regardless of the agent or location of the infection. In most cases a traumatic episode allows the organisms to cross the mucosal or epithelial surface of the mouth or lower gastrointestinal tract. Aspiration of the organisms may lead to pulmonary or thoracic actinomycosis. In deeper tissue the organisms grow anaerobically, elicit a cellular infiltrate, and spread by expansion to contiguous tissue. Multiple pyogenic lesions become joined by interconnecting sinuses. If unchecked, this process continues, and draining sinus tracts may erupt to the skin surface. The organisms are contained within the pyogenic or, subsequently, granulomatous lesions and within granules in the sinus channels. The granules, which are also called grains or sulfur granules, are composed of tissue elements and the organisms.

The pathogenetic determinant(s) of the agents of actinomycosis is not understood. Numerous, similar endogenous bacteria do not cause disease. Although formation of granules reflects both host and microbial responses, granules appear to protect the bacteria from phagocytosis by the many neutrophils that they elicit. Furthermore, several studies have indicated that most actinomycotic granules are colonized by gram-negative bacteria, which may combine with the actinomycete to enhance pathogenicity.

Clinical Manifestations

CERVICOFACIAL ACTINOMYCOSIS. Cervicofacial disease accounts for at least half the cases of actinomycosis. A trauma to the oral mucosa permits these endogenous bacteria to breach the normal defenses of the intact mucosa. Most cases follow dental caries or gingival disease, and the lower jaw region becomes involved. With growth of the bacteria, the area becomes swollen and discolored. Patients experience discomfort but little pain, and if detected early, the prognosis is good. Pyogenic abscesses may develop, with the formation of interconnecting sinuses that contain the granules. Because these bacteria can penetrate the cortex of any bone and produce osteomyelitis, the potential for bone involvement is very high.

THORACIC ACTINOMYCOSIS. Either extension of the cervicofacial form or aspiration of the agent may lead to pulmonary infection. The symptoms, which often resemble those of subacute pulmonary infection, are mild fever, cough, and purulent sputum. Eventually, lung tissue is destroyed, sinus tracts develop, and invasion of the ribs or vertebrae may occur.

ABDOMINAL ACTINOMYCOSIS. Abdominal infection is initiated by a traumatic perforation of the intestinal mucosa, most often resulting from a ruptured appendix or an ulcer. The symptomatology is determined by the location of the lesion and the organs that are involved. The disease progresses slowly and insidiously. Involvement of the liver may produce jaundice, whereas spread to the urinary tract can cause cystitis or pyelonephritis. The vertebrae may become infected, and sinuses may erupt through the abdominal wall. Radiography often reveals an indistinct tumorlike mass.

GENITAL ACTINOMYCOSIS. Genital actinomycosis has been described in women using intrauterine devices. In most cases, diagnosis is based on histologic evidence of infection with actinomycetous bacteria, and granules are uncommon. Subclinical colonization of intrauterine devices with actinomycetes may occur more frequently.

Laboratory Diagnosis

DIRECT EXAMINATION. Sputum, pus collected from draining sinuses, tissue sections, and cervical exudates should be examined for the presence of granules. The usual size and color of actinomycetous granules are indicated in Table 32–3. The yellowish appearance of these sulfur granules probably is due to the abundance of macrophages containing lipid vacuoles. Actinomycotic granules are up to 1 mm in size, lobulated, and composed of tissue cells and bacterial filaments 1 μm in width (Fig. 32–3). These filaments often appear clubshaped at the periphery of the granule. The clubs are filaments that have been enlarged or swollen by the deposition of calcium phosphate on the cell walls. The clubs, as does the granule itself, develop only during infection and result from the interaction between the host and the bacteria. Crushed granules should be examined for gram-positive, nonacid-fast diphtheroids (Fig.

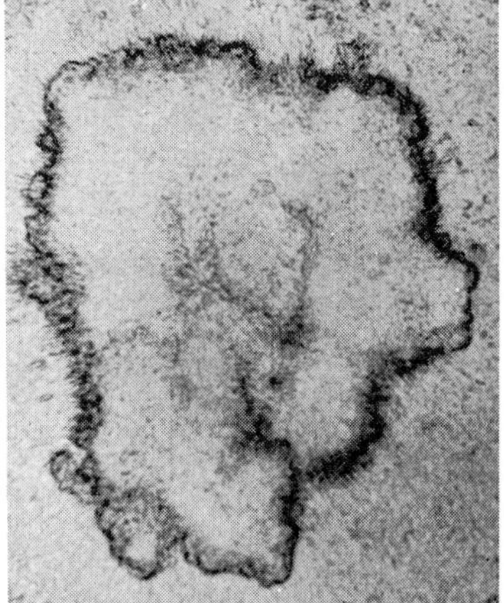

Fig. 32–3. *Actinomyces israelii.* Granule in pus. × 350. *(From Conant et al: Manual of Clinical Mycology, ed 3. Saunders, 1971.)*

TABLE 32–3. GRANULES IN ACTINOMYCETOUS INFECTIONS

Disease	Agents	Granule Presence	Granule Color	Granule Size (mm)	Peripheral Clubs
Actinomycosis	*Actinomyces israelii*	+	White to yellow	Small (0.1–0.3)	+
	Actinomyces naeslundii	Rare	White to yellow	Small (0.1–0.3)	+
	Arachnia propionica	+	White to yellow	Small (0.1–0.3)	+
	Bifidobacterium dentium	–			
Nocardiosis	*Nocardia asteroides*	–			
	Nocardia brasiliensis	+	White	Small (<0.2)	±
	Nocardia otitidiscaviarum	Rare	White to yellow	Small (<0.2)	±
Actinomycetoma	*Actinomadura madurae*	+	White, yellow, or pink	Large (1–10)	+
	Actinomadura pelletierii	+	Red	Small (0.3–1)	–
	N. asteroides	Rare	White	Small (<0.2)	–
	N. brasiliensis	+	White	Small (<0.2)	±
	N. otitidiscaviarum	+	White to yellow	Small (<0.2)	±
	Nocardiopsis dassonvillei	+	White to yellow	Large (0.5–2)	–
	Streptomyces somaliensis	+	Yellow to brown	Large (0.5–2)	–

+, granule production; –, granule or clubs not normally formed; ±, clubs may or may not be seen.

32–4). Typical granules are not produced by *B. dentium* or *A. odontolyticus.* Granulelike structures, lacking clubs, are occasionally seen with other bacteria such as *Staphylococcus aureus* in subcutaneous or visceral botryomycosis.

If cultures are not positive or definitive, specific fluorescent antibody stains have been used to recognize the presence of *Actinomyces* species or *A. propionica* in smears or sections.

CULTURE. Specimens of tissue or exudate are cultured on enriched media and incubated anaerobically in the presence of carbon dioxide. In thioglycollate broth *A. israelii* produces compact and discrete colonies, whereas colonies of other species of *Actinomyces* grow more diffusely and produce a homogeneous turbidity. With the exception of *A. viscosus*

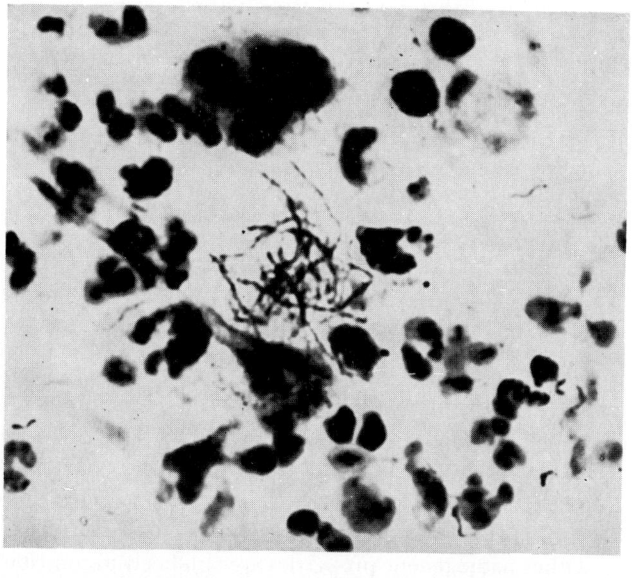

Fig. 32–4. *Actinomyces israelii.* Gram stain of crushed granule, showing gram-positive branching filaments. × 1300. *(From Conant et al: Manual of Clinical Mycology, ed 3. Saunders, 1971.)*

(Table 32–2), the catalase test can be used to distinguish these agents from *Corynebacterium, Mycobacterium,* and *Propionibacterium,* which are catalase positive.

Actinomycosis often is associated with a mixed bacterial flora. Pyogenic aerobic and anaerobic species may be recovered. In severe or chronic cases of cervicofacial actinomycosis, *A. israelii* usually is accompanied by *Actinobacillus actinomycetemcomitans.*

Treatment. The drug of choice for the treatment of actinomycosis is penicillin G, which is administered parenterally or orally for a period of several weeks. Lesions may also require surgical excision and drainage. A variety of other antibiotics including tetracycline, erythromycin, clindamycin, and sulfonamide derivatives, have also been used successfully.

Nocardiosis

Nocardiosis is caused by infection with *Nocardia asteroides,* or less frequently, *Nocardia brasiliensis* or *Nocardia otitidiscaviarum.* An older species, *Nocardia farcinica,* is now considered a subgroup of *N. asteroides.* All species of *Nocardia* are found in nature in the soil and aquatic environments. Nocardiosis is initiated in animals and in humans by inhalation of the bacteria. The infection is rarely acute but usually runs a chronic course. It may be subclinical and confined to the lung or may disseminate hematogenously to any organ, but preferentially to the central nervous system.

Morphology and Staining

Species of *Nocardia* are aerobic, gram-positive, partially acid-fast bacilli. Within the genus, filamentation and branching are highly developed. *Nocardia* produce both substrate and aerial filaments (also called *hyphae* or *mycelia*) about 1 μm wide. Cells of the substrate filaments separate into beaded forms, and aerial filaments undergo fragmentation to yield unicellular,

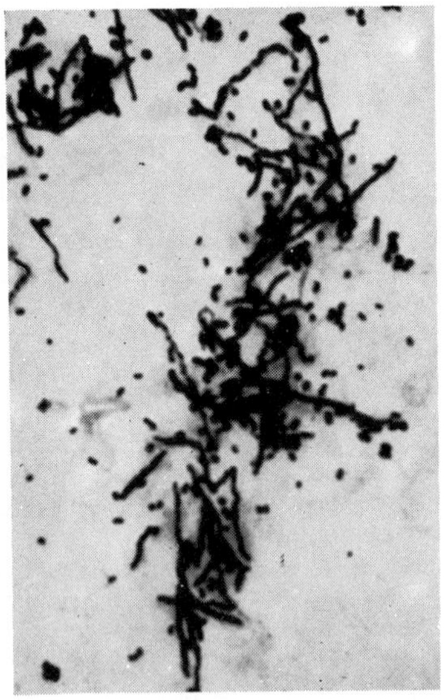

Fig. 32–5. *Nocardia asteroides.* Gram-stained smear of culture on Sabouraud agar. × 1000.

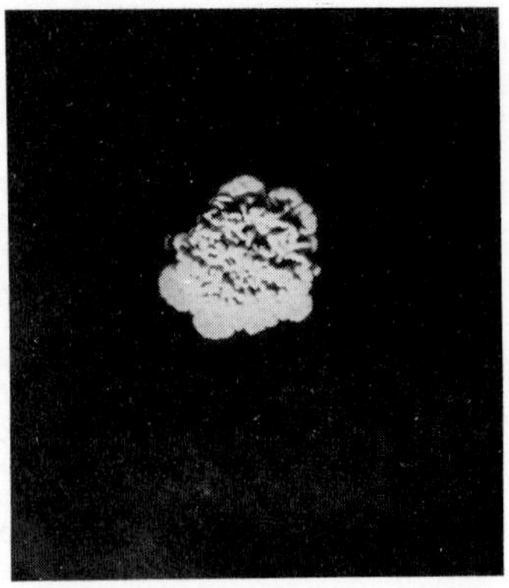

Fig. 32–6. *Nocardia asteroides.* Culture on Sabouraud agar at room temperature for 12 days.

sporelike cells that are readily dispersed and aerosolized (Fig. 32–5).

As with *Mycobacterium, Rhodococcus,* and *Corynebacterium,* the cell walls of *Nocardia* possess mycolic acids, called *nocardic acids.* Mycolic acids are long α-branched, β-hydroxy fatty acids, usually saturated or monounsaturated. As discussed in Chapter 6, the acid-fastness of *Mycobacterium* species is correlated with the presence in the cell wall of mycolic acids with chain lengths of 50 to 90 carbon atoms. Nocardic acids are about 50 carbons long, and corynemycolic acids have 32 to 36 carbons. *Corynebacterium* species are nonacid-fast, and *Nocardia* are weakly or partially acid-fast when stained with carbolfuchsin according to Kinyoun's method. If decolorized with 1% to 4% sulfuric acid instead of the stronger, acid-alcohol decolorant, most strains of *Nocardia* will stain acid-fast. However, some isolates never exhibit acid-fastness, and others lose this property after prolonged culture in the laboratory.

Fractions of the cell walls of some *Nocardia* and related species such as the mycobacteria enhance the antimicrobial and antitumor activities of macrophages. Currently, investigations are exploring the immunoadjuvant and anticancer potential of these cell wall preparations.

Physiology

Cultural Characteristics. *Nocardia* grow readily on a variety of laboratory media. On agar media, colonies appear within 3 days. After 7 to 10 days, colonies are heaped, irregular, waxy, shiny, and several millimeters in diameter (Fig. 32–6). As aerial filaments are formed, the colony surface becomes dull and fuzzy. Colonies of *N. asteroides* vary considerably in pigmentation and may be yellow, orange, red, or mixtures of these hues.

Differential Metabolic Properties. *Nocardia* can be distinguished from similar genera by their ability to decompose and utilize paraffin as a source of carbon and energy. This property permits selective isolation of *Nocardia* from mixed cultures. One method of paraffin baiting for *Nocardia* involves the use of paraffin-coated glass rods prepared by immersing a glass rod in melted paraffin. When the rod is removed and cooled, a thin film of paraffin wax coats the glass. The rods can be placed in natural soil or water, and *Nocardia* species, if present, will grow around the paraffin-coated glass rod. Using this technique, pathogenic and saprophytic *Nocardia* species have been isolated from a wide variety of soils, freshwater, and seawater worldwide. The quantity of *Nocardia* in soil has been estimated to exceed 10^3/g of dry weight of soil. Ecologic studies tend to correlate the prevalence of a particular strain of *N. asteroides* in the environment with its incidence of infection in the indigenous population. In addition to paraffin digestion, *Nocardia* species produce catalase and urease. Although similar to *Nocardia* in morphology, the genus *Actinomadura* lacks mycolic acids and is unable to digest paraffin or urea. Unlike those of *Nocardia,* the substrate filaments of *Actinomadura* do not fragment after formation (Table 32–1).

The three etiologic agents of nocardiosis—*N. asteroides, N. brasiliensis,* and *N. otitidiscaviarum* (*N. caviae*)—can be speciated by testing the ability of each to decompose casein, gelatin, hypoxanthine, tyrosine, and xanthine. Media are prepared with coagulated or crystalline forms of these substrates; the media support the growth of all species, but if the *Nocardia* species being tested can utilize the substrate, a clear zone develops in the medium around the colony. As indicated in Table 32–4, *N. asteroides* is uniformly negative, whereas *N. brasiliensis* digests all but xanthine, which distinguishes *N. otitidiscaviarum.* Because of the high variability, colony pigmentation is not a reliable aid to identification.

Determinants of Pathogenicity

Studies of host-microbial interactions from the laboratory of B. L. Beaman have shown that logarithmically growing cells of *N. asteroides* are more virulent than stationary phase cells and are more resistant to phagocytosis and intracellular killing by alveolar macrophages. This increased virulence is associated with differences in the nocardial cell wall and inhibition of the fusion of macrophage lysosomes and phagosomes that contain the engulfed bacteria. The mechanism of this inhibition may be related to the presence in nocardial cell walls of large amounts of cord factor, or trehalose dimycolate, which inhibits calcium-induced fusion between liposomes.

Other pathogenetic properties are also likely to contribute to the virulence of strains of *N. asteroides.* In vitro experiments demonstrated that virulent *N. asteroides* grow within and destroy macrophages, whereas avirulent organisms are able to

TABLE 32–4. CHARACTERISTICS OF AGENTS OF ACTINOMYCETOMA

Character	*N. asteroides*	*N. brasiliensis*	*N. otitidiscaviarum*	*Nocardiopsis dassonvillei*	*A. madurae*	*A. pellitieri*	*S. somaliensis*
Colony pigment	Yellow to orange-red	Colorless or orange-red	Colorless or white	White to orange-brown	White to gray	Red-brown	White
Mycolic acids	+	+	+	−	−	−	−
Lysozyme resistance	+	+	+	−	−	−	−
Substrates hydrolyzed							
Casein	−	+	−	+	V	−	+
Gelatin	−	+	−	+	+	+	+
Hypoxanthine	−	+	+	+	+	V	−
Tyrosine	−	+	−	+	+	+	+
Xanthine	−	−	+	+	−	−	−

+, 90% or more of strains are positive for hydrolysis or resistance to lysozyme; −, 10% or less of strains are positive; V, 11-89% of strains are positive

survive intracellularly as L-forms. Activated macrophages are better able to withstand challenge with virulent *N. asteroides*, but maximal host resistance is associated with intact cell-mediated immunity. The resistance of *N. asteroides* to the oxidative killing mechanisms of human neutrophils and monocytes may be attributable to the high levels of nocardial catalase and cell-surface-bound superoxide dismutase. Beaman and associates have correlated increased levels of these enzymes with the murine virulence of log-phase cells and their resistance to hydrogen peroxide, superoxide, singlet oxygen, and hydroxyl radicals.

The remarkable neurotropism of *N. asteroides* remains to be elucidated. Surface components may promote the attachment of bacteria to cells or tissue in the central nervous system, the bacteria may elude certain host defenses by invading the brain, or components in the brain may enhance the production of cord factor or other nocardial virulence factors.

Clinical Infection

Epidemiology. More than half the patients who develop nocardiosis are in some way compromised. Thirty percent of patients have a history of receiving steroids or immunosuppressive therapy or both, but chronic and pulmonary infections and cancer, with or without its attendant therapies, also provide the setting for opportunistic nocardiosis. Approximately 6% of patients have previous or concurrent tuberculosis. Other categories of high risk include transplant recipients and patients with chronic alcoholism. In those patients in whom no underlying condition prevails the prognosis is considerably better. The frequency of nocardiosis in the United States was estimated in 1976 as 500 to 1000 cases per year. Since then, nocardiosis has been recognized more frequently as an opportunistic infection. The infection is diagnosed and treated earlier. Since 0.5% to 2% of patients with acquired immunodeficiency disease (AIDS) acquire nocardiosis, several hundred new cases occur every year. Nocardiosis is not transmitted among humans or animals, although rare outbreaks among compromised patients have been reported.

Most cases of nocardiosis, whether pulmonary only or disseminated, occur in males. Ten years ago, the fatality rates for pulmonary and disseminated nocardiosis were approximately 40% and 80% respectively. Today, more rapid diagnosis and treatment have reduced the mortality rate considerably.

The opportunistic nature of nocardiosis is exemplified by a retrospective study of a specific group of patients at risk at the Stanford University Medical Center. Between 1968 and 1978, 13% of the cardiac transplant recipients developed opportunistic nocardiosis. In most cases, infection involved the lung, symptoms were nonspecific, and onset occurred 1½ months to 3 years after the surgery. No particular risk factor or source of infection was identified. With rapid diagnosis and long-term treatment with sulfisoxazole, the prognosis was excellent. After resolution of the nocardiosis, one fourth of these patients subsequently developed nontuberculous mycobacterial infections.

Clinical Manifestations. Nocardiosis begins as chronic lobar pneumonia after inhalation of the etiologic agent, which in 80% to 90% of the cases is *N. asteroides*. At least 75% of reported cases have this initial presentation, but a variety of signs and symptoms may be observed, including fever, weight loss, or chest pain. The presenting complaints are not distinctive and mimic tuberculosis and other infections. Pulmonary consolidations may develop, but granuloma formation and caseation are rare.

From the lung, metastatic foci of infection may appear anywhere, but most frequently they involve the central nervous system. Abscesses develop in the brain. The meninges usually are not inflamed enough to cause diagnostic changes in the spinal fluid. The onset of lesions can be sudden or gradual, and patients may present with headache, lethargy, convulsions, or more severe symptoms of central nervous system dysfunction.

Another frequently involved site is the kidney, where either the cortex or medulla may be involved. In more than half the cases caused by *N. brasiliensis* localized lesions develop in the skin and subcutaneous tissue.

Regardless of the tissue infected or the specific agent, the pathology of nocardiosis is the same, namely, abscess formation. Multiple abscesses, characterized by central necrosis and dense infiltration of neutrophils, are indistinguishable from infections caused by pyogenic bacteria. Although nocardiosis resembles tuberculosis in chronicity and symptomatology, the pathology is not granulomatous but pyogenic.

Laboratory Diagnosis

DIRECT EXAMINATION. Specimens of sputum, skin lesions, tissue biopsies, or surgical material should be examined mi-

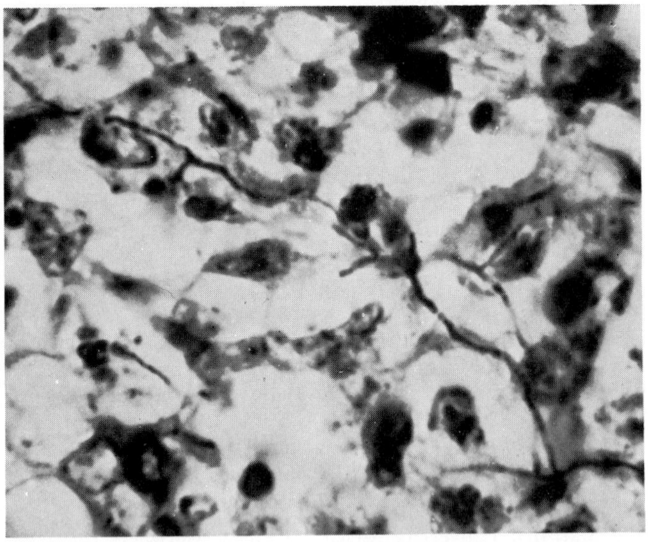

Fig. 32–7. *Nocardia asteroides.* Gram-stained section of brain abscess showing gram-positive branching filaments. × 1300. *(From Conant et al: Manual of Clinical Mycology, ed 3. Saunders, 1971.)*

croscopically and cultured. The direct microscopic examination of positive sputum or tissue smears reveals delicate, multiply branched and beaded filaments that are gram-positive and partially acid-fast (Fig. 32–7). The organisms are very difficult to see in tissue stained with hematoxylin and eosin. Granules are not usually observed with systemic lesions.

CULTURE. *Nocardia* will grow aerobically on most laboratory media. Colonies, which appear within 3 to 7 days, are composed of branching filaments that usually stain acid-fast when decolorized with 1% to 4% H_2SO_4 instead of acid alcohol. Because of the formation of an abundance of substrate filaments, colonies cling tenaciously to the agar. Both substrate and aerial filaments may fragment to form beadlike chains and coccobacillary cells. The genus and species identifications are confirmed by the production of urease and the tests indicated in Table 32–4. On Löwenstein-Jensen medium, *N. asteroides* may be identical macroscopically to atypical mycobacteria, but *Nocardia* can be differentiated from *Mycobacterium* because the latter are strongly acid-fast and exhibit minimal branching. If *N. asteroides* is suspected, cultures of nonsterile specimens can be incubated at 40C to 50C to inhibit growth of most of the other bacteria.

Treatment. Although *N. asteroides* is susceptible to a number of newer antibiotics, the sulfonamides still are effective against nocardiosis. Sulfa blood levels of 10 to 20 mg/mL should be maintained during treatment. Despite the rare occurrence of treatment failures, the treatment of choice for nocardiosis is the trimethoprim-sulfamethoxazole (TMP-SMX) combination, which penetrates the central nervous system better than sulfa alone. Recently, amikacin and imipenem have also shown promise in the treatment of nocardiosis. In vitro, both drugs displayed synergy in combination with TMP-SMX, and optimal combinations of these or other antibiotics may be recommended in the future.

Actinomycetoma

Mycetoma (Madura foot) is a chronic suppurative and granulomatous infection of the subcutaneous tissue. The lesions are characterized by the formation of tumefaction and abscesses, with interconnecting and draining sinuses that contain granules. Actinomycotic mycetoma, or actinomycetoma, is caused by traumatic inoculation of exogenous actinomycetes that normally dwell in soil and aquatic environments. The most common agents are members of the genera *Actinomadura, Streptomyces,* and *Nocardia* (see Table 32–3). Mycetoma may also be caused by a variety of fungi that are also normally found in the environment (Chap. 83). Similar lesions due to *A. israelii, A. propionica,* and other endogenous actinomycetes are considered to be cases of actinomycosis.

Morphology and Cultural Characteristics

The agents associated with actinomycetoma are listed in Table 32–4. In addition to its acid-fastness, *Nocardia* can be differentiated from the other agents of actinomycetoma with the lysozyme tolerance test. The pathogenic species of *Nocardia* are able to grow in nutrient broth containing lysozyme, whereas species of *Actinomadura* and *Streptomyces somaliensis* are inhibited.

ACTINOMADURA. The genus *Actinomadura* closely resembles *Nocardia* in culture and microscopic appearance (p. 532). Both genera are gram-positive and produce catalase, but *Actinomadura* cannot break down urea or paraffin and is nonacid-fast. Furthermore, their cell wall chemotypes are different (Table 32–1), and the filaments of *Actinomadura* do not fragment. The colony of *Actinomadura madurae* is whitish, smooth, and waxy; *Actinomadura pelletieri* produces a pink to red colony and granule. Table 32–3 compares the granules produced by pathogenic actinomycetes.

OTHER SPECIES. Colonies of *S. somaliensis* are initially white but become brown to black; the granules are yellow to brown. Filaments of *S. somaliensis* do not fragment. *Nocardiopsis dassonvillei* produces long aerial filaments that develop distinctive zig-zag chains of spores.

Clinical Infection

Epidemiology. Most of the agents of actinomycetoma are ubiquitous soil saprophytes. The agents and infection are more common in the subtropical and tropical regions. Ecologic studies of the prevalence of specific agents tend to reflect the incidence of infection. The likelihood of walking barefoot and the risk of traumatic inoculation is also greater in warmer climates. In the United States, *A. madurae* is the most frequently isolated agent.

Clinical Manifestations. Regardless of the actinomycete involved, the infection follows trauma to the subcutaneous tissue and contamination by soil containing the organism. Exposed areas of the extremities are most often involved, especially the foot or hand, although any body surface may become infected. The infection progresses slowly. An initial subcutaneous nodule develops, enlarges, and ulcerates, and

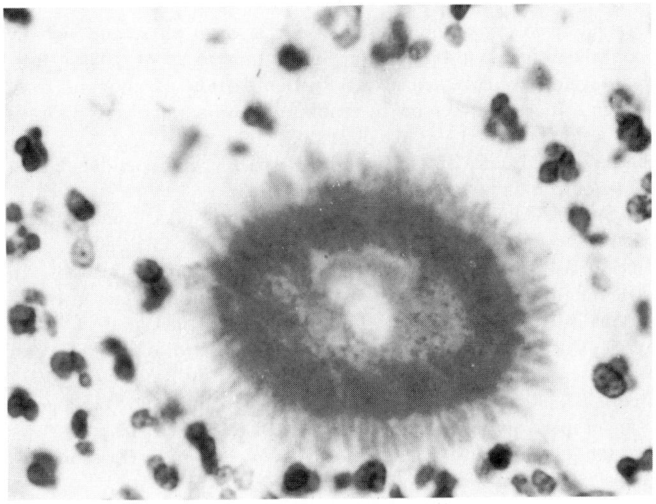

Fig. 32–8. *Nocardia brasiliensis.* Tissue section of actinomycetoma granule, showing peripheral clubs. × 212. *(Courtesy of Dr. L. Linares.)*

satellite lesions develop that become connected by sinus tracts. If unchecked, the infection progresses to cause deformation of the involved tissue with destruction of underlying muscle and bone.

Laboratory Diagnosis

DIRECT EXAMINATION. Pus or exudate expressed from lesions should be examined for the presence of granules. The shape, color, size, and microscopic appearance of the granule usually will confirm the bacterial etiology. Figure 32–8 depicts a typical actinomycotic granule with peripheral clubs.

CULTURE. These bacteria can be isolated on most routine bacteriologic media and identified on the basis of morphology, physiologic characteristics, and cell wall composition.

Treatment. Complete eradication of the infection requires both surgical débridement and long-term antibiotic therapy. The recommended chemotherapy is daily, intramuscular injections of 1 g streptomycin sulfate for 1 month, coupled with daily TMP-SMX or dapsone. *A. pelletieri* responds better to TMP-SMX, and *A. madurae,* to dapsone. *S. somaliensis* and *Nocardia* species respond to either regimen. Infections that do not respond can be treated with a combination of streptomycin and either rifampin or sulfadoxine and pyrimethamine.

Other Actinomycetous Diseases

Dermatophilosis

Dermatophilosis, or streptothricosis, is a skin infection caused by *Dermatophilus congolensis. D. congolensis* produces branching filaments that divide by longitudinal as well as transverse septa to yield coccoid cells that are motile. These flagellated cells initiate filaments that expand and divide to repeat this cycle. *D. congolensis* is an obligate pathogen of the uncornified, mammalian epidermis. Dermatophilosis is most common among cattle, sheep, and similar animals. The lesion causes a pustular, exudative dermatitis that eventually becomes crusty and flakes off. Human infection is acquired from animals and is very rare. The organisms are short, branched, irregular filaments in the cutaneous tissue. Topical treatment with metallic compounds is recommended, although *D. congolensis* is susceptible to many antibiotics, including penicillin, streptomycin, erythromycin, and the tetracyclines.

Farmer's Lung

Farmer's lung is an allergic disease induced by inhalation of thermophilic actinomycetes. The usual agents are *Faenia rectivirgula* or *Thermoactinomyces vulgaris. F. rectivirgula* develops chains of spores from both substrate and aerial filaments. Species of *Thermoactinomyces* also develop extensive, branching aerial and substrate filaments, both of which bear lateral spores. Growth is optimal at 50C. A similar allergy is induced by *Thermoactinomyces sacchari,* which is associated with sugar cane. This condition is bagassosis (Chap. 81).

F. rectivirgula and *T. vulgaris* thrive in haystacks, composts, and grain storage silos at temperatures of 45C to 60C. Farmer's lung apparently is mediated by type I or type III hypersensitivity reactions to bacterial surface antigens. In dry places these bacteria are easily aerosolized, and inhalation of the bacterial allergens by sensitive individuals induces an asthmatic reaction. As the name implies, farmer's lung is an occupational disease of persons in frequent contact with stored grain and similar reservoirs for these bacteria. This condition is treated with antiallergic drugs and by avoiding exposure.

FURTHER READING

Books and Reviews

Bradley SG: Significance of nucleic acid hybridization to systematics of actinomycetes. Adv Appl Microbiol 19:59, 1975

Bradley SG, Bond JS: Taxonomic criteria for mycobacteria and nocardiae. Adv Appl Microbiol 18:131, 1974

George LK: Agents of human actinomycosis. In Balows A, Dehaan RM, Guze LB, et al (eds): Anaerobic Bacteria. Springfield, Ill, Charles C Thomas, 1974, p 237

Goodfellow M, Minnikin DE: Nocardioform bacteria. Annu Rev Microbiol 31:159, 1977

Goodfellow M, Mordarski M, Williams ST (eds): The biology of the actinomycetes. London, Academic Press, 1984

Gordon MA: Aerobic pathogenic *Actinomycetaceae.* In Lennette EH, Balows A, Hausler WJ Jr, Shadomy HJ (eds): Manual of Clinical Microbiology, ed 4. Washington, DC, American Society for Microbiology, 1985, p 249

Kalakoutskii LV, Agre NS: Comparative aspects of development and differentiation in actinomycetes. Bacteriol Rev 49:469, 1976

Land GA, Staneck JL: The aerobic actinomycetes. In Wentworth BB (ed): Diagnostic Procedures for Mycotic and Parasitic Infections, ed 7. Washington, DC, American Public Health Association, 1988, p 271

Lerner PI: The lumpy jaw. Cervicofacial actinomycosis. Infect Dis Clin North Am 2:203, 1988

Lloyd DH, Sellers KC. *Dermatophilus* Infection in Animals and Man. London, Academic Press, 1976

Mariat F, Destombes P, Segretain G: The mycetomas: Clinical features,

pathology, etiology and epidemiology. Contrib Microbiol Immunol 4:1, 1977
McGinnis MR, Fader RC: Mycetoma: A contemporary concept. Infect Dis Clin North Am 1988, p 939
Segretain G, Mariat F: Mycetoma. In Warren KS, Mahmoud AAF (eds): Tropical and Geographical Medicine. New York, McGraw-Hill, 1984, p 934
Slack JM, Gerencser MA. *Actinomyces,* Filamentous Bacteria. Biology and Pathogenicity. Minneapolis, Burgess, 1975
Sneath PHA, Mair NS, Sharpe ME, Holt JG (eds): Bergey's Manual of Systematic Bacteriology, vol 2. Baltimore, Williams & Wilkins, 1986
Williams ST, Sharpe ME, Holt JG (eds): Bergey's Manual of Systematic Bacteriology, vol 4. Baltimore, Williams & Wilkins, 1989

Selected Papers

Angeles AM, Sugar AM: Identification of a common immunodominant protein in culture filtrates of three *Nocardia* species and use in etiologic diagnosis of mycetoma. J Clin Microbiol 25:2278, 1987
Bach MC, Sabath LD, Finland M: Susceptibility of *Nocardia asteroides* to 45 antimicrobial agents in vitro. Antimicrob Agents Chemother 3:1, 1973
Barnicoat MJ, Wierzbicki AS, Norman PM: Cerebral nocardiosis in immunosuppressed patients: Five cases. Q J Med 72:689, 1989
Beaman BL, Burnside J, Edwards B, et al: Nocardial infections in the United States, 1972–1974. J Infect Dis 134:286, 1976
Beaman BL, Moring SE: Relationship among cell wall composition, stage of growth, and virulence of *Nocardia asteroides* GUH-2. Infect Immun 56:557, 1988
Beaman L, Beaman BL: Monoclonal antibodies demonstrate that superoxide dismutase contributes to protection of *Nocardia asteroides* within the intact host. Infect Immun 58:3122, 1990
Beradi RS: Abdominal actinomycosis. Surg Gynecol Obstet 149:257, 1979
Berd D: Laboratory identification of clinically important aerobic actinomycetes. Appl Microbiol 25:665, 1973
Berkey P, Bodey GP Sr: Nocardial infection in patients with neoplastic disease. Rev Infect Dis 11:407, 1989
Boiron P, Provost F: Use of partially purified 54-kilodalton antigen for diagnosis of nocardiosis by Western blot (immunoblot) assay. J Clin Microbiol 28:328, 1990
Brock DW, Georg LK, Brown JM, et al: Actinomycosis caused by *Arachnia propionica:* Report of 11 cases. Am J Clin Pathol 59:66, 1973
Brown JR: Human actinomycosis. A study of 181 subjects. Hum Pathol 4:319, 1973
Brownell GH, Belcher KE: DNA probes for the identification of *Nocardia asteroides.* J Clin Microbiol 28:2082, 1990
Butler WR, Kilburn JO, Kubica GP: High-performance liquid chromatography analysis of mycolic acids as an aid in laboratory identification of *Rhodococcus* and *Nocardia* species. J Clin Microbiol 25:2126, 1987
Causey WA: *Nocardia caviae:* A report of 13 new isolations with clinical correlation. Appl Microbiol 28:193, 1974
Chapman SW, Wilson JP: Nocardiosis in transplant recipients. Semin Respir Infect 5:74, 1990
Coleman RM, Georg LK, Rozzell AR: *Actinomyces naeslundii* as an agent of human actinomycosis. Appl Microbiol 18:420, 1969
Davis-Scibienski C, Beaman BL: Interaction of alveolar macrophages with *Nocardia asteroides:* Immunological enhancement of phagocytosis, phagosome-lysosome fusion, and microbicidal activity. Infect Immun 30:578, 1980
Davis-Scibienski C, Beaman BL: Interaction of *Nocardia asteroides* with rabbit alveolar macrophages: Effect of growth phase and viability on phagosome-lysosome fusion. Infect Immun 29:24, 1980
de Magaldi SW, Mackenzie DWR: Comparison of antigens from agents of actinomycetoma by immunodiffusion and electrophoresis procedures. J Med Vet Mycol 28:363, 1990
Filice GA: Resistance of *Nocardia asteroides* to oxygen-dependent killing by neutrophils. J Infect Dis 148:861, 1983
Filice GA, Beaman BL, Remington JS: Effects of activated macrophages on *Nocardia asteroides.* Infect Immun 27:643, 1980
Filice GA, Simpson GL: Management of *Nocardia* infections. In Remington JS, Swartz MN (eds): Current Clinical Topics in Infectious Diseases, ed 5. New York, McGraw-Hill, 1984, p 49
Frazier AR, Rosenow ED III, Roberts GD: Nocardiosis. A review of 25 cases occurring during 24 months. Mayo Clin Proc 50:657, 1975
Georg LK, Roberstad GW, Brinkman SA, et al: A new pathogenic anaerobic *Actinomyces* species. J Infect Dis 115:88, 1965
Gordon RE, Mihm JM: Identification of *Nocardia caviae* (Erikson) *nov. comb.* Ann N Y Acad Sci 98:628, 1967
Heffner JE: Pleuropulmonary manifestations of actinomycosis and nocardiosis. Semin Respir Infect 3:352, 1988
Holmberg K, Nord C-E: Numerical taxonomy and laboratory identification of *Actinomyces* and *Arachnia* and some related bacteria. J Gen Microbiol 91:17, 1975
Hsu CT, Roan CH, Rai SY, et al: Actinomycosis affecting the fallopian tube and ovary: Report of 3 cases, with special reference to 2 cases following IUD application. Asia Oceania J Obstet Gynaecol 14:275, 1988
Knouse MC, Lorber B: Early diagnosis of *Nocardia asteroides* endophthalmitis by retinal biopsy: Case report and review. Rev Infect Dis 12:393, 1990
Kramer MR, Uttamchandani RB: The radiographic appearance of pulmonary nocardiosis associated with AIDS. Chest 98:382, 1990
Kruk VA, Stinson EB, Remington JS: *Nocardia* infection in heart transplant patients. Ann Intern Med 82:18, 1975
Kurup PV, Randwana HS, Mishra SK: Use of parrafin bait technique in the isolation of *Nocardia asteroides* from sputum. Mycopathol Mycol Appl 40:363, 1970
Law BJ, Marks MI: Pediatric nocardiosis. Pediatrics 70:560, 1982
Levine LA, Doyle CJ: Retroperitoneal actinomycosis: A case report and review of the literature. J Urol 140:367, 1988
McNeil MM, Brown JM, Jarvis WR, et al: Comparison of species distribution and antimicrobial susceptibility of aerobic actinomycetes from clinical specimens. Rev Infect Dis 12:778, 1990
Mishra SK, Gordon RE, Barnett DA: Identification of nocardiae and streptomycetes of medical importance. J Clin Microbiol 11:728, 1980
Nichols DR: Actinomycosis: Results in therapy in 156 patients. Probl Antimicrob Anticancer Chemother 11:8, 1970
Poland GA, Jorgensen CR, Sarosi GA: *Nocardia asteroides* pericarditis: Report of a case and review of the literature. Mayo Clin Proc 65:819, 1990
Reiner SL, Harrelson JM, Miller SE, et al: Primary actinomycosis of an extremity: A case report and review. Rev Infect Dis 9:581, 1987
Rose HD, Varkey B, Kesavan Kutty CP: Thoracic actinomycosis caused by *Actinomyces meyerii.* Am Rev Respir Dis 125:251, 1982
Schofield GM, Schaal KP: A numerical taxonomic study of members of the *Actinomycetaceae* and related taxa. J Gen Microbiol 127:237, 1981
Schwartz JG, McGough DA, Thorner RE, et al: Primary lymphocutaneous *Nocardia brasiliensis* infection: Three case reports and a review of the literature. Diagn Microbiol Infect Dis 10:113, 1988
Schwartz JG, Tio FO: Nocardial osteomyelitis: A case report and review of the literature. Diagn Microbiol Infect Dis 8:37, 1987

Seeliger HP: Immunologic aspects in actinomycetes and actinomycetomas. Mycoses 31:20, 1988

Shawar RM, Moore DG, LaRocco MT: Cultivation of *Nocardia* spp. on chemically defined media for selective recovery of isolates from clinical specimens. J Clin Microbiol 28:508, 1990

Simpson GL, Stinson EB, Egger MJ, et al: Nocardial infections in the immunocompromised host: A detailed study in a defined population. Rev Infect Dis 3:492, 1981

Smego RA Jr: Actinomycosis of the central nervous system. Rev Infect Dis 9:855, 1987

Smego RA Jr, Gallis HA: The clinical spectrum of *Nocardia brasiliensis* infection in the United States. Rev Infect Dis 6:164, 1984

Smego RA Jr, Moeller MB, Gallis HA: Trimethoprim-sulfamethoxazole therapy for *Nocardia* infections. Arch Intern Med 143:711, 1983

Stackebrandt E, Charfreitag O: Partial 16S rRNA primary structure of five *Actinomyces* species: Phylogenetic implications and development of an *Actinomyces israelii*–specific oligonucleotide probe. J Gen Microbiol 136:37, 1990

Stenhouse D, MacDonald DG, MacFarlane TW: Cervico-facial and intra-oral actinomycosis: A 5-year retrospective study. Br J Oral Surg 13:172, 1975

Sugar AM, Schoolnik GK, Stevens DA: Antibody response in human nocardiosis: Identification of two immunodominant culture-filtrate antigens derived from *Nocardia asteroides*. J Infect Dis 151:895, 1985

Tight RR, Bartlett MS: Actinomycetoma in the United States. Rev Infect Dis 3:1139, 1981

Valicenti JF Jr, Pappas AA, Graber CD, et al: Detection and Prevalence of IUD-associated *Actinomyces* colonization and related morbidity: A prospective study of 69,925 cervical smears. JAMA 247:1149, 1982

Wallace RJ Jr, Septimus EJ, Williams TW Jr, et al: Use of trimethoprim-sulfamethoxazole for treatment of infections due to *Nocardia*. Rev Infect Dis 4:315, 1982

Wallace RJ Jr, Tsukamura M, Brown BA, et al: Cefotaxime-resistant *Nocardia asteroides* strains are isolates of the controversial species *Nocardia farcinica*. J Clin Microbiol 28:2726, 1990

Weese WC, Smith IM: A study of 57 cases of actinomycosis over a 36-year period. A diagnostic "failure" with good prognosis after treatment. Arch Intern Med 135:1562, 1975

Wilson JP, Turner HR, Kirchner KA, et al: Nocardial infections in renal transplant recipients. Medicine 68:38, 1989

Young LS, Armstrong D, Blevins A, et al: *Nocardia asteroides* infection complicating neoplastic disease. Am J Med 50:356, 1971

CHAPTER 33

Enterobacteriaceae: General Characteristics

The family Enterobacteriaceae is composed of a large number of closely related species that are found in soil, water, decaying matter, and the large intestines of humans, animals, and insects. Because of their normal habitat in humans, these organisms are referred to as the "enteric bacilli" or "enterics." Included in this family are some of the most important causes of gastrointestinal disease: the agents of typhoid fever and bacillary dysentery. Most species are not intestinal pathogens, however, but opportunistic organisms that can infect any body site when given an altered host. In fact, the enterics are responsible for the majority of nosocomial (hospital-acquired) infections seen today. The medical and economic implications of these nosocomial infections becomes apparent when one considers that an estimated 2 million patients per year (5% to 10% of the total hospital population) in the United States will acquire an infection while hospitalized. The seriousness of the problem is further complicated by the fact that many of the organisms isolated from nosocomial infections are resistant to multiple antimicrobial agents.

Taxonomy

The taxonomy of the Enterobacteriaceae has been studied more than any other group of microorganisms. New species are being described and named at a seemingly rapid rate. In 1972 there were only 26 named species of Enterobacteriaceae; currently there are 86 named species and 11 clusters of organisms referred to as enteric groups, which need further study before assigning a species designation. Fortunately, only approximately 25 of the 97 described enterics either are important human pathogens or are frequently isolated from clinical specimens. The other 72 organisms either have not been isolated from human sources or as a group account for only 1% to 2% of clinical isolates. Table 33–1 lists all members of the family, and Table 33–2 depicts the more important human pathogens and the more frequently isolated enteric species that are discussed in Chapters 34 and 35. Although the genus *Yersinia* belongs in the family Enterobacteriaceae, it is discussed separately in Chapter 38 because of the historic and epidemiologic importance of one species, *Y. pestis,* the cause of bubonic plague.

Morphology

The Enterobacteriaceae are small (0.5 by 3.0 μm), gram-negative, non-spore-forming rods. They may be motile or nonmotile. When motile, locomotion is by means of peritrichous flagella, a property that aids in differentiating the enterics from the polar flagellated Pseudomonadaceae (Chapter 37) and Vibrionaceae (Chapter 36). Two genera, *Shigella* and *Klebsiella,* are characteristically nonmotile.

Enteric bacilli may possess a well-defined capsule, as seen with the genus *Klebsiella,* or a loose, ill-defined coating referred to as a slime layer, or they may lack either structure. Fimbriae or pili are present in most species and are responsible for the attachment of the bacterial cells to other bacteria, host cells, and bacteriophages. The cell wall is composed of murein, lipoprotein, phospholipid, protein, and lipopolysaccharides

TABLE 33–1. CLASSIFICATION OF THE FAMILY ENTEROBACTERIACEAE[a]

Buttiauxella agrestis[b]	*Obesumbacterium proteus*[b]
Cedecea davisae	*Proteus mirabilis*
C. lapagei	*P. myxofaciens*[b]
C. neteri	*P. penneri*
C. species 3	*P. vulgaris*
C. species 5	
	Providencia alcalifaciens
Citrobacter amalonaticus	*P. rettgeri*
C. amalonaticus biogroup 1	*P. rustigianii*
C. diversus	*P. stuartii*
C. freundii	
	Rhanella aquatilis
Edwardsiella hoshinae[b]	
E. ictaluri[b]	*Salmonella* subgroup 1
E. tarda	*S.* subgroup 2
E. tarda biogroup 1	*S.* subgroup 3a
	S. subgroup 3b
Enterobacter aerogenes	*S.* subgroup 4
E. agglomerans	*S.* subgroup 5
E. amnigenus biogroup 1	
E. amnigenus biogroup 2[b]	*Serratia ficaria*
E. asburiae	*S. fonticola*
E. cloacae	*S. liquifaciens*
E. dissolvens[b]	*S. marcescens*
E. gergoviae	*S. marcescens* biogroup 1
E. hormaechei[b]	*S. odorifera* biogroup 1
E. intermedium[b]	*S. odorifera* biogroup 2
E. nimipressuralis[b]	*S. plymuthica*
E. sakazakii	
E. taylorae	*Shigella* groups A, B, C[c]
	S. sonnei[c]
Escherichia blattae[b]	
E. coli	*Tatumella ptyseos*
E. fergusonii	
E. hermanii	*Xenorhabdus luminescens*[b]
E. vulneris	*X. nematophilus*[b]
Ewingella americana	*Yersinia enterocolitica*
	Y. frederiksenii
Hafnia alvei	*Y. intermedia*
H. alvei biogroup 1[b]	*Y. kristensenii*
	Y. pestis
Klebsiella group 47	*Y. pseudotuberculosis*
K. oxytoca	*Y. rukeri*[b]
K. ozaenae	
K. planticola	Enteric group 41
K. pneumoniae	Enteric group 45
K. rhinoscleromatis	Enteric group 57
K. terrigena[b]	Enteric group 58
	Enteric group 59
Kluyvera abscorbata	Enteric group 60
K. cyrocrescens	Enteric group 63[b]
	Enteric group 64[b]
Morganella morganii	Enteric group 68
M. morganii biogroup 1	Enteric group 69[b]

Adapted from Farmer, Davis, Hickman-Brenner, et al: J Clin Microbiol 21:46, 1985, and other publications on individual organisms.
[a] All organisms have been isolated from human sources except as indicated.
[b] These organisms have not been isolated from human sources.
[c] These organisms are genetically indistinguishable from *E. coli* but are recognized as distinct human pathogens.

TABLE 33–2. ENTEROBACTERIACEAE MOST FREQUENTLY ISOLATED FROM CLINICAL SPECIMENS OR THAT ARE IMPORTANT HUMAN PATHOGENS

Citrobacter diversus	*Proteus mirabilis*
C. freundii	*P. vulgaris*
Enterobacter aerogenes	*Providencia alcalifaciens*
E. agglomerans	*P. rettgeri*
E. cloacae	*P. stuartii*
Escherichia coli	*Salmonella,* all subgroups
Hafnia alvei	*Serratia marcescens*
	S. liquifaciens
Klebsiella pneumoniae	
K. oxytoca	*Shigella,* all species
Morganella morganii	*Yersinia enterocolitica*
	Y. pestis

Adapted from Farmer, Davis, Hickman-Brenner, et al: J Clin Microbiol 21:46, 1985.

(LPS) and is arranged in layers. The murein-lipoprotein layer constitutes approximately 20% of the cell wall and is responsible for cellular rigidity. The remaining 80% of the cell wall is joined to the lipid of the lipoprotein to form a lipid bilayer. LPS contains the specific polysaccharide side chains that determine the antigenicity of the various species and is the portion of the cell responsible for endotoxic activity (p. 541).

Physiology

Biochemical and Cultural Characteristics. Enterobacteriaceae are biochemically diverse, facultative organisms. When grown in anaerobic or low-oxygen atmospheres, they ferment carbohyrates; but when given sufficient oxygen, they utilize the tricarboxylic acid cycle and the electron transport system for energy production. By definition, all members of the family ferment glucose, reduce nitrates to nitrites, but do not liquify alginate, and are oxidase negative. Most enterics ferment glucose by the mixed acid pathway, but members of the genera *Klebsiella, Enterobacter,* and *Serratia* utilize the butanediol fermentative pathway (Chap. 4). Various species differ in the carbohydrates they ferment, and these differences, together with the variations in end-product production and substrate utilization, form the basis for speciation within this family. The important biochemical features of the various genera may be found in the chapters dealing with individual organisms.

On nondifferential or nonselective media, such as blood agar or infusion agars, the various species cannot be distinguished from each other and appear as moist, smooth, gray colonies. Smooth to rough variations can occur. Some strains of certain genera are β-hemolytic. A variety of selective and differential media has been devised for the isolation and differentiation of this family (Table 33–3). The selective media originally were designed to isolate the enteric pathogens of the genera *Salmonella* and *Shigella* from fecal material, whereas the differential media were designed to selectively inhibit gram-positive organisms and to separate the enterics into broad categories by their ability to ferment selected carbohydrates such as lactose.

TABLE 33–3. COMMONLY USED MEDIA FOR THE ISOLATION OF ENTERIC BACILLI

Media	Carbohydrates	H_2S Detection
Differential media—permit most species to grow		
MacConkey agar	Lactose	No
Eosin methylene blue	Lactose, sucrose	No
Isolation media for intestinal pathogens		
Hektoen enteric agar	Lactose, sucrose, salicin	Yes
Xylose lysine deoxycholate (XLD) agar	Lactose, sucrose, xylose	Yes

Genetics. The Enterobacteriaceae are useful tools for geneticists and are the organisms most often used in the developing recombinant DNA industry. Most of the information concerning bacterial genetics, gene mapping, and gene transfer described in Chapters 7 and 8 has been derived from studies with these organisms. These studies have shown that genetic information can be transferred among distantly related genera, as well as among closely related genera, by transduction or conjugation. This transfer of genetic material occasionally gives rise to hybrids with altered biochemical or structural properties. Such hybrids are not only products of laboratory experimentation but are also observed in the hospital environment. For example, most *Escherichia coli* do not produce hydrogen sulfide, but some strains have acquired plasmids from *Salmonella* that enable the *E. coli* to produce this gas. From a practical viewpoint this requires that the clinical laboratory employ more detailed identification procedures for the enterics than is used for some of the other clinically significant bacteria. Changes in antimicrobial susceptibility also occur when a resistant organism possessing the resistance transfer factor (RTF) transfers the genes encoding for the antimicrobial resistance to a previously sensitive organism. The pathogenicity of an organism can also be altered with the acquisition of genetic material (e.g., the plasmids' encoding for enterotoxin production [p. 546]).

A number of enterics harbor plasmids that encode for the production of antibacterial substances known as bacteriocins. Different bacteriocins attack different molecular sites such as sites of nucleic acid or protein synthesis or ATP formation. Bacteriocins generally are active only against susceptible organisms of the same species. This selectivity provides a useful epidemiologic tool for subdividing or typing a species. For example, if all the *Proteus mirabilis* strains isolated from wounds of patients on a particular hospital ward had the same bacteriocin type, they probably originated from the same source or had a common means of transmission.

Resistance. Since the enteric bacilli do not produce spores, they are destroyed relatively easily by heat and low concentrations of common germicides and disinfectants. Phenolics, formaldehyde, β-glutaraldehyde, and halogen compounds are bactericidal, but quarternary ammonium compounds may be only bacteriostatic, depending on the particular formulation and the situation in which they are used. Chlorination of water has been effective in controlling the dissemination of intestinal pathogens, such as the agent of typhoid fever. The enterics are also relatively sensitive to drying but can survive for long periods of time if provided adequate moisture. Moisture-laden respiratory care and anesthesia equipment have been sources of enterobacterial infections in the hospital setting, and organisms have been isolated from snow and ice after several months, providing a mechanism of contaminating water supplies during spring thaws. Control of these organisms in foods can be achieved by pasteurization, thorough cooking, and proper refrigeration.

Antigenic Structure

With certain species of Enterobacteriaceae the antigenic structure plays an important role in epidemiology and classification. This is particularly true with the intestinal pathogens of the genera *Salmonella* and *Shigella*. The O, H, and K antigens are the major components used in the serologic typing of the family. In addition to these primary antigens the enterics share a common antigen (ECA) that is present on the outer surface of the bacterial cell. This antigen is useful in taxonomic and epidemiologic studies.

Capsular (K) Antigens. The term *K antigen* comes from the German *Kapsule* and was used to describe the polysaccharide capsular antigens of enteric bacilli. The K antigen of *Klebsiella* species is a well defined polysaccharide capsule as is seen in the pneumococcus (Chap. 3). In other genera the K antigen represents an amorphous slime layer surrounding the bacterial cell. Recent studies have shown that certain K antigens of *E. coli* are proteins, not polysaccharides, and form fimbriae of certain strains. The K88 and K99 fimbriae of animal isolates and the colonizing factor antigens (CFA) of human isolates are examples of nonpolysaccharide K antigens. The Vi antigen of *Salmonella typhi* and certain *Citrobacter* is a type of K antigen that originally was believed the virulence determinant for *S. typhi*.

Flagellar (H) Antigens. The flagellar, or H, antigens are proteins. The antigenic variation of the various flagellar types is due to the differences in amino acid sequences. Serologic typing of flagellar antigens helps form the basis of antigenic typing of the *Salmonella*.

Somatic (O) Antigens. The LPS of the cell wall of the enterics is composed of three distinct regions. The O-specific or cell wall antigen is contained in region I and is a polymer of repeating oligosaccharide units of three or four monosaccharides. Within certain genera such as *Escherichia, Salmonella,* and *Shigella,* these polymers vary with different isolates, allowing for serologic subgrouping of the genera. Attached to the O antigen is region II, which consists of a core polysaccharide that is constant within a particular enterobacterial genus but differs between genera. The lipid A moiety, or region III, is attached to region II through a unique eight-carbon sugar, 2-keto-3-deoxyoctonate (KDO). The basic unit of lipid A is a diasaccharide attached to five or six fatty acids. Structurally, lipid A joins the LPS to the murein-lipoprotein layer of the cell wall. Besides being useful as a serologic marker, LPS may serve as an important virulence factor in that it is toxic (see Endotoxin below). In addition, the O antigen may enhance the establishment of the organism in the host. In certain species of enterics the carbohydrates in region I of LPS appear to be involved in both the attachment of the bacteria to host tissues during infection and the protection of the organism from the natural killing of complement in serum. The LPS molecule is discussed further in Chapters 3 and 6.

Determinants of Pathogenicity

Endotoxin. The LPS of the cell wall is also referred to as endotoxin since it is associated with the bacterial cell and is toxic to animals. The toxicity of LPS resides in the lipid A portion of the molecule. After their injection into animals, endotoxins produce a variety of effects such as fever, fatal shock, leukocytic alterations, regression of tumors, alterations in host response to infection, the Sanarelli-Shwartzman reaction, and various metabolic changes. The cellular targets of endotoxin are varied, and the exact mechanism of action of endotoxin has not been clearly delineated. For further information concerning the cellular targets of endotoxin, see the reviews by Bradley and Morrison and the symposium edited by Kaas and Wolff.

Although the role of endotoxin in urinary tract or wound infections remains unclear, it is evident that endotoxin contributes to the high mortality rate in patients with gram-negative bacteremia. Approximately 30% of patients with enteric bacteremia will develop a condition known as endotoxin shock, and an estimated 40% to 90% of the patients in shock will die. This percentage translates to an estimated 18,000 to 100,000 deaths per year. The exact nature of endotoxin shock has not been determined, but the chief defect is a pooling of blood in the microcirculation, which in turn causes cellular hypoxia and metabolic failure due to the inadequacy of blood in vital organs. Survival is directly proportional to the length of time needed to recognize the bacteremia and to institute adequate treatment for the infection as well as the shock syndrome.

Enterotoxins. Enterotoxins are toxins that usually affect the small intestines, causing a transduction of fluid into the intestinal lumen and subsequent diarrhea. The use of the techniques developed in studies on cholera (Chap. 36) has demonstrated that a number of Enterobacteriaceae, including *Salmonella, Shigella,* and strains of *E. coli, K. pneumoniae, Citrobacter freundii,* and *Enterobacter,* produce a variety of enterotoxins. Some of these enterotoxins are similar to the cholera toxin, whereas others differ significantly in structure and mode of action.

Enterotoxin-producing *E. coli* are major causes of traveler's diarrhea and diarrhea in children in developing countries, whereas the incidence of disease caused by the enterotoxin-producing *Citrobacter, Klebsiella,* and *Enterobacter* species is unknown. The role of enterotoxins in salmonellosis and shigellosis is still unclear since other factors such as tissue penetration are important in the pathology of these diseases. A more detailed description of the enterotoxins is found in the chapters dealing with the specific organisms.

Shiga Toxins and Shigalike Toxins (Verotoxins). Members of the genus *Shigella* produce a toxin that interferes with protein synthesis of mammalian cells. Also, certain *E. coli* strains produce similar toxins, which were first called *verotoxins* because of their action on Vero (African green monkey) tissue culture cells. The role of these toxins in shigellosis is still unclear, but verotoxin-producing *E. coli* (VTEC) are important causes of hemolytic diarrhea and hemolytic uremic syndrome. In some locations, VTEC are the third or fourth leading cause of diarrhea, with the incidence of VTEC diarrhea exceeding that of shigellosis. A more complete description of these toxins is found in Chapters 34 and 35.

Colonization Factors. The cellular surface properties of certain enterics are important in the establishment of the organisms in the host. The capsule of *Klebsiella pneumoniae* functions in a manner similar to that of the pneumococcal capsule to prevent phagocytosis. Although another type of K antigen, the "Vi" antigen of *S. typhi,* does not prevent phagocytosis of the organism, it may function in some protective manner to prevent intracellular destruction of the bacterial cell. Fimbriae such as the CFA antigens of human isolates and the K88 and K99 antigens of animal strains of *E. coli* are necessary for the attachment of the organism to target tissues. The O antigen may also bind the organism to certain tissue receptor sites. Experiments with *Salmonella typhimurium* show that the loss of O-specific side chains is associated with an increase of the lethal dose (LD_{50}) in mice.

Other Factors. Members of the genus *Shigella* and certain enteropathogenic *E. coli* penetrate the epithelial lining of the intestinal tract. Whether these organisms elaborate a toxin or possess unique surface characteristics has not been clearly determined. However, tissue penetration is an important feature of shigellosis and occurs even with enterotoxin-producing strains. Similarly, *Salmonella* are able to penetrate the epithelial lining of the large intestines, and they also can invade tissues beyond the epithelium and survive intracellularly in a variety of host cells.

A number of enterics produce additional toxins, enzymes, and hemolysins that produce a variety of effects in various experimental systems. The role of these factors is discussed in the chapters dealing with specific organisms.

Clinical Infection

Types of Infection. In the United States the Enterobacteriaceae are the leading causes of bacteremia and urinary tract infections. In addition, they can invade any body site and can cause wound infections, pneumonia, meningitis, and various gastrointestinal disorders. The nature of these diseases and their epidemiology are discussed in the chapters dealing with the individual organisms. It is useful, however, to think of the infections caused by organisms other than *Salmonella, Shigella, Yersinia,* and enteropathogenic *E. coli* as opportunistic or secondary infections. The opportunistic infections usually occur outside of the intestine and require an alteration of the host by some mechanical, physiologic, or infectious process before they can cause disease. *Salmonella, Shigella,* and *Yersinia* are considered to be true enteric pathogens, and their isolation from intestinal sources implies either a diseased or carrier state. Although *E. coli* can cause either intestinal disease or opportunistic infections, most of the infections seen in the United States are nonintestinal or opportunistic. Regardless of the site of initial infection, the one potential danger with enterobacterial infections is the development of secondary bacteremia and endotoxin shock.

Laboratory Diagnosis. Specimens submitted for the isolation of the enterobacteria include sputum, tissue, pus, body fluids, rectal swabs, or feces. These specimens must be cultured immediately or placed in an appropriate transport medium such as Stuart's or Amies medium in order to prevent desiccation of the specimen and to prevent organism overgrowth, which will distort the true microbial nature of the specimen.

The medium used for the isolation of the enteric bacilli depends on the clinical source of the specimen. With nonfecal specimens any enteric could be a pathogen; therefore these specimens are plated on media that will permit the growth of all enterics but that will inhibit the growth of gram-positive bacteria. With fecal specimens the laboratory is seeking to isolate the intestinal pathogens, *Salmonella, Shigella,* or *Yersinia.* The isolation of enteropathogenic *E. coli* is difficult, and the techniques for detecting these organisms are not readily available to the routine hospital laboratory. Regardless of the purpose, most enteric media contain various carbohydrates and acid-base indicators to differentiate between the various species of organism growing on the media. One can readily distinguish a fermentative colony from a nonfermentative colony by the color changes produced from the interaction of fermentative acids with the acid-base indicator. The most commonly used carbohydrate is lactose, and in laboratory jargon the organisms are referred to as "lactose fermenters" and "nonlactose fermenters." This terminology arose during the time when the primary purpose of enteric isolation was to differentiate the nonfermentative colonies of intestinal pathogens from the fermentative colonies of the major inhabitants of the intestinal tract, *Escherichia, Enterobacter,* and *Klebsiella.* Other carbohydrates and methods for detecting H_2S production have been used in several different media in order to aid in the colonial differentiation of various enteric colonies. Table 33–3 lists several of the commonly used enteric isolation media and their purpose.

Once the individual organisms are isolated, they are speciated by various biochemical tests. Because of the complexity of the family, many different biochemical schema have been devised to help identify these organisms. The reader is referred to the chapters on the individual organisms, the *Manual of Clinical Microbiology,* or the text by Ewing for detailed biochemical information. In addition to biochemical reactions, the clinical laboratory also uses serologic grouping of the O, H, and K antigens to characterize certain enteric isolates. When dealing with the genera *Salmonella* and *Shigella,* serologic characterization is necessary for the complete identification of the organism; with other organisms, serologic grouping is used primarily for epidemiologic purposes.

Treatment. Despite the discovery of newer antimicrobial agents, adequate treatment of enterobacterial infections remains a major therapeutic problem. Several factors contribute to the difficulty of treating these infections. One of the most important factors is the underlying disease of the patient. Studies on patients with gram-negative bacteremia show that despite appropriate antibiotic therapy, the fatality rate is closely linked to the underlying disease. Patients who have rapidly fatal underlying disease (death occurring within 1 year) have an 85% mortality when they are bacteremic with enteric organisms, whereas the mortality rate for bacteremia patients with ultimately fatal diseases (death within 5 years) is 42%. This compares to a 10% mortality rate in bacteremic patients who have nonfatal underlying disease.

Another important factor is the emergence of resistant organisms. This resistance has been attributed to the indiscriminate use of antibiotics that tend to select for resistant forms and the ability of these resistant forms to transfer their genes to previously sensitive organisms. The biochemical nature and the genetics of resistance factors and their transfer are discussed in Chapters 8 and 9. Besides developing new antibiotics to control resistant organisms, some researchers have attempted to neutralize the bacterial defenses against the antibiotic. The most successful approaches have been to incorporate the β-lactamase-binding agents clavulanic acid and sulbactam with a penicillin. These binding agents inactivate the bacterial β-lactamase, leaving the penicillin intact to kill the organism.

TABLE 33–4. ANTIMICROBIALS USEFUL IN TREATMENT OF ENTEROBACTERIAL DISEASES

Penicillins	Polymyxins
Amoxicillin	Colistin
Ampicillin	Polymyxin B
Carbenicillin	Quinolones
Mezlocillin	Sulfonamides
Pipercillin	Tetracyclines
Ticarcillin	Other antibiotics
Penicillins with β-lactamase inhibitors	Chloramphenicol
Amoxicillin and clavulanic acid	Imipenem
Ampicillin and sulbactam	Nitrofurantoin
Ticarcillin and clavulanic acid	Trimethoprim-sulfamethoxazole
Cephalosporins	
Aminoglycosides	
Amikacin	
Gentamicin	
Kanamycin	
Netilmicin	
Tobramycin	

Table 33–4 lists some of the antibiotics that have been developed to treat gram-negative infections. Because of the variability of sensitivity patterns in individual organisms, the appropriate antibiotic must be chosen by careful evaluation of the isolate's susceptibility pattern, the condition of the host, and the site of infection.

Patients who develop endotoxin shock require prompt, vigorous treatment of both the infection and the shock. Treatment of shock centers on the cardiovascular system and includes restoration of the intravascular volume, digitalization, and the administration of isoproterenol. Some patients may require additional treatment with other agents such as steroids, pressor amines, and norepinephrine.

FURTHER READING

Books and Reviews

Acar JF: Problems and changing patterns of resistance with gram-negative bacteria. Rev Infect Dis 7(suppl 4):S545, 1985

Allan JD, Moellering RC Jr: Management of infections caused by gram-negative bacilli: The role of antimicrobial combinations. Rev Infect Dis 7(suppl 4):S559, 1985

Bradley SG: Cellular and molecular mechanisms of action in bacterial endotoxins. Ann Rev Microbiol 33:67, 1979

Bryan CS, Reynolds KL, Brenner ER: Analysis of 1186 episodes of gram-negative bacteremia in non-university hospitals: The effects of antimicrobial therapy. Rev Infect Dis 5:629, 1983

Cohen PS, Maguire JH, Weinstein L: Infective endocarditis caused by gram-negative bacteria: A review of the literature 1945–1977. Prog Cardiovasc Dis 22:205, 1980

DuPont HL: Enteropathogenic organisms. New etiologic agents and concepts of disease. Med Clin North Am 62:945, 1978

Ewing WH: Edwards and Ewing's Identification of Enterobacteriaceae, ed 4. New York, Elsevier, 1986

Kaas EH, Wolff SM (eds): Bacterial lipopolysaccharides: Chemistry, biology and clinical significance of endotoxin. J Infect Dis 128 (July suppl):1, 1973

Kelly MT, Brenner DJ, Farmer JJ III: Enterobacteriaceae. In Lennette EH, Balows A, Hausler WJ, Shadomy HJ (eds): Manual of Clinical Microbiology, ed 4. Washington DC, American Society for Microbiology, 1985, p 263

Konisky J: Colicins and other bacteriocins with established modes of action. Ann Rev Microbiol 36:125, 1982

Lindberg F, Normark S: Contribution of chromosomal beta-lactamases to beta-lactam resistance in enterobacteria. Rev Infect Dis 8(suppl 3):S292, 1986

Makela PH, Mayer H: Enterobacterial common antigen. Bacteriol Rev 40:591, 1976

Morrison DC: Bacterial endotoxins and pathogenesis. Rev Infect Dis 5 (suppl 4):S733, 1983

Orskov I, Orskov F, Jann B, Jann K: Serology, chemistry, and genetics of O and K antigens of *Escherichia coli.* Bacteriol Rev 41:667, 1978

Ottow JCG: Ecology, physiology and genetics of fimbriae and pili. Ann Rev Microbiol 29:79, 1975

Qureshi N, Takayama K: Structure and function of Lipid A. In Iglewski BH, Clark VL (eds): The Bacteria, vol XI: Molecular Basis of Bacterial Pathogenesis. San Diego, Academic Press, 1990, p 319

Roberts JA: Urinary tract infections. Am J Kidney Dis IV:103, 1984

Smith-Keary PF: Molecular genetics of *Escherichia coli.* New York, Guilford Press, 1989

Sutherland IW: Biosynthesis and composition of gram-negative bacterial extracellular and wall polysaccharides. Ann Rev Microbiol 39:243, 1985

von Graevenitz A: The role of opportunistic bacteria in human disease. Ann Rev Microbiol 31:447, 1977

Weinstein L: Gram-negative bacterial infections: A look at the past, a view of the present, and a glance at the future. Rev Infect Dis 7(suppl 4):S538, 1985

Young LS: Treatment of infections due to gram-negative bacilli: A perspective of past, present, and future. Rev Infect Dis 7(suppl 4):S572, 1985

Selected Papers

Bartlett JG, O'Keefe P, Tally FP, et al: Bacteriology of hospital-acquired pneumonia. Arch Intern Med 146:868, 1986

Bauernfeind A, Petermuller C, Schneider R: Bacteriocins as tools in analysis of nosocomial *Klebsiella pneumoniae* infections. J Clin Microbiol 14:15, 1981

Beachey EH: Bacterial adherence: Adhesion-receptor interactions mediating the attachment of bacteria to mucosal surfaces. J Infect Dis 143:325, 1981

Berk SL, McCabe WR: Meningitis caused by gram-negative bacilli. Ann Intern Med 93:253, 1980

Brenner DJ, McWhorter AC, Kai A, et al: *Enterobacter asburiae* sp. nov., a new species found in clinical specimens and reassignment of *Erwinia dissolvens* and *Erwinia nimipressuralis* to the genus *Enterobacter* as *Enterobacter dissolvens* comb. nov. and *Enterobacter nimipressuralis* comb. nov. J Clin Microbiol 23:1114, 1986

Farmer JJ III, Davis BR, Hickman-Brenner FW, et al: Biochemical identification of new species and biogroups of *Enterobacteriaceae* isolated from clinical specimens. J Clin Microbiol 21:46, 1985

Karnad A, Alvarez S, Berk SL: Pneumonia caused by gram-negative bacilli. Am J Med 79(suppl 1A):61, 1985

McCue JD: Improved mortality in gram-negative bacillary bacteremia. Arch Intern Med 145:1212, 1985

O'Hara CM, Steigerwalt AG, Hill BC, et al: *Enterobacter hormaechei,* a new species of the family Enterobacteriaceae formerly known as enteric group 75. J Clin Microbiol 27:2046, 1989

CHAPTER 34

Opportunistic Enterobacteriaceae

Historically the Enterobacteriaceae have been divided into the opportunistic pathogens and the intestinal pathogens. The intestinal pathogens traditionally have included the members of the genera *Salmonella, Shigella,* and *Yersinia,* and the opportunistic pathogens included all the other genera. However, recent developments in the genetic relationships of *Escherichia coli* and *Shigella,* coupled with the discoveries in mechanisms of diarrheal disease, have made this distinction less clear-cut. Although the statement can no longer be made that a particular species is an opportunistic or an enteric pathogen, it is still clinically useful to make this distinction since the vast majority of infections caused by the organisms discussed in this chapter do not involve the gastrointestinal tract. All of the opportunistic enteric bacilli are capable of causing similar diseases, but the epidemiology, frequency, severity, and treatment of these diseases differ for the various species.

Genus *Escherichia*

The genus *Escherichia* contains the one bacterium, *E. coli,* that has been the object of more scientific research than any other microorganism. This organism is the major facultative inhabitant of the large intestine and is unique among normal flora organisms in that it is also the most commonly isolated human pathogen causing urinary tract and wound infections, pneumonia, meningitis, and septicemia. Recent studies have demonstrated that certain strains of *E. coli* are also important intestinal pathogens, causing a wide variety of gastrointestinal diseases. In addition to *E. coli,* the genus *Escherichia* includes several other species that rarely are isolated from human disease.

Taxonomy. As noted in Chapter 33, DNA homology studies show that the genus *Escherichia* includes the *Shigella;* however, the clinical importance of bacillary dysentery requires that the *Shigella* be considered as separate entities, and as such they are discussed in Chapter 35. Excluding the *Shigella,* the genus *Escherichia* includes six species, five of which have been associated with human disease. *E. coli* is responsible for virtually all the clinically significant infections caused by the genus, whereas the other species account for less than 1% of the clinical isolates of the genus. *Escherichia adecarboxylata,* a rare human isolate, has also been classified as enteric group 41 by the Centers for Disease Control (CDC) and as *Enterobacter agglomerans* by others. *Escherichia hermannii,* formerly classified as enteric group 11, has been isolated from blood and spinal fluid, although it is primarily found in wound infections and feces. *Escherichia vulneris,* formerly enteric group 21, API group 2, and Alma group 1, has also been isolated from wound infections. *Escherichia fergusonii,* formerly enteric group 10, has been isolated from blood and urine but primarily has been isolated from feces and animals. *Escherichia blattae* has not been isolated from human sources but has been isolated only from cockroach intestines. Because of their rare isolation from human infections, species other than *E. coli* are not discussed further.

Biochemical and Cultural Characteristics. *E. coli* grows well on commonly used media. On enteric isolation media (Chap. 33) most strains appear as lactose-fermenting colonies. Some strains, particularly those associated with urinary tract infections, are β-hemolytic on blood agar. The majority of isolates are nonpigmented and motile and are biochemically characterized by the production of lysine decarboxylase, the use of acetate as a carbon source, and the hydrolysis of tryptophan to indole.

Antigenic Structure. Serologic typing of *E. coli* is based primarily on the determination of the O antigen type, H antigen type, and when applicable, the K antigen type. There are more than 164 O antigens, 100 K antigens, and 50 H antigens described for *E. coli.* The H antigens can be further subdivided into the L, A, and B subgroups. Determination of the antigenic profile of the various strains is useful in epidemiologic studies, and several studies have linked particular antigenic types to various diarrheal diseases. For example, serotype O157:H7 produces a Shigalike toxin (see below) that is responsible for hemorrhagic colitis, and nearly all O78:H11 and O78:H12 isolates are enterotoxigenic. Other antigenic types such as O111a,111b:H2 have been associated with infantile diarrhea, and O124:H30 strains are enteroinvasive and cause a bacillary dysentery similar to that caused by *Shigella.* Many other antigenic types in addition to the ones listed above are linked to the various diseases; the reader is referred to the text by Ewing and the reviews by Evans and Evans and by Levine and Edelman for a complete listing of these serotypes.

Determinants of Pathogenicity

The descriptive term *E. coli* encompasses a diverse group of organisms that can infect any host system and produce a vast number of virulence factors, ranging from structural features to excreted toxins. The relative importance of each of these factors depends not only on the genetics of a particular strain of organism but also on the site of infection and the underlying condition of the host.

Surface Factors. In both the United States and Europe *E. coli* and group B streptococci are the primary causes of neonatal meningitis, and 80% of all *E. coli* isolated from individuals with this disease produce a polysialic acid capsule termed *K1.* Organisms possessing this capsular type also are more likely to cause neonatal sepsis. Interestingly, this capsule is identical to the group B polysaccharide capsule of *Neisseria meningitidis* (Chap. 26). The K1 capsule is unique among the capsular antigens of *E. coli* in that it enables the organism to resist killing by both human neutrophils and normal serum in various in vitro assays. Other capsular types inhibit the killing power of normal serum, particularly when associated with smooth LPS, but fail to protect organisms from phagocytic death. The K1 capsule may also aid in the survival of the organism in the blood and spinal fluid of neonates because of its similarity to the embryonic form of the polysialic acid of the neural cell adhesion molecule (N-CAM). Some authors believe that this structural similarity prevents the neonate from forming opsonizing antibodies to the K1 antigen. However, the presence of K1 antigen is not sufficient to explain all of the virulence of *E. coli* in neonatal disease. The type of O antigen of the infecting organism also appears to be important, as does production of S fimbriae, which have a predilection for binding to receptors present on the vascular endothelium and the epithelial lining of the choroid plexus and the ventricules of the brains of neonatal mice.

In addition to the S type fimbriae, *E. coli* produce a number of different types of fimbriae that enable the organism to attach to various host tissues. These fimbriae have been divided into two large groups termed *mannose resistant* and *mannose sensitive.* The mannose-sensitive fimbriae bind to mannose-containing receptors in host cells, and their ability to bind to these receptors is reduced when the bacterial cells are pretreated with D-mannose. Mannose-sensitive or type I fimbriae are also called *common pili* because they are found on most *E. coli.* Although type I fimbriae attach to a wide variety of eucaryotic cells, no pathogenic function has been defined for them, since there is no correlation between the presence or absence of type I fimbriae and disease. However, some authors believe that these fimbriae are important in the colonization of the bladder in the absence of other fimbriae. Furthermore, type I fimbriae are believed to play a major role in colonization by binding the organism to the mucosa of the large intestines, buccal cavity, and vaginal tract.

The surface factors involved with mannose-resistant adhesion are more complex than the type I fimbriae. Included in this group of surface-adherent factors are fimbriae and other surface properties termed *adhesins.* Regardless of the nature of these adhesive factors, they all appear to be important in the establishment of pathogenic strains of *E. coli* in various host tissues, and the genetic information for a number of them is found closely associated with other virulence factors. One such mannose-resistant adherence factor is the type S fimbriae described above as a cofactor with K1-encapsulated *E. coli.* Another major mannose-resistant fimbriae group is that of the P fimbriae, so-named because of their ability to bind to the human P blood group antigens. These antigens contain a Gal(α1-4)Galβ moiety, which is also found in a number of other human cells, including those of the kidney and bladder. Uropathogenic *E. coli* frequently contain the P fimbriae that bind to these sites, and organisms containing P fimbriae are more likely to be associated with complicated urinary tract infections. Approximately 70% of *E. coli* strains isolated from patients with pyelonephritis possess P fimbriae, compared to only 36% of strains from cystitis patients and 19% of fecal strains. Another group of heterologous adhesins, termed *X factors,* may also be important in the uropathogenicity of *E. coli,* although their exact role has not yet been determined. They appear to bind sites other than the P blood group antigen and mannose-containing moieties. They include the adhesins that appear to bind to the Dr blood group antigen, the adhesin associated with the M blood group antigen, the nonfimbrial protein antigens NFA 1 and NFA 2, and the F1C and G fimbriae.

Mannose-resistant fimbriae and adhesins are also important adherence factors in intestinal infections caused by *E. coli.* In animals the F4 (formerly K88), F5 (formerly K99), 987P, and F41 fimbriae are necessary for the establishment of the enteropathogenic strains in the gastrointestinal tract. The CFA1 and CFA2 (CS1, CS2, CS3) fimbriae perform the same function in human enterotoxigenic *E. coli* (ETEC). Enteropathogenic *E. coli* (EPEC), enteroadherent *E. coli* (EAEC), and verotoxin-producing *E. coli* (VTEC) produce nonfimbrial adhesins that attach the organisms to their target cells in a closer association than is seen with other means of attachment. Some of these adhesins appear to be bacterial surface proteins, but the mechanism by which they attach the bacterial cell to the host cell is not clear. Once attached to the target cell, the EPEC and EAEC produce modifications in the host cellular structure, and this alteration is thought to be responsible for the changes in cellular permeability, leading to diarrhea. Whether the adhesin alone is responsible for the structural alteration or whether other bacterial products are produced is not known. The binding of VTEC to target cells is thought to provide a means of allowing transfer of the toxin directly to the target cells. The genetic information for the majority of these adhesins appears to be contained on plasmids.

The precise role of other surface antigens is not known. As noted in the sections on antigenic determinants and clinical manifestations, certain O serotypes have been associated with different diseases. Whether the genetic location of a pathogenic determinant is merely close to the genetic loci for antigenic specificity or whether the surface antigens are truly necessary for establishing the organism in the host has not been determined. However, intact O antigens protect the organism from the effects of the complement. Furthermore, the lipid A portion of the lipopolysaccharide (LPS) is responsible for the endotoxic effects seen in bacteremic patients (Chap. 6).

Enterotoxins. Various *E. coli* strains play a significant role in gastrointestinal disease, and the pathogenic mechanisms of *E. coli* diarrhea are varied and complex. One of these pathogenic mechanisms involves the production of a wide variety of enterotoxins, some of which are associated with human disease, whereas others are primarily associated with animal infections. However, given the goals and space constraints of this text, the animal enteroxins are not discussed. Regardless of the host system, the target organ of *E. coli* enterotoxins is the small intestine, and the result is a watery diarrhea caused by the outpouring of fluids and electrolytes. The ability to produce the majority of these toxins is dependent on the presence of plasmids encoding for toxin production.

E. coli strains possessing the necessary plasmid produce a heat-labile enterotoxin (LT) that is similar to the enterotoxin of *Vibrio cholerae* (Chap. 36). As with cholera toxin (CT), LT stimulates adenyl cyclase activity in the epithelial cells of the small intestinal mucosa, which in turn increases the permeability of the intestinal lining, resulting in a loss of fluids and electrolytes. The B subunits of both the CT and LT bind to the ganglioside GM_1 of intestinal cells. The A subunit is then hydrolyzed and the A_1 fragment enters the host cell and enzymatically catalyzes the transfer of adenosine diphosphate (ADP)-ribose from nicotinamide adenine dinucleotide (NAD) to the regulatory subunit of adenyl cyclase, thereby increasing the level of cyclic AMP. This increase in cyclic AMP causes a loss of electrolytes and fluid from the cells. Although CT and LT are structurally similar and produce the same effects in tissue culture and animal models, they have slightly different antigenic structures, and the potency of the LT is about 100-fold less than the cholera toxin in animal models. The overall amino acid and nucleotide homology of the two toxins is approximately 80%.

A second class of LT, LT-II, which does not share immunologic reactivity or nucleotide homology with either CT or LT, has been identified. The LT-II class contains at least two different toxins, LT-IIa and LT-IIb. The genes encoding for the B subunits of LT-IIa and LT-IIb are 66% homologous with each other, but they share no significant homology with the LT-I or CT. The genes encoding for the A subunit of both the LT-IIa and LT-IIb are 71% homologous with each other and 57% homologous with the genes of LT-I and CT, with most of the homology occurring in the region encoding for the A_1 subunit. Although the mode of action of LT-IIa and LT-IIb is similar to that of CT and LT, they do not cause fluid accumulation in the ligated adult rabbit intestine model, nor do they bind to the ganglioside GM_1. Furthermore, the genetic information for these toxins is encoded on the bacterial chromosome, not on plasmids. The importance of these toxins in human disease is not known.

In addition to the LT, *E. coli* can produce two heat-stable (ST) enterotoxins, ST_a (ST-I) and ST_b (ST-II). ST_a is a polypeptide with a molecular weight of 1500 to 2000 Da, is methanol soluble, and is active in suckling mice and neonatal pigs. ST_a has a tightly coiled secondary structure that appears to be required for activity as evidenced by its high content of cysteine, its inactivation by reducing agents, and its alkaline pH. ST_b is not methanol soluble and is active only in weaned pigs. The two toxins are also different in amino acid sequence. ST_a binds tightly to specific intestinal receptors and then rapidly activates a particulate guanylate cyclase in intestinal mucosa cells, causing a secretory response primarily by inhibiting sodium and chloride absorption by the brush border membrane. The mechanism of action of ST_b is not known, but it does not involve cylic nucleotide production. Although ST_a-producing *E. coli* strains do cause diarrhea in humans, one study did not report the detection of any ST_b-producing *E. coli* in stools of patients from Brazil and Bangladesh. The ability to produce ST_a is encoded on two plasmids, one of which also encodes for LT and the other for ST only, and probe studies have revealed that there are at least two distinct ST_a genes, ST_a-I and ST_a-II.

Verotoxins (Shigalike Toxins). *E. coli* produces at least two human-derived and one porcine-derived cytotoxin, termed *verotoxins* because of their irreversible cytotoxic effect on Vero tissue culture cells, a cell line developed from African green monkey kidney cells. VTEC have been associated with three human syndromes: diarrhea, hemorrhagic colitis, and hemolytic uremic syndrome (HUS). Because of the similarities of verotoxins to Shiga toxin (Chap. 35), these toxins have also been referred to as Shigalike toxins (SLT); the term *SLT-I* is interchangeable with VT1, and VT2 is referred to as *SLT-II* by other authors. Both VT1 and VT2 inhibit protein synthesis in eucaroytic cells in the same manner as Shiga toxin, but they differ from each other and Shiga toxin in immunologic reactivity and biologic activities in animal and tissue culture models. VT1 is almost identical to Shiga toxin, both in structure and mode of action, but it differs in molecular weight, and the two toxins differ in their activities in animal models. VT2 has similar biologic properties to VT1 but is not neutralized by Shiga-toxin antibody. The two verotoxins share a 58% homology in nucleotide sequence in their encoding genes and a 56% homology in amino acid composition. VT2 appears to differ from VT1 in the spacing of the subunits and in the DNA restriction pattern. The level of toxin production is important in development of disease. High-level VTEC produce large amounts of toxin in supernatant fluids of cultures and have been linked to hemorrhagic colitis, diarrhea, and HUS. Low- and trace-level-producing VTEC do not have easily detected amounts of toxin in supernatant fluids and do not appear to be associated with disease production. VTEC are infected with either one or both bacteriophages that encode for the production of either VT1 or VT2 or both VT1 and VT2. Although a number of *E. coli* strains can become infected with these bacteriophages and thus produce verotoxins, the majority of VTEC isolates in outbreaks in the United States and Canada have been attributed to the O157:H7 serotype.

Other Factors. Enteroinvasive *E. coli* strains are similar to *Shigella* and penetrate the epithelial lining of the intestinal tract (Chap. 35). These organisms possess large plasmids that encode for O antigens, which may be important in the binding of the organisms to host cells and subsequent intracellular survival.

Hemolytic *E. coli* strains are isolated more commonly from nonintestinal infections than from fecal specimens, and hemolytic strains appear to be more nephropathogenic. The hemolysis is due to the production of a filterable hemolysin, which not only lyses the erythrocytes of a variety of species but also is cytotoxic for leukocytes and chicken and mouse fibroblasts. The lytic action of hemolysin appears to be due to the insertion of hemolysin molecules into lipid membranes, producing a cation-selective channel that increases the permeability of the membrane to calcium, potassium, mannose, and sucrose. Some authors believe that the hemolysin contributes to inflammation, tissue injury, and impaired host defenses by acting either directly on tissue cells or indirectly by lysis of monocytoctes and granulocytes. Hemolysin production may be encoded by chromosomal genes or by the presence of a 41 MDa plasmid. Studies with hemolysin plasmid-containing strains show that the loss of the plasmid is associated with a loss of nephropathogenicity. Interestingly, a number of hemolytic strains also produce P fimbriae, which may aid in the colonization of these organisms in the renal system. The role of the hemolysin in relation to the bacterial cell may be to provide a means of acquiring iron in the host environment where most of the iron is tightly bound to protein molecules or is present in very low concentrations.

Another means of acquiring iron for *E. coli* is through the production of the iron-chelating siderophore aerobactin. There appears to be a reciprocal relationship between aerobactin and hemolysin production, and some authors have proposed that different strains use aerobactin and hemolysin as two alternative means of obtaining iron.

Hemolytic strains frequently produce a cytotoxic necrotizing factor (CNF). This 110,000 Da protein causes necrosis in rabbit skin and induces the formation of multinucleated cells in tissue culture. In one survey 63% of hemolytic strains produced CNF, whereas none of the nonhemolytic strains produced this toxin. The exact role of CNF in disease and its relationship to the hemolysin is not yet known, although some researchers believe that it is responsible for some of the tissue damage observed in some infections.

Clinical Infection

Clinical Manifestations. In the United States *E. coli* is the leading cause of both nosocomial and community-acquired urinary tract infections. The spectrum of disease ranges from cystitis to pyelonephritis. Females are more likely to have urinary tract infections at a younger age because of differences in anatomic structure, sexual maturation, the changes that occur during pregnancy and childbirth, and the presence of tumors. After the age of 45, the male with prostatic hypertrophy is more likely to have a urinary tract infection. Catheterization or other mechanical manipulation of the urinary tract, obstruction, diabetes, and failure to empty the bladder completely during urination are other factors that predispose individuals to urinary tract infections with *E. coli* and other microorganisms.

E. coli can also cause pulmonary infections. In some institutions *E. coli* was the cause of 50% of nosocomial pneumonia, whereas in other hospitals the incidence of *E. coli* pneumonia was as low as 12%. Most patients with *E. coli* pneumonia are more than 50 years of age and have one or more underlying chronic diseases. Endogenous aspiration of oral secretions containing *E. coli* appears to be the main source of the infection, although patients with *E. coli* bacteremia may seed the lung with septic emboli. Empyema can occur, especially in patients who have had pneumonia for more than 6 days.

E. coli is an important cause of neonatal meningitis but is rarely seen as a cause of meningitis in older populations. The mortality rate in patients with this disease is between 40% and 80% and the majority of survivors have subsequent neurologic or developmental abnormalities.

E. coli can also be isolated from wound infections, particularly those occurring in the abdomen. Peritonitis caused by *E. coli* and other bowel organisms is a frequent complication of ruptured appendices.

As with other opportunistic pathogens, *E. coli* can invade the bloodstream from any of the primary infection sites listed above. In most hospitals it is the most frequent cause of gram-negative sepsis and, in fact, is usually the leading blood culture isolate. As noted in Chapter 33, one of the leading dangers of gram-negative sepsis is the development of endotoxic shock.

The role of *E. coli* in diarrheal disease is not yet completely understood because the methods for detecting the enteropathogenic organisms are not readily available in the routine hospital laboratory. Furthermore, the mechanisms by which *E. coli* can cause diarrhea are complex. One estimate puts the incidence of *E. coli* diarrhea in the United States at 4%. In tropical countries, however, enteropathogenic *E. coli* are important causes of childhood diarrhea. ETEC have been associated with 11% to 15% of childhood diarrhea in developing countries and are major causes of the traveler's diarrhea seen in visitors to these countries. ETEC have been responsible for approximately 30% to 45% of traveler's diarrhea in visitors to Mexico. Studies in other countries indicate that ETEC may be the cause of 11% to 72% of traveler's diarrhea. EAEC appear to be another major cause of traveler's diarrhea, with these organisms causing up to 30% of the disease in some studies.

EPEC are a special group of adherent organisms associated with outbreaks of infantile diarrhea. Traditionally this term has been reserved for the classic serotypes: O:26:H11, O:26:NM, O55:NM, O55:H6, O:55:H7, O86:NM, O86:H34, O86:H2, O111:NM, O111:H2, O111:H12, O111:H21, O114:H2, O119:H6, O125ac:H21, O128ab:H2, O142:H6 and O158:H23. These organisms are common causes of diarrhea in infants in day and hospital nurseries in the United Kingdom, Canada, and Israel. The incidence in the United States is not known since most hospitals stopped screening for these organisms in the mid-1970s when the ETEC were discovered and many individuals thought that enterotoxin production was the key to determining if an organism is an enteropathogen. In Brazil, where screening for EPEC has continued, these organisms are the leading cause of infantile diarrhea in the community.

Enteroinvasive *E. coli* (EIEC) cause bacillary dysentery in all age groups. The disease caused by these organisms is indistinguishable from shigellosis. In a survey of 410 Thai children with diarrhea EIEC was responsible for 4% of the diarrhea as compared to 23% from *Shigella.* The role of this group of organisms in diarrheal disease in other countries is not known.

In the United States and Canada VTEC have caused a number of outbreaks of diarrhea, hemorrhagic colitis, and HUS. Hemorrhagic colitis is a self-limiting, acute, bloody diarrheal illness that is characterized by abdominal cramps, watery diarrhea, and a hemorrhagic discharge. HUS is characterized by acute renal failure, microangiopathic hemolytic anemia, and thrombocytopenia. Both hemorrhagic colitis and HUS are complications of a mild and common diarrhea that is seen primarily in child-care institutions or in kindergarten-aged children and elderly patients. The source of the infections is probably meat and animal products such as milk and hamburger. Serotype O157:H7 is a high producer of verotoxin and has been implicated in several outbreaks; however, several other serotypes of VTEC have also been isolated by Canadian workers. In several prospective studies in the United States and Canada VTEC were the third or fourth leading cause of diarrhea, and the number of VTEC isolates was exceeded only by the isolates of *Campylobacter* and *Salmonella.*

Laboratory Diagnosis. *E. coli* grows readily on the media described in Chapter 33, and most strains are identified easily by the methods used in clinical laboratories. However, the mere isolation of *E. coli* from contaminated specimens, such as sputum and wounds, does not mean that it is the cause of the patient's infection. Careful consideration must be given to patient factors and other organisms that are isolated. For example, a patient given penicillin for a pneumococcal pneumonia may have a heavy growth of *E. coli* in subsequent sputum cultures because the penicillin killed the normal respiratory flora, allowing the *E. coli* to colonize the upper respiratory tract.

The recent developments in the study of the causes of diarrhea demonstrate that in the absence of known enteropathogens, *E. coli* must be considered in the diagnosis. However, the routine hospital laboratory does not have the techniques for detecting many of these organisms. Most of the published reports implicating *E. coli* in diarrheal disease are from investigations of outbreaks by public health groups or from designed prospective studies by teams of specialized investigators. However, recent developments in the area of nucleic acid probes and monoclonal antibodies may provide the hospital laboratory with the ability to detect ETEC. Techniques that may aid in the detection of other forms of EPEC are being developed and may soon become routine. In fact, potential VTEC can now be detected with commercially available reagents. VTEC of serotype O157:H7 do not ferment sorbitol, and this fact was used to design a medium that substitutes sorbitol for lactose in MacConkey agar. Once sorbitol-negative isolates are obtained, they can be tested for the O157:H7 antigens. This method will not detect other sorbitol-fermenting serotypes of VTEC, nor will it confirm that the isolates produce verotoxins. However, for a patient with a history of bloody diarrhea and the isolation of a potential pathogen, the diagnosis of verotoxin-caused disease is highly probable. Serologic typing of diarrhea-producing *E. coli* is available, but clinicians and laboratorians must develop an awareness of the importance of detecting these organisms before these procedures become part of the routine screening of stools from neonates.

Treatment. Most organisms isolated from community-acquired infections are usually sensitive to most of the antibiotics listed in Chapter 33. Resistant forms do occur, especially in patients with a history of prior antibiotic treatment. Each individual isolate should be tested to determine which antibiotics would be most effective. The best treatment for diarrhea appears to be the management of the fluid and electrolyte imbalance, although infantile diarrhea and bacillary dysentery do respond to antibiotic treatment. Prophylactic treatment with trimethoprim-sulfamethoxazole reduces the incidence of traveler's diarrhea; however, some clinicians believe that prophylaxis may only serve to select for resistant organisms and to potentiate the carrier state in persons infected with *Salmonella* rather than *E. coli.*

Genus *Klebsiella*

The most commonly isolated member of the genus *Klebsiella* is *K. pneumoniae* (Friedländer's bacillus). As its name implies, it can cause pneumonia and was originally thought to be the cause of classic lobar pneumonia, the true agent of which is *Streptococcus pneumoniae.* Like other opportunistic Enterobacteriaceae, *K. pneumoniae* can infect other sites besides the respiratory tract. Other species of *Klebsiella* can cause similar diseases but are isolated less frequently.

Taxonomy. As with all Enterobacteriaceae, there has been a dramatic shift in the taxonomy of the *Klebsiella.* Based on DNA-relatedness studies, the genus consists of five species: *K. pneumoniae, K. oxytoca, K. planticola, K. terrigena,* and *Klebsiella* group 47. Two former species, *K. ozaenae* and *K. rhinoscleromatis,* are biochemically inactive strains of *K. pneumoniae;* however, because of their association with specific human diseases and the need to simplify reporting, the Enteric Bacteriology Section of the CDC continues to use the species

TABLE 34–1. CHARACTERISTICS OF THE GENUS *KLEBSIELLA*

Test	*K. pneumoniae*	*K. ozaenae*	*K. rhinoscleromatis*	*K. oxytoca*	*K. planticola*	*K.* group 47
Indole	−	−	−	+	±	+
Voges-Proskauer	+	−	−	+	+	±
Ornithine decarboxylase	−	−	−	−	−	+
Malonate	+	−	+	+	+	+
Growth at 5C	−	−	−	−	+	+

designation for these two organisms. *K. terrigena* has been isolated only from environmental sources and is not considered further. *K. planticola* is also an environmental organism; however, it has been implicated in human urinary tract and wound infections. *Klebsiella* group 47 has been isolated primarily from the respiratory tract and occasionally from blood. *K. oxytoca* was formerly classified as indole-positive *K. pneumoniae* and causes the same spectrum of diseases as *K. pneumoniae,* albeit at a much lower frequency. Group K, or *K. trevisanii,* has been proposed as another species by some authors, but this group appears to be similar to *K. planticola.*

Biochemical and Cultural Characteristics. With the exception of *K. rhinoscleromatis* and most strains of *K. ozaenae, Klebsiella* species appear as lactose-fermenting colonies on differential enteric isolation media. All *Klebsiella* species are nonmotile. The presence of a large capsule causes colonies of *Klebsiella* growing on agar to appear large, moist, and mucoid. Table 34–1 lists some of the differentiating characteristics of the members of this genus.

Antigenic Structure. *Klebsiella* possess O and K antigens. The polysaccharide K antigens are the most useful in serologic typing. All species share the same capsular antigens and thus can be typed with the same set of antisera. There are 77 K antigens described, and no one serotype appears to be more likely to cause a particular type of infection or to be more virulent than another serotype. Nevertheless, serologic typing provides a useful epidemiologic tool for investigating individual outbreaks caused by these organisms.

Determinants of Pathogenicity. The capsule enables the organism to resist phagocytosis and the killing power of normal serum. Encapsulated strains are more virulent than nonencapsulated organisms in animal models. With the exception of endotoxin, no other toxin that plays a role in opportunistic infections has been identified in *Klebsiella* species. Enterotoxin-producing strains of *K. pneumoniae* have been isolated from patients with tropical sprue. These toxins are similar, if not identical, to the ST and LT of *E. coli,* and the ability to produce enterotoxin is plasmid mediated. A filterable cytotoxin that affects a variety of tissue culture cells has been reported in several isolates of *K. oxytoca* obtained from patients with hemorrhagic colitis. The exact nature of this toxin and its role in disease are not known.

Clinical Infection. *K. pneumoniae* can cause a primary community-acquired pneumonia as well as a nosocomial pneumonia. The typical patient is a middle- or older-aged man with underlying medical problems such as alcoholism, chronic bronchopulmonary disease, or diabetes mellitus. Approximately 25% to 75% of patients produce a thick, nonputrid, bloody sputum. Necrosis and abscess formation are more likely with *K. pneumoniae* infections than with any other bacterial pneumonia, and blood cultures are positive in approximately 25% of patients. The mortality rate is between 25% and 50% despite adequate antibiotic coverage, and it closely correlates with the development of bacteremia.

In addition to pneumonia, *K. pneumoniae* can cause urinary tract and wound infections, bacteremia, and meningitis. In some hospitals, *K. pneumoniae* has replaced *E. coli* as the leading blood culture isolate. A 5-year review of one institution showed that *K. pneumoniae* was responsible for 15% of the gram-negative meningitis, with most isolates coming from neurosurgery patients who had infections at other sites.

The role of enterotoxigenic and cytotoxic organisms in patients with diarrhea is difficult to assess. There have been no major systematic studies looking for these organisms in diarrhea patients, and most isolates have been obtained from tropical countries where diarrhea is a chronic problem.

K. oxytoca resembles *K. pneumoniae* in its disease spectrum and from a clinical viewpoint can be considered to be the same organism. *K. ozaenae* causes a chronic atrophic rhinitis characterized by a fetid odor. Similarly, *K. rhinoscleromatis* infects the nose and pharynx, producing a granulomatous destruction of these structures. Nasal and pharyngeal infections by these two organisms are rare in the United States and are primarily seen in immigrants from endemic regions such as Central and Eastern Europe and South America. The majority of isolates of *K. ozaenae* and *K. rhinoscleromatis* in the United States are obtained from patients with urinary tract and soft tissue infections and from cases of secondary bacteremia.

Treatment. The majority of *K. pneumoniae* isolates produce β-lactamase, which inactivates ampicillin and carbenicillin but not cephalosporin antibiotics. Other antibiotics listed in Chapter 33 are also usually effective against this organism, although isolates from nosocomial infections are often resistant to treatment with multiple antibiotics. In one prospective study of antimicrobial susceptibility 18% of the isolates from patients who remained in the hospital 15 days or longer were resistant to several antibiotics, whereas only 4% of community isolates displayed multiple resistance.

Genus *Enterobacter*

The genus *Enterobacter* (formerly *Aerobacter*) contains 12 species that inhabit soil and water and, to a lesser extent, the large intestines of man and animals. Two species, *E. amnigenus* and *E. intermedium,* are environmental organisms that are isolated

TABLE 34–2. CHARACTERISTICS OF *ENTEROBACTER* ISOLATED FROM HUMAN SPECIMENS

Test	*E. cloacae*	*E. aerogenes*	*E. agglomerans*	*E. gergoviae*	*E. sakazakii*	*E. taylorae*
Lysine decarboxylase	−	+	−	+	−	−
Arginine dihydrolase	+	−	−	−	+	+
Ornithine decarboxylase	+	+	−	+	+	+
Urease	±	−	±	+	−	−
Fermentation						
Adonitol	±	+	−	−	−	−
Sorbitol	+	+	±	−	−	−
Sucrose	+	+	±	+	+	−

from soil and water and are not known to cause human infections, although *E. amnigenus* has been isolated from clinical specimens.

Taxonomy. The eight species of *Enterobacter* that have been associated with human disease are *E. cloacae, E. aerogenes, E. agglomerans, E. gergoviae, E. sakazakii, E. taylorae, E. asburiae,* and *E. hormaechii.* It is recognized that *E. agglomerans* is a complex group that may include as many as 12 DNA homology groups or species. One organism, which was formerly classified as *E. hafniae,* has been given a separate genus status as *Hafnia alvei.*

Biochemical and Cultural Characteristics. *Enterobacter* are motile organisms that readily grow on media used for the isolation of enterics. Most of the commonly isolated species are rapid lactose fermenters and present as pigmented colonies on enteric media. With the exception of *E. agglomerans,* all species decarboxylate ornithine. The characteristics used to differentiate the more commonly isolated species are listed in Table 34–2. *E. sakazakii* can be distinguished from other members of the genus and other enterics by the yellow pigment it produces.

Antigenic Structure. Antigenic subgrouping of the *Enterobacter* is not as developed as that of *E. coli* and *K. pneumoniae.* Two schemas have been developed for typing *E. cloacae.* One schema uses 53 O antigens and 57 H antigens, and the other schema consists of 28 O antigen types. Some strains are encapsulated, and some of them cross-react with antisera for the *Klebsiella* capsules. *Klebsiella* capsular antisera are also useful in typing *E. aerogenes.* In one study 90% of *E. aerogenes* isolates reacted with *Klebsiella* antisera, and two thirds were lysed by *Klebsiella* bacteriophages. Typing schemas for the other species are limited or have not yet been devised.

Clinical Infection. *Enterobacter* are isolated less frequently than *Klebsiella* and *E. coli,* and although they are capable of infecting any tissue in the body, they are most frequently associated with urinary tract infections. Most infections occur in patients with underlying problems, many of which are nosocomial. Older patients with complicating diseases are more likely to acquire *Enterobacter* infections. Long-term hospitalization, placement of intravenous catheters, respiratory colonization, and prior use of antibiotics, particularly cephalosporins, are indicators of high risk for development of *Enterobacter* bacteremia.

E. cloacae causes the majority of infections, followed by *E. aerogenes* and *E. agglomerans.* In the 1970s *E. agglomerans* and *E. cloacae* were responsible for 150 cases of bacteremia and nine deaths in a nationwide epidemic associated with contaminated intravenous fluids. These organisms were isolated from fluids in eight hospitals scattered through seven states. Enterotoxigenic *E. cloacae* have been isolated from jejunal aspirates of patients with tropical sprue. As with enterotoxigenic *Klebsiella,* the toxins are similar to LT and ST of *E. coli,* and the overall significance of these findings is not clear. *E. gergoviae* has been associated with nosocomial urinary tract infections and has been isolated from respiratory specimens and blood. *E. sakazakii* most commonly is isolated from wounds and the respiratory tract but also causes meningitis, brain abscesses, and bacteremia in neonates. *E. taylorae* is a relatively new species of *Enterobacter,* and its clinical significance is not known since the majority of isolates have been obtained from specimens with mixed bacterial flora such as wounds, stool, and sputum. The spectrum of *H. alvei* infections is similar to that of the *Enterobacter* species, and their frequency is similar to that of *E. agglomerans.*

As with all enterics, resistance patterns of individual isolates of *Enterobacter* vary. Most of the commonly isolated species produce a potent cephalosporinase that inactivates ampicillin and first-generation cephalosporins. However, a number of the second- and third-generation cephalosporins and most of the antimicrobials listed in Chapter 33 are useful in the treatment of *Enterobacter* infections.

Genus *Serratia*

Organisms of the genus *Serratia* form the third and last group of organisms that formerly were classified in the tribe Klebsielleae or that were referred to as the K-E-S (*Klebsiella, Enterobacter, Serratia*) group. *Serratia* were at one time thought to be harmless saprophytes, and pigmented variants of *Serratia marcescens* were used as markers to trace air currents in both the environment and hospitals. These organisms have emerged as major entities in nosocomial infections. In nature they are found widely distributed in soil and water and are found associated with a large number of plants and animals, including insects, for which they may be pathogenic.

Taxonomy. The genus *Serratia* presently consists of nine species, some of which may be actually composed of two or more DNA homology groups. The majority of human disease is caused by one species, *S. marcescens. S. liquifaciens* formerly

TABLE 34–3. DIFFERENTIATION OF SELECTED *SERRATIA* SPECIES

Test	*S. marcescens*	*S. liquifaciens*	*S. rubidaea*	*S. odorifera* Biogroup 1	*S. odorifera* Biogroup 2
DNase	+	±	+	+	+
Lysine decarboxylase	+	+	±	+	+
Ornithine decarboxylase	+	+	−	+	−
Fermentation					
Arabinose	−	+	+	+	+
Adonitol	±	−	+	±	±
Sorbitol	+	+	−	+	+

was classified in the genus *Enterobacter* and may contain four different groups of organisms. It is the second most frequently isolated *Serratia* species in the United States, and in Great Britain it is isolated more frequently than *S. marcescens*. *S. rubidaea* has also been referred to as *S. marinorubra* by some workers. It was originally isolated from seawater and is a rare, but not unusual human isolate. *S. ficaria* is associated ecologically with the fig wasp and is transmitted to the plant by this wasp during pollination. Its role in human infections is not known, although it has been isolated from patients known to have eaten figs. *S. fonticola* is tentatively classified in the *Serratia* and in all likelihood will be moved in future classification schemes. It is widely distributed in water, and its role in human disease is questioned. *S. grimesii* is also found in a variety of environmental sources, and its significance in human disease is not known, although it has been isolated from blood cultures. *S. odorifera* may in fact be two species, and some classification schemes separate the species into two biogroups. Like other nonmarcescens species, *S. odorifera* has been isolated occasionally from human infections. *S. plymuthica* is an extremely rare human isolate, and although its clinical significance is uncertain, it has been reported to have caused at least one case of nosocomial bacteremia and one case of osteomyelitis. *S. proteamaculans* is not known to occur in human specimens.

Biochemical and Cultural Characteristics. *Serratia* can be distinguished from other Enterobacteriaceae by their ability to produce extracellular deoxyribonuclease (DNase), lipase, and gelatinase and by their resistance to colistin and cephalothin. Only *S. fonticola* does not share these properties. Other tests that differentiate the members of the genus are listed in Table 34–3. The majority of *S. rubidaea* form a red to pink pigment, as do some strains of *S. marcescens*. Pigment production of *S. marcescens* is enhanced by incubation at room temperature. *S. odorifera* are characterized by the production of a very musty, pungent odor that permeates the incubator in which the organism is growing.

Antigenic Structure. The O and H antigens of *Serratia* are important epidemiologic markers. Approximately 120 serotypes of *Serratia* have been described, and approximately 95% of the isolates can be serologically typed.

Clinical Infection. Almost all *Serratia* infections are associated with underlying disease, changing physiologic patterns, immunosuppressive therapy, or mechanical manipulations of the patient. In several studies 75% to 90% of all *Serratia* infections were hospital acquired. *S. marcescens* is the most frequently isolated member of the genus, and it has been associated with a number of nosocomial outbreaks of urinary tract and wound infections, pneumonia, and septicemia. Contaminated respiratory equipment and lapses in catheterization techniques are major factors involved in development of *Serratia* infections in hospitals. As with all enteric infections, secondary bacteremia is a major complication of *Serratia* infections. In intensive care units respiratory and rectal colonization is an indicator of high risk for the development of *Serratia* bacteremia.

The role of other species in human disease is not completely clear. *S. liquifaciens* has been isolated from a number of clinical specimens, and the disease spectrum appears to be the same as that of *S. marcescens*. Other species have been isolated primarily from microbially mixed clinical specimens, and their role in human disease is not clearly defined.

Amikacin, gentamicin, chloramphenicol, ciprofloxacin, and the combination trimethoprim-sulfamethoxazole are usually effective against *S. marcescens;* however, there is considerable strain-to-strain variation, particularly in outbreak situations.

Proteeae

Ewing divided the Enterobacteriaceae into tribes consisting of closely related genera. Although this division is not currently accepted by most taxonomists, this concept is useful for describing the genera discussed in this section: *Proteus, Morganella,* and *Providencia*. The majority of isolates from this tribe are from urine, although infections of other body sites frequently occur. The members of this tribe are frequent clinical isolates and may account for 10% to 15% of the nosocomial infections seen in the United States.

Taxonomy. The genus *Proteus* consists of two frequently isolated pathogens, *P. mirabilis* and *P. vulgaris;* one very rare human pathogen, *P. penneri;* and *P. myxofaciens,* which has been isolated only from gypsy moths. *Morganella morganii* is the only species in the genus *Morganella,* although some taxonomists believe there are two biogroups within the species. This organism was formerly classified as *Proteus morganii*. The genus *Providencia* consists of four species, one of which, *P. rettgeri,* was classified previously in the genus *Proteus*. The other three species of *Providencia* are *P. alcalifaciens, P. stuartii,* and *P. rustigianii.*

TABLE 34–4. BIOCHEMICAL CHARACTERISTICS OF THE PROTEEAE

Test	*Proteus mirabilis*	*Proteus vulgaris*	*Proteus penneri*	*Morganella morganii*	*Providencia alcalifaciens*	*Providencia stuartii*	*Providencia rettgeri*	*Providencia rustigianii*
Urease	+	+	+	+	−	±	+	−
Ornithine decarboxylase	+	−	−	+	−	−	−	−
Indole	−	+	−	+	+	+	+	+
Fermentation								
Adonitol	−	−	−	−	+	±	±	−
Trehalose	+	±	±	±	−	+	−	−

Biochemical and Cultural Characteristics. *P. mirabilis* and *P. vulgaris* are actively motile at 37C, producing a translucent sheet of growth on nonselective media such as blood agar. This phenomenon is referred to as swarming. These two species also produce hydrogen sulfide from sodium thiosulfate, which may cause colonies of these organisms to be confused with those of the enteric pathogens *Salmonella*. All members of the tribe can be distinguished from other enterics by their ability to produce phenylalanine deaminase. All *Proteus* species, *M. morganii, P. rettgeri,* and some strains of *P. stuartii* produce a powerful urease that rapidly hydrolyzes urea to ammonia and carbon dioxide. In contrast to other members of the Proteeae, *P. mirabilis* does not hydrolyze tryptophan to indole, and this characteristic has been used in the medical literature to divide the organisms into indole-positive and indole-negative *Proteus*. Other major biochemical reactions that are useful in identifying the members of the tribe are listed in Table 34–4.

Antigenic Structure. All members of the tribe possess O, H, and K antigens. There have been several attempts to organize the various antigenic types into some type of serologic scheme that would prove to be epidemiologically useful; however, the antisera are not readily available, and antigen typing is used by only a few select laboratories. The major clinical use of the antigen typing of *Proteus* species has been the diagnosis of rickettsial disease. Certain *P. vulgaris* strains (OX-19, OX-K, and OX-2) share antigens with the *Rickettsia*, which allows them to be used as the antigens for the detection of rickettsial antibodies in the Weil-Felix test (Chap. 49).

Clinical Infection. *P. mirabilis* accounts for the majority of human infections seen with this group of organisms. It is the second leading cause of community-acquired urinary tract infections and is a major cause of nosocomial infections. All members of the tribe can cause urinary tract and wound infections, pneumonia, and septicemia. *Providencia* infections are almost exclusively nosocomial, and most isolates are resistant to multiple antibiotics. Urinary tract infections caused by the urease-producing members of the tribe are characterized by an alkaline pH. This increase in pH causes precipitation of calcium and magnesium salts from the urine and results in the formation of urinary calculi. The alkaline pH also damages renal epithelial cells. Patients with long-term indwelling urinary catheters are prone to developing bladder colonization with *P. mirabilis* and *P. stuartii.* Besides being a problem for the individual patient, this colonization provides a reservoir of organisms for outbreaks in long-term care facilities. Secondary bacteremias are common in debilitated patients, and the mortality rate is high.

P. mirabilis differs from other members of the tribe in that it is sensitive to ampicillin and cephalosporin antibiotics. All Proteeae are resistant to tetracycline. Most isolates are sensitive to aminoglycoside antibiotics and the combination of trimethoprim-sulfamethoxazole. The *Providencia* generally have greater resistance to more antibiotics than other Proteeae; however, considerable variation in susceptibility patterns occurs, necessitating testing of each individual isolate.

Genus *Citrobacter*

Citrobacter species formerly were classified as the Bethesda-Ballerup Group and have been included in the tribe Salmonelleae. These organisms have been isolated from a number of environmental sources and from the feces of man and lower animals. They have been implicated in a wide variety of human infections, ranging from urinary tract infections to neonatal meningitis.

Taxonomy. There are currently three species in the genus *Citrobacter: C. freundii, C. diversus,* and *C. amalonaticus. C. amalonaticus* has also been classified as *Levinea amalonatica* by some workers, but this classification has not gained acceptance in the United States. *C. amalonaticus* is also divided into two biotypes by the workers at CDC. *C. diversus* formerly was classified as *Levinea malonatica* and *C. koseri.*

Biochemical and Cultural Characteristics. *Citrobacter* grow well on enteric isolation media. *C. freundii* produces hydrogen sulfide from sodium thiosulfate, but the other species do not. Most isolates produce a weak urease that will hydrolyze urea within 2 days. Other characteristics of typical isolates are shown in Table 34–5.

Antigenic Structure. *Citrobacter* possess many O, H, and K antigens. The antigens of *C. freundii* are closely related to the antigens of many *Salmonella* and *Escherichia*. Some strains also possess the Vi antigen of *S. typhi* (Chap. 35). About 70% of clinical isolates can by typed with existing antisera.

Clinical Infection. These organisms are typical opportunistic pathogens and can infect any body site. The majority of the isolates, however, are from the urinary tract. In one review, 75% of the patients with clinically significant infections

TABLE 34–5. REACTIONS OF *CITROBACTER*

Test	*C. amalonaticus*	*C. freundii*	*C. diversus*
Indole	+	−	+
H_2S	−	+	−
Growth in KCN	+	+	−
Malonate	−	+	±

had underlying diseases or other predisposing factors. *C. diversus* comprised 42% of the isolates in this study, *C. freundii* accounted for 29% of isolates, and an additional 29% of isolates were identified as *Citrobacter* species.

C. diversus has been identified as an important cause of neonatal meningitis and brain abscesses. Isolates of *C. diversus* obtained from patients in an outbreak of neonatal meningitis in Maryland possessed a 32 kDa outer membrane protein that was not found in other isolates. In a newborn rat model strains with this protein were more likely to cause bacteremia, meningitis, and death. However, strains lacking this protein were still virulent and produced ventriculitis and brain abscesses. The importance of *C. diversus* as a neonatal pathogen is not limited to meningitis since at least one hospital has reported a high incidence of neonatal septicemia without meningitis. This same report indicates that this organism has become the leading nosocomial pathogen in the neonatal intensive care unit.

Enterotoxigenic *C. freundii* have been isolated from patients with diarrhea. In one study 46 of 328 patients with diarrhea had *C. freundii* isolated from their stools. Of the 46 isolates produced, 3 had an enterotoxin similar to the ST_a of *E. coli.* As with the other noncoli enterics, it is difficult to assess the relative importance of this finding.

Most isolates are sensitive to the aminoglycoside antibiotics, tetracycline, and chloramphenicol. Resistant forms do occur and are more likely to be isolated from patients who have been hospitalized for extended periods and who have had previous antibiotic therapy. In most hospitals *C. freundii* tends to be more resistant to antimicrobials than *C. diversus.*

Other Organisms

As noted in Chapter 33, a large number of enteric organisms such as *Cedecea, Kluyvera,* and *Edwardsiella* have been isolated from a variety of opportunistic infections; however, they constitute a small percentage of the isolates seen in the United States. The overall significance of these organisms depends on the circumstances in which they are isolated. No one would question the significance of multiple isolates from normally sterile sites such as blood or spinal fluid; however, the importance of isolates obtained from potentially mixed cultures of wounds and respiratory secretions must be carefully evaluated for each patient. In previous editions of this text *Arizona hinshawii* was listed in this chapter. However, present classification systems place this organism in the genus *Salmonella,* and it is discussed in Chapter 35.

FURTHER READING

Books and Reviews

Aronoff SC: The emergence of beta-lactam resistance among strains of *Enterobacter cloacae* and *Pseudomonas aeruginosa.* Pediatr Infect Dis J 8(suppl 9):S100, 1989

Arroyo JC, Sonnenwirth AC, Liebhaber H: *Proteus rettgeri* infections: A review. J Urol 117:115, 1977

Cavalieri SJ, Bohach GA, Snyder IS: *Escherichia coli* α-hemolysin: Characteristics and probable role in pathogenicity. Microbiol Rev 48:326, 1984

Cooke EM: *Escherichia coli*—An overview. J Hyg (Camb) 95:523, 1985

DuPont HL, Pickering LK: Infections of the Gastrointestinal Tract: Microbiology, Pathophysiology, and Clinical Features. New York, Plenum, 1980, pp 61, 129, 195

Evans DJ, Evans DG: Classification of pathogenic *Escherichia coli* according to serotype and production of virulence factors, with special reference to colonization-factor antigens. Rev Infect Dis 5(suppl 4):S692, 1983

Ewing WH: Edwards and Ewing's Identification of Enterobacteriaceae, ed 4. New York, Elsevier, 1986

Farmer JJ III, Davis BR, Hickman-Brenner FW, et al: Biochemical identification of new species and biogroups of Enterobacteriaceae isolated from clinical specimens. J Clin Microbiol 21:46, 1985

Farthing MJK, Keusch GT (eds): Enteric Infection. Mechanisms, Manifestations, and Management. New York, Raven Press, 1989

Fekety R: Recent advances in the management of bacterial diarrhea. Rev Infect Dis 5:246, 1983

Gaastra W, DeGraaf FK: Host-specific fimbrial adhesions of noninvasive enterotoxigenic *Escherichia coli* strains. Microbiol Rev 46:129, 1982

Grimont PAD, Grimont F: The genus *Serratia.* Ann Rev Microbiol 32:221, 1978

Gross RJ: *Escherichia coli* diarrhoea. J Infect 7:177, 1983

Hawkey PM: *Providencia stuartii:* A review of a multiply antibiotic-resistant bacterium. J Antimicrob Chemother 13:209, 1984

John JK Jr, Sharbaugh RJ, Bannister ER: *Enterobacter cloacae* bacteremia, epidemiology, and antibiotic resistance. Rev Infect Dis 4:13, 1982

Johnson JR: Virulence factors in *Escherichia coli* urinary tract infection. Clin Microbiol Rev 4:80, 1991

Karmali MA: Infection by verotoxin-producing *Escherichia coli.* Clin Microbiol Rev 2:15, 1989

Kelly MT, Brenner DJ, Farmer JJ III: Enterobacteriaceae. In Lennette EH, Balows A, Hausler WJ Jr, Shadomy HJ (eds): Manual of Clinical Microbiology, ed 4. Washington DC, American Society for Microbiology, 1985, p 263

Levine MM, Edelman R: Enteropathogenic *Escherichia coli* of classic serotypes associated with infant diarrhea: Epidemiology and pathogenesis. Epidemiol Rev 6:31, 1984

Rao MC: Toxins which activate guanylate cyclase: Heat-stable enterotoxins. In Ciba Foundation Symposium 112: Microbial toxins and Diarrhoeal Disease. London, Pittman, 1985, p 74

Roberts JA: Urinary tract infections. Am J Kidney Dis 4:103, 1984

Silver RP, Vimr ER: Polysialic acid capsule of *Escherichia coli* K1. In Iglewski BH, Clark VL (eds): The Bacteria, vol XI: Molecular Basis of Bacterial Pathogenesis. San Diego, Academic Press 1990, p 39

Tennent JM, Hultgren S, Marklund B, et al: Genetics of adhesin expression in *Escherichia coli.* In Iglewski BH, Clark VL (eds): The Bacteria, vol XI: Molecular Basis of Bacterial Pathogenesis. San Diego, Academic Press 1990, p 79

Varaldo PE, Biavasco F, Manelli S, et al: Distribution and antibiotic susceptibility of extraintestinal clinical isolates of *Klebsiella, Enterobacter* and *Serratia* species. Eur J Clin Microbiol Infect Dis 7:495, 1988

Warren JW: *Providencia stuartii:* A common cause of antibiotic resistant bacteremia in patients with long-term indwelling catheters. Rev Infect Dis 8:61, 1986

Weikel CS, Guerrant RL: STb enterotoxin of *Escherichia coli:* Cyclic nucleotide-independent secretion. In Ciba Foundation Symposium 112: Microbial Toxins and Diarrhoeal Disease. London, Pittman, 1985, p 94

Wilfert CM: *E. coli* meningitis: K1 antigen and virulence. Ann Rev Med 29:129, 1978

Yu VL: *Serratia marcescens*—Historical perspective and clinical review. N Engl J Med 300:887, 1979

Selected Papers

Adegbola RA, Old DC, Senior BW: The adhesins and fimbriae of *Proteus mirabilis* strains associated with high and low affinity for the urinary tract. J Med Microbiol 16:427, 1983

Burchard KW, Barrall DT, Reed M, Slotman GJ: *Enterobacter* bacteremia in surgical patients. Surgery 100:857, 1986

Cahoon FE, Thompson JS: Frequency of *Escherichia coli* O157:H7 isolation from stool specimens. Can J Microbiol 33:914, 1987

Caprioli A, Falbo V, Ruggeri FM, et al: Cytotoxic necrotizing factor production by hemolytic strains of *Escherichia coli* causing extraintestinal infections. J Clin Microbiol 25:146, 1987

Darfeuille-Michaud A, Forestier C, Joly B, et al: Identification of a nonfimbrial adhesive factor of an enterotoxigenic *Escherichia coli* strain. Infect Immun 52:468, 1986

Davis TJ, Matsen JM: Prevalance and characteristics of *Klebsiella* species: Relation to association with the hospital environment. J Infect Dis 130:402, 1974

Deb M, Bhujwala RA, Singh S, et al: *Klebsiella pneumoniae* as the possible cause of an outbreak of diarrhoea in a neonatal special care unit. Ind J Med Res 71:359, 1980

de la Torre MG, Romero-Vivas J, Martinez-Beltran J, et al: Klebsiella bacteremia: An analysis of 100 episodes. Rev Infect Dis 7:143, 1985

Drelichman V, Band JD: Bacteremias due to *Citrobacter diversus* and *Citrobacter freundii.* Incidence, risk factors, and clinical outcome. Arch Intern Med 145:1808, 1985

Dreyfus LA, Jaso-Friedmann L, Robertson DC: Characterization of the mechanism of action of *Escherichia coli* heat-stable enterotoxin. Infect Immun 44:493, 1984

Golstein EJC, Lewis RP, Martin WJ, et al: Infections caused by *Klebsiella ozaenae:* A changing disease spectrum. J Clin Microbiol 8:413, 1978

Graham DR, Band JD: *Citrobacter diversus* brain abscess and meningitis in neonates. JAMA 245:1923, 1981

Higaki M, Chida T, Takano H, Nakaya R: Cytotoxic component(s) of *Klebsiella oxytoca* on Hep-2 cells. Microbiol Immunol 34:147, 1990

Hodges GR, Degener CE, Barnes YWG: Clinical significance of *Citrobacter* isolates. Am J Clin Pathol 70:37, 1978

Holmes RK, Twiddy EM, Pickett CL: Purification and characterization of type II heat-labile enterotoxin of *Escherichia coli.* Infect Immun 53:464, 1986

Jones BD, Lockatell CV, Johnson DE, et al: Construction of a urease-negative mutant of *Proteus mirabilis:* Analysis of virulence in a mouse model of ascending urinary tract infection. Infect Immun 58:1120, 1990

Klipstein FA, Engert RF: Purification and properties of *Klebsiella pneumoniae* heat-stable enterotoxin. Infect Immun 13:373, 1976

Klipstein FA, Engert RF: Partial purification and properties of *Enterobacter cloacae* heat-stable enterotoxin. Infect Immun 13:1307, 1976

Klipstein FA, Engert RF, Short HB: Enterotoxigenicity of colonizing coliform bacteria in tropical sprue and blind loop syndrome. Lancet 2:342, 1978

Korhonen TK, Valtonen MV, Parkkinen J, et al: Serotypes, hemolysin production, and receptor recognition of *Escherichia coli* strains associated with neonatal sepsis and meningitis. Infect Immun 48:486, 1985

MacDonald KL, O'Leary MJ, Cohen ML, et al: *Escherichia coli* O157:H7, an emerging gastrointestinal pathogen. Results of a one-year, prospective, population-based study. JAMA 259:3567, 1988

Mathewson JJ, Johnson PC, DuPont HL, et al: A newly recognized cause of traveler's diarrhea: Enteroadherent *Escherichia coli.* J Infect Dis 151:471, 1985

Mathewson JJ, Johnson PC, DuPont HL, et al: Pathogenicity of enteroadherent *Escherichia coli* in adult volunteers. J Infect Dis 154:524, 1986

McConnell MM, Chart H, Scotland SM, et al: Properties of adherence factor plasmids of enteropathogenic *Escherichia coli* and the effects of host strain on the expression of adherence to Hep-2 cells. J Gen Microbiol 135:1123, 1989

Mikhail IA, Hyams KC, Podgore JK, et al: Microbiologic and clinical study of acute diarrhea in children in Aswan, Egypt. Scand J Infect Dis 21:59, 1989

Miller RH, Shulman JB, Canalis RF, et al: *Klebsiella rhinoscleromatis:* A clinical and pathogenic enigma. Otolaryngol Head Neck Surg 87:212, 1979

Minam J, Okabi A, Shiode J, Hayashi H: Product of unique cytotoxin by *Klebsiella oxytoca.* Microb Pathog 7:203, 1989

Mobley HT, Green DM, Trifillis AL, et al: Pyelonephritogenic *Escherichia coli* and killing of cultured human renal proximal tubular epithelial cells: Role of hemolysin in some strains. Infect Immun 58:1281, 1990

Neto U, Ferreira V, Patricio FRS, et al: Protracted diarrhea: Importance of the enteropathogenic *E. coli* (EPEC) strains and *Salmonella* in its genesis. J Pediatr Gastroenterol Nutr 8:207, 1988

Nowicki B, Labigne A, Moseley S, et al: The Dr hemagglutinin, afimbrial adhesins AFA-I and AFA-II, and F1845 fimbriae of uropathogenic and diarrhea-associated *Escherichia coli* belong to a family of hemagglutinnins with the DR receptor. Infect Immun 58:279, 1990

Opal SM, Cross AS, Gemski P, Lyhte LW: Aerobactin and α-hemolysin as virulence determinants in *Escherichia coli* isolated from human blood, urine, and stool. J Infect Dis 161:794, 1989

Overturf GD, Wilkins J, Ressler R: Emergence of resistance of *Providencia stuartii* to multiple antibiotics: Speciation and biochemical characteristics of *Providencia.* J Infect Dis 129:353, 1974

Peerbooms PGH, Verweij AMJJ, MacLaren DM: Uropathogenic properties of *Proteus mirabilis* and *Proteus vulgaris.* J Med Microbiol 19:55, 1985

Pickett CL, Twiddy EM, Coker C, Holmes RK: Cloning, nucleotide sequence, and hybridization studies of type IIb heat-labile enterotoxin gene of *Escherichia coli.* J Bacteriol 171:4945, 1989

Ryan CA, Tauxe RV, Hoesk GW, et al: *Escherichia coli* O157:H7 diarrhea in a nursing home: Clinical, epidemiological, and pathological findings. J Infect Dis 154:631, 1986

Saito H, Elting L, Bodey GP, Berkey P: *Serratia* bacteremia: Review of 118 cases. Rev Infect Dis 11:912, 1989

Senior BW: *Proteus morganii* is less frequently associated with urinary tract infections than *Proteus mirabilis*—An explanation. J Med Microbiol 16:317, 1983

Simoons-Smitt AM, Verwij-Van Vught AMJJ, MacLaren DM: The role of K antigens as virulence factors for *Klebsiella.* J Med Microbiol 21:133, 1986

Taylor DN, Echeverria P, Sethabutr O, et al: Clinical and microbiologic features of *Shigella* and enteroinvasive *Escherichia coli* infections detected by DNA hybridization. J Clin Microbiol 26:1362, 1988

Waldman SA, Kuno T, Kamisaki Y, et al: Intestinal receptor for heat-stable enterotoxin of *Escherichia coli* is tightly coupled to a novel form of particulate guanylate cyclase. Infect Immun 51:320, 1986

Weikel CS, Tiemens KM, Moseley SL, et al: Species specificity and lack of production of STb enterotoxin by *Escherichia coli* strains isolated from humans with diarrheal illness. Infect Immun 52:323, 1983

Williams WW, Mariano J, Spurrier M, et al: Nosocomial meningitis due to *Citrobacter diversus* in neonates: New aspects of the epidemiology. J Infect Dis 150:229, 1984

CHAPTER 35

Enterobacteriaceae: Salmonella and Shigella, Intestinal Pathogens

Among the very young, the old, the malnourished, and those living in marginal conditions, diarrhea represents a serious, life-threatening situation. As many as one third of pediatric deaths in developing countries are attributed to diarrhea and the resulting dehydration. There are an estimated 3 to 5 billion cases of diarrhea, with 5 to 10 million deaths, each year in Africa, Asia, and Latin America. For the adult population of well-developed countries diarrhea generally represents, at most, an inconvenience; however, healthy hosts placed in closely housed situations with suboptimal sanitization, such as in prisons, mental institutions, or cruise ships, can develop a debilitating diarrhea. Even the course of military history has been altered when large numbers of men were incapacitated and unfit for battle because of diarrheal diseases. The family Enterobacteriaceae contains two genera, *Salmonella* and *Shigella*, which are among the leading causes of bacterial diarrhea. Although they are classified in the same family and infect the same organ system, these organisms differ greatly in their microbiologic, epidemiologic, and pathologic properties.

Shigella

Shigella species are the major causes of bacillary dysentery, a disease characterized by severe abdominal cramps and the frequent, painful passage of low-volume stools containing blood and mucus. Most disease is seen in the pediatric age group, with the majority of infections occurring in children 1 to 10 years of age. In the United States *Shigella* have been estimated to cause 15% of pediatric diarrhea, whereas in developing countries these organisms are leading causes of infant diarrhea and mortality.

Taxonomy

Genetically, *Shigella* are indistinguishable from *Escherichia coli,* and most taxonomists believe that they are the same species. However, since most strains of *Shigella* cause bacillary dysentery and most *E. coli* do not, the majority of clinical microbiologists continue to use the two genus designations. The *Shigella* are divided into four major serogroups, which have been given species names: serogroup A, *S. dysenteriae;* serogroup B, *S. flexneri;* serogroup C, *S. boydii;* and, serogroup D, *S. sonnei.* Serogroups A, B, and C are biochemically similar, whereas serogroup D is biochemically distinct. All *Shigella* can cause bacillary dysentery, but the severity of the disease, mortality, and epidemiology vary for each species.

Physiology

Biochemical Properties and Cultural Characteristics. *Shigella* appear as non-lactose-fermenting colonies on the differential media used to isolate enteric bacteria (Chap. 33). All species are nonmotile, do not produce H_2S, and with the exception of *S. flexneri* serotype 6, do not produce gas from glucose. These factors distinguish them from most *Salmonella.* In contrast to most *E. coli,* they do not produce lysine decarboxylase, do not utilize acetate as a carbon source, and do not ferment lactose rapidly (within 18 to 24 hours). However, *S. sonnei* will ferment lactose on extended incubation. Table 35–1 depicts the characteristics that will commonly separate the four serogroups.

Resistance to Physical and Chemical Agents. *Shigella* are less resistant than other enterics to physical and chemical agents, and most common disinfectants will kill the organisms at the concentrations usually employed. High concentrations of acids are detrimental, necessitating the use of well-buffered media for the transport of specimens and growth of the organisms. *Shigella* can tolerate low temperatures if adequate moisture is present, and they can survive for more than 6 months in water at room temperature.

Antigenic Structure

The *Shigella* are divided into four major O antigenic groups, designated A, B, C, and D. In addition to the major O antigens, groups A, B, and C contain minor O antigens, which allow for subgrouping. The subgroups are designated by arabic numbers. At the present time there are 12 serologic types of group A, 6 serologic types of group B, 18 serologic types of group C, and 1 serotype in group D. Some strains possess K or envelope antigens, which are not important for serologic typing but, when present, may interfere with the serologic reactions of the O antigen. This interference can be removed by boiling the cell suspension before typing the organism. Fimbriae have been demonstrated in serotypes 1 to 5 of serogroup B but not in serotype 6 or other *Shigella.* All fimbriae antigens are immunologically identical. Since all *Shigella* are nonmotile, there are no H antigens.

TABLE 35–1. TESTS USEFUL IN SPECIATION OF *SHIGELLA*

Test	*S. dysenteriae*	*S. flexneri*	*S. boydii*	*S. sonnei*
O antigen group	A	B	C	D
Mannitol	−	+	+	+
Jordan tartrate	±	−	−	+
Raffinose—with prolonged incubation	−	±	−	±

Determinants of Pathogenicity

The events involved in bacillary dysentery are complex and not fully understood at the molecular level. Pathogenic organisms must survive the passage through the upper gastrointestinal tract, attach to colonic cells, and penetrate the epithelial cells. Once inside the cells, they multiply and pass from cell to cell. Bacterial multiplication leads to inflammation, epithelial cell death, ulceration, impaired colonic fluid absorption, and discharge of blood, mucus, and pus. During the first 24 to 48 hours approximately 50% of patients present with watery diarrhea and fever.

Surface Properties. The ability to survive the passage through the host defenses may be due to the O antigens. The importance of a smooth lipopolysaccharide (LPS) structure, termed *phase I colony type,* has been demonstrated best with *S. sonnei* and *S. flexneri.* These organisms possess a large, 120 to 140 MDa plasmid that encodes for O-specific side chains. Loss of this plasmid results in a phase II or rough-colony formation and avirulent organisms. Further evidence for the importance of the specific side chains was obtained from experiments involving hybrids of *Shigella* and *E. coli* that were virulent only when the *Shigella* O side chains were expressed. It is not known if these side chains only allow for passage of the organisms through the host or if they may also be responsible for the attachment of the bacteria to specific host cell receptors.

Invasiveness. Virulent *Shigella* penetrate the mucosa and epithelial cells of the colon in an uneven manner. They rarely penetrate beyond the epithelial cells into the lamina propria. The attachment of the organisms may involve divalent cations such as calcium. The internalization of the bacteria may be the result of a receptor-mediated endocytosis or the production of some bacterial product that causes a host cell response. Both the host cells and the bacterial cells must be metabolically active for internalization of the *Shigella.* Initially the organisms are contained in phagosomes, but virulent organisms disrupt the phagosome and multiply in the cytoplasm. This is in contrast to the situation seen with *Salmonella,* which remain in the host vacuoles. *Shigella* probably disrupt the phagosomal membrane with the plasmid-encoded contact hemolysin, a hemolytic component that requires that the organism be in direct contact with the host cellular membranes. Although the term *hemolysin* is used because hemolysis was the first effect to be described, most researchers believe that its major function is to lyse other types of cellular membranes. Avirulent mutants that penetrate the cell but do not multiply intracellularly have been isolated and are associated with a mild inflammation but not fully developed disease. Intracellular multiplication leads to invasion of adjacent cells, inflammation, and cell death. The genetics of the invasion process is complex and involves at least three chromosomal loci, as well as five loci on the large 140 kilobase plasmid. The chromosomal loci appear to be associated with the intracellular survival of the bacteria, whereas the plasmid genes—ipaB, ipaC, and ipaD—encode for polypeptides that may play a role in binding of the bacteria to host cells. The virF gene controls the transcriptional expression of both the ipa genes and the virG gene, which is responsible for the intracellular spread of bacteria to adjacent cells in tissue cultures.

Toxins. Cellular death probably is due to the cytotoxic properties of the Shiga toxin, which interferes with protein synthesis. *Shigella* carry the gene for the toxin on the chromosome, and the organisms that produce higher levels of toxin cause more severe disease. This toxin has a multiplicity of effects and is neurotoxic, cytotoxic, and enterotoxic.

The intact Shiga toxin has a molecular weight of 70 kDa, and consists of one subunit A, molecular weight 32 kDa, and five subunit B fragments, with a molecular weight of 6.5 kDa each. Subunit A can be divided further into A_1 and A_2. The A_1 peptide (molecular weight 28 kDa) is enzymatically active in protein synthesis and irreversibly inactivates the 60S ribosomal subunit by removing the adenine base at position 4324 of the 28S ribosomal RNA by an *N*-glycosidase activity. This leaves the phosphoribose backbone intact but susceptible to chemical cleavage in vitro. This is the same mode of action as that of the toxic plant protein ricin. In fact, Shiga toxin and the Shigalike toxins of *E. coli* (Chap. 34) have the same mechanism and site of action as ricin, and all four toxins have regions of amino acid homology. The subunit B may serve as a binding factor as observed with other bacterial toxins. The binding sites for Shiga toxin are the glycolipids globotriosylceramide and galbiosyl-ceramide. These receptors are probably polyvalent and may represent multiple, closely associated digalactosyl chains. From these binding sites the toxin enters susceptible cells through receptor-mediated endocytosis from coated pits. From here the toxin A fragment is translocated to the Golgi apparatus and subsequently to the cytosol.

The role of this toxin in classic dysentery is not completely understood because toxin-negative strains are still capable of producing disease in volunteers and toxin-producing, noninvasive mutants are nonvirulent. Animal studies indicate that this toxin may be chiefly responsible for microvascular damage to the intestine, resulting in hemorrhage. In fact, a major hallmark of the disease caused by *E. coli* producing Shigalike toxins is a bloody diarrhea. The explanation of this conflicting data may be that bacillary dysentery is a two-stage disease that appears to involve both the small and large intestines. The watery diarrhea seen in the early stages of the disease in many patients may be attributed to the enterotoxic properties of the Shiga toxin, which are well documented in rabbit models. One could postulate that the *Shigella* multiply in a noninvasive manner in the jejunum and produce the toxin, which is taken up by small bowel receptors, resulting in an activated secretory process. The second phase of the illness would then involve the large intestine and the tissue invasion phase in which the action of the Shiga toxin would increase the severity of the disease. These theories are supported by monkey experiments, which demonstrate that dysentery and ulceration only occur in animals infected intracecally, whereas animals infected orally first demonstrate a watery diarrhea, then dysentery. The enterotoxic effect of Shiga toxin is to block absorption of electrolytes, glucose, and amino acids from the intestinal lumen rather than to increase the secretion of chloride ions, as is seen with the enterotoxins of *E. coli* and *Vibrio cholerae* (Chaps. 34 and 36).

Clinical Infection

Epidemiology. During 1989, there were 25,010 cases of shigellosis reported to the Centers for Disease Control. *S. sonnei* caused 80% of these infections, with the majority of other infections caused by *S. flexneri.* These data are unchanged from the 105,832 cases reported from 1964 to 1973, when *S. boydii* and *S. dysenteriae* caused less than 2% of all *Shigella* infections. In developing countries, where hygiene is poor, the isolation pattern is reversed: *S. dysenteriae* and *S. boydii* are more frequently isolated, followed by *S. flexneri* and then *S. sonnei.* Interestingly, the reservoir of *S. flexneri* in the United States seemingly has shifted to the men in the age group 20 to 49. In 1970 only 5.5% of all *S. flexneri* isolates came from men 20 to 49. In 1985 this age group accounted for 23% of all isolates. The exact reason for this shift is not known, but in San Francisco 66% of the patients with shigellosis were homosexual or bisexual men, and 82% of all reported cases of *Shigella* were *S. flexneri.* It remains to be established whether sexual practices are the true reason for the increased incidence of *Shigella* infections in this group of patients or whether there are some other extenuating factors.

Only higher primates are infected naturally with *Shigella;* therefore the spread of *Shigella* is from human to human through the fecal-oral route. The reservoir is the carrier who sheds the organism in his feces. The carrier state usually lasts for 1 to 4 weeks, although long-term carriers have been described in confined environments. From the carriers the organisms can be spread by flies, fingers, food, or feces. *Shigella* can be isolated from clothing, toilet seats, or water contaminated by infected individuals. Because of their oral habits, children under the age of 5 account for almost one half of all cases, and children under 10 account for two thirds of all reported cases.

Outbreaks involving many people occur in closed groups, such as families, mental hospitals, Indian reservations, daycare nurseries, prisons, or cruise ships. Secondary transmission is high, with children less than 1 year of age being most susceptible and having an infection rate of 60% compared to 20% for other ages. The high communicability is attributed to the low infective dose needed to produce disease. Studies in healthy human volunteers indicate that as few as 200 organisms are needed to produce disease in some individuals. The percentage of infected individuals increases as the number of infecting organisms increases.

Pathogenesis. As with most diseases, the spectrum of shigellosis symptoms varies from asymptomatic infection to severe bacillary dysentery with high fever, chills, convulsions, abdominal cramps, tenesmus, and frequent bloody stools. The typical patient presents initially with fever and a watery diarrhea that changes on the second day to frequent but small-volume stools with blood and mucus. Human volunteer studies show that the organisms multiply in the small bowel to a concentration of 10^8/mL. During this phase, abdominal cramps and fever are common. After 1 to 3 days the organisms cannot be cultured from the small intestines but are isolated from the colon. The patient then develops the symptoms of dysentery. In previously healthy adults spontaneous cure can occur in 2 to 7 days. In the young or old and in malnourished individuals the disease is longer lasting, and the mortality due to dehydration and electrolyte imbalance is higher. Death is most likely to occur in the pediatric population and when *S. dysenteriae* is the causative agent.

Rarely do the organisms penetrate the intestinal wall and spread to other parts of the body. One study reported 11 cases of septicemia in 569 South African children with shigellosis. Of the 11 children, 9 were suffering from kwashiorkor or marasmus. The rate of bacteremia in uncompromised individuals is not known.

Laboratory Diagnosis. The best specimen for diagnosis of shigellosis is a rectal swab of an ulcer taken by sigmoidoscopic examination. Feces can also be used; however, since the *Shigella* are sensitive to the acids present in fecal material, the specimen must be placed on isolation media or in a buffered transport medium as quickly as possible. Clinical specimens should be placed on the media listed in Chapter 33. Identification of suspected *Shigella* isolates is based on biochemical reactions and serologic typing (Table 35–1).

Treatment. As with other diarrheal diseases, the immediate concern in shigellosis is the patient's state of hydration. In severe cases of dehydration, intravenous fluids are administered rapidly (i.e., isotonic fluid 20 to 30 mL/kg over 1 hour). Oral solutions are used when mild or moderate dehydration occurs. In contrast to *Salmonella* gastroenteritis (p. 563), *Shigella* infections respond to antibiotic treatment with a decrease in fever, diarrhea, and duration of the carrier state. Prompt treatment also reduces secondary cases. Ampicillin or its analogue amoxicillin is the drug of choice for sensitive isolates. Trimethoprim-sulfamethoxazole is the drug of choice when the sensitivity is unknown or the patient is allergic to penicillin-type antibiotics. Adult patients can also be treated with either norfloxacin or ciprofloxacin. As with other enteric organisms, resistant forms are isolated, particularly in epidemic situations and endemic countries.

Control. Since humans represent the only reservoir of *Shigella,* adequate sanitization and detection and treatment of carriers remain the only effective control measures. If possible, patients should be kept on enteric isolation until cultures are negative. Carriers should be treated and not allowed to handle food. Proper sewage disposal and chlorination of water are important measures in controlling the spread of *Shigella* and other gram-negative intestinal pathogens. Breast-feeding through the first year of life has also been effective in reducing shigellosis in children. Several types of vaccines, including hybrids with other organisms, have been developed and are in various stages of testing. However, to date there is no effective vaccine that prevents shigellosis.

Salmonella

In contrast to *Shigella,* the genus *Salmonella* is composed of a more biochemically and serologically diverse group of microorganisms. In addition to humans, they infect many animals and are capable of invading extraintestinal tissue and causing enteric fevers, the most severe of which is typhoid fever. In the United States the number of reported *Salmonella* infections is approximately twice the number of reported cases of shigellosis.

Taxonomy

The taxonomy of the *Salmonella* is complicated by the development and use of several different nomenclatures over the years. The Kauffmann-White antigenic scheme gave rise to more than 2000 "species" of *Salmonella* because each antigenic type that was discovered was given a species designation, such as *S. typhimurium.* Ewing and coworkers then proposed that there were only three species of *Salmonella: S. choleraesuis, S. enteritidis,* and, *S. typhi.* All other species or serotypes were defined as serotypes of *S. enteritidis.* Under this scheme *S. typhimurium* of the Kauffmann-White scheme became *S. enteritidis* serotype typhimurium. This three-species designation was used by the National Salmonella Center at the Enteric Reference Laboratory of the Centers for Disease Control (CDC) from 1972 to 1983 but was not used by other countries or in reports of the Bureau of Epidemiology at CDC. Since that time genetic studies have revealed that all *Salmonella* and organisms formerly classified in the genus *Arizona* belong to the same species in a genetic, phylogenic, and evolutionary sense. Any differences in antigenic types, biochemical reactions, and host or geographic distributions were due to divergence within a single species, *S. enterica.* Within this one species there are now six subgroups based on DNA hybridization studies. They are referred to as: *Salmonella* subgroup 1, with subspecies designation *enterica; Salmonella* subgroup 2, with subspecies designation *salamae; Salmonella* subgroups 3a and 3b, with subspecies designations *arizonae* and *diarizonae,* respectively; *Salmonella* subgroup 4, with subspecies designation *houtenae; Salmonella* subgroup 5, with subspecies designation *bongori;* and *Salmonella* subgroup 6, with subspecies designation *indica.* Although any organism can be associated with human disease, the majority of human isolates are found in subgroup 1. The major use of these designations will be in scientific publications. The CDC and clinical laboratories are reporting organisms as serotypes, such as *Salmonella* serotype *typhimurium,* rather than using the taxonomically correct, but more cumbersome, *Salmonella enterica* subspecies *enterica* serotype typhimurium.

Physiology

Biochemical Properties and Cultural Characteristics. *Salmonella,* with the exception of a rare isolate, do not ferment lactose. Most strains are motile and produce H_2S from the inorganic sulfur source, thiosulfate. With the exception of the typhi serotype, most isolates produce gas from glucose. Tests that help distinguish the various subgroups and commonly isolated bioserotypes are listed in Tables 35–2 and 35–3.

Resistance to Physical and Chemical Agents. *Salmonella* are capable of tolerating relatively larger concentrations of bile than most other enterics, a property that is used in designing media for the isolation of these organisms from fecal material. The members of this genus are typical enterics with respect to their resistance to other physical and chemical agents. Serotype choleraesuis is used as a standard test organism for determining the efficacy of disinfectants.

Antigenic Structure

The O and H antigens are the major antigens used to serotype the *Salmonella.* The O antigens are similar to the O antigens of other Enterobacteriaceae, but the H antigens are different in that they are diphasic (i.e., the H antigens can exist in either of two major antigenic phases—phase 1, specific phase;

TABLE 35–2. PROPERTIES USED TO DISTINGUISH THE SUBGROUPS OF *SALMONELLA*

Property	Subgroup 1 *enterica*	Subgroup 2 *salamae*	Subgroup 3a *arizonae*	Subgroup 3b *diarizonae*	Subgroup 4 *houtenae*	Subgroup 5 *bongori*
Usual phase of flagellar antigen	Diphasic	Diphasic	Monophasic	Diphasic	Monophasic	Monophasic
KCN	−	−	−	−	+	+
ONPG[a]	−	−	+	+	−	+
Malonate	−	+	+	+	−	−
Fermentation						
Dulcitol	+	+	−	−	−	+
Lactose	−	−	±	±	−	−
Salicin	−	−	−	−	+	−
Mucate	+	+	+	−	−	+

Adapted from Farmer et al: J Clin Microbiol 21: 46, 1985; Edward and Ewing's Identification of Enterobacteriaceae, ed 4. Elsevier, 1986.
[a] *O*-nitrophenyl-β-d-galactopyranoside.

or phase 2, nonspecific phase). Phase 1 antigens are shared by only a few organisms and react only with homologous antisera, but phase 2 antigens are shared by many organisms and react with heterologous antisera. The numerous antigenic types of *Salmonella* were organized by White to form a logical classification scheme that was useful for epidemiologic typing of these organisms. This scheme was revised and perfected by Kauffmann into the present day Kauffmann-White format that divides the *Salmonella* into major serologic groups, designated by the capital letters A to I, on the basis of common O antigens. Subdivision into individual serotypes is accomplished by determining the remaining O antigens and the phase 1 and phase 2 H antigens of a particular isolate.

Because of the large number of serotypes, only reference centers are capable of completely typing the *Salmonella*. However, only 38% of the 2000 known serotypes account for 95% of all clinical isolates, greatly simplifying the number of antisera needed to identify clinical isolates. In a study of more than 500,000 *Salmonella* isolates in the United States, serogroup B accounted for 47% of all isolates. Serogroups C_1, C_2, D, and E_2 accounted for 13%, 7%, 24%, and 4.4% of all the remaining isolates, respectively.

The capsular antigens play a minor role in the classification of the genus, but they may have a pathogenic significance. The Vi (virulence) antigen of serotype typhi may prevent the intracellular destruction of the organism. This antigen is rarely found in other serotypes of *Salmonella*.

TABLE 35–3. TESTS USED TO CHARACTERIZE CLINICALLY IMPORTANT *SALMONELLA ENTERICA* SUBSPECIES *ENTERICA* (SUBGROUP 1)

Test	Bioserotype *choleraesuis*	Bioserotype *typhi*	Other Common Bioserotypes
Citrate	−[a]	−	+
Ornithine decarboxylase	+	−	+
Gas from glucose	+	−	+
Fermentation			
Dulcitol	−	−	+
Trehalose	−	+	+

Adapted from Ewing: Edwards and Ewing's Identification of Enterobacteriaceae, ed 4. Elsevier, 1986.
[a] Reactions after 1 to 2 days incubation.

Determinants of Pathogenicity

Salmonella are complex organisms that produce a variety of virulence factors, including surface antigens, factors contributing to invasiveness, endotoxin, cytotoxins, and enterotoxins. The role of each of these factors in the pathogenesis of *Salmonella* infections probably varies with the individual serotype causing the infection and the host system being studied because *Salmonella* are capable of causing different syndromes in different hosts. In fact, many serotypes are adapted to specific hosts. For example, *S. typhimurium* causes a syndrome similar to typhoid fever in its natural host, the mouse, but in humans it is associated mainly with a self-limiting gastroenteritis. Similarly, *S. typhi* is uniquely limited to humans and does not cause disease in animals when given orally. These differences in host response probably lie in the ability of the various organisms to survive intracellularly in the host's phagocytic cells. This intracellular capability, coupled with their ability to grow in extracellular environments, has led some researchers to use the term *facultative intracellular parasites* to describe the pathogenesis of these organisms.

Surface Antigens. The ability of *Salmonella* to attach to host receptor cells and to survive intracellularly may be due to the O antigenic side chains or, in the case of the typhi serotype, to the presence of Vi antigen. As with *Shigella*, rough colonial variants deficient in O-specific side chains are avirulent, and smooth colonial variants are virulent. Similarly, studies in human volunteers show that those organisms containing Vi antigen are clearly more virulent than those lacking this antigen. The O antigen of *Salmonella* apparently is important in determining the susceptibility of some serotypes to complement, to host cationic proteins, and to an interaction with host macrophages. Organisms with intact O antigens are more resistant than "rough" variants to the complement-mediated killing of normal serum. The resistance to killing by normal serum probably is due to the shielding of the complement-activating lipid A and LPS core polysaccharides by the polysaccharides of the O antigen. The uptake of the organisms by macrophages also is affected by the deposition of complement on the organisms. Different O antigens prevent the activation and subsequent deposition of complement factors on bacterial surfaces to varying degrees. This in turn leads to the observed differences in the phagocytosis of the various serotypes. The ability of the O antigen to protect an organism against the effects of complement and phagocytosis may also be a function of the serotype because O-antigen deficient choleraesuis mutants were of equal virulence with parent strains when given intraperitoneally or intravenously but were avirulent when given orally. It is postulated that the O antigen for this serotype is more important for intestinal survival than survival in serum.

Differences in phagocytosis rates have also been attributed to the presence of the Vi antigen. The physiologic role of the Vi antigen has not been determined; however, one group has shown that typhi strains with the Vi antigen were not phagocytized by polymorphonuclear leukocytes as readily as organisms without the Vi antigen because of the decrease in binding of C3b caused by the Vi antigen.

Type 1 or mannose-binding fimbriae have been described in some *Salmonella.* However, fimbriate organisms are only slightly more virulent than are nonfimbriate organisms. The ability to bind to host cells may be due to the presence of some undefined adhesion factor. It previously was thought that high-molecular-weight plasmids were necessary for the adherence and invasiveness of *Salmonella.* Further work has shown that these plasmids control the ability of the organism to spread beyond the intestinal cells to invade other tissues and that they do not control the initial attachment of the intestinal cells. Whether these plasmids encode for changes in the surface properties of *Salmonella* that in turn facilitate the spread of the organisms is unknown.

Invasiveness. Like *Shigella,* virulent *Salmonella* penetrate the epithelial lining of the small bowel. However, unlike the *Shigella,* the *Salmonella* do not merely reside in the epithelial lining but penetrate into the subepithelial tissue. Recent evidence has shown that the organisms synthesize new bacterial proteins when grown in the presence of mammalian cells and that these new proteins are necessary for the adherence and penetration of the mammalian cells. Further studies have revealed that organisms grown in an atmosphere of 0 to 1% oxygen are almost 70% more adherent and invasive than those bacteria grown in 20% oxygen. The oxygen level may be the environmental cue the organisms use to produce these new proteins. As the bacteria approach the epithelium, the brush border begins to degenerate, and the bacteria enter the cell where they are immediately surrounded by inverted cytoplasmic membranes similar to phagocytic vacuoles. They then pass through the epithelial cells into the lamina propria. Occasionally, epithelial penetration occurs at an intercellular junction. After penetration the organisms multiply and may spread to other body sites. Epithelial destruction occurs during later stages of the disease. Whether this destruction is due to a cytotoxin or the host cell response is not known. The importance of the O antigens for cell penetration into eucaryotic cells appears to vary with the serotype. Serotype typhimurium does not require intact O antigen for penetration in cell cultures, whereas the host-adapted serotypes choleraesuis and typhi, which lack intact O antigens, cannot enter cell monolayers.

Differences in the type of disease caused by the various serotypes of *Salmonella* may be due to the type of host cell that is invaded. For example, in humans serotypes causing gastroenteritis penetrate and proliferate in epithelial cells, whereas the target cell for serotype typhi is the macrophage. The ability to survive in macrophages is due to the production of bacterial proteins that enable the organisms to withstand both the oxygen-dependent and the non-oxygen-dependent killing mechanisms of these "professional" phagocytic cells. The oxygen-dependent mechanisms include the production of hydrogen peroxide and superoxide, and the oxygen-independent mechanisms include the production of antibacterial, cationic proteins known as defensins. The genetic control of the proteins that protect the bacteria from defensins resides in the *phoP* locus. The product of this gene appears to effect the pleiotropic control of a large number of genes on the bacterial chromosome. The molecular basis of this process and its role in the survival of these organisms in macrophages has yet to be determined.

Endotoxin. As with all enteric bacilli, endotoxin may play a role in the pathogenesis of *Salmonella* infections, especially during the bacteremic stages of enteric fevers. Presumably, endotoxin is responsible for the fever seen in patients with these diseases. Whether the fever is produced by the endotoxin acting directly or indirectly through the release of endogenous pyrogens from leukocytes is not known. Endotoxin activation of the chemotactic properties of the complement system may cause the localization of leukocytes in the classic lesions of typhoid fever. However, the true role of endotoxin remains unclear since endotoxin-tolerant volunteers infected with the typhoid bacillus still display all the classic signs of typhoid fever.

Other Factors. Enterotoxins similar to both the heat-labile (LT) and heat-stable enterotoxins (ST) of *E. coli* have been demonstrated in several *Salmonella* species; however, the role of these enterotoxins in disease is not clearly defined, since, like shigellosis, the major target tissue of salmonellosis is the colon, and the enterotoxins appear to affect the small bowel. Furthermore, the enterotoxin is cell associated and is not excreted extracellularly, as are the enterotoxins of *E. coli* and *V. cholerae* (Chaps. 34 and 36). The role of these enterotoxins may vary with the infecting organism. Serotype typhimurium produces a severe ileitis in experimental animals that is not seen with other *Salmonella* and produces enterotoxin. Whether these toxins are produced intracellularly by organisms infecting the colon is not known.

Salmonella also produce a cytotoxin that is distinct from the enterotoxins. This toxin appears to be associated with the outer bacterial membrane, which may mean that the toxin is important in cellular invasion as well as cellular destruction. In a study of 131 strains of *Salmonella,* all strains were found to produce cytotoxins, but there was a quantitative difference in the amount of toxin produced by the various strains. The choleraesuis and enteritidis serotypes always produced the most cytotoxin, whereas the typhi serotype produced the least amount of toxin. This difference may again reflect the differences in the disease spectrum caused by the various serotypes of *Salmonella.* Although the toxins produced by all *Salmonella* were genetically and immunologically distinct from the Shiga toxin and the SLT-I and SLT-II of *E. coli,* the mechanism of action of both groups of cytotoxins is similar in that the protein synthesis of Vero cells is inhibited.

Clinical Infection

Epidemiology

Typhoid Fever. *Salmonella* serotype typhi is uniquely adapted to humans, and human carriers represent the sole source of these organisms. Carriers can be either convalescent carriers who excrete the organism for a short period of time or chronic carriers who shed the organism for longer than 1 year. Approximately 3% of the typhoid fever patients become chronic carriers. The majority of chronic carriers are older women with gallbladder disease. The organism resides in gallstones or scars in the biliary tree and is excreted in large numbers. Other individuals are infected by ingesting food or water contaminated by the carrier. The epidemiology of a typhoid fever outbreak in a migrant worker camp in Florida in 1973 serves as an example of the spread of *Salmonella* through contaminated water. This outbreak involved 225 individuals and was the largest outbreak of typhoid fever in the United States since 1939. It is suspected that a faulty sewage system permitted contamination of well water by a typhoid carrier. A nonfunctioning chlorinator failed to purify the water and contributed to the spread of the organism.

Food-borne outbreaks also occur, as evidenced by the largest restaurant outbreak in more than 50 years. In this 1981 San Antonio outbreak 80 persons were infected by one female employee who was involved in food preparation. She had gallstones, and a culture of the stones and her gallbladder grew the organism. Large-scale outbreaks in Scotland (515 cases) and Germany (344 cases) involved contaminated corned beef and potato salad, respectively.

The control of carriers, chlorination of water, and proper sewage disposal have reduced the number of typhoid fever cases in the United States from more than 5000 in 1942 to 460 in 1989. Seventy percent of all U.S. cases are acquired during travel in endemic regions. In developing countries without adequate control measures typhoid fever remains a major health problem involving thousands of people. In these regions water represents the major vehicle of transmission.

Other *Salmonella* Infections. Salmonellosis represents a major communicable disease problem in the United States, with 47,812 cases reported in 1989. The actual number of cases has been estimated to be closer to 2 million because most of the gastrointestinal infections are not reported. Although any *Salmonella* serotype can cause disease, the majority of cases in the United States have been caused by serotype typhimurium. This may be changing in the future because the number of infections caused by serotype enteritidis is increasing in the United States and other parts of the world. In 1989 serotype enteritidis was the cause of 20% of all reported *Salmonella* infections in the United States, whereas serotype typhimurium was the causative agent in 21% of the reported cases. The number of countries reporting serotype enteritidis as the leading *Salmonella* isolate rose from 2 in 1979 to 21 in 1987. There is some evidence that this increase may be due to the consumption of eggs and poultry that harbor this organism.

As with typhoid fever, contaminated food and water are the vehicles of transmission for other *Salmonella* infections. However, in contrast to typhoid fever, for which the human carrier is the sole source of the organism, contaminated animals and animal products are the major sources of other *Salmonella*. In countries where intensive animal husbandry practices are carried out, 50% of a herd or flock may harbor *Salmonella*. A number of these organisms are also resistant to antibiotics because of the indiscriminate use of antibiotics as growth factors in animal feeds. Many investigators believe that these resistant organisms represent a major health hazard and advocate that the use of antibiotics in feeds be curtailed. Poultry and beef products represent the largest sources of nontyphoid *Salmonella* in the United States. Meat products are contaminated with fecal material during slaughter. Improper storage or undercooking then allows the organisms to proliferate to the necessary infective dose of about 10^6 organisms. Eggs and dried egg products that do not reach killing temperatures during the drying process serve to contaminate other products such as cake mixes.

Dogs and other pets harbor *Salmonella* for extended periods. Cold-blooded animals are also efficient carriers of the organisms and have served as sources of infection. Before the restrictions on the sale of pet turtles, these animals were significant sources of infection in children.

The human carrier serves as a source of secondary infections with *Salmonella*. Patients with gastroenteritis shed the organism for several weeks after recovering from the infection. In direct contrast to *Shigella* infections, antibiotic treatment of *Salmonella* gastroenteritis prolongs the carrier state. In the United States carriers are the source of small-scale outbreaks involving a select group, such as those eating at a particular restaurant or picnic. The general level of hygiene in this country usually limits the role of the carrier to these groups. In developing countries where food-handling practices and water standards are lower, human carriers represent a major source for *Salmonella* infections.

Clinical Manifestations and Pathogenesis

Salmonella infections may present as any of three distinct clinical entities: a self-limiting gastroenteritis, a septicemia with focal lesions, or an enteric fever such as typhoid fever.

Gastroenteritis. *Salmonella* gastroenteritis represents an actual infection of the colon and usually occurs 18 to 24 hours after ingestion of the organism. The disease is characterized by diarrhea, fever, and abdominal pain. It is usually self-limiting, lasting from 2 to 5 days. In extreme cases the disease may last for several weeks. In most cases the individual does not seek medical attention and attributes the symptoms to "stomach flu." Dehydration and electrolyte imbalance constitute the major threats in severe cases and in the very young and old. Although the organism can be isolated from the feces for several weeks, the occurrence of chronic carriers is rare.

Typhoid Fever and Other Enteric Fevers. The prototype and most severe enteric fever is typhoid fever, which is caused by serotype typhi. Other *Salmonella*, particularly serotypes paratyphi A and paratyphi B, can also cause enteric fevers, but the symptoms are milder, and the mortality is lower.

The number of organisms in ingested food and water is important in determining the infection rate with the typhoid bacillus. Volunteer studies show that only 25% of people become infected on ingestion of 10^5 organisms, with the infection rate increasing to 95% when the infecting dose increases to 10^9 viable organisms. During the first week of infection the symptoms of lethargy, fever, malaise, and general aches and pains can be confused with a variety of other illnesses, particularly by physicians in countries with low rates of typhoid fever. Constipation rather than diarrhea is the rule. During this time the organism is penetrating the intestinal wall and infecting the regional lymphatic system. Some organisms also invade the bloodstream and infect other parts of the reticuloendothelial system. At both sites the organisms are ingested by monocytes but are not killed, and they undergo multiplication. During the second week of illness they reenter the bloodstream, causing a prolonged bacteremia. Infection of the biliary tree and other organs occurs at this time. The patient is severely ill with a sustained fever of about 104F and is often delirious. The abdomen is tender and may have the typical rose-colored spots. Diarrhea begins during the second to third week of illness. At this time the organisms are reinfecting the intestinal tract from the gallbladder and may cause necrosis of Peyer's patches. After the third week the patients are exhausted and still febrile but continue to show improvement if no complications occur. Complications include intestinal perforation, severe bleeding, thrombophlebitis, cholecystitis, pneumonia, and abscess formation. The death rate ranges from 2% to 10% and is lowest when supportive therapy is readily available. Approximately 20% of patients relapse.

Septicemia. *Salmonella* septicemia is prolonged and characterized by fever, chills, anorexia, and anemia. Focal lesions may develop in any tissue, producing secondary osteomyelitis, pneumonia, pulmonary abscess, meningitis, or endocarditis. Gastroenteritis is minor or even absent, and the organism is rarely cultured from feces. Serotype choleraesuis is a frequent cause of this syndrome and is particularly associated with osteomyelitis in patients with sickle cell trait.

A chronic bacteremia has also been described in patients with schistosomiasis. The *Schistosoma* carry the bacterium, so cure of the bacteremia is not achieved until the underlying parasitic infection is cured.

Laboratory Diagnosis

Isolation of the organism constitutes a positive laboratory diagnosis of salmonellosis or the carrier state. During the acute stages of gastroenteritis the number of organisms in feces is large, and the stool represents the specimen of choice. Blood is the best specimen for the detection of septicemia and enteric fevers during the first week of illness. Approximately 80% of typhoid fever patients have positive blood cultures during the first week of illness, with only 25% of patients having positive blood cultures by the fourth week. In contrast, fecal specimens are positive in only 25% of typhoid fever patients during the first week; however, by the third week feces are positive in 85% of all patients. Urine and other specimens, such as sputum or spinal fluid, are appropriate for the diagnosis of complications of *Salmonella* infections.

Salmonella can be isolated on any of the media used to isolate other enterics. Serologic typing of organisms biochemically characterized as *Salmonella* is important for complete identification and for epidemiologic studies.

Treatment

Antibiotic treatment of uncomplicated *Salmonella* gastroenteritis only serves to prolong the carrier state and increase the likelihood of secondary cases. Treatment of gastroenteritis should center around supportive therapy and maintaining fluid and electrolyte balance.

In cases of enteric fever or septicemia, ampicillin or chloramphenicol is the drug of choice. In 1972 an epidemic in Mexico was caused by a chloramphenicol-resistant strain of the typhoid bacillus. Ampicillin resistance also occurred in a number of isolates. Approximately 50 cases involving this strain were imported into the United States. Trimethoprim-sulfamethoxazole proved an effective treatment. Ampicillin, not chloramphenicol, is the drug of choice for treatment of chronic carriers of the typhi serotype. Cholecystectomy may also be required to cure the chronic carrier state completely. Ampicillin together with surgery produces an 85% cure rate in carriers when gallstones or gallbladder disease is present.

Control

Prevention of salmonellosis requires that water standards be observed and that food be properly cooked and stored. Temperatures below 40F halt the proliferation of *Salmonella* in foods, whereas temperatures above 140F kill the organism. It is critical that the center of the food reach these temperatures to prevent the organisms from multiplying in the center of the food and then spreading throughout the food at a later time. Commercial kitchens are required to keep the food stored in shallow pans to allow proper temperature distribution throughout the entire volume of food. Keeping separate surfaces for the preparation of different types of foods is also important. Using for salads the same wooden cutting board that was used to cut poultry results in contamination of the salads with organisms. Simple washing is not sufficient to remove all organisms from the cracks of such boards.

Detection and treatment of carriers are the major control mechanisms for typhoid fever. Removal of persons who are known carriers or who are recovering from gastroenteritis from food-handling duties is necessary to prevent the occurrence of secondary cases of salmonellosis.

The use of vaccines in the control of typhoid fever has had mixed results. The most promising was an oral vaccine of an attenuated typhoid bacillus, Ty21a. In a field trial in Alexandria, Egypt, involving 32,000 children, the infection rate was 0/100,000 in the vaccinated group as compared to 126/100,000 in the placebo group and 133/100,000 of non-vaccinated children. However, a larger trial involving 82,543 children in Santiago, Chile, did not confirm the results of the Egyptian trial. The efficacy of the vaccine in the Chilean children was only 59% for the first 2 years, and there was no protection after 3 years. In addition, this vaccine was not effective in reducing the incidence of typhoid fever in travelers to India. Whether there was a difference in vaccines, a difference in the virulence of the indigenous organism, a difference in susceptibilities of the population tested, or a combination of factors not completely understood requires further study. At present there is no readily available vaccine for the prevention of typhoid fever. Efforts for the development of an effective vaccine continue, but progress is hampered by the lack of an acceptable animal model in which the pathogenic and immunologic characteristics of the organism can be studied.

FURTHER READING

Books and Reviews

Brunton JL: The Shiga toxin family: Molecular nature and possible role in disease. In Iglewski BH, Clark VL (eds): The Bacteria, vol

XI: Molecular Basis of Bacterial Pathogenesis. San Diego, Academic Press, 1990, p 377
Buchwald DS, Blaser MJ: A review of human salmonellosis: II. Duration of excretion following infection with nontyphi *Salmonella*. Rev Infect Dis 6:345, 1984
Chiodini RJ, Sundberg JP: Salmonellosis in reptiles, a review. Am J Epidemiol 113:494, 1981
Cohen ML, Tauxe RV: Drug-resistant *Salmonella* in the United States: An epidemiologic perspective. Science 234:964, 1986
DuPont HL: *Shigella*. Infect Dis Clin North Am 2:599, 1988
DuPont HL, Pickering LK: Infections of the Gastrointestinal Tract: Microbiology, Pathophysiology and Clinical Features. New York, Plenum, 1980, pp 61, 83
Ewing WH: Edwards and Ewing's Identification of Enterobacteriaceae, ed 4. New York, Elsevier, 1986, pp 137, 181, 247, 319
Farmer JJ III, Davis BR, Hickman-Brenner FW, et al: Biochemical identification of new species and biogroups of Enterobacteriaceae isolated from clinical specimens. J Clin Microbiol 21:46, 1985
Finlay BB, Falkow S: Common themes in microbial pathogenicity. Microbiol Rev 53:210, 1989
Finlay BB, Falkow S: *Salmonella* as an intracellular parasite. Mol Microbiol 3:1833, 1989
Formal SB, Hale TL, Kapfer C: *Shigella* vaccines. Rev Infect Dis 11(suppl 3):S547, 1989
Formal SB, Hale TL, Sansonetti PJ: Invasive enteric pathogens. Rev Infect Dis 5(suppl 4):S702, 1983
Groisman EA, Fields PI, Heffron F: Molecular biology of *Salmonella* pathogenesis. In Iglewski BH, Clark VL(eds): The Bacteria, vol XI: Molecular Basis of Bacterial Pathogenesis. San Diego, Academic Press, 1990, p 251
Groisman EA, Saier MH Jr: *Salmonella* virulence new clues to intramacrophage survival. Trends Biochem Sci 15:30, 1990
Guerrant RL: Microbial toxins and diarrhoeal disease: Introduction and overview. In 1985 Microbial Toxins and Diarrhoeal Diseases. Ciba Foundation Symposium 112, London, Pittman, 1985, p 1
Gulig PA: Virulence plasmids of *Salmonella typhimurium* and other salmonellae. Microbial Pathog 8:3, 1990
Hackett J: *Salmonella*-based vaccines. Vaccine 8:5, 1990
Jimenez-Lucho VE, Leive LL: Role of the O-antigen of lipopolysaccharide in *Salmonella* in protection against complement action. In Iglewski BH, Clark VL (eds): The Bacteria, vol XI: Molecular Basis of Bacterial Pathogenesis. San Diego, Academic Press, 1990, p 339
Keusch GT, Donohue-Rolfe A, Jacewicz M: Shigella toxin and the pathogenesis of shigellosis. In 1985 Microbial Toxins and Diarrhoeal Diseases. Ciba Foundation Symposium 112, London, Pittman, 1985, p 193
Kopecko DJ, Baron LS, Buysse J: Genetic determinants of virulence in *Shigella* and dysenteric strains of *Escherichia coli:* Their involvement in the pathogenesis of dysentery. Curr Top Microbiol Immunol 118:71, 1985
Levine MM: Bacillary dysentery mechanisms and treatment. Med Clin North Am 66:623, 1982
Levine MM, Edelman R: Future vaccines against enteric pathogens. Infect Dis Clin North Am 4:105, 1990
Rosenberg ML, Weissman JB, Gangarosa EJ, et al: Shigellosis in the United States: Ten year review of nationwide surveillance, 1964–1973. Am J Epidemiol 104:543, 1976
Ryder RW, Merson MJ, Pollard RA, et al: Salmonellosis in the United States, 1968–1974. J Infect Dis 133:483, 1976
Stephen J, Wallis TS, Starkey WG, et al: Salmonellosis: In retrospect and prospect. In 1985 Microbial Toxins and Diarrhoeal Diseases. Ciba Foundation Symposium 112, London, Pittman, 1985, p 175
Stocker BAD, Makela PH: Genetic determination of bacterial virulence, with special reference to *Salmonella*. Curr Top Microbiol Immunol 118:149, 1985
Takeuchi A: Electron microscope observation on the pentration of the gut epithelial barrier by *Salmonella typhimurium*. In Schlessinger D (ed): Microbiology—1975. Washington, DC, American Society for Microbiology, 1975, p 174

Selected Papers

Ashkenazi S, Cleary TG, Murray BE, et al: Quantitative analysis and partial characterization of cytotoxin production by *Salmonella* strains. Infect Immun 56:3089, 1988
Black RE, Craun GF, Blake PA: Epidemiology of common-source outbreaks of shigellosis in the United States, 1961–1975. Am J Epidemiol 108:47, 1978
Black RE, Levine MM, Ferreccio C, et al: Efficacy of one or two doses of Ty21a *Salmonella typhi* vaccine in enteric-coated capsules in a controlled field trial. Vaccine 8:81, 1990
Blaser MJ, Feldman RA: *Salmonella* bacteremia: Reports to the Centers for Disease Control, 1968–1979. J Infect Dis 143:743, 1981
Butler T, Mahmoud AAF, Warren KS: Algorithms in the diagnosis and management of exotic diseases. XXIII. Typhoid fever. J Infect Dis 135:1017, 1977
Butler T, Mahmoud AAF, Warren KS: Algorithms in the diagnosis and management of exotic diseases. XXVII. Shigellosis. J Infect Dis 136:465, 1977
Buysse JM, Venkatesan M, Mills JA, Oaks EV: Molecular characterization of a trans-acting, positive effector (ipaR) of invasion plasmid antigen synthesis in *Shigella flexneri* serotype 5. Microbial Pathog 8:197, 1990
Cleric P, Baudry B, Sansonetti PJ: Plasmid-mediated contact haemolytic activity in *Shigella* species: Correlation with penetration into HeLa cells. Ann Inst Past Microbiol 137A:267, 1986
Eiklid K, Olsnes S: Animal toxicity of *Shigella dysenteriae* cytotoxin: Evidence that the neurotoxic, enterotoxic, and cytotoxic activities are due to one toxin. J Immunol 130:380, 1983
Feldman SB, Baine WB, Nitzkin JL, et al: Epidemiology of *Salmonella typhi* infection in migrant labor camp in Dade County, Florida. J Infect Dis 130:334, 1974
Finlay BB, Heffron F, Falkow S: Epithelial cell surfaces induce *Salmonella* proteins required for bacterial adherence and invasion. Science 243:940, 1989
Fontaine A, Arondel J, Sansonetti PJ: Role of Shiga toxin in the pathogenesis of bacillary dysentery, studied by using toxmutant of *Shigella dysenteriae* 1. Infect Immun 56:3099, 1988
Formal SB, Baron LS, Kopecko DJ, et al: Construction of a potential bivalent vaccine strain: Introduction of *Shigella sonnei* form I antigens into the gal E *Salmonella typhi* Ty 21a typhoid vaccine strain. Infect Immun 34:746, 1981
Helmuth R, Stephan R, Bunge C, et al: Epidemiology of virulence-associated plasmids and outer membrane protein patterns within seven common *Salmonella* serotypes. Infect Immun 48:175, 1985
Hirschel B, Wuthrich R, Somaini B, et al: Inefficacy of the commercial live oral Ty 21a vaccine in the prevention of typhoid fever. Eur J Clin Microbiol 4:295, 1985
Jacewicz M, Keusch GT: Pathogenesis of shigella diarrhea. VIII. Evidence for a translocation step in the cytotoxic action of Shiga toxin. J Infect Dis 148:844, 1983
Jones GW, Rabert DK, Svinarich DM, et al: Association of adhesive, invasive, and virulent phenotypes of *Salmonella typhimurium* with autonomous 60-megadalton plasmids. Infect Immun 38:476, 1982
Kawahara K, Haraguchi Y, Tsuchimoto M, et al: Evidence of corre-

lation between 50-kilobase plasmid of *Salmonella choleraesuis* and its virulence. Microbial Pathog 4:155, 1988

Lee CA, Falkow S: The ability of *Salmonella* to enter mammalian cells is affected by the bacterial growth state. Proc Natl Acad Sci USA 87:4304, 1990

Little TWA, Sojka WJ, Wray C: Consequenses on emergence of resistant bacteria from the use of antibacterials in animal husbandry. Scand J Infect Dis Suppl 49:124, 1986

Looney RJ, Steigbigel RT: Role of the Vi antigen of *Salmonella typhi* in resistance to host defense in vitro. J Clin Med 108:506, 1986

Mroczenski-Wildey MJ, DiFabio JL, Cabello FC: Invasion and lysis of HeLa cell monolayers by *Salmonella typhi:* The role of lipopolysaccharide. Microbial Pathog 6:143, 1989

Nnalue NA, Lindberg AA: *Salmonella choleraesuis* strains deficient in O antigen remain fully virulent for mice by parenteral inoculation but are avirulent by oral administration. Infect Immun 58: 2493, 1990

Olsnes S, Reisbig R, Eiklid K: Subunit structure of *Shigella* cytotoxin. J Biol Chem 256:8732, 1981

Reisbig R, Olsnes S, Eiklid K: The cytotoxin activity of *Shigella* toxin evidence for catalytic inactivation of the 60S ribosome subunit. J Biol Chem 256:8739, 1981

Reitmeyer JC, Peterson JW, Wilson KJ: *Salmonella* cytotoxin: A component of the bacterial outer membrane. Microbial Pathog 1:503, 1986

Rodrigue DC, Tauxe RV, Rowe B: International increase in *Salmonella enteritidis:* A new pandemic? Epidemiol Infect 105:21, 1990

Sakai T, Sasakawa C, Yoshikawa M: Expression of four virulence antigens of *Shigella flexneri* is positively regulated at the transcriptional level by the 30 kilodalton virF protein. Mol Microbiol 2:589, 1988

Sandvig K, Olsnes S, Brown JE, et al: Endocytosis from coated pits of Shiga toxin: A glycolipid-binding protein from *Shigella dysenteriae* 1. J Cell Biol 108:1331, 1989

Sansonetti PJ, Kopecko DJ, Formal SB: *Shigella sonnei* plasmids: Evidence that a large plasmid is necessary for virulence. Infect Immun 34:75, 1981

Sansonetti PJ, Ryter A, Clerc P, et al: Multiplication of *Shigella flexneri* within HeLa cells: Lysis of the phagocytic vacuole and plasmid-mediated contact hemolysis. Infect Immun 51:461, 1986

Scragg JN, Rubidge CJ, Appelbaum PC: *Shigella* infection in African and Indian children with special reference to *Shigella* septicemia. J Pediatr 93:796, 1978

Speelman P, Kabir I, Islam M: Distribution and spread of colonic lesions in shigellosis: A colonoscopic study. J Infect Dis 150:899, 1984

Tauxe RV, McDonald RC, Hargrett-Bean N, Blake PA: The persistance of *Shigella flexneri* in the United States: Increasing role of adult males. Am J Public Health 11:1432, 1988

Tauzon CU, Nash T, Cheever A, et al: Influence of *Salmonella* and other gram-negative bacteria on survival of mice infected with *Schistosoma japonicum.* J Infect Dis 154:179, 1986

Taylor DN, Echeverria P, Tibor Pal, et al: The role of *Shigella* spp., enteroinvasive *Eschericha coli,* and other enteropathogens as causes of childhood dysentery in Thailand. J Infect Dis 153:1132, 1986

Taylor JP, Shandera WX, Betz TG, et al: Typhoid fever in San Antonio, Texas: An outbreak traced to a continuing source. J Infect Dis 149:553, 1984

Watanabe H, Nakamura A: Large plasmids associated with virulence in *Shigella* species have a common function necessary for epithelial cell penetration. Infect Immun 48:260, 1985

Wahdan MH, Serie CH, Germanier R, et al: A controlled field trial of live oral typhoid vaccine. Bull WHO 58:469, 1980

Wilkins EGL, Roberts C: Extraintestinal salmonellosis. Epidemiol Infect 100:361, 1988

Williamson CM, Baird GD, Manning EJ: A common virulence region on plasmids from eleven serotypes of *Salmonella.* J Gen Microbiol 134:975, 1988

CHAPTER 36

Vibrionaceae

Vibrio, Aeromonas, and *Plesiomonas* are the three genera of the family Vibrionaceae that have clinical significance for humans. The two major pathogens of the family, *Vibrio cholerae* and *Vibrio parahaemolyticus,* are among the leading causes of gastrointestinal infections. In addition to these organisms, nine other *Vibrio* species, three *Aeromonas* species, and *Plesiomonas shigelloides* have been implicated in human disease, causing sporadic cases of diarrhea and soft tissue infections. All members of this family are aquatic organisms that are frequently associated with the zooplankton. They are widely distributed throughout the world, with the *Vibrio* being more commonly found in brackish or salt water and *Aeromonas* and *Plesiomonas* being more frequently associated with fresh water. Soft tissue infections with these organisms are usually the result of being injured while in a marine environment, whereas gastrointestinal infections are the result of ingesting food or water containing large numbers of organisms.

The members of this family are gram-negative, facultative organisms that do not have exacting nutritional requirements. Like the Enterobacteriaceae (Chaps. 33, 34, 35), the Vibrionaceae have a fermentative and respiratory metabolism. However, they can be differentiated from the enterics by their positive oxidase reaction and the presence of polar, rather than peritrichous, flagella. Additional identifying characteristics may be found in the sections dealing with the individual organisms and in Tables 36–1 and 36–2.

Vibrio

The genus *Vibrio* is a diverse group of marine organisms that contains 34 species, 11 of which cause human disease. Included in this genus are *V. cholerae,* the cause of epidemic asiatic cholera, and *V. parahaemolyticus,* the leading cause of summer diarrhea in Japan.

Vibrio cholerae

Cholera is endemic in the Bengal region of India and Bangladesh, and it has spread from this region to other parts of the world in a series of pandemics. Since 1817 there have been seven cholera pandemics, the most recent occurring from the 1960s through the 1980s and involving Africa, Western Europe, the Philippines, and other areas of Southeast Asia. This pandemic has provided the impetus for successful research efforts in elucidating the pathogenic mechanisms of the organism as well as providing significant advances in the treatment of the disease. In addition, the research methods developed for the study of cholera have proven useful in the study of other causes of bacterial diarrhea.

TABLE 36–1. BIOCHEMICAL PROPERTIES OF THE PATHOGENIC VIBRIOS

Test	*V. cholerae*	*V. alginolyticus*	*V. damsela*	*V. fluvialis*	*V. hollisae*	*V. mimicus*	*V. parahaemolyticus*	*V. vulnificus*
Sensitivity to O/129	+	d	+	d	d	+	+	+
Oxidase	+	+	+	+	+	+	+	+
Arginine dihydrolase[a]	–	–	+	+	–	–	–	–
Lysine decarboxylase[a]	+	+	d	–	–	+	+	+
Ornithine decarboxylase[a]	+	d	–	–	–	+	+	d
Voges-Proskauer[a]	d	+	+	–	–	–	–	–
ONPG	+	–	–	d	–	+	–	d
Sucrose fermentation	+	+	–	+	–	–	–	d
Growth in NaCl								
0%	+	–	–	–	–	+	–	–
1%	+	+	+	+	+	+	+	+
6%	–	+	+	+	+	–	+	d
8%	–	+	–	d	–	–	d	–
10%	–	d	–	–	–	–	–	–

d, different reactions; ONPG, *O*-nitrophenyl-β-D-galactopyranosidase.
[a] with 1% NaCl.

Taxonomy

The taxonomy of *V. cholerae* has been confusing because of attempts to link the nomenclature to the various distinct serologic and pathologic entities. Classic epidemic cholera is caused by organisms that agglutinate in antisera directed against the O1 antigen and that produce disease primarily by means of a specific enterotoxin. These organisms can be distinguished further biochemically into the cholerae and el tor biotypes. A second group of organisms is biochemically similar to the O1 organisms and type with the O1 antisera. However, they do not produce the classic cholera enterotoxin. A third group of organisms does not agglutinate in O1 antisera but is indistinguishable from the O1 group both biochemically and genetically. In the past, this last group has been referred to as the nonagglutinating vibrios (NAG) or noncholera vibrios (NCV). All three groups of organisms have been shown to be genetically similar and are now classified as *V. cholerae.* The accepted convention is to refer to these organisms as *V. cholerae* O1, atypical or nontoxigenic *V. cholerae* O1, and non-O1 *V. cholerae,* respectively.

Morphology

The cholera vibrios are short (0.5 μm by 1.5 to 3.0 μm), gram-negative rods that appear to be comma-shaped on initial isolation. In fact, Koch initially named his isolates the *Kommabacillus.* Upon serial transfers, the organisms revert to straight forms. Motility is by means of a single, thick, sheathed, polar flagellum.

Physiology

Biochemical and Cultural Characteristics. *V. cholerae* is a facultative organism with an optimum growth temperature ranging from 18C to 37C. Its metabolism is both respiratory and fermentative. Cholera vibrios will grow on a wide variety of simple media when provided with a source of carbohydrate, inorganic nitrogen, sulfur, phosphorus, minerals, and adequate buffering. They grow best at pH 7.0 but can tolerate alkaline conditions to pH 9.0—a trait that is used in the design of cholera isolation media. They are extremely sensitive to acid pH, and a pH of 6.0 or less will sterilize cultures. When grown on meat extract agar, fresh isolates develop an iridescent green to red-brown color that is best seen when viewed at low magnification with oblique lighting. When initially isolated, the colonies are translucent, but with age and when passed on laboratory media, they become opaque and corrugated (rugose variant). Most strains will grow on MacConkey agar. However, a number of isolation media have been developed to enhance the selection of vibrio colonies from fecal material. These selective media include tellurite taurocholate gelatin agar (TTGA) and thiosulfate citrate bile sucrose agar (TCBS).

As with other members of the genus, the cholera vibrios can be differentiated from other oxidase-positive, fermentative, gram-negative rods by their sensitivity to O129 (2,4 diamine-6,7-diisopropyl pteridine). The cholera vibrios can be distinguished from other members of the genus by the tests listed in Table 36–1. The O1 cholera vibrios can be further subdivided into the el tor and cholerae or classic biotypes. This differentiation is useful for epidemiologic studies and was based originally on the hemolysis of sheep erythrocytes by the el tor biotype. However, recent epidemics have been caused by a nonhemolytic el tor strain. Identification of nonhemolytic strains is based on a positive Voges-Proskauer reaction and the agglutination of chicken erythrocytes. Further differentiation of the biotypes is based on the sensitivity of the cholerae biotype to polymyxin B and classic IV bacteriophage.

Genetics. Unlike the genes of the closely related *Escherichia coli* LT (Chap. 34), the genes for cholera enterotoxin are found on the chromosome rather than plasmids. The arrangement and number of these genes also differ for the el tor and cholerae biotypes. With the cholerae biotype, there is a nontandem duplication of the toxin genes in identical positions and orientation, whereas most el tor strains have a single copy of the gene, and the strains that have two copies have the copies arranged in tandem. In all strains of both biotypes, the toxin genes appear to be part of a larger, highly conserved DNA sequence. Included in this sequence is a genetic element that encodes for a toxin-coregulated pilus colonization factor (TCP). Enterotoxigenic *V. cholerae* may also contain a second gene cluster, the accessory colonization factor (ACF), which encodes for additional proteins or pili that may aid in colonization of the intestinal tract. The expression of toxin production, TCP, and ACF appear to be under the control of a *toxR* gene, which in turn is activated by a combination of environmental signals and the action of a *toxS* gene. The *toxR* and *toxS* genes also appear to control the type of outer membrane proteins that may play a role in attachment of the organism to host cells.

Antigenic Structure

The important antigens for serologic typing of the cholera vibrios are the O or somatic antigens. All *V. cholerae* appear to share a common flagellar antigen. There are six O antigen groups, which include some 70 serovarieties. Serogroup O1 contains the el tor and cholerae biotypes, which are responsible for classic epidemic cholera. Serologically, both biotypes can be subdivided into the serotypes ogawa, inaba, and hikojima. Conversion among the ogawa, inaba, and hikojima serotypes can occur in natural and experimental infections and appears to be related to the development of agglutinating antibody. The other five serogroups of *V. cholerae* are associated with sporadic and milder forms of diarrhea and apparently have limited epidemic potential.

The O antigens of the cholera vibrios are part of the lipopolysaccharide (LPS) component of the cell wall and are structurally similar to other gram-negative organisms in that they contain lipid A, a common core region of polysaccharides and O-specific side chains of polysaccharides that are responsible for antigenic differences within the species. However, the LPS of the vibrios lacks 2-keto-3-deoxyoctonate (KDO).

Determinants of Pathogenicity

Enterotoxins. The major pathogenic factor produced by *V. cholerae* O1 is a potent, extracellular enterotoxin that acts on the cells of the small intestine. This enterotoxin was the first of many similar toxins to be discovered and is very closely related to the LT of *E. coli* (Chap. 34) in both structure and function.

The cholera toxin (CT), or choleragen, is a complex, protein molecule with a molecular weight of approximately 84,000 Da. It is composed of two major subunits, subunit A, which is responsible for the biologic activity, and subunit B, which is responsible for the cellular binding of the toxin. Subunit A consists of two polypeptides linked together by a single disulfide bond. The toxic activity resides in A_1, whereas A_2 serves as the link to subunit B. The B subunit consists of five identical peptides with a molecular weight of 11,500 Da each. Subunit B binds rapidly and irreversibly to the GM_1 monosialoganglioside molecules of the cells of the small intestines. Subunit A then disassociates from subunit B and penetrates the cellular membrane. Activation of A_1 occurs with the reduction of the disulfide bond. The activated A_1 enzymatically transfers the adenosine diphosphate ribose from nicotinamide adenine dinucleotide (NAD) to a guanosine triphosphate (GTP)-binding protein that regulates adenylcyclase activity. This action inhibits the GTP turnoff mechanism of adenylcyclase activity and increases adenylcyclase activity. The increased adenylcyclase activity produces increased levels of intracellular cyclic AMP (cAMP), which in turn cause a rapid secretion of electrolytes into the lumen of the small bowel. The electrolyte loss is due to the increased sodium-dependent chloride secretion and the prevention of sodium and chloride absorption across the brush border by the sodium chloride cotransport mechanism. The resulting secretion is an isotonic fluid with a bicarbonate level twice the concentration of normal plasma and a potassium 4 to 8 times that of normal plasma. Fluid losses may be as high as 1 L per hour, and all the effects seen in patients can be attributed directly to this extreme fluid and electrolyte loss.

Recent research has indicated that the CT-B subunit of the classic biotype is markedly conserved, whereas the el tor biotype CT-B subunit is genetically diverse outside the GM_1 binding site, with at least five unique epitopes described thus far. These variations may explain some of the differences seen in infections caused by the two biotypes and also may play an important role in the efforts to develop effective vaccines. Other researchers have shown that the amount of toxin production is influenced greatly by the salinity and organic substrate concentration, indicating that environmental factors may play an important role in the epidemiology and pathogenicity of enterotoxinogenic *V. cholerae.*

The classic enterotoxin described above is clearly associated with the O1 cholera strains. However, it has been increasingly evident that non-O1 cholera vibrios can cause diarrhea in humans and that the disease caused by these organisms can take two forms, one that is indistinguishable from classic cholera and one that is characterized by fever and bloody diarrhea. It is now known that some strains of non-O1 *V. cholerae* can produce the classic enterotoxin, whereas other strains may produce a heat-stable enterotoxin (NAG-ST) that may be similar to the ST of *E. coli* (p. 546). This heat-stable toxin is active in the suckling mouse assay. However, the pathogenicity of non-O1 *V. cholerae* may not be attributed solely to NAG-ST production, since there are various reports of these organisms producing other factors, including shiga-like toxins, cytotoxins, and hemolysins, which may play a role in disease. The importance of NAG-ST may vary with the geographic site from which the organism was isolated. A survey of 371 non-O1 isolates from Calcutta failed to find any organisms that produced NAG-ST. Another group showed that 7 of 103 isolates from Thailand contained the genetic information for NAG-ST production, whereas neither the 31 isolates from Mexico nor the 47 isolates from the United States tested positive for NAG-ST genes.

When genetically engineered laboratory strains of *V. cholerae* were used as vaccines in human volunteers, about one third of the volunteers developed a mild diarrhea. These organisms were shown to produce a new cholera toxin (NCT), which differs from CT. The overall importance of this enterotoxin in the pathogenesis of cholera or disease caused by nontoxinogenic *V. cholerae* O1 has yet to be determined.

Adherence. Enterotoxin production alone is not the sole factor in the pathogenesis of cholera. Virulent, O1 *V. cholerae* must also establish themselves in the intestinal tract by attaching to the intestinal lining. Studies on adherence show that virulent cells penetrate the intestinal mucus and attach to the microvilli at the brush border of the epithelial cells. However, the nature of the attachment of virulent organisms to intestinal cells is unclear. Motility may be involved in the adherence of *V. cholerae,* since nonmotile, toxinogenic strains are unable to produce the disease. Several investigators have demonstrated that the flagella act as adhesins and bind the bacteria to cellular surfaces, whereas other studies indicate that the somatic antigens and slime layers may be responsible for the attachment of the vibrios to host cells. Recent studies have shown that O1 organisms isolated directly from animal models contain at least 7 to 8 envelope antigens that are not produced by organisms grown in vitro. In addition, at least two different pili types have been described, and the genes for one type (TCP) have been found to coexist with the genes encoding for enterotoxin production. Chemotaxis may be important because motile strains that respond to chemotaxic stimuli are better able to survive in animals than are motile, nonchemotaxic strains. Virulent *V. cholerae* also produce a mucinase that may enable the organism to penetrate the mucus lining of the small intestine. What role each of these factors plays in the pathogenesis of the nontoxinogenic O1 and the non-O1 *V. cholerae* has not been determined, although human volunteer studies show that in order to cause diarrhea, strains producing NAG-ST must also possess colonizing factors.

Clinical Infection

Epidemiology. Both the el tor and cholerae biotypes of serogroup O1 are capable of causing widespread disease involving large numbers of people. There have been seven pandemics described since 1817, and until the development of effective treatment during the seventh, and still ongoing outbreak, there has been a high mortality associated with the disease. A 1947 epidemic in Egypt involved 33,000 persons, with 20,000 deaths. In the United States, there were 150,000 cholera deaths during the second pandemic (1832–1849), and 50,000 died in the United States during the pandemic of 1866. The cholerae biotype was responsible for the majority of cases seen in the fifth and sixth pandemics. However, the seventh pandemic has been caused by the el tor biotype. The replacement of the cholerae biotype by the el tor strain has been attributed to the greater ability of the el tor strain to survive in the environment and the higher incidence of asymptomatic carriers with el tor infections. However, there has been an increase in the isolation rate of the cholerae biotype in Bangladesh since 1982.

Although *V. cholerae* can exist naturally in the environment, the role of these naturally occurring organisms is difficult to assess in the regions with endemic cholera. Because these areas lack adequate sanitation facilities, the human carrier may be more important than the environment as a source of new cholera cases. Large numbers of organisms are shed in the carrier's feces, which contaminate water and food supplies. There are two types of carriers, the convalescent and the chronic carrier. The convalescent carrier is one recovering from the disease and is generally under 50 years of age. This carrier sheds the organism for several months to 1 year after the illness. In contrast, the chronic carrier is usually over 50 years of age and sheds organisms intermittently over a period of years. The chronic carrier seems to harbor the organism in the gallbladder and sheds the organism when there is a natural purging resulting from some other intestinal disorder. Usually, the index case of new outbreaks is a member of the household of the chronic carrier. The carrier rate in endemic areas varies greatly from under 1% to over 20%. The spread of the organism from endemic areas is greatly facilitated by modern international travel and the presence of carriers. In the early 1980s alone, there were 79,000 cases of cholera in 34 countries reported in a 2-year period. The potential for spread is magnified when one examines the case/asymptomatic carrier rate. During one outbreak in Bangladesh involving both biotypes of O1, the clinical case/carrier rate was 1:36 for the el tor biotype and 1:4 for the cholerae biotype.

Idiopathic, tropical hypochlorhydria may be a major factor in the spread of the disease in endemic areas. Persons with cholera in endemic areas frequently have achlorhydria or hypochlorhydria, and their digestive juices do not kill the organism. Experimental studies in volunteers show that the infective dose is lowered at least fivefold when the stomach acidity is lowered with bicarbonate.

During the past 15 years, there has been an increase in the number of cases of cholera in the United States. These cases appear to be caused by indigenous organisms rather than being imported cases. The first case of indigenous cholera since 1911 was described in a Texas man in 1973. Since that time there have been several outbreaks in the Texas–Louisiana coastal area. All U.S. O1 isolates have been hemolytic el tor biotype, serotype inaba. Most cases have been associated with raw or undercooked shellfish or crabs. A number of non-O1 cholera infections in the United States have also been associated with ingestion of raw oysters. Although it is clear that most cases of *V. cholerae* gastroenteritis in the United States are caused by non-O1 organisms, the true incidence of non-O1 disease is difficult to assess because the severity of the disease usually does not require the patient to seek medical attention. However, seven hospitals in the Gulf Coast states reported only 7 isolates from 11,000 stools that were screened for vibrios.

Pathogenesis and Clinical Manifestations. Classic asiatic cholera is one of the most devastating human diseases. The incubation period may be hours or days, with a mean of 2 to 3 days. There is an abrupt onset of diarrhea and vomiting. Fluid losses in severe cases approach 15 to 20 L per day. The fluid is watery, odorless, and without enteric organisms. Hypovolemic shock and metabolic acidosis result from the fluid loss. The eyes and cheeks of patients appear sunken, skin turgor is diminished, and the hands have a washerwoman's appearance. The untreated case fatality rate is over 60%. Milder forms of the disease do occur, and these patients are less likely to be hospitalized.

Non-O1 cholera diarrhea is usually of a milder disease, without the huge fluid loss seen in classic cholera. These organisms are isolated also from other body sites, causing localized wound infections and otitis media. Septicemia has been described in patients with underlying diseases.

Laboratory Diagnosis. The laboratory diagnosis of cholera depends on the isolation and identification of the organism. Because of the organism's sensitivity to acid and desiccation, clinical specimens should be cultured quickly or placed in a suitable transport medium, such as Amies or Cary-Blair modification of Stuart's transport medium. Selective media, such as TCBS and alkaline peptone broth, are used to facilitate the isolation and differentiation of *Vibrio* species from other enteric organisms. Once the organism is isolated, experienced workers in endemic countries can identify the organism with minimal test procedures, such as darkfield motility and the string test. In countries where the disease is rare, organisms are identified with a series of biochemical and serologic tests (Table 36–1). Distinction between the O1 cholera and non-O1 cholera organisms requires serologic typing of isolates. Several in vitro tests for toxin production have been developed, but the overall usefulness of these procedures has not been determined in the routine clinical laboratory.

Direct fluorescent antibody procedures on stools obtained during outbreaks in the Philippines and India showed over 90% correlation with culture methods, but efforts to apply this method for the detection of carriers were unsuccessful.

Treatment. Recent advances in treatment have reduced the mortality of cholera to less than 1%. Prompt replacement of fluid and electrolyte losses causes a rapid response and reversal of the patient's condition within a matter of hours. In severe cases, intravenous infusion of sodium chloride and bicarbonate solutions at a rate of 2 L per hour is required. After initial recovery from shock, fluid and electrolyte balance can be maintained with oral solutions of electrolytes and glucose. Oral therapy alone can be used to treat milder cases and is effective because the absorptive powers of the colon are unaffected by the disease. Oral therapy also has the advantage of being able to be administered by paramedical personnel in rural areas.

Tetracycline lowers the number of infecting organisms and, thereby, lowers the fluid loss by 60%. Tetracycline also is effective in reducing the carrier rate because it is concentrated in bile. Antibiotic therapy reduces the number of subsequent cases in household contacts of index cases. However, the emergence of tetracycline-resistant forms in Africa raises questions about the usefulness of mass prophylaxis in epidemic situations.

Prevention and Control. The primary defense in the control of cholera is the maintenance of adequate sewage treatment and water purification systems. Detection and treatment of carriers is important in endemic areas. The risk of infection in countries like the United States can be lowered by not eating raw or improperly cooked shellfish. Studies during a recent Louisiana outbreak involving crabs demonstrated that the crabs must be boiled at least 10 minutes to destroy *V. cholerae.* Steaming does not destroy the organism. Travelers to endemic countries are cautioned against eating uncooked vegetables and unpeeled fruits and drinking unbottled water.

Parenteral vaccines have been in existence for many years, but they do not offer protection beyond 6 months, and they require injections that are not practicable in the endemic regions. Because of the enteric nature of the disease, the focus of all cholera vaccine efforts has been to develop oral vaccines that offer ease of administration and provide stimulation of the local IgA system of the intestinal tract. However, attempts to develop an effective oral vaccine have met with mixed success. Attenuated *V. cholerae* strains, termed Texas Star-SR, have been used in volunteer studies. The overall efficacy of the vaccine was 61% in challenge studies, and those vaccinees who contracted the disease had lower stool volumes than the nonvaccinated group. However, 24% of the vaccinees also experienced loose stools after receiving the vaccine. Other workers have combined inactivated, whole organisms with the B subunit of the enterotoxin to form an oral vaccine. Trials of this vaccine in Bangladesh showed an 85% overall efficacy for the first 6 months after administration. In persons over 5 years of age, this protection lasted for more than 3 years, but in children under 5, the protection decreased to under 40% after 2 years. Other vaccine strategies involve the use of live genetically engineered organisms that colonize the intestinal tract but lack the toxic potential to produce disease. One strain, CVD103-HgR, has produced good immunologic responses in volunteers with minimal side effects, but its overall efficacy awaits large-scale trials in endemic areas.

Vibrio parahaemolyticus

V. parahaemolyticus is a marine organism that is found in estuaries throughout the world. It is a major cause of gastroenteritis associated with seafood.

Morphology and Physiology. *V. parahaemolyticus* resembles other *Vibrio* species in its structural and staining characteristics. When grown in liquid media and when grown on media of pH 8.5 or higher, the organisms produce a single, sheathed flagellum. However, when grown on solid media, unsheathed, peritrichous flagella also are produced.

As with other members of the genus, the nutritional requirements of *V. parahaemolyticus* are simple, and the organism grows best at alkaline conditions between pH 7.6 and 9.0. Unlike cholera vibrios, members of this species are halophilic, or salt-loving, and require at least 2% NaCl for growth. The sodium ion appears to be required for protein synthesis as well as for osmotic regulation. When provided with the appropriate conditions for growth, the generation time for this species is between 9 and 15 minutes, a property that is important in the epidemiology of the disease. Biochemical characteristics of this organism are listed in Table 36–1.

Antigenic Structure. The O and K antigens of *V. parahaemolyticus* are useful for serologic grouping. Currently, 12 O types and 59 K types are recognized. However, no particular serotype appears to be more prevalent or more virulent than any other serotype.

Determinants of Pathogenicity. The pathogenic mechanisms of *V. parahaemolyticus* have not been defined or clearly elucidated. Unlike *V. cholerae,* no clearly defined enterotoxin has been discovered. However, hemolysis on Wagatsuma agar has been used to identify pathogenic strains (Kanagawa phenomenon). Over 95% of human isolates exhibit the Kanagawa phenomenon, whereas less than 1% of environmental isolates are hemolytic. Hemolysis is due to at least four factors: a heat-stable direct hemolysin, a heat-labile direct hemolysin, a phospholipase A, and a lysophospholipase. The Kanagawa-positive strains typically possess the heat-stable hemolysin, whereas the heat-labile hemolysin is found more frequently in Kanagawa-negative strains. The heat-stable hemolysin is a protein and is lethal when injected into mice, but its role in intestinal disease is not clear. Some authors have described enterotoxic activity with the heat-stable hemolysin, but others have not. High numbers of organisms must be ingested before disease is seen, and there is evidence that the organism invades intestinal tissue. However, the usual tests for invasiveness are negative with this organism. Recent studies have shown that some pathogenic strains produce pili, and other studies describe the production of hemagglutinins other than pili that appear to be responsible for attachment of the organism to intestinal tissue in vitro. The role of either of these factors in the establishment of the organism in humans requires further investigation.

Clinical Infection

EPIDEMIOLOGY. *V. parahaemolyticus* is found in brackish waters of estuaries and coastal waters but not in open seawater. It can adsorb onto chitin and frequently is associated with shellfish and zooplankton. In temperate climates, the organism appears to be confined to the sediment in winter, but as the temperature rises in the spring, the organism levels in water increase. There is some evidence that the organism is susceptible to lysis by *Bdellovibrio* and that the seasonal variation may be keyed to the presence of this organism.

The number of cases of parahaemolyticus infections increases during the summer months and is due to the increase in numbers of organisms. Most cases of gastrointestinal disease are attributed to the ingestion of raw or improperly cooked seafood. In Japan, *V. parahaemolyticus* is the most common cause of diarrhea in the summer and is most commonly associated with eating of sushi. Outbreaks in the United States have been traced to mixing of raw and cooked seafood, improperly refrigerated seafood, and recontamination of cooked seafood by using seaweed as a packaging or ornamental feature. The rapid generation time of the organism allows the organism burden in food to achieve the infective dose of 10^6 organisms in a relatively short time. *V. parahaemolyticus* also causes wound infections in patients who receive traumatic injuries during exposure to marine environments.

CLINICAL MANIFESTATIONS. *V. parahaemolyticus* gastroenteritis is usually self-limiting but can mimic cholera. Diarrhea is explosive and watery, with little blood or mucus, although a dysentery syndrome has been described. Headache, abdominal cramps, nausea, vomiting, and fever may be present and may persist for 10 days. There is a fatty infiltration and cloudy swelling in the liver. Septicemia has been described in a patient with underlying liver disease, and pneumonia with bacteremia has been described in a patient who worked in a plant that makes products from fish.

LABORATORY DIAGNOSIS. Fecal material should be cultured onto TCBS agar and in alkaline peptone broth supplemented with 3% NaCl. On isolation of the organism, final identification is made using the tests outlined in Table 36–1.

TREATMENT. Most common cases of gastroenteritis are mild and self-limiting, and the patient does not seek medical treatment. Severe cases require fluid and electrolyte replacement and antibiotic therapy. Tetracycline, chloramphenicol, and the cephalosporin antibiotics usually are effective. Wound infections also are treated with antibiotics and debridement as needed.

CONTROL. The ubiquitous nature of the organism prevents its elimination from the environment. Control measures should be aimed at keeping the number of organisms below the infective dose. Refrigeration of raw seafood is essential, and efforts should be made to prevent recontamination of cooked seafood that is served chilled. The International Commission on Microbiological Specification for Foods has set a limit of 100 colony-forming units of *V. parahaemolyticus* per gram of raw shrimp, although there is a question about the efficiency of the recovery methods used to detect the vibrios from environmental sources. This concern is due to the belief that *V. cholerae* may enter a resting "viable but not culturable" state. Some investigators believe that other vibrios may have a similar state.

Other *Vibrio* Species

In addition to *V. cholerae* and *V. parahaemolyticus*, nine other species of *Vibrio* have been described as human pathogens. With the exception of *Vibrio mimicus*, all are found naturally in saltwater and require NaCl for growth in the laboratory. Table 36–1 lists some of the characteristics used to speciate these organisms.

Vibrio alginolyticus is a marine *Vibrio* that has been isolated from extraintestinal sites, such as wounds and ears of patients in contact with seawater. Septicemia has occurred in at least one person who was severely burned in a boating mishap, and there are case reports of the organism being isolated from the blood of patients with various malignancies. In contrast to most of the other members of the genus, *V. alginolyticus* has not been associated with gastroenteritis. Most isolates are susceptible to aminoglycosides, tetracycline, chloramphenicol, and trimethoprim-sulfamethoxazole but are resistant to ampicillin because of the production of a β-lactamase.

Vibrio damsela is another marine organism that infects wounds of persons exposed to brackish or seawater, with most cases resulting from lacerations received while swimming or handling fish. Wounds infected with this organism appear to require surgical debridement as well as antibiotic therapy. There are case reports of individuals in whom the infection had spread beyond the initial site of infection to involve entire limbs, which required amputation to stop the spread. This organism produces a potent extracellular cytolysin that may play a role in its pathogenicity. Most isolates are sensitive to tetracycline, cephalothin, gentamicin, and chloramphenicol. Previously classified as CDC group EF-5, *V. damsela* derives its name from the fact that it was originally isolated from skin ulcers of a damselfish.

Vibrio fluvialis was described originally as group F or CDC group EF-6. These organisms cause a diarrhea characterized by vomiting, abdominal pain, fever, and moderate to severe dehydration. Most patients are children or young adults. Although the majority of the reported cases have occurred in Asia, the disease has been described in the United States. The organism produces several enterotoxins that appear to be responsible for the symptoms. Fluid replacement, supplemented with antibiotics in severe cases, is the treatment of choice. A closely related species, *Vibrio furnissii*, also has been isolated from outbreaks of gastroenteritis. This organism was thought originally to be an aerogenic variant of *V. fluvialis* but subsequently has been shown to be a genetically distinct organism. Both species are found in marine environments.

Vibrio hollisae is another *Vibrio* species that has been described as a cause of human gastroenteritis. The number of cases is limited, but most of the patients have had a history of recent ingestion of raw seafood. As with other *Vibrio* infections, the disease is characterized by vomiting, diarrhea, fever, and abdominal pain. One patient had a bloody diarrhea, and one patient with hepatic cirrhosis had a bacteremia and died shortly after being hospitalized. This organism may produce a thermostable hemolysin similar to that of *V. parahaemolyticus* and a heat-sensitive enterotoxin.

A nonmarine *Vibrio,* which originally was thought to be a variant of non-O1 *V. cholerae,* has been classified as *V. mimicus.* The disease spectrum of this organism appears to be similar to that of the non-O1 *V. cholerae.* The two organisms can be distinguished by the tests listed in Table 36–1. Like the non-O1 cholera *Vibrio, V. mimicus* can produce two types of enterotoxin, one of which is similar to CT.

Vibrio vulnificus is a lactose-fermenting, marine *Vibrio* that causes three distinct forms of human disease. One is a wound infection characterized by swelling and erythema, which may progress with the formation of vesicles and bullae. Patients with wound infections usually have had contact with seawater or were handling shellfish. The second syndrome is a primary septicemia characterized by malaise, fever, chills, and prostration. Vomiting, diarrhea, and hypotension are seen in 20% to 30% of the septic patients, and metastatic cutaneous lesions that become necrotic appear in 75% of septic patients within 2 days. The mortality rate is 50%, with most deaths occurring within 1 day of the initiation of therapy. Most septic patients have become infected by ingesting raw oysters, and 75% of these patients had preexisting liver disease. The third syndrome is an acute, self-limiting diarrhea similar to other *Vibrio* infections and is usually a result of ingesting raw oysters. The incubation period for all forms of the infection can be less than 1 day, with a median of 18 hours. A heat-labile, cytolytic toxin has been isolated and may be responsible for the symptoms seen with this organism. In addition, this organism possesses a capsule that may aid in its survival in the bloodstream. In contrast to *V. cholerae,* it is resistant to complement-mediated lysis by human serum. Although the organism is susceptible to many antibiotics in vitro, tetracycline is the drug of choice together with aggressive supportive therapy and debridement and amputation if necessary.

Vibrio meschnikovii has been isolated from the blood of one patient with cholecystitis. Although this organism has also been isolated from human feces, it has not been defined clearly as a cause of gastroenteritis. This organism was formerly classified as CDC group 16.

Vibrio cincinnatiensis is the most recent member of the genus isolated from human infections. It was isolated from the spinal fluid of an alcoholic, elderly individual. The patient responded to moxalactam therapy, and there were no sequelae. The source of this isolate was not determined.

Aeromonas

The genus *Aeromonas* contains several species that are found free-living in water. Although they have been isolated from saltwater-freshwater interfaces, they generally are considered to be freshwater organisms. They are pathogens of cold-blooded animals, such as frogs and snakes. Human infections may take several forms: wound infections after exposure to water or soil, acute and chronic diarrhea, or opportunistic infections of blood or other body sites.

There are some differences in the literature concerning the taxonomy of the genus and the relative importance of the various species to human infections. DNA homology studies indicate that there are several hybridization groups within each of the designated species, but there is a lack of correlating phenotypic properties that provide a clear distinction between the groups. The literature is also difficult to interpret, since most clinical laboratories do not speciate the motile aeromonads. Furthermore, a number of previous reports have attributed all pathogenic properties to one species, *Aeromonas hydrophilia.* There appear to be some geographical differences in the relative distribution of the various organisms. Nevertheless, most investigators agree that the motile species, *A. hydrophilia, Aeromonas caviae,* and *Aeromonas sobria,* are the organisms associated with human disease, whereas the nonmotile species have not been isolated from human infections. All motile species possess a single polar flagellum. All *Aeromonas* are oxidase-positive, fermentative, gram-negative rods that grow on common laboratory media. They can be differentiated from the *Vibrio* and *Plesiomonas* by their resistance to O129. The distinguishing features of the motile isolates are shown in Table 36–2.

The pathogenic species produce a variety of toxins and hemolysins that may play a role in human disease. The symptoms of gastroenteritis may be due to one or both of the two types of enterotoxins that have been isolated. One enterotoxin appears to be similar to the LT of *E. coli* and the enterotoxin of *V. cholerae.* The other enterotoxin is a cytotoxin similar to that of *Shigella dysenteriae.* Two hemolysins, α and β, are lethal for experimental animals and are cytotoxic for various cell systems. Recent evidence suggests that the hemolytic, cytotoxic, and enterotoxic properties can all be found on a single polypeptide, but the polypeptides from different isolates may be chemically and immunologically different.

Human infections with *Aeromonas* increase from May to November and appear to be due to increased contact with the aquatic environment. The role of aeromonads in gastrointestinal disease is hampered by the lack of good epidemiologic markers and a clear case definition. Studies in Peace Corps volunteers in Thailand indicated a higher isolation rate in patients with diarrhea, but there was no difference in isolation rates among native Thais living in the same area. Studies in Australia showed a 10% isolation rate in diarrhea patients compared with no isolations from healthy individuals. A similar study by the CDC in the United States showed an association of aeromonad isolation with the presence of persistent diarrhea in patients with a history of drinking contaminated water and with the use of antibiotics that were not effective against *Aeromonas.* However, attempts to produce disease in human volunteers with organisms isolated from diarrhea patients have failed. Nevertheless, in countries with

TABLE 36–2. BIOCHEMICAL CHARACTERISTICS OF PATHOGENIC *AEROMONAS* AND *PLESIOMONAS* SPECIES

Test	*A. hydrophilia*	*A. caviae*	*A. sorbia*	*P. shigelloides*
Oxidase	+	+	+	+
Ornithine decarboxylase	−	−	−	+
DNase	+	+	+	−
Voges-Proskauer	+	−	d	−
Salicin fermentation	+	+	−	d

d, different reactions.

a low intestinal colonization rate, most clinicians would consider the isolation of *Aeromonas* in the absence of other enteric pathogens to be significant.

Skin and wound isolates generally occur in the lower extremities and typically occur as cellulitis, with purulent drainage and fever. Sepsis is usually seen in patients with underlying malignancies. Meningitis, peritonitis, osteomyelitis, arthritis, and urinary tract and eye infections also are described in both adult and pediatric populations. Most isolates are sensitive to the aminoglycoside antibiotics, tetracycline, cefamandole, and trimethoprim-sulfamethoxazole. They are resistant to the β-lactam antibiotics, penicillin, ampicillin, cephalothin, and carbenicillin.

Plesiomonas

Plesiomonas shigelloides is an aquatic organism that shares many phenotypic characteristics with *Vibrio* and *Aeromonas* species but is probably more closely related to the Proteeae of the family Enterobacteriaceae (Chap. 34). However, at present most taxonomists prefer its remaining in the family Vibrionaceae. It resembles other members of the Vibrionaceae in that it is an oxidase-positive, fermentative, gram-negative rod. Two characteristics that help differentiate *Plesiomonas* from other members of the family are its ability to ferment inositol and the presence of lophotrichous flagella.

The role of *Plesiomonas* in human disease is similar to that of *Aeromonas* in that both organisms have been isolated from opportunistic infections and both have been implicated in gastrointestinal disease. The extraintestinal spectrum of *Plesiomonas* infections includes septicemia, endophthalmitis, septic arthritis, meningitis, cellulitis, and cholecystitis. Like *Aeromonas,* the causal evidence of *Plesiomonas* involvement in gastrointestinal disease is circumstantial. Epidemiologic evidence indicates that *Plesiomonas* has been associated with at least two outbreaks of diarrhea in Japan, and a case controlled study in the United States shows a high correlation of *Plesiomonas* isolation, a history of seafood ingestion followed by clinical symptoms, and a recent travel history to Mexico. Additional evidence for intestinal pathogenicity includes the finding by several investigators of enterotoxic activity. Other workers, however, have failed to find either toxic or adhesive properties in their isolates. Attempts to produce disease in human volunteers have been unsuccessful. These conflicting results, however, may be explained by the discovery of seven strains that produced enterotoxin activity only after serial passage in rabbit intestine. On subculture to media, these organisms quickly lost this activity. This study may indicate a host factor requirement for enterotoxin production. Growth in an iron-poor medium also is necessary for the detection of enterotoxin activity. Further studies on the role of *Plesiomonas* in diarrheal disease are needed. At present, however, in developed countries, and as in the case of *Aeromonas* gastroenteritis, the isolation of *Plesiomonas* from fecal samples of patients with diarrhea is considered significant by most laboratories and clinicians.

Most isolates of *Plesiomonas* are resistant to the penicillins but are sensitive when a penicillin is combined with a β-lactamase inhibitor. In vitro studies show that most isolates are also susceptible to the cephalosporins, aminoglycosides, imipenem, and ciprofloxacin.

FURTHER READING

Books and Reviews

Betley MJ, Miller VL, Mekalanos JJ: Genetics of bacterial enterotoxins. Annu Rev Microbiol 40:577, 1986

Black RE: Prophylaxis and therapy of secretory diarrhea. Med Clin North Am 66:611, 1982

Brenden RA, Miller MA, Janda JM: Clinical disease spectrum and pathogenic factors associated with *Plesiomonas shigelloides* infections in humans. Rev Infect Dis 10:303, 1988

Carpenter CCJ: The pathophysiology of secretory diarrheas. Med Clin North Am 66:597, 1982

Craig JP, Benenson AS, Hardegree MC, et al (eds): The structure and functions of enterotoxins. J Infect Dis 133:S1, 1976

DiRita VJ, Peterson KM, Mekalanos JJ: Regulation of cholera toxin synthesis. In Iglewski BH, Clark VL (eds): The Bacteria, vol XI: Molecular Basis of Bacterial Pathogenesis. San Diego, Academic Press, 1990, p 355

DuPont HL, Pickering LK: Infections of the Gastrointestinal Tract. Microbiology, Pathophysiology and Clinical Features. New York, Plenum, 1980, p 129

Edelman R, Pierce NF: Summary of the 19th United States-Japan joint cholera conference. J Infect Dis 149:1014, 1984

Farmer JJ III, Hickman-Brenner FW, Kelly MT: *Vibrio.* In Lennette EH, Balows A, Hausler WJ Jr, et al (eds): Manual of Clinical Microbiology, ed 4. Washington, DC, American Society for Microbiology, 1985, p 282

Hill MK, Sanders CV: Localized and systemic infection due to *Vibrio* species. Infect Dis Clin NA 1:687, 1987

Holmgren J, Clemens J, Sack DA, Svennerholm A: New cholera vaccines. Vaccine 7:94, 1989

Janda JM, Powers C, Bryant RG, Abbott SL: Current perspectives on the epidemiology and pathogenesis of clinically significant *Vibrio* spp. Clin Microbiol Rev 1:245, 1988

Joseph SW, Colwell RR, Kaper JB: *Vibrio parahaemolyticus* and related halophilic vibrios. CRC Crit Rev Microbiol 10:77, 1982

Kardori N, Fainstein V: *Aeromonas* and *Plesiomonas* as etiological agents. Annu Rev Microbiol 42:395, 1988

Morris JG Jr, Black RE: Cholera and other vibrioses in the United States. N Engl J Med 312:343, 1985

Richards KL, Douglas SD: Pathophysiological effects of *Vibrio cholerae* and enterotoxinogenic *Escherichia coli* and their exotoxins on eucaryotic cells. Microbiol Rev 42:592, 1978

Rodrick GE, Hood MA, Blake NJ: Human *Vibrio* gastroenteritis. Med Clin North Am 66:665, 1982

von Graevenitz A: *Aeromonas* and *Plesiomonas.* In Lennette EH, Balows A, Hausler WJ Jr, et al (eds): Manual of Clinical Microbiology, ed 4. Washington, DC, American Society for Microbiology, 1985, p 278

West PA: The human pathogenic vibrios—A public health update with environmental perspectives. Epidemiol Infect 103:1, 1989

Selected Articles

Almedia RJ, Hickman-Brenner FW, Sowers EG, et al: Comparison of a latex agglutination assay and an enzyme-linked immunosorbent assay for detecting cholera toxin. J Clin Microbiol 28:128, 1990

Arita M, Takeda T, Honda T, Miwatani T: Purification and characterization of *Vibrio cholerae* non-O1 heat-stable enterotoxin. Infect Immun 52:45, 1986

Attridge SR, Rowley D: The role of the flagellum in adherence of *Vibrio cholerae.* J Infect Dis 147:864, 1983

Attridge SR, Rowley D: The specificity of *Vibrio cholerae* adherence and the significance of the slime agglutinin as a second mediator of in vitro attachment. J Infect Dis 147:873, 1983

Blake PA, Allegra DT, Snyder JD, et al: Cholera—A possible epidemic focus in the United States. N Engl J Med 302:305, 1980

Brayton PR, Bode RB, Colwell RR, et al: *Vibrio cincinnatiensis* sp. nov., a new human pathogen. J Clin Microbiol 23:104, 1986

Brenner DJ, Hickman-Brenner FW, Lee JV, et al: *Vibrio furnissii* (formerly aerogenic biogroup of *Vibrio fluvialis*), a new species isolated from human feces and the environment. J Clin Microbiol 18:816, 1983

Chintis DS, Sharma KD, Kamat RS: Role of somatic antigen of *Vibrio cholerae* in adhesion to intestinal mucosa. J Med Microbiol 15:53, 1982

Chopra AK, Houston CW, Genaux CT, et al: Evidence for production of an enterotoxin and cholera toxin cross-reactive factor by *Aeromonas hydrophila*. J Clin Microbiol 24:661, 1986

Chowdhury MAR, Aziz KMS, Kay BA, Rahim Z: Toxin production by *Vibrio mimicus* strains isolated from human and environmental sources in Bangladesh. J Clin Microbiol 25:2200, 1987

Clark RB, Lister PD, Arneson-Rotert L, Janda JM: In vitro susceptibilities of *Plesiomonas shigelloides* to 24 antibiotics and antibiotic-β-lactamase-inhibitor combinations. Antimicrob Agents Chemother 34:159, 1990

Cook WL, Wachsmuth K, Johnson SR, et al: Persistence of plasmids, cholera toxin genes, and prophage DNA in classical *Vibrio cholerae* O1. Infect Immun 45:222, 1984

Craig JP, Yamanoto K, Takeda Y, et al: Production of cholera-like enterotoxin by a *Vibrio cholerae* non-O-1 strain isolated from the environment. Infect Immun 34:90, 1981

Datta-Roy K, Banerjee K, De SP, Ghose AC: Comparative study of expression of hemagglutinins, hemolysins, and enterotoxins by clinical and environmental isolates of non-O1 *Vibrio cholerae* in relation to their enteropathogenicity. Appl Environ Microbiol 52:875, 1986

Freter R, O'Brien PCM, Macsai MS: Role of chemotaxis in the association of motile bacteria with intestinal mucosa: In vivo studies. Infect Immun 34:234, 1981

Garner SE, Fowlston SE, George WL: Effect of iron on production of a possible virulence factor by *Plesiomonas shigelloides*. J Clin Microbiol 28:811, 1990

Garner SE, Fowlston SE, George WL: In vitro production of cholera toxin-like activity by *Plesiomonas shigelloides*. J Infect Dis 156:720, 1987

Gray LD, Kreger AS: Purification and characterization of an extracellular cytolysin produced by *Vibrio vulnificus*. Infect Immun 48:62, 1985

Gyobu Y, Kodama H, Uetake H: Production and partial purification of a fluid-accumulating factor of non-O1 *Vibrio cholerae*. Microbiol Immunol 32:565, 1988

Herrington DA, Hall RH, Losonsky G, et al: Toxin, toxin-coregulated pili and the toxR regulon are essential for *Vibrio cholerae* pathogenesis in humans. J Exp Med 168:1487, 1988

Herrington DA, Tzipori S, Robins-Browne RM, et al: In vitro and in vivo pathogenicity of *Plesiomonas shigelloides*. Infect Immun 55:979, 1987

Hoge CW, Sethabutr O, Bodhidatta L, et al: Use of a synthetic oligonucleotide probe to detect strains of non-serovar O1 *Vibrio cholerae* carrying the gene for heat-stable enterotoxin (NAG-ST). J Clin Microbiol 28:1473, 1990

Hoge CW, Watsky D, Peeler RN, et al: Epidemiology and spectrum of *Vibrio* infections in a Chesapeake Bay community. J Infect Dis 160:985, 1989

Holmberg SD, Wachsmuth IK, Hickman-Brenner FW, et al: *Plesiomonas* enteric infections in the United States. Ann Intern Med 105:690, 1986

Howard-Jones N: Robert Koch and the cholera vibrio: A centenary. Br Med J 288:379, 1984

Iijima Y, Yamada H, Shinoda S: Adherence of *Vibrio parahaemolyticus* and its relation to pathogenicity. Can J Microbiol 27:1252, 1981

Iwanaga M, Nakasone N, Ehara M: Pili of *Vibrio cholerae* O1 biotype El Tor: A comparative study on adhesive and non-adhesive strains. Microbiol Immunol 33:1, 1989

Johnson G, Svennerholm A, Holmgren J: *Vibrio cholerae* expresses cell surface antigens during intestinal infection which are not expressed during in vitro culture. Infect Immun 57:1809, 1989

Klontz KC, Lieb S, Schreiber M, et al: Syndromes of *Vibrio vulnificus* infections. Clinical and epidemiologic features in Florida cases, 1981–1987. Ann Intern Med 109:318, 1988

Kothary MH, Kreger AS: Purification and characterization of an extracellular cytolysin produced by *Vibrio damsela*. Infect Immun 49:25, 1985

Kreger A, Lockwood D: Detection of extracellular toxin(s) produced by *Vibrio vulnificus*. Infect Immun 33:583, 1981

Levine MM, Black RE, Clements ML, et al: Evaluation in humans of attenuated *Vibrio cholerae* El Tor Ogawa strain Texas Star-SR as a live oral vaccine. Infect Immun 43:515, 1984

Lowry PW, McFarland LM, Peltier BH, et al: *Vibrio* gastroenteritis in Louisiana: A prospective study among attendees of a scientific congress in New Orleans. J Infect Dis 160:978, 1989

Matthews BG, Douglas H, Guiney DG: Production of a heat-stable enterotoxin by *Plesiomonas shigelloides*. Microbiol Pathol 5:207, 1988

Migasena S, Pitisuttitham P, Prayurahong B, et al: Preliminary assessment of the safety and immunogenicity of live oral cholera vaccine strain CVD 103-HgR in healthy Thai adults. Infect Immun 57:3261, 1989

Miyamoto Y, Obara Y, Nikkawa T, et al: Simplified purification and biophysiochemical characteristics of Kanagawa phenomenon-associated hemolysin of *Vibrio parahaemolyticus*. Infect Immun 28:567, 1980

Morris JG Jr, Takeda T, Tall BD, et al: Experimental non-O group 1 *Vibrio cholerae* gastroenteritis in humans. J Clin Invest 85:697, 1990

Nair GB, Oku Y, Taeda Y, et al: Toxin profiles of *Vibrio cholerae* non-O1 from environmental sources in Calcutta, India. Appl Environ Microbiol 54:3180, 1988

Nakasone N, Iwagnaga M: Pili of a *Vibrio parahaemolyticus* strain as a possible colonization factor. Infect Immun 58:61, 1990

Papers presented at the Second International Workshop on *Aeromonas* and *Plesiomonas*. J Diarrhoeal Dis Res 6:77, 1988

Peterson KM, Mekalanos JJ: Characterization of the *Vibrio cholerae* *ToxR* regulon: Identification of novel genes involved in intestinal colonization. Infect Immun 56:2822, 1988

Reinhardt JF, George WL: Comparative in vitro activities of selected antimicrobial agents against *Aeromonas* species and *Plesiomonas shigelloides*. Antimicrob Agents Chemother 27:643, 1985

Research on *Aeromonas* and *Plesiomonas*. Papers presented at the First International Workshop on *Aeromonas* and *Plesiomonas*. Experientia 43:347, 1987

Rose JM, Houston CW, Coppenhaver DH, et al: Purification and chemical characterization of a cholera toxin cross-reactive cytolytic enterotoxin produced by a human isolate of *Aeromonas hydrophilia*. Infect Immun 57:1165, 1989

Saha S, Sanyal SC: Immunobiological relationships among new cholera toxin produced by CT gene-negative strains of *Vibrio cholerae* O1. J Med Microbiol 28:33, 1989

Sanyal SC, Huq MI, Neogy PKB, et al: Experimental studies on the pathogenicity of *Vibrio mimicus* strains isolated in Bangladesh. Aust J Exp Biol Med Sci 62:515, 1984

Schneider DR, Parker CD: Purification and characterization of mucinase of *Vibrio cholerae.* J Infect Dis 145:474, 1982

Shehabi AA, Drexler H, Richardson SH: Virulence mechanisms associated with clinical isolates of non-O1 *Vibrio cholerae.* Zentralbl Bakt Hyg [A] 261:232, 1986

Tacket CO, Brenner F, Blake PA: Clinical features and an epidemiological study of *Vibrio vulnificus* infections. J Infect Dis 149:558, 1984

Tamplin ML, Colwell RR: Effects of microcosm salinity and organic substrate concentration on the production of *Vibrio cholerae* enterotoxin. Appl Environ Microbiol 52:297, 1986

Tamplin ML, Ahmed MK, Jalali R, Colwell RR: Variation in epitopes of the B subunit of el tor and classical biotype *Vibrio cholerae* O1 cholera toxin. J Gen Microbiol 135:1195, 1989

Wall VW, Kreger AS, Richardson SH: Production and partial characterization of a *Vibrio fluvialis* cytotoxin. Infect Immun 46:773, 1984

Yamamoto K, Takeda Y, Miwatani T, et al: Purification and some properties of a non-O1 *Vibrio cholerae* enterotoxin that is identical to cholera enterotoxin. Infect Immun 39:1128, 1983

Yamamoto T, Yokota T: Adherence targets of *Vibrio parahaemolyticus* in human small intestines. Infect Immun 57:2410, 1989

Yoh M, Honda T, Miwatani T: Comparison of hemolysins of *Vibrio cholerae* non-O1 and *Vibrio hollisae* with the thermostable direct hemolysin of *Vibrio parahaemolyticus.* Can J Microbiol 34:1321, 1988

CHAPTER 37

Pseudomonas

The genus *Pseudomonas* is a complex of many species of gram-negative, nonfermentative, aerobic bacilli that inhabit soil and water. In their natural habitat, these widely distributed organisms play an important role in the decomposition of organic matter. Several species are pathogens of plants and animals, and although most *Pseudomonas* do not infect humans, some are important opportunistic pathogens that infect individuals with impaired host defenses. Human infections usually are severe and difficult to treat because of the organisms' resistance to many of the commonly used antibiotics and the underlying condition of the host.

Pseudomonas aeruginosa

Pseudomonas aeruginosa is the most frequently isolated human pathogen of the genus *Pseudomonas*. In a number of hospitals, it is the third most common cause of nosocomial infections being surpassed by only *Staphylococcus aureus* and *Escherichia coli*. *P. aeruginosa* is a major pathogen and a leading cause of death in patients with cystic fibrosis, neoplastic disease, and severe burns.

Morphology and Ultrastructure

P. aeruginosa is a gram-negative rod, measuring 0.5 to 1.0 μm by 3 to 4 μm. Most cells possess a single polar flagellum, but occasionally some may have two or three flagella. Isolates obtained from clinical specimens frequently have pili that promote the attachment of the organism to host cells. An extracellular slime layer, similar to a capsule, is produced. This layer has been referred to as the glycocalyx or mucoid substance and is composed of alginate, an anionic polymer of β-1,4-linked mannuronic acid and L-guluronic acid in which some of the mannuronate residues are mono-O-acetylated and others are di-O-acetylated. Although alginates can be isolated from many biologic sources, they differ in the proportions of mannuronate and guluronate residues and in the tertiary structure formed by polymers of these residues. The alginate of *P. aeruginosa* is unlike other alginates in that it lacks polyguluronate blocks, which makes the overall structure more elastic and less brittle. Organisms isolated from cystic fibrosis patients produce an abundance of the glycocalyx and are extremely mucoid in appearance.

The structure and composition of the cell wall of *P. aeruginosa* resemble those of the gram-negative organisms of the family Enterobacteriaceae (Chap. 33). Like the enteric bacteria, *P. aeruginosa* cell wall lipopolysaccharide (LPS) is composed of core polysaccharides that are common to all strains and side chain polysaccharides that are strain specific. Also, the LPS inner core of both groups of organisms contain 2-keto-3-deoxyoctonic acid (KDO) and lipid A. However, the LPS of *P. aeruginosa* has more phosphorus and contains a distinctive amide-linked L-alanine and the amino sugars fucosamine, quinovosamine, and, occasionally, D-bacillosamine. The lipid A of *P. aeruginosa* lacks the β-hydoxymyristic acid found in the enterobacteria.

Physiology

Biochemical and Cultural Characteristics. *P. aeruginosa* is an extremely adaptable organism that can use over 80 organic compounds for growth. In nature, it lives in a variety of moist environments and can even grow in distilled water. In the laboratory, it can be isolated on virtually any medium. It grows on the media used for the isolation of the enterobacteria, as well as the alkaline media used to isolate *Vibrio* species. Although an aerobic organism, *P. aeruginosa* can use nitrate as a terminal electron acceptor and grow under anaerobic conditions. Arginine can be used anaerobically via the arginine dihydrolase pathway to generate adenosine triphosphate (ATP) by substrate-level phosphorylation. The optimal temperature for growth is 35C, but growth can occur from 10C to 42C.

Clinical isolates are frequently β-hemolytic when grown on blood agar plates. Hemolysis is due to the production of two distinct hemolysins, a heat-labile phospholipase C and a heat-stable glycolipid. Phosphorylase C is a lecithinase that frees phosphorylcholine from lecithin, whereas the hemolytic glycolipid functions as a detergent that acts in combination with a phosphatase to degrade lipids and lecithins in cell membranes. *P. aeruginosa* is the only gram-negative organism that produces the blue phenazine pigment pyocyanin. About 50% of *P. aeruginosa* strains produce this pigment, which is responsible for the characteristic blue pus seen in wounds infected with this organism. Pyocyanin is an antibiotic that may allow the *P. aeruginosa* to exist in nature. It also may play a role in nutrition by functioning as a means of acquiring inorganic phosphate. Other pigments, such as pyoverdin and pyochelin, may play a role in nutrition by accumulating iron.

Energy obtained from the use of carbohydrates is derived from oxidative rather than fermentative pathways. Since the amount of acid produced by oxidative pathways is less than that produced by fermentation, special media, such as the O-F medium of Hugh and Leifson, must be used for diagnostic tests. The carbohydrate utilization tests listed in Table 37–1 used this basal medium. Also listed in Table 37–1 are the biochemical reactions useful for identification of *P. aeruginosa* and other selected *Pseudomonas* species.

Resistance. *P. aeruginosa* is one of the most adaptable vegetative bacteria known. When adequate moisture is provided, it can survive with only minimum nutrients. It can be isolated from a number of sites in the hospital environment, such as respiratory care equipment, baths, water faucets, cold water humidifiers, bed pans, and floors. *P. aeruginosa* is very resistant to chemical disinfection and has even grown in certain types of quaternary ammonium compounds, hexachlorophene soaps, and iodine solutions. Phenolics and β-gluteraldehyde usually are effective disinfectants for *Pseudomonas.* Boiling water kills the organism, as does desiccation. Most of the commonly used antibiotics, particularly the penicillins and first generation cephalosporins, are not effective against *Pseudomonas.*

Genetics. Gene transfer between *P. aeruginosa* strains can occur through conjugation, transduction, and transformation. Strain differences can be detected by serologic typing of the O antigen, phage typing, and pyocin (bacteriocin) typing. Lysogeny is common, and most strains are lysogenic for at least one prophage. Comparisons of genetic maps of pseudomonads to that of the enteric bacteria demonstrate fundamental differences in the arrangement of functionally related genes. The gene arrangement of the pseudomonads is noncontiguous, whereas the enterics have a contiguous arrangement of similar genes. Furthermore, bacteriocinogenic determinants found in plasmids of the Enterobacteriaceae are inserted into the *Pseudomonas* chromosome.

Antigenic Structure

The somatic, or O, antigens have been used to group various strains for epidemiologic purposes. Serologic typing of the O antigen is a less cumbersome and less variable system of strain characterization than is pyocin or phage typing, although the latter systems may be necessary for complete characterization of strains isolated during outbreaks. Various vaccines using commonly isolated O types have been developed for prevention of *Pseudomonas* infections (see p 580). In addition to O antigens, most, if not all, *P. aeruginosa* strains harbor a polyagglutinable antigen (PA). The slime layer of *P. aeruginosa* also is immunogenic and may play a role in protecting the organism from phagocytosis. Active and passive immunization against the slime layer protects animals from the toxic and lethal effects of challenge with live organisms.

Determinants of Pathogenicity

P. aeruginosa is an extremely complex organism that possesses an almost bewildering array of virulence factors that play a

TABLE 37–1. BIOCHEMICAL REACTIONS OF SELECTED *PSEUDOMONAS* SPECIES

Test	*P. aeruginosa*	*P. cepacia*	*P. fluorescens*	*P. mallei*	*P. maltophilia*	*P. pseudomallei*	*P. putida*
Oxidase	+	+	+	d	–	+	+
Oxidation of[a]							
Glucose	+	+	+	+	+	+	+
Maltose	–	+	d	+	+	+	d
Lactose	–	+	d	+	d	+	d
Mannitol	d	+	d	d	–	+	d
Nitrate to N_2 gas	d	–	–	–	–	+	–
Pyocyanin	d	–	–	–	–	–	–
Lysine decarboxylase	–	+	–	–	+	–	–
Ornithine decarboxylase	–	d	–	–	–	–	–
Arginine dihydrolase	+	–	+	+	–	+	+
Growth at 42C	+	d	–	–	d	+	–

+, greater than 90% of strains positive; –, less than 10% of strains positive; d, Between 11% and 89% of strains positive.
[a] Organisms grown at 30C in O-F medium of Hugh and Leifson.

role in human disease. There are anatomic features that aid in the establishment and maintenance of the organism in various host systems and a variety of extracellular products that induce numerous pathologic changes. The exact role of each of these factors probably differs with the site of infection and the underlying condition of the host.

P. aeruginosa exists in nature in two forms, a freely motile swimming form and a microcolony form encased in an enlarged glycocalyx. It has been postulated that these forms, which enable the organism to survive in an aquatic environment, also play an important role in the establishment and dissemination of the organism in human infections. Motility is important in the establishment of the organism and dissemination to new sites. Both motile and nonmotile organisms are fully capable of infecting and proliferating in burn sites, but the incidence of secondary bacteremia and systemic invasion is less in infections caused by nonmotile forms. Passive immunization with antiflagellar antibody also decreases systemic invasion and sepsis in animals infected with motile forms. The microcolony appears to be the means by which the organism exists in the lungs of cystic fibrosis patients. Electron micrographs of postmortem lung tissue of cystic fibrosis patients provide direct evidence for the existence of the microcolonies in tissue, and the organisms isolated from these patients produce extremely mucoid colonies. Similar evidence points to the existence of microcolonies in bladders of catheterized patients with *Pseudomonas* infections. The glycocalyx encasing the microcolony protects the organism from antibodies directed against the O antigens, and the size of the microcolony prevents phagocytosis. The glycocalyx may serve to initiate attachment of the organism to the mucins produced in cystic fibrosis patients, and the flexibility of the microcolony may allow it to conform to the lung during coughing, thereby preventing it from being dislodged and removed.

In addition to the glycocalyx, there are other factors, such as pili, that enable the organism to attach to host cells. Interestingly, the attachment of organisms to tracheal cells requires prior injury to the cells. Such injuries can be caused mechanically by the intubation procedures common on intensive care units and with surgery, chemically by acids from aspirations of stomach contents, or from other infectious agents, such as influenza viruses. Enzymatic injury has been proposed as a mechanism of altering host cells. Fibronectin normally protects cells from bacterial attachment and frequently is lost when there is an increase in the level of salivary proteases. The colonization of cystic fibrosis patients by *P. aeruginosa* may be due to this mechanism, since these patients have increased levels of proteases and decreased levels of fibronectin. Colonization of the respiratory tract also may be enhanced by the production of the pigment pyocyanin, which has been shown to decrease the beating of respiratory cilia.

The cell wall LPS or endotoxin of *P. aeruginosa* may play an important role in the pathogenesis of human infections. Because *Pseudomonas* endotoxin is not as toxic as the endotoxin of the Enterobacteriaceae, some researchers do not believe that the toxic properties of endotoxin are as important as other toxins in pseudomonal disease. However, LPS may be important in establishing infection, since LPS antibody is highly protective against infection in experimental models, and mutants deficient in high molecular weight polysaccharides are 1000 times less virulent than the parent strains.

Once established in the host, *P. aeruginosa* produces a number of extracellular enzymes and toxins that may be important in human disease. One of the toxins that is thought to play a major role in *Pseudomonas* infections is exotoxin A. This toxin is lethal for animals and produces a number of pathologic effects in animal models. There is indirect evidence that this toxin is produced also during human infections. Elevated antibody titers to exotoxin A are produced during infection, and antibody to exotoxin A appears to be important for the survival of immunocompromised patients. Furthermore, patients who are bacteremic with exotoxin A-producing strains have a higher mortality than patients bacteremic with non-toxin-producing strains.

The mode of action of exotoxin A is identical to that of *Corynebacterium diphtheriae* (Chap. 30). Both toxins have ADP-ribosyl transferase activity, which inactivates the elongation factor 2 (EF-2) of eucaryotic cells by catalyzing the transfer of ADP from NAD to a modified histidine residue in EF-2, causing a cessation of protein synthesis and cell death. Both toxins bind to cell surface receptors and then enter coated pits in the cells, known as endocytic vesicles. These vesicles rapidly acidify, exposing hydrophobic residues that probably assist the toxins in inserting into the membrane. From this site, the toxins enter the cytosol as enzymatically active fragments that inactivate EF-2. Although the two toxins are similar in many respects, there are differences. The target organ of exotoxin A is the liver, whereas diphtheria toxin affects the heart. The molecular receptor sites for the two toxins also differ. Both toxins have similar molecular weights, but their amino acid sequences are similar only in regions that bind NAD and that catalyze the ADP-ribosylation reactions. Exotoxin A is synthesized intracellularly as a 638 amino acid precursor. A 25 amino acid residue at the amino terminus of the precursor molecule is thought to be responsible for the secretion of the toxin from *P. aeruginosa*. The active form of exotoxin A is a single-chain polypeptide consisting of 613 amino acid residues divided into three functional domains. The amino-terminal end comprises the domain responsible for binding to eucaryotic cell receptors, the middle domain is responsible for translocation, and the carboxyterminal end contains the domain with enzymatic activity.

P. aeruginosa produces many other toxins besides exotoxin A that may play a role in human infections. One of these toxins, exoenzyme S, is a second distinct ADP-ribosyl transferase that is produced by approximately 40% of clinical isolates. The target of exoenzyme S, however, is not elongation factor 2 but rather one or more proteins in eucaryotic cells. The exact role of exoenzyme S has not been delineated clearly, but studies in animal models indicate that this toxin enhances the severity of the infection. Purified exoenzyme S produces extensive gross changes in rat lungs within 2 hours, and treatment of monolayers of bronchial fibroblasts results in vacuolation and membrane damage. These findings suggest that exoenzyme S may play a role in the characteristic necrotic injury seen in *P. aeruginosa* pneumonia. In the burnt-mouse model, exotoxin S-producing strains are more likely to become disseminated in the blood than are non-toxin-producing strains.

The phosphorylase C hemolysin also may contribute to the invasiveness of the organism by destroying pulmonary surfactant and attacking pulmonary tissue to produce atelectasis and necrosis. Several proteases are produced by most strains of *P. aeruginosa*. These enzymes may be responsible for the hemorrhagic skin lesions observed in some patients. One protease, elastase, also plays an important role in corneal infections and enhances the effects of exotoxin A in lung infections. Elastase has been shown to degrade immunoglobulins, complement, coagulation factors, and α-proteinase. These properties may enable the organism to survive in the bloodstream. *P. aeruginosa* also produces a cytotoxin. Although this toxin was originally described as a leukocidin, it is toxic to most eucaryotic cells studied. An enterotoxin, which may play a role in the diarrhea seen in some patients, has been isolated.

Clinical Infection

Epidemiology. *P. aeruginosa* infections occur in patients with altered host defenses, traumatic wounds, or burns or who require catheterization or entubation. Epidemiologic investigations have shown that *P. aeruginosa* is responsible for 10% of all nosocomial infections, 11% of all blood isolates, but only 4% of nosocomial epidemics. In specialty units, such as burn or cancer centers, *P. aeruginosa* is the leading gram-negative isolate and may cause 30% of all infections. Nonhospitalized individuals also acquire pseudomonal infections. Intravenous drug abusers are prone to pseudomonas endocarditis and osteomyelitis. Folliculitis occurs in patients exposed to improperly maintained hot tubs and swimming pools. This population is also prone to an external otitis known as *swimmer's ear*. Corneal infections have been attributed to contaminated contact lens fluid, cosmetics, and trauma to the eye.

The ubiquitous nature of *P. aeruginosa* enhances its spread. It is present not only in soil and water but also on the skin of some normal individuals and in approximately 10% of normal stools. Colonization of patients increases with the length of hospital stay. In one study, 19% of patients admitted to an intensive care unit from the community were colonized, whereas 34% of patients admitted to the unit from other parts of the hospital were colonized. By the seventh day on the unit, 90% of all patients were colonized. The loss of normal flora by use of broad-spectrum antibiotics enhances the colonization rate. Contaminated respiratory care equipment, catheters, intravenous fluids, and even soaps have been vehicles for transmission of the organism. The presence of *Pseudomonas* on lettuce has led some experts to ban this food on oncology and bone marrow transplant units to lessen the chances for colonizing the gastrointestinal tracts of patients on these services.

Pathogenesis and Clinical Manifestations. *P. aeruginosa* can infect almost any tissue or body site. Localized lesions occur in burns or wounds, corneal tissue, urinary tract, or lungs. The organisms can spread from the localized lesions via the hematogenous route, causing septicemia and focal lesions in other tissue. Mortality in septic patients is high and may approach 80% in immunocompromised patients. Approximately 30% of patients with *P. aeruginosa* septicemia will have ecthyma gangrenosum.

Pseudomonas pneumonia is associated with a high mortality, which approaches 70% compared to the 35% seen with other gram-negative pneumonias. Patients experience toxicity, confusion, and progressive cyanosis. Empyema is common, and x-rays of lower lobes reveal infiltrates and nodules that may necrose with abscess formation. The virulent form of *Pseudomonas* pneumonia is seen most frequently in cancer patients and patients on intensive care units. In cystic fibrosis patients, *Pseudomonas* pneumonia is a chronic process with progressive lung destruction. Death in these patients is usually a result of pulmonary insufficiency and anoxia and not generalized dissemination of the organism. The major factor in controlling the spread of the organism is a functioning phagocytic system, which most cystic fibrosis patients have. Neutropenic patients with granulocyte counts below 500 have the highest mortality with pneumonia and other pseudomonal infections.

P. aeruginosa urinary tract infections also are common, particularly in patients who have had bladder manipulations, such as cystoscopy or catheterization. Pyelonephritis is a frequent complication of ascending infections, although it can also be a result of hematogenous spread of the organism. Cure of urinary tract infections often is hindered by the underlying conditions of the host, which may require prolonged catheter use. The urinary tract often serves as an important source of organisms for infections in other parts of the body.

P. aeruginosa is the second leading cause of burn infections, ranking behind *S. aureus*. The organisms proliferate in the eschar, and when the organism density exceeds 10^5/g of tissue, they spread to the blood and cause a lethal bacteremia. In one burn institute, *Pseudomonas* bacteremia was associated with a 28% increase in mortality.

Pseudomonas endocarditis is a complication of bacteremia that is seen most frequently in intravenous drug abusers. The tricuspid valve is involved most frequently, although other valves may be affected. Left-sided endocarditis requires surgery as well as medical treatment. Complications include embolic lesions in the lung that frequently cavitate.

Intravenous drug abusers also are susceptible to developing *Pseudomonas* osteomyelitis of the vertebrae or clavicle. Vertebral osteomyelitis has occurred in patients with urinary tract infections. The spread of the organism from the urinary tract is thought to occur through the lumbar paravertebral veins that communicate with the veins of the pelvis. Osteomyelitis also occurs in children as a complication of puncture wounds to the foot. An osteomyelitis of the temporal bone at the site where cranial nerves exit can develop in elderly patients with underlying disease, such as diabetes. This disease is known as malignant otitis, since the organism gains access to the deep tissue via the external auditory canal through defects in the anatomic structure of the canal. Extension of the infection to the petrous ridge with subsequent development of brain abscess is a complication seen in some patients.

Pseudomonas eye infections usually result from an abrasion from contact lens, eye pads, surgery, or some other trauma. The first indication is an ulcer at the site of infection. This ulcer may progress rapidly to a panophthalmitis, with destruction of the eye by the proteases. A blepharoconjunctivitis may develop following the application of mascara.

The recreational use of hot tubs has caused an increase in dermatologic infections with *P. aeruginosa*. A unique syndrome, characterized by a vesicular or pustular rash, malaise, fatigue, and otitis externa, develops within hours after exposure to contaminated tubs or spas. Mastitis can occur in 10% of people, and urinary tract infections and pneumonia have developed in some patients. In most patients, the folliculitis is self-limiting.

Laboratory Diagnosis. Diagnosis of *Pseudomonas* infections is made by the isolation of the organism. This process does not require any unusual procedures. Since the organism grows on most commonly used media, it can be isolated from any properly collected and transported specimen. It can be differentiated from the enterics by a positive oxidase test and its oxidative metabolism. Differentiation from other pseudomonads can be made by the tests listed in Table 37–1.

Treatment. Most of the commonly used antibiotics are not effective in the treatment of *P. aeruginosa* infections. Prevention of colonization, control of the underlying disease, and a functioning phagocytic system are the most important factors in the survival of patients with infections caused by this organism.

A majority of *P. aeruginosa* strains are susceptible to the aminoglycosides (amikacin, gentamicin, and tobramycin) and the extended-spectrum penicillins (azlocillin, carbenicillin, mezlocillin, piperacillin, and ticarcillin) on initial isolation. However, resistance develops if the duration of therapy is long and when the penicillins are used alone. Combinations of high-dose aminoglycosides and extended-spectrum penicillins are recommended for life-threatening infections. Third-generation cephalosporins, such as ceftazidime and cefoperazone, have antipseudomonal activity. These antibiotics appear to have an advantage in neurologic infections and are useful in patients with impaired renal function. However, resistant strains also develop. Two newer types of antibiotics with antipseudomonal activity, the quinolones and the carbapenems, are now being marketed. Ciprofloxacin is an example of a quinolone with good antipseudomonal activity, and imipenem is the first practical carbapenem. The usefulness of these newer agents requires evaluation over a period of time, since resistant forms occur with extended use.

Therapy of burn infections is aimed at keeping the organism burden below 10^5/g of tissue to prevent septicemia, since it appears to be impossible to prevent the colonization of the burn by *P. aeruginosa.* Topical application of Sulfamylon cream, silver sulfadiazine cream, or silver nitrate soaks is the most commonly accepted form of therapy for burns.

Immunologic therapy in the form of hyperimmune gamma globulin and granulocyte transfusion has been used with some success in the treatment of patients with neoplastic disease.

Control. Control measures should be aimed at preventing colonization of patients with *Pseudomonas.* Elimination of the organism from the environment would be impossible, but proper care of respiratory care equipment and other invasive instruments will reduce the spread of the organism via these objects. Prevention of moisture accumulation also will reduce the organism burden.

At least two manufacturers have prepared vaccines of cell wall preparations of *P. aeruginosa.* The success of these vaccines is mixed. A 3-year prospective vaccine trial in cystic fibrosis patients failed to show a difference in colonization rate or progression of disease in the vaccinated group as compared to the control group. In another study conducted in burn patients in New Delhi, there was a fourfold reduction of mortality in the vaccinated adult population and a twofold reduction in the mortality of the vaccinated children. These results have not been duplicated in other countries. Also, these vaccines have frequent side effects and require multiple injections.

The side effects seen with the older vaccines appear to be due to the LPS content. Other vaccines with lower LPS content have been developed and seem to have a lower incidence of adverse side reactions. Combination vaccines composed of the more purified vaccine with toxoid of exotoxin A produce high levels of antibody in volunteers for an extended period. Other investigators are developing vaccines directed at the outer membrane protein-F, *Pseudomonas* flagella, or glycocalyx. Instead of attempting to vaccinate patients with pseudomonal infections, some investigators have attempted to use passive immunization to obtain protection. Promising results have been obtained both in animal studies and in pilot clinical trials. The usefulness of these newer immunologic approaches has yet to be determined in large-scale controlled trials.

Other *Pseudomonas* Species

A number of other *Pseudomonas* species have been isolated from clinical specimens and the hospital environment. When they are isolated from clinical specimens, careful evaluation of the clinical condition of the patient must be made, since these organisms may represent contaminants or colonizers rather than etiologic agents of disease. Like *P. aeruginosa,* most of the other members of the genus are found in soil and water. *Pseudomonas mallei,* however, appears to be a specialized animal pathogen. The laboratory characteristics of the more common or important pathogens are listed in Table 37–1.

Pseudomonas cepacia. One of the more frequently isolated pseudomonads is *P. cepacia,* formerly classified as EO-1, *Pseudomonas kingii,* and *Pseudomonas multivorans.* It has been associated with endocarditis, septicemia, and wound and urinary tract infections. Most infections occur in patients who are debilitated or immunosuppressed or whose host defenses are compromised by instrumentation or trauma. Nosocomial infections have been traced to the use of contaminated medications, antiseptics, and instruments. Several cystic fibrosis centers have reported increased rates of isolation of *P. cepacia* from their patients. As in *P. aeruginosa* infections, two clinical situations occur with cystic fibrosis patients who acquire *P. cepacia* in their lungs. In one group of patients, the organism appears only to colonize the lung without any apparent change in clinical status. However, in the other group of patients, there is rapid clinical deterioration. One study showed that the severity of the underlying disease, the use of aminoglycoside antibiotics, and having a sibling with cystic fibrosis were risk factors for *P. cepacia* colonization. Another study showed a sharp decline in *P. cepacia* colonization in cystic fibrosis patients when strict infection control methods were employed, indicating that there is patient-to-patient transfer of the organism. The epidemiology of *P. cepacia* cystic fibrosis infections may become clear as investigators apply the newer subgrouping methods of fatty acid composition, chromosome analysis, and serologic and bacteriocin typing. A better understanding of the true incidence of *P. cepacia* infections will be obtained as more laboratories use the selective media developed to isolate the organism from contaminated specimens, such as sputum.

An extracellular protease, which has properties similar to the elastase of *P. aeruginosa,* has been isolated from culture filtrates of *P. cepacia.* It produces a bronchopneumonia with leukocyte infiltration and proteinaceous exudates in rats. The role of this enzyme in cystic fibrosis and other pulmonary infections requires further investigation.

Treatment of *P. cepacia* infections is difficult because of the innate resistance of the organism to most antibiotics. However, most strains on initial isolation are sensitive to chloramphenicol and the combination of trimethoprim-sulfamethoxazole. Ceftazidime, a third-generation cephalosporin, has shown some promise as an effective agent. Most strains are sensitive in laboratory tests, and some patients who have failed conventional therapy have shown clinical improvement with ceftazidime.

***Pseudomonas maltophilia* (*Xanthomonas maltophilia*).** There is some question about the taxonomic placement of this organism, and some authors have proposed that it be placed in the genus *Xanthomonas* as *X. maltophilia.* However, since the majority of the clinical literature uses the name *Pseudomonas maltophilia,* it is discussed in this chapter. Like most of the other organisms of the genus, *P. maltophilia* is found in soil and water. In addition, it frequently colonizes the oropharynx of normal adults. Therefore, the laboratory isolation of this organism requires careful evaluation of the clinical situation before determining its role in the patient's disease. Nonetheless, *P. maltophilia* infections of wounds, lung, cerebrospinal fluid, urinary tract, and blood have been documented. As with infections caused by other *Pseudomonas* species, most infections occur in patients whose host defenses are compromised. Clusters of nosocomial infections have been described. In one outbreak of urinary tract infections, transmission of the organism was attributed to the use of a contaminated disinfectant solution. Antimicrobial susceptibility varies with the strain isolated, but most isolates are susceptible to trimethoprim-sulfamethoxazole. Resistance to β-lactam antibiotics is attributed both to a low outer membrane permeability to the drugs and to the production of two broad-spectrum β-lactamases.

Pseudomonas mallei. This organism appears to be a specialized animal pathogen, causing the disease glanders in horses and donkeys. Humans are infected by direct contact through skin abrasions and inhalation of the organism. Since this disease has been eliminated from the equine population of the United States and Canada, the disease rarely is seen in these countries.

Pseudomonas pseudomallei. This organism is a common inhabitant of the soil of the tropics and subtropics between latitudes 20 N and 20 S. It causes melioidosis, a glanderslike disease, in humans. In a report from a 1000-bed hospital in Thailand, there were approximately 100 cases of culture-proven melioidosis each year, with the majority of cases occurring during the rainy season. About 150 cases were diagnosed in U.S. servicemen during the Vietnam war, with about one third of the cases occurring in helicopter crews. The organism gains entrance to the body by inhalation, ingestion, or through skin abrasions.

The disease may take one of four forms: acute, subacute, chronic, or latent. In the acute form, septicemia occurs with abscess formation in virtually every organ of the body. Clinically, it cannot be distinguished from other gram-negative septic episodes. The mortality remains at 30% in spite of antibiotic therapy. The subacute form is characterized by a prolonged course, with abscess formation in various organs, a milder bacteremia, and pneumonia. The chronic form has a benign pulmonary course, mimicking primary tuberculosis or a fungal infection. Some patients may have prostatitis. Serologic evidence shows that approximately 30% of the adult population in endemic areas have antibodies to *P. pseudomallei,* indicating a latent or asymptomatic infection. Both the chronic and latent forms may be reactivated to a symptomatic form after many years. Reactivation may be triggered by the development of other diseases, such as cancer. This delay has given the disease the nickname *Vietnamese timebomb.* At the time of reactivation, the organism can be isolated from blood, pus, sputum, or urine.

P. pseudomallei produces a lethal exotoxin that inhibits protein and DNA synthesis in macrophages. This toxin may be responsible for the abscess formation that characterizes this disease. The organism can survive and proliferate intracellularly in polymorphonuclear and mononuclear leukocytes, which may be responsible for the organism's ability to survive in vivo for extended periods of time.

The treatment of choice is trimethoprim-sulfamethoxazole for an extended course, although in vitro studies show that these drugs are only inhibitory for the organism. Most strains are sensitive also to tetracycline, chloramphenicol, and sulfadiazine. In vitro studies indicate that imipenem is the most effective drug, with concentrations between 0.5 and 1 μg/mL killing most isolates. However, no clinical data on the usefulness of imipenem are available at this time. The organism is resistant to the aminoglycoside antibiotics.

Other Species. Other *Pseudomonas* species are isolated from clinical material. Frequently, they are not the etiologic agents of disease but rather represent colonization. However, many of these organisms have been shown to be the causes of opportunistic infections similar to those of the more frequently isolated pseudomonads.

FURTHER READING

Books and Reviews

Clarke PH, Richmond MH (eds): Genetics and Biochemistry of Pseudomonas. London, Wiley, 1975

Cryz SJ: Current topic: *Pseudomonas aeruginosa* infections. Eur J Clin Microbiol 4:153, 1985

Döring G, Holder IA, Botzenhart K: Basic research and clinical aspects of *P. aeruginosa.* Antibiot Chemother 39:1, 1987

Gacesa P, Russell NJ (eds): Pseudomonas Infection and Alginates. London, Chapman and Hall, 1990

Gilardi GL: *Pseudomonas.* In Lennette EH, Balows A, Hausler WJ Jr, et al (eds): Manual of Clinical Microbiology, ed 4. Washington, DC, American Society for Microbiology, 1985, p 350

Goldman DA, Klinger JD: *Pseudomonas cepacia:* Biology, mechanisms of virulence, epidemiology. J Pediatr 108:806, 1986

Gustafson TL, Band JD, Hutcheson RH Jr, et al: Pseudomonas folliculitis: An outbreak and review. Rev Infect Dis 5:1, 1983

Hiby N, Pedersen SS, Shand GH, et al: *Pseudomonas aeruginosa* infection. Antibiot Chemother 42:1, 1989

Holloway DE, Morgan AF: Genome organization in *Pseudomonas.* Annu Rev Microbiol 40:79, 1986

Hornick DB: Pulmonary host defense: Defects that lead to chronic inflammation of the airway. Clin Chest Med 9:669, 1988

Howe C, Sampath A, Spontnitz M: The pseudomallei group: A review. J Infect Dis 124:598, 1971

Kanai K, Dejsirilert S: *Pseudomonas pseudomallei* and melioidosis with special reference to the status in Thailand. Jpn J Med Sci Biol 41:123, 1988

Martone WJ, Osterman CA, Fisher KA, et al: *Pseudomonas cepacia:* Implications and control of epidemic nosocomial colonization. Rev Infect Dis 3:708, 1981

Neu HC: The role of *Pseudomonas aeruginosa* in infections. J Antimicrob Chemother 11(suppl B):1, 1983

Pastan I, FitzGerald D: *Pseudomonas* exotoxin: Chimeric toxins. J Biol Chem 264:15157, 1989

Pennington JE: *Pseudomonas aeruginosa* vaccines and immunotherapy. Infect Dis Clin North Am 4:259, 1990

Pier GB: Pulmonary disease associated with *Pseudomonas aeruginosa* in cystic fibrosis: Current status of the host–bacterium interaction. J Infect Dis 151:575, 1985

Pitt TL: Epidemiological typing of *Pseudomonas aeruginosa.* Eur J Clin Microbiol Infect Dis 7:238, 1988

Ramphal R, Vishwanath S: Why is *Pseudomonas* the colonizer and why does it persist? Infection 15:281, 1987

Sadoff JC, Sanford JP (eds): Symposium on *Pseudomonas aeruginosa* infections. Rev Infect Dis 5(suppl 5):S833, 1983

Vasil ML: *Pseudomonas aeruginosa:* Biology, mechanisms of virulence, epidemiology. J Pediatr 108:800, 1986

von Graevenitz A: Clinical role of infrequently encountered nonfermenters. In Gilardi, GL (ed): Glucose Nonfermenting Gram-Negative Bacteria in Clinical Microbiology. West Palm Beach, CRC Press, 1978, p 119

Wieland M, Lederman MM, Kline-King C, et al: Left-sided endocarditis due to *Pseudomonas aeruginosa:* A report of 10 cases and review of the literature. Medicine 65:180, 1986

Woods DE, Iglewski BH: Toxins of *Pseudomonas aeruginosa:* New perspectives. Rev Infect Dis 5(suppl 4):S715, 1983

Selected Articles

Baltch AL, Hammer MC, Smith RP, et al: Effects of *Pseudomonas aeruginosa* cytotoxin on human serum and granuloyctes and their microbiocidal, phagocytic, and chemotactic functions. Infect Immun 48:498, 1985

Baltimore RS, Christie CD, Smith GJ: Immunohistopathologic localization of *Pseudomonas aeruginosa* in lungs from patients with cystic fibrosis. Implications for the pathogenesis of progressive lung deterioration. Am Rev Respir Dis 140:1650, 1989

Carson LA, Tablan OC, Cusick LB, et al: Comparative evaluation of selective media for isolation of *Pseudomonas cepacia* from cystic fibrosis patients and environmental sources. J Clin Microbiol 26:2096, 1988

Chaudhary VK, Jinno Y, FitzGerald D, Pastan I: *Pseudomonas* exotoxin contains a specific sequence at the carboxyl terminus that is required for cytotoxicity. Proc Natl Acad Sci USA 87:308, 1990

Chaudhary VK, Jinno Y, Gallo MG, et al: Mutagenesis of *Pseudomonas* exotoxin in identification of sequences responsible for the animal toxicity. J Biol Chem 265:16306, 1990

Cross AS, Sadoff JC, Iglewski BH, et al: Evidence for the role of toxin A in the pathogenesis of infections with *Pseudomonas aeruginosa.* J Infect Dis 142:538, 1980

Cryz SJ Jr, Pitt TL, Furer E, et al: Role of lipopolysaccharide in virulence of *Pseudomonas aeruginosa.* Infect Immun 44:508, 1984

Cryz SJ Jr, Sadoff JC, Ohman D, Furer E: Characterization of the human immune response to *Pseudomonas aeruginosa* O-polysaccharidetoxin A conjugate vaccine. J Lab Clin Med 111:701, 1988

Dance DAB, Wuthiekanun V, Chaowagul W, White NJ: The antimicrobial susceptibility of *Pseudomonas pseudomallei.* Emergence of resistance in vitro and during treatment. J Antimicrob Chemother 24:295, 1989

Drake D, Montie TC: Flagella, motility and invasive virulence of *Pseudomonas aeruginosa.* J Gen Microbiol 134:43, 1988

Fisher MC, Long SS, Roberts EM, et al: *Pseudomonas maltophilia* bacteremia in children undergoing open heart surgery. JAMA 246:1571, 1981

Hamood AN, Olson JC, Vincent TS, Iglewski BH: Regions of toxin A involved in toxin A excretion in *Pseudomonas aeruginosa.* J Bacteriol 171:1817, 1989

Holder IA: Experimental studies of the pathogenesis of infections owing to *Pseudomonas aeruginosa:* Elastase, an IgG protease Can J Microbiol 30:1118, 1984

Iglewski BH, Sadoff J, Bjorn MJ, et al: *Pseudomonas aeruginosa* exoenzyme S: An adenosine diphosphate ribosyltransferase distinct from toxin A. Proc Natl Acad Sci USA 75:3211, 1978

Kreger AS, Gray LD: Purification of *Pseudomonas aeruginosa* proteases and microscopic characterization of pseudomonal protease-induced rabbit corneal damage. Infect Immun 19:630, 1978

Kulczski LL, Murphy TM, Bellanti JA: *Pseudomonas* colonization in cystic fibrosis a study of 160 patients. JAMA 240:30, 1978

Langford DT, Hiller J: Prospective, controlled study of a polyvalent pseudomonas vaccine in cystic fibrosis—Three-year results. Arch Dis Child 59:1131, 1984

Leppla SH, Martin OC, Muehl LA: The exotoxin of *P. aeruginosa:* A proenzyme having an unusual mode of action. Biochem Biophys Res Commun 81:532, 1978

McEniry DW, Gillespie SH, Felmingham D: Susceptibility of *Pseudomonas pseudomallei* to new β-lactam and aminoglycoside antibiotics. J Antimicrob Chemother 21:171, 1988

McKevitt, AI, Bajaksouzian S, Klinger JD, Woods DE: Purification and characterization of an extracellular protease from *Pseudomonas cepacia.* Infect Immun 57:771, 1989

Mett H, Rosta S, Schacher B, Frei R: Outer membrane permeability and β-lactamase content in *Pseudomonas maltophilia* clinical isolates and laboratory mutants. Rev Infect Dis 10:765, 1988

Mohamed R, Nathan S, Embi N, et al: Inhibition of macromolecular synthesis in cultured macrophages by *Pseudomonas pseudomallei* exotoxin. Microbiol Immunol 33:811, 1989

Mukwaya GM, Welch DF: Subgrouping of *Pseudomonas cepacia* by cellular fatty acid composition. J Clin Microbiol 27:2640, 1989

Nicas TI, Bradley J, Lochner JE, et al: The role of exoenzyme S infections with *Pseudomonas aeruginosa.* J Infect Dis 152:716, 1985

Olson B, Weinstein RA, Nathan C, et al: Epidemiology of endemic *Pseudomonas aeruginosa:* Why infection control efforts have failed. J Infect Dis 150:808, 1984

Pennington JE: Lipopolysaccharide pseudomonas vaccine: Efficacy against pulmonary infection with *Pseudomonas aeruginosa.* J Infect Dis 140:72, 1979

Pier GB, Thomas DM: Characterization of the human response to a polysaccharide vaccine from *Pseudomonas aeruginosa.* J Infect Dis 148:206, 1983

Pollack M, Young LS: Protective activity of antibodies to exotoxin A and lipopolysaccharide at onset of *Pseudomonas aeruginosa* septicemia in man. J Clin Invest 63:276, 1979

Pruksachartvuthi S, Aswapokee N, Thankerngpol K: Survival of *Pseudomonas pseudomallei* in human phagocytes. J Med Microbiol 31:109, 1990

Rabkin CS, Jarvis WR, Anderson RL, et al: *Pseudomonas cepacia* typing systems: Collaborative study to assess their potential in epidemiologic investigations. Rev Infect Dis 11:600, 1989

Ramphal R, Sadoff JC, Pyle M, et al: Role of pili in the adherence of *Pseudomonas aeruginosa* to tracheal epithelium. Infect Immun 44:38, 1984

Ramphal R, Small PM, Shands JW Jr, et al: Adherence of *Pseudomonas aeruginosa* to tracheal cells injured by influenza infection or endotracheal entubation. Infect Immun 27:614, 1980

Sokol PA, Dennis JJ, MacDougall PC, et al: Cloning and expression of the *Pseudomonas aeruginosa* exoenzyme S toxin gene. Microbiol Pathogen 8:243, 1990

Sokol PA, Iglewski BH, Hager TA, et al: Production of exoenzyme S by clinical isolates of *Pseudomonas aeruginosa.* Infect Immun 34:147, 1981

Suryanarayanan V, Ramphal R: Adherence of *Pseudomonas aeruginosa* to human tracheobronchial mucin. Infect Immun 45:197, 1984

Swings J, de Vos P, Van den Mooter M, et al: Transfer of *Pseudomonas maltophilia* Hugh 1981 to the genus *Xanthomonas* as *Xanthomonas maltophilia* (Hugh 1981) comb. nov. Int J Syst Bacteriol 33:409, 1983

Tablon OC, Chorba TL, Schidlow DV, et al: *Pseudomonas cepacia* colonization in patients with cystic fibrosis: Risk factors and clinical outcome. J Pediatr 107:382, 1985

Thomassen MJ, Demko CA, Doershuk CF, et al: *Pseudomonas cepacia:* Decrease in colonization in patients with cystic fibrosis. Am Rev Respir Dis 134:669, 1986

Van Wye JE, Collins MS, Baylor M, et al: *Pseudomonas* hyperimmune globulin passive immunotherapy for pulmonary exacerbations in cystic fibrosis. Pediatr Pul 9:7, 1990

Vasil ML, Iglewski BH: Comparative toxicities of diphtheria toxin and *Pseudomonas aeruginosa* exotoxin A: Evidence for different cell receptors. J Gen Microbiol 108:333, 1979

White NJ, Dance DAB: Clinical and laboratory studies of malaria and melioidosis. Trans R Soc Trop Med Hyg 82:15, 1988

Wilson R, Pitt T, Taylor G, et al: Pyocyanin and 1-hydroxyphenazine produced by *Pseudomonas aeruginosa* inhibit the beating of human respiratory cilia in vitro. J Clin Invest 79:221, 1987

Woods DE, Hwang WS, Shahrabadi MS, Que JU: Alteration of pulmonary structure by *Pseudomonas aeruginosa* exoenzyme S. J Med Microbiol 26:133, 1988

Woods DE, Que JU: Purification of *Pseudomonas aeruginosa* exoenzyme S. Infect Immun 55:579, 1987

Woods DE, Strauss DC, Johnson WJ Jr, et al: Role of pili in adherence of *Pseudomonas aeruginosa* to mammalian buccal epithelial cells. Infect Immun 29:1146, 1980

CHAPTER 38

Yersinia

The genus *Yersinia* contains three species of facultatively intracellular bacteria that are pathogenic for humans—*Yersinia pestis, Yersinia enterocolitica,* and *Yersinia pseudotuberculosis.* These are primarily animal pathogens, and humans are accidental hosts for infection. *Y. pestis* is the etiologic agent of plague. *Y. enterocolitica* and *Y. pseudotuberculosis* cause an enteritis that can vary in severity from a mild disease to a severe gastrointestinal illness that mimics acute appendicitis. In addition to these pathogens, the genus also contains *Yersinia intermedia, Yersinia kristensenii,* and *Yersinia frederiksenii,* which behave more like opportunistic pathogens. Previously classified in the genus *Pasteurella,* these organisms are now a separate genus in the family Enterobacteriaceae. They express the enterobacterial common antigen, and their physiologic characteristics and lipid composition are similar to those of other Enterobacteriaceae species.

Yersinia pestis

History. Fragments of early writing suggest that plague was present in the western world more than 2000 years ago, but the extent of the disease at that time is unknown. The first documented pandemic occurred during the reign of the Byzantine emperor Justinian I in AD 542. It probably began in Egypt or Ethiopia, spread widely, and lasted 60 years. Approximately 100 million persons died of the infection, and many towns were completely decimated.

The second pandemic, known as the Black Death, started in the fourteenth century. The disease originated in Central Asia and became rampant throughout Europe, the Near East, India, and China. Both rats and infectious droplets from pneumonic victims played a prominent role in transmission of the disease. In Europe alone, 25 million persons died, one fourth of the entire population. After the second pandemic, the disease became endemic among urban rat populations in many of the affected areas. Periodic smaller epidemics continued to occur through the seventeenth century, but from that time until the end of the nineteenth century, the disease was relatively quiescent.

The third pandemic originated in Burma, spread to China in 1894, and from Hong Kong was carried to other continents, including North America, via rat-infested ships. The United States was invaded for the first time. The toll in India was especially high, with more than 10 million recorded deaths during the next 20 years. During this last pandemic, foci of plague became firmly established among wild commensal rodents in large rural areas. These foci currently give rise to sporadic cases of plague that have a potential for dissemination even in countries with high standards of public health. The third pandemic, however, appears to be approaching quiescence. In 1989, 770 human plague cases were reported to the World Health Organization from 11 countries. Forty-nine percent of these were from Vietnam, and 23% were from Madagascar.

Morphology and Physiology

The causative agent of plague, *Y. pestis,* is a gram-negative, nonmotile coccobacillus (Fig. 38–1). It shows marked bipolar staining, especially in tissue impressions, bubo aspirates, and pus stained with Wayson's stain. The cells have a safety pin appearance, with the polar bodies staining blue and the remainder staining light blue to reddish. Freshly isolated virulent organisms are enveloped.

Yersinia are facultative anaerobes. They are anaerogenic and usually do not ferment lactose. They are oxidase-negative and produce catalase.

Cultural Characteristics. *Y. pestis* can grow over a wide temperature range, from 0C to 43C, the optimal temperature for growth being 28C. Several phenotypic characteristics are best expressed at room temperature. It can grow on ordinary laboratory media even from small inocula. On nutrient agar plates, small mucoid colonies appear in 1 to 2 days. On deoxycholate agar, very small red colonies may be seen on the second day of incubation. No hemolysis is produced on blood agar.

Strain Identification. Three biotypes have been identified on the basis of their ability to reduce nitrates to nitrites and to ferment glycerol. These biotypes have been designated orientalis, mediaevalis, and antigua, and are characterized by differences in their geographic distribution. Orientalis is the biotype associated with infections in the western states of the United States and was the biotype associated with the 1894 pandemic. *Y. pestis* strains are characterized also by quantitative differences in their antigens, as described below.

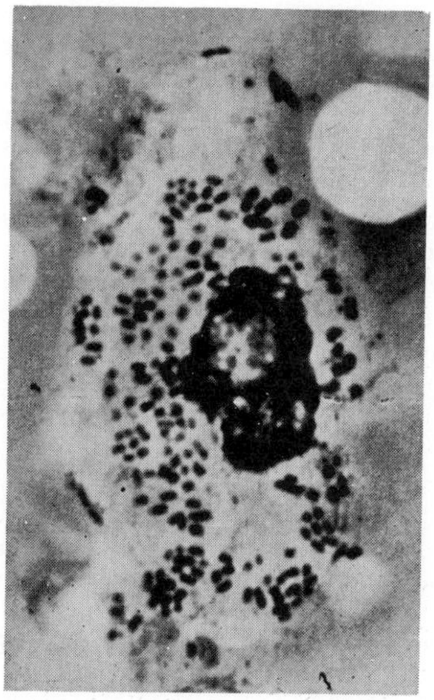

Fig. 38–1. *Yersinia pestis* in monocyte from mouse lung tissue. Giesma stain. × 1500. *(From Meyer: J Immunol 64:139, 1950.)*

Antigenic Structure

At least 20 different antigens have been detected in *Y. pestis* by gel diffusion and biochemical analysis, many of which are shared with *Y. pseudotuberculosis* and *Y. enterocolitica.* Quantitative differences occur in the amount of some of these antigens, which vary independently from one isolate to another. Variations also exist in the protein patterns of isolates from different areas. Common enterobacterial antigen is found in all strains of the three *Yersinia* species. Several of the antigens are virulence determinants, some of which are plasmid encoded. Among the major virulence-associated antigens are the F-1 envelope antigen, the V and W antigens, and a set of outer membrane proteins (Yops).

Determinants of Pathogenicity

Yersinia are facultative intracellular parasites. Virulence is thus assumed to reflect the organisms' ability to proliferate within mammalian cells. Most of the virulence factors that have been defined are primarily associated either with resistance to intracellular killing or with invasive properties that permit the organism to gain access to favored sites of replication in fixed macrophages. Mutant methodologies have been employed to study the phenotypic properties of *Y. pestis* that contribute to its virulence. Among the most fundamental of the findings was the discovery that expression of many of the virulence determinants in *Y. pestis* is under the control of an intricate global regulatory network, responsive to changes in temperature and Ca^{2+} levels. Some of the factors that have been identified as virulence-associated factors are (1) Ca^{2+} dependency, (2) V and W antigens, (3) outer membrane proteins (Yops), (4) F-1 envelope antigen, (5) pesticin, coagulase, and fibrinolysin production, and (6) pigment absorption.

The importance of each of these factors is difficult to assess separately. The V and W antigens develop early in infection and appear to confer on *Y. pestis* the ability of small numbers of bacilli to establish infection in animals. Once infection is established, the F-1 envelope antigen, pesticin, coagulase, and fibrinolysin contribute to its rapid extension. Determinants for F-1 antigen and pigment receptors are controlled by chromosomal genes, whereas plasmid DNA controls the expression of V and W antigens and of pesticin and its attendant invasive enzymes.

Ca^{2+} Dependency. A major virulence determinant of *Y. pestis* is associated with expression in vitro of a nutritional requirement for Ca^{2+} (2.5 mMl) at host temperature but not at room temperature. This effect is potentiated by $MgCl_2$ (20 mMl). When deprived of Ca^{2+}, cells undergo an ordered metabolic stepdown with the shutdown of net protein synthesis and restriction of growth. Accompanying this low-calcium response (Lcr^+) is the coordinate expression of several virulence-related proteins, the V and W antigens, and several outer membrane proteins (Yops). The conditions that provoke the Lcr^+ phenotype simulate the mammalian intracellular environment with respect to Ca^{2+} and Mg^{2+} and provide signals necessary for adaptation to intracellular survival. The low Ca^{2+} response in *Y. pestis* is mediated by a 75-kilobase (kb) plasmid (pCD1) that encodes the regulatory protein, the virulence-associated V antigen, and the Yops.

V and W Antigens. These antigens are always produced together. The V antigen consists of a 38 kDa peptide, and the W antigen is a 145 kDa lipoprotein. Bacteria that express these antigens are Vwa$^+$. Vwa$^+$ is encoded by a 45-megadalton plasmid. The V antigen is cytoplasmic, and the W antigen is an envelope constituent. They are found also in *Y. enterocolitica* and *Y. pseudotuberculosis* but appear to be unique to this genus. The phenotypic expression of V and W is controlled by the Lcr operon on the Lcr plasmids.

In vivo, the V and W antigens correlate with pathogenicity and with the ability of *Y. pestis* to proliferate rapidly and to cause overwhelming septicemia. However, there is no definitive evidence of a pathogenic role for these substances because no mutants are available that lack only the two antigens.

Outer Membrane Proteins. Another property mediated by the 75 kb Lcr virulence plasmid of *Y. pestis* is the expression of a set of Yops. The transcription of these proteins is regulated by temperature and Ca^{2+}, being maximally expressed at 37C in the absence of Ca^{2+}. The phagolysosome of the resident macrophage may provide the proper environment for their expression in vivo. There are 11 Yops in *Y. pestis* (Yops B, C, D, E, F, H, J, K, L, M, and N). In *Y. pestis* grown in vitro, Yops are rapidly degraded by a proteolytic enzyme encoded by the plasminogen activator-coagulase gene on a plasmid unique to *Y. pestis*. This has hampered the in vitro assessment of the possible roles for Yops in the pathogenesis of *Y. pestis*. Yops E, K, and L have been shown to be essential for full virulence in mice. Yersiniae lacking these Yops are compromised in their ability to initiate rapid growth in the liver and spleen, resulting in clearance from the spleen.

Envelope Antigen. F-1 antigen, or envelope antigen, is a soluble antigen contained within the bacterial envelope. It consists of two immunologically identical complexes: a protein complexed with polysaccharides (fraction 1A), which contain *N*-acetyglucosamine and hexuronic acid, and a component protein (fraction 1B). F-1 apparently consists of a series of serologically identical molecular aggregates. Maximal production occurs at 37C, the temperature of the mammalian host, and none is produced at ambient temperatures that exist in the flea. During the incubation period of the infection, the antigen is produced by organisms replicating in mononuclear cells and in the regional lymph nodes. As much as 7% of the dry weight of the organism may be F-1 antigen. The F-1 antigen appears to be antiphagocytic and prevents phagocytosis by professional phagocytes, thus potentiating the rapid evolution of septicemia that characterizes the clinical disease. The antigen is highly immunogenic, and the antibodies to it appear to be protective in both humans and experimental animals.

Pigment Binding and Iron-regulated Surface Proteins. In *Yersinia*, the importance of iron in the degree of pathogenicity has been known for many years. In the mammalian host, iron is complexed to proteins, such as transferrin in blood and lactoferrin in secretions, and is not readily available as a free ion. In yersiniae, avirulent and low-pathogenicity strains require iron overload to produce septicemia in humans or lethality in mice. Highly pathogenic species do not depend on an exogenous iron supply to produce the same effects.

The demonstration of high-molecular-weight proteins (HMWPs) located in the outer membrane of highly pathogenic strains of *Yersinia* has provided a better understanding of the role of iron in pathogenicity and an explanation of earlier observations with pigmented strains. Virulent strains of *Y. pestis* absorb exogenous hemin and basic aromatic dyes during growth on solid media at 26C, thereby forming intensely colored or pigmented colonies (Pgm$^+$). Mutational loss of this chromosomally mediated function results in white colonies, loss of a major outer membrane peptide, and avirulence in mice after intraperitoneal injection. Avirulent nonpigmented organisms may be restored to their original expression of virulence for mice by providing an excess of free serum iron. *Y. pestis* can use hemin as a sole source of iron and also can accumulate Fe^{3+} by an inducible, siderophore-independent, cell-bound, high-affinity transport system. The Pgm$^+$ determinant is thought to serve merely as a mechanism to store the cation.

Under conditions of iron starvation, highly pathogenic species of *Yersinia* synthesize two HMWPs located in the outer membrane. The expression of the novel siderophores is controlled by chromosomal genes.

Pesticin I, Coagulase, and Plasminogen Activator. The production of these components is genetically linked. Pesticin I is a bacteriocin produced by *Y. pestis* that inhibits the growth of *Y. pseudotuberculosis* as well as some strains of *Escherichia coli* and *Y. enterocolitica*. Pesticin is a monomeric 65 kDa protein that converts sensitive bacteria to nonviable osmotically stable spheroplasts. The production of pesticin, coagulase, and plasminogen-activator (fibrinolysin) is mediated by a 9.5-kb plasmid. Strains of *Y. pestis* lacking these enzymes are infectious for the mouse or guinea pig, but lethality is attenuated significantly. It is thought that these enzymes, especially the plasminogen activator, promote dissemination of the bacteria from the primary site of infection and may contribute to the highly invasive fulminant character of the disease.

Other Virulence-associated Factors. A number of additional factors have been proposed as virulence factors—a murine toxin, endotoxin, and a protein antigen, the pH 6 Ag. For rats and mice the LD_{50} dose of murine toxin is less than 1 μg, but for other animals, the toxin is relatively atoxic—hence the name murine toxin. It is a protein that acts as a β-adrenergic blocking agent and inhibits the β-receptor responses of catecholamines, leading to blockade of stress-induced fatty acid mobilization and sensitivity to temperature-induced hypothermia.

The role of *Y. pestis* endotoxin in the disease process is ill-defined. A biphasic febrile response, induced tolerance, and both localized and generalized Shwartzman reactions are produced by the lipopolysaccharide of the cell wall. Endotoxin shock is produced in sensitive animals.

The pH 6 Ag is synthesized by *Y. pestis* at a temperature of 37C and at pH levels similar to those in macrophage phagolysosomes or abscesses. The antigen is composed of aggregates of an immunoreactive 15 kDa subunit. Mutation in the chromosomal gene encoding the pH 6 Ag results in a 100-fold reduction in the intravenous LD_{50} lethal dose of *Y. pestis* in mice, thus implicating it in the pathogenesis of plague.

Clinical Infection

Epidemiology. At the present time, over 90% of the total world incidence of plague occurs in Southeast Asia, especially in South Vietnam, Burma, Nepal, and Indonesia. Another major active focus is in Brazil. Outbreaks in the current pandemic, however, have been less extensive than in the past.

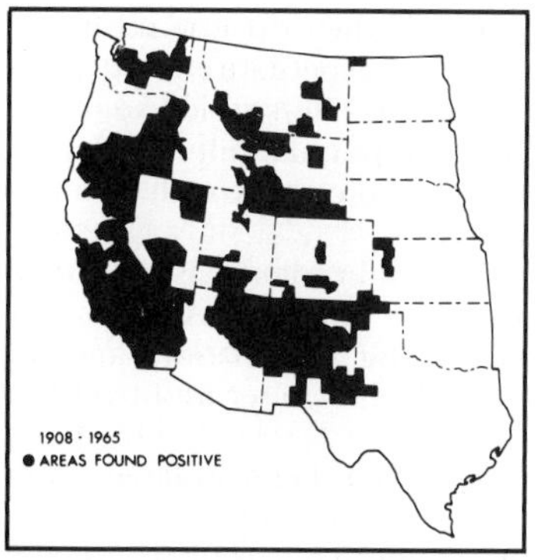

Fig. 38–2. Areas of the United States in which foci of sylvatic plague have been identified. *(Courtesy of the Centers for Disease Control.)*

Plague was introduced into the United States from China in 1900, when the first human case of the disease was reported in San Francisco. Within the next decade, studies showed the presence of infected wild rodents, especially ground squirrels, in wide areas south of San Francisco. In 1907–1908, a major epidemic with 167 cases occurred in San Francisco. Permanent foci of plague now exist that involve at least 57 wild rodent species and their fleas. These extend as far east as Kansas, Oklahoma, and Texas and to approximal areas of Canada and Mexico (Fig. 38–2). The disease does not have natural foci in North America east of these areas. At present, infected fleas are the major mechanism for transmission.

Plague is perpetuated by three cycles: (1) natural foci among commensal rodents with transmission by fleas (sylvatic plague, wild plague), (2) urban rat plague, which is transmitted by the rat flea (domestic plague, urban plague), and (3) human plague, which may be acquired by contact with either of the former cycles and which may be transmitted by pneumonic spread or, rarely, by the bite of a human flea (Fig. 38–3).

SYLVATIC PLAGUE. This is the only form prevalent in the United States. Wild rodent plague in the area west of the 100th meridian is one of the largest world reservoirs. A major factor in the restriction of plague to the western United States is the presence of dense colonies of rodents, such as prairie dogs, in the western areas.

Flea-related Factors. In nature, the flea is essential for perpetuation of plague. At least four flea-related factors influence the epidemic potential of plague.

1. Fleas vary greatly in their vector efficiency. Most wild rodent fleas are relatively inefficient in the transmission of disease to humans. However, the Oriental rat flea, *Xenopsylla cheopis,* is highly efficient and has been the classic vector in urban rat-borne epidemics.
2. The restricted feeding habits of most wild rodent fleas limit their threat to humans. However, the spread of infection within rodent populations, especially among different species that commingle, is facilitated by the transfer of fleas from one rodent host to another. Humans occasionally have been infected when wild rodent deaths during an epizootic left hungry fleas in search of a new host. Dog and cat fleas are very poor vectors and have been associated with individual cases of human plague but not with outbreaks.

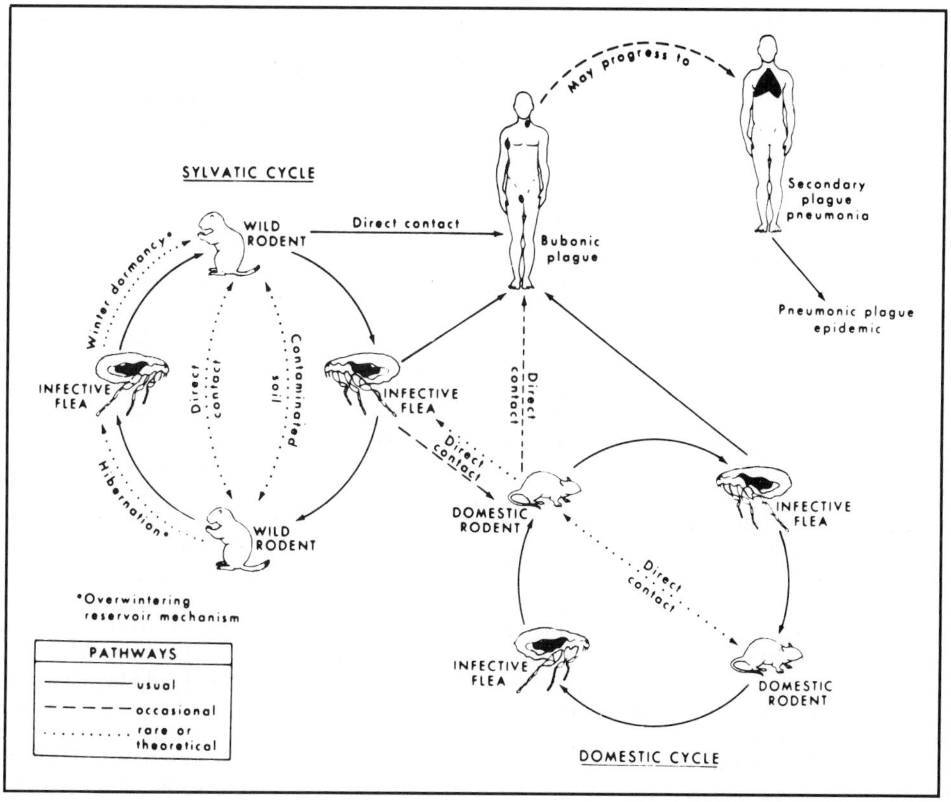

Fig. 38–3. Epidemiologic cycles of plague. *(From Kartman: Am J Public Health 56:1554, 1966.)*

3. Some infective wild rodent fleas survive in burrows for long periods of time even after the rodent hosts have died. Survival of fleas for as long as 15 months has been shown.
4. The development of dichlorodiphenyltrichloroethane (DDT)-resistant fleas in some areas may influence the epidemic potential of plague. This occurred in some instances concomitant with widespread DDT spraying during malaria control programs.

Transmission of plague by fleas may occur in several ways. The most efficient involves ingestion of the organism by the flea during a blood meal from a bacteremic host. In the flea stomach, the infected blood is coagulated by coagulase, an enzyme produced by *Y. pestis* when in contact with an enzyme from the flea stomach. Bacteria are thus trapped in a matrix of fibrin, which fixes them to the spines of the fleas' proventriculus. As the bacteria multiply, the proventriculus is occluded, causing blockage. The time between ingestion and blockage is the extrinsic incubation time, and for *X. cheopis* it is usually about 2 weeks. During subsequent attempts to obtain a blood meal, regurgitation of infected material results in infection of the new host. The hungry flea also becomes less fastidious about his host and will readily attack humans. Hot, dry weather adversely affects all stages in the life cycle of the flea, explaining the subsidence of many epidemics at the beginning of a hot and dry season. Blockage of the proventriculus is enhanced at temperatures below 26C. Above 27C, the fibrinolytic factor of *Y. pestis* and the trypsinlike activity of the flea stomach enzyme are activated, destroying the fibrin meshwork needed for blockage. Decreased blockage results in decreased vector efficiency.

Mechanical transmission via contaminated mouth parts of the flea is also important in the transmission of plague, especially in wild plague. The fleas of many wild rodents do not become blocked or may be poor vectors even when blocked. Mechanical transmission by such fleas, which are highly prevalent, may be the primary means by which enzootics and epizootics occur.

Wild Rodent-related Factors. The essential components of a natural focus for wild plague include the presence of *Y. pestis* organisms of sufficient virulence to cause infection, a dense population of rodents that may develop bacteremia when infected, and a high index and infestation rate of fleas that are capable of transmitting the infection. Over 200 species of rodents and other small animals may be infected during an enzootic. Ten rodent and two rabbit genera are especially important and include squirrels, field mice, prairie dogs, chipmunks, and voles. Populations of wild rodents vary widely in their susceptibility to plague. The introduction of disease into a population may cause a catastrophic dying off of almost the entire population or may cause extensive infection without apparent illness. This variation in susceptibility to plague is a function of the experience of the population with former outbreaks of plague and is genetically determined. Animals that are genetically highly susceptible are unlikely to survive the disease to manifest an immune response. Inherently resistant animals, however, may survive and demonstrate serologic evidence of exposure.

Reservoirs of Infection. The maintenance of plague foci is enhanced by a commingling of rodents or other mammals of differing susceptibility. The relatively resistant species act as a reservoir of infection. Although they do not succumb, they develop bacteremia that serves to perpetuate a population of infected fleas. The relatively susceptible species augment the level of infectivity of the local flea population, and deaths among this species may bring them into contact with humans or domestic animals.

The hibernating habits of some wild rodents also facilitate survival of plague during the winter months. Animals are much more resistant to plague during hibernation, and an infected animal may survive through the winter and transmit disease again in the spring.

Attenuated *Y. pestis* organisms have been isolated from natural foci. These organisms may produce infection without causing death and provide another mechanism for perpetuation of the disease. It is not known at present whether these attenuated strains reacquire virulence. Perpetuation of the infection is facilitated also by the ability of *Y. pestis* to survive for long periods in the soil of animal burrows.

Human Infection. The transmission of infection from wild plague foci to humans is an accidental occurrence. From 1908 to 1968, 120 cases were attributed to wild sources. In 1988, 15 cases were reported to the Centers for Disease Control. Currently, the fatality rate remains at about 15%. Disease is usually sporadic and most often bubonic in character. Cases often occur in areas where there is extensive mortality among the rodent populations. Most of the cases occur from June through August, and many patients are children. Other victims are hunters and other persons who come into professional or avocational contact with wild animals.

A particularly high-risk group is the Native Americans of the Southwest, especially the Navajos, whose cultural patterns bring them into close contact with prairie dogs. In 1965, an epidemic among the Navajos was associated with an extensive epizootic of the local prairie dog colonies. Dogs associated with these outbreaks developed antibody to F-1 antigen without experiencing serious disease. Domestic dogs and cats bring infected wild rodents and their fleas into areas of human habitation, increasing the danger of infection among domestic rodents and humans.

URBAN PLAGUE. Urban plague has been the principal cause of the massive epidemics of plague in recent history. The characteristics of this form of plague are quite distinct from those of wild plague, although there has been extensive interaction between the two forms. Urban plague is characterized by an accompanying epizootic of plague among the rodents, particularly the black rat that lives in close proximity to human habitations. An epizootic occurs when there is a sufficiently dense population of susceptible domestic rats, a high index of parasitism with fleas capable of transmitting disease (the flea index), adequate climatic conditions, and introduction of disease. Centers for commerce, especially seaports, have been frequent sites of explosive disease. During the eras of epidemic human plague, the natural history of the epidemic included a gradual onset of fatal disease among the domestic rodents. As the infected fleas moved from the dead or dying rodents to other living rodents, the rate of death among the rodents increased. Human cases could be expected when approximately 10% of the rats were infected. Human cases usually began as bubonic disease, and usually there was only one or a few cases per family. The disease was seasonal, and the onset of adverse climatic conditions would curtail an epidemic. The disease was also cyclical, with severe disease following seasons of no disease or mild disease.

Initial epizootics characteristically caused the death of essentially the entire population of domestic rodents. Subsequent generations of rodents, however, were relatively more resistant to plague. After several such epizootics, the rodents developed herd resistance and did not die of the disease, with the result that the severity of subsequent epidemics gradually declined. This probably accounts in large part for the fact that epidemic urban plague during the current pandemic has been declining for many decades. Repopulation of an urban area by a susceptible species of rodent, however, as occurred in Bombay in 1948 with susceptible bandicoots, may again lead to extensive epizootic and epidemic disease.

RURAL PLAGUE. Urban plague commonly has been disseminated to rural areas through lines of commerce. Grain shipment in Vietnam probably played a role in the establishment of new foci. In rural areas, the disease first affects domestic rats. It is then spread to commensal wild rodents, thereby establishing a focus of sylvatic plague. In contrast to urban plague, sylvatic plague causes small numbers of sporadic human cases. There is little tendency for rural plague to disappear because the constant influx of susceptible rodents from wild sources precludes the development of effective herd immunity.

INTERHUMAN TRANSMISSION. Pneumonic plague is the clinical form of the disease with the greatest potential for rapid dissemination. It occurs after close contact with a victim of bubonic plague who has developed secondary pulmonary involvement and exhales the organism in droplets. This form of disease may be widespread and rapid in onset and is the only form of plague that is directly contagious. Epidemiologic characteristics of pneumonic plague show that familial spread is most common, and disease is most frequent in areas of overcrowding. Cold weather with high humidity fosters the disease. Although most epidemics are predominantly either bubonic or pneumonic in clinical presentation, recent epidemics in Vietnam have been mixed. Factors that determine whether an epidemic will be predominantly bubonic or pneumonic are not well understood.

Clinical Manifestations. The various clinical forms of plague overlap but may be grouped as predominantly bubonic, septicemic, or pneumonic.

BUBONIC PLAGUE. Bubonic plague is essentially the only form of disease that occurs in humans after infection from a wild focus. The bubo represents the infected regional lymph node that drains the area of skin through which the organism was introduced. The groin is the region most commonly affected, with axillary and cervical nodes less frequently. Buboes in more than one site are extremely rare. The incubation period of bubonic plague is usually less than a week, and the bubo may be preceded by prodromata of chills, fever, malaise, confusion, nausea, and pains in the limbs and back. Onset of disease usually is sudden. Patients may experience pain at the site of the future bubo before it is palpable. The lesion itself is tender, the node is enlarged and may suppurate, and erythema of the surrounding tissues is common. The bubo of plague cannot be distinguished clinically from other causes of acute lymphadenitis. Bacteremia usually is present even in mild cases. Approximately one half of early blood cultures will yield the organism. The level of bacteremia, however, is usually low, and organisms are seldom seen on direct observation of stained buffy coat smears.

Pulmonary involvement is common in all severe cases of plague and is often the immediate cause of death. Hemorrhagic and edematous effusions predominate, probably associated with emboli that may be septic and originate from the bubo. Endotoxin-mediated effects are observed. Another primary manifestation of bubonic plague is congestion of the vessels of the conjunctivae. The three clinical findings that traditionally have been most useful in the diagnosis of plague are a rapid rise in temperature, regional buboes, and conjunctivitis. In very mild plague, the only clinical finding may be vesiculation at the site of inoculation. Slightly more active disease, with local buboes but without systemic signs of disease, is termed *pestis minor*.

SEPTICEMIC PLAGUE. At the opposite extreme is septicemic plague. In the United States, approximately 20% of cases are septicemic, and the fatality rate is very high. In this form of disease, the patient experiences a high level of bacteremia early in the course of the disease before local buboes evolve. The mortality rate in both treated and untreated cases is high, with rapid peripheral vascular collapse. A prominent finding in this form, as well as in other forms of plague, is disseminated intravascular coagulation with a generalized Shwartzman phenomenon. Purpuric lesions with intravascular thrombi occur in all areas of the body.

PNEUMONIC PLAGUE. This form of plague usually arises from septic embolization to the lungs. Patients also may acquire the pneumonic form following pharyngeal plague and direct extension into the lung from the cervical or tonsillar buboes. Inhalation of organisms in droplet nuclei dispersed by another person with plague also provides a mechanism for direct inoculation of the lung parenchyma. This was probably the etiology of the highly fatal fulminant epidemics in China in the late 1890s. In untreated patients with pneumonic plague, the average length of time from the first appearance of symptoms to death is less than 2 days. The disease is highly contagious. Marked central nervous system abnormalities, including convulsions, incoordination, stupor, and delirium, usually accompany the disease.

PLAGUE MENINGITIS. Plague meningitis is an infrequent complication. Clinical evidence suggests that it is most common in persons who experience an attenuated form of infection, as occurs in the partially immune patient or after inadequate treatment. The clinical findings are those of an acute bacterial meningitis.

Laboratory Diagnosis. Clinical materials containing *Y. pestis* may be hazardous. Suspicious cultures or specimens should be sent immediately to a laboratory with facilities for making a rapid definitive identification. Aspirates from buboes, pus from the area of the flea bite, sputum, throat swabs, or blood should be collected carefully and placed in Cary-Blair transport medium for transfer to the laboratory.

SEROLOGIC DIAGNOSIS. Antibodies to the F-1 antigen may be detected by use of the agglutination test or the complement-fixation test. The complement-fixation test also may be used for detecting the F-1 antigen either in tissue extracts or in the organism itself. Complement-fixing antibodies decrease rapidly after recovery from plague. The passive hemagglutination test, which uses tanned erythrocytes coated with F-1 antigen or murine toxin, is also a sensitive indicator of *Y. pestis* antigen or antibody. A serologic response is apparent by day 5, with a peak by day 14. This antibody may persist for several years after recovery from plague and is a sensitive test for identifying a quiescent plague focus.

Precipitin tests are useful in the detection of F-1 antigen in dried and decomposed carcasses of animals. An immunofluorescence test using F-1 antibody is a rapid and generally accurate method of identifying *Y. pestis,* although cross-reaction with *Y. pseudotuberculosis* may occur in a small percentage of cases.

Treatment. Streptomycin is bactericidal and highly effective for most strains. Resistant organisms have been observed in the Far East but not in the United States. Alternative treatment is tetracycline or chloramphenicol. Kanamycin appears to be equally as effective as streptomycin and shows no cross-resistance. Penicillin is inadequate, and the sulfonamides are not uniformly effective. Sulfamethoxazole-trimethoprim has been used successfully in the treatment of a small number of patients, but further evaluation is necessary.

Prevention. A vaccine for immunization against plague is available. During the war in Vietnam, only a small number of cases of plague occurred in U.S. military personnel stationed in that country in spite of widespread plague among Vietnamese civilians. The plague vaccine that is licensed for use in the United States at present is inactivated with formalin, and its efficacy appears to be directly proportional to the content of F-1 antigen. The primary immunization series consists of three doses of vaccine given on days 0 and 30 and 3 to 6 months after dose 2. A booster dose should be given at 6 months and at 1 year. Persons at continued risk should receive boosters at 1- to 2-year intervals. Severe reactions to the vaccine have not been common, although immediate and generalized urticaria and anaphylaxis may occur.

Immunization is recommended for persons who (1) are working in the laboratory or field with *Y. pestis* strains that are resistant to antimicrobials, (2) are engaged in aerosol experiments with *Y. pestis,* and (3) are engaged in field operations in areas with enzootic plague where prevention of exposure cannot be achieved. There is no evidence that vaccine protects against pneumonic plague, and the efficacy in prevention of bubonic disease under field conditions also is uncertain. Therefore, if a person has had a definite exposure, prophylactic antibiotics may be indicated even if the person has received vaccine.

Control. Plague is one of the internationally quarantinable diseases, and reporting of cases is mandatory. Public health authorities may institute enforced quarantine and disinfection of persons, ships, and aircraft arriving with known or suspected infected persons or animals. Efforts to prevent plague have been directed toward preventing transportation of rats, especially by ships and airplanes. Current methods of shipping and docking make the classic importation of shipboard rats into western countries unlikely, but the possibility of spreading diseased rats by container shipping may still exist.

Control of urban plague has proceeded along the principles of flea control, which should precede rat control, rodent extermination, treatment or quarantine of cases or both, quarantine of contacts of pneumonic plague, restriction of movement in highly infected areas, thorough garbage disposal, and application of good personal hygiene.

Yersinia pseudotuberculosis and *Yersinia enterocolitica*

The term *yersiniosis* denotes infection with *Yersinia* species other than *Y. pestis,* namely, *Y. pseudotuberculosis* and *Y. enterocolitica.* These are zoonotic diseases, and human infection appears to be acquired accidentally from disease cycles in wild and domestic animals.

Morphology and Physiology

Unlike the plague bacillus, *Y. pseudotuberculosis* and *Y. enterocolitica* are motile. The flagella are paripolar or peritrichous in location and are produced during growth at 22C but not at 37C. A microscopically visible capsule is not produced.

Both species may be isolated from clinical material by culture on blood agar and the usual media used for the enteric bacteria. They are characterized by urease production, an acid slant and acid butt on triple sugar iron agar, and no hydrogen sulfide production. Growth requirements and metabolic pathways are similar to those of the other Enterobacteriaceae. Differentiation of *Y. enterocolitica* and *Y. pseudotuberculosis* is based on biochemical differences between the species (Table 38–1). The results of many of these tests are affected markedly by temperature, a property that should be noted when interpreting test results.

TABLE 38–1. DISTINGUISHING PROPERTIES OF HUMAN DISEASE-ASSOCIATED *YERSINIA* SPECIES

Characteristics	*Y. pestis*	*Y. pseudotuberculosis*	*Y. enterocolitica*
Motility (25C)	−	+	+
Ornithine decarboxylase (Møller)	−	−	+
Urease	−	+	+
β-Xylosidase[a]	+	+	−
Voges-Proskauer test, 25C	−	−	+
Indole production	−	−	d
γ-Glutamyl transferase	−	d	+
Acid production from			
Rhamnose	−	+	−
Sucrose	−	−	+
Cellobiose	−	−	+
Melibiose	d	+	−
Sorbose	−	−	+
Sorbitol	−	−	+

Adapted from Bercovier and Mollaret: In Krieg and Holt (eds): Manual of Systematic Bacteriology, vol 1. Williams & Wilkins, 1984, p 503.
d, different reactions.
[a] Using *p*-nitrophenyl-β-D-xylopyranoside as a substrate.

Antigenic Structure

Yersinia pseudotuberculosis. There are six serotypes of *Y. pseudotuberculosis*, each of which is characterized by type-specific O and H antigens. The O-antigen specificity is conferred by 3,6-dideoxyhexoses, some of which also are present in the cell walls of *Salmonella* groups B and D and are responsible for cross-reactions with these organisms. Serotyping can be performed by agglutination or hemagglutination methods.

The V and W antigens of *Y. pestis* are also present in virulent *Y. pseudotuberculosis*.

Yersinia enterocolitica. Organisms currently regarded as *Y. enterocolitica* are serologically heterogeneous. Twenty-seven serotypes have been identified on the basis of their O and H antigens. Certain serologic types are consistently associated with human infection. *Y. enterocolitica* serotypes 0:3 and 0:9 are the most common cause of human infection in Europe, Japan, and Canada, whereas serotype 0:8 strains are responsible for most infections in the United States.

Y. enterocolitica bears little antigenic relationship to other *Yersinia* but cross-reacts with *Brucella*. Most species of *Brucella* show complete cross-reaction with *Y. enterocolitica* serotype 0:9. For diagnostic purposes, it should be kept in mind that a positive *Brucella* agglutination titer may represent a *Y. enterocolitica* 0:9 infection. The antigenic determinant responsible for this cross-reactivity is probably cell wall lipopolysaccharide. There is also antigenic similarity between some *Y. enterocolitica* strains and *Vibrio cholerae* serotype inaba.

Determinants of Pathogenicity

Invasion and intracellular survival are important aspects of the virulence of *Y. pseudotuberculosis* and *Y. enterocolitica*. These organisms are transmitted by the fecal-oral route. They invade the intestinal epithelium and gain access to the reticuloendothelial system, where they multiply and from which they may be disseminated throughout the body. Organisms internalized by cells enter singly, enclosed within a vacuole, but the vacuoles do not appear to coalesce. They appear to spend much of their time within macrophages. As in *Y. pestis*, novel mechanisms are required for life within this niche.

A study of the genetic determinants that enable *Y. pseudotuberculosis* and *Y. enterocolitica* to invade cultured animal cells has identified two chromosomal genes that are necessary for cell entry. The *inv* (invasion) gene encodes a large surface protein (ca 108 kDa) that promotes adherence to and invasion of cells by these organisms. A second gene in *Y. enterocolitica*, designated *ail* (attachment-invasion locus), encodes a novel cell entry factor (15 kDa) that is distinct from invasion. A complete understanding of the roles that these proteins play in vivo for *Yersinia* invasion is lacking at present, but there is considerable evidence that they are important in the overall pathogenesis of these species. Mutation in the genes encoding them results in strains impaired in their ability to invade tissue culture cells. The application of *inv* and *ail* DNA probes has provided an excellent method for the detection of pathogenic *Yersinia* species among clinical isolates. Epidemiologically, there is excellent correlation between the presence of DNA homologous to these genes and the presence of *Y. enterocolitica* clinical disease.

Some of the virulence traits produced by *Y. pestis* are also present in *Y. pseudotuberculosis* and *Y. enterocolitica*. Plasmids approximately 70 kb in size that are required for expression of virulence are found in the three pathogens. These plasmids share large regions of homology and contain three recognized elements: (1) a set of regulatory genes that control the expression of other genes on the plasmid in response to Ca^{2+} concentration and temperature (Fig. 38–4), (2) the V antigen, and (3) a set of genes encoding outer membrane proteins. The conserved maintenance of these three regions in all pathogenic *Yersinia* suggests that the gene products expressed are important in pathogenicity.

The V and W antigens of *Y. pseudotuberculosis* and *Y. enterocolitica* are antigenically similar to those of *Y. pestis*, as are most of the Yops produced by the three species. All of the Yops as well as the V and W antigens are expressed maximally during growth at 37C in the absence of Ca^{2+} except Yop 1, which is temperature-regulated but not Ca^{2+}-regulated. The Yop 1 protein is produced by *Y. pseudotuberculosis* and *Y. enterocolitica* but not by *Y. pestis* or nonpathogenic species. Yop 1 is a HMWP forming a fibrillar matrix on the bacterial surface. It confers resistance to the bactericidal activity of human serum, confers autoagglutinability and mannose-resistant hemagglutination properties, and promotes intestinal colonization in mice.

Two additional virulence traits have been identified in *Y. pseudotuberculosis* and *Y. enterocolitica*. These are HMWPs located in the outer membrane and synthesized de novo only by highly pathogenic strains under conditions of iron starvation. The synthesis of the HMWPs is controlled by chromosomal genes. The finding of these virulence factors is impor-

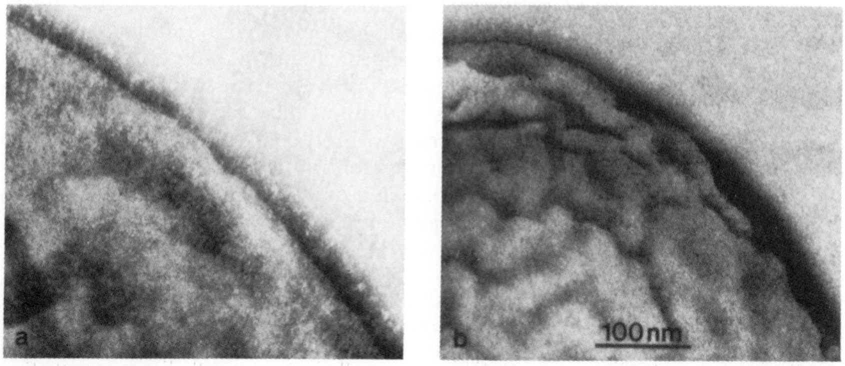

Fig. 38–4. Electron micrographs of *Y. enterocolitica* showing temperature-inducible surface fibrillae (**left**) and plasmid-cured strain with disappearance of fibrillae (**right**). *(From Kapperud: Infect Immun 47:561, 1985.)*

tant in providing an understanding of earlier clinical observations. Normally, iron is complexed to host proteins, such as transferrin in blood, and is not readily available as a free ion. Only highly pathogenic species of *Yersinia* can cause septicemia in these individuals. In patients with iron overload as a result of hemochromatosis, thalassemia, or oral overdose, however, low pathogenicity strains can produce septicemia.

Enterotoxin is produced by *Y. enterocolitica.* Since its synthesis is not limited to strains associated with human infections, however, the role of enterotoxin in the organism's pathogenicity is uncertain at present. Its physicochemical and antigenic properties and mode of action are similar to those of the heat-stable toxin of *E. coli.*

Clinical Infection

Epidemiology. The yersinioses have been recognized in wild and domestic mammals, birds, invertebrates, and amphibians. Clinically apparent disease with both species has occurred in humans in all areas of the world, but the majority of cases have come from northern Europe, especially France, Germany, and the Scandinavian countries.

In the United States, *Y. pseudotuberculosis* has been identified in six species of domestic mammals and several wild mammals, including deer, rabbits, and rodents. Wild birds also are reservoirs of *Y. pseudotuberculosis.* Fecal-oral spread of both *Y. enterocolitica* and *Y. pseudotuberculosis* appears to be the major natural method of transmission.

Sources of infection in humans are poorly defined. Direct contamination of food or water by infected animals may account for cases in which identical strains have been obtained from an owner and a pet or domestic animal, frequently a dog or pig, in *Y. enterocolitica*–related disease. Most reports are of individual cases or small family outbreaks. Secondary cases are common, as is a high attack rate. A single school outbreak of *Y. enterocolitica* enteritis in Japan involved 20% of the entire student body. Person to person spread within related families and between personnel on hospital wards has demonstrated the potential for rapid transmission under appropriate conditions. It most commonly occurs in persons from rural areas.

Contamination of water supplies by *Y. enterocolitica* has been demonstrated. Survival of both organisms in various types of water is shortest in the spring and summer and longest in the fall and winter, a finding probably attributable to the ability of the organisms to grow at the lower temperature. The majority of human infections occur during the winter and early spring. The incidence of infection with both organisms is the same for males and females. Large outbreaks have been traced to contaminated tofu, chocolate milk, and other chocolate milk products.

The relative clinical importance of *Y. enterocolitica* and *Y. pseudotuberculosis* as causes of gastrointestinal disease in the United States is considerable. Surveys of routine stool cultures suggest that rarely are the organisms found in normal persons. In some areas, these *Yersinia* species are as common a cause of serious gastrointestinal disease as are *Shigella.* It is expected that as physicians and laboratories in the United States become more familiar with these organisms, they will be recognized more frequently.

Pathogenesis. The primary lesion results from invasion of the wall of the small intestine, usually in the area of the ileum. Ulcers of the intestinal mucosa at the site of lymphoid tissue may develop and lead to extensive loss of blood and fluid, strongly resembling the intestinal findings in typhoid fever. The mesenteric nodes usually are the most extensively involved structures. Enlarged nodes may become confluent. Histopathologic differentiation of these lesions from gastrointestinal infection with *Francisella tularensis, Salmonella* species, and cat-scratch fever occasionally may be difficult.

Although infection usually is restricted to the gastrointestinal tract, invasion of the portal system with liver involvement and generalized septicemia resulting in colonization in other body sites may occur.

Clinical Manifestations. A short prodromal period of approximately 1 day precedes symptoms of gastrointestinal disease. The majority of naturally acquired human cases present primarily with gastrointestinal symptoms, including diarrhea and mesenteric lymphatic involvement. Systemic symptoms usually accompany the focal gastrointestinal complaints and consist of headache, which may be severe, malaise, and fever associated with convulsions. Both organisms produce severe abdominal pain, which together with enlarged mesenteric nodes has resulted, in many instances, in exploratory surgery in the expectation of appendicitis. The uncomplicated case of gastroenteritis caused by either *Y. enterocolitica* or *Y. pseudotuberculosis* is not clinically distinguishable from that caused by *Salmonella* or *Shigella.*

Complications consisting of septicemia and hepatic abscesses may occur in a small number of patients, most of whom have preexisting liver disease, are less than 1 year old, have a hemoglobinopathy, are diabetics, or are receiving corticosteroids. An arthritis–erythema nodosum syndrome also has been reported extensively by Scandinavian physicians but is observed infrequently in the United States or Canada. Patients with this syndrome are predominantly females in the 15- to 45-year age group. The arthritis, which usually is preceded by abdominal pain and diarrhea and often affects multiple large joints sequentially, occurs primarily in persons who are HLA-B27 positive.

Laboratory Diagnosis. A definitive diagnosis can be made only by culture of the organism. For isolation of *Yersinia* from noncontaminated samples, blood agar or nutrient agar can be used, and the culture is incubated for 48 hours at 28C or at 37C for 24 hours, followed by 24 hours at room temperature. The organisms can be isolated from mesenteric lymph nodes, feces, blood (in generalized septicemia), effusions from serous cavities, and organ specimens. For selective enrichment and holding, the specimen should be placed in isotonic saline with or without potassium tellurite and promptly refrigerated. The Widal-type agglutination test is the most specific serologic test for evaluation. The agglutinins have immunologic specificity and seldom cross-react with other gram-negative organisms. A titer of 1:160 or greater is significant and indicative of infection by *Y. enterocolitica* or *Y. pseudotuberculosis* depending on the specific antigen employed.

Treatment. The susceptibility of *Y. enterocolitica* and *Y. pseudotuberculosis* to ampicillin, tetracycline, and other commonly used antibiotics is variable, necessitating sensitivity testing of each isolate. Most strains are susceptible to the aminoglycosides and to trimethoprim-sulfamethoxazole. Other forms of supportive care, such as maintenance of fluid and electrolyte balance, are essential in the care of the severely ill patient.

FURTHER READING

Acker G, Bitter-Suermann D, Meier-Dieter U, et al: Immunocytochemical localization of enterobacterial common antigen in *Escherichia coli* and *Yersinia enterocolitica* cells. J Bacteriol 168:348, 1986

Bolin I, Portnoy DA, Wolf-Watz H: Expression of the temperature-inducible outer membrane proteins of yersiniae. Infect Immun 48:234, 1985

Brubaker RR: The Vwa$^+$ virulence factor of yersiniae: The molecular basis of the attendant nutritional requirement for Ca^{++}. Rev Infect Dis 5(suppl):748, 1983

Butler T: A clinical study of bubonic plague. Am J Med 53:268, 1972

Carniel E, Antoine J-C, Guiyoule A, et al: Purification, location, and immunological characterization of the iron-regulated high-molecular-weight proteins of the highly pathogenic yersiniae. Infect Immun 57:540, 1989

Cavanaugh DC: Specific effect of temperature upon transmission of the plague bacillus by the oriental rat flea, *Xenopsylla cheopis*. Am J Trop Med Hyg 20:264, 1971

Centers for Disease Control: Imported bubonic plague—District of Columbia. MMWR 39:895, 1990

Clark VL: Environmental modulation of gene expression in gram-negative pathogens. In Iglewski BH, Clark VL (eds): The Bacteria, vol XI. Molecular Basis of Pathogenicity. New York, Academic Press, 1990. p. 111

Cornelis G, Laroche Y, Balligand G, et al: *Yersinia enterocolitica*, a primary model for bacterial invasiveness. Rev Infect Dis 9:64, 1987

Cover TL, Aber RC: *Yersinia enterocolitica*. N Engl J Med 321:16, 1989

Delor I, Kaeckenbeeck A, Wauters G, Cornelis GR: Nucleotide sequence of *yst*, the *Yersinia enterocolitica* gene encoding the heat-stable enterotoxin, and prevalence of the gene among pathogenic and nonpathogenic yersiniae. Infect Immun 58:2983, 1990

Forsberg Å, Wolf-Watz H: Genetic analysis of the *yopE* region of *Yersinia* spp.: Identification of a novel conserved locus, *yerA*, regulating *yopE* expression. J Bacteriol 172:1547, 1990

Gutman LT, Ottesen EA, Quan TT, et al: An interfamilial outbreak of *Yersinia enterocolitica* enteritis. N Engl J Med 288:1372, 1973

Hudson BW, Quan SF, Goldenberg MI: Serum antibody responses in a population of *Microtus californicus* and associated rodent species during and after *P. pestis* epizootics in the San Francisco Bay area. Zoonoses Res 3:15, 1964

Hull HF, Montes JM, Mann JM: Septicemic plague in New Mexico. J Infect Dis 155:113, 1987

Isberg RR: Determinants for thermoinducible cell binding and plasmid-encoded cellular penetration detected in the absence of the *Yersinia pseudotuberculosis* invasin protein. Infect Immun 57:1998, 1989

Isberg RR, Voorhis DL, Falkow S: Identification of invasin: A protein that allows enteric bacteria to penetrate cultured mammalian cells. Cell 50:769, 1987

Kapperud G, Namork E, Skurnik M, Nesbakken T: Plasmid-mediated surface fibrillae of *Yersinia pseudotuberculosis* and *Yersinia enterocolitica:* Relationship to the outer membrane protein YPO1 and possible importance for pathogenesis. Infect Immun 55:2247, 1987

Kartman L: Historical and ecological observation on plague in the United States. Trop Geogr Med 22:257, 1970

Lassen J, Kapperud G: Serotype-related HEp-2 cell interaction of *Yersinia enterocolitica*. Infect Immun 52:85, 1986

Legters LJ, Cottingham AJ, Hunter DH: Clinical and epidemiologic notes on defined outbreak of plague in Viet Nam. Am J Trop Med Hyg 19:639, 1970

Lindler LE, Klempner MS, Straley SC. *Yersinia pestis* pH 6 antigen: Genetic, biochemical and virulence characterization of a protein involved in the pathogenesis of bubonic plague. Infect Immun 58:2569, 1990

Mehigh RJ, Sample AK, Brubaker RR: Expression of the low calcium response in *Yersinia pestis*. Microbial Pathogen 6:203, 1989

Michiels T, Wattiau P, Brasseur R, et al: Secretion of Yop proteins by yersiniae. Infect Immun 58:2840, 1990

Miller VL, Falkow S: Evidence for two genetic loci in *Yersinia enterocolitica* that can promote invasion of epithelial cells. Infect Immun 56:1242, 1988

Miller VL, Farmer JJ, Hill WE, et al: The *ail* locus is found uniquely in *Yersinia enterocolitica* serotypes commonly associated with disease. Infect Immun 57:121, 1989

O'Loughlin EV, Gall DG, Pai CH: *Yersinia enterocolitica:* Mechanisms of microbial pathogenesis and pathophysiology of diarrhoea. J Gastroenterol Hepatol 5:173, 1990

Pepe JC, Miller VL: The *Yersinia enterocolitica inv* gene product is an outer membrane protein that shares epitopes with *Yersinia pseudotuberculosis* invasin. J Bacteriol 172:3780, 1990

Perry RD, Brubaker RR: Vwa$^+$ phenotype of *Yersinia enterocolitica*. Infect Immun 40:166, 1983

Perry RD, Harmon PA, Bowmer WS, Straley SC: A low-Ca^{2+} response operon encodes the V antigen of *Yersinia pestis*. Infect Immun 54:428, 1986

Pollitzer R: Plague. WHO Monograph Series, No. 22. Geneva, World Health Organization, 1954

Portnoy DA, Blank HF, Kingsbury DT, Falkow S: Genetic analysis of essential plasmid determinants of pathogenicity in *Yersinia pestis*. J Infect Dis 148:297, 1983

Price SB, Straley SC: *lcrH*, a gene necessary for virulence of *Yersinia pestis* and for the normal response of *Y. pestis* to ATP and calcium. Infect Immun 57:1491, 1989

Price SB, Leung KY, Barve SS, Straley SC: Molecular analysis of *lcrGVH*, the V antigen operon of *Yersinia pestis*. J Bacteriol 171:5646, 1989

Sikkema DJ, Brubaker RR: Resistance to pesticin, storage of iron, and invasion of HeLa cells by yersiniae. Infect Immun 55:572, 1987

Skurnik M: Expression of antigens encoded by the virulence plasmid of *Yersinia enterocolitica* under different growth conditions. Infect Immun 47:183, 1985

Sodeinde OA, Sample AK, Brubaker RR, Goguen JD: Plasminogen activator/coagulase gene of *Yersinia pestis* is responsible for degradation of plasmid-encoded outer membrane proteins. Infect Immun 56:2749, 1988

Straley SC, Brubaker RR: Cytoplasmic and membrane proteins of yersiniae cultivated under conditions simulating mammalian intracellular environment. Proc Natl Acad Sci USA 78:1224, 1981

Straley SC, Cibull ML: Differential clearance and host-pathogen interactions of YopE$^-$ and YopK$^-$ YopL$^-$ *Yersinia pestis* in BALB/c mice. Infect Immun 57:1200, 1989

Straley SC, Harmon PA: *Yersinia pestis* grows within phagolysosomes in mouse peritoneal macrophages. Infect Immun 45:655, 1984

Une T, Brubaker RR: In vivo comparison of avirulent Vwa$^-$ and Pgm$^-$ and Pst r phenotypes of yersiniae. Infect Immun 43:895, 1984

Velimirovic B, Velimirovic H: Plague in Vienna. Rev Infect Dis 11:808, 1989

World Health Organization. Human plague in 1989. Weekly Epidemiol Rec 65:321, 1990

Yother J, Chamness JW, Goguen JD: Temperature-controlled plasmid regulon associated with low calcium response in *Yersinia pestis*. J Bacteriol 165:443, 1986

Zahorchak RJ, Brubaker RR: Effect of exogenous nucleotides on Ca^{++} dependence and V antigen synthesis in *Yersinia pestis*. Infect Immun 38:953, 1982

Leisure Time Reading

Burnet M, White DO: Natural History of Infectious Diseases, ed 4. Cambridge, Cambridge University Press, 1972

Cravens G, Marr JS: The Black Death. New York, Ballantine Books, 1977

Tuchman BW: A Distant Mirror. The Calamitous 14th Century. New York, Knopf Pub, 1978

CHAPTER 39

Francisella

Tularemia is a major zoonotic disease indigenous to many areas of the United States. It is caused by *Francisella tularensis,* which is transmitted to humans by insect vectors or by the handling or ingestion of infected animals or animal products. Human disease, often referred to as deerfly fever or rabbit fever, is characterized by a focal ulcer at the site of entry of the organisms and enlargement of the regional lymph nodes.

Most of the early work on the etiology and epidemiology of tularemia was carried out by epidemiologists in the United States. The organism was first isolated in 1911 by McCoy and Chapin from ground squirrels in Tulare County, California—hence the name, tularemia. These workers found animals in the area to be infected with a plaguelike organism that caused disease and produced lesions resembling those of plague. Human cases were recognized under circumstances that implicated rabbits as the source of infection. Extensive studies by Francis and colleagues of the United States Public Health Service resulted in a classic description of the human disease and a bacteriologic description of the causative organism.

Previously classified as *Bacterium tularense, Brucella tularense,* and *Pasteurella tularensis,* the organism is currently classified in the genus *Francisella. Francisella novicida,* isolated from water, is the only other member of the genus and is not known to infect humans.

Francisella tularensis

Morphology and Physiology

F. tularensis is a small, weakly staining, gram-negative coccobacillus, 0.2 by 0.2 to 0.7 μm in size. It is nonmotile and displays bipolar staining with polychrome stains, such as Giemsa. A relatively thick capsule surrounds virulent organisms, and loss of this capsule is accompanied by loss of virulence. In young cultures, the cells are relatively uniform in appearance, but older cultures are characterized by extreme pleomorphism (Fig. 39–1). *F. tularensis* is an obligate aerobe and is weakly catalase-positive. Carbohydrates are dissimilated slowly, with the production of acid but no gas. Biochemical characterization, however, is of little value in identification.

DNA hybridization studies indicate that the genus *Francisella* is not closely related to *Pasteurella, Yersinia,* or the coliform organisms. Also, in *F. tularensis,* the lipid concentration in the capsule and cell wall (50% and 70%, respectively) is unusually high for gram-negative organisms. The lipid composition is also unlike other bacteria, with relatively large amounts of long-chain saturated and monoenoic C_{20} to C_{26} fatty acids as well as α-OH and β-OH fatty acids.

Cultural Characteristics. Growth of *F. tularensis* occurs over a temperature range of 24C to 39C, with an optimal temperature of 37C. The survival rate of the organisms is best at lower temperatures. *F. tularensis* is a slow-growing organism with a growth requirement for cysteine or cystine. No growth is obtained on routine culture media, but 1 to 4 mm unpigmented colonies are obtained after 2 to 4 days on glucose-cysteine-blood agar (GCBA) or peptone-cysteine agar (PCA). On media containing blood, a greenish discoloration surrounds the colony, but no true hemolysis occurs.

Determinants of Pathogenicity

A general correlation exists among a smooth colonial morphology, high degree of virulence for experimental animals, acriflavin reaction, acid agglutination, and staining with crystal violet. Fresh isolates of the organism produce smooth colonies, but repeated passage on artificial media results in a change from the smooth to the rough form and loss of the capsule, which is a major determinant of pathogenicity.

Francisella are facultative intracellular parasites. Although attenuated and avirulent strains of *F. tularensis* are both ingested and killed by human polymorphonuclear leukocytes,

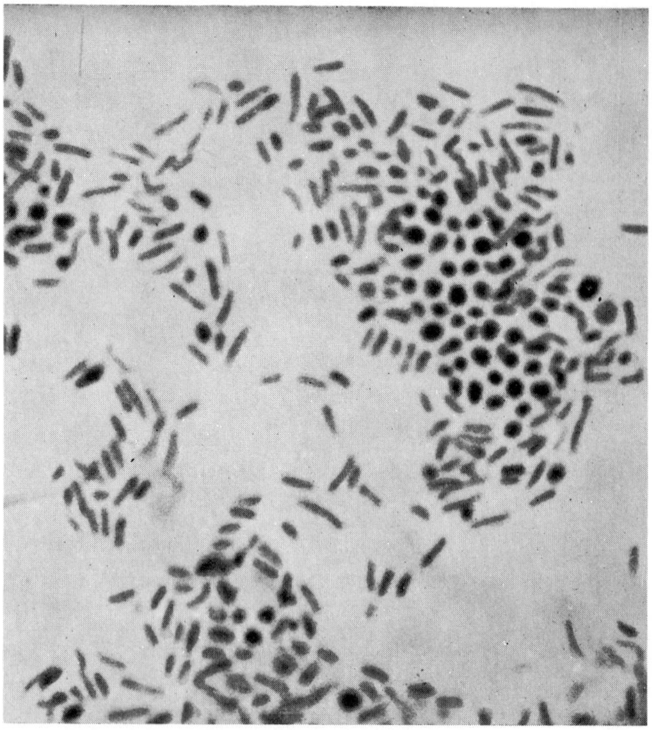

Fig. 39–1. *Francisella tularensis* from culture on glucose cystine agar, showing coccoid and bacillary forms in the same field. Approx. × 5000. *(From the U.S. Army Medical Museum. Courtesy of Edward Francis, U.S. Public Health Service.)*

wild virulent strains undergo phagocytosis but evade intracellular killing. The mechanism of intracellular survival is unclear, but wild strains have been shown to be resistant to polymorphonuclear lysosomal oxidants, including hypochlorous acid.

In addition to changes in virulence that accompany colonial variation, inherent differences exist among the wild strains of *F. tularensis*. There are two biovars of *F. tularensis*. Strains with high virulence for humans are most often associated with tick-borne tularemia of rabbits, exhibit citrulline ureidase activity, and ferment glycerol. These strains are the major type in the United States, occur only in North America, and are termed Jellison type A, or *F. tularensis* biovar *tularensis*. Strains of lesser virulence for humans are associated with water-borne disease of rodents, seldom ferment glycerol, and do not exhibit citrulline ureidase activity (Jellison type B, or *F. tularensis*, biovar *palaearctica*). These strains are found mainly in the eastern states of the United States and are the predominant type in Europe, Russia, and the Far East. In some areas, both types are present.

Antigenic Structure

There is a single immunologic type of *F. tularensis*. Therefore, immune sera produced with whole organisms react with and can be absorbed by all strains. Only living vaccines are effective immunogens against infection of susceptible hosts. Three major antigens have been obtained from all strains tested: (1) a polysaccharide antigen that produces an immediate wheal and erythematous skin reaction in patients recovering from tularemia, (2) cell wall and envelope antigens that contain the immunizing antigen and are responsible for endotoxin activity, and (3) a protein antigen that causes a delayed-hypersensitivity reaction in patients with the disease. A common protein antigen is shared by *F. tularensis* and members of the genus *Brucella*.

Clinical Infection

Epidemiology. Tularemia is a reportable disease in the United States. Since 1939 when 2291 cases were reported, there has been a steady decline in the annual number of reported cases. Throughout the 1980s, about 200 cases were reported yearly, with the largest number of cases occurring in the Midwest. The majority of the cases are from rural areas, with adult males accounting for 65% to 75% of the tick-borne and rabbit-associated infections. Women and children, however, commonly acquire the infection while skinning a rabbit. Two seasonal incidence peaks occur, one in the spring and summer months in areas where tick-borne cases predominate and another in the winter months in areas where rabbit-associated infections are prevalent.

Tularemia is enzootic in all areas of the continental United States, as well as most other areas of the northern hemisphere, with the exception of the British Isles. *F. tularensis* has been isolated from approximately 100 types of wildlife and from natural waters in areas frequented by these animals. In the United States, the most important reservoir hosts are rabbits and ticks. Other wild and domestic animals susceptible to tularemia include deer, fox, mink, hare, raccoon, opossum, beaver, mouse, rat, mole, dog, sheep, cat, and horse. Many species of birds also probably are naturally infected.

Of the two biovars that occur in the United States, biovar *tularensis* accounts for approximately 80% of the recognized human cases in North America, is highly virulent for humans, and usually is tick-borne and rabbit-associated. Biovar *palaearctica* occurs among sheep kids, may be transmitted to humans by mosquitoes or ticks, is less virulent for humans, and usually is associated with disease of water-dwelling rodents, such as muskrats, and with associated contamination of streams. The source of disease in muskrats and beavers is probably an epizootic of tularemia in a neighboring, highly susceptible rodent population, leading to a dying off of the rodents in the area adjacent to the water, contamination of the water, and disease of the larger rodents. Apparent disease from tularemia among rodent species ranges from asymptomatic disease to bacteremia with survival or to the rapid death of the entire colony.

F. tularensis has been recovered from over 54 arthropod species, half of which are known to have transmitted the disease to humans. At least 10 species of ticks, especially *Dermacentor andersoni, Dermacentor variabilis*, and *Amblyomma americanum*, transmit tularemia and are the most common arthropod vectors, but other bloodsucking arthropods may be involved, including deerflies, mites, blackflies, mosquitoes, and occasionally lice. *F. tularensis* may be transmitted directly from an infected female tick to her offspring, an example of transovarial passage of infection.

The most common methods by which humans become infected with *F. tularensis* are by contact with infected animals or through the bite of an arthropod vector. Other methods of infection include ingestion of inadequately cooked infected meat, usually rabbit, leading to primary cervical or gastrointestinal tularemia, which presents without a lesion of the skin. *F. tularensis* is a hardy organism and retains its viability on fomites, which may serve as a vehicle for the transmission of infection. Two examples of this latter mode of transmission are (1) laboratory-acquired infections, which are common and from which a great deal has been learned concerning the natural history of the disease, and (2) inhalation of dust that has been contaminated with infected vole feces during an epizootic. Other methods of acquiring the disease include direct inoculation into the skin from an infected animal bite or scratch, such as from a cat and, rarely, direct spread from an infected person. This is known to have occurred only in the case of a pathologist who accidentally contaminated himself while handling infected material. Under normal circumstances, person-to-person transfer does not occur. Congenital infection has been reported.

In humans, tularemia is usually a sporadic disease, but it may be epidemic in situations that favor the arthropod vector, such as the deerfly, or when water or food supplies are contaminated. Regional differences in the ecology of the reservoirs of tularemia markedly affect its epidemiologic characteristics. No other disease is more varied in its reservoir, vectors, and ecology.

Pathogenesis. The infective dose for highly susceptible animals, such as mice and guinea pigs, is one organism. For humans, the intradermal infective dose is 10 organisms, and 10 to 50 organisms will produce disease after exposure to infectious aerosols. Macrophages of the fixed reticuloendothelial system and circulating mononuclear phagocytes ingest and harbor the organism. Approximately 2 weeks after infection, specific T lymphocytes are activated, and macrophages ingest and kill the organism. Peripheral polymorphonuclear leukocytes phagocytize *F. tularensis* only in the presence of immune serum. Infected tissue is characterized by invasion of macrophages, necrosis, and granuloma formation.

In the original description of tularemia, Francis recognized at least four clinical forms: glandular, ulceroglandular, oculoglandular, and typhoidal. Tularemic meningitis, gastrointestinal disease, bacterial endocarditis, pharyngitis, and pneumonia were described subsequently. These variations in presentation depend largely on the method by which the person has acquired the infection, the virulence of the organism, and the individual's resistance to tularemia.

Most infections in the United States are acquired by direct inoculation or from the bite of a contaminated arthropod, usually a tick, deerfly, or mosquito, which leads to the ulceroglandular form of disease. Ulceration at the site of inoculation and regional lymphadenitis are similar following the arthropod bite or direct inoculation, such as occurs during the dressing of an infected rabbit. At the site of inoculation, a single punched-out ulcer develops within 1 to 3 days. Lymphangitic spread from the ulcer to the draining nodes may be apparent as induration and erythema. These painful and swollen regional nodes may be the first noticeable sign of disease. Abscess formation with caseation is typical of involved nodes.

Clinical Manifestations. In the United States, approximately 75% of cases are ulceroglandular, and the rest are typhoidal in presentation. There is an abrupt onset of disease that occurs early in the course of illness, with systemic manifestations, such as back pain, anorexia, headache, chills and fever, sweating, and prostration. Nonproductive cough, nausea, vomiting, and abdominal pain also are common. Over 10% of patients develop a rash that may be macular, papular, or blotchy, is painless, is not pruritic, and lasts for approximately a week.

In untreated ulceroglandular cases, the primary ulcer often suppurates and heals with scarring in 4 to 7 weeks. Lymphadenopathy is often of long duration, and convalescence usually extends from 3 to 6 months. Suppuration sometimes continues for years, and relapses are frequent. Before specific therapy became available, the mortality rate was about 10%, but it is now less than 1%. In areas of the world where less virulent disease is prevalent, such as Russia and Japan, low mortality rates always have prevailed.

Oculoglandular disease, which is usually acquired during the skinning of a rabbit, accounts for less than 5% of the cases and is similar to the ulceroglandular forms except that the conjunctival sac is the primary site of inoculation. In the early stages, a papule may develop in the conjunctiva, and the histopathology is that of a granulomatous conjunctivitis that may suppurate. Involved lymph nodes are the preauricular, parotid, submaxillary, and cervical. Although blindness is uncommon, the disease often is accompanied by severe systemic signs of disease and may be fatal.

The two forms of the disease that do not have a primary ulcer are glandular and typhoidal tularemia. Glandular disease presents with adenopathy. Typhoidal disease is characterized by general and severe systemic symptoms and must be differentiated from typhoid fever, brucellosis, tuberculosis, and other generalized bacterial diseases. Hepatosplenomegaly is common, and the mortality rate is particularly high. Diagnosis is more difficult because there is no history of contact with an appropriate vector or source. Blood and sputum cultures most frequently yield *F. tularensis*.

Pulmonary disease commonly accompanies tularemia and may be the dominant feature. Roentgenographic findings, which are not specific for tularemia, include bronchopneumonia, pleural effusion, hilar adenopathy, nodular infiltrations, and peribronchial thickening. The etiology of these changes probably includes hematogenous spread to the lung parenchyma, extension from involved hilar lymph nodes, and, occasionally, inhalation of bacteria. Most of the reported cases of laboratory-acquired tularemia have been assumed to have resulted from inhaled infected particles. Persons with tularemic pulmonary involvement, however, seldom disseminate disease to other persons, and secondary spread is extremely rare. Other rare forms of tularemia have included meningitis following septicemia, gastrointestinal disease following ingestion of infected food, and congenital infection.

Immunity. Humoral antibodies usually are found in the serum by the second to third week of the primary infection. Both IgM and IgG agglutinating antibodies are formed, and both typically persist indefinitely. Therefore, the presence of IgM antibody to *F. tularensis* does not necessarily indicate a recent infection. The agglutinating and precipitating antibodies to *F. tularensis* confer incomplete protective immunity to virulent strains. Humans and animals with high titers of these antibodies after immunization subsequently have acquired the disease. The epitopes for agglutinating antibody are carbohydrate antigens located on the surface of encapsulated *F. tularensis*.

The major factor in acquired resistance to tularemia appears to be a cellular immune mechanism involving an activated macrophage population. Evidence for this has come from several observations, among the most important of which is the finding that peritoneal macrophages from immune animals exhibit enhanced destruction of *F. tularensis* and prolonged cell viability after phagocytosis as compared with cells from nonimmune animals. This phenomenon is influenced negligibly by specific antibody. Significant also is the finding that protective immunity to *F. tularensis* may be conferred by the transfer of macrophages from immune animals. These and other observations are thus consistent with the concept that *F. tularensis* is a facultative intracellular parasite of the reticuloendothelial system and that development of protective immunity is coincident with the development of cell-mediated immunity.

A more precise definition of the cell population responsible for delayed hypersensitivity to *F. tularensis* and protection against disease has indicated that T lymphocytes are centrally involved. Membrane polypeptides of *F. tularensis* cause immunospecific stimulation of T lymphocytes, which are capable of presenting the antigen to macrophages and thereby initiating the cycle leading to delayed hypersensitivity.

Another important aspect of host resistance to arthropod-borne tularemia is the correlation that exists between host resistance to tick infestation and the transmission of *F. tularensis*. Sheep and other animals that have been sensitized to ticks have a greatly decreased death rate when exposed to tularemia-infected ticks, as compared with animals that have not been sensitized to ticks.

SKIN TEST. A skin test using phenolized and diluted vaccine gives a delayed reaction within 7 days of the onset of disease in approximately 90% of persons with known tularemia. This skin test has been useful in epidemiologic studies on the prevalence of tularemia in endemic areas and in hazardous occupations. A reactive status persists for many years after infection or vaccination, long after circulating antibody has greatly decreased. The tularemia skin test does not elicit a response in persons previously infected with *Brucella* species without *F. tularensis* infection. The skin test also is more sensitive than most serologic tests, being reactive earlier in infection and lasting longer. In one study, 72% of persons with a delayed hypersensitivity reaction had demonstrable circulating antibody. At the present time, skin test antigen is not commercially available.

Laboratory Diagnosis

CULTURE. Diagnosis of tularemia by culture of *F. tularensis* is uncommon because of the requirement for special media and frequent overgrowth by other organisms. Overgrowth may be controlled partially by the use of selective inhibitors, such as penicillin G and cycloheximide. Another obstacle in the recovery of *F. tularensis* from clinical specimens is the reluctance of many laboratories to attempt isolation because of the high rate of laboratory-acquired disease. This is especially true when animal inoculation is used. In one review of 2465 laboratory-associated infections in the United States, tularemia was second only to brucellosis in frequency. Even in laboratories well equipped to attempt isolation, the proportion of isolates to suspected cases is low when compared with most bacterial diseases. In patients with pulmonary foci of disease, direct culture of pharyngeal secretion and morning gastric aspirates may yield an isolate, as may the primary ulcer and regional lymph node. Although the organism is infrequently isolated from blood, at least 3 mL of blood (without anticoagulant) should be cultured on one of the recommended cysteine agar media. Serologic confirmation of *F. tularensis* isolates is accomplished by slide agglutination with specific antiserum.

SEROLOGIC TESTS

Direct Examination. The examination of gram-stained clinical specimens by the ordinary light microscope is unproductive for *F. tularensis*. However, using the direct or indirect fluorescent antibody techniques, a rapid and specific identification of the organism in exudates, tissue impressions, and sections may be made, even when the organisms are nonviable. Under such circumstances, a thermostable antigen may be extracted from organisms or infected tissue and identified by a precipitin reaction using appropriate antibody.

Agglutination Test. The agglutination test is the most commonly used serologic method for the clinical diagnosis of tularemia. It usually becomes positive by the second to fourth week of disease, at which time the titer rises sharply to a maximum of over 1:1280 in 4 to 8 weeks and persists for a variable time. Agglutination titers that are considered to be diagnostic of tularemia are set arbitrarily by each laboratory. A single assay with titer greater than 1:160 is diagnostic of past or current infection; two assays with a fourfold increase in titer are highly associated with disease that is characteristic of tularemia or of culture-proven tularemia. The skin test usually becomes positive before the agglutination test and remains positive longer. The serologic assay for agglutinating antibody to *F. tularenis* usually is not included in screening studies for febrile agglutinins.

Recently developed tests for the diagnosis of tularemia include an enzyme-linked immunosorbent assay (ELISA) and lymphocyte stimulation assays. The ELISA test appears to be reactive earlier in the illness than the agglutination assay, and after infection, both types of assay remain positive for years to decades. The ELISA test appears not to be more sensitive except during the first week of illness. No assay permits correlation of serum titer with severity of disease, since illnesses of all severities induce similar mean antibody responses.

The antibody response to infection or to vaccination with attentuated or killed *F. tularensis* includes production of agglutinins that cross-react with *Brucella abortus* and *Brucella melitensis*. The agglutinating titer to *Brucella* that is stimulated by *F. tularensis* is usually two to four dilutions lower than that to *F. tularensis*.

Treatment. Streptomycin is the recommended treatment for tularemia. Bactericidal concentrations are achieved readily, and there is little clinical tendency to relapse. In contrast, clinical studies with both chloramphenicol and tetracyclines have demonstrated recurrent disease and failure of these drugs to eradicate subcutaneous deposits of bacteria. Treatment during early infection is more likely to result in eradication of organisms than is treatment of chronic tularemia. Strains naturally resistant to streptomycin, chloramphenicol, or tetracycline are exceedingly rare. Penicillin is inefficacious.

Prevention. Prevention involves avoidance of animals likely to be infected, especially rabbits, protection from biting arthropods, and provision of clean water supplies. The natural foci of disease appear to be stable and are unlikely to be eradicated. Rabbits sick with tularemia are caught more easily by dogs or cats and may, therefore, be brought into contact with humans. Persons at risk include rabbit hunters, all persons who handle wet skins of potentially infected animals, such as muskrats and beavers, sheepshearers, and persons in endemic areas whose field work brings them into contact with rodents. Precautionary measures may include wearing clothing with secure ankles and wrists to protect against attachment of ticks.

At high risk are all laboratory personnel handling cultures of *F. tularensis* and infected laboratory animals. Persons likely to be exposed in this way, including the animal handlers, are candidates for immunization with live vaccine. Chemoprophylaxis is not recommended.

IMMUNIZATION. Attenuated live tularemia vaccine is available through the Centers for Disease Control. Experimental and clinical experience with the use of this vaccine has been acquired in Russia, Japan, and the United States. The tularemia vaccine and the vaccine of the bacillus of Calmette and Guerin (BCG) for tuberculosis are the only currently licensed live bacterial vaccines. Use of the tularemia vaccine is restricted to persons whose risk of exposure is high, such as sheepherders, sheepshearers, trappers, and laboratory personnel.

The vaccine, which is usually administered by scarification, produces a papular-vesicular lesion at the site of the injection, similar to that in smallpox vaccination. Reactions to the vaccine are not severe, but regional lymphadenitis does occur. The vaccine stimulates a cellular immune response manifested by the development of cutaneous delayed hypersensitivity. Most vaccines produce an antibody response that reaches a peak within 1 month for 50% of the vaccinees and within 2 months in the remainder. In vaccinated persons, the infective dose of *F. tularensis* is estimated to be 10 to 50 virulent organisms, which is several logarithms higher than it is for nonimmune individuals. When clinical disease does occur in previously vaccinated individuals, it is modified in severity.

FURTHER READING

Anthony LSD, Skamene E, Konigshavn PAL: Influence of genetic background on host resistance to experimental murine tularemia. Infect Immun 56:2089, 1988

Bell JF, Stewart SJ, Wikel SK: Resistance to tick-borne *Francisella tularensis* by tick-sensitized rabbits: Allergic klendusity. Am J Trop Med Hyg 28:876, 1979

Bevanger L, Maeland JA, Haess A: Agglutinins and antibodies to *Francisella tularensis* outer membrane antigens in the early diagnosis of disease during an outbreak of tularemia. J Clin Microbiol 26:433, 1988

Buchanan TM, Brooks GF, Brachman PS: The tularemia skin test: 325 skin tests in 210 persons: Serologic correlation and review of the literature. Ann Intern Med 74:336, 1971

Francis E: Symptoms, diagnosis and pathology of tularemia. JAMA 91:1155, 1928

Jellison WL, Owen CR, Bell JF: Tularemia and animal populations: Ecology and epizoology. Wildlife Dis 17:22, 1961

Lofgren S, Tärnvik A, Thore M, Carlsson J: A wild and an attenuated strain of *Francisella tularensis* differ in susceptibility to hypochlorous acid: A possible explanation of their different handling by polymorphonuclear leukocytes. Infect Immun 43:730, 1984

Pike RM: Laboratory associated infections: Summary and analysis of 3,921 cases. Health Lab Sci 13:105, 1976

Sandström G, Löfgren S, Tärnvik A: A capsule-deficient *Francisella tularensis* LVS exhibits enhanced sensitivity to killing by serum but diminished sensitivity to killing by polymorphonuclear leukocytes. Infect Immun 56:1194, 1988

Surcel H-M: Diversity of *Francisella tularensis* antigens recognized by human T lymphocytes. Infect Immun 58:2664, 1990

Sutinen S, Syrjala H: Histopathology of human lymph node tularemia caused by *Francisella tularensis* var *palaearctica*. Arch Pathol Lab Med 110:42, 1986

Syrjala H, Herva E, Ilonen J, et al: A whole-blood lymphocyte stimulation test for the diagnosis of human tularemia. J Infect Dis 150:912, 1984

Syrjala H, Koskela P, Ripatti T, et al: Agglutination and ELISA methods in the diagnosis of tularemia in different clinical forms and severities of the disease. J Infect Dis 153:142, 1986

Tärnvik A: Nature of protective immunity to *Francisella tularensis*. Rev Infect Dis 11:440, 1989

Young LS, Bicknell DS, Archer BG, et al: Tularemia epidemic: Vermont, 1968. Forty-seven cases linked to contact with muskrats. N Engl J Med 280:1253, 1969

CHAPTER 40

Pasteurella and Miscellaneous Gram-Negative Bacilli

Pasteurella

Organisms of the genus *Pasteurella* are primarily parasites of domestic and wild animals and birds, but they also are capable of producing a variety of diseases in humans. The genus comprises an extremely heterogeneous group of organisms, with six currently recognized species (Table 40–1). *Pasteurella multocida* is the species most frequently associated with human infections. The organism derives its name *multocida* (*many killings*) from its wide host spectrum and now includes as biovars those organisms previously classified as different species because of their isolation from different animal hosts.

Pasteurella multocida

Morphology and Physiology

Pasteurella are small, nonmotile, coccobacillary or rod-shaped organisms 0.3 to 1.0 μm by 1.0 to 2.0 μm in size. They are gram-negative and show bipolar staining, especially in preparations from infected tissue. In cultures from clinical material, they occur singly or in pairs and, occasionally, in short chains. Some strains of *P. multocida*, however, exhibit marked pleomorphism on primary cultures. Virulent organisms produce a capsule that may be demonstrated in Giemsa-stained smears of purulent exudates.

Pasteurella species are facultatively anaerobic. They are catalase-positive and usually oxidase-positive. Their metabolism is fermentative, and acid is produced by most strains from glucose, mannitol, and sucrose. Distinguishing properties of *P. multocida* are shown in Table 40–1.

Cultural Characteristics. *Pasteurella* will grow on standard laboratory media containing blood or hematin. On blood agar, *P. multocida* is nonhemolytic but may produce a brownish discoloration of the medium in areas of confluent growth. The optimum temperature for growth is 37C, with growth occurring between 25C and 40C. *P. multocida* will not grow in bile-containing media (e.g., MacConkey's agar).

Colonies of the various species in this genus are similar in appearance—round, grayish, and from 1 to 3 mm in diameter after 24 hours. Some strains of *P. multocida*, especially isolates from the respiratory tract, produce a large hyaluronic acid capsule that imparts a watery to mucoid character to the colonies. Other virulent strains of *P. multocida* produce smooth iridescent colonies that, on subculture, readily dissociate to smooth noniridescent and rough blue colony forms. The latter two colonial variants are nonencapsulated and avirulent.

Antigenic Structure

Multiple antigenic types of *P. multocida* can be distinguished based on the capsular and somatic antigens. On the basis of polysaccharide capsular antigens, there are four different serotypes, designated A, B, D, and E. Types A and D are the most frequent types associated with human infections. A number of different O, or somatic, antigen types also have been demonstrated, which together with the capsular serotypes have provided systems for identifying more than 16 somatic O groups, or serovars. The serovar of a strain is designated by a number that indicates the O type, followed by a letter indicating the capsular type, for example, serovar 1:A.

Determinants of Pathogenicity

Encapsulated organisms usually are pathogenic for mice, but other ill-defined factors, including the somatic antigens, play an important role in pathogenicity. The cell walls of *Pasteurella* have significant endotoxin activity, but no exotoxin has been demonstrated. Neuraminidase activity is present in *P. multocida* and *Pasteurella haemolytica,* and fimbriae that function as adhesins in type A *P. multocida* are believed to play a role in colonization and infection of nasopharyngeal mucosa. Some strains produce hyaluronidase, especially isolates that come from animals with hemorrhagic septicemia.

Clinical Infection

Epidemiology. *Pasteurella* species are present as normal flora in many domestic animals. *P. multocida* occupies an ecologic niche in the nasopharynx of the cat similar to that of α-hemolytic *Streptococcus* in humans. It survives poorly in soil and water and is transmitted most commonly by direct contact, usually a bite. The tonsils of dogs are a site commonly colonized with *P. multocida.* The organism is more common in young male dogs, and the rate of colonization is higher in the cold seasons. Rates of colonization for the dog vary, but the majority of cats harbor *P. multocida,* as do many other domestic animals. Colonized animals generally are asymptomatic, and the disease usually occurs during stressful situations, such as the shipping of cattle, when highly virulent organisms may be recovered from diseased animals. *P. multocida* is responsible for outbreaks of cholera of domestic or wild fowl, hemorrhagic septicemia of cattle, and primary and secondary pneumonias.

P. multocida types A and D are widely distributed in nature, and most respiratory tract disease in humans is caused by type A. Types B and C have been recovered primarily from cattle, bison, and buffalo. Organisms recovered from human disease following dog or cat bite or scratch usually are nontypable and rough and lack pathogenicity for mice.

Pathogenesis and Clinical Manifestations. Human disease caused by *P. multocida* or by other members of the genus that are rarely pathogenic for humans may be of three types: (1) infection via bites or scratches, (2) superinfection of a chronically diseased lung, and (3) other foci of disease that are secondary to septicemia.

Animal bites are common and frequently require medical attention. *P. multocida* can be recovered from approximately half of infected animal bites. In addition, half of the wounds that initially are colonized with *P. multocida* develop frank infection. Wounds that have been sutured are particularly prone to develop infection with the organism. Complications of bites infected with *P. multocida* are common. Cat bites may progress to pyarthrosis, necrotizing synovitis, and osteomyelitis of the underlying bone, presumably due to the depth of the bite and associated trauma of adjacent tissue. Regional lymphadenitis, with severe local pain, swelling, and discoloration, follows the often sudden onset of signs of infection.

Septicemia occurs primarily in persons with underlying disease that impairs reticuloendothelial function, such as cirrhosis of the liver and rheumatoid arthritis, but also has been reported in apparently normal persons.

The second most common form of human disease with *P. multocida* is infection of the lung in patients with preexisting chronic pulmonary disease. These patients usually are middle-aged or older. Lower respiratory tract diseases associated with recovery of *P. multocida* are bronchiectasis, bronchogenic carcinoma, chronic bronchitis, emphysema, pulmonary abscess, and pneumonia, including sinusitis, mastoiditis, and chronic otitis media. *P. multocida* also has been recovered from upper respiratory tract infections. Disease with *P. multocida* in these settings of previously chronic disease may occur with asymptomatic colonization and insidious progression to apparent pulmonary disease or with an acute or fulminant onset.

TABLE 40–1. DIFFERENTIAL PROPERTIES OF *PASTEURELLA* SPECIES

Property	*P. multocida*	*P. pneumotropica*	*P. haemolytica*	*P. ureae*	*P. aerogenes*	*P. gallinarum*
β-Hemolysis on blood agar	−	−	+	−	−	−
Growth on MacConkey's agar	−	−	+	−	+	−
Indole production	+	+	−	−	−	−
Urease activity	−	+	−	+	+	−
Gas from carbohydrates	−	−	−	−	+	−
Acid production from						
Glucose	+	+	+	+	+	+
Lactose	−	d	d	−	−	−
Mannitol	+[a]	−	+	+	−	−

From Carter: In Krieg and Holt (eds): Bergey's Manual of Systematic Bacteriology, vol 1. Williams & Wilkins, 1984.
+, 90% or more of strains are positive; −, 90% or more of strains are negative; d, 11%–89% of strains are positive.
[a] Strains from dogs and cats may be negative.

Other sites of infection with *P. multocida* are unusual and represent either hematogenous dissemination during bacteremia or local extension. Examples are meningitis, chorioamnionitis with premature delivery, cerebellar abscess, and infectious endocarditis.

Laboratory Diagnosis. Identification of the causative agent requires culture of appropriate specimens from the patient, depending on the area of involvement. Early morning sputum, bronchial washing, nasal swabs from respiratory tract infections, purulent exudate from animal bites, spinal fluid, and repeated blood cultures are appropriate for this purpose.

Treatment and Prevention. Among the gram-negative rods, *Pasteurella* species are unusual in their uniform sensitivity to penicillin, which is the drug of choice. The mean inhibitory concentrations of tetracycline, ampicillin, and benzyl penicillin are less than 0.5 μg/mL. As with other pyogenic infections, localized abscesses must be drained. After an animal bite the wound should be meticulously cleaned, and suturing should be avoided. Initiation of treatment with penicillin or tetracycline at the time of the bite is recommended by many physicians, but the value of prophylactic administration of antibiotics has not been evaluated adequately.

There are no effective means of preventing human *Pasteurella* infections at the present time other than limiting contact with wild and domestic animals. A number of vaccines and antisera preparations have been used in the past in an attempt to control veterinary disease caused by these organisms, but these lacked efficacy and are no longer used.

Actinobacillus

Except for *Actinobacillus actinomycetemcomitans,* most members of the genus are found both as pathogens and as commensal organisms in domestic mammals and birds. As commensals, the actinobacilli are present in the respiratory, alimentary, and genital tracts of normal animals, in which they cause sporadic opportunistic infections. *A. actinomycetemcomitans* is a strictly human parasite. Its name was derived from the Greek *actis* (ray), *mycetis* (fungus), and Latin *comitans* (accompanying) because of its early isolation in association with *Actinomyces* in actinomycotic and actinomycotic-like lesions.

Morphology and Physiology. The cells of this organism are spherical or rod-shaped, 0.3 to 0.5 μm by 0.6 to 1.4 μm in size. They are nonencapsulated and nonmotile. *A. actinomycetemcomitans* is a facultative anaerobe, but growth is better under microaerophilic conditions in an atmosphere of 10% CO_2. Metabolism is fermentative, and acid but no gas is produced from glucose and fructose. The organism will not grow on MacConkey's agar but requires an enriched medium, such as blood or serum agar (Table 40–2). Colonies reach their maximal size of 1 mm after 2 to 3 days at 37C, are starlike in appearance, and adhere to the agar.

Clinical Infection. Although earlier isolates were obtained from lesions also infected with *Actinomyces* species, in the majority of clinical isolations since, *A. actinomycetemcomitans* has been the sole isolate. Most systemic clinical isolates have been from infected blood and bone. It is a part of the normal mouth flora and has been isolated in high numbers from subgingival plaque samples from patients with juvenile periodontitis. The majority of *A. actinomycetemcomitans* strains are able to selectively destroy isolated human polymorphonuclear neutrophils (PMN), whereas other subgingival plaque isolates lack this ability. The destruction of PMNs by the leukotoxin produced by this organism is believed to play an important role in the pathogenesis of inflammatory periodontal disease. Persons with prosthetic heart valves or structural heart abnormalities are at risk of developing *Actinobacillus* endocarditis after dental manipulation or in association with periodontal disease. In addition to culture from patients with endocarditis, the organism has been isolated in pure culture from cases of brain abscess, pneumonia, urinary tract infections, thyroid abscess, and osteomyelitis. The apparent etiology of some cases of human *Actinobacillus* disease is related to impaired host defenses, as in such diseases as malignant lymphoma and leukemias.

Isolates are variable in their susceptibility to penicillin but are uniformly susceptible to tetracycline and chloramphenicol. Infective endocarditis attributable to this organism has been

TABLE 40–2. DIFFERENTIAL PROPERTIES OF *ACTINOBACILLUS* AND OTHER MORPHOLOGICALLY OR PHYSIOLOGICALLY SIMILAR GENERA

Property	*Actinobacillus*	*Haemophilus*	*Gardnerella*	*Capnocytophaga*	*Cardiobacterium*
Oxidase test	−	D	−	−	+
Catalase test	+	D	−	+	−
Yellow-orange pigmented colonies	−	−	−	+	−
Nitrate to nitrite	+	+	−	D	−
Growth on blood agar, 37C					
In air	−	−	+	−	d
In air + CO_2	+	−[a]	+	+	+
β-Hemolysis, 5% human blood agar	−	−	+	−	−
Mol% G + C of DNA	40–43	38–44	42–44	33–41	59–60

Adapted from Greenwood and Pickett: In Krieg and Holt (eds): Bergey's Manual of Systematic Bacteriology, vol 1. Williams & Wilkins, 1984.
+, typically positive; −, typically negative; D, differs among species; d, differs among strains of a genus with a single species; G + C, guanine plus cytosine.
[a] One species, *H. aphrophilus*, can grow on blood agar.

treated successfully with a combination of penicillin G and streptomycin or with ampicillin alone.

Streptobacillus

Rat-bite fever is a clinical term for a systemic febrile disease that is acquired by direct contact with rats or other small rodents. It can be caused by either *Streptobacillus moniliformis* or *Spirillum minus* (Chap. 46), which are present as part of the normal flora of the nasopharynx of wild and laboratory rats. Distinguishing features of the organisms and the clinical diseases with which they are associated are summarized in Table 40–3.

Morphology and Physiology. *S. moniliformis* is a nonencapsulated, nonmotile, gram-negative bacillus, 0.3 to 0.7 μm by 1 to 5 μm in length. Its cell morphology is extremely variable and is markedly affected by the age and condition of culture. The organism frequently occurs in long chains and filaments 10 to 150 μm long. It often is extremely pleomorphic and may produce a series of elongated bulbous swellings giving the appearance of a string of beads (Fig. 40–1). It is a facultative anaerobe with a fermentative type of metabolism. Glucose is fermented with acid but no gas. The most distinguishing characteristic of the organism is the spontaneous development of L-phase variants during in vitro culture (Fig. 40–2). The designation L-phase was first used by Klieneberger-Nobel to refer to the pleuropneumonia-like organism associated with *S. moniliformis* in cultures. It is now known that most bacteria and fungi are capable of similar changes, but this organism remains the prototype of this phenomenon.

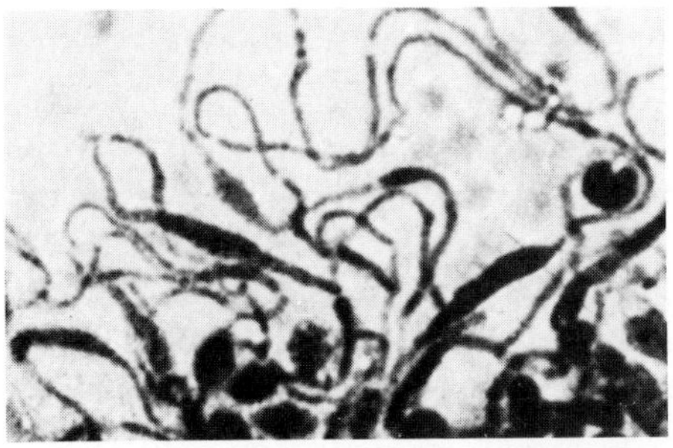

Fig. 40–1. Edge of a colony of *Streptobacillus moniliformis*. × 3000. *(From Sharp: The Role of Mycoplasmas and L Forms of Bacteria in Disease. Springfield, Ill, Charles C Thomas, 1970.)*

TABLE 40–3. DISTINGUISHING CHARACTERISTICS OF TWO CAUSES OF RAT-BITE FEVER IN HUMANS

Characteristic	*Streptobacillus moniliformis*	*Spirillum minor*
Bacteriology	Microaerophilic gram-negative pleomorphic bacillus	Gram-negative spiral organism
Diagnostic serology	Agglutinins	Not available
Incubation period	Usually 1–3 days	Usually more than 7 days
Source of human disease	Animal bite from wild or laboratory rat, animal bite from mouse, cat, dog, contaminated food	Animal bite from rat or cat
Rash	Morbiliform, maculopapular, or petechial on palms, soles, extremities	Violaceous macules become confluent on palms, soles, extremities
Fever	Usually septic	Usually relapsing, with fever lasting 3–4 days occurring at irregular intervals
Epidemiology	Poor sanitation with heavy rodent infestation, occupational exposure	Same as *S. moniliformis*
Treatment	Penicillin or tetracycline	Same as *S. moniliformis*

Culture of *S. moniliformis* requires a medium supplemented with serum or blood, increased CO_2, and a humid environment. After 3 days on serum agar, typical bacterial colonies are 1 to 2 mm in diameter and are smooth, grayish, and butyrous in consistency. L-phase colonies are considerably smaller, 300 to 500 nm in diameter, and exhibit a characteristic fried-egg appearance, with a dense center that extends into the agar and a lacy peripheral portion. In liquid media, the bacterial form produces typical puffballs of growth in the bottom of the tube.

Clinical Infection. Human disease caused by *S. moniliformis* is worldwide in its occurrence and, because of the usual rodent vector, is associated with poor or primitive living conditions, especially urban areas with a large rat population. In the United States, the disease is uncommon.

S. moniliformis is a common inhabitant of the nasopharynx of wild and laboratory rats. Although the disease usually is acquired by the bite of a rat or other rodent, it also may be transmitted by means of milk, water, and food. Human consumption of milk contaminated with *S. moniliformis* is believed to have been the cause of the disease known as

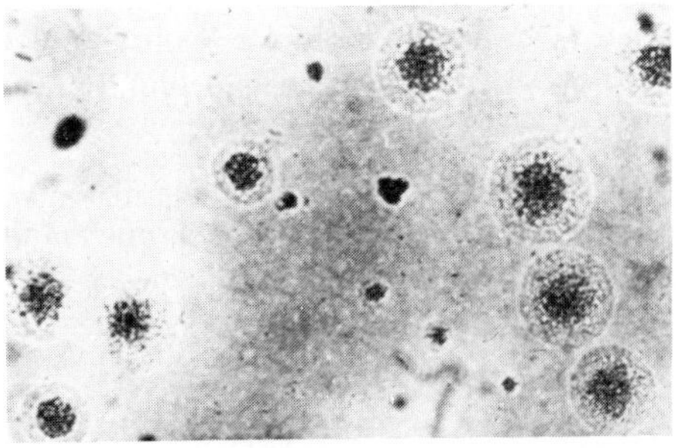

Fig. 40–2. L-form colony of *Streptobacillus moniliformis* produced spontaneously. × 100. *(From Sharp: The Role of Mycoplasmas and L Forms of Bacteria in Disease. Springfield, Ill, Charles C Thomas, 1970.)*

Haverhill fever. This disease frequently is recognized in laboratory workers who have been bitten by a rat or other rodent and in children who live amidst poor sanitary conditions that would allow them to be bitten by rats. Cases also have been reported of rat-bite fever developing in the absence of an actual bite but after close contact with dogs, cats, pigs, or rats.

The disease begins 1 to 5 days after introduction of the organism. The onset is abrupt, with chills, fever, vomiting, headache, and severe pain in the joints. A maculopapular rash develops within the first 48 hours, and one or more joints become swollen and painful. The rash characteristically is morbilliform, maculopapular, or petechial and involves the palms, soles, and extremities. Acute arthritis is a characteristic and persistent symptom. Endocarditis, pneumonia, and multiple abscesses in many organ systems characterize severe forms of the disease.

LABORATORY DIAGNOSIS. Diagnosis is made by isolation of the organism from the blood or from joint fluids and pus. Agglutinins appear in the patient's serum within 10 days and reach a maximum in 3 to 4 weeks. A titer of 1:80 is considered diagnostic, and a fourfold rise in titer is significant.

TREATMENT. Penicillin is the drug of choice. Tetracycline, streptomycin, chloramphenicol, and erythromycin also have been used successfully in treatment. If the disease is not treated, the mortality rate may be as high as 10%.

Calymmatobacterium

The genus *Calymmatobacterium* contains a single species, *Calymmatobacterium granulomatis*, the etiologic agent of donovanosis (granuloma inguinale). This is a chronic, mildly infectious disease characterized by ulcerating lesions of the skin and mucosa of the genital and inguinal areas.

Morphologic and Cultural Characteristics. The generic name of the organism is derived from the Greek word *calymma*, meaning sheath or mantle. *C. granulomatis* is a pleomorphic, gram-negative, nonmotile rod, 1 to 2 μm in length. It usually is heavily encapsulated and exhibits single or bipolar condensation of chromatin, a property that gives rise to the characteristic appearance of a safety pin when gram-stained. For primary isolation, the organism can be cultured on fresh egg yolk media or in the yolk sac of embryonated chicken eggs. *C. granulomatis* is antigenically similar to but not identical with *Klebsiella* species. Its taxonomic relationships to other bacterial genera have not been sufficiently defined, however, to associate the genus with any established family.

Within the host, *C. granulomatis* replicates intracellularly. The pathognomonic cell is a large, histiocytic endothelial cell containing numerous encapsulated bacilli, the Donovan bodies. These were first described in 1905 by Donovan, who observed them in epithelial cells of the skin of infected persons in India.

Clinical Infection. The disease associated with *C. granulomatis*, donovanosis, usually is classified as one of the minor venereally transmitted diseases. However, evidence of direct transmission by sexual contact is poor, and primary lesions have been diagnosed in skin areas other than the genital area. It is an inhabitant of the intestinal tract, and it is possible that skin disease is contracted through poor hygiene and abrasions of the skin in anal and perineal regions. It is primarily a disease of tropical and subtropical areas but occasionally is diagnosed in the southern United States. Communicability is apparently not high, since the disease is rarely transmitted to sexual partners. It occurs primarily in persons who are promiscuous and have had other venereally transmissible diseases. Although experimental infection in animals has not been achieved, infection in humans has been obtained by inoculation of diseased tissue or exudate.

The initial lesions of granuloma inguinale may occur in any of the pubic areas. They begin as painless papules that develop into spreading, ulcerating lesions, which may bleed and become secondarily infected. The lesions spread by direct extension or by contact of one skin area with another, such as between the scrotum and thigh. The patient is unlikely to have constitutional symptoms and remains afebrile. However, the infection may progress very slowly for long periods of time and heal with scarring. The scarring may lead to genital elephantiasis if treatment is not provided. Metastatic lesions to joints, bones, and liver have been reported.

Diagnosis depends on demonstration of Donovan bodies by direct examination of biopsy material that has been stained with the Wright or Giemsa stain. Culture may be attempted, but initial isolation is difficult.

Treatment consists of tetracycline, ampicillin, or trimethoprim-sulfamethoxazole.

Gardnerella vaginalis

The taxonomic position of this organism has for some time remained unresolved. On the basis of either superficial growth characteristics or morphology, *Gardnerella vaginalis* was classified as a member of the genus *Haemophilus* or the genus *Corynebacterium*. DNA-DNA hybridization studies, however, failed to show a close relationship to these or other recognized genera and led to the establishment of a new genus, *Gardnerella*.

Morphologic and Cultural Characteristics. Morphologically, the organism appears as pleomorphic bacilli approximately 0.5 μm in diameter and 1.5 to 2.5 μm in length. It is gram-negative to gram-variable, with retention of the gram stain being more pronounced in young cultures 8 to 12 hours old. Club forms and metachromatic granules often are present. The organism is nonmotile and nonencapsulated. Most strains of *Gardnerella* are facultatively anaerobic and are fastidious in their nutritional requirements. Unlike *Haemophilus* species, however, *Gardnerella* requires neither hemin nor nicotinamide adenine nucleotides. On human blood agar, a diffuse β-hemolysis is produced. Other distinguishing properties of the genus are shown in Table 40–2.

Clinical Infection. The clinical significance of *G. vaginalis* remains controversial, but it appears to act in concert with certain anaerobes to cause nonspecific vaginitis. It is present in the vagina of 40% of asymptomatic women but is found in large numbers in over 95% of patients with vaginitis. Masses of bacteria may be found on the surface of epithelial cells in the discharge. These cells observed in wet mounts are referred to as *clue cells* and are considered characteristic of *G. vaginalis* infection. Oral metronidazole has been used successfully to eliminate both organisms in the infection.

G. vaginalis also has been associated with septic abortion, puerperal fever with bacteremia, and neonatal bacteremia.

Other Gram-Negative Bacilli

A number of other facultative, gram-negative organisms may be encountered in the clinical microbiology laboratory, often from compromised patients or from patients with hospital-acquired infections. These organisms constitute a heterogeneous group whose taxonomy is currently in a state of flux and whose isolation from clinical materials frequently causes problems of identification.

Cardiobacterium

The only species in this genus is *Cardiobacterium hominis,* a gram-negative rod, 0.5 to 0.75 μm wide and 1 to 3 μm long, arranged singly or in pairs, short chains, or clusters. On blood agar containing yeast extract, organisms stain homogeneously and are uniform in size, but in the absence of yeast extract, pleomorphic forms with enlarged ends, rosette clusters, or serpentine forms may occur.

C. hominis is microaerophilic and grows well on enriched medium, such as trypticase soy agar, chocolate agar, or heart infusion agar, at 30C to 37C and in an atmosphere of 3% to 5% carbon dioxide. A high-humidity requirement is growth limiting. Growth is characteristically very slow, with minute punctiform colonies visible after 24 hours and attaining a maximum size of 1 to 2 mm in 3 to 4 days. No hemolysis is observed, but in areas of heavy growth, a slight greening of the blood agar may develop. *C. hominis* does not grow on MacConkey's agar and other selective media used for the isolation of the Enterobacteriaceae. *C. hominis* is oxidase-positive, catalase-negative, and nonmotile. It is fermentative and produces acid throughout triple sugar iron (TSI) medium. Its production of indole is an especially important biochemical clue to its recognition in the clinical microbiology laboratory. Other biochemical properties are listed in Table 40–2.

C. hominis is a part of the normal flora of the human upper respiratory tract and also has been recovered from cervical and vaginal cultures of a few asymptomatic individuals. Infection occurs primarily in compromised individuals and has been described most frequently in association with endocarditis and bacteremia. In cases of endocarditis, the infection usually has been chronic and has manifested itself in patients with damaged or prosthetic heart valves. Other diseased sites from which *C. hominis* has been cultured with increasing frequency include the cervix, vagina, empyema fluid, spinal fluid, mandible, and sputum. Penicillin and ampicillin have been used successfully in the treatment of *C. hominis* infection.

Chromobacterium

Organisms in this genus are gram-negative, motile rods resembling certain nonfluorescent pseudomonads. They produce the pigment violacein, which is responsible for the violet color of colonies on suitable media. On blood agar, the colonies may appear to be black. Two species are recognized, *Chromobacterium violaceum* and *Chromobacterium fluviatile,* but only the former has been associated with human infection. *C. violaceum* grows on ordinary peptone medium and on MacConkey's agar. Most strains can be identified readily by pigmentation and the fermentative utilization of glucose and certain other carbohydrates.

C. violaceum is an inhabitant of soil and water and is especially common in tropical countries. Although usually considered to be nonpathogenic, it has been shown to cause severe pyogenic or septicemic infections of mammals, including humans. Infection with this organism has been confined primarily to tropical and subtropical regions, and in the United States, all cases have occurred in the southeast. The organism usually is introduced through injury to the skin resulting in localized abscesses and a very slowly evolving systemic disease. Infection usually is characterized by liver abscess, sepsis, and death. *C. violaceum* also may gain entry to the body via the gastrointestinal tract and is associated with diarrhea. The organism is sensitive to aminoglycosides, chloramphenicol, and tetracycline.

Capnocytophaga

These recently characterized oral organisms are fastidious gram-negative flexible rods, fusiform in shape, and with a gliding motility. They have a fermentative metabolism, are oxidase- and catalase-negative, and grow under anaerobic or aerobic conditions in the presence of 5% to 10% CO_2 (Table 40–2). Increased CO_2 is essential for aerobic growth. On blood agar at 37C, growth is characteristically slow. Colonies invisible to the unaided eye at 24 hours become 2 to 3 mm in diameter after 2 to 4 days. The genus has been divided into three distinct species that infect man based on physiologic and morphologic properties: *Capnocytophaga ochracea* (formerly *Bacteroides ochracea*), *Capnocytophaga sputigena,* and *Capnocytophaga gingivalis.* Group-specific and type-specific antigens have been identified, and various cell envelope components have been shown to have immunomodulating activity.

Considerable interest has focused recently on *Capnocytophaga* because it has been shown to be a predominant cultivable organism in the advancing front of periodontal lesions in individuals with juvenile-onset diabetes and those with defects in neutrophil adherence, chemotaxis, or both. It has been shown also to be capable of causing periodontal disease, including bone loss, when implanted into gnotobiotic rats. The organism has been recognized increasingly as a cause of bacteremia in immunocompromised granulocytopenic patients, and more recently it has been reported in nonimmunocompromised patients as a cause of sepsis and local infections. Isolation of the organism frequently has been associated with other flora in polymicrobial infection.

Eikenella corrodens

This is a small, 0.3 to 0.4 μm by 1.5 to 4.0 μm, gram-negative, facultatively anaerobic rod previously called *Bacteroides corrodens.* It is nonmotile and possesses no flagella, but a form of surface translocation termed *twitching motility* attributable to piluslike structures occurs with some strains. Hemin is required for aerobic growth but not for growth under anaerobic conditions. It does not grow on MacConkey's agar or other similar selective media. Growth, which is enhanced in an

TABLE 40–4. BIOCHEMICAL PROPERTIES OF *EIKENELLA CORRODENS*

Test or Substrate	Reaction
Oxidase	+
Catalase	−
Growth on	
MacConkey's agar	−
Salmonella-Shigella agar	−
Oxidation-fermentation test	I
Urease	−
Indole	−
Motility	−
Nitrate to nitrite only	+
Pigment (pale yellow)	+

From Rubin et al: In Lennette et al (eds): Manual of Clinical Microbiology, ed. 4. American Society for Microbiology, 1985, p 330.
+, 90% or more positive; −, no reaction in 90% or more; I, inactive, 100%.

atmosphere of 3% to 10% CO_2, is characteristically slow, with small pinpoint colonies usually visible after 24 hours of aerobic incubation on blood or chocolate agar. A distinctive feature observed with about 45% of the isolates is a pitting or corroding of the agar under the colony after several days of growth. The organism is nonhemolytic, but a slight greening may occur around colonies on blood media. It is oxidase-positive but is biochemically inactive, lacking both oxidative and fermentative capabilities (Table 40–4).

E. corrodens is a part of the indigenous flora of the mouth and upper respiratory tract as well as other mucosal surfaces of the human body. It is isolated most commonly from respiratory specimens but also may be isolated from a variety of other materials, such as blood, spinal fluid, abscesses, or joint aspirates. *E. corrodens* usually is associated with polymicrobic infections frequently involving the head and neck or abdominal area. It may be the sole cause of infection. Infections are usually the result of predisposing factors that compromise the body's host defense mechanisms and permit the organism to penetrate surrounding tissue. Hematogenous spread from this primary infection and establishment of foci in other body sites may then occur. *E. corrodens* has been reported from cases of meningitis, brain abscesses, endocarditis, osteomyelitis, and soft-tissue abscesses, among others. More than 60 documented cases of infection of human bites also have been reported. *E. corrodens* is sensitive to penicillin, tetracycline, colistin, and chloramphenicol but is resistant to clindamycin.

Flavobacterium

The genus *Flavobacterium* is a taxonomically heterogeneous group that currently is undergoing revision. Members of the genus appear to have closer similarities biochemically and chemotaxonomically to organisms within the family Cytophagaceae than to any other group. The clinically important members of the genus include *Flavobacterium meningosepticum*, *Flavobacterium indologenes* (King group II b), *Flavobacterium breve, Flavobacterium odoratum,* and *Flavobacterium multivorum. F. meningosepticum* is the species most commonly associated with human infection.

As currently defined, the genus *Flavobacterium* includes nonmotile gram-negative rods with rounded ends 0.5 μm wide and 1.0 to 3.0 μm long. They are aerobic, oxidase-positive, and very weakly fermentative and produce chromogenic colonies on solid media. Blood agar or chocolate agar is recommended for primary isolation from clinical materials. After 18 to 24 hours of incubation on blood agar, the organisms produce colonies 1 mm in diameter and cause a distinctive lavender-green discoloration of the red cells. In contrast to the intense yellow color of most *Flavobacterium* colonies, those of *F. meningosepticum* usually have only a slight yellow pigment, which can be intensified by growth on nutrient agar at room temperature.

The flavobacteria are widely distributed in nature in soil and water and normally are not a part of the indigenous human flora. They often are found in the hospital environment and have been isolated from a number of reservoirs, such as humidifiers, ice machines, waterbaths, saline solutions, respiratory equipment, incubators, and indwelling catheters, all of which may serve as a source for nosocomial infections. Most of these infections are caused by *F. meningosepticum* and occur primarily in neonates. Meningitis is the primary manifestation, and the mortality rate is high. In meningitis, blood cultures usually are positive. By contrast, infection in adults generally is mild and usually follows operative or manipulative procedures. The pathogenicity of the other *Flavobacterium* species is less well documented. They have been recovered from clinical specimens, such as blood, urine, and wound exudates, and have been reported as rare causes of meningitis and bacteremia in immunocompromised patients. Clinical isolates of *Flavobacterium* species usually are resistant to most antimicrobial agents. In vitro studies indicate that erythromycin, rifampin, and trimethoprim-sulfamethoxazole might prove useful in therapy.

FURTHER READING

Books and Reviews

Krieg NR, Holt JG (eds): Bergey's Manual of Systematic Bacteriology, vol 1. Baltimore, Williams & Wilkins, 1984

Balows A, Hausler WJ Jr, Herrman KL, et al (eds): Manual of Clinical Microbiology, ed 5. Washington, DC, American Society for Microbiology, 1991

Selected Articles

PASTEURELLA

Carter GR, Chengappa MM: Hyalunonidase produced by type B *Pasteurella multocida* from cases of hemorrhagic septicemia. J Clin Microbiol 11:94, 1980

Feder HM, Shanley JD, Barbera JA: Review of 59 patients hospitalized with animal bites. Pediatr Infect Dis J 6:24, 1987

Foged NT: Quantification and purification of the *Pasteurella multocida* toxin by using monoclonal antibodies. Infect Immun 56:1901, 1988

Glorioso JC, Jones GW, Rush HG, et al: Adhesion of type A *Pasteurella multocida* to rabbit pharyngeal cells and its possible role in rabbit respiratory tract infections. Infect Immun 35:1103, 1982

Heddleston KL, Wessman G: Characteristics of *Pasteurella multocida* of human origin. J Clin Microbiol 1:377, 1975

Hubbert WT, Rosen MN: I. *Pasteurella multocida* infection due to animal bite. II. *Pasteurella multocida* infection in man unrelated to animal bite. Am J Public Health 60:1103, 1109, 1970

Lu Y-S, Afendis SJ, Pakes SP: Identification of immunogenic outer membrane proteins of *Pasteurella multocida* 3:A in rabbits. Infect Immun 56:1532, 1988

Lu Y-S, Lai WC, Pakes SP, Nie LC. A monoclonal antibody against a *Pasteurella multocida* outer membrane protein protects rabbits and mice against pasteurellosis. Infect Immun 59:172, 1991

Murata M, Horiuchi T, Namioka S: Studies on the pathogenicity of *Pasteurella multocida* for mice and chickens on the basis of O-groups. Cornell Vet 54:294, 1964

Oberhofer TR: Characteristics and biotypes of *Pasteurella multocida* isolates from humans. J Clin Microbiol 13:566, 1981

Petersen SK, Foged NT: Cloning and expression of the *Pasteurella multocida* toxin gene, *tox A*, in *Escherichia coli.* Infect Immun 57:3907, 1989

Smith JE: Studies of *Pasteurella septica.* I. The occurrence in the nose and tonsils of dogs. J Comp Pathol 65:239, 1955

Truscott WM, Hirsch DC. Demonstration of an outer membrane protein with antiphagocytic activity from *Pasteurella multocida* of avian origin. Infect Immun 56:1538, 1988

ACTINOBACILLUS

Affias SA, West A, Stewart J, et al: *Actinobacillus actinomycetemcomitans* endocarditis. Can Med Assoc J 118:1256, 1978

Baehni P, Tsai C-C, McArthur WP, et al: Interaction of inflammatory cells and oral microorganisms. VIII. Detection of leukotoxic activity of a plaque-derived gram-negative microorganism. Infect Immun 24:233, 1979

Baehni PC, Tsai CC, McArthur WP, et al: Leukotoxic activity in different strains of the bacterium *Actinobacillus actinomycetemcomitans* isolated from juvenile periodontitis in man. Arch Oral Biol 26:671, 1981

Clark RA, Leidal KG, Taichman NS: Oxidative inactivation of *Actinobacillus actinomycetemcomitans* leukotoxin by the neutrophil myeloperoxidase system. Infect Immun 53:252, 1986

Ellner JJ, Rosenthal MS, Lerner PI, et al: Infective endocarditis caused by slow-growing, fastidious, gram-negative bacteria. Medicine 58:145, 1979

Hammond BF, Lillard SE, Stevens RH: A bacteriocin of *Actinobacillus actinomycetemcomitans.* Infect Immun 55:686, 1987

Holt SC, Tanner ACR, Socransky SS: Morphology and ultrastructure of oral strains of *Actinobacillus actinomycetemcomitans* and *Haemophilus aphrophilus.* Infect Immun 30:588, 1980

King EO, Tatum HW: *Actinobacillus actinomycetemcomitans* and *Haemophilus aphrophilus.* J Infect Dis 111:85, 1962

Nowotny A, Behling UH, Hammond B, et al: Release of toxic microvesicles by *Actinobacillus actinomycetemcomitans.* Infect Immun 37:151, 1982

Stevens RH, Hammond BF, Lai CH: Characterization of an inducible bacteriophage from a leukotoxic strain of *Actinobacillus actinomycetemcomitans.* Infect Immun 35:343, 1982

Taichman NS, Dean RT, Sanderson CJ: Biochemical and morphological characterization of the killing of human monocytes by a leukotoxin derived from *Actinobacillus actinomycetemcomitans.* Infect Immun 28:258, 1980

Vandepitte J, DeGeest H, Jousten P: Subacute bacterial endocarditis due to *Actinobacillus actinomycetemcomitans.* Report of a case with review of the literature. J Clin Pathol 30:842, 1977

STREPTOBACILLUS

Cole JS, Stoll RW, Bulger RJ: Rat-bite fever: Report of three cases. Ann Intern Med 71:979, 1969

Holden FA, MacKay JC: Rat-bite fever—An occupational hazard. Can Med Assoc J 91:78, 1964

Raffin BJ, Freemark M: Streptobacillary rat-bite fever: A pediatric problem. Pediatrics 64:214, 1979

Roughgarden JW: Antimicrobial therapy of rat-bite fever. Arch Intern Med 116:39, 1965

Rumley RL, Patrone NA, White L. Rat-bite fever as a cause of septic arthritis: A diagnostic dilemma. Ann Rheum Dis 46:793, 1987

CALYMMATOBACTERIUM

Anderson K: The cultivation from granuloma inguinale of a microorganism having the characteristics of Donovan bodies in the yolk sac of chick embryos. Science 97:560, 1943

Davis CM: Granuloma inguinale. A clinical, histological and ultrastructural study. JAMA 211:632, 1970

Kuberski T: Granuloma inguinale (donovanosis). Sex Transmit Dis 7:29, 1980

Kuberski T, Papadimitriou JM, Phillips P: Ultrastructure of *Calymmatobacterium granulomatis* in lesions of granuloma inguinale. J Infect Dis 142:744, 1980

Latif AS, Mason PR, Paraiwa E. The treatment of donovanosis (granuloma inguinale). Sex Transmit Dis 15:27, 1988

GARDNERELLA

Boustouller YL, Johnson AP, Taylor-Robinson D: Pili on *Gardnerella vaginalis* studied by electron microscopy. J Med Microbiol 23:327, 1987

Cano RJ, Beck MA, Grady DV: Detection of *Gardnerella vaginalis* on vaginal smears by immunofluorescence. Can J Microbiol 29:27, 1983

Greenwood JR, Pickett MJ: Transfer of *Haemophilus vaginalis* Gardner and Dukes to a new genus, *Gardnerella: G. vaginalis* (Gardner and Dukes) comb nov. Int J Syst Bacteriol 30:170, 1980

Josephson S, Thomason J, Sturino K, et al: *Gardnerella vaginalis* in the urinary tract: Incidence and significance in a hospital population. Obstet Gynecol 71:245, 1988

McCarthy LR, Mickelsen PA, Smith EG: Antibiotic susceptibility of *Haemophilus vaginalis* (*Corynebacterium vaginale*) to 21 antibiotics. Antimicrob Agents Chemother 16:186, 1979

Piot P, vanDyck E, Totten PA, et al: Identification of *Gardnerella* (*Haemophilus*) *vaginalis.* J Clin Microbiol 15:19, 1982

Reimer LG, Reller LB: *Gardnerella vaginalis* bacteremia: A review of thirty cases. Obstet Gynecol 64:170, 1984

Rottini G, Dobrina A, Forgiarini O, et al: Identification and partial characterization of a cytolytic toxin produced by *Gardnerella vaginalis.* Infect Immun 58:3751, 1990

Scott TG, Smyth CJ, Keane CT: In vitro adhesiveness and biotype of *Gardnerella vaginalis* strains in relation to the occurrence of clue cells in vaginal discharges. Genitourin Med 63:47, 1987

OTHER GRAM-NEGATIVE BACILLI

Cabrera HA, Davis GH: Epidemic meningitis of the newborn caused by flavobacteria. I. Epidemiology and bacteriology. Am J Dis Child 101:289, 1961

Coyle-Gilchrist MM, Crewe P, Roberts G: *Flavobacterium meningosepticum* in the hospital environment. J Clin Pathol 29:824, 1976

Dorff GJ, Jackson LJ, Rytel MW: Infections with *Eikenella corrodens:* Newly recognized human pathogen. Ann Intern Med 80:305, 1974

Frandsen EVG, Reinholdt J, Kilian M: Enzymatic and antigenic characterization of immunoglobulin Al proteases from *Bacteroides* and *Capnocytophaga* spp. Infect Immun 55:631, 1987

Geraci JE, Greipp PR, Wilkowske CJ, et al: *Cardiobacterium hominis* endocarditis: Four cases with clinical and laboratory observations. Mayo Clin Proc 53:49, 1978

Jackson FL, Goodman YE: Transfer of the facultatively anaerobic organism *Bacteroides corrodens* Eiken to a new genus, *Eikenella.* Int J Syst Bacteriol 22:73, 1972

Johnson WM, DiSalvo AV, Steuer PR: Fatal *Chromobacterium violaceum septicemia.* Am J Clin Pathol 56:400, 1971

Kagermeier A, London J: Identification and preliminary characterization of a lectinlike protein from *Capnocytophaga gingivalis* (emended). Infect Immun 51:490, 1986

Leadbetter ER, Holt SC, Socransky SS: *Capnocytophaga:* New genus of gram-negative gliding bacteria. I. General characteristics, taxonomic considerations and significance. Arch Microbiol 122:9, 1979

Murayama Y, Muranishi K, Okada H, et al: Immunological activities of *Capnocytophaga* cellular components. Infect Immun 36:876, 1982

Newman MG, Sutter VL, Pickett MJ, et al: Detection, identification, and comparison of *Capnocytophaga, Bacteroides ochraceus,* and DF-1. J Clin Microbiol 10:557, 1979

Olsen H, Frederiksen WC, Sibbon KE: *Flavobacterium meningosepticum* in 8 nonfatal cases of postoperative bacteremia. Lancet 1:1294, 1965

Parenti DM, Snydman DR: *Capnocytophaga* species: Infections in non-immunocompromised and immunocompromised hosts. J Infect Dis 151:140, 1985

Rubenstein JE, Leiberman MF, Gadoth N: Central nervous system infection with *Eikenella corrodens:* Report of two cases. Pediatrics 57:264, 1976

Rubin SJ, Granato PA, Wasilauskas BL: Glucose-nonfermenting gram-negative bacteria. In Lennette EH, Balows A, Hausler WJ Jr, et al (eds): Manual of Clinical Microbiology, ed 4. Washington, DC, American Society for Microbiology, 1985, p 330

Savage DD, Kagan RL, Young NA, et al: *Cardiobacterium hominis* endocarditis: Description of two patients and characterization of the organism. J Clin Microbiol 5:75, 1977

Slotnick IJ, Dougherty M: Further characterization of an unclassified group of bacteria causing endocarditis in man: *Cardiobacterium hominis.* Leeuwenhoek 30:261, 1964

Stamm WE, Colella JJ, Anderson RL, et al: Indwelling arterial catheters as a source of nosocomial bacteremia. An outbreak caused by *Flavobacterium* species. N Engl J Med 292:1099, 1975

Stevens RH, Hammond BF, Lai CH: Group and type antigens of *Capnocytophaga.* Infect Immun 23:532, 1979

Weaver RE, Hollis DG, Bottone EJ: Gram-negative fermentative bacteria and *Francisella tularensis.* In Lennette EH, Balows A, Hausler WJ Jr, et al (eds): Manual of Clinical Microbiology, ed 4. Washington, DC, American Society for Microbiology, 1985, p 309

Wilson ME, Jonak-Urbanczyk JT, Bronson PM, et al: *Capnocytophaga* species: Increased resistance of clinical isolates to serum bactericidal action. J Infect Dis 156:99, 1987

Wormser GP, Bottone EJ: *Cardiobacterium hominis:* Review of microbiologic and clinical features. Rev Infect Dis 5:680, 1983

Zinner SH, Daly AK, McCormack WM: Isolation of *Eikenella corrodens* in a general hospital. Appl Microbiol 24:705, 1973

CHAPTER 41

Brucella

Malaise, anorexia, fever, and profound muscular weakness characterized a debilitating illness first recognized by Marston in 1861 as "gastric remittent fever." The responsible organism, *Micrococcus melitensis,* was isolated in 1887 by Sir David Bruce. The organism derived its species name from Melita, the Roman name for the Isle of Malta, where the disease was recognized. The classic description of the clinical illness by Hughes in 1897 altered its designation to the more frequently used term, *undulant fever.*

Recognition of infections with other members of the genus *Brucella* occurred independently. Nocard, in 1862, first recognized the presence of bacteria between the fetal membranes and the wall of the uterus of the pregnant cow, but it remained for Bang, a Danish veterinarian, to isolate the organism, *Brucella abortus.* In a report of his findings in 1897, Bang linked the organisms to infectious abortions in animals. The third member of the genus was identified in 1914 when Traum isolated *Brucella suis* from a premature pig. As a result of the observations of Alice Evans, the relationship of these organisms was recognized and the genus *Brucella* was named in honor of Sir David Bruce.

Brucellae are facultatively intracellular pathogens. They are mammalian parasites and pathogens with a relatively wide host range. Human infection is a zoonosis that is acquired from animals or animal products. Six species are currently recognized: *B. melitensis, B. abortus, B. suis, B. ovis, B. neotomae* (isolated from desert wood rats), and *B. canis. B. neotomae* has not yet been found to cause disease in man.

Morphology and Physiology

Brucellae are small, usually coccobacillary gram-negative nonmotile rods, with a size range of 0.5 to 0.7 μm by 0.6 to 1.5 μm. *Brucella* frequently take the counterstain poorly and require a minimum of 3 minutes for good definition. Organisms occur singly or in groups, and true capsules are not produced. The ultrastructure is similar to that of other gram-negative organisms, but the inner electron-dense peptidoglycan layer of the cell wall is much more prominent than in *E. coli. B. melitensis* has been shown to release outer membrane fragments during exponential growth. The major proteins in these fragments are group 3 structural proteins analogous to the Omp A protein in the outer membrane of *Escherichia coli.* It contains phosphatidylcholine, which is an uncommon membrane constituent of bacteria.

The brucellae are strict aerobes. They produce catalase and are usually oxidase positive. Brucellae grow slowly and require complex media containing serum or blood for primary isolation. Many strains of *B. abortus* also require supplementary CO_2 for growth. Colonies of *Brucella* are spheroidal in shape, 2 to 7 mm in diameter, but reach maximum size only after 5 to 7 days. The colony morphology may be altered by the conditions of growth, but usually colonies are moist, translucent, and slightly opalescent.

The members of this genus comprise a closely knit genetic group as defined by DNA hybridization studies. Gas liquid chromatography of the fatty acid methyl esters can be used for the differentiation of the six *Brucella* species. Differentiation of *B. abortus, B. melitensis,* and *B. suis* is based on quantitative differences in several physiologic tests: (1) requirement of increased CO_2 for growth, (2) H_2S production, and (3) growth in the presence of basic fuchsin and thionin. Within each of these three species of *Brucella,* a number of strains or biovars have been recognized on the basis of these and additional biochemical properties (Table 41–1)

Antigenic Structure

Serial propagation in the laboratory of *B. abortus, B. melitensis,* and *B. suis* results in a change in antigenicity of the organism,

TABLE 41–1. DIFFERENTIAL CHARACTERISTICS OF SPECIES AND BIOTYPES IN THE GENUS *BRUCELLA*

				Growth on Dye Media[a]			Agglutination in Monospecific Sera	
Species	Biotypes	CO_2 Required	H_2S Produced	Basic Fuchsin 1:100,000	1:25,000	1:100,000	*B. abortus*	*B. melitensis*
B. melitensis	1	−	−	+	−	+	−	+
	2	−	−	+	−	+	+	−
	3	−	−	+	−	+	+	+
B. abortus	1	±	+	+	−	−	+	−
	2	+	+	−	−	−	+	−
	3	±	+	+	+	+	+	−
	4	±	+	+	−	−	−	+
	5	−	−	+	−	+	−	+
	6	−	±	+	−	+	−	+
	7	−	±	+	−	+	+	−
	8	+	−	+	−	+	+	+
	9	±	+	+	−	+	−	+
B. suis	1	−	+	−	+	+	+	−
	2	−	−	−	−	+	+	−
	3	−	−	+	+	+	+	−
	4	−	−	+	+	+	+	+
B. neotomae		−	+	−	−	+	+	−
B. ovis		+	−	+	+	+	−	−
B. canis		−	−	−	+	+	−	−

Modified from WHO Tech Rep Ser 464:71, 1971.
[a] Species differentiation is obtained on albimi or tryptose agar with graded concentrations of dyes. Interpretation should be controlled with the reference strains of each species.

with visible alterations in colonial morphology and a reduction in virulence for laboratory animals. Rigorous monitoring of the cultures during laboratory propagation is necessary to assure accurate identification and consistent antigens for use in serologic testing. There are at least two antigenic determinants—A (abortus) and M (melitensis)—present on the lipopolysaccharide (LPS) protein complex, which constitutes the major agglutinogen of fresh or smooth isolates.

Quantitative agglutinin-absorption tests differentiate among the antigens of the three species. Monospecific antisera are produced by adsorption of heterologous antisera. *B. melitensis* adsorption leaves serum reactive only with *B. abortus* and *B. suis,* which are indistinguishable by agglutination tests. Adsorption of a second aliquot with *B. abortus* leaves serum specific for *B. melitensis.* Since *B. canis* and *B. ovis* exist only in the rough form, differentiation from other *Brucella* species is a problem only when those species are also present in the rough form. A 19-carbon cyclopropane acid is common to all species except *B. canis.* This provides a means for rapid identification by gas-liquid chromatography. There is some antigenic cross-reaction between smooth *Brucella* species with other organisms, such as *Yersinia enterocolitica* 0:9, *Francisella tularensis, Salmonella* 0:3, *Escherichia coli* 0:157, and *Vibrio cholerae.*

Determinants of Pathogenicity

The intracellular survival and multiplication of *Brucella* is a property associated with virulence, since it is essential to the organism's ability to gain access to nodes and tissues. Organisms are opsonized by normal human serum, which promotes their phagocytosis. *Brucella* are partially protected in the phagolysosome. *B. abortus* releases 5′guanosine monophosphate (GMP) and adenine, which are capable of inhibiting the degranulation of peroxidase-positive granules of polymorphonuclear leukocytes (PMNLs). This would decrease the release of myeloperoxidase enzyme into the phagolysosome and reduce the iodination of proteins. The myeloperoxidase–hydrogen peroxide–halide antibacterial system is inhibited, and the intracellular survival of the organism is facilitated. Smooth *Brucella* are ingested less readily than rough organisms, although both can survive within PMNLs or macrophages until the macrophages are activated. Mononuclear cells from immune animals can kill ingested organisms, thereby eliminating infection.

Normal human serum has a heat-labile bactericidal effect on *B. abortus* that is not complement dependent. Since *B. melitensis* is serum resistant and is more virulent in man, serum sensitivity has been suggested as a virulence determinant.

B. melitensis, B. abortus, and *B. suis* are virulent in the smooth phase but lose the ability to cause disease or establish persistent infection in the preferred natural host when they mutate to rough-phase organisms. In *B. canis* and *B. ovis,* however, where no smooth form exists, the rough phase is virulent but the organism has a narrower host range than other *Brucella* species.

Recent in vitro work has shown that rough strains bind immunogloublin (IgG) and other serum proteins nonspecifically, whereas smooth strains do not. This is consistent with the hypothesis that outer membrane proteins are exposed as the organisms become rough. It is possible that these surface changes contribute to the loss of virulence by increasing the accessibility of the organisms to specific and nonspecific IgG.

Characterization of the outer membrane proteins of *B. abortus* suggests that group 2 and group 3 proteins are analogous to the matrix porins and OMP A of *E. coli*, respectively. The group 2 proteins resemble *E. coli* porins in their amino acid composition and their strong association with the peptidoglycan layer. The *Brucella* porin channels have been characterized in liposome reconstitution assays as "open," and detectable differences in the channel diameter have been observed between *Brucella* species. The differences may explain the differential sensitivity of the various species to the diagnostic dyes (basic fuchsin, thionine, threomine blue).

Another potential virulence factor of *Brucella* is a cell wall carbohydrate that is responsible for binding to human B lymphocytes. Although all *Brucella* can bind to lymphocytes, species pathogenic for humans exhibit greater activity. The binding appears to result from interaction between a lectin on the lymphocyte and a specific carbohydrate on the bacterial cell wall.

Studies of cell envelope components of smooth *B. abortus* and attenuated rough organisms do not show any ultramicroscopically detectable differences. The LPS composition, however, varies as shown by the presence of both phenol- and water-soluble LPS fractions in smooth-phase organisms, but the absence of phenol-soluble LPS in rough organisms. The fatty acid composition of *Brucella* LPS is distinct from that of enterobacterial LPS. A native hapten (NH), or second polysaccharide, is present in endotoxin preparations from smooth-phase *Brucella*. Polysaccharide B, present in the cytoplasmic fraction, is also nontoxic and nonimmunogenic when extracted from rough organisms. It has been proposed that the situation in *Brucella* is analogous to that in *E. coli* and *Salmonella*, where the nontoxic hapten is thought to be an incompletely assembled cytoplasmic precursor of the O-polysaccharide chain of the smooth LPS.

B. abortus exhibits a characteristic predilection for fetal bovine tissue. Quantitation of the tissue distribution of organisms has shown that 60% to 85% of the organisms extracted from the tissues of infected animals are present in fetal cotyledons. The 4-carbon polyhydric alcohol erythritol ($OHCH_2$—CHOH—CHOH—CH_2OH) appears to be a fetal product measurable in placental tissue and amniotic and allantoic fluids from normal bovine fetuses. This alcohol functions efficiently as a carbohydrate source in a basal medium for virulent *B. abortus* but not for attenuated or rough organisms. It also enhances the intracellular growth of the organisms in an in vitro system employing phagocytes and *B. abortus*. There is, therefore, a significant correlation of the organotropism in cattle, sheep, and goats with the presence of erythritol. The absence of such tissue localization in human disease correlates with the absence of large amounts of erythritol in these organs.

Clinical Infection

Epidemiology

Brucella organisms are distributed throughout the world, and human infection is a direct result of contact with infected animals or animal products. The pathogenesis of infection in the various animal species is similar. Under natural conditions, goats harbor *B. melitensis*, cattle harbor *B. abortus*, swine harbor *B. suis*, and sheep harbor *B. melitensis* or, less frequently, *B. ovis*. Infrequently, dogs may be reservoirs of any of these three species if they come in contact with infected animals. *B. canis* has been identified as a significant pathogen in dogs, particularly in kennels of beagles. Other animals that may be infected with brucellae include buffalo and the Bactrian camel (*B. abortus*), as well as reindeer and caribou (*B. suis*). Other farm animals, such as horses and poultry, may become infected with brucellae in very unusual situations, but they do not constitute a large reservoir or significant source of human infections.

Infection of animals occurs through the gastrointestinal tract, skin, and mucous membranes, including the conjunctivae. Animal food substances may come in contact with *Brucella*-infected materials and, when ingested by the animal, result in infection. *B. ovis*, *B. suis*, and *B. canis* are also transmitted with some frequency from an infected male to a female at the time of breeding.

Infection of lymph nodes nearest the portal of entry is followed by bacteremia, which in the pregnant or lactating animal can lead to massive multiplication of the organism in the uterus and mammary glands. Brucellae localize in chorionic epithelial cells and cause necrosis of placental cotyledons. The animal fetus may become infected or may be aborted because of asphyxia.

Animals usually recover spontaneously but excrete the bacteria for varying intervals of time in vaginal secretions, urine, and milk, which are infectious. *B. melitensis* is excreted for months in the milk of infected goats, but sheep tend to excrete the organisms for a shorter time. The organisms are extremely long lived under the proper environmental conditions. Survival is altered by pH and temperature, and exposure to sunlight will kill the organisms after a few hours. *B. melitensis* has been shown to survive in damp soil for as long as 72 days, in milk for 17 days, and in seawater for 25 days.

Pathogenesis

The disease is similar in its pathogenesis in humans. Organisms are acquired through contact with infected materials. Within the United States, 90% of brucellosis is now due to contact with infected materials rather than to ingestion of contaminated fresh milk and milk products. The occurrence of disease principally in men between the ages of 20 and 50 years reflects the occupational hazard to persons in the meat-processing industry. There is no adequate means of detecting infected meat. Prevention is possible only by elimination of the infection in cattle and swine. Movement of animals allows the organism to be reintroduced into uninfected herds. Other workers at risk because of animal contact include veterinarians, livestock producers, farmers, dairy workers, and laboratory personnel working with the organism.

Organisms can enter through abraded skin, where they gain access to the lymphatics and lymph nodes. There is often local lymphadenopathy with subsequent bloodstream invasion secondary to the bacterial multiplication and dissemination from the primary node. The subsequent localization of the organisms occurs particularly in the reticuloendothelial system. Intracellular organisms are protected from antibodies and antibiotics. Infected tissues may have granulomas, microabscesses, and in rare cases caseation. The spleen is heavily infected, and the bone marrow frequently has detectable granulomas. Hepatic involvement is very common, and bacteria may be present despite normal liver function tests. Microscopic examination most often reveals granulomas, but diffuse hepatitis or microabscesses may be present.

Clinical Manifestations

The incubation period of disease may be as short as 3 days but is sometimes several months in duration. More commonly, there is a time period of approximately 3 weeks after known exposure to organisms before the onset of symptoms. Weakness is seen in the vast majority of patients and is the most outstanding complaint. Fatigue results in the inability to perform normal activities. Chills, sweats, and anorexia are seen in approximately three fourths of the patients with acute illness, and more than one half of the patients report generalized muscle aching, headache, and backache. These nonspecific symptoms may be accompanied by associated mental depression and increased nervousness.

The findings on physical examination are minimal in contrast to the multiple complaints. More than 90% of patients have fever, but only 10% to 20% have palpable splenomegaly or lymphadenopathy. This organomegaly is more common in children. The fever tends to be intermittent, with characteristic diurnal variation. Illness may begin either insidiously or with a rather abrupt onset. The majority of patients with infection due to *B. abortus* have a self-limited disease. *B. melitensis* is the most invasive species in humans, and illness due to *B. melitensis* or *B. suis* may be more severe or chronic.

Complications resulting from *Brucella* infections are usually attributable to the granulomas that occur in various organs and tissues. Debilitating neuropsychiatric disorders, infection of a bone or joint (including the vertebral column), and in unusual cases endocarditis due to *Brucella* has been seen. Other viscera, such as spleen and liver, and bone marrow may have evidence of infection for a significant period of time.

Immunity

After natural infection in both humans and animals there is an initial IgM antibody response, followed by an IgG antibody response. The agglutination test measures antibody directed at *Brucella* LPS antigens. Macrophages from immune animals more efficiently destroy the intracellular organisms and undoubtedly contribute to eradication of this infection by the host.

Laboratory Diagnosis

The clinical illness is often nonspecific when considered in the individual patient. Therefore, evaluation of patients often includes a number of tests dictated by the differential diagnosis. When a patient is suspected of having brucellosis, at least one blood specimen should be taken for culture. Other materials, including bone marrow and tissues, can also be examined. Bone marrow cultures have been positive more often than blood cultures, especially when patients have taken antibiotics. The intracellular localization of *Brucella* within reticuloendothelial cells may account for the positive cultures from bone marrow aspirates at a time when blood cultures from the same patient are negative. Isolation of *Brucella* organisms provides the definitive diagnosis. Isolation of organisms from the tissues of infected animals may also be important.

Culture. In vitro growth of *Brucella* from patient specimens requires careful and informed laboratory processing of materials. For primary culture, direct inoculation of materials on solid media is recommended to facilitate recognition and isolation of the developing colonies and to limit the establishment of nonsmooth mutants. The Castañeda technique, involving a biphasic (solid and liquid) medium in the same bottle, is recommended for the culture of blood and other body fluids. For the solid phase, trypticase soy agar, tryptose agar, or brucella agar may be used; the liquid phase consists of the same basal medium without agar. Incubation should be in an atmosphere of 5% to 10% CO_2 at 35C to 37C. *Brucella* colonies usually appear after 4 to 5 days, but cultures should be kept for 30 days before they are discarded as negative. Commercial blood culture bottles may also be used for culturing *Brucella;* however, subcultures must be made every 4 to 5 days. Laboratory processing of materials, such as animal tissue or milk that may be heavily contaminated with other microorganisms, requires either animal inoculation or the use of selective media containing antibiotics.

Serologic Diagnosis. The enzyme-linked immunosorbent assay (ELISA) employing commercially available reagents for measurement of total IgG and IgM anti-*Brucella* antibodies have been tested on human sera. These tests eliminate the prozone phenomena and are replacing previous serologic tests. Longitudinal measurements of antibody in infected patients by ELISA have shown a steady decline in antibody over periods of 2 months in treated patients. Treated patients maintained detectable low titers. Patients with chronic illness or relapse had sporadic increases in their IgG titers; antibiotic therapy does halt this rise in antibody titer. The ELISA test has been found to be more sensitive and specific than agglutination tests. However, there is cross-reactivity with *Yersinia enterocolitica* 09, and blocking assays or a modified *Y. enterocolitica* 09 LPS will be required to establish the correct diagnosis.

The serologic diagnosis of infection by the standard tube agglutination test is sensitive and reproducible. The success of the agglutination test has depended largely on the selection and standardization of the antigen. The antigen from *B. abortus* (strain 1119) has been used to diagnose disease with any one of the three commonly encountered species of *Brucella.* For the diagnosis of disease caused by *B. canis,* it is necessary to use either specific antigen or antigen from *B. ovis.* There is a low level of cross-reactivity between the serum agglutinins of *Brucella* and those of *F. tularensis, V. cholerae,* and *Yersinia* species. The homologous titer, however, is considerably higher than that of the heterologous species.

There is a prozone phenomenon in the measurement of agglutinating antibodies to *Brucella* organisms, which apparently is due to the presence of blocking antibodies. During the acute phase of illness, when IgM agglutinating antibodies predominate, it is easy to detect agglutination. However, IgG antibodies are formed during the course of the infection, and some of them bind with antigen, thus preventing agglutination by the larger IgM molecule. A modified Coombs (antiglobulin) test has been used to increase the efficiency of serologic diagnosis. With the use of antiglobulin to bind the IgG antibody and antigen, agglutination can again be detected.

Comparative serologic studies by Buchanan indicate that a single titer of greater than 1:160 by the standard tube agglutination test is presumptive evidence of current or recent infection with *Brucella* organisms. A fourfold rise in agglutinins is seen in the first 3 months of infection in more than 90% of patients with cultures positive for *Brucella.*

Other serologic tests include complement fixation (CF) and the 2-mercaptoethanol (2 ME) agglutination test. The 2 ME test has been reliable in demonstrating IgG (2 ME-resistant) agglutinins. The absence of such agglutinins militates against active disease, which is helpful in evaluation for chronic brucellosis. Persistence of IgM agglutinating antibody titers for years in patients without active infection confuses serologic evaluation.

Skin Test. The *Brucella* skin test is a measurement of sensitization to the antigens of the organism at an undetermined time. It is not used for diagnosis of acute infection because it may remain positive for years after infection, even after the agglutination test becomes negative.

Treatment

Oral doxycycline plus rifampin for 30 days is now the preferred therapy for adults because of its safety and efficacy in acute illness and because relapses following therapy are infrequent. Trimethoprim-sulfamethoxazole for 3 weeks and intramuscular gentamicin for 5 days are used in children less than 8 years of age. Children more than 8 years of age should receive doxycycline or oxytetracyline for 3 weeks with gentamicin. Infection of the bone requires 2 to 3 weeks of streptomycin or gentamicin therapy in addition to two oral agents. Endocarditis has a high mortality, and surgical removal of the valve may be imperative. Streptomycin or gentamicin must be included in the therapy. Intracellular killing of *Brucella,* which is essential for the final eradication of the bacteria, is dependent on the normal mechanisms of the phagocyte. Since rifampin penetrates cells, it may be helpful in eradication of organisms. Relapses occur in fewer than 5% of cases when therapy is instituted early and maintained for 6 weeks. Relapses usually occur within 3 to 10 months and respond to a second course of therapy.

Prevention

Control of Animal Disease. There has been a decline in the reported cases of brucellosis in the United States, from 3510 in 1950 to 95 in 1989. There is approximately 0.04 case per 100,000 population annually. The continued decline of recognized illness is a result of controls exerted on the animal reservoirs of infection. The majority of human cases of disease in the United States are associated with the meat-processing industry. Thus this infection is no longer primarily food borne but is an occupational hazard of those in contact with infected cattle or swine.

An effective vaccine is available for animal immunization. An attenuated *B. abortus* strain is used for cattle, and a *B. melitensis* strain for sheep and goats. In animals immunized during the first 6 to 8 months of life, abortion is prevented, organisms are not excreted in the milk, and the animal has a permanent immunity against natural infection.

Prophylaxis in Humans. Prevention of human brucellosis is primarily dependent on control of the animal sources of infection. Modifications in processing of milk and dairy products, as well as animal surveillance and animal immunization, have greatly reduced the dangers of this disease within the United States. The population at risk consists almost exclusively of persons in contact with animals or their contaminated products. Available vaccines are suitable only for animals. The disease remains one of economic importance in many countries of the world, where control of infected animal herds has not been readily accomplished.

FURTHER READING

Books and Reviews

Alton CG, Jones LM: Laboratory techniques in brucellosis. In Buchanan RE, Gibbons NE (eds): World Health Organization monograph series no. 55. Geneva, WHO, 1967

Thimm BH: Brucellosis: Distribution in Man, Domestic and Wild Animals. New York, Springer-Verlag, 1982

Young EJ: Human brucellosis. Rev Infect Dis 5:821, 1983

Selected Papers

Anaj GF, Lulu AR, Saadah MA, et al. Evaluation of ELISA in the diagnosis of acute and chronic brucellosis in human beings. J Hyg (Camb) 97:457, 1986

Buchanan TM, Baber LC, Feldman RA: Brucellosis in the United States, 1960–72: An abattoir-associated disease. Part I. Clinical features and therapy. Medicine 53:403, 1974

Buchanan TM, Sulzer CR, Frix MK, et al: Brucellosis in the United States, 1960–72: An abattoir-associated disease. Part II. Diagnostic aspects. Medicine 53:415, 1974

Buchanan TM, Hendricks SL, Patton CM, et al: Brucellosis in the United States, 1960–72: An abattoir-associated disease. Part III. Epidemiology and evidence for acquired immunity. Medicine 53:427, 1974

Canning PC, Roth JA, Tabatabai LB, Deyoe BL: Isolation of components of *Brucella abortus* responsible for inhibition of function in bovine neutrophils. J Infect Dis 152:913, 1985

Canning PC, Roth JA, Deyoe BL: Release of 5′-guanosine monophosphate and adenine by *Brucella abortus* and their role in the intracellular survival of the bacteria. J Infect Dis 154:464, 1986

Douglas JT, Rosenberg EY, Nikaido H, et al: Porins of *Brucella* species. Infect Immun 44:16, 1984

Gazapo E, Lahoz JG, Subiza JL, et al: Changes in IgM and IgG antibody concentrations in brucellosis over time: Importance for diagnosis and followup. J Infect Dis 159:219, 1989

Gotuzzo E, Carillo C, Guerra J, Llosa L: An evaluation of diagnostic methods for brucellosis: The value of bone marrow culture. J Infect Dis 153:122, 1986

Hall WH. Modern chemotherapy for brucellosis in humans. Rev Infect Dis 12:1060, 1990

Klerk ED, Anderson R: Comparative evaluation of the enzyme-linked immunosorbent assay in the laboratory diagnosis of brucellosis. J Clin Microbiol 21:381, 1985

Luban MM, Dudin KL, Sharda DC, et al: A multicenter therapeutic study of 1100 children with brucellosis. Pediatr Infect Dis J 8:75, 1989

Moreno E, Jones LM, Berman DT: Immunochemical characterization of rough *Brucella* lipolysaccharides. Infect Immun 43:779, 1984

Moreno E, Speth SL, Jones LM, et al: Immunochemical characterization of *Brucella* lipopolysaccharides and polysaccharides. Infect Immun 31:214, 1981

Sippel JE, El-Masry NA, Farid Z: Diagnosis of human brucellosis with ELISA. Lancet 2:19, 1982

Smith H, Keppie J, Pearce JH, et al: The chemical basis of the virulence of *B. abortus*. I. Isolation of abortus from bovine foetal tissue. B J Exp Pathol 42:631, 1961

Smith H, Keppie J, Pearce JH, et al: Erythritol: A constituent of bovine foetal fluids which stimulates the growth of *B. abortus* in bovine phagocytes. Br J Exp Pathol 43:31, 1962

Smith H, Keppie J, Pearce JH, et al: Foetal erythritol a cause of the localization of *B. abortus* in pregnant cows. Br J Exp Pathol 43:530, 1962

Verstreate DR, Creasy MT, Caverney NT, et al: Outer membrane proteins of *B. abortus:* Isolation and characterization. Infect Immun 35:979, 1982

Wise RI: Brucellosis in the United States: Past, present and future. JAMA 244:2318, 1980

Young EJ, Borchert M, Knetzer FL, Musher DM: Phagocytosis and killing of *Brucella* by human polymorphonuclear leucocytes. J Infect Dis 151:682, 1985

CHAPTER 42

Bacillus

The Genus *Bacillus*

The genus *Bacillus* is comprised of large, gram-positive rods characterized by their ability to produce endospores. The genus is a large one, containing both strict aerobes and facultative anaerobes. Only a single species, *Bacillus anthracis*, is a major cause of disease in man and mammals. Numerous other species within the genus are widely distributed in nature and are found in most soil, water, and dust samples. Many of the distinctive properties of members of this genus are attributable to their quest for survival under the adverse conditions encountered in their diverse native habitats.

Historically, considerable attention was early focused on the genus *Bacillus* because of the economic importance of anthrax, the disease caused by *B. anthracis*. Anthrax was one of the first bacterial infections whose cause was definitively established. It was in studies on anthrax that Koch demonstrated for the first time a set of criteria or postulates that must be satisfied before an organism can be identified as the etiologic agent of a specific infection. Another significant achievement resulting from studies with anthrax was the development by Pasteur of active immunization against the disease by inoculation with heat-attenuated cultures, the first instance of a bacterial vaccine. Also, in his pioneering work on phagocytosis, Nobel Prize winner Metchnikoff studied virulent and attenuated strains of *B. anthracis*, which he found to be phagocytized at different rates.

In *Bergey's Manual of Systematic Bacteriology*, 34 different species of *Bacillus* are recognized. One of the distinctive features of the genus, in contrast to most bacterial genera, is the wide range of the guanine plus cytosine (G + C) content of the DNA of the various species—32 to 62 mol%. This reflects the tremendous heterogeneity of the organisms within the genus. There is diversity of metabolic type, nutritional requirements, and composition and structure of the vegetative cell walls. Psychrophiles, mesophiles, and thermophiles, as well as alkalophilic, neutrophilic, and acidophilic species are included in the genus. Also, virtually all of the currently recognized species secrete a variety of soluble extracellular enzymes, which reflect the diversity of the parental habitats.

Certain members of the genus *Bacillus* have assumed importance as producers of antibiotics, some of which (polymyxin and bacitracin) have been clinically useful. Other species within the genus are significant because of their use in the industrial production of solvents, alcohols, enzymes, and vitamins. As a result of intense interest in these industrial applications, there has accumulated a wealth of basic knowledge on the genetics and physiology of the *Bacillus* cell.

In the clinical microbiology laboratory, species of *Bacillus* are primarily encountered as contaminants. However, the recognition of their etiologic role in food poisoning, as a cause of sepsis in heroin addicts, and as a significant pathogen in the compromised host should make the clinical microbiologist wary of labeling *Bacillus* isolates as contaminants or of not reporting them at all.

Bacillus anthracis

Anthrax is primarily a disease of herbivorous animals, particularly sheep and cattle and, to a lesser extent, horses, hogs, and goats. It is caused by *B. anthracis*, a gram-positive, aerobic, spore-forming bacillus that was first isolated by Robert Koch in 1877. Humans accidentally encounter this disease in an agricultural setting, usually with the development of a local skin infection that may become generalized. The disease also may be acquired in an industrial setting during the processing of hides or animal hair with resultant inhalation of anthrax and the production of a virulent type of pneumonia. Rarely, the disease may be acquired by ingestion. Widespread immunization of animals has markedly diminished outbreaks of anthrax in herds, with the result that the illness is now rare in humans.

Morphology and Physiology

B. anthracis is a straight rod, 3 to 5 μm long and 1 to 1.2 μm wide. When examined in smears from the blood or tissues of an infected animal, the organisms usually are found singly or in pairs. Their ends appear square, and the corners are often so sharp that the bacilli in the chains are in contact at these points, leaving an oval opening between the organisms. Unlike most members of the genus, *B. anthracis* is nonmotile. Bacilli are encapsulated during growth in the infected animal, but capsules cannot be demonstrated in vitro unless the organisms are cultured on a bicarbonate-containing medium in the presence of 6% CO_2. Spores are formed in culture, in the soil, and in the tissues and exudates of dead animals but not in the blood or tissues of living animals. They are ellipsoidal or oval and are centrally located.

Cultural Characteristics. The organisms grow well on most common laboratory media, but for demonstration of characteristic colonial morphology, specimens should be inoculated on 5% blood agar plates, prepared with blood free of antibiotics. Maximal growth is obtained at pH 7.0 to 7.4 under aerobic conditions, but growth does occur, albeit sparsely, in the absence of oxygen. The optimal temperature for maximal growth is 37C, but growth occurs over a wide temperature range of 15C to 40C. After 24 hours of incubation on simple laboratory media, the organisms produce large, raised, opaque, grayish white, plumose colonies, 2 to 3 mm in diameter, with an irregular, fringelike edge. Tangled masses of long hairlike curls can be seen with a colony microscope. The colony is membranous in consistency and emulsifies with difficulty. No hemolysis is produced.

Laboratory Identification. The identification of typical virulent strains of *B. anthracis* isolated from clinical material is relatively simple, but the identification of strains from nonclinical material may be more difficult. Differential properties useful in the identification of *B. anthracis* are listed in Table 42–1. Neither morphologic features nor the usual cultural characteristics will differentiate *B. anthracis* from nonmotile strains of *Bacillus cereus,* the organism most easily mistaken for *B. anthracis.* Virulent strains of *B. anthracis,* however, are the only organisms that produce rough colonies when grown in the absence of increased CO_2, and mucoid colonies when grown on sodium bicarbonate medium in an atmosphere of 5% CO_2.

The differential susceptibility of *B. anthracis* and *B. cereus* to penicillin is the basis for the string-of-pearls reaction that separates virulent and avirulent *B. anthracis* from other aerobic spore formers. This reaction is most dramatic and can be demonstrated after a 3- to 6-hour incubation of *B. anthracis* on the surface of a solid medium containing penicillin, 0.5 μg/mL. The cells become large and spherical and occur in chains that, when viewed on the agar surface, resemble a string of pearls. Another useful test for differentiating *B. anthracis* and *B. cereus* is based on the susceptibility of *B. anthracis* to a variant bacteriophage, γ-phage; no lysis of *B. cereus* occurs. Confirmation of the identity of an isolate may be obtained by the inoculation of a mouse with a suspension of organisms from an agar plate. Death from anthrax infection usually occurs within 2 to 5 days, and organisms can be recovered from the heart blood. API (Analytab Products, Inc.) tests have been used successfully to differentiate *B. anthracis* from other *Bacillus* species and are especially useful in identifying slightly virulent and avirulent strains.

Resistance. Because of its ability to produce spores, the anthrax bacillus is extremely resistant to adverse chemical and physical environments. A temperature of 120C for 15 minutes will inactivate the spore. The vegetative cell is comparable in resistance to other non-spore-forming bacteria and is de-

TABLE 42–1. PROPERTIES OF *B. ANTHRACIS* AND RELATED *BACILLUS* SPECIES

Property	*B. anthracis*	*B. cereus*	*B. mycoides*	*B. thuringiensis*
Capsule formation	Variable	−	−	−
Agglutinated by *Glycine max* lectin	+	−	+	−
Hydrolysis of *p*-nitrophenyl-β-D-*N*-acetylglucosamine	−	+	−	+
Sensitivity to penicillin	Sensitive	Resistant	Resistant	Resistant
Motility	−	+	−	+
β-hemolysis on sheep blood agar	Variable	Variable	Variable	Variable
Growth at 45C	Slight	Rapid	None	Slight
Enhanced hydrolysis of *p*-nitrophenyl-α-D-glucoside in presence of 1% Triton X-100	+	−	−	−
Percentage G + C	32–40	32–40	32–40	32–40
Lysis of bacteriophage	+	−	Variable	−
Pathogenesis in animals (skin reactions)	+	+	−	+
Colonial morphology	MH[a]	MH	MH	MH

Adapted from Lennette, Balows, Hausler, Shadomy (eds): Manual of Clinical Microbiology, ed 4. American Society for Microbiology, 1985.
+, 90% or more of reactions are positive; −, less than 10% of reactions are positive; variable, 10% to 90% of reactions are positive.
[a] MH, Medusa head or serrated outgrowth from the periphery of the colony.

stroyed in 30 minutes by a temperature of 54C. Spores remain viable for years in contaminated pastures and remain a source of infection for long periods of time.

Antigenic Structure

Three antigens of *B. anthracis* have been partially characterized: (1) the capsular polypeptide, (2) a polysaccharide somatic antigen, and (3) a complex protein toxin. Unlike most bacterial capsules, the capsule of *B. anthracis* is a polypeptide of high molecular weight consisting exclusively of D-glutamic acid. There appears to be a single antigenic capsular type. The somatic polysaccharide antigen is a component of the cell wall and contains equimolar amounts of *N*-acetylglucosamine and D-galactose. It cross-reacts with human blood group A material and with type 14 pneumococcus polysaccharide. Antibodies to this antigen are not protective.

Anthrax toxin, derived from the thoracic and peritoneal exudates of infected animals, is a complex exotoxin consisting of three protein components: protective antigen, lethal factor, and edema factor. Each of the separate components is serologically active and distinct and is also immunogenic (see below).

Determinants of Pathogenicity

The pathogenesis of *B. anthracis* depends on two important virulence factors: a poly (D-glutamic acid) capsule and an exotoxin. Fully virulent organisms have two large plasmids that code for these products. The capsule interferes with phagocytosis and is especially important during the early stages of infection. Antibodies against the capsular antigen are produced, but they are not protective against the disease.

The symptoms of anthrax are attributable to toxin that gradually accumulates in the infected animal, with a maximum accumulation at the time of death. The pathophysiology of the bacillary disease and the toxemia from sterile toxin are very similar. In both cases and in all animal hosts tested, respiratory failure and anoxia result from action of the toxin on the central nervous system.

The lethal effects of *B. anthracis* are due to an exotoxin consisting of three distinct and serologically active proteins: protective antigen (PA), edema factor (EF), and lethal factor (LF). These proteins act synergistically to produce the characteristic systemic effects of anthrax (Table 42–2); individually, the three proteins have no known toxic activity. However, PA in combination with EF produces localized edema in the skin of test animals, whereas PA in combination with LF produces death in test animals. Anthrax toxin is actually two toxins and resembles staphylococcal leukocidin and botulinum C_2 toxin in having receptor-binding and effector domains on separate proteins. The PA protein binds to a receptor on the cell surface and is subsequently cleaved by a cellular protease. The larger C-terminal piece of PA remains bound to the receptor and then binds either EF or LF, which enters the cell by endocytosis. The EF protein is an adenylate cyclase that is active only in the presence of the eucaryotic cofactor, calmodulin. The adenylate cyclase of *B. anthracis* is immunologically related to the adenylate cyclase of *Bordetella pertussis*, a taxonomically very distinct organism. At present, these are the only known examples of procaryotic enzymes activated by calmodulin. The molecular action of LF is unknown.

TABLE 42–2. TOXIC AND IMMUNOLOGIC ACTIVITIES OF *B. ANTHRACIS* TOXIN COMPONENTS

Factor	Toxic Activity	Immunologic Activity
Edema factor (EF)	Inactive	Serologically active, nonimmunizing
Protective antigen (PA)	Inactive	Serologically active, nonimmunizing
Lethal factor (LF)	Inactive	Serologically active, weakly immunizing
EF + PA	Gross local edema	Strongly immunizing
EF + LF	Inactive	Weakly immunizing
PA + LF	Lethal	Immunizing
EF + PA + LF	Edema, lethal	Immunizing

From Hambleton, Carman, Melling: Vaccine 2:125, 1984.

Clinical Infection

Epidemiology

IN ANIMALS. The ultimate reservoir of anthrax infection is the soil. During the terminal stages of the disease, bacilli are shed in large numbers from all orifices of the infected animal. The organisms sporulate in the soil and remain a source of infection for many decades. Anthrax has been detected in nearly every country. It has especially been a problem in the Mediterranean region, Africa, and Asia. Animal products, especially goat hair and bone meal imported from these areas, are likely to be contaminated. Sporadic cases continue to occur in the United States, especially in states where anthrax foci still exist (Louisiana, Oklahoma, Colorado, and California). The incidence of infection in these areas appears to increase as a result of drought or overgrazing when there is a greater likelihood of animals ingesting contaminated forage.

In animals, anthrax is severe and usually takes the form of a septicemia. Although it is impossible to determine the precise time of infection in a case of spontaneous anthrax, it is certain that the infected animal remains free of symptoms until a few hours before death. The mortality rate in herbivorous animals is about 80%.

IN HUMANS. In spite of the wide distribution of *B. anthracis*, the incidence of anthrax in humans is low. Human cases fall into two groups: agricultural cases that result from direct contact with animals dying of anthrax and industrial cases that result from contact with contaminated animal products, such as hides, goat hair, wool, and bones imported from Africa, the Middle East, and Asia. A wide variety of finished products have been linked to human infection, including such items as shaving brushes, ivory piano keys, bongo drums, and wool products. At present most cases occur in unvaccinated employees in textile and felt mills. The widespread use of vaccines among this group of workers has markedly reduced morbidity, but the only method of completely eliminating potential exposure is to discontinue the use of imported goat hair. Although an effective vaccine for anthrax in cattle is available, the sporadic occurrence of bovine anthrax fails to provide ranchers with incentive to vaccinate their livestock routinely.

Pathogenesis. Humans become infected in one of three ways:

1. Cutaneous route. Organisms gain access through small abrasions or cuts and multiply locally with a rather dramatic inflammatory response.
2. Inhalation. Organisms are inhaled, multiply in the lung, and are swept to the draining hilar lymph nodes, where marked hemorrhagic necrosis may occur.
3. Ingestion. Rarely, organisms are ingested in infected meat, with resultant invasion and ulceration of the gastrointestinal mucosa.

From all three surface areas, invasion of the bloodstream and profound toxemia may occur. Metastatic infections, such as meningitis, may complicate the primary process.

Clinical Manifestations. Anthrax presents in one of three ways, depending on the mode of infection. Cutaneous anthrax accounts for more than 95% of human cases. It begins 2 to 5 days after infection as a small papule that develops within a few days into a vesicle filled with dark bluish black fluid. Rupture of the vesicle reveals a black eschar at the base, with a very prominent inflammatory ring of reaction around the eschar. This is sometimes referred to as a malignant pustule. The lesion is classically found on the hands, forearms, or head and is painless. It is rarely found on the trunk or lower extremities. The pulmonary infection, known as wool-sorter's disease, occurs in patients who handle raw wool, hides, or horsehair and acquire the disease by the inhalation of spores. The patient's symptoms are typically those of a respiratory infection with fever, malaise, myalgia, and an unproductive cough. Within several days, however, it rapidly progresses to a very severe infection with marked respiratory distress and cyanosis. With the sudden worsening of the illness, death usually occurs within 24 hours. In the gastrointestinal form of anthrax, infection is associated with nausea, vomiting, and diarrhea. Occasionally there is loss of blood, either through hematemesis or in the stools. This is associated with profound prostration, eventual shock, and death. In all three of these surface infections, there may be invasion of the bloodstream and localization in the meninges, with a resultant fatal meningitis.

Anthrax infection in humans provides permanent immunity; second attacks are rare.

Laboratory Diagnosis. Specimens for culture should be obtained from a malignant pustule, the sputum, or blood. A Gram stain and a fluorescent-antibody stain are useful in making a presumptive diagnosis. The organism will grow readily on most laboratory media. However, the greatest problems encountered in establishing a diagnosis are the frequency with which nonpathogenic species of bacilli, such as *B. cereus*, are confused with *B. anthracis* and the fact that most laboratory personnel have never seen *B. anthracis*.

Antibodies to the organism can be demonstrated by the Ouchterlony gel diffusion, microhemagglutination, and enzyme-linked immunosorbent assay (ELISA) procedures. Acute and convalescent sera of suspect cases should be obtained and submitted to the Centers for Disease Control for confirmation of infection.

Treatment. *B. anthracis* is quite susceptible to penicillin, which is curative for cutaneous anthrax. The major difficulty is the lack of clinical suspicion of anthrax because of its rarity. For this reason, cutaneous anthrax may be misdiagnosed and an antibiotic inappropriate for anthrax given. With pulmonary anthrax the diagnosis is usually made postmortem, as is the case with gastrointestinal anthrax. If the diagnosis of pulmonary anthrax is made in sufficient time, large intravenous doses of penicillin should be instituted as quickly as possible. In patients allergic to penicillin, tetracycline or erythromycin may be used. If a skin lesion is mistakenly identified as a staphylococcal infection, incision and drainage may be attempted. This can lead to disastrous results because of widespread dissemination of the organism.

Prevention. Control of human anthrax ultimately depends on control of the disease in animals. Animals with known or suspected anthrax should be handled with care and their carcasses buried deeply to prevent the spread of spores to new pastures. Wool, horsehair, and hides coming from areas where epidemic anthrax is present should be gas sterilized. A vaccine is available for control of outbreaks of human anthrax in an industrial setting.

IMMUNIZATION. Active immunization is the only known method of preventing anthrax in herbivorous animals in areas where the pasture land is already contaminated with spores. Pasteur's famous attenuated living anthrax vaccine was effective but difficult to maintain at a desired level of virulence. It has been superseded by a living spore vaccine derived from a nonencapsulated strain of *B. anthracis* (Sterne strain). The widespread use of a living spore vaccine in South Africa has reduced the incidence of anthrax in the cattle of this area by more than 99%. For the protection of humans in high-risk work situations, a nonliving vaccine consisting of aluminum hydroxide–adsorbed supernatant material from fermentor cultures of a toxigenic but nonencapsulated strain of *B. anthracis* is used. This antigen appears to be effective but requires multiple doses over long periods of time. Studies are now being directed toward the formulation of a new nonliving vaccine containing appropriate mixtures of the purified components of anthrax toxin.

Other Aerobic Spore-Forming Bacilli

Bacillus cereus. *B. cereus* is an infrequently recognized cause of food-borne illness in the United States. It is similar to *B. anthracis* in cellular morphology, but unlike *B. anthracis*, it is usually motile and is not susceptible to penicillin or γ-phage (Table 42–1).

B. cereus food poisoning can cause two clinical syndromes. The first has a short incubation period of 4 hours. It is characterized clinically by severe nausea and vomiting and is frequently mistaken for staphylococcal food poisoning. Epidemics have been described after the ingestion of such foods as fried rice in which extensive multiplication of the organisms had occurred. The second syndrome has a longer incubation period (17 hours) and is characterized by abdominal cramping and diarrhea. It is commonly confused with clostridial food poisoning. *B. cereus* food poisoning is initiated when the spore forms survive cooking and the contaminated food is allowed to reach temperatures that permit germination of the spore and elaboration of an enterotoxin. Strains of *B. cereus* produce at least two enterotoxins with different actions in experimental animals, depending on the nature of the outbreak from which the strains were initially isolated. Proof of the cause of *B. cereus* food poisoning usually depends on the isolation of the same type of organism from the food and from the stools of infected patients.

In addition to food poisoning, *B. cereus* has also been implicated in serious infections associated with impairment of host defense mechanisms primarily by foreign bodies, prosthetic devices, or restricted blood supply. In patients who have serious underlying diseases, such as acute leukemia, or who are immunosuppressed because of transplantation surgery overwhelming bacteremia, endocarditis, or meningitis can develop. Also, because these organisms are resistant to the β-lactam antibiotics, they may be selected for by the prior use of antibiotics for therapeutic or prophylactic purposes.

Clindamycin is the drug of choice. Usually the organism is also susceptible to the aminoglycosides, vancomycin, tetracycline, and erythromycin.

Other *Bacillus* Species. *Bacillus subtilis* is present in the air, dust, brackish water, and infusion of vegetable matter. It is usually a common laboratory contaminant but, like *B. cereus*, is capable of producing infection in the compromised host. It has also been seen in overwhelming bacteremias and eye infections in heroin addicts and has been cultured from street heroin. *B. subtilis* infections usually respond to therapy with the β-lactam antibiotics. Another species of interest is *Bacillus stearothermophilus*, the spores of which are used to evaluate the efficacy of autoclaving and other sterilization procedures. Several species produce disease in insects and in some cases have been used in insect control. The best studied of these is *Bacillus thuringiensis*, which is pathogenic for the larvae of *Lepidoptera*. This species is distinguished from *B. cereus* by the production of a crystalline protein body or, rarely, by two or three bodies in the cell during sporulation. This body separates readily from the liberated spore, and toxin is released from the crystal by enzymatic action in the larval gut.

FURTHER READING

Books and Reviews

Davey RT Jr, Tauber WB: Post traumatic endophthalmitis: The emerging role of *Bacillus cereus* infection. Rev Infect Dis 9:110, 1987

Farrar WE: Serious infections due to "nonpathogenic" organisms of the genus *Bacillus:* Review of their status as pathogens. Am J Med 34:134, 1963

Hambleton P, Carman JA, Melling J: Anthrax: The disease in relation to vaccines. Vaccine 2:125, 1984

Lincoln RE, Fish DC: Anthrax toxin. In Montie TC, Kadis S, Ajl SJ (eds): Microbial Toxins, vol 3. New York, Academic Press, 1970, p 361

Schlessinger D (ed): Bacilli: Biochemical genetics, physiology and industrial applications. In Microbiology—1976. Washington, DC, American Society for Microbiology, 1976, p 5

Turnbull PCB: *Bacillus cereus* toxins. Pharmacol Ther 13:453, 1981

Selected Papers

Allured VS, Case LM, Leppla SH, McKay DB: Crystallization of the protective antigen protein of *Bacillus anthracis*. J Biol Chem 260:5012, 1985

Bekemeyer WB, Zimmerman GA: Life threatening complications associated with *Bacillus cereus* pneumonia. Am J Respir Dis 131:466, 1985

Berke E, Collins WF, Von Graevenitz A, et al: Fulminant postsurgical *Bacillus cereus* meningitis. J Neurosurg 55:637, 1981

Blaustein RO, Koehler TM, Collier RJ, Finkelstein A: Anthrax toxin: Channel-forming activity of protective antigen in planar phospholipid bilayers. Proc Natl Acad Sci USA 86:2209, 1989

Brachman PS: Anthrax. Ann NY Acad Sci 174:577, 1970

Brachman PS: Inhalation anthrax. Ann NY Acad Sci 353:83, 1980

Centers for Disease Control: Animal anthrax in California. MMWR 17:279, 1968

Centers for Disease Control: Anthrax in humans—United States, 1978. MMWR 28:160, 1979

Centers for Disease Control: Human cutaneous anthrax—North Carolina, 1987. MMWR 37:413, 1988

Coonrod JD, Leadley PJ, Eickhoff TC: Antibiotic susceptibility of *Bacillus* species. J Infect Dis 123:102, 1971

Escuyer V, Duflot E, Sezer O, Danchin A, Mock M: Structural homology between virulence-associated bacterial adenylate cyclases. Gene 71:293, 1988

Ezzell JW, Ivins BE, Leppla SH: Immunoelectrophoretic analysis, toxicity, and kinetics of in vitro production of the protective antigen and lethal factor components of *Bacillus anthracis* toxin. Infect Immun 45:761, 1984

Fitz-James PC, Young IE: Comparison of species and varieties of the genus *Bacillus*. J Bacteriol 78:743, 755, 765, 1959

Friedlander AM: Macrophages are sensitive to anthrax lethal toxin through an acid-dependent process. J Biol Chem 261:7123, 1986

Gianella RA, Brasile L: A hospital food-borne outbreak of diarrhea caused by *Bacillus cereus:* Clinical, epidemiologic and microbiologic studies. J Infect Dis 139:366, 1979

Gold H: Treatment of anthrax. Fed Proc 26:1563, 1967

Gordon MA, Moody MD, Barton AM, et al: Industrial air sampling for anthrax bacteria. Arch Indust Hyg Occup Med 10:16, 1954

Hambleton P, Carman JA, Melling J: Anthrax: The disease in relation to vaccines. Vaccine 2:125, 1984

Iacono-Connors LC, Schmaljohn CS, Dalrymple JM: Expression of the *Bacillus anthracis* protective antigen gene by baculovirus and vaccinia virus recombinants. Infect Immun 58:366, 1990

Ihde DC, Armstrong D: Clinical spectrum of infection due to *Bacillus* species. Am J Med 55:839, 1973

Ivins BE, Ezzell JW Jr, Jemski J, et al: Immunization studies with attenuated strains of *Bacillus anthracis*. Infect Immun 52:454, 1986

Ivins BE, Welkos SL: Cloning and expression of the *Bacillus anthracis* protective antigen gene in *Bacillus subtilis*. Infect Immun 54:537, 1986

Jones WI Jr, Klein F, Walker JS, et al: Growth of anthrax bacilli in resistant, susceptible, and immunized hosts. J Bacteriol 94:600, 1967

Klein F, DeArmon IA Jr, Lincoln RE, et al: Immunity against *Bacillus anthracis* from protective antigen live vaccine. J Immunol 88:15, 1962

Labruyere E, Mock M, Ladant D, et al: Characterization of ATP and calmodulin-binding properties of a truncated form of *Bacillus anthracis* adenylate cyclase. Biochemistry 29:4922, 1990

Leppla SH: Anthrax toxin edema factor: A bacterial adenylate cyclase that increases cyclic AMP concentrations in eukaryotic cells. Proc Natl Acad Sci USA 79:3162, 1982

Leppla SH: Production and purification of anthrax toxin. Methods Enzymol 165:103, 1988

Little SF, Knudson GB: Comparative efficacy of *Bacillus anthracis* live spore vaccine and protective antigen vaccine against anthrax in the guinea pig. Infect Immun 52:509, 1986

Little SF, Leppla SH, Friedlander AM: Production and characterization of monoclonal antibodies against the lethal factor component of *Bacillus anthracis* lethal toxin. Infect Immun 58:1606, 1990

Logan NA, Carman JA, Melling J, Berkeley RCW: Identification of *Bacillus anthracis* by API tests. J Med Microbiol 20:75, 1985

Makino S-I, Uchida I, Terakado N, et al: Molecular characterization and protein analysis of the *cap* region, which is essential for encapsulation in *Bacillus anthracis*. J Bacteriol 171:722, 1989

Metchnikoff E: Concerning the relationship between phagocytes and anthrax bacilli. Rev Infect Dis 6:761, 1984

Mock M, Labruyere E, Glaser P, et al: Cloning and expression of the calmodulin-sensitive *Bacillus anthracis* adenylate cyclase in *Escherichia coli*. Gene 64:277, 1988

Nungester WJ: Proceedings of the Conference on Progress in the Understanding of Anthrax. Fed Proc 26:1491, 1967

O'Brien JO, Friedlander A, Dreier T, et al: Effects of anthrax toxin components on human neutrophils. Infect Immun 47:306, 1985

Sliman R, Rehm S, Shlaes DM: Serious infections caused by *Bacillus* species. Medicine 66:218, 1987

Terranova W, Blake PA: *Bacillus cereus* food poisoning. N Engl J Med 298:143, 1978

Tuazon CU, Murray HW, Levy C, et al: Serious infections from *Bacillus* species. JAMA 241:1137, 1979

Turnbull PC, Broster MG, Carman JA, et al: Development of antibodies to protective antigen and lethal factor components of anthrax toxin in humans and guinea pigs and their relevance to protective immunity. Infect Immun 52:356, 1986

Turnbull PC, Jorgensen K, Kramer JM: Severe clinical infections associated with *Bacillus cereus* and the apparent involvement of exotoxin. J Clin Pathol 32:289, 1979

Weller PF, Nicholson A, Braslow N: The spectrum of *Bacillus* bacteremia in heroin addicts. Arch Intern Med 139:293, 1979

Wright GG: Anthrax toxin. In Schlessinger D (ed): Microbiology—1975. Washington, DC, American Society for Microbiology, 1975, p 292

CHAPTER 43

Introduction to the Anaerobic Bacteria: Non-Spore-Forming Anaerobes

Anaerobic Bacteria

Recognition of the anaerobic nature of certain species of microorganisms is credited to Pasteur, who noted in 1863 that motility of certain bacteria was lost on exposure to air. By 1900, a variety of bacteria had been isolated that would grow only in gaseous environments having substantially reduced oxygen tensions. The study of anaerobic bacteria lagged, however, because of their sensitivity to oxygen, their generally fastidious growth requirements, and their frequent occurrence in complex mixtures of anaerobic and facultative species. Provision of anaerobic environments for culture was technically difficult, making it almost impossible to obtain pure cultures for study. Improved anaerobic technology, however, has demonstrated a high incidence of anaerobic organisms in clinical specimens, and a better understanding of these organisms has evolved.

The anaerobic bacteria are widespread in nature. They constitute the predominant part of our normal indigenous flora on skin and membrane surfaces and outnumber facultatively anaerobic bacteria in the gut by a factor of 1000:1. On the skin, in the mouth, in the upper respiratory tract, and often in the female lower genital tract, they outnumber facultatively anaerobic bacteria by a factor of 5:1 to 10:1. Many of these anaerobic organisms, previously considered to be harmless commensals of our indigenous flora, are now recognized as opportunistic pathogens that may produce disease when the host's resistance is reduced.

Types of Anaerobic Organism

The anaerobic bacteria include many different types, both gram-positive and gram-negative. In *Bergey's Manual of Systematic Bacteriology*, anaerobic bacteria are classified in different sections on the basis of their Gram stain reactions, cellular morphology, ability to form spores, and intolerance to oxygen. DNA homology and other biochemical and serologic techniques have increased our understanding of relatedness among anaerobes, but a need still exists for further work on classification and for simplification of procedures for cultivation and identification. The same organism may have a variety of names, which were coined over the years, and reference to authoritative manuals on anaerobic bacteriology is helpful in reading some of the older literature.

Primarily on the basis of differences in the types of disease produced, anaerobic bacteria conveniently may be divided into (1) the clostridia, which form spores, and (2) the non-spore-forming anaerobic bacteria. The pathogenic exotoxin-producing clostridia and other species of Clostridium are covered separately in Chapter 44. Certain of these clostridia, however, also occur in combination with the non-spore-forming anaerobes in infections of the types that are discussed in the present chapter. The general aspects of morphology, physiology, laboratory culture, and identification of medically significant anaerobes discussed in the first part of this chapter also pertain to the clostridia. The pathogenic mechanisms and types of infection especially associated with non-spore-forming anaerobes and many of the particular genera and species with a recognized role in human infection (Table 43–1) are discussed in the remainder of the chapter. Additional information on anaerobic or microaerophilic organisms is found in Chapters 32, 45, 46, and 47 on *Actinomyces, Treponema, Borrelia, Campylobacter,* and oral microbiology, respectively.

TABLE 43–1. MAJOR NON-SPORE-FORMING ANAEROBIC BACTERIA OF CLINICAL SIGNIFICANCE[a]

Species	Former Designation
Gram-Negative Bacilli	
Bacteroides	
(*B. fragilis* group)	*B. fragilis*
fragilis	ssp *fragilis*
thetaiotaomicron	ssp *thetaiotaomicron*
distasonis	ssp *distasonis*
vulgatus	ssp *vulgatus*
ovatus	ssp *ovatus*
ureolyticus	*B. corrodens*
gracilis	
Prevotella	*Bacteroides*
bivia	*bivius*
disiens	*disiens*
oris	*oris*
buccae	*buccae*
intermedia	*intermedius*
corporis	*corporis*
melaninogenica	*melaninogenicus*
denticola	*denticola*
loescheii	*loescheii*
Porphyromonas	*Bacteroides*
asaccharolytica	*asaccharolyticus*
gingivalis	*gingivalis*
Fusobacterium	
nucleatum	
necrophorum	
mortiferum	
Gram-Positive Bacilli	
Actinomyces israelii	
Eubacterium	
lentum	
nodatum	
Propionibacterium acnes	
Mobiluncus	
mulieris	
curtisii	
Gram-Positive Cocci	
Peptostreptococcus	
anaerobius	
magnus	*Peptococcus magnus*
prevotii	*Peptococcus prevotii*
asaccharolyticus	*Peptococcus asaccharolyticus*
tetradius	*Gaffkya anaerobia*
Gemella morbillorum	*Streptococcus morbillorum*
Gram-Negative Cocci	
Veillonella parvula	

[a] Includes some microaerophilic species. Also, numerous species of *Clostridium*, histotoxic and others, can occur with the non-spore-formers (see Chap. 46). *Treponema* and *Borrelia* are covered in Chapter 47.

Morphology

The anaerobic bacteria include a variety of morphologic types, including bacilli, cocci, comma-shaped organisms, and spiral-shaped organisms. Some species are motile by means of flagella. Although the clostridia generally stain boldly with the Gram stain, many of the non-spore-forming anaerobic bacteria stain poorly, are pale in appearance, and may be gram-variable. Better definition may be obtained with the use of Kopeloff's modification of the Gram stain. Observation of certain of the anaerobes (or microaerophilic organisms), including *Campylobacter, Treponema,* and *Borrelia,* may require phase contrast or darkfield microscopy.

As a group, anaerobic bacteria are more pleomorphic in appearance than most aerobic or facultatively anaerobic bacteria, a property that may be useful in their recognition from clinical material or in culture (Figs. 43–1 through 43–4). Pleomorphism, however, is quite variable, depending on species and strain differences and on the chemical environment present in infected material or in artificial culture, and thus is not always apparent.

Colony morphology of anaerobic bacteria on solid and in liquid media is helpful in recognition of certain anaerobes, but for many species colonies are not sufficiently unique to aid appreciably in identification. Characteristics helpful in some instances include production of turbid, granular, or flocculent growth in liquid culture and the size, shape, color, and consistency of colonies on solid media. Hemolysis does not aid in the identification of these organisms to the same extent that it does with certain facultatively anaerobic bacteria. Colony morphology, like cellular morphology, is extremely dependent on the cultural environment.

Physiology

Anaerobiosis. Oxygen intolerance among anaerobic bacteria is not completely understood at present. Various factors play

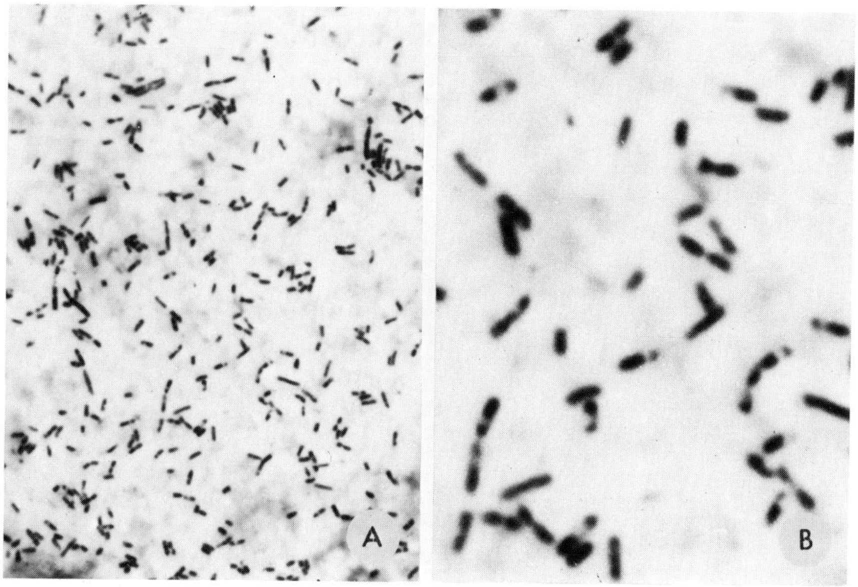

Fig. 43–1. *Bacteroides fragilis* from supplemented thioglycolate. Pleomorphism, which may be considerably more or less apparent than shown here, is highly dependent on the cultural environment and on strain differences. **A.** × 1000. **B.** × 3000. Note vacuoles present within cells.

a role, but no single mechanism has received total acceptance by investigators. Among the proposals are the following:

1. O_2 has a direct toxic effect.
2. O_2 is indirectly toxic by specific mediators, such as H_2O_2 or free radicals.
3. An appropriately low oxidation-reduction potential that appears to be required for many anaerobic bacteria is unachievable in the presence of normal O_2 tensions.
4. Essential sulfhydryl-containing enzymes are oxidized and therefore inactivated by O_2.
5. O_2 inhibits metabolism by reaction with flavoproteins and reduced nicotinamide adenine dinucleotide (NADH) oxidases, thereby critically lowering the reducing power of the cell.

The most popular theories advanced to explain the toxicity of O_2 for anaerobic bacteria have been based on their lack of the enzymes catalase (or peroxidase) and superoxide dismutase, which thereby allows accumulation of toxic levels of H_2O_2 or superoxide ions, respectively. Although undoubtedly important, experimentation has not substantiated the hypothesis that the absence of any one of these enzymes is solely responsible for the toxicity of oxygen. Also, catalase, superoxide dismutase, or both have been detected in certain species, especially in the more aerotolerant clinical isolates. The simultaneous presence of both enzymes in sufficient quantities might be required. Indeed, a single mechanism may not be applicable to all anaerobes, and different mechanisms may also apply under different environmental conditions.

Anaerobes are not equally intolerant of O_2. Maximum

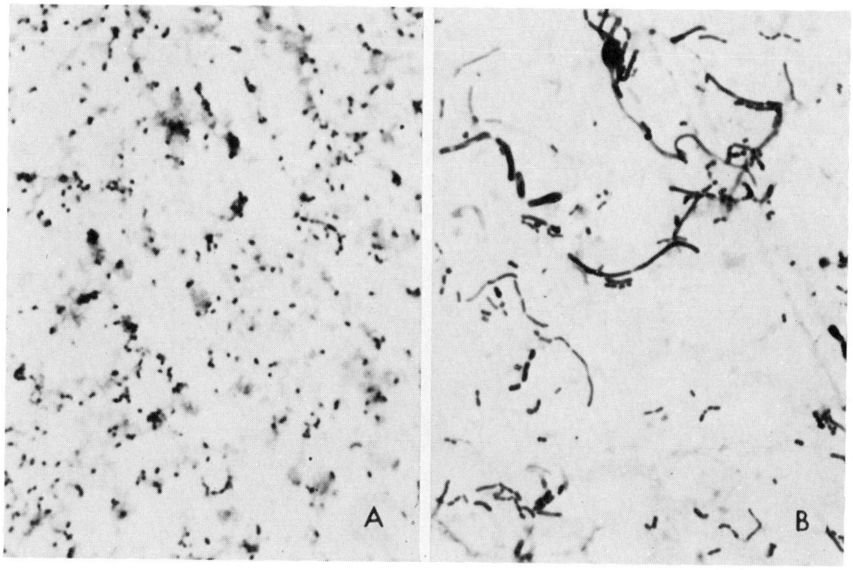

Fig. 43–2. **A.** *Prevotella intermedia* from supplemented thioglycolate, 24 hours. As shown here, the organism often appears as small coccobacilli. × 1000. **B.** *Prevotella intermedia* from chopped-meat medium with carbohydrate, 24 hours. × 1000. The same strain is shown in **A** and **B** to demonstrate variation in morphology dependent on the culture medium. Pleomorphism is also observed within a single culture, as demonstrated in **B.**

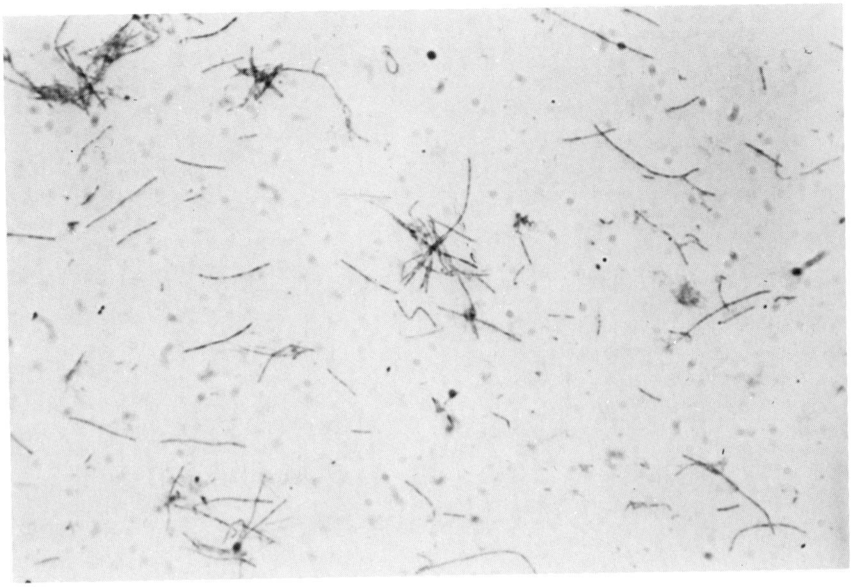

Fig. 43–3. *Fusobacterium nucleatum* from sheep's blood agar plate. As shown here, this organism may appear as thin bacilli, often with very tapered ends, or may form long thin filaments. It stains palely gram-negative. × 1000.

growth occurs at a Po_2 equal to or less than 0.5% for strict anaerobes and equal to or less than 3% for moderate anaerobes. Thus most anaerobic bacteria will not grow on the surface of blood agar plates exposed to air. Anaerobic gaseous environments also commonly include 5% or more of CO_2, which is stimulatory, or a requirement for many anaerobic (or microaerophilic) bacteria. There is much overlap with regard to classification of the gaseous requirements of organisms for growth. A genus such as *Clostridium* primarily includes obligate anaerobes, but certain strains (or species) of clostridia grow sparsely under aerobic conditions. Conversely, genera such as *Lactobacillus* and *Streptococcus* mostly are made up of strains or species that are facultatively anaerobic, but certain members within these genera are obligately anaerobic. Also, it has been common practice to include among anaerobic classification schemes genera encompassing mostly microaerophilic species or strains, e.g., *Campylobacter,* and mostly CO_2-requiring species or strains, e.g., *Actinomyces,* that grow in the presence of nearly ambient Po_2 if the atmosphere is CO_2-enriched. Microaerophilic organisms prefer an O_2 environment of 5% to 10%. Many such strains show the most luxuriant growth or are isolated initially only under anaerobic conditions with the usual clinical laboratory procedures. More precise determination of the relationships of organisms to O_2 and CO_2 would aid in our overall understanding of the gaseous requirements for survival and growth and probably would be useful in species identification.

Growth Requirements. In addition to the provision of a CO_2-enriched anaerobic atmosphere, anaerobes generally are

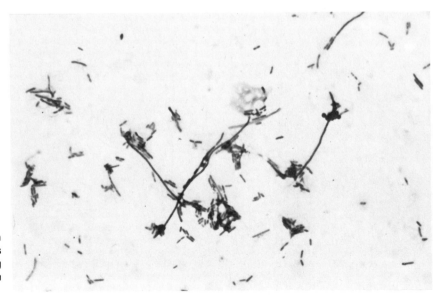

Fig. 43–4. *Fusobacterium necrophorum* from chopped-meat medium with carbohydrate. This organism may be highly pleomorphic, appearing as short, long, or filamentous bacilli, often with bulbous swellings and round bodies. × 1000.

nutritionally very fastidious and require an enriched medium for growth. Growth factor requirements usually may be met by the addition of yeast extract, blood (for solid media), serum or ascites fluid (for liquid medium), vitamin K, hemin, and a fermentable carbohydrate to the basal medium, although other additives, such as cystine or arginine, may be required for some strains. Solid media (or broth) prepared from an enriched base such as Brucella, brain-heart infusion, or Schaedler are preferable. Cooked chopped-meat medium containing carbohydrate is an excellent broth medium, but supplemented thioglycolate and other broths also work well. Selective plates are helpful for isolation and aid in presumptive identification of anaerobes from clinical specimens, which often include multiple species of facultative and anaerobic bacteria.

Solid and liquid media should be either freshly prepared, prestored in an anaerobic environment overnight or longer, or sterilized and maintained under anaerobic conditions. These steps reduce the quantities of oxygen or oxidized components, thus shortening the lag phase and providing for more optimal growth of anaerobes.

Laboratory Culture and Identification

Anaerobic Culture Systems

At present the primary types of anaerobic culture systems available include the anaerobic jar or small O_2-impermeable plastic bag, the roll-tube (Hungate) system, and the anaerobic glove chamber. They all provide an anaerobic atmosphere for incubation of growth media, and for the roll-tube and glove chamber methods an anaerobic atmosphere is also provided during primary inoculation, subculture, and examination steps. A mixture of gases containing 10% H_2, 5% to 10% CO_2, and a balance of N_2 usually is used, although 100% CO_2 or N_2 is used for certain applications. Anaerobic atmospheres are achieved through various combinations of mechanical and chemical methods with the use of pressurized gas cylinders or other anaerobic gas sources (e.g., disposable generator packet), often a vacuum source, and a catalyst such as palladium to chemically reduce O_2. Palladium catalyst reacts with residual oxygen in the presence of hydrogen to form water.

Each of these anaerobic systems has certain advantages and disadvantages. Although the roll tube and anaerobic glove chamber systems yield a higher number of isolates of the more oxygen-sensitive species, the anaerobic bacteria associated with clinical infections usually are less sensitive to oxygen than many other anaerobic members of the indigenous flora, and optimal anaerobic jar techniques work well.

Isolation and Identification

When specimens arrive in the laboratory for culture, an immediate Gram stain of the material is often valuable in the selection of appropriate media and methods for culture and as a quality control for the types of bacteria that laboratory culture should reveal. Specimens should be cultured as soon as possible to minimize exposure to oxygen. Also, since many anaerobic infections are polymicrobic, the nutritive material present in most clinical specimens will tend to support growth of the least fastidious, most rapidly growing bacteria at the expense of other strains that may be present in high proportions in the original material. Delay in transporting specimens to the laboratory and in inoculating media and culturing initially only in broth (without directly streaking plates) may significantly alter the relative concentrations of species as they exist in the infection, thus giving misleading results.

It is generally characteristic of anaerobes to grow more slowly than facultative or aerobic species do because of the lower energy yield of their fermentative metabolism. Ideally, plates should be checked at 18 to 24 hours for faster-growing species (e.g., *Clostridium perfringens* and *Bacteroides fragilis*) and daily thereafter up to 5 to 7 days to isolate strains that grow slowly (e.g., certain *Actinomyces, Eubacterium,* and *Propionibacterium* species).

Once an organism has been isolated in pure culture and is determined to be anaerobic rather than facultative, a number of procedures are available for its identification. The proper genus usually can be determined by Gram stain reaction, cellular morphology, and gas-liquid chromatography of growth media for the presence of particular short-chained fatty acids (e.g., propionic, butyric, lactic, succinic) and alcohols produced as end products of metabolism. Tests for motility also may be necessary at times. Species determination is based on fermentation of various sugars, detection of particular enzymes, and other biochemical reactions similar to those used for aerobic or facultative bacteria. Commercial miniaturized identification kits are available and are suitable for identification of clinical isolates. While gas liquid chromatography usually is not required for species identification, its inclusion considerably increases accuracy.

Other techniques appear promising for increased accuracy and speed of identification of anaerobic bacteria directly in clinical material or in pure culture. For example, DNA hybridization (probe techniques) and antigen detection by monoclonal or polyclonal antibodies using immunofluorescence or an ELISA technique have been applied successfully, mostly on an experimental basis, for species of various genera. Fluorescent-antibody conjugates have been used clinically for specific staining of species of *Bacteroides, Fusobacterium, Clostridium, Actinomyces,* and *Propionibacterium.* Protein electrophoresis of whole cells or components has been applied mostly in taxonomic and microbial flora studies but has not been adapted for convenient clinical use. High-resolution gas chromotography of cellular fatty acids appears to provide accurate species identifications based on computerized analysis and comparison with known species, but it is used primarily in research at present.

Further details on media, anaerobic systems for cultivation, and identification of anaerobes can be found in the various manuals on anaerobic bacteriology listed in the Further Reading section of this chapter.

Determinants of Pathogenicity

Specific Virulence Factors. Information on the mechanisms of pathogenicity among non-spore-forming anaerobic bacteria is limited because of the delay in recognition of their medical importance. No toxins produced by the non-spore-forming anaerobes are comparable to the potent toxins of certain clostridia. Yet, the existence and importance of virulence factors are apparent from the unequal pathogenicity observable with various species or strains of anaerobes. For example, certain organisms, such as *B. fragilis* (Fig. 43–1), are frequently isolated in infection but are found in the indigenous flora in much lower numbers than other prevalent endogenous organisms that are rarely associated with infection.

Lipopolysaccharide has been demonstrated in strains of

Fusobacterium, Prevotella, Porphyromonas, Wollinella, Bacteroides, and *Veillonella.* However, the endotoxins of strains of *Bacteroides* tested have an altered chemical structure compared with the endotoxins of aerobic and facultative gram-negative bacteria, and many of the biologic activities of this lipopolysaccharide are weak. Nevertheless, the lipopolysaccharide of *B. fragilis* appears to promote abscess formation in experimental animals. Also, enhanced coagulation (decreased clotting time) has been demonstrated in mice injected with whole bacteria, lipopolysaccharide, or lipid A from strains of *Bacteroides* and *Fusobacterium.* When similar extraction methods were used, certain biologic activities of the lipopolysaccharide of *Porphyromonas gingivalis* were comparable in degree to those of *Escherichia coli. Fusobacterium* species have structurally typical lipopolysaccharide and in many aspects are more potent biologically than *Bacteriodes* species.

A polysaccharide capsule has been demonstrated to be an important virulence factor for strains of *B. fragilis* (see section on *B. fragilis*). Capsules also have been observed on other species among *Bacteriodes, Prevotella,* and *Porphyromonas.* The presence of capsular material is frequently, but not always, correlated with production of abscesses in experimental animals and, at least in *B. fragilis,* is more active in this regard than is lipopolysaccharide. Capsular material apparently protects anaerobic bacteria from phagocytosis and killing by polymorphonuclear leukocytes, much as it protects aerobic and facultative bacteria.

Various enzymes that may serve as virulence factors have been detected in different strains of anaerobic bacteria. These include collagenase, heparinase, hyaluronidase, fibrinolysin, gelatinase, aminopeptidases, and other proteolytic enzymes, lecithinase, phospholipase, lipase, chondroitin sulfatase, deoxyribonuclease, phosphatase, neuraminidase, and elastase. Although a role in virulence is hypothetical for many, some enzymes have been demonstrated to be active in disease production. Examples are the collagenase of strains of *P. gingivalis;* the heparinase of certain *Bacteroides* species, which may be an alternate mechanism to that of endotoxin for the development of thrombophlebitis and septic emboli; and various hemolysins and lipases associated with strains of *Fusobacterium necrophorum.* In a general sense, oxygen-protective enzymes such as superoxide dismutase, peroxidase, and catalase can be thought of as virulence factors because they enhance survival of anaerobes in tissue environments prior to establishment of a low oxygen tension and oxidation-reduction potential.

Certain of the short-chained fatty acids produced as metabolic end products by most of the anaerobic bacteria may act as virulence factors. Butyrate at concentrations found to be present in dental plaque or in the supernatant fluid of a broth culture of a strain of *Porphyromonas* is toxic for mammalian cells in culture. Also, succinic acid at concentrations corresponding to those measured in abscesses significantly reduces phagocytic killing of *E. coli* by human polymorphonuclear leukocytes and decreases their chemotatic migration. All species of *Bacteroides* produce succinate.

Synergy. The endogenous anaerobic bacteria are opportunists, causing disease when factors combine to produce an environment in tissue that promotes their growth. Individual strains of anaerobic bacteria generally lack the full complement of virulence factors that provides for invasion of tissue, resistance to host defense mechanisms, growth in tissue, and injury to host tissue. The deficiencies in individual strains can be compensated for by other species, however, so that, collectively, a mixture of organisms has a full complement of virulence factors. Thus, although infections do occur with a single species, mixed infection, either with a variety of anaerobic species or with a combination of facultative and anaerobic species, is most common. Deficiencies in individual bacteria may also be compensated for by compromised host defenses, as discussed below.

Well-documented early studies pioneered work on the polymicrobic nature of many anaerobic infections and the combined pathologic activities of organisms in synergistic mixtures. Intratracheal inoculation of pyorrhea exudate from humans containing a fusospirochetal mixture of oral anaerobic bacteria—spirochetes, fusiform bacilli, streptococci, and usually vibrios—was shown to produce aspiration pneumonia and lung abscess in laboratory animals as a model of human disease after aspiration. Subsequent studies in a variety of laboratory animals have demonstrated production of infection by synergistic mixtures of two or more anaerobic species or, more commonly, by facultative and anaerobic species that were noninfective or less infective individually. These have included models of veterinary infections and human infections, such as appendicitis peritonitis, genital infections, soft tissue infections, periodontal disease, skin necrosis, and intrahepatic and intra-abdominal abscesses. However, the specific contributions of each strain essential to the infective mixture have rarely been determined. Examples of specific determinants that were essential in the particular model system studied are (1) the requirement for a naphthaquinone produced by a gram-positive species such as a diphtheroid for the growth of *P. gingivalis,* which was itself required for infectivity of a mixture of strains from periodontal disease, and (2) the ability of succinate to replace the requirement of *Klebsiella pneumoniae* for infectivity of *P. gingivalis.*

Other interactions among species in a mixture that could have clinical significance are (1) the inhibition of phagocytosis and intracellular killing by polymorphonuclear leukocytes of facultative gram-negative rods in the presence of certain *Bacteroides, Prevotella,* or *Porphyromonas* species by competition for opsonins, inhibition by capsular material or metabolic products, or by other mechanism(s); (2) the protection of antibiotic-susceptible strains in mixtures by destruction of penicillin or cephalosporins by β-lactamase-producing anaerobes; and (3) the use of oxygen by facultative species that aids in producing a suitable environment for growth of anaerobes.

Clinical Infection

A number of features under discussion characterize the majority of infections involving the non-spore-forming anaerobic bacteria (Table 43–2) and distinguish them, in particular,

TABLE 43–2. FEATURES ASSOCIATED WITH INFECTIONS INVOLVING ANAEROBES

Caused by endogenous opportunistic pathogens, usually not transmissible
Occur in settings of compromised host defense, particularly local reduction in tissue Po_2
Usually polymicrobic, synergistic mixtures of aerobes and anaerobes or exclusively anaerobes
Abscess formation and tissue necrosis frequently present
Broad-spectrum antimicrobial therapy generally required

from certain more classic infectious diseases that are consistent with Koch's postulates. Most important, perhaps, is that most of the anaerobic bacteria that cause infection are members of our normal indigenous flora and therefore do not meet the criterion that the organism must be found only in the presence of disease. Skin and membrane surfaces of the upper respiratory tract, the gastrointestinal tract, and the genitourinary tracts are populated with a varied and great abundance of anaerobic organisms (Table 43–3). Other features also are frequently present:

1. Infections often develop slowly and may become chronic, although acute episodes, such as gram-negative septicemia or necrotizing fasciitis, occur.
2. Anaerobic bacteria frequently produce a putrid odor in infected material or in vitro culture because of certain end products of their metabolism.
3. Gas may be present in tissue or in loculations, although it may occur also with certain facultative bacteria.

Pathogenesis

The pathogenesis of infection with non-spore-forming anaerobes is not completely understood, although the clinical settings that predispose to invasion by endogenous anaerobic bacteria are clear. Tissues normally are well oxygenated and resistant to invasion of anaerobes. A change from the normal, apparently benign host-parasite relationship occurs most often in settings of reduced oxygen tension and oxidation-reduction potential.

Reduction of the normal oxidation-reduction potential of tissue (approximately +120 mV) and a lowered oxygen tension may stem from an impaired blood supply, necrosis of tissue, or growth of facultative bacteria. These conditions may be associated with vascular disease, trauma, surgery, presence of foreign bodies, malignancy, radiation therapy, injection of vasoconstrictive agents such as epinephrine, shock, cold, or edema. In these settings not only is an appropriate anaerobic environment provided, but other local host defenses also are impaired, enabling these opportunists to initiate growth. Foreign bodies and blood products (e.g., hemin, Fe^{+++}, fibrin) have an adjuvant effect, reducing the inoculum required to produce infection, or increasing the severity, or both. Although local factors usually are more significant, as with other opportunists, a generalized compromise of host defenses that accompanies administration of immunosuppressive drugs, steroids, and cytotoxic agents or that occurs in the presence of diseases such as diabetes mellitus also may predispose to infection with anaerobes. The introduction of very high numbers of anaerobic bacteria already in a milieu of low oxidation-reduction potential, such as fecal material spilled into the peritoneal cavity, can overwhelm even normal host defenses and result in infection without direct tissue damage. Also, the low oxygen tension present in anaerobic infections may interfere with oxygen-dependent pathways of phagocytic killing.

In these settings, anaerobic bacteria may initiate infection by direct extension from membrane or cutaneous surfaces into normally sterile adjacent tissue or may be carried to more distant sites by hematogenous or other mechanisms of spread. Thus, disturbance of the natural balance between tissue resistance and endogenous flora is basic in the pathogenesis of these infections. Once introduced into the affected site, the production of toxins, enzymes, and other virulence factors is obviously significant, but their specific role in the overall disease process requires further clarification in many instances, as discussed previously.

Aerobic or facultative bacteria most often are present in infections involving anaerobes and usually are derived from the same endogenous source. Their presence is not required for infection to occur, as long as conditions in tissue are appropriate for anaerobic growth and the pure or mixed species of anaerobes possess the necessary complement of virulence factors. Nevertheless, mixed aerobic-anaerobic species may be more efficient in initiating and maintaining infection; there are numerous examples of how the one may complement the activity of the other.

Clinical Manifestations

The types of infection produced and the particular anaerobic species involved are related to the endogenous habitat on the skin and in the upper respiratory, gastrointestinal, and genitourinary tracts (Table 43–3). Of the tremendous variety of indigenous species, only relatively few are common as opportunistic pathogens (Table 43–1). Many species are ubiquitous,

TABLE 43–3. INCIDENCE OF ANAEROBIC BACTERIA AS INDIGENOUS FLORA IN HUMANS

	Cocci		Bacilli										
			Gram-positive						Gram-negative				
Anatomic Site	*Gram-positive*	*Gram-negative*	*Clostridium*	*Actinomyces*	*Bifidobacterium*	*Eubacterium*	*Lactobacillus*[a]	*Propionibacterium*	*Bacteroides*	*Prevotella*	*Porphyromonas*	*Fusobacterium*
Skin	1	0	0	0	0	U	0	2	0	0	0	0
Upper respiratory tract[b]	1	1	0	1	0	±	0	1	0	2	1	1
Mouth	2	2	±	1	1	1	1	±	0	2	2	2
Intestine	2	1	2	±	2	2	1	±	2	1	1	1
External genitalia	1	0	0	0	0	U	±	U	1	1	±	0
Urethra	±	U	±	0	0	U	±	±	±	±	±	0
Vagina	2	1	±	±	±	±	2	±	±	2	1	±

Modified from Sutter, Citron, Edelstein, Finegold: Wadsworth Anaerobic Bacteriology Manual, ed 4. Star Publishing, 1985.

[a] Includes anaerobic microaerophilic, and facultative strains.

[b] Includes nasal passages, nasopharynx, oropharynx and tonsils.

U, unknown; 0, not found, rare; ±, irregular; 1, usually present; 2, usually present in large numbers.

but some are most typically etiologic in particular body sites. For example, *B. fragilis,* which is not a usual member of the upper respiratory tract and mouth flora but is present in the gastrointestinal tract, is very common in abdominal infections and, to a lesser degree, pelvic infections. *Prevotella bivia,* which is a prevalent species in the vaginal flora, is common in genital tract infections but considerably less common in infections in other sites. Facultative organisms that frequently may accompany anaerobes in mixed infections are *E. coli, Klebsiella, Enterobacter, Proteus, Streptococcus, Staphylococcus* (usually not *Staphylococcus aureus*), and diphtheroids, depending also on the body site.

The incidence of anaerobic bacteria in the infections they are most commonly associated with is shown in Table 43–4. The major types of infection are briefly discussed below.

TABLE 43–4. SELECTED INFECTIONS TYPICALLY INVOLVING NON-SPORE-FORMING ANAEROBIC BACTERIA

Site	Approximate Incidence of Anaerobes (%)	Approximate Percentage of Anaerobe-Positive Sites With Anaerobes Exclusively
Septicemia	15	80
Central nervous system		
Brain abscess	89	66
Head, neck, dental, and orofacial		
Chronic otitis media	50	10
Chronic sinusitis	52	80
Postoperative wound infection	95	<10
Peritonsillar abscess	76	20
Dental, periodontal, orofacial, root canal abscess or infection	≥95	40–70
Thoracic		
Aspiration pneumonia	85	30–50[a]
Lung abscess	89	66
Bronchiectasis	76	33
Empyema (nonsurgical)	62	50
Intra-abdominal		
Intra-abdominal infection (general)	90	20
Liver abscess (pyogenic)	52	33
Appendicitis with peritonitis	96	<10
Postoperative infections	93	20
Biliary tract	43	<10
Obstetric-gynecologic		
Vulvovaginal abscess	75	25
Salpingitis and pelvic peritonitis	50	20
Tubo-ovarian and pelvic abscess	90	50
Septic abortion and endometritis	75	20
Postoperative wound infection	67	25
Other sites, soft tissue or abscess		
Necrotizing fasciitis	81	<10
Cellulitis	92	10
Diabetic foot ulcers	95	<10
Osteomyelitis	40	10
Perirectal abscess	80	40

Adapted from Sutter, Citron, Edelstein, Finegold: Wadsworth Anaerobic Bacteriology Manual, ed 4. Star Publishing, 1985.
[a] Rate for solely community-acquired aspiration pneumonia is higher.
Note: Numerous species of *Clostridium*, histotoxic and others, may accompany the non-spore-formers, particularly in abdominal infections, necrotizing fasciitis, and cellulitis.

Intra-abdominal Infections. Infectious complications generally derive from spillage of fecal matter into the peritoneal cavity in such settings as penetrating abdominal trauma, surgery, appendicitis, diverticulitis, inflammatory bowel disease, or cancer. The first clinical manifestation is generally peritonitis, which in survivors is followed by abscess formation and localization of the infection. Infectious complications that follow disruption of the integrity of the lower bowel and colon are more frequent than those of the upper bowel because of the higher concentrations of bacteria, especially anaerobes (10^{11}/g feces), in the colon. On average, five species—three anaerobic and two facultative—are isolated from abdominal infections. Species of *Bacteroides,* particularly *B. fragilis* and related organisms, *Clostridium, Fusobacterium,* and anaerobic gram-positive cocci are the most frequent anaerobic isolates.

Obstetric and Gynecologic Infections. Anaerobes play an important role in salpingitis, tuboovarian and pelvic abscesses, vaginal cuff infections following hysterectomy, pelvic cellulitis, endometritis, postabortal sepsis, chorioamnionitis, and other infections. Especially associated with infection are premature rupture of membranes, prolonged labor, extensive manipulations and hemorrhage during delivery, nonelective cesarean section, nonmedical abortion, malignancy, gonococcal salpingitis, and intrauterine contraceptive devices. Endometritis may be limited or may spread to produce tuboovarian infection, peritonitis, pelvic abscess, and septicemia. Chronic pelvic infections may subsequently develop. Likewise, salpingitis may extend and produce generalized pelvic infections with such sequelae as chronic pelvic pain, infertility, ectopic pregnancy, and recurrent infection. Multiple anaerobic and facultative species are common, as in abdominal infections. *Prevotella,* particularly *P. bivia* and *P. disiens,* various black-pigmenting anaerobic gram-negative rods, and anaerobic gram-positive cocci are frequently isolated. *Streptococcus pyogenes* is no longer a common etiologic agent in puerperal sepsis as it was in the past.

Pleuropulmonary Infections. Anaerobic bacteria are important causes of pneumonitis (pulmonary infiltrate without cavity formation), lung abscess, necrotizing pneumonia, and empyema but not of lobar pneumonia or chronic bronchitis. Aspiration of mouth flora, as may occur in alcoholism or general anesthesia, generally is the inciting event for these diverse pleuropulmonary infections. Other common underlying conditions are dental infections or other extrapulmonary anaerobic disease, bronchogenic carcinoma, pulmonary embolus with infarction, and bronchiectasis. As in other anaerobic infections, pleuropulmonary foci yield mixed species of bacteria, usually three or four but ranging to more than 10 species per specimen. In these settings, the common anaerobic isolates are *Fusobacterium nucleatum* (Fig. 43–3), pigmenting prevotella, *Porphyromonas,* and gram-positive cocci. *B. fragilis* is isolated in approximately 20% of these infections, which are usually complicated cases, even though it is not present in the normal flora of the oral cavity.

Upper Respiratory Tract Infections. Chronic forms of a wide variety of infections of the upper respiratory tract are associated with anaerobes. These include periodontal disease, various fusospirochetal diseases, actinomycosis, peritonsillar abscesses, otitis media, mastoiditis, and sinusitis. Species of *Porphyromonas* and *Prevotella* contribute significantly to the pathogenesis of many of these infections.

The association of anaerobic bacteria with chronic otitis media, mastoiditis, and sinusitis doubtlessly accounts for the contiguous spread of these organisms into the central nervous system and their high incidence in nontraumatic brain abscesses. Hematogenous spread from anaerobic pleuropulmonary infections and sepsis after dental extractions are also sources of brain abscess.

Soft Tissue Infections. Anaerobic infections of the skin and soft tissues usually evolve from traumatic injury, surgery, or ischemia associated with vascular disease or diabetes mellitus. The specific anaerobes involved depend largely on the site of infection or the source of the infecting bacteria. For example, human bites that can develop into serious infections usually involve the indigenous facultative and anaerobic flora of the mouth. These diverse anaerobic infections usually produce extensive tissue necrosis with extension along subcutaneous and fascial planes, gas, and a foul odor. The better characterized of these infections include the following:

1. Progressive bacterial synergistic gangrene
2. Chronic undermining ulcer of Meleney
3. Synergistic necrotizing cellulitis
4. Necrotizing fasciitis
5. Streptococcal gangrene, usually caused by *S. pyogenes* and less frequently by anaerobic gram-positive cocci.

Septicemia. Anaerobic septicemias generally stem from abdominal and pelvic infections and most often involve anaerobic gram-positive cocci, certain *Prevotella,* and *Bacteroides,* particularly *B. fragilis* from abdominal sources. These septicemias may be associated with jaundice, septic thrombophlebitis, and suppuration at distant sites from metastases. The overall mortality associated with anaerobic septicemia is 25% to 35%, but large differences are found relative to the patient population. Bacteremia stemming from abdominal infections, particularly with underlying diseases, is associated with a high mortality and poorer prognosis than bacteremia in obstetric patients.

Laboratory Diagnosis

Specimen Collection and Reporting. Because of their endogenous nature (Table 43–3), the bacteriologic diagnosis of infections involving anaerobic bacteria differs from those with exogenously derived aerobic or facultative pathogens. Thus isolation of anaerobic bacteria may be clinically meaningless or uninterpretable unless the specimen is derived from an appropriate source (Table 43–5), a closed loculation or a site that is normally sterile. The following specimens are generally unacceptable for anaerobic culture because the collection sites are colonized or because contamination with indigenous flora often occurs: expectorated sputum, throat swabs, nasotracheal or bronchoscopy aspirates, gastrointestinal contents, feces (except for *Clostridium difficile*), vaginal or endocervical secretions, midstream urine, and skin or superficial wound swabs.

TABLE 43–5. APPROPRIATE SPECIMENS FOR ANAEROBIC CULTURE

Normally sterile tissues	Endometrium (lochia)[a]
Body fluids: bile, pleural, sinus, joint, pericardial, peritoneal	Culdocentesis fluid
Abscess contents	Urine—catheterized or suprapubic aspirate (only in complicated cases)
Blood cultures	
Deep aspirates of wounds	
Transtracheal aspirates	Cerebrospinal fluid (only in complicated cases)
Bronchoscopy aspirates[a]	
Amniotic fluid—at cesarean section, amniocentesis, amniotomy	

[a] When collected with a device that protects the sampling portion (e.g., swab, brush, aspirator) from contamination with endogenous flora en route to a normally sterile area being cultured.

Aspirated or tissue specimens are preferable to swabs whenever feasible, because better survival of pathogens, greater quantity of specimen, and less contamination with extraneous organisms are often achieved. Ideally, specimens should be placed in an anaerobic transport device that consists of a tube or vial containing an anaerobic gas mixture substituted for air, which protects the organisms from O_2-exposure and drying during transport to the laboratory. Specimens should be delivered immediately (within 20 minutes) for culture; this is particularly important if anaerobic transport is not used.

Culture reports for anaerobic bacteria generally require more time than for facultative organisms, as many anaerobes grow more slowly and usually must be isolated from complex mixtures of species. A direct Gram stain of the specimen read by a trained person can be a significant aid to the clinician in determining the types of organisms involved and thus in the choice of initial antibiotic therapy.

Communication between clinician and microbiologist is important in securing appropriate specimens and in the reporting of anaerobic cultures. Most combinations of species isolated/specimen source are readily interpretable, but other situations are highly dependent on numerous clinical parameters. For example, *Propionibacterium acnes* usually is considered a contaminant (of blood, spinal fluid, or other cultures) because it is part of the normal flora of the skin. In certain clinical settings, however, it may assume the role of a pathogen.

Susceptibility Testing. Routine antimicrobial susceptibility testing of anaerobic isolates has not been performed in many clinical laboratories because of the polymicrobic nature of most anaerobic infections, delayed testing and reporting because of the generally slower growth of anaerobes, and the necessity for special methods. Increasing resistance among anaerobic bacteria, particularly the gram-negative bacilli, and the current availability of a wider variety of antimicrobials for which susceptibility is less predictable require more testing. Susceptibility testing of anaerobes should be performed in case of life-threatening infections, in critical sources such as blood, cerebrospinal fluid, and surgical osteomyelitis specimens, when there is no response to antimicrobial therapy, and whenever serious sequelae are likely. Reference dilution tests for determination of the minimum inhibitory concentration of antimicrobials have been developed for anaerobes under the auspices of the National Committee for Clinical Laboratory Standards (USA).

Treatment

In many circumstances, surgical drainage and resection of necrotic tissue are therapeutic mainstays for anaerobic infections. Even where surgery or percutaneous needle aspiration is appropriate, however, effective concurrent antimicrobial therapy is important. In nonsurgical settings, antimicrobial selection may be critical, because the most common clinical isolate, *B. fragilis,* and strains of many other *Bacteroides* and *Prevotella* are resistant to some of the more frequently used antibiotics. In anaerobic septicemias, especially those involving *Bacteroides,* the mortality among patients treated with antimicrobials active against the infecting anaerobes is 12% to 16%, compared with 60% among patients who receive inappropriate drugs. Parenteral therapy usually is required to attain adequate drug levels in necrotic tissue and abscesses where high concentrations of anaerobic bacteria usually are present. Chronic infections, such as lung or liver abscesses, must be treated for prolonged periods to prevent relapse.

A key element of a drug's performance is activity against the *B. fragilis* group (see discussion of *B. fragilis*) and certain *Prevotella* species, because these organisms are usually or often resistant to many commonly used antimicrobials. *Bacteroides thetaiotaomicron* and *Bacteroides ovatus* among the *B. fragilis* group are even more antibiotic resistant than is *B. fragilis.* These bacteria constitutively produce β-lactamases that can inactivate penicillins and the older cephalosporin antibiotics. Certain of the newer cephalosporins and penicillins are more active against these resistant *Bacteroides* because of increased resistance to β-lactamase degradation, or the higher blood levels achievable, or both. Other mechanisms of resistance are active, depending on the nature of the drug, but for β-lactam drugs, resistance also can occur through blocked penetration.

Genetic transfer of drug resistance among *Bacteroides* apparently has a limited clinical impact at present but is worrisome because of the high frequency of these organisms in infection and the high concentrations in our endogenous flora. Resistance transfer, most intensively studied with *B. fragilis* strains, has been observed for tetracycline, clindamycin, erythromycin, cefoxitin, and high-level penicillin and ampicillin resistance. Certain resistance determinants are also transferrable to *E. coli.*

The antimicrobials with the highest activities against anaerobic bacteria, indicated both by in vitro susceptibility tests and clinical efficacy, are primarily metronidazole, imipenem, β-lactam drug with β-lactamase inhibitor combinations, clindamycin, and chloramphenicol, followed by cefoxitin, piperacillin, and mezlocillin. Other agents are less effective in vitro or less clinical data are available.

Metronidazole has specific activity for anaerobes and is mostly inactive against aerobic and facultative bacteria. It is bactericidal for most obligately anaerobic strains, which includes the *Bacteroides,* but less frequently encountered organisms—aerotolerant or microaerophilic strains of *Streptococcus, Actinomyces, Propionibacterium,* and certain other gram-positive bacilli—are often resistant. Metronidazole penetrates the blood-brain barrier and is effective in anaerobic brain abscess. Imipenem is a newer highly active broad-spectrum antimicrobial that has been used primarily for serious infections. It is highly stable in the presence of β-lactamases, and anaerobic bacteria are almost uniformly susceptible to the drug in vitro. Combination agents such as ampicillin plus sulbactam and ticarcillin plus clavulanic acid are active against a broad spectrum of bacteria including most of the anaerobes. The β-lactamase inhibitors, sulbactam and clavulanic acid, prevent destruction by bacterial β-lactamases of the β-lactam drugs, so that organisms normally resistant because of these enzymes remain susceptible. Clindamycin has high activity against most anaerobic bacteria, including *B. fragilis,* although some other members of the *B. fragilis* group can be resistant. It has proved clinical effectiveness in body sites other than the central nervous system, where it does not penetrate. Limited instances of plasmid-mediated resistance of *B. fragilis* to clindamycin have been reported. Chloramphenicol is widely active in vitro against anaerobic bacteria, including *B. fragilis,* and was previously the major drug available for treatment of anaerobic brain abscesses. Occasional failure of the drug in vivo may relate to its decreased penetration of abscesses as compared to clindamycin and metronidazole or inactivation of the drug by high concentrations of *Bacteroides* and *Clostridium.* The serious side effects of the drug, although quite infrequent, have generally restricted its use to severe or life-threatening infection.

Members of the *B. fragilis* group are resistant to the usual clinical levels of penicillin G, ampicillin, nafcillin, methicillin, and cephalothin. Despite previous generalizations, resistance to these drugs has not been limited to the *B. fragilis* group. Resistance also is apparently increasing among many species, however, and certain other *Bacteroides* and *Prevotella,* notably *P. bivia, P. disiens,* and *P. oris,* are frequently resistant or only moderately susceptible. The high association of *B. fragilis* and other resistant *Bacteroides* and *Prevotella* with anaerobic infections of the abdomen and pelvis precludes widespread use of penicillin or the other drugs noted above for serious anaerobic infections in these sites. Penicillin G has been the drug of choice for infections involving anaerobic bacteria in the upper and lower respiratory tract because of the infrequent presence of organisms of the *B. fragilis* group. Recently, however, penicillin has been demonstrated to be less effective than clindamycin in the treatment of anaerobic lung abscess and persistent tonsillar infections. Penicillin G, ampicillin, and cephalothin, nonetheless, are highly active against a variety of other anaerobes, including certain of the *Prevotella* and most fusobacteria and anaerobic gram-positive cocci and bacilli.

Almost all anaerobic bacteria are resistant to the aminoglycoside antibiotics, making such drugs as streptomycin, neomycin, kanamycin, gentamicin, tobramycin, and amikacin useless against anaerobes in infection. Many anaerobes were sensitive to tetracycline in the past, but increasing resistance has been noted and presently about two thirds of clinical isolates of *B. fragilis* are resistant. Two tetracycline derivatives—doxycycline and minocycline—are active against 65% to 75% of *B. fragilis* strains, in addition to many other anaerobes.

Knowledge of the usual pathogens in specific sites of infection and a direct Gram stain of the specimen aid in the choice of initial therapy, but changes may be necessary when the laboratory obtains the isolates from culture. Since mixed infections containing both anaerobic and facultative species frequently occur, two or even three antibiotics may be required for coverage of known pathogens unless one of the more broad-spectrum agents, which also covers the facultatively anaerobic species, is appropriate. For example, clindamycin and metronidazole are not active against facultative gram-negative rods and must be combined with an aminoglycoside or a cephalosporin to cover such organisms as *E. coli*, especially in pelvic and abdominal infection.

Hyperbaric oxygen theoretically could be an alternate mode of therapy for anaerobic infections, but it has been primarily evaluated only for clostridial myonecrosis (Chap. 44). The bacteriostatic and bactericidal effects of high oxygen tensions on anaerobic bacteria, achievable by hyperbaric oxygenation, might be useful clinically as an adjunct to conventional antimicrobial and surgical therapy or as an alternate to surgery for inoperable patients.

Clinically Significant Non-Spore-Forming Anaerobic Bacteria

This section presents a brief description of some of the species of clinically significant non-spore-forming anaerobic bacteria. The following genera, listed in approximately decreasing order of incidence, are isolated from the types of infection discussed in this chapter: *Bacteroides, Prevotella, Peptostreptococcus, Porphyromonas, Clostridium* (a spore-former), and *Fusobacterium,* primarily; followed by *Eubacterium, Propionibacterium, Wollinella, Streptococcus, Actinomyces, Lactobacillus, Veillonella, Mobiluncus,* and *Bifidobacterium. Treponema, Borrelia,* and *Campylobacter,* not included in this list, are covered in Chapters 45 and 46.

Anaerobic Gram-Negative Bacilli

Bacteroides

Bacteroides fragilis. Previously, *B. fragilis* was divided into five subspecies: *fragilis, thetaiotaomicron, distasonis, vulgatus,* and *ovatus.* These now have been designated as separate species on the basis of DNA homology studies, but they are frequently referred to collectively as the *B. fragilis* group (Table 43–1). These species, as identified by phenotypic characteristics, also were found to contain additional homology groups that have been named but are very uncommon in clinical specimens compared with the five species already mentioned.

Among this group of saccharolytic intestinal *Bacteroides, B. fragilis* is by far the most common isolate from infections, yet it is present in relatively lower concentrations in the normal fecal flora. *B. thetaiotaomicron* is the next most frequent from clinical sources among this group and, as pointed out earlier, tends to be more resistant to antibiotics. These *Bacteroides* are associated primarily with intra-abdominal infections or septicemias derived from this site. Although *B. fragilis* and the other former subspecies are infrequently present in the vagina and cervix of healthy women, they are isolated from some, usually serious, genital tract infections where they probably gain access from the perineal region or perhaps by translocation across the gut wall. All of the *B. fragilis* group are generally resistant to ordinary doses of penicillin and older cephalosporin antibiotics and share many characteristics. However, since *B. fragilis* is clinically most important and possesses some unique characteristics, it will be discussed separately in the remainder of this section.

MORPHOLOGY AND PHYSIOLOGY. *B. fragilis* may appear as pleomorphic bacilli with vacuoles and swellings, which are particularly apparent when the organisms are stained from broth containing fermentable carbohydrate (Fig. 43–1). Colonies of *B. fragilis* are low convex, white to gray, semiopaque, and glistening, and some strains may be hemolytic. The organisms grow more rapidly than most non-spore-forming anaerobes, and growth is stimulated by bile. *B. fragilis* is a moderate anaerobe, growing maximally in Po_2 less than 3%, but it is capable of surviving prolonged exposures to oxygen, particularly in the presence of blood. The organism produces superoxide dismutase and also a catalase (in the presence of hemin).

ANTIGENIC STRUCTURE. Thermolabile protein and thermostable lipopolysaccharide antigens have provided a basis for serologic classification of *B. fragilis.* Strains of the five former subspecies of *B. fragilis* can be divided into corresponding serotypes on the basis of agglutination, gel diffusion, and fluorescent-antibody assays. Commercial pooled antisera are available for fluorescent-antibody detection of the *B. fragilis* group (all former subspecies).

A species-specific capsular polysaccharide antigen has been demonstrated for strains of *B. fragilis.* The capsule is characteristic of clinical strains of *B. fragilis* and may be lost or diminished by continued culture (passage) in the laboratory.

The antibody response of patients with various infections, including septicemia, soft tissue infections, or abscesses due to members of the Bacteroidaceae, has been investigated to study the pathologic significance of bacteroides in mixed infections and possibly to devise a clinically useful method of detecting bacteroides infections. Precipitin and agglutination techniques have detected antibodies to *B. fragilis* in the sera of infected patients that are absent in control sera. With the use of a sensitive radioactive antigen-binding assay, antibody response to *B. fragilis* capsular polysaccharide has been demonstrated in experimental animals with abscesses induced with an encapsulated strain of *B. fragilis* and in women with pelvic infection.

DETERMINANTS OF PATHOGENICITY. As previously mentioned, the lipopolysaccharide of the outer membrane of *B. fragilis* lacks certain characteristics of classic endotoxin and has less biologic activity. Yet purified *B. fragilis* lipopolysaccharide produces sterile abscesses in experimental animals and thus probably constitutes a virulence factor. The polysaccharide capsule of *B. fragilis* especially appears to confer added virulence to this species, as evidenced from experimental studies in animals by (1) increased virulence of encapsulated strains, (2) production of abscesses by heat-killed encapsulated *B. fragilis* or purified capsular polysaccharide, and (3) protection against challenge with encapsulated *B. fragilis* through prior immunization with capsular polysaccharide. It has been shown that T cells mediate immunity to *B. fragilis* abscesses and that a soluble cell-free factor derived from the T cells of mice previously immunized with purified capsular polysaccharide from *B. fragilis* can protect mice from developing abscesses after challenge with *B. fragilis.* Mechanisms by which the capsule enhances virulence are not totally understood but may include interference with chemotaxis, with phagocytosis and opsonophagocytic killing by neutrophils, and possibly also with clearance of the organism through enhanced adherence of encapsulated organisms to peritoneal mesothelium. Yet the role of cellular versus supernatant factors is not completely clear, and soluble bacterial products such as succinate may account wholly or partially for some of the interactions with neutrophils.

Strains of *B. fragilis* that produce an enterotoxin recently have been described. These enterotoxigenic strains are pathogenic in experimental rabbit model assays and are significantly associated with diarrheal disease in humans and livestock lacking other recognized enteric pathogens.

Pigmenting Gram-Negative Bacilli

All bacilli that produced tan to black pigmentation of colonies on blood agar previously were classified as subspecies of *Bacteroides melaninogenicus.* By DNA homology, DNA base composition, and other studies, these organisms have been shown to be heterogeneous, even within the former subspecies groups, and the better-characterized homology groups have been elevated to species rank and reclassified into two new genera: *Porphyromonas* and *Prevotella* (Table 43–1). The new genus *Prevotella,* however, also contains some nonpigmented species. The natural habitat and the sites of occurrence in clinical infections are not completely known for all of the newly designated species. *Prevotella melaninogenica, Prevotella denticola, Prevotella loescheii, Prevotella intermedia, Porphyromonas endodontalis,* and *Porphyromonas gingivalis* are indigenous in the gingival crevice, and most are known to occur in various dental infections, including periodontitis, and in other sites primarily in the head, neck, and respiratory tract. The natural habitat of *Porphyromonas asaccharolytica* and *Prevotella corporis* does not appear to be the mouth but probably at least includes the lower genital tract; these species usually are found in nonoral sites of infection.

The cellular morphology of these organisms differs somewhat according to species, but strains often appear as small coccobacilli, usually with longer rod forms also present (see Fig. 43–2). Colonies on blood agar usually are convex, smooth, circular, sometimes β-hemolytic, and usually pigmented, becoming tan to black in 2 to 21 days. Vitamin K and hemin are required or are highly stimulatory for the growth of most strains.

These species can be separated on the basis of serologic tests. A polysaccharide capsular antigen that is species-specific for *P. gingivalis* has been isolated. As in *B. fragilis,* the lipopolysaccharide present in the outer membrane of these pigmented species is biochemically distinct from that of facultative gram-negative organisms; its biologic potency varies, depending on the parameter being assayed. Collagenase and apparently a polysaccharide capsule are virulence factors for certain strains. These organisms are important agents in oral, pulmonary, pelvic, intra-abdominal, and various soft tissue infections. Clinical isolates may produce β-lactamase, and some strains are resistant to penicillin and certain cephalosporins.

Prevotella bivia

P. bivia usually appears as a small coccobacillus, often occurring in pairs or short chains. Hemin is required for growth. *P. bivia* is an anaerobic gram-negative rod prevalent in the vaginal flora, particularly in the presence of bacterial vaginosis. It is most commonly isolated from genital tract infections, particularly obstetric infections, although it also can be pathogenic in other body sites. Many strains produce β-lactamase and are resistant to penicillin G and the older cephalosporins.

Fusobacterium

Fusobacterium nucleatum is the most common of the fusobacteria isolated from infections. *F. nucleatum* characteristically is thin with pointed ends and may resemble scattered wheat straw or appear as very long, thin filaments (see Fig. 43–3). Colonies sometimes are α-hemolytic and may be convex and translucent, with internal flecking or mottling, or more umbonate, heaped, dull, and opaque. *F. nucleatum* is present in the normal flora of the mouth and occasionally in the urogenital tract. It is an important agent in oral infections, lung abscesses, other pleuropulmonary infections, and amniotic fluid infections in the presence of intact membranes and preterm gestation.

Another species, *F. necrophorum,* is an important animal pathogen and is found in a variety of human infections, particularly abdominal infections and liver abscesses. These bacilli are generally broad, usually with rounded ends, and may be short, long, or filamentous, often with bulbous swellings and round bodies (Fig. 43–4). Colonies may be α- or β-hemolytic. A lipase and a partially characterized leukocidal toxin are produced. The organism's normal habitat is probably the gastrointestinal tract. Most of the fusobacteria are susceptible to penicillin G and the older cephalosporins in addition to the more active antianaerobe agents.

Anaerobic Gram-Positive Bacilli

Eubacterium, Propionibacterium, Lactobacillus, Actinomyces, Mobiluncus, and *Bifidobacterium*

Many of these organisms grow slowly in contrast to *Clostridium,* the spore-forming anaerobic bacilli. Strains within *Propionibacterium, Lactobacillus, Bifidobacterium,* and *Actinomyces* may show sparse to good growth in a CO_2 incubator or even aerobically, while other strains are obligately anaerobic. Many gram-positive rods are isolated, that cannot be identified by present schemes.

Eubacterium lentum is the most common of the eubacteria isolated from nonoral clinical specimens. It is a coccobacillus that often is found with *B. fragilis,* but little is known of its pathogenic role, if any. It is part of the normal flora of the gastrointestinal tract. Three newly described species of *Eubacterium—E. brachy, E. timidum,* and *E. nodatum—*are prevalent in periodontitis. Their relatively slow and minimal growth on artificial media retarded their recognition from dental and other body sites. These species generally are isolated from pulmonary, head, and neck infections, relating to their source in the mouth. *E. nodatum* strongly resembles *Actinomyces* in cellular and often in colonial morphology and, like *Actinomyces,* also is isolated from the upper and lower female genital tract in association with use of an intrauterine contraceptive device.

The *Actinomyces* are covered separately in Chapter 32. Previously, their characteristically slow growth resulted in their affiliation with diagnostic mycology rather than bacteriology laboratories.

Propionibacterium acnes and *Propionibacterium granulosum* are normal inhabitants of the gastrointestinal tract and, primarily, of the skin. Consequently, they occur most frequently as contaminants in cultures of blood and cerebrospinal fluid, but rarely they are causally associated with infections. They were previously classified as anaerobic members of the genus *Corynebacterium*. *Propionibacterium* may closely resemble *Actinomyces* since the cells are pleomophic and may be branched, diphtheroidal, or both.

Strains of *Lactobacillus* are normal flora in the mouth and gastrointestinal tract, and in many women they are the predominant flora in the vagina. Most species apparently have minimal pathogenic potential, but *Lactobacillus catenaforme* is occasionally associated with pleuropulmonary infections.

Mobiluncus is a newly designated genus consisting of motile, curved anaerobic bacilli. These organisms have a gram-positive type of cell wall, but strains frequently stain gram-negative or gram-variable. *Mobiluncus mulieris* and *Mobiluncus curtisii* are highly associated with the presence of bacterial vaginosis (previously termed nonspecific vaginitis) in women, although their role in this entity is unclear. Initial isolation is complicated by their slow growth and small colonies on plated media in the frequent presence of multiple other species.

Bifidobacteria are infrequently involved in infection. *Bifidobacterium dentium* (previously *Actinomyces eriksonii* or *Bifidobacterium eriksonii*) has been isolated from a variety of sites. Various bifidobacteria are normal flora in the mouth and occasionally in the urogenital tract, and they occur in large numbers in the gastrointestinal tract.

Anaerobic Gram-Positive Cocci

Peptostreptococcus and *Streptococcus*

The anaerobic gram-positive cocci are commonly found in clinical infections. The obligately anaerobic species most frequently isolated are *Peptostreptococcus anaerobius, Peptostreptococcus tetradius, Peptostreptococcus magnus, Peptostreptococcus asaccharolyticus,* and *Peptostreptococcus prevotii* (Table 43–1). The latter three species previously were classified in the genus *Peptococcus*. Other cocci, strains of which often are anaerobic only when initially isolated, are *Streptococcus intermedius* and *Streptococcus constellatus*. The nomenclature of these organisms is controversial at present, but they are generally included in the *Streptococcus milleri* group. Another, *Gemella morbillorum* (previously *Streptococcus morbillorum*), is considered anaerobic to aerotolerant. After subculture(s) in the laboratory most strains of these three species are able to grow in a CO_2 incubator or, rarely, in air. All of these streptococci produce lactic acid as their major end product.

The cellular morphology of the anaerobic cocci varies, depending on the genus, species, and strain, and includes singles, pairs, tetrads, irregular clumps, and chains. Various ones among these species of cocci are indigenous flora in the mouth, gastrointestinal tract, and genital tract. They are prevalent in a wide variety of human infection but are particularly important in pleuropulmonary disease, brain abscesses, and obstetric and gynecologic infections. Most of these species are susceptible to β-lactam antibiotics and to other drugs used to treat anaerobic infections. Certain strains, usually microaerophilic or aerotolerant, among the streptococci, however, are resistant to metronidazole.

Anaerobic Gram-Negative Cocci

Veillonella

Veillonella parvula is isolated from clinical specimens, but little is known of its role in the production of infection. *Veillonella*, organisms are small cocci that occur in pairs, short chains, and clumps. They are present in the normal flora of the mouth in particular and in the gastrointestinal and genital tracts.

FURTHER READING

Books, Manuals, and Reviews

Appelbaum PC: Anaerobic infections: nonsporeformers. In Wentworth BB (coord ed): Diagnostic Procedures for Bacterial Infections, ed 7. New York, American Public Health Association, Inc., 1988, vol 2, p 45

Balows A, DeHaan RM, Dowell VR Jr, et al (eds): Anaerobic Bacteria: Role in Disease. Springfield, Ill, Charles C. Thomas, 1974

Brook I: Encapsulated anaerobic bacteria in synergistic infections. Microbiol Rev 50:452, 1986

Dowell VR Jr, Allen SD: Anaerobic bacterial infections. In Balows A, Hausler WJ (eds): Diagnostic Procedures for Bacterial, Mycotic and Parasitic Infections, ed 6. New York, American Public Health Association, Inc, 1981, p 171

Dowell VR Jr, Lombard GL: Pathogenic members of the genus *Bacteroides*. In Starr MP, Stolp H, Truper HG, et al (eds): The Prokaryotes: A Handbook on Habitats, Isolation, and Identification of Bacteria. New York, Springer-Verlag, 1981, p 1425

Dowell VR Jr, Lombard GL, Thompson FS, et al: Media for Isolation, Characterization, and Identification of Obligately Anaerobic Bacteria. Atlanta, DHEW Public Health Service, Centers for Disease Control, 1977

Finegold SM: Anaerobic Bacteria in Human Disease. New York, Academic Press, 1977

Finegold SM, Shepherd WE, Spaulding EH: Practical Anaerobic Bacteriology, Cumitech 5. Washington, DC, American Society for Microbiology, 1977

Finegold SM: National Committee for Clinical Laboratory Standards Working Group on Anaerobic Susceptibility Testing. Susceptibility testing of anaerobic bacteria. J Clin Microbiol 26:1253, 1988

George WL, Kirby BD, Sutter VL, et al: Gram-negative anaerobic bacilli: Their role in infection and patterns of susceptibility to antimicrobial agents. II. Little-known *Fusobacterium* species and miscellaneous genera. Rev Infect Dis 3:599, 1981

Gorbach SL, Bartlett JG: Anaerobic infections. N Engl J Med 290:1177, 1237, 1289, 1974

Hill GB: The anaerobic cocci. In Starr MP, Stolp H, Truper HG, et al (eds): The Prokaryotes: A Handbook on Habitats, Isolation, and Identification of Bacteria. New York, Springer-Verlag, 1981, p 1631

Hill GB: Bacteriology of the vagina. Scand J Urol Nephrol 86:23, 1985

Hofstad T: Virulence determinants in nonsporeforming anaerobic bacteria. Scand J Infect Dis 62(suppl):15, 1989

Hofstad T: Current taxonomy of medically important nonsporing anaerobes. Rev Infect Dis 12:S122, 1990

Holdeman LV, Cato EP, Moore WEC: Anaerobe Laboratory Manual, ed 4. Blacksburg, Virginia, Anaerobe Laboratory, Virginia Polytechnic Institute and State University, 1977

Holt JG, Krieg NR (eds): Bergey's Manual of Systematic Bacteriology, vol 1. Baltimore, Williams & Wilkins, 1984

Holt JG, Sneath PHA, Mair NS, et al (eds): Bergey's Manual of Systematic Bacteriology, vol 2. Baltimore, Williams & Wilkins, 1986

Kirby BD, George WL, Sutter VL, et al: Gram-negative anaerobic bacilli: Their role in infection and patterns of susceptibility to antimicrobial agents. I. Little-known *Bacteroides* species. Rev Infect Dis 2:914, 1980

Lennette EH, Balows A, Hausler WJ Jr, et al (eds): Manual of Clinical Microbiology, ed 4. Washington, DC, American Society for Microbiology, 1985

MacLaren DM, Namavar F, Verweij-Van Vught AMJJ, et al.: Pathogenic synergy: Mixed intra-abdominal infections. Antonie van Leeuwenhoek 50:775, 1984

Moore LVH, Cato EP, Moore WEC: Anaerobe Lab Manual Update. Blacksburg, Virginia, Anaerobe Laboratory, Virginia Polytechnic Institute and State University, 1987

Moore WEC, Cato EP, Holdeman LV: Anaerobic bacteria of the gastrointestinal flora and their occurrence in clinical infections. J Infect Dis 119:641, 1969

National Committee for Clinical Laboratory Standards: Methods for Antimicrobial Susceptibility Testing of Anaerobic Bacteria, ed 2. Villanova, Pa, The Committee, 1989

Phillips I: New methods for identification of obligate anaerobes. Rev Infect Dis 12:S127, 1990

Rotstein OD, Pruett TL, Simmons RL: Mechanisms of microbial synergy in polymicrobial surgical infections. Rev Infect Dis 7:151, 1985

Sabbaj J, Sutter VL, Finegold SM: Anaerobic pyogenic liver abscess. Ann Intern Med 77:629, 1972

Smith LdS, Williams B: The Pathogenic Anaerobic Bacteria, ed 3. Springfield, Ill, Charles C Thomas, 1984

Styrt B, Gorbach SL: Recent developments in the understanding of the pathogenesis and treatment of anaerobic infections. N Engl J Med 321: 240, 298, 1989

Sutter VL, Citron DM, Edelstein MAC, Finegold SM: Wadsworth Anaerobic Bacteriology Manual, ed 4. Belmont, Calif, Star Publishing Co, 1985

van Winkelhoff AJ, van Steenbergen TJM, DeGraaff J: The role of black-pigmented *Bacteroides* in human oral infections. J Clin Periodontol 15:145, 1988

Selected Papers

Altemeier WA: The pathogenicity of the bacteria of appendicitis peritonitis. Surgery 11:374, 1942

Aranki A, Freter R: Use of anaerobic glove boxes for the cultivation of strictly anaerobic bacteria. Am J Clin Nutr 25:1329, 1972

Bartlett JG: Anti-anaerobic antibacterial agents. Lancet 2:478, 1982

Bartlett JG, Finegold SM: Anaerobic infections of the lung and pleural space. Am Rev Respir Dis 110:56, 1974

Brook I: The role of β-lactamase-producing bacteria in the persistence of streptococcal tonsillar infection. Rev Infect Dis 6:601, 1984

Brook I: A 12 year study of aerobic and anaerobic bacteria in intra-abdominal and postsurgical abdominal wound infections. Surg Gynecol Obstet 169:387, 1989

Brook I: Pathogenicity of the *Bacteroides fragilis* group. Ann Clin Lab Sci 19:360, 1989

Brown WJ: National Committee for Clinical Laboratory Standards agar dilution susceptibility testing of anaerobic gram-negative bacteria. Antimicrob Agents Chemother 32:385, 1988

Carter B, Jones CP, Alter RL, et al: *Bacteroides* infections in obstetrics and gynecology. Obstet Gynecol 1:491, 1953

Chow AW, Guze LB: Bacteroidaceae bacteremia: Clinical experience with 112 patients. Medicine 53:93, 1974

Connolly JC, McLean C, Tabaqchali S: The effect of capsular polysaccharide and lipopolysaccharide of *Bacteroides fragilis* on polymorph function and serum killing. J Med Microbiol 17:259, 1984

Cornick NA, Cuchural GJ, Syndman DR, et al.: The antimicrobial susceptibility patterns of the *Bacteroides fragilis* group in the United States, 1987. J Antimicrob Chemother 25:1011, 1990

Coykendall AL, Kaczmarek FS, Slots J: Genetic heterogeneity in *Bacteroides asaccharolyticus* (Holdeman and Moore 1970) Finegold and Barnes 1977 (approved lists, 1980) and proposal of *Bacteroides gingivalis* sp. nov. and *Bacteroides macacae* (Slots and Genco) comb. nov. Int J Syst Bacteriol 30:559, 1980

Del Bene VE, Carek PJ, Twitty JA, et al: In vitro activity of cefbuperazone compared with that of other new β-lactam agents against anaerobic gram-negative bacilli and contribution of β-lactamase to resistance. Antimicrob Agents Chemother 27:817, 1985

Dowell VR Jr: Comparison of techniques for isolation and identification of anaerobic bacteria. Am J Clin Nutr 25:1335, 1972

Ezaki T, Yamamoto N, Ninomiya K, et al: Transfer of *Peptococcus indolicus, Peptococcus asaccharolyticus, Peptococcus prevotii* and *Peptococcus magnus* to the genus *Peptostreptococcus* and proposal of *Peptostreptococcus tetradius* sp. nov. Int J Syst Bacteriol 33:683, 1983

Finegold SM, Bartlett JG, Chow AN, et al: Management of anaerobic infections. Ann Intern Med 83:375, 1975

Gorbach SL, McGowan K: Comparative clinical trials in treatment of intra-abdominal sepsis. J Antimicrob Chemother 8(suppl D):95, 1981

Gregory EM, Kowalski JB, Holdeman LV: Production and some properties of catalase and superoxide dismutase from the anaerobe *Bacteroides distasonis.* J Bacteriol 129:1298, 1977

Hill GB: Enhancement of experimental anaerobic infections by blood, hemoglobin, and hemostatic agents. Infect Immun 19:443, 1978

Hill GB, Ayers OM, Kohan AP: Characteristics and sites of infection of *Eubacterium nodatum, Eubacterium timidium, Eubacterium brachy,* and other asaccharolytic *Eubacteria.* J Clin Microbiol 25:1540, 1987

Hill GB, Osterhout S, Pratt PC: Liver abscess production by nonsporeforming anaerobic bacteria in a mouse model. Infect Immun 9:599, 1974

Holdeman LV, Cato EP, Burmeister JA, et al: Descriptions of *Eubacterium timidum* sp. nov., *Eubacterium brachy* sp. nov., and *Eubacterium nodatum* sp. nov. isolated from human periodontitis. Int J Syst Bacteriol 30:163, 1980

Holdeman LV, Cato EP, Moore WEC: Taxonomy of anaerobes: Present state of the art. Rev Infect Dis 6(Suppl 1):S3, 1984

Holdeman LV, Johnson JL: *Bacteroides disiens* sp. nov. and *Bacteroides bivius* sp. nov. from human clinical infections. Int J Syst Bacteriol 27:337, 1977

Holdeman LV, Johnson JL: Description of *Bacteroides loescheii* sp. nov. and emendation of the descriptions of *Bacteroides melaninogenicus* (Oliver and Wherry) Roy and Kelly 1939 and *Bacteroides denticola* Shah and Collins 1981. Int J Syst Bacteriol 32:399, 1982

Holdeman LV, Moore WEC, Churn PJ, et al: *Bacteroides oris* and *Bacteroides buccae,* new species from human periodontitis and other human infections. Int J Syst Bacteriol 32:125, 1982

Ingham HR, Sisson PR, Middleton RL, et al: Phagocytosis and killing of bacteria in aerobic and anaerobic conditions. J Med Microbiol 14:391, 1981

Ingham HR, Sisson PR, Selkon JB: Current concepts of the pathogenetic mechanisms of non-sporing anaerobes: Chemotherapeutic implications. J Antimicrob Chemother 6:173, 1980

Johnson JL: Taxonomy of the bacteroides. I. Deoxyribonucleic acid homologies among *Bacteroides fragilis* and other saccharolytic *Bacteroides* species. Int J Syst Bacteriol 28:245, 1978

Johnson JL, Holdeman LV: *Bacteroides intermedius* comb. nov. and descriptions of *Bacteroides corporis* sp. nov. and *Bacteroides levii* sp. nov. Int J Syst Bacteriol 33:15, 1983

Kasper DL, Onderdonk AB, Polk BF, et al: Surface antigens as virulence factors in infection with *Bacteroides fragilis.* Rev Infect Dis 1:278, 1979

Koga T, Nishihara T, Fujiwara T, et al: Biochemical and immunobiological properties of lipopolysaccharide (LPS) from *Bacteroides gingivalis* and comparison with LPS from *Escherichia coli.* Infect Immun 47:638, 1985

Loesche WJ: Oxygen sensitivity of various anaerobic bacteria. Appl Microbiol 18:723, 1969

Mansheim BJ, Onderdonk AB, Kasper DL: Immunochemical characterization of surface antigens of *Bacteroides melaninogenicus.* Rev Infect Dis 1:263, 1979

Mayrand D, McBride BC: Ecological relationships of bacteria involved in a simple, mixed anaerobic infection. Infect Immun 27:44, 1980

McCord JM, Keele BB Jr, Fridovich I: An enzyme-based theory of obligate anaerobiosis: the physiological function of superoxide dismutase. Proc Natl Acad Sci USA 68:1024, 1971

McDonald JB, Sutton RM, Knoll ML, et al: The pathogenic components of an experimental fusospirochetal infection. J Infect Dis 98:15, 1956

McGowan K, Gorbach SL: Anaerobes in mixed infections. J Infect Dis 144:181, 1981

Meleney FL: Bacterial synergism in disease process. Ann Surg 94:961, 1931

Namavar F, Verweij-Van Vught AMJJ, Vel WAC, et al: Polymorphonuclear leukocyte chemotaxis by mixed anaerobic and aerobic bacteria. J Med Microbiol 18:167, 1984

Nichols RL, Smith JW, Fossedal EN, et al: Efficacy of parenteral antibiotics in the treatment of experimentally induced intraabdominal sepsis. Rev Infect Dis 1:302, 1979

Nord CE, Olsson B, Dornbusch K: β-lactamases in *Bacteroides.* Scand J Infect Dis (suppl) 13:27, 1978

O'Keefe JP, Tally FP, Barza M, et al: Inactivation of penicillin G during experimental infection with *Bacteroides fragilis.* J Infect Dis 137:437, 1978

Onderdonk AB, Markham RB, Zaleznik DF, et al: Evidence for T cell-dependent immunity to *Bacteroides fragilis* in an intraabdominal abscess model. J Clin Invest 69:9, 1982

Onderdonk AB, Kasper DL, Cisneros RL, et al: The capsular polysaccharide of *Bacteroides fragilis* as a virulence factor: Comparison of the pathogenic potential of encapsulated and unencapsulated strains. J Infect Dis 136:82, 1977

Onderdonk AB, Kasper DL, Mansheim BJ, et al: Experimental animal models for anaerobic infections. Rev Infect Dis 1:291, 1979

Roberts DS: Editorial: Synergistic mechanisms in certain mixed infections. J Infect Dis 120:720, 1969

Rotstein OD, Nasmith PE, Grinstein S: The *Bacteroides* by-product succinnic acid inhibits neutrophil respiratory burst by reducing intracellular pH. Infect Immun 55:864, 1987

Rotstein OD, Wells CL, Pruett TL, et al: Succinic acid production by *Bacteroides fragilis.* Arch Surg 122:93, 1987

Rudek W, Haque R: Extracellular enzymes of the genus *Bacteroides.* J Clin Microbiol 4:458, 1976

Salyers AA, Wong J, Wilkins TD: Beta-lactamase activity in strains of *Bacteroides melaninogenicus* and *Bacteroides oralis.* Antimicrob Agents Chemother 11:142, 1977

Shah HN, Collins DM: Proposal for reclassification of *Bacteroides asaccharolyticus, Bacteroides gingivalis* and *Bacteroides endontalis* in a new genus, *Porphyromonas.* Int J Syst Bacteriol 38:128, 1988

Shah HN, Collins DM: *Prevotella,* a new genus to include *Bacteroides melaninogenicus* and related species formerly classified in the genus *Bacteroides.* Int J Syst Bacteriol 40:205, 1990

Shapiro ME, Kasper DL, Zaleznik DF, et al: Cellular control of abscess formation: Role of T cells in the regulation of abscesses formed in response to *Bacteroides fragilis.* J Immunol 137:341, 1986

Simon GL, Klempner MS, Kasper DL, et al: Alterations in opsonophagocytic killing by neutrophils of *Bacteroides fragilis* associated with animal and laboratory passage: effect of capsular polysaccharide. J Infect Dis 145:72, 1982

Singer RE, Buckner BA: Butyrate and propionate: Important components of toxic dental plaque extracts. Infect Immun 32:458, 1981

Smith DT: Experimental aspiratory abscess. Arch Surg 14:231, 1927

Socransky SS, Gibbons RJ: Required role of *Bacteroides melaninogenicus* in mixed anaerobic infections. J Infect Dis 115:247, 1965

Sonnenwirth AC: Antibody response to anaerobic bacteria. Rev Infect Dis 1:337, 1979

Speigel CA, Roberts M: *Mobiluncus* gen. nov., *Mobiluncus curtisii* subsp. *curtisii* sp. nov., *Mobiluncus curtisii* subsp. *holmesii* subsp. nov., and *Mobiluncus mulieris* sp. nov., curved rods from the human vagina. Int J Syst Bacteriol 34:177, 1984

Steffen EK, Hentges DJ: Hydrolytic enzymes of anaerobic bacteria isolated from human infections. J Clin Microbiol 14:153, 1981

Sweet RL: Treatment of mixed aerobic-anaerobic infections of the female genital tract. J Antimicrob Chemother 8(suppl D):105, 1981

Tally FP, Cuchural GJ Jr, Malamy MH: Mechanisms of resistance and resistance transfer in anaerobic bacteria: Factors influencing antimicrobial therapy. Rev Infect Dis 6(suppl 1):S260, 1984

Tally FP, Goldin BR, Jacobus NV, et al: Superoxide dismutase in anaerobic bacteria of clinical significance. Infect Immun 16:20, 1977

Thadepalli H, Gorbach SL, Broido P, et al: A prospective study of infections in penetrating abdominal trauma. Am J Clin Nutr 25:1405, 1972

Tofte RW, Peterson PK, Schmeling D, et al: Opsonization of four *Bacteroides* species: Role of the classical complement pathway and immunoglobulin. Infect Immun 27:784, 1980

Wade BH, Kasper DL, Mandell GL: Interactions of *Bacteroides fragilis* and phagocytes: studies with whole organisms, purified capsular polysaccharide and clindamycin-treated bacteria. J Antimicrob Chemother 17(suppl C):51, 1983

Weinstein WM, Onderdonk AB, Bartlett JG, et al: Antimicrobial therapy of experimental intraabdominal sepsis. J Infect Dis 132:282, 1975

Weinstein WM, Onderdonk AB, Bartlett JG, et al: Experimental intraabdominal abscesses in rats: development of an experimental model. Infect Immun 10:1250, 1974

Zaleznik DF, Zhang Z, Onderdonk AB, et al: Effect of subinhibitory doses of clindamycin on the virulence of *Bacteroides fragilis:* Role of lipopolysaccharide. J Infect Dis 154:40, 1986

CHAPTER 44
Clostridium

Clostridium

The clostridia are anaerobic, spore-forming bacilli that usually stain gram-positive. Most species are obligate anaerobes, but a few species are aerotolerant and will grow minimally in air at atmospheric pressure. The pathogenic species produce soluble toxins, some of which are extremely potent. Some species are saccharolytic, producing acid and gas from carbohydrates; many are proteolytic. The clostridia are widely distributed in nature and are present in soil and in the intestinal tract of humans and animals.

The pathogenic clostridia can be divided into four major groups, according to the types of diseases they produce:

1. The histotoxic clostridia characteristically cause a variety of tissue infections, usually subsequent to wounds or other types of traumatic injury.
2. The enterotoxigenic clostridia produce food poisoning and more severe forms of gastrointestinal disease.
3. *Clostridium tetani,* the causative agent of tetanus, causes disease through a potent exotoxin that is produced during limited growth within tissue.
4. *Clostridium botulinum* is the etiologic agent of botulism, which results from the ingestion of a powerful exotoxin previously formed by the organism in contaminated food.

Histotoxic Clostridia

The histotoxic clostridia cause a severe infection of muscle, clostridial myonecrosis. Older and frequently used synonyms for this infection are *gas gangrene* and *clostridial myositis.* The term *gas gangrene,* however, is misleading since the presence of gas in the infected tissues may be a late or variable manifestation of the disease, and *clostridial myositis* suggests muscle inflammation rather than the actual pathologic condition, necrosis. The most important histotoxic clostridia are *Clostridium perfringens, C. novyi,* and *C. septicum.* Three other organisms of lesser importance also are capable alone of producing clostridial myonecrosis: *C. histolyticum, C. sordellii,* and *C. fallax.* All of these histotoxic clostridia produce a variety of toxins of different potencies, and for each species toxins are designated by Greek letters in order of importance or discovery. Thus, the α-toxins of different species are not identical. None of these histotoxic clostridia is a highly invasive pathogen; each plays an opportunistic role that requires a special set of conditions within tissue to initiate infection. A spectrum of clinical involvement is seen in clostridial wound infections, ranging from simple contamination of wounds to the most serious type of infection, myonecrosis.

Because the clostridia are so widely distributed in nature, contamination of wounds with these bacteria is very common. Often more than one of the clostridia are present, including both saprophytic and histotoxic species. An average of 2.6 species of clostridia were isolated from cases of clostridial myonecrosis during World War II; higher numbers would probably have been demonstrated with the improved anaerobic culture techniques currently available. Reported figures for clostridial contamination of wounds in civilian life range up to 39%, and contamination during warfare is considerably higher. Only a small proportion of wounds contaminated with *C. perfringens* or other histotoxic clostridia, however, evolve into true clostridial myonecrosis. The incidence of the disease in civilian life is difficult to establish, with considerable variation according to the precipitating incident and geographic location. Its incidence during warfare is from 10 to 100 times greater than during peacetime, occurring in 0.2% to 1% of war casualties. An important corollary to the high rate of clostridial contamination of wounds is that the isolation of histotoxic clostridia from wounds or drainage material does *not* by itself indicate clostridial myonecrosis. Diagnosis of clostridial myonecrosis must be made on clinical grounds; the bacteriology laboratory contributes to a careful differential diagnosis by demonstrating histotoxic clostridia or the presence of other bacteria that are associated with a different disease with similar symptoms.

Clostridium perfringens

C. perfringens is cultured from 60% to 90% of cases of clostridial myonecrosis. There are five types of *C. perfringens,* A to E, separated according to their production of four major lethal toxins (Table 44–1). *C. perfringens* type A is the organism primarily responsible for diseases in humans: clostridial myonecrosis, less severe wound infections, and a common form of food poisoning. *C. perfringens* type A has been found in the intestinal tract of almost every animal that has ever been cultured for this organism, but is a less common cause of disease in animals than in humans. In contrast, types B, C, D, and E, which occur in the intestinal tracts of animals and only occasionally in humans, produce a variety of naturally occurring diseases of domestic animals; these types do not permanently inhabit the soil, as does type A.

Morphology

C. perfringens usually appears as a short, plump, strongly gram-positive rod (Fig. 44–1). The organisms are uniform in appearance, 2 to 4 μm long and 1 to 1.5 μm wide. The length varies according to the stage of growth, as well as the nutritional and ionic composition of the medium. Rapidly growing organisms may appear almost coccoid or cubical, whereas more elongated cells occur in older cultures. Unlike the other pathogenic clostridia, *C. perfringens* is nonmotile. Also, it does not produce spores in ordinary media; special media normally must be used to demonstrate sporulation. Capsules may be observed by direct examination of smears from wounds but are not uniformly demonstrable in culture.

Physiology

C. perfringens is an aerotolerant anaerobe, especially when streaked on blood agar plates, and will survive and even grow in oxygen tensions that are inhibitory to most other anaerobes. Some strains produce superoxide dismutase. Anaerobic culture methods suitable for *C. perfringens* and other clostridia are discussed in Chapter 43. It will grow over a pH range of 5.5 to 8.0 and a temperature range of 20C to 50C. Although *C. perfringens* is usually grown at 37C, a temperature of 45C is optimal for many strains and reduces the generation time to as little as 10 minutes.

Cultural Characteristics. Surface colonies that are produced on blood agar after 24 hours of incubation are circular and smooth, 2 to 4 mm in diameter. However, as the colonies increase in size with age, the periphery often loses symmetry and projections on the periphery suggest the appearance of a colony of motile bacteria showing swarming. Variation in colonial morphology occurs, depending on the degree of encapsulation and smooth to rough transition.

The rapid growth of *C. perfringens* in chopped-meat media at 45C can be used to isolate it from mixtures of bacteria. As *C. perfringens* will outgrow most other organisms during the first 4 to 6 hours of incubation, blood agar plates streaked after that time and incubated at 37C will have proportionally

TABLE 44–1. TOXINS AND SOLUBLE ANTIGENS OF *CLOSTRIDIUM PERFRINGENS*

Type	Group	Disease	Major Lethal Toxins[a]				Minor Antigens[b]				
			α	β	ε	τ	δ	θ	κ	λ	μ
A		Gas gangrene in humans and animals Food poisoning in humans[c]	++	−	−	−	−	++	++	−	++
B	1	Lamb dysentery Enterotoxemia of foals	++	++	++	−	−	++	−	++	++
	2	Enterotoxemia of sheep and goats (Iran)	++	++	++	−	−	++	++	−	−
C	1	Enterotoxemia (struck) of sheep	++	++	−	−	++	++	++	−	−
	2	Enterotoxemia of calves and lambs (Colorado)	++	++	−	−	−	++	++	−	−
	3	Enterotoxemia of piglets	++	++	−	−	−	++	+	−	+
	4	Necrotic enteritis (pig-bel) of humans (New Guinea)	++	++	−	−	−	++	+	−	++
	5	Necrotic enteritis of humans and fowl (Germany)[c]	++	++	−	−	−	−	−	−	−
D		Enterotoxemia of sheep, lambs, goats, and cattle	++	−	++	−	−	++	++	+	++
E		Isolated from sheep and cattle; pathogenicity doubtful	++	−	−	++	−	++	++	++	+

Modified from Kadis, Montie, Ajl (eds): Microbiol Toxins, vol 2A. Bacterial Protein Toxins, Academic Press, 1971.
++, Produced by all or most strains; +, produced by less than 50% of strains; −, not produced.
[a] Lethal antigens primarily responsible for pathogenicity and type designation.
[b] Lower order of toxicity; some may be involved in pathogenicity.
[c] Some strains produce heat-resistant spores.

higher numbers of *C. perfringens.* Heat treatment (80C to 100C) of mixed cultures is an aid in the isolation of many clostridial species that sporulate well, but this method is not recommended for *C. perfringens.* Cultures of clinical isolates of this organism usually contain few spores, and the heat resistance of the spores appears to be inversely related to the toxigenicity of the vegetative forms.

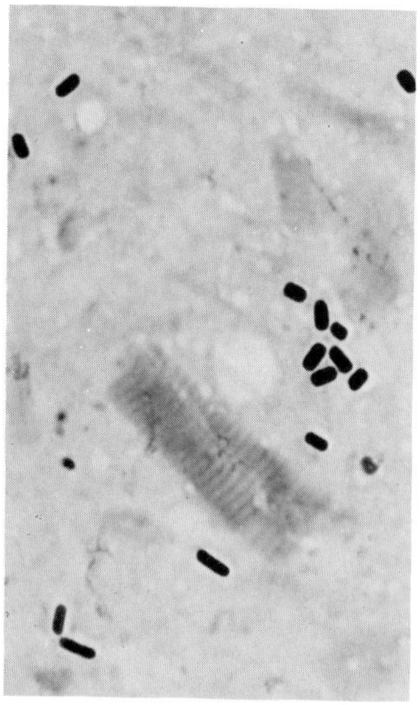

Fig. 44–1. *Clostridium perfringens* directly smeared from infected muscle in clostridial myonecrosis, demonstrating short, plump bacilli that lack spores. A variety of other bacteria, including other clostridia, may also be present, but polymorphonuclear leukocytes are characteristically absent. Note the disintegrated muscle tissue. ×1000.

Laboratory Identification

A few easily observable characteristics aid in the identification of *C. perfringens.* In chopped-meat glucose media there is abundant growth with gas formation; in vivo toxicity testing may be carried out with supernates from this medium. *C. perfringens* also produces a characteristic pattern of hemolysis on blood agar plates, precipitation (opalescence) in serum or egg yolk media, and "stormy" fermentation in milk media. After overnight incubation on rabbit, sheep, ox, or human blood agar, colonies of most strains demonstrate a characteristic target hemolysis resulting from a narrow zone of complete hemolysis due to the θ-toxin and a much wider zone of incomplete hemolysis due to the α-toxin. This double-zone pattern of hemolysis may fade with longer incubation. *C. perfringens* also produces a characteristic pattern of synergistic β-hemolysis when streaked alongside *Streptococcus agalactiae* (the reverse CAMP test).

A dense opalescence in human serum is produced by growing organisms or by the supernatant fluid from an overnight culture. This reaction (the Nagler reaction) is caused by the α-toxin (a lecithinase C) and is specifically inhibited by *C. perfringens* antitoxin. Opalescence, produced by the toxin, is more easily observable in egg yolk agar. This medium can be inoculated directly with wound specimens for screening purposes and is helpful in the identification of pure cultures of *C. perfringens* and other clostridia that produce a lecithinase (or a lipase). *C. perfringens* can be presumptively identified by covering one half of an egg yolk agar plate with *C. perfringens* antitoxin, streaking the organisms over the entire plate, and then observing for the inhibition of opalescence on the antitoxin-treated portion after incubation. This reaction, however, is not totally specific for *C. perfringens* since the lecithinases produced by *Clostridium bifermentans*, *C. sordelli*, and *Clostridium baratii* are antigenically similar and are partially inhibited by antitoxin to *C. perfringens* α-toxin. These organisms can be separated by other tests.

In milk media, most strains of *C. perfringens* produce "stormy" fermentation, in which the fermentation of the lactose in milk produces a large amount of acid, causing the protein (casein) to coagulate. This acid clot is then disrupted and torn apart by the large volume of gas formed from the lactose fermentation. This action in milk media is useful in the identification of *C. perfringens*, but when used alone is not diagnostic because the reaction also may be produced by a number of other clostridial species, including *C. septicum*. Fermentation reactions and other biochemical tests used in the identification of *C. perfringens* are covered in greater detail in the reference manuals listed in the Further Reading section of this chapter.

Antigenic Structure

Strains of *C. perfringens* produce at least 12 different soluble substances or toxins, all of which are protein in nature and antigenic (Table 44–1). Of the four major lethal antigens, α-, β-, ε-, and ι-toxins, the most important is the α-toxin, which is produced by all five types of *C. perfringens*. All of the toxins are exotoxins.

Many of the other soluble substances or minor antigens are enzymes with defined substrates. These substances are nonlethal and should not be referred to as toxins, as has been customary in the past. Examples of these substances are collagenase (κ-antigen), deoxyribonuclease (ν-antigen), and hyaluronidase (μ-antigen).

In general, serotyping with somatic antigens has not been practical in the further subdivision of *C. perfringens*, although a large number of serologic types exist. One application, however, has been for epidemiologic studies of outbreaks of food poisoning, where a correlation was found between the serotypes of heat-resistant (100C for 1 hour) *C. perfringens* type A isolated from the feces of patients and the serotype from the incriminated food.

Determinants of Pathogenicity

The toxin of primary importance in the pathogenesis of clostridial myonecrosis is the α-toxin, which initially was described in terms of its lethal, dermonecrotic, and hemolytic activities. The toxin is a lecithinase C (or phospholipase C), which splits lecithin to phosphorylcholine and a diglyceride. The toxin is activated by Ca^{2+} and Mg^{2+} ions; it also hydrolyzes sphingomyelin. Titration of α-toxin can be performed with in vivo lethality testing and with in vitro procedures, which are dependent on its enzymatic action against lecithin-containing substrates such as egg yolk emulsion, human serum, or erythrocytes of certain animal species. α-Toxin is an excellent antigen; in vivo protection or therapy of animals is dependent entirely on the α-antitoxin titer. The in vivo action of α-toxin is apparently on lecithin-containing lipoprotein complexes in the cell membrane and probably on mitochondria. Disruption or leakage of cell membranes alone can explain the lysis of erythrocytes, destruction of tissue, and edema observed in this disease. Its local activity in the muscle lesion is obvious, but the basis for the generalized toxicity or systemic manifestations and death seen in clostridial myonecrosis is not fully explained. Other substances, such as θ-, κ-, or μ-antigens, apparently exert an ancillary role in abetting the local spread of the infection through tissue and providing nutrients for the proliferation of the organism. At low concentrations θ-toxin is toxic for human leukocytes and may be primarily responsible for the unusual absence of obvious polymorphonuclear leukoytes in infected muscle tissue.

Clinical Infection

Wound and Soft Tissue Infection

EPIDEMIOLOGY. *C. perfringens* is ubiquitous; type A strains are commonly found in the intestinal tracts of humans and animals and are numerous in the soil in both the vegetative and the spore forms. Infection may be due to endogenous or exogenous clostridia. In traumatic injuries, either accidental or during warfare, the source of clostridia is usually soil carried into the tissues; the incidence of contamination and infection depends on the concentration of *C. perfringens* in the soil, which varies with the geographic location. Endogenous infections stem from fecal flora present on the skin or on particles of clothing carried into the wound or from clostridia escaping from the bowel when its integrity is disrupted by disease, traumatic injury, or surgery.

One of the essential factors predisposing to clostridial myonecrosis is trauma associated with deep and lacerated or crush wounds of muscle and with vascular damage of major vessels and capillary beds. If ischemia and necrosis are present deep within the muscle, however, the trauma need not have been severe, for example, intramuscular injections of vasoconstrictive agents such as epinephrine. The basis for the requirement of trauma with ischemic or necrotic areas is the anaerobic nature of the clostridia, which require a reduced oxygen tension and oxidation-reduction potential for growth (see also Chap. 43). Clostridia are unable to initiate infection in healthy tissues in which the oxidation-reduction potential is normal. Even with the high frequency of pathogenic clostridia in wounds, the incidence of gas gangrene remains relatively low because of these growth restrictions.

The principal settings for infections of this type occur during periods of war, when massive wounds of muscle contaminated with soil, clothing, and metal fragments are common. Before the early 1950s, evacuation and medical care of the wounded following injury was delayed, providing optimal conditions for the histotoxic clostridia to initiate infection. More recently, however, rapid evacuation of the wounded and early medical care have drastically reduced the wartime incidence of clostridial myonecrosis. In civilian life, settings that may lead to this disease include automobile and motorcycle accidents, gunshot wounds, compound fractures, industrial accidents, surgical complications, septic abortion, and injections of medications such as epinephrine. A reduced blood supply stemming from edema, cold, or shock, and the presence in the wound of facultative organisms also predisposes to clostridial infection.

PATHOGENESIS. When *C. perfringens* is introduced into tissue, the primary requirement for initiation of infection is a lowered oxidation-reduction potential. In areas of reduced oxygen tension the pyruvate of muscle is incompletely oxidized and lactic acid accumulates, causing a drop in pH. The combination of lowered oxidation-reduction potential and a drop in pH may activate endogenous proteolytic enzymes, resulting in tissue autolysis. This release of nutrients and the lowered oxidation-reduction potential combine to produce conditions suitable for growth of anaerobic organisms.

Proliferation of the organisms is accompanied by the production of soluble toxins. In true clostridial myonecrosis, these toxins diffuse from the initial site of growth and attack healthy muscle and surrounding tissues. These tissues are in turn destroyed by the toxins, thus permitting spread of the infection into new necrotic areas. The edema fluid produced by action of the clostridial toxins and enzymes on tissue components and gas accumulated from the metabolism of the organism also increase the pressure within muscle bundles so that circulation is impaired, further decreasing the oxidation-reduction potential and pH and providing new areas within muscle suitable for growth of the clostridia. The disease progresses in this manner, with the organisms moving into new areas behind the destructive action of their toxins. The local infection and its extension into healthy tissues is well understood. Still unknown, however, are the cause of the generalized systemic toxicity and the immediate cause of death in clostridial myonecrosis, although the α-toxin is recognized as an essential element in their pathogenesis. Both α- and θ-toxins, as well as a lethal toxin, inhibit myocardial function in an experimental animal model, which may relate to the profound shock that usually accompanies *C. perfringens* myonecrosis.

CLINICAL MANIFESTATIONS. Wound infections can be divided into three categories of increasing levels of severity: (1) simple wound contamination, (2) anaerobic cellulitis, and (3) clostridial myonecrosis. Two additional clinical settings—uterine infections and clostridial septicemia—are special types of wound and soft tissue infection with certain unique features. The symptoms of the three catogories, however, may overlap, and an infection may evolve from a cellulitis into true clostridial myonecrosis. The essential clinical features of wound infections are given in Table 44–2.

Simple Wound Contamination. In simple wound contamination one or more histotoxic clostridia may be present without an obvious pathologic process. Either the clostridia present may be nontoxicogenic or the environmental conditions in the wound may be unsuitable for toxin production and the initiation of a progressive infection by toxigenic strains.

Anaerobic Cellulitis. Anaerobic cellulitis is a more serious form of wound infection, in which the clostridia infect tissue that is already severely compromised or frankly necrotic as a result of ischemia or direct trauma. The organisms in this case spread through subcutaneous tissue and along fascial planes between muscles but do not invade healthy, intact muscle. Growth of *C. perfringens* within the necrotic tissue is extensive, and gas is normally a prominent feature. Patients, however, are not in an extremely toxic condition, and the overall prognosis is considerably better than for clostridial myonecrosis. Careful distinction between this level of infection and true clostridial myonecrosis is necessary to avoid the sometimes extreme surgical measures that are unnecessary for anaerobic cellulitis but often are required for treatment of clostridial myonecrosis.

Clostridial Myonecrosis. The term *clostridial myonecrosis* should be limited to use in characteristic anaerobic infections of muscle in which organisms are *invasive* and the infection is associated with profound toxemia, extensive local edema, variable amounts of gas, massive tissue damage, and death in untreated cases.

After injury there is an incubation period, usually of 12 to 48 hours, before symptoms suddenly appear. The characteristic initial symptom is pain in the affected area, which increases in severity as the infection spreads. There is local edema and a thin, blood-stained exudate. The pulse rate rises disproportionately more than the temperature. If the disease remains untreated, the process advances rapidly, with increasing toxemia and extension of the infection. With increased exudation from the area, gas usually becomes obvious, but it is a variable symptom. Skin color changes and finally may become black. Necrosis of large muscle masses is associated with severe shock and prostration. Infrequently, intravascular

TABLE 44–2. DIFFERENTIATION OF GASSY INFECTIONS OF SOFT TISSUES AND WOUNDS

Criterion	Infected Vascular Gangrene	Anaerobic Cellulitis	Clostridial Myonecrosis	Streptococcal Myonecrosis
Incubation	Over 5 days, usually longer	Almost always over 3 days	Usually under 3 days	3 to 4 days
Onset	Gradual	Gradual	Acute	Subacute or insidious
Toxemia	None or minimal	None or slight	Very severe	Severe only after some time
Pain	Variable	Absent	Severe	Variable, usually fairly severe
Swelling	Often marked	None or slight	Marked	Marked
Skin	Discolored, often black and desiccated	Little change	Tense, often very white	Tense, often with coppery tinge
Exudate	None	None or slight	Variable, may be profuse, serous, and blood stained	Very profuse; seropurulent
Gas	Abundant	Abundant	Rarely pronounced, except terminally	Very slight
Smell	Foul	Foul	Variable, may be slight, often sweetish	Very slight, often sour
Muscle	Dead	No change	Marked change	Little change at first, except edema

Modified from MacLennan: Bacterial Rev 26:177, 1962.

hemolysis occurs, producing hemoglobinemia, hemoglobinuria, and renal failure. Death occurs rapidly in untreated cases.

Uterine Infection. Uterine infections are a special type of clostridial myonecrosis, usually involving the gravid uterus. Before abortion was legalized many cases followed illegal attempts at mechanically induced abortion by nonmedical practitioners. They may occasionally occur as puerperal infections. The source of *C. perfringens* may be exogenous or endogenous. As in wound infections, there may be different levels of clinical involvement. In contrast to clostridial myonecrosis from wounds, septicemia and intravascular hemolysis are common in uterine myonecrosis and lead to secondary renal failure. The disease progresses rapidly and has a high mortality rate.

Clostridial Septicemia. Invasion of the bloodstream may occur in association with malignancy and may involve a localized myonecrosis in addition to a fulminating clostridial septicemia. There usually is no history of external trauma. The organisms apparently migrate out of the patient's intestinal tract, which is altered as a consequence of the malignant process. Septicemia also may follow biliary tract or gastrointestinal surgery. *C. septicum* or *C. perfringens* is usually the etiologic agent. Rapid diagnosis and treatment are essential, because death may occur in untreated cases in less than 24 hours after the onset of symptoms.

LABORATORY DIAGNOSIS. An early diagnosis of clostridial myonecrosis is essential and, as previously stated, must be made primarily on clinical grounds. Bacteriologic confirmation of the organisms present in the infection is important, however. Usually a direct smear and Gram stain of material from deep within the wound (Fig. 44–1) provide valuable and timely information to aid in a differential diagnosis. Cultures and smears (from tissue, aspirates, or deep swabs) should be taken from affected muscle, preferably at a site between the advancing border and the initial site of the wound or trauma. Cultures from two or three sites may be advantageous if the infected area is extensive. Cultures of involved areas in cases of clostridial cellulitis are done similarly. More than one clostridial species is usually present; other organisms also are commonly found and include *Staphylococcus, Streptococcus, Escherichia, Proteus, Bacillus, Bacteroides,* and other anaerobes. Gram stain and culture assist in differentiating clostridial myonecrosis from rare cases of anaerobic streptococcal myonecrosis or other mixed anaerobic infections (Table 44–2).

TREATMENT. Simple wound infections with *C. perfringens* can be treated by removal of necrotic tissue and by cleansing. Administration of antibiotics is rarely required. Anaerobic cellulitis, which is a more serious infection, usually can be treated by opening the involved area, removing all necrotic tissue, cleansing thoroughly, and administering antibiotics. These infections must be carefully monitored.

For clostridial myonecrosis, intensive and immediate therapy is indicated. Mortality rates vary from approximately 15% to 30% and are highly dependent on the anatomic location of the infection. Among the standard treatment modalities of surgery, antibiotics, and supportive measures, the surgical removal of all infected and necrotic tissue is of prime importance. Intensive antibiotic and antitoxin therapy is partially effective, but if all infected muscles are not excised because of their anatomic location or for other reasons, the results obtained with antibiotic and antitoxic therapy alone are poor. Patients who survive this infection usually require extensive surgery and amputation. Clostridial myonecrosis is more common in areas of the body that have large masses of muscle, such as the buttock, thigh, and shoulder, and mortality from infections in these sites is higher. In addition, treatment is more difficult because of spread of the infection to the trunk and involvement of areas that cannot be excised.

Although antibiotic therapy alone is ineffective in treating clostridial myonecrosis, there is general agreement on its therapeutic effectiveness as an ancillary agent. Penicillin in high doses still is the drug of choice, but clindamycin or metronidazole can be substituted for patients with penicillin allergy. There has been an isolated report of one group of *C. perfringens* strains with increased resistance, but most strains apparently remain quite susceptible to penicillin. Secondary infection with facultative gram-negative organisms such as *Escherichia coli* must be treated with gentamicin or tobramycin. In addition, metronidazole, clindamycin, or some other anti-anaerobe agent is indicated when *Bacteroides* is suspected or demonstrated. Although the value of antitoxin, which is available commercially as a polyvalent serum, has been disputed, it is probably a valuable therapeutic adjunct to surgery when used in adequate dosage. In spite of the risk of hypersensitivity reactions, antitoxin therapy is generally employed in a setting of extreme toxemia, particularly with intravascular hemolysis.

Hyperbaric oxygen was introduced in 1961 as an adjunct in the therapy of clostridial myonecrosis. Its therapeutic effectiveness is supported by clinical use and by experimental observations in animals, but controlled therapeutic trials in human disease that might conclusively demonstrate its efficacy in the reduction of mortality are not available. However, patients with clostridial myonecrosis involving the trunk, usually a lethal infection, more often survive (approximately 50%) when treated with hyperbaric oxygen in addition to the standard modes of therapy, which again suggests the effectiveness of this adjunct. The administration of hyperbaric oxygen also appears to have eliminated the necessity for early radical amputation of limbs or excision of tissue in an attempt to check surgically the irreversible spread of infection. Initial surgery can be limited to debridement and removal of frankly necrotic tissue, with hyperbaric oxygen used to halt further spread of the infection and improve oxygenation of marginally viable tissue.

When hyperbaric oxygen is administered, the patient is given seven intermittent exposures to 100% O_2 in a chamber pressurized to 3 atmospheres of absolute pressure. The first treatment is given as soon as possible after diagnosis, and further treatments are tightly sequenced to prevent further spread of infection. Hyperbaric oxygen exerts a direct inhibitory action on the organism and on toxin production, although preformed α-toxin is not inactivated. Indirect effects include an increase in the oxidation-reduction potential of the tissues surrounding the infection, which probably prevents spread of the organisms.

Clostridial septicemia complicating malignancy is amenable to antibiotic therapy with penicillin if initiated early. If localized myonecrosis develops, additional appropriate treatment is required.

PREVENTION. The most important preventive measure against clostridial myonecrosis is early and adequate wound debridement. The incidence of the disease markedly increases with delay in debridement. Adequate cleansing, removal of necrotic tissue, delay in primary closure of large, ragged wounds, maintenance of drainage, and avoidance of tight packing are all of prime importance in prevention. Administration of prophylactic antibiotic (penicillin) probably reduces the risk of an anaerobic infection, particularly if administered shortly after wounding.

Food Poisoning. A mild form of food poisoning has been recognized with increasing frequency since its association with *C. perfringens* was first demonstrated in 1945. The organisms usually involved are strains of type A that produce heat-resistant spores and minimal amounts of theta toxin, although more typical type A strains also may cause the disease. Between 8 and 24 hours after ingestion of contaminated food, acute abdominal pain and diarrhea develop. Nausea may occur, but vomiting is uncommon, as are other signs of infection, such as fever and headache. Symptoms normally last for 12 to 18 hours, and recovery usually is complete except for rare instances of death in elderly or debilitated patients.

The symptoms are attributable to enterotoxin that may exist in more than one biochemical form and that usually is synthesized during sporulation of the organism. Properties of the enterotoxin(s) are erythema after intracutaneous injection, fluid accumulation in intestinal loops, and lethality for mice. Clinical symptoms probably are due to the action of enterotoxin on the intestinal mucosa, producing leakage in the plasma membranes of cells and disrupting the osmotic equilibrium. Repeated attacks occur, indicating absence of immunity.

This type of food poisoning usually results from the ingestion of meat dishes, such as roasts, poultry, fish, and stews, that are heavily contaminated with *C. perfringens*. Contamination of food may occur at any time, as this organism is widespread in the environment. Raw meat may be contaminated at slaughter, through handling during preparation, or by exposure to flies and dust. The initial heating or cooking of the food may produce germination of heat-resistant spores, or food may become contaminated after cooking. The clostridia multiply during cooling of the meat or during a storage period and will produce food poisoning if the food is served cool or is inadequately reheated. Symptoms occur only if the organisms multiply to a concentration of 10^6 to 10^7 viable cells per gram of food, so that 10^8 to 10^9 viable bacteria are ingested. A diagnosis can be made from isolation of *C. perfringens* in higher than normal numbers from the feces of infected patients and, if possible, from samples of the ingested food. A more specific diagnosis is possible by use of an enzyme-linked immunosorbent assay (ELISA) to detect *C. perfringens* enterotoxin in the feces of affected persons.

Enteritis Necroticans (Necrotizing Jejunitis, Necrotic Enteritis). Enteritis necroticans is caused by type C strains of *C. perfringens* and is more severe than *C. perfringens* type A food poisoning. After an incubation period of less than 24 hours, the onset is sudden, with severe abdominal pain, diarrhea, and in some patients loss of intestinal mucosa with bleeding into the stool. The disease may be fatal, with peripheral circulatory collapse or intestinal obstruction and peritonitis. Although strains causing this disease were originally designated as a new type of *C. perfringens*, type F, they are now considered to be an atypical type C strain that produces heat-resistant spores (Table 44–1). In addition to sporadic cases, major outbreaks have been reported from New Guinea, where it is associated with the ingestion of contaminated and inadequately cooked pork (pig feasting) and where the disease is called pig-bel. In New Guinea the disease occurs in four forms, varying in severity and degree of toxicity but having an overall mortality rate of 35% to 40%. The β-toxin produced by *C. perfringens* type C is responsible for the symptoms; the administration of *C. perfringens* type C antitoxin to patients with enteritis necroticans significantly reduces the mortality rate.

Other Histotoxic Clostridia

Clostridium septicum

C. septicum is closely related to *Clostridium chauvoei,* and both species are widely distributed in nature and in the intestinal tracts of humans and animals. *C. chauvoei* is pathogenic in animals only, but *C. septicum* is pathogenic in humans and other animals. Because this organism can escape from the intestinal tracts of humans and animals and invade tissues shortly after death, the presence of *C. septicum* in pathologic specimens must be interpreted with caution. *C. septicum* is 0.8 μm in diameter and 3 to 5 μm long; it is motile by means of peritrichous flagella. Colonies on blood agar are surrounded by zones of complete hemolysis, and swarming across the surface of plates may be marked. The major toxin produced by *C. septicum* is α-toxin, which is lethal, necrotizing, hemolytic, and possibly leukocidic. The organism also produces deoxyribonuclease, hyaluronidase, and an oxygen-labile hemolysin. The percentage of *C. septicum* isolates from cases of clostridial myonecrosis ranges from 5% to 20%, according to different reports. Endogenous *C. septicum* from the patient's own intestinal tract may produce septicemia and occasionally localized myonecrosis in patients with underlying focal carcinoma or leukemia. This association is strong enough that if this species is isolated, a thorough examination of the patient for an occult malignancy, particularly of the intestinal tract, should be performed.

Clostridium novyi

C. novyi has been differentiated into three major types—A, B, and C—on the basis of the soluble antigens present in toxic filtrates of the organism. These bacteria (especially type A) are found in the soil and in the livers (types A and B) of a variety of apparently healthy animals. *C. novyi* type A is 4 to 8 μm in length and 1 μm in width; type B organisms are even larger. These bacteria have oval subterminal spores; peritrichous flagella make them motile, with swarming on the surface of blood agar plates.

C. novyi type A, rather than type B, causes most of the clostridial myonecrosis and other wound infections in humans. Both types produce an α-toxin that is necrotizing, lethal, and the most potent toxic substance in filtrates of *C. novyi* cultures. The α-toxin apparently increases capillary permeability and produces the intense gelatinous edema in muscle tissue that is characteristic of clostridial myonecrosis caused by *C. novyi*. β (type B) and γ (type A) toxins are lecithinase C enzymes, which are hemolytic, necrotizing, and, in the case of β-toxin, lethal. These toxins produce lecithinase reactions on egg yolk agar plates. Type A also produces a lipase (ε-antigen) that gives a pearly layer effect (similar to oil on water) on and around colonies on egg yolk agar plates.

The production of the lethal α-toxin by *C. novyi* appears

to be bacteriophage-dependent. A toxigenic *C. botulinum* type C cured of its prophage becomes a nontoxigenic strain; this organism, if infected with another specific bacteriophage, then is converted from a nontoxigenic strain into toxigenic *C. novyi* type A, which produces the lethal α-toxin. Continued toxigenicity and interconversion of species of toxigenic *C. botulinum* type C and *C. novyi* type A thus depend on the presence of specific bacteriophages.

The percentage of clostridial myonecrosis due to *C. novyi* varies in different reported series but was approximately 42% during World War II. As this organism, especially type B, is extremely fastidious and oxygen sensitive, its true occurrence may be greater than reported. Clostridial myonecrosis caused by *C. novyi* generally is characterized by a high mortality rate and large amounts of edema fluid, with little or no observable gas in the infected tissue.

Clostridium histolyticum

C. histolyticum has been isolated from the human gastrointestinal tract and from the soil. It is an aerotolerant species and produces limited growth on blood agar plates incubated under aerobic conditions, although improved growth is produced in an anaerobic environment. The organism is markedly proteolytic, digesting a variety of native proteins. Several soluble antigens are produced, of which the most important are the α- and β-toxins, which are lethal and necrotizing. The β-toxin is a collagenase that causes the destruction of collagen fibers and marked disruption of tissues observed in cases of clostridial myonecrosis caused by this organism. The incidence of *C. histolyticum* in cases of clostridial myonecrosis during World War II was between 3% and 6%.

Clostridium sordellii

Although *C. bifermentans* and *C. sordellii* are very similar and for a time were considered a single species, there are sufficient serologic and physiologic differences to justify their separation into different species. *C. sordellii* is inhibited by 1% mannose and produces sialidase and usually urease, tests for which *C. bifermentans* is negative. *C. sordellii* usually is pathogenic, but nonpathogenic strains also exist; *C. bifermentans* usually is nonpathogenic, but pathogenic strains are occasionally isolated. Both organisms are found in the soil and as part of the normal intestinal flora of humans and other animals. Both species produce proteolytic enzymes and usually a lecithinase that is serologically related to the α-toxin of *C. perfringens* and is therefore partially inhibited by *C. perfringens* antitoxin. Pathogenic strains of *C. sordellii* also produce a lethal toxin. Clostridial myonecrosis involving *C. sordellii* is characterized by large amounts of edema and thus may resemble infection with *C. novyi*. The incidence of *C. sordellii* in clostridial myonecrosis is about 4%.

Clostridium fallax

Although MacLennan considers *C. fallax* capable by itself of causing clostridial myonecrosis, there are few cases on record, and the organism is rarely encountered. *C. fallax* is a strict anaerobe that rapidly loses virulence after isolation and artificial cultivation. Its natural habitat is not known.

Other Clostridia in Tissue Infections

Various other species of clostridia are commonly encountered in soft tissue infections, abscesses, wound infections, anaerobic cellulitis, and clostridial myonecrosis. These organisms are usually considered to be nonpathogenic, but there are unanswered questions regarding their possible role in the development of infection. Many probably should be considered as opportunistic pathogens.

There is a correlation between the incidence in wound infections of the various species of clostridia, both pathogenic and nonpathogenic, and their occurrence in the soil, but the source also may be endogenous organisms on the skin and clothing. Alteration of the integrity of the intestinal wall by disease, surgery, or trauma also may release a variety of endogenous bacteria, including these so-called nonpathogenic clostridial species, which may then be isolated from subsequent infections such as peritonitis, intra-abdominal abscesses, and occasionally bacteremia. It is important to remember that rarely *C. tetani* and *C. botulinum* also may be present in a wound in addition to the histotoxic and other clostridial species.

Of the clostridia currently labeled as nonpathogenic, *C. sporogenes* is frequently encountered in wound infection, along with *C. bifermentans* and *C. tertium*. *C. tertium*, in particular, has been isolated from the bloodstream of neutropenic patients. This organism is aerotolerant and may not be recognized from blood cultures as a clostridium with medical significance. Additional organisms that may be isolated from wound sources are *C. innocuum*, *C. ramosum*, *C. subterminale*, *C. limosum*, *C. butyricum*, *C. sphenoides*, *C. cadaveris*, *C. putrificum*, and *C. paraputrificum*. Although *C. sporogenes* does not appear to produce toxins, there is some evidence that the organism, when associated with frank pathogens such as *C. perfringens* or *C. novyi*, may play a synergistic role in clostridial myonecrosis. Its presence with either of these organisms is correlated with a high mortality rate.

Clostridium difficile and Antibiotic-associated Colitis

A variety of gastrointestinal disorders, ranging from mild to severe, have been recognized as side effects of the administration of antibiotics. *Clostridium difficile* recently has been found to be responsible for virtually all severe complications (e.g., pseudomembranous enterocolitis) and a portion of the less severe manifestations, such as diarrhea. Studies of the fatal hemorrhagic cecitis that can be induced in guinea pigs and hamsters by administration of penicillin, clindamycin, and other antibiotics helped significantly in the elucidation of *C. difficile* as the etiologic agent in human disease.

Characteristics of *C. difficile*. *C. difficile* is an obligate anaerobe that is saccharolytic and weakly proteolytic, producing a complex array of acid fermentation products detectable by gas-liquid chromatography. A selective agar medium containing cefoxitin, cycloserine, fructose, and egg yolk significantly aids in its isolation from feces. The organism has been isolated from both human and animal feces. Six serologic groups have been described which were detectable by agglutination tests. Particular serogroups were associated with toxicogenicity and type of host population. Electrophoretic patterns of cellular proteins and bacteriophage-bacteriocin typing methods also have been useful for studying the epidemiology of *C. difficile.*

C. difficile produces two major protein toxins that are important in antibiotic-associated colitis and are antigenically distinct. Toxin B, or cytotoxin, produces a cytopathic effect in vitro on tissue culture cells, a procedure that has been used for the detection of toxin from feces of patients and from cultures of *C. difficile.* The cytopathic effect of this toxin can be inhibited by specific antisera to purified toxin B or, because of antigenic cross-reactivity, by the *C. sordellii* antitoxin component of polyvalent gas gangrene antitoxin. It initially was assumed that this toxic moiety was entirely responsible for enterotoxic activity. Purification studies, however, led to the detection of a second toxic component, toxin A, which produced significantly more disease in some model biologic assay systems but had much less cytotoxic activity for tissue culture cells than toxin B. Toxin A is a potent enterotoxin, which causes severe damage to the intestinal mucosa and an excess fluid response. The toxin apparently is a strong chemoattractant for human granulocytes, causing a transient rise in their intracellular calcium concentration. These activated granulocytes then release inflammatory mediators within the lamina propria that damage the epithelial cells of the gut mucosa. Toxigenic strains of *C. difficile* usually produce both toxins A and B, and protection experiments in animals immunized against either toxin alone or both toxins indicate that both moieties are involved in disease. Each of these toxins is lethal for experimental animals when small amounts are injected intraperitoneally or subcutaneously, and toxin A alone given intragastrically to healthy hamsters results in intestinal pathology, diarrhea, and death.

Clinical Manifestations and Epidemiology. Clinical disease associated with administration of antibiotics may be only diarrhea or it may be colitis, of which pseudomembranous colitis is a more severe form. Pseudomembranous enterocolitis is a severe, potentially lethal, disease of the gastrointestinal tract characterized by exudative plaques with underlying necrosis of the mucosal surface of the intestine. The plaques may coalesce, forming large pseudomembranes, and sloughing may occur. This pathologic entity had been described in a variety of clinical settings, particularly with gastrointestinal tract surgery, before the antibiotic era, but an increased incidence and a higher predilection for involvement of the colon became apparent with antibiotic-associated disease. Diarrhea or colitis may develop when antibiotics are being administered, or they can occur even weeks after antibiotics have been discontinued. Pseudomembranous colitis, as confirmed by gross appearance on sigmoidoscopy or by biopsy and that occurs in association with antibiotic administration, is highly correlated with the presence of *C. difficile* by culture and detection of the cytotoxin (96%) from feces. Diarrhea, which usually resolves spontaneously, is a much more frequent adverse reaction after administration of antibiotics than is colitis. Only approximately one third or fewer of the patients with antibiotic-associated diarrhea have been found to be positive for *C. difficile* or the cytotoxin.

Risk factors for development of *C. difficile*–related enteric disease are antibiotic exposure, primarily (and occasionally, exposure to antineoplastic drugs), older age, female sex, and probably impaired intestinal motility. A wide variety of antibiotics have been associated with the development of diarrhea or colitis, although the drugs most frequently linked to colitis are ampicillin, clindamycin, and the cephalosporins. The *C. difficile* strain isolated from a patient with pseudomembranous colitis may be resistant or susceptible to the implicated antimicrobial(s), so it has become apparent that the mechanism of disease production is not simply overgrowth by resistant strains of *C. difficile.* Yet alteration of the normal microbial ecology of the gastrointestinal tract and suppression of prevalent endogenous organisms are obviously important in allowing *C. difficile* to colonize or in predisposing to its proliferation and toxin production. Gastrointestinal procedures, in particular, may precipitate the disease without prior antimicrobial exposure, although much less frequently.

The source of an infecting strain of *C. difficile* can be either endogenous or exogenous. *C. difficile* can be isolated from the feces of 3% or less of healthy adults. Infants, however, may acquire *C. difficile* early in the neonatal period, with isolation rates as high as 64% reported for infants up to 8 months of age. It appears that environmental spread of *C. difficile* in nurseries is an important reason for the high colonization in this age group. Typing schemes for clinical isolates of *C. difficile* have been the key to demonstrating instances of nosocomial spread of the organism in nursery outbreaks and in hospitalized adult populations. This anaerobic microorganism can survive on contaminated surfaces in an ambient air environment because of its ability to form spores.

Laboratory Diagnosis. Colonoscopy and sigmoidoscopy with biopsy often has been used as diagnostic procedures for colitis, but although these techniques are useful, they are invasive and must be used judiciously. Laboratory diagnosis of *C. difficile*–related enteric disease has depended primarily on demonstration of cytotoxic activity (toxin B) in stool specimens taken from patients with an appropriate clinical history, signs, and symptoms. Culture of stool specimens for *C. difficile,* while sometimes helpful, is less specific than cytotoxin assay for diagnosis, since up to 21% of hospitalized patients who have no symptoms (no diarrhea or colitis) are colonized with *C. difficile.* Cytotoxin assay alone is insufficient for positive diagnosis because cytotoxin has been detected, although infrequently, from feces of patients who have received antibiotics but did not have diarrhea or colitis. The high frequency of *C. difficile* in neonates has confounded understanding of the role of this organism in gastrointestinal disorders in this population. The organism and cytotoxin have been detected in infants with necrotizing enterocolitis but also in a significant proportion of healthy neonates. Thus, even high cytotoxin levels in feces do not always correlate with the presence of diarrhea or colitis.

There has been interest in developing immunoassays for diagnosis (based on detection of toxin A or toxin B) to avoid the necessity of the tissue culture assay. ELISA tests for toxin A and B have been studied. At present, however, it appears that a microtiter cytoxicity assay (toxin B) is the best overall test, considering both sensitivity and specificity, although an ELISA test for toxin A is highly specific. A latex agglutination test is available commercially and is useful as a rapid screening test, which can be followed by a test with higher specificity whenever clinically warranted.

Treatment. Treatment of *C. difficile* enterocolitis consists of (1) discontinuing the implicated antimicrobial agent(s) or substituting better-tolerated drugs, whenever possible, (2) maintaining fluid and electrolyte balance, (3) avoiding drugs that slow intestinal motility, and (4) administering an anti–*C. difficile* drug for those patients who have mild cases of the disease but do not respond to the aforementioned supportive management or who are sufficiently ill that specific therapy is deemed necessary. Vancomycin is considered the treatment of choice and probably should be used in the most severe cases or in patients who have suffered relapse. Metronidazole and bacitracin also have been shown to be effective, and they are less expensive. All agents are administered orally, so that high antimicrobial levels are achieved in the intestinal tract. Approximately 20% to 39% of the patients experience a relapse after treatment, some patients on multiple occasions. These patients usually respond to subsequent treatments. An antibody response often is absent or delayed in those patients with relapses after antimicrobial therapy for *C. difficile* colitis, and successful resolution appears to be coincidental with the production of antibodies. Among adults over 30 years of age, 70% to 80% have neutralizing antibodies to toxins A and B. Other therapeutic modalities are under study, including the possibility of reestablishing a normal gut flora with the use of fecal organisms or establishing colonization with nontoxigenic strains of *C. difficile*.

For prevention of *C. difficile*–related enteric disease, it is important to be aware of the potential for mild to severe gastrointestinal disease associated with administration of antimicrobial agents. Documentation of five or more loose stools per day without other apparent cause in patients receiving antimicrobial drugs commonly has been used as an indication to discontinue antibiotic therapy, if appropriate, or to substitute alternate antimicrobial agents believed to be less frequently associated with diarrhea and colitis sequelae.

Clostridium tetani

Clostridium tetani is the causative agent of tetanus, a disease that is now relatively rare in well-developed countries. In developing countries, however, where many unimmunized mothers give birth to children in whom umbilical cord care is neglected, neonatal tetanus has a significant impact on overall mortality. In the adult, the disease classically follows a puncture wound and is characterized by severe muscle spasms, the most characteristic being that of the jaw; hence the term *trismus* or *lockjaw*. Despite many advances in treatment, the mortality rate is quite high, especially in the very young and the very old.

The anaerobic nature of *C. tetani* was in part responsible for the delay in its discovery and isolation, which was accomplished by Kitasato in 1889. Clinical recognition that a small local infection produced by this organism could result in profound toxemia with neuromuscular manifestations led to the discovery of tetanus toxin and the detection shortly after of its specific antitoxin. Although antitoxin is quite effective when administered prophylactically, it is less effective when used therapeutically. The discovery, however, that the toxin can be converted to a toxoid, which is an excellent immunizing agent, provided a remarkably effective method for the prevention of tetanus. Widespread use of the toxoid has resulted in a marked reduction in incidence of the disease.

Morphology and Physiology

Morphology. The tetanus bacillus is quite long and thin when compared with other pathogenic clostridia. Individual bacilli range from 2 to 5 μm in width and 3 to 8 μm in length. Young cultures of the organism usually stain gram-positive, but in older cultures and in smears made from wounds the organisms frequently stain gram-negative. Under appropriate cultural conditions the organism produces a spore that is terminally located and of considerably greater diameter than the vegetative cell, giving a characteristic drumstick appearance. The spore does not stain with the Gram stain and appears as a colorless round structure. With prolonged incubation the vegetative cells autolyze, leaving behind either the spore with a portion of the vegetative cell attached or free spores. Most isolates of *C. tetani* possess numerous peritrichous flagella that convey active motility to the organism.

Cultural Characteristics. *C. tetani* is an obligate anaerobe, moderately fastidious in its requirement for anaerobiosis. The optimal temperature for growth is 37C, and the optimal pH is 7.4. Nutritional requirements of *C. tetani*, like those of other clostridia, are complex and include a number of amino acids and vitamins. These requirements, however, can be readily met by blood agar or cooked-meat broth. Since swarming of the organisms occurs on blood agar plates, the isolation of surface colonies is difficult. The edge of the colony appears as a translucent, finely granular sheet with a delicate filamentous advancing edge. This pronounced motility, especially in the presence of condensed moisture, has been used to advantage in isolating the organism from mixed cultures containing bacteria that are less motile than *C. tetani*. Where isolated colonies can be obtained, faint β-hemolysis is observed. In cooked-meat broth a small amount of growth can be detected in 48 hours; no digestion of the meat is noted. The organism does not ferment any carbohydrates.

Resistance. The spore of *C. tetani* conveys to the organism considerable resistance to the various disinfectants and to heat. It is not destroyed by boiling for 20 minutes. For practical purposes, autoclaving at 120C for 15 minutes is the preferred method for sterilizing contaminated materials.

Laboratory Identification. Clinical materials for culture should be transported to the laboratory in vessels containing carbon dioxide. They should be planted immediately both on prereduced solid media and on anaerobic liquid culture media, such as chopped meat, and incubated under anaerobic conditions. Sometimes isolation of the organism is difficult because of the presence of other organisms in the mixture. In such cases heating the culture at 80C for 20 minutes after an initial 24-hour incubation period will kill non-spore-forming organisms and permit recovery of *C. tetani*. The rapid motility of the organism may also be useful in its isolation. One half of a culture plate is inoculated with a culture. The remaining half is left uninoculated and after 24 hours is examined for a thin film of the motile *C. tetani*. Final proof of the isolation of a toxin-producing *C. tetani* rests on the in vivo demonstration of toxin production when injected into mice and its neutralization in mice previously inoculated with antitoxin.

Antigenic Structure

Flagella (H), somatic (O), and spore antigens have been demonstrated in *C. tetani.* The spore antigens are different from the H and O antigens of the somatic cell. Strains of the organism have been differentiated into ten types on the basis of their flagellar antigens. There is a single somatic agglutination group for all strains that permits identification of the organism by use of fluorescein-labeled antisera. Of tremendous practical importance, however, is the production of a single antigenic type of toxin by all strains of *C. tetani* and its neutralization by a single antitoxin.

Determinants of Pathogenicity

Very little is known about the conditions that allow the tetanus bacillus to survive within the human host. *C. tetani* has little invasive ability and when present alone rarely produces an invasive cellulitis. Frequently, however, it is found in association with other bacteria that play a more significant role in the local infection and that lower the oxidation-reduction potential at the site of injury.

Tetanus Toxin. All of the symptoms in tetanus are attributable to an extremely toxic neurotoxin, tetanospasmin, which is an intracellular toxin released by cellular autolysis. The structural gene for the toxin is located on a 75 kb plasmid.

PROPERTIES. The purification of intracellular toxin is best accomplished by its extraction from cells in the late exponential phase of growth before there is appreciable toxin detectable in the culture medium. The toxin is a heat-labile protein that may be inactivated by heating for 20 minutes at 60C. The primary structure of the toxin molecule has been defined and shown to be significantly homologous to some of the toxins of *Clostridium botulinum.* The toxin is synthesized by *C. tetani* as a single polypeptide chain composed of three domains—A, B, and C—each with a molecular weight of approximately 50 kDa. On release from the bacterium, the toxin is cleaved by clostridial proteases to yield two subunits—a light chain, designated A, and a heavy chain, designated BC—linked by a single disulfide bond. Separated, the heavy and light chains are nontoxic, thus conforming to the usual activity pattern of A-B dichain toxins. By analogy to these toxins, it is thought that tetanus toxin is taken up by receptor-mediated endocytosis and that the low pH in the endosomal lumen causes the toxin to insert itself into the lipid bilayer and cross the membrane to reach the cytosol. The toxicity of intact tetanus toxin is associated with the A light chain. Purified fragment B of the heavy chain forms channels in lipid membranes, while a ganglioside-binding site is located on the fragment C domain. Although gangliosides can be shown to tightly bind tetanus toxin, there is some question as to whether they represent the true tissue receptor. Several studies suggest that tetanus toxin might bind to and use the receptor-uptake system normally used by thyroid-stimulating hormone. Tetanus toxin binds to membrane receptors from thyroid cells with characteristics quite similar to those for thyrotropin binding.

Tetanus toxin is one of the most poisonous substances known; only botulinum toxin and *Shigella* dysentery toxin are comparable in toxicity. There is no simple in vitro test for determining its activity; toxicity must be assayed by observing its lethal effect on an experimental animal. In quantitating the toxin, the most meaningful dose is the lethal dose for 50% of the animals injected (LD_{50}), since this level of toxin lies on the steepest part of the dose-response curve. Animals vary in their susceptibility to the toxin. Man and the horse are probably the most susceptible, while birds and cold-blooded animals are usually quite resistant. In mice, pure toxin preparations have a potency of about 30 million minimum lethal doses (MLDs) per milligram of protein. Although toxin constitutes about 5% to 10% of the bacterial weight, the physiology of its production and function in the parent organism is largely unknown.

Although toxin forms nontoxic dimers spontaneously, production of toxoid with formaldehyde increases the degree of polymerization and produces a more stable and reliable product. This material is useful in immunization against the disease. Toxoid is nontoxic but retains the antigenic determinants of tetanus toxin that give rise to antitoxin antibody. The tetanus toxin molecule contains at least 20 distinct antigenic determinants, and antibodies to at least nine different determinants are each capable of neutralizing the toxicity of the toxin. Also, different combinations of two, three, or four monoclonal antibodies to these determinants are synergistic in their effect and enhance neutralization to an extent equivalent to that exhibited by a standard unit of tetanus antitoxin.

MODE OF ACTION. The molecular basis for the action of tetanus toxin is unknown. Part of its mechanism of action, however, involves binding to peripheral nerve endings followed by internalization and transport intra-axonally against the flow (retrograde intra-axonal transport). When it reaches the region of the nucleus, it is transported to the inhibitory interneurons, where it inhibits the release of inhibitory transmitters. Small amounts of the toxin injected locally in experimental animals result in local tetanospasm followed by ascending tetanus and the development of increasing muscle spasticity above the site of the injection. Intravenous injection of the tetanus toxin produces descending tetanus characterized by spasticity in the head and neck that spreads to the back and limbs and is followed by generalized tetanic convulsions. Localization of radiolabeled tetanus toxin injected intravenously suggests that generalized tetanus results from the summation of innumerable forms of local tetanus. The inhibition of the release of inhibitory transmitter substances allows the more powerful muscles to prevail. In the human, this can be seen in the form of muscle spasms of the masseter muscles with trismus flexion of the upper extremities and extension of the lower extremities with arching of the back (opisthotonus).

Clinical Infection

Epidemiology. Although the incidence of tetanus is decreasing in parts of the world where standards of living are high, it remains a common and uncontrolled disease in the developing world. Some climates, soils, and agricultural economies are associated with higher risk than others. In unimmunized rural populations tetanus develops at higher rates than in urban populations. In the United States, tetanus is a sporadic disease that is seen most frequently in the southern, southeastern, and midwestern states. It has become increasingly a disease of older persons because of the failure to be immunized with tetanus toxoid during childhood or in military service. Recently, addiction to heroin has been associated with increased numbers of cases in large urban centers.

Pathogenesis. The spores of *C. tetani* are ubiquitous. They have been found in 20% to 64% of soil samples taken for culture and are present in even higher yields in cultivated lands. They are present in the gastrointestinal tracts of humans and other animals. If one carefully cultures traumatic wounds, *C. tetani* can also be demonstrated fairly frequently. It is quite uncommon, however, for tetanus to develop from these wounds. The most significant feature of the pathogenesis of tetanus is the setting of the wound where the oxidation-reduction potential must be properly poised to permit multiplication of the organism and toxigenesis. Classically, the wounds seen in practice are the simple puncture wounds from a nail, splinter, or thorn. Other settings, however, such as compound fractures, "skin popping" by drug addicts, decubitus and varicose ulcers, external otitis, and dental extractions, also provide the proper conditions. The most feared form of tetanus, tetanus neonatorum, is a significant cause of morbidity and mortality in developing nations. This form of tetanus usually results from cutting the umbilical cord with unsterile instruments or from improper care of the umbilical stump. In the United States most neonatal cases have resulted from unattended home deliveries. Tetanus may also follow operative procedures, but with modern hospital facilities this is rare.

The lowering of the oxidation-reduction potential is associated with tissue necrosis after traumatic injuries or the injection of necrotizing substances. An important contributing factor is the presence of aerobic bacteria that will grow to the point of removing oxygen and then continue to grow facultatively as anaerobes. This growth will effectively reduce the oxidation-reduction potential to the point where tetanus spores may germinate. After germination of the spores, toxin is elaborated and gains entrance to the central nervous system. The infection with *C. tetani* remains localized and inconspicuous, with minimal reaction unless other organisms are present. In any collection of cases of tetanus, there are always a few cases that give no preceding history of injury.

Clinical Manifestations. Following implantation of spores into an appropriate site, there is an incubation period of 4 to 10 days. In rare instances tetanus may occur in a localized form, developing in muscles adjacent to the site of inoculation. More frequently, however, it is generalized in nature. The earliest manifestation is muscle stiffness, followed by spasm of the masseter muscles (trismus or lockjaw). This is the classic symptom of tetanus. As the disease progresses, tetanospasms cause clenching of the jaw, producing a grimace referred to as risus sardonicus, arching of the back (opisthotonos), flexion of the arms, and extension of the lower extremities. These tetanospasms are relatively brief in duration but may be frequent and exhausting. Recently attention has been brought to the sympathetic effects of tetanus toxin—hypotension-hypertension, tachycardia, and cardiac disturbance. Respiratory complications such as aspiration pneumonia and atelectasis are common. Occasionally the spasms will be of sufficient intensity to produce bone fractures.

It takes several weeks for the disease to run its course; death may ensue during one of these spasms. Poor prognosis is associated with a short incubation period between injury and seizure, rapid development from muscle spasm to tetanospasms, injury close to the head, extremes of age, and frequency and severity of convulsions. Patients who recover usually return to a completely normal state after a variable period of stiffness. Except for possible damage to the lungs from pulmonary complications or bone fracture, tetanus leaves no permanent residua.

Immunity. There is no evidence that the natural disease confers immunity against subsequent tetanus infection. The tetanus toxin is so toxic that an amount sufficient to cause clinical tetanus is too small to be immunogenic. Recurrent attacks are not uncommon, and for this reason patients who recover from the disease should be actively immunized with toxoid to prevent possible exogenous reinfection or recurrence of infection from spores of *C. tetani* retained within the body. Adequate immunization of pregnant patients is extremely important to ensure passive immunity for the newborn and thereby diminish the likelihood of tetanus neonatorum. This maternally transmitted immunity will last until active immunization has been started during the first year of life.

Laboratory Diagnosis. The diagnosis of tetanus is made on clinical grounds because isolation of the organism can occur in the absence of disease and also because it is possible to have the disease but be unable to isolate the organism. If the local lesion can be detected and Gram-stained, one can occasionally demonstrate thin gram-positive or gram-negative rods and sometimes spores with varying amounts of the vegetative cell attached. Most such attempts to demonstrate the organisms directly, however, have been unsuccessful. Material from a known wound should be transported to the microbiology laboratory in transport vessels that have been filled with carbon dioxide for culture under anaerobic conditions.

Treatment. The treatment of tetanus varies with the severity of the disease. In general, however, it is designed to prevent the further elaboration and absorption of toxin. Antitoxin is administered, and because of the immediate and delayed complications from antitoxin prepared in a horse or sheep, human immune globulin from pooled hyperimmune donors is recommended. The use of intrathecal human globulin is not officially approved, but reports concerning its efficacy when it is used early have been enthusiastic. In addition, dèbridement of the wound and removal of any foreign bodies are recommended unless the extent or location precludes such a surgical approach. Large doses of penicillin should also be given; if the patient is allergic to penicillin, tetracycline or metronidazole may be considered. Mild tetanospasm may be controlled with barbiturates and diazepam. With severe tetanospasms, however, a curare-like agent may be used to completely paralyze the patient's muscles so that respiratory function may be maintained by means of a positive pressure breathing apparatus. To minimize respiratory complications, tracheostomy should be performed after the onset of the first tetanospasm. To minimize the frequency and severity of the tetanospasms, good supportive care of the patient should also include careful control of the environment to reduce auditory and visual stimuli. With improved control of tetanospasms and respiratory complications, greater attention has been paid to controlling the sympathetic effects of the toxin. Morphine and labetalol have been reported to be useful.

Prevention. Tetanus is almost completely preventable with properly applied active or passive immunization. During World War II only 12 cases of tetanus occurred in 2,735,000 hospital admissions for wounds and injuries in soldiers who had been previously immunized. This successful experience resulted in the passage by most state legislatures in the United

TABLE 44–3. ROUTINE DIPHTHERIA, TETANUS, AND PERTUSSIS IMMUNIZATION SCHEDULE SUMMARY FOR CHILDREN UNDER 7 YEARS OLD—UNITED STATES, 1985

Dose	Age and Interval[a]	Product
Primary 1	6 weeks old or older	DTP[b]
Primary 2	4–8 weeks after first dose[c]	DTP[b]
Primary 3	4–8 weeks after second dose[c]	DTP[b]
Primary 4	6–12 months after third dose[c]	DTP[b]
Booster	4–6 years old, before entering kindergarten or elementary school (not necessary if fourth primary immunizing dose administered on or after fourth birthday)	DTP[b]
Additional boosters	Every 10 years after last dose	Td

From Centers for Disease Control: Ann Intern Med 103:896, 1985.
DTP, diphtheria and tetanus toxoids and pertussis vaccine adsorbed; Td, tetanus and diphtheria toxoids adsorbed.
[a] Customarily begun at 8 weeks of age, with second and third doses given at 8-week intervals.
[b] Diphtheria and tetanus toxoids adsorbed (DT) if pertussis vaccine is contraindicated. If the child is 1 year of age or older at the time the primary dose is given, a third dose 6 to 12 months after the second completes primary immunization with DT.
[c] Prolonging the interval does not require restarting series.

TABLE 44–4. SUMMARY GUIDE TO TETANUS PROPHYLAXIS IN ROUTINE WOUND MANAGEMENT—UNITED STATES, 1985

History of Adsorbed Tetanus Toxoid (Doses)	Clean, Minor Wounds		All Other Wounds[a]	
	Td[b]	TIG	Td[b]	TIG
Unknown or less than 3	Yes	No	Yes	Yes
3 or more[c]	No[d]	No	No[e]	No

From Centers for Disease Control: Ann Intern Med 103:896, 1985.
Td, Tetanus and diphtheria toxoids adsorbed; TIG, tetanus immune globulin.
[a] Such as, but not limited to, wounds contaminated with dirt, feces, soil, saliva, puncture wounds; avulsions; and wounds resulting from missiles, crushing, burns, and frostbite.
[b] For children under 7 years old; diphtheria and tetanus toxoids and pertussis vaccine adsorbed (diphtheria and tetanus toxoids if pertussis vaccine is contraindicated) is preferred to tetanus toxoid alone. For persons 7 years old and older, tetanus and diphtheria toxoids adsorbed is preferred to tetanus toxoid alone.
[c] If only three doses of fluid toxoid have been received, a fourth dose of toxoid, preferably an adsorbed toxoid, should be given.
[d] Yes, if more than 10 years since last dose.
[e] Yes, if more than 5 years since last dose. (More frequent boosters are not needed and can accentuate side effects.)

States of laws making admission to primary school contingent upon adequate immunization with tetanus toxoid. Compliance has resulted in a steady decline in the incidence of tetanus. It is especially important that infants and children, pregnant women, and the elderly be immunized.

ACTIVE IMMUNITY. Routine immunization with tetanus toxoid should begin at the age of 1 to 3 months and should involve the administration of a combination of tetanus and diphtheria toxoid and pertussis vaccine (DPT). Three doses of DPT should be given at intervals of 3 or 4 weeks, with booster doses 1 and 4 years later. Immunity to tetanus can be maintained with a single booster dose of toxoid every 10 years. Because young children are very prone to lacerations and puncture wounds, in the past they were exposed repeatedly to booster shots when brought to emergency rooms. Also, requirements of schools, camps, and the armed forces have led to an inordinate exposure to tetanus toxoid. For this reason, patients coming to an emergency room with a history of the basic immunizing series and a booster injection within a 4-year period probably do not need to receive a booster injection at the time of injury. Persons who come to the emergency room with no history of immunization or with partial immunization should receive the human immune globulin in one arm and the first of a series of toxoid injections in the other arm in order to prevent future tetanus (Tables 44–3 and 44–4).

PASSIVE IMMUNITY. Passive immunity may be conferred by the administration of antitoxin. This form of immunity was developed during World War I, when it was recognized that a small dose of tetanus antitoxin prepared in a horse was impressively protective when administered at the time of injury. Because of the risk of anaphylaxis and serum sickness associated with the use of a foreign serum, human tetanus immune globulin is recommended for passive immunization. The prophylactic administration of a single 250-unit dose of antitoxin should be reserved for patients with tetanus-prone wounds who have no record of immunization, for those who have received only one dose of tetanus toxoid, and for those who are not seen until 48 hours after the injury. Penicillin or tetracycline also should be given, along with appropriate surgical care. Such persons receiving antitoxin should also be given alum-absorbed toxin, administered at the same time at a different site, and a second dose of toxoid 1 month later.

Clostridium botulinum

C. botulinum produces the most potent exotoxin known. The toxin, which is a neurotoxin, is the cause of botulism, a severe neuroparalytic disease characterized by sudden onset and swiftness of course, terminating in profound paralysis and pulmonary arrest. Although disease caused by *C. botulinum* toxin is rare in humans, it is much more common in animals. Unlike tetanus toxin, there are eight serologically distinct botulinum toxins, designated A, B, C_1, C_2, D, E, F, and G. Table 44–5 gives the animal species affected in outbreaks caused by the various types.

The most common form of botulism is foodborne botulism, an intoxication caused by the ingestion of preformed botulinum toxin in contaminated food. The disease botulism received its name from the Latin *botulus* (sausage), a term introduced in 1870 to describe a fatal food-poisoning syndrome associated with the eating of sausage. Although of historical interest, the name has lost much of its significance because fish and other animal proteins also transmit the disease and because in the United States plants are more common vehicles than animal products. The canning industry's use of autoclaving at temperatures sufficient to kill the spores has reduced the relative importance of commercially canned food

TABLE 44–5. ANIMAL SPECIES SUSCEPTIBLE TO *CLOSTRIDIUM BOTULINUM* TYPES

Type	Species	Sites of Outbreaks
A	Human	United States, Soviet Union
B	Human, horse	United States, Northern Europe, Soviet Union
C_α[a]	Birds, turtles	Worldwide
C_β[b]	Cattle, sheep, horses	Worldwide
D	Cattle, sheep	Australia, South Africa
E	Human, birds	Northern Europe, Canada, United States, Japan, Soviet Union
F	Human	Denmark, United States
G	No outbreaks have been recognized	

From Smith: Botulism. Charles C Thomas, 1977.
[a] Major toxin produced by type C_α is C_1 (see below).
[b] Major toxin produced by type C_β is C_2.

TABLE 44–6. SOME CULTURAL CHARACTERISTICS OF *CLOSTRIDIUM BOTULINUM*

	Physiologic Group			
Characteristic	**I**	**II**	**III**	**IV**
Digestion of coagulated protein	+	–	–[a]	+
Fermentation of glucose	+	+	+	–
Fermentation of mannose	–	+	+	–
Hydrolysis of gelatin	+	+	+	+
Formation of lipase	+	+	+	+
Production of indol	–	–	–	–
Reduction of nitrate	–	–	–	–
Fermentation products	A, P, IB, B, IV	A, B	A, P, B	A, P, IB, B, IV

From Smith: Botulism. Charles C Thomas, 1977.
A, Acetic acid; B, butyric; IB, isobutyric; IV, isovaleric; P, propionic.
[a] Weak proteolysis by some strains.

as a source of disease except where procedural errors have occurred. Because the toxin is destroyed by heat, the routine cooking of home-canned food limits the frequency of this type of food poisoning.

In addition to food-borne botulism, the disease also occurs when toxin is produced by *C. botulinum* organisms contaminating traumatic wounds (wound botulism) and when toxin is elaborated within the gastrointestinal tracts of infants (infant botulism).

Morphology and Physiology

Morphology. *C. botulinum* is a straight to slightly curved gram-positive rod with rounded ends. Although it exhibits marked variation in size, depending on cultural conditions and serologic type, the size falls within the range of 3.4 to 8.6 μm by 0.5 to 1.3 μm. Involution forms on artificial media are frequently observed. *C. botulinum* is motile with peritrichous flagella. It produces heat-resistant spores that are oval and subterminal and that tend to distend the bacillus. These are produced more consistently when the organism is grown on alkaline glucose gelatin media at 20C to 25C; spores usually are not produced at higher temperatures.

Cultural Characteristics. *C. botulinum* is a strict anaerobe that is easily cultured in an anaerobic environment on routine media. On blood agar, all strains except those of type G are β-hemolytic. The nutritional requirements of the organism are complex, especially those of the nonproteolytic strains. Although initially classified into two groups—proteolytic and nonproteolytic—the species has subsequently been divided into four groups. Some of the physiologic properties used to separate the groups are listed in Table 44–6.

Resistance. The heat resistance of the spores of *C. botulinum* is greater than that of any other anaerobe; the degree of resistance to various physical and chemical factors depends on the specific strain and serologic type of the organism. Type A is more resistant than types B, C, and D; type E is the least heat resistant, but variants of this type that are exquisitely resistant to heat have been obtained. In general, the spores may survive several hours at 100C and up to 10 minutes at 120C. The spores are also resistant to irradiation and can survive temperatures of −190C.

Antigenic Structure

Exotoxin. The species *C. botulinum* includes a very heterogeneous group of strains that have been divided into eight serologically distinct types—A, B, C_α, C_β, D, E, F, and G—on the basis of the type of toxin produced. Immunologic differences between these types are constant and clear cut and are of epidemiologic significance. Except for strains of types C and D, a single toxin is produced by each type. Strains of types C and D are complex and produce three different toxins. Strains that produce predominantly C_1 and C_2 toxins are designated C_α and C_β, respectively; type D strains produce D toxin in the greatest amount.

Somatic Antigens. The antigenic composition of vegetative cells of *C. botulinum* is very complex and has not been completely defined for most of the types. Types A and B have been divided into six subgroups on the basis of their heat-labile antigens. These strains of *C. botulinum* share one heat-stable antigen with *C. tetani, C. histolyticum,* and *C. sporogenes.* The fluorescent antibody technique has been used to demonstrate cross-reactions among the strains of A, B, and F and between strains of C and D. There are different heat-stable and heat-labile agglutinating antigens among strains of type E. These strains, however, appear to be homogeneous and distinct and do not cross-react with strains of other types. For each of the types, spore antigens appear to be more specific than antigens of the vegetative cells.

Determinants of Pathogenicity

Properties of Botulinum Toxin. The clinical manifestations of botulism are attributable to the toxin of *C. botulinum* that is present in the ingested food, in the gastrointestinal tracts of infants, or in wounds. Botulinum toxin is one of the most potent toxins known. One microgram of the purified toxin contains about 200,000 MLDs for a 20 g mouse.

The optimal temperature for toxin production varies greatly both within and across types, with maximum production between 30C and 38C except for *C. botulinum* type E, which has an optimum of 25C to 28C. Initiation of growth and toxin production occurs only over a narrow pH range of 7.0 to 7.3. Although *C. botulinum* can be grown on a completely defined synthetic medium, maximum toxin production is obtained on more complex culture media.

Botulinum toxin is usually classified as an exotoxin because of its high potency and antigenicity. It differs, however, from a classic exotoxin in that it is not released during the life of the organism but appears in the medium only after death and autolysis of the organism. The role played by the toxin in the metabolism of *C. botulinum* is not known; the organism may be rendered nontoxigenic without any discernible effect on the growth rate. The toxin is synthesized by *C. botulinum* in seven antigenically distinct forms. Each of these is produced as a low-toxicity single-chain polypeptide with a molecular weight of approximately 150 kDa. Cleavage or nicking of the molecule by bacterial proteases in the course of its release from the cell yields a dichain molecule composed of a heavy chain and a light chain (approximately 100 and 50 kDa, respectively) held together by noncovalent bonds and one disulfide bond. Conversion to the dichain is accompanied by an increase in toxicity. In the laboratory, toxin can be activated with trypsin. Most clostridia are proteolytic and are thus capable of converting the single-chain progenitor toxin to the active dichain molecule. Type E *C. botulinum,* however, is nonproteolytic and requires the use of proteolytic enzymes within the gastrointestinal tract for activation of toxin. The oral toxicity of the larger-molecular-weight aggregates of botulinum toxin is greater than that of smaller ones. This may be attributable to the greater stability of the larger aggregates against prolonged exposure in the gastrointestinal tract to enzymes that reduce their ultimate toxicity.

The production of botulinum toxin is governed by specific bacteriophages. Curing *C. botulinum* of toxigenic bacteriophages renders the organism nontoxigenic. It is also possible to convert one type of toxin-producing *C. botulinum* to another by reinfecting cured strains with a different bacteriophage. Of special importance also is the observation that bacteriophage infection of certain strains of *C. botulinum* can convert that organism to a different clostridial species, *Clostridium novyi,* a causative agent of gas gangrene.

Biologic Activity of Botulinum Toxin. Botulinum toxin gains access to the peripheral nervous system, where it acts preferentially on cholinergic nerve endings to block the release of the neurotransmitter, acetylcholine, from the nerve terminals of neuromuscular junctions. Experimental findings suggest that the toxin acts in three distinct sequential steps: (1) binding between toxin and a receptor on the surface of the plasma membrane with no obvious effects on neuromuscular transmission, (2) translocation or internalization of toxin, and (3) an intracellular event, the end result of which is a blockade of nerve stimulus–induced release of acetylcholine. Structure-function relationships of the botulinum toxin have not been firmly established, but there is strong evidence that the heavy chain mediates binding. The nature of the cell surface receptor for the heavy chain and the mechanism of cell entry of the light chain are not known. The light chain of botulinum C_2 toxin has ADP-ribosylating activity. The protein substrate is nonmuscle actin. Like other microbial toxins that have ADP-ribosylating activity, the botulinum C_2 toxin has glycohydrolase activity and splits nicotinamide adenine dinucleotide into ADP-ribose and nicotinamide. The pathophysiologic relevance of actin ADP-ribosylation has not been established for either botulinum C_2 toxin or other toxin types.

Inactivation of Toxin. The susceptibility of toxin to inactivation by various chemical and physical agents is of practical importance because of its role in food poisoning. The resistance of botulinum toxin to various deleterious agents is determined by its serologic type, as well as temperature, pH, and the presence of extraneous materials. Thermostability depends on the solute of the toxin. All toxin types are inactivated completely by boiling for 1 minute or by heating at 75C to 85C for 5 to 10 minutes. At room temperature toxin retains its activity for several days in tap water, an important observation that suggests the potential for prolonged contamination of water supplies. Toxin is destroyed by direct sunlight within 5 days unless it is protected from air, in which case its inactivation proceeds at a slower rate. A low pH of 3.5 to 6.8 favors preservation of the toxin, while an alkaline pH accelerates detoxification. Substances that usually are found in putrifying canned foods have no effect on the toxin's activity.

Laboratory Detection of Toxin. The incrimination of *C. botulinum* as the cause of food poisoning is based on the demonstration of toxin in the food or in the sera or gastric contents of the patient. The most commonly used method is the mouse toxicity and neutralization test, which can detect amounts as small as 10 μg of toxic protein. Other methods, such as the ELISA, are available, but, except for radioimmunoassay, their sensitivity is not as great. Also, the fact that immunoassays detect protein but not biologic activity is a recognized drawback to their use.

Clinical Intoxication

Ecology. *C. botulinum* causes a lethal type of food poisoning in several animal species. In general, food poisoning in a particular animal species is usually associated with certain types of the organism. The reason for this specificity is not known. Humans are susceptible to types A, B, E, and F; birds primarily to A and C; ruminants to C and D; and mink to A, B, C, and E (Table 44–6). *C. botulinum* has been isolated from many sources, including the sediments of lakes and rivers, virgin and cultivated terrestrial soil, the intestinal tracts of fish, and the intestinal tracts, spleens, and livers of a variety of animals. In general, *C. botulinum* is isolated more frequently from soil containing silt and is more easily cultured from manured than from nonmanured land.

Table 44–6 shows the major geographic areas associated with each type of *C. botulinum.* Data such as this are based on reports of disease in animals and humans caused by the different types and on isolation of the organisms from animals and the soil in various parts of the world. Although there is an observed prevalence of certain types of *C. botulinum* food poisoning in various localities, this does not exclude the possibility that other spore types may be present in a particular locality. In the United States, types A and B are widely distributed and have been associated with most outbreaks of human botulism. Type A is the predominant type in the Pacific Coast states, in the Rocky Mountains, and in Maine, New York, and Pennsylvania. The strains found in the soil of the Mississippi River Valley, the Great Lakes region, and New Jersey, Delaware, Maryland, Georgia, and South Carolina are predominantly type B. In recent years, type E has been isolated in several parts of the United States, but it is especially prevalent in the Great Lakes area.

Disease in Animals. A number of characteristic paralytic diseases of birds and mammals are caused by the ingestion of botulinum toxin in the animals' food. The best-known examples include grass or fodder sickness of horses, silage disease in cattle, limberneck in chickens, lamziekte of cattle, and dust sickness in wild birds. Outbreaks of botulism in animals reflect the geographic distribution of the organism, susceptibility of the animal species to the different toxins, and other predisposing factors. Thus lamziekte in cattle is restricted to areas in which the soil and herbage are markedly deficient in phosphorus. In such areas the cattle are prone to eat putrid bones and carcasses of small animals that are often toxic as a result of *C. botulinum* in the intestinal tract. Botulism in sheep results from bone chewing and is associated with periods of drought or with overgrazed ranges. Forage poisoning in cattle and horses occurs in many parts of the world as a result of the ingestion of toxic hay or silage. The toxin in the hay originates from an animal carcass. Carcasses of small animals, especially cats, found in a herd's food or bedding have been shown to contain as much as 3000 MLDs of toxin per gram. This toxin diffuses out into the hay or silage.

Type C botulinum toxin is the cause of large epidemics of botulism in aquatic and shore birds. Wild ducks are most frequently involved in these epidemics, which may affect thousands of birds. The disease is the major natural cause of death of ducks in the western United States. Outbreaks have also occurred in domestic ducks, gulls, loons, and sandpipers. Such outbreaks are thought to have their origin in strong coastal winds that uproot aquatic plants and lead to their decay. Invertebrates that are present in the decaying vegetation die because of lack of oxygen, and *C. botulinum* proliferates in their bodies. While searching for food among the masses of decaying vegetation, ducks ingest these toxic bodies of the invertebrates. After the duck's death the carcass is invaded by the organisms; the carcass itself becomes toxic and serves to perpetuate the outbreak. The carcass becomes flyblown and the fly larvae pick up a considerable amount of toxin, both in their exterior slimy coating and by ingestion. The ingestion by ducks of only a few of these fly larvae results in death; the dead ducks are invaded by *C. botulinum* and become flyblown, thus furnishing toxic larvae to poison more ducks. Botulism in pheasants follows a similar pattern.

Carrion eaters, such as the vulture, are almost completely resistant to botulinum toxin. The mechanism of this resistance is not known, but apparently it cannot be attributed to the presence of antitoxin in the animal's blood.

Disease in Humans

TYPES OF BOTULISM. In the United States, cases of botulism are now classified into four categories:

1. Food-borne botulism is a lethal food poisoning that results from ingestion of the neurotoxin in incompletely processed food contaminated with the organisms.
2. Infant botulism is related to the ingestion by infants of *C. botulinum* spores, the multiplication of organisms within the gastrointestinal tract, and subsequent absorption of toxin.
3. Wound botulism, which is the least common, is a neuroparalytic illness associated with wounds that show little clinical evidence of active infection.
4. Unclassified botulism occurs in persons over the age of 1 year who have symptoms of clinical botulism with no identifiable vehicle of transmission.

EPIDEMIOLOGY. The geographic distribution of botulism is primarily in the northern hemisphere between 30 and 65 degrees north latitude—north of the Gulf of Mexico, the Mediterranean Sea, the Persian Gulf, and the Bay of Bengal. Most of the outbreaks occur in seven countries: Canada, France, Germany, Japan, Poland, the Soviet Union, and the United States. In the United States, outbreaks occur at a rate of 10 per year, a rate that has varied little since records have been kept.

At the present time most cases of food-borne botulism occur in relatively circumscribed outbreaks after the consumption of home-preserved food. Sterilization procedures employed by commercial canneries use pressure apparatus in which canned products are held at a temperature of 121.1C for 30 minutes. As a result, outbreaks of botulism are rarely associated with commercially canned food. In recent years, however, there have been outbreaks from canned tuna and from vichyssoise as well as from smoked fish. The home-canned food most often incriminated as the source of botulism is green beans, which may have only a slightly sharp taste, prompting the housewife to rinse the contents of the jar of beans and serve them in a salad. Highly acidic foods, such as tomatoes and citrus fruits, are rarely the source because the organisms do not grow and release toxin at the low pH's encountered. Because of increased use of home freezers, meat has become an extremely rare source of *C. botulinum* in the United States. Although in its early descriptions botulism followed the ingestion of contaminated sausage and meat products, botulism of this type is now uncommon. Specialized foods eaten by certain ethnic groups are often responsible for the prevalence of a particular type of botulism poisoning in a given locality. In Japan, sushi (fermented raw fish salad) is often implicated; among the Indians of the northwest Pacific Coast, salmon egg cheese or stink eggs are responsible. The Alaskan Eskimos prepare muklak by soaking beluga flippers in seal oil for an extended period before eating. In all of these foods, conditions are suitable for *C. botulinum* growth and toxin production.

Since the recognition in 1976 of infant botulism as a disease entity, this syndrome has been recognized with increased frequency. According to statistics from the Centers for Disease Control, since 1979 this has been recognized as the predominant form of botulism in the United States. There appears to be no seasonality of its occurrence or of toxin type. An important feature of the disease is its propensity for afflicting children 2 to 6 months of age. In a significant number of cases the syndrome has followed the ingestion of honey that was contaminated with botulinum spores, strongly supporting this source as one method of intoxication. Most epidemiologic features of this syndrome, however, remain unknown.

Pathogenesis

Human botulism usually results from the ingestion of preformed botulinum toxin in contaminated foods. After ingestion the toxin is absorbed primarily from the stomach and small bowel, but toxin reaching the colon may be slowly absorbed, perhaps accounting for the delayed onset and prolonged duration of symptoms seen in many patients. The toxin appears in the lymphatics draining the intestine before it is found in the bloodstream. After an incubation period that is inversely related to dose, botulinum intoxication leads to a functional disturbance of the peripheral nervous system resulting from inhibition of the release of acetylcholine. The toxin acts at the myoneural junction to produce complete paralysis of the cholinergic nerve fibers at the point of release of acetylcholine. Botulinum toxin affects both sets of cholinergic transmission points in the autonomic system—the synaptic ganglia and the parasympathetic motor end plates peripherally located in the junction between the nerve and cell fibers.

In wound botulism, *C. botulinum* contaminates a traumatic wound. The rarity of this form of botulism is probably due to the inability of *C. botulinum* spores to germinate readily in tissues. The inhalation of aerosolized toxin can also lead to clinical botulism, as has been demonstrated after exposure within the setting of the experimental laboratory.

Less clear is the role of infection in the gastrointestinal tract as a source of botulism. Infants are especially susceptible to colonization of their intestinal tracts with *C. botulinum* and elaboration of the toxin in vivo. Both *C. botulinum* and botulinum toxin have been regularly demonstrated in the stools of these infants. In addition, toxin has been found in the serum of a number of confirmed cases of infant botulism. Until recently only type A and B organisms have been associated with this form of the disease. In 1986, however, two cases caused by type E botulinum toxin were reported. These cases are of special interest because the bacterium that produced the type E toxin was not *C. botulinum* but *C. butyricum*. *C. butyricum* is capable of colonizing the intestinal tracts of human infants, but its association with disease had not been previously demonstrated.

Evolutionary changes in diet and microbial intestinal flora are credited with the relative resistance of the adult to intestinal colonization. However, cases of the infant-type botulism are now being observed in adults, especially in persons with underlying abnormalities of the gastrointestinal tract resulting from inflammatory bowel disease or surgery. Alterations of the normal gut flora as a result of achlorhydria or the administration of broad-spectrum antibiotics are additional risk factors for infection of the intestinal tract with *C. botulinum* and the sustained production of toxin in vivo. It is thought that at least some of the patients with the fourth (unclassified) type of botulism have intestinal infection with secondary intoxication such as occurs in infants.

Clinical Manifestations

The incubation period and clinical manifestations are similar for all types of botulinum toxin. Because the length of the incubation period can be related to the dose of toxin, the shorter the incubation period, the poorer the prognosis. Characteristically, symptoms begin 12 to 36 hours after ingestion of the contaminated food or as late as 8 days after. Type E botulism appears to have a shorter incubation period than do types A and B. Severe nausea and vomiting are frequently observed with type E intoxication but are less common with types A and B. Weakness, lassitude, and dizziness are often early complaints. There is usually no diarrhea, but constipation is common. The early symptoms of botulism would rarely bring a patient to a physician's attention. Cranial nerve palsies are usually the presenting symptom: classically, diplopia (double vision), dysphagia (difficulty in swallowing), and dysphonia (difficulty in speaking). The pupils are dilated and the tongue is very dry and furry. In type E intoxication, abdominal distention is especially common, leading to a mistaken diagnosis of acute abdomen. Fever is rarely observed, and the mental processes remain intact. As the disease progresses, weakness of muscle groups (particularly of the neck, proximal extremities, and respiratory musculature) is often observed, leading ultimately to sudden respiratory paralysis, airway obstruction, and death. The mortality rate is affected by the type of toxin consumed, the distribution of toxin in the food, and the speed with which the disease is diagnosed and antitoxin therapy is initiated. Recent mortality is about 32% for type A, 17% for type B, and 40% for type E toxin.

Clinically, infant botulism is an acute flaccid paralysis that manifests as weakness of head, face, and throat musculature and then extends symmetrically to involve the muscles of the trunk and extremities. Death results from paralyzed tongue or pharyngeal muscles occluding the airway, from paralysis of the diaphragm and intercostal muscles, or from secondary complications. Fulminant forms may resemble the sudden infant death syndrome (SIDS or crib death). The age distribution rises rapidly after the first week of life, peaking at 1 to 2 months and gradually subsiding, with only a small number of cases occurring beyond the age of 6 months. Most adult cases of this form of the disease occur in compromised persons after recent gastrointestinal surgery coupled with perioperative antibiotic therapy.

The neurologic diseases most frequently confused with botulism are myasthenia gravis, Guillain-Barré syndrome, and cerebrovascular accidents.

Laboratory Diagnosis

The rapid diagnosis of botulism and the early establishment of the type of botulinum toxin affecting the patient are crucial. Unfortunately, however, the disease is difficult to diagnose because at its onset the symptoms of botulism are often confused with the symptoms of other diseases and because few physicians are familiar with the disease. Diagnosis in an isolated case may be extremely difficult, and by the time the nature of the disease is apparent it is usually too late for therapy.

As soon as botulism is suspected on clinical grounds, a specimen of the patient's blood should be drawn immediately and allowed to clot. Specimens of stool and gastric washings should also be obtained if possible. The State Health Department should be immediately contacted for assistance in microbiologic diagnosis and for release of antitoxin for treatment.* Collected specimens should be refrigerated until arrangements are made to send them by air express to the reference laboratory in Atlanta. If at all possible, the original food specimen should be obtained for similar study, but all

* If a representative of the State Health Department cannot be reached, the Centers for Disease Control in Atlanta, Ga. should be contacted. Telephone (404) 329-2888 (24 hours).

too frequently the ingested food has been discarded. Since it is imperative to begin specific treatment as quickly as possible, the diagnosis must be made clinically and then confirmed by laboratory methods.

Infant botulism has presented a problem in diagnosis since the toxin is usually not detectable in the patient's serum. Diagnosis rests on identification of the toxin or isolation of the organism from the stool. Isolation of the organism has been facilitated by recognition that *C. botulinum* is resistant to cycloserine, sulfamethoxazole, and trimethoprim. Addition of these agents to an egg yolk agar medium has provided a selective tool for its isolation. Rapid identification of colonies producing toxin is accomplished by the ELISA technique.

Electromyography also may provide supporting information, as it can demonstrate a characteristic finding of abundant brief small-amplitude motor unit potentials.

Treatment

The treatment of botulism leaves much to be desired. Immediate administration of antitoxin has been the cornerstone of therapy for adult botulism, but its efficacy, especially in well-developed cases of neuroparalytic disease, has been questioned. Antitoxin in the type E syndrome, however, has received enthusiastic reports. The presently used antitoxin (polyvalent A, B, E available through the Centers for Disease Control) is of equine origin and thus carries the risk of potential side effects of immediate anaphylaxis and serum sickness. Skin testing for hypersensitivity to horse serum must be performed before administration of the antitoxin. In addition to antitoxin, the physiologic support of the patient is critical; this calls for management in an intensive care unit where the support of respiratory, cardiovascular, and renal services is available. Saline enemas have been recommended. Other therapeutic considerations include guanidine hydrochloride, which enhances acetylcholine release. Variable success has been encountered with the use of this agent, but caution is required in its use because of potentially serious side effects. Experimentally, aminopyridines have given interesting results in animal models and may provide clinically useful drugs in the future. Unless there are infectious complications, antibiotics are not recommended. There is one report of aminoglycoside potentiation of the paralytic effects of botulism.

Prevention

Although existing preventive measures for the control of botulism are simple and effective when properly carried out, the fact that a number of outbreaks still occur each year indicates the need for improved methods of control. The homemaker should be alerted to the necessity of using sterilized containers and pressure cookers in the canning of all foods so as to kill any *C. botulinum* spores that may be on the food. Also, before any home-canned food is eaten it should be boiled for 1 minute or heated at 80C for 5 minutes to destroy any toxin that might have been produced in the anaerobic environment provided.

The safety record of the canning industry during the past 40 years has been impressive. Unfortunately, however, minor breaks in technique do occur, and unless rigid controls are constantly monitored, there will continue to be sporadic outbreaks. A bulging or defective can should be discarded immediately.

Because botulism is a relatively rare disease, immunization of the entire population is impractical. An effective toxoid is available, however, for laboratory workers in high-risk situations. The recommended schedule for the establishment of active immunity in humans is two injections of toxoid, either absorbed on aluminum sulfate or mixed with an equal volume of Freund's adjuvant, given at 0 and at 10 weeks, with a booster injection 52 weeks later.

Economically, botulism in animals is a very important disease, causing the death of many thousands of animals and birds each year. For range cattle, immunization with toxoid is the most practical method for prevention. In addition, lamziekte in cattle may be controlled by keeping the feeding area free of carcasses and by providing a diet adequate in phosphorus. Botulism in sheep can be prevented by supplementing the diet with carbohydrates and protein. Forage poisoning in cattle and horses may be prevented by keeping food and bedding free of carcasses of small animals.

FURTHER READING

Books and Reviews

HISTOTOXIC AND ENTEROTOXIC CLOSTRIDIA

Balows A, DeHaan RM, Dowell VR Jr, et al (eds): Anaerobic Bacteria—Role in Disease. Springfield, Ill, Charles C Thomas, 1974

George WL, Sutter VL, Finegold SM: Antimicrobial agent–induced diarrhea—A bacterial disease. J Infect Dis 136:822, 1977

Hill EO: The genus *Clostridium* (medical aspects). In Starr MP, Stolp H, Truper HG, et al (eds): The Prokaryotes: A Handbook on Habitats, Isolation, and Identification of Bacteria. New York, Springer-Verlag, 1981, p 1756

Holdeman LV, Moore WEC: Anaerobic Bacteriology Manual, ed 4. Anaerobe Laboratory, Blacksburg, Virginia Polytechnic Institute and State University, 1977

Holt JG, Sneath PHA, Mair NS, et al (eds): Bergey's Manual of Systematic Bacteriology, vol 2. Baltimore, Williams & Wilkins, 1986

Kadis S, Montie TC, Ajl SJ (eds): Microbial Toxins. Bacterial Protein Toxins, vol IIA. New York, Academic Press, 1971

Lennette EH, Balows A, Hausler WJ Jr, et al: Manual of Clinical Microbiology, ed 4. Washington DC, American Society for Microbiology, 1985

Lyerly DM, Krivan HC, Wilkins TD: *Clostridium difficile:* Its disease and toxins. Clin Microbiol Rev 1:1, 1988

MacLennan JD: The histotoxic clostridial infections of man. Bacteriol Rev 26:177, 1962

Rolfe RD: Diagnosis of *Clostridium difficile*–associated intestinal disease. CRC Crit Rev Clin Lab Sci 24:235, 1986

Smith LDS: The Pathogenic Anaerobic Bacteria, ed 3. Springfield, Ill, Charles C Thomas, 1984

Sutter VL, Citron DM, Edelstein MAC, et al: Wadsworth Anaerobic Bacteriology Manual, ed 4. Belmont, Calif, Star Publishing, 1985

Willis AT: Clostridia of Wound Infection. London, Butterworth, 1969

Clostridium tetani

Bizzini B: Tetanus Toxin. Bacteriol Rev 43:224, 1979

Dowell VR Jr: Botulism and tetanus: Selected epidemiologic and microbiologic aspects. Rev Infect Dis 6 (suppl 1):202, 1984

Schofield F: Selective primary health care: Strategies for control of disease in the developing world. XXII. Tetanus: A preventable problem. Rev Infect Dis 8:144, 1986

Simpson LL: Molecular pharmacology of botulinum toxin and tetanus toxin. Ann Rev Pharmacol 26:427, 1986

Smith LD, Holdeman LV: The Pathogenic Anaerobic Bacteria. Springfield, Ill, Charles C Thomas, 1968

Stanfield JP, Galazka A: Neonatal tetanus in the world today. Bull WHO 62:647, 1984

Van Heyningen S: Tetanus toxin. Pharmacol Ther 11:141, 1980

Veronesi R: Tetanus—Important New Concepts. Amsterdam, Excerpta Medica, 1981

Willis AT: Clostridia of Wound Infections. London, Butterworths, 1969

Clostridium botulinum

Arnon SS, Damus K, Chin J: Infant botulism: Epidemiology and relation to sudden infant death syndrome. Epidemiol Rev 3:45, 1981

Feldman RA (ed): A seminar on infant botulism. Rev Infect Dis 1:607, 1979

Lewis GE Jr (ed): Biomedical Aspects of Botulism. New York, Academic Press, 1981

Simpson LL: Botulinum Neurotoxin and Tetanus Toxin. New York, Academic Press, 1989

Simpson LL: Molecular pharmacology of botulinum toxin and tetanus toxin. Ann Rev Pharmacol Toxicol 26:427, 1986

Smith LDS: Botulism. Springfield, Ill, Charles C Thomas, 1977

Sugiyama H: *Clostridium botulinum* neurotoxin. Microbiol Rev 44:419, 1980

Selected Papers

HISTOTOXIC AND ENTEROTOXIC CLOSTRIDIA

Alpern BJ, Dowell VR Jr: *Clostridium septicum* infections and malignancy. JAMA 209:385, 1969

Altemeier WA, Fuller WD: Prevention and treatment of gas gangrene. JAMA 217:806, 1971

Aronsson B, Mollby R, Nord CE: Antimicrobial agents and *Clostridium difficile* in acute enteric disease: Epidemiological data from Sweden, 1980–1982. J Infect Dis 151:476, 1985

Aronsson B, Mollby R, Nord CE: Occurrence of toxin-producing *Clostridium difficile* in antibiotic-associated diarrhea in Sweden. Med Microbiol Immunol (Berl) 170:27, 1981

Bartlett JG, Gorbach SL: Pseudomembranous enterocolitis (antibiotic-related colitis). Adv Intern Med 22:455, 1977

Brown RA, Fekety R Jr, Silva J Jr, et al: The protective effect of vancomycin on clindamycin-induced colitis in hamsters. Johns Hopkins Med J 141:183, 1977

Cato EP, Hash DE, Holdeman LV, et al: Electrophoretic study of *Clostridium* species. J Clin Microbiol 15:688, 1982

Cato EP, Holdeman LV, Moore WEC: *Clostridium perenne* and *Clostridium paraperfringens:* Later subjective synonyms of *Clostridium barati.* Int J Syst Bacteriol 32:77, 1982

Dasgupta BR, Pariza MW: Purification of two *Clostridium perfringens* enterotoxin-like proteins and their effects on membrane permeability in primary cultures of adult rat hepatocytes. Infect Immun 38:592, 1982

Delmee M, Homel M, Wauters G: Serogrouping of *Clostridium difficile* strains by slide agglutination. J Clin Microbiol 21:323, 1985

Eklung MW, Poysky FT, Meyers JA, et al: Interspecies conversion of *Clostridium botulinum* type C to *Clostridium novyi* type A by bacteriophage. Science 186:456, 1974

George WL, Rolfe RD, Finegold SM: *Clostridium difficile* and its cytotoxin in feces of patients with antimicrobial agent–associated diarrhea and miscellaneous conditions. J Clin Microbiol 15:1049, 1982

George WL, Sutter VL, Citron D, et al: Selective and differential medium for isolation of *Clostridium difficile.* J Clin Microbiol 9:214, 1979

Hauschild AHW, Nolo L, Dorward WJ: The role of enterotoxin in *Clostridium perfringens* type A enteritis. Can J Microbiol 17:987, 1971

Hobbs BC, Smith ME, Oakley CL, et al: *Clostridium welchii* food poisoning. J Hyg (Lond) 51:75, 1953

Holland JA, Hill GB, Wolfe WG, et al: Experimental and clinical experience with hyperbaric oxygen in the treatment of clostridial myonecrosis. Surgery 77:75, 1975

Holst E, Helin I, Mardh PA: Recovery of *Clostridium difficile* from children. Scand J Infect Dis 13:41, 1981

Jackson SG, Yip-Chuck DA, Brodsky MH: Evaluation of the diagnostic application of an enzyme immunoassay for *Clostridium perfringens* type A enterotoxin. Appl Environ Microbiol 52:969, 1986

Kim KH, Fekety R, Batts DH, et al: Isolation of *Clostridium difficile* from the environment and contacts of patients with antibiotic-associated colitis. J Infect Dis 143:42, 1981

Libby JM, Jortner BS, Wilkins TD: Effects of the two toxins of *Clostridium difficile* in antibiotic-associated cecitis in hamsters. Infect Immun 36:822, 1982

Lyerly DM, Lockwood DE, Richardson SH, et al: Biological activities of toxins A and B of *Clostridium difficile.* Infect Immun 35:1147, 1982

Lyerly DM, Sullivan NM, Wilkins TD: Enzyme-linked immunosorbent assay for *Clostridium difficile* toxin A. J Clin Microbiol 17:72, 1983

Macfarlane MG: On the biochemical mechanism of action of gas gangrene toxins. Symp Soc Gen Microbiol 5:57, 1955

Macfarlane MG, Knight BCJG: The biochemistry of bacterial toxins. I. The lecithinase activity of *C. welchii* toxins. Biochem J 35:884, 1941

Marrie TJ, Haldane EV, Swantee CA, et al: Susceptibility of anaerobic bacteria to nine antimicrobial agents and demonstration of decreased susceptibility of *Clostridium perfringens* to penicillin. Antimicrob Agents Chemother 19:51, 1981

Nguyen VK, Rihn B, Heckel C, et al: Enzyme immunoassay (ELISA) for detection of *Clostridium difficile* toxin B in specimens of faeces. J Med Microbiol 31:251, 1990

Pierce PF Jr, Wilson R, Silva J Jr, et al: Antibiotic-associated pseudomembranous colitis: An epidemiologic investigation of a cluster of cases. J Infect Dis 145:269, 1982

Popoff MR, Guillou JP, Carlier JP: Taxonomic position of lecithinase-negative strains of *Clostridium sordellii.* J Gen Microbiol 131:1697, 1985

Pothoulakis C, Sullivan R, Melnick DA, et al: *Clostridium difficile* toxin A stimulates intracellular calcium release and chemotactic response in human granulocytes. J Clin Invest 81:1741, 1988

Roggentin P, Gutschker-Gdaniec G, Schauer R, et al: Correlative properties for a differentiation of two *Clostridium sordellii* phenotypes and their distinction from *Clostridium bifermentans.* Zentralbl Bakteriol Mikrobiol Hyg [A] 260:319, 1985

Rolfe RD, Helebian S, Finegold SM: Bacterial interference between *Clostridium difficile* and normal fecal flora. J Infect Dis 143:470, 1981

Sherertz RJ, Sarubbi FA: The prevalence of *Clostridium difficile* and toxin in a nursery population: A comparison between patients with necrotizing enterocolitis and an asymptomatic group. J Pediatr 100:435, 1982

Speirs G, Warren RE, Rampling A: *Clostridium tertium* septicemia in patients with neutropenia. J Infect Dis 158:1336, 1988

Stern M, Warrock GH: The types of *Clostridium perfringens.* J Pathol Bacteriol 88:279, 1964

Stevens DL, Mitten J, Henry C: Effects of α and θ toxins from *Clostridium perfringens* on human polymorphonuclear leukocytes. J Infect Dis 156:324, 1987

Stevens DL, Troyer BE, Merrick DT, et al: Lethal effects and cardiovascular effects of purified α- and θ-toxins from *Clostridium perfringens.* J Infect Dis 157:272, 1988

Tabaqchali S, O'Farrell S, Nash JQ, et al: Vaginal carriage and neonatal acquisition of *Clostridium difficile.* J Med Microbiol 18:47, 1984

Taylor NS, Thorne GM, Bartlett JG: Comparison of two toxins produced by *Clostridium difficile.* Infect Immun 34:1036, 1981

Thaler M, Gill V, Pizzo PA: Emergence of *Clostridium tertium* as a pathogen in neutropenic patients. Am J Med 81:596, 1986

Viscidi R, Willey S, Bartlett JG: Isolation rates and toxigenic potential of *Clostridium difficile* isolates from various patient populations. Gastroenterology 81:5, 1981

Walker PD, Murrell TGC, Nagy LK: Scanning electronmicroscopy of the jejunum in enteritis necroticans. J Med Microbiol 13:445, 1980

Walker RC, Ruane PJ, Rosenblatt JE, et al: Comparison of culture, cytotoxicity assays, and enzyme-linked immunosorbent assay for toxin A and toxin B in the diagnosis of *Clostridium difficile*–related enteric disease. Diagn Microbiol Infect Dis 5:61, 1986

Clostridium tetani

Black RE, Huber DH, Curlin GT: Reduction in neonatal tetanus by mass immunization of non-pregnant women: Duration of protection provided by one and two doses of aluminum adsorbed tetanus toxoid. Bull WHO 58:927, 1980

Centers for Disease Control, Immunization Practices Advisory Committee: Diphtheria, tetanus, and pertussis: Guidelines for vaccine prophylaxis and other preventive measures. Ann Intern Med 103:896, 1985

Centers for Disease Control: Tetanus—United States, 1985–86. MMWR 36:477, 1987

Crutchley DR, Habig WH, Fishman PH: Re-evaluation of the role of gangliosides as receptors for tetanus toxin. J Neurochem 47:213, 1986

Edsall G, Elliott MW, Peebles TC, Levine L, Eldred MC: Excessive use of toxoid boosters. JAMA 202:17, 1967

Eisel U, Jarsch W, Goretzki K: Tetanus toxin: Primary structure, expression in *E. coli* and homology with botulinum toxins. EMBO J 5:2495, 1986

Erdman G, Hanauske A, Wellhouer HH: Intraspinal distribution and reaction to grey matter with tetanus toxin of intracisternally injected anti-tetanus toxin F(ab')2 fragments. Brain Res 211:367, 1980

Halpern JL, Habig WH, Neale EA, Stibitz S: Cloning and expression of functional fragment C of tetanus toxin. Infect Immun 58:1004, 1990

Halpern JL, Smith LA, Seamon KB, et al: Sequence homology between tetanus and botulinum toxins detected by an antipeptide antibody. Infect Immun 57:18, 1989

Helting TB, Zwisler O: Structure of tetanus toxin. I. Breakdown of the toxin molecule and discrimination between polypeptide fragments. J Biol Chem 252:187, 1977

Helting TB, Zwisler O, Wiegandt H: Structure of tetanus toxin. II. Toxin binding to ganglioside. J Biol Chem 252:194, 1977

Hortnagel H, Brucke T, Hackl JM: The involvement of the sympathetic nervous system in tetanus. Klin Wochenschr 57:383, 1979

Laird WJ, Aaronson W, Silver RP, Habig WH, Hardegree MC: Plasmid associated toxigenicity in *Clostridium tetani.* J Infect Dis 142:623, 1980

Lin CS, Habig WH, Hardegree MC: Antibodies against the light chain of tetanus toxin in human sera. Infect Immun 49:111, 1985

Matsuda M, Lei D-L, Sugimoto N, et al: Isolation, purification, and characterization of fragment B, the NH_2-terminal half of the heavy chain of tetanus toxin. Infect Immun 57:3588, 1989

Mellanby J, Green J: How does tetanus toxin act? Neuroscience 6:281, 1981

Murphy SG, Miller KD: Tetanus toxin and antigenic derivatives. I. Purification of the biologically active monomer. J Bacteriol 94:580, 586, 1967

Olsen KM, Hiller FC: Management of tetanus. Clin Pharmacol 6:570, 1987

Price DL, Griffin J, Young A, et al: Tetanus toxin: Direct evidence for retrograde intraaxonal transport. Science 188:945, 1975

Robinson JP, Picklesimer JB, Puett D: Tetanus toxin—Effect of chemical modifications on toxicity, immunogenicity, and conformation. J Biol Chem 250:7435, 1975

Ruben FL, Nagel J, Fireman P: Antitoxin response in the elderly to tetanus-diphtheria (Td) immunization. Am J Public Health 108:145, 1978

Schiavo G, Papini E, Genna G, Montecucco C: An intact interchain disulfide bond is required for the neurotoxicity of tetanus toxin. Infect Immun 58:4136, 1990

Van Heyningen S: Binding of ganglioside by the chains of tetanus toxin. FEBS Lett 68:5, 1976

Volk WA, Bizzini B, Snyder RM, et al: Neutralization of tetanus toxin by distinct monoclonal antibodies binding to multiple epitopes on the toxin molecule. Infect Immun 45:604, 1984

Zacks SI, Sheff MF: Tetanus toxin: Fine structure localization of binding sites in striated muscle. Science 159:643, 1968

Clostridium botulinum

Aktories K, Wegner A: ADP-ribosylation of actin by clostridial toxins. J Cell Biol 109:1385, 1989

Arnon SS: Infant botulism: Anticipating the second decade. J Infect Dis 154:201, 1986

Arnon SS, Midura TF, Clay SA, et al: Infant botulism: epidemiological, clinical, and laboratory aspects. JAMA 237:1946, 1977

Arnon SS, Midura TF, Damus K, et al: Honey and other environmental factors for infant botulism. J Pediatr 94:331, 1979

Aureli P, Fenicia L, Pasolini B, et al: Two cases of type E infant botulism caused by neurotoxigenic *Clostridium butyricum* in Italy. J Infect Dis 154:207, 1986

Bandyopadhyay S, Clark AW, DasGupta BR, Sathyamoorthy V: Role of the heavy and light chains of botulinum neurotoxin in neuromuscular paralysis. J Biol Chem 262:2660, 1987

Black JD, Dolly JO: Interaction of 125-I-labeled botulinum neurotoxins with nerve terminals. I. Ultrastructural audioradiographic localization and quantitation of distinct membrane acceptors for types A and B on motor nerves. J Cell Biol 103:521, 1986

Boroff DA, Nyberg S, Hoglund S: Electron microscopy of the toxin and hemagglutinin of type A *Clostridium botulinum.* Infect Immun 6:1003, 1972

Boroff DA, Reilly JRV: Prophylactic immunization of pheasants and ducks against avian botulism. J Bacteriol 77:142, 1959

Boroff DA, Shu-Chen G: Radioimmunoassay for type A toxin of *Clostridium botulinum.* Appl Microbiol 25:545, 1973

Bott TL, Johnson J Jr, Foster EM, Sugiyama H: Possible origin of high incidence of *Clostridium botulinum* type E in an inland bay (Green Bay of Lake Michigan). J Bacteriol 95:1542, 1968

Cardella MA, Duff JT, Wingfield BH, Gottfried C: VI. Purification and detoxification of type D toxin and immunologic response to toxoid. J Bacteriol 79:372, 1960

Chia JK, Clark JB, Ryan CA, Pollack M: Botulism in an adult associated with food-borne intestinal infection with *Clostridium botulinum.* N Engl J Med 315:239, 1986

Craig JM, Pilcher KS: *Clostridium botulinum* type F isolated from salmon from the Columbia River. Science 153:311, 1966

DasGupta BR, Sugiyama H: Molecular forms of neurotoxins in proteolytic *Clostridium botulinum* type B cultures. Infect Immun 14:680, 1976

Dezfulian M, Dowell VR: Cultural and physiological characteristics and antimicrobial susceptibility of *Clostridium botulinum* isolates from food-borne and infant botulism cases. J Clin Microbiol 11:604, 1980

Eklund MW, Poysky FT: Interconversion of type C and D strains of *Clostridium botulinum* by specific bacteriophages. Appl Microbiol 27:251, 1974

Eklund MW, Poysky FT, Reed SM, Smith CA: Bacteriophage and the toxigenicity of *Clostridium botulinum* type C. Science 172:480, 1971

Kitamura M, Iwamori M, Nagai Y: Interaction of *Clostridium botulinum* neurotoxin and gangliosides. Biochem Biophys Acta 628:328, 1980

Kozaki S, Kamata Y, Nagai T, et al: The use of monoclonal antibodies to analyze the structure of *Clostridium botulinum* type E derivative toxin. Infect Immun 52:786, 1986

Kozaki S, Miki A, Kamata Y, et al: Immunological characterization of papain-induced fragments of *Clostridium botulinum* type A neurotoxin and interaction of the fragments with brain synaptosomes. Infect Immun 57:2634, 1989

Kozaki S, Miyazaki S, Sakaguchi G: Development of antitoxin with each of two complementary fragments of *Clostridium botulinum* type B derivative toxin. Infect Immun 18:761, 1977

MacDonald KL, Cohen ML, Blake PA: The changing epidemiology of adult botulism in the United States. Am J Epidemiol 124:794, 1986

Merson MH, Dowell VR: Epidemiologic, clinical and laboratory aspects of wound botulism. N Engl J Med 289:1005, 1973

Miyazaki S, Iwasaki M, Sakaguchi G: *Clostridium botulinum* type D toxin: Purification, molecular structure, and some immunological properties. Infect Immun 17:395, 1977

Oguma K: Stability of toxigenicity in *Clostridium botulinum* type C and type D. J Gen Microbiol 92:67, 1976

Ohishi I: Response of mouse intestinal loop to botulinum C_2 toxin: Enterotoxic activity induced by cooperation of nonlinked protein components. Infect Immun 40:691, 1983

Ohishi I, Sakaguchi G: Activation of botulinum toxins in the absence of nicking. Infect Immun 17:402, 1977

Pickett J, Berg B, Chaplain E, Brunsletter-Shafer MA: Syndrome of botulism in infancy: Clinical and electrophysiologic study. N Engl J Med 295:770, 1976

Sathyamoorthy V, Dasgupta BR: Separation, purification, partial characterization and comparison of the heavy and light chains of botulinum neurotoxin types A, B, and E. J Biol Chem 260:10461, 1985

Scott AB: Botulinum toxin injection into extraocular muscles as an alternative to strabismus surgery. Ophthalmology 87:1044, 1980

Simpson LL, Schmidt JJ, Middlebrook JL: Isolation and characterization of the botulinum neurotoxins. Methods Enzymol 165:76, 1988

Tacket CO, Shandera WX, Mann JM, et al: Equine antitoxin use and other factors that predict outcome in type A foodborne botulism. Am J Med 76:794, 1984

Takagi A, Kawata T, Yamamoto S: Electron microscope studies on ultrathin sections of spores of the *Clostridium* group with special reference to the sporulation and germination process. J Bacteriol 80:37, 1960

Terranova W, Breman JG, Lacey RP, Speck S: Botulism type B: Epidemiologic aspects of an extensive outbreak. Am J Epidemiol 108:150, 1978

Tsuzuki K, Kimura K, Fujii N, et al: Cloning and complete nucleotide sequence of the gene for the main component of hemagglutinin produced by *Clostridium botulinum* type C. Infect Immun 58:3173, 1990

Wainwright RB, Heyward WL, Middaugh JP, et al: Food-borne botulism in Alaska, 1947–1985: Epidemiology and clinical findings. J Infect Dis 157:1158, 1988

Williams-Walls NJ: Type E botulism isolated from fish and crabs. Science 162:375, 1968

Wonnacott S, Marchbanks RM: Inhibition by botulinum toxin of depolarization-evoked release of (^{14}C)acetylcholine from synaptosomes in vitro. Biochem J 156:701, 1976

CHAPTER 45

The Spirochetes

Spirochaetales

The spirochetes are motile, slender, helically coiled, flexible organisms with one or more complete turns in the helix. They are gram-negative and are 0.1 to 3.0 μm wide and 5 to 250 μm in length. Multiplication is by transverse fission. Their most distinctive morphologic property is the presence of axial fibrils (also referred to as axial filaments, periplasmic flagella, and endoflagella), which are wound around the helical protoplasmic cylinder and are encased in an outer sheath. These fibrils are believed to be responsible for locomotion of the organisms, but the mechanism is not clear. Cellular motility includes rapid rotation around the long axis, flexation of cells, and locomotion along a helical path. Unlike other flagellated bacteria, spirochetes are locomotory even in environments of high viscosity.

TABLE 45–1. PROPERTIES OF THE FAMILIES OF THE ORDER SPIROCHAETALES

Property	Spirochaetaceae	Leptospiraceae
Cell diameter	0.1–3.0 μm	0.1 μm
Cell hooked at end	−	+
Diamino acid in peptidoglycan	L-ornithine	Diaminopimelic acid
Metabolism	Anaerobic, facultatively anaerobic, or microaerophilic	Aerobic
Carbon and energy source	Carbohydrates and/or amino acids	Long-chain fatty acids or alcohols
Genera	*Spirochaeta, Cristispira, Treponema, Borrelia*	*Leptospira*

Taxonomy. Spirochetes belong to the order Spirochaetales, which contains two families, Spirochaetaceae and Leptospiraceae. Some members of both families are free-living in soil, freshwater, or marine habitats, whereas others are parasitic and may be pathogenic for humans and animals. Morphologic and physiologic differences between the two families are listed in Table 45–1. Of the four genera in the family Spirochaetaceae, only *Treponema* and *Borrelia* contain species that cause major human illness. The family Leptospiraceae contains a single genus, *Leptospira*. *Leptospira interrogans* is the only species in this genus that is pathogenic for humans.

The three *Treponema* species that are pathogenic for humans have not been cultured in vitro. *Treponema pallidum* is the cause of venereal and endemic syphilis (Table 45–2). *Treponema pertenue* causes yaws, and *Treponema carateum* is the cause of pinta. Differentiation of these pathogenic *Treponema* species is difficult and is based solely on mode of infection, severity of infection, and infectivity for laboratory animals. *Bergey's Manual of Systematic Bacteriology* has recently changed the treponemal nomenclature of the human species to reflect their relatedness. *T. pallidum* is now termed *T. pallidum* subspecies *pallidum; T. pertenue* is now termed *T. pallidum* subspecies *pertenue;* and the new term *T. pallidum* subspecies *endemicum* has been given to the *T. pallidum* variant associated with endemic syphilis. In this chapter, however, the older, more familiar terminology will be adhered to. In addition to these pathogenic, nonculturable *Treponema* species, a number of culturable treponemes have been identified as part of the normal flora of the oral cavity and genital tract. They are seldom major human pathogens, but some may cause disease of the oral cavity.

TABLE 45–2. TREPONEMAL SPECIES PATHOGENIC FOR HUMANS

Organism	Human Disease	Differentiating Characteristics
T. pallidum	Syphilis	Cutaneous lesions in rabbits
	Endemic syphilis	No cutaneous lesions in hamsters or guinea pigs
T. pertenue	Yaws	Cutaneous lesions in rabbits and hamsters; no cutaneous lesions in guinea pigs
T. carateum	Pinta	No cutaneous lesions in rabbits, hamsters, or guinea pigs

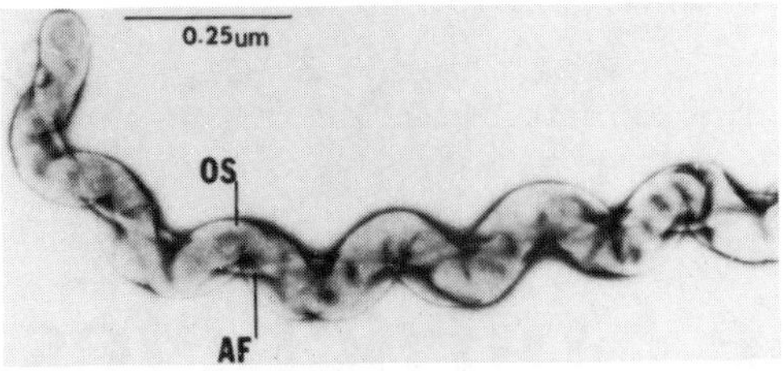

Fig. 45–1. *Leptospira interrogans*, showing regular, tight coils and hooked end. The outer sheath (OS) and axial fibrils (AF) are indicated. *(From Holt: Microbiol Rev 42:114, 1978.)*

Borrelia species cause endemic and relapsing fever in humans, as well as the recently recognized syndrome Lyme disease. Methods for the speciation of *Borrelia* are primitive and are based on the arthropod vector with which they are associated. Many have been cultured on complex media. Unlike *Treponema* and *Leptospira, Borrelia* species stain readily and can be observed with conventional microscopy. *Leptospira* species cause human and animal leptospirosis and are characterized by their motion, hooking or bending of one or both ends, and the presence of two fibrils that do not cross at the midsection. There are two recognized species, *Leptospira interrogans* and *Leptospira biflexa. L. interrogans* includes known human and animal pathogens, whereas *L. biflexa* includes free-living saprophytes.

Ultrastructure. The basic cellular components of a spirochetal cell are the outer sheath that encompasses the cell, the axial fibril, and the protoplasmic cylinder, which includes the cell wall, cell membrane, and the enclosed cytoplasmic contents (Fig. 45–1). The outer sheath appears to be a unit membrane, which may be separated from the cell for examination by electron microscopy. The structure of the outer membrane varies from one species to another and also may be altered by fixation techniques. Although the precise chemical composition is uncertain, carbohydrates, proteins, and phospholipids are present. The function of the outer sheath is not known, but in *Leptospira interrogans canicola,* the outer sheath is immunogenic and antibodies to it may be protective.

The axial fibril is morphologically similar to a flagellum. In spite of this similarity, however, an unequivocal role in motility has not been demonstrated. The axial fibril consists of a shaft and its covering sheath and an insertion apparatus. The shaft resembles a bacterial flagellum in substructure and is composed entirely of protein. It lies between the outer sheath and the outermost layer of the protoplasmic cylinder and is, therefore, an internal structure of the bacterium. One or more axial fibrils wind around the protoplasmic cylinder and may overlap at the center of the cell in *Treponema* and *Borrelia,* but not in *Leptospira.* The diameter of the axial fibril

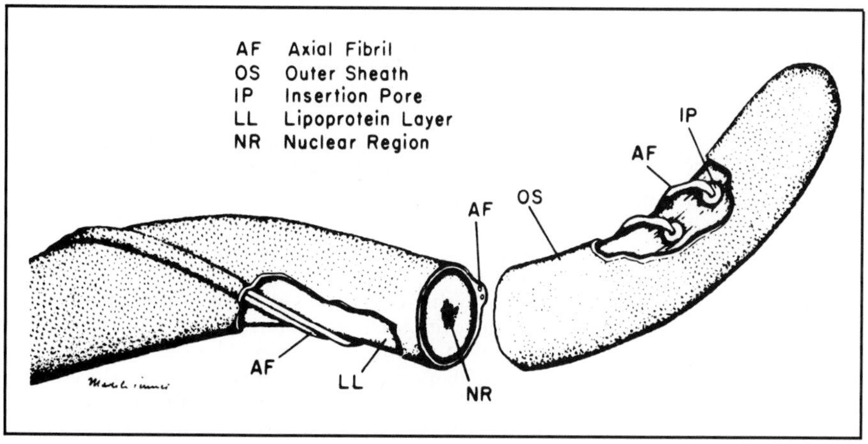

Fig. 45–2. Diagrammatic representation of a typical spirochete as interpreted from electron micrographs. An outer sheath envelops the cell. The axial fibrils are between the outer sheath and layers of the protoplasmic cylinder (seen here as lipoprotein layers) and insert into the cylinder by way of an insertion pore. *(From Holt: Microbiol Rev 42:114, 1978.)*

in most species of Spirochaetales is approximately 15 to 20 μm. The sheath covering the shaft of the axial filament often appears to have a striated substructure (Fig. 45–2). The number of axial fibrils per cell end is a morphologic characteristic of each species; for *Treponema* that are pathogenic for humans the number is 3, it varies for *Borrelia* from 7 to 30, and for *Leptospira* it is 1.

The insertion apparatus of the axial fibril consists of a proximal hook and insertion discs. The proximal hook is an extension of the shaft and bends sharply toward and into the protoplasmic cylinder. The insertion discs are platelike structures, approximately 20 to 40 μm in diameter, which are inserted into a hole or depression near the end of the cell (Fig. 45–3). The number of insertion discs varies depending on the genus, *Leptospira* having three to five, *Borrelia* having two, and *Treponema* having one.

The protoplasmic cylinder lies directly beneath the outer envelope and consists of the cytoplasmic membrane and cell wall. The cell wall–cell membrane complex is similar to that of other gram-negative bacteria, consisting of two electron-dense layers separated by an electron-transparent layer. The cell wall of *Treponema* and *Borrelia* species contains ornithine in the peptidoglycan component, whereas *Leptospira* contain diaminopimelic acid.

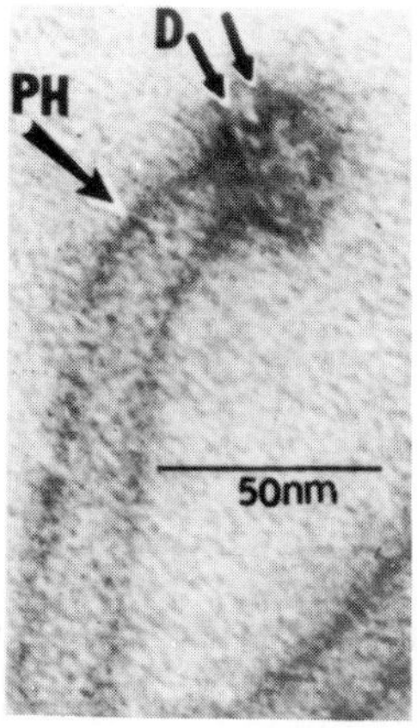

Fig. 45–3. Spirochetal axial fibrils that are seen to be continuous with the proximal hook (PH), which terminate with the insertion disks (D). *(From Holt: Microbiol Rev 42:114, 1978.)*

Treponema pallidum

Morphology and Physiology

The name *Treponema* is derived from the Greek words *trepo* and *nema,* meaning *turning thread.* Individual organisms of *T. pallidum* are 5 to 20 μm in length and 0.09 to 0.5 μm in diameter; the ends are finely tapered. Cells appear to have a flat wave with one or more planes per cell, giving it the appearance of a helical coil. There are 8 to 14 evenly distributed waves per cell. Motility is sluggish, with a drifting motion and graceful, flexuous movements. Motility is most pronounced in an environment of relatively high viscosity.

The structure of *T. pallidum* is in general similar to that of the other Spirochaetaceae and consists of a multilayer cytoplasmic membrane, flagella-like fibrils, the cell wall, and outer sheath (outer cell envelope). Pathogenic *T. pallidum* also have a capsulelike outer coat that is not present in the nonpathogenic species. Most *Treponema* species contain intracytoplasmic microtubules, which extend along the inner layer of the cytoplasmic membrane. These fibrils, which occur in clusters of six to eight, appear to be unique to the genus and have not been demonstrated in other Spirochaetales. Pathogenic *Treponema* have a tapered end, which is oriented toward the host cell surfaces during attachment.

Until recently, *T. pallidum* could not be grown in vitro although it could be maintained for 4 to 7 days at 25C in an anaerobic medium containing albumin, sodium bicarbonate, pyruvate, cysteine, and a bovine serum ultrafiltrate. By use of special tissue culture techniques and a carefully monitored reduced oxygen tension, it has been shown that the organism can multiply through several generations in primary tissue cultures of rabbit epithelial cells. In this system, virulence is maintained but the organisms have not been passed in subculture. Virulent strains (e.g., the Nichols strain) are propagated by intratesticular inoculation of rabbits. Primary and secondary infections in the rabbit are similar to human infections. In experimental chancres in rabbits, the division time of organisms is about 30 hours, and division is by transverse fission.

T. pallidum is microaerophilic and survives for a longer

period of time in an atmosphere of 3% to 5% oxygen. The uptake of oxygen and a functional electron transport system have been demonstrated. Oxygen uptake is glucose dependent, and the oxidation of pyruvate occurs only when oxygen is present.

Hyaluronidase is produced by pathogenic species of *Treponema,* but there is little additional information on specific virulence determinants of the organism. The inability to continuously cultivate *T. pallidum* in vitro has greatly hampered experimental analyses for study of virulence properties and immunogenic determinants. Several cell surface protein antigens have been identified, as well as a unique class of extracellular protein antigens. Certain of these proteins are among the earliest recognized by IgG antibodies after experimental infection of rabbits with *T. pallidum.* Recombinant DNA technology currently is being applied to the study of these proteins in order to produce sufficient quantities so that their role in pathogenesis and their applicability as vaccinogens or serodiagnostic reagents can be determined.

Clinical Infection

History. Syphilis was first recognized in Europe at the end of the fifteenth century, when the disease first appeared in the Mediterranean areas and rapidly reached epidemic proportions at that time. One theory concerning the origin of syphilis is that it is of New World origin and that Columbus's crew acquired syphilis while in the West Indies and introduced it into Spain upon their return. Alternatively, the disease that had been endemic for centuries in Africa may have been transported to Europe at that time during the migration of armies and civilian populations. The relatively benign African diseases, yaws and bejel, may have been transformed in the susceptible population of Europe into a highly virulent disease with high mortality rates.

Syphilis initially was called the *Italian disease,* the *French disease,* and the *great pox* as distinguished from smallpox. Its venereal transmission was not recognized until the eighteenth century. Delineation of the characteristics of syphilis was hindered by confusion of its symptoms with those of gonorrhea. In 1767, John Hunter, a great English experimental biologist and physician, inoculated himself with uretheral exudate from a patient with gonorrhea. Unfortunately, the patient also had syphilis, and the subsequent symptoms experienced by Hunter convinced two generations of physicians of the unity of gonorrhea and syphilis. The separate nature of gonorrhea and syphilis was demonstrated in 1838 by Ricord, who reported his observations on more than 2500 human inoculations. Recognition of the stages of syphilis followed, and in 1905 Schaudinn and Hoffman discovered the causative agent. The following year Wassermann introduced the diagnostic serologic test that bears his name.

Epidemiology

Syphilis is not a highly contagious disease; a person who has had sexual contact with an infected partner has approximately one chance in 10 of acquiring disease. The disease also has a relatively long incubation period during which time the contact is noninfectious. For these reasons, tracing and treating contacts of persons with infectious forms of syphilis has been an effective means of controlling spread of the disease. However, there has been a sharp recent increase in the number of cases of infectious syphilis. The rate of primary and secondary syphilis in the United States in 1985 was about 14/100,000 population, and more than 25,000 cases were reported. By 1989 the rate was almost 20/100,000, more than 44,000 cases had been reported, and the numbers were continuing to escalate (Fig. 45–4). As is typical of patients with other venereal diseases, persons who acquire syphilis often have had sexual contact with an average of five other persons during the incubation period. The increased rates of infectious syphilis that occurred during the early 1980s were due primarily to male-to-male transmission. There has been a relative decline of infection in the male population and a recent increase among women. The groups that are most significantly affected are drug users; prostitution for drugs or for money to purchase drugs represents the central epidemiologic aspect of the problem.

An increase in the rate of other venereal diseases also has occurred in the same period. For example, in one area of the United States, 8% of persons with gonorrhea also had concomitant syphilis. Because many of these persons with dual diseases are treated in the preprimary stage of syphilis, gonorrhea may never become manifest clinically or serologically.

Transmission

T. pallidum has the capacity to invade the intact mucous membranes or skin in areas of abrasions. Direct inoculation

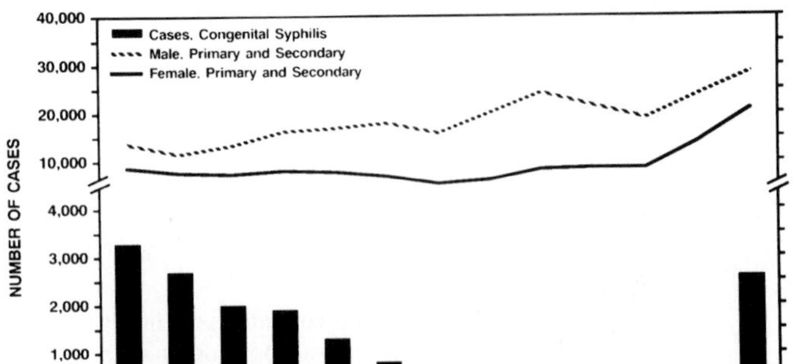

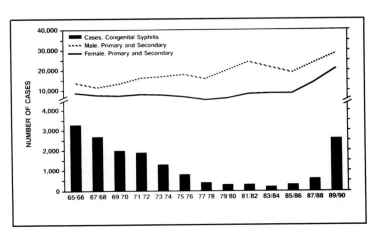

Fig. 45–4. Primary and secondary syphilis and congenital syphilis in the United States, 1965–1990. *(Data from the Centers for Disease Control.)*

from contact with an infected person is necessary for infection inasmuch as survival of the organism outside the host is limited. Sexual contact is the common method of transmission, and the site of inoculation usually is on the genital organs, the vagina or the cervix in females and the penis in males. Other sites include lips, which can be infected by kissing, and other areas of the skin, which can be infected through abrasions. Examining physicians or pathologists may be infected in this way if appropriate barrier protection is not provided.

Pathogenesis

Syphilis is a disease of blood vessels and of the perivascular areas. After invasion the organisms undergo rapid multiplication and are widely disseminated. Spread through the perivascular lymphatics and then the systemic circulation occurs before development of the primary lesion. Ten to ninety days later, but usually within 3 to 4 weeks, the patient manifests an inflammatory response to the infection at the site of the inoculation. The resulting lesion, the chancre, is characterized by profuse shedding of spirochetes; by accumulation of mononuclear leukocytes, lymphocytes, and plasma cells; and by swelling of capillary endothelia. The regional lymph nodes are enlarged, and the cellular infiltrate resembles that of the primary lesion. Resolution of the primary lesion is by fibrosis.

In experimental systems, pathogenic *T. pallidum* may be shown both in vitro and in vivo to attach avidly to a wide range of cell lines and tissue specimens. *Treponema* organisms that attach to cultivated cell lines in vitro have a prolonged survival time. The organisms attach by their tapered ends, as shown in Figure 45–5. They are able to penetrate through the hyaluronic acid–containing extracellular matrix that joins capillary endothelial cells. After attachment of the treponemes, an alteration of host cell membrane properties serves to block attachment of additional organisms. Specific host membrane ligands function as mediators of attachment. Cell surface adherence involves attachment with specific treponemal ligands and is an energy-requiring process. Antibody to the protein fragment that appears to serve as the treponemal ligand for mammalian cell cytadherence will block the organism's adherence to cells. Adherence of treponemes to mammalian cells is potentiated by the coating of the organisms with fibronectin. Fibronectin priming of the treponemes results in greatly enhanced attachment of the organisms to the extracellular matrix or to bound fibronectin. Avirulent strains of *Treponema* species do not attach to cultured cells.

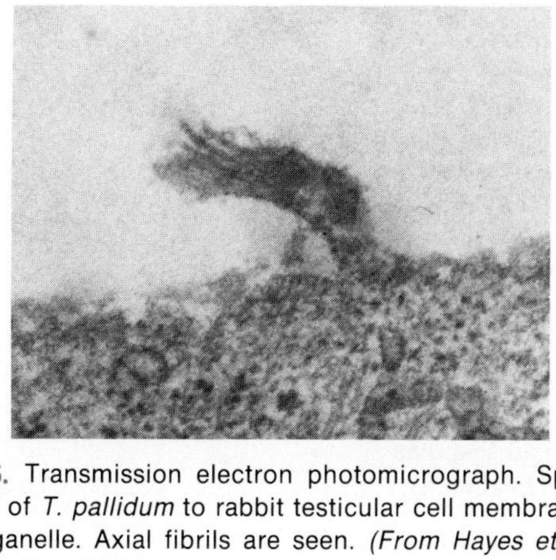

Fig. 45–5. Transmission electron photomicrograph. Specific attachment of *T. pallidum* to rabbit testicular cell membrane by terminal organelle. Axial fibrils are seen. *(From Hayes et al: Infect Immun 17:174, 1977.)*

Secondary lesions develop when tissue of ectodermal origin, such as skin, mucous membranes, and central nervous system, participate in an inflammatory response. Mucous patches in the mouth are due to local vasculitis. The cellular infiltrate resembles that of the primary lesion, with a predominance of plasma cells. There is little or no necrosis, and healing is without scarring but may include pigmentary changes.

Tertiary syphilis may involve any organ system and often is asymmetric. Gummas are lesions typified by extensive necrosis, few giant cells, and paucity of organisms. They commonly occur in internal organs, bone, and skin. The other major form of tertiary lesion—a diffuse chronic inflammation with plasma cells and lymphocytes but without caseation—may result in aneurysm of the aorta, paralytic dementia, or tabes dorsalis. Chronic swelling of the capillary endothelium and fibrosis result in the characteristic tissue changes.

Clinical Manifestations

Primary Disease. The chancre of primary syphilis typically is a single lesion, nontender and firm, with a clean surface, raised border, and reddish color. It may be overlooked by women, in whom it frequently is situated on the cervix or vaginal wall, or by either sex if it is within the anal canal. Systemic signs or symptoms are absent, but the draining lymph nodes frequently are enlarged and nontender.

Secondary Disease. Two to ten weeks after the primary lesion, the patient may experience secondary disease (Fig. 45–6). Prominent findings include fever, sore throat, generalized lymphadenopathy, headache, and rash. Involvement of palms and soles is common, in contradistinction to many other dermatologic conditions. On mucous membranes the lesions may appear as white mucous patches. Condylomata lata occur around moist areas, such as the anus and vagina. All secondary lesions of the skin and mucous membranes are highly infectious.

Other signs of this stage of disease may be secondary to the generalized immunologic response. Nephrotic syndrome with immune complex nephritis results from deposition of antigen-antibody complexes within the glomerular basement membrane. Arthritis and arthralgias may have a similar cause. Involvement of other systems also occurs.

After the last episode of secondary disease, the patient enters the stage of latent disease, the first 4 years of which are considered early latent and the subsequent period late latent. By definition, persons in the late latent stage of disease have no signs or symptoms of active syphilis but remain seroreactive. If therapy for syphilis is first given during this stage, the patient is unlikely to show regression of nontreponemal antibody determinations. Approximately 60% of untreated patients in the late latent stage continue to have a symptom-free course, whereas symptoms of late disease develop in 40%. Progression of disease from late latent to late symptomatic syphilis usually is prevented if appropriate antimicrobial therapy is given at this stage.

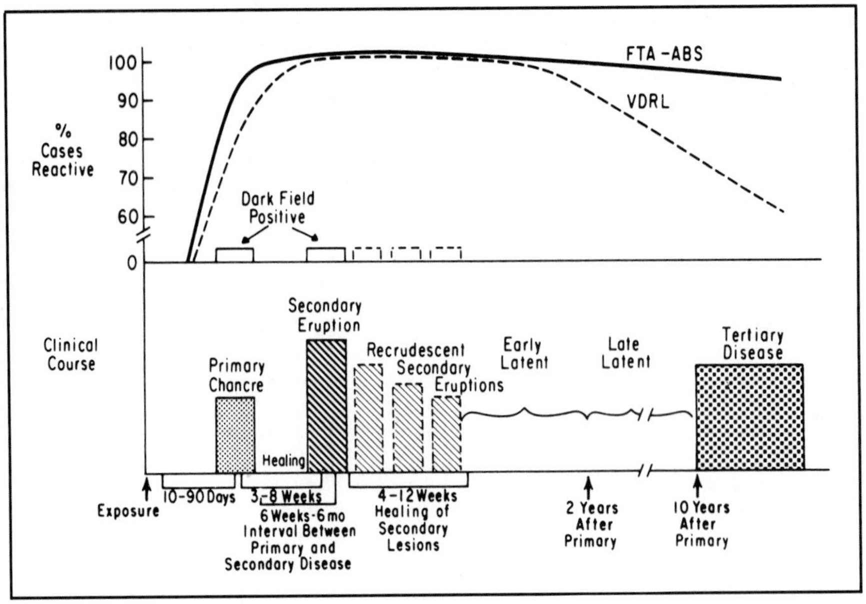

Fig. 45–6. The course of untreated syphilis.

Tertiary Disease

GUMMAS. Three to ten years after the last evidence of secondary disease, the patient may develop nonprogressive, localized lesions of the dermal elements or supporting structures of the body, which are called *gummas.* Because these lesions are relatively quiescent, the term *benign tertiary syphilis* often is used. Spirochetes are extremely sparse or absent. The gummatous reaction is primarily a pronounced immunologic reaction of the host.

NEUROSYPHILIS. During the early stages of syphilis, approximately one third of all patients have involvement of the central nervous system, but only half of these, if untreated, develop late neurosyphilis. The interval between primary disease and late neurosyphilis usually is more than 5 years. Late neurosyphilis may present in a variety of ways. Classic presentations include paralytic dementia, tabes dorsalis, amyotropic lateral sclerosis, meningovascular syphilis, seizures, optic atrophy, and gummatous changes of the cord. Neurosyphilis may resemble virtually any other neurologic disease.

CARDIOVASCULAR SYPHILIS. Approximately 10 to 40 years after primary syphilis occurs, signs of cardiovascular involvement may develop in the untreated patient. The most commonly involved organs are the great vessels of the heart, where syphilitic aortic and pulmonary arteritis develop. The inflammatory reaction also may cause stenosis, with resulting angina, myocardial insufficiency, and death.

Congenital Syphilis. Congenital syphilis results from transplacental infection of the developing fetus and often is a severe and mutilating form of the disease. In spite of widespread programs to examine all pregnant women, in 1984 there were 326 reported cases of early congenital syphilis in the United States; there were 700 by 1988. There are approximately two cases of early congenital syphilis per 100 cases of primary or secondary syphilis in women of childbearing age.

At the onset of congenital syphilis, *T. pallidum* is liberated directly into the circulation of the fetus, resulting in spirochetemia with widespread dissemination. The mortality rate of untreated congenital syphilis is approximately 25%, and an additional 40% of children suffer from late stigmata (Table 45–3). Abortion because of congenital syphilis usually occurs during the second trimester of pregnancy, and histopathologic reactions to *T. pallidum* rarely are found in fetal tissue before that time. It has been generally thought that the fetus is protected from congenital infection until the sixteenth week of pregnancy, when the Langhans' layer of the chorion atrophies. There also is evidence, however, that infection of the fetus may occur earlier but that the typical inflammatory response that results in tissue injury and fetal death does not

TABLE 45–3. STIGMATA OF LATE CONGENITAL SYPHILIS

Stigmata	Percentage of Total Patients[a]
Frontal bossae of Parrott	87
Short maxilla	84
High palatal arch	76
Hutchinson's triad	75
Hutchinson's teeth	63
Interstitial keratitis	9
Eighth-nerve deafness	3
Saddle nose	73
Mulberry molars	65
Higouménakis' sign	39
Relative protuberance of mandible	26
Rhagades	7
Saber shin	4
Scaphoid scapulae	0.7
Clutton's joint	0.3

Adapted from Fiumara: Arch Dermatol 102:78, 1970.
[a] An analysis of 271 patients.

occur until the fetus becomes immunologically competent. Pregnant women with syphilis who have not been treated may transmit the infection to the fetus at any clinical stage of their disease. In general, the greater the time that has elapsed since the woman's primary or secondary infection, the less likely she is to transmit disease to the fetus. Almost all pregnant women with untreated primary syphilis, 90% of women with secondary syphilis, and approximately 30% of women with early latent syphilis may infect their fetuses.

The manifestations of congenital syphilis are highly variable in both signs and intensity. Especially prominent early symptoms include hepatosplenomegaly, jaundice, hemolytic anemia, pneumonia, and multiple long bone involvement. Snuffles, skin lesions, and testicular masses are common.

Late manifestations of congenital syphilis result both from scars of the active disease and from the progression of active disease (Table 45–3). Some changes may be prevented by early treatment, but others often progress despite therapy.

Immunity

Immune Response. The fundamental question in the study of syphilis is how the organism is capable of establishing persistent infection for decades in spite of a vigorous host response. This question remains largely unanswered. There is a vigorous immunologic response by the host to the infection, and yet the infection is neither fully controlled nor eradicated. During the initial infection with *T. pallidum,* humoral IgG and IgM antibody is detectable by the time the chancre appears. Thereafter both IgG and IgM antibodies persist for long periods in the untreated patient. If the patient is adequately treated, IgM antibody declines during the next 1 to 2 years, but IgG antibody usually persists throughout the lifetime of the patient. If the patient is not treated, the stages of syphilis will evolve in spite of humoral antibody response.

The outer layers of virulent treponomal strains possess a dense coat that appears to protect the organism against the effects of specific antibody attachment. This coat of surface-associated protein is composed at least in part of host protein, including fibronectin. It is strongly adherent to the treponemal envelope and may be removed only with vigorous trypsinization. Host transferrin and ceruloplasmin may be found in this host protein outer coating. The function of this coat is unknown, but it could serve to mask the bacterial antigen from the host response.

Polymorphonuclear neutrophils (PMNs) are attracted to pathogenic *Treponema* and ingest them. After phagocytosis, the organisms are enclosed within a phagocytic vacuole, degranulation occurs, and the *Treponema* are digested. The entire phagocytic cycle thus appears to be functional and intact. There are, however, preliminary indications that small numbers of organisms may evade PMN detection. In addition, PMNs appear to have difficulty ingesting very long organisms because of physical factors. Therefore the host defenses in initial disease are modified.

Inhibition of cell-mediated immunity occurs in early syphilis. Lymphocytes from persons with syphilis show reduced or absent response specifically to treponemal antigens. Paracortical areas of syphilitic lymph nodes in early stages of disease are correspondingly depleted of lymphocytes. There is a particularly marked depression of natural killer cell activity in patients with secondary syphilis. The effect appears to be mediated primarily by autologous serum and is found in the immunoglobulin fraction. The suppressive factor may be immune complexes. There is a correlation between poor lymphocyte transformation of lymphocytes from patients with syphilis and the presence of elevated levels of immune complexes. These alterations in cellular immune response abate during the disease. Persons with late secondary syphilis and tertiary syphilis exhibit cell-mediated immunity to treponemal antigen. In addition, there is experimental evidence of nonspecific activation of macrophages several weeks after infection with *T. pallidum.*

Natural Immunity. The progressive decline in severity of syphilis between its introduction into Europe at the end of the fifteenth century and the present time indicates that there has occurred a change in the virulence of the organism or the development of relative resistance by affected human populations, or both. Natural humoral or cell-mediated immunity sufficient to protect against disease has not been demonstrated, and the infective dose for 50 percent infection (ID_{50}) for humans in an experimental situation has been estimated to be as few as 57 organisms.

Acquired Immunity. Persons with untreated syphilis have a relative resistance to reinfection, so that the development of a chancre with second infection is unusual and probably depends on the challenge inoculum. After reexposure, untreated persons may develop an increased humoral antibody level.

In persons who have been treated for syphilis, especially if treatment was given during the secondary or earlier stages, the protective effect of prior disease is minor, and active disease after reinfection is common. This applies to persons who maintain a reactive nontreponemal antibody test (serofast), as well as to those who are serononreactive. In summary, although active or prior syphilis modifies the response of the patient to subsequent reinfection, protection is only relative and is unreliable.

Serologic Tests

There are two basic types of serologic tests for syphilis, the nontreponemal antigen tests and the tests that use treponemal antigen (Table 45–4). Although the latter tests indicate experience with a treponemal infection, they cross-react with antigens other than those of *T. pallidum;* thus no test is specific for syphilis. Because yaws and pinta are rare diseases in the United States, however, the treponemal tests generally provide a reliable indication of syphilitic infection.

Nontreponemal Tests. The original test for syphilis, as described by Wassermann, used syphilitic tissue as a complement-fixing antigen for the detection of antibody (reagin) that is induced by *T. pallidum.* Extracts of normal tissue, however, such as beef heart, have similar properties, and the purification and standardization of these materials led to the use as antigen of a preparation containing cardiolipin and lecithin in cholesterol.

Two types of tests use cardiolipin-lecithin as antigen: (1) complement-fixation tests, including the Wassermann and Kolmer tests, and (2) flocculation tests, including the Venereal Disease Research Laboratory (VDRL), Hinton, and rapid reagin tests. These tests provide similar clinical information and have similar advantages. They are inexpensive to perform, demonstrate rising and falling antibody titers, and correlate

TABLE 45–4. SEROLOGIC TESTS FOR SYPHILIS

Antigen	Antigen Source	Test	Reactivity (%) Primary Stage	Secondary Stage	Tertiary Stage
Nontreponemal	Extracts of tissue (cardiolipin-lecithin-cholesterol)	Complement fixation (Wassermann, Kolmer)			
		Flocculation (VDRL, Hinton, Kahn)	78	90	77
Treponemal	*T. pallidum* Reiter strain	RPCF	61	85	72
	T. pallidum	TPI	56	94	92
		FTA-ABS	85	99	96
		MHA-TP	85	98	95

RPCF, Reiter protein complement fixation; TPI, *T. pallidum* immobilization test; FTA-ABS, fluorescent treponemal antibody absorption; MHA–TP, microhemagglutination–*T. pallidum*.

somewhat with the clinical status of a patient. Disadvantages include a relatively high proportion of biologic acute and chronic false-positive reactions and an increasing proportion of false-negative reactions in the later stages of untreated syphilis. The technical difficulties include a negative reaction due to the prozone phenomenon when only undiluted serum is tested.

Treponemal Tests

TREPONEMA PALLIDUM IMMOBILIZATION (TPI). This test is based on the capacity of reaginic antibody and complement to immobilize a suspension of living and motile treponemes maintained in rabbit testes. The effect of the test serum on the motility of the spirochetes is determined by darkfield microscopy. The test is difficult and expensive, requires living organisms, and is also positive in the nonvenereal treponematoses, bejel, yaws, and pinta. The TPI test now is performed in only a few research laboratories, primarily for comparison with and evaluation of other tests. It also retains a useful clinical role in distinguishing between syphilis and biologic false-positive reactions in patients who have collagen vascular disease with abnormal serum globulin levels.

REITER PROTEIN COMPLEMENT FIXATION. Antigen for this test is an extract from a nonvirulent treponeme, the Reiter strain, which may be cultured in vitro. The test detects group antigen; therefore both false-positive and false-negative results are not uncommon. Nonvirulent treponemal organisms in the oral cavity may stimulate the production of cross-reacting antibody. The test frequently is nonreactive in late stages of syphilis.

FLUORESCENT ANTIBODY TESTS. The most significant development of the past two decades in the serology of syphilis is the detection of treponemal antibody by fluorescein-labeled antihuman antibody. The tests are used to confirm the validity of a positive reaginic test, to diagnose congenital syphilis, and to diagnose late stages of syphilis. The tests are both sensitive and reliable.

Fluorescent treponemal antibody (FTA) tests use lyophilized Nichols strain organisms as antigen. Antigen is fixed on a slide, and the test serum is applied, allowing reaction of antitreponemal antibody with antigen. The slide is then layered with fluorescein isothiocyanate-labeled antihuman gamma globulin, and the presence or absence of antibody is determined by fluorescence microscopy.

The currently used modification of this method is the fluorescent treponemal antibody absorption (FTA-ABS) test in which test sera are preabsorbed with sorbent to eliminate group antibody.* The test thus is rendered relatively specific for disease with virulent treponemal species, usually *T. pallidum*.

The FTA-ABS test is expensive and time-consuming. Therefore it is recommended not for general screening but for confirmation of positive nontreponemal tests and diagnosis of later stages of syphilis in which the results of nontreponemal tests frequently are falsely negative.

HEMAGGLUTINATION TESTS. A hemagglutination method, the microhemagglutination assay–*T. pallidum* (MHA-TP), for serodiagnosis of syphilis has been automated and is both technically easy to perform and inexpensive. It is as sensitive as the FTA-ABS tests, except in primary syphilis, and is highly specific. This is a relatively newly developed test that recently has received standard technique status. Like the FTA-ABS test, the test is unlikely to revert to a nonreactive state after treatment of the patient unless treatment is given very early. The test usually is also reactive in persons with nonsyphilitic treponematoses.

IgM-FTA-ABS TEST. In the diagnosis of congenital syphilis it is necessary to differentiate between passive transplacental transfer of maternal antibody to the fetus and production by the fetus of endogenous antitreponemal antibody. Because antibodies of the IgG but not of the IgM class cross the placenta, detection of specific IgM antibody in the fetal circulation usually indicates antibody production by the fetus as a result of active fetal infection. The FTA-ABS test will detect immunoglobulin of both the IgG and IgM classes and thus will not distinguish between active infection and passive transfer. This problem stimulated the development of a fluorescent antihuman antibody that is specific for IgM class antitreponemal antibody, the IgM-FTA-ABS test. A reactive test result with infant blood is strong evidence of active congenital disease. However, the test may be nonreactive in infants with congenital syphilis if the disease was transmitted to the infant

* Sorbent originally consisted of sonicate of Reiter treponemes; other substances may be used.

late in pregnancy, as often is the case. Furthermore, there are indications that a reactive test does not always absolutely confirm the diagnosis of congenital syphilis. Therefore the test is not highly reliable and has been abandoned by many laboratories.

False-Positive Reactions. All the available serologic tests for syphilis produce occasional positive reaction results in patients for whom there is no other evidence of syphilitic infection. These reactions usually are called *biologic false positive* (BFP), as distinct from positive reactions due to technical errors. The majority of BFP reactions occur with nontreponemal tests; approximately 1% of normal adults will have a BFP reaction by nontreponemal antigen tests. Reaginic antibody is reactive with at least 200 antigens other than those of *T. pallidum*, and although the specific stimulus for this antibody in syphilis, as well as other diseases, is unknown, it may represent antibody to cellular lipoidal antigens of the host that are liberated during various diseases. For clinical purposes, BFP reactions may be classified as acute, in which the reactivity resolves within 6 months, or chronic, in which reactivity is persistent.

ACUTE BIOLOGIC FALSE POSITIVE REACTIONS. Most BFP reactions are detected by nontreponemal tests and occur in patients with other acute illnesses, especially pneumonia, hepatitis, vaccinations, and viral exanthematous disease. The prognosis for the patient's health is not affected by the finding. The titer of antibody usually is low, less than 1:8, and in most instances the FTA-ABS test is nonreactive. Approximately two thirds of patients with BFP reactions have acute reactions, and reactivity subsides in 6 months or less.

CHRONIC BIOLOGIC FALSE POSITIVE REACTIONS. Drug addiction, chronic hepatitis, old age, leprosy, and collagen vascular disease are highly associated with chronic BFP reactions. The antibody detected by the VDRL test in chronic BFP reactions is predominantly IgM, whereas in syphilis it is mainly IgG. Patients with chronic BFP reactions and systemic lupus erythematosus commonly also have a reactive FTA-ABS response. The TPI test may be helpful in the differential diagnosis in these instances.

Laboratory Diagnosis

Efforts to diagnose infectious syphilis are hampered by the lack of a method to culture the organism on laboratory media. Three methods are useful in the diagnosis of syphilis: (1) direct visualization of the organism by darkfield microscopy, by fluorescent antibody technique, or by special stains of infected tissue, (2) animal inoculation, and (3) demonstration of serologic reactions typical of syphilis.

Syphilis in patients with a primary chancre, as well as with active secondary lesions, may be diagnosed by darkfield microscopy. Inasmuch as this depends on direct visualization of motile spirochetes, the organisms must be active and viable. Prior use of many antibiotics rapidly destroys the motility of the organisms, as do many topical disinfectants. Serous fluid from the base of the lesion should be collected for darkfield examination. Syphilitic lesions of the mouth may harbor indigenous treponemes whose morphologic similarity to pathogenic species can confuse the interpretation of findings. The technique, however, is particularly helpful in making a diagnosis early in the disease before the development of seroreactivity. If darkfield microscopy is unavailable, a direct fluorescent antibody stain for *T. pallidum* may be made. Exudate is collected in capillary tubes or on slides and stained with specific antibody. Syphilis that has progressed beyond the primary stage is diagnosed in most patients by serologic methods.

TECHNIQUES UNDER DEVELOPMENT. Although continuous in vitro cultivation of virulent strains of *T. pallidum* has not been possible, 10 to 100 generations of organisms may replicate in a modified tissue culture medium by use of rabbit epithelial cells. This technique has allowed some assessment of the in vitro sensitivity of strains of virulent *T. pallidum* to various antimicrobial agents.

Investigation of the major immunogens of *T. pallidum* has indicated that outer membrane proteins are potential virulence determinants. One of these proteins, a 47 kDa antigen, has been identified as an epitope for treponemicidal activity of immune serum and has been detected as an early antigen in sera of infants with congenital syphilis.

Treatment

Because *T. pallidum* cannot be grown in vitro, estimates of the sensitivity of strains to antimicrobial agents depend on the results of treatment of experimental animals, especially rabbits. The minimal inhibitory concentration of penicillin for *T. pallidum* is approximately 0.004 U/mL, making it one of the most sensitive of human pathogens. There is no evidence that the resistance of the organism to penicillin has increased during the past three decades of penicillin use. For these reasons, penicillin has remained the single most widely and successfully used antimicrobial agent for treatment of all stages of syphilis.

Essential requirements for effective therapy include maintenance of at least 0.03 units of penicillin per milliliter of serum for 7 to 10 days in early syphilis and avoidance of penicillin-free intervals during therapy. Provision of treatment for an individual patient may require frequent injections of short-acting penicillin preparations or the use of long-acting preparations. If the disease is beyond the early stages, the patient should receive adequate doses of penicillin for at least 21 days.

Successful eradication of active disease also has been achieved with erythromycin, tetracyclines, and cephaloridine. However, infected women have delivered syphilitic infants after treatment with these forms of therapy, possibly because of the relatively poor passage of erythromycin and tetracycline from the mother into the fetal circulation.

Specific treatment recommendations are subject to revision. Current recommendations are periodically reviewed by the Centers for Disease Control.*

In most patients who receive appropriate therapy during the primary or secondary stage, active disease is totally and permanently arrested. Persistent seroreactivity as measured by FTA-ABS may be avoided if treatment is given during the preprimary stage but seldom thereafter. Nevertheless, progression to tertiary disease seldom, if ever, occurs. Similarly, therapy during early or late latent syphilis averts the devel-

* For recent recommendations, see *Morbidity and Mortality Weekly Report* 38(suppl 8), 1989; and Zenker PN, Rolfs RT: Treatment of syphilis, 1989. Rev Infect Dis 12:S590, 1990.

opment of symptomatic tertiary disease. Antimicrobial therapy for symptomatic neurosyphilis, optic neuritis, and cardiovascular syphilis may not be followed by significant clinical improvement, and established damage to vital organs may fail to resolve.

Syphilis Associated with Human Immunodeficiency Virus (HIV) Infections. Because of the epidemiologic associations between acquisition of infectious syphilis and exposure to persons who are substance abusers, who are prostitutes, who are homosexual or bisexual males, and who have other sexually transmitted diseases (STDs), many persons with syphilis also are infected with HIV. Recent evaluation of the courses of syphilis in persons who are HIV-positive have shown that early onset of neurosyphilis may occur, relapse of secondary syphilis may occur in spite of standard courses of therapy, failure of therapy to control secondary disease may occur, and serologic response to therapy may be slow. Because of the concerns regarding the efficacy of therapy of syphilis in persons with HIV, intensive therapy, with particularly careful follow-up observation, is indicated.

Jarisch-Herxheimer Reaction. Two to twelve hours after the treatment of active syphilis with either heavy metals or penicillins, a variable proportion of patients develop an acute focal and systemic reaction usually consisting of headache, malaise, and fever 38C or higher. The reaction most commonly is observed in the early stages of syphilis and does not affect the course of recovery. Most reactions in late syphilis are clinically insignificant, but an occasional reaction may produce damage to the central nervous system or the cardiovascular system.

Prevention

Methods to control the spread of syphilis have relied extensively on treatment of case contacts. Persons with acute syphilis are interviewed to identify all sexual contacts that may have occurred during the incubation period. The contacts are examined, and if they are not infectious, they receive treatment appropriate for primary syphilis. Advantage thus is taken of the long incubation period of syphilis by preventing disease in contacts before they themselves can transmit infection.

Other forms of prevention include barrier methods such as the use of a condom, in which prevention of direct contact between infected mucous membranes is achieved. For male-to-male spread of disease, prevention by use of "safe sex" techniques has accompanied a decline in incidence in some communities.

Other Treponemal Diseases

Yaws (Frambesia)

Yaws is a spirochetal disease of the tropics caused by *T. pertenue,* an organism very closely related to *T. pallidum* (Table 45–2). The two organisms are serologically and morphologically indistinguishable and are differentiated by the type of lesions produced in experimental animals. No serologic test distinguishes human yaws from syphilis. DNA–DNA hybridization studies with *T. pallidum* and *T. pertenue* show a 100% homology between the two organisms. On the basis of these results, these two species have been combined and are considered as subspecies of *T. pallidum.*

Yaws is endemic in tropical forest regions of Africa, in parts of South America, India, and Indonesia, and on many of the Pacific Islands. In these areas it is most commonly acquired in childhood and by direct contact other than sexual contact. The disease rarely occurs congenitally, because most infected children have passed the early stages of disease by the age of sexual maturity.

The course of yaws resembles that of syphilis. The initial lesion is called the *mother yaw* or *framboise* and occurs about a month after the primary infection. It is a painless erythematous papule that heals during the subsequent 1 or 2 months. Secondary lesions that resemble the primary lesion occur 6 weeks to 3 months later. Recurrent disease may continue to occur for several years. Tertiary lesions are most likely to involve the skin and bones with gummatous ulcerations. Infection of the feet causes a crippling form of disease called *crab yaws.*

Yaws is readily treated with penicillin. Eradication of yaws has accompanied the general improvement in sanitation and standard of living in most areas of the world.

Pinta

Pinta is a disease of tropical areas of Central and South America, caused by *T. carateum.* This organism is serologically and morphologically similar to both *T. pallidum* and *T. pertenue* and is distinguished by failure to produce cutaneous lesions in rabbits, hamsters, or guinea pigs (Table 45–2). Chimpanzees, however, may be experimentally infected.

Human pinta is acquired by person-to-person contact and rarely by sexual intercourse. The primary and secondary lesions are flat, erythematous, and nonulcerating. The healing lesion first becomes hyperpigmented and later, as scarring occurs, will be depigmented. The lesions most commonly occur on the hands, feet, and scalp. Tertiary disease, such as occurs in syphilis, is uncommon in pinta. Treatment with penicillin is highly efficacious.

Bejel

Bejel is a disease that closely resembles yaws both epidemiologically and in its clinical manifestations. It is considered to be a form of endemic syphilis and occurs in areas of the Middle East. Bejel is caused by a variant of *T. pallidum,* now given a subspecies designation (*T. pallidum* subspecies *endemicum*). Poor hygienic conditions are important in perpetuating these infections, which are decreasing in incidence in most areas. Bejel is transmitted by direct contact, usually during early childhood, and results uniformly in serologic reactions that are indistinguishable from those of syphilis.

Borrelia

Relapsing Fever

The disease in humans known as *relapsing fever* is caused by spirochetes of the genus *Borrelia.* This is an acute infection characterized by febrile episodes that subside spontaneously but tend to recur over a period of weeks. The organisms are transmitted by ticks or by the human body louse. Other terms used to describe this disease are *tick fever, borreliosis,* and *famine fever.*

Relapsing fever has been known to the Western world since the time of Hippocrates. In recent times it has been associated with poverty, crowding, and warfare. After World War I, louse-borne relapsing fever was disseminated through large areas of Europe, carried by louse-infested dislocated civilians, soldiers, and prisoners. A high mortality rate occurred in these debilitated populations who often were also experiencing epidemic typhus.

Separation of the genus *Borrelia* from other members of the Spirochaetaceae is based on their characteristic morphology as revealed by the electron microscope (Table 45–5). The speciation of *Borrelia* is based primarily on the arthropod vector.

Morphology and Physiology

Borrelia are helical organisms 0.2 to 0.5 μm wide and 3 to 20 μm in length, with 3 to 30 uneven coils. Spirals are coarser and more irregular than those of the treponemes or leptospires and usually can be seen with light microscopy in preparations stained with aniline dyes, such as Wright's or Giemsa stains. Borreliosis is the only disease in which spirochetes may be demonstrated in the peripheral blood by direct stain, and the presence of morphologically typical forms is adequate for diagnosis. In fresh blood the organisms are actively motile; they move in forward and backward waves and in a corkscrew-like motion. Observed variations in morphology depend on the parasitized host and on the stage of the disease.

Borrelia are microaerophilic. Special culture media containing natural animal proteins are available, and propagation of cultures of several species has been accomplished. Little is known of the nutritional requirements of the organisms other than the fact that long-chain fatty acids are required for growth. Very little is known about the endotoxin content of the organisms. The optimum temperature for growth is 28C to 30C, and the generation time is about 18 hours.

Borrelia that cause relapsing fever typically have 15 to 30 periplasmic flagella per cell end, whereas the species that causes Lyme disease has 7 to 11. The borreliae causing Lyme disease also differ from those isolated from relapsing fever sources in the guanine-plus-cytosine (G + C) ratios and in the extent of DNA–DNA homology. These results support the distinction of the *Borrelia* organisms causing Lyme disease into a separate species, *B. burgdorferi* (p. 670). The endoflagellae of *Borrelia* species are unsheathed, in contrast to *Trepenoma* species, which have sheathed endoflagellae.

In vitro and in vivo culture of relapsing fever strains for diagnostic purposes is difficult and not always successful. If inoculation of experimental animals is attempted, great care should be taken to ensure that the animals are free from preexisting borreliosis. Suckling or 21-day-old mice may be inoculated subcutaneously or intraperitoneally and smears of peripheral blood subsequently examined for *Borrelia.* Chick embryo cultures have been irregularly successful, as have tissue culture techniques.

Speciation of relapsing fever strains is based on two considerations: (1) the species responsible for louse-borne disease is designated *Borrelia recurrentis,* as opposed to all tick-borne strains, and (2) for tick-borne strains, the close vector-strain relationship has led to the definition of most species by the tick vector. For example, *Borrelia hermsii* is associated with the tick *Ornithodoros hermsi* (Fig. 45–7). The type species is *Borrelia anserina,* which is the cause of avian spirochetosis. There are 19 recognized species of *Borrelia,* 10 of which cause relapsing fever in humans and all of which have an arthropod vector. The principal species of *Borrelia* in North America are

TABLE 45–5. PHENOTYPIC CHARACTERISTICS OF SPIROCHETES

	Borrelia burgdorferi	Other *Borrelia*	*Treponema*	*Leptospira*
Cell diameter	0.18–0.25	0.2–0.5	0.1–0.4	0.1
Cell length	4–30	3–20	5–20	4–20
Number of periplasmic flagella per cell end	7–11	15–30	1–8	1
Overlapping of periplasmic flagella at cell center	Present	Present	Present	Absent
Cytoplasmic tubules	Absent	Absent	Present	Absent
Diamino amino acid in peptidoglycan	Ornithine	Ornithine	Ornithine	α,ε-diaminopimelic acid
Conditions for conversion to spherical forms	Hypotonic	Hypotonic	Hypotonic	Hypertonic
Oxygen requirements	Microaerophilic	Microaerophilic	Anaerobic	Aerobic
Catalase production	Absent	Absent	Absent	Present
Major carbon and energy source	Carbohydrate	Carbohydrate	Carbohydrate and/or amino acids	Long-chain fatty acids
Long-chain fatty acid requirement	Present	Present	Present	Present
Capacity to degrade long-chain fatty acids	Absent	Absent	Absent	Present
Metabolic end products	Lactic acid	Lactic acid	Several organic acids	Acetic acid
Tick-transmitted	+	+	–	–
Associated human disease	Lyme arthritis	Relapsing fever	Syphilis, yaws, bejel, pinta	Leptospirosis

From Johnson et al: Yale J Biol Med 57:529, 1984.

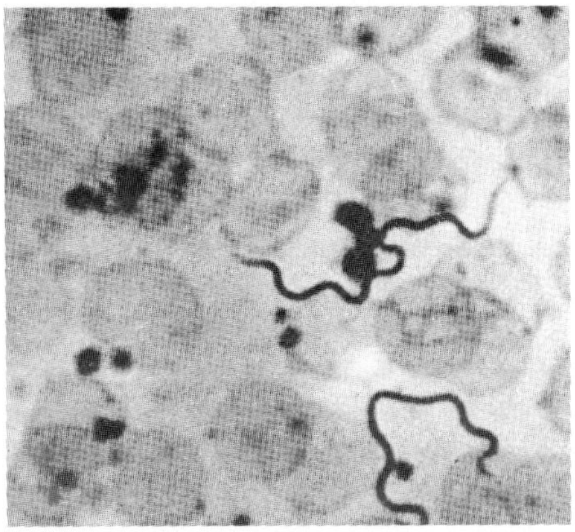

Fig. 45–7. *Borrelia hermsii* from *Ornithodoros hermsi*, collected at Broune Mountain. Giemsa-stained smear of mouse blood. × 2300 *(From Thompson: JAMA 210:1045, 1969.)*

B. hermsii, Borrelia parkeri, and *Borrelia turicatae.* There is evidence by DNA homology studies that these strains represent a single species.

Antigenic Structure

The most striking property of relapsing fever is the capacity of *Borrelia* to undergo several antigenically distinct variations within a given host during the course of a single infection. Early studies of experimental infection of rats with *B. hermsii* showed the presence of major serotypes that represented antigenic shifts. These shifts were observed to occur in a regular sequence, were most readily determined by immunofluorescent methods, and were accompanied by appropriate antibody responses in the host. The organisms disappeared from the peripheral blood coincident with appearance of specific antibody and reappeared after antigenic variation had occurred.

Recent studies have shown that a single strain of *B. hermsii* can give rise to progeny that represent at least 26 separate serotypes when studied by indirect immunofluorescent methods. These strain variations occur both in vitro and in vivo and are not dependent on the selective pressure of the host immunologic response. During relapses, the host typically demonstrates spirochetemia with several different serotypes of organisms at a time. In animals, conversions from one serotype to another occur constantly and are independent of relapses. Switching from one antigenic type to the next occurs at a rate of approximately 10^{-4} to 10^{-3} per cell per generation. Each antigenic variation is associated with a change in the variable major protein (VMP), the protein coat that is externally exposed in these organisms and that occurs in relatively large quantities. The molecular weights and peptide maps of the VMP of *B. hermsii* are unique for each of the 26 serotypes.

Research on the mechanism of antigenic variation indicates that the genes for expression of VMP lie on linear extrachomosomal elements and that there are silent or expressed genes for each of the antigenic types. VMPs contain regions of partial amino acid homology that are common to multiple strains, as well as regions unique to each strain. These findings probably represent a previously unrecognized pathogenic mechanism and currently are under intense investigation.

In human relapsing fever, immobilizing antibody to both autologous and heterologous strains develops in most patients. Studies also have demonstrated that a low level of protection against subsequent relapse strains is afforded by antigenic stimulation with the initial strains of the infection and that there is a frequent lack of cross-protection. The actual method of elimination of borreliosis from infected mammals is uncertain. The complement-dependent lytic pathway is not necessary for recovery and elimination of infection. Also, recovery appears to be independent of T cell function.

The technical problems associated with antigenic variation and the recognition of the coexistence of mixed populations of *Borrelia* have precluded the development of a reliable serologic test for borreliosis. Although several experimental systems are being evaluated, all lack adequate standards. Agglutination of *Proteus* OX-K at moderate titers has been observed in the majority of patients with louse-borne relapsing fever and in one study of an outbreak of tick-borne disease. The test is nonspecific but may be marginally helpful.

Clinical Infection

Epidemiology

TICK-BORNE DISEASE. The vectors of tick-borne borreliosis are ticks of the genus *Ornithodoros,* which comprise the soft ticks (argasid ticks).

In the United States, tick-borne disease may be transmitted by *Ornithodoros turicatae, Ornithodoros parkeri,* and *O. hermsi.* Throughout the world, more than 15 species of *Ornithodoros* ticks have been found to transmit borreliosis. *Ornithodoros* species feed exclusively on blood, often at night. They usually have a painless bite and feed for a short time (usually less than 1 hour), after which they spontaneously leave the host. An individual is therefore frequently unaware of having received a bite.

When the tick bites a *Borrelia* host, the *Borrelia* penetrate the tick's coelomic cavity. There is a predilection for the coxal and salivary glands and gonads, enabling transovarian passage to occur. The infected tick may survive for years without food in environments of low humidity. The infection is transmitted by ticks both by contamination of the bite with coxal fluid and by the salivary fluid. The life span of the tick is not shortened by carrying *Borrelia.* Many *Ornithodoros* species will feed on a variety of hosts.

B. hermsii and its vector are found primarily at elevations above 3000 feet and are associated with tree squirrels and chipmunks, which may carry the ticks into cabins, where they become established. *O. turicatae* parasitizes goats, sheep, and rodents and is found in caves and animal burrows mainly in Florida and Mexico. *O. parkeri* inhabits the homes of ground squirrels and prairie dogs at lower elevations than does *O. hermsi* and is widely distributed geographically. Numerous other small mammals also serve as reservoirs for tick-borne *Borrelia,* including rats, mice, rabbits, opossums, and hedgehogs. Birds have not been implicated. Once infected, the tick may harbor the disease for many years. Tick-borne disease is not rapidly spread, however, and in the United States is responsible only for sporadic cases.

In the United States, relapsing fever is a disease limited to persons who have come in contact with infected ticks. This most commonly results from vacationing in a tick-infested summer cottage. In one recent outbreak, 11 of 42 members of a Boy Scout troop contracted relapsing fever. Most of those infected had slept in a rodent-infested cabin, whereas the scouts who were younger had slept in tents and did not become infected. The spring and summer distribution of disease coincides with the season of maximal tick activity and the avocational invasion of humans into tick-infested areas. In the United States, foci of tick-borne borreliosis occur mainly in the western states, particularly Oklahoma, California, New Mexico, Colorado, Washington, Texas, and Kansas, which may reflect the distribution of *Ornithodoros* ticks.

In some areas of Africa, inhabitation of the home by *Ornithodoros moubata* is considered to be good luck and has resulted in introduction of disease.

LOUSE-BORNE DISEASE. The human body and head lice, *Pediculus humanus corporis* and *Pediculus humanus capitis*, are the vectors of epidemic relapsing fever caused by *B. recurrentis*, although there is some evidence that bedbugs may occasionally also transmit the disease. After the louse ingests *Borrelia*, the organisms pass exclusively into the hemolymph and central ganglion. Because other organs are not invaded, there occurs neither transovarian transmission nor direct infection during the feeding by an intact louse. *Borrelia* escape the louse to infect the host only when the louse is injured, as may occur during scratching. A single louse, therefore, can infect only one person. The infected louse remains infectious for its life span, which is approximately 10 to 60 days. Lice may rapidly and widely disseminate disease. Epidemics usually occur in the cold seasons, among the crowded and poor, and in homes with inadequate hygiene. Because of a narrow temperature preference, the louse typically leaves a febrile patient in search of a new host, potentiating rapid spread of an epidemic. Although *B. recurrentis* is considered to be the louse-borne species, tick-borne *Borrelia* also may be transmitted by lice. No natural animal reservoir of *B. recurrentis* is known. Currently, *B. recurrentis* is endemic, primarily in areas of Ethiopia.

Relapsing fever occasionally may be acquired by means other than louse or tick infestation. For example, transplacental transmission has caused congenital disease, and infected blood may be the cause of laboratory accidents leading to infection.

Pathogenesis. During the entire course of borreliosis, there is a constant spirochetemia, which worsens during febrile periods and wanes between recurrences. Specific pathogenic factors are ill defined. The organisms, however, appear to contain a heat-stable pyrogen that is not endotoxin. Skin biopsy specimens from infected persons have shown that there is no inflammatory response around the spirochetes that are within the dermis and that the dermal vessels show no thrombosis or other evidence of vasculitis, as would be expected if endotoxin were produced.

Borrelia are actively phagocytized by PMNs of humans. Immune serum both enhances phagocytosis and exerts a direct effect on *B. hermsii*, causing decreased motility and viability and increased agglutination.

Clinical Manifestations. Before the development of effective antimicrobial agents, fever induction was used in the therapy of tertiary syphilis. Induced infection with *Borrelia* often was selected for this purpose, and much of our present knowledge concerning prodromata, incubation period, natural history, and complications stems from these experiences.

The symptoms and severity of relapsing fever depend on the immune status of the host, geographic location, strain of *Borrelia*, and phase of the epidemic. There also may be consistent differences between some characteristics of louse-borne disease and tick-borne disease, but both forms will be described together (Table 45–6).

TABLE 45–6. CLINICAL MANIFESTATIONS IN RELAPSING FEVER

Manifestation	Mean Value of Incidence	
	Tick-Borne Disease[a]	Louse-Borne Disease[b]
Incubation period (days)	~7	
Duration of primary febrile attack (days)	3.1	5.5
Duration of afebrile interval (days)	6.8	9.25
Duration of relapses (days)	2.5	1.9
Number of relapses	3	1
Maximum temperature (primary attack)	~40.5C (105F)	
Splenomegaly (%)	41	77
Hepatomegaly (%)	17–18	66
Jaundice (%)	7	36
Rash (%)	28	8
Respiratory symptoms (%)	16	34
CNS involvement (%)	8.9	30

Adapted from Southern and Sanford: Medicine 48:129, 1969.
[a] Based on review of 1105 reported cases.
[b] Based on review of 2073 reported cases.

The natural history of a course of relapsing fever includes the incubation period, the primary attack, the afebrile interval, and subsequent attacks. In epidemic, endemic, and therapeutically induced disease, few prodromata have been noted. The incubation period is approximately 6 days, with a range of 2 to 14 days. Late in the incubation period the patient may experience chills. The onset usually is very sudden and accompanied by fever, headache, tachycardia, and muscle pain. The initial attack usually lasts 3 to 7 days, may be longer for louse-borne than for tick-borne disease, and ends by crisis. The fever usually is continuous.

A macular rash is seen in varying numbers of patients and usually appears near the end of the first paroxysm. Hepatosplenomegaly, jaundice, nausea, and vomiting are common. In the United States, bronchitis and bronchopneumonia are frequent. Meningeal signs with and without encephalitic disease may affect up to 30% of some groups of patients, and ocular disease is common.

The crisis is coincidental with the immune response. Occasionally, the crisis is associated with shock. Usually, the temperature returns to normal, and the patient is symptom-free until the subsequent attack. The interval between initial and subsequent attacks usually is shorter with louse-borne disease, 5 to 9 days, than with tick-borne disease, which lasts approximately 14 days.

Data from the period 1921 to 1941 described the course of untreated tick-borne disease as follows: no relapse, 16%; one relapse, 20%; two relapses, 27%; three relapses, 17%; and four or more relapses, 18% of cases. A similar distribution of relapses has occurred in some outbreaks of louse-borne disease.

Subsequent attacks usually are shorter in duration, less severe, and with increasingly shorter apyrexial periods between attacks but are otherwise clinically similar to the initial episode. Most physicians fail to diagnose relapsing fever until one or more relapses have occurred.

Treatment and Prevention. Treatment of relapsing fever includes general supportive measures, such as fluid and electrolyte therapy. Evaluation of efficacy of antimicrobial therapy has been inhibited by the lack of information on in vitro sensitivity. The most clinically effective antimicrobial agents appear to be tetracyclines and chloramphenicol. Streptomycin has been found to modify the disease, although it may fail to prevent relapses.

Prevention of relapsing fever depends on control of exposure to the arthropod vectors. In tick-borne borreliosis, this includes wearing protective clothing and careful cleaning of rodent-infested cabins, followed by spraying with appropriate insecticides, such as aldrin, benzene hexachloride, or malathion. Louse-borne relapsing fever is controlled by the application of good personal and public standards of hygiene.

Lyme Disease

The discovery or emergence of a newly recognized illness is a particularly exciting event in the history of infectious diseases. In 1975 a newly recognized syndrome consisting of an illness that was associated with a unique skin lesion, erythema chronicum migrans (ECM), was recognized in a cluster of rural children in Lyme, Connecticut. This illness, now known as Lyme disease, also is referred to as erythema chronicum migrans, Lyme arthritis, and Bannwarth's syndrome. The causative agent of Lyme disease is a new species of *Borrelia*, *B. burgdorferi*, named for Dr. Burgdorf, the microbiologist who isolated and identified the agent. The rapid elucidation of the etiology, diagnosis, sequelae, and treatment of this major disease represents one of the recent and exciting events in clinical microbiology and epidemiology.

Borrelia burgdorferi

Morphology. *B. burgdorferi*, which is a microaerophilic organism, resembles other members of the family Spirochaetaceae in its general morphology. It is similar in size to *Treponema* species. It has 7 to 11 periplasmic flagella per cell end, which is less than the number for other *Borrelia* species, which contain 15 to 30 (Table 45–5). *Borrelia* harbor plasmids, one of which contains the genes that encode for the two major surface proteins, OspA and OspB. These plasmids also may encode for other virulence factors.

Attributes of *B. burgdorferi* that led to its classification as a *Borrelia* species include its transmission by ticks, its microaerophilic metabolism, and its in vitro culture in the Barbour-Stoenner-Kelly medium used for other *Borrelia* species. The chromosomal DNA nucleotides of *B. burgdorferi* show mol% G + C ranges that are similar to those of other North American borreliae and that differ from those of *Leptospira* and *Treponema* species. DNA homology studies similarly indicate considerable homology between *B. burgdorferi* strains of other North American *Borrelia*.

European forms of the disease caused by *B. burgdorferi* have a lower incidence of arthritis and a higher incidence of neurologic disease compared with disease in the United States. To examine possible reasons for these dissimilarities, antigenic components of strains from a wide variety of sources have been examined. Analysis by polyacrylamide gel electrophoresis of the major exposed proteins of the spirochetal surface, the OspA proteins, has revealed differences between the strains in the United States and those of most European countries. It is not yet known whether *B. burgdorferi* resembles other *Borrelia* species in its capacity for antigenic variation.

Clinical Infection

Epidemiology. *B. burgdorferi* is transmitted through the bite of a tick. Ticks that are known to harbor and transmit Lyme disease to humans include *Ixodes pacificus* on the West Coast, *Ixodes dammini* on the East Coast and in the Midwest, *Ixodes ricinus* in Europe, and *Ambylomma americanum*, the Lone Star tick that also is a vector of tularemia and Rocky Mountain spotted fever. The preferred host for nymphal *Ixodes* ticks is the deer mouse, and for adult ticks it is deer. Human disease is transmitted mainly by nymphal ticks, which are very small and aggressive.

In the United States there are three major foci of recognized cases of Lyme disease: the midsection of the West Coast, Minnesota and Wisconsin, and the North Eastern coast. However, almost 30 states, as well as Europe and Asia, have reported cases.

Clinical Manifestations. The clinical disease commonly presents as three consecutive stages of illness. In the initial stage there is a highly characteristic expanding skin lesion, which usually shows a papule at the site of the tick bite, has sharply demarcated borders, often shows relatively minimal involvement of the skin centrally, and often is accompanied by various constitutional symptoms such as malaise, fever, headache, and stiff neck. The lesion may reach a large size, may fade over several months, may periodically recur, and may be associated with multiple other annular lesions at other sites.

The subsequent stage of the disease is estimated to occur in about 5% to 15% of patients and is characterized by the onset of neurologic or cardiac involvement, usually within a few months or less of the initial lesion. Headache, Bell's palsy, radiculoneuropathy, myocarditis, and arrhythmias are common presentations.

The third recognized stage of disease primarily involves migrating episodes of arthritis and occurs weeks to months after the tick bite. Each event may last as long as several months, remits, and may be followed by another attack in another joint. These episodes may continue to be associated with fever and may last for several years. The arthritis is not destructive, and joints are relatively normal after resolution.

Immunologic Response. Human mononuclear leukocytes appear to be the most efficient cell type in the phagocytosis of *B. burgdorferi*, although neutrophils also are active and both cells kill the spirochete after ingestion. Antibody facilitates but is not required for phagocytosis. Spirochetes may be demonstrated in skin biopsy material from lesions and from infected synovial tissue by Dieterle's silver stain. The pathology of involved areas includes a plasma cell and lymphocytic infiltrate, as well as microvascular injury. The local neutrophilic response is minimal.

During the first 10 days after infection patients exhibit an IgM response to the spirochete, followed by an IgG response that persists for years if untreated. The indirect immunofluorescence assay and an enzyme-linked immunosorbent assay (ELISA) test for antibody currently are available for diagnostic purposes. An assay based on the augmentation of the OspA antigen by the polymerase chain reaction also has been developed and is being evaluated.

There have been significant difficulties in the serologic diagnosis of Lyme disease. In the early stages of the disease, the diagnostic test results may be negative or equivocal because the patient's antibody response is delayed or nonspecific. In the later stages of Lyme disease, cross-reactions with antibody produced against other spirochetes also may result in equivocal or false-positive responses. The development of assays that are reliable, sensitive, and specific is greatly needed.

Treatment and Prevention. The acute illness usually is adequately treated with phenoxymethylpenicillin or tetracycline for 2 to 3 weeks. Many patients who receive therapy early in the initial stages of illness will not have later manifestations of disease. Patients with neurologic or synovial disease may be successfully treated with longer courses of oral penicillin or amoxicillin or with parenteral penicillin for 10 to 20 days. However, as many as 50% of patients who are treated during postacute stages of disease have had continued signs and symptoms of disease. The optimal therapy for the various stages of borreliosis has not been defined, and even the methods for determining sensitivities to antimicrobial agents are not well standardized.

Prevention of Lyme disease depends on proper precautions against tick exposure and on recognition and treatment of early disease.

Leptospira

Leptospirosis, an acute illness associated with febrile jaundice and nephritis, was first recognized by Weil in 1886 as a clinical entity distinct from other icteric fevers. Commonly referred to since that time as *Weil's disease,* the infection is caused by a leptospira transmitted to humans from a wide variety of animal hosts.

By 1948 more than 300 cases of human leptospirosis had been reported, most of which were clinically severe and accompanied by jaundice. Recognition of other forms of leptospirosis, however, was exceedingly slow in spite of indications in Europe and other parts of the world that clinically milder and nonicteric forms of leptospirosis were common and that animal reservoirs were not restricted to rodents. In 1938 Meyer described canicola fever in dogs and humans. Infection in cattle was reported in 1948, and shortly thereafter human infection by this same strain (serovar *pomona*) was recognized in Georgia. Human leptospirosis is now known to be caused by infection with a family of organisms. These organisms may be classified into multiple serogroups and serotypes. The various serogroups of *Leptospira* cause diseases that are extremely varied in their clinical presentations.

Evidence of widespread leptospiral disease among cattle, swine, horses, and other livestock led to appreciation of the economic losses attributable to these infections, as well as to their threat to human health. By the early 1950s, several public health laboratories were capable of evaluating serologic evidence of infection with an increasing number of leptospiral serogroups; syndromes, such as pretibial fever (Fort Bragg fever), aseptic meningitis, and other mild febrile illnesses, were attributed to leptospiral infection. Commonly used terms for leptospirosis include swineherd's disease, Fort Bragg fever, pretibial fever, Weil's disease, canicola fever, and autumnal fever.

Morphology

The family Leptospiraceae contains the one genus *Leptospira,* which is characterized by fine coiling of the primary spirals. The name is derived from the Greek word *lepto,* meaning *thin* or *fine* spiral. *Leptospira* organisms are helicoidal, usually 6 to 20 μm in length and 0.1 μm in diameter. The coils are 0.2 to 0.3 μm in overall diameter and 0.5 μm in pitch. In liquid media, one or both ends usually are hooked. In the living state the organisms are clearly visible by darkfield microscopy and much less clearly by phase-contrast microscopy.

Ultrastructure. *Leptospira* organisms consist of a helicoidal protoplasmic cylinder, two axial filaments, and an outer envelope. The outer envelope is composed of three to five layers and surrounds the whole organism. Located between the outer envelope and the cytoplasmic membrane are two independent axial filaments, each of which is inserted by one end subterminally at opposite ends of the protoplasmic cylinder. The free ends are directed toward the center of the cell, where they usually do not overlap. During cellular reproduction, septal wall formation occurs at the middle region of the organism, leading to transverse division.

Lipids comprise 18% to 28% of the dry weight of the leptospiral cell and are composed of approximately 70% phospholipid and 30% free fatty acids. The composition of fatty acids is a reflection of those present in the culture medium, because with few exceptions *Leptospira* can neither synthesize fatty acids de novo nor elongate chains.

The major compounds of the leptospiral cell wall are polysaccharide and peptidoglycan. Alanine, glutamic acid, diaminopimelic acid, glucosamine, and muramic acid are the predominant amino acids and sugars. The diaminopimelic acid content of *Leptospira* serves to differentiate these organisms from *Treponema* and *Borrelia,* which instead contain ornithine.

Physiology

Leptospira are obligate aerobes and have a respiratory type of metabolism, with oxygen utilized as the final electron acceptor. They are oxidase-positive and catalase- or peroxidase-positive or both. *Leptospira* grow well at pH 7.2 to 7.4 in rabbit serum or Tween 80 albumin media. The generation time of pathogenic species cultivated in laboratory media is 12 to 16 hours, and 4 to 8 hours in inoculated animals. Long-chain unsaturated fatty acids serve as the major source of carbon and energy and are required by the parasitic strains. *Leptospira* can use inorganic ammonium salts as a source of nitrogen.

Characterization of Species

The genus *Leptospira* comprises two species, *L. interrogans* and *L. biflexa. L. interrogans* includes pathogenic organisms, whereas *L. biflexa* includes saprophytic or water *Leptospira* that com-

TABLE 45–7. *LEPTOSPIRA* SEROGROUPS AND SEROVARS COMMONLY ISOLATED FROM HUMANS AND DOMESTIC ANIMALS IN THE UNITED STATES

Serogroup	Serovar	Host
Autumnalis	*fort-bragg*	Human
Canicola	*canicola*	Human, cattle, dog, swine
Grippotyphosa	*grippotyphosa*	Cattle, swine
Hebdomadis	*szwajizak*	Cattle
	georgia	Human
	hardjo	Cattle
Icterohaemorrhagiae	*icterohaemorrhagiae*	Human, cattle, dog, swine
	copenhageni	Human, dog
Illini	*illini*	Cattle
Pomona	*pomona*	Human, cattle, dog, goat, horse, swine
Australis	*bratislava*	Dog, raccoon, fox
Ballum	*ballum*	Mouse, pig, skunk

monly occur in fresh, surface waters. Distinguishing characteristics of the two species, other than their ability to infect animals, include the inhibition of growth of *L. interrogans* by 8-azaguanine, growth of *L. interrogans* at 13C, and serologic characteristics. The two species also are distinguishable genetically. On the basis of DNA–DNA annealing tests, there is no genetic homology between *L. interrogans* and *L. biflexa*. The taxonomy of *Leptospira* remains provisional, however, until further advances in the basic microbiology of these complex organisms make more accurate speciation possible.

Antigenic Structure

Each species of *Leptospira* includes a large number of serologically distinct serogroups as determined by cross-agglutination and microscopic agglutinin-absorption tests. Strains that share major agglutinogens are arbitrarily assembled into serogroups. The serogroup is not a recognized taxon and serves primarily serodiagnostic purposes. The basic taxon is the serovar. Serovars have been characterized by the use of factor sera, in which cross-absorption with related strains has yielded a serum with a narrow range of agglutination. Attempts to identify serovars also have included use of DNA base composition analysis, immunodiffusion analysis of axial filament antigen, enzymatic characteristics, and restriction endonuclease analysis. The standard method of characterizing serogroups and serovars of *Leptospira* has remained, however, the difficult microscopic agglutination assay.

Among the parasitic leptospiras, more than 150 serovars are now recognized and classified into approximately 19 serogroups, all of which are characterized by very wide distribution both in variety of animal species affected and in geographic occurrence. Table 45–7 indicates serogroups and serovars isolated from humans and domestic animals in the United States. Between 1974 and 1978, of the 498 cases of human leptospirosis in the United States, 332 were found to have been caused by 1 of 17 serogroups.

Determinants of Pathogenicity

Although mechanisms of virulence remain uncertain, a number of biologic properties characterize the pathogenic strains of *Leptospira*.

1. Both complement and specific immune sera are required for lysis of *Leptospira*. Avirulent strains are relatively more sensitive to this leptospirocidal effect of immune serum than are virulent strains. Human macrophages and polymorphonuclear leukocytes fail to ingest virulent *Leptospira* in the presence of normal serum but do so in the presence of immune serum. Complement does not appear to be required for phagocytosis although serotype-specific antibody is essential for host defense to virulent leptospirosis by opsonization. Macrophages are capable of ingesting and killing saprophytic leptospiras even in the absence of homologous antibody.
2. Some virulent strains of *Leptospira* produce a soluble hemolysin that appears to be important in the manifestations of leptospirosis in a number of animal species. The hemolysin is thermolabile and probably protein in nature. Previous infection with a hemolytic serotype confers immunity to subsequent hemolytic disease.
3. Some of the clinical manifestations of leptospirosis, such as conjunctival irritation and iritis, probably are caused by cell-mediated sensitivity to leptospiral antigen.
4. Some strains of *Leptospira* appear to contain small amounts of endotoxin. Clinical findings in animals with leptospirosis suggest the presence of endotoxemia.

Clinical Infection

Epidemiology. Leptospirosis is a zoonotic disease with a wide range of host reservoirs. The predominant natural reservoirs of pathogenic *Leptospira* are wild mammals, although domestic animals, such as dogs, cattle, swine, sheep, goats, and horses, also may be major sources of human infections. The improved ability of regional laboratories to group *Leptospira* has resulted in the recognition of the large number of serovars endemic in the United States, as well as the extent of infections in a variety of animal species. Nevertheless, it is an infrequently diagnosed human disease. In the period 1980 to 1989, there were 40 to 93 cases per year reported to the Centers for Disease Control.

The major mode of transmission between animals and humans is by indirect contact with urine infected with virulent *Leptospira* from an animal with leptospiruria. *Leptospira* from infected soil, food, and water enter the body through a break in the skin and through mucous membranes. Survival of *Leptospira* outside the host is fostered by a temperature of 22C or above, moisture, and a neutral to slightly alkaline environment. *Leptospira* are readily killed by temperatures above 60C, detergents, desiccation, and acidity.

Because of its prevalence in rodents and domestic animals, leptospirosis has been primarily a disease of persons in occupations that involve direct or indirect contact with animals or animal products, such as sewer workers, swineherders, veterinarians, abattoir workers, and farmers. Also at risk are persons living in rodent-infested housing, such as urban slums.

The convoluted renal tubules of animal reservoirs harbor viable *Leptospira,* which are passed in the urine, and the duration of asymptomatic urinary shedding varies with the animal species. There is a higher incidence of disease in men than in women. At present the majority of cases occur in the summer and fall in teen-agers and young adults. Avocational exposure has become increasingly common.

In the United States dogs are the most important reservoir for bringing humans into contact with leptospirosis. A sizable (15% to 40%) proportion of dogs are infected, and the majority of human cases are associated with intimate contact with a dog. Immunization of a dog to leptospirosis may fail to prevent renal shedding.

Common source outbreaks attributed to contaminated ponds or slowly moving streams are numerous; more than 14 instances have been reported in the United States since 1939. A high attack rate, summer season, young age-group, and the proximity of animals to the water typify most of these outbreaks. In some areas of the world, the run-off during flooding also is highly infectious.

Forms of transmission other than direct and indirect contact with contaminated urine are rare. Lactating animals shed *Leptospira* in milk, but whole milk is leptospirocidal after a few hours, and no known human cases have occurred in this manner. *Leptospira* are not shed in saliva, and animal bites are therefore not a direct source of infection. Person-to-person transmission has not been reported and probably is rare. Humans rarely shed *Leptospira* for more than a few months.

Pathogenesis. The organism probably invades the human through small breaks in the skin or intact mucosa. The initial sites of multiplication are unknown. Nonspecific host defenses fail to contain *Leptospira* to any significant extent, and leptospiremia occurs rapidly after infection and continues through the initial acute illness. A local lesion at the site of entry does not develop.

Leptospira usually infect the kidneys. The major renal lesion, common to all forms of leptospirosis and present even in patients with normal renal function, is an interstitial nephritis with associated glomerular swelling and hyperplasia. Studies of infections in experimental mice have demonstrated that the earliest lesion of the kidney is interstitial edema, which occurs by the second day after infection. This is followed by a thickening of the basement membrane of the proximal tubules. By the tenth day *Leptospira* can be identified in areas adjoining tubular epithelial cells. The glomerulus apparently is not involved. Late manifestations of this disease may be caused by the host immunologic response to the infection.

Clinical Manifestations. The severity of human leptospirosis varies greatly and is determined to a large extent by the infecting strain and by the general health of the host. Severe icteric disease with a high fatality rate occurs in a small proportion of patients and frequently is associated with serogroup Icterohaemorrhagiae serovars. Less severe and anicteric disease is far more prevalent and commonly is caused by serovars of serogroups Australis and Pyrogenes; disease due to those of Canicola, Ballum, and Pomona is often mild. There is, however, no absolute correlation between severity of disease or clinical syndrome with infecting serogroups. Leptospirosis is a disease that is unusually protean in its clinical manifestations.

The incubation period usually is 10 to 12 days but ranges from 3 to 30 days after inoculation. Prominent presenting signs include an abrupt onset of fever, chills, headache, conjunctival suffusion, myalgias, and gastrointestinal complaints. The clinical presentations of leptospirosis often suggest other disease processes, most commonly hepatitis, viral meningitis, fever of unknown cause, and encephalitis.

Clinical illness is biphasic, the first leptospiremic stage lasting approximately 7 days in most instances. The appearance of humoral antibody coincides with the termination of fever and leptospiremia. A few days after the initial defervescence, a second and shorter febrile period may occur. Routine laboratory studies usually do not aid in the diagnosis.

Infection of the kidneys results in the excretion of organisms in the urine. Renal failure in Weil's disease is not rare and is the cause of death in most fatal cases. With the availability of extracorporeal dialysis, however, the mortality rate is very low, and there is complete return of renal function after recovery.

Hepatic injury with hepatocellular disease is common in leptospirosis. The pathogenesis of the liver disease is not certain but may be due to the vasculitis that generally is present. Jaundice may be extensive and may be due to both conjugated and unconjugated bilirubin. Electron microscopic changes in hepatocytes during leptospirosis include increases in smooth endoplasmic reticulum, destruction of mitochondria, and abnormalities in cell wall structure.

Certain presentations and complications of leptospirosis require attention. Meningeal irritation is common and probably a frequent cause of undiagnosed aseptic meningitis. Approximately half the patients examined during the second week of illness may have a cerebrospinal fluid lymphocytosis associated with a moderate elevation of cerebrospinal fluid protein. *Leptospira* may be isolated from the cerebrospinal fluid early in the disease. The later onset of symptoms of central nervous system involvement may reflect an untoward antigen-antibody reaction. Permanent neurologic sequelae are exceedingly rare.

An infectious agent from patients with a syndrome named Fort Bragg fever (pretibial fever), first described in 1943 at Fort Bragg, North Carolina, was identified in 1952 as pathogenic *Leptospira* (serovar *fort bragg*) in the Autumnalis serogroup. Sporadic cases have subsequently been reported from other parts of the United States, including the Pacific Northwest. Clinical characteristics of this syndrome include an unusual symmetric rash limited to the pretibial areas. The lesions resemble erythema nodosum but are urticarial in a few cases. Fever, headache, a palpable spleen, and leukopenia are prominent. A similar syndrome may occur with other *Leptospira* serovars.

Immunity. In all patients with leptospiral bacteremia, homologous agglutinating antibodies develop. During the initial immunologic response the antibody is of the IgM class. It is detectable within 1 week after onset of disease and may persist in high titer for many months. IgG antibodies also may develop in some patients a month or more after onset of illness. Human convalescent serum contains protective and agglutinating antibodies that persist in a patient's serum for many years. The capacity of sera to protect against disease is best correlated with titer of agglutinating antibody, which may be of either the IgG or the IgM class.

Laboratory Diagnosis

CULTURE. During the acute phase of the disease, *Leptospira* can be readily cultured from the blood or cerebrospinal fluid.

After the first week of disease and for several months thereafter, *Leptospira* may be shed intermittently in the urine by a large proportion of patients and may be demonstrated by cultural means.

Isolation of *Leptospira* may be accomplished by direct inoculation of laboratory media or by animal inoculation. Commonly used media include Fletcher's and Stuart's media, which contain rabbit serum. Ellinghausen's medium is semisolid and also provides an effective method of recovery. Isolation of *Leptospira* from contaminated specimens may be accomplished by the use of a selective inhibitor, such as 5-fluorouracil, or by intraperitoneal inoculation of young hamsters or guinea pigs.

DIRECT EXAMINATION. The direct demonstration of *Leptospira* by darkfield microscopy, fluorescent antibody, silver impregnation, or staining with aniline dyes is successful in only a small portion of cases. It is not recommended as a single diagnostic procedure because of the frequently mistaken identification of artifacts as *Leptospira*.

SEROLOGIC TESTS. The macroscopic slide agglutination test, which employs formalinized antigen, is a safe and rapid screening test for the detection of leptospiral antibody. Determination of serovar-specific antibody, however, is accomplished with the very sensitive microscopic agglutination test using live organisms. The microscopic agglutination test (agglutination-lysis) was the original method for determining antibody response to leptospirosis and remains the reference method. Use of living organisms gives the most specific reaction, with highest titer and fewer cross-reactions. Formalinized antigen also may be used. Results are read by low-power, darkfield microscopy. These tests require maintenance of appropriate living or formalinized antigen, may be dangerous and arduous to perform, and are available only in reference laboratories. Because agglutinating antibodies persist for long periods after the acute episode, these tests are useful in determining the past experience of a community with leptospirosis.

Recent advances in leptospirosis diagnosis have led to the development of an IgM-specific dot ELISA test. The antigen used in this test is a broadly reactive antigen from *L. interrogans* serovar *sejroe*. The results of the dot ELISA test compare very favorably with the microscopic agglutination test in both sensitivity and specificity. This test is usually positive for IgM and IgG antibody within 4 to 5 days of onset of clinically apparent disease.

It should be noted that even though animals are shedding virulent *Leptospira* in their urine, they may fail to demonstrate serologic evidence of leptospirosis. The absence of a positive serologic test should thus not be interpreted as having proved an animal to be free of leptospirosis.

Treatment and Prevention. Penicillin, streptomycin, tetracycline, and the macrolide antibiotics are active against *Leptospira* in vitro and in experimentally infected animals. Recovery of human cases appears to be hastened if therapy is initiated during the first 2 days after onset. When therapy is initiated after the fourth day of illness, the course of the disease usually may not be altered. A placebo-controlled study with penicillin, begun within 4 days of onset of illness, indicated that the illness was shortened in treated patients.

Vaccines have been effectively used in veterinary medicine for humans in endemic areas. Protection is serovar specific. Short-term prophylaxis may be accomplished by administration of tetracycline.

FURTHER READING

Books and Reviews

TREPONEMA PALLIDUM

Baughn RE: Role of fibronectin in the pathogenesis of syphilis. Rev Infect Dis 9(suppl 4):S372, 1987

Canale-Parola E: Physiology and evolution of spirochetes. Bacteriol Rev 41:181, 1977

Canale-Parola E: Family I. Spirochaetaceae. In Krieg NR, Holt JG (eds): Bergey's Manual of Systematic Bacteriology, vol 1. Baltimore, Williams & Wilkins, 1984, p 39

Clark EG, Danbolt N: The Oslo study of the natural course of untreated syphilis. Med Clin North Am 48:613, 1964

Holt SC: Anatomy and chemistry of spirochetes. Microbiol Rev 42:114, 1978

Johnson RC (ed): The Biology of Parasitic Spirochetes. New York, Academic Press, 1976

Musher D, Schell R (eds): The Immunology of Treponemal Infection. New York, Marcel Dekker, 1982

Pavia CS, Folds JD, Baseman JB: Cell-mediated immunity during syphilis. A review. Br J Vener Dis 54:144, 1978

Zenker PN, Rolfs RT: Treatment of syphilis, 1989. Rev Inf Dis 12:S590, 1990

BORRELIA

Barbour AG: Antigenic variation of a relapsing fever *Borrelia* species. Annu Rev Microbiol 44:155, 1990

Barbour AG, Hayes SF: Biology of *Borrelia* species. Microbiol Rev 50:381, 1986

Ciesielski CA, Markowitz LE, Horsley R, et al: Lyme disease surveillance in the United States, 1983–1986. Rev Infect Dis 11:S1435, 1989

Luft BJ, Gorevic PD, Halperin JJ, et al: A perspective on the treatment of Lyme borreliosis. Rev Infect Dis 11:S1518, 1989

LEPTOSPIRA

Johnson RC, Faine S: Family II. Leptospiraceae. In Krieg NR, Holt JG (eds): Bergey's Manual of Systematic Bacteriology, vol 1. Baltimore, Williams & Wilkins, 1984, p 62

Selected Papers

TREPONEMA PALLIDUM

Alderete JF, Baseman JB: Surface-associated host proteins on virulent *Treponema pallidum*. Infect Immun 26:1048, 1979

Alderete JF, Baseman JB: Surface characterization of virulent *Treponema pallidum*. Infect Immun 30:814, 1980

Baughn RE: Demonstration and immunochemical characterization of natural, autologous anti-idiotypic antibodies throughout the course of experimental syphilis. Infect Immun 58:766, 1990

Baughn RE, McNeely MC, Jorizzo JL, Musher DM: Characterization of the antigenic determinants and host components in immune complexes from patients with secondary syphilis. J Immun 136:1406, 1986

Clark EG, Danbolt N: The Oslo study of the natural course of untreated syphilis. Med Clin North Am 48:613, 1964

Dallas WS, Ray PH, Leong J, et al: Identification and purification of a recombinant *Treponema pallidum* basic membrane protein expressed in *Escherichia coli*. Infect Immun 55:1106, 1987

Fieldsteel AH, Cox DL, Moeckli RA: Cultivation of virulent *Treponema pallidum* in tissue culture. Infect Immun 32:908, 1982

Fitzgerald TJ, Repesh LA: The hyaluronidase associated with *Treponema pallidum* facilitates treponemal dissemination. Infect Immun 55:1023, 1987

Gjestland T: The Oslo study of untreated syphilis—An epidemiologic investigation of the natural course of untreated syphilis based on a restudy of the Boeck-Bruusgaard material. Acta Derm Venerol [suppl] (Stockh) 1955

Musher DM, Hague-Park M, Gyorkey F, et al: The interaction between *Treponema pallidum* and human polymorphonuclear leukocytes. J Infect Dis 147:77, 1983

Musher DM, Hamill RJ, Baughn RE: Effect of human immunodeficiency virus (HIV) infection on the course of syphilis and on the response to treatment. Ann Intern Med 113:872, 1990

Norris SJ, Edmondson DG: In vitro culture system to determine MICs and MBCs of antimicrobial agents against *Treponema pallidum* subsp *pallidum* (Nichols strain). Antimicrob Agents Chemother 32:68, 1988

Rolfs RT, Goldberg M, Sharrar RG: Risk factors for syphilis: Cocaine use and prostitution. Am J Public Health 80:853, 1990

Sanchez PJ, McCracken GH, Wendel GD, et al: Molecular analysis of the fetal IgM response to *Treponema pallidum* antigens: Implications for improved serodiagnosis of congenital syphilis. J Infect Dis 159:508, 1989

Steiner BM, Sell S, Schell RF: *Treponema pallidum* attachment to surface and matrix proteins of cultured rabbit epithelial cells. J Infect Dis 155:742, 1987

Thomas DD, Baseman JB, Alderete JF: Enhanced levels of attachment of fibronectin-primed *Treponema pallidum* to extracellular matrix. Infect Immun 52:736, 1986

BORRELIA

Barbour AG, Carter CJ, Burman N, et al: Tandem insertion sequence-like elements define the expression site for variable antigen genes of *Borrelia hermsii*. Infect Immun 59:390, 1991

Barbour AG, Hayes SF, Heiland RA, et al: A *Borrelia*-specific monoclonal antibody binds to a flagellar epitope. Infect Immun 52:549, 1986

Barstad PA, Coligan JE, Raum MG, Barbour AG: Variable major proteins of *Borrelia hermsii*. Epitope mapping and partial sequence analysis of CNBr peptides. J Exp Med 161:1302, 1985

Boyer KM, Munford RS, Maupin GO, et al: Tickborne relapsing fever: An interstate outbreak originating at Grand Canyon National Park. Am J Epidemiol 105:469, 1977

Bryceson ADM, Parry EHO, Perine PL, et al: Louse-borne relapsing fever. A clinical and laboratory study of 62 cases in Ethiopia and a reconsideration of the literature. Q J Med 39:129, 1970

Meier JT, Simon MI, Barbour AG: Antigenic variation is associated with DNA rearrangements in a relapsing fever borrelia. Cell 41:403, 1985

Paster B, Stackebrand JE, Hespell RB, Hahn CM: The phylogeny of spirochetes. Syst Appl Microbiol 5:337, 1984

Plasterk RHA, Simon MI, Barbour AG: Transposition of structural genes to an expression sequence on a linear plasmid causes antigenic variation in the bacterium *Borrelia hermsii*. Nature 318:257, 1985

Southern PM, Sanford JP: Relapsing fever. A clinical and microbiological review. Medicine 48:129, 1969

Spagnuolo PJ, Butler T, Bloch EH, et al: Opsonic requirements for phagocytosis of *Borrelia hermsii* by human polymorphonuclear leukocytes. J Infect Dis 145:358, 1982

Stoenner HG, Dodd T, Larsen C: Antigenic variation of *Borrelia hermsii*. J Exp Med 156:1297, 1982

LYME DISEASE

Barbour AG, Heiland RA, Howe TR: Heterogenicity of major proteins in Lyme disease borreliae: A molecular analysis of North American and European isolates. J Infect Dis 152:478, 1985

Benach JL, Coleman JL, Skinner RA, Bosler EM: Adult *Ixodes dammini* on rabbits: A hypothesis for the development and transmission of *Borrelia burgdorferi*. J Infect Dis 155:1300, 1987

Dattwyler RJ, Halperin JJ, Pass H, Luft BJ: Ceftriaxone as effective therapy in refractory Lyme disease. J Infect Dis 155:1322, 1987

Johnson RC, Hyde FW, Rumpel CM: Taxonomy of Lyme disease spirochetes. Yale J Biol Med 57:529, 1984

Magnarelli LA, Anderson JF, Fish D: Transovarial transmission of *Borrelia burgdorferi* in *Ixodes dammini* (Acari: Ixodidae). J Infect Dis 156:234, 1987

Magnarelli LA, Anderson JF, Johnson RC: Cross-reactivity in serological tests for Lyme disease and other spirochetal infections. J Infect Dis 156:183, 1987

Malloy DC, Nauman RK, Paxton H. Detection of *Borrelia burgdorferi* using the polymerase chain reaction. J Clin Microbiol 28:1089, 1990

Peterson PK, Clawson CC, Lee DA, et al: Human phagocyte interactions with the Lyme disease spirochete. Infect Immun 46:608, 1984

Wilkes B, Schierz G, Preac-Mursic V, et al: Intrathecal production of specific antibodies against *Borrelia burgdorferi* in patients with lymphocytic meningoradiculitis (Bannwarth's syndrome). J Infect Dis 153:304, 1986

LEPTOSPIRA

Adler B, Fain S: The antibodies involved in the human immune response to leptospiral infection. J Med Microbiol 11:387, 1978

Banfi E, Cinco M, Bellini M, et al: The role of antibodies and serum complement in the interaction between macrophages and leptospiras. J Gen Microbiol 128:813, 1982

Chapman AJ, Adler B, Faine S. Antigens recognized by the human immune response to infection with *Leptospira interrogans* serovar *hardjo*. J Med Microbiol 25:269, 1988

Faine S, Stallman ND: Amended descriptions of the genus *Leptospira* Noguchi 1917 and the species *L. interrogans* (Stimson 1907), Wenyon 1926 and *L. biflexa* (Wolbach and Binger 1914) Noguchi 1918. Inter J Syst Bacteriol 32:461, 1982

Fairbrother JM: Serological interrelationship of *Leptospira* serovar and genus-specific antigens by enzyme-linked immunosorbent assay. J Clin Microbiol 20:1089, 1984

Marshall RB, Wilton BE, Robinson AJ: Identification of *Leptospira* serovars by restriction-endonuclease analysis. J Med Microbiol 14:163, 1981

Martone WJ, Kaufman AF: Leptospirosis in humans in the United States, 1974–1978. J Infect Dis 140:1020, 1979

McGrath H, Adler B, Vinh T, Faine S: Phagocytosis of virulent and avirulent leptospires by guinea-pig and human polymorphonuclear leukocytes in vitro. Pathology 16:243, 1984

Swart KS, Wilks CR, Jackson KB, Hayman JA: Human leptospirosis in Victoria. Med J Aust 1:460, 1983

Wang B, Sullivan JA, Sullivan GW, Mandell GL: Role of specific antibody in interaction of leptospires with human monocytes and monocyte-derived macrophages. Infect Immun 46:809, 1984

Watt G, Alquiza LM, Padre P, et al: The rapid diagnosis of leptospirosis. A prospective comparison of the dot enzyme-linked immunosorbent assay and genus-specific microscopic agglutination test at different stages of illness. J Infect Dis 157:840, 1988

CHAPTER 46

Campylobacter, Helicobacter, and Spirillum

The genera *Campylobacter, Helicobacter,* and *Spirillum* include motile gram-negative bacteria that are helical or vibrioid in form. They are aerobic or microaerophilic. The genera *Campylobacter* and *Helicobacter* consist of well-defined groups of organisms, some of which cause diarrhea, gastritis, and systemic infections in humans in all parts of the world. As currently defined, there is no recognized species of the genus *Spirillum* that is a human pathogen. *Spirillum minus,* which is one cause of rat-bite fever in humans, does not belong to the genus *Spirillum,* but a new taxonomic position has not been assigned. It does, however, exhibit some morphologic and physiologic similarities to *Campylobacter* and other aerobic or microaerophilic gram-negative organisms that are motile and helical or vibrioid in shape. This loose assemblage of organisms composes Section 2 of *Bergey's Manual of Systematic Bacteriology.*

Campylobacter

Morphology and Physiology. The genus name *Campylobacter* is derived from the Greek word *campylo,* meaning *curved.* Organisms in the genus are slender, gram-negative, helically curved rods, 0.2 to 0.5 μm wide and 0.5 to 5 μm long. Several morphologic forms of *Campylobacter* have been reported, including spirals, S shapes, gull-winged forms, commas, and coccoid shapes (Fig. 46–1). They are characteristically comma-shaped when seen in infected tissues but are filamentous or coccoid after laboratory isolation. The spiral forms are more abundant in young cultures, whereas coccoid forms predominate in old cultures. The organisms have a distinctive cork-screw-darting type of motility, which is best observed with phase contrast or darkfield microscopy. Most species have a single unipolar or bipolar flagellum.

Campylobacter are microaerophilic and require a low oxygen tension (3% to 15%) and an increased CO_2 level (3% to 5%) for growth. They are extremely sensitive to hydrogen peroxide and superoxide ions that appear in the culture medium when it is exposed to air and light. The candle jar provides an adequate atmosphere for some strains of *Campylobacter,* but others will not grow in it unless a supplement is added that will enhance the organism's tolerance for oxygen. The campylobacters are unable to use sugars either oxidatively or fermentatively.

Taxonomy. Because of conflict in classification schemes and difficulties encountered in biochemically and serologically differentiating among strains, there has been considerable taxonomic and epidemiologic confusion. The initial isolate of this genus, made in 1909, was classified as *Vibrio fetus* because

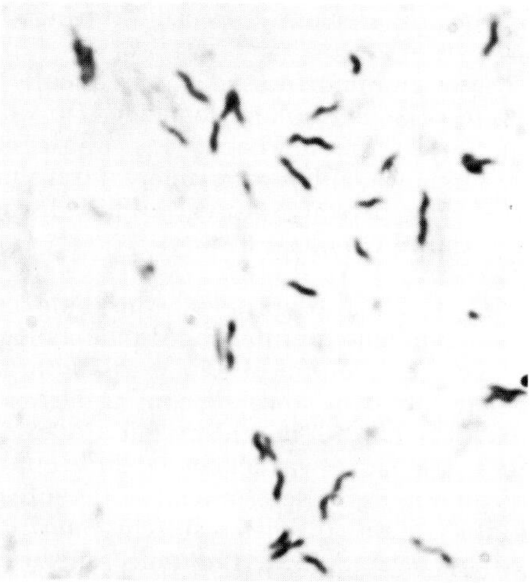

Fig. 46–1. *Campylobacter jejuni.* Note curved and serpentine forms.

of its morphology. A new genus, *Campylobacter,* was created to include *V. fetus* when it was recognized to be unrelated to vibrios in the family Vibrionaceae on the basis of its different nucleotide base composition, as well as its inability to use sugars either oxidatively or fermentatively. In 1947 the first human infection was recognized, and subsequently isolations of *C. fetus* and other *Campylobacter* were made from blood, spinal fluid, and feces. Current taxonomy recognizes four *Campylobacter* species as human pathogens: *C. jejuni, C. coli, C. laridis,* and *C. fetus. C. jejuni, C. coli,* and *C. laridis* differ only by minor properties. The genus also includes a number of other species that are associated with animals, either as commensals or as the cause of disease.

TABLE 46–1. PROPERTIES OF *CAMPYLOBACTER* AND *HELICOBACTER* SPECIES THAT ARE MAJOR HUMAN PATHOGENS

	C. jejuni	*C. coli*	*C. fetus*	*H. pylori*
Urease	−	−	−	+
Oxidase	+	+	+	+
Catalase	+	+	+	
Growth at				
25C	−	−	+	+
37C	+	+	+	+
42C	+	+	−	+
Cephalothin sensitive	R	R	S	S
Nalidixic acid sensitive	S	S	R	R
Hippurate hydrolysis	+	−	−	−
Growth anaerobically at 37C	+	+	+	−
Nitrate reduction	+	+	+	−
Motility from agar plate	+	+	+	−

R, resistant; S, sensitive.

Campylobacter jejuni, Campylobacter fetus, Campylobacter coli, and *Campylobacter laridis*

Laboratory Identification. Isolation of *C. jejuni* from rectal and stool specimens has been facilitated by the development of selective media, without which isolation is infrequent. Appropriate selective media include Butzler's, Skirrow's, and Campy-BAP plating media. These media contain various antibiotics to inhibit overgrowth of competing rectal flora. Inoculated plates are incubated at 42C in an atmosphere containing 5% O_2, 10% CO_2, and 85% N_2. Although *C. jejuni* will grow at 37C, the higher temperature suppresses the normal competing intestinal flora while permitting the thermophilic *Campylobacter* to grow. Colonies are fully developed at 24 to 48 hours. Some important properties for the identification of pathogenic *Campylobacter* species are found in Table 46–1.

Campylobacter species most often associated with human infections are catalase-positive. *C. jejuni, C. coli,* and *C. laridis* are thermophilic, with a temperature optimum of 42C. Resistance to nalidixic acid is the test for distinguishing *C. jejuni* from *C. laridis.*

Inasmuch as *C. fetus* is an opportunistic pathogen and is more likely to be involved in extraintestinal infections, cultures of blood or normally sterile body fluids should be made on nonselective blood agar plates or in liquid blood culture medium. Microaerophilic conditions of incubation are required, but a temperature of 25C should be used because some strains of *C. fetus* will not grow at 42C. If patients show diarrheal symptoms, culture should be made on selective media without cephalosporin antibiotics.

Antigenic Structure. Most of the studies on the antigenic configuration of *Campylobacter* species have focused on the surface structures of *C. jejuni.* This species appears to be antigenically diverse as indicated by the demonstration of at least 50 heat-stable serotypes based on lipopolysaccharide (LPS) and more than 36 serotypes based on flagellar antigens. Attempts to find a single specific surface or outer membrane protein (OMP) that is solely responsible for serotypic specificity have been unsuccessful. A likely candidate for inclusion in a *Campylobacter* vaccine is a surface protein that appears to be common to strains of a variety of heat-labile serotypes. Another possible candidate for a vaccine is a major OMP that exhibits considerable antigenic relatedness to major OMPs of campylobacters of diverse serotypes. This protein probably is a porin molecule since it is transmembrane and peptidoglycan associated.

The surface structure of *C. fetus* differs markedly from that of *C. jejuni* and other thermophilic species. *C. fetus* possesses a protein antigen that appears as a variously described "microcapsule," or S layer, composed of regular surface protein arrays taking the form of crystalline lattices that cover the cell surface. The layer is antiphagocytic and plays a central role in the pathogenesis of *C. fetus. C. fetus* is resistant to the bactericidal effect of normal or immune human or rabbit serum, whereas *C. jejuni* is sensitive. The basis of serum resistance is a high molecular weight protein that is a constituent of the bacterial capsule and is a part of the "S protein" surface array proteins. These proteins prevent binding of C3b, which thus leads to defective opsonization.

The LPS of *C. jejuni* is of the low molecular weight lipooligosaccharide type and appears to be antigenically diverse, which accounts for the large number of serotypes. In *C. fetus* the polysaccharide O antigen chains are of intermediate length and, in contrast to the long heterogeneous chains of the Enterobacteriaceae, are homogeneous in chain length. The characteristics of the LPS may determine in part whether a strain is sensitive to the bactericidal action of normal human serum. Serum resistance usually is associated with a smooth-type LPS.

The flagella of *Campylobacter* also are important surface antigens. Flagellins prepared from *C. jejuni* of different heat-labile serogroups are structurally similar and differ from *C. fetus* flagellin. Immunochemical analysis of these flagellins reveals the presence of both internal and surface-exposed epitopes. Both serospecific and antigenically cross-reactive epitopes have been demonstrated.

TYPING. Serotyping of *C. jejuni* and *C. coli* is useful for epidemiologic studies. Two of the methods currently in use are the Penner method for soluble heat-stable antigens, with an indirect hemagglutination technique, and the Lior method for heat-labile antigens with a slide agglutination technique.

Clinical Infection

Epidemiology. Campylobacters are found worldwide as commensals in the intestinal tract of a large number of wild and domesticated animals. In veterinary medicine, infections caused by these organisms are of primary interest because of the serious economic losses to farmers that result from abortions and infertility of infected cattle and sheep. Infection of animals is venereally transmitted, and the organisms may be harbored asymptomatically in the genitourinary and intestinal tracts for long periods of time. *C. jejuni* has the broadest animal reservoir, which includes poultry, dogs, cats, sheep, and cattle; *C. coli* is found primarily in swine; *C. fetus* is isolated from sheep and cattle, and *C. laridis* from seagulls. With the exception of *C. laridis,* these sources provide reservoirs for human infections.

Large outbreaks of human infections have been traced to the consumption of contaminated milk, water, and food, which provide the major vehicle for the transmission of the organisms to humans. Human-to-human spread, however, through a fecal-oral route also has been demonstrated. *C. jejuni* infects persons of all ages, but diagnosis is more frequent in children than in adults. The care of small children with *C. jejuni* diarrhea carries a risk of infection for their adult caretakers. Outbreaks in day-care centers may be spread in this way. The incidence of infection is greater in the summer and fall months. *C. laridis* appears to be epidemiologically, clinically, and microbiologically similar to *C. jejuni.*

Because of the lack of definitive surveillance data, the precise incidence of *Campylobacter* infections is unknown. Hospital-based studies in the United States and other developed countries indicate, however, that *C. jejuni* causes as much enteric disease in humans as do *Salmonella* and *Shigella.* According to some data, the incidence of *C. jejuni* in persons with diarrhea is similar to that of *Yersinia enterocolitica,* about 9% of diagnosed cases. *C. jejuni* frequently causes acute diarrheal diseases in travelers visiting developing countries. In striking contrast to the findings in developed countries, in the Third World countries *C. jejuni* is much more commonly isolated from healthy persons, especially during the first 5 years of life.

C. fetus causes an opportunistic and frequently fatal septicemic illness in persons who are debilitated, in women who are pregnant, or in the newborn. The sources of these infections are unknown, although a venereal transmission has been suggested. Few persons with bacteremic disease due to *C. fetus* have a known exposure history.

Pathogenesis. There appears to be considerable variation in individual susceptibility to infection. Epidemiologic studies have shown that the ingestion of as few as 500 organisms in milk will initiate illness in some persons, whereas in others the ingestion of less than 10^6 organisms fails to cause diarrhea. Variation in the relative virulence of different strains is probably also an important determinant of the infective dose.

Enteric infection with *C. jejuni* results in a mucosal invasion characterized by ulceration of the mucosal surface, crypt abscesses, and hemorrhagic necrosis of the ileum and jejuneum. Examination of the stools during infection reveals bloody diarrhea in a large proportion of cases, and fecal leukocytes usually are present, even in young children. The degree of parasitism of the small bowel has not been adequately investigated, but *C. jejuni* has been isolated from a jejunal aspirate. In addition to causing ulcerative disease of the mucosa, *C. jejuni* also invades the lamina propria, resulting in disease of regional lymph nodes and occasional dissemination of infection.

Three potentially pathogenic properties have been identified for *C. jejuni:* invasiveness, enterotoxin production, and cytotoxin production. Colonization of the mucous lining of the gastrointestinal tract appears to play a major role in the organism's ability to produce disease. Crucial for colonization are the flagella that enhance attachment and by virtue of their motility allow the organisms to penetrate the mucous layer covering the gut surface. Strains of *Campylobacter* isolated from patients with watery diarrhea produce a heat-labile enterotoxin that is structurally and immunologically related to the cholera enterotoxin. The toxin causes a secretory diarrhea by stimulating adenylate cyclase activity in the intestinal mucosa and disrupting the normal ion transport in the enterocytes. A cytotoxin also is produced by some isolates of *C. jejuni* and *C. coli.* It injures a variety of mammalian cells, but its role in human diarrheal disease is unknown.

Immunity. Patients who have been infected with *C. jejuni* develop strain-specific antibody responses that may be measured by agglutination, bactericidal activity, and complement fixation techniques. Patients with IgA deficiency may suffer from relapsing *C. jejuni* disease. After acute illness, normal persons demonstrate rising titers of IgG, IgM, and IgA antibodies as measured by enzyme-linked immunosorbent assay (ELISA). Bactericidal antibodies are dependent on the classic complement pathway, and ingestion and killing of *C. jejuni* by polymorphonuclear leukocytes depend on homologous antibody. *C. jejuni* may survive ingestion by mononuclear phagocytes for several days, which may be a mechanism used by the organism for survival and persistence. Specific antibodies to the identified *Campylobacter* toxins also have been demonstrated after acute illness.

Clinical Manifestations. *C. jejuni* infection can be manifest in several different forms. Acute enteritis is the most common presentation, with symptoms lasting from 1 day to 1 week or longer. The incubation period is variable (1 to 7 days), with prodromal symptoms of fever, headache, and myalgia often occurring 12 to 24 hours before onset of the intestinal symptoms. Diarrhea may vary from loose stools to massive watery stools or stools containing blood and inflammatory cells. Abdominal pain is a common symptom and is cramping in nature. Infection also may manifest as an acute colitis with fever, abdominal cramps, and bloody diarrhea. Tenesmus is a common symptom, and in the severest forms patients have a toxic appearance. Occasionally, acute abdominal pain, usually in the right lower quadrant, may be the major or only symptom of infection. Likewise, extremely high and persistent fever may be the sole manifestation of infection.

Bacteremia occurs in less than 1% of patients with *C. jejuni.* Although extraintestinal infections are rare, cases of meningitis, cholecystitis, and urinary tract infections have been reported. Both *C. jejuni* and *C. coli* are associated with inflammatory proctitis in male homosexuals. Persons who are HLA-27 genotype and who have *C. jejuni* diarrhea are at considerable risk of developing a postinfection–reactive arthritis.

Unlike *C. jejuni, C. fetus* is associated less frequently with enteric disease but manifests as an acute febrile bacteremic infection. Bacteremic disease in older men with cirrhosis, malignancies, and cardiovascular disease may lead to localized infection of the meninges, pleural space, lungs, joints, pericardium, and peritoneum. *C. fetus* appears to have a tropism for vascular sites and causes vascular necrosis in patients with endocarditis and pericarditis. The fatality rate in newborns with central nervous system infections due to *C. fetus* is high, but infection in this age-group is rare. Women in the third trimester of pregnancy also are susceptible to bacteremic disease, manifested by upper respiratory symptoms, pneumonitis, and fever.

Treatment. Most *C. jejuni* strains are sensitive in vitro to erythromycin, aminoglycosides, tetracycline, and chloramphenicol. Treatment with erythromycin shortens fecal excretion. Most infections, however, are self-limited, and antimicrobial therapy is not always indicated. Relapses after cessation of therapy are not rare.

Helicobacter pylori

In 1989 *Campylobacter pylori* (formerly *C. pyloridis*) was reclassified in a new genus, *Helicobacter pylori.* Since 1983 considerable interest has focused on *Helicobacter pylori,* which was observed on the surface of gastric antral epithelium in patients with active chronic gastritis. Although a complete understanding of the organism and the nature of its association with disease is incomplete, gastritis appears to predispose to gastric ulcers because the damaged cells are more susceptible to acid and peptic digestion.

Morphology and Physiology. In tissue sections the organisms can be most easily seen with silver stain, but in many cases they also can be demonstrated directly in Gram-stained smears of the tissue. They appear closely associated with the surface of epithelial cells and in the lumen, under the mucous layer (Fig. 46–2). In tissue the organisms are curved and stain gram-negative, whereas in culture they often are more rodlike, and bizarre U-shaped and circular cells are present. *H. pylori* strains have a number of characteristics that distinguish them from *Campylobacter* species. *Campylobacter* organisms have a single polar flagellum, whereas *H. pylori* has a tuft of polar flagella that are sheathed; axial filaments are not present. Optimal motility, which is corkscrew in nature, is exhibited in a highly viscous milieu such as occurs in the gastric mucous sheath. Unlike the cell wall of *C. jejuni,* which has a wrinkled appearance, the wall of *H. pylori* is smooth and contains unusual fatty acids. Other traits of *H. pylori* that separate it from *Campylobacter* species include its very high urease and catalase activity and the absence of the respiratory quinone, methylated menaquinone-6. It is because of these differences that *C. pylori* was reclassified in the new genus *Helicobacter.*

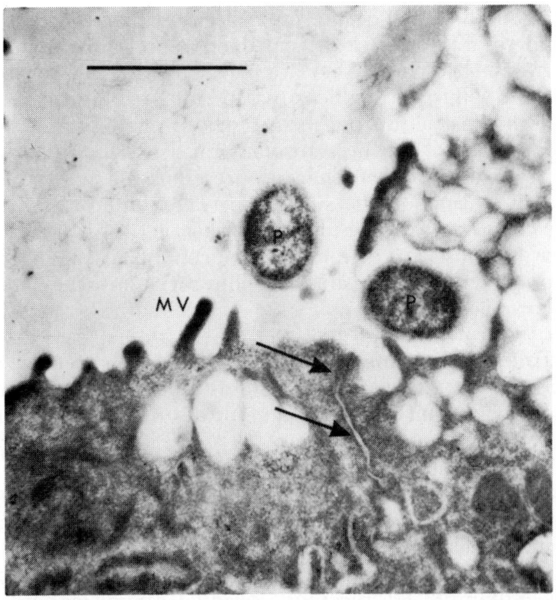

Fig. 46–2. Electron micrograph showing the location of *H. pylori* (P) close to the intracellular junction (arrows) of mucus-secreting gastric epithelial cells. Bacteria can be seen in among the microvilli (MV). *(Reprinted with the kind permission of Professor S. L. Hazell. From Hazell et al: J Infect Dis 153:658, 1986.)*

H. pylori is microaerophilic and, if the humidity is high, will grow at 37C in standard CO_2 incubators containing 10% CO_2. It grows on media containing whole or lysed blood, producing circular, translucent, nonpigmented colonies with a maximal size of 0.5 mm. No sugars are metabolized.

Clinical Infection

Epidemiology. The recent interest in *H. pylori* was prompted by studies of gastric biopsy specimens derived from patients with acute and chronic gastritis, gastric and duodenal ulcers, and other gastrointestinal conditions. For several decades, outbreaks of multiple cases of acute gastritis were observed to occur after gastric endoscopy, presumably as an infectious disease. Since 1982 when *H. pylori* was first isolated from biopsy material, the association of *H. pylori* with antral gastritis and of antral gastritis with gastric and duodenal ulcers has been repeatedly demonstrated. Placebo-controlled therapeutic studies of the efficacy of treatment of *H. pylori* in volunteers with *H. pylori*–associated gastritis also has shown a significantly better response in the treated group.

Pathogenesis. The organisms are acid-sensitive and appear to reside as a layer of organisms deep in the mucous coating that lines the stomach. They are highly motile and are closely associated with gastric mucus-secreting cells. They appear to invade the gastric mucosa in the regions of the intercellular junctions and to produce large amounts of ammonium ions and carbon dioxide from the urea present at the site. Presence of the organisms on the surface, between enterocytes, deep inside antral pits, and inside enterocytes results in an inflammatory response that includes polymorphonuclear leukocytes. Loss of microvilli in parasitized regions occurs in some patients with chronic gastritis.

Treatment. Treatment of ulcers with antibacterial compounds, such as bismuth compounds alone or with an antibiotic, has resulted in lower relapse rates than has treatment with cimetidine alone. In vitro, *H. pylori* is susceptible to a number of antibiotics, including erythromycin, tetracycline, penicillin, cephalosporin, and metronidazole. Of special interest is the susceptibility of *H. pylori* to bismuth, a component of some over-the-counter remedies for gastritis and gas, but the organism is not susceptible to cimetidine and antagonists of the histamine H_2 receptor. Residual organisms and the associated gastritis and duodenitis that follow therapy with the latter agents are believed to be responsible for the recurrence of ulcerative disease and gastritis.

Spirillum minus

Morphology. *S. minus* is a short, thick organism with tapering ends, 0.2 to 0.5 μm in size. It has two or three spirals that are thick and regular. It is gram-negative but can best be visualized in blood smears with phase-contrast microscopy or with Giemsa or Wright's stains. Silver impregnation methods, such as that of Fontana-Tribondeau, stain the polytrichous polar flagella. Darkfield illumination of a drop of blood containing the organism is the best method for demonstrating its rapid motility, spiral structure, and flagella.

Laboratory Identification. *S. minus* has not been cultured on artificial media. Proof that the organism produces rat-bite fever has been obtained by experimental inoculation of humans with blood containing the organisms. The diagnosis of rat-bite fever is based on the demonstration of the organisms in animals inoculated with the patient's blood, exudate from initial lesion, serum expressed from exanthematous patches, lymph node aspirates, or ground-up tissue from lesions. White mice or guinea pigs are useful for this purpose. Because mice often harbor *S. minus,* it is essential that animals be free of spirilla before inoculations are made. Alternatively, diagnosis may be made by examination of blood and exudate from lesions by darkfield illumination and by stains. The organism rarely has been detected with certainty in the blood of humans but may be demonstrated in material from the lesions.

Clinical Infection

Rat-bite fever is an acute bacteremic infection caused by *S. minus* or by *Streptobacillus moniliformis,* both of which are present in the normal oropharyngeal flora of rodents. Differences in clinical manifestations between the two forms, however, permit differentiation of the two diseases. Rat-bite fever caused by *S. minus* is commonly referred to as *sodoku fever.* (See Table 40–3).

Epidemiology. Rat-bite fever is primarily a disease of wild rats that is transmissible to rats, various other animals, and humans by the bite of an infected animal. Fleas and other insects are not vectors, and there is no record of transmission of the disease from human to human by contact, excreta, or fomites. Cases attributed to the bites of cats, ferrets, and weasels have been reported.

The infecting organisms are carried into the wound of the bite by the rat's teeth. Spirilla have not been found in the saliva of the rats. They may get into the mouth and on the teeth in blood from injured gums, lesions in the mouth, infectious conjunctival exudate that drains through the lacrimal ducts, or exudate from pulmonary lesions. When several persons are bitten by an infected rat, often only the first victim will contract the disease.

Pathogenesis. Rat-bite fever begins as a wound that may be infected with organisms other than *S. minus.* A variety of cocci, bacilli, and actinomycetes have been found in these conditions.

There are few recorded autopsies of cases of rat-bite fever. The local lesion, which is a granuloma without suppuration, shows necrosis of the epithelium and dense round cell infiltration of the corium. Similar round cell infiltration with dilated vessels occurs in the lesions of the skin eruption.

Clinical Manifestations. In a case uncomplicated by mixed or secondary infection, the wound of the bite heals promptly. After an incubation period of 5 to 14 days, the site of the wound swells and becomes purplish and painful. A chancre-like indurated ulcer with a black crust may develop at this site and may reach a diameter of 5 to 10 cm. The regional lymphatics are inflamed, and the adjacent lymph nodes become enlarged and tender. The development of the local lesion is accompanied by malaise and headache and a sharp rise in temperature, usually with a chill. After this, periods of fever alternate with afebrile periods. The temperature rises abruptly, remains elevated for 24 to 48 hours, and falls rapidly to normal within about 36 hours. The intervening afebrile periods last from 3 to 9 days. In untreated cases this relapsing type of fever may continue for weeks or months, gradually subsiding.

Within the first week of the beginning of the fever, a characteristic purplish maculopapular eruption of the skin of the arms, legs, and trunk, and occasionally on the face and scalp, usually appears. The skin lesions do not ulcerate. They fade somewhat during the afebrile periods but reappear, with new patches of eruption, during the paroxysms of fever.

The major serious complication is subacute bacterial endocarditis. In the preantibiotic era, the mortality rate was estimated to be about 10% and usually was due to secondary pyogenic infection. Some patients develop a false-positive reaction to treponemal antigens.

Treatment. Penicillin is the drug of choice. Streptomycin also has been used successfully.

FURTHER READING

Campylobacter

Black RE, Levine MM, Clements ML, et al: Experimental *Campylobacter jejuni* infection in humans. J Infect Dis 157:472, 1988

Blaser MJ, Hopkins JA, Perez-Perez GI, et al: Antigenicity of *Campylobacter jejuni* flagella. Infect Immun 53:47, 1986

Blaser MJ, Perez-Perez G, Smith PF, et al: Extra-intestinal *Campylobacter jejuni* and *Campylobacter coli* infections. Host factors and strain characteristics. J Infect Dis 153:552, 1986

Blaser MJ, Smith PF, Kohler PF: Susceptibility of *Campylobacter* isolates to the bactericidal activity of human serum. J Infect Dis 151:227, 1985

Blaser MJ, Smith PF, Repine JF, et al: Pathogenesis of *Campylobacter fetus* infections. Failure of encapsulated *Campylobacter fetus* to bind C3b explains serum and phagocytosis resistance. J Clin Invest 81:1434, 1988

Chow AW, Patten V, Bednorz D: Susceptibility of *Campylobacter fetus* to twenty-two antimicrobial agents. Antimicrob Agents Chemother 13:416, 1978

Guerrant RL, Wanke CA, Pennie RA, et al: Production of a unique cytotoxin by *Campylobacter jejuni.* Infect Immun 55:2526, 1987

Karmali MA, Penner JL, Fleming PC, et al: The serotype and biotype distribution of clinical isolates of *Campylobacter jejuni* and *Campylobacter coli* over a three-year period. J Infect Dis 147:243, 1983

Kiehlbauch JA, Albach RA, Baum LL, et al: Phagocytosis of *Campylobacter jejuni* and its intracellular survival in mononuclear phagocytes. Infect Immun 48:446, 1985

Konkel ME, Babakhani F, Joens LA: Invasion-related antigens of *Campylobacter jejuni.* J Infect Dis 162:888, 1990

Korlath JA, Osterholm MT, Judy LA, et al: A point-source outbreak of campylobacteriosis associated with consumption of raw milk. J Infect Dis 152:592, 1985

Lee A, O'Rourke JL, Barrington PJ, et al: Mucus colonization as a determinant of pathogenicity in intestinal infection by *Campylobacter jejuni:* A mouse cecal model. Infect Immun 51:536, 1986

Logan SM, Trust TJ: Outer membrane characteristics of *Campylobacter jejuni.* Infect Immun 38:898, 1982

Morrison VA, Lloyd BK, Chia JKS, Tuazon V: Cardiovascular and bacteremic manifestations of *Campylobacter fetus* infection: Case report and review. Rev Infect Dis 12:387, 1990

Pei Z, Blasser MJ: Pathogenesis of *Campylobacter fetus* infections. Role of surface array proteins in virulence in a mouse model. J Clin Invest 85:1036, 1990

Pennie RA, Pearson RD, Barrett LJ, et al: Susceptibility of *Campylobacter jejuni* to strain-specific bactericidal activity in sera of infected patients. Infect Immun 52:702, 1986

Perez-Perez GI, Blaser MJ: Lipopolysaccharide characteristics of pathogenic campylobacters. Infect Immun 47:353, 1985

Simor AE, Karmali MA, Jadavji T, Roscoe M: Abortion and perinatal sepsis associated with *Campylobacter* infection. Rev Infect Dis 8:397, 1986

Tauxe RV, Patton CM, Edmonds P, et al: Illness associated with *Campylobacter laridis,* a newly recognized *Campylobacter* species. J Clin Microbiol 21:222, 1985

Walker RI, Caldwell MB, Lee EC, et al: Pathophysiology of *Campylobacter* enteritis. Microbiol Rev 50:81, 1986

Helicobacter

Barthel JS, Everett ED: Diagnosis of *Campylobacter pylori* infection: The "Gold Standard" and alternatives. Rev Infect Dis 12(suppl):S107, 1990

Blaser MJ: Epidemiology and pathophysiology of *Campylobacter pylori* infections. Rev Infect Dis 12(suppl):S99, 1990

Buck GE, Gourley WK, Lee WK, et al: Relation of *Campylobacter pyloridis* to gastritis and peptic ulcer. J Infect Dis 153:664, 1986

Dooley CP, Cohen H, Fitzgibbons PL, et al: Prevalence of *Helicobacter pylori* infection and histologic gastritis in asymptomatic persons. N Engl J Med 321:1562, 1989

Drumm B, Sherman P, Cutz P, et al: Association of *Campylobacter pylori* on the gastric mucosa with antral gastritis in children. N Engl J Med 316:1557, 1987

Hazell SL, Lee A, Bradley L, et al: *Campylobacter pyloridis* and gastritis: Association with intracellular spaces and adaptation to an environment of mucus as important factors in colonization of the gastric epithelium. J Infect Dis 153:658, 1986

Marshall BJ: *Campylobacter pylori:* Its link to gastritis and peptic ulcer disease. Rev Infect Dis 12(suppl):S87, 1990

Marshall BJ, Goodwin CS: Revised nomenclature of *Campylobacter pyloridis.* Int J Syst Bacteriol 37:68, 1987

Perez-Perez GI, Blaser MJ: Conservation and diversity of *Campylobacter pyloridis* major antigens. Infect Immun 55:1256, 1987

Smoot DT, Mobley HLT, Chippendale GR, et al: *Helicobacter pylori* urease activity is toxic to human gastric epithelial cells. Infect Immun 58:1992, 1990

Spirillum

Bayne-Jones S: Rat-bite fever in the United States. Int Clin [41st ser] 3:235, 1931

Brown TM, Nunemaker JC: Rat-bite fever: A review of the American cases with reevaluation of etiology: Report of cases. Bull Johns Hopkins Hosp 70:201, 1942

Gilbert GL, Cassidy JF, Bennett N McK: Rat-bite fever. Med J Aust 2:1131, 1971

Jellison WL: Rat-bite fever (soduku and Haverhill fever). In Hull (ed): Diseases Transmitted from Animals to Man, 5th ed. Springfield, Ill, Charles C Thomas, 1963, p 652

Krieg NR: Genus *Aquaspirillum.* In Krieg NR, Holt JG (eds): Bergey's Manual of Systematic Bacteriology, vol 1. Baltimore, Williams & Wilkins, 1984, p 72

Place EH, Sutton LE: Erythema arthriticum epidemicum (Haverhill fever). Arch Intern Med 54:659, 1934

Roughgarden JW: Antimicrobial therapy of rat-bite fever. Arch Intern Med 116:39, 1965

Watkins CG: Rat-bite fever. J Pediatr 28:429, 1946

CHAPTER 47

Oral Microbiology

An important responsibility of physicians is to recognize the presence of oral diseases in their patients and to refer them for proper care as needed, just as the same responsibility exists for dentists with regard to systemic diseases in their patients.

The most common oral infections are dental decay (dental caries) and diseases of the gingiva and alveolar bone that support the teeth (periodontal disease). Although these diseases are not normally life threatening, virtually the entire population is affected at some time by one or both conditions. Other oral infections include endodontic infections that involve the pulp of the tooth after trauma or carious exposure and periapical infections resulting from extension of bacteria from infected pulp through the apex of the tooth. Abscesses may form from periapical infections or from deep periodontal pockets. Mild to severe pyogenic infections, which are potentially life threatening, can result from all these sources or from heavy contamination of tissues during oral surgery.

Of additional significance to systemic health is the potential for oral bacteria to induce endocarditis in susceptible heart valves or for chronic oral infection to affect the course of some systemic diseases such as diabetes. Conversely, some systemic conditions (e.g., pregnancy, diabetes) enhance oral inflammation or destructive processes of periodontal disease. Patients undergoing radiation therapy that affects salivary glands often experience severe oral complications, including rampant tooth decay.

Other infections of the tongue and oral mucosa include those caused by herpes simplex virus, types 1 and 2, and various fungi. *Candida albicans* may infect the tongue and mucosa after antibiotic therapy, especially with tetracyclines. Oral infections by the herpes viruses and by *Candida* species commonly occur in patients infected with the human immunodeficiency virus (HIV). Another lesion, termed *hairy leukoplakia,* has been found to occur only in persons infected with HIV. It is manifested as an epithelial hyperplasia affecting primarily the lateral borders of the tongue and is associated with the presence in the tissue of Epstein-Barr virus.

Rarely, chronic granulomatous lesions caused by *Cryptococcus neoformans, Histoplasma capsulatum, Coccidioides immitis,* or oral *Actinomyces* species occur in the mouth. These infections may be encountered with about the same frequency as oral carcinoma, from which they must be differentiated. The agents of these infections are described in Chapters 32, 82, and 85.

In addition, in certain systemic infections such as measles and herpes zoster, the oral mucosa exhibits lesions characteristic of the specific infection. Details of these infections may be found in more comprehensively referenced texts.

Oral Microbial Flora

Large masses of bacteria develop in different ecologic niches within the mouth—on the epithelial surfaces of the tongue and cheek and on the teeth (especially in occlusal fissures, approximal areas, and surfaces along the gingival margin). Dental plaque accumulations contain more than 10^{11} microorganisms per gram wet weight, and saliva contains approximately 10^8 bacteria per milliliter (Table 47–1). The organisms present in saliva do not represent a resident population but are organisms that have been dislodged from the oral surfaces, especially the tongue.

The oral cavity usually is sterile at birth, but within the first day, possibly coinciding with the first feeding, resident flora begin to colonize the mouth. Within a week *Streptococcus salivarius* and *Streptococcus mitior* are detected, probably acquired from the parents or attendants, and *Veillonella* and other anaerobic species appear shortly thereafter. With the emergence of teeth and the provision of a more suitable anaerobic environment, an increase occurs in the number of anaerobic organisms, such as *Fusobacterium* and *Bacteroides*.

Also detectable after the eruption of teeth are certain facultative organisms distinctive of the adult flora, *Streptococcus mutans* and *Streptococcus sanguis*. By the end of the first year the overall flora of infants is similar to that of adults. Two important groups, however—the oral spirochetes and *Bacteroides melaninogenicus* and related species that colonize the gingival crevice—usually are not present in the oral cavity until the time of puberty.

Flora of Different Parts of the Mouth

Within the oral cavity are several diverse ecosystems, each with its characteristic collection of bacteria. *S. salivarius*, for example, preferentially colonizes the dorsal surface of the tongue, whereas *S. sanguis* colonizes the smooth surfaces of the teeth and *S. mutans* may colonize occlusal pits and fissures of crowns. *S. mitior* is the predominant organism on the buccal mucosa, whereas *B. melaninogenicus* and oral spirochetes prefer the gingival crevice area.

Ecologic and Environmental Influences

The ecology and intraoral distribution of the various bacterial types indigenous to the mouth are regulated by a number of physical, chemical, and mechanical factors.

These factors include selection of an anaerobic bacterial flora in plaque as the redox potential (E_h) drops from +140 mV on clean tooth surfaces to −200 mV after 7 days of plaque growth near the gingival margin. Well-developed plaque in the gingival crevice exhibits large proportions of anaerobic forms. Table 47–1 contrasts the proportions of anaerobic and air-tolerant bacteria in various oral environments. Adherence of *S. salivarius* by means of pili to mucosal epithelial cells accounts for its predominance on tongue mucosa. Other adherence factors are involved in colonization of teeth and in plaque development. Frequency of fermentable dietary carbohydrates and acid production plays a decisive role in selection of aciduric and acidogenic bacteria in plaque that contribute to caries.

Dental Plaque

Formation of Dental Plaque. The bacterial colonization of teeth results in the formation of dental plaque, a layer of bacteria on the erupted surfaces of teeth and in the gingival crevice. The presence of plaque with specific bacterial species may lead to the development of caries and periodontal disease. Between the bacterial plaque and the enamel surface is a thin amorphous film less than 1 μm in thickness, the *acquired pellicle*. This layer consists primarily of salivary anionic glycoproteins that absorb selectively to the enamel surface within seconds after it is cleaned. Because of their affinity for these saliva glycoproteins, cells of *S. sanguis* are first to colonize the pellicle. These are followed by *S. mitior, Neisseria*, and *Veillonella*, within the first few days and unbranched and branched gram-positive rod forms, *Rothia, Eubacterium, Leptotrichia, Nocardia*, and *Actinomyces*, within the first 14 days. Approaching 21 days without disruption, dental plaque at the gingival margin also will exhibit anaerobic, motile spirochetal and curved rod forms. Thus continued bacterial growth results in a confluent microbial layer composed of organisms held together by a matrix consisting primarily of salivary constituents and carbohydrate polymers of bacterial origin.

Bacterial colonization of plaque is a selective process dependent on the specific ability of bacteria to attach to pellicle, to matrix, or to other bacteria. Synergistic interactions have been demonstrated that involve the production of peroxidase by facultative streptococci, catalase by *Actinomyces viscosus*, and superoxide dismutase by most facultative species. These enzymes eliminate toxic peroxides formed from oxygen, thereby permitting anaerobic species to grow in the plaque. Lactic, formic, and isobutyric acids and polyamines serve as nutrients for various anaerobic gram-negative bacteria such

TABLE 47–1. COUNTS OF BACTERIA ON ORAL SURFACES AND IN SALIVA

	Coronal Plaque	Gingival Plaque	Saliva	Tongue Epithelial Cells	Cheek Epithelial Cells
Direct microscopic count	2.5×10^{11}/g	1.7×10^{11}/g		100/cell	10–20/cell
Total cultivable count—anaerobic incubation	4.6×10^{10}/g	4.0×10^{10}/g	1.1×10^{8}/ml		
Total cultivable count—aerobic incubation	2.4×10^{10}/g	1.6×10^{10}/g	4.0×10^{7}/ml		

From Gibbons and van Houte: In Shaw et al (eds): Textbook of Oral Biology. Saunders, 1978.

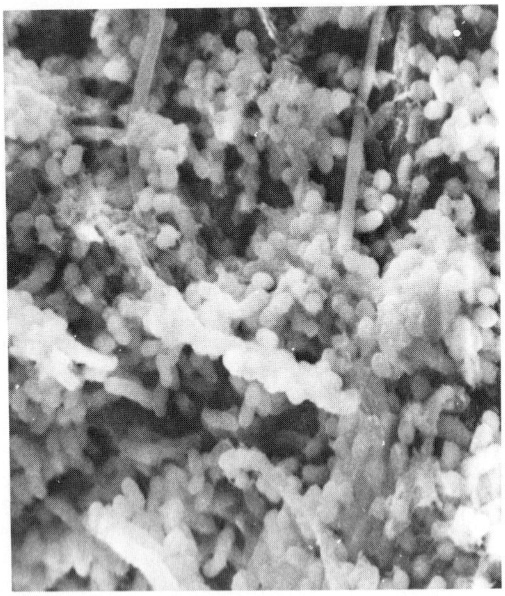

Fig. 47–1. Two-day plaque. Some of the filaments are covered by cocci resembling a corncob formation in an area demonstrating an increasing degree of structural complexity. × 4000 scanning electron microscopy (SEM). *(From Löe: J Periodont Res 12:85, 1977.)*

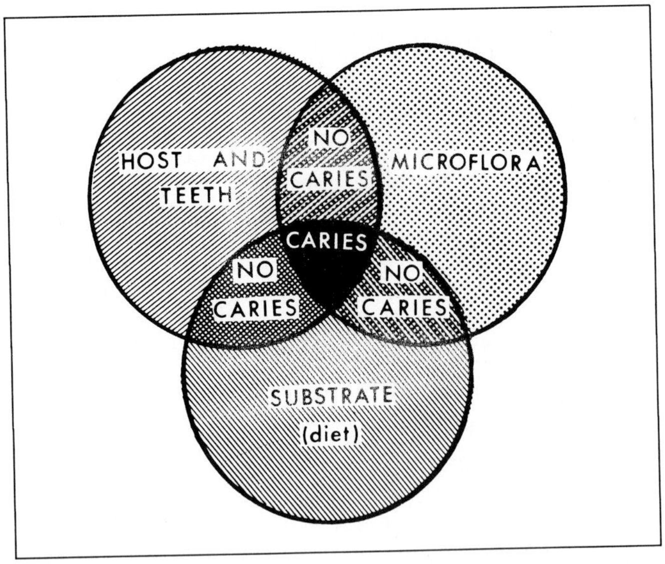

Fig. 47–2. Overlapping circles depicting factors responsible for caries activity. *(Courtesy of Dr. P. H. Keyes, National Institute of Dental Research.)*

as *Veillonella* species, *Eikenella corrodens*, and vibrio and spirochetal forms. Vitamin K, which is required by gram-negative anaerobic *B. melaninogenicus*, is produced by early appearing gram-positive facultative plaque bacteria. Also, levans or other surface polysaccharides produced by *A. viscosus* will aggregate *Veillonella* and certain strains of *S. sanguis* and appear to be responsible for the formation of "corncob" structures seen in well-developed plaque (Fig. 47–1).

Dental Caries and Periodontal Diseases

Dental Caries

The past 20 years have witnessed a drastic decrease in caries incidence because of impressive progress in understanding etiologic factors and in the widespread application of fluorides and other preventive measures. This decrease also has been attributed in part to widespread use of antibiotics to treat other infections. Development of a vaccine to protect against dental caries has been extensively studied and vaccination is now a real possibility.

Etiology

Caries is the result of acid demineralization of tooth structure that occurs only when interdependent factors coincide, as illustrated in Figure 47–2. Factors contributing to susceptibility of a tooth to dental caries include low fluoride content and surface irregularities such as pits and fissures or margins of restorations. These areas can be readily colonized by plaque bacteria that are difficult to dislodge with regular oral hygiene procedures.

Dietary sucrose is the major substrate for bacterial acid production by plaque bacteria and also is used by *S. mutans* as a substrate for the synthesis of adherent polysaccharides (Fig. 47–3) that thicken plaque and prolong the maintenance of a low pH on the tooth surface. The length of time that this acidic environment is sustained in critical sites has a significant effect on caries occurrence. Other carbohydrates, including

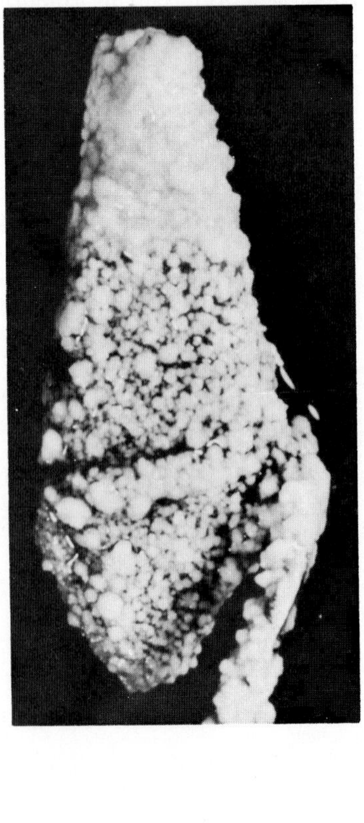

Fig. 47–3. Demonstration of extensive bacterial plaque-like matts or deposits that can form on a tooth incubated in sucrose broth culture of *Streptococcus mutans* for 24 hours and transferred to fresh broth medium daily for 4 or more days. *(Courtesy of Dr. P. H. Keyes, National Institute of Dental Research.)*

starches, also may be metabolized, although more slowly than sucrose. Such foods that are retained in pits and fissures thereby may contribute significantly to caries in these areas.

Dietary lipids such as cheese and proteins such as peanuts have been shown to limit pH changes resulting from carbohydrate metabolism by plaque bacteria. The quantity and quality of saliva significantly influence the occurrence and progression of dental caries. When the salivary flow rate is significantly reduced, a dramatic increase in caries may occur. This is due to reductions in mechanical cleansing effects and in buffering capacity of saliva, which leads to a shift toward more acidogenic bacteria. Salivary flow rate is affected by radiation therapy to the head and neck area and by numerous drugs, including those used for cancer chemotherapy. Various natural and acquired defense factors in saliva such as lysozyme, lactoferrin, peroxidase, secretory immunoglobulin, and other antimicrobial components may contribute to caries inhibition, but their role at present remains undefined.

Enamel Caries

Caries that initiate in pits and fissures on biting surfaces of molars and premolars are classified as *occlusal caries,* and caries affecting other enamel surfaces are referred to as *smooth-surface caries.* Factors contributing to the etiology of caries may differ in significance according to the type of tooth surface affected.

Bacteriologic Basis. Evidence is overwhelming that *S. mutans* is the primary etiologic agent in enamel caries in humans. There is evidence, however, that other acidogenic bacteria, especially *Lactobacillus* species, may play an important secondary role in the caries process.

MUTANS STREPTOCOCCI. Mutans streptococci (Table 47–2) are those streptococci found in dental plaque that ferment mannitol and usually sorbitol and that produce extracellular glucans from sucrose. These streptococci have in the past been referred to collectively as *Streptococcus mutans* but currently are separated into five species on the basis of differences in nucleic acid base content and sequence. Most of the species of mutans streptococci are cariogenic in animal models, with *S. mutans* accounting for 70% or more of human mutans streptococci isolates. The remainder of human isolates are almost entirely from *Streptococcus sobrinus.* Seven serovars have been identified for mutans streptococci on the basis of their carbohydrate antigens. *S. mutans* strains possess c, e, or f antigens, with c being most common in humans.

In humans the occurrence of caries correlates highly with the presence of *S. mutans.* Although this organism comprises only a small proportion of total plaque samples, the proportions are much greater on carious or precarious pits and fissures than on adjacent sound surfaces of the same tooth. Various animal models have demonstrated conclusively that mutans streptococci alone can induce dental caries that are transmissible to other animals.

Important to the virulence of *S. mutans* are its acidogenic potential and aciduric nature. It produces lactic acid from sucrose and other carbohydrates more rapidly than do other oral bacteria.

Another property highly correlated with cariogenicity is the synthesis of high molecular weight insoluble glucans (Fig. 47–3). This is a sucrose-dependent reaction involving first the cleavage of sucrose by a cell surface enzyme glucosyltransferase, followed by the subsequent polymerization of the glucose moiety into branched glucans with primarily $\alpha 1 \rightarrow 3$ and $\alpha 1 \rightarrow 6$ linkages. *S. mutans* cells also contain on their cell surfaces lectinlike protein receptor sites, referred to as *surface protein antigen A* (SPaA), which enable the cells to bind to the tooth surface. Receptor sites for glucans also are present. These promote the aggregation of *S. mutans* and the establishment of an insoluble plaque. This plaque acts as a barrier, separating buffering agents in saliva from acids on the tooth surface. The combination of acidogenic or aciduric capacity and the production of insoluble glucans in the presence of sucrose enables *S. mutans* to colonize new fissure sites and produce pH levels approaching 5.0, which are then sufficient to induce enamel demineralization.

Contributing to the persistence of *S. mutans* is its ability to hydrolyze salivary mucins and to use the carbohydrate released as a nutrient source. In addition, cariogenic strains of *S. mutans* are able to convert excess sucrose to intracellular storage polysaccharides (Fig. 47–4) and to use these storage depots as exogenous energy sources are depleted, thus perpetuating a low pH.

In the absence of sucrose, *S. sanguis* and other bacteria less acidogenic than *S. mutans* will colonize newly erupted teeth. Thus the child's teeth will harbor a caries-resistant plaque. Even if dietary sucrose is increased and *S. mutans* is readily available, these surfaces remain more resistant to caries than do teeth that erupt after the dietary change. The timing of *S. mutans* infection with respect to tooth eruption thus can have a long-term effect on caries rates. Thus infants and young children in families in which there are significant *S. mutans* infections are likely to incorporate *S. mutans* into their oral flora early and then be at high risk for caries.

OTHER BACTERIA. Before the emergence of interest in *S. mutans* as a cariogenic agent in the 1970s, diagnostic and research efforts were devoted to investigating the role of the highly acidogenic *Lactobacillus* species. Observations indicated that the extent of dental caries could be correlated with the numbers of lactobacilli present. Their strong acidogenic and aciduric properties and consistent association with dental caries made the lactobacilli likely candidates as primary etiologic agents. It is now recognized that lactobacilli are important secondary agents in dental caries and are of particular importance in smooth surface caries and in carious lesions that have progressed into the dentin of the tooth.

Other acidogenic bacteria in the oral cavity include *S. sanguis, S. mitior,* and *Streptococcus milleri.* These species are not as aciduric or as acidogenic as *S. mutans,* but they may contribute to acid demineralization, particularly in occlusal caries.

Control and Prevention. Efforts to prevent dental caries have been directed toward control of one or more components of the etiologic triad: improvement of tooth resistance by incorporation of fluoride into communal water supplies and by topical fluoride application; control of dietary carbohydrate intake; and daily removal of dental plaque. Although the impact of such preventive approaches is apparent, optimal levels of control have not been attained in all individuals, and high-risk groups still persist. Currently, efforts are being concentrated on the identification of safe and effective antimicrobial approaches.

A variety of plaque-inhibiting agents such as chlorhexidine have been identified and are available by prescription in the United States for short-term use. Although shown to be

TABLE 47–2. SUMMARY OF SOME BASIC DIFFERENCES WITHIN THE *MUTANS* GROUP OF STREPTOCOCCI

	S. mutans serovars			*S. rattus serovar*
	c	e	f	b
Genotype, mol% G + C		36–38		42–43
Antigenic serovar determinant	Glucose-(α) (1–4)glucose	Glucose-(β) (1–4)glucose	Glucose-(α) (1–6)glucose	(β) galactose
Cell wall carbohydrate		Glucose, rhamnose		Galactose, rhamnose
Fermentation				
Mannitol	+	+	+	+
Sorbitol	+	+	+	+
Raffinose	+	+	+	+
Melibiose	+	+/−	+	+
NH_3 from arginine	−	−	−	+
Growth in bacitracin[a]	+	+	−	+

From Newbrun: Cariology, ed 3. Quintessence Pub Co, Inc., 1989, Table 3–3, p. 78.
G + C, guanosine plus cytosine; ND, not determined.
[a] 0.2 U/ml.

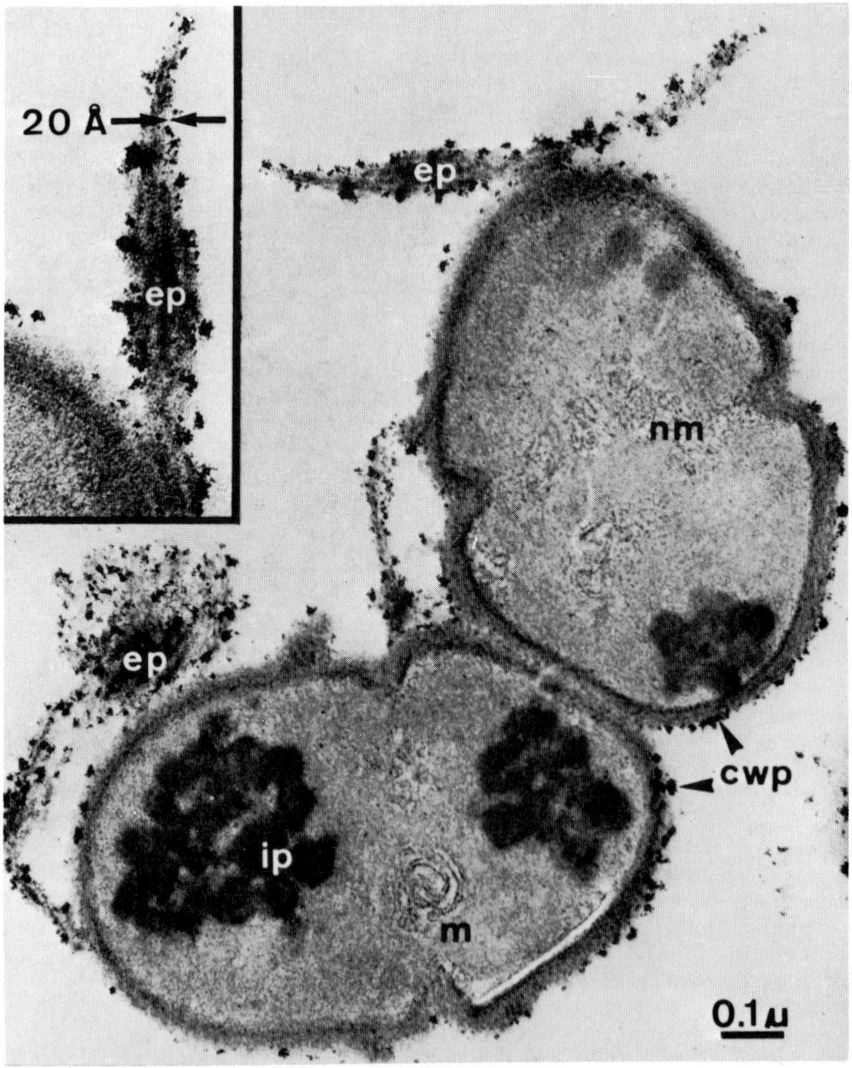

Fig. 47–4. Sucrose-grown cells of streptococci contrasted with "osmium black." Heavily electron-dense granules of intracellular polysaccharides (ip), mesosomes (m), and nuclear material (nm) are shown in detail. The cell wall has a dense middle layer; its outer surface carries strongly dense osmiophilic particles labeling sites of polysaccharides (cwp, arrows). In direct continuation with the cell wall there are extracellular polysaccharides (ep). This material consists of very fine protofibrils approximately 20 nm thick (inset). × 99,000; inset, × 165,000. *(From Guggenheim and Schroeder: Helv Odont Acta 11:131, 1967.)*

S. sobrinus serovars			*S. cricetus* serovar	*S. ferus* serovar
d	g	h	a	c
	44–45		43–44	44
Galactose-(β) (1–6)glucose	(β)-galactose	ND	Glucose-(β) (1–6)glucose	ND
	Glucose, galactose, rhamnose		Glucose, galactose, rhamnose	Glucose, rhamnose
+	+	+	+	+
+/−	+/−	−	+	+
−	−	−	+	−
−	−	+	+	ND
−	−	−	−	−
−	+	−	−	−

effective against *S. mutans,* these agents are approved only for control of plaque and gingivitis in adults. Thus their use as a potential caries control agent is limited at the present time.

The development and application of an effective anticaries vaccine have been demonstrated in animal models. These experimental vaccines have all utilized constituents of *S. mutans* as the immunogen. Immunization with glucosyltransferase, for example, has been found to effectively diminish the synthesis of glucans and decrease caries although not necessarily reduce the numbers of *S. mutans.* In humans, adult volunteers who ingested capsules of formalin-killed *S. mutans* cells developed significant specific salivary IgA antibody levels with no change in serum antibody levels.

More recent studies have successfully utilized purified cell wall antigens or ribosomal preparations from *S. mutans* as immunogens in animal models. Local application of a preparation of monoclonal antibodies formed against an *S. mutans* cell wall antigen was found to decrease colonization of the teeth by *S. mutans* and to prevent caries development in monkeys. Although effective and presumably safe vaccines have been developed, their use is questionable, given the nonlethal nature of dental caries and the general reduction in caries that already has occurred. It has been suggested that the most likely implementation of a caries vaccine will be in developing countries, where caries in children is emerging as a major health problem.

The use of salivary counts of *S. mutans* and lactobacilli has been advocated for detection of patients at high risk for the development of caries. Predictive value for these tests is enhanced when other caries risk factors also are evaluated. For individual dental patients, salivary bacterial counts are useful to supplement clinical examinations and to monitor treatment.

Caries in Nursing Infants. In Western cultures, nursing caries affects about 5% of the infant population. Prevalence in other cultures often is much higher. Nursing caries is a form of rampant dental decay affecting primarily maxillary incisors as a result of prolonged use of the nursing bottle as the infant goes to sleep. The etiology involves the same interplay of factors discussed earlier in this chapter, with *S. mutans* being the primary microbial factor. The presence of *S. mutans* and the extended exposure of affected tooth surfaces to sucrose, lactose, or other fermentable carbohydrate results in a rapid caries process that may extend to other teeth as they erupt. Usually, mandibular incisors are protected by the tongue during nursing and are not affected. Prevention of this condition involves reduction of exposure time and use of sucrose-free liquids.

Root Surface Caries

A significant dental problem in older persons is decay of cementum root surfaces, exposed mainly by gingival recession related to periodontal pathology. Cementum is much less mineralized than is enamel and consequently is susceptible to decay under less stringent requirements than is enamel.

S. mutans and lactobacilli have been implicated as important etiologic agents in root surface caries, as well as coronal caries. Also, consistently associated are *Actinomyces* species such as *A. viscosus* and *Actinomyces naeslundii.* These actinomycetes have a predilection for colonizing the cervicoradicular area of a tooth, are mildly acidogenic, and produce soluble extracellular polysaccharides.

Prevention of root caries is not unlike that of enamel caries but usually requires a more intensified application, that is, avoidance of sucrose and soft foods, meticulous oral hygiene, and regular fluoride exposure. Obtaining salivary counts of *S. mutans* may help in managing root caries.

Radiation Caries

Of particular concern to medical personnel is the potential for rampant and severe dental decay in patients in whom xerostomia (dry mouth) develops as a result of radiation therapy that damages salivary glands. This severe reduction in salivary flow results in multiple oral problems; thus prior consultation with a knowledgeable dentist is critical to the patient's oral health and comfort during radiation therapy. Teeth in questionable condition sometimes are extracted to prevent problems of discomfort or infection likely to ensue during therapy. If appropriate preventive measures are not instituted, severe decay may affect all tooth surfaces, even those not normally susceptible such as incisal edges of anterior teeth. The reduction of salivary flow results in a drastic increase in acidity in the oral environment. There is an increase in acidogenic aciduric bacteria such as *S. mutans*, lactobacilli, and also *Candida* and *Staphylococcus* species, with a concurrent decrease in *S. sanguis, Neisseria,* and *Fusobacterium,* which are normal constituents of the oral cavity. Thus a major shift in microbial balance occurs that predisposes the patient to multiple problems. The risk of orofacial infections, particularly osteomyelitis, is significantly increased, especially if the individual has dental disease at the outset.

As mentioned, prevention may involve extraction of compromised teeth before radiation therapy. Diagnosis, prevention, and therapy are based on symptoms rather than on bacteriologic testing. If teeth are retained, a rigorous program of fluoride therapy, including daily self-application, is essential for the prevention of radiation caries. This should be accompanied by good oral hygiene, dietary sucrose restriction, and use of artificial saliva.

Periodontal Diseases

The attachment of the gingiva to the teeth represents a unique interface between mineralized and soft tissue. Most periodontal diseases occur at this junction. Periodontal disease affects the vast majority of adults and is the primary cause of tooth loss in this population. Bacterial plaque products rather than bacterial invasion account for the majority of the diseases (Table 47–3). The interaction of the plaque products with the host defense mechanisms results in inflammation. This inflammation can cause loss of connective tissue, which allows apical migration of the epithelial attachment and formation of a periodontal pocket. As the inflammation spreads, there is loss of adjacent supporting bone.

Although bacterial plaque is the primary etiologic factor in periodontal diseases, the precise nature of the relationship is unclear. Initially it was postulated that the plaque mass or quantity of plaque was responsible for the inflammatory changes. In the 1970s a specific hypothesis was formulated in which certain bacterial species were implicated as causative factors. This specific theory may allow for a protective role by certain commensal gram-positive cocci within dental plaque.

TABLE 47–3. POSSIBLE MICROBIAL MECHANISMS OF TISSUE DESTRUCTION IN PERIODONTAL DISEASE

Direct Effects	Indirect Effects
Bacterial enzymes	Host enzymes
Collagenase	Collagenase
Hyaluronidase	Hyaluronidase
Chondroitin sulfatase	Antibody-mediated
Proteases	Pathogenic effects
DNAase	Anaphylactic
RNAase	Cytotoxic
Neuraminidase	Immune complex
Others	Delayed hypersensitivity
Cytotoxic agents	Lymphokines
Endotoxin[a]	Activation of complement
Peptidoglycans[b]	Chemotaxis of polymorphonuclear neutrophils
Ammonia	
Hydrogen sulfide	
Toxic amines	
Organic acids	

[a] Gram-negative organisms.
[b] Gram-positive organisms.

Bacterial plaque is a dynamic ecosystem in which colonies of facultative cocci, rod forms, anaerobic cocci, and fusobacteria adhere to the teeth at the tooth-tissue junction. If plaque is left undisturbed, an environment suitable for anaerobic rods, vibrios, spirochetes, or other potentially pathogenic forms may develop. If the early bacterial flora in dental plaque such as cocci and short rods continue to predominate, the conditions needed for the growth of pathogenic forms possibly may be precluded. Recently it has been theorized that pathogenic bacteria that initiate periodontal infections may be from an exogenous source rather than an endogenous change of normal flora. This has yet to be demonstrated conclusively. However, it is a logically plausible mechanism of disease transmission.

Gingivitis

Plaque-associated gingivitis is the most common of periodontal diseases. It consists of inflammation within the marginal tissues without loss of connective tissue attachment or alveolar bone support.

Experimental Early Gingivitis in Adults. The potential for plaque bacteria to harm the gingiva has been established in an adult human model. After an ideal degree of gingival health with no evidence of inflammation is achieved, brushing and flossing are suspended for 1 month. The following changes are noted: After only 1 day, exposed surfaces of teeth just above the gingiva become colonized with a film of cocci (mainly *S. sanguis*) roughly 20 cells thick. Extensive numbers of filamentous forms and fusobacteria accumulate within 4 to 7 days, followed by a proliferation of vibrios and spirochetes at the marginal gingiva in about 2 weeks. Histologic changes are present in the gingival tissues within 2 to 3 days of plaque accumulation. Within 2 weeks of plaque accumulation a plasma cell infiltrate is noted with dissolution of subepithelial connective tissue. This established lesion is characterized by bleeding on gentle probing. It occurs within a few days after spirochetes become abundant within the plaque. This plaque mass has been found to be approximately 100 to 300 bacteria thick. Restoring daily brushing and flossing to disrupt and remove the plaque permits restoration of gingival health within 2 to 3 days. Bacteriologic evaluation by culture in experimental gingivitis demonstrates that associated plaques are composed almost entirely of gram-positive bacteria, with about 50% being *Actinomyces* species. Morphologic evaluation would note an increase in spirochetes, vibrios, and gram-negative forms, as compared with initially healthy gingiva.

Long-Standing Gingivitis. In long-standing gingivitis often found in dental patients, the flora is similar but approximately 25% of the bacteria may be gram-negative, including species of *Fusobacterium, Veillonella, Campylobacter,* and *Bacteroides intermedius.* Erythematous margins, bleeding upon manipulation, and edematous gingiva are characteristic. The patient usually is unaware or has only minor discomfort associated with this disease process. Treatment is directed toward removal of the bacterial plaque or calculus deposits and oral hygiene instruction. This results in the resolution of the inflammatory disease process.

Acute Necrotizing Ulcerative Gingivitis. Acute necrotizing ulcerative gingivitis (ANUG) is a potentially recurring acute gingival infection. It is characterized clinically by punched-out-appearing interdental papillae. There usually is significant discomfort, bleeding, and a fetid odor. The condition usually occurs in persons under stress who also have deficient oral hygiene. ANUG is characterized by a predominance of spirochetes and fusiform bacteria. Medium-sized spirochetes penetrate the tissues and infect the gingiva. *B. intermedius* has been consistently cultured from plaque associated with this lesion.

Treatment of ANUG consists of débridement of plaque, calculus, and necrotic tissue by gentle scaling, chlorhexidine rinses, restoration of good oral hygiene, rest, and an improved diet. Antibiotic therapy of penicillin or metronidazole is effective if systemic manifestations are present. Antibiotic therapy without local débridement should be avoided, because temporary suppression of the infection without removing the causative factors allows recurrence of the disease, with potential for more extensive tissue damage. If ANUG is unresponsive to therapy, evaluation of a potential systemic disease should be pursued.

Pharyngitis (Vincent's angina) caused by fusospirochetal bacteria is uncommon but may resemble diphtheria. Phase-contrast or darkfield examination of a wet-mount preparation can be used to identify the disease. Anaerobic cultures are not helpful.

Steroid Hormone-induced Gingivitis. Elevation of steroid hormone allows for increased levels of steroid in the transudate called the *gingival crevicular fluid.* It appears that the steroid provides nutritional factors that encourage growth of a flora high in *Bacteroides* organisms, which is potentially pathogenic for periodontal tissues. This is the type of gingivitis represented by pregnancy gingivitis, puberty gingivitis, and gingivitis associated with birth-control medication or steroid therapy. Because the inflammation is plaque induced, attention to meticulous plaque removal should result in resolution of the disease state.

Medication-influenced Gingival Overgrowth. Phenytoin, cyclosporin, and nifedipine can all result in an overgrowth of gingival tissue. Phenytoin may be associated with plaque-induced inflammation. Patients should be carefully monitored during therapy that includes these medications.

Periodontitis

Periodontitis is the plaque-derived inflammation at the tooth-gingiva margin that has resulted in loss of subjacent connective tissue with downgrowth of epithelium, loss of attachment to the tooth, and loss of alveolar bone. It usually is diagnosed by increased pocket probing depths and radiographic evidence of bone loss. There are four major forms of the disease.

Adult Periodontitis. Adult periodontitis is the most common form of periodontitis. Subgingival plaque bacteria become established in areas of loss of attachment. Bacteria associated with those lesions vary according to the rate of destruction, level of disease activity, and host resistance. Periodontitis usually becomes clinically evident during the patient's mid-30s. Prevalence and severity increase with age; however, the disease is episodic, with periods of quiescence and repair. Subgingival plaque in the patient with periodontitis has a component attached to the tooth that is usually composed of *Actinomyces israelii, A. naeslundii,* and *A. viscosus.* There is an unattached portion adjacent to the soft tissues composed primarily of spirochetes and gram-negative rods. Studies of cultivable bacteria during periods of disease activity implicate *Bacteroides gingivalis, B. intermedius,* and *Actinobacillus actinomycetemcomitans* as potential periodontal pathogenic bacteria. Other bacteria and groups of bacteria also have been implicated as pathogens. There are no bacteria or groups of bacteria that fulfill Koch's postulates in the microbial etiology of periodontitis.

Treatment primarily relates to the mechanical removal of plaque, calculus, and plaque-derived products, such as endotoxin, from the root portion of the teeth. Surgical access may be necessary for proper instrumentation on the root surface and in an attempt at repair or regeneration of the defect. Antibiotics are often used in situations in which the disease is refractory to mechanical therapy.

Rapidly Progressive Periodontitis. Rapidly progressive periodontitis is an uncommon disease that is noted in young adults in their early 20s through mid-30s. It manifests as severe marginal inflammation with rapid loss of bony support. Approximately two thirds of the patients have depressed neutrophil chemotaxis. Bacteria associated with the rapidly progressive disease include *B. gingivalis, B. intermedius, Bacteroides capillus, Eikenella corrodens, Eubacterium brachy, Fusobacterium nucleatum,* and *Wolinella recta.*

Gingivitis and periodontitis associated with HIV infection are included in this rapidly progressive disease group. In these cases there is significant destruction not commensurate with etiologic factors present. The bacteriology of HIV periodontitis appears to be similar to that usually found in adult periodontitis except that additional microorganisms may be present. *Candida* species are present in the subgingival plaque of a high proportion of these patients. Antibiotic therapy often is used to augment conventional therapy in rapidly progressive disease.

Localized Juvenile Periodontitis. Localized juvenile periodontitis (LJP) is a rare condition noted around puberty. It usually is characterized by severe angular bony defects around first permanent molars and incisor teeth. Plaque is minimal, and the level of gingival inflammation usually is not consistent with the presence of the extensive underlying defects. Depressed neutrophil chemotaxis often is noted with this disease. Predominant subgingival organisms associated with juvenile periodontitis are *A. actinomycetemcomitans, Capnocytophaga ochracea, B. intermedius,* and *E. corrodens.*

A. actinomycetemcomitans is of particular interest because of its significant potential for pathogenicity. It is present in the plaque of a high percentage of patients with LJP, as compared with healthy and adult periodontitis groups. Although the prevalence of LJP varies among studies, persistence of the organism after therapy correlates with continued disease activity while elimination of the organism results in resolution of the inflammatory state.

Recommended therapy involves surgical débridement of the bony defects augmented by tetracycline therapy.

Prepubertal Periodontitis. Prepubertal periodontitis is a rare condition affecting the primary dentition. The generalized form of the disease is characterized by severe gingival inflammation, rapid bone loss, and tooth loss in both primary and secondary dentitions. There are defects in both polymorphonuclear and mononuclear leukocytes. These patients are subject to other infections such as otitis media and upper respiratory tract infections. The localized form of the disease affects only the primary teeth and is not as invasive as the generalized disease. Defects may be noted in either PMN leukocytes or mononuclear leukocytes, but not both. This disease is associated with a subgingival microflora dominated by *B. intermedius* and *Capnocytophaga sputigena.*

Laboratory Diagnosis

Periodontal disease is diagnosed primarily by clinical evaluation. No clinical criteria, however, allow accurate prediction of disease activity. A number of factors hinder microbial assessment. Periodontal diseases are episodic, and microbial evaluation may not coincide with a period of disease activity.

Culturing is the reference method for evaluating the microbial composition of plaque samples. It is laborious and technique sensitive. There are approximately 325 different bacterial species that may be isolated from the mouth. These vary at different sites within the same mouth and among individuals. A significant number of these organisms are difficult to culture because of nutritional or anaerobic requirements. Selective media or the use of DNA probes have reduced the cost and complexity of analysis of plaque samples. Both techniques, however, limit the evaluation of the total bacterial flora. In addition, the DNA probes do not allow for evaluation of antibiotic sensitivity of the organism.

Morphologic evaluation by darkfield or phase contrast microscopy has been advocated. Present periodontopathic organisms such as *A. actinomycetemcomitans* or *B. gingivalis,* however, are neither motile nor detectable by cell morphology. Problems related to technique such as site sampling, dispersion, and morphologic classification have detracted from the reliability of this procedure. Evaluation of spirochetes and motile forms has been shown to be an unreliable predictor of gingivitis.

Most cases of adult periodontitis are well controlled by conventional therapy and do not require antibiotic treatment. Patients whose periodontitis is refractory to conventional therapy may benefit from concomitant antibiotic therapy. Microbial evaluation by culture permits determination of both the specific organisms and their antibiotic sensitivity. It has been reported that one third of patients with refractory disease had yeasts, enteric rods, or pseudomonads in their oral flora. Without antibiotic sensitivity testing it would be difficult to determine the appropriate antibiotic treatment regimen.

Pyogenic Oral Infections

The complexity and severity of many pyogenic infections of orofacial tissues present a serious and difficult challenge to the physician, dentist, and clinical microbiologist. Acute or chronic infections such as periodontal abscesses, periapical infections, or pericoronitis may be painful but mild, with no progression nor systemic involvement, and may respond well to appropriate dental treatment. Approximately 10% of outpatients treated in surgical dental clinics may exhibit moderate to severe odontogenic infections, of which nearly half are postsurgical infections. Severe infections are progressive, associated with fatigue, malaise, fever, lymphadenopathy, or an elevated blood neutrophil count, and require immediate antimicrobial and clinical therapy.

Source of Infections. Infections result from displacement or extension of plaque flora into tissues. Bacteria can spread into tissues from infected dental pulps, from periodontal pockets, from infected pericoronal tissues, or from traumatic injuries. Plaque also may be forced into tissues during invasive dental treatments such as tooth extraction.

Pathogenesis of resulting infections involves the same mechanisms as those proposed for other mixed anaerobic infections.

Extension of Odontogenic Infections

Progressive pyogenic odontogenic infections are of serious concern because they can precipitously extend along fascial planes to the head or neck. *Bacteroides melaninogenicus,* one of the most common of the agents in these mixed infections, produces heparinase that can induce thrombi in small vessels. In maxillary infections, thrombi can be carried by venous return to the vasculature surrounding the brain. Resulting brain abscesses are detected by neurologic symptoms. Cavernous sinus thrombophlebitis, a potential consequence, causes a rare but usually fatal occlusion of the major blood sinus beneath the brain. Mandibular infections can spread to the neck to produce suffocation (Ludwig's angina) or to the thorax to cause fatal pericarditis. Because of these possible complications, it is essential to provide immediate aggressive clinical and antimicrobial therapy for all orofacial infections that appear to be progressive or produce signs of systemic involvement, or both.

Management. Management of severe or progressive, pyogenic orofacial infections involves several critical steps: (1) collection of a specimen for culture, drainage of exudate, and removal of necrotic bone and tissue debris, (2) immediate antibiotic therapy, (3) treatment of the source of infection, such as removal or treatment of the offending tooth, and (4) provision of supportive care and pain control as needed. Because of the critical nature of some orofacial infections, hospitalization should be considered early for debilitated or medically compromised patients.

Laboratory Diagnosis

Specimen Collection. Methods for specimen collection and transport are much the same as those routinely used for anaerobic infections in other parts of the body (Chap. 43). Except for research purposes, samples need not be collected under a continuous flow of oxygen-free gas. Pathogens of concern readily survive ordinary collection procedures if they can immediately be introduced into an anaerobic environment or be cultured within a few minutes after collection.

Exudates (0.5 to 1 ml) are best collected with a syringe and large needle before the lesion is incised and should be carefully transferred to anaerobic tubes or vials to avoid oxygen contamination. Both aerobic and anaerobic species will survive transport in a reduced atmosphere. Swabs of exudate may be collected from incised intraoral lesions if saliva contamination is kept to a minimum. An adequate amount of exudate can be collected because counts of bacteria in exudates often equal or exceed those in saliva. Samples should be transported to the laboratory immediately and should be called to the attention of the technologist who will culture them, with an explanation of their importance and the kinds of information needed. The better the communication, the better and more useful the results are likely to be. This specificity may avoid a useless report such as "only normal oral flora detected."

Culture. The major value of culturing acute, severe infections is to confirm the effectiveness of the antibiotic in use or to guide any changes in therapy if the infection is not responding in 48 to 72 hours. Time is therefore crucial. Exudates are inoculated on blood agar plates under conditions suitable for cultivation of *Bacteroides* species and then incubated anaerobically. Gram-stained smears of exudates are examined primarily to confirm detection of all major forms visible in such smears.

In the treatment of acute, progressive orofacial infection, it is critical that descriptions of the predominant organisms be reported within the first 24 to 48 hours. If indicated, other slower growing organisms can be detected and reported later. For antibiotic sensitivity testing the number of organisms and antibiotics tested should be determined by consultations with the clinician. Predominant gram-positive, facultative, and gram-negative anaerobic species or any definite pathogens need to be tested. "Normal oral flora" never is an appropriate or acceptable report of results from an aerobic or anaerobic culture of exudate. All bacteria obtained from normally sterile tissues are pathogens.

Microbiology of Pyogenic Infections. As seen in Table 47–4 most of the bacteria found in odontogenic infections are facultative and anaerobic species similar to those found in plaque. Mixtures in which two to six species predominate frequently are encountered. The most common mixtures include *Streptococcus faecalis* or other indigenous viridans streptococci, *Eikenella*, and the anaerobic *Bacteroides, Fusobacterium, Veillonella*, or *Propionibacterium* species. Predominating pathogens usually are those that grow within 48 hours. The finding of slow-growing *Actinomyces* species in acute pyogenic infections of a few days' duration does not indicate actinomycosis in the absence of clinical indications of actinomycosis.

Among the anaerobic gram-negative rods, *B. melaninogenicus* is one of the most common isolates. *Bacteroides fragilis* may be detected less frequently. It is more common in patients with severe, persistent infections that require hospitalization. Facultative pathogens are also sometimes important. *Staphylococcus aureus* is found in fewer than 10% of all oral infections; *Streptococcus pyogenes* is found in fewer than 1%. Coliform bacteria, especially *Enterobacter* species, may be found as secondary invaders in about 14% of all infections.

Orofacial infections are difficult diagnostic problems for the dentist, physician and microbiologist. Because they are mixed infections involving both anaerobic and facultative species, almost all the species detectable in a patient's plaque or saliva may also be present in some orofacial infections. Laboratory identification, therefore, usually is limited to the predominating two to four species. An additional obstacle is that laboratory personnel usually attribute no importance to facultative streptococci and consider them contaminants, just as they would from throat cultures. Nevertheless, *S. mitior, S. sanguis, S. mutans, Enterococcus faecalis* and possibly even *S. salivarius* are significant when obtained in abundance from exudates or blood where they should not exist. On a routine basis, these need not be identified to species. For effective guidance of therapy, however, the antibiotic susceptibility of the most abundant organism strains must be determined and rapidly reported, together with that of other rapidly growing anaerobic species.

Treatment and Prevention

Penicillin and erythromycin are the initial drugs of choice for outpatient therapy. For hospitalized patients, some clinicians prefer to use broader-spectrum antibiotics, including clinda-

TABLE 47–4. PREDOMINANT ORGANISMS IN ACUTE OROFACIAL ABSCESSES

Anaerobic Organism	Number of Lesions[a] (%)	Aerobic Organism	Number of Lesions[a] (%)
Bacteroides melaninogenicus	16 (35)	*Streptococcus mitior*	1 (2)
Bacteroides melaninogenicus		*Streptococcus viridans*	26 (57)
ss *melaninogenicus*[b]	3 (7)	*Enterococcus faecalis*	1 (2)
ss *intermedius*[c]	1 (2)	*Streptococcus* group B	1 (2)
Bacteroides asaccharolyticus[d]	2 (4)	*Staphylococcus aureus*	1 (2)
Bacteroides uniformis	1 (2)	*Klebsiella pneumoniae*	3 (7)
Bacteroides sp	19 (41)		
Fusobacterium nucleatum	2 (4)		
Fusobacterium sp	1 (2)		
Veillonella parvula	3 (7)		
Streptococcus intermedius	2 (4)		
Peptostreptococcus parvulus	1 (2)		
Peptostreptococcus anaerobius	1 (2)		
Peptostreptococcus micros	1 (2)		
Peptostreptococcus sp	1 (2)		
Anaerobic gram-positive rods	2 (4)		

[a] Total number of infections is 46, some of which contained a mixture of organisms.
[b] Presently separated into *Bacteroides denticola, B. melaninogenicus*, and *B. loescheii* (p. 622).
[c] Presently separated into *B. corporis* and *B. intermedius* (p. 622).
[d] See page 622.

mycin, and to carefully monitor for possible drug side effects (e.g., pseudomembranous ulcerative colitis). Other antimicrobial agents such as second- and third-generation cephalosporins and metronidazole have been used in resistant infections. In practice, however, and with the aid of drug susceptibility tests, an acceptable dose of a common antibiotic or an elevated dose of penicillin G usually provides adequate therapy and can provide rapid control of severe orofacial infections. Commonly used drugs include penicillin and its derivatives, erythromycin, cephalosporins, vancomycin, doxycycline, and metronidazole.

Early treatment of decayed, periodontally diseased, or nonvital teeth; good training of all patients in plaque control, especially those with conditions that compromise their resistance; and removal of plaque before dental, and especially before surgical, treatments will all help to reduce risks of orofacial infections that can become life threatening.

FURTHER READING

Books and Reviews

Crawford JJ: Periapical infections and infections of oral facial tissues. In McGhee JR, Michalek SM, Cassell GH (eds): Dental Microbiology. Philadelphia, Harper & Row, 1982, p 786

Curtiss R III: Genetic analysis of *Streptococcus mutans* virulence. Curr Top Microbiol Immunol 118:253, 1985

Guggenheim B (ed): Cariology Today. Proceedings of International Congress on Cariology, 1983. Zurich, Switzerland, Karger, 1984

Hamada S, Michalek SM, Kiyono H, et al (eds): Molecular Microbiology and Immunobiology of *Streptococcus mutans*. Amsterdam, Elsevier, 1986

Kleinberg I, Ellison SA, Mandel ID: Proceedings: Saliva and Dental Caries. Microbiology Abstracts [special suppl], 1979

Kolenbrander PE: Intergeneric coaggregation among human oral bacteria and ecology of dental plaque. Annu Rev Microbiol 42:627, 1988

Krasse B: Biological factors as indicators of future caries. Int Dent J 38:219, 1988

Lobene RR: Clinical studies of plaque control agents: An overview. J Dent Res 58:2381, 1979

Loesche WJ: Role of *Streptococcus mutans* in human dental decay. Microbiol Rev 50:353, 1986

Maiden MFJ, Carmen RJ, Curtis MA, et al: Detection of high-risk groups and individuals for periodontal diseases: Laboratory markers based on the microbiological analysis of subgingival plaque. J Clin Periodontol 17:1, 1990

McFarlane TW: Plaque related infections. J Med Microbiol 29:161, 1989

McGhee JR, Michalek SM: Immunobiology of dental caries: Microbial aspects and local immunity. Annu Rev Microbiol 35:595, 1981

McGhee JR, Michalek SM, Cassell GH (eds): Dental Microbiology. Philadelphia, Harper & Row, 1982

Nevins M, Becker W, Kornman K: Proceedings of the World Workshop in Clinical Periodontics. Princeton, NJ, American Academy of Periodontology, 1989

Newbrun E: Sucrose in the dynamics of the carious process. Int Dent J 32:13, 1982

Newbrun E: Cariology, ed. 3. Carol Stream, Ill, Quintessence, 1989

Newman HN: Plaque and chronic inflammatory periodontal disease. A question of etiology. J Clin Periodontol 17:533, 1990

Newman MG, Nisengard R: Oral Microbiology and Immunology. Philadelphia, Saunders, 1988

Ripa LW: Nursing caries: A comprehensive review. Pediatr Dent 10:268, 1988

Shaw JH: Causes and control of dental caries. N Engl J Med 317:996, 1987

Shaw JH, Sweeney EA, Cappucino CC, et al (eds): Textbook of Oral Biology. Philadelphia, Saunders, 1978

Slots J, Dahlen G: Subgingival microorganisms and bacterial virulence factors in periodontitis. Scand J Dent Res 93:119, 1985

Smith GE: Tooth decay in the developing world: Could a vaccine help prevent caries? Perspect Biol Med 31:440, 1988

VanDyke TE, Levine MJ, Genco RJ: Neutrophil function and oral disease. J Oral Pathol 14:95, 1985

Virginia Polytechnic Institute Anaerobe Laboratory: Outline of Clinical Methods in Anaerobic Bacteriology. Blacksburg, Virginia Polytechnic Institute and State University of Virginia, 1971

Selected Papers

Bowen WH, Amsbaugh SM, Monell-Torrens S, et al: A method to assess the cariogenic potential of foodstuffs. J Am Dent Assoc 100:677, 1980

Brown LR, Dreizen S, Handler S, et al: Effect of radiation-induced xerostomia on human oral microflora. J Dent Res 54:741, 1975

Chassy BM, Beall JR, Bielawski RM, et al: Occurrence and distribution of sucrose-metabolizing enzymes in oral streptococci. Infect Immun 14:408, 1976

Christersson LA, Slots J, Rosling BG, et al: Microbiological and clinical effects of surgical treatment of localized juvenile periodontitis. J Clin Periodontol 12:465, 1985

Crawford J, Sconyers J, Moriarty J, et al: Bacteremia after tooth extractions studied with the aid of prereduced anaerobically sterilized culture media. Appl Microbiol 27:927, 1974

Dzink JL, Tanner ACR, Haffajee A, et al: Gram negative species associated with active periodontal lesions. J Clin Periodontol 12:648, 1985

Ellen RP, Banting DW, Fillery ED: *Streptococcus mutans* and *Lactobacillus* detection in the assessment of dental root surface caries risk. J Dent Res 64:1245, 1985

Germaine GR, Schachtele CF: *Streptococcus mutans* dextransucrase: Mode of interaction with high-molecular-weight dextran and role in cellular aggregation. Infect Immun 13:365, 1976

Heimdahl A, Von Konow L, Satch T, et al: Clinical appearance of orofacial infections of odontogenic origin in relation to microbiological findings. J Clin Microbiol 22:299, 1985

Holt RG, Abiko Y, Saito S, et al: *Streptococcus mutans* genes that code for extracellular proteins in *Escherichia coli* K-12. Infect Immun 38:147, 1982

Hunt DE, Meyer RA: Continued evolution of the microbiology of oral infections. J Am Dent Assoc 107:26, 1983

Keene HJ, Daly T, Brown LR, et al: Dental caries and *Streptococcus mutans* prevalence in cancer patients with irradiation-induced xerostomia: 1–13 years after radiotherapy. Caries Res 15:416, 1981

Listgarten MA, Schifter CC, Laster L: Three-year longitudinal study of the periodontal status of an adult population with gingivitis. J Clin Periodontol 12:225, 1985

Löe H, Theilade E, Jensen SB: Experimental gingivitis in man. J Periodontol 36:177, 1965

Meiers JC, Wirthlin MR, Shklair IL: A microbiological analysis of human early carious and non-carious fissures. J Dent Res 61:460, 1982

Milnes AR, Bowden GHW: The microflora associated with developing lesions of nursing caries. Caries Res 19:289, 1985

Shklair IL, Gaugher RW: Glucan synthesis by the oral bacterium *Streptococcus mutans* from caries-active and caries-free naval recruits. Arch Oral Biol 26:683, 1981

Singletary MM, Crawford JJ, Simpson DM: Darkfield microscopic monitoring of subgingival bacteria during periodontal therapy. J Periodontol 53:671, 1982

Slots J, Bragd L, Wilkstrom M, et al: The occurrence of *Actinobacillus actinomycetemcomitans, Bacteroides gingivalis* and *Bacteroides intermedius* in destructive periodontal disease in adults. J Clin Periodontol 13:570, 1986

Slots J, Rains TE, Listgarten MA: Yeasts, enteric rods and pseudomonads in the subgingival flora of severe adult periodontitis. Oral Microbiol Immunol 3:47, 1988

Tanzer JM: Essential dependence of smooth surface caries on, and augmentation of fissure caries by, sucrose and *Streptococcus mutans* infection. Infect Immun 25:526, 1979

CHAPTER 48

Legionellaceae

During the summer of 1976 a fulminant pneumonia occurred in 221 persons attending an American Legion convention in Philadelphia. The cause of this epidemic was a previously undescribed bacterium that genetically was unrelated to any known human pathogen. The bacterium was named *Legionella pneumophila* to honor the victims of this outbreak. Subsequent examination of tissue and sera saved from other undiagnosed cases of respiratory illness revealed that *L. pneumophila* was the cause of at least three major outbreaks before 1976.

In the 14 years since the discovery of *L. pneumophila,* 29 additional species of *Legionella* and several *Legionella*-like organisms have been described in the literature (Table 48–1). Because of their unrelatedness to other known bacterial species and their unique lipid content, they have been placed in a separate new family, Legionellaceae. Legionella species are primarily environmental organisms and are found widely distributed throughout the world—inhabiting lakes, cooling towers, and water supplies of hospitals and hotels. Human pulmonary infections appear to result from contact with aerosols from these environmental sources. These infections can range from a mild flulike illness termed *Pontiac fever* to a severe pneumonia with systemic involvement. Despite the relatively recent discovery of these organisms, several studies have indicated that *Legionella* are common causes of both community-acquired and nosocomial infections.

Legionella pneumophila

Although more than half the described *Legionella* species have been implicated in human disease, *L. pneumophila* serotype 1 accounts for approximately 70% of all infections.

Morphology

L. pneumophila is a rod-shaped organism 0.3 to 0.9 μm in width and 2 to 3 μm long; forms more than 20 μm in length also occur, especially after in vitro cultivation. Motility is observed in fresh isolates and occurs by means of flagella. Pili also are present. Electron microscopic examination reveals typical procaryotic cells resembling known gram-negative bacteria. The organism is surrounded by two triple-layer unit membranes separated by the periplasmic space. Lipid vacuoles are present, and organisms grown on artificial media reveal Sudan black B staining inclusions that appear to be poly-β-hydroxybutyrate.

The organism is difficult to stain with the usual bacterial stains and consequently is missed with conventional examination of clinical material. *L. pneumophila* is not acid-fast and does not stain with hematoxylin and eosin. *Legionella* will faintly stain gram-negative if the safranin is left on for an extended period of time or if a dilute solution of carbolfuchsin is used as a counterstain. The organism can be visualized in tissue by Dieterle's silver impregnation stain and direct fluorescent antibody methods.

Physiology

Biochemical and Cultural Characteristics. *L. pneumophila* was first grown on the artificial agar medium of Mueller-Hinton supplemented with hemoglobin and IsoVitaleX in an atmosphere of 5% CO_2. While several other media have been developed for cultivating *L. pneumophila* in the laboratory, charcoal yeast extract agar (CYE) buffered with *N*-(2-acetamido)-2-aminoethanesulfonic acid (ACES) has proved to be a superior medium for the growth of all *Legionella.* The role of carbon dioxide for growth appears to depend on the medium used. With buffered CYE, recovery of *L. pneumophila* was the same in a room-air atmosphere as in a candle jar. Carbon dioxide concentrations exceeding 5% may inhibit the growth of *Legionella.* Growth is slow, requiring 3 to 5 days of incu-

TABLE 48–1. SPECIES WITHIN THE FAMILY LEGIONELLACEAE

Isolated From Human Sources[a]	Isolated Only From Environmental Sources
L. pneumophila	*L. brunensis*
L. anisa	*L. erythra*
L. bozemanii	*L. gratiana*
L. birminghamensis	*L. israelensis*
L. cherrii	*L. jamestowniensis*
L. cincinnatiensis	*L. moravica*
L dumoffii	*L. parisiensis*
L. feeleii	*L. quinlivanii*
L. gormanii	*L. rubrilucens*
L. hackeliae	*L. santicrucis*
L. jordanis	*L. spiritensis*
L longbeachae	*L. steigerwaltii*
L. maceahernii	
L. micdadei	
L. oakridgensis	
L. sainthelensi	
L. tucsonensis	
L. wadsworthii	

[a] Species that have been isolated from human disease or that have been serologically implicated in human infections.

bation. The generation time is from 2 to 6 hours, depending on the growth conditions. The optimal temperature for growth is 37C. Although the organisms can survive temperatures of 65C, they do not grow in temperatures above 42C. *Legionella* are unusual in that they use amino acids as the major source of carbon and energy and in that they require cysteine for growth on artificial media.

L. pneumophila hydrolyzes starch, gelatin, and hippurate; it is catalase positive and weakly oxidase positive. In contrast to some *Legionella, L. pneumophila* does not fluoresce blue-white or red when exposed to long-wave UV light. Like most members of the family, *L. pneumophila* produces a brown pigment when grown on media containing tyrosine. However, although useful in distinguishing this organism from non-*Legionella* species, this characteristic is shared by most members of the family. A surprising lack of useful laboratory procedures that can be used to characterize these organisms has resulted in an opinion by some experts that *Legionella* can be speciated only by serogrouping or DNA hybridization.

The fatty acid composition of Legionellaceae is unique among gram-negative bacteria. All species contain a predominance of branched-chained cellular fatty acids and have a relatively small amount of ester-linked hydroxy acids. The genus also has ubiquinones with 9 to 14 isoprene units. It has been proposed that the cellular fatty acid and quinone compositions of the family be used as a rapid means of grouping and classifying these organisms. The function of the fatty acids may be to protect the organism in thermophilic environments inasmuch as similar fatty acid profiles can be found in thermophilic gram-positive bacteria. The lipid A structure of the lipopolysaccharide of *L. pneumophila* is a complex structure, which differs from that found in enteric bacteria, consisting of a pattern of 19 3-hydroxy fatty acids, 13 to 23 carbons in length, 2 dihydroxy fatty acids, and 8 ester-linked nonhydroxylated fatty acids.

Resistance. *L. pneumophila* may survive as long as 139 days at room temperature in distilled water and for more than 1 year in tap water, with growth, not just survival, occurring in the tap water. The organism can survive in aerosols and has been found at a distance of 200 m from the aerosol source. Proteinaceous matter and extracts of blue-green algae stabilize the organism in aerosols. Various disinfectants, such as chlorinated phenolic thioether, may be useful in temporary control of the number of organisms in cooling towers. Hyperchlorination has been effective in reducing organism counts in potable water supplies. The organism load in water supplies also can be reduced by heating to temperatures higher than 60C; however, organism counts return to previous levels if heating is not continued.

Antigenic Structure

There are currently 14 distinct serogroups of *L. pneumophila* as defined by direct immunofluorescent staining of whole bacterial cells. The complexity of antigenic types and corresponding DNA relatedness studies have led some investigators to propose dividing *L. pneumophila* into at least three subspecies. In addition to the various serogroup antigens there are a number of antigens that are common to all *L. pneumophila* serogroups and other species of *Legionella*. All *Legionella* species have a single, common flagellar antigen.

Clinical Infection

Epidemiology. Legionnaires' disease is widespread, with cases being reported worldwide. The disease occurs sporadically, as well as in well-defined epidemic clusters. Although infections occur throughout the year, the majority of cases appear in the summer months. Risk factors are of two types: patient associated and environmental. Patients who smoke, have chronic pulmonary disease, whose alcohol consumption is high, or who are immunosuppressed are more susceptible to infection. Renal transplant patients or persons requiring dialysis also are at increased risk for the disease. The male to female ratio is 2.6:1. Most cases occur in persons 50 years of age or older, but cases have been seen in most age-groups. Pontiac fever is more likely to occur in healthy individuals.

Investigations of epidemics point to continuing common-source airborne exposure. Person-to-person spread has not been documented. Exposure to air conditioning cooling towers or evaporative condensers is postulated as the cause of numerous outbreaks of *Legionella* pneumonia and Pontaic fever. Potable water supplies have been found to be the source of several nosocomial outbreaks of legionellosis. Airborne spread of the organism from potable water may occur in showers or whirlpools. Nebulizers filled with tap water have been implicated as the source of infection in one study of nosocomial legionellosis.

L. pneumophila can grow and multiply in a variety of protozoa. The role of this association has not been clearly elucidated, but several authors have postulated that this may provide a means of survival in thermophilic environments and may explain the intracellular nature of the organism in human infections.

Clinical Manifestations. There are two distinct clinical diseases caused by *L. pneumophila*, pneumonia (legionnaires' disease) and Pontiac fever. The syndrome of Pontiac fever was first described in a 1968 epidemic that occurred in a county health department in Pontiac, Michigan. It is a self-limited illness that occurs primarily in healthy individuals and is characterized by the abrupt onset of fever, chills, headache, and myalgias. It is similar to influenza and other viral illnesses. The incubation period is less than that for *Legionella* pneumonia, and cough occurs only in approximately 50% to 60% of patients.

Legionnaires' disease or pneumonia varies in severity from a mild pneumonia to an adult respiratory distress syndrome accompanied by major extrapulmonary manifestations. The incubation period is 2 to 10 days (median 4 days) and is followed by an abrupt onset of high fever, nonproductive cough, chills, and headache or myalgias. Frequently, the patients show signs of toxicity. Central nervous system symptoms, confusion, and delirium develop in about one third of patients, which suggests the presence of a diffuse encephalopathy. Diarrhea has been reported in 36% of cases. Within 3 or 4 days the cough becomes productive with small amounts of nonpurulent sputum. Pneumonic infiltrates are found in almost all patients. A patchy or segmented alveolar infiltrate is found in one lobe, with consolidation of the involved lobe being the most common pattern of progression. Radiographic resolution is slow to occur and in the majority of patients may take more than 8 weeks. In some series, pleural effusions have been described in as many as half the patients.

Empyema, pneumothorax, and respiratory failure can occur, particularly in patients not treated appropriately. Hyponatremia occurs in half the patients. The organism may spread to other parts of the body, with dissemination occurring more frequently in immunosuppressed patients. There are case reports of organisms being isolated from blood, kidney, liver, spleen, brain, myocardium, ascitic fluid, and a hemodialysis fistula. In untreated cases, mortality varies from 10% to 20%.

Pathogenesis. Autopsy findings demonstrate an acute fibrinopurulent pneumonia, with exudation of neutrophils, macrophages, and large amounts of fibrin in the alveolar spaces. Electron microscopic examination of human biopsy specimens and experimental animal studies show that the capillaries are damaged, causing leakage of edema fluid and fibrin. The exudation interferes with gas exchange and is responsible for hypoxia.

L. pneumophila appears to be a facultative intracellular parasite and is capable of growing in human leukocytes as well as protozoa. The organisms are phagocytized by both neutrophils and pulmonary macrophages, but they survive and grow intracellularly. Antibody to *Legionella* enhances phagocytosis but does not lead to intracellular killing of the organism. Activated macrophages, however, kill ingested organisms, indicating that cellular immunity may play an important role in the prevention of disease. Genetic studies have resulted in the discovery of a gene that encodes a 24 kDa surface protein that appears to enhance the ability of the organism to infect explanted human alveolar macrophages. The gene has been designated the *mip* gene for macrophage infectivity potentiator. This surface protein may help the organism establish itself in the lung. Intracellular multiplication of *Legionella* may be attributed to one or more of the recently discovered toxins that interfere with the biochemical functions of polymorphonuclear leukocytes. One toxin is an extracellular protease that is toxic for tissue culture cells and that hemolyzes canine and guinea pig erythrocytes. However, the role that this and other recently discovered toxins and enzymes play in cell death or disease has yet to be clearly defined. Prevention of lysosome-phagosome fusion in *Legionella*-infected macrophages also has been demonstrated and may be responsible for the intracellular survival of the organism in these cells. Multiplication of the organisms intracellularly can lead to cell death and lysis with the release of host cell enzymes and factors that may be responsible for the damage to lung tissue.

Laboratory Diagnosis. Laboratory confirmation of Legionnaires' disease is made by direct demonstration of the organism in clinical specimens, culture of the organism, detection of specific antibodies in the patient's sera, or by the use of specific DNA probes.

L. pneumophila can be detected in tissue specimens by modified Dieterle's silver stain. When this stain is used, it is important that the tissue be negative for bacteria with the usual histologic stains because Dieterle's stain also will detect other bacteria. Specific identification of *Legionella* in clinical specimens can be made by direct immunofluorescent staining of the sample. The sensitivity of direct immunofluorescent detection varies from 50% to 80%, whereas the specificity is approximately 95% in most studies.

Culture of *Legionella* species has been greatly enhanced by the development of buffered CYE media, and the addition of antibiotics to this medium facilitates isolation of the organism from contaminated specimens, such as sputum. The sensitivity of culture is about 70%. Some workers have reported enhanced isolation rates from contaminated specimens when the samples are first washed with an acid solution.

Serologic diagnosis still remains the primary method of diagnosis of Legionnaires' disease for a number of hospital laboratories, albeit retrospective in many cases. The indirect immunofluorescence assay (IFA) is the primary test used, although enzyme-linked immunosorbent assays (ELISA) also have been developed. The demonstration of a fourfold rise in IFA titers to a level of at least 1:128 indicates recent infection. Seroconversion, however, may require 6 to 8 weeks. Antibody never develops in about 25% of patients with culture-documented legionellosis.

ELISA and radioimmunoassay methods for detecting serogroup 1 antigen in urine have been developed as diagnostic aids. These tests can detect approximately 75% of the patients with serogroup 1 infections but are not useful with other serogroups or species of *Legionella.* The antigen can be detected as early as 1 to 3 days after symptoms begin, and the test reaction remains positive for as long as 42 days after treatment has begun.

Nucleic acid probe technology has become commercially available for the detection of *Legionella* in clinical specimens. The sensitivity for this technique appears to be approximately 60% to 80%. Whereas the initial studies have shown that this technique has a high degree of specificity, there is at least one report of a high incidence of positive results in the absence of any other evidence of *Legionella* infection. The overall reliability of this assay has yet to be determined over a longer period of time.

Treatment. Erythromycin is the drug of choice for Legionnaires' disease. The use of rifampin in combination with tetracycline has met with reasonable success as an alternative therapy. Cephalosporin and penicillins are ineffective because of the production of β-lactamase. Respiratory therapy often is required for the seriously ill patient.

Control. Elimination of *Legionella* from the environment is not possible. However, elimination or reduction of the number of organisms in closed systems, such as hospital and hotel water supplies and cooling towers, has been achieved by means of hyperchlorination or the use of disinfectants. Some studies have reported that high heating of the hot water supplies and removal of contaminated shower heads and gaskets also have temporarily reduced the numbers of organisms. The prevalence of antibody in healthy individuals indicates that the patient factors probably are of more importance than is the environmental presence of organisms in determining infection rates and the severity of disease.

Other *Legionella* Species

The techniques used to discover and characterize *L. pneumophila* have led to the establishment of 29 additional species within the genus *Legionella* (Table 48–1). Fifty percent of these organisms have been isolated from clinical materials, as well as from environmental sources. Although the remaining species have been isolated only from the environment, there is serologic evidence that some may be involved in human infections. The disease caused by non–*L. pneumophila* organisms is similar to that caused by *L. pneumophila,* and the treatment is the same.

Legionella micdadei. In 1979 an organism was isolated from the lung tissue of two renal transplant recipients in whom an acute purulent pneumonia had developed. The organism was acid-fast in tissues and was named the *Pittsburgh pneumonia* agent. This organism subsequently was shown to be identical to both the TATLOCK agent isolated by Tatlock in 1943 from the blood of a patient with Fort Bragg fever and the HEBA agent isolated by Bozeman in 1959 from the blood of a patient with pityriasis rosea. These organisms were phenotypically similar to *L. pneumophila* but were genetically and serologically distinct. Although the names *Tatlockia micdadei* and *Legionella pittsburgensis* have been proposed, these organisms currently are referred to as *L. micdadei* in honor of McDade who first isolated *L. pneumophila* from materials obtained in the 1976 Philadelphia epidemic.

In addition to serologic differentiation, *L. micdadei* can be distinguished from *L. pneumophila* by its inability to hydrolyze hippurate, by the absence of β-lactamase, and by its inability to produce a brown pigment on tyrosine-containing media.

L. micdadei is second to *L. pneumophila* as the leading cause of legionellosis, causing approximately 58% of documented non–*L. pneumophila* infections. The pneumonia caused by *L. micdadei* is similar to that of *L. pneumophila,* but it is most likely to occur in immunosuppressed patients or in patients with other underlying illnesses. Almost 76% of the reported *L. micdadei* infections have been hospital acquired. Of the 26 reported cases of community-acquired *L. micdadei* infections, 11 occurred in nonimmunosuppressed patients; 10 of the 11, however, were elderly men. Mixed infections with both *L. pneumophila* and *L. micdadei* have been reported. As with *L. pneumophila* infections, erythromycin therapy is the treatment of choice.

Legionella bozemanii. In 1959 Bozeman and co-workers isolated an organism, termed WIGA, from lung tissue of a patient who had died of pneumonia. After the discovery of *L. pneumophila,* similar organisms were isolated from a number of patients with pneumonia. These isolates and the WIGA agent subsequently were found to be related to, but distinct from, *L. pneumophila.* The name *L. bozemanii* was given to this group of organisms, although some workers favored the genus name *Fluoribacter* because of the blue-white fluorescence produced when colonies on agar are exposed to long-wave UV light. *L. bozemanii* is variable in its ability to produce oxidase and β-lactamase, but it does produce a brown pigment on tyrosine-containing media.

Disease caused by *L. bozemanii* is similar to that caused by other members of this family and is treated with erythromycin. In contrast to *L. micdadei* infections, 81% of reported *L. bozemanii* infections were community acquired. *L. bozemanii* is the third leading cause of legionellosis, with 45 cases having been reported through November 1988.

Other Species. Several other species of *Legionella* have been isolated from clinical material obtained from persons with pneumonia similar to that of *L. pneumophila. L. dumoffii* was one of the first non–*L. pneumophila* species to be described. It has been isolated from water and human lung tissue. Like *L. bozemanii, L. dumofii* produces a blue-white fluorescence when exposed to UV light and its inclusion in the proposed genus *Fluoribacter* has been favored by some taxonomists. It is the fourth leading cause of legionellosis, with 23 cases reported through 1988.

L. feeleii was isolated from a factory in which 317 cases of Pontiac fever occurred. Although the organism was not isolated from the patients, serologic evidence indicated that it was the causative agent. *L. feeleii* also has been isolated from a *Legionella*-like pneumonia in at least six patients. *L. hackeliae* was isolated from a bronchial biopsy specimen of a patient with pneumonia. *L. jordanis* originally was isolated from environmental sources but recently has been isolated from lung tissue and has been serologically implicated in other cases of human pneumonia. *L. longbeachae* has been isolated only from human sources and consists of two serogroups. *L. wadsworthii* also has been described as a cause of pneumonia in immunosuppressed patients. Table 48–1 lists other species that have been implicated in human disease either directly by isolation of the organism or indirectly by serologic evidence. The relative importance of these organisms in the total picture of legionellosis is as yet unclear because most of them have been implicated as human pathogens only in a single publication to date. It also is likely that a number of the environmental strains and a number of similar, still unnamed, organisms eventually will be isolated from human infections.

FURTHER READING

Books and Reviews

Balows A, Fraser DW (eds): International Symposium on Legionnaires' Disease. Atlanta, Centers for Disease Control, Nov 13–15, 1978. Ann Intern Med 90:489, 1979

Bartlett CLR, Macrae AD, Macfarlane JT: Legionella Infections. London, Edward Arnold, 1986

Cianciotto N, Eisenstein BI, Engleberg NC, Shuman H: Genetics and molecular pathogenesis of *Legionella pneumophila,* an intracellular parasite of macrophages. Mol Biol Med 6:409, 1989

Cunha BA (ed): Legionnaires' disease. Semin Respir Infec 2:189, 1987
Edelstein PH: Laboratory diagnosis of infections caused by legionellae. Eur J Clin Microbiol 6:4, 1987
Fang GD, Yu VL, Vickers RM: Disease due to *Legionellaceae* (other than *Legionella pneumophila*): Historical, microbiological, clinical and epidemiological review. Medicine 68:116, 1989
Katz SM (ed): Legionellosis, vols I and II. Boca Raton, Fla, CRC Press, 1985
Meyer RD: Legionella infections: A review of five years research. Rev Infect Dis 5:258, 1983
Muder RR, Yu VL, Woo AH: Mode of transmission of *Legionella pneumophilia:* A critical review. Arch Intern Med 146:1607, 1986
Muder RR, Yu VL, Zuravleff JJ: Pneumonia due to the Pittsburgh agent: New clinical perspective with a review of the literature. Medicine 62:120, 1983
Thornsberry C, Balows A, Feeley JC, Jakubowski W (eds): Legionella: Proceedings of the 2nd International Symposium. Washington, DC, American Society for Microbiology, 1984
Winn WC Jr: Legionella and Legionnaires' disease: A review with emphasis on environmental studies and laboratory diagnosis. CRC Crit Rev Clin Lab Sci 21:323, 1985
Winn WC Jr, Myerowitz RL: The pathology of *Legionella* pneumonias, a review of 74 cases and the literature. Hum Pathol 12:401, 1981

Selected Papers

Barbaree JM, Fields BS, Feeley JC, et al: Isolation of protozoa from water associated with a legionellosis outbreak and demonstration of intracellular multiplication of *Legionella pneumophila.* Appl Environ Microbiol 51:422, 1986
Benson RF, Thacker WL, Waters RP, et al: *Legionella quinlivanii* sp. nov. isolated from water. Curr Microbiol 18:195, 1989
Berendt RF: Influence of blue-green algae (Cyanobacteria) on survival of *Legionella pneumophila* in aerosols. Infect Immun 32:690, 1981
Best M, Goetz A, Yu VL: Heat eradication measures for control of nosocomial Legionnaires' disease. Am J Infect Control 12:26, 1984
Bolin GE, Plouffe JF, Para MF, Hackman B: Aerosols containing *Legionella pneumophila* generated by shower heads and hot-water faucets. Appl Environ Microbiol 50:1128, 1985
Borenstein N, Marmet D, Surgot M, et al: *Legionella gratiana* sp. nov. isolated from French spa water. Res Microbiol 140:541, 1989
Brenner DJ, Steigerwalt AG, Gorman GW, et al: *Legionella bozemanii* sp. nov. and *Legionella dumoffii* sp. nov.: Classification of two additional species of *Legionella* associated with human pneumonia. Curr Microbiol 4:111, 1980
Brenner DJ, Steigerwalt AG, Groman GW, et al: Ten new species of *Legionella.* Int J Syst Bacteriol 35:50, 1985
Broome CV, Cherry WB, Winn WC, et al: Rapid diagnosis of Legionnaires' disease by direct immunofluorescent staining. Ann Intern Med 90:1, 1979
Chandler FW, Blackmon JA, Hicklin MD, et al: Ultrastructure of the agent of Legionnaires' disease in tissue. N Engl J Med 297:1218, 1977
Cherry WB, Gorman GW, Orrison LH, et al: *Legionella jordanis:* A new species of *Legionella* isolated from water and sewage. J Clin Microbiol 15:290, 1982
Cianciotto NP, Eisenstein BI, Mody CH, Engleberg NC: A mutation in the *mip* gene results in an attenuation of *Legionella pneumophila* virulence. J Infect Dis 162:121, 1990
Edelstein PH, Brenner DJ, Moss CW, et al: *Legionella wadsworthii* species nova: A cause of human pneumonia. Ann Intern Med 97:809, 1982
England AC III, Fraser DW: Sporadic and epidemic legionellosis in the United States. Epidemiologic features. Am J Med 70:707, 1981
England AC III, Fraser DW, Plikaytis BD, et al: Sporadic legionellosis in the United States: The first thousand cases. Ann Intern Med 94:164, 1981
Fields BS, Shotts EB, Feeley JC, et al: Proliferation of *Legionella pneumophila* as an intracellular parasite of the ciliated protozoan *Tetrahymena pyriformis.* Appl Environ Microbiol 47:467, 1984
Fraser DW, Tsai TF, Orenstein W, et al: Legionnaires' disease: Description of an epidemic pneumonia. N Engl J Med 297:1189, 1977
Friedman RL, Iglewski BH, Miller RD: Identification of a cytotoxin produced by *Legionella pneumophila.* Infect Immun 29:271, 1980
Freidman RL, Lochner JE, Bigley RH, Iglewski BH: The effects of *Legionella pneumophila* toxin on oxidative processes and bacterial killing of human polymorphonuclear leukocytes. J Infect Dis 146:328, 1982
Glick TH, Gregg MB, Berman B, et al: Pontiac fever—epidemic of unknown etiology in a health department. I. Clinical and epidemiological findings. Am J Epidemiol 107:149, 1978
Griffith ME, Lindquist DS, Benson RF, et al: First isolation of *Legionella gormanii* from human disease. J Clin Microbiol 26:380, 1988
Herbert GA, Steigerwalt AG, Brenner DJ: *Legionella micdadei* species nova: Classification of a third species of *Legionella* associated with human pneumonia. Curr Microbiol 3:225, 1980
Herwaldt LA, Gorman GW, McGrath T, et al: A new *Legionella* species, *Legionella feeleii* species nova, causes Pontiac fever in an automobile plant. Ann Intern Med 84:333, 1984
Keen MG, Hoffman PS: Characterization of a *Legionella pneumophila* extracellular protease exhibiting hemolytic and cytotoxic activities. Infect Immun 57:732, 1989
Lambert MA, Moss CW: Cellular fatty acid compositions and isoprenoid quinone contents of 23 *Legionella* species. J Clin Microbiol 27:465, 1989
McDade JE, Shepard CC, Fraser DW, et al: Legionnaires' disease: Isolation of a bacterium and demonstration of its role in other respiratory disease. N Engl J Med 297:1197, 1977
McKinney RM, Porschen RK, Edelstein PH, et al: *Legionella longbeachae* species nova, another etiologic agent of human pneumonia. Ann Intern Med 94:739, 1981
Meyer RD: Legionnaires' disease: Aspects of nosocomial infection. Am J Med 76:657, 1984
Morris GK, Steigerwalt AG, Feeley JC, et al: *Legionella gormanii* sp nov. J Clin Microbiol 12:718, 1980
Moss CW, Lambert-Fair MA: Reevaluation of the cellular fatty acid composition of *Legionella micdadei* Bari 2/158. J Clin Microbiol 28:389, 1990
Pasculle AW, Myerowitz RL, Rindaldo CR Jr: New bacterial agent of pneumonia isolated from renal-transplant recipients. Lancet 2:58, 1979
Rechnitzer C, Diamant M, Pedersen BK: Inhibition of human natural killer cell activity by *Legionella pneumophila* protease. Eur J Clin Microbiol Infect Dis 8:989, 1989
Reingold AL, Thomason BM, Blake BJ, et al: Legionella pneumonia in the United States: The distribution of serogroups and species causing human illness. J Infect Dis 149:819, 1984
Rodgers FG: The role of structure and invasiveness on the pathogenicity of legionella. Zbl Bakt Hyg I Abt Org A 255:138, 1983
Rowbotham TJ: Preliminary report on the pathogenicity of *Legionella pneumophila* for fresh water and soil amoebae. J Clin Pathol 33:1179, 1980
Rowbatham TJ: Isolation of *Legionella pneumophila* from clinical spec-

imens via amoebae and the interaction of these and other isolates with amoebae. J Clin Pathol 36:978, 1983

Skaliy P, Thompson TA, Gorman GW, et al: Laboratory studies of disinfectants against *Legionella pneumophila*. Appl Environ Microbiol 40:697, 1980

Snyder MB, Siwicki M, Wireman J, et al: Reduction in *Legionella pneumophila* through heat flushing followed by continuous supplemental chlorination of hospital hot water. J Infect Dis 162:127, 1990

Sonesson A, Jantzen E, Bryn K, et al: Chemical composition of a lipopolysaccharide from *Legionella pneumophila*. Arch Microbiol 153:72, 1989

Soracco RJ, Gill HK, Fliermans CB, Pope DH: Susceptibilities of algae and *Legionella pneumophila* to cooling tower biocides. Appl Environ Microbiol 45:1254, 1983

Thacker WL, Benson RF, Hawes L, et al: Characterization of a *Legionella anisa* strain isolated from a patient with pneumonia. J Clin Microbiol 28:122, 1990

Thacker WL, Benson RF, Schifman RB, et al: *Legionella tucsonensis* sp. nov. isolated from a renal transplant recipient. J Clin Microbiol 27:1831, 1989

Thacker WL, Benson RF, Staneck JL, et al: *Legionella cincinnatiensis* sp. nov. isolated from a patient with pneumonia. J Clin Microbiol 26:418, 1988

Thacker WL, Wilkinson HW, Benson RF, et al: *Legionella jordanis* isolated from a patient with fatal pneumonia. J Clin Microbiol 26:1400, 1988

White HJ, Felton WW, Sun CN: Extra pulmonary histopathologic manifestations of Legionnaires' disease. Evidence for myocarditis and bacteremia. Arch Pathol Lab Med 104:287, 1980

Wilkinson HW, Draser V, Thacker WL, et al: *Legionella moravica* sp. nov. and *Legionella brunensis* sp. nov. isolated from cooling-tower water. Ann Inst Pasteur Microbiol 139:393, 1988

Wilkinson HW, Sangster N, Ratcliff RM, et al: Problems with identification of *Legionella* species from the environment and isolation of six possible new species. Appl Environ Microbiol 56:796, 1990

Wilkinson HW, Thacker WL, Benson RF, et al: *Legionella birminghamensis* sp. nov. isolated from a cardiac transplant recipient. J Clin Microbiol 25:2120, 1987

Wong KH, Feeley JC: Antigens and toxic components of Legionella in pathogenesis and immunity. Zbl Bakt Hyg I Abt Org A 255:132, 1983

Yee RB, Wadowsky RM: Multiplication of *Legionella pneumophila* in unsterilized tap water. Appl Environ Microbiol 43:1330, 1982

CHAPTER 49

Rickettsiae

Rickettsiaceae

TABLE 49–1. CLASSIFICATION OF THE RICKETTSIAS AND CHLAMYDIAS

	Species
Order I: Rickettsiales	
Family: Rickettsiaceae	
Tribe: Rickettsieae	
Genus: *Rickettsia*	*rickettsii, akari, prowazekii, typhi, tsutsugamushi*
Rochalimaea	*quintana*
Coxiella	*burnetii*
Tribe: Ehrlichieae	
Genus: *Ehrlichia*	*sennetsu, canis, equi, phagocytophila, risticii*
Family: Bartonellaceae	
Genus: *Bartonella*	*bacilliformis*
Order II: Chlamydiales	
Family: Chlamydiaceae	
Genus: *Chlamydia*	*trachomatis, psittaci*

Rickettsial infections have been significant factors in the history of Western civilization. Epidemic typhus, recognized as a distinct clinical entity since the sixteenth century, has always been intimately associated with war, famine, and human suffering. In fact, typhus played a decisive role in the outcome of several major European wars. Charles I abandoned his plan to march on London in 1643 because of an epidemic of typhus fever. In 1741 Prague fell to the French army after 60,000 defenders had died from typhus. During an 1816 to 1819 epidemic in Ireland there were 600,000 cases of typhus among the population of 6,000,000. In both World Wars, typhus killed or caused great suffering in hundreds of thousands of people. Scrub typhus was a major problem for both Allied and Japanese armies during World War II. Its occurrence and control were factors in military strategy in the Pacific.

In spite of these and many other devastating epidemics, the first microbiologic description of *Rickettsia* did not occur until the first decade of the twentieth century, when Howard Ricketts described the etiologic agent of Rocky Mountain spotted fever, cultivated the organism in laboratory animals, and deduced its natural ecology and epidemiology. Using similar experimental approaches, other investigators rapidly obtained a basic microbiologic understanding of typhus and other spotted fevers. The name *Rickettsiaceae* honors Ricketts for his brilliant experiments, which were performed with modest funds and simple laboratory equipment. Ricketts and a number of early rickettsiologists eventually were killed by the disease agents they were studying.

After Rickett's discoveries, the importance of arthropod vectors in the transmission of other rickettsial diseases was appreciated, and outbreaks of the typhus fevers were curbed by sanitary and vector control measures. Later, the introduction of tetracycline and chloramphenicol further brought the rickettsioses under human control. In spite of these accomplishments, Hans Zinsser's comment in his book *Rats, Lice and History* is as appropriate today as it was 55 years ago:

> Typhus is not dead. It will continue to break into the open whenever human stupidity and brutality give it a chance, as most likely they occasionally will. But its freedom of action is being restricted and more and more it will be confined, like other savage creatures, in the zoologic gardens of controlled diseases.

The family Rickettsiaceae, one of the three members of the order Rickettsiales, is composed of three tribes (Rickettsieae, Ehrlichieae, and Wolbachieae). The tribe Rickettsieae in turn contains three genera that infect man: *Rickettsia, Rochalimaea,* and *Coxiella* (Table 49–1). Rickettsiaceae may be parasitic or mutualistic. Parasitic forms are associated with the reticuloendothelial and vascular endothelial cells of vertebrates. Mutualistic forms are intracellularly associated with arthropod tissues. With one exception, *Rochalimaea quintana,* the causative agent of trench fever, species pathogenic for man have not been cultured in cellfree media. Rickettsiaceae morphologically resemble other prokaryotic bacteria but are unique in the obligatory nature of their intracellular parasitic life. Interest in the Rickettsiaceae stems both from the diseases they produce and from the challenges they provide investigators seeking a better understanding of host-parasite relationships. All members of the family Rickettsiaceae are phylogenetically related to the purple bacteria. The three members of the genus *Rickettsia* have closely related rRNA sequences and belong within the alpha subdivision of the purple bacteria, as do Ehrlichieae. *Coxiella* are classified as members of the gamma subdivision of purple bacteria and have a specific but distinct relationship to the genus *Legionella.*

Morphology and Physiology

RICKETTSIA AND *ROCHALIMAEA.* Rickettsiae belonging to these genera are pleomorphic, rodshaped to coccoid organisms ranging in size from 0.3 to 0.6 μm in width to 0.8 to 2.0 μm in length. They stain poorly with Gram's stain but can be visualized with both the Giemsa and Macchiavello methods.

Their morphology is similar to that of gram-negative bacteria (Fig. 49–1). All contain a trilaminar cell membrane consisting of a cytoplasmic membrane and a double leaflet cell wall. Rickettsiae lack flagella and pili. Typhus and spotted fever group rickettsiae have a thick inner cell wall leaflet; scrub typhus rickettsiae have a thick outer leaflet and a thin inner leaflet. Attached to the outer leaflet of their cell wall is a slime (glycocalix) layer. This slime layer has not yet been purified or characterized because it is rapidly lost while separating rickettsiae from host cell components. The relationship of the slime layer to virulence is still conjectural.

COXIELLA. Coxiella are smaller than organisms of the genus *Rickettsia* and exhibit greater variation in morphology. Two distinct cell types, designated large and small cell variants (LCV and SCV), can be separated by density gradient centrifugation. Both types are infectious; both are capable of transverse binary fission. When cultured separately, *Coxiella* organisms convert to a mixture of cell types. SCV originate from the LCV by forming an electron-dense "cap" in the large periplasmic space of the LCV. This cap progressively develops into a sporelike SCV, which eventually is released during lysis of the LCV. Such a developmental cycle in *Coxiella burnetii* is comparable, but not identical, to a cycle of sporogenesis and vegetative cell differentiation.

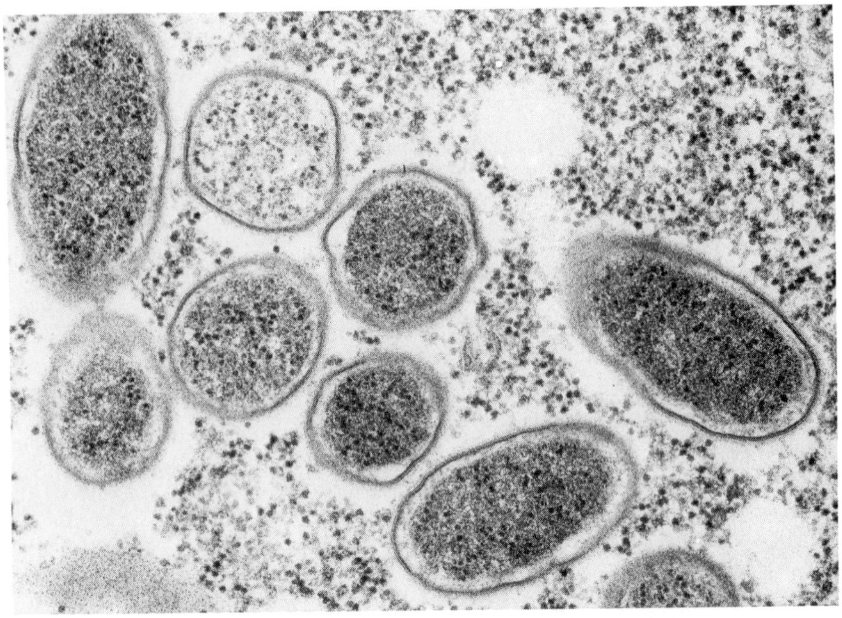

Fig. 49–1. *Rickettsia rickettsii*, the causative agent of Rocky Mountain spotted fever, in ovarian tissue of *Dermacentor andersoni*. × 66,000. *(Courtesy Dr. Lyle Brinton; Rocky Mountain Laboratory, USPHS, Hamilton, Mont.)*

Cultivation and Growth. Except for *R. quintana*, all rickettsiae require living cells for growth. *R. quintana* can be cultivated aerobically in host cellfree media. When grown in a cell culture, *Rochalimaea* adhere to the outer surface of the cells.

Other rickettsiae can be propagated in embryonated eggs, various tissue culture systems, and laboratory animals and in certain arthropods. *Rickettsia rickettsii* has been isolated and propagated in primary bone marrow cells and monocyte cultures. Because of well-known dangers of infection of laboratory personnel, cultures should be processed only in specially equipped facilities.

In their natural hosts rickettsiae preferentially enter endothelial cells lining small blood vessels. Entry requires interaction of viable rickettsiae and viable host cells. Rickettsiae enter both professional and nonprofessional phagocytes by parasite-directed phagocytosis (induced phagocytosis). After cell entry, members of the genus *Rickettsia* quickly escape from phagosomes and exist in the cytoplasm, free of host cell membranes. Phospholipase is involved in this escape from phagosomes. In fact, phospholipase activity may be responsible for host cell membrane damage that occurs as rickettsiae enter and exit cells. The virulence of some strains (e.g., Breinl and E strains of *Rickettsia prowazekii*) may be related to their ability to escape from phagosomes after cell entry. *R. prowazekii* multiplies in irradiated chicken embryo cells at 34C, with a generation time of about 9 hours. When large numbers of rickettsiae have accumulated intracellularly, host cells lyse. The nucleus is not invaded. In *R. rickettsii* infection, a high rickettsial intracytoplasmic density is not attained. *R. rickettsii* escapes into extracellular spaces early in infection and rapidly infects adjacent host cells. Occasionally, *R. rickettsii* invades and multiplies within the nucleus. The infection cycle of *Rickettsia tsutsugamushi* is similar to that of *R. prowazekii* except that organisms are extruded in projections from the surface of intact cells and are released with the surrounding host cell membrane. These membrane-bound rickettsiae in turn enter other host cells; nonenveloped organisms do not.

In contrast to *Rickettsia* and *Rochalimaea, Coxiella* grows preferentially within host membrane-bound vacuoles containing lysosomal enzymes (phagolysosomes). When grown in chicken embryo yolk sacs, *Coxiella* undergoes a cycle of development that includes the formation of an endospore-like body (p. 701). *C. burnetii* also undergoes phase variation. In nature or in laboratory animals *Coxiella* exists in phase I. With repeated passage through embryonated eggs, phase I organisms convert to the phase II state. However, injection of a phase II organism into laboratory animals results in rapid reversion to phase I.

The genus *Ehrlichia* parasitizes circulating leukocytes of humans and a variety of wild and domestic animals. *Ehrlichia sennetsu* has a predilection for mononuclear leukocytes, as does the closely related species, *Ehrlichia canis*. Both exist within the cytoplasm in membrane-bound vacuoles that form inclusions containing variable numbers of organisms. Three developmental stages are observed microscopically. The earliest stage forms are called elementary bodies. They in turn become the slightly larger initial bodies, which finally give rise to even larger inclusion bodies.

Metabolism. The intracellular location of rickettsiae in host cell cytoplasm provides them with an extensive array of preformed metabolites. To exploit their intracytoplasmic niche, rickettsiae have evolved carrier-mediated transport systems for key phosphorylated compounds. The most studied of these is an exchange transport system for ADP and ATP functionally similar to that used by mitochondria. It provides for the exchange of intracellular and extracellular adenine nucleotides on a one-for-one basis. It does not catalyze the net transport of nucleotides and is highly specific for ADP or ATP. Rickettsiae fulfill most of their energy requirements by coupling the phosphorylation of ADP to ATP with the oxidation of glutamate via the tricarboxylic acid cycle, mainly to aspartate, carbon dioxide, and ammonia. Glutamate is essential for the maintenance of a high adenylate energy charge. Glucose and glucose-6-phosphate are not catabolized by either

TABLE 49–2. DIFFERENTIAL PROPERTIES OF THE GENERA OF THE TRIBE RICKETTSIEAE

Property	*Rickettsia*	*Rochalimaea*	*Coxiella*
Axenic cultivation	−	+	−
Growth in eucaryotic cells			
In cytoplasm or nucleus	+	−	−
In phagolysosomes	−	−	+
Epicellular	−	+	−
Presence of endosporelike forms	−	−	+
Metabolism[a]			
Optimal pH	7.0	7.0	4.5
CO_2 produced from			
Glucose	−	−	Weak
Glutamate	+	Weak	+
Succinate	Weak	+	+
Mol% G and C of DNA	29–33	39	43

From Weiss, Moulder. In Krieg and Holt (eds): Bergey's Manual of Systematic Bacteriology, vol 1. Williams & Wilkins, 1984.
G + C, guanine-plus-cytosine content.
[a] When separated from host cells.

intact cells or extracts (Table 49–2). *R. rickettsii* has the ability to synthesize proteins in the absence of protein synthesis by host cells.

The location of *Coxiella* within phagolysosomes requires adaptation to an acidic environment. Intact cells of *C. burnetii* utilize glucose and glutamate slowly at pH 7, but they transport and metabolize both substrates quite vigorously at pH 5. As in the other rickettsiae, ATP generated by the aerobic oxidation of glutamate appears to be the chief source of energy.

Resistance. Rickettsiae remain viable for long periods when stored at −70C or lyophilized from appropriate media. Members of the genus *Rickettsia* are unstable extracellularly under ordinary environmental conditions. Special techniques are required to isolate organisms from body fluids and tissue. In contrast, *C. burnetii* is resistant to heat and drying, a characteristic important in understanding its ecology and epidemiology. The presence of endospore-like structures in *C. burnetii* may explain this resistance.

Antigenic Structure

Differences in antigenic composition of pathogenic rickettsiae have made possible their classification into genera, groups, and species. There is no common antigen for all members of the family Rickettsiaceae or for the tribe that contains the genera *Rickettsia, Rochalimaea,* and *Coxiella.* Pathogenic rickettsiae are divided into five serogroups or biotypes: spotted fever, typhus, scrub typhus, Q fever, and trench fever. The spotted fever group has six pathogenic *Rickettsia* species (*R. rickettsii, R. sibirica, R. conorii, R. australis, R. japonica,* and *R. akari*) and numerous nonpathogenic *Rickettsia* species (e.g., *R. rhipicephali* and *R. montana*). The typhus group has two *Rickettsia* members (*R. prowazekii* and *R. typhi*). The remaining three groups each have one species (*R. tsutsugamushi, C. burnetii,* and *R. quintana*). A second species of *Rochalimaea* has been described (*R. vinsonii*), but at this time it is not proven to be a human pathogen.

Two major kinds of antigens have been detected in rickettsiae: (1) ether-soluble group-specific antigens representing stripped-off capsular material and (2) type-specific antigens associated with the cell wall. Antigenic differences permit further speciation within the first two groups. Additional methods of separating various biotypes include cross-protection tests in laboratory animals, DNA base ratio analysis, and reactivity to monoclonal antibodies. The essential protective antigens of *R. prowazakii* and *R. typhi* are species specific and heat labile. Homologous, water-soluble, 120 kDa polypeptides constitute the microcapsular protein layer lying outside the rickettsial outer membrane. This 120 kDa antigen and a second surface protein (155 kDa) have been identified as major protective antigens in the humoral response to experimental infection.

Members of the spotted fever and typhus group rickettsiae all contain a 17 kDa antigenic protein. Genes encoding this protein from various pathogenic species have been cloned, sequenced, and compared. All exhibit a high degree of sequence homology. However, selected sequences of the genes of 17 kDa antigens are unique to the spotted fever group and have been used to synthesize primers for use in polymerase chain reaction technology.

Phase variation analogous to S → R variation in other bacteria has been observed in *C. burnetii* but in no other rickettsiae. In *C. burnetii* there are two main surface antigens; the presence or absence of phase I antigen causes the phase variations. Organisms isolated from natural infections of humans and animals are in phase I, but after repeated passage in the yolk sac, the lipopolysaccharide (LPS) antigen appears, and organisms move into phase II. Transition between phases may occur when one or more carbohydrates from the LPS moiety are no longer synthesized. Since the polysaccharide phase I antigen interferes with immune phagocytosis and antibody production, it may serve to conceal the organism from the immune system of its natural host and permit inapparent infections of long duration.

Serologic Diagnosis. Specific antibodies develop in response to rickettsial infection. Demonstration of an immune response during convalescence remains the most widely used method of confirming a clinical diagnosis. Antibody may not be detectable in cases early after onset or in fulminant cases with a fatal outcome. Separation of antibody into IgM and IgG may help in elucidating whether infection is recent or remote. Complement-fixing antibodies are useful in identifying infection due to rickettsiae of different genera and groups but are not highly sensitive and thus are no longer used for diagnosis in the United States. Highly purified reagents can minimize confusion resulting from cross-reactions. A wide array of serologic procedures, including microagglutination, indirect hemagglutination, and fluorescent antibody techniques, are available to diagnose rickettsial infections. The indirect fluorescent antibody technique is most commonly used to diagnose Rocky Mountain spotted fever in the United States. In patients with Rocky Mountain spotted fever, fluorescent antibody identification of intracellular rickettsiae in punch biopsies of skin has yielded the earliest diagnosis. However, this procedure lacks sensitivity and can be hazardous if done with frozen sections. Detection of *R. rickettsii* and *R. typhi* DNA in clinical specimens using polymerase chain reaction technology is also possible. Thus far such technology remains investigational; its sensitivity and specificity for clinical diagnosis are still unknown.

Weil-Felix Reaction. The Weil-Felix reaction is based on the cross-reactions between rickettsial antigens and *Proteus* polysaccharide O antigen. The test is simple to perform and is inexpensive; however, its specificity and sensitivity are low. *Proteus* agglutinins usually do not appear until the second week of illness, limiting their usefulness in early diagnosis. Some rickettsial diseases (e.g., rickettsialpox and Q fever) are not associated with Weil-Felix antibody rises, and *Proteus* bacterial infections such as urinary tract infection, bacteremia, and wound infections can give rise to false-positive results. Thus the Weil-Felix reaction is of limited clinical use and has been supplanted by more sensitive and specific tests such as the microimmunofluorescent antibody test.

Determinants of Pathogenicity

The microscopic pathology of rickettsial diseases is characteristic. Members of the genus *Rickettsia* appear to have tropism for endothelial cells. Multiplication of the organisms in endothelial cells lining capillaries and small blood vessels causes endothelial proliferation and perivascular infiltration, resulting in leakage and thrombosis. *R. rickettsii* is also unique in its ability to invade and damage vascular smooth muscle cells and the endothelium of larger blood vessels. Centripetal spread from capillaries to arterioles and veins may occur. The result is widespread infectious vasculitis with rash and organ dysfunction. Chick embryos, tissue cultures, small laboratory animals, and human umbilical vein endothelial cell cultures have been successfully used as experimental models for rickettsial infection. Although such models have provided useful information on penetration and multiplication of rickettsiae in host cells, little is known about mechanisms by which rickettsiae actually damage the host cell.

Only viable rickettsiae are capable of penetrating host cells; organisms inactivated by heat, formalin, or ultraviolet irradiation lose infectivity for mice. Rickettsial infection of an individual host cell is a two-stage process. Absorption to cholesterol-containing receptors precedes cell penetration. Both steps are dependent on energy produced by the infecting rickettsiae. Once inside host cells, rickettsiae cause little detectable damage to the parasitized cell until cell rupture. However, when large numbers of viable rickettsiae are injected into mice, death occurs within 8 hours. This effect can be blocked by the administration of type-specific antibody but not by the antirickettsial drugs tetracycline or chloramphenicol. To be effective, immune serum must be administered before infection, suggesting the elaboration of a toxin and that attachment of the toxin to its primary binding site of action occurs very rapidly. Although the isolation and chemical characterization of a true rickettsial toxin have not been accomplished, there is experimental evidence that at least one rickettsial component possesses endotoxic activity. Typhus fever rickettsiae are capable of hemolyzing erythrocytes of several animal species. This hemolytic activity is correlated with infectivity of the rickettsiae and their metabolic activities. The role of these phenomena in human rickettsial disease remains conjectural.

The microscopic pathology of human *Coxiella* infections is poorly understood since Q fever is rarely fatal and few tissue specimens from infected humans have been studied. *Coxiella* produce microscopic changes similar to those of most bacterial pneumonias. Granulomatous inflammation may occur in the liver of humans with Q fever. The cellular mechanisms for such changes remain unknown.

Different isolates of the same rickettsial species vary in virulence. More than 40 years ago, Spencer and Parker showed that when ticks infected with a virulent strain of *R. rickettsii* are refrigerated for several months, rickettsiae lose virulence for guinea pigs, although they still immunize animals against challenge with virulent strains. This phenomenon is not due to a spontaneous mutation or to differences in the number of rickettsiae. Despite refrigeration, *R. rickettsii* retains its virulence for chick embryos, and a single egg passage reestablishes virulence for guinea pigs. The use of monoclonal antibodies to surface proteins has demonstrated the presence of surface antigens in high-virulence strains not found in low-virulence strains.

Little is known concerning the mechanism of variations in virulence in naturally occurring human infections. Rhesus monkeys infected with *R. rickettsii* develop a clinical illness similar to that of humans; this model has been used to study the pathogenesis of human *R. rickettsii* infection. Such studies suggest that the duration of the incubation period and the severity of the disease are related to the size of the inoculum of *R. rickettsii.*

Coxiella contain plasmids affecting their virulence and, possibly, the composition and antigenicity of their surface lipopolysaccharides. Three general groups of *Coxiella* have been described. One contains a QpRS plasmid, the second contains a QpH1 plasmid, and a third lacks plasmids. The first and last groups have been associated with chronically infected patients and animals; the second with acute infections. Strains containing the QpH1 plasmid are highly susceptible in vitro to chloramphenicol and tetracycline; those with the QpRS plasmid are not.

Host Defenses

Both humoral and cell-mediated immunity are important in recovery from rickettsial infection. However, the relative importance of various host defense mechanisms in infected humans remains uncertain. Delayed hypersensitivity to typhus group antigens develops after human *R. prowazekii* infection. Similar lymphocyte-mediated hypersensitivity can be demonstrated after vaccination or infection with *C. burnetii.* Lymphocytes collected from humans previously infected with *R. rickettsii* undergo blast transformation after in vitro exposure to spotted fever group antigens. An interaction between humoral antibody (opsonins) and macrophages is required for effective killing of *R. prowazekii* by human macrophages. Similarly, antibody-treated *R. rickettsii* organisms are phagocytized and destroyed by guinea pig peritoneal macrophages, whereas untreated rickettsiae replicate and destroy peritoneal phagocytic cells. Experimentally, resistance to *R. typhi* infection is not transferred by immune serum, but resistance to intradermal challenge with *R. typhi* can be transferred using immune spleen cells. In addition, even unopsonized rickettsiae are destroyed by macrophages that have been preexposed to lymphokines from rickettsial antigen-treated mouse spleen cells. Such lymphokine activity has been attributed to gamma interferon, a soluble product of T lymphocytes. This may be an important host defense against intracellular growth of rickettsiae. The immune elimination of *R. prowazekii* may involve a similar combination of antibody and macrophages.

Clinical Infection

Diverse clinical illnesses produced by rickettsiae include primary pneumonia (Q fever), fulminant vasculitis (Rocky Mountain spotted fever), febrile illness associated with vesicular rash (rickettsialpox), asymptomatic infection (trench fever), recrudescent infection appearing years or decades after primary infection (Brill-Zinsser disease), and endocarditis (Q fever) (Table 49–3). Endothelial damage secondary to angiitis is a common finding in rickettsial infections, particularly those due to spotted fever and typhus group organisms.

Spotted Fever Group

The basic pathologic process in the spotted fever group is widespread vasculitis involving the skin (with production of a rash) and internal organs (producing dysfunctions of the brain, heart, lungs, and kidneys).

Rocky Mountain Spotted Fever (Tick-borne Typhus)

Epidemiology. Rocky Mountain spotted fever has been recognized as a distinct clinical entity for almost a century. First recognized in the Rocky Mountain region, the same illness was later recognized throughout the Midwest, South, and Eastern United States. The name *Rocky Mountain spotted fever* is misleading. The illness currently is most prevalent in the southwestern (Oklahoma) and southeastern (North Carolina) United States (Fig. 49–2), but cases continue to be reported annually in varying numbers from almost every state. Between 600 and 1000 cases of Rocky Mountain spotted fever (incidence 0.3/100,000 per year) are reported annually in the United States to the Centers for Disease Control (Fig. 49–3). Undoubtedly many cases are either not reported, not recognized, or never confirmed serologically. Rocky Mountain spotted fever accounts for more than 95% of the reported cases and for most of the deaths due to rickettsial disease in humans in the United States.

Most cases of Rocky Mountain spotted fever occur in children and adolescents, whereas most fatalities occur in adults. Fatalities are also more common in blacks and males. The explanation for these phenomena are still incompletely studied. The seasonal distribution of Rocky Mountain spotted fever is related to the activities of its tick vector. Disease typically appears in endemic regions in April and continues through August. However, Rocky Mountain spotted fever may also occur in the fall or, rarely, in the winter in endemic regions. People living in rural and suburban locations are at higher risk of infection than are urban dwellers, but rare cases have been described in such improbable areas as New York City.

ECOLOGY. *R. rickettsii*, the etiologic agent of Rocky Mountain spotted fever, is cycled in nature through ticks, small rodents, and larger wild and domestic animals. Humans are only accidentally infected. The ecology and epidemiology of spotted fever are directly related to the life cycle of four species of ixodid (hard) ticks: the Rocky Mountain wood tick (*Dermacentor andersoni*), the American dog tick (*Dermacentor variabilis*), the Lone Star tick (*Amblyomma americanum*), and the rabbit tick (*Haemaphysalis leporispalustris*). *D. andersoni* is the major vector in the Rocky Mountain region; the American dog tick is the major vector in the eastern and southeastern United States. The rabbit tick is found throughout the continental United States but rarely attaches to humans. It is thought to be important in maintaining a reservoir of infection in nature.

TABLE 49–3. EPIDEMIOLOGIC FEATURES OF SELECTED RICKETTSIOSES

Disease	Etiologic Agent	Geographic Distribution	Arthropod Vector	Animal Reservoir
Spotted Fever Group				
Rocky Mountain spotted fever	*R. rickettsii*	North and South America	Tick	Wild rodents, dogs
Rickettsialpox	*R. akari*	Worldwide	Mite	Mouse
Boutonneuse fever	*R. conorii*	Mediterranean countries, Africa, India	Tick	Wild rodents, dogs
Queensland tick typhus	*R. australis*	Australia	Tick	Wild rodents, marsupials
North Asian tick typhus	*R. sibirica*	Siberia, Mongolia	Tick	Wild rodents
Typhus Group				
Epidemic typhus	*R. prowazekii*	Worldwide	Body louse	Humans, flying squirrel
Brill-Zinsser	*R. prowazekii*	Worldwide	None	Humans (recrudescence)
Murine typhus	*R. typhi*	Worldwide	Rat flea	Small rodents
Scrub typhus	*R. tsutsugamushi*	Asia, Australia, South Pacific	Mite	Wild rodents
Others				
Q fever	*C. burnetii*	Worldwide	Tick (inhalation of organism)	Cattle, sheep, goats
Trench fever	*R. quintana*	Europe, Middle East, North Africa, Mexico	Body louse	Humans
Sennetsu rickettsiosis	*E. sennetsu*	Japan, Malaysia (?), Philippines (?)	Unknown	Humans

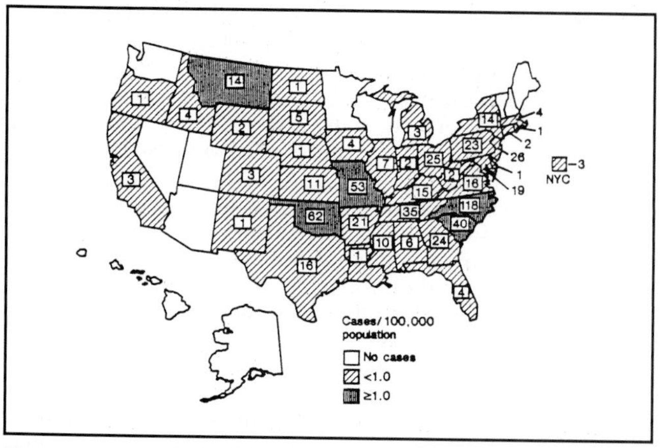

Fig. 49–2. Rocky Mountain spotted fever. Reported cases and rates by state in the United States, 1989. *(From CDC: MMWR 39:281, 1990.)*

Ixodid ticks pass through four stages in their life cycle. If infected by feeding on a rickettsemic animal, they may in turn transmit infection to their progeny transovarially. Thus infected ticks function both as a reservoir and as a vector of spotted fever rickettsiae.

TRANSMISSION. Most but by no means all patients give a history of a recent tick bite. Infection may also occur through contamination of fingers while removing ticks feeding on animals or on another person. Except for rare reports of infections associated with needle-stick injuries and blood transfusions, human transmission of spotted fever does not occur. Acquisition of infection by laboratory workers handling *R. rickettsii* is a well-known occurrence, and in the preantibiotic era it killed a number of investigators.

Pathogenesis. *R. rickettsii* infection produces widespread endothelial damage, resulting in occlusion of small vessels, microthrombi, microhemorrhages, secondary fluid and electrolyte changes, and in severe cases, necrosis, shock, and death. However, the precise mechanism by which rickettsial infection produces endothelial damage is still largely unknown. Activation of the kallikrein-kinin system has been observed in humans with Rocky Mountain spotted fever. It has been suggested that kinins play a role in the pathophysiology of the vasculitis and disseminated intravascular coagulation sometimes present in patients with severe infection.

Clinical Manifestations. The incubation period ranges from 2 to 12 days. Disease typically begins abruptly with headache, fever, and malaise. Chills may occur. Diffuse myalgias are common. Usually a rash appears 2 to 4 days after onset; in many cases it first appears on the ankles and wrists and then becomes generalized. The rash is usually initially maculopapular but may later become petechial or hemorrhagic. Involvement of palms and soles is common. Onset of rash may be delayed in some patients, particularly adults, for up to 7 days. Rarely, rash may be absent, including in those patients with severe or fulminant infection.

Gastrointestinal complaints, arthralgias, conjunctivitis, stiff neck, and periorbital edema may be dominant symptoms, leading to diagnostic confusion and delays in recognition. In fact, early and pronounced gastrointestinal signs and symptoms have led to laparotomy and the erroneous diagnosis of cholecystitis or appendicitis. Splenomegaly is detected in approximately 25% of cases. Hyponatremia and thrombocytopenia are common findings. Severe disease can be associated with features suggesting disseminated intravascular coagulation. Petechial and purpuric skin manifestations rarely evolving to gangrene of digits or the scrotum may occur. Vasculitis involving the brain, heart, liver, and kidneys may produce clinical complications, including seizures, coma, congestive heart failure, jaundice, and acute renal failure.

Reported fatality rates have declined from approximately 20% in the 1940s to 3% to 10% in the past few years. Factors associated with an increased mortality rate include increasing age, increasing length of time from onset to institution of effective chemotherapy, nonwhite race, and male sex. An association of glucose-6-phosphate dehydrogenase with fulminant disease has been reported.

Laboratory Diagnosis. Initial diagnosis and treatment of

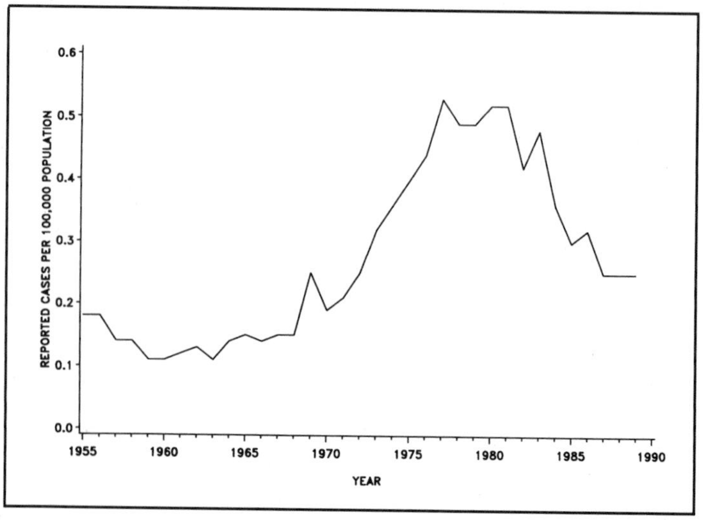

Fig. 49–3. Rocky Mountain spotted fever (tick-borne typhus fever). Rates, by year, in the United States, 1955–1989. A total of 623 cases were reported in 1989. *(From CDC: MMWR 38(54):48, 1989.)*

Rocky Mountain spotted fever must be made on clinical grounds and never delayed until laboratory confirmation is obtained. An appropriate constellation of symptoms is sufficient justification to begin treatment even in those with no history of a tick bite. In endemic regions it may be appropriate to suspect and empirically treat febrile patients lacking a rash if no other diagnosis is apparent and spotted fever is considered possible on clinical and epidemiologic grounds.

R. rickettsii can be isolated from blood, but this is expensive and requires trained personnel and specialized facilities available in only a few locations. In most cases diagnosis is confirmed by the demonstration of specific convalescent antibodies in serum. Two to three samples of the patient's blood should be taken: one drawn as soon as possible after onset of illness, one at the end of week 2, and one at the end of week 4 after onset.

The Weil-Felix test lacks specificity and sensitivity and is no longer recommended as a diagnostic test. The microimmunofluorescent antibody (IFA) test is the most widely used serologic test to diagnose Rocky Mountain spotted fever in the United States. A fourfold rise in titer is evidence of recent rickettsial infection. A single convalescent titer of 1:64 or greater, although considered diagnostic of infection with spotted fever group rickettsiae, is weaker evidence of acute infection; such findings do not exclude remote infection. Because of poor sensitivity, the complement-fixation test is no longer used by most laboratories. Enzyme-linked immunosorbent assay (ELISA) techniques are highly sensitive but are not widely available in the United States because of the lack of commercially available purified rickettsial antigens. Indirect hemagglutination, latex agglutination, and microagglutination tests are available in some state health laboratories in the United States. The latter two tests lack sensitivity for late convalescent serum samples.

Punch biopsies of skin stained with fluorescent conjugates of antirickettsial serum are useful in diagnosing Rocky Mountain spotted fever in its early stages. However, this test lacks sensitivity; it may fail to diagnose spotted fever accurately in as many as 50% of cases. Thus a negative biopsy does not exclude the diagnosis. Prior chemotherapy or the absence of a rash may further reduce the sensitivity or utility of this procedure. Also, this test is limited to a relatively few properly equipped laboratories.

Polymerase chain reaction technology has been successfully adapted to the diagnosis of *R. rickettsii* infection. However, the sensitivity, specificity, and clinical utility of such methods are unknown.

Treatment. The mortality rate for untreated Rocky Mountain spotted fever has varied from 20% to 80% but averages about 25%. Both chloramphenicol and tetracycline are effective against *R. rickettsii.* They remain the only two approved antimicrobials for the treatment of Rocky Mountain spotted fever.

Because the clinical presentation of meningococcemia and Rocky Mountain spotted fever overlaps, chloramphenicol is the drug of choice when these two diseases cannot be clinically differentiated. Intensive care may be necessary to combat problems of fluid loss, hypoxemia, congestive heart failure, and bleeding—all secondary to widespread vasculitis.

Prevention. Traditional measures of vector control are generally not practical. Protective clothing such as boots, leggings, and tightly buttoned shirts may be helpful in preventing tick attachment in persons exposed to heavily infested environments.

Individuals exposed to ticks and tick-infested environments should inspect their bodies regularly and carefully remove attached ticks. Experimental studies have shown that a period of reactivation is required from the time an infected tick attaches and begins feeding until it transmits pathogenic rickettsiae. Therefore even infected ticks removed within several hours of attachment may not transmit rickettsiae. Forceps and gentle traction are recommended for tick removal. Ticks can also be removed by hand, using paper or cloth to protect fingers. Care should be taken during removal to prevent crushing the arthropod and contaminating fingers because both tick tissues and tick feces are potentially infectious.

At present there is no commercially available vaccine for Rocky Mountain spotted fever. Previously available killed vaccines were withdrawn by the Food and Drug Administration because they were ineffective.

In areas where the disease occurs frequently, both the public and physicians should be periodically reminded of the signs, symptoms, and epidemiologic features of the disease.

Rickettsialpox.

Rickettsialpox is characterized by a local eschar, a papulovesicular rash, and a benign clinical course. The causative agent, *R. akari,* is a member of the spotted fever group.

Epidemiology. Rickettsialpox was first recognized in New York City in 1946. Sporadic cases subsequently have been recognized in many urban areas of the United States. The mite vector of the disease (*Allodermanyssus sanguineus*) is found throughout a large part of the United States. Rickettsialpox is typically a mild disease. Exact morbidity figures are not available since few cases have been reported. Whether this reflects true infrequency of disease, lack of recognition, or lack of reporting is unknown.

An organism identical to *R. akari* has been isolated in urban areas in Russia, where the epidemiology and clinical features of the disease appear to be similar to rickettsialpox in the United States. *R. akari* has also been isolated from a wild Korean rodent (*Microtus fortis pelliceus*), implying occurrence of a rural cycle of transmission.

ECOLOGY. *R. akari* infects its mite vector, which in turn is an ectoparasite of the common house mouse. Mites infect their progeny transovarially. As in several other rickettsial diseases, humans only accidentally enter this cycle of infection. Human infections are more likely to occur when the rodent population is suddenly reduced by vermin control programs. When murine hosts are scarce, *A. sanguineus* readily attacks humans. Most reported cases of rickettsialpox have been from urban areas where the density of both the murine mites and humans is high.

Pathogenesis. Little is known concerning the pathogenesis of *R. akari* infection. Microscopically, the rash of rickettsialpox shows mononuclear perivascular infiltrates and necrosis of epithelial cells, resulting in intraepidermal vesicles.

Clinical Manifestations. The clinical hallmarks of rickettsialpox are a vesicular rash and a local eschar associated with regional lymphadenopathy. The incubation period is not precisely known since patients typically are unaware of a mite bite. The first sign of disease is usually a local erythematous papule that evolves to a vesicle and then an eschar. Approximately 3 to 7 days after the appearance of an eschar, chills and fever begin abruptly, often in association with headache, malaise, and myalgia. Within 72 hours of the appearance of fever, a generalized maculopapular rash becomes apparent and quickly evolves into a vesicular eruption. Differentiation of the rash of rickettsialpox from chickenpox may be difficult. Unlike chickenpox, rickettsialpox is associated with a primary eschar, and its cutaneous vesicles are surrounded by papular rings. In contrast, the rash of chickenpox is entirely vesicular, and patients lack a primary lesion.

No fatalities attributable to rickettsialpox have been reported. Although a small scar may occur at the site of the primary lesion, the vesiculopapular eruption typically heals without scarring.

Laboratory Diagnosis. Weil-Felix antibodies do not appear after infection with *R. akari.* Cross-reacting antibodies to *R. rickettsii* typically occur after *R. akari* infections, but the two diseases are usually easily distinguishable on clinical grounds. Specific *R. akari* antigens for serologic testing are available only at the Centers for Disease Control or through research laboratories.

R. akari can be isolated from the blood and the vesicular fluid from lesions of infected persons. Such isolations require the technical facilities of specially equipped laboratories.

Treatment and Prevention. Both tetracycline and chloramphenicol produce rapid defervescence and clinical improvement.

Measures aimed at controlling both rodent populations and their mite ectoparasites will prevent transmission of *R. akari* to humans. Human-to-human transmission does not occur.

Other Tick-borne Diseases

Other species of spotted fever group rickettsiae cause tick-borne diseases resembling Rocky Mountain spotted fever (Table 49–3). *R. sibirica* is the causative agent of North Asian tick typhus; *R. australis* causes Queensland tick typhus; *R. conorii* causes boutonneuse fever, and *Rickettsia japonica* is the causative agent of a recently recognized illness, Japanese spotted fever. North Asian tick typhus occurs in central Asia, Mongolia, and the Siberian region of the Union of Soviet Socialist Republics. Queensland tick typhus occurs throughout eastern Australia, and boutonneuse fever occurs in the Mediterranean region, Africa, and India. Boutonneuse fever has also been called South African tick bite fever, Kenya tick typhus, Indian tick typhus, and Mediterranean spotted fever.

All spotted fever group rickettsiae are maintained in nature in both ixodid ticks and wild animals. Humans only accidentally enter their natural cycle of infection.

Diseases caused by these rickettsiae may cause local eschars at the site of tick attachment and regional lymphadenopathy. All four species typically produce disease milder than Rocky Mountain spotted fever, although they have many of the same basic symptoms: fever, headache, myalgia, malaise, and maculopapular eruptions that may become petechial. Fatalities occur but are uncommon even without treatment. During the last several years there has been a resurgence of boutonneuse fever in the Mediterranean countries.

Infection with any of these four rickettsiae is followed by the production of group-specific antibodies and inconsistently by *Proteus* OX-19 or OX-2 agglutinating antibodies. Type-specific complement-fixing antibodies can be measured after infection, although serologic cross-reactivity with other members of the spotted fever group occurs. This is usually not a diagnostic problem since the geographic ranges of individual spotted fever group rickettsiae rarely overlap (with the exception of *R. akari* and *R. rickettsii*). However, with rapid international travel and the increasing popularity of outdoor and "adventure" vacations, these rickettsial diseases may actually manifest in locations far removed from the site of acquisition. All spotted fever group rickettsiae are sensitive to both chloramphenicol and tetracycline.

Rickettsiae Not Associated with Human Disease

Rickettsia parkeri, Rickettsia montana, Rickettsia helvetica, Rickettsia heilongjangi and *Rickettsia rhipicephali* are nonpathogenic rickettsiae serologically related to the spotted fever group. They do not have the ability to cause disease in animals and presumably are nonpathogenic for humans as well.

R. parkeri, originally referred to as the "maculatum agent," first was isolated from Gulf Coast ticks (*Amblyomma maculatum*) removed from cattle in eastern Texas. Subsequent isolations of this rickettsia were made from the same tick species in Mississippi and Georgia. To date, *R. parkeri* has not been isolated from any other ticks or from other parts of the world. The reason for this host specificity is unclear, but an interference phenomenon has been invoked as an explanation.

R. montana initially was isolated from ticks in eastern Montana; subsequent isolations in other states suggest that it is widely distributed in natural cycles involving small rodents and ticks. *R. montana* is a natural parasite of the major tick hosts of *R. rickettsii* but is antigenically distinct from other spotted fever group rickettsiae. Guinea pigs immunized with *R. montana* are almost completely protected against challenge with *R. rickettsii.*

R. rhipicephali has been isolated from brown dog ticks (*Rhipicephalus sanguineus*) in several southeastern states. *R. rhipicephali* differs biologically and antigenically from *R. rickettsii.* There is no evidence of pathogenicity for the dog or for man, but it has been hypothesized that both this species and *R. montana* provide dogs with partial protection against *R. rickettsii* infection. Serologic surveys in several areas of the United States indicate that antibodies against *R. rhipicephali* are prevalent in canines.

Typhus Group

Typhus group rickettsiae cause epidemic typhus (and its recrudescent infection, Brill-Zinsser disease) and murine typhus. Typhus group organisms are characterized by intracytoplasmic growth and a common, soluble, group-specific, complement-fixing antigen.

Epidemic Typhus (Louse-borne Typhus)

Epidemic typhus is a louse-borne disease caused by *R. prowazekii,* a rickettsia named after the Polish investigator, von Prowazek, who died of typhus contracted in the course of his studies. Epidemic typhus has had a tremendous impact on the history of man. According to Zinsser, Napoleon's retreat from

Moscow "was started by a louse." In World War I, typhus was responsible for the death of more than 150,000 Serbians and more than 3 million Russians and caused nonfatal illness in additional millions.

Epidemiology. Epidemic typhus, once worldwide in occurrence, has disappeared from areas with high standards of hygiene. There has not been an outbreak of epidemic typhus in the United States since 1922. *R. prowazekii* infection occasionally occurs in the United States, however, in its recrudescent form (Brill-Zinsser disease) or sporadically secondary to a sylvatic cycle of infection. At present, the most important foci of epidemic typhus are in Africa. Minor foci also exist in Central and South America.

ECOLOGY AND TRANSMISSION. *R. prowazekii* can infect both the human body louse (*Pediculus humanus corporis*) and the head louse (*Pediculus humanus capitis*). The former is the more significant vector. Body lice feed only on humans. All three stages of their life cycle (egg, nymph, and adult) may occur on the same host.

Lice become infected after a blood meal from a rickettsemic human. Several days later infective rickettsiae appear in the arthropod's feces. If an infected louse encounters a susceptible human at this point, transmission of *R. prowazekii* may occur. During each blood meal the louse defecates. The feeding process is irritating to the host; scratching produces minor excoriations that in turn become portals of entry for rickettsiae in the louse's feces. Lice do not transmit *R. prowazekii* to their progeny but succumb to their infections within 1 to 3 weeks.

Louse-human-louse transmission thrives under conditions in which individuals wear the same clothes continuously in crowded environments. Thus it is not surprising that major epidemics have occurred in association with war, poverty, and famine. Persons in cold climates are more likely to acquire epidemic typhus, particularly if they are forced by hard circumstances to wear the same clothes for long periods of time.

Lice actively seek locations where the temperature is approximately 20C, a temperature often found in the folds of clothing. Lice will abandon a host with a body temperature of 40C or greater, as well as the body of a dead person.

Recently a sylvatic cycle of *R. prowazekii* has been recognized in the United States. Flying squirrels (*Glaucomys volans*) in the southeastern United States and their ectoparasites (both lice and fleas) may be naturally infected with *R. prowazekii*. The mechanisms by which *R. prowazekii* infection is transmitted from flying squirrels to humans remain unknown. More than 35 cases of human *R. prowazekii* infection have been confirmed in the United States since 1976. Most have occurred in the eastern United States in rural environments during the colder months of the year when flying squirrels may temporarily nest in the attics of human dwellings. Serosurveys of flying squirrels have demonstrated persistent enzootic foci of infection and a maximum incidence of seroconversions in serially trapped animals during the fall and winter months.

Restriction DNA analysis of *R. prowazekii* strains isolated from flying squirrels in the United States differs slightly from that of those strains isolated from epidemic typhus patients from Europe. The significance of these differences remains conjectural.

Clinical Manifestations. The incubation period typically ranges from 10 to 14 days. Prodromal symptoms of headache, malaise, and fever sometimes occur. Usually the onset is abrupt, with generalized myalgias, chills, fever, and headache. The latter is characteristically frontal, severe, and unremitting. Other symptoms such as gastrointestinal complaints, weakness, and cough may also be present and lead to diagnostic confusion. Meningismus may be present, but spinal fluid is typically, but not invariably, normal.

One of the hallmarks of epidemic typhus, skin rash, usually appears from 4 to 7 days after onset. It may first appear as patchy cutaneous erythema and later progress to maculopapular, petechial, or hemorrhagic forms. In contrast to that of Rocky Mountain spotted fever, rash in typhus patients characteristically appears first on the trunk and later spreads to the extremities. A wide variety of complications may occur in severe cases, including hypotension, oliguria, azotemia, and, rarely, gangrene of the skin, genitalia, and digits. The name *typhus* is derived from the Greek word for smoke (*typhos*), underscoring the fact that stupor, delirium, or other forms of altered sensorium may be prominent features in patients with typhus.

Untreated, epidemic typhus may last up to 3 weeks. Its mortality rate has varied from 10% to 40%. Case fatality ratios increase with increasing age. Survivors of epidemic typhus are generally immune for years after their primary infection, although mild recurrences of illness (Brill-Zinsser disease) may occur years to decades later.

Laboratory Diagnosis. Treatment should be instituted before laboratory confirmation. Laboratory substantiation of a clinical diagnosis can be achieved serologically or by isolation of *R. prowazekii*. However, the latter is difficult, potentially dangerous, expensive and requires specialized personnel and equipment.

As in patients with Rocky Mountain spotted fever, patients convalescent from typhus produce Weil-Felix antibodies that agglutinate *Proteus vulgaris* OX polysaccharide antigens. These agglutinins usually appear in the second week after onset. However, their sensitivity and specificity are so low that specific serologic tests such as the microimmunofluorescent antibody test should be used instead. These antibodies typically appear late in the second week after onset.

As with *R. rickettsii*, primers for use in polymerase chain reaction technology have been synthesized and have been used to diagnose typhus in a laboratory worker infected in a laboratory accident.

Treatment. Both chloramphenicol and tetracycline produce prompt defervescence and clinical improvement when given early in the course of the illness. As in patients ith Rocky Mountain spotted fever, patients who develop circulatory and renal complications before receiving specific treatment may require intensive care and may die even with the best available care.

Prevention and Control. It is possible to interrupt epidemic louse-human-louse transmission of *R. prowazekii* by using insecticides. However, some populations of lice, especially in Africa, have become increasingly resistant to insecticides (including DDT and malathion). Once free of lice, patients with typhus are not infectious. In poorly controlled studies typhus vaccine prepared from infected yolk sacs lessened the severity and shortened the course of clinical disease. Two doses of vaccine given 4 weeks apart are recommended for primary immunization. It is advised that booster doses be given every 6 to 12 months during periods of exposure.

Brill-Zinsser Disease

Individuals who previously have had epidemic typhus may develop recrudescent *R. prowazekii* years or decades later. This phenomenon, Brill-Zinsser disease, is named for Nathan Brill, who first recognized and described the clinical features, and Hans Zinsser, who in 1934 suggested that the illness was actually a relapse of a prior epidemic typhus infection. Epidemiologic, serologic, clinical, and experimental data subsequently confirmed Zinsser's hypothesis.

Epidemiology. In the United States, recrudescent typhus occurs primarily in immigrants from previously endemic areas such as Eastern Europe. Brill-Zinsser disease may occur in an individual living in a lousefree environment decades after initial infection with *R. prowazekii*. Lice feeding on such patients may in turn become infected. If local conditions are favorable for louse-human-louse transmission, an outbreak of epidemic typhus may result. Latent human infection thus represents an interepidemic reservoir for *R. prowazekii*.

Clinical Manifestations. Brill-Zinsser disease is a milder illness than classic epidemic typhus. Skin rash is rarely seen, and the duration of disease is shorter (less than 2 weeks). Fever may be erratic instead of sustained. As in epidemic typhus and other rickettsial diseases, headache, malaise, and myalgias are common symptoms. Complications and fatalities are rare.

Laboratory Diagnosis. In the United States, Brill-Zinsser disease should be suspected if fever of obscure origin occurs in a foreign-born person from an area where epidemic typhus has occurred and if an intense headache and a maculopapular skin rash develop on the fourth to sixth day of illness.

Weil-Felix agglutinins often do not develop in patients with Brill-Zinsser disease. As a general rule, the sooner recrudescent infection occurs after the primary infection, the less likely it is that Weil-Felix antibodies are present. Complement-fixing or microimmunofluorescent antibodies may be detected during the second week after onset, which is earlier than in patients with epidemic typhus. Since some typhus patients may have detectable complement-fixing antibodies years after the primary infection, an isolated convalescent serum sample may yield confusing results. Therefore a fourfold antibody rise should be sought in patients suspected of having recrudescent typhus.

Patients with epidemic typhus initially have an IgM antibody response followed by an IgG antibody response, whereas patients with Brill-Zinsser disease initially have an anamnestic IgG antibody response. The microimmunofluorescence test using IgM and IgG reagents is the most sensitive and reliable laboratory method for differentiating Brill-Zinsser disease from primary epidemic typhus.

Treatment and Prevention. As in epidemic typhus, both tetracycline and chloramphenicol are effective. Prevention of Brill-Zinsser disease is necessarily dependent on prevention of epidemic typhus. If recrudescent typhus occurs in an environment in which lice rarely infest humans, no special precautionary public health measures are required. In areas where the potential for louse-human-louse transmission exists, delousing patients and their contacts may prevent an outbreak of epidemic typhus.

Murine Typhus (Endemic Typhus, Flea-borne Typhus, Rat Typhus)

Murine typhus is a flea-borne illness caused by *R. typhi*. Typically, it is a mild illness characterized by fever, headache, and a generalized skin rash.

Epidemiology

PREVALENCE. Murine typhus is endemic in many countries, including the United States, where it occurs primarily in the Southeast and Gulf Coast region. It is also endemic in parts of Central America and Mexico. Previously, most cases occurred in the United States in individuals working in rat-infested shipyards and harbors. More recently, cases have occurred in inland rural locations where infected rats exist in large numbers near grain and feed storage areas. In the past decade nearly three fourths of all reported cases in the United States have occurred in Texas, where cases may occur any month of the year. However, the onset of 40% of all cases was in April, May, or June. Annual incidence increases with age. The incidence of murine typhus has gradually decreased in the past two decades. Whether this decrease is real or due to lack of recognition or reporting is unknown.

ECOLOGY. *R. typhi* is cycled in nature by the rat and two of its ectoparasites, the Oriental rat flea (*Xenopsylla cheopis*) and the rat louse (*Polyplax spinulosus*). The former is the most important vector. As with Rocky Mountain spotted fever, humans enter this arthropod-vertebrate-arthropod cycle accidentally. *X. cheopis* acquires *R. typhi* infection by feeding on a rickettsemic mouse or rat. Once infected, fleas may infect other susceptible rodents. Thus a natural cycle of flea-rodent-flea infection may become established. Rodents infected with *R. typhi* do not succumb to their infection despite the presence of viable rickettsiae in rodent brains for periods up to several months. Fleas do not transmit *R. typhi* transovarially.

TRANSMISSION. Transmission of *R. typhi* may occur when infected fleas infesting humans or a rodent take a blood meal and defecate on their host. The host in turn inoculates rickettsia-containing feces into small excoriations by scratching. Flea feces are also infective if accidentally transmitted to mucosal surfaces such as the conjunctivae.

Clinical Manifestation. Murine typhus is usually a mild illness with a mortality rate of less than 2%. The incubation period ranges from 1 to 2 weeks. Hallmarks of disease are abrupt onset of fever, headache, malaise, myalgias, and, in most cases, a macular or maculopapular, nonpruritic skin rash. Rash usually appears on the trunk on the third to fifth day of illness. Later it spreads to the extremities. This exanthem may be fleeting or absent in some cases and is not apparent in blacks unless a careful inspection is made. Chills or chilliness, cough, nausea, vomiting, arthralgias, weakness, and extreme prostration may also occur. Untreated, illness may last up to 2 weeks. Defervescence may occur either abruptly (by crises) or gradually (by lysis). Fatalities are uncommon but do occur rarely in the old and infirm. Fatality may be heralded by peripheral vascular collapse and central nervous system dysfunction such as stupor and coma.

Clinical confusion between murine typhus and Rocky Mountain spotted fever may occur. Spotted fever is usually a more severe illness. Unlike murine typhus it is often associated with an antecedent tick bite. The rash of murine typhus begins first on the trunk and spreads to the extremities; the opposite evolution occurs with Rocky Mountain spotted fever. However, because precise information about the evolution of the rash often is unavailable, this differential point is often not helpful. In older immigrant patients confusion between murine typhus and Brill-Zinsser disease may also occur (p. 710). Since the treatment for all rickettsial diseases is identical, diagnostic confusion should not affect treatment.

Laboratory Diagnosis. Weil-Felix agglutinins to *Proteus* OX-19 or OX-2 antigens appear in the second week of infection; but as in other rickettsial diseases, such antibodies lack specificity and sensitivity. Serologic cross-reactions among members of the typhus group are common using complement-fixation and microimmunofluorescent antibody tests. Patients with murine typhus develop higher antibody titers against *R. typhi* than against *R. prowazekii* antigens. Only special reference laboratories such as those at the Centers for Disease Control can distinguish serologically between *R. prowazekii* and *R. typhi* infections.

Treatment and Prevention. Both tetracycline and chloramphenicol are effective against *R. typhi,* but rarely relapses do occur. For instance, patients with laboratory-acquired murine typhus treated with chloramphenicol within 2 to 4 days of onset have experienced clinical relapses despite the presence of antirickettsial antibodies. Such relapses respond to reinstitution of the same antimicrobials. Insecticides and rodenticides are effective in reducing rat-flea-human transmission in endemic areas.

Rickettsia canada Infections

R. canada was first isolated from rabbit ticks collected in Ontario, Canada, in 1967. Antigenically, *R. canada* belongs to the typhus group biotype. However, it grows in both the cytoplasm and the nuclei of infected cells, a characteristic of the spotted fever group.

R. canada has not been isolated from human sources, although serologic evidence of *R. canada* infection has been reported in four patients with symptoms typical of Rocky Mountain spotted fever. *R. canada* appears to circulate between wild rabbits and the rabbit tick (*Haemaphysalis leporispalustris*). Its relationship to other typhus group rickettsiae is still controversial. DNA studies have suggested it may not belong in the typhus group biotype.

Cross-reactions by complement-fixation techniques occur using *R. canada, R. prowazekii,* and *R. typhi* antigens. In experimental infections in guinea pigs, *R. canada* produces fever but no scrotal reaction. The epidemiology and clinical manifestations of human *R. canada* infection are unknown.

Scrub typhus (Chigger-borne Typhus), Tsutsugamushi Disease

R. tsutsugamushi (*Rickettsia orientalis*) produces a characteristic clinical illness in humans despite the fact that different strains of the same organisms possess markedly different surface antigens. The name *tsutsugamushi* is derived from two Japanese words: *tsutsuga* (something small and dangerous) and *mushi* (creature). The appellation *scrub typhus* is derived from the fact that infection commonly occurs in endemic areas after exposure to terrain with secondary (scrub) vegetation. However, *R. tsutsugamushi* infection also occurs in habitats that cannot be described as scrub, including sandy beaches, mountain deserts, and equatorial rain forests. Thus scrub typhus is a misnomer; "chigger-borne typhus" is a more descriptive and accurate name.

Three major antigenic types of *R. tsutsugamushi* (Karp, Gilliam, and Kato) exist. Immune cross-reactions occur among the three types. Patients surviving infection with one strain are immune to all strains for a few months; however, immunity is durable for longer periods only to the homologous strain.

Epidemiology

PREVALENCE. Chigger-borne typhus is endemic in a triangular geographic area that includes Australia, Japan, Korea, India, and Vietnam. In World War II, it caused morbidity and mortality in both Japanese and American soldiers. In peacetime it occurs predominantly as a sporadic endemic illness. Epidemics may occur, however, when groups of people are brought into endemic mite-infested areas. Chigger-borne typhus occurred sporadically in American troops stationed in Vietnam.

ECOLOGY. Several species of trombiculid mites are the vectors of chigger-borne typhus. These mites have four-stage life cycles (egg, larva, nymph, and adult). The larva (chigger) is the only stage that feeds on vertebrates. After engorgement on a vertebrate host, chiggers detach and metamorphose: first into eight-legged nymphs and then into adults. The latter two stages are free-living in the soil. Transmission of *R. tsutsugamushi* occurs both transstadially (from larva to nymph to adult) and transovarially (from adult to egg). Thus trombiculid mites function as both vector and reservoir of chigger-borne typhus.

In endemic areas a natural cycle of *R. tsutsugamushi* transmission occurs between chiggers and small mammals such as field mice and rats. Ground-feeding birds may also enter into this zoonotic cycle of infection and function as transporters of *R. tsutsugamushi* over long distances. In chigger-borne typhus, as in rickettsialpox, Rocky Mountain spotted fever, and murine typhus, humans only accidentally enter the natural cycle of rickettsial infection. Areas such as savannas, forest clearings, riverbanks, grassy fields, and gardens may provide conditions allowing infected mites to thrive, resulting in foci of high risk to humans. Such mite-infested foci, which may be as small as a few meters in diameter, have been called "scrub typhus islands." The term *zoonotic tetrad* describes the coexistence and intimate relationship among *R. tsutsugamushi,* chiggers, rats, and secondary or transitional forms of vegetation. All four are essential components of a scrub typhus island.

The seasonal incidence of disease varies with climate, occurring more frequently during the rainy season in the summer or fall.

Person-to-person transmission of infection has not been reported.

Clinical Manifestations. Approximately 1 to 3 weeks after being bitten by an infected chigger, humans abruptly develop chills, fever, and headache. Any or all of the following additional symptoms may also occur: cough, nausea, vomiting, myalgia, abdominal pain, and sore throat. The skin rash of scrub typhus is classically but not invariably heralded by a local cutaneous lesion or eschar. Such lesions may evolve from a small indurated papule or vesicle into an ulcerated lesion covered by a black scab. Lymphadenopathy is often prominent in the area proximal to the eschar. Five to eight days after the onset of fever, a macular or maculopapular eruption may appear on the trunk and later become generalized. Eschar and skin rash are not always present. Only 46% of American servicemen in Vietnam with scrub typhus had an identifiable eschar; fewer (34%) had a skin rash. Splenomegaly, conjunctivitis, and pharyngitis sometimes are seen with chigger-borne typhus. In severe cases, deterioration in mental status (stupor, delirium), or pneumonia, or circulatory failure, or all three may occur. Some patients experience a second attack of scrub typhus. This is not surprising since infection with one strain of *R. tsutsugamushi* does not confer lasting protection against other strains.

Fatality rates during epidemics have varied from 0 to 50% in untreated patients. However, with prompt recognition and early appropriate treatment, fatality rates are almost nil.

Laboratory Diagnosis. Serologic tests are of less value in the diagnosis of scrub typhus than in the diagnosis of infection due to rickettsiae of the spotted fever and typhus groups because different strains have different surface antigens that may not cross-react with each other. Thus a minimum of three different antigens (representing the Karp, Gilliam, and Kato strains) must be used. Weil-Felix agglutinins to *Proteus* OX-K (but not OX-2 and OX-19) antigens appear in the convalescent sera of many but not all patients with scrub typhus. As in other rickettsial diseases, such agglutinins are of low utility because they lack specificity and sensitivity. A fluorescent antibody test using pooled conjugates made from the three major strains of *R. tsutsugamushi* may be a useful technique. As with all rickettsial serologic tests, paired sera should be collected to demonstrate a significant (fourfold) titer rise.

R. tsutsugamushi can be isolated by inoculating white mice with blood samples from ill patients.

Treatment. Both tetracycline and chloramphenicol are effective against scrub typhus and usually produce prompt defervescence and clinical improvement. Relapses may occur when antibiotics are discontinued too quickly, especially in patients treated within a few days of onset. In patients first treated in their second week of illness, tetracycline or chloramphenicol can be discontinued 1 to 2 days after defervescence occurs. Fluorescent antibody levels are lower in patients given early antibiotic treatment.

Prevention. Because of strain variations, an effective scrub typhus vaccine has not been developed. In endemic or hyperendemic areas, measures to prevent chigger bites (protective clothing, insect repellents) and to control mite populations (insecticides, clearing of vegetation, and chemical treatment of the soil) can prevent chigger-human-chigger transmission.

Other Rickettsioses

Trench Fever (Shinbone Fever)

Trench fever is caused by *Rochalimaea quintana* and is transmitted by the body louse (*Pediculus humanus corporis*) in a human-louse-human cycle of infection. *R. quintana* is the only *Rickettsia* that can be grown on cellfree media (p. 702).

Trench fever was first recognized in World War I as a 5- to 6-day febrile illness associated with pains in the shins. It caused large epidemics in both German and Allied armies. By the end of the war a wider spectrum of clinical illness and the louse-borne transmission of the infection had been recognized. Trench fever disappeared during the next two decades only to reappear in epidemic form in the armies on the Eastern Front during World War II. It has been rarely reported since 1945.

Epidemiology. Trench fever has occurred in England, France, Yugoslavia, Italy, Russia, Germany, and several other countries in eastern Europe. *R. quintana* has been isolated from lice in Mexico, an area where clinical trench fever has not yet been recognized.

ECOLOGY. The body louse acquires infection by feeding on a rickettsemic human. Once infected, lice excrete *R. quintana* fecally for the remainder of their lives, which are not shortened by rickettsial infection. Unlike all other members of the tribe Rickettsieae, *R. quintana* proliferates extracellularly in the lumen of the gut rather than within the intestinal epithelial cells of its arthropod host. Transovarial transmission of *R. quintana* to the louse's offspring does not occur.

No animal reservoir other than humans has been identified. Thus a louse-human-louse cycle of infection like that of epidemic typhus occurs. Little is known about the prevalence and distribution of *R. quintana* in nonepidemic intervals. *R. quintana* has been isolated from apparently healthy patients years after their original attack.

Clinical Manifestations. The incubation period of trench fever in volunteers given intradermal inoculations of *R. quintana* ranges from 8 to 10 days. Clinical manifestations are highly variable, ranging from a mild afebrile illness to a moderately severe febrile disease with multiple relapses. Onset may be gradual or abrupt. Other symptoms include headache, malaise, chilliness, myalgias, and bone pain (especially in the tibial region). Fever curves vary widely among patients. A macular rash resembling the rose spots of typhoid fever may occur.

Laboratory Diagnosis. Laboratory animals such as guinea pigs, rabbits, or mice are not suitable for the isolation of *R. quintana.* In the past, xenodiagnosis (the feeding of uninfected lice on an infected patient and the later demonstration of rickettsia in the louse tissue) and primary isolation on enriched blood-agar media have been used for diagnosis. Like other members of the tribe Rickettsieae, the organism can also be grown in yolk sacs of embryonated hens' eggs. Complement-fixation, passive hemagglutination antibody, and indirect immunofluorescent antibody tests have been developed but are available only through a few reference and research laboratories. Now that suitable primers have been synthesized, diagnosis using polymerase chain reaction technology is possible.

Treatment. Data on the efficacy of tetracycline and chloramphenicol in the treatment of trench fever are not available. Based, however, on in vitro sensitivity testing and the near-universal susceptibility of other rickettsiae to these agents, both drugs are likely to be effective.

Prevention and Control. Measures to control human louse infestation will control the transmission of louse fever.

Q Fever

The name *Q fever* (Q for "query") was first used in 1937 to describe a mysterious febrile illness in Brisbane, Australia, packinghouse workers. The causal agent was isolated from infected workers and later was identified as a rickettsia. Almost simultaneously, the same organism was identified in wood ticks collected in Montana. Cox, an American, and Burnet, an Australian, were honored for their early work with this organism by the selection of the name *Coxiella burnetii.* Along with trench fever and epidemic typhus, Q fever caused epidemics in the armies fighting in Europe in World War II. In the ensuing years, *C. burnetii* was found to have a worldwide distribution and a complex ecology and epidemiology.

Epidemiology

PREVALENCE. Exact morbidity figures on the incidence of Q fever are not available; surveys, however, have demonstrated that many people throughout the world have serologic evidence of past infection with *C. burnetii.* In most such surveys the incidence of positive serologic tests exceeded the incidence of clinical Q fever. The disease has been recognized in at least 51 countries on five continents. In the United States, outbreaks of Q fever, all associated with livestock or livestock products, have occurred in California, Texas, and Illinois.

ECOLOGY. In nature there are two cycles of infection of *C. burnetii.* One involves arthropods (especially ticks) and a variety of vertebrates. The other cycle is maintained among domestic animals. The significance of arthropod-vertebrate transmission is conjectural. Although humans are not directly infected by ticks, arthropods may transmit infection to domestic animals, especially sheep and cattle. Domestic animals have inapparent infections but may shed large quantities of infectious organisms in their urine, milk, feces, and, especially, their placental products. Because *C. burnetii* is unique among Rickettsieae in its resistance to desiccation and light or temperature extremes, infectious organisms in placental products of domestic animals may become aerosolized after parturition, causing widespread outbreaks in humans and other animals miles from the place of origin. Dust in sheep or cattle sheds may become heavily contaminated and function as a source of infection for susceptible humans and animals. Once established, animal-to-animal spread is maintained primarily through airborne transmission.

Outbreaks of Q fever in humans have been traced to consumption of infected milk, handling of contaminated wool or hides, soil contaminated by infected animal feces, infected straw, and even to dusty clothing. Q fever is an occupational risk in abattoir workers, sheep shearers, dairy and other farm workers, workers in tanneries, wool, and felt plants, and laboratory workers, especially those using sheep and goats for experimental purposes. *C. burnetii* may enter the body through the skin (e.g., a contaminated minor abrasion), lungs (e.g., inhalation of infectious aerosols), mucous membranes (e.g., conjunctival contact with infectious materials), or gastrointestinal tract (e.g., ingestion of contaminated raw milk). Although rare, human-to-human transmission of Q fever has occurred. Immunologic evidence indicates that placental transfer of *C. burnetii* may result in human fetal infection. Asymptomatic recrudescence of infection may occur during pregnancy.

Clinical Manifestations. Clinical findings in patients with Q fever are diverse. *C. burnetii* is capable of causing inapparent infection, an influenza-like illness, pneumonia, prolonged fever, endocarditis, and hepatitis.

C. burnetii isolates associated with acute and chronic human infection apparently are genetically distinct. Isolates from patients with a chronic infection contain a plasmid (QpRS) that is 2 to 3 kb larger than the plasmid (QpH1) found in strains causing acute disease. Furthermore, these strains have differences in the composition and antigenicity of their surface lipopolysaccharides and in their in vitro antimicrobial susceptibilities. Thus different disease syndromes caused by *C. burnetii* may be partially or completely caused by differences in the infecting organism rather than by the condition of the human host.

Undiagnosed mild or subclinical cases frequently occur. Like most rickettsial diseases, clinically recognized Q fever usually begins abruptly with fever, chills or chilliness, headache, malaise, and myalgia. However, unlike most other rickettsial diseases, skin rash is not a part of the clinical syndrome, although evanescent macular rashes have been reported in a few cases. Patients may complain of nonspecific gastrointestinal symptoms, sore throat, chest pain, nonproductive cough, and painful eyes.

Physical findings may include hepatosplenomegaly, rales, rhonchi or dullness to chest percussion, and a relative bradycardia. Unilateral or bilateral lower-lobe infiltrates appearing on chest X-ray film that are similar to infiltrates seen in patients with viral and mycoplasma pneumonia and with psittacosis may be present. Liver function tests are often minimally abnormal, but granulomatous hepatic lesions have been documented even in patients with mild or minimal liver function test abnormalities.

Q fever endocarditis may occur months or years after acute illness and should be suspected when routine blood cultures are negative and no response occurs with antimicrobial therapy in a clinical setting strongly suggestive of bacterial endocarditis. Q fever endocarditis usually occurs on previously damaged heart valves, often the aortic valve. Until recently *C. burnetii* endocarditis was usually fatal.

Laboratory Diagnosis. The most definitive diagnostic procedure, isolation of *C. burnetii* from clinical specimens, can be accomplished by intraperitoneal inoculation of guinea pigs, mice, or embryonated hens' eggs. However, unless there are available experienced personnel working in specialized facilities with stringent safeguards to prevent accidental infection of laboratory personnel, primary isolation should not be attempted.

Complement-fixation tests using purified antigens are available through some state health departments. Since *C. burnetii* exists in two phases, complement-fixing reagents prepared using phase I and phase II antigens can be useful in distinguishing an acute from a chronic (e.g., endocarditis) or past infection (p. 703). A microagglutination test has also been developed. Both the complement-fixation and microagglutination tests are sensitive and specific. Weil-Felix antibodies are not elicited in response to infection with *C. burnetii.*

Treatment. Even though many patients with mild or subclinical illnesses recover without antimicrobial therapy, all clinically diagnosed cases should be treated. Tetracycline and chloramphenicol are effective against *C. burnetii,* but Q fever patients treated with these drugs do not respond as uniformly and as quickly as do patients with other rickettsial diseases. Tetracycline is the preferred drug. In vitro susceptibility to rifampin and 4-fluoroquinolones has been described, but clinical trials with these agents have not been reported.

Successful treatment of Q fever endocarditis has been reported after prolonged (10 months) therapy with tetracycline and with a combination of tetracycline and trimethoprim-sulfamethoxazole. Relapse after apparently successful long-term treatment may occur. Surgical replacement of the infected valve may be necessary since antibiotic therapy alone often is unsuccessful.

Prevention and Control. A completely satisfactory vaccine has not been developed. Both live and killed Q fever vaccines elicit complement-fixing antibodies that are protective in guinea pigs. Vaccine use in humans, however, has been hampered by the high rate of adverse reactions.

Measures to identify and decontaminate infected areas and to vaccinate domestic animal populations are difficult, expensive, and impractical. Milk-borne transmission can be prevented by pasteurization.

Ehrlichiosis

Of the six species of the genus *Ehrlichia,* only two have been associated with human infection. *Ehrlichia sennetsu* is the causative agent of human "sennetsu rickettsiosis"; *Ehrlichia canis* causes tropical canine pancytopenia in dogs.

Sennetsu Rickettsiosis. Sennetsu rickettsiosis (sennetsu fever) is characterized by three cardinal findings: fever, lymphadenopathy, and atypical lymphocytosis. The disease is localized to Japan and Malaysia where it has been called a variety of names, including infectious mononucleosis, glandular fever, hyuganetsu, and kagaminetsu.

E. sennetsu originally was misclassified as *Rickettsia sennetsu* (*sennetsu* from Japanese, meaning glandular fever). It has been isolated from blood, lymph nodes, and bone marrow of infected humans. *E. sennetsu* also shares antigens with *E. canis* but is not antigenically related to other rickettsiae of medical importance.

EPIDEMIOLOGY. The mode of transmission of *E. sennetsu* is unknown. Seasonal occurrence of illness in summer and fall suggests transmission by an invertebrate vector such as ticks. The occurrence of latent infections in dogs after experimental infection raises the possibility of a role for the dog in the perpetuation of this agent.

CLINICAL MANIFESTATIONS. The incubation period for *E. sennetsu* is about 14 days. Typically, onset is sudden and is heralded by fever and chills. Fever may fluctuate widely, with peaks occurring in late afternoon with morning remissions. Headache, chills, muscle pain, sore throat, back and joint pain, and sleeplessness are common in the acute febrile stage. Generalized lymphadenopathy usually develops 5 to 7 days after onset. Involved lymph nodes may be tender, but suppuration does not occur. Skin rash rarely occurs. An eschar has not been described.

Tetracycline is effective, but even untreated disease is benign. No fatal cases, serious complications, or sequelae have been reported.

LABORATORY DIAGNOSIS. Confirmation of the clinical diagnosis of sennetsu rickettsiosis may be made by (1) isolation of the organism from mice inoculated intraperitoneally or (2) specific immunoserologic techniques. Complement-fixing and immunofluorescent antibody titers reach their maximum 2 to 3 weeks after onset.

***Ehrlichia canis* Infection.** *E. canis,* the causative agent of canine ehrlichiosis, was originally isolated in Algeria in 1935. During the 1960s *E. canis* caused outbreaks of ehrlichiosis among military dogs at U.S. bases in Vietnam. Since that time numerous cases of canine ehrlichiosis have been reported throughout the United States and in other parts of the world, especially the tropics and subtropics. *E. canis* is now recognized as an important canine infectious disease in the United States, with cases occurring in nearly every state where the vector, the brown dog tick *Rhipicephalus sanguineus,* exists. Three phases of infection are recognized: acute, subclinical, and chronic. Dogs with chronic infection develop pancytopenia and frequently die of hemorrhage or secondary infection.

The first well-substantiated report of a human infection with *E. canis* appeared in 1986. In this case the patient visited Arkansas before his illness and had onset of his illness 12 to 14 days after receiving multiple tick bites. His illness resembled Rocky Mountain spotted fever except that there was no rash. A diagnosis of *E. canis* infection was based on the presence of characteristic intracytoplasmic inclusions in leukocytes and on a convalescent rise in titer to *E. canis* antigens.

Since this original case report, more than 50 cases of human ehrlichiosis have been described in the United States. A prospective study in Georgia suggested that ehrlichiosis is more common than Rocky Mountain spotted fever. Cases have been described from Oklahoma, Texas, Missouri, Arkansas, and seven states east of the Mississippi River, mostly in the southeastern region.

The incubation period for patients recalling a tick bite ranges from 7 to 21 days, with an average of 12 days. Typically illness begins abruptly. Symptoms resemble those of Rocky Mountain spotted fever. However, far fewer patients with ehrlichiosis have a skin rash. When present, the rash may be maculopapular or petechial. Leukopenia and thrombocytopenia sometimes occur, along with a history of tick bite, representing important clinical clues to the diagnosis. Chronic infection analogous to that seen in canines has not been described in humans.

The tick vector for human ehrlichiosis is unknown. The reservoir of *E. canis* may be chronically infected dogs. Thus far no isolates of *Ehrlichia* have been reported from humans. Until this is accomplished, it remains unknown if *E. canis* or a closely related species causes human disease. All cases diagnosed in humans have been based on the finding of intracytoplasmic inclusions in lymphocytes, monocytes, or neutrophils or by detecting antibodies to *E. canis* antigens. Tetracycline, the treatment of choice for canine ehrlichiosis, is the recommended treatment for humans. Information on the use of chloramphenicol is unavailable.

Bartonellaceae

Members of the family Bartonellaceae are parasites of the erythrocytes of man and other vertebrates. The only organism of medical significance is *Bartonella bacilliformis*, the etiologic agent of bartonellosis, or Carrión's disease, which is confined geographically to a small area on the western slopes of the Andes Mountains in South America. Bartonellosis is arthropod borne and encompasses two very different syndromes: Oroya fever and verruga peruana. Oroya fever is characterized by severe hemolytic anemia associated with bartonellae both in and on erythrocytes. Verruga peruana is a benign cutaneous erythematous nodular eruption. The homology of the two syndromes was first demonstrated in 1885 by a Peruvian medical student, Daniel Carrión, in a dramatic but tragic experiment. Carrión inoculated himself with material from the skin lesions of a patient with verruga peruana and developed fatal Oroya fever. In 1926, Noguchi isolated identical organisms from patients with Oroya fever and from others with verruga peruana. Using either isolate, he produced Oroya fever in rhesus monkeys. Subsequently, he reisolated the organism in pure culture, fulfilling Koch's postulates.

Although *B. bacilliformis* is the only definite human pathogen in this family, other erythrocyte-associated organisms in the families Bartonellaceae and Anaplasmataceae are found in animals. There are scattered reports of human disease associated with as yet unidentified hemotropic organisms exhibiting similarities to various members of this diverse group.

Morphology

Bartonella are small, exceedingly polymorphic, motile, gram-negative bacteria. They range in shape from small coccoid and ring-shaped structures to long angular forms in chains and clusters. They usually appear in erythrocytes as short rods ranging from 1 to 3 μm in length by 0.25 to 0.5 μm in width (Fig. 49–4). Organisms stain weakly with aniline dyes but appear bright red to purple with Wright's or Giemsa stain. They are not acid or alcohol fast. The cultured organisms possess a tuft of 1 to 10 unipolar flagella (Fig. 49–5), but flagella have not been seen in fresh preparations of human clinical specimens.

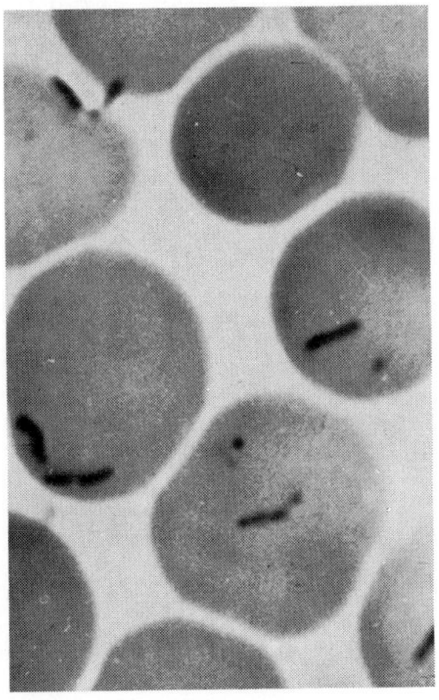

Fig. 49–4. *Bartonella bacilliformis.* Human blood stained with Giemsa stain. × 3000. *(From Wigand et al: Z Tropenmed Parasitol 4:539, 1953.)*

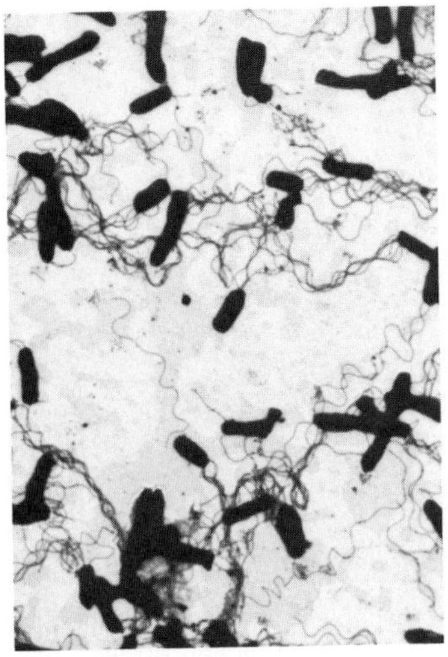

Fig. 49–5. Aggregates of *B. bacilliformis* showing flagella of centrifuged bacteria viewed by transmission electron microscopy. *(From Benson et al: Infect Immun 54:347, 1986.)*

Physiology

Cultural Characteristics. *B. bacilliformis* is an obligate aerobe. Growth and maintenance in serial passage in the laboratory may be achieved in cellfree semisolid media containing agar, fresh rabbit serum, and rabbit hemoglobin. Growth occurs at temperatures of 28C and 37C, with greater longevity at 28C. Cultures remain viable for long periods when stored at −70C. In semisolid agar colonies are 1 to 5 mm puffs of white that appear 1 to 2 weeks after inoculation. Two *Bartonella* colonial morphologies have been described, T1 and T2. These colony types differ in their adherence properties, but because of the absence of a suitable nonprimate in vivo model, the relative virulence of the two colony types is unknown. *Bartonella* can also be grown in the yolk sac and the chorioallantoic fluid of an embryonated hen's egg and in a variety of tissue culture systems. In the latter the organisms grow in the cytoplasm and extracellularly.

In media containing a variety of sugars, neither acid nor gas is produced. Hemolysin production in vitro has not been demonstrated.

All strains appear to be similar in respect to morphology, growth characteristics, and antigenic reactivity. Organisms are agglutinated and complement is fixed by immune serum derived either from naturally infected humans or from inoculated laboratory animals.

Cell Entry. Under natural conditions *B. bacilliformis* is found in or on erythrocytes and in the cytoplasm of reticuloendothelial and vascular endothelial cells.

Entry of the organisms into erythrocytes appears to be the result of a process of forced endocytosis. In vitro studies show that the binding of *B. bacilliformis* to human erythrocytes results in substantial and long-lasting deformations in the erythrocyte membranes (Fig. 49–6). The polar flagella probably provide the deforming force. Deep invaginations containing bacteria are observed, and membrane fusion at the necks of the invaginations results in the formation of intracellular vacuoles containing bacteria.

Clinical Infection

Epidemiology. Outbreaks of Oroya fever may occur when nonimmune persons arrive in sharply demarcated endemic

Fig. 49–6. Scanning electron microscopy showing deformation of erythrocytes by *B. bacilliformis*, with the production of deep pits that result from bacteria's pushing into the erythrocyte membrane. (From Benson et al: Infect Immun 54:347, 1986.)

areas of the western slopes of the Andes. In 1871 such an occurrence resulted in the first reported cases of the hemolytic disease when expatriate laborers were employed to build a railroad from Lima to the city of Oroya. Hundreds of cases occurred. Case fatality rate reached 40%. The eruptive form of the disease subsequently appeared in some survivors and in other individuals not initially observed to have had fever. Subsequent epidemics have been similar. Recognized endemic foci have been notable for their stability over many years.

Transmission of bartonellosis is restricted by the habits and ecology of the vector, the *Phlebotomus* fly. Its endemic area extends from 2° north of the equator to 13° south latitude, a distance of approximately 1600 km. It is further confined to a rather narrow band 800 to 2600 m above sea level, generally less than 160 km wide, on the western slopes of the Andes in Peru, Colombia, and Ecuador. Conditions of temperature and humidity inimical to the vector limit transmission further. Transmission occurs at night when female flies take blood meals. Before full understanding of insect transmission, disease was prevented in susceptible railroad workers by removing them from known endemic areas before nightfall.

Humans are the only known vertebrate reservoir. In some endemic areas, bacteremia may be detected in up to 5% of apparently healthy individuals. Duration of the bacteremia in such asymptomatic persons may be as long as a year.

Unsolved problems persist in understanding the epidemiology of bartonellosis. Experimental transmission has been achieved using flies captured in endemic areas, transported to nonendemic areas, and fed on laboratory monkeys. However, most transmission experiments have been unsuccessful and hampered by the difficulty of colonizing *Phlebotomus* in laboratories and by the incomplete expression of *Bartonella* infection in laboratory animals.

Pathogenesis. The erythrocytes of patients with Oroya fever contain large numbers of bartonellae. Infected red blood cells are hemolyzed by unknown mechanisms. Organisms may also be found in large clusters distending the cytoplasm of blood and lymphatic capillary endothelial cells. In patients with verruga peruana, organisms are found less easily, but they may be demonstrable in properly fixed and Giemsa-stained sections of the verruga lesions. The proliferative response of verruga lesions may be so intense that it occasionally may be misdiagnosed on biopsy as sarcoma. Insect transmission and invasion of and growth within erythrocytes and capillary endothelial cells by a bacterium such as *Bartonella* are unusual. Such properties more often are associated with protozoa and viruses.

Clinical Manifestations. Without treatment, Oroya fever is often lethal. Oroya fever is characterized clinically by fever, diffuse bone and muscle pain, and anemia. Most signs and symptoms are directly attributable to rapidly progressive hemolysis and resultant profound anemia. An incubation period of 2 to 5 weeks, hepatosplenomegaly, and terminal secondary infection with *Salmonella* further typify the disease.

Verruga peruana is a chronic nonfatal illness. It may develop in people surviving Oroya fever or in others with no prior clinical evidence of bartonellosis. Verruga peruana is characterized by localized or generalized angiomatous warts varying in size and degree of superficiality. Superficial lesions may appear bright red and reach the size of an egg. Fever, generalized pain, and malaise occur, although less frequently than in patients with Oroya fever. Skin lesions may last from 1 month to 2 years; most average 4 to 6 months in duration.

Infection with *B. bacilliformis* results in an immunologic response that includes the production of complement-fixing antibodies and varying degrees of resistance to subsequent disease and infection. Oroya fever is believed to occur in the fully susceptible individual, whereas verruga peruana probably signifies a state of partial immunity.

Laboratory Diagnosis. Bartonellosis can be confirmed by demonstration of organisms in erythrocytes in Giemsa-stained films of peripheral blood or by blood culture. Complement-fixing and agglutinating antibodies may be detectable in convalescent serum samples but are less useful than visualization or growth of the causative organism.

Treatment. Penicillin, streptomycin, tetracyclines, and chloramphenicol have each been reported to dramatically improve the course of patients with Oroya fever. Bacteremia, however, may not be eliminated with antimicrobial therapy. Transfusions are often useful. Antibiotics are less beneficial in patients with verruga peruana.

Control. *Phlebotomus* flies are exquisitely sensitive to DDT and can be controlled by its use. Antivector measures using insecticides such as DDT and antimicrobial treatment of ill individuals are the best control measures and serve to limit spread of the disease.

Vaccine development ceased in the 1940s when it became evident that antibiotics were curative and that the vector could be locally controlled by DDT.

FURTHER READING

Books and Reviews

RICKETTSIACEAE

Avakyan AA, Popov VL: Rickettsiaceae and Chlamydiaceae: Comparative electron microscopic studies. Acta Virol 28:159, 1985

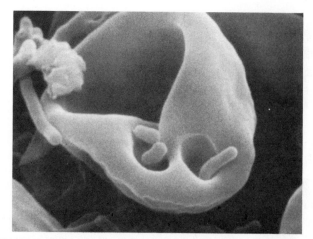

Baca OG, Paretsky D: Q fever and *Coxiella burnetii:* A model for host-parasite interactions. Microbiol Rev 47:127, 1983

Brettman LR, Lewin S, Holzman RS, et al: Rickettsialpox: Report of an outbreak and a contemporary review. Medicine 60:363, 1981

Burgdorfer W, Anacker RL (eds): Rickettsiae and Rickettsial Diseases. New York, Academic Press, 1981, p 3

Font-Creus B, Bella-Cueto F, Espejo-Arenas E, et al: Mediterranean spotted fever: A cooperative study of 227 cases. Rev Infect Dis 7:635, 1985

Hase T: Developmental sequence and surface membrane assembly of rickettsiae. Ann Rev Microbiol 39:69, 1985

Kakoma I, Ristic M, Winkler H: Leukocytic rickettsiae of humans and animals. In Leive L (ed): Microbiology—1986. Washington, DC, American Society for Microbiology, 1986, p 181

Kirk JL, Fine DP, Sexton DJ, Muchmore HG: Rocky Mountain spotted fever. A clinical review based on 48 confirmed cases 1943–1986. Medicine 69:35, 1990

Marchette NJ: Ecological Relationships and Evolution of the Rickettsiae. Cleveland, CRC Press Inc, 1982, vols I, II

McDade JE, Newhouse VF: Natural history of *Rickettsia rickettsii.* Ann Rev Microbiol 40:287, 1986

Moulder JW: Comparative biology of intracellular parasitism. Microbiol Rev 49:298, 1985

Ormsbee RA: Rickettsiae as organisms. Acta Virol 29:432, 1985

Osterman JV: Rickettsiae and hosts. Acta Virol 29:166, 1985

Samuel JE, Frazier ME, Mallavia LP: Correlation of plasmid type and disease caused by *Coxiella burnetii.* Infect Immunol 49:775, 1985

Walker DH: Rocky Mountain spotted fever: A disease in need of microbiologic concern. Clin Microbiol Rev 2:227, 1989

Walker DH: The role of host factor in the severity of spotted fever and typhus rickettsioses. Ann NY Acad Sci 590:10, 1990

Weiss E: The biology of rickettsiae. Ann Rev Microbiol 36:345, 1982

Weiss E, Moulder JW: Rickettsiales. In Krieg NR and Holt JG (eds): Bergey's Manual of Systematic Bacteriology, vol 1. Baltimore, Williams & Wilkins, 1984, p 687

Williams JC, Winkler HH: Molecular biology of rickettsiae. In Leive L, Schlessinger D (eds): Microbiology—1984. Washington DC, American Society for Microbiology, 1984, p 239

Zdrodovski P, Golinevich R: The Rickettsial Diseases. New York, Pergamon Press, 1960

Zinsser H: Rats, Lice and History. Boston, Little & Brown, 1935

BARTONELLACEAE

Colichon HF, DeBedon C: Enfermedad de Carrión II. Nutrientes utillizables para el crecimiento de la *Bartonella bacilliformis.* Rev Latinoam Microbiol 15:75, 1973

Dooley JR: Bartonellosis. In Binford CH, Conner DH (eds): Pathology of Tropical and Extraordinary Diseases. Washington, Armed Forces Institute of Pathology, 1976, p 192

Kreier JP, Dominquez N, Krampitz HE, et al: The hemotropic bacteria: The families Bartonellaceae and Anaplasmataceae. In Starr MP, Stolp H, Truper HG, et al (eds): The Prokaryotes—A Handbook on Habitats, Isolation and Identification of Bacteria. New York, Springer-Verlag, 1981

McDade JE, Fishbein DB: Rickettsiaceae: The rickettsiae. In Balows A, Hausler WJ, Lennette EH: Laboratory Diagnosis of Infectious Diseases Principles and Practice, vol II. New York, Springer-Verlag, 1988, p 865

Weinman D: Infectious anemias due to bartonella and related red cell parasites. Am Philos Soc 33(part 3); 1944

Weinman D: Bartonellosis. In Weinman D, Ristic M (eds): Infectious Blood Diseases of Man and Animals. New York, Academic Press, 1968, Chap 15

Selected Papers

RICKETTSIACEAE

Amano K-I, Williams JC: Sensitivity of *Coxiella burnetii* peptidoglycan to lysozyme hydrolysis and correlation of sacculus rigidity with peptidoglycan-associated proteins. J Bacteriol 160:989, 1984

Amano K-I, Williams JC: Chemical and immunological characterization of lipopolysaccharides from phase I and phase II *Coxiella burnetii.* J Bacteriol 160:994, 1984

Anacker RL, List RH, Mann RE, et al: Antigenic heterogeneity in high and low virulence strains of *Rickettsia rickettsii* revealed by monoclonal antibodies. Infect Immun 51:653, 1986

Anacker RL, McCaul TI, Burgdorfer W, et al: Properties of selected rickettsiae of the spotted fever group. Infect Immun 27:468, 1980

Anderson BE, Tzianabost T: Comparative sequence analysis of a genus-common rickettsial antigen gene. J Bacteriol 171:5199, 1989

Atkinson WH, Winkler HH: Transport of AMP by *Rickettsia prowazekii.* J Bacteriol 161:32, 1985

Bozeman FM, Elisberg BL, Humphries JW, et al: Serologic evidence of *Rickettsia canada* infection of man. J Infect Dis 121:367, 1970

Brezina R: Diagnosis and control of rickettsial diseases. Acta Virol 29:338, 1985

Carl M, Vaidya S, Robbins F-M, et al: Heterogeneity of CD4-positive human T-cell clones which recognize the surface protein antigen of *Rickettsia typhi.* Infect Immun 57:1276, 1989

Centers for Disease Control: Q fever among slaughterhouse workers—California. MMWR 35:223, 1986

Dawson JE, Fishbein DB, Eng TR, et al: Diagnosis of human ehrlichiosis with the indirect fluorescent antibody test: Kinetics and specificity. J Infect Dis 162:91, 1990

Duma RJ, Sonenshine DE, Bozeman FM, et al: Epidemic typhus in the United States associated with flying squirrels. JAMA 245:2318, 1981

Feng HM, Walker DH, Wang JG: Analysis of T-cell-dependent and -independent antigens of *Rickettsia conorii* with monoclonal antibodies. Infect Immun 55:7, 1987

Fishbein DB, Kemp A, Dawson JE, et al: Human ehrlichiosis: Prospective active surveillance in febrile hospitalized patients. J Infect Dis 160:803, 1989

Hackstadt T, Williams JC: Biochemical stratagem for obligate parasitism of eukaryotic cells by *Coxiella burnetii.* Proc Natl Acad Sci USA 78:3240, 1981

Hanson B: Identification and partial characterization of *Rickettsia tsutsugamushi* major protein immunogens. Infect Immun 50:603, 1985

Harden VA: Rocky mountain spotted fever: Research and the development of the insect vector theory, 1900–1930. Bull Hist Med 59:449, 1985

Harell GT: Rocky Mountain spotted fever. Medicine 28:333, 1949

Harkess JR, Ewing SA, Crutcher JM, et al: Human ehrlichiosis in Oklahoma. J Infect Dis 159:576, 1989

Hart RJ: The epidemiology of Q fever. Postgrad Med J 49:535, 1973

Hechemy KE, Stevens RW, Gasowski S, et al: Discrepancies in Weil-Felix and micro-immunofluorescence test results for Rocky Mountain spotted fever. J Clin Microbiol 9:292, 1979

Helmick CG, Bernard KW, D'Angelo LJ: Rocky Mountain spotted fever: Clinical, laboratory, and epidemiological features of 262 cases. J Infect Dis 150:480, 1984

Jerrells TR: Immunosuppression associated with the development of chronic infections with *Rickettsia tsutsugamushi:* Adherent suppressor cell activity and macrophage activation. Infect Immun 50:175, 1985

Koster FT, Williams JC, Goodwin JS: Cellular immunity in Q fever: Specific lymphocyte unresponsiveness in Q fever endocarditis. J Infect Dis 152:1283, 1985

Krause DC, Winkler HH, Wood DO: Cosmid cloning of *Rickettsia prowazekii* antigens in *Escherichia coli* K-12. Infect Immun 47:157, 1985

Lange JV, Walker DH: Production and characterization of monoclonal antibodies to *Rickettsia rickettsii.* Infect Immun 46:289, 1984

Maeda K, Markowitz N, Hawley RC, et al: Human infection with *Ehrlichia canis,* a leukocytic rickettsia. N Engl J Med 316:853, 1987

McCaul TF, Williams JC: Developmental cycle of *Coxiella burnetii:* Structure and morphogenesis of vegetative and sporogenic differentiation. J Bacteriol 147:1063, 1981

McDonald GA, Anacker RL, Garjian K: Cloned gene of *Rickettsia rickettsii* surface antigen: Candidate vaccine for Rocky Mountain spotted fever. Science 235:83, 1987

Meiklejohn G, Reimer LG, Graves PS, et al: Cryptic epidemic of Q fever in a medical school. J Infect Dis 144:107, 1981

Mitchell C, Martin EE, Dasch GA: Human T helper cells specific for antigens of typhus group rickettsiae enhance natural killer cell activity in vitro. Infect Immun 54:297, 1986

Murray ES, Baehr G, Shwartzman G, et al: Brill's disease. I. Clinical and laboratory diagnosis. JAMA 142:1059, 1950

Murray ES, Gaon JA, O'Connor JM, et al: Serologic studies of primary endemic typhus and recrudescent typhus. J Immunol 94:723, 1965

Newhouse VF, Shepard CC, Redus MD, et al: A comparison of the complement-fixation, indirect fluorescent antibody and microagglutination test for the serologic diagnosis of rickettsial diseases. Am J Trop Med Hyg 28:387, 1979

Oaks EV, Rice RM, Kelly DJ, Stover CK: Antigenic and genetic relatedness of eight *Rickettsia tsutsugamushi* antigens. Infect Immun 57:3116, 1989

Okada T, Tange Y, Kobayashi Y: Causative agent of spotted fever group rickettsiosis in Japan. Infect Immun 58:887, 1990.

Palmer BA, Hetrick FM, Jerrells TR: Gamma interferon production in response to homologous and heterologous strain antigens in mice chronically infected with *Rickettsia tsutsugamushi.* Infect Immun 46:237, 1984

Parker RR: Rocky Mountain spotted fever. JAMA 110:1185, 1938

Petersen LR, Sawyer LA, Fishbein DB, et al: An outbreak of ehrlichiosis in members of an army reserve unit exposed to ticks. J Infect Dis 159:562, 1989

Rapmund G: Rickettsial diseases of the far east: New perspectives. J Infect Dis 149:330, 1984

Relman DA, Loutit JS, Schmidt TM, et al: The agent of bacillary angiomatosis: An approach to the identification of uncultured pathogens. N Engl J Med 323:1573, 1990

Rohrbach BW, Harkess JR, Ewing SA, et al: Epidemiology and clinical characteristics of persons with serologic evidence of *E. canis* infection. Am J Public Health 80:442, 1990

Rollwagen FM, Dasch GA, Jerrells TR: Mechanisms of immunity to rickettsial infections: Characterization of a cytotoxic effector cell. J Immunol 136:1418, 1986

Samuel JE, Frazier ME, Mallavia LP: Correlation of plasmid type and disease caused by *Coxiella burnetii.* Infect Immun 49:775, 1985

Silverman DJ, Santucci LA: Potential for free radical-induced lipid peroxidation as a cause of endothelial cell injury in Rocky Mountain spotted fever. Infect Immun 56:3110, 1988

Silverman DJ, Wisseman CL, Waddell AD, et al: External layers of *Rickettsia prowazekii* and *Rickettsia rickettsii:* Occurrence of a slime layer. Infect Immun 22:233, 1978

Slater LN, Welch DF, Hensel D, Coody DW: A newly recognized fastidious gram-negative pathogen as a cause of fever and bacteremia. N Engl J Med 323:1587, 1990

Stuart BM, Pullen RM: Endemic murine typhus fever: Clinical observations. Ann Intern Med 23:520, 1945

Taylor JP, Betz TG, Fishbein DB, et al: Serological evidence of possible human infection with *Ehrlichia* in Texas. J Infect Dis 158:217, 1988

Taylor JP, Betz TG, Rawlings JA: Epidemiology of murine typhus in Texas 1980 through 1984. JAMA 255:2173, 1986

Todd WJ, Burgdorfer W, Wray GP: Detection of fibrils associated with *Rickettsia rickettsii.* Infect Immun 41:1252, 1983

Traub R, Wisseman CL Jr: The ecology of chiggerborne rickettsiosis (scrub typhus). J Med Entomol 11:237, 1974

Walker TS: Rickettsial interactions with human endothelial cells in vitro: Adherence and entry. Infect Immun 44:205, 1984

Walker DH, Cain BG: A method for specific diagnosis of Rocky Mountain spotted fever on fixed, paraffin-embedded tissue by immunofluorescence. J Infect Dis 137:206, 1978

Weisburg WG, Woese CR, Dobson ME, Weiss E: A common origin of rickettsial and certain plant pathogens. Science 230:556, 1985

WHO Working Group on Rickettsial Diseases and Rickettsioses: A continuing disease problem. Bull WHO 60:157, 1982

Winkler HH, Daugherty RM: Acquisition of glucose by *Rickettsia prowazekii* through the nucleotide intermediate uridine 5′-diphosphoglucose. J Bacteriol 167:805, 1986

Winkler HH, Daugherty RM: Phospholipase A activity associated with the growth of *Rickettsia prowazekii* in L929 cells. Infect Immun 57:36, 1989

Wisseman CL Jr, Waddell A: Interferonlike factors from antigen- and mitogen-stimulated human leukocytes with antirickettsial and cytolytic actions on *Rickettsia prowazekii.* J Exp Med 157:1780, 1983

Woodward TE: A historical account of rickettsial diseases with a discussion of unsolved problems. J Infect Dis 127:583, 1973

Yamada T, Harber P, Pettit GW, et al: Activation of the kallikrein-kinin system in Rocky Mountain spotted fever. Ann Intern Med 88:764, 1978

Yeaman MR, Roman MJ, Baca OG. Antibiotic susceptibilities of two *Coxiella burnetii* isolates implicated in distinct clinical syndromes. Antimicrob Agents Chemother 33:1052, 1989

BARTONELLACEAE

Benson LA, Kar S, McLaughlin G, Ihler GM: Entry of *Bacillus bacilliformis* into erythrocytes. Infect Immun 54:347, 1986

Dooley JR: Haemotropic bacteria in man. Lancet 2:1237, 1980

Ristic M, Kreir JP: Hemotropic bacteria. N Engl J Med 301:937, 1979

Schultz MG: A history of bartonellosis (Carrión's disease). Am J Trop Med Hyg 17:503, 1968

Walker TS, Winkler HH: *Bartonella bacilliformis:* Colonial types and erythrocyte adherence. Infect Immun 31:480, 1981

Weisburg WG, Dobson ME, Samuel JE, et al: Phylogenetic diversity of the rickettsiae. J Bacteriol 171:4202, 1989

CHAPTER 50

Chlamydiae

Chlamydia

Chlamydiaceae is a family of obligate intracellular bacterial parasites with a tropism for columnar epithelial cells lining the mucous membranes. Because of their strict intracellular parasitism, the chlamydiae for many years were thought to be viruses. However, like other bacteria, they (1) possess a cell envelope similar to that of gram-negative bacteria, (2) contain both DNA and RNA, (3) possess procaryotic ribosomes and synthesize their own proteins, nucleic acids, and lipids, and (4) are susceptible to a wide range of antibiotics.

Chlamydia infect a wide spectrum of vertebrate hosts within three major ecologic niches: birds, mammals, and humans. Human diseases commonly caused by these organisms include trachoma, inclusion conjunctivitis, various urogenital tract infections of both males and females, infantile pneumonia, lymphogranuloma venereum, and psittacosis. Humans are also occasionally infected with *Chlamydia* that normally are associated with diseases of other animals, such as feline pneumonitis.

Three distinct species of *Chlamydia* are recognized: (1) *Chlamydia trachomatis*, which is inhibited by sulfonamides and produces iodine-staining cytoplasmic inclusions, (2) *Chlamydia psittaci*, and (3) *Chlamydia pneumoniae*, both of which are not inhibited by sulfonamides and do not produce iodine-staining inclusions. There is significant DNA homology within each species but little homology among the three, suggesting a long-standing evolutionary separation.

Morphology

There are two morphologically distinct forms of chlamydiae: elementary body (EB) and reticulate body (RB) (Fig. 50–1). The EB is a small, dense spherical body, 0.2 to 0.4 μm in diameter, which rivals mycoplasma for the designation "smallest of the procaryotes." It is the infectious form of the organism, responsible for attaching to the target host cell and promoting its entry. The rigidity of the cell wall permits survival of the EB during its limited extracellular existence. This rigidity is believed to be due more to disulfide bond cross-linking among the major outer membrane proteins rather than to an extensively cross-linked classic peptidoglycan matrix. Freeze-fracture studies reveal a thin wall layer between the outer membrane and the cytoplasmic membrane, but chemical analyses detect little to no muramic acid, although D-alanine is present. As with most gram-negative bacteria, the chlamydiae possess a lipopolysaccharide, but it is truncated, resembling the Re chemotype.

The DNA is compactly organized in a central nucleoid and is a closed circular molecule with a molecular weight of 660 kDa. A molecule of this size could provide information for about 600 different proteins, which is approximately one fourth the amount provided by the *Escherichia coli* genome. Both *C. psittaci* and *C. trachomatis* contain a 4.4 MDa cryptic

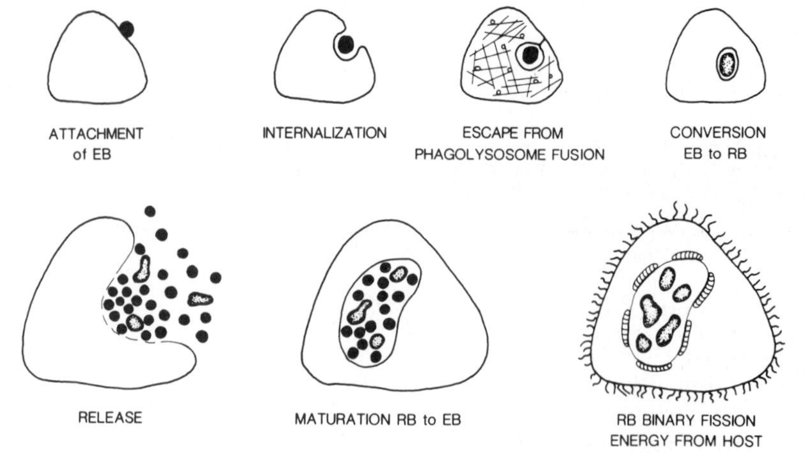

Fig. 50–1. Schematic diagram of the developmental cycle of chlamydiae. EB, elementary body; RB, reticulate body.

plasmid, but there is no homology between the two plasmids. The EB also contains procaryotic ribosomal RNA with sedimentation coefficients of 21S, 16S, and 4S.

The RB is the intracellular, metabolically active form that divides by binary fission. It is larger than the EB, approximately 0.6 to 1.0 μm in diameter, and is osmotically fragile. The RBs synthesize their own DNA, RNA, and proteins, but some of their metabolic capabilities are limited. For example, they cannot complete the pentose cycle and do not utilize pyruvate by way of the tricarboxylic acid cycle. Furthermore, the RBs cannot generate high-energy phosphate bonds. Thus their adaptation for an intracellular habitat is due apparently to their total dependency on eucaryotic cells for energy. Mitochondrial ATP is acquired by growing RB by means of a chlamydial ATP-ADP translocase. The ATP is broken down to ADP by a specific RB ATPase, and the resultant protonmotive force helps drive the transport of nutrients.

The chlamydiae are nonmotile, lacking flagella, and nonpiliated. They do, however, possess unusual cylindric surface projections, averaging 18 in number and arranged in a hexagonal array (Fig. 50–2D). The projections are anchored in the cytoplasmic membrane and protrude through holes in the envelope. Current evidence suggests that the projections of developing chlamydiae penetrate the endosome membrane that surrounds the chlamydial microcolony, permitting uptake of nutrients from the host cytoplasm.

Developmental Cycle

A unique developmental cycle characterizes the growth of these intracellular bacteria in their host cells (Figs. 50–1 and 50–2). The cycle consists essentially of five major phases: (1) attachment and penetration of the EB, (2) transition of the metabolically inert EB into metabolically active RB, (3) growth and division of the RB, producing many progeny, (4) maturation of the noninfectious RB into infectious EB, and (5) release of EB from the host cell.

The initial event in the infectious process begins with attachment of the EB to microvilli of a susceptible columnar epithelial cell (Fig. 50–2A). The EB travels down the microvilli and localizes in indentations of the host-cell plasma membrane resembling coated pits (Fig. 50–2B). One method of internalization resembles the receptor-mediated endocytosis-like pathway of viruses but may also be, in part, parasite specified. In addition, cytochalasin-D-sensitive, microfilament-dependent phagocytic entry mechanisms have been described. For a parasite whose survival depends on growth within its target host cell, multiple strategies for gaining entry no doubt exist. Specific adhesions and receptors have yet to be identified. *C. psittaci* EB-containing endosomes escape interaction with lysosomes and proceed to the nuclear hof area. In contrast, *C. trachomatis* EB-containing endosomes begin to fuse with one another and perhaps with lysosomes. In both cases the chlamydiae remain bounded and protected by the endosome membrane throughout their intracellular development. The EBs undergo changes in their cell wall that result in a spheroplastlike transition to the RB form. DNA, RNA, and protein synthesis are initiated, permitting growth of the RB and division by binary fission (Fig. 50–2C). At some point in the developmental cycle, host-cell mitochrondria migrate to and are positioned against the enlarging endosome, and RB parasitize the ATP. The developing chlamydial microcolony is termed an *inclusion* (Fig. 50–2E and F) and may contain anywhere from 100 to 500 progeny, depending on the species. Presumably when nutrients have been depleted, the RBs mature into EBs and are released from the host cell. In the case of *C. psittaci* the host cell is usually severely damaged, and release of chlamydiae is by lysis within 48 hours. The *C. trachomatis* inclusion appears to be exocytosed in 72 to 96 hours, and a scar forms in the surviving host cell. In one provocative study, *C. trachomatis* inclusions in cultured human endometrial cells were observed to undergo division, followed by segregation of divided inclusions into daughter epithelial cells at the time of eukaryotic cell division. Should this event occur in the basal cells, which are not lost at menstruation and from which the endometrium regenerates, it could provide one explanation for chlamydial persistent infection in vivo in the female genital tract.

Chlamydiae-specific lipopolysaccharide (LPS) is exported to the surface of the infected cell concomitant with active RB growth. Whether this antigenic material plays a role in the perpetuation of disabling chlamydial disease as a result of prolonged inflammatory response and immune-mediated pathology remains a controversial issue. However, since oral

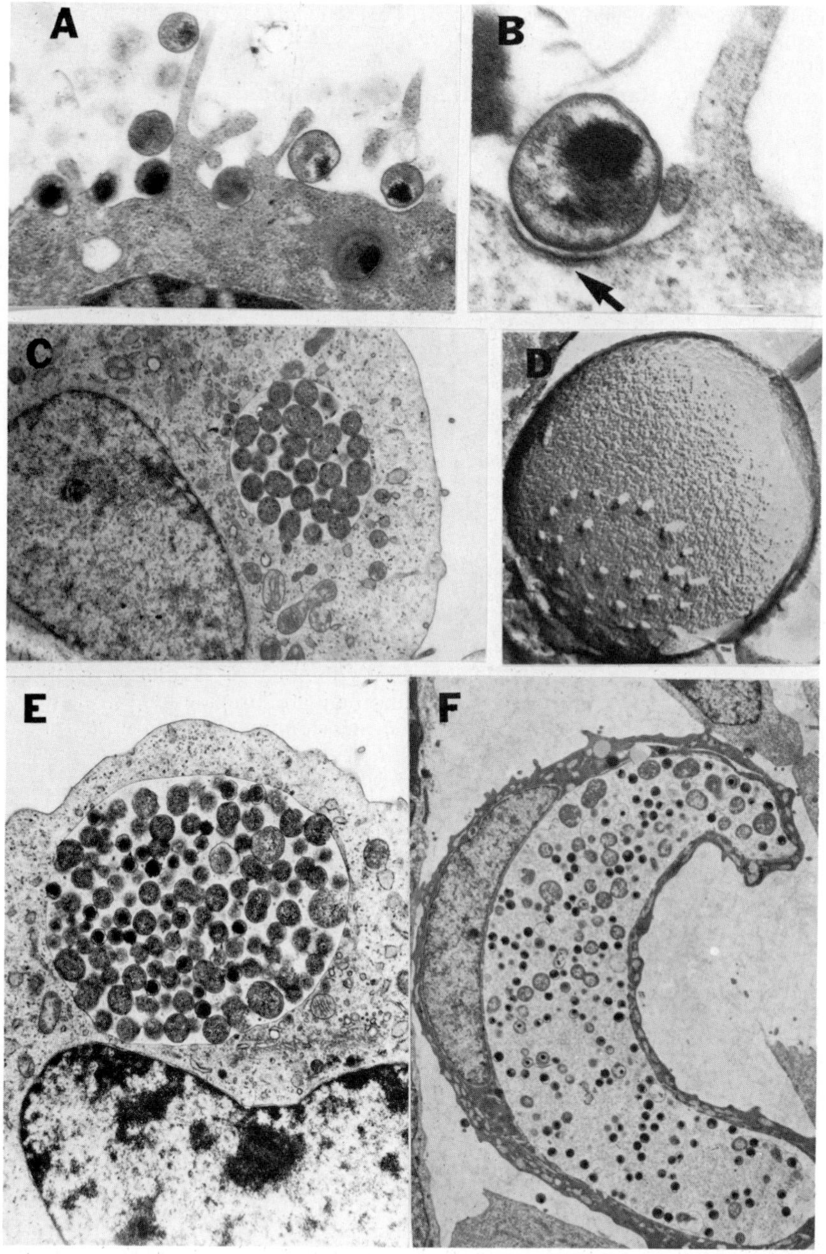

Fig. 50–2. Electron photomicrographs illustrating various stages of the chlamydial developmental cycle. **A.** Attachment of elementary body (EB) to the microvilli of a susceptible eucaryotic cell. **B.** Localization of an EB in a coated pit. **C.** A developing inclusion containing an actively growing reticulate body (RB). **D.** Freeze-fracture preparation of chlamydia revealing surface projections. **E.** *C. psittaci* inclusion. **F.** *C. trachomatis* inclusion.

immunization of cynomolgus monkeys with a recombinant vaccine expressing chlamydial LPS fails to protect against chlamydial eye infection, LPS may not be an important antigen for stimulating immunity against chlamydiae. An interesting hypothesis has been advanced for a role of the chlamydial exoglycolipid in pathogenesis: The accumulation of this material in the eucaryotic plasma membrane decreases membrane fluidity, which may in turn compromise the efficiency of immune recognition and cytotoxic T cell onslaught, thereby protecting chlamydiae in their intracellular niche. More recently, a 57 kDa protein, with genus specificity, possible "common antigen" epitopes, and potential heat-shock reactivity, has been shown to induce delayed conjunctival hypersensitivity in ocular immune guinea pigs. The histopathologic findings appear virtually identical to those found in individuals suffering from trachoma.

Laboratory Diagnosis

The laboratory diagnosis of *Chlamydia* infections can be accomplished by (1) direct examination of clinical specimens for chlamydial inclusions, antigens, or nucleic acids, (2) isolation of the organisms, or (3) detection of specific antibodies against these bacteria. Because these procedures differ considerably in sensitivity, depending on the type and handling of individual specimens, selection of a practical method must be carefully evaluated by the clinical laboratory.

Specimen Collection. The utility of any diagnostic procedure for the detection of chlamydiae depends on the proper collection of specimens. Columnar epithelial cells must be obtained; exudates or discharges are not adequate and should be removed from the site before sampling. Specimens should be collected from the involved sites by vigorous swabbing or scraping with plastic- or metal-shafted swabs of rayon, Dacron, or cotton or with cytologic sampling devices. Calcium alginate and wooden-shafted swabs may be inhibitory to chlamydiae or toxic to the cells that support their growth and should not be used when isolation of the organism is necessary. All specimens submitted for culture should be placed immediately in an appropriate transport medium, refrigerated at 4C during transport and storage, and processed within 48 hours of collection. If there will be a delay in processing of more than 48 hours, the specimen should be stored at −70C. Repeated freezing and thawing should be avoided. The most commonly used transport media for chlamydiae include 2-sucrose phosphate and sucrose-phosphate-glutamate. The addition of protein additives such as bovine serum albumin to the medium may preserve chlamydial viability in specimens stored at −70C. Vancomycin, gentamicin, and amphotericin B are frequently added in combination to the transport medium. Ocular, urogenital, rectal, nasopharyngeal, and throat specimens can be tested for *C. trachomatis*. Improved recovery rates from the endocervix may be obtained using a cytologic brush, collecting multiple samples, or pooling specimens from the cervix and urethra. For women with salpingitis or endometritis, fallopian tube biopsies or endometrial aspirates may be used. Blood, sputum, and biopsy tissue specimens are used for the detection of *C. psittaci*, and urogenital and lymph node or bubo aspirates are acceptable for lymphogranuloma venereum (LGV) strains of *C. trachomatis*. Swabs of the posterior oropharynx should be obtained for the detection of *C. pneumoniae*.

Direct Cytopathologic Examination. *C. trachomatis* develops compact, clearly defined, glycogen-containing, intracellular microcolonies or inclusions. These are found in infected yolk sac preparations, infected animal tissue, inoculated tissue culture cells, and conjunctival scrapings of persons with active trachoma or inclusion conjunctivitis. They are basophilic and gram negative; they stain a mahogany color with iodine and may also be detected by FA (fluorescent antibody) or Giemsa stain. Direct microscopic examination of Giemsa-stained smears has long been recognized as the standard procedure for the detection of chlamydial inclusions in certain clinical specimens. This technique is simple to perform and inexpensive and provides a permanent preparation. It is most useful in the diagnosis of neonatal inclusion conjunctivitis in which many inclusions are produced, but it has limited to no value in diagnosing adult inclusion conjunctivitis or genital tract infections.

Iodine staining for glycogen-containing inclusions of *C. trachomatis* is a rapid and simple method for screening many slides in a relatively short period of time. The iodine-stained slide can be counterstained by the Giemsa method and can be preserved indefinitely. However, the sensitivity of this method is poor, and it is unreliable since glycogen is present only during certain periods in the developmental cycle. Its primary usefulness is in the rapid staining of tissue culture monolayers used for the isolation of *C. trachomatis* from clinical specimens. Inclusions of *C. psittaci* are not stained by the iodine technique since this organism produces no glycogen during its development.

Rapid Antigen Detection Methods. Within the last decade, direct FA staining and enzyme immunoassays (EIA) have been used with increasing frequency, either alone or in conjunction with standard tissue culture methods, for the rapid identification of *C. trachomatis* in clinical specimens. These assays are available in a kit format from a number of commercial sources. The kits are easy to use and provide standardized technology to laboratories unable to perform cell culture. Such techniques are equal to or more sensitive than conventional direct-staining methods and have the advantage of detecting small amounts of specific antigens or intact organisms. These procedures are equivalent in sensitivity and specificity to cell culture in certain clinical settings and provide for a simple, rapid, and readily available diagnosis of chlamydial infections. For patients with minimally symptomatic infections, culture is recommended.

In general, FA staining requires considerable experience and thoughtful interpretation, is not well suited for processing large numbers of specimens, and requires the use of a fluorescence microscope. However, it does allow for determining the adequacy of the specimen by direct observation of the number of columnar epithelial cells present. EIA is automated and can be applied to large numbers of samples; it requires minimal training and equipment and provides objective, quantitative results. The recent development of rapid monoclonal antibody-based membrane culture EIA devices may offer further advantages in sensitivity and ease of performance for the detection of chlamydial antigen. The greatest application of FA and EIA methods is in the direct detection of *C. trachomatis* from infected cervical or urethral specimens and conjunctival scrapings of adults. They have also been successfully used to identify *C. trachomatis* in nasopharyngeal and conjunctival specimens from infants with chlamydial conjunctivitis and pneumonitis.

Recently, testing for *Chlamydia* antigens by either FA or EIA in urine sediments of men has proved equal in sensitivity to culture of the male urethra. Rarely do these specimens contain intact intracellular inclusions that can be detected by other staining methods. They do, however, contain extracellular elementary bodies that can be detected readily in clinical specimens by either direct FA staining or EIA. Also, the use of FA staining or EIA for the detection of inclusions in tissue culture cells is more sensitive than iodine staining, which permits the rapid and accurate screening of numerous clinical specimens for infected cells. FA tests using monoclonal antibodies specific for *C. pneumoniae* and *C. psittaci* have also been described but have been used primarily as research tools.

DNA hybridization techniques have also been developed for the detection of chlamydial nucleic acids from clinical specimens and cultured cells. Both DNA and RNA probes to chromosomal DNA and the cryptic plasmid found in all isolates of *C. trachomatis* have been used in standard sandwich and dot-blot hybridizations. The specificity of these tests is good, but the sensitivity varies considerably, depending on the hybridization and probe-labeling conditions used in the assays. In general, these methods are considered less sensitive than isolation techniques for the detection of chlamydiae. Cloned chlamydial plasmid has also been used as a probe in in situ hybridizations to detect chlamydiae in tissue biopsies and cervical smears. A commercial nucleic acid probe assay has been developed that uses a nonisotopically labeled, chemiluminescent DNA probe to detect conserved sequences of ribosomal RNA found in high copy number in chlamydial cells. This assay is highly specific and has demonstrated comparable sensitivity with FA staining, EIA, and culture. Amplification of chlamydial target sequences using the polymerase chain reaction has also been described. Because chlamydiae are present in small numbers in most clinical specimens, this method offers a major advance in increasing the sensitivity of probe technology by amplifying small amounts of nucleic acid to levels readily detected by standard hybridization techniques. With the continued development of nucleic acid probe technology, such assays will be available for widespread diagnostic testing. At the present time, however, these methods are costly, require skilled personnel, and are not readily adapted to all laboratories.

Isolation of *Chlamydia*. Traditionally the isolation of *Chlamydia* has been accomplished by the inoculation of infected material into either embryonated eggs, experimental animals, or selected tissue culture cell lines. All known strains of *Chlamydia* will infect the chick embryo, and group-specific antigen and characteristic inclusions can be found in yolk sac material from infected 6- to 8-day embryos. However, this procedure is impractical for use by clinical laboratories since it is tedious, time-consuming, and less sensitive than tissue culture.

Some strains of *Chlamydia* will infect mice, and it is possible to partially characterize a strain by the route of inoculation by which the infection may be established. LGV strains usually will infect mice inoculated intracerebrally, but other *C. trachomatis* strains will not infect mice by any route of infection. They will, however, cause a rapid toxic death in mice if injected intravenously. Mice can be protected against toxic death by prior immunization with the same strain. *C. psittaci* can be isolated from intracerebrally and subcutaneously inoculated mice. Mouse inoculation for the isolation of chlamydiae, however, is less sensitive than either cell culture or inoculation of embryonated eggs.

Cell culture is still considered the most sensitive and specific method for the isolation and identification of *Chlamydia*. Cell lines commonly used to isolate *Chlamydia* include McCoy, HeLa 229, BHK-21, L 929, and Buffalo green monkey kidney cells. Both genital and ocular strains of *C. trachomatis* tend to vary widely in their infectivity for cell cultures. Propagation of *C. pneumoniae* in cell culture has proven to be difficult. HeLa 229 cells and, more recently, the heteroploid HL cell line have been described as being more sensitive than McCoy cells for the isolation of this organism. Egg culture methods may be necessary for the growth of certain fastidious strains. *C. psittaci* can be isolated from infected material by methods similar to those used for other *Chlamydia*. The organism grows best in L 929 cells. However, suitable isolation or containment facilities should be available for this extremely infectious human pathogen; laboratory-acquired infections are common.

In the standard culture method used for *Chlamydia*, clinical specimens are inoculated by centrifugation onto cell monolayers. These monolayers are grown in shell vials on glass coverslips or on the surface of multiwell microculture plates. They usually are irradiated or pretreated with such chemicals as 5-iodo-2-deoxyuridine, cytochalasin B, or cycloheximide to enhance chlamydial replication and to allow easier recognition of inclusions. Pretreatment of the cells with diethylaminoethyl-dextran (DEAE-dextran) or centrifugation of the chlamydiae onto the host cells increases contact between the infectious chlamydial particles and the host cell monolayer, with a subsequent increase in infectivity. After incubation of the cultures for 48 to 72 hours, chlamydial inclusions are visualized, using either Giemsa stain, iodine, or fluorescein-labeled monoclonal antibodies. Of the three methods, immunofluorescence is the most sensitive for identifying inclusion bodies after primary cell culture.

Serologic Diagnosis. The diagnosis of chlamydial infections can be accomplished by either the complement-fixation (CF) test or the microimmunofluorescence (micro-IF) technique. The utility of these methods varies considerably with the particular disease, and neither serologic test can be used for all human chlamydial infections. Antibody can be detected in the serum, tears, and genital secretions of individuals with chlamydial infections. However, the value of local antibody detection is uncertain. The CF test uses the genus-specific antigen (LPS) and is applicable for the diagnosis of infections caused by *C. psittaci*, *C. pneumoniae*, and the LGV strains of *C. trachomatis*. This method has little value in diagnosing trachoma and genital infections. The test also is technically demanding and requires rigid standardization for proper performance. A fourfold rise in CF antibody titers in acute and convalescent serum of patients is diagnostic. However, many patients without documented disease are seropositive by CF, which decreases the sensitivity of this test. Therefore a titer of 1:64 or greater is generally recommended for diagnosis of LGV or psittacosis by the CF procedure.

The micro-IF test has been widely used in the diagnosis of ocular and genital infections caused by *C. trachomatis*. The method is more sensitive than the CF test and, in contrast, measures immunotype-specific antibody either to each of the 15 serovars of the organism or to antigenically related groups of pooled immunotype antigens. Measurements of IgG, IgM, and local antibody in various secretions can be accomplished. Micro-IF is the method of choice for the diagnosis of pneumonia in infants in whom a serum IgM titer of 1:32 or greater is diagnostic of chlamydial infection. In the majority of patients for whom the identity of the infecting serovar of *C. trachomatis* is known, there is a type-specific antibody response with a titer of 1:8 or greater. Exceptions include patients with LGV, in whom the antibody is frequently reactive with more than one serovar. This results in extremely high titers (i.e., $\geq$1:1000). Early antibody formation is of the IgM class and persists for approximately 1 month before being replaced by IgG. In the few instances in which serial antibody determinations have been made, type-specific antibody has decreased fairly rapidly after primary infection, often within 1 or 2 months. Reinfection with the same serovar results only in a rise of IgG antibody, whereas reinfection with a new serovar results in increased IgM titers to the new serovar and in elevated levels of IgG to the previous immunotype. The level of seropositivity for uninfected individuals is high. Therefore recommendations for the serologic diagnosis of *C. trachomatis* infections by micro-IF include (1) demonstration of seroconversion, (2) a fourfold increase in titer to a specific serovar, or (3) the presence of IgM antibody.

The micro-IF test can also be used to diagnose infections caused by *C. pneumoniae*. A serum IgM titer of 1:32 or greater or an IgG titer of 1:64 or greater is indicative of recent infection. Although the micro-IF test appears to have practical application in the diagnosis of certain chlamydial infections, the test is labor intense and available in only a few laboratories.

Variations of the micro-IF test have been described and include whole inclusion immunofluorescence and whole inclusion immunoperoxidase assays. The antigen source for both methods are tissue culture cells containing chlamydial inclusions. The tests can detect both genus- and species-specific antibodies and demonstrate a broad reactivity to a variety of chlamydial infections. However, such assays have had limited application as diagnostic tests.

Enzyme immunoassays using whole EBs or RBs as the antigen have been described for the detection of chlamydial antibody. These tests detect genus-specific antibodies, and measurements of IgG and IgM can be accomplished. They are comparable in sensitivity to the micro-IF test but may have limited specificity. The utility of the EIA as a serologic test for the diagnosis of chlamydial infections is unclear. However, such assays are attractive because they are rapid and automated and can easily test large numbers of specimens. The assay has been used successfully to detect chlamydial IgM in infants with pneumonia and can be readily applied to large epidemiologic studies.

The Frei test is an intradermal skin test that detects a delayed hypersensitivity response to chlamydial antigen. The test has been used for the diagnosis of LGV and uses antigens of generic specificity prepared from infected chick embryo yolk sac material. The assay is neither sensitive nor specific for LGV and has been replaced by CF and the micro-IF tests. At present, the Frei test has few diagnostic indications and is seldom used.

Antigenic Structure

Because of the difficulty of obtaining large quantities of organisms for conventional physicochemical fractionation, most of the information on the molecular architecture and chemistry of chlamydial antigens has been obtained indirectly from serologic studies. Three major groups of antigens have been identified: genus-specific antigens, species-specific antigens, and serotype-specific antigens.

The heat-stable genus-specific antigen common to all *Chlamydia* is LPS, with an acidic polysaccharide as the antigenic determinant. The immunodominant group, 2-keto-3-deoxyoctanoic acid, is similar to but not identical with the LPS of *Salmonella.* The antigen, which is present throughout the developmental cycle, can be detected by the complement-fixation test, SDS polyacrylamide gel electrophoresis, and by polyclonal or epitope specific monoclonal antibodies.

Several species-specific antigens have been detected on or near the envelope surface. These protein antigens are shared by all members of a chlamydial species. At least 18 species-specific antigens are present in *C. trachomatis* and 15 in *C. psittaci.*

Serotype-specific determinants are common only to certain isolates within a species. The *C. trachomatis* species responsible for human diseases is subdivided into two biologic variants (biovars): LGV and trachoma. Each biovar contains a number of serologically distinct types of serovars. There are three serovars of biovar LGV (LGV1, LGV2, and LGV3) and 12 serovars of the trachoma biovar. Serovars A, B, Ba, and C have been isolated primarily from the eyes of persons with trachoma in trachoma endemic areas. Isolation of these types from genital sites is rare. Serovars D through K have been isolated from the eyes of persons in areas where trachoma is nonendemic and most frequently from the genital tracts of adults. They also represent isolates obtained from the eyes and lungs of infants born to mothers with cervical infection. These serovars were originally identified by the micro-IF test. More recently, serovar specific monoclonal antibodies have been developed. There are conflicting reports concerning the chemical nature of the serovar antigens, but they are probably surface exposed, are part of the major outer membrane protein (MOMP), and seem to play a major role in the development of protective immunity.

Chlamydia trachomatis

Human infections caused by *C. trachomatis* primarily involve the eyes and genital tract. Trachoma is the leading cause of preventable blindness in the world today, afflicting an estimated 500 million people. Chlamydia is also the leading cause of sexually transmitted diseases in the United States and Europe. In men the disease begins as urethritis and can spread to the epididymis. In women, infection begins in the cervix; ascending spread to the endometrium and fallopian tubes can result in pelvic inflammatory disease and infertility. Infants born to a mother with cervicitis often develop inclusion conjunctivitis and pneumonitis. The slow growth of these organisms in their protected intracellular niche results in a clinically indolent disease course that allows many cases to go untreated. The medical and economic consequences are considerable.

Ocular Infections

Trachoma. Trachoma is a chronic keratoconjunctivitis caused by *C. trachomatis* serotypes A, B, or C. The name *trachoma,* derived from the Greek word *trakhus* (rough), refers to the pebbled appearance of the infected conjunctiva.

EPIDEMIOLOGY. Trachoma is a disease of poverty and squalor and continues to persist in the less developed areas of Africa, the Middle East, Afghanistan, India, Southeast Asia, and the Pacific Islands. In the United States, American Indians are the group most frequently infected. In endemic areas, children act as the main reservoir for transmission of the disease. In these areas clinically active trachoma is found in infants only 2 to 3 months of age, and in preschool children the prevalence of active disease may be as high as 70% to 100%. Most children, however, are free of active disease by the age of 10 to 15 years. Within a community where blinding trachoma is hyperendemic, individuals living in the most poverty-stricken households are the most severely affected. Extended families living together and the consequent overcrowding are among the most significant disease risk factors. Such conditions promote eye-to-eye transmission of infection by droplets, hands, and contaminated clothing. In certain communities, seasonal episodes of acute conjunctivitis appear to be associated with certain eye-seeking flies.

PATHOGENESIS. *C. trachomatis* replicates preferentially on mucosal surfaces within columnar or transitional epithelial cells. The organisms stimulate a brisk infiltration of polymorphonuclear cells, especially early in infection. Submucosal lymphocytic infiltration is also impressive, leading to lymphoid follicle formation and fibrotic changes.

Experimental studies in monkeys have provided a more precise understanding of the histopathology of *C. trachomatis* ocular infection and have emphasized the importance of repeated reinfection for the development of chronic trachoma. A single inoculation of monkeys with viable *C. trachomatis* produces an episode of inclusion conjunctivitis, whereas repeated inoculations are essential for the establishment and maintenance of chronic disease. In the monkey, lymphoid follicles with germinal centers develop only after repeated infection and are associated with areas of intracellular injury and an inflammatory response from plasma cells, polymorphonuclear leukocytes, lymphocytes, and mast cells. Macrophages are present in the germinal centers.

IMMUNITY. The immune response to chlamydial infection seems to confer partial protection against subsequent infection, yet the immune response appears responsible for much of the pathology and tissue destruction seen in patients with trachoma. Both local ocular and systemic humoral immune response to chlamydial eye infection have been well characterized, although the precise role of antibody-mediated immunity is unclear. Many patients with *C. trachomatis* infections show hyperimmunoglobulinemia with polyclonal activation and secretion of IgM, IgG, and IgA in tears and serum. Although neutralizing antibody plays a protective role in experimental infection, antibodies are not totally protective since disease persists as long as reinoculation continues. The antibody's role in vivo may be to limit the extent of chlamydial multiplication rather than to effect a cure.

Recurrent mucosal disease with *C. trachomatis*, as occurs with ocular trachoma, appears to be associated with enhanced suppressor T cell activation, enhanced humoral antibody response, and enhanced fibrosis. Worsening disease after recurrent challenge in endemic regions has also occurred after vaccination with whole killed elementary body vaccines. One current concept of the chronicity of diseases due to *C. trachomatis* biovars is that there is a disorder of immunoregulation in some individuals, leading to failure of eradication or to scarring sequelae.

CLINICAL MANIFESTATIONS. According to the internationally accepted MacCallan classification of trachoma, there are four major stages of disease. Stage I, or incipient, trachoma may be relatively asymptomatic, with little if any conjunctival exudate. Minimal keratitis is usually present. Stage II is established trachoma, with follicular and papillary hypertrophy. Trachomatous pannus accompanies corneal infiltration. Stage III includes cicatricial complications, with scarring of the conjunctiva; trichiasis, entropion, and further pannus develop. Stage IV represents healed trachoma without evidence of active inflammation. If no complications of trachoma develop during active infection, this stage may be asymptomatic.

Long periods of latent infection occur, and superinfection with other bacteria contributes to more advanced forms of the disease. Trachomatous persons living in hygienic conditions experience a mild course or clinical resolution of infection. Repeated exposure to infection, however, is associated with an increased incidence of marginal infiltration and neovascularization. This may have a late onset after inclusions are no longer detectable in conjunctival scrapings and represents host response to chlamydial antigen, which then contributes to the severe ocular damage resulting in impairment of vision. Recurrences often occur after apparent healing.

TREATMENT AND PREVENTION. Antibiotics may be used topically and systemically. Although systemically administered tetracyclines and sulfonamides cause regression of clinical trachomatous activity, infection persists, and subclinical disease may continue to occur. Nevertheless, treatment may limit complications and should be administered. Vaccines that are efficacious and safe are not available, and since the protection afforded by most vaccines is of a relatively low order and duration, vaccines are usually not used in programs to control trachoma. Current research on the development of a more effective vaccine is in progress. Basic, however, to the ultimate control of trachoma, are good standards of hygiene that accompany improvement in standards of living.

Inclusion Conjunctivitis

IN INFANTS. In the infant, inclusion conjunctivitis is a disease of the newborn eye that is derived from passage through the infected maternal birth canal. It is generally caused by *C. trachomatis* of serotypes D through K. Because of its close relationship to the agent causing ocular trachoma, the term *TRIC agent* historically encompassed both and referred to "Trachoma inclusion conjunctivitis" (Table 50–1). The incidence of chlamydial infection of the eyes of infants depends on the prevalence of cervical infection in the mothers.

The disease in the newborn usually becomes clinically apparent 5 to 12 days after birth. It is characterized by a sticky exudate and conjunctivitis and may be unilateral. Vulvovaginitis, ear infection, and mucopurulent rhinitis may accompany ocular disease. Many children with neonatal inclusion conjunctivitis are premature, and infection of the mother is associated with a variety of perinatal complications for both mother and child.

Inclusion conjunctivitis of the newborn eye has a high incidence of micropannus, conjunctival scars, and late recurrence, which can be prevented by treatment.

TABLE 50–1. HUMAN DISEASES CAUSED BY *CHLAMYDIA TRACHOMATIS*

Biovar	Serovar	Clinical Disease or Syndrome	Geographic Distribution
Trachoma	A, B, Ba, C	Trachoma	Primarily endemic in Asia and Africa
	D–K	Inclusion conjunctivitis Pneumonia in infants Nongonococcal urethritis Other genital infections	Worldwide
Lymphogranuloma venereum (LGV)	LGV1, LGV2, LGV3	LGV	Worldwide

Neonatal Pneumonia. *C. trachomatis* is a prevalent cause of pneumonitis in infants. The children characteristically become ill at 4 to 16 weeks of age, have prominent respiratory symptoms of wheezing and cough, and lack systemic findings of fever or toxicity. They may be eosinophilic and have elevated serum IgG and IgM, with a very pronounced titer to the infecting serovar. Chlamydial neonatal conjunctivitis often precedes the onset of the pneumonia.

IN ADULTS. Inclusion conjunctivitis in the adult is usually sporadic but may be epidemic following contamination of unchlorinated swimming pools. Inclusion conjunctivitis must be differentiated from epidemic keratoconjunctivitis, which is a viral disease.

Genital Tract Infections

C. trachomatis infections of the genital tract are of two types: (1) those caused by the oculogenital serotypes D through K and (2) LGV caused by serotypes L1, L2, and L3.

Chlamydial Urogenital Infections. Recovery of biovar trachoma and serologic evidence of infection with *Chlamydia* of serotypes D through K occurs in approximately 20% of males with nongonococcal urethritis and in half of their sexual contacts. It occurs in men with a history of other venereal diseases and promiscuity and frequently in the consorts of women with cervical chlamydial infection.

Infections in adult women include chronic cervicitis and urethritis. Postpartum fever in infected mothers is common. In addition, maternal cervical infection is associated with an increased rate of premature delivery and perinatal morbidity. Ectopic pregnancies, many apparently secondary to chlamydial salpingitis, have increased in incidence in the past decade.

REITER'S SYNDROME. Patients with Reiter's syndrome characteristically exhibit a triad of recurring symptoms, including conjunctivitis or iridocyclitis, polyarthritis, and genital inflammation. The disease usually occurs in young white males and apparently is initiated by an infection at a site distant from the affected joints. Recognized precipitating infections include genital and gastrointestinal infections. A number of organisms have been etiologically associated with Reiter's syndrome, but in the United States where genital infections are the most commonly recognized initiators of reactive arthritis, nongonococcal genital infections (NGGI) are regarded as the only important group. Approximately 50% to 65% of patients with Reiter's syndrome have acute *C. trachomatis* genital infection at the time of onset of their arthritis. A higher proportion of these patients also have increased humoral reactivity to chlamydial antigens as compared to patients with gonorrhea or uncomplicated *C. trachomatis* genital infections. Other infectious agents are probably also capable of initiating this genetically programmed reaction pattern.

Lymphogranuloma Venereum (LGV). Lymphogranuloma inguinale, climatic bubo, tropical bubo, and esthiomene are synonyms of this sexually transmissible disease that is worldwide in distribution. LGV should not be confused with granuloma inguinale, which is caused by *Calymmatobacterium granulomatis*. Humans are the sole natural hosts of this infection caused by the LGV biovar of *C. trachomatis* (Table 50–1).

CLINICAL INFECTION

Epidemiology. Currently in the United States, the incidence of LGV is less than 300 reported cases per year. The disease occurs more commonly in blacks and is more frequently recognized in males than in females. In the United States, male homosexuals are especially likely to experience LGV infection and constitute a major reservoir of disease. Patients with LGV commonly have other concomitant venereal diseases, especially syphilis; therefore all patients with LGV should be thoroughly examined for evidence of other sexually transmitted diseases.

Little is known about the infectivity of LGV or the duration of infection when untreated. The frequency of relapse and the observation that a man may infect a new sexual partner many years after his initial infection indicate that it may be a very long, indolent, and chronically active disease.

Pathogenesis. LGV serovars are more invasive than are other serovars of *C. trachomatis*. The preferred site of multiplication for biovar LGV is the regional lymph nodes, whereas that of biovar trachoma is squamocolumnar epithelial cells.

Autopsies of patients with chronic LGV infection reveal lesions of the lymph nodes composed of aggregations of large mononuclear cells forming abscesses surrounded by epithelial cells. A few giant cells of the Langhans type may be found, and numerous plasma cells may invade the granuloma formation. Occasionally in disease of long duration, the lesions are necrotic with few or no granulocytes but are surrounded by giant cells. Fibrosis with bands of granulation and connective tissue and thickened capsule is observed.

Hyperglobulinemia is common in early infection and may be accompanied by a positive reaction for rheumatoid factor, cryoglobulins, and elevated IgA.

Clinical Manifestations. The usual incubation period of LGV is 1 to 4 weeks. Early constitutional symptoms such as fever, headache, and myalgia are common. The primary lesion is painless, small, inconspicuous, and vesicular and often escapes notice. Characteristically the presenting complaint concerns the enlarged matted inguinal and femoral lymph nodes, which are moderately painful and firm and may become fluctuant. Aspiration of fluctuant nodes may be therapeutic and provide diagnostic material.

Women commonly experience proctitis, presumably because the lymphatic drainage from the vagina is perirectal. Symptoms may include diarrhea, purulent rectal drainage, tenesmus, anemia, abdominal pain, and the formation of infected sinuses. Rectal stricture and rectal perforation are recognized late sequelae to LGV proctitis.

The course of the disease is variable. It may cause progressive destruction of the vulva and urethra. Lymphatic obstruction in women can lead to elephantiasis of the vulva, called *esthiomene*. Vulvar carcinoma is reported as increased in women who have had LGV. An unknown percentage of persons have asymptomatic infections or heal without complications.

The Frei test is an intradermal skin test, previously used for the diagnosis of LGV. Antigens of generic specificity are responsible for a positive Frei test, which demonstrates delayed hypersensitivity to chlamydial infection with antigen (lygranum) prepared from infected chick embryo yolk sac material. At present, the test has few diagnostic indications.

Treatment. Treatment may include sulfadiazine or tetracycline; penicillin has proved effective when other drugs have failed. Meticulous follow-up for relapse or the development of complications is essential.

Chlamydia psittaci

Chlamydia psittaci is the etiologic agent of psittacosis, an infection of birds that is transmissible to humans. The human infection was first recognized in 1879 by a Swiss physician who described an unusual pneumonia that developed in patients after contact with tropical birds. The infection attracted worldwide interest in 1929 to 1930 when an epidemic of pneumonia involving more than 750 cases appeared in 12 different countries, including the United States. The etiology of the infection was established, and the main source of infection in the epidemic was traced to shipments of infected parrots from South America. Subsequently, psittacosis has been shown to cause endemic disease not only in parrots and parakeets but in a wide range of other birds, including ducks, chickens, and turkeys. Infection of flocks of turkeys in the United States in the 1950s caused considerable human disease. Because many birds other than the psittacine species can harbor the causative agent, the more general term *ornithosis* has been suggested as a more accurate designation for the infection.

Etiology

Four characteristics distinguish *C. psittaci* from *C. trachomatis:* (1) The intracellular microcolonies contain little glycogen and do not stain recognizably with iodine. (2) The inclusions are more diffuse and irregular in shape and do not indent the nucleus of the host cell as they do in *C. trachomatis.* These inclusions, the LCL (Levinthal-Cole-Lillie) bodies, stain with the Giemsa and Macchiavello stains. (3) The development of inclusions is not inhibited by sulfadiazine or cycloserine. (4) The DNA base composition differs from that of strains of *C. trachomatis,* and for those strains studied the degree of homology is low (Table 50–2).

Clinical Infection

Epidemiology. The general prevalence of psittacosis is unknown, but a study of sera referred for diagnostic studies on patients with respiratory disease found that 2.8% were positive for chlamydia. Since 1956 when there were 568 cases reported, the number of cases of psittacosis in the United States has declined steadily, with a total of 172 cases in 1984. The incidence of infection is highest during the autumn.

The respiratory tract is the main portal of entry, and infection usually is acquired by inhalation of organisms from infected birds and their droppings. Many patients, but not all, give a clear history of exposure to psittacine birds. Since pigeons, turkeys, chickens, and wild birds may also harbor the disease, a patient may not recognize a possible exposure. In addition, person-to-person transmission occurs. Exposure to patients who will die of psittacosis in the next 1 or 2 days is especially likely to propagate a very severe or fatal secondary infection.

SPONTANEOUS DISEASE IN ANIMALS. In parrots the naturally acquired disease is characterized by apathy, shivering, weakness, diarrhea, and respiratory symptoms. At necropsy, multiple areas of necrosis are found in the liver and spleen and occasionally in the lungs. Subclinical infections occur in birds of the psittacine group and even more frequently in non-psittacine birds. In Colorado, sheep have a polyarthritic type of infection from which *Chlamydia* organisms have been isolated. Many other mammals experience arthritis, abortion, encephalitis, and conjunctivitis when infected with these agents.

Pathogenesis. *C. psittaci* gains access to the body through the respiratory tract, rapidly enters the blood, and is transported to the reticuloendothelial cells of the liver and spleen. It replicates in these sites, producing focal areas of necrosis with a predominance of mononuclear cells. The organisms then invade the lung and other organs by hematogenous seeding. In the lung the inflammatory response is predominantly lymphocytic. Consolidation occurs, characterized by thickening of alveolar walls, infiltration of mononuclear cells, and a gelatinous alveolar exudate, which also contains mononuclear cells.

Clinical Manifestations. Psittacosis was originally believed to be severe, with a 20% mortality rate, but it is now recognized that the signs, symptoms, and severity vary greatly. Most cases are heralded by constitutional signs of fever, myalgia, and often a severe frontal headache. They precede the pulmonary signs of the disease, which include nonproductive cough, rales, and consolidation. Radiologic examination of the chest may suggest bronchopneumonia or mycoplasma pneumonia. If inadequately treated, patients may suffer repeated episodes of pneumonia.

The second most frequently involved organ system is the central nervous system. Symptoms are usually no more pronounced than a severe headache, but encephalitis, coma, convulsions, and death may occur. The cause usually is thought to be a toxic encephalitis rather than direct invasion of the central nervous system by *Chlamydia,* although typical inclusions have been identified in the meninges of involved cases.

Patients with psittacosis may also develop carditis, subacute bacterial endocarditis, hepatitis with or without formation of hepatic granulomata, erythema nodosum, and follicular keratoconjunctivitis. During the early phase of the illness, an acute false-positive test for syphilis may develop in one third of the patients.

TABLE 50–2. CHARACTERISTICS OF SPECIES OF THE GENUS *CHLAMYDIA*

Characteristic	*C. trachomatis*	*C. psittaci*	*C. pneumoniae*
Inclusion morphology	Oval, vacuolar	Variable, dense	Oval, dense
Elementary body morphology	Round	Round	Pear shaped
Folate biosynthesis	+	–	–
Glycogen in inclusions	+	–	–
Number of serovars[a]	15	NA	1

[a] Based on microimmunofluorescence determination.

Treatment. Results of treatment of psittacosis are imperfect. Tetracycline may be used with some success, and although a good response has been achieved by the use of erythromycin, pulmonary findings persist for weeks. Asymptomatic persistence of infection in patients with psittacosis has not been well studied, but one patient is reported to have shed the organism in his sputum for 12 years.

Prevention. Prophylactic treatment of psittacine birds with antibiotic-supplemented feed reduces the risk of disease in bird handlers. The recognition, however, that *C. psittaci* can infect many avian and mammalian species, sometimes causing subclinical communicable disease with occasional outbreaks involving human beings, widens the need for careful epidemiologic investigation of each case. Workers in poultry processing plants should have stringent environmental protection, as they are especially at risk of heavy exposure to this infection.

Chlamydia pneumoniae

In 1986, Grayston and colleagues reported a series of isolations of a new strain of *C. psittaci* from acute respiratory tract infections. The strain was called *TWAR*, an acronym reflecting the history of the first two isolates, *Taiwan*, and *acute respiratory*. In 1989 it was identified as a separate species and is now classified as *Chlamydia pneumoniae*. Unique properties that characterize this species are listed in Table 50–2. Isolates grow poorly in tissue culture systems, but direct fluorescent staining with monoclonal antibody makes possible the detection and direct passage of strains. Direct fluorescent antibody staining of clinical specimens has also been diagnostically successful.

C. pneumoniae can cause a relatively mild upper respiratory infection, but its most characteristic presentation to date is pneumonia in young adults. Although most cases are usually mild, some patients require hospitalization, especially if there is an associated underlying disease. Sore throat, low-grade fever, and persistent cough are common symptoms. Unlike most human disease caused by *C. psittaci*, pneumonia associated with *C. pneumoniae* is transmitted from human to human with no intervening avian or mammalian host. The disease has been recognized in situations where young adults are grouped, such as military camps and college campuses. Chronically malnourished children may be severely affected.

Treatment. Isolates of *C. pneumoniae* are sensitive to erythromycin and tetracycline. Clinical results of therapy with these agents have not been evaluated fully.

FURTHER READING

Books and Reviews

Barnes RC: Laboratory diagnosis of human chlamydial infections. Clin Microbiol Rev 2:119, 1989

Barron AL: Microbiology of Chlamydia. Boca Raton, Fla, CRC Press, 1988

Bowie WR, Caldwell HD, Jones RB, et al (eds): Human Chlamydial Infections. Cambridge, Cambridge University Press, 1990

Holmes KK, Mardh PA, Sparling PF, et al: Sexually Transmitted Diseases. New York, McGraw-Hill, 1990

Kunimoto D, Brunham RC: Human immune response and *Chlamydia trachomatis* infection. Rev Infect Dis 7:665, 1985

Moulder JW: The rickettsias and chlamydiae. In Krieg N, Holt JG (eds): Bergey's Manual of Systematic Bacteriology, vol 1. Baltimore, Williams & Wilkins, 1984, p 729

Moulder JW: Comparative biology of intracellular parasitism. Microbiol Rev 49:298, 1985

Oriel JD, Ridgway G, Schacter J, et al (eds): Human Chlamydial Infections. Cambridge, Cambridge University Press, 1986

Reeve P (ed): Chlamydial Infections. New York, Springer-Verlag, 1987

Schachter J: *Chlamydiaeceae:* The *Chlamydiae.* In Lennette EH, Halonen P, Murphy FA (eds): Laboratory Diagnosis of Infectious Diseases: Principles and Practice. vol II, Viral, Rickettsial, and Chlamydial Diseases. New York, Springer-Verlag, 1988, p 847

Smith TF: Chlamydia. In Schmidt NJ, Emmons RW (eds): Diagnostic Procedures for Viral, Rickettsial, and Chlamydial Infections, ed 6. New York, American Public Health Association, 1989, p 1165

Storz J: *Chlamydia* and *Chlamydia*-Induced Diseases. Springfield, Ill, Charles C Thomas, 1971

Selected Papers

Brunham RC, Kuo CC, Cles L, et al: Correlation of host immune response with quantitative recovery of *Chlamydia trachomatis* from the human endocervix. Infect Immun 39:1491, 1983

Caldwell HD, Schachter J: Antigenic analysis of the major outer membrane protein of *Chlamydia* sp. Infect Immun 35:1024, 1982

Campbell LA, Kuo C-C, Wang S-P, Grayston JT: Serological response to *Chlamydia pneumoniae* infection. J Clin Microbiol 28:1261, 1990

Centers for Disease Control: *Chlamydia trachomatis* infections: Policy guidelines for prevention and control. MMWR 34:67, 1985

Centers for Disease Control: *Chlamydia trachomatis* infections. MMWR 34(suppl):535, 1985

Cooper MD, Rapp J, Jeffery-Wiseman C, et al: *Chlamydia trachomatis* infection of human fallopian tube organ cultures. J Gen Microbiol 136:1109, 1990

Eissenberg LG, Wyrick PB, David CH, et al: *Chlamydia psittaci* elementary body envelopes: Ingestion and inhibition of phagolysosome fusion. Infect Immun 40:741, 1983

Grayston JT, Kuo C-C, Campbell LA, Wang S-P: *Chlamydia pneumoniae* sp. nov. for *Chlamydia* sp. strain TWAR. Int J Syst Bacteriol 39:88, 1989

Grayston JT, Kuo C-C, Wang SP, Altman J: A new *Chlamydia psittaci* strain, TWAR, isolated in acute respiratory tract infections. N Engl J Med 315:161, 1986

Grayston JT, Wang SP: New knowledge of chlamydiae and the diseases they cause. J Infect Dis 132:87, 1975

Kleemola M, Saikku P, Visakorpi R, et al: Epidemics of pneumonia caused by TWAR, a new *Chlamydia* organism, in military trainees in Finland. J Infect Dis 157:230, 1988

Kuo C-C, Grayston JT: In vitro drug susceptibility of *Chlamydia* sp strain TWAR. Antimicrob Agents Chemother 32:257, 1988

Ladany S, Black CM, Farshy CE, et al: Enzyme immunoassay to determine exposure to *Chlamydia pneumoniae* (strain TWAR). J Clin Microbiol 27:2778, 1989

Martin DH, Koutsky L, Eschenbach DA, et al: Prematurity and perinatal mortality in pregnancies complicated by maternal *Chlamydia trachomatis* infection. JAMA 247:1585, 1982

Morrison RP, Lyng K, Caldwell HD: Chlamydial disease pathogenesis. J Exp Med 169:663, 1989

Newhall WJ, Batteiger B, Jones RB: Analysis of the human serological response to proteins of *Chlamydia trachomatis.* Infect Immun 39:1181, 1982

Patton DL, Taylor HR: The histopathology of experimental trachoma: Ultrastructural changes in the conjunctival epithelium. J Infect Dis 153:870, 1986

Saikku P, Ruutu P, Leinonen M, et al: Acute lower-respiratory tract infection associated with chlamydial TWAR antibody in Filipino children. J Infect Dis 158:1095, 1988

Williams DM, McGee DM, Bonewald LF, et al: A role in vivo for tumor necrosis factor alpha in host defense against *Chlamydia trachomatis.* Infect Immun 58:1572, 1990

Yong EC, Klebanoff SJ, Kuo C-C: Toxic effect of human polymorphonuclear leukocytes on *Chlamydia trachomatis.* Infect Immun 37:422, 1982

CHAPTER 51

Mycoplasma

The Mycoplasmas

Mycoplasmas are the smallest procaryotes capable of self-replication. The unique property that characterizes these simple forms and separates them from the true bacteria is the absence of a cell wall. Mycoplasmas are members of the class Mollicutes (*mollis,* soft; *kutis,* skin), a taxon that contains small procaryotic organisms bounded by a single trilaminar cell membrane. The term *mycoplasmas* is used rather loosely to denote any species in this class.

Mycoplasmas are ubiquitous organisms occurring as saprophytes or as parasites in many animal and plant species. A number of them are pathogenic and play a proven primary role in certain infectious diseases. The first recorded isolation of a mycoplasma was from cattle with contagious bovine pneumonia, thus its name, the *pleuropneumonia organism* (PPO). Similar organisms subsequently isolated from a variety of animals, both from the carrier and the disease state, were referred to as pleuropneumonia-like organisms (PPLO) because of their similarity to the original isolate. Although known for a number of years to be a part of the normal flora of the human respiratory and genitourinary tracts, the first clearly proven association of a mycoplasma with human disease was in 1962 with the identification of a mycoplasma as a frequent causative agent of the clinical syndrome known as primary atypical pneumonia. This group of pneumonias differed from the typical bacterial lobar pneumonias in their radiographic appearance and in their low mortality. Three important observations helped to define the illness clinically: (1) the finding that cold agglutinins, nonspecific antibodies that agglutinate human red blood cells in the cold, appear in the convalescent serum of infected patients, (2) the availability of penicillin, which had no effect on this particular infection but served to distinguish it from the typical pneumonias; and (3) the frequency of the disease in the military personnel during World War II. The causative organism, initially isolated in hamsters and referred to as the *Eaton agent,* was subsequently isolated in embryonated eggs and on artificial media. Definitive proof was provided that it was a mycoplasma, and it was given the name *Mycoplasma pneumoniae.*

TAXONOMY. Three families of the class Mollicutes are currently recognized, based on nutritional and morphologic criteria and on differences in genome size. The establishment of a fourth family for the presently unassigned anaerobic mycoplasmas has been proposed but has not been officially approved (Table 51–1).

Morphology. Mycoplasmas are very small pleomorphic cells bounded by a trilaminar membrane 8 to 10 nm thick. They range in size from 0.2 to 0.8 μm in diameter and are capable of passing through a membrane filter of 450 nm pore size. Because they lack a rigid cell wall, they assume a number of morphologic forms, ranging from spherical or pear-shaped structures to filamentous cells with branching or with terminal structures. Replication is basically by binary fission, but genome replication is not necessarily synchronized with cell division and accounts for the budding forms and chains of beads often observed (Fig. 51–1). Whereas many mycoplasma species can be distinguished by their characteristic morphology, cell shape also depends on the nutritional quality and osmotic pressure of the growth medium and on the growth phase of the culture. Phase-contrast and darkfield microscopy of young logarithmic-phase cultures are recommended for the microscopic examination of mycoplasmas because they produce minimal distortions of the plastic cells. The real cell shape can be observed best by examination of cells growing in a liquid medium but attached to a glass surface. Gram-stained preparations are of limited usefulness except in dif-

TABLE 51–1. MAJOR CHARACTERISTICS OF MEMBERS OF THE CLASS MOLLICUTES

Classification	Genome Size (MDa)	Sterol Requirement	Special Features	Habitat
Mycoplasmataceae				
Mycoplasma	≈500	+		Humans and animals
Ureaplasma	≈500	+	Urease activity	Humans and animals
Acholeplasmataceae				
Acholeplasma	≈1,000	−		Humans, animals, and plant surfaces
Spiroplasmataceae				
Spiroplasma	≈1,000	+	Helical and motile filaments	Arthropods and plants
Anaeroplasmataceae				
Anaeroplasma	≈1,000(?)	Some + Some −	Strict anaerobes	Rumens of cattle and sheep

From Razin: Microbiol Rev 49:419, 1985.

ferentiating mycoplasmas from bacteria in contaminated broth cultures. In many *Mycoplasma* species, electron microscopy reveals a fuzzy layer or a nap covering all or part of the cell surface. Internally, the mycoplasma cell contains ribosomes interspersed with fine strands of the nucleoid, but there is no evidence of mesosomes or other intracellular membranous structures.

Some mycoplasmas, including *M. pneumoniae*, exhibit a gliding motility on liquid-covered surfaces. In these species, specialized tip structures have been differentiated to serve both as an attachment site and as the leading edge of the cell during movement. In the helical spiroplasmas there is a rapid rotary motion, and the flectional movements resemble those of spirochetes. The isolation of an actinlike protein from this group of organisms suggests the presence in mycoplasmas of contractile proteins and a primitive cytoskeleton.

Physiology. The *Mycoplasma* genome consists of a circular double-stranded DNA molecule, which in *Mycoplasma* and *Ureaplasma* is 500 MDa, and is the smallest for any known self-replicating cell. This is consistent with the organism's limited biosynthetic capabilities and requirement for highly complex culture media. The *Mycoplasma* genome also differs from that of other procaryotes in its low guanine-plus-cytosine

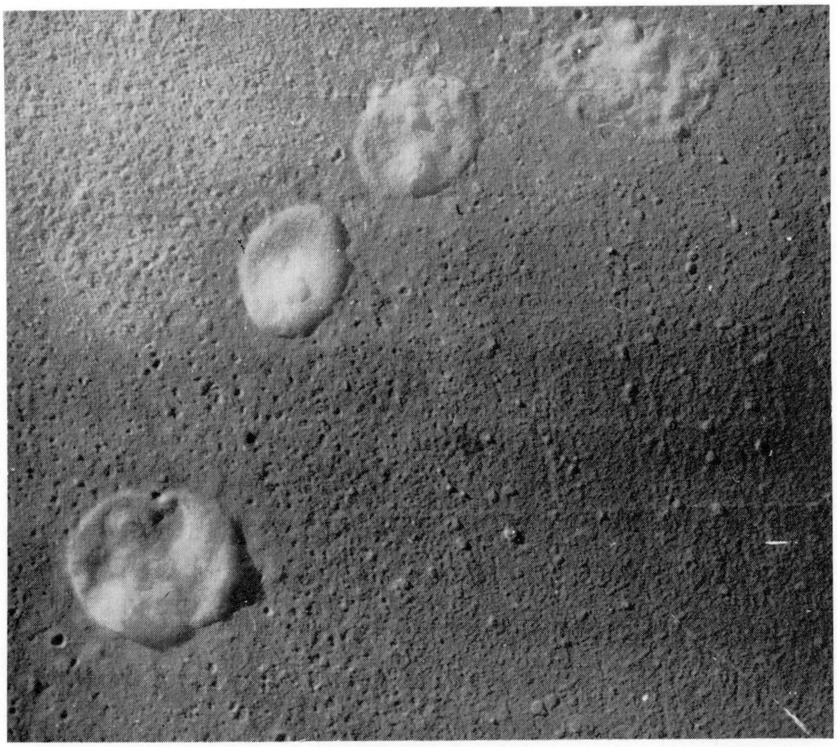

Fig. 51–1. Electron micrograph of *Mycoplasma*. Note the obvious plasticity of the organism and the lack of a definite cell wall. × 20,000. *(From Morton et al: J Bacteriol 68:697, 1954.)*

content, imposing further restrictions on the amount of genetic information available to mycoplasma cells. Genetic evidence indicates that mycoplasmas arose by degenerate evolution from a branch of the eubacterial phylogenetic tree containing gram-positive eubacteria with DNA of low guanine-plus-cytosine content. Ribosomal transfer-RNA analysis suggests a relationship to bacteria of the genus *Clostridium.* During the major genome reductions accompanying mycoplasma evolution, the heat-response genes have been conserved, suggesting that the system plays an essential role in cell physiology.

CULTURAL CHARACTERISTICS. Most mycoplasmas have a unique requirement among procaryotes for cholesterol and related sterols for membrane synthesis. They also lack the enzymatic pathways for the synthesis of purines and pyrimidines. Complex culture media such as beef-heart infusion broth supplemented with horse serum, yeast extract, and nucleic acids are thus required for in vitro culture. The purine and pyrimidine requirement for growth provides the basis of a useful technique for detecting *Mycoplasma*-infected tissue culture systems since purines and pyrimidines are not taken up by tissue culture cells.

When grown on solid media, mycoplasmas slowly form a dome-shaped colony on the surface of the agar. The central part of the colony grows down into the agar, producing a more dense central core. When viewed from above, the colony resembles a fried egg in appearance. The colonies are extremely small and often require a dissecting microscope for visualization (Fig. 51–2). Although the *Mycoplasma* culture follows a bacterial growth curve pattern, the organism's doubling time of 1 to 6 hours means that up to 3 weeks may be required before colony formation is visible. Because bacterial L-phase variants share with mycoplasmas the fried-egg colony shape, it is necessary to transfer the isolated colony to a penicillin-free medium to rule out the possibility that the fried-egg-shaped colonies are those of L-phase variants induced by the penicillin included in most mycoplasma media.

METABOLISM. Most species are facultative anaerobes, although growth is better in an aerobic environment. Mycoplasmas can be divided into two broad physiologic groups: the fermentative and the nonfermentative. In the fermentative organisms, adenosine triphosphate (ATP) is derived from sugars via glycolysis, whereas in nonfermentative mycoplasmas the arginine dihydrolase pathway is probably the major source for ATP. ATPase is associated with the cell membrane of all mycoplasmas. Most of the enzymes involved in membrane lipid biosynthesis in mycoplasmas are also membrane bound.

Determinants of Pathogenicity. Since most mycoplasmas produce surface infections and rarely invade the bloodstream and tissues, the ability to adhere to cell surfaces is important for colonization. Intimate contact of the mycoplasmas with their host cells is required to furnish nutrients and specific growth factors, especially nucleic acid precursors, which mycoplasmas are unable to synthesize. Mycoplasmas attach to the mucous membranes of the respiratory, gastrointestinal, and genitourinary tracts. Specific receptor proteins have been identified, and a specific receptor tip on some mycoplasmas has been demonstrated.

The mechanisms by which mycoplasmas cause disease in humans and animals are ill defined. A number of extracellular products that contribute to their disease-inciting ability are produced, but except for the neurotoxin produced by *Mycoplasma neurolyticum,* attempts to detect toxins produced by the other species have been unsuccessful. Although neurotoxic symptoms similar to those caused by the *M. neurolyticum* exotoxin are also observed after intravenous inoculation with *Mycoplasma gallisepticum,* in the latter case the neurotoxic effects are associated with viable mycoplasma cells and not with a

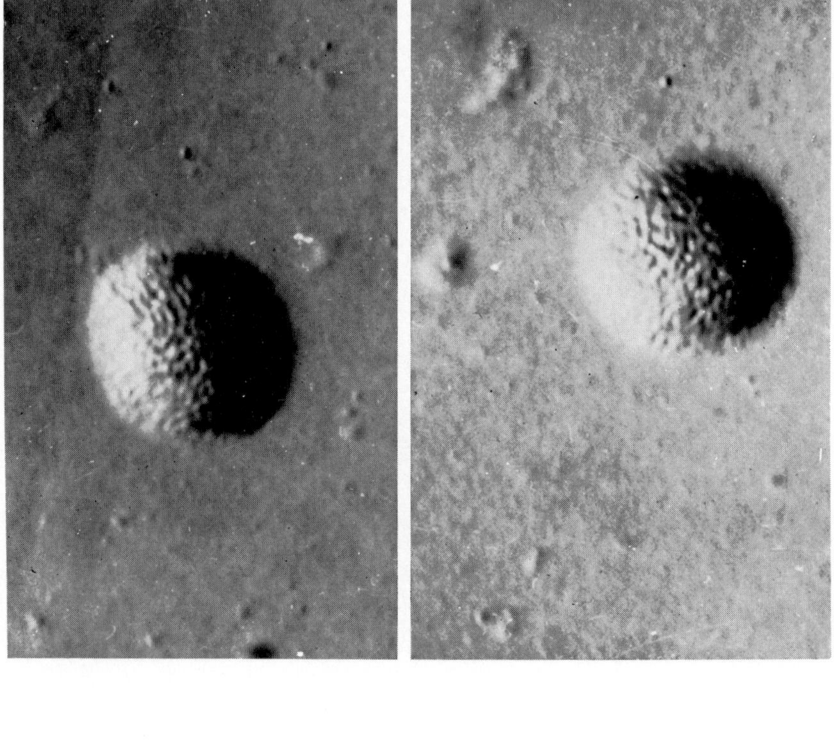

Fig. 51–2. Colonies of *M. pneumoniae.* Note the granular appearance. The organisms grow down into the agar beneath the surface colony. *M. pneumoniae,* on initial isolation, frequently does not have surrounding surface growth. *(From Chanock et al: Proc Natl Acad Sci USA 48:41, 1962.)*

soluble exotoxin. *Mycoplasma mycoides* produces and excretes a galactan that aggregates around the exterior cell surface and is shed into the medium. The galactan produces a pathologic response in animals in the absence of organisms and is thought to play a pathogenic role analogous to the endotoxin of gram-negative bacteria, although biochemically different. Lipoglycans from a number of *Mycoplasma* and *Acholeplasma* species also have endotoxin-like activity, but evidence that any of these lipopolysaccharide (LPS)-like molecules mediates the pathogenicity of any mycoplasmal disease is inconclusive.

A local accumulation of certain mycoplasmal metabolites, including enzymes, hydrogen peroxide, superoxide radicals, and ammonia, may participate either individually or in concert with other factors to produce tissue damage. The cytopathic effects are reflected in changes in the metabolism of the infected tissues. Among the most prominent biochemical changes are a depletion of arginine and alterations in host nucleic acid metabolism. Further discussion of determinants of pathogenicity in *M. pneumoniae* is found below.

Mycoplasma pneumoniae

Of the 10 accepted human species of the genus *Mycoplasma*, only *M. pneumoniae* has been clearly proven to produce disease (Table 51–2). It is not a part of the normal flora as are most of the other human mycoplasmal isolates but accounts for as much as 10% of the total x-ray-proven pneumonia.

Morphology and Physiology. *M. pneumoniae* varies in shape from small coccoidal to short, branched filamentous cells. The most distinctive feature of its morphology is a bulbous enlargement with a differentiated tip structure that can be seen in young filamentous cells grown in broth cultures. *M. pneumoniae* can attach to glass surfaces, red cells, and respiratory epithelial cells by this differentiated pole. When so attached, the organisms show a gliding movement.

The organism is more fastidious and grows more slowly than most other mycoplasmas, with colonies appearing 5 to 10 days after inoculation. The colony is more compact than that of most *Mycoplasma* colonies, is 50 to 100 μm in diameter, and has a minimal skirt, giving more of a mulberry-colony appearance. With repeated transfer and adaptation to artificial media, growth is more rapid, and colonies have the typical fried-egg appearance. The optimal temperature for growth is 36C to 38C. *M. pneumoniae* adsorbs to and agglutinates erythrocytes from various species, a property not shared by other human respiratory mycoplasmas. This property thus makes it possible to rapidly identify *M. pneumoniae* colonies on agar medium by microscopic examination after flooding the plate with an erythrocyte suspension, decanting, and rinsing.

Determinants of Pathogenicity. Both organism-related and host-related factors are involved in the pathogenesis of *M. pneumoniae* and its subsequent complications. Essential to the initiation of disease is the ability of the organism to attach to and establish an intimate association with respiratory mucosal cells while evading phagocytosis and modulating the immune response. *M. pneumoniae* is a surface parasite colonizing the epithelial linings of the respiratory tract. It has a predilection for the lower respiratory tract, with invasion of the bloodstream a rare event. It is unclear how *M. pneumoniae* penetrates the mucous gel coating of the respiratory epithelium, but it is believed that the gliding motility of the organism facilitates penetration, and its minute size and plastic nature enable it to adapt its shape to conform to the contours of the host cell surface. Filamentous forms with their differentiated terminal attachment organelle permit the organisms to locate in crypts and folds of the host cell membrane and in between microvilli and cilia where they are protected from phagocytosis. Direct contact between the mycoplasmal membrane and that of the host cell creates a condition that theoretically could

TABLE 51–2. DIFFERENTIAL PROPERTIES OF RESPIRATORY AND UROGENITAL MYCOPLASMAS

Species	Arginine or Sugar Utilization	Hemadsorption of Guinea Pig Red Blood Cells	Aerobic Reduction of Tetrazolium	Urease Activity
Respiratory Organisms				
Mycoplasma pneumoniae	Glucose	+	+	–
M. salivarium	Arginine	–	–	–
M. orale	Arginine	–	–	–
M. buccale	Arginine	–	–	–
M. faucium	Arginine	–	–	–
M. lipophilum	Arginine	–		–
M. primatum	Arginine	–	–	–
Acholeplasma laidlawii	Glucose	–	+	–
Urogenital Organisms				
Ureaplasma urealyticum	–	–[a]	–	+
Mycoplasma hominis	Arginine	–	–	–
M. fermentans	Arginine and glucose	–	–	–
M. genitalium	Glucose	+		–

[a] All strains negative except serotype 3, which does hemadsorb.

lead to the fusion of the two membranes. Although data to support the occurrence of fusion are lacking, the transfer of host membrane antigens to the membrane of attached mycoplasmas has been demonstrated. An event of this type could trigger immunologic responses with serious consequences to the host.

M. pneumoniae adheres to a variety of surfaces, including erythrocytes, HeLa cells, spermatozoa, tracheal epithelial cells and organ cultures, and inert substances such as glass. The attachment of the organism to erythrocytes and epithelial cells is mediated by the sialic acid moieties of membrane glycoconjugate receptors that are destroyed by pretreatment with neuraminidase. The mycoplasmas appear to attach to the host cells by a combination of hydrophobic and ionic bonds.

A high-molecular-weight protein, designated *protein P1*, has been identified as a major *M. pneumoniae* adhesin. Cytoadsorption of the organism is inhibited if the 170 kDa protein P1 is enzymatically cleaved by trypsin or is coated with monospecific anti-P1 antibody. The positioning of P1 in the mycoplasmal membrane appears to be precisely regulated. In avirulent hemadsorption-negative mycoplasmas, it is sparsely distributed over the entire surface, whereas in virulent hemadsorption-positive organisms, P1 molecules are greatly enriched in the specialized tip structure. Patients with mycoplasmal pneumonia consistently develop antibodies to P1, an observation in support of the idea of using purified P1 protein as a vaccinogen.

Antigenic Structure. The surface antigens presented to the infected host are components of the cell membrane and consist of glycolipids and proteins. The glycolipid antigens of *M. pneumoniae* are major membrane antigens found in the lipid fraction. The purified glycolipids act as antigens in the complement-fixation test and other in vitro antigen-antibody reactions but are poor immunogens in vivo unless attached to proteins. On the surface membrane, galactosyl and glycosyl diglycerides appear to be the antigens that stimulate humoral immunity. Serologically active lipids also occur in *M. pneumoniae* and a number of other species of *Mycoplasma*. The organism cross-reacts with the urogenital species, *Mycoplasma genitalium*, but is antigenically distinct from other species of human origin as determined by agglutination, complement fixation, and other serologic procedures. *M. pneumoniae* strains show marked genetic homogeneity by restriction endonuclease, DNA hybridization, and electrophoretic patterns of cell proteins.

During the course of infection a number of protein antigens are recognized. Among them are two major surface antigens, one of which is the P1 protein that mediates attachment. Antibody to these surface proteins is found consistently in convalescent human sera and in respiratory secretions by radioimmunoprecipitation, gel electrophoresis, and Western blot analysis. A large number of intracellular protein antigens are also present in patients with *M. pneumoniae* and are revealed to the host immune system through phagocytosis and degradation of the organisms. These antigens play an important role in stimulating T lymphocyte reactions that may generate lymphocytic cellular infiltrates, as in the delayed hypersensitivity reaction.

The cold agglutinins that are induced in patients with *M. pneumoniae* infection are directed against the I antigen determinant of erythrocytes, which is also present on the surface of other blood cells. The receptors for *M. pneumoniae* on human erythrocyte membranes are sialylated oligosaccharides, giving support to the concept that the stimulus for the production of cold agglutinins in *M. pneumoniae* infection is the interaction of *M. pneumoniae* with the host antigen I, thus rendering the I antigen antigenic. Shared idiotypic antigens have been demonstrated on cold agglutinins from patients with *M. pneumoniae* infection and probably provide the basis for the autoimmune responses seen in association with infection by this organism. These responses include the development of antibody to lung, smooth muscle, brain, and human lymphocytes.

Clinical Infection

Epidemiology. *M. pneumoniae* is worldwide in its distribution. The infection is endemic in the population throughout the year, with epidemics occurring at 4- to 6-year intervals. Spread is usually quite slow, however, and true epidemics are rare except in confined populations of persons such as in schools, families, and army barracks. Spread appears to occur first among school-aged children who then introduce the infection into the family unit. Spread is slow and appears to require close contact with an ill person. Although transmission by aerosol droplets may occur and is responsible for some point-source outbreaks, it is not the major method of spread. Infection with *M. pneumoniae* is common in children less than 5 years of age, but the illness is usually mild, with coryza and wheezing but without fever and pneumonia. Infection rates are greatest in school-aged children and young adults, and *M. pneumoniae* pneumonia is most commonly encountered in the 5- to 20-year-old group. Thus after infection, illness is more likely to occur and to be more severe with increasing age, leading to the speculation that part of the clinical illness may result from the host's reaction to the pathogen.

Immunity. In a primary *M. pneumoniae* infection, resistance at mucosal surfaces provides the first line of defense and consists of such nonspecific factors as complement and phagocytic cells. Early in infection before a specific immune response has been generated, complement is activated by the alternative pathway or by cross-reacting IgM antibody that is present in "normal" sera, and it appears to play an important role in controlling infection. Later, as the infection proceeds, complement acts to amplify the protective effects of IgG. Subsequent to mycoplasmal infection an antibody response is induced that follows the usual course of IgM, IgG, and IgA. In respiratory secretions IgA predominates, followed by IgG, with IgM present in lesser amounts as compared with sera. This local accumulation of antibody is more important in recovery from mycoplasmal infection. Serum antibody, however, can be a useful measure of immunity. A variety of techniques have demonstrated that immunity to mycoplasmal infection is associated with the presence and magnitude of serum antibody to the organism.

The development of a delayed hypersensitivity reaction to *M. pneumoniae* appears to correlate with the severity of disease and to explain the observed differences between infection in young children and adults. Specific antigens to which the host may be responding have not been identified but possibly are polysaccharide-protein complexes. Current concepts also suggest that the complications of mycoplasmal disease have an immunologic basis. The development of antibodies for normal tissues provides a basis for autoimmune reactions and an explanation for disease at distant sites.

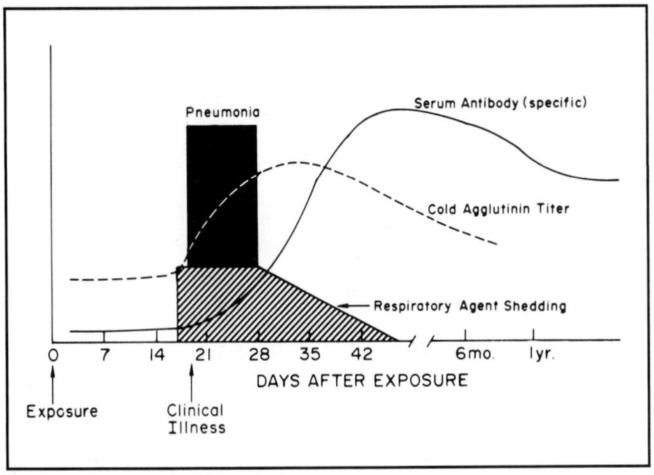

Fig. 51–3. The course of *Mycoplasma pneumoniae* infection.

Circulating antigen-antibody complexes during acute illness have been described.

Clinical Manifestations. After infection with *M. pneumoniae,* only about one third of the infected persons develop pneumonia. The most common clinical syndrome is tracheobronchitis, which accounts for approximately 70% to 80% of mycoplasmal infections. Pharyngitis alone may occur and cannot be distinguished from pharyngitis caused by viruses and group A streptococci. Pneumonia caused by *M. pneumoniae* is generally mild. Following an incubation period of 2 to 3 weeks after exposure, there is a gradual onset of fever, with malaise, headache, and a persistent nonproductive hacking cough. Physical examination in the early stages of the illness frequently does not reveal many chest findings, in contrast to x-ray examination, which usually reveals a unilateral bronchopneumonia of a lower lobe but sometimes shows bilateral feathery infiltrates. As the disease progresses, loud rales become prominent, with little physical findings of consolidation. The peripheral white blood count during the early stages of the illness is usually within normal limits, although as the disease progresses, it may become elevated (Fig. 51–3). Microscopic examination and culture of the sputum on routine culture media yield only normal flora. Without treatment the disease may last up to 3 weeks but is usually of much shorter duration. The cold agglutinins commonly found in convalescent sera occasionally are associated with hemolytic anemia or cold acrocyanosis. A fatal outcome is extremely rare.

Rarely, other organ systems have been implicated, resulting in otitis media and bullous myringitis, meningoencephalitis, or myocarditis. Pulmonary infections occasionally are complicated by a bullous eruption of the skin and mucous membranes, the Stevens-Johnson syndrome.

The illness must be differentiated from a large number of other atypical pneumonias caused by a variety of different agents: viral infection (e.g., influenza, adenovirus, respiratory syncytial virus), psittacosis, Q fever, and legionellosis.

Laboratory Diagnosis. In the early stages of infection the diagnosis must be made on clinical grounds since no rapid specific tests have gained widespread acceptance. Immunofluorescence microscopy using monoclonal antibodies has been used experimentally to localize mycoplasma in infected animals but has not been applied to clinical situations. However, antigen detection by nucleic acid hybridization has been introduced recently as a diagnostic tool and promises to be useful in rapid diagnosis of *Mycoplasma* infection. In the evaluation of a commercial probe test based on hybridization of a ^{125}I-labeled DNA probe with the ribosomal RNA of *M. pneumoniae,* the test proved both sensitive and specific for lower respiratory tract *M. pneumoniae* infection.

CULTURE. Isolation of *M. pneumoniae* is accomplished best from sputum, but throat swabs may also be cultured if they are placed in transport media containing protein to protect them from drying. A selective diphasic culture medium containing broth over agar is preferable to solid agar, but ideally both media should be inoculated. The addition of penicillin and thallium to the culture medium inhibits overgrowth by the routine bacterial species. When positive, most specimens will show typical small colonies on the agar medium and spherules (fluid medium colonies) and acid production in broth by days 10 to 12. For confirmation of the identity of the colonies as *M. pneumoniae,* the original agar isolation plate is overlaid with a thin layer of agar containing guinea pig erythrocytes. After overnight incubation, a small zone of hemolysis develops around the colonies of *M. pneumoniae.* Definitive identification is accomplished subsequently by demonstration of the inhibition of colonial growth with specific antiserum.

SEROLOGIC TESTS. During the acute phase of the illness, no diagnostic serologic tests are available. A frequently used nonspecific serologic test that has been helpful in establishing diagnosis is the cold agglutination reaction. Cold agglutinins are measured in both the acute and convalescent phases of the illness to demonstrate a rising titer. This test is easily performed by mixing dilutions of the patient's serum with a standard concentration of washed human type O cells and incubating the mixture overnight at 4C. The test is based on the development of hemagglutination, which can be reversed by placing the tubes at 37C.

The complement-fixation test with either whole organisms or lipid antigen is effective for the detection of infections in mycoplasmal pneumonia patients. The lipid antigen used in this test, however, is a mixture of relatively simple glycolipids that appear to be widely distributed in nature in a variety of substances, including normal mammalian tissue, bacteria, and spinach. Use of this lipid antigen results in the generation of false-positive reactions and is the basis for the finding that persons with proven bacterial meningitis often have significant increases in antibody to *M. pneumoniae* antigens. A more sensitive test based on the ability of antibodies from patients' convalescent sera to inhibit the growth of mycoplasma in vitro has been devised. In this test, growth inhibition is a function of the inhibition of glucose fermentation or tetrazolium reduction. Complement-mediated mycoplasmacidal and radioimmunoprecipitation tests are also more sensitive techniques, but like the growth inhibition test, they require personnel experienced in mycoplasmal cultivation technique. If a more purified and commercially available antigen can be obtained, the enzyme-linked immunosorbent assay (ELISA) would be especially useful since it can distinguish between IgM and IgG antibodies.

Treatment. Treatment of *M. pneumoniae* pneumonia is usually instituted on the basis of a clinical impression. Penicillin has no effect on the natural history of the disease. The tetracyclines and erythromycin reduce the clinical course of the illness in terms of fever, number of hospital days, and resolution based on x-ray films. Interestingly, however, the drugs do not alter the shedding of the agent from the respiratory tree. Erythromycin sometimes is preferred in older patients because of its effectiveness against both *Mycoplasma* and *Legionella pneumophila.* In the pediatric age group, pneumonia is seen more commonly in upper respiratory tract syndromes, and is usually treated symptomatically.

Prevention. There is no commonly accepted method available for preventing *M. pneumoniae* infection other than avoiding close contact with acutely ill patients. One approach to prophylaxis is the use of antibiotics in persons at high risk of infection. Use of prophylactic tetracycline in members of families with an index case of infection has been reported to cause a significant reduction in clinical illness, although the incidence of infection is only minimally reduced.

Formalin-inactivated vaccines and living attenuated vaccines have been tested in humans, but the results have been disappointing. Cell-free component vaccines (tip protein, polysaccharides, and glycolipids) are presently under investigation for use as vaccinogens.

Ureaplasma urealyticum and *Mycoplasma hominis*

U. urealyticum and *M. hominis* are the mycoplasmas most frequently isolated from the urogenital tract (Table 51–2). *Mycoplasma hominis,* a large colony-forming *Mycoplasma* 200 to 300 μm in diameter with a characteristic fried-egg appearance, was the first of these wall-less organisms to be isolated from a human subject. *U. urealyticum* organisms originally were referred to as T-strain mycoplasmas (*T* for tiny) because of the small colonies (15 to 60 μm) they produce. They also differ from all other mycoplasmas because of their unique ability to metabolize urea, with the production of ammonia. A more recent isolate, *Mycoplasma genitalium,* has been isolated from urethral specimens of patients with nongonococcal urethritis, but technical problems have impeded large-scale surveys to determine its prevalence. *M. genitalium* is of especial interest because it shares extensive serologic cross-reactivity with *M. pneumoniae* and possesses an attachment mechanism and surface protein similar to that of *M. pneumoniae.*

M. hominis and ureaplasmas have been associated with a large variety of clinical conditions. At least 60% of apparently healthy sexually experienced women carry *U. urealyticum,* and about 20% carry *M. hominis* in their vagina. Both organisms appear to be effective opportunists in internal sites. *M. hominis* has been implicated in postpartum fever, postabortal fever, pelvic inflammatory disease, and pyelonephritis. *U. urealyticum* and *M. genitalium* probably contribute to a small percentage of nongonococcal urethritis. Ureaplasmas may also play a role in perinatal mortality. Although mycoplasmas have been demonstrated as the unequivocal etiologic agents of arthritis in animals, there is not as yet convincing evidence that they are the etiologic agent in human illness.

FURTHER READING

Books and Reviews

Archer DB: The structure and function of the *Mycoplasma* membrane. Int Rev Cytol 69:1, 1981

Barile MF, Razin S (eds): Cell biology. The Mycoplasmas, vol I. New York, Academic Press, 1979

Baseman JB, Quackenbush RL: Preliminary assessment of AIDS-associated mycoplasma. Am Soc Microbiol News 56:319, 1990

Cassell GH, Cole BC: Mycoplasmas as agents of human disease. N Engl J Med 304:80, 1981

Dallo SF, Chavoya A, Baseman JB: Characterization of the gene for a 30-kilodalton adhesin-related protein of *Mycoplasma pneumoniae.* Infect Immun 58:4163, 1990

Dascher CC, Poddar SK, Maniloff J: Heat shock response in mycoplasmas, genome-limited organisms. J Bacteriol 172:1823, 1990

Denny FW: Atypical pneumonia and the Armed Forces Epidemiological Board. J Infect Dis 143:305, 1981

Kleemola SRM, Karjalainen JE, Räty RKH: Rapid diagnosis of *Mycoplasma pneumoniae* infection: Clinical evaluation of a commercial probe test. J Infect Dis 162:70, 1990

Lo SC, Dawson DM, Newton PB III, et al: Identification of *Mycoplasma incognitus* infection in patients with AIDS: An immunohistochemical, *in situ* hybridization and ultrastructural study. Am J Trop Med Hyg 41:601, 1989

Loveless RW, Feizi T: Sialo-oligosaccharide receptors for *Mycoplasma pneumoniae* and related oligosaccharides of poly-*N*-acetyllactosamine series are polarized at the cilia and apical microvillar domains of the ciliated cells in human bronchial epithelium. Infect Immun 57:1285, 1985

Maniloff J: Evaluation of wall-less prokaryotes. Annu Rev Microbiol 37:477, 1983

Razin S (ed): Mycoplasma infections. Isr J Med Sci 17:509, 1981

Razin S: Molecular biology and genetics of mycoplasmas (Mollicutes). Microbiol Rev 49:419, 1985

Razin S, Barile MF: Mycoplasma pathogenicity. The Mycoplasmas, vol 4. New York, Academic Press, 1985

Razin S, Freundt EA: The mycoplasmas. In Krieg NR, Holt JG (eds): Bergey's Manual of Systematic Bacteriology, vol 1. Baltimore, Williams & Wilkins, 1984

Razin S, Kahane I, Banai M, Bredt W: Adhesion of mycoplasmas to eukaryotic cells. In Adhesion and Microorganism Pathogenicity. Ciba Foundation Symposium 80. Tunbridge Wells, Pitman Medical, 1981, p 98

Razin S, Tully JG (eds): Mycoplasma characterization. Methods in Mycoplasmology, vol 1. New York, Academic Press, 1983

Saillard C, Carle P, Bove JM, et al: Genetic and serologic relatedness between *Mycoplasma fermentans* and a mycoplasma recently identified in tissues of AIDS and non-AIDS patients. Res Virol 385, 1990

Stuart PM, Cassell GH, Woodward JG: Differential induction of bone marrow macrophage proliferation by mycoplasmas involves granulocyte-macrophage colony-stimulating factor. Infect Immun 58:3558, 1990

Sugama K, Kuwano K, Furukawa M, et al: Mycoplasmas induce transcription and production of tumor necrosis factor in a monocytic cell line, THP-1, by a protein kinase C-independent pathway. Infect Immun 58:3564, 1990

Taylor-Robinson D, Gourlay RN: Genus II. Ureaplasma. In Krieg NR, Holt JG (eds): Bergey's Manual of Systematic Bacteriology, vol 1. Baltimore, Williams & Wilkins, 1984, p 770

Taylor-Robinson D, McCormack WM: The genital mycoplasmas. N Engl J Med 302:1003, 1063, 1980

Tully JG, Razin S (eds): Diagnostic mycoplasmology. Methods in Mycoplasmology, vol 2. New York, Academic Press, 1983

Tully JG, Whitcomb RF (eds): Human and animal mycoplasmas. The Mycoplasmas, vol 2. New York, Academic Press, 1979

Selected Papers

Broughton RA: Infections due to mycoplasmas in childhood. Pediatr Infect Dis 5:71, 1986

Hu PC, Cole RM, Huang YS, et al: *Mycoplasma pneumoniae* infection: Role of a surface protein in the attachment organelle. Science 216:313, 1982

Hu PC, Schaper U, Collier AM, et al: A *Mycoplasma genitalium* protein resembling the *Mycoplasma pneumoniae* attachment protein. Infect Immun 55:1126, 1987

Kohler RB: Antigen detection for rapid diagnosis of *Mycoplasma* and *Legionella pneumoniae*. Diagn Microbiol Infect Dis 4:475, 1986

Krause DC, Baseman JB: *Mycoplasma pneumoniae* proteins that selectively bind to host cells. Infect Immun 37:382, 1982

Kundsin RB, Driscoll S, Pelletier PA: *Ureaplasma ureolyticum* incriminated in perinatal morbidity and mortality. Science 213:474, 1981

Morrison-Plummer J, Lazzell A, Baseman JB: Shared epitopes between *Mycoplasma pneumoniae* major adhesin protein P1 and a 140-kilodalton protein of *Mycoplasma genitalium*. Infect Immun 55:49, 1987

Thomsen AC, Lindskov HO: Diagnosis of *Mycoplasma hominis* pyelonephritis by demonstration of antibodies in urine. J Clin Microbiol 9:681, 1979

Trevino LB, Haldenwang WG, Baseman JB: Expression of *Mycoplasma pneumoniae* antigens in *Escherichia coli*. Infect Immun 53:129, 1986

Weisburg WG, Tully JG, Rose DL, et al: A phylogenetic analysis of the mycoplasmas: Basis for their classification. J Bacteriol 171:6455, 1989

Woese CR, Maniloff J, Zablen LB: Phylogenetic analysis of the mycoplasmas. Proc Natl Acad Sci USA 77:494, 1980

SECTION IV

BASIC VIROLOGY

CHAPTER 52

The Nature, Isolation, and Measurement of Animal Viruses

Many important infectious diseases that afflict humankind are caused by viruses. Some are important because they frequently are fatal, such as AIDS, poliomyelitis, hepatitis, rabies, hemorrhagic fevers, and encephalitic diseases. Others are important because they cause acute discomfort, such as influenza, the common cold, measles and mumps, infections with various herpesviruses, and respiratory-gastrointestinal disorders. Still other viruses, such as rubella and cytomegalovirus, can cause congenital abnormalities. Finally, there are viruses that can cause tumors and cancer.

There is little that can be done to interfere with the growth of viruses, since they multiply only within cells, using the cells' synthetic capabilities. Only a limited number of highly specialized reactions are under their own control. It is hoped that the selective inhibition of these reactions will form the basis for a rational system of antiviral chemotherapy, thereby permitting viral infections to be controlled, just as antibiotics control most bacterial infections.

In addition to their medical importance, viruses provide simple model systems for many basic problems in biology. The reason is that viral genomes are very much smaller than the genomes of higher organisms: they encode, depending on the virus, from fewer than 10 to about 200 genes, compared with the roughly 100,000 genes in the human genome. Viruses, therefore, afford unrivaled opportunities for studying the arrangement, replication, and expression of genetic material. Knowledge gained from these studies is fundamental to an understanding of human genetics, growth and development, the operation of differentiated functions, and many other fields. Such knowledge is not only directly applicable to but also essential for the successful practice of medicine.

Nature of Viruses

Viruses are a heterogeneous class of agents. They vary in size and morphology, complexity, host range, and how they affect their hosts. However, certain characteristics are shared by all viruses:

1. They consist of a genome, either RNA or DNA, that is surrounded by a protective protein shell. Frequently, this shell is itself enclosed within an envelope that contains both protein and lipid.
2. They multiply only in living cells. They are absolutely dependent on the host cells' energy-yielding and protein-synthesizing apparatus. They are parasites at the genetic level.
3. Their multiplication cycles include, as an initial step, the separation of their genomes from their protective shells.

In essence, viruses are nucleic acid molecules that can invade cells and replicate within them and that encode proteins capable of forming protective shells around them.

Given this definition, are viruses to be regarded as living

organisms or as lifeless arrangements of molecules? The answer to this question depends on whether one is concerned with viruses as extracellular particles or as infectious agents. Isolated virus particles are arrangements of nucleic and protein molecules with no metabolism of their own; they are no more alive than isolated chromosomes. Within cells, however, virus particles are capable of reproducing their own kind abundantly. Considered in this light, viruses may indeed be said to possess at least some of the attributes of life. However, such terms as *organism* and *living* are not really applicable to viruses. It is preferable to refer to viruses as being functionally active or inactive rather than alive or dead.

Origin of Viruses

The origin of viruses poses a fascinating problem. There are two likeliest hypotheses: (1) Viruses are the products of regressive evolution of free-living cells. An evolutionary pathway of this type has been suggested for mitochondria, which still retain vestiges of cellular organization as well as mechanisms for replicating, transcribing, and translating genetic information. The largest animal viruses, the poxviruses, are so complex that one could imagine them also to be derived from a cellular ancestor. (2) Viruses are derived from cellular genetic material that has acquired the capacity to exist and function independently. Today the latter hypothesis is considered much more likely for all viruses (with the possible exception of poxviruses).

Detection of Animal Viruses

The presence of viruses is recognized by the manifestation of some abnormality in host organisms or host cells. In the organism, symptoms of infection vary widely, from inapparent infections (detectable only by the formation of antibody) or the development of local lesions or mild disease characterized by light febrile response to progressively more severe disease culminating in death. In cells the symptoms of viral infection vary from changes in morphology and growth patterns to cytopathic effects such as rounding, breakdown of cell organelles, the development of inclusion bodies, and general necrotic reactions, finally resulting in complete disintegration.

Characteristics of Cultured Animal Cells

The medical practitioner must understand not only how viruses affect the patient as a whole but also how viruses interact with various individual types of cells. This understanding can be acquired only by studying cloned cells, cultured and infected in vitro. Animal virology provided the primary impetus for the development of the technique of tissue culture, that is, culturing and growing cells in vitro. Cultured cells are now used extensively in many fields of biologic and biomedical research. Since knowledge concerning normal cells is crucial to an understanding of the virus-cell interaction, we examine briefly the characteristics of animal cells cultured in vitro.

Establishment of Animal Cell Strains

Cells of many organs can be grown in vitro. As a rule, small pieces of the tissue in question are dissociated into single cells by treatment with a dilute solution of trypsin, and the resulting single cell suspension is placed into a flask, bottle, or Petri dish. There the cells attach to the flat surface and multiply, provided that they are supplied with a growth medium. The essential constituents of growth media are physiologic concentrations of the 13 essential amino acids, vitamins, salts, glucose, and a buffering system that generally consists of bicarbonate in equilibrium with an atmosphere containing about 5% carbon dioxide. This medium is supplemented to the extent of about 5% with serum, the source of which is not predicated by the animal species from which the cells were derived. Horse, calf, and fetal calf serum are those most commonly employed. Antibiotics, such as penicillin and streptomycin, usually are added also in order to minimize the growth of bacterial contaminants, and a dye, such as phenol red, generally is included as a pH indicator. This medium, or more complex versions of it, will permit most cell types to multiply with a division time of 24 to 48 hours.

When cells are brought into contact with a surface, they generally attach firmly and flatten so as to occupy the maximum surface area. The only time when they are not maximally extended is during mitosis, when they become round and are, therefore, easily dislodged from the substratum. Cells multiply until they occupy all available surface area—that is, until they are confluent—but no further. The reason for this is that cells cease dividing when they make contact with neighboring cells, a phenomenon known as *contact inhibition* (Chap. 59).

Animal cells can be cloned just like bacterial cells, although the efficiency of cloning is usually less than 100%. Many genetically pure cell strains are now available. They fall into two morphologic categories, epithelial cells with a polygonal outline and fibroblasts with a narrow spindlelike shape (Fig. 52–1).

The first cultures after tissue dispersion are known as *primary cultures*. When such cultures are confluent, they are passaged by dislodgment from the surface by treatment with trypsin or the chelating agent ethylene diamine tetraacetate (EDTA) and reseeding into several new containers, in which they form secondary cultures. Passaging can be continued in this manner, provided that an adequate supply of growth medium is supplied at regular intervals.

The overall properties of cell strains generally are stable on continuous culturing. However, mutations do occur constantly, so that one particular mutant, or variant, usually emerges as the dominant population component under any given set of conditions. As a result, the same cell strain cultured in different laboratories may exhibit detectable phenotypic differences.

Multiplication Cycle

The multiplication of individual cells conforms to a regular pattern that can be thought of as a cycle (Fig. 52–2). According to this scheme, the interval between successive mitoses is

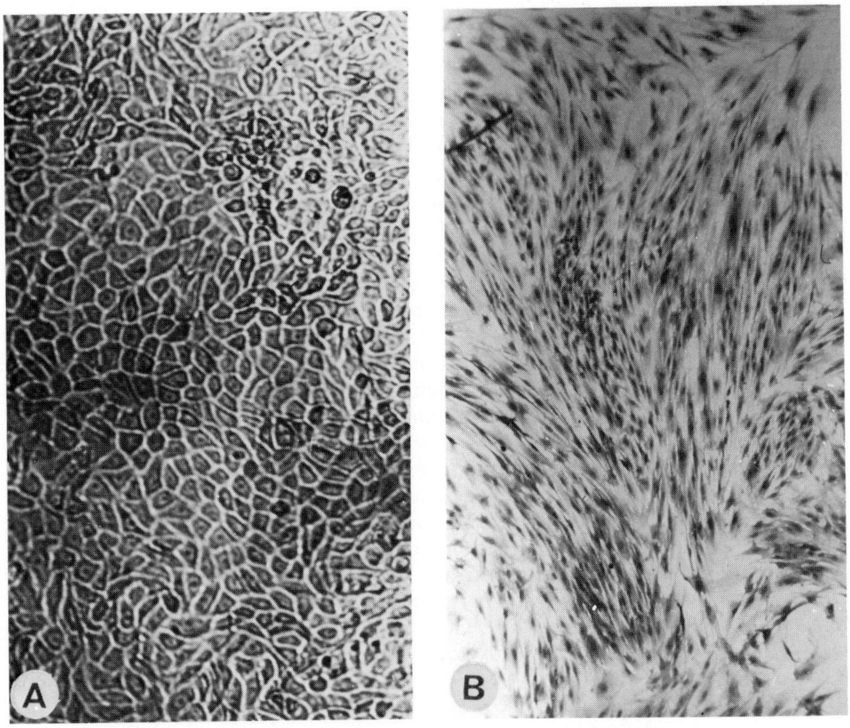

Fig. 52–1. Cultured mammalian cells. **A.** Unstained monkey kidney cells, which exhibit typical epithelioid morphology. **B.** Chick embryo fibroblasts (Giemsa stain). Note characteristic spindle shape and orderly alignment. *(**A** from Eagle and Foley: Cancer Res 18:1017, 1958; **B** courtesy of Dr. R. E. Smith.)*

divided into three periods: the G1 period, which precedes DNA replication, the S period, during which DNA replicates, and the G2 period, during which the cell prepares for the next mitosis. RNA and protein are not synthesized while mitosis proceeds—that is, during metaphase—but otherwise are synthesized throughout the multiplication cycle. Nongrowing cells usually are arrested in the G1 period. The resting state is often referred to as G0 (G zero). Under conditions of normal growth, the individual cells of a growing culture pass through this multiplication cycle in an unsynchronized fashion, so that cells at all stages of the cycle are present.

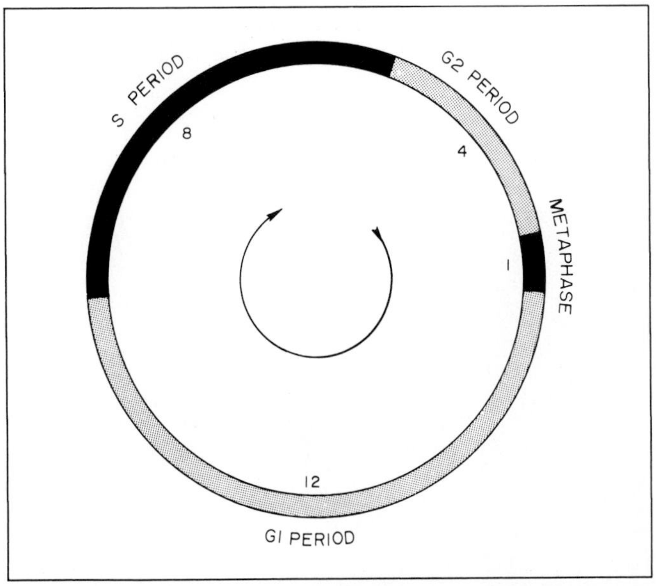

Fig. 52–2. Cell multiplication cycle. The duration of the cycle illustrated here is 25 hours. The average length (in hours) of each individual period of the cycle is indicated by the numbers inside the circle.

Aging of Cell Strains

Cells derived from normal tissues cannot be passaged indefinitely. Instead, after about 50 passages, which generally occupy about 1 year, their growth rate inevitably begins to slow. The amount of time that they spend in G0 after each mitosis gradually increases, fewer and fewer cells enter the S period, and the cells' karyotype (i.e., their chromosomal complement) changes from the euploid (diploid) pattern of normal cells to an aneuploid one, characterized by the presence of translocations (in which portions of chromosomes are exchanged by breakage and reunion), supernumerary chromosomes (i.e., extra copies of certain chromosomes), and chromosome fragments. Finally, the cell strain dies out. Loss of cell strains in this manner generally is guarded against by growing large numbers of cells during the early passages and storing them at −196C, the boiling point of liquid nitrogen.

Continuous Cell Lines

Whereas cells derived from normal tissues have the properties described thus far, malignant tissues give rise to aneuploid cell lines that have an infinite life span and are referred to as *continuous cell lines*. Infrequently such cell lines seem to arise from euploid cell strains, but the possibility that malignant or premalignant cells were not present originally is difficult to rule out. In addition to being aneuploid and immortal, continuous cell lines usually have two other significant properties: they form tumors when transplanted into animals, and they can grow in suspension culture like bacteria. Cells growing in suspension are used extensively for studies of virus multiplication, since they are easier to handle experimentally than cells growing as monolayers.

Patterns of Macromolecular Biosynthesis

Since virus multiplication consists essentially of nucleic acid and protein synthesis, a brief description of the patterns of macromolecular synthesis in normal, uninfected animal cells is relevant. The essential feature of the animal cell is its compartmentalization. The DNA of the animal cell is restricted to the nucleus at all stages of the cell cycle except during metaphase, when no nucleus exists. All RNA is synthesized in the nucleus. Much of it remains there, but messenger RNA and transfer RNA migrate to the cytoplasm. Ribosomal RNA is synthesized in the nucleolus. The two ribosomal subunits are assembled partly in the nucleolus and partly in the nucleus, and then they also migrate to the cytoplasm. All protein synthesis proceeds in the cytoplasm. The only exception to this brief summary concerns the mitochondria, which are located only in the cytoplasm and which contain DNA-synthesizing, RNA-synthesizing, and protein-synthesizing systems of their own.

Isolation of Animal Viruses

Many techniques have been developed for isolating viruses. The source of virus may be excreted or secreted material, the bloodstream, or some tissue. Samples are collected and, unless processed immediately, sheltered from heat, preferably by storage at −70C, the temperature of dry ice. If necessary, a suspension is then prepared by homogenizing or sonicating in the presence of cold buffer solution, and this is then centrifuged to remove large debris and contaminating microorganisms.

This suspension is then tested for the presence of virus by injecting it back into the original host species in order to determine whether the first noted abnormality is produced. It is also injected into other animal species in order to establish whether there exist more susceptible hosts in which the disease develops more rapidly, more severely, or in a more easily recognizable manner. Newborn or suckling animals (often mice or hamsters) or developing chick embryos are hosts that permit many viruses to multiply more extensively than do adult animals and that accordingly are widely used for virus isolation. A search is usually conducted for a cultured animal cell strain or line in which the virus will multiply well, so that it may be grown in quantity, isolated and characterized. Cells also are needed in which the virus rapidly elicits readily observable cytopathic effects that can be used to assay it. It is also essential to make certain that only a single unique virus is being isolated. This may be accomplished either by limiting serial dilution, when the virus suspension is diluted to such an extent that only one of several aliquots inoculated into cells used to detect it gives a positive response, or by plaque isolation (see below). The latter is preferable, since plaques originate from single virus particles.

Adaptation and Virulence

During the isolation of viruses, there may emerge variants capable of multiplying more efficiently in the host cells used for this purpose than the original wild-type virus. This phenomenon is known as *adaptation*. Often such variants damage the original host less severely than the wild-type virus and are, therefore, said to be less virulent. Viruses are often purposely adapted in order to alter growth and virulence characteristics. An example is provided by the attenuated vaccine virus strains, which are obtained by repeated passaging of virus virulent for one host in some other host, until virus strains with decreased virulence for the original host have been selected.

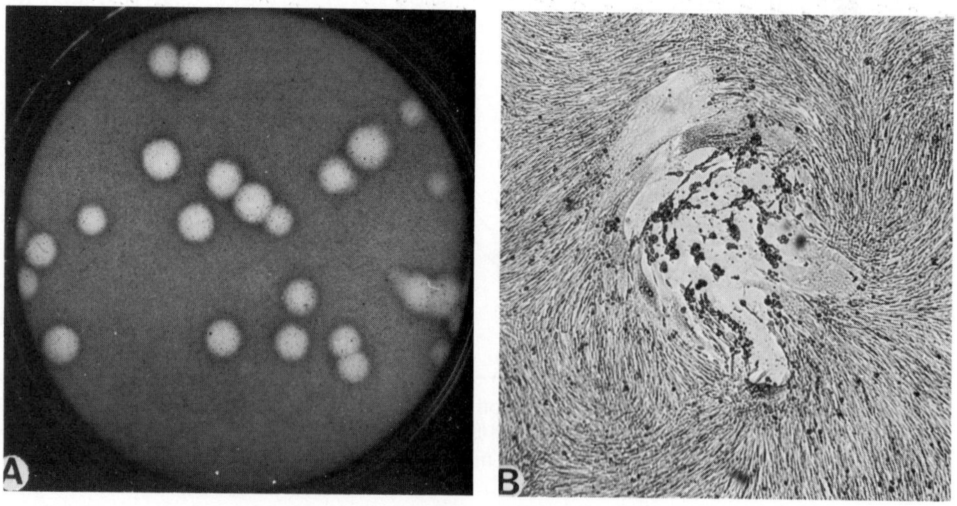

Fig. 52–3. Virus plaques. **A.** Plaques of influenza virus on monolayers of chick embryo cells, 4 days after inoculation. The monolayers were stained with neutral red on day 3. **B.** Photograph showing the microanatomy of a herpesvirus plaque on BHK 21 cells. *(**A** courtesy of Dr. G. Appleyard; **B** courtesy of Dr. S. M. Brown.)*

Measurement of Animal Viruses

Viruses are measured by several methods that can be divided into two categories. First, viruses may be measured as infectious units, that is, in terms of their ability to infect, multiply, and produce progeny. Second, viruses may be measured as virus particles, irrespective of their function as infectious agents.

Measurement of Viruses as Infectious Units

Measurement of the amount of virus in terms of the number of infectious units per unit volume is known as titration. There are several ways of determining the titer of a virus suspension,

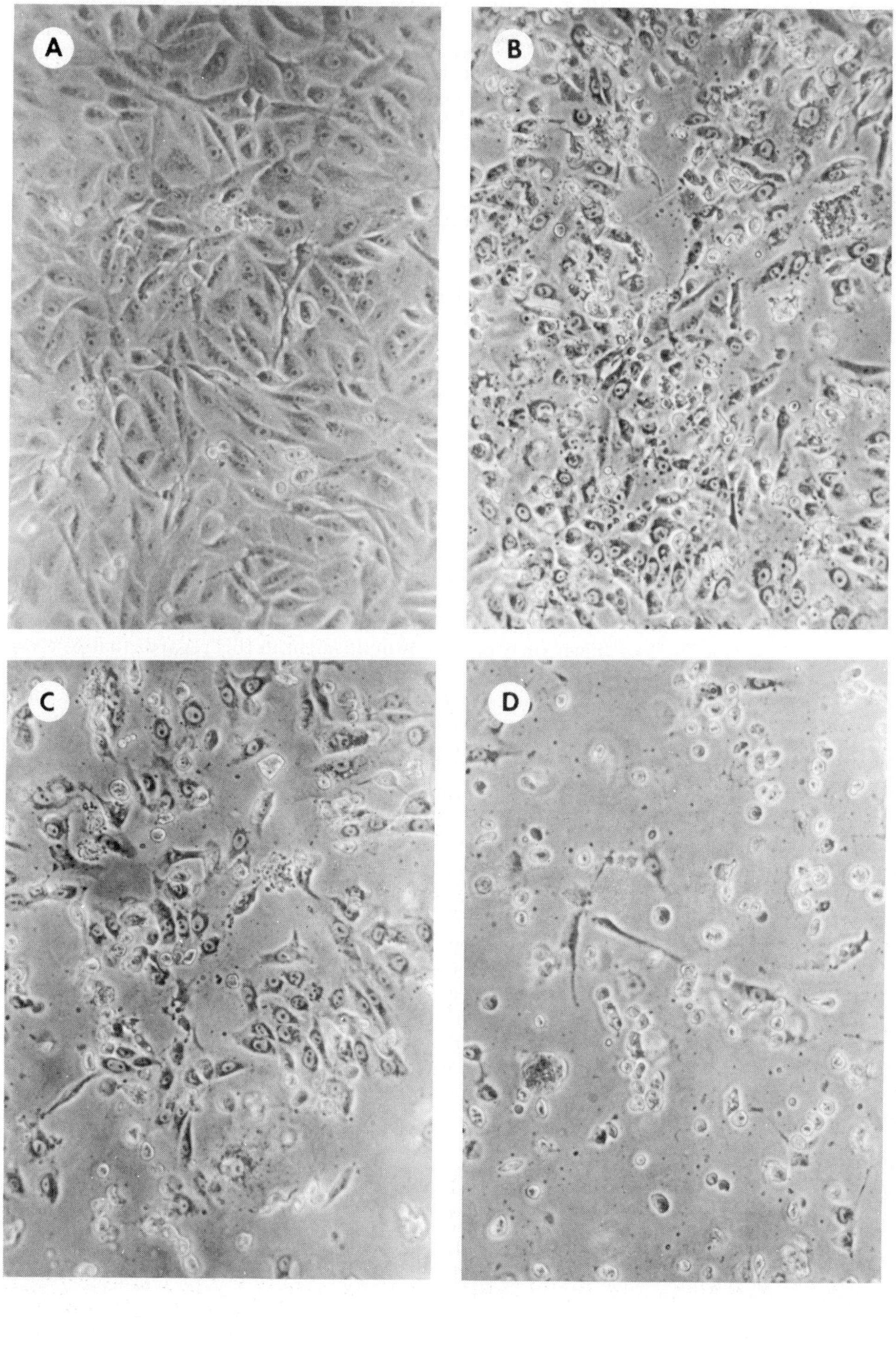

Fig. 52–4. The cytopathic effects caused by reovirus serotype 3 in Vero monkey kidney cells. **A.** Normal cell monolayer. **B.** Partial cell destruction at 20 hours after infection. **C.** 36 hours after infection. **D.** 48 hours after infection. × 125. *(Courtesy of Dr. E. C. Hayes.)*

all of them involving infection of host or target cells in such a way that each particle that causes productive infection elicits a recognizable response.

Plaque Formation

In this method, monolayers of susceptible cells are inoculated with small aliquots of serial dilutions of the virus suspension to be titrated. Wherever virus particles infect cells, progeny virus particles are produced and released and then immediately infect adjoining cells. This process is repeated until, after a period ranging from 2 to 12 days or more, areas of infected cells develop that can be seen with the naked eye. These are called *plaques*. In order to ensure that progeny virus particles liberated into the medium do not diffuse away and initiate separate (or secondary) plaques, agar is frequently incorporated into the medium.

The fundamental prerequisite for this method of enumerating infectious units is that the infected cells must differ in some recognizable manner from noninfected cells. For example, they must either be completely destroyed, become detached from the surface on which they grow, or possess staining properties different from those of normal cells. In practice, the most common method of visualizing plaques is to apply the vital stain neutral red to infected cell monolayers and to count the number of areas that do not stain (Fig. 52–3). Titers are expressed in terms of numbers of plaque-forming units (PFU) per milliliter.

There is a linear relationship between the amount of virus and the number of plaques produced; that is, the dose-response curve is linear. This indicates that each plaque is caused by a single virus particle. The virus progeny in each plaque are clones, and virus stocks derived from single plaques are said to be *plaque purified*. Plaque purification is an important technique for isolating pure virus strains.

Plaque formation is often the most desirable method of titrating viruses. It is economical of cells and virus, as well as technically simple. However, not all viruses can be measured in this way because there may be no cells that develop the desired cytopathic effects. For these viruses, alternate titration methods must be used.

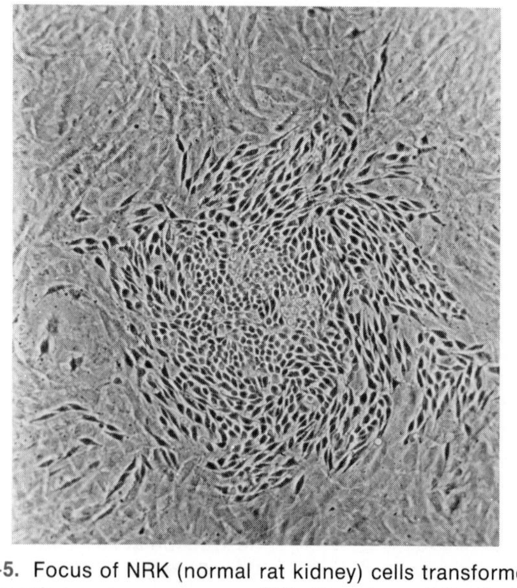

Fig. 52–5. Focus of NRK (normal rat kidney) cells transformed by Kirsten murine sarcoma virus. × 200. *(Courtesy of Dr. S. A. Aaronson.)*

Serial Dilution End Point Method

Some viruses destroy the cells that they infect but do not produce the type of cytopathic effects necessary for visible plaque formation. Such viruses may be titrated by means of the serial dilution end point method. In this method, serial dilutions of virus suspensions are inoculated into cell monolayers, which are then incubated until the cell sheets show clear signs of cell destruction (Fig. 52–4). The end point is that dilution that gives a positive (cell-destroying) reaction, and the titer is calculated assuming that the last positive dilution originally contained at least one infectious unit.

Focus Formation

Many tumor viruses do not destroy the cells in which they multiply and, therefore, produce no plaques. Instead, they cause cells to change morphology and to multiply at a faster rate than uninfected cells. Such cells are called *transformed cells*. Colonies of transformed cells often develop into foci large enough to be visible to the naked eye (Fig. 52–5). Assay by focus formation (counting the number of focus-forming units, or FFU) is analogous to assay by plaque formation.

Enumeration of Total Number of Virus Particles: Hemagglutination Assay

The most common technique for measuring the total number of virus particles is the hemagglutination assay. Many animal viruses adsorb to the red blood cells of various animal species. Each virus particle is multivalent in this regard; that is, it can adsorb to more than one cell at a time. In practice, the maximum number of cells with which any particular virus particle can combine is two, because red cells are far bigger than virus particles. In a virus-cell mixture in which the number of cells exceeds the number of virus particles, the small number of cell dimers that may be formed generally is not detectable, but if the number of virus particles exceeds the number of cells, a lattice of agglutinated cells is formed that settles out in a highly characteristic manner readily distinguishable from the settling pattern exhibited by unagglutinated cells.

The hemagglutination assay is performed by determining the virus dilution that will just agglutinate a standard number of red cells (Fig. 52–6). Since the number of virus particles necessary for this is readily calculated (it is slightly more than the number of cells), hemagglutination serves as a highly accurate and rapid method of quantitating virus particles.

Significance of Infectious Unit/Virus Particle Ratio

For animal viruses the number of virus particles in any given preparation always exceeds the number of infectious units. Usually the ratio of virus particles to infectious units is in the

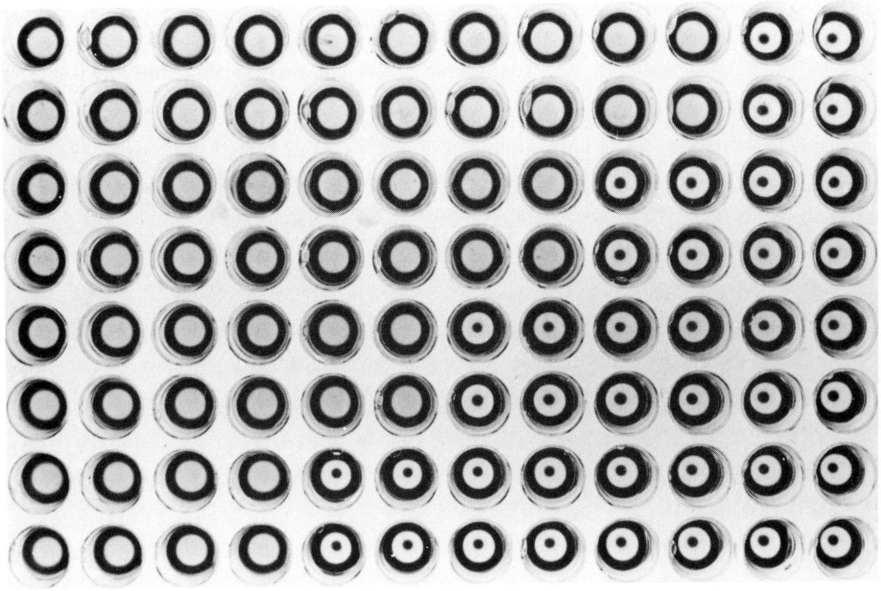

Fig. 52–6. Hemagglutination titration of influenza virus. In the top two rows a sample of influenza virus was diluted in serial twofold steps from left to right. In the next two rows the amount of virus in the first well was the same as in the third well in the top row, and so on down. The same number of red blood cells was then added to each well, and after mixing, the tray was kept at 4C for 2 hours. Unagglutinated cells form a dark button. Cells agglutinated by virus form a lattice that has a quite different appearance. *(Courtesy of Dr. E. C. Hayes.)*

range of 10 to 1000 or even greater. Sometimes the reason for this situation is that the virus preparation contains a large excess of noninfectious particles. However, more commonly the explanation is that although all virus particles in a given preparation are capable of causing productive infection, only a small proportion of them actually succeed in doing so. Two lines of evidence support this view. The first is that the titers of virus preparations often vary markedly depending on the nature of the assay system. For example, titers often differ depending on the route of inoculation if assays are carried out in whole animals or with cell type if cultured cells are used. Second, before a virus particle can manifest itself as a plaque or focus, it must initiate a productive infection cycle which requires numerous reactions, many of which have a low probability of occurring (Chap. 55). Therefore, the number of infectious units cannot equal the total number of virus particles. In fact, the ratio of the number of infectious units to the number of virus particles may generally be regarded as a measure of the probability with which the particular virus particles achieve productive infection.

FURTHER READING

Books

VIRUSES

Fenner FJ, Gibbs A: Portraits of Viruses: A History of Virology. Basel, Karger, 1988
Fields BN, et al (eds): Virology. New York, Raven Press, 1990
Fields BN, Knipe DM (chief eds): Fundamental Virology, ed 2. New York, Raven Press, 1991
Fraenkel-Conrat H, Kimball PC, Levy JA: Virology. Englewood Cliffs, NJ, Prentice-Hall, 1988
Hull R, Brown F, Payne C: Virology: Directory and Dictionary of Animal, Bacterial and Plant Viruses. London, Macmillan, 1989
Kucera LS, Myrvik QN: Fundamentals of Medical Virology. Philadelphia, Lea & Febiger, 1985
Porterfield JS (ed): Andrewes' Viruses of Vertebrates, ed 5. London, Bailliere Tindall, 1989
Rothschild H, Cohen JC (eds): Virology in Medicine. New York, Oxford University Press, 1986

CELLS

Alberts B, Bray D, Lewis J, et al: Moecular Biology of the Cell, ed 2. New York, Garland Publishing, Inc., 1989
Baserga R (ed): Cell Growth and Division: A Practical Approach. New York, Oxford University Press, 1989
Becker WM: The World of the Cell. Menlo Park, Calif., Benjamin-Cummings, 1986
Bubel A: Microstructure and Function of Cells. New York, Wiley, 1989
Darnell J, Lodish H, Baltimore D: Molecular Cell Biology. New York, Scientific Books, Freeman, 1990
Matlin KS, Valentich JD (eds): Functional Epithelial Cells in Culture. New York, Alan R Liss, 1989
Pollard JW, Walker JM (eds): Animal Cell Culture. Clifton, NJ, Humana Press, 1990
Swanson CP, Webster PL: The Cell. Englewood Cliffs, NJ, Prentice-Hall, 1985
van Holde KE. Chromatin. New York, Springer-Verlag, 1989
Widnell CC, Pfenninger KH: Essential Cell Biology. Baltimore, Williams & Wilkins, 1990

Selected Reviews and Articles

Denhardt DT, Edwards DR, Parfett CLJ: Gene expression during the mammalian cell cycle. Biochim Biophys Acta 865:83, 1986
Franke WW: Nuclear lamins and cytoplasmic intermediate filament proteins: A growing multigene family. Cell 48:3, 1987
Gray MW: Origin and evolution of mitochondrial DNA. Annu Rev Cell Biol 5:25, 1989
Griffiths G, Simons K: The trans Golgi network: Sorting at the exit site of the Golgi complex. Science 234:438, 1986
Gruenberg J, Howell K: Membrane traffic in endocytosis: Insights

from cell-free assays. Annu Rev Cell Biol 5:453, 1989
Hynes RO: Integrins: A family of cell surface receptors. Cell 48:549, 1987
Kelly RB: Microtubules, membrane traffic, and cell organization. Cell 61:5, 1990
Laskey RA, Fairman MP, Blow JJ: S phase of the cell cycle. Science 246:609, 1989
Lewin B: Driving the cell cycle: M phase kinase, its partners and substrates. Cell 61:743, 1990
Maniatis T, Goodbourn S, Fischer JA: Regulation of inducible and tissue-specific gene expression. Science 236:1237, 1987
Metcalf D: The molecular control of cell division, differentiation commitment and maturation in haematopoietic cells. Nature 339:27, 1989
Pardee AB: G1 events and regulation of cell proliferation. Science 246:603, 1989
Simons K, Wandinger-Ness A: Polarized sorting in epithelia. Cell 62:207, 1990
Smith JR, Hayflick L: Variation in the life span of clones derived from human diploid strains. J Cell Biol 62:48, 1974
Stack SN, Brown DB, Dewey WC: Visualization of interphase chromosomes. J Cell Sci 26:281, 1977
Stillman B: Initiation of eukaryotic DNA replication in vitro. Annu Rev Cell Biol 5:246, 1989
Watt FM, Harris H: Microtubule organizing centers in mammalian cells in culture. J Cell Sci 44:103, 1980
Weintraub H, Roberts J, Cross F: Simple and complex cell cycles. Annu Rev Cell Biol 5:341, 1989

CHAPTER 53

Structure, Components, and Classification of Viruses

Morphology of Animal Viruses

Although animal viruses differ widely in shape and size, they are nevertheless constructed according to certain common principles. Basically, viruses consist of nucleic acid and protein. The nucleic acid is the genome that contains the information necessary for multiplication; the protein is arranged around the genome in the form of a layer or shell that is termed the *capsid*. The structure consisting of shell plus nucleic acid is the *nucleocapsid*. Many animal virus particles consist of naked nucleocapsids, while others possess an additional envelope that is usually acquired as nucleocapsids bud from host cells. The complete virus particle is known as the *virion*, a term that denotes both intactness of structure and the property of infectiousness.

Capsids

The essential feature of capsids is that they are composed of repeating subunits—identical or belonging to only a few different species—arranged in precisely defined patterns. The simplest subunits are single protein molecules. More complex forms are morphologic subunits termed *capsomers* that can be seen with the electron microscope and that consist of several either identical or different protein molecules. Using only a few types of subunits for capsid construction has two noteworthy consequences: (1) it minimizes the amount of genetic information necessary to specify capsids, and (2) it ensures that they will be assembled efficiently. Capsid proteins exhibit a strong tendency to associate with each other, and much of the information necessary for nucleocapsid morphogenesis is inherent in their amino acid sequence.

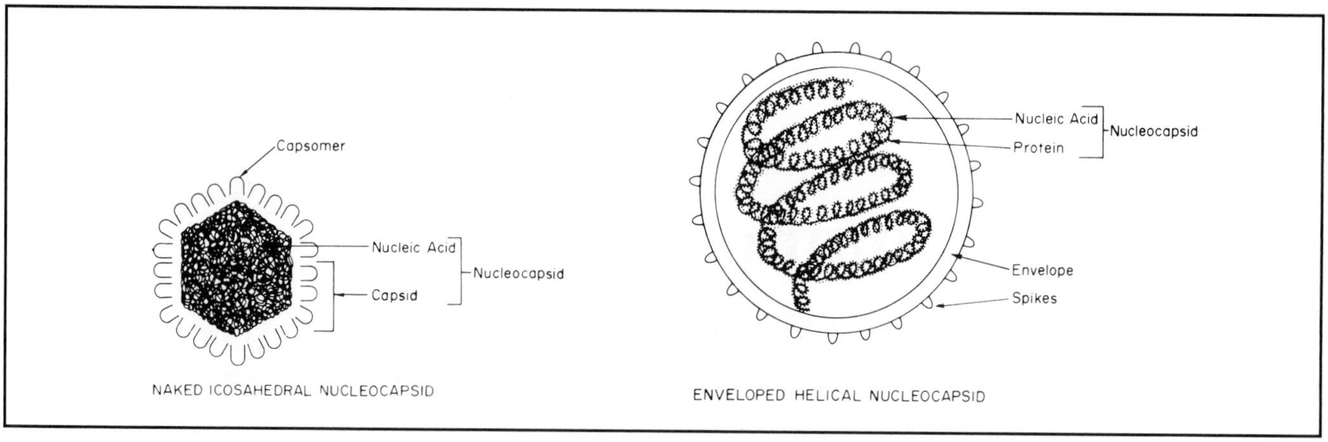

Fig. 53–1. The two basic patterns of animal virus structure. **Left.** The condensed genome is enclosed by a shell of capsomers arranged so as to display 5:3:2 rotational symmetry. **Right.** The extended genome is sheathed by protein molecules arranged so as to display helical symmetry. The resultant structure, the nucleocapsid, is enclosed in an envelope to whose outer surface glycoprotein spikes are attached.

Capsids (and envelopes) have a dual function. The first is to protect viral genomes from potentially destructive agents in the extracellular environment. The second is to introduce viral genomes into host cells. The necessity for the latter function stems from the fact that viral nucleic acids often are longer than cell diameters and cannot penetrate into cells by themselves. Capsids (and envelopes), on the other hand, adsorb readily to cells and can enter cells by several mechanisms (Chap. 55).

Envelopes

Only seven families of animal viruses exist as naked nucleocapsids. In all others, the nucleocapsids are enclosed by membrane-containing envelopes that are acquired as the nucleocapsids bud through special patches of cell membrane—either in outer plasma cell membranes or in vacuolar membranes–on their way to the exterior of the cell. The membrane patches through which nucleocapsids bud are virus-modified in that the cell-specified proteins in them are more or less completely replaced with virus-specified proteins. Thus, viral envelopes consist of lipid bilayers directly derived from some host cell membrane, the outer surface of which is studded with virus-encoded glycoproteins. These glycoproteins are anchored in the lipid bilayer by means of hydrophobic regions close to one of their ends; only a few amino acids, generally no more than 30, extend into the interior of the virus particle. The glycoprotein molecules are usually associated with each other in the form of oligomers (dimers, trimers, or tetramers) that are easily visible in the electron microscope and are known as *spikes*. Sometimes the spikes are very prominent, as in the case of coronaviruses, where they are large and club-shaped and surround the virus particles like a corona (hence the name) (see Fig. 53–8); at other times, they are visualized only with difficulty, as in the case of many retroviruses. As a rule, they are not arranged in regular patterns, but the spikes of bunyaviruses, influenza C virus, and certain togaviruses are arranged in characteristic hexagonal lattice patterns (see below).

The inner surfaces of viral envelopes are usually associated with virus-encoded proteins known as *membrane* or *matrix proteins*. Many of these proteins possess several hydrophobic domains, which suggests that they traverse the bilayer repeatedly. They appear to make specific contact with the internal regions of spike glycoproteins on the one hand and with nucleocapsid proteins on the other.

Viral envelopes generally lack rigidity. Therefore they

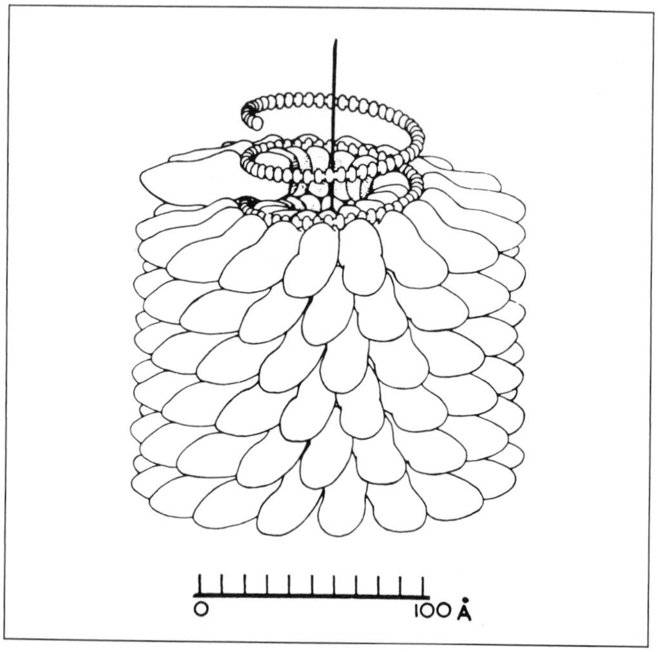

Fig. 53–2. Schematic representation of tobacco mosaic virus. As can be seen in the cutaway section, the ribonucleic acid helix is associated with protein molecules in the ratio of one protein molecule for every three nucleotides. *(From Klug and Caspar: Adv Virus Res 7:225, 1960.)*

usually appear heterogeneous in shape and size when fixed for electron microscopy, and enveloped viruses are thus often said to be pleomorphic. There is little doubt, however, that in their native state most enveloped viruses are spherical. However, two types of enveloped viruses are not spherical. These are the rhabdoviruses, which possess a highly characteristic bullet-like shape, rounded at one end and flat at the other, and certain strains of influenza virus type C, which are long and filamentous (see below).

Herpesvirus Tegument

Herpesvirus nucleocapsids are enveloped, but here a featureless layer of material termed the *tegument* is interposed between the nucleocapsid and the envelope (see Fig. 53–11). The thickness of the tegument is variable; in thin sections, it is often distributed asymmetrically. It is composed of proteins encoded by the virus. Its function is not clear.

Nucleocapsids

Viral nucleocapsids are constructed according to only a few basic patterns. Two of them have been studied in great detail at both the structural and the molecular level. In one, the nucleic acid is extended; in the other, it is condensed (Fig. 53–1). Superimposed on these two patterns are variations dictated both by the size of the genome and by the nature of the capsid proteins.

Nucleocapsids with Helical Symmetry

The prototype of nucleocapsids in which the nucleic acid exists as an extended filament is a plant virus, tobacco mosaic virus (TMV), the structure of which has been studied extensively by x-ray diffraction. In this virus the extended nucleic acid molecule is surrounded by protein molecules arranged helically so as to yield a structure with a single rotational axis (Fig. 53–2). The ortho- and paramyxoviruses, rhabdoviruses, bunyaviruses, filoviruses, arenaviruses, and coronaviruses possess nucleocapsids constructed in this manner, each with its own characteristic length, width, periodicity, flexibility, and stability (Fig. 53–3). It should be noted that these nucleocapsids are not the complete virus particles. The particles of these viruses consist of the nucleocapsids coiled within envelopes; that is, these virus particles are enveloped nucleocapsids (Figs. 53–4 to 53–8).

Nucleocapsids with Icosahedral Symmetry

In the second pattern of virus structure, the nucleic acid is condensed and forms the central portion of a quasispherical nucleocapsid. Here the capsid consists of a shell of protein

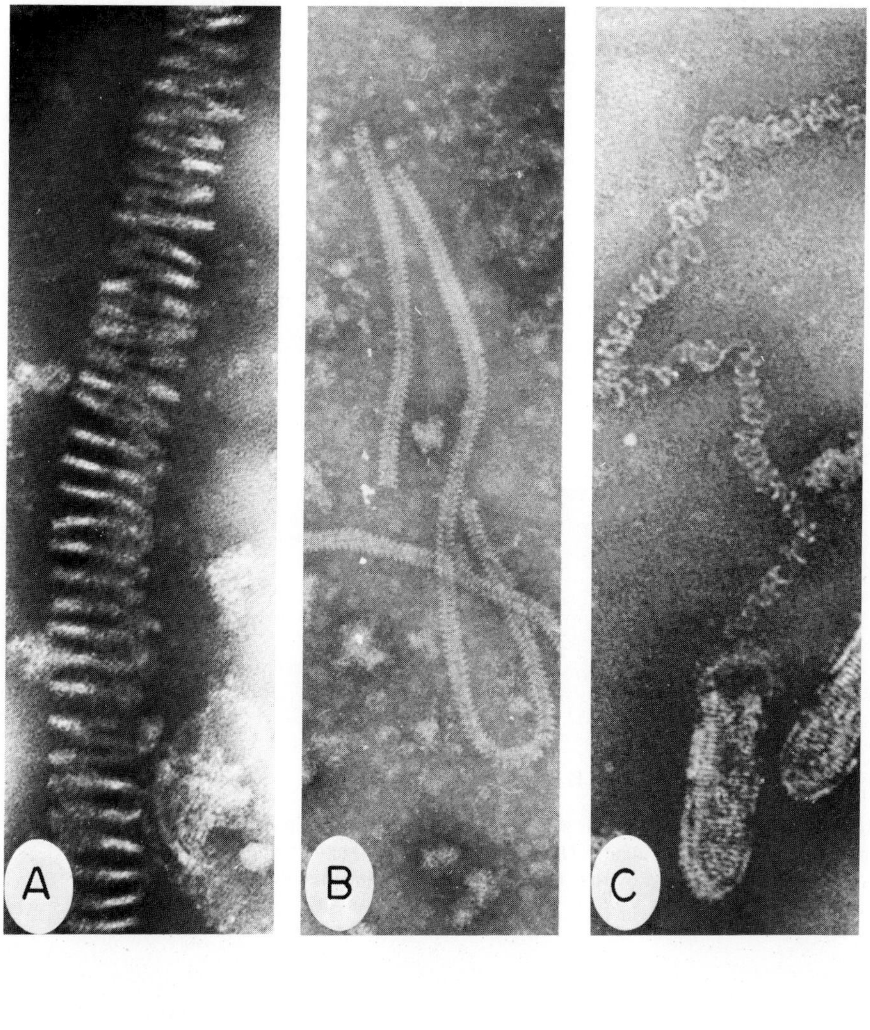

Fig. 53–3. The nucleocapsids of **(A)** the orthomyxovirus influenza A virus strain PR8 (× 225,000), **(B)** the paramyxovirus measles virus (× 150,000), and **(C)** the rhabdovirus vesicular stomatitis virus (VSV) (× 160,000). The last is emerging from a damaged virus particle. *(**A** from Almeida and Waterson. In Barry and Mahy (eds): The Biology of Large RNA Viruses, Academic Press, 1970; **B** from Finch and Gibbs: J Gen Virol 6:144, 1970; **C** from Simpson and Hauser: Virology 29:660, 1966.)*

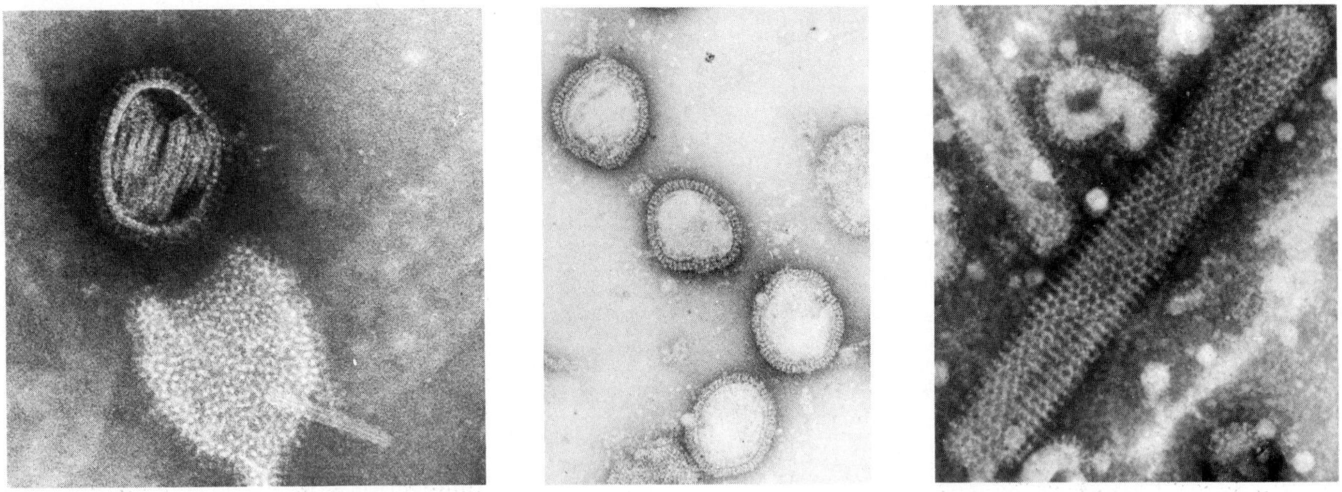

A B C

Fig. 53–4. The structure of influenza virus. **A.** Influenza virus A_2, stained with phosphotungstate. One particle is penetrated by the strain, thereby revealing the arrangement of its internal nucleocapsid. × 155,000. *(Courtesy of Dr. M. V. Nermut.)* **B.** Influenza virus A_o/WSN, stained with phosphotungstate, revealing the characteristic arrangement of spikes on the particle surface. There are two types of spikes; hemagglutinin (HA) spikes are about six times more numerous than neuraminidase (NA) spikes. HA spikes are distributed uniformly on the viral surface, but NA spikes are concentrated in discrete areas that may correspond to the region where the membrane of the budding virus particle separates from the plasma cell membrane. Location of NA in that position may facilitate release of virus (see p. 825). × 135,000. *(Courtesy of Dr. I. T. Schulze.)* **C.** A filamentous particle of an influenza C strain. Note the regular subunit (glycoprotein spike) surface pattern. × 115,000. *(From Apostolov and Flewett: J Gen Virol 4:366, 1969.)*

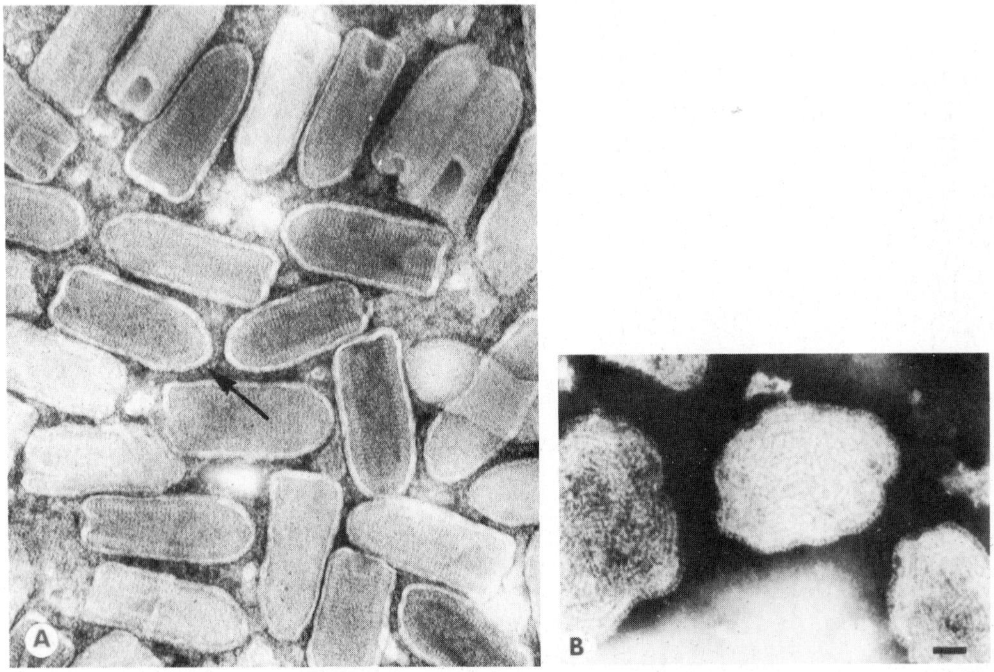

Fig. 53–5. **A.** Highly characteristic bullet-shaped vesicular stomatitis virus (VSV) particles, some penetrated by stain, revealing the tightly coiled nucleocapsids. Note glycoprotein spikes (arrow). *(Courtesy of Dr. Erskine Palmer.)* **B.** Sendai virus, a paramyxovirus. Note the tightly coiled nucleocapsids. × 73,500. *(From Maeno et al: J Virol 6:492, 1970.)*

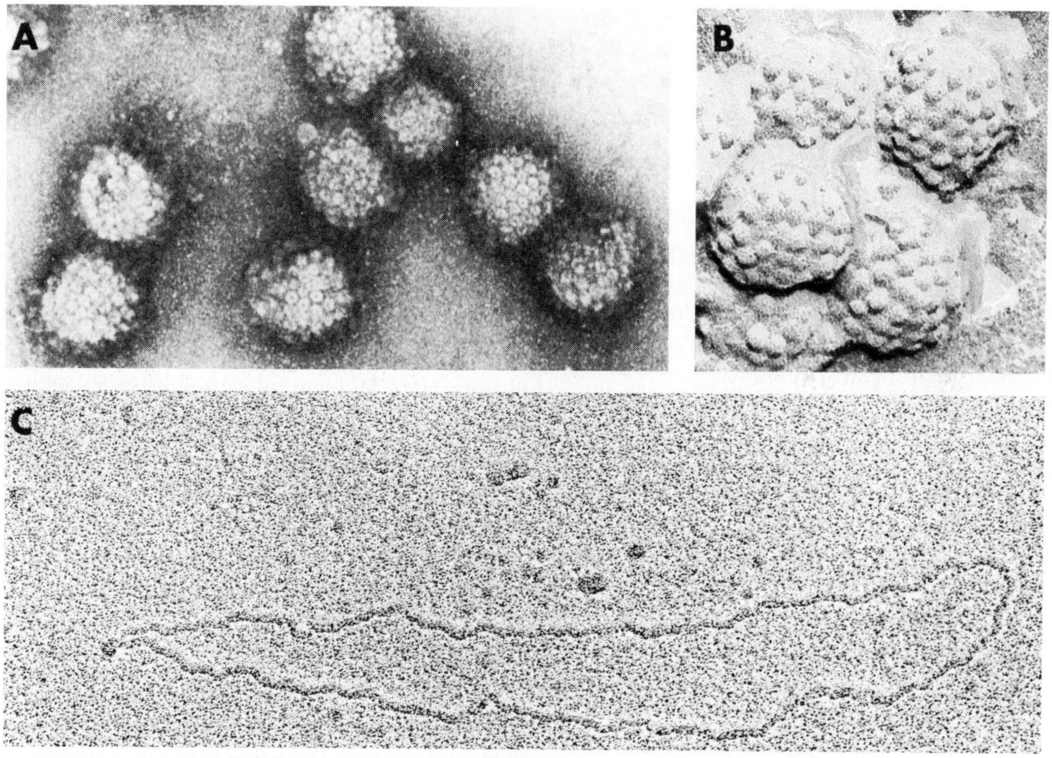

Fig. 53–6. The structure of Uukuniemi virus, a bunyavirus. **A.** Virus particles fixed with glutaraldehyde and negatively stained with uranyl acetate. × 100,000. **B.** Freeze-etched, glutaraldehyde-fixed virus particles. Note the hexagonal arrangement of surface projections (spikes) (see also Fig. 53–4C). × 180,000. **C.** Circular nucleocapsid of this virus, shadowed with platinum. Nucleocapsids are released from virus particles by treatment with the nonionic detergent Triton X-100. They are circular because the viral RNA possesses inverted terminal complementary repeated sequences that base-pair with each other. × 60,000. *(From von Bonsdorff: J Virol 16:1296, 1975.)*

A B C
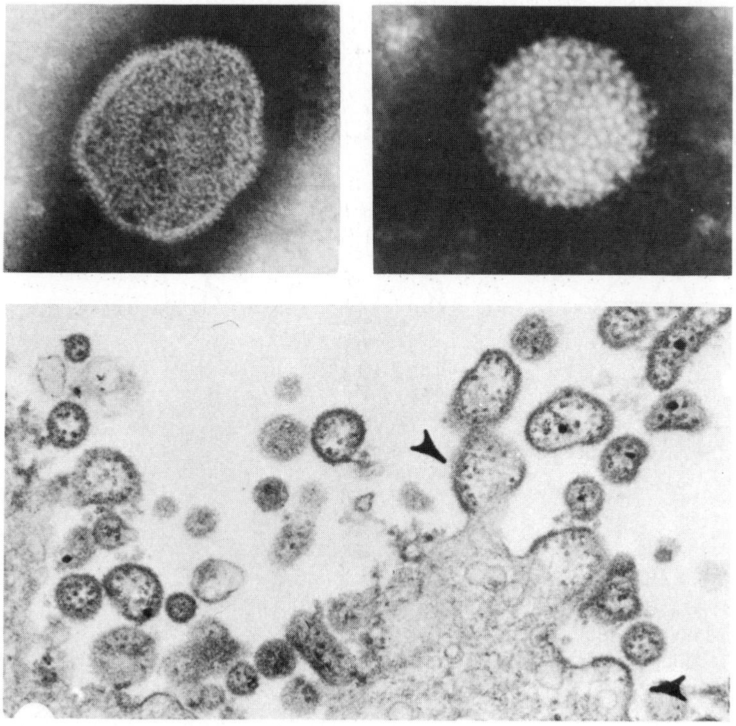

Fig. 53–7. Tacaribe virus, an arenavirus. **A, B.** Two virus particles, one of which has been partially penetrated by negative contrast medium, showing the glycoprotein spikes that cover their surface. × 135,000 and × 235,000, respectively. **C.** Thin section of Paraña virus particles, another arenavirus, budding from the plasma membrane of Vero African green monkey kidney cells. Note the characteristic dense granules, which resemble grains of sand (hence the name, Latin *arenosus*, sandy); they are ribosomes. × 45,000. *(From Murphy et al: J Virol 6:507, 1970.)*

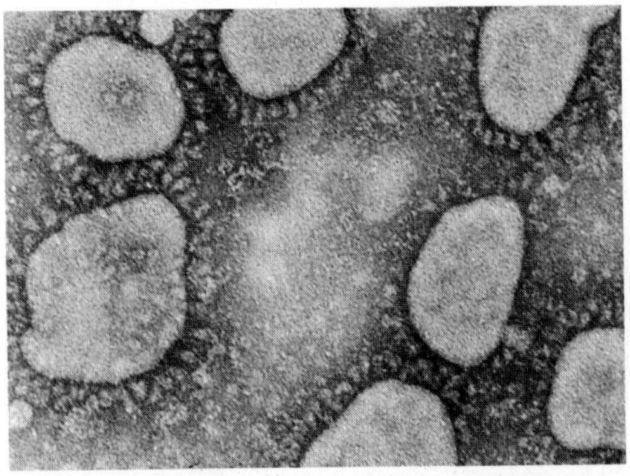

Fig. 53–8. Coronavirus particles. Note the characteristic large, widely spaced club- or pear-shaped surface projections, or spikes, also referred to as peplomers, that are dimers or trimers of a large glycoprotein. × 144,000. *(From Kapikian. In Lennette and Schmidt (eds): Diagnostic Procedures for Viral and Rickettsial Infections, ed 4. American Public Health Association, 1969.)*

molecules that are clustered into small groups called *capsomers*, with the bonds between molecules within capsomers being stronger than those between capsomers. Capsomers are morphologic units that often can be seen with the electron microscope. They vary in size and shape from virus to virus.

X-ray diffraction analysis indicates that in this type of nucleocapsid the capsomers are arranged very precisely in icosahedral patterns characterized by 5:3:2-fold rotational symmetry (Fig. 53–9). Two such patterns are found among animal viruses. The first is exhibited most clearly by adenoviruses. The adenovirus capsid is constructed in the shape of an icosahedron, with six capsomers along each edge and 252 capsomers altogether (Fig. 53–10). Of these, 240 are spherical and are situated along the edges and on the faces of the icosahedron. Each has six nearest neighbors and is known as a *hexon*. The remaining 12 are situated at the 12 vertices of the icosahedron and have five nearest neighbors; these are known as *pentons*. Adenovirus pentons have a highly characteristic shape, consisting of a spherical base and a long fiber that serves as the cell attachment organ. The capsids of two other virus families are constructed similarly. Iridovirus capsids possess 10 capsomers along each edge, and there are 1112 capsomers altogether—1100 hexons and 12 pentons. Herpesvirus capsids possess five capsomers along each edge and 162 capsomers altogether—150 prism-shaped hexons and 12 pentons (Fig. 53–11).

The second pattern is exhibited most clearly by picornaviruses. Here 60 identical capsomers, each composed of four different proteins, are situated equidistantly from a common center, which results in a spherical capsid (Fig. 53–12). Similarly, papovavirus capsids consist of 72, parvovirus capsids of 32, and birnavirus capsids of 92 identical capsomers (Fig. 53–13).

Reoviruses are unique in possessing two capsids shells (Fig. 53–14). Both possess icosahedral symmetry, but it has so far proved impossible to discern either the total number of capsomers or the precise manner in which they are arranged. The capsid shells of some members of this family, such as the orbiviruses and the rotaviruses, appear to be composed of 32 large ring-shaped capsomers. It is more likely, however, that this type of capsid is composed of numerous small subunits arranged in ring-shaped (or hexagonal) patterns and that many of these subunits are shared by adjacent rings so that what is visible is 32 holes, rather than 32 capsomers. Reovirus capsids are probably structured similarly, although here the rings are less prominent.

Another unique situation is presented by the retroviruses, which possess apparently icosahedral capsids that contain concentrically coiled, probably helical nucleocapsids (Fig. 53–15).

In the case of the picornaviruses, caliciviruses, birnaviruses, adenoviruses, papovaviruses, parvoviruses, and reoviruses, the virus particles are the naked nucleocapsids. How-

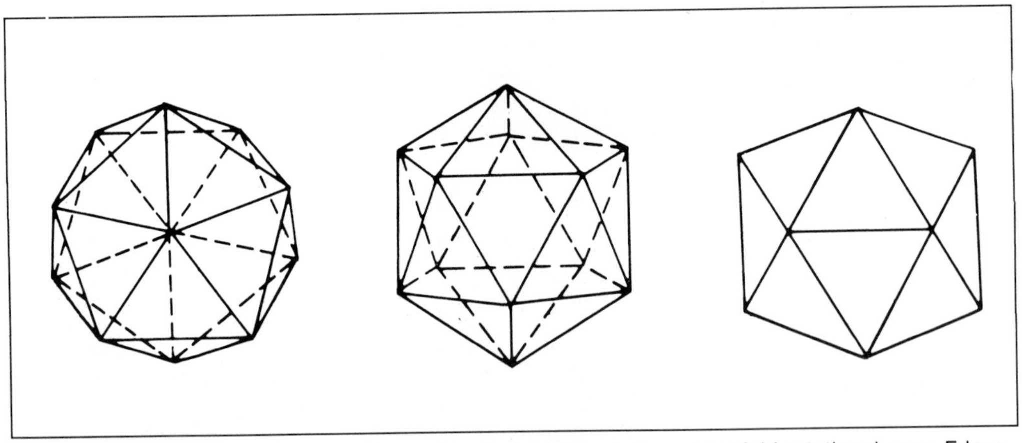

Fig. 53–9. The icosahedron viewed normal to fivefold, threefold, and twofold rotational axes. Edges of the upper and lower surfaces are drawn in solid and broken lines, respectively. The fivefold rotational axes pass through the vertices (left); the threefold rotational axes pass through the centers of the triangular faces (center); and the twofold rotational axes pass through the edges (right). In this view the edges on the upper and lower surfaces coincide. Note that the icosahedron possesses 12 vertices, 20 triangular faces, and 30 edges.

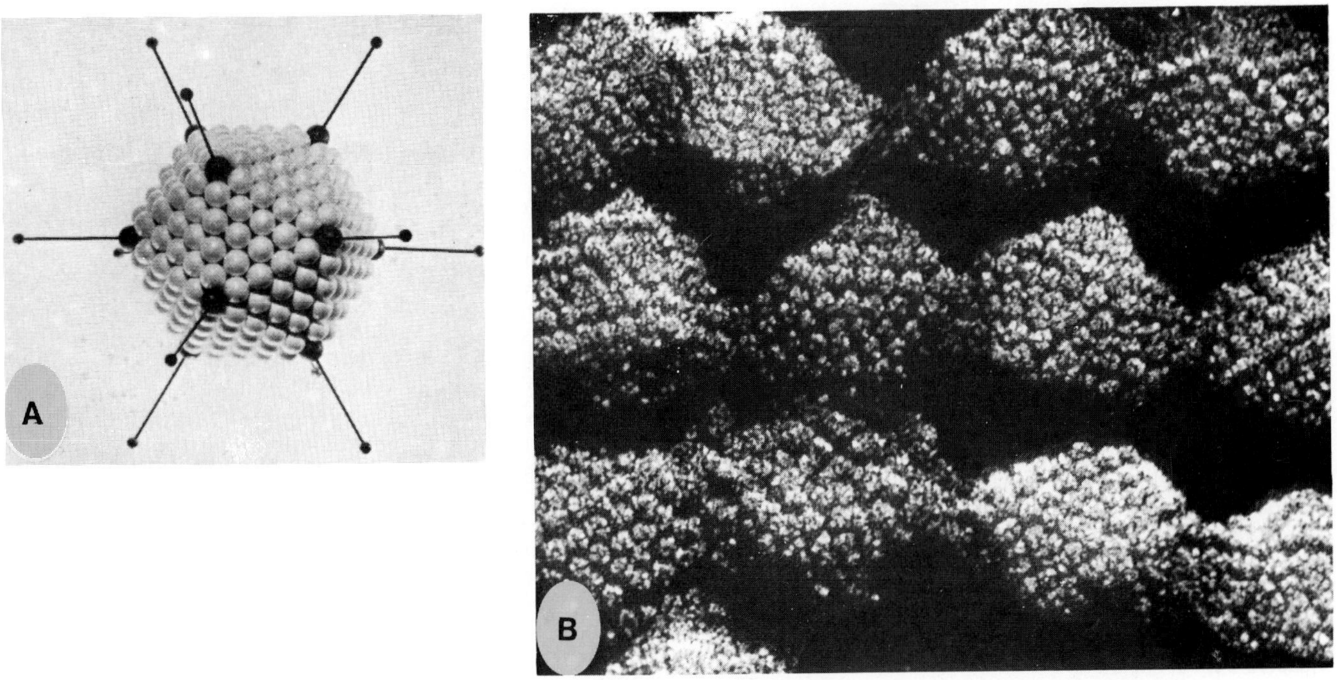

Fig. 53–10. **A.** Model of the adenovirus particle constructed by R.C. Valentine. **B.** Adenovirus freeze-dried and shadowed with platinum. × 400,000. *(Courtesy of Dr. M. V. Nermut.)*

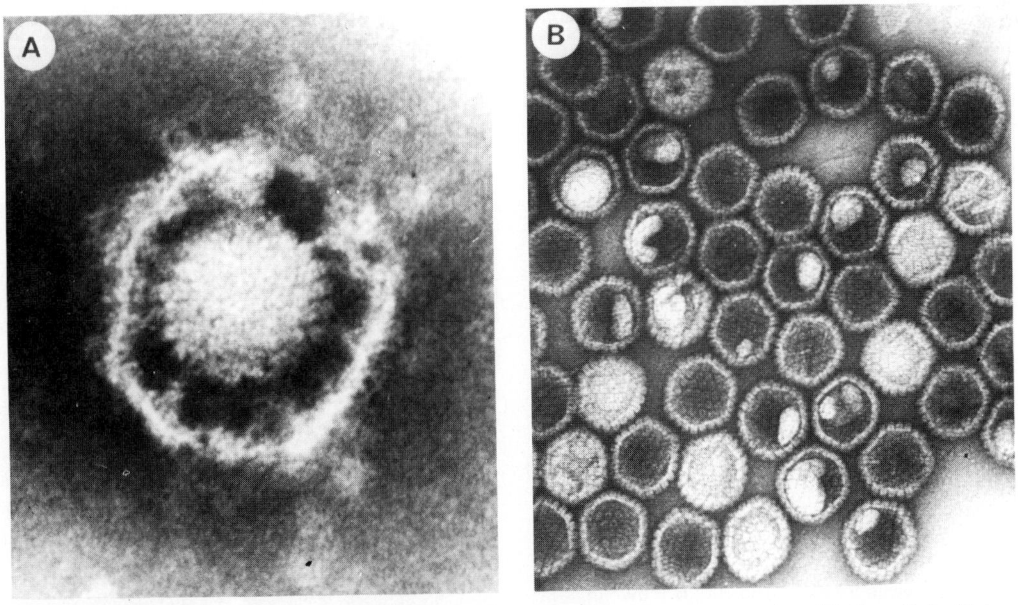

Fig. 53–11. The morphology of herpesviruses. **A.** Enveloped equine abortion virus (EAV) particle. Note the large amount of tegument between the envelope and the nucleocapsid. × 125,000. **B.** EAV particles from which the envelope and tegument have been removed by treatment with detergent. × 75,000. *(From Abodeely, Lawson, Randall: J Virol 5:513, 1970.)*

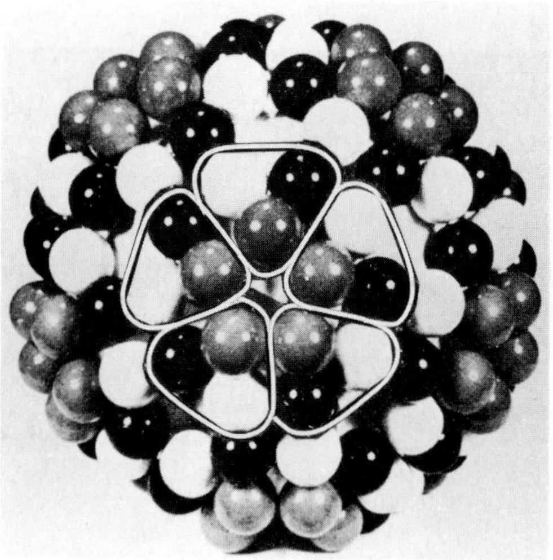

Fig. 53–12. Model of the picornavirus capsid. There are 60 capsomers, each consisting of three protein molecules, represented here by white, gray, and black balls. (In fact, in the mature virion, one of these protein molecules is cleaved into a larger and a smaller fragment, both of which remain in position.) Groups of five capsomers (as outlined) form units that are intermediates during morphogenesis; the capsid is composed of 12 of these "groups of five." *(Adapted from Johnston and Martin: J Gen Virol 11:77, 1971.) See also Figure 55–32 for the structure of poliovirus as deduced from x-ray crystallography.*

ever, there are several viruses whose icosahedral nucleocapsids are not infectious by themselves; here the infectious virus particles are again enveloped (this time icosahedral) nucleocapsids. These are the herpesviruses, the togaviruses (Fig. 53–16), the retroviruses, the flaviviruses (for the nucleocapsids of which icosahedral symmetry is inferred but not yet demonstrated conclusively), as well as the only iridovirus that is a mammalian virus, namely, African swine fever virus.

Structure of Poxviruses, Hepadnaviruses, and Some As Yet Unclassified Viruses

Poxviruses are the largest and most complex of all animal viruses. Morphologically, there are two major classes of poxviruses. Most poxvirus particles are prolate ellipsoids that are brick-shaped when fixed for electron microscopy. They possess an outer layer that consists of a membrane that is covered with tubules or filaments arranged in a characteristic whorled or mulberry pattern (Fig. 53–17). This outer layer encloses a DNA-containing nucleoid or core bounded by a layer of well-defined protein subunits, as well as two large lateral bodies of unknown composition and function.

Parapoxviruses are somewhat smaller, ovoid rather than brick-shaped, and are covered on their outer surface by tubules or filaments similar to those that cover the particles just described, except that they are arranged in a highly regular, crisscross pattern that is probably caused by one continuous filament wound round each particle in 12 to 15 left-handed turns (Fig. 53–18). The internal components of parapoxvirus particles are similar to those of poxvirus particles.

Hepatitis B virus particles possess a lipid-containing outer layer or envelope that encloses an electron-dense DNA-containing spherical core or nucleocapsid about the same size as a picornavirus particle (Fig. 53–19). The components of the outer layer, also known as the *surface antigen*, possess a strong tendency to associate with each other to form either spherical (22 nm diameter) or rod-shaped particles that lack cores and are often present in patient sera in very large numbers (more than 10^{13}/mL), outnumbering virus particles (the 42 nm Dane particles) by factors of 10,000 or more.

Finally, there are several viruses that have not yet been assigned to any virus family. Among these are the non-A, non-B hepatitis viruses (HCV and HEV), the delta hepatitis virus (HDV), the astroviruses, the toroviruses, the Borna disease virus, and the chronic infectious neuropathic agents (see Table 53–4).

The relative sizes of some important animal viruses are illustrated in Figure 53–20. Their morphology is summarized in Table 53–1.

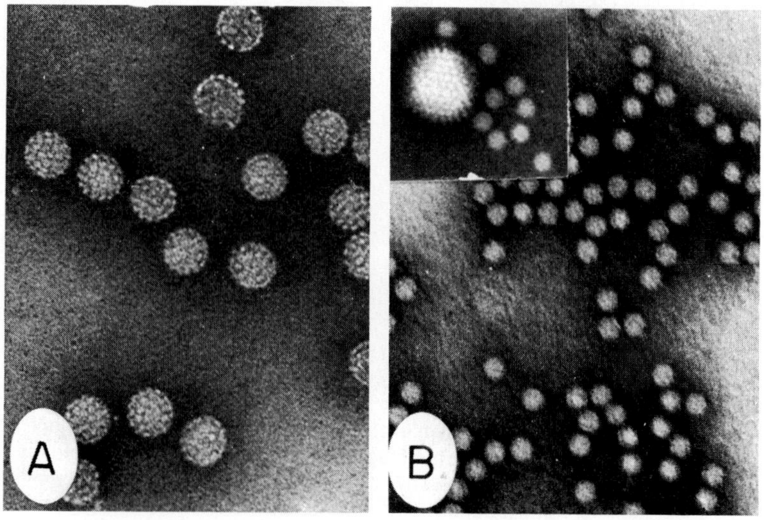

Fig. 53–13. **A.** The papovavirus SV40. × 160,000. **B.** The parvovirus adenoassociated virus (AAV) type 4. × 150,000. **Insert.** Particle of the simian adenovirus SV15, which enabled the AAV to multiply (Chap. 55). *(Courtesy of Dr. Heather Mayor.)*

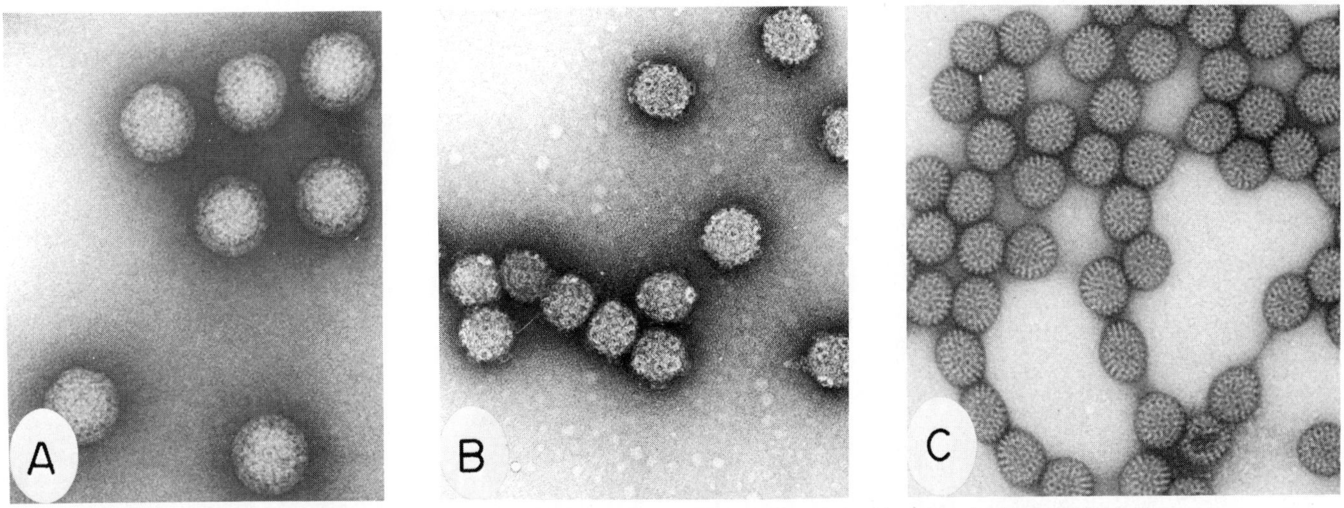

Fig. 53–14. Morphology of reovirus and human rotavirus. **A.** Reovirus. Note the double capsid shell. The arrangement of capsomers is clearly discernible at the periphery. × 120,000. **B.** Reovirus cores. Cores are derived from reovirus particles by digesting their outer capsid shell with chymotrypsin. Note the large spikes. There are 12, located as if situated on the 12 vertices of an icosahedron. They are hollow so as to permit messenger RNA molecules that are formed inside the virus particles to be liberated (Chap. 55). **C.** Human rotavirus. The morphology of rotaviruses and of orbiviruses is similar. × 136,000 *(**A,B** courtesy of Drs. R. B. Luftig and W. K. Joklik; **C** courtesy of Dr. Erskine Palmer, Centers for Disease Control, Atlanta.)*

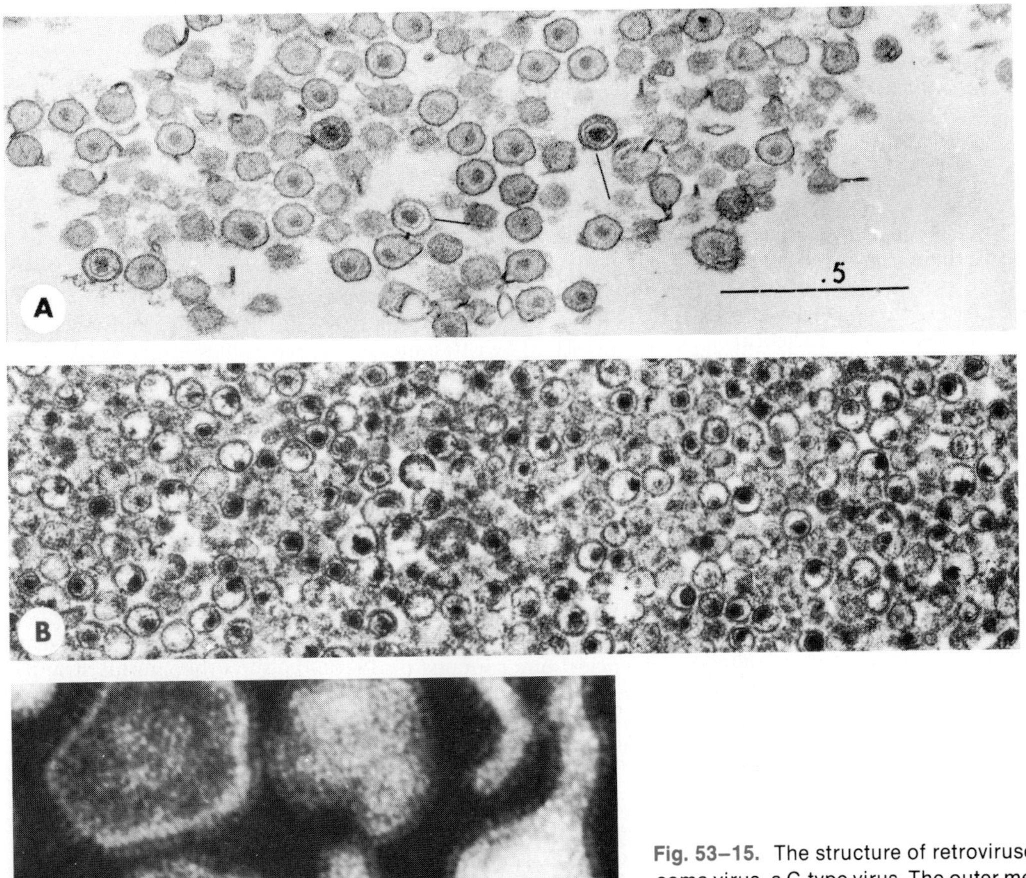

Fig. 53–15. The structure of retroviruses. **A.** Thin section of Rous sarcoma virus, a C-type virus. The outer membrane as well as the nucleoid are clearly visible (arrows). Note the central location of the nucleoid. × 52,000. **B.** Thin section of mouse mammary tumor virus, a B-type retrovirus. Note the eccentric location of the nucleoid. **C.** Mouse mammary tumor virus stained with phosphotungstate. Note the prominent glycoprotein spikes. *(**A** from Courington and Vogt: J Virol 1:400, 1967; **B, C** courtesy of Dr. D. Moore.)* See also Figures 59–7 and 59–8.

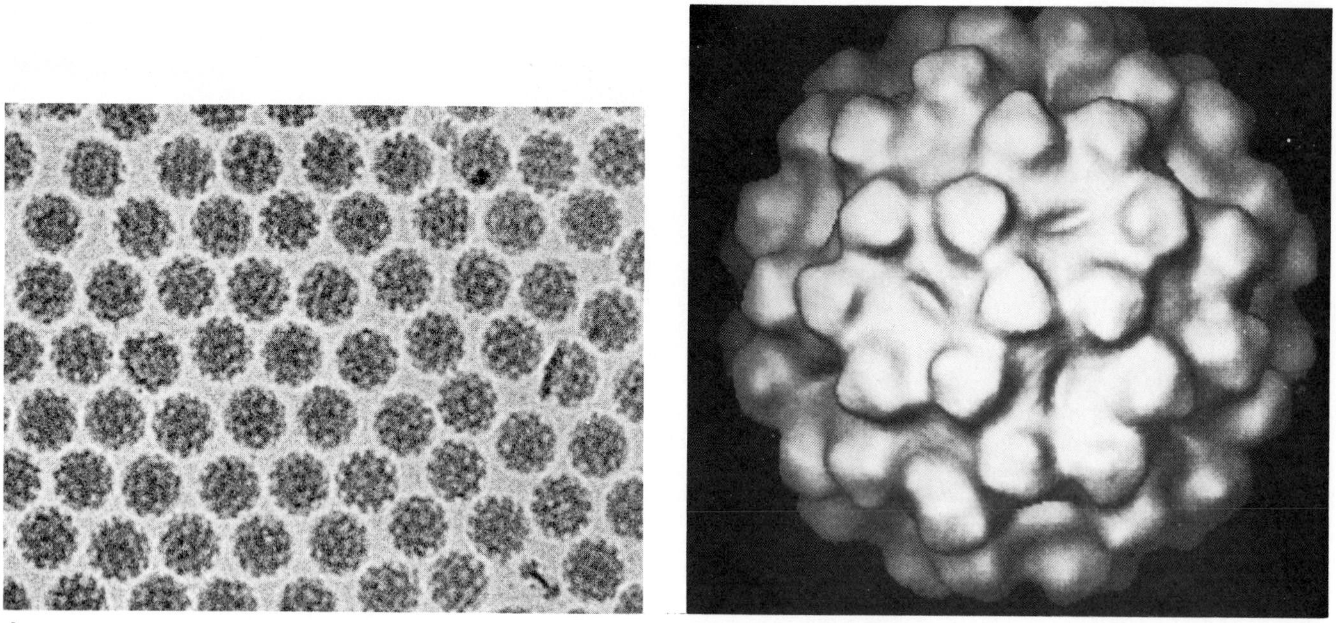

Fig. 53–16. A. Cryoelectron micrograph (unstained) of the togavirus Semliki Forest virus. × 140,000. The icosahedral arrangement of subunits is clearly visible. **B.** Surface representation of the very similar togavirus Sindbis virus as revealed by three-dimensional reconstruction of cryoelectron micrographs. Note the fivefold and sixfold axes of symmetry. See also Figure 55–35. *(Courtesy of Dr. S. D. Fuller.)*

Viral Nucleic Acids

The nucleic acids of animal viruses are astonishingly diverse. Some are DNA, others RNA; some are double-stranded, others single-stranded; some are linear, others circular; some have plus polarity, others minus polarity. Information concerning these and other properties of viral nucleic acids is essential for an understanding of the key reactions during virus multiplication cycles.

Size of Viral Nucleic Acids

The genome sizes of animal viruses vary over an almost 100-fold range. The smallest is that of hepatitis B virus; the largest are those of the poxviruses and of the herpesviruses (Fig. 53–21). Interestingly, the sizes of the genomes of RNA-containing viruses vary far less than those of DNA-containing viruses. Almost all are either 6 to 9 kb or 11 to 16 kb long (Table 53–2).

Structure of Viral Nucleic Acids

Strandedness

Both double-stranded and single-stranded DNA, as well as RNA, can act as the genome of animal viruses (Table 53–2).

Polarity

The single-stranded RNA molecules present in picornavirus, calicivirus, togavirus, coronavirus, and retrovirus particles can be translated by ribosomes and serve as messenger RNA. This is not the case for the RNA molecules present in ortho- and paramyxovirus, rhabdovirus, filovirus, bunyavirus, and arenavirus particles. These RNAs must first be transcribed into RNA strands of the opposite polarity, and it is these transcripts that are then translated by ribosomes. Because the polarity of messenger RNA is generally designated as plus, RNAs in the former group of viruses are said to be plus-stranded, and those in the latter group negative-stranded.

The adeno-associated satellite viruses, which belong to the parvovirus family and contain single-stranded DNA, present a unique situation. There are two kinds of these virus particles; one contains plus strands, the other minus strands. These two kinds of particles are produced in equal amounts. For other parvoviruses the proportion of particles that contain plus strands is much smaller, sometimes approaching zero.

Segmentation

Most viral genomes consist of single nucleic acid molecules, but the genomes of some viruses are segmented. In particular, the genomes of reoviruses and rotaviruses consist of 10 and 11 segments of double-stranded RNA, respectively (Fig. 53–22), and the genomes of influenza viruses, bunyaviruses, and arenaviruses consist of eight, three, and two single-stranded RNA molecules, respectively. One of the conse-

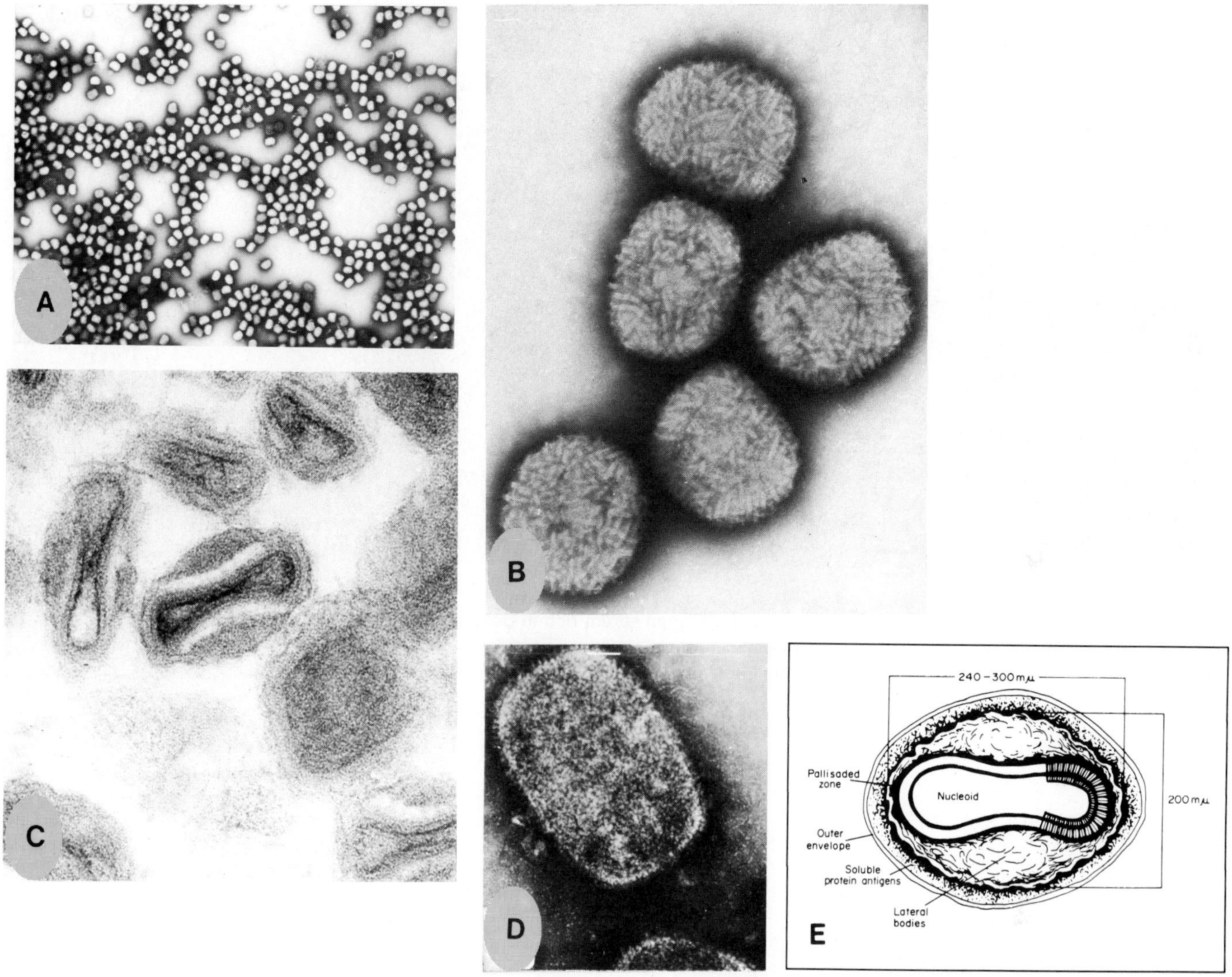

Fig. 53–17. The structure of vaccinia virus. **A.** A purified virus preparation. Note characteristic brick shape. × 6000. **B.** Vaccinia virus particles stained with phosphotungstate to reveal surface structure. Note the characteristic arrangement of rodlets or tubules. × 60,000. **C.** Cross-section of vaccinia virus particle. × 70,000. **D.** An isolated core, showing regular surface elements. × 90,000. **E.** A model of the vaccinia virus particle. *(**A, B, C** courtesy of Dr. Samuel Dales; **D** from Easterbrook: J Ultrastr Res 14:484, 1966; **E** adapted from Westwood et al: J Gen Microbiol 34:67, 1964.)*

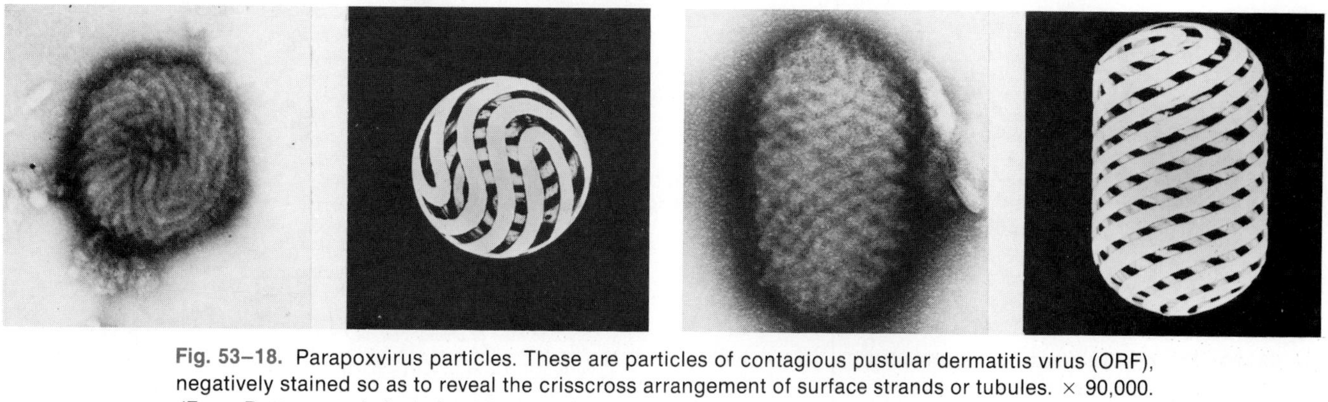

Fig. 53–18. Parapoxvirus particles. These are particles of contagious pustular dermatitis virus (ORF), negatively stained so as to reveal the crisscross arrangement of surface strands or tubules. × 90,000. *(From Buttner et al: Arch Ges Virusforsch 14:657, 1964.)*

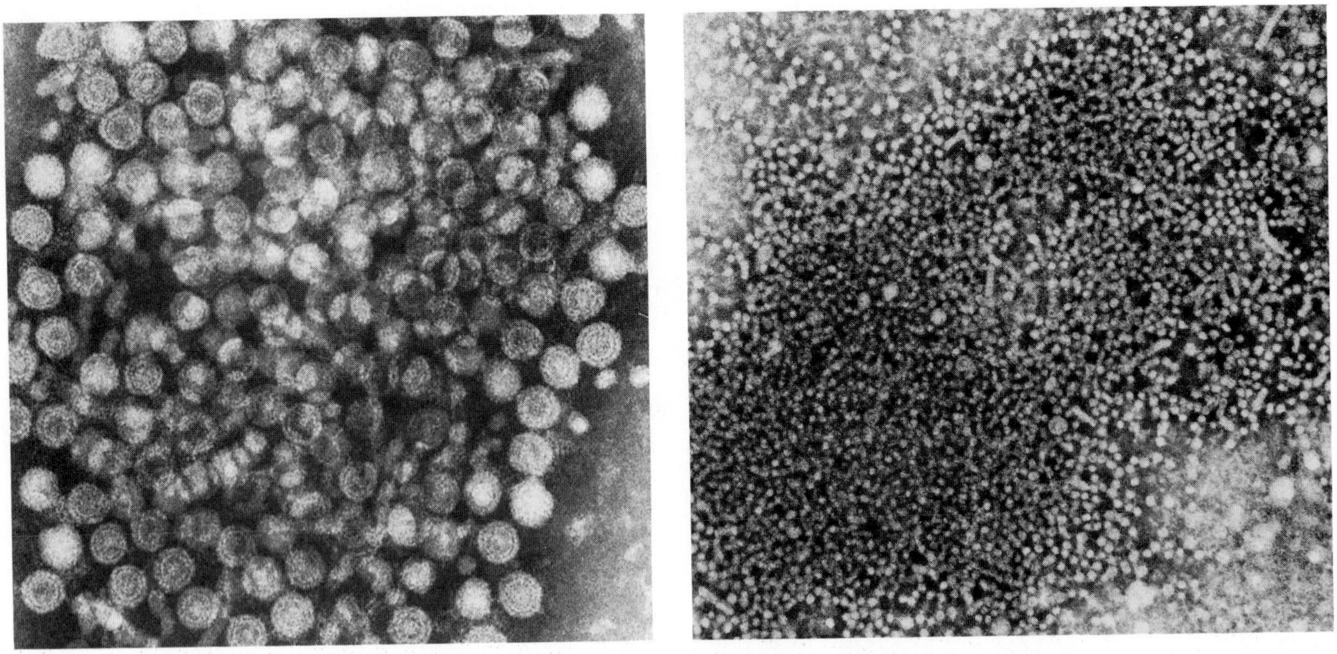

A B

Fig. 53–19. Hepatitis B virus (HBV). **A.** Human serum rich in Dane particles, the infectious virus particles. × 155,000. **B.** Human plasma showing primarily HBsAg (surface antigen) particles, some HBV (Dane) particles, and some filamentous forms. × 60,000. *(Courtesy of Dr. E. H. Cook.)*

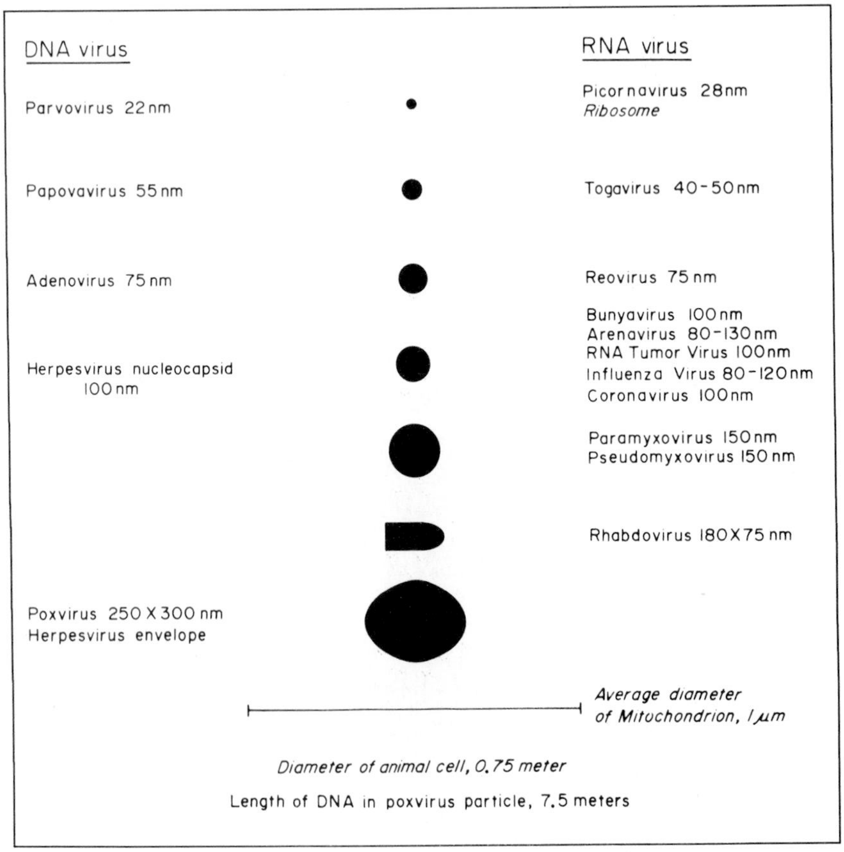

Fig. 53–20. The relative sizes of the principal families of animal viruses. Unless otherwise indicated, the scale is the same for all.

TABLE 53–1. THE MORPHOLOGY OF HUMAN VIRUSES

Virus Family	Morphology
DNA viruses	
Poxvirus	Complex
Herpesvirus	Enveloped icosahedral nucleocapsid
Adenovirus	Naked icosahedral nucleocapsid
Papovavirus	Naked icosahedral nucleocapsid
Hepadnavirus	Enveloped nucleocapsid
Parvovirus	Naked icosahedral nucleocapsid
RNA viruses	
Picornavirus	Naked icosahedral nucleocapsid
Calicivirus	Naked icosahedral nucleocapsid
Togavirus	Enveloped icosahedral nucleocapsid
Flavivirus	Enveloped icosahedral (?) nucleocapsid
Coronavirus	Enveloped helical nucleocapsid
Reovirus	Naked icosahedral nucleocapsid
Rhabdovirus	Enveloped helical nucleocapsid
Filovirus	Enveloped helical nucleocapsid
Paramyxovirus	Enveloped helical nucleocapsid
Orthomyxovirus	Enveloped helical nucleocapsid
Bunyavirus	Enveloped helical nucleocapsid
Arenavirus	Enveloped helical nucleocapsid
Retrovirus	Enveloped icosahedral (?) nucleocapsid

quences of segmentation is highly efficient genetic recombination caused by random reassortment of segments in multiply infected cells (Chaps. 55 and 57).

Circularity and Supercoiling

Most viral nucleic acids are linear, but papovavirus DNA exists in the form of supercoiled double-stranded circles. The reason why papovavirus DNA circles are supercoiled is as follows. Papovavirus DNAs, like SV40 DNA, exist in virus particles in the form of minichromosomes, that is, associated with nucleosomes (Fig. 53–23), like the chromatin of eucaryotic cells. Nucleosomes consist of two molecules of each of the four histones H3, H4, H2A, and H2B, and the DNA is wound around them. There are about 24 nucleosomes per SV40 DNA molecule. Because it is about 5200 base airs long, there are about 220 base pairs per nucleosome, 180 of which are intimately associated with each nucleosome, and 40 are present in the space between adjacent nucleosomes. Coiling the circular double-stranded DNA molecule around the nucleosomes requires a reduction in the number of helix turns per unit length if the resulting structure is to be devoid of strain. Therefore, when the nucleosomes are removed and the naked

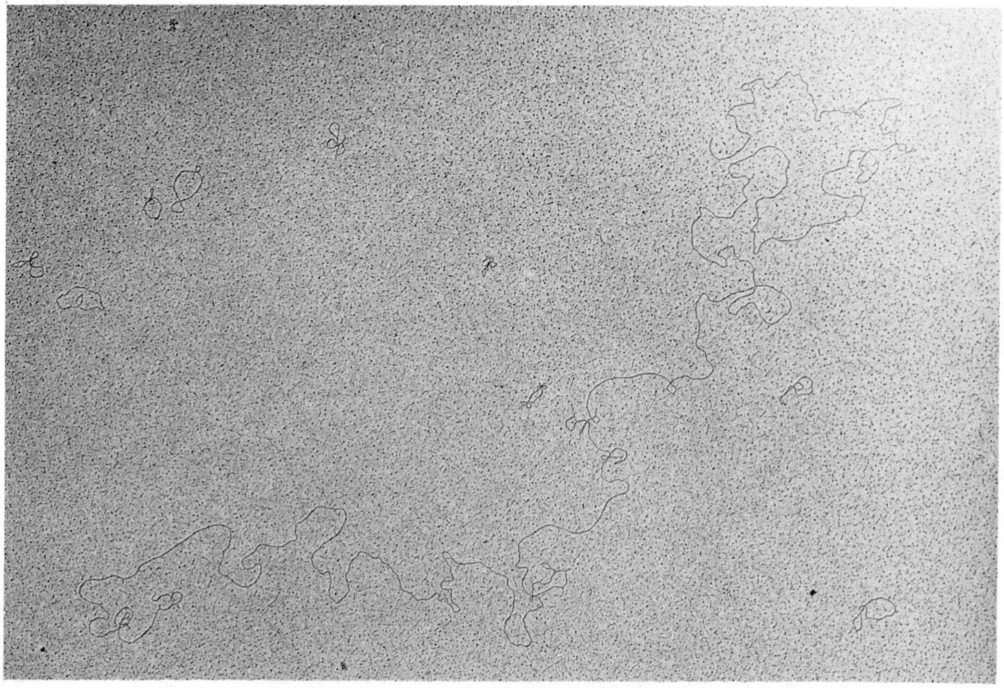

Fig. 53–21. Electron micrograph of an intact herpesvirus DNA molecule. It is about 44 μm long. The small circular molecules are intact DNA molecules of the bacteriophage ΦX 174 (Chap. 60), which were added to provide a size marker. *(Courtesy of Dr. Edward K. Wagner.)*

TABLE 53–2. CHARACTERISTICS OF THE NUCLEIC ACIDS OF HUMAN VIRUSES

Virus	Nature of Nucleic Acid	Size (kb or kbp)	Strandedness	Structure	Number of Segments	Polarity	Infectivity of Naked Nucleic Acid
Poxvirus	DNA	130–280	Double	Linear, crosslinked	1		−
Herpesvirus	DNA	130–220	Double	Linear	1		+
Adenovirus	DNA	36	Double	Linear	1		+
Papovavirus	DNA	5,8[a]	Double	Supercoiled circular	1		+
Hepadnavirus	DNA	3	Double	Linear, cohesive ends	1		−
Parvovirus	DNA	5	Single	Linear	1	+ and −[b]	+
Picornavirus	RNA	7	Single	Linear	1	+	+
Calicivirus	RNA	8	Single	Linear	1	+	+
Togavirus	RNA	12	Single	Linear	1	+	+
Flavivirus	RNA	11	Single	Linear	1	+	+
Coronavirus	RNA	27	Single	Linear	1	+	+
Reovirus	RNA	23	Double	Linear	10,11[c]		+
Rhabdovirus	RNA	11	Single	Linear	1	−	−
Filovirus	RNA	13	Single	Linear	1	−	−
Paramyxovirus	RNA	15	Single	Linear	1	−	−
Orthomyxovirus	RNA	14	Single	Linear	8	−	−
Bunyavirus	RNA	14	Single	Linear, cohesive ends	3	−	−
Arenavirus	RNA	11	Single	Linear, cohesive ends	2	−	−
Retrovirus	RNA	5–9	Single	Linear	2[d]	+	−

[a] 8 kb for papillomaviruses, 5 kb for all others.
[b] Genus *Parvovirus*, 50%–99% −, remainder +; genus *Dependovirus* (adeno-associated virus, AAV) and genus *Densovirus*, 50% −, 50% +.
[c] Orthoreoviruses and orbiviruses, 10 segments; rotaviruses, 11 segments.
[d] The genome is not segmented, but diploid; the two molecules are identical.

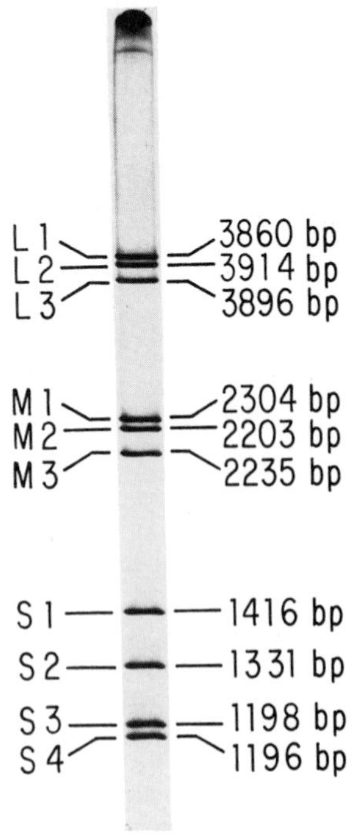

Fig. 53–22. The structure of the reovirus genome. RNA extracted from reovirus particles by treatment with the detergent sodium dodecyl sulfate (SDS) was subjected to electrophoresis in a polyacrylamide gel. In such gels, molecules of various sizes migrate as discrete bands, the smallest ones moving fastest. The direction of migration in the gel shown here was from top to bottom. Bands of RNA were visualized by autoradiography. Each band corresponds to a reovirus genome segment. The reovirus genome is seen to consist of 10 molecular species that fall into three size classes, designated L, M, and S. Because the rate of migration is inversely proportional to the square of the molecular weight, estimates of relative molecular weights can be made by measuring the distances traveled by the various bands. The sizes of the 10 reovirus genes are indicated at the right of the gel.

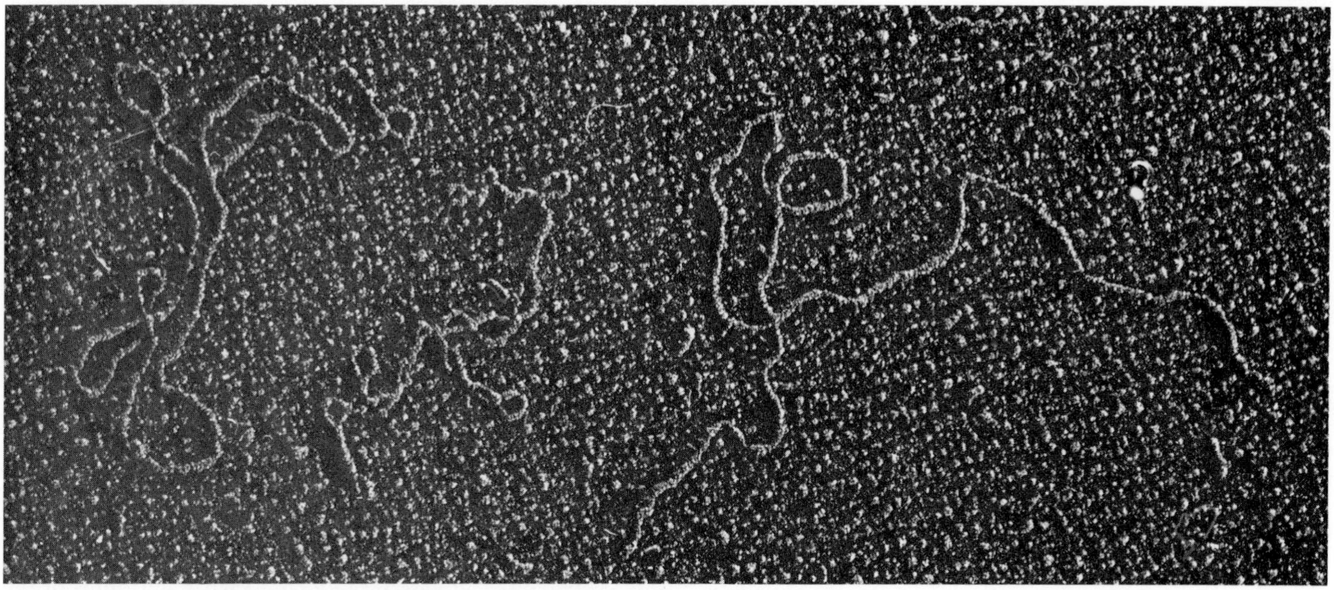

A

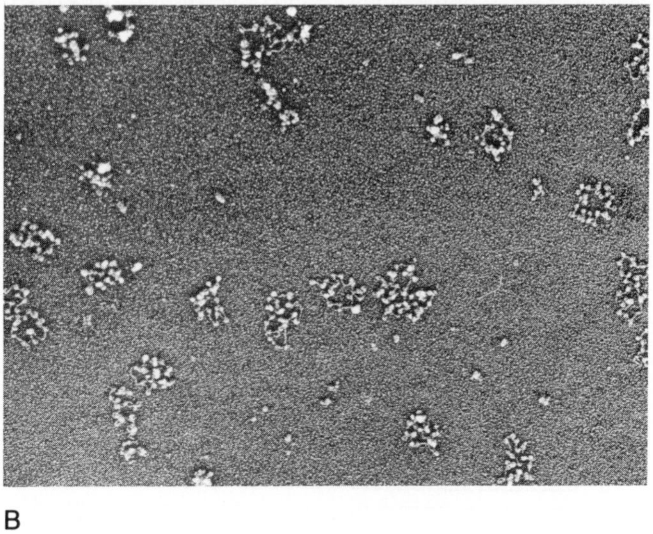

B

Fig. 53–23. A. The three forms of papovavirus DNA. In the center is a supercoiled twisted circular molecule, which is the form in which the DNA exists within the virus. To the left is a relaxed circular molecule, in which one strand has been nicked by treatment with deoxyribonuclease, thereby relieving the supercoiling by permitting free rotation of the remaining intact strand. On the right is a linear molecule, generated by the introduction of nicks close to one another in both strands. × 66,000. *(Courtesy of Dr. H. J. Bujard.)* **B.** Electron micrograph of the SV40 DNA nucleoprotein complex in the chromatinlike beads-on-a-string nucleosome conformation. × 50,000. *(From Keller and Mueller: Science 201:406, 1978.)*

DNA is examined in pure form, it is supercoiled, the supercoiling being due to the deficiency in helical turns. For the SV40 DNA molecule, the deficiency is about 24 helical turns. The negative supercoils are introduced into the DNA by the enzyme DNA gyrase, which is a topoisomerase, a class of enzymes that catalyze adenosine triphosphate-dependent changes in the linking number of circular DNA; that is, they coil the DNA helix axis by causing DNA strands to pass "through" DNA strands by transiently breaking them. Supercoiling is relieved by the action of untwisting enzymes, which are also topoisomerases (DNA gyrase being the only topoisomerase that *introduces* supercoils), or of nucleases that nick one strand, or by the intercalation of substances such as ethidium bromide (Fig. 53–24).

Terminal Redundancy

The nucleic acids of several animal viruses are terminally redundant; that is, their base composition may be represented as A, B, C. . . . X, Y, Z, A, where A, B, C, and so on are nucleotide sequences. The presence of terminal repeats is most readily demonstrated, in the case of double-stranded DNAs, by treating them briefly with bacteriophage λ exonuclease, which digests DNA strands from their 5′-phosphate-containing termini. In this way, one end of one strand and the other end of the other strand are digested. On melting and reannealing, DNA digested in this manner circularizes, indicating that the two single-stranded regions at the two ends are complementary and, hence, that the sequences must be repeats of each other (Fig. 53–25). Both herpesvirus DNA

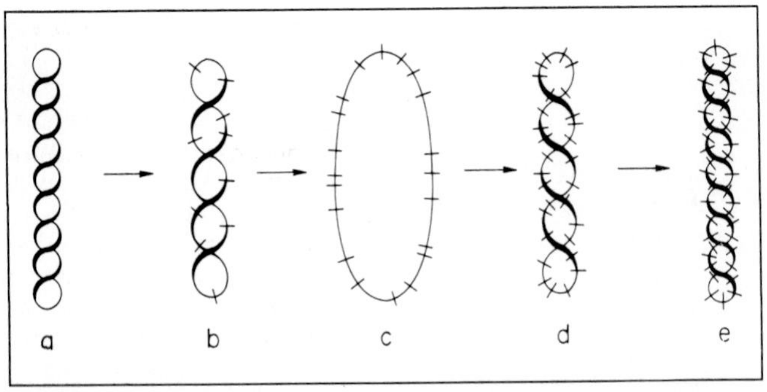

Fig. 53–24. Diagrammatic representation of the removal and reversal of supercoiling turns by intercalation of ethidium bromide. The Watson-Crick helix is here represented as a single continuous line. The number of supercoiling turns in the original molecule **(a)** decreases as ethidium bromide molecules (represented by bars perpendicular to the helix axis) bind to the DNA and intercalate between base pairs **(b)**. At equivalence, the accumulated untwisting due to the number of intercalated drug molecules balances the initial number of supercoiling turns **(c)**. Intercalation of further drug molecules **(d)** leads to the introduction of supercoiling turns in the opposite sense **(e)**. *(From Crawford and Waring: J Gen Virol 1:387, 1967.)*

and retrovirus RNA possess repeated sequences of this type that are about 500 and 50 to 200 residues long, respectively.

Adenovirus, parvovirus, and poxvirus DNAs, as well as rhabdovirus, bunyavirus, and arenavirus RNAs, are also terminally redundant, but here the repeated sequences are the inverted or reversed complements of each other; that is, their structure is of the form 5′-GATCAT . . . ATGATC-3′. This is demonstrated, for those viral genomes that are double-stranded DNA, by the fact that here single-stranded DNA circles form on melting and reannealing (Fig. 53–26). The length of inverted terminal repeats (ITRs) generally varies from 20 to 150 residues, but for poxvirus DNAs may exceed 10,000 base pairs (more than 5% of the length of the genome).

The significance of the various forms of terminal redundancy is no doubt related to the mode of replication and expression of these nucleic acids. Examples of situations in which the reasons for terminal redundancy seem clear are described in Chapters 59 and 60.

Crosslinking

The DNAs of poxviruses are unique in being crosslinked covalently at their ends. This is shown by the fact that when these DNAs are melted, single-stranded circles are generated whose circumference is twice the length of the linear double-stranded poxvirus DNA molecules. The structure of the ends of vaccinia virus DNA is shown in Figure 53–27.

Covalent Linkage with Protein

Several viral nucleic acids are linked covalently to protein molecules. For example, the RNA of picornaviruses like poliovirus is linked at its 5′-terminus to the tyrosine residue of a 22 amino acid-long protein, and each 5′-terminus of the double-stranded DNA of adenoviruses is linked to a protein with a molecular weight of about 55 kDa. The 5′-terminus of calicivirus RNA, of the minus strand of hepatitis B virus DNA, and of parvovirus DNA also is linked to protein. These proteins function as primers in the replication of these nucleic acids and/or as packaging signals.

Infectivity of Viral Nucleic Acids

Viral nucleic acids contain all the information necessary for the formation of virus particles. This was first shown by Hershey and Chase in 1952, when they found that the

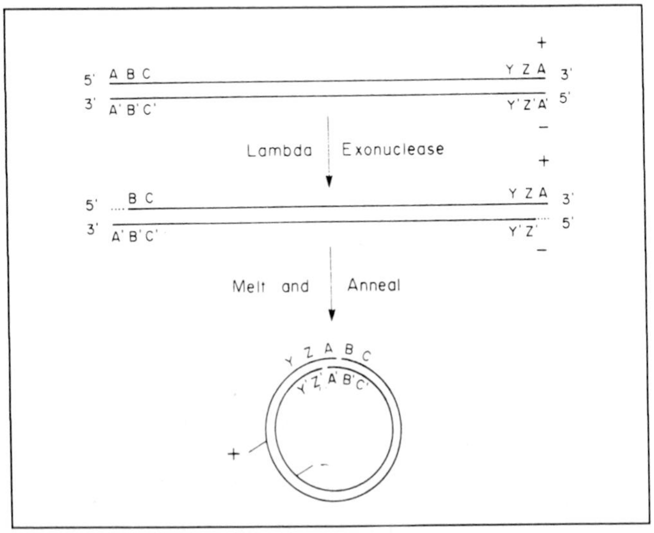

Fig. 53–25. Demonstration of terminal repeats in double-stranded DNA. Note that the A–A′ sequences that are paired in the circularized molecule were located originally at opposite ends of the linear molecule.

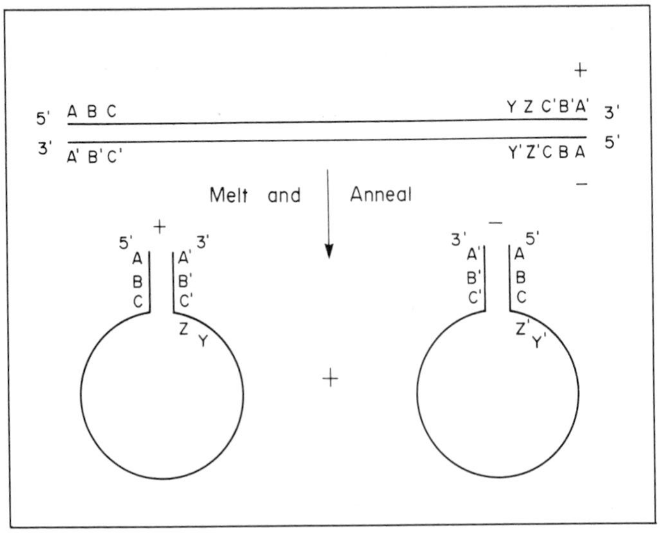

Fig. 53–26. Demonstration of the presence of inverted terminal repeats (ITRs).

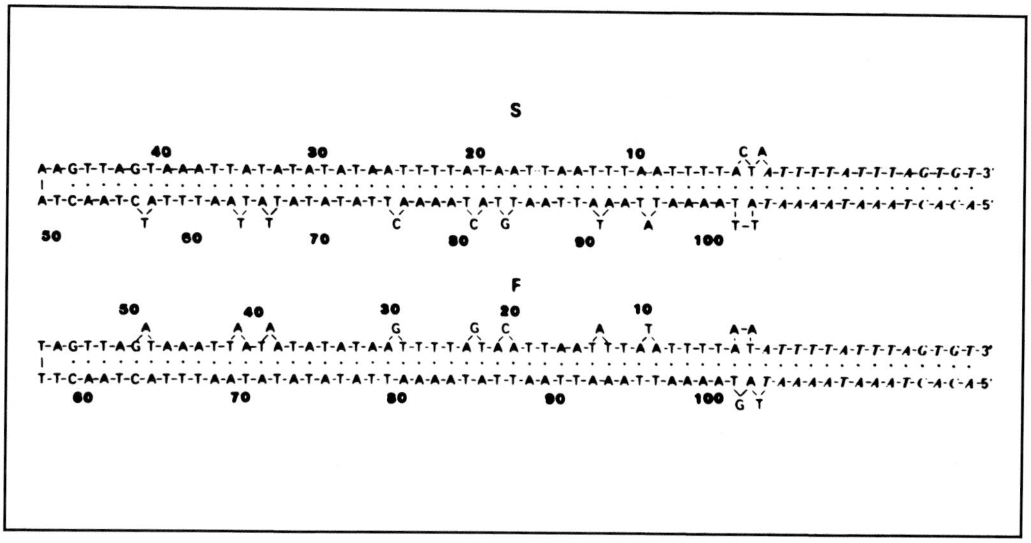

Fig. 53–27. The structure of the ends of the DNA of vaccinia virus strain WR. The terminal region, to the left of the sequences in italics, exists in two equally abundant forms, S and F, which are inverted complements of each other. These sequences can be written in the form of the two almost, but not quite, perfectly base-paired continuous structures shown here. Since vaccinia virus DNA possesses inverted terminal repeats, its two ends are identical. *(From Baroudy et al: Cell 28:315, 1982; Pickup et al: Virology 124:215, 1983.)*

introduction of naked bacteriophage DNA into bacterial cells resulted in the formation of progeny virus particles. Later, in 1956, Gierer and Schramm showed that the same was true for RNA when they found that RNA extracted from tobacco mosaic virus particles was infectious.

The nucleic acids of several groups of animal viruses, such as the picornaviruses, togaviruses, flaviviruses, coronaviruses, parvoviruses, papovaviruses, adenoviruses, and herpesviruses, also are infectious (Table 53–2). These are all nucleic acids that either can act as messenger RNA themselves or are transcribed into messenger RNA by cellular RNA polymerases. Viral nucleic acids that are transcribed into messenger RNA by *virus-coded* polymerases (see below), such as the negative-stranded RNAs of ortho- and paramyxoviruses, rhabdoviruses, bunyaviruses, and arenaviruses, and the double-stranded DNAs of poxviruses, are not infectious, since they cannot express themselves in cells.

In all cases, the naked nucleic acids are less infectious by factors ranging from 10^3 to 10^6 than the virus particles from which they were extracted. There are two principal reasons for this. First, naked viral nucleic acids are quickly degraded by nucleases, which are generally present in extracellular fluids, as well as on outer cell membranes; second, naked nucleic acids are taken up very poorly by cells. Uptake can be increased significantly by complexing naked nucleic acids with polycations such as protamine or DEAE-dextran, adsorbing them to precipitated calcium phosphate, which is taken up well by cells, or by lipofecting them into cells on liposomes. The inefficiency with which naked viral nucleic acids penetrate into cells emphasizes the role of the viral capsid in this vital function.

The host range of naked viral nucleic acids is much broader than that of the respective virus particles. This stems from the fact that viral host range is restricted by the specificity of the interactions between virus particles and their cell surface receptors (Chap. 55). This is not the case for naked viral nucleic acids. For example, whereas poliovirus can infect and therefore multiply only in cells of human or primate origin, poliovirus RNA can also infect chick cells and mouse cells.

Presence of Host Cell Nucleic Acids in Virus Particles

As a rule, virus particles contain only viral nucleic acids. Sometimes, however, segments of host nucleic acid become encapsidated instead. For example, particles exist that contain, within a papovavirus capsid, a linear piece of host DNA roughly the same size as papovavirus DNA. Each such particle, known as a *pseudovirion*, contains a different segment of host DNA. Pseudovirions usually make up only a small fraction of the virus yield, but in some cell lines the majority of progeny polyomavirus particles are pseudovirions.

Viral Proteins

The principal constituent of all animal viruses is protein. All such proteins are referred to as structural proteins, since their primary function is to serve as virus particle building blocks. They are almost always encoded by the viral genome.

Structural viral proteins vary widely in size, from less than 10 to more than 150 kDa. They also vary in number, some virus particles containing as few as three species, others more than 50. Viral proteins are characterized most conveniently by dissociating highly purified virus preparations with detergent and subjecting the resulting protein mixtures to electrophoresis in polyacrylamide gels. The most commonly used detergent is sodium dodecyl sulfate (SDS), which not only destroys the secondary structure of proteins but also forms complexes with them. These complexes carry numerous strong negative charges, so that on electrophoresis in polyacrylamide gels, they migrate primarily according to size. As a result, SDS-PAGE (polyacrylamide gel electrophoresis) provides a very convenient technique for determining not only the number of different protein species that make up virus particles, but also their sizes. The SDS-PAGE profile of vaccinia virus proteins is shown in Figure 53–28.

All members of the same virus family display the same or almost the same highly characteristic electrophoretic protein patterns. The patterns of reovirus, rhinovirus, murine encephalomyelitis (ME) virus, and Sendai virus (a paramyxovirus) proteins are illustrated in Figure 53–29.

Glycoproteins

Viral envelopes usually contain glycoproteins in the form of spikes or projections. As a rule, these spikes are oligomers. For example, the two types of spikes on the surface of influenza virus particles are trimers and tetramers, respectively, of the hemagglutinin and neuraminidase proteins (see below). The

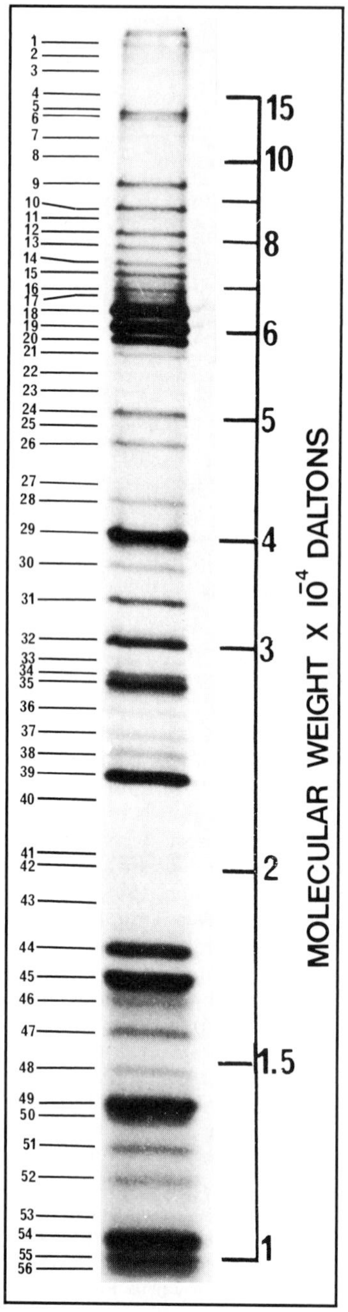

Fig. 53–28. SDS-PAGE of vaccinia virus structural proteins. Vaccinia virus labeled with ^{35}S-methionine was dissociated in a buffer containing sodium dodecyl sulfate and electrophoresed in a 10% polyacrylamide gel. An autoradiogram was then prepared from it by exposing it to x-ray film. The direction of electrophoresis was from top to bottom. Over 50 proteins are clearly visible. There is evidence that the vaccinia virus particle may comprise as many as 100 different species of proteins. (*From Dales: Virology 95:355, 1979.*)

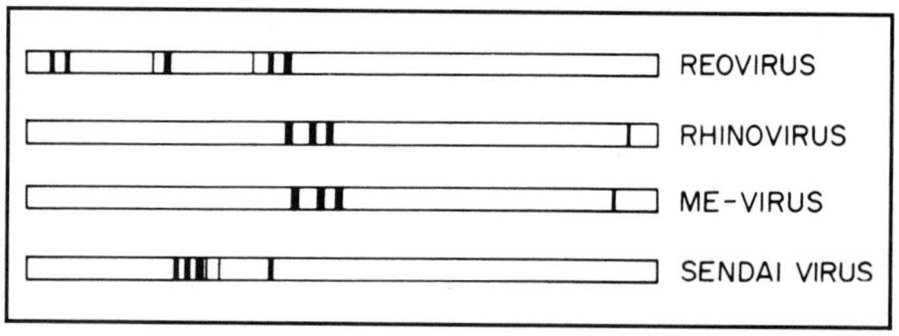

Fig. 53–29. Drawings of polyacrylamide gel patterns of the proteins of reovirus, rhinovirus, murine encephalomyelitis (ME) virus, and Sendai virus. Highly purified preparations of these viruses were dissolved in buffer containing sodium dodecyl sulfate (SDS). The illustration shows gels in which the SDS complexes of the proteins of these four viruses had been electrophoresed from left to right. The location of each band is a measure of its molecular weight. Thus the largest protein shown is the leftmost protein of reovirus (mol wt about 145 kDa); the smallest, the rightmost protein of rhinovirus (mol wt about 7 kDa). The relative amount of each protein is indicated by the thickness of the band representing it. It is clear from the gel patterns shown that the protein complements of rhinovirus and ME virus, both picornaviruses, are very similar and that they are quite different from those of reovirus and Sendai virus.

carbohydrate moieties of the glycoproteins consist of oligosaccharides comprising 10 to 15 monosaccharide units that are linked to the protein backbone through N- and O-glycosidic bonds involving asparagine and serine or threonine, respectively. Their principal components are generally galactose and galactosamine, glucose and glucosamine, fucose, mannose, and sialic acid, which always occupies a terminal position.

It was long thought that the structure of the oligosaccharides of viral glycoproteins is specified solely by the nature and relative abundance of the various host cell glycosyl transferases that assemble them from their monosaccharide components. This is certainly an important factor, but it now appears that the nature of the protein that is being glycosylated also influences oligosaccharide structure. As a result, the oligosaccharides of viral glycoproteins may differ from those of cellular glycoproteins. Further, the oligosaccharides of glycoproteins of different viruses grown in the same cell are probably not identical, and the oligosaccharides of the glycoproteins of the same virus grown in different cells are also probably different, although no doubt closely related. The structure of the oligosaccharide of the spike glycoprotein of vesicular stomatitis virus is shown in Figure 53–30.

Viral Proteins with Specialized Functions

Some viral proteins have specialized properties and functions. Among them are the following.

Hemagglutinins

Many animal viruses, both naked and enveloped, agglutinate the red blood cells of certain animal species. This property, which is called *hemagglutination*, reflects the fact that such red cells possess receptors for certain surface components of virus particles that function as cell attachment proteins. In the case of ortho- and paramyxoviruses, these viral surface components, called hemagglutinins, are glycoprotein spikes present

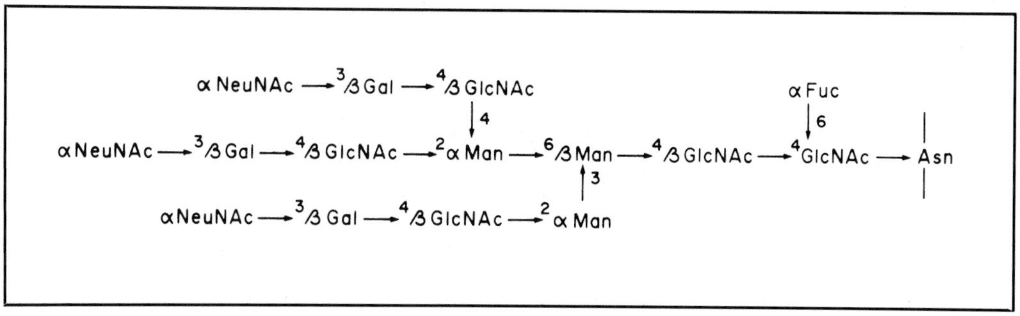

Fig. 53–30. The structure of the oligosaccharide unit of the vesicular stomatitis virus spike glycoprotein. There are two of these units per protein molecule. Asn, asparagine; GlcNAc, *N*-acetylglycosamine; Man, mannose; Gal, galactose; NeuNAc, *N*-acetyl-neuraminic acid; Fuc, fucose. (*From Reading et al: J Biol Chem: 253:5600, 1978.*)

on the virus particle surface (see Fig. 53–4). The ability to hemagglutinate can be used to quantitate viruses (Chap. 52).

Enzymes

Virus particles often contain enzymes (Table 53–3). Among them are the following.

1. Orthomyxovirus and paramyxovirus particles contain an enzyme, neuraminidase, that hydrolyzes the galactose-*N*-acetylneuraminic acid bond at the ends of the oligosaccharide chains of glycoproteins and glycolipids, thereby liberating *N*-acetylneuraminic acid. Like the hemagglutinin, this enzyme forms glycoprotein spikes. Orthomyxoviruses possess two types of spikes, one with hemagglutinin and the other with neuraminidase activity. Paramyxoviruses also possess two types of spikes, on one of which both activities are located. The primary function of neuraminidase appears to be to facilitate the release of virus particles from the cells in which they were formed. The reason why the release of these viruses requires a special enzyme is that their hemagglutinins possess strong affinity for the sialic acid (*N*-acetylneuraminic acid) residues at the ends of oligosaccharide chains. By hydrolyzing them, the enzyme permits the liberation of virus particles that would otherwise not not be released, readsorb immediately after being liberated, or aggregate with each other.

   Influenza C virus strains do not possess neuraminidase. Instead, they contain an acetyl esterase that cleaves the acetyl group from 9-0-acetylated neuraminic acid. Coronaviruses possess a similar enzyme.
2. Many virus particles contain RNA polymerases. The necessity for such enzymes stems from the fact that viral genomes must be able to express themselves once they have gained access to the interior of host cells. If viral genomes can act as messenger RNA, like picornavirus or togavirus RNA, there is no problem. If they cannot, either because they are double-stranded or negative-stranded RNA, or because they are DNA, RNA with plus polarity must first be synthesized. There are two possible sources for the enzymes necessary for this purpose. The first is enzymes existing in host cells. Herpesvirus, adenovirus, and papovavirus DNAs are transcribed into messenger RNA by DNA-dependent RNA polymerases specified by host cells. Alternatively, the virus particle itself must contain the enzyme. Examples of this type are the poxviruses that possess a DNA-dependent RNA polymerase, reoviruses that possess an RNA-dependent RNA polymerase, and negative RNA-stranded viruses that contain RNA polymerases that transcribe plus RNA strands from the minus RNA strands present within them. These enzymes are usually not active in intact virus particles but are activated when the envelope or capsid is partially degraded, which generally occurs very soon after infection.
3. Retroviruses possess a DNA polymerase, the so-called reverse transcriptase, which transcribes their single-stranded RNA into double-stranded DNA, which is then integrated into the host cell genome (Chap. 59).

TABLE 53–3. ENZYMES IN HUMAN VIRUSES

Virus	Enzyme
DNA Viruses	
Poxvirus	DNA-dependent RNA polymerase Messenger RNA capping enzymes Poly (A) polymerase Nicking–joining enzyme DNA-dependent nucleotide phosphohydrolase Topoisomerase Protein kinase
Herpesvirus	None
Adenovirus	None
Papovavirus	None
Hepatitis virus	DNA polymerase
Parvovirus	None
RNA Viruses	
Picornavirus	None
Calicivirus	None
Togavirus	None
Flavivirus	None
Coronavirus	Acetyl esterase
Reovirus	RNA-dependent RNA polymerase Nucleotide phosphohydrolase Messenger RNA capping enzymes
Rhabdovirus	RNA-dependent RNA polymerase
Paramyxovirus	Neuraminidase RNA-dependent RNA polymerase
Orthomyxovirus	Neuraminidase or acetyl esterase RNA-dependent RNA polymerase
Bunyavirus	RNA-dependent RNA polymerase
Arenavirus	RNA-dependent RNA polymerase
Retrovirus	RNA-dependent DNA polymerase (reverse transcriptase) Ribonuclease H Endonuclease (integrase?) Protease

Furthermore, hepatitis B virus contains a DNA polymerase capable of transcribing both DNA and RNA into DNA (Chap. 55).

All these enzymes are virus-specified. The evidence for this conclusion is provided by the existence of virus strains that contain variant enzymes and the fact that the enzymes in question often simply do not exist in uninfected cells.

Viruses often also contain other enzymes. Among them are the enzymes that modify both ends of the messenger RNA molecules synthesized by their polymerases, notably the capping enzymes and poly(A) polymerase. Further, retroviruses contain a protease that functions during maturation, as well as nucleases that function during reverse transcription and during integration of proviral DNA into the cellular genome. The complex poxviruses also contain deoxyribonucleases, DNA-dependent phosphohydrolases, and a topoisomerase that probably function during DNA replication.

Viral Lipids

Viral envelopes contain complex mixtures of neutral lipids, phospholipids, and glycolipids. As a rule, the composition of these mixtures resembles that of the membranes of the host cells in which the virus multiplied. As the lipid composition of membranes varies markedly from one cell strain to another and even for the same cell strain depending on the composition of the medium, this means that the same virus grown in different cell strains may have different neutral lipid, phospholipid, and glycolipid complements, even though its biologic properties are identical.

The nature and extent of the differences in composition that are encountered are well illustrated by the example of the paramyxovirus SV5. On average, this virus contains about 20% total lipid, of which roughly 25% and 5% are cholesterol and triglycerides, respectively; 55% are phospholipids, and 15% are glycolipids. If grown in cells the membranes of which have a molar ratio of cholesterol to phospholipid of 0.81, the ratio for the viral envelope is 0.89; if the cellular ratio is 0.51, that for the viral envelope is 0.60. The same holds for the relative amounts of several phospholipids. If the ratio of phosphatidylcholine to phosphatidylethanolamine in host cell membranes is 3.55, the ratio in the viral envelops is 2.55; if the ratio in host cell membranes is 0.8, the ratio in the viral envelope is 0.6. However, for one cell the ratio is 1.6, whereas that in the viral envelope derived from it is 0.6, which suggests that a limited degree of lipid selection is possible.

Classification of Animal Viruses

Attempts to devise a system of classification for animal viruses began almost as soon as their importance as pathogens became apparent. However, the criteria on which to base such a system have changed with advances in our knowledge of their nature and properties. For example, host range cannot be such a criterion; not only is each animal species subject to infection by a wide variety of viral agents, but also numerous viruses infect several different animal species. Similarly, the pattern of pathogenesis of the disease that is caused is an unreliable foundation on which to base a system of classification.

Criteria for Virus Classification

Viruses are classified according to a three-level system. Virus strains that are recognizably different in more than one gene (i.e., excluding mutants and variants) are designated species, species that exhibit readily apparent genetic similarity are grouped together into genera, and genera are grouped into families based on morphology, on the physical and chemical nature of viral components, and on the molecular strategies used by viral genomes to express themselves and to replicate.

Morphology

The primary criterion for classification is morphology. It is easy to apply because it does not require purified virus. Virus particles can be examined either within cells, that is, in thin sections of infected tissue, or in their extracellular state. Morphologic detail is usually brought out by shadowing with thin films of some heavy metal, such as uranium or tungsten, by staining with osmic acid or uranyl acetate, or by negative staining with phosphotungstic acid.

Physical and Chemical Nature of Viral Components

Morphologic similarity correlates closely with similarity of viral components. For example, all viruses with the morphology of adenoviruses contain double-stranded DNA genomes about 35 kbp long; all togaviruses contain plus-stranded RNA genomes, and all reoviruses contain segmented double-stranded RNA genomes about 23 kbp long. In fact, a system of virus classification based on the structure and size of viral genomes yields the same grouping as one based on morphology. Similarly, viruses with similar morphology are composed of similar populations of proteins, and a classification system based on polyacrylamide gel patterns, such as illustrated in Figures 53–28 and 53–29, again yields the same grouping.

Strategies Used for Gene Expression and Replication

Classification according to morphology and nature of virion components correlates exactly with yet a third viral characteristic: the strategy used by viral genomes to express themselves and to replicate. For example, although picornaviruses, togaviruses, and coronaviruses all possess plus-stranded RNA genomes, the strategies used by each to express the information encoded by them are quite different. On the other hand, reoviruses and rotaviruses are unrelated as judged by nucleic acid base sequence and immunologic criteria, but they possess a similar morphology and similar nucleic acid and protein components judged by size, number of species, and function, and they use the same strategies for gene expression and replication; both are therefore Reoviridae.

Major Families of Animal Viruses

Table 53–4 presents a summary of the distinguishing characteristics of the major families of animal viruses, together with a list of the most important animal and human pathogens in each. It is based in large part on recommendations made by the International Committee on Taxonomy of Viruses.

TABLE 53–4. THE MAJOR FAMILIES OF ANIMAL VIRUSES

DNA-containing Viruses

Poxviridae

- All genera except *Parapoxvirus*: Brick-shaped complex particles, whorled surface filament pattern
- Dimensions: 225 × 300 nm
- *Parapoxvirus*: Ovoid complex particles, regular surface filament pattern
- Dimensions: 150 × 200 nm

Strains pathogenic for many animal species exist. There are eight genera approved by the International Committee for the Taxonomy of Viruses (ICTV). The members of each are closely related antigenically but share only one major antigen with members of the others. Poxviruses multiply in the cytoplasm.

Subfamily	*Host*	*Symptoms in Humans*
Chordopoxvirinae (poxviruses of vertebrates)		
Genus *Orthopoxvirus*		
Variola major	Humans	Smallpox
Variola minor	Humans	Alastrim
Monkeypox	Monkey, humans	Smallpoxlike disease
Vaccinia	Cattle	—
Cowpox	Cattle, humans	Vesicular eruption of the skin
Ectromelia (mousepox)	Mouse	—
Buffalopox	Buffalo	—
Genus *Leporipoxvirus*		
Myxoma	Rabbit	—
Rabbit fibroma	Rabbit	—
Hare fibroma	Hare	—
Squirrel fibroma	Squirrel	—
Genus *Avipoxvirus*		
Fowlpox	Chicken	—
Other birdpox viruses	Various birds	—
Genus *Capripoxvirus*		
Sheeppox	Sheep	—
Goatpox	Goat	—
Lumpy skin disease	Cattle	—
Genus *Suipoxvirus*		
Swinepox	Pig	—
Genus *Parapoxvirus*		
Orf (contagious pustular dermatitis, CPD)	Sheep, goats, humans	Nodules on hands
Pseudocowpox (milker's nodule virus)	Cattle, humans	Nodules on hands
Bovine papular stomatitis	Cattle	—
Genus *Molluscipoxvirus*		
Molluscum contagiosum	Humans	Benign epidermal tumors
Genus *Yatapoxvirus*		
Yaba monkey tumor virus	Monkeys, humans	Benign epidermal tumors that soon regress
Tanapox	Monkeys, humans	Acute febrile illness with pox-like localized skin lesions
Entomopoxvirinae (poxviruses of insects)		
Various strains	Coleoptera, lepidoptera, diptera	—

Herpesviridae

- Enveloped icosahedral nucleocapsids
- Diameter of enveloped particles: 180–250 nm
- Diameter of naked nucleocapsids: 100 nm

The classification of herpesviruses is based both on biologic properties and on genome structure. Alphaherpesviruses are neurotropic viruses with either GC-rich (66%–68% GC) (genus *Simplexvirus*) or AT-rich (46% GC) (genus *Varicellavirus*) coding sequences. Alphaherpesviruses have a variable host range (from very wide to very narrow); usually have a relatively short replication cycle; are often highly cytopathic in cultured cells; frequently establish latent infections in sensory ganglia; and possess a genome that is about 150 kbp long. Betaherpesviruses are the salivary gland inclusion viruses. Cells infected with them often become enlarged (cytomegaly); hence the name. Their coding sequences are GC-rich (55%–60% GC). They have a narrow host range and a relatively long replication cycle; are less cytopathic than alphaviruses; frequently establish latent infections in secretory glands (salivary gland) and other tissues, including lymphoreticular cells and kidneys; and possess a genome that is about 230 kbp long. Gammaherpesviruses include the GC-rich (60% GC) lymphotropic viruses of humans and Old World monkeys and the AT-rich (36% GC) lymphotropic viruses of New World monkeys and lower vertebrates. Gammaherpesviruses have a narrow host range; a predilection for lymphoblastoid cells in which they frequently establish latent infections but which they can also transform (i.e., they can cause tumors); are specific for either T or B lymphocytes; and possess genomes that are about 150 kbp long.

Few herpesviruses are closely related to each other as judged by DNA–DNA hybridization, but most show some relatedness (2%–10% cross-hybridization). Almost all herpesviruses possess some common antigenic determinants. Herpesviruses cause type A nuclear inclusions (single large acidophilic inclusion bodies separated from basophilic marginated chromatin by a nonstaining halo).

(continued)

TABLE 53–4. THE MAJOR FAMILIES OF ANIMAL VIRUSES (*continued*)

DNA-containing Viruses		
Herpesviridae (continued) *Subfamily*	*Host*	*Symptoms in Humans*
Alphaherpesvirinae		
Genus *Simplexvirus*		
Human herpesvirus 1 (herpes simplex virus type 1, HSV1)	Humans	Infections of the oropharynx, eye, skin and genitalia; generalized systemic disease; severe and generally fatal encephalitis
Human herpesvirus 2 (herpes simplex virus type 2, HSV 2)	Humans	Primarily genital infections
Cercopithecine herpesvirus 1 (B virus)	Humans, monkeys	Fatal encephalitis
Bovine herpesvirus 2 (bovine mammillitis virus)	Cattle	—
Genus *Varicellovirus*		
Human herpesvirus 3 (varicella-zoster virus, VZV)	Humans	Chickenpox, herpes zoster
Suid herpesvirus 1 (pseudorabies virus)	Swine	—
Equid herpesvirus 1 (equine rhinopneumonitis virus, also known as equine abortion virus, EAV)	Horse	—
Equid herpesvirus 4 (coital-exanthema virus)	Horse	—
Bovine herpesvirus 1 (infectious bovine rhinotracheitis, IBRT)	Cattle	—
Betaherpesvirinae		
Genus *Cytomegalovirus*		
Human herpesvirus 5 (human cytomegalovirus, HCMV)	Humans	Jaundice, hepatosplenomegaly, brain damage, death
Various cytomegaloviruses	Monkeys, horse, cat, swine	—
Genus *Muromegalovirus*		
Murid herpesvirus 1 (mouse CMV)	Mouse	
Various cytomegaloviruses	Guinea pig, hamster, rat, ground squirrel	—
Gammaherpesvirinae		
Genus *Lymphocryptovirus*		
Human herpesvirus 4 (Epstein-Barr virus, EBV)	Humans	Infectious mononucleosis, Burkitt lymphoma, nasopharyngeal carcinoma
Various herpesviruses of primates	Baboon, chimpanzee, orangutan, gorilla	—
Various herpesviruses	Monkeys	—
Genus *Rhadinovirus*		
Ateline herpesvirus 2 (herpesvirus ateles)	Spider monkey	—
Saimirine herpesvirus 2 (herpesvirus saimiri)	Squirrel monkey	—
Various herpesviruses	Wildebeest, hare	—
Genus *Thetalymphocryptovirus*		
Gallid herpesvirus 2 (Marek's disease virus, MDV)	Chicken	—
Maleagrid herpesvirus 1 (turkey herpesvirus)	Turkey	—
Unassigned		
Human herpesvirus 6 (human β-lymphotropic virus)	Humans	Exanthem Subitum (roseola infantum, Duke disease, Fourth disease)
Infectious rhinotracheitis virus	Cat	—
Infectious laryngotracheitis virus (ILTV)	Chicken	—
Various herpesviruses	Spider monkey, vervet monkey, macaque, marmoset	—
Various herpesviruses	Dog, sheep, goat	—
Herpesviruses of amphibians (such as Lucké virus and frog virus 4)	Frog	—
Channel catfish virus	Channel catfish	—
Herpesviruses of fish	Carp, turbot, salmon	—

(continued)

TABLE 53–4. THE MAJOR FAMILIES OF ANIMAL VIRUSES *(continued)*

DNA-containing Viruses

Adenoviridae

• Naked icosahedral nucleocapsids
• Diameter: 70 nm

Adenoviruses can be isolated from many species of animals. The family is divided into two genera, one for mammalian adenoviruses, the other for avian ones. Members of each genus share a group-specific antigen; there is no common antigen that characterizes the whole family. There are 42 human adenovirus serotypes that are grouped into seven subgenera on the basis of antigenic cross-reactivity, DNA hybridization characteristics, ability to transform cells of various animal species, and ability to agglutinate rhesus monkey and rat erythrocytes. Viruses of subgenus A possess 48% GC and regularly cause tumors in newborn hamsters (high tumorigenicity). Those in subgenus B possess 51% GC and sometimes cause tumors in newborn hamsters (low tumorigenicity), and members of subgenera C to G possess 58% GC and do not cause tumors but transform cultured cells. Members of subgenus A exhibit about 60% homology with each other; for members of the other subgenera, this value is 90%–100%. The extent of homology between subgenera is 10%–20%. Recombination occurs only within, not among, subgenera. Adenoviruses produce intranuclear type B inclusions (basophilic masses sometimes connected to the nuclear periphery by strands of chromatin).

	Host	*Symptoms in Humans*
Genus *Mastadenovirus*		
Human adenoviruses	Humans	
42 serotypes		
Subgenus A		
Serotypes 12, 18, and 31		No known pathogenicity; regularly isolated from feces of apparently healthy individuals; high incidence of antibodies
Subgenus B		
Serotypes 3, 7, 11, 14, 16, 21, 34, 35		Acute respiratory disease (3, 7, 14, 21); pharyngitis (3, 7, 14); acute hemorrhagic cystitis in children (11, 21); epidemic keratoconjunctivitis (11); persistent infections of the urinary tract in AIDS and immunosuppressed patients (34, 35); low incidence of antibodies
Subgenus C		
Serotypes 1, 2, 5, 6		Acute febrile pharyngitis; pneumonia (1, 2); hepatitis in infants and children with liver transplants (1, 2, 5)
Subgenus D		
Serotypes 8, 9, 10, 13, 15, 17, 19, 22, 23, 24, 26, 27, 29, 30, 32, 33, 36, 37		Epidemic keratoconjunctivitis (8, 11, 19, 37); low incidence of antibodies
Subgenus E		
Serotype 4		Acute respiratory disease, pneumonia
Subgenus F		
Serotype 40, 41, 42		Gastroenteritis in children (40, 41)
Simian adenoviruses	Monkey	—
23 serotypes		
Canine adenoviruses (infectious canine hepatitis, ICH)	Dog	—
Adenoviruses of	Cattle, pigs, sheep, frogs,	—
Genus *Aviadenovirus*		
Avian adenoviruses (CELO, chicken-embryo-lethal-orphan; GAL, gallus-adeno-like)	Chicken, quail, other birds	—

Papovaviridae

• Naked icosahedral nucleocapsids
• Diameter: 55 nm (papillomaviruses)
44 nm (all other papovaviruses)

Papovaviruses (*pa*pilloma-*po*lyoma-simian *va*cuolating agent) fall into two distinct groups on the basis of size; members of the genus *Papillomavirus* possess both larger capsids and larger genomes than members of the genus *Polyomavirus*. There are other significant differences. For example, papillomaviruses infect surface epithelia, polyomaviruses internal organs; papillomaviruses cause benign tumors that may become malignant, polyomaviruses set up persistent lytic infections that may become malignant; papillomavirus genomes are usually not integrated into host cell genomes in transformed cells, polyomavirus genomes are integrated. Most papovaviruses produce tumors in animals; all produce latent and chronic infections in their natural hosts. Most humans acquire antibodies against BK virus and JC virus before age 12 to 16 years; both viruses persist in kidney epithelium.

(continued)

TABLE 53–4. THE MAJOR FAMILIES OF ANIMAL VIRUSES (*continued*)

DNA-containing Viruses

Papovaviridae (continued) *Subfamily*	*Host*	*Symptoms in Humans*
Subfamily Papillomavirinae		
Genus *Papillomavirus*		
Human papillomaviruses (HPV) 1–58	Humans	
HPV 1, 2, and 4	Humans	Plantar warts (verruca plantaris)
HPV 2 and 4	Humans	Common warts (verruca vulgaris)
HPV 3, 10	Humans	Flat warts (verruca plana)
HPV 5, 8, 9, 12, 14, 15, 17, 19–25, 46, 47, 50	Humans	Epidermodysplasia verruciformis (EV) (potential for malignancy, 5, 8, 14, 17, 20)
HPV 6, 11, 54	Humans	Anogenital warts (condylomata acuminata), laryngeal papilloma
HPV 7	Humans	Meat-handlers' warts
HPV 13	Humans	Oral focal hyperplasia
HPV 16, 18, 31, 33, 35, 39, 45, 51, 52	Humans	Genital tract cancers, including invasive carcinomas of the cervix
HPV 41	Humans	Disseminated warts, cutaneous squamous cell carcinomas
Bovine papillomaviruses 1–5	Cattle	—
Shope rabbit papillomavirus	Rabbit	—
Various viruses pathogenic for other animal species		—
Genus *Polyomavirus*		
Polyomavirus	Mouse	—
K virus	Mouse	—
Hamster papovavirus (HapV)	Hamsters	
Rabbit kidney vacuolating agent (RKV)	Rabbit	—
Simian vacuolating agent (SV40)	Monkey, humans	?
BK virus	Humans	Isolated from the urine of renal transplant patients
JC virus	Humans	Isolated from brains of patients with progressive multifocal leukoencephalopathy (PML)
Lymphotrophic papovavirus (LPV)	African green monkey, humans (?)	Multiplies only in monkey and human B lymphoblasts; about 30% of humans have antibody against it
Simian agent 12 (SA12)	Baboon	—
Budgerigar fledgling disease	Budgerigar	—

Parvoviridae

- Naked icosahedral nucleocapsids
- Diameter: 22 nm

Parvoviruses contain single-stranded DNA. Members of the genus *Parvovirus* encapsidate negative-stranded DNA preferentially (50%–99%), but particles of members of the *Dependovirus* and *Densovirus* genera encapsidate plus-stranded and minus-stranded DNA with equal efficiency. The replication of parvoviruses tends to be dependent on helper functions, which for members of the genus *Parvovirus* are supplied by rapidly growing (not resting) cells, which explains why they are often found associated with tumors and possess oncolytic properties, and for members of the genus *Dependovirus* by coinfection with adenoviruses, herpesviruses, or poxviruses. The essential function that must be supplied is most probably activation of the transcription of the parvovirus genome. Members of the genus *Parvovirus* are 70%–90% related genetically; those of the genus *Dependovirus* 60%–70%. The rodent parvoviruses are unrelated immunologically to FPLV, CPV, and MEV, which are themselves closely related immunologically. Parvoviruses generally have narrow host ranges. Parvoviruses can establish latent infections; cells latently infected possess parvovirus genomes integrated into their DNA but are not transformed and exhibit no discernible change in phenotype.

	Host	*Symptoms in Humans*
Genus *Parvovirus*		
Parvovirus-like agent (PVLA) Strain B19	Humans	Erythemia infectiosum (fifth disease); aplastic crisis in hemolytic anemia/sickle cell anemia; polyarthralgia

(continued)

TABLE 53–4. THE MAJOR FAMILIES OF ANIMAL VIRUSES *(continued)*

DNA-containing Viruses

Subfamily	*Host*	*Symptoms in Humans*
Lu-111	Humans	No known disease
Feline panleukopenia virus (FPLV)	Cat	—
Canine parvovirus (CPV)	Dog	—
Mink enteritis virus (MEV)	Mink	—
Hamster osteolytic viruses (H-1, H-3, x-14)	Rat, hamster	—
Kilham rat virus (KRV)	Rat	—
Minute virus of mice (MVM)	Rat	—
Aleutian mink disease virus	Mink	—
Bovine parvovirus (BPV)	Cattle	—
Porcine parvovirus	Pig	—
Genus *Dependovirus*		
Adeno-associated virus (AAV)	Humans	Antibodies very prevalent; no known symptoms
Serotypes 1, 2, 3, 5		
Serotype 4	Monkeys	—
Genus *Densovirus*	Insects	—
Densonucleosis viruses		

Hepadnaviridae

- Enveloped icosahedral nucleocapsids
- Diameter: 42 nm

Hepadnavirus genomes are the smallest human or animal virus genomes known (about 3 kbp). Their lipoprotein envelope (surface antigen, HbsAg) possesses an extraordinary tendency for self-association, forming spherical or rodlike particles (diameter 22 nm) that are often present in the sera of infected individuals in 10,000-fold excess over the 42 nm virions, also known as Dane particles. HbsAg possesses several epitopes, some of which are group-specific, whereas others are not only type-specific but subtype-specific; thus 8 allelic subtypes of human HBV have been described. The epitopes on the core component (HbcAg) are partially group-specific. The replication of hepadnavirus DNA involves reverse transcription of RNA into DNA. Hepadnaviruses exhibit tissue tropism for hepatocytes. Persistent infections are common. Hepadnavirus DNA is capable of integrating into cellular DNA.

	Host	*Symptoms in Humans*
Hepatitis B virus	Humans	Acute and chronic hepatitis; cirrhosis; hepatocellular sarcoma; immune complex disease; polyarteritis; glomerulonephritis; infantile papular acrodermatitis; aplastic anemia
Woodchuck hepatitis B virus (WHBV)	Eastern woodchuck	—
Ground squirrel hepatitis B virus	Ground squirrel	—
Tree squirrel hepatitis B virus (TSHBV)	Tree squirrel	—
Duck hepatitis B virus (DHBV)	Peking duck	—

RNA-containing Viruses

Picornaviridae

- Naked icosahedral nucleocapsids
- Diameter: 25–30 nm

Picornaviruses comprise a large number of virus strains pathogenic for many animal species. They are subdivided into four genera: *Enterovirus* and *Cardiovirus*, whose members are acid-stable, and *Rhinovirus* and *Aphthovirus*, whose members are acid-labile.

	Host	*Symptoms in Humans*
Genus *Enterovirus*		
Human enteroviruses		
Poliovirus	Humans, monkey	Poliomyelitis
3 serotypes		
Coxsackie virus A	Humans, mouse	Primarily general striated muscle damage; herpangina (2–6, 8, 10); aseptic meningitis (2, 4, 7, 9, 10); common cold syndrome (21, 24); epidemic myalgia (11); exanthema (4, 5, 6, 9, 16); infantile diarrhea (18, 20, 21, 22, 24); acute hemorrhagic conjunctivitis (24)
23 serotypes (1–24; A23 is ECHO virus 9)		

(continued)

TABLE 53–4. THE MAJOR FAMILIES OF ANIMAL VIRUSES (*continued*)

RNA-containing Viruses

Picornaviridae (continued)

	Host	Symptoms in Humans
Coxsackie virus B 6 serotypes	Humans, mouse	Primarily fatty tissue and CNS damage; undifferentiated febrile illness; pleurodynia (Bornholm disease); aseptic meningitis; severe systemic illness of newborns; pericarditis, myocarditis; upper respiratory illness and pneumonia (4, 5); rash (5)
ECHOviruses (*e*nteric *c*ytopathogenic *h*uman *o*rphan) 32 serotypes	Humans	Paralysis; aseptic meningitis; encephalitis; exanthema; respiratory disease
Human enteroviruses 68–71	Humans	Lower respiratory illness (68); acute hemorrhagic conjunctivitis (70); meningitis (71)
Simian enteroviruses 18 serotypes	Monkey	—
Murine encephalomyelitis (ME) viruses	Mouse	—
Poliovirus muris (Theiler's virus) GDVII strain and others	Mouse	—
Bovine enteroviruses 7 serotypes	Cattle	—
Porcine enteroviruses 11 serotypes	Swine	—
Genus *Cardiovirus*		
Encephalomyocarditis virus (EMC) (several closely related viruses, including Mengovirus, ME virus, EMC virus, MM virus, and Columbia SK virus)	Primarily mouse, various other species, including humans	Mild febrile illness
Genus *Rhinovirus*		
Human rhinoviruses 113 serotypes	Humans	Common cold, bronchititis, croup, bronchopneumonia
Other rhinoviruses	Strains pathogenic for horses, cattle	—
Genus *Aphthovirus*		
Foot-and-mouth disease virus (FMDV) 7 serotypes	Cattle, swine, sheep, goats	—
Unassigned		
Human hepatitis A virus (HAV) (human enterovirus 72)	Humans	Infectious hepatitis, jaundice
Various insect viruses, including cricket paralysis virus and *Drosophila* C virus	Insects	—

Caliciviridae

- Naked icosahedral nucleocapsids
- Diameter: 35–40 nm

Caliciviruses differ significantly from picornaviruses in size and structure, as well as in strategy for genome expression. Vesicular exanthema virus and San Miguel sea lion virus are very closely related; feline caliciviruses are related to them to the extent of about 10% as judged by RNA hybridization analysis.

	Host	Symptoms in Humans
Vesicular exanthema of swine virus (VE)	Swine	—
San Miguel sea lion virus (SMSV)	Seals	—
Feline caliciviruses	Cat	—
Probable caliciviruses	Humans	—
Norwalk agent	Humans	Epidemic viral gastroenteritis
Hepatitis E virus (HEV)	Humans	Endemic hepatitis

Togaviridae

- Enveloped icosahedral nucleocapsids
- Diameter: 60–70 nm

The togavirus family includes many plus-stranded RNA-containing viruses that are enveloped icosahedral nucleocapsids. It is made up of three genera. By far the largest is the genus *Alphavirus*, which encompasses the old group A arboviruses (*ar*thropod-*bo*rne). They multiply in bloodsucking insects as well as in vertebrates; in their natural environment they alternate between an insect vector (usually a mosquito or tick) and a vertebrate reservoir, rarely producing disease in either. Many cause subclinical infections in humans, particularly in the tropics, but several cause severe and frequently fatal disease. They are commonly named for the geographic site where they were isolated.

(continued)

TABLE 53–4. THE MAJOR FAMILIES OF ANIMAL VIRUSES (*continued*)

RNA-containing Viruses

	Reservoir/Host	*Symptoms in Humans*
Genus *Alphavirus* (mosquito-borne)		
Eastern equine encephalitis (EEE)	Birds	Encephalitis: frequently fatal
Western equine encephalitis (WEE)	Birds	Encephalitis
Venezuelan equine encephalitis (VEE)	Rodents	Systemic febrile illness (encephalitis)
Sindbis	Monkeys	Fever, rash, arthritis
Semliki Forest virus	Monkeys	Encephalitis (rare)
Chikungunya	Monkeys	Myositis-arthritis
O'Nyong-Nyong	?	Fever, arthralgia, rash
Ross River virus	Mammals	Fever, rash, arthralgia
Genus *Rubivirus*		
Rubella virus	Humans	Severe deformities of fetuses in first trimester of pregnancy
Genus *Arterivirus*		
Equine arteritis virus	Horse	—
Unclassified togavirus		
Riley's lactic dehydrogenase elevating virus (LDHV)	Mouse	—

Flaviviridae

- Enveloped icosahedral nucleocapsids
- Diameter: 45–55 nm

The flavivirus family (from Latin *flavus*, yellow, for yellow fever virus, the prototype virus) comprises the old group B arboviruses, which were, until recently, the genus *Flavivirus* of the Togaviridae. The reason why this genus was reconstituted as a separate family was the gradual realization, as information became available, that the strategy according to which they express their information is quite different from that employed by togaviruses; in particular, there is no subgenomic mRNA species. Some flaviviruses are mosquito-borne, others tick-borne. They infect a wide range of vertebrate hosts and cause primarily encephalitis and hemorrhagic fevers. Some of the most lethal viruses known, such as yellow fever virus and Japanese encephalitis virus, are flaviviruses.

It should be noted that the genus *Pestivirus* is here assigned to the Flavoviridae family. This genus is officially still grouped with the Togaviridae. However, recent evidence indicates quite clearly that the strategy of virus replication employed by pestiviruses closely resembles that of the flaviviruses and is quite different from that used by the togaviruses.

	Reservoir/Host	*Symptoms in Humans*
Mosquito-borne		
Yellow fever virus	Monkey	Hemorrhagic fever, hepatitis, nephritis, often fatal
Dengue virus (4 serotypes)	Humans	Fever, arthralgia, rash
West Nile virus	Birds	Fever, arthralgia, rash
Kunjin virus	Birds	—
St. Louis encephalitis	Birds	Encephalitis
Japanese encephalitis	Birds	Encephalitis; frequently fatal
Murray Valley encephalitis	Birds	Encephalitis
Tick-borne		
Central European tick-borne encephalitis (biphasic meningoencephalitis)	Rodents, hedgehog	Encephalitis
Far Eastern tick-borne encephalitis (Russian spring-summer encephalitis, RSSE)	Rodents	Encephalitis
Kyasanur forest virus	Rodents	Hemorrhagic fever
Louping ill	Sheep	Encephalitis
Powassan	Rodents	Encephalitis
Omsk hemorrhagic fever virus	Mammals	Hemorrhagic fever
Genus *Pestivirus*		
Mucosal disease virus (bovine virus diarrhea virus)	Cattle	—
Hog cholera virus (European swine fever)	Pig	—
Border disease virus	Sheep	—
Possible flavivirus		
Simian hemorrhagic fever virus	Monkeys	—

(continued)

TABLE 53–4. THE MAJOR FAMILIES OF ANIMAL VIRUSES (*continued*)

RNA-containing Viruses

Coronaviridae

- Enveloped helical nucleocapsids
- Diameter: about 120 nm

The distinctive features of coronaviruses are large (up to 20 nm long), well-separated, petal-shaped spikes or *peplomers* attached to the envelope and possession of a helical nucleocapsid that contains plus-stranded RNA. Coronaviruses cause a wide spectrum of disease in animals, including respiratory, enteric, and neurologic infections, hepatitis, peritonitis, nephritis, pancreatitis, and adenitis. The family is not subdivided into genera, but into antigenic groups. Human coronaviruses grow well in cultured cells only after extensive adaptation by passage. The two best-studied established strains, 229E and OC43, belong to two different antigenic groups.

	Host	*Symptoms in Humans*
Antigenic group 1		
Human Coronavirus strain HCV-229E	Humans	Upper respiratory disease
Porcine transmissible gastroenteritis virus (TGEV)	Swine	—
Canine coronavirus (CCV)	Dog	—
Feline enteric coronavirus (FECV)	Cat	—
Feline infectious peritonitis virus (FIPV)	Cat	—
Antigenic group 2		
Human coronavirus strain HCV-OC43	Humans	Upper respiratory disease
Mouse hepatitis virus (MHV)	Mouse	—
Porcine hemagglutinating encephomyelitis virus (HEV)	Swine	—
Bovine coronavirus (BCV)	Cattle	
Rabbit coronavirus (RbCV)	Rabbit	—
Antigenic group 3		
Avian bronchitis virus (IBV)	Chicken	—
Antigenic group 4		
Turkey coronavirus (TCV)	Turkey	—

Reoviridae

- Naked nucleocapsids that possess two capsid shells (except cytoplasmic polyhedrosis virus), each with icosahedral symmetry
- Diameter: 75 nm

The name is an acronym based on *r*espiratory-*e*ntero. The primary criterion for inclusion in this family is possession of a genome consisting of 10, 11, or 12 segments of double-stranded RNA. There are six genera with widely differing host ranges and somewhat differing morphologies. The vertebrate reoviruses possess two clearly defined capsid shells; the orbiviruses (many of which are transmitted by arthropods and are functionally arboviruses) possess a structurally featureless outer shell and an inner shell composed of 32 large ring-shaped capsomers (hence the name, Latin *orbis*, ring; however, see p. 751). the cytoplasmic polyhedrosis viruses possess only one capsid shell with clearly defined icosahedral symmetry. Phytoreoviruses closely resemble the orthoreoviruses, while Fijiviruses possess a structure more reminiscent of cytoplasmic polyhedrosis viruses. Rotaviruses present a wheellike appearance (see Fig. 53–14) (Latin *rota*, wheel). The members of the six genera are not related antigenically.

	Host/Reservoir	*Symptoms in Humans*
Genus *Orthoreovirus*		
Mammalian reoviruses 3 serotypes	Humans, other mammals	Pathogenicity not established
Avian reoviruses 5 serotypes	Chicken, duck	—
Genus *Orbivirus*		
Bluetongue virus	Culicoides, sheep	—
Eubenangee virus	Mosquitoes	—
Kemerovo	Ticks	—
African horse sickness virus	Culicoides, horse	—
Colorado tick fever virus	Ticks, mammals	Encephalitis
Genus *Cypovirus*		
Cytoplasmic polyhedrosis viruses Numerous strains	*Bombyx mori* (silkworm) and other Lepidoptera, Diptera, and Hymenoptera	—
Genus *Phytoreovirus*		
Wound tumor virus	Plants, leaf hoppers	—
Rice dwarf virus	Plants, leaf hoppers	—

(continued)

TABLE 53–4. THE MAJOR FAMILIES OF ANIMAL VIRUSES (*continued*)

RNA-containing Viruses

	Host/Reservoir	*Symptoms in Humans*
Genus Fijivirus		
Maize rough dwarf virus	Plants, leaf hoppers	—
Fiji disease virus	Plants, leaf hoppers	—
Genus *Rotavirus*		
Human rotavirus	Humans	Acute infantile gastroenteritis
Calf rotavirus (Nebraska calf diarrhea virus)	Calf	—
Murine rotavirus (epizootic diarrhea of infant mice, EDIM)	Mouse	—
Simian rotavirus (SA11)	Monkey	—
Bovine or ovine rotavirus ("O" agent)	Cattle or sheep	—
Numerous other rotaviruses	Guinea pig, goat, horse, deer, antelope, rabbit, dog, duck	—

Rhabdoviridae

- Bullet-shaped enveloped helical nucleocapsids
- Dimensions: 180 × 75 nm

This family comprises all viruses with the unique bullet-shaped morphology, as well as some that are baciliform (rounded at both ends). It includes vesicular stomatitis virus (VSV), rabies, and some viruses isolated from insects that infect birds and mammals, including humans, without causing clinical disease.

	Host	*Symptoms in Humans*
Genus *Vesiculovirus*		
Vesicular stomatitis virus (VSV)	Cattle, horse, swine	Mild febrile illness; sometimes with herpeslike vesicular lesions in the mouth
Chandipura virus	Isolated from humans	—
Flanders-Hart Park virus	Mosquitoes, birds	—
Kern Canyon virus	Bats	—
Mount Elgon bat virus	Bats	—
Genus *Lyssavirus*		
Rabies virus	All warm-blooded animals	Encephalitis, almost invariably fatal
Other Rhabdoviruses		
Numerous fish rhabdoviruses like Spring viremia of carp	Fish	—
Drosophila sigmavirus	*Drosophila*	—
Numerous plant rhabdoviruses	Plants	—

Filoviridae (proposed family)

- Enveloped helical nucleocapsids.
- The virus particles exist as filaments with uniform diameter (80 nm) but very variable length (up to 14,000 nm); the unit length is probably about 800 nm. They are also very pleomorphic; branched, circular, and U-shaped forms are commonly found.

There are only two members of this proposed new family; the reason for placing them into a family of their own is their unique morphology. The two viruses are among the most lethal of human viruses; they can be studied under only the most stringent containment conditions. Their natural hosts are probably monkeys. They probably infect humans only rarely except in certain areas, where the incidence of antibodies against them among the local population is high. The two viruses are not related antigenically.

	Host	*Symptoms in Humans*
Marburg virus	Humans	Acute hemorrhagic fever; frequently fatal
Ebola virus	Humans	Acute hemorrhagic fever; frequently fatal

Paramyxoviridae

- Enveloped helical nucleocapsids
- Diameter: about 150 nm

Members of this family were until recently grouped with the orthomyxoviruses in the family Myxoviridae. They have now been placed into a separate family because their genomes are not segmented and because they employ a different molecular strategy for gene expression and gene replication; in fact, this strategy closely resembles that employed by rhabdoviruses. Like orthomyxoviruses, members of the genus *Paramyxovirus* possess two types of glycoprotein spikes, but one possesses both hemagglutinin and neuraminidase activities, while the other possesses membrane-fusing activity. Members of the *Morbillivirus* and *Pneumovirus* genera possess no neuraminidase activity, and members of the genus *Pneumovirus* possess no hemagglutinin activity either.

(continued)

TABLE 53–4. THE MAJOR FAMILIES OF ANIMAL VIRUSES (*continued*)

RNA-containing Viruses

Paramyxoviridae (continued)	*Host*	*Symptoms in Humans*
Genus *Paramyxovirus*		
Parainfluenza viruses types 1 to 4	Humans and other animals	Respiratory tract infections
Sendai virus (murine parainfluenza virus type 1 [hemagglutinating virus of Japan, HVJ])	Mouse	
SV5 (canine parainfluenza virus type 2)	Dog	—
Newcastle disease virus (NDV)	Chicken	—
Mumps	Humans	Parotitis, orchitis, meningoencephalitis
Genus *Morbillivirus*		
Measles	Humans	Measles; chronic degeneration of the central nervous system (SSPE)
Distemper	Dog	—
Rinderpest	Cattle	—
Genus *Pneumovirus*		
Respiratory syncytial virus (RSV)	Humans	Pneumonia and bronchiolitis in infants and children; common cold syndrome
Bovine respiratory syncytial virus	Cattle	—
Pneumonia virus of mice (PVM)	Mouse	—

Orthomyxoviridae

- Enveloped helical nucleocapsids
- Diameter: 80–120 nm

The term *myxovirus* was coined to denote the unique affinity of influenza viruses for glycoproteins. Nowadays, members of this family are characterized by possession of nucleocapsids with helical symmetry surrounded by envelopes, to whose outer surface two types of glycoprotein spikes are attached, the hemagglutinin and the neuraminidase. Influenza virus strains of type C differ from those of type A and type B in that they possess only one type of glycoprotein spike, which is a hemagglutinin and binds to receptors that are different from those that bind influenza A and B strains, as well as a receptor-destroying enzyme that is not a neuraminidase but an acetyl esterase. There are 13 serotypes of type A hemagglutinin in nature (H1–H13), and 9 serotypes of neuraminidase (N1–N9).

	Host	*Symptoms in Humans*
Genus *Influenza virus*		
Influenza virus type A		
Human subtypes	Humans	
A_0 (H1N1) 1933–47 and 1977–present		Acute respiratory disease
A_1 (H1N1) 1947–57		Acute respiratory disease
A_2 (H2N2) 1957–68 (Asian)		Acute respiratory disease
A_2 (H3N2) 1968–present (Hong Kong)		Acute respiratory disease
Swine influenza virus	Swine	Acute respiratory disease
Avian subtypes		
Fowl plague virus and numerous other strains	Chicken, duck, turkey, and others	—
Equine subtypes	Horse	—
Influenza virus type B		
Human subtypes		
B_0 1940–1945	Humans	Acute respiratory disease
B_1 1945–1955		Acute respiratory disease
B_2 1962–1964		Acute respiratory disease
B_3 1962–present (Taiwan)		Acute respiratory disease
Influenza virus type C (possible separate genus)	Humans	Respiratory disease

Bunyaviridae

- Enveloped helical nucleocapsids
- Diameter: about 100 nm

Bunyaviruses include all former group C arboviruses, as well as previously ungrouped arboviruses. They form a homogeneous family that is divided into four genera, members of each of which cross-react serologically. Although members of the various genera are not so related, they share numerous other characteristics.

(continued)

TABLE 53–4. THE MAJOR FAMILIES OF ANIMAL VIRUSES *(continued)*

RNA-containing Viruses

	Host	*Symptoms in Humans*
Genus *Bunyavirus* (16 serogroups)		
Bunyamwera and related viruses	Mammals	Fever, rash (rare)
California encephalitis group, including La Crosse, Tahyna, and Snowshoe hare virus	Mammals	Encephalitis
Genus *Phlebovirus* (8 serogroups)		
Sandfly fever virus	Sandfly, mammals	Fever, facial erythema
Rift Valley fever virus	Humans, sheep, cattle	Fever, arthralgia, retinitis (sometimes fatal)
Genus *Nairovirus* (6 serogroups)		
Crimean-Congo hemorrhagic fever (CCHF) 2 serotypes	Mammals	Hemorrhagic fever
Five other serotypes, including Nairobi sheep disease virus	Mammals	Acute febrile illness (relatively rare)
Genus *Uukuvirus* (1 serogroup)		
Uukuniemi and related viruses	Birds, mammals	—
Genus *Hantavirus* (1 serogroup)		
Hantaan virus (Korean hemorrhagic fever)	Rodents	Hemorrhagic fever with renal syndrome (may be fatal)

Arenaviridae

- Enveloped helical nucleocapsids
- Diameter: 110–130 nm

This family comprises viruses characterized by well-defined envelopes that bear closely spaced projections and enclose, beside two helical nucleocapsids, a variable number of electron-dense granules about 25 nm in diameter that are ribosomes. They share a group-specific antigen, but antisera do not cross-neutralize. They include several viruses that cause frequently fatal hemorrhagic fevers.

	Host	*Symptoms in Humans*
Lymphocytic choriomeningitis virus (LCM)	Mouse, humans	Fever, meningitis (sometimes fatal)
Tacaribe virus complex		
Several viruses, including Argentinian (Junin) and Bolivian (Machupo) hemorrhagic fever	Rodents, humans	Hemorrhagic fever, frequently fatal
Lassa virus	Rodents	Hemorrhagic fever, frequently fatal

Retroviridae (RNA tumor viruses)

- Enveloped particles containing a coiled nucleocapsid within a probably icosahedral core shell
- Diameter: about 100 nm

The retrovirus family comprises a large group of viruses characterized by a common morphology, a genome that consists of two identical plus-stranded RNA molecules, and possession of reverse transcriptase. There are three subfamilies. The first, the Oncovirinae, comprises the C-, B-, and D-type retroviruses. These viruses are oncogenic; they cause leukemias, lymphomas, and mammary and neuronal tumors. The second subfamily, the Lentivirinae, comprises the Visna group of viruses and the human immunodeficiency virus (HIV). They resemble the Oncovirinae with respect to morphology, nature of the genome, and possession of a reverse transcriptase, but do not transform cells. The third subfamily, the Spumavirinae, comprises the foamy viruses, which are found in spontaneously degenerating kidney (and other) cell cultures, causing the formation of multinucleated vacuolated giant cells that have a highly characteristic appearance.

Subfamily	*Host*	*Symptoms in Humans*
Oncovirinae		
Genus *Oncornavirus C*		
Subgenus Oncornavirus C avian		
Endogenous leukemia/leukosis viruses (RAV-0, RAV-1, RAV-2, etc.)	Chicken	—
Nondefective avian sarcoma viruses (ASV) (Rous sarcoma virus)	Chicken	—
Defective sarcoma/acute leukemia viruses	Chicken	—
Numerous viruses, including		
Fujinami sarcoma virus (FSV)		
Avian myeloblastosis virus (AMV)		
Avian erythroblastosis virus (AEV)		
Avian myelocytomatosis virus (MC29)		
Reticuloendotheliosis virus (REV)	Chicken, duck	—

(continued)

TABLE 53–4. THE MAJOR FAMILIES OF ANIMAL VIRUSES (*continued*)

RNA-containing Viruses

Retroviridae (RNA tumor viruses) (continued) *Subfamily*	*Host*	*Symptoms in Humans*
Subgenus Oncornavirus C mammalian		
Endogenous leukemia viruses, numerous strains	Mammals	—
Defective sarcoma/acute leukemia viruses	Rodents	—
Numerous strains, including		
Abelson murine leukemia virus		
Murine sarcoma viruses (Harvey, Kirsten, Moloney, Rasheed)		
Feline sarcoma viruses	Cats	—
(Snyder, Theilen, Gardner-Arnstein, McDonough and other strains)		
Simian sarcoma virus	Monkeys	—
Subgenus *Oncornavirus* (reptilian)		
Numerous viruses	Reptiles	—
Genus *Oncornavirus B*		
Mouse mammary tumor virus (Bittner virus) (milk factor)	Mouse	—
Viruses of guinea pigs, baboons, and other mammals	Mammals	—
Genus *Oncornavirus D*		
Mason-Pfizer monkey virus (MPMV)	Rhesus monkey	—
Viruses from primates	Primates	?
Guinea pig virus	Guinea pig	—
SAIDS virus	Monkeys	—
Genus (unnamed)		
Human T cell leukemia (or lymphotropic) virus		
HTLV-I	Humans	Adult T cell leukemia
HTLV-II	Humans	Isolated from a T cell line established from a patient with a variant of hairy cell leukemia
Bovine leukemia virus	Cattle	—
Lentivirinae		
Visna	Sheep	—
Maedi	Sheep	—
Progressive pneumonia virus	Mice	—
Equine infectious anemia virus	Horse	—
Caprine arthritis-encephalitis virus (CAEV)	Goat	—
Human immunodeficiency virus (HIV) (HIV-1 and HIV-2)	Humans	Acquired immunodeficiency syndrome (AIDS)
Simian immunodeficiency virus (SIV)	Monkeys	—
Feline immunodeficiency virus	Cats	—
Spumavirinae		
Human foamy virus	Human cells	—
Simian foamy viruses 9 serotypes	Monkey kidney cells	—
Canine foamy virus	Dog kidney cells	—
Bovine syncytial virus	Bovine kidney cells	—
Feline syncytial virus	Feline cells	—
Hamster syncytial virus	Hamster cells	—

Miscellaneous Viruses	Several viruses do not fit into any of the families listed so far. The following are the most important:
Toroviridae	A new family has been proposed for enveloped viruses characterized by (1) the tubular morphology of their nucleocapsids (which may be bent into an open torus, which confers a biconcave disk- or kidney-shaped morphology onto the virus particles [120–140 nm], or straight, which results in rod-shaped [35 × 170 nm] particles), and (2) the fact that their glycoprotein spikes are large and drumstick-shaped, like the peplomers of coronaviruses. The virus particles comprise three proteins besides the spike glycoprotein, namely, a matrix protein, a nucleocapsid protein, and a phosphoprotein, and a single large plus-stranded RNA molecule about 20,000 nucleotides long. Five major subgenomic polyadenylated RNA species have been detected in infected cells, which, like coronavirus messenger RNAs (Chap. 55), form a nested set. Possession of the very large genome, the nested transcript set, and the prominent peplomers characterizes these viruses as coronavirus-like. All toroviruses so far described cause enteric infections in horses, cattle, and humans. The prototype virus is the Berne virus, an equine virus.

(continued)

TABLE 53–4. THE MAJOR FAMILIES OF ANIMAL VIRUSES *(continued)*

	RNA-containing Viruses
Norwalk Group of Viruses	During the past decade, the Norwalk group of viruses has emerged as an important cause of epidemic viral gastroenteritis in adults. They are probably caliciviruses.
Non-A, non-B Hepatitis, Parenterally Transmitted (PT-NA/NBH) (Hepatitis C Virus, HCV)	Ninety percent of posttransfusion hepatitis in the United States is caused by this virus. It is related to the togaviruses and the flaviviruses.
Non-A, non-B Hepatitis, Enterically Transmitted (ET-NA/NBV) (Hepatitis E virus, HEV)	This virus was formerly referred to as water-borne or endemic hepatitis. It causes very large epidemics via the fecal-oral route in areas with inadequate sanitation and undernourished populations. It is probably a calicivirus.
Delta hepatitis virus	Hepatitis D virus, also known as HDV or the delta virus. Its unique characteristic is that it requires HBV as helper virus; the virus particle possesses an envelope composed of HBsAg, the HBV surface component, and its genome is a very small viroid-like RNA molecule (Chap. 55).
The Astroviruses	Characteristically star-shaped, 27–30 nm diameter particles visualized by electron microscopy in fecal specimens from humans, calves, dogs, swine, lambs, ducks, and turkeys. There are five antigenically distinct groups of human astroviruses. Their genome is RNA of a size similar to that of poliovirus.
Borna disease Virus (BDV)	BDV causes a rare neurologic disease in horses and sheep characterized by behavioral disturbances and the accumulation of specific proteins in limbic system neurones. Borna disease can be transmitted to birds, rodents, and primates. No infectious particle has yet been identified. Using a subtraction complementary cDNA expression library, three RNA species have been tentatively identified as being BDV-specific.
Chronic Infectious Neuropathic Agents (CHINAs)	These agents have preclinical periods lasting months to several years, succeeded by a slowly progressing, usually fatal disease. They include the agents that cause Kuru and Creutzfeldt-Jakob disease in humans, scrapie in sheep, and transmissible mink encephalopathy in mink. All are slow degenerative disorders of the central nervous system marked by ataxia and wasting, and end in death. The etiologic agents have been transmitted but not yet isolated or even visualized. They may, in fact, not be viruses as commonly defined, but they are certainly infectious.

FURTHER READING

Books and Reviews

STRUCTURE AND CLASSIFICATION

Acharya R, Fry E, Stuart D, et al: The three-dimensional structure of foot-and-mouth disease virus at 2.9 A resolution. Nature 337:709, 1989

Aiken JM, Marsh RF: The search for scrapie agent nucleic acid. Microbiol Rev 54:242, 1990

Arnold E, Rossmann MG: Analysis of the structure of a common cold virus, human rhinovirus 14, refined at resolution of 3·0 A. J Mol Biol 211:763, 1990

Casjens S (ed): Virus Structure and Assembly. Boston, Jones and Bartlett, 1985

Caspar DLD, Klug A: Physical principles in the construction of regular viruses. Cold Spring Harbor Symp Quant Biol 27:1, 1962

Fields BN, Knipe DM (chief eds): Fundamental Virology, ed 2. New York, Raven Press, 1991

Harris JR, Horne RW: Viral Structure. New York, Academic Press, 1986

Harrison SC: Virus structure: High-resolution perspectives. Adv Virus Res 28:175, 1986

Kingsbury DW: Biological concepts in virus classification. Intervirology 29:242, 1988

Matthews REF: Viral taxonomy for the nonvirologist. Annu Rev Microbiol 39:451, 1985

Rossmann MG, Johnson JE: Icosahedral RNA virus structure. Annu Rev Biochem 58:533, 1989

Schrag JD, Prasad BVV, Rixon FJ, Chiu W: Three dimensional structure of the HSV1 nucleocapsid. Cell 56:651, 1989

Staczek J: Animal cytomegaloviruses. Microbiol Rev 54:90, 1990

Stewart M, Vigers G: Electron microscopy of frozen-hydrated biological material. Nature 319:631, 1986

Wimmer E: Genome-linked proteins of viruses. Cell 29:199, 1982

DNA-CONTAINING VIRUSES

Anderson MJ, Pattison JR: The human parvovirus. Arch Virol 82:137, 1984

Baxby D: Jenner's Smallpox Vaccine: The Riddle of Vaccinia Virus and Its Origin. London, Heineman, 1981

Behoni M: The smallpox story: Life and death of an old disease. Microbiol Rev 47:455, 1983

Berns KI (ed): The Parvoviruses. New York, Plenum, 1984

Chorba T, Coccia P, Holman RC, et al: The role of parvovirus B19 in aplastic crisis and erythema infectiosum (Fifth disease). J Infect Dis 154:383, 1986

de Palo G, Rilke F, zur Hausen H (eds): Herpes and Papillomaviruses. New York, Raven Press, 1986

Fenner F, Wittek R, Dumbell KR: Orthopoxviruses: Unorthodox Viruses. San Diego, Academic Press, 1989

Howard CR: The biology of hepadnaviruses. J Gen Virol 67:1215, 1986

Howley PM, Broker TR: Papillomaviruses: Molecular and Clinical Aspects. New York, Liss, 1985

Marion PL, Robinson WS: Hepadnaviruses: Hepatitis B and related viruses. Curr Top Microbiol Immunol 105:99, 1983

McGeoch DJ: The genomes of the human herpesviruses: Contents, relationships, and evolution. Annu Rev Microbiol 43:235, 1989

Nermut MV: The architecture of adenoviruses: Recent views and problems. Arch Virol 64:175, 1980

Takahashi M: Chickenpox virus. Adv Virus Res 28:286, 1986

RNA-CONTAINING VIRUSES

Calisher CH, Thompson WH (eds): California Serogroup Viruses. New York, Liss, 1983

Cheevers WP, McGuire TC: The lentiviruses: Maedi/visna, caprine arthritis-encephalitis, and equine infectious anemia. Adv Virus Res 34:189, 1988

Cukor G, Blacklow NR: Human viral gastroenteritis. Microbiol Rev 48:157, 1984
Diener TO: PrP and the nature of the scrapie agent. Cell 49:719, 1987
Estes MK, Palmer EL, Obijeski JF: Rotaviruses: A review. Curr Top Microbiol Immunol 105:123, 1983
Horzinek MC, Flewett TH, Saif LJ, et al: A new family of vertebrate viruses: Toroviridae. Intervirology 27:17, 1987
Joklik WK (ed): The Reoviridae. New York, Plenum, 1983
Kolakofsky P, Mahy B (eds): Genetics and Pathogenicity of Negative-Strand Viruses. Amsterdam, New York, Oxford, Elsevier, 1989
Krug RM (ed): The Influenza Viruses. The Viruses, vol 6. New York, Plenum Press, 1989
Narayan O, Clements JE: Biology and pathogenesis of lentiviruses. J Gen Virol 70, 1617, 1989
Oldstone MBA: Arenaviruses. Curr Top Microbiol Immunol 133:1, 1987
Prince AM: Non-A, non-B hepatitis viruses. Annu Rev Microbiol 36:217, 1983
Prusiner SB: Molecular structure, biology, and genetics of prions. Adv Virus Res 35:83, 1988
Prusiner SB: Scrapie prions. Annu Rev Microbiol 43:345, 1989
Putnak JR, Phillips BA: Picornaviral structure and assembly. Microbiol Rev 45:287, 1981
Racaniello VR (ed): Picornaviruses. Curr Top Microbiol Immunol 161:1, 1990
Siddell S, Wege H, ter Meulen V: The biology of coronaviruses. J Gen Virol 64:761, 1983
Vogt P (ed): Human T-cell leukemia virus. Curr Top Microbiol Immunol 115:1, 1984
Vogt P, Koprowski H (eds): Mouse mammary tumor virus. Curr Top Microbiol Immunol 106:1, 1983
Vogt PK, Koprowski H (eds): Retroviruses 1, 2, 3 and 4. Curr Top Microbiol Immunol 103, 1983; 107, 1983; 112, 1984; 123, 1986
Wagner RR (ed): The Rhabdoviruses. New York, Plenum Press, 1987

Selected Papers

Structure

Brown P, Liberski PP, Wolff A, Gajdusek DC: Resistance of scrapie infectivity to steam autoclaving after formaldehyde fixation and limited survival after ashing at 360°C: Practical and theoretical implications. J Infect Dis 161:467, 1990
Fuller SD: The T=4 envelope of Sindbis virus is organized by interactions with a complementary T=3 capsid. Cell 48:923, 1987
Luo M, Rossmann MG, Palmenberg AC: Prediction of three-dimensional models for foot-and-mouth disease virus and hepatitis A virus. Virology 166:503, 1988
Luo M, Vriend G, Kamer G, et al: The atomic structure of Mengo virus at 3.0 Å resolution. Science 235:182, 1987
Palmer E, Martin ML, Goldsmith C, Switzer W: Ultrastructure of human immunodeficiency virus type 2. J Gen Virol 69:1425, 1988
Prasad BVV, Wang GJ, Clerx JPM, Chiu W: Three-dimensional structure of rotavirus. J Mol Biol 199:269, 1988
Rossmann MG: Constraints on the assembly of spherical virus particles. Virology 134:1, 1984
Ruigrok RWH, Calder LJ, Wharton SA: Electron microscopy of the influenza virus submembranal structure. Virology 311:316, 1989

Genome Structure and Classification

de la Torre JC, Carbone KM, Lipkin WI: Molecular characterization of the Borna disease agent. Virology 179:853, 1990
Kiley MP, Cox NJ, Elliott LH, et al: Physicochemical properties of Marburg virus: Evidence for three distinct virus strains and their relationship to Ebola virus. J Gen Virol 69:1957, 1988
Snijder EJ, Horzinek MC, Spaan WJM: A 3′-coterminal nested set of independently transcribed mRNAs is generated during Berne virus replication. J Virol 64:331, 1990
Snijder EJ, den Boon JA, Horzinek MC, Spaan WJM: Comparison of the genome organization of toro- and coronaviruses: Evidence for two nonhomologous RNA recombination events during Berne virus evolution. Virology 179:448, 1990

CHAPTER 54

Viruses and Viral Proteins as Antigens

Many viral proteins are good antigens. This is of vital significance both medically and scientifically. Although great strides have been made in defining the biochemistry and molecular biology of virus multiplication, antiviral chemotherapy is not yet available for most viral diseases. In fact, with few exceptions, viral infections cannot be controlled. Instead, it is necessary to rely on the natural ability of the host to form antibodies against the invading virus. When the spread of infection to essential organs is too rapid or when for some reason antibody formation does not take place early enough, the patient may succumb. Gamma globulin from hyperimmune sera is sometimes administered as a last resort. Even then, one must rely on antibodies, not on drugs. By the same token, the only practical form of antiviral prophylaxis at present is provided by antibodies produced in response to vaccines (Chap. 58).

Structural viral proteins stimulate the formation of antibodies not only as components of virus particles but also as components of virus particle subunits, such as capsomers and nucleocapsids, and in the free state. The principal antigenic determinants are often the same in all three forms, but extra antigenic sites are sometimes generated when individual proteins become part of more complex structures. For example, adenovirus hexons exhibit antigenic determinants not expressed by the free hexon protein, and the capsids of picornaviruses possess antigenic specificities that are not exhibited by their component structural proteins.

The range of antiviral antibodies formed under conditions when viruses can and cannot multiply differs greatly. If a virus *cannot* multiply, either because it has been inactivated or because the host is not susceptible, only antibodies against surface components of the virus particle are usually formed. However, if the virus *can* multiply, not only is far more antibody formed because progeny virus will also act as antigen, but also the range of antibodies produced is much wider. This is because antibodies are then also formed against the unassembled and partially assembled virus components that are synthesized as a result of virus multiplication, as well as against the nonstructural virus-coded proteins. For example, antisera against inactivated vaccinia virus contain only a few species of antibody, most of which are directed against its surface components, but antisera from animals in which vaccinia virus has multiplied contain antibodies against at least 30 different viral proteins in readily detectable amounts.

The antigenic determinants of virus-coded proteins are of great importance for virus classification. Viruses that belong to the same genus or major antigenic group share common determinants, the group-specific antigens, that are generally located on *internal* virus components. By contrast, the most specific, or individual, viral antigenic determinants are usually located on *external*, or surface, components of virus particles; these are the type-specific antigens that identify individual virus strains.

Possession of group- and type-specific antigenic determinants provides an important tool for epidemiology. Newly isolated virus strains are usually characterized on the basis of their ability to react with antisera of known specificity. This reveals the nature of their group- and type-specific antigens. It is also possible to determine whether a given human or animal population has been exposed to a particular virus strain by testing serum samples for the presence of antibodies against it.

The interaction of viruses and viral proteins with antibodies can be recognized and measured in several ways. The four most important ways are described.

Interaction of Virus with Neutralizing Antibodies

Antibodies against viral surface components neutralize infectivity; these are the neutralizing antibodies that protect against disease. They usually persist in the body for many years, probably because the viruses are not totally eliminated from the body but set up inapparent persistent infections that generate small amounts of viral antigens that continue to stimulate antibody production (see below). When antibody levels drop, a secondary or anamnestic response to virus generally boosts their titers to very high levels very rapidly, so that no second cycle of infection ensues. This explains the fact that animals generally contract any particular viral disease only once. Exceptions, such as the common cold and influenza, are due to special circumstances. The reason for the frequent recurrence of the common cold syndrome is that it is elicited by many viruses, among which are rhinoviruses, enteroviruses, adenoviruses, ortho- and paramyxoviruses, and coronaviruses. The reason for the recurrent epidemics caused by influenza virus is the emergence of new antigenic variants (Chaps. 55 and 57).

The reaction between neutralizing antibody and virus follows first-order kinetics, which has been assumed to indicate that one antibody molecule inactivates one virus particle. However, this is not necessarily the case. In fact, there is little doubt that neutralization often requires at least two and probably more antibody molecules. It should also be remembered that nonneutralizing antibodies exist, that is, antibody molecules that bind but do not inhibit infectivity.

Combination with neutralizing antibody interferes with initial events in virus multiplication cycles. There are three likely mechanisms. The first is steric hindrance; that is, virus particles combined with antibody molecules may be unable to react with their receptors on cell surfaces. Since each virus particle contains multiple antigenic sites and multiple cell attachment sites (from a minimum of 12 to more than 1000), this mechanism would be expected to operate only with very small viruses combined with several antibody molecules. The second mechanism is interference with uncoating by single bivalently attached antibody molecules that would, in effect, cross-linked capsomers and in that way stabilize viral capsids. Small viruses, such as picornaviruses, may be neutralized in this manner. The third mechanism is inhibition of uncoating by preventing the intraendosomal acid-catalyzed membrane fusion that results in the liberation of naked nucleic acids and nucleocapsids into the cytoplasm (Chap. 55). This mechanism probably applies to all but the smallest icosahedral viruses and probably requires the binding of several antibody molecules per virus particle.

Nature of Viral Protein Epitopes

Knowledge concerning the nature of the antigenic sites, or epitopes, on viral proteins is of great interest. Not only is it essential for understanding how viruses interact with antibodies, but it is also important for studies of the molecular basis of serotyping, that is, differentiating and classifying virus strains by immunologic means, and for the development of antiviral vaccines (Chap. 58).

The primary technique for identifying epitopes on viral proteins is the characterization of immunologic escape mutants, that is, variant virus strains capable of growing in the presence of monoclonal antibodies that inhibit, by neutralization (see below), the multiplication of the parent virus. When proteins of such variants are sequenced, it is found that mutation to resistance almost universally involves replacement of single amino acids in clustered 10 to 15 amino acid-long sequence segments. These are the epitopes. Interestingly, it might be thought that mutations far removed from antibody-binding sites might affect affinity for antibody by altering protein conformation, but this is not the case. Mutations in escape mutants are almost always located in the epitopes themselves. The reason is that epitopes are located in sequences that form protruding ridges on protein surfaces, the conformation of which is insensitive to changes in overall protein conformation.

Viral proteins generally possess from three to five epitopes. This does not mean that no other regions of these proteins are antigenic, only that the epitopes identified by the techniques described above are the immunodominant ones. Nor does replacement of every amino acid in these epitopes yield escape mutants. On the contrary, some replacements fail to affect antibody-binding affinity, others merely reduces it, and only some cause complete loss of antibody-binding ability.

Studies along these lines have been carried out on several viral spike glycoproteins, notably the hemagglutinin of influenza virus, and on the capsid proteins of poliovirus, rhinovirus, and foot-and-mouth disease virus. Since the atomic structure of some of these proteins has been established as a result of x-ray crystallographic analyses, the location of several major, that is, immunodominant, epitopes of these viral proteins is now known.

Complement-fixing Antigens and Antibodies

Complexes of viral protein and antibody often fix complement. Since sensitive methods for titrating complement are available, this provides a convenient and accurate method of measuring the amount of either viral antigens or antibody against such antigens (complement-fixing antigen or antibody, CFA). This method of quantitating viral proteins is particularly useful for detecting abortive viral infections when only part of the genetic information present in the viral genome is expressed and no virus particles are produced (Chap. 56). It is also of great importance in epidemiology because it is often far easier to identify newly isolated virus strains by determining whether extracts of cells infected with them fix complement with antisera of known specificity than by measuring the ability of such antisera to neutralize infectivity.

Hemagglutination Inhibition

As described in Chapter 52, many viruses can agglutinate red blood cells. They do so because their cell attachment proteins interact with receptors on the red blood cell surface. Antibody molecules prevent such interaction, and specific antisera, therefore, inhibit hemagglutination. The antigens involved here are viral surface components, which, as pointed out above, possess the most type-specific antigenic determinants. Hemagglutination-inhibition, therefore, provides a highly specific means of characterizing viruses. Because it is also very easy to perform, this technique is very useful for identifying viruses and in epidemiology.

Gel Immunodiffusion and Immunoelectrophoresis

Under appropriate conditions of antigen-antibody equivalence, antigen-antibody complexes are insoluble. This property is used in gel immunodiffusion and gel immunoelectrophoresis, techniques that are used widely for resolving mixtures of viral antigens in extracts of infected cells.

The most widely used version of gel immunodiffusion is the Ouchterlony method, which employs Petri plates containing agar into which are cut several wells, one being situated centrally and the others equidistantly from it and from each other. Antiserum or antibody is placed into the center well; antigen is placed into the outer ones, and diffusion is then allowed to proceed. Where the concentration of antigen-antibody complexes exceeds their solubility product, precipitin lines form, the location of which depends on the relative diffusion rates, and therefore on the relative sizes, of antigen and antibody. Identity of antigens is revealed by fusion of precipitin lines (Fig. 54–1).

In the gel immunoelectrophoresis technique, antigens are not separated by free diffusion but by electrophoresis in agar slabs, after which antiserum is applied in a trough cut parallel to the direction of electrophoresis. After diffusion, precipitin lines form as above (Fig. 54–2). The concentrations of antibody and antigen used in both these techniques are generally adjusted so that the precipitin lines are very thin, thus permitting great resolution.

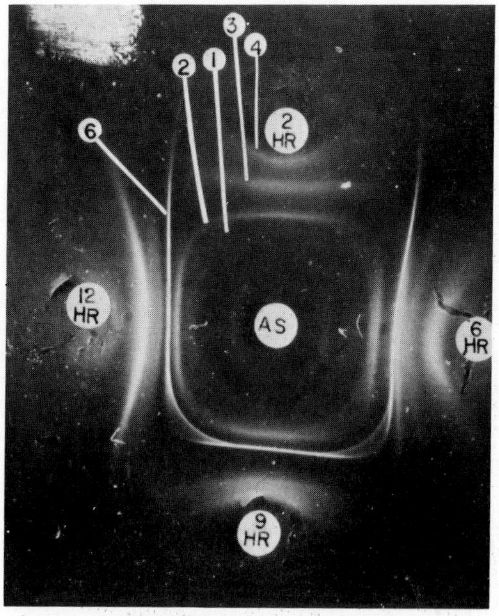

Fig. 54–1. The use of gel diffusion to detect virus-specified proteins in extracts of infected cells. Antiserum to vaccinia virus was placed into the center well (AS) of a Petri dish containing a layer of agar. Extracts of HeLa cells infected for 2, 6, 9, and 12 hours, respectively, with vaccinia virus were placed into the other four wells, and the antibodies and antigens were allowed to diffuse toward each other. Precipitin lines, formed as described in the text, were then stained with Poinceau S. The pattern becomes increasingly complex with increasing time after infection, as more virus-specified proteins are synthesized. The advantage of this method is that virus-specified proteins are revealed without having to be purified. *(From Salzman and Sebring: J Virol 1:16, 1967.)*

Visualization of Viral Antigens Using Tagged Antibodies

There are many occasions when direct visual localization of viral antigens is desired. This can be achieved by using antibody that is tagged, conjugated, or labeled with some material that can be visualized with either the light microscope or the electron microscope. The two best ways of labeling antibody so that it can be seen with the light microscope are either to label it with the dye fluorescein, after which it fluoresces brightly when viewed with a microscope equipped with a source of ultraviolet light (Fig. 54–3); or to conjugate it with peroxidase, when it can be localized readily following the addition of hydrogen peroxide and 3,3′-diamino benzidine, which is converted to a dark brown precipitate. Antibody labeled in this manner is a sensitive research tool in viral pathogenesis—that is, in studies of the route of infection and the spread of virus within an organism—because it can reveal the presence of a few infected cells among large numbers of uninfected cells. It can also serve as a rapid diagnostic tool, since small amounts of infected biopsy material can be treated with fluorescein- or peroxidase-labeled antibodies against several suspected viruses, one of which may cause the infected cells to fluoresce or be stained. Finally, because antibody labeled in this manner can also reveal the pattern of viral antigen distribution within infected cells and because this pattern is often highly characteristic (nuclear or cytoplasmic, diffuse or highly localized), it can also serve as a useful adjunct to virus identification.

Antibody molecules can also be tagged with large molecules or particles that can be seen with the electron microscope. The two best suited for this purpose are ferritin, a large iron-containing protein, or colloidal gold particles, both of which are very electron-dense and, therefore, easily visible. Use of such antibody tagged in this manner permits exquisitely detailed observation of the distribution of viral antigens in infected cells and is invaluable in studies aimed at establishing the exact location of the sites of synthesis, accumulation, and assembly of viral protein components (Fig. 54–4).

Detection of Minute Amounts of Viral Antigens and Antibodies

Appropriate patient management frequently depends on the early detection of viral infections or on the recognition of persistent viral infections. In both situations, diagnosis requires the correct and rapid identification of minute amounts of viral antigens and antibodies. In recent years, great strides have been made in the development of extremely sensitive techniques for this purpose. Two such techniques are as

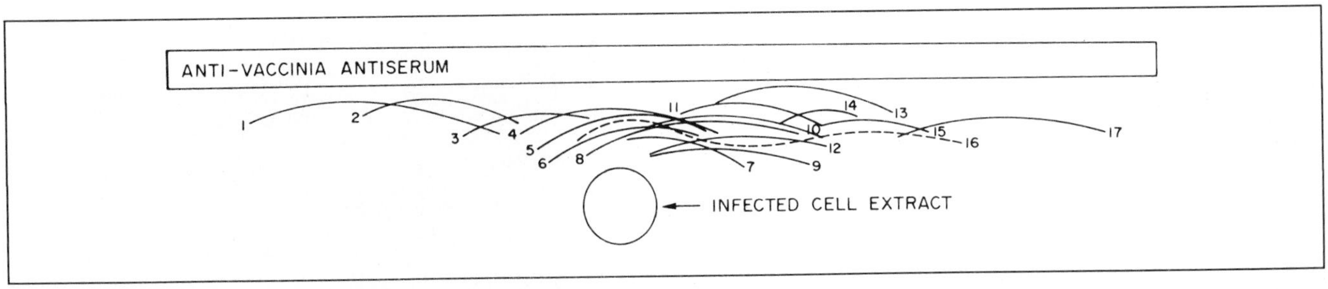

Fig. 54–2. Diagrammatic representation of an immunoelectrophoretic pattern of virus-specified proteins present in an extract of chick cells infected with vaccinia virus. In this technique the cell extract is placed into a circular well cut into an agar slab and an electric field is applied, causing antigens to migrate at rates governed by their charge and size. After electrophoresis, antiserum against vaccinia virus is placed into a trough cut parallel to the direction of electrophoresis and allowed to diffuse toward the separated cell extract components. Virus-specified proteins able to react with antibodies in the antiserum form precipitin lines. Seventeen such proteins can be detected in the extract shown here. *(From Rodriguez-Burgos et al: Virology 30:569, 1966.)*

follows. The first is radioimmunoassay. Not only is this technique capable of detecting extremely small amounts of virus-encoded proteins, but it is also very useful for assessing serologic relatedness because one can measure the efficiency with which unknown antigens can prevent antibody from precipitating standard labeled test antigens—the closer the serologic relationship, the more efficient the competition.

The second technique is the enzyme-linked immunosorbent assay (ELISA), in which antigen is immobilized on some surface, such as the wells of a plastic microtiter plate (see Fig. 52–6), and specific antiserum coupled with alkaline phosphatase or peroxidase is then added. Following extensive washing, substrate is added, and the reaction product that is formed by the antibody-linked enzyme bound to the antigen is measured colorimetrically. This technique can be made to be over 100 times more sensitive than complement-fixation assays.

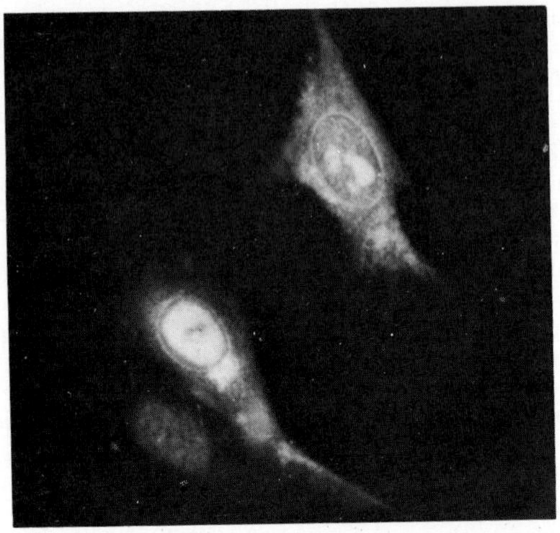

Fig. 54–3. Visualization of viral antigens by means of immunofluorescence. Cells infected with herpes simplex virus were washed, fixed with acetone, and allowed to react either with herpesvirus antibody conjugated with fluorescein isothiocyanate (direct immunofluorescence) or with herpesvirus antibody prepared in rabbits, followed by antirabbit globulin conjugated with fluorescein isothiocyanate (indirect immunofluorescence). Cells were then examined under ultraviolet light. The cells shown here were stained by the indirect method. The top cell shows fluorescent nuclear patches as well as fluorescence at the nuclear membrane and some diffuse cytoplasmic fluorescence. The other cell shows bright fluorescence of practically the whole nucleus, as well as cytoplasmic fluorescence. × 550. *(From Ross et al: J Gen Virol 2:115, 1968.)*

A further dimension has recently been added to these techniques by the use of protein A, which is present in the cell walls of certain strains of *Staphylococcus* and possesses high affinity for the Fc portion of most mammalian IgGs. Cells of such strains, or isolated A protein coupled to inert particles such as agarose, can be used to adsorb minute amounts of antigen-antibody complexes from complex mixtures, and the antigens in them can then be analyzed.

Virus-encoded Proteins Located on Cell Surfaces

As described in Chapters 55 and 59, virus-specified antigenic determinants frequently appear on the surfaces (outer plasma membranes) of infected cells. In the case of enveloped viruses, these proteins become, in due course, part of viral envelopes. In the case of nonenveloped viruses, they are early nonstructural or sometimes also structural proteins. In either case, virus-encoded proteins located on the cell surface provide signals to the immune mechanism that the cells are infected.

Immune Response to Viral Infection

Viral infections elicit both humoral and cell-mediated responses from the immune system. Usually the destruction of infected cells is beneficial to the host. However, sometimes such destruction is harmful. As a rule, the number of cells destroyed is not large enough to cause serious problems for the host organism, but there are exceptions. An example is provided by lymphocytic choriomeningitis virus (LCM), which causes encephalitis in mice (and also, rarely, in humans). LCM,

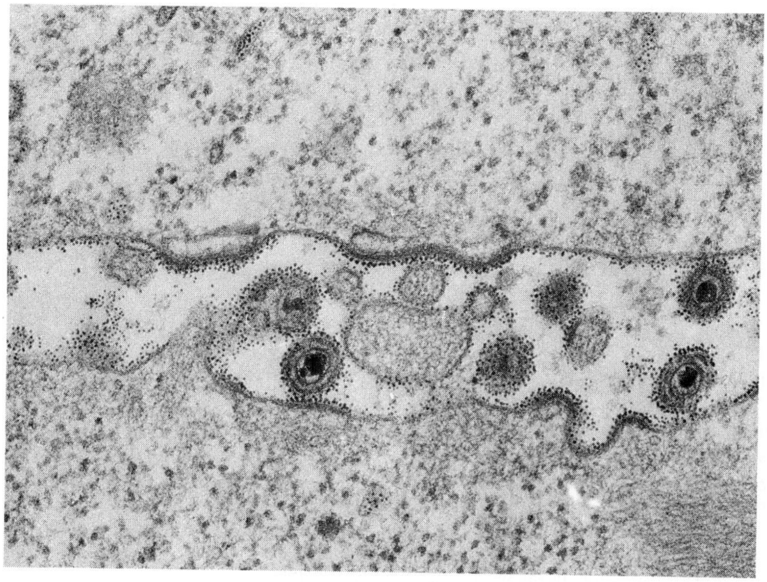

Fig. 54–4. Visualization of viral antigens by means of ferritin-conjugated antibody. This electron micrograph reveals the localization of virus-specified proteins on the surfaces of cells infected with herpes simplex virus. Infected cells were allowed to react with herpesvirus antibody conjugated with ferritin; the cells were then washed, fixed, embedded, and sectioned. The surfaces of two adjacent cells are seen, both with intensely labeled patches. Budding virus particles and detached cytoplasmic fragments are also labeled. × 48,000. *(From Nii et al: J Virol 1:1172, 1968.)*

an enveloped virus, is not a very lytic virus, and cells infected with it are not severely damaged and may survive for long periods of time. In mice, LCM produces no overt disease if the immune mechanism is not operative (in tolerant or immunosuppressed animals). However, in immunologically competent mice, LCM causes a fatal meningitis within a week, that is, as soon as antibody begins to be formed, death being due to the destruction of infected cells by activated macrophages. Thus the disease is not caused by the destruction of the host's cells by the virus but by the destruction of infected cells by the host's immune mechanism. A similar interaction between immune lymphocytes and virus-specified cell surface antigens may account for the symptoms associated with some viral diseases of humans, such as hepatitis.

The same is true for the second mechanism for destroying infected cells, namely, combination with antibody and complement, which will destroy infected cells long before cells break down as a direct result of viral infection. This mechanism also, though no doubt generally valuable as a defense against infection, may cause severe damage to the host. For example, it appears that the sometimes fatal hemorrhagic shock syndrome associated with dengue fever is caused by sudden increases in vascular permeability that may be triggered by the interaction of immune complexes with the complement and clotting systems.

Yet another example is provided by the phenomenon of immune enhancement. It turns out that several flaviviruses, in particular dengue virus, grow to much higher titers, and therefore set up much more serious infections in individuals who have already been exposed to the virus and who therefore possess some antibody against it, than in individuals who have never been infected. The reason is that infectious virus-antibody complexes are formed on reinfection that adsorb to susceptible cells via Fc receptors much more efficiently than virus alone interacting with its own specific receptors.

Although virus-antibody complexes are usually eliminated from the body without difficulty either before or after combination with complement, they may cause diseases quite unrelated to those caused by virus alone. This realization has come primarily from studies of animals infected with LCM and lactic dehydrogenase elevating virus (LDHV). Infection with these viruses results in the presence of large amounts of virus-antibody complexes in the bloodstream; it is also characterized by the development of glomerulonephritis caused by the presence of large amounts of virus-antibody-complement complexes in kidney capillaries. Similar observations have been made with respect to Aleutian mink disease and equine infectious anemia, in which the inflammatory changes are not confined to the kidneys but also involve blood vessels (with the development of arteritis) and other parts of the body. Some forms of human glomerulonephritis may also be caused by virus-antibody complexes.

FURTHER READING

Books and Reviews

Carter MJ, ter Meulen V: The application of monoclonal antibodies in the study of viruses. Adv Virus Res 29:95, 1986

Dimmock NJ: Mechanisms of neutralization of animal viruses. J Gen Virol 65:1015, 1984

Huppert J, Wild TF: Virus-related pathology: Is the continued presence of the virus necessary? Adv Virus Res 31:357, 1986

Katz D, Kohn A: Immunosorbent electronmicroscopy for detection of viruses. Adv Virus Res 29:169, 1986

Kennedy RC, Dreesman GR: Immunoglobulin idiotypes: Analysis of viral antigen-antibody systems. Prog Med Virol 31:168, 1985

Laver WG, Air GM, Webster RG, Smith-Gill SJ: Epitopes on protein antigens: Misconceptions and realities. Cell 61:553, 1990

Matsui SM, Mackow ER, Greenberg HB: Molecular determinant of rotavirus neutralization and protection. Adv Virus Res 36:181, 1989

McCullough KC: Monoclonal antibodies: Implications for virology. Arch Virol 87:1, 1986

Porterfield JS: Antibody-dependent enhancement of viral infectivity. Adv Virus Res 31:335, 1986

Rossmann MG: Neutralization of small RNA viruses by antibodies and antiviral agents. FASEB J 3:2335, 1989

Rossmann MG: The canyon hypothesis. J Biol Chem 264:14587, 1989

Schochetman G, Epstein JS, Zuck TF: Serodiagnosis of infection with the AIDS virus and other human retroviruses. Annu Rev Microbiol 43:629, 1989

Underwood PA: Measurement of the affinity of antiviral antibodies. Adv Virus Res 34:283, 1988

van Regenmortel MHV, Neurath AR (eds): Immunochemistry of Viruses II: The Basis for Serodiagnosis and Vaccines. Amsterdam, Elsevier, 1990

Selected Papers

INDUCTION OF THE IMMUNE RESPONSE AGAINST VIRUSES

Anders EM, Kapaklis-Deliyannis GP, White DO: Induction of immune response to influenza virus with anti-idiotypic antibodies. J Virol 63:2758, 1989

Bennink JR, Yewdell JW, Smith GL, Moss B: Anti-influenza virus cytotoxic T lymphocytes recognize the three viral polymerases and a nonstructural protein: Responsiveness to individual viral antigens is major histocompatibility complex controlled. J Virol 61:1098, 1987

Galloway DA, Jenison SA: Characterization of the humoral immune response to genital papillomaviruses. Mol Biol Med 7:59, 1990

Hom RC, Finberg RW, Mullaney S, Ruprecht RM: Protective cellular retroviral immunity requires both CDr^{++} and $CD8^{+}$ immune T cells. J Virol 65:220, 1991

Moskophidis D, Lehmann-Grube F: Virus-induced delayed-type hypersensitivity reaction is sequentially mediated by $CD8^{+}$ and $CD4^{+}$ T lymphocytes. Proc Natl Acad Sci USA 86:3291, 1989

Openshaw PJM, Anderson K, Wertz GW, Askonas BA: The 22,000-kilodalton protein of respiratory syncytial virus is a major target for K^d-restricted cytotoxic T lymphocytes from mice primed by infection. J Virol 64:1683, 1990

Puddington L, Bevan MJ, Rose JK, Lefrancois L: N protein is the predominant antigen recognized by vesicular stomatitis virus-specific cytotoxic T cells. J Virol 60:708, 1986

Reay PA, Jones IM, Gotch FM, et al: Recognition of the PB1, neuraminidase, and matrix proteins of influenza virus A/NT/60/68 by cytotoxic T lymphocytes. Virology 170:477, 1989

Urbanelli D, Sawada Y, Roskova J, et al: C-terminal domain of the adenovirus E1A oncogene product is required for induction of cytotoxic T lymphocytes and tumor-specific transplantation immunity. Virology 173:607, 1989

Whitton JL, Southern PJ, Oldstone MBA: Analyses of the cytotoxic T lymphocyte responses to glycoprotein and nucleoprotein components of lymphocytic choriomeningitis virus. Virology 162:321, 1988

MECHANISM OF THE IMMUNE RESPONSE AGAINST VIRUSES

Kingsford L, Boucquey KH, Cardoso TP: Effects of specific monoclonal antibodies on La Crosse virus neutralization: Aggregation, inactivation by fab fragments, and inhibition of attachment to baby hamster kidney cells. Virology 180:591, 1991

Lewis RM, Cosgriff TM, Griffin BY, et al: Immune serum increases arenavirus replication in monocytes. J Gen Virol 69:1735, 1988

Outlaw MC, Armstrong SJ, Dimmock NJ: Mechanisms of neutralization of influenza virus in tracheal epithelial and BHK cells vary according to IgG concentration. Virology 178:478, 1990

Poumbourios P, Brown LE, White DO, Jackson DC: The stoichiometry of binding between monoclonal antibody molecules and the hemagglutinin of influenza virus. Virology 179:768, 1990

Rigg RJ, Carver AS, Dimmock NJ: IgG-neutralized influenza virus undergoes primary, but not secondary uncoating in vivo. J Gen Virol 70:2097, 1989

Wohlfart C: Neutralization of adenoviruses: Kinetics, stoichiometry, and mechanisms. J Virol 62:2321, 1988

VIRAL PROTEIN EPITOPES

Boege U, Kobasa D, Onodera S, et al: Characterization of Mengo virus neutralization epitopes. Virology 181:1, 1991

Luo L, Li Y, Snyder RM, Wagner RR: Point mutations in glycoprotein gene of vesicular stomatitis virus (New Jersey serotype) selected by resistance to neutralization by epitope-specific monoclonal antibodies. Virology 163:341, 1988

Niesters HGM, Bleumink-Pluym NMC, Osterhaus ADME, et al: Epitopes on the peplomer protein of infectious bronchitis virus strain M41 as defined by monoclonal antibodies. Virology 161:511, 1987

Parekh BS, Buchmeier MJ: Proteins of lymphocytic choriomeningitis virus: Antigenic topography of the viral glycoproteins. Virology 153:168, 1986

Roivainen M, Närvänen A, Korkolainen M, et al: Antigenic regions of poliovirus type 3/Sabin capsid proteins recognized by human sera in the peptide scanning technique. Virology 180:99, 1990

Weber EL, Buchmeier MJ: Fine mapping of a peptide sequence containing an antigenic site conserved among arenaviruses. Virology 164:30, 1988

CHAPTER 55

The Virus Multiplication Cycle

Virus particles represent the static or inert form of viruses. The very existence of viruses is recognizable only in terms of their interaction with cells, which is the central theme of virology.

The interaction of virus and cell generates a novel entity, the infected cell, the fate of which varies widely because it depends both on the nature of the cell and on the nature of the virus. The two most commonly observed virus-cell interactions are (1) the lytic interaction, which results in virus multiplication and lysis of the host cell, and (2) the transforming interaction, which results in the integration of the viral genome into the host genome and the permanent transformation or alteration of the host cell with respect to morphology, growth habit, and the manner in which it interacts with other cells with which it comes into contact.

In studying the virus-host interaction, one can focus primarily either on the fate and functioning of the invading virus particle and on the production of virus progeny or on the reaction of the host cell to viral infection. Both approaches are of fundamental importance to the medical practitioner. The former is particularly relevant to the development of a rational approach to antiviral chemotherapy; the latter to an understanding of chronic viral infection and cancer. This chapter focuses on the invading virus particle, and Chapter 56 focuses on the response of the cell.

Lytic Virus-Cell Interaction

The lytic virus-cell interaction is best thought of in terms of a cycle—the infection or multiplication cycle—during which the virus enters cells, multiplies, and is released. This cycle is repeated many times when a virus particle infects an organism, until, for one reason or another, further multiplication is arrested or the host dies.

One of the principal goals of virology is to define in molecular terms all the various reactions that proceed during the virus multiplication cycle. As an example, when a poliovirus particle infects a cell, one RNA molecule and about 200 protein molecules are introduced into it. How does this RNA molecule replicate? What are the proteins that it encodes, and what are their functions? How are mature virus particles assembled? What is the fate of the 200 parental protein molecules? What effect do they have on the host cell? What are the reactions that cause the host cell to die?

It is impossible to answer these and many other questions by studies in the intact organism. Instead, simple experimental systems that can be manipulated at will are required. Such systems are provided by cloned strains of animal cells that are capable of growing in vitro and that can be infected with pure (plaque-purified) strains of virus. Among their many advantages is that they permit focusing on one multiplication cycle rather than on many repeated cycles, which is achieved by infecting all cells at the same time. In fact, one of the major conceptual breakthroughs in virology occurred about 50 years ago when Ellis and Delbrück demonstrated how very much simpler analysis of the one-step growth cycle is than that of numerous successive unsynchronized cycles. In populations of cultured cells infected at high multiplicity—that is, with many virus particles per cell—so as to ensure that infection commences at the same time in all cells, the various reactions that together comprise virus multiplication proceed synchronously according to a strictly regulated progressive pattern that is amenable to study by the techniques of biochemistry and molecular biology.

One-step Growth Cycle: General Aspects

The virus multiplication cycle can be divided into several periods, using events of critical importance as markers (Fig. 55–1). As discussed below, the infectivity of virus particles is destroyed or eclipsed when they adsorb. The initial period of the multiplication cycle is, therefore, often referred to as the *eclipse period*. This period ends with the formation of the first mature progeny virus particle, which marks the beginning of the *rise period*. Alternatively, the synthesis of the first progeny genome is often regarded as dividing the multiplication cycle into early and late periods. The eclipse and early periods and the rise and late periods overlap substantially, with the interval between the beginning of the late and rise periods representing the average time necessary for the incorporation of a viral genome into a mature virus particle.

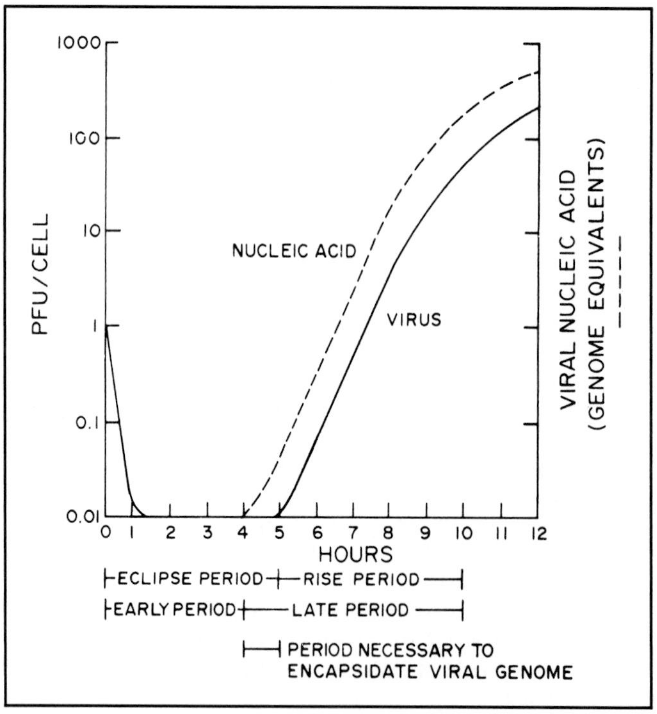

Fig. 55–1. The one-step growth cycle. Its essential features are: Following adsorption, infectivity is abolished or "eclipsed"; this is caused by uncoating of the infecting virus particles. During the eclipse or early period, which can last from a few minutes to many hours, the stage is set for viral nucleic acid replication. The appearance of the first progeny genome marks the beginning of the late period, and the appearance of the first mature progeny virus particle marks the beginning of the rise period. The lengths of all periods, as well as the extent of virus multiplication, vary greatly for different viruses and different cells.

Eclipse Period

Adsorption

The first step of the virus-cell interaction is adsorption, which can itself be separated into several stages. The first of these is ionic attraction. Both cells and virus particles are negatively charged at pH 7, and positive ions are, therefore, required as counter-ions. As a rule this requirement is met most efficiently by magnesium ions. The second stage involves the interaction of virus particles with specific receptors. Indirect evidence for the existence of specific virus receptors has been available for some time. For example, poliovirus adsorbs only to cells of human or primate origin. In fact, in the body, poliovirus adsorbs only to cells of the central nervous system and to cells lining the intestinal tract. Other human and primate cells develop the ability to adsorb poliovirus only after being cultured in vitro.

Most virus receptors appear to be glycoproteins. Several have been identified: Thus the cell adhesion molecule ICAM-1 is the major cell surface receptor for human rhinoviruses; another new member of the immunoglobulin superfamily is the cellular receptor for poliovirus; the CD4 T cell antigen is the receptor for the human immunodeficiency virus (HIV); the type 2 complement receptor on B lymphocytes, CD21, is the receptor for the Epstein-Barr virus; and the acetylcholine receptor may be the receptor for rabies virus. Whereas these viruses apparently recognize both the carbohydrate as well as the protein moieties of their receptors, other viruses, such as the orthomyxoviruses, recognize only their sialic acid–containing carbohydrate moieties; and the receptors for herpes simplex virus appear to be heparin sulfate proteoglycans.

The time course of virus adsorption follows first-order kinetics. The rate of adsorption is independent of temperature but directly proportional to the amount of surface to which virus can adsorb, that is, to cell concentration. The kinetics of adsorption are described by the relation

$$\frac{V_t}{V_0} = e^{-Ktc}$$

where V_0 and V_t are the concentrations of free virus at time 0 and after t minutes, respectively; t is the time in minutes; c is the cell concentration; and K is the adsorption rate constant.

The number of virus particles or infectious units adsorbed per cell is referred to as the multiplicity of infection (moi). Animal cells are generally capable of adsorbing very large amounts of virus. The number of receptors for most viruses ranges from 100,000 to 500,000 per cell (Fig. 55–2). It is known, however, that the number of virus receptors per cell can vary over a 10-fold range and is greatest during the exponential growth phase.

Penetration and Uncoating

The second stage of the virus multiplication cycle involves penetration and uncoating. Penetration concerns the entry of the virus particle into the cytoplasm. It may be observed directly by means of electron microscopy or indirectly by measuring the loss of ability of antiviral antiserum to arrest the initiation of virus multiplication. The reason for this is that as long as virus particles remain outside the cell, combination with antibody decreases their ability to initiate productive infection; but once the particles have penetrated into the cell, they are no longer accessible to antibody.

Uncoating signifies the physical separation of viral genomes from their capsids or, in the case of negative-stranded RNA viruses, the disruption of envelopes followed by liberation of the nucleocapsids. Uncoating is of taxonomic significance because viruses are the only intracellular infectious agents or parasites for which this is an obligatory step of their multiplication cycle.

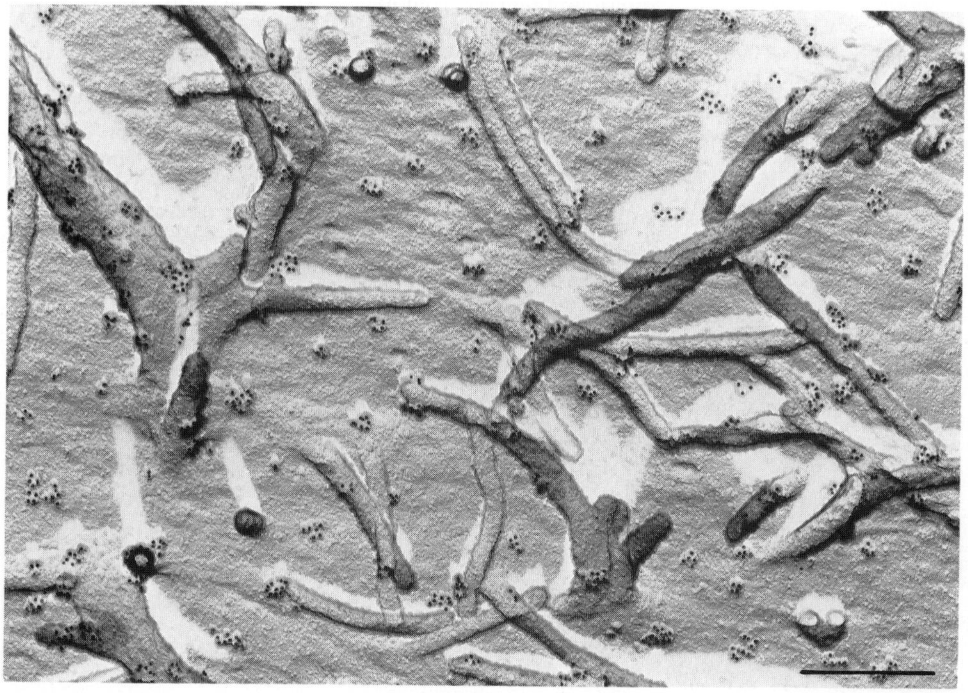

Fig. 55–2. Transmission electron microscope image of a platinum-carbon replica prepared from a HeLa cell surface showing the patchlike localization of the poliovirus receptor labeled with monoclonal antibodies directed against the receptor. Immunogold markers. ×49,000. Bar: 0.5 μm. *(From Mannweiler et al: J Gen Virol 71:2737, 1990.)*

Uncoating is best assessed by measuring physical and chemical changes in the adsorbed virus particles. Among these changes are progressive labilization of the capsid structure as judged by loss of its ability to shield the viral genome from hydrolysis by nucleases, development of susceptibility to reagents such as urea to which intact virus particles are resistant, loss of antigenic determinants, and progressive loss of capsid protein. The total time from adsorption to final uncoating ranges from several minutes to several hours.

The actual pathways of penetration and uncoating differ markedly for the various types of virus particles, a fact not surprising in view of their structural diversity. The essential features of this process are as follows. Virus particles usually bind to receptors on microvilli, elongated projections extending from cell surfaces. They then move down the microvillus shafts toward the body of the cell, where they encounter coated pits. These are specialized regions of the cell membrane that are coated on their cytoplasmic, or inner, side with a large protein known as clathrin. In these coated pits the plasma membrane flows over and around the virus particles, thereby engulfing them (endocytosis) and transporting them into the interior of the cell. After the clathrin is removed from the outside of these coated vesicles, they fuse with endosomes, and it is within the resulting endosomal vesicles that virus particles are uncoated or that the uncoating process begins. In the case of most enveloped viruses, the low pH within endosomal vesicles causes the viral envelope to fuse with the endosomal membrane, thereby liberating the nucleocapsid into the cytoplasm. The fusing activity is a property of one end of one of the spike glycoproteins that is normally buried within the spike but that becomes exposed at pH 5 to 6. Since these ends are usually very hydrophobic, they possess membrane fusing activity. The one exception to this chain of events is infection with paramyxoviruses, which possess a glycoprotein, the F protein (see p. 823), which is capable of fusing virus envelopes and host plasma cell membranes directly, so that paramyxovirus nucleocapsids are introduced into the cytoplasm without the intervention of clathrin-coated and endoplasmic vesicles.

For nonenveloped viruses, uncoating proceeds via variations of the pathway just described. For example, adenoviruses are also transported into cells through clathrin-coated and endoplasmic vesicles that are disrupted by the fusogenic fibers. The 12 pentons are then removed, which results in partially uncoated virus particles being released into the cytoplasm. These particles then migrate to the nucleus where adenovirus DNA is fully uncoated (Fig. 55–3). Similarly, the outer region of poxvirus particles is degraded in endosomal vesicles, and cores are liberated into the interior of the cell, but here core degradation requires the synthesis of a special virus-encoded uncoating protein (Fig. 55–4). Finally, in the case of reoviruses, the outer capsid shell is partially digested after endoplasmic vesicles fuse with lysosomes, and subviral particles that consist of the core to which about one half of the components of the outer capsid shell are still attached are released into the cytoplasm, where they remain throughout the multiplication cycle, naked reovirus RNA never being liberated (see p. 830).

Eclipse

Adsorption, penetration, and uncoating result in loss of infectivity, which is referred to as eclipse. The only residual infectivity is that due to the viral nucleic acid itself (or to the nucleocapsid, as the case may be), which, however, is never more than a small fraction (less than 0.1%) of that of the virus particles themselves.

The first three stages of infection are usually inefficient processes. Virus particles often adsorb to portions of the cell surface at which penetration will not proceed, viral genomes may be damaged by ribonucleases, which are frequently associated with plasma cell membranes, and uncoated virus particles may fail to be released from endoplasmic vesicles. All these inefficiencies account in large part for the fact that the ratio of infectious to total animal virus particles is almost always far less than 1 (Chap. 52).

Synthetic Phase of the Virus Multiplication Cycle

Once the viral genome is uncoated, the synthetic phase of the multiplication cycle commences. In essence, this encompasses, in a precisely regulated program, the replication of the viral genome, the synthesis of viral proteins, and the formation of progeny virus particles.

The location of viral genome replication is characteristic for each virus (Table 55–1). There is no correlation between this location and any other property, such as chemical nature

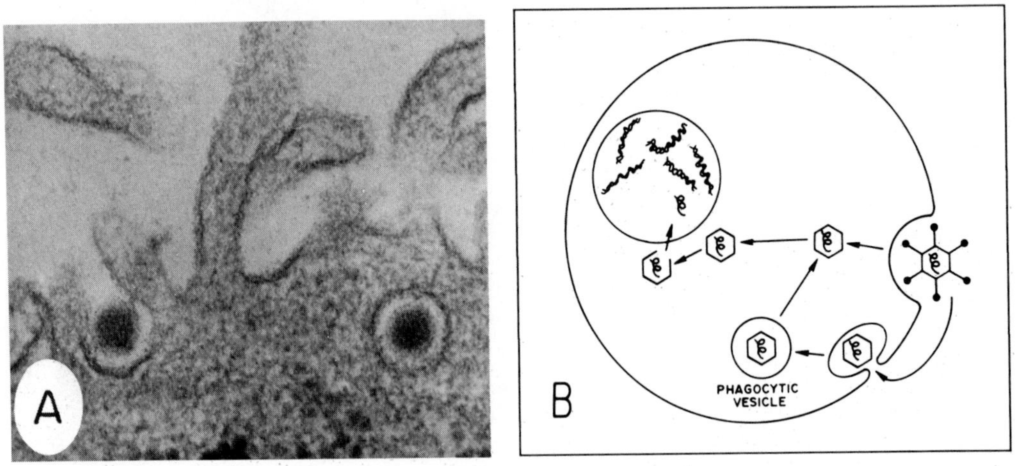

Fig. 55–3. The uptake of adenovirus particles into cells. **A.** One virus particle is about to be engulfed into a clathrin-coated pit; another is inside a coated vesicle. *(From Chardonnet and Dales: Virology 40:462, 1970.)* **B.** Diagrammatic representation of the uptake and uncoating of adenovirus particles.

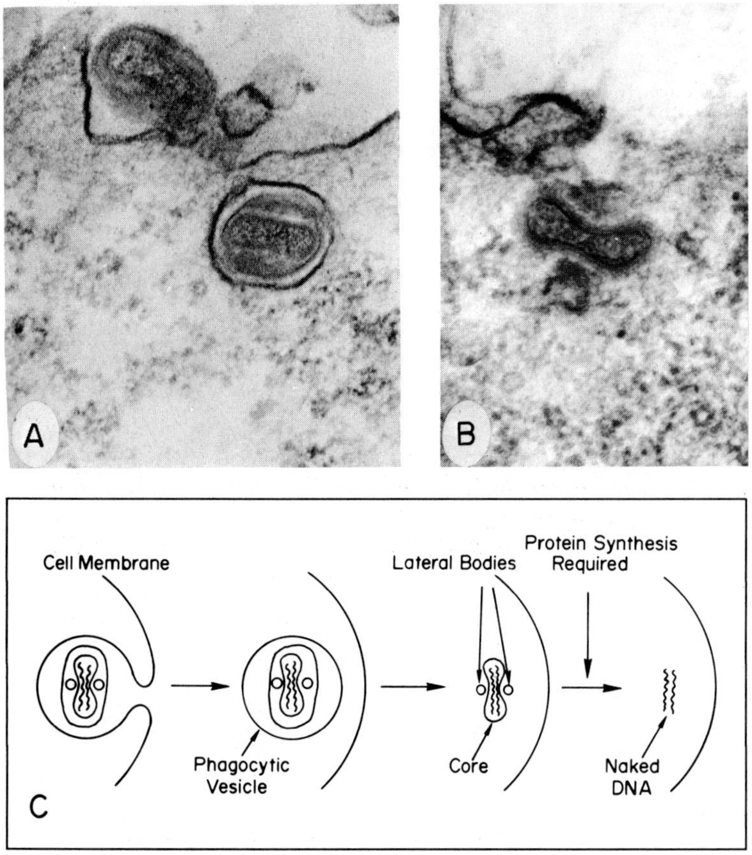

Fig. 55–4. The penetration and uncoating of vaccinia virus. Three stages are shown. **A.** One of the two virus particles is in a coated pit; the other is already in the cytoplasm within a coated vesicle. **B.** The vesicle has broken down, as has the virus particle's outer protein coat. The core is now free, and the two laterial bodies have moved some distance away. The final stage of uncoating is the breakdown of the core, which results in liberation of the DNA. This step is not achieved if protein synthesis is inhibited. This indicates that the synthesis of a special uncoating protein is required. Poxviruses are the only viruses that require the synthesis of a special protein for uncoating. The whole process is depicted diagrammatically in **C.** **A** and **B**, × 80,000. (**A, B** from Dales: J Cell Biol 18:63, 1963; **C** adapted from Joklik: J Mol Biol 8:277, 1964.)

TABLE 55–1. UNCOATING, VIRAL GENOME REPLICATION, AND VIRUS MATURATION

Virus	Uncoated to	Genome Replication	Virion Maturation
Poxviruses	DNA	Cytoplasm	Cytoplasm
Herpesviruses	DNA	Nucleus	At nuclear membrane
Adenoviruses	DNA	Nucleus	Nucleus
Papovaviruses	DNA	Nucleus	Nucleus
Hepadnaviruses	DNA	Nucleus	Cytoplasm
Parvoviruses	DNA	Nucleus	Nucleus
Picornaviruses	RNA	Cytoplasm	Cytoplasm
Togaviruses	RNA	Cytoplasm	At membranes
Flaviviruses	RNA	Cytoplasm	At membranes
Coronaviruses	RNA	Cytoplasm	At membranes
Reoviruses	Subviral particle	Cytoplasm	Cytoplasm
Rhabdoviruses	Nucleocapsid	Cytoplasm	At membranes
Paramyxoviruses	Nucleocapsid	Cytoplasm	At membranes
Orthomyxoviruses	Nucleocapsids	Nucleus	At membranes
Bunyaviruses	Nucleocapsids	Cytoplasm	At membranes
Arenaviruses	Nucleocapsids	Cytoplasm	At membranes
Retroviruses	Nucleocapsids	Nucleus	At membranes

or size of the genome. Viral protein is always synthesized in the cytoplasm on polyribosomes composed of virus messenger RNA, host cell ribosomes, and host cell transfer RNA. In the case of RNA-containing viruses, most, if not all, of their genetic information is expressed soon after uncoating. In the case of the double-stranded DNA-containing viruses, however, the multiplication cycle can be divided into clearly defined early and late periods, with the onset of viral DNA replication marking the beginning of the late period (Fig. 55–1).

Early Period

The early period of the synthetic phase is devoted primarily to the activation of reactions that are prerequisite for initiating viral genome replication. This activation proceeds as a result of viruses exercising certain early functions. Among them are (1) inhibition of host DNA, RNA, and protein synthesis—which may involve the synthesis of virus-encoded proteins that either inhibit or alter the specificities of the DNA-replicating, RNA-transcribing, and protein-synthesizing systems—so that viral rather than host cell genetic information is processed, (2) the synthesis of proteins that form the matrix of inclusions, either in the nucleus or in the cytoplasm, within which viral nucleic acids replicate and viral morphogenesis proceeds, and (3) the synthesis of enzymes that synthesize viral DNA and RNA.

The extent to which early functions are expressed varies greatly from virus to virus. Some viruses possess so little genetic information that only very few early functions are expressed; others possess so much that they may express from 30 to 50 early functions. Early functions are expressed through (early) proteins that are transcribed from early viral messenger RNA species. Viral genomes that are plus-stranded RNA serve directly as messenger RNA; for all other viruses, messenger RNAs must first be transcribed from parental genomes by means of polymerases either associated with virus particles or preexisting in the host cell.

Late Period

During the late period, the late viral functions are expressed. The late viral proteins are primarily virus particle components (structural proteins) and enzymes and other nonstructural proteins that function during viral morphogenesis. They are encoded by late viral messenger RNA molecules that are transcribed from regions of the viral genomes different from the early ones. Late messenger RNA molecules are transcribed primarily from progeny genomes, and because there are always more progeny than parental genomes, many more late messenger RNA molecules are formed than early ones. Therefore, much greater amounts of late proteins than of early proteins are always synthesized. Activation of the regions of the viral genome that encode late functions may or may not be accompanied by deactivation of the regions that encode early ones. In either case, a mechanism exists that specifies that one set of genes (the early set) is transcribed from parental genomes and that another set (the late set) is transcribed only from progeny genomes. There are several ways in which this could be accomplished. The basis of one that is used by certain bacteriophages lies in the specificity of the enzymes that transcribe DNA: the DNA-dependent RNA polymerase is modified several times during infection, which enables it to recognize successively new classes of promoters and, therefore, transcribe, in turn, several classes of early and late genes (Chap. 60). Animal viruses, such as vaccinia virus, herpes simplex virus, adenovirus, and others, use a different mechanism. Here the DNA-dependent RNA polymerase remains the same, but the transcription factors change in cascadelike fashion, each factor (or factors) binding to a new set of promoters, thus causing the genes that they control to be transcribed.

During the late period the newly formed viral genomes and capsid proteins are assembled into progeny virus particles, a process known as *morphogenesis*. This is a spontaneously occurring process, since most of the information for virus assembly resides in the amino acid sequences of the capsid proteins. Nucleic acid performs no essential function during morphogenesis, a fact demonstrated by the occurrence among the yield of most icosahedral viruses of empty virus particles—that is, virus particles that contain no nucleic acid—that are morphologically indistinguishable from mature virus particles.

The duration of the late period is generally limited by the ability of the host cell to supply energy for macromolecular biosynthesis. This is a critical factor because infection with lytic viruses invariably interferes with the functioning of the host cell by multiple mechanisms, which are discussed in Chapter 56. As a result, the synthesis of viral nucleic acids and proteins slows down progressively, thereby limiting the amount of viral progeny.

Release of Progeny Virus

The final step of the infection cycle is the release of progeny virus. There is no special mechanism for the release of unenveloped viruses. Infected cells simply disintegrate more or less rapidly, liberating the viral progeny that has accumulated within them. The amount of cell-associated virus, therefore, exceeds the amount of released virus until the very last phase of the multiplication cycle (Fig. 55–5). A special mechanism does, however, exist for the enveloped viruses, for which release is the final stage of morphogenesis. Here virus-encoded envelope proteins are incorporated into certain areas of the host cell membrane while nucleocapsids are being synthesized. The nucleocapsids then bud through the modified membrane patches and are enveloped by them (p. 855).

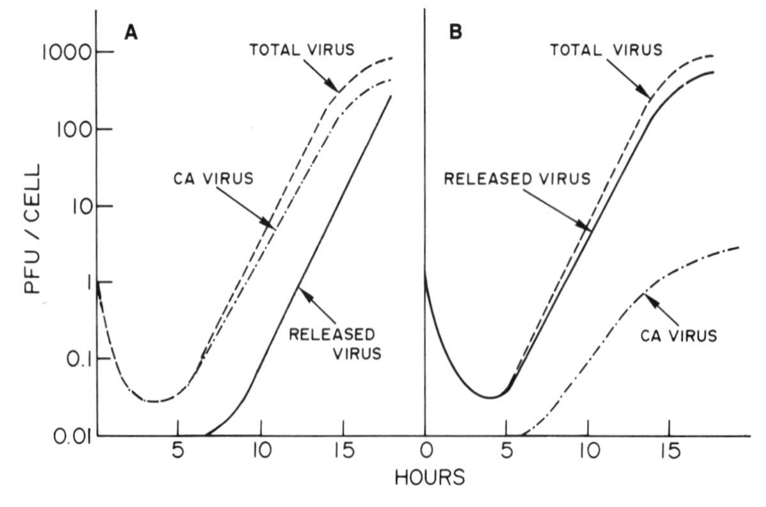

Fig. 55–5. The relationship between virus multiplication and release. **A.** This graph refers to viruses with icosahedral nucleocapsids. Such viruses are not released readily from cells. Viral progeny accumulates within cells, so that for much of the rise period, the amount of cell-associated (CA) virus greatly exceeds the amount of released virus. Release of virus occurs only when cells break down at the end of the rise period. **B.** This graph refers to enveloped viruses. Such viruses mature only in the process of being released, since it is only then that they acquire their envelope. The amount of liberated virus, therefore, always greatly exceeds the amount of CA virus. The only CA virus particles are those in the process of budding from the plasma membrane and those that bud into intracytoplasmic vacuoles.

TABLE 55–2. APPROXIMATE DURATION OF THE ECLIPSE PERIOD AND OF THE ENTIRE MULTIPLICATION CYCLE

Virus	Eclipse Period (hours)	Total Multiplication Cycle (hours)
Poxvirus: vaccinia virus	4	24
Herpesvirus: herpes simplex virus	3–5	24–36
Adenovirus	8–10	48
Papovavirus: polyoma virus	12–14	48
Poliovirus	1–2	6–8
Togavirus: Sindbis virus	2	10
Reovirus	3	15
Orthomyxovirus: influenza virus	3–5	18–36
Rhabdovirus: vesicular stomatitis virus	2	8–10

Budding occurs both at the outer plasma cell membrane and also, less frequently, at membranes lining intracytoplasmic vacuoles, which then transport the virus to the exterior of the cell. These viruses do not exist in mature infectious form within cells (except for the virus that has budded into the intracytoplasmic vacuoles), and the amount of extracellular virus, therefore, greatly exceeds the amount of cell-associated virus at all stages of the multiplication cycle (Fig. 55–5).

The duration of the various phases of the virus multiplication cycle varies greatly depending on the nature of the virus and on the nature of the host cell. Table 55–2 lists the average lengths of the eclipse periods and of the complete multiplication cycles of some well-studied viruses.

Multiplication Cycles of Several Important Viruses

Of the many facets of virus multiplication, the two that are central are (1) the nature of the information encoded in viral genomes and (2) the manner in which this information is expressed. Not only does description of a virus in this manner define it in its most fundamental terms, but it also provides the framework of knowledge essential for a rational approach to antiviral chemotherapy.

Knowledge concerning viral multiplication cycles has expanded enormously in recent years as a result of the advent of recombinant DNA technology. This technology has been of crucial importance in several vital areas. For example, it has permitted the cloning of viral RNA genomes, that is, their conversion to the double-stranded DNA form. As a result, it is now possible to map all viral genomes using bacterial restriction endonucleases. These enzymes, which are components of the restriction-modification systems in bacteria, cleave DNA at palindromic sequences that are highly specific for each enzyme. These sequences, which possess twofold rotational symmetry, may be as simple as

5′ . . . GGCC . . .

. . . CCGG . . . 5′

or as complex as

5′ . . GCCNNNNNNGGC . . .

. . . CGGNNNNNNCCG . . . 5′

Clearly, the simpler the recognition site, the more often will it occur and the more often will the DNA be cut. The fragments that result may be ordered or mapped by digesting DNA under conditions when it is only partially cleaved and analyzing the incompletely hydrolyzed pieces for neighboring fragments. Figure 55–6 shows the 6 *Hin*dIII restriction endonuclease fragments of SV40 DNA, and Figure 55–7 shows the order in which they are arranged, that is, the *Hin*dIII restriction map. Several other restriction endonuclease maps of SV40 DNA are also shown. Such maps—and more than 100 restriction endonucleases are now available—are physical maps because here the viral DNA is treated as a sequence of nucleic acid bases. Physical maps can be correlated by a variety of techniques with genetic maps that define the order of the various genes that comprise the viral genome. The ultimate aim of this type of analysis is to define exactly where each gene is located in the viral genome, when it is transcribed during the virus multiplication cycle, how frequently it is transcribed, and, finally, what controls or regulates the transcription program.

Another area that has profited from the advent of recombinant DNA technology is that of sequencing. Many viral genomes have by now been sequenced, and many others are in the process of being sequenced. Finally, there is also the area of site-specific mutagenesis. It is now possible to introduce

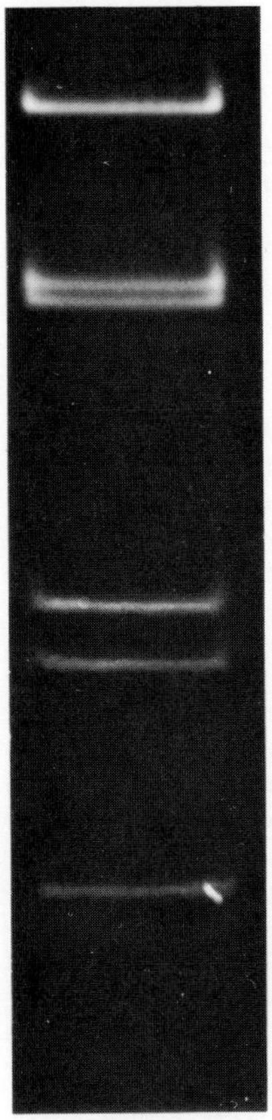

Fig. 55–6. Autoradiogram of a polyacrylamide gel in which the six fragments were electrophoresed that result when circular ^{32}P-labeled SV40 DNA is digested with restriction endonuclease *HindIII*. *(Courtesy of Drs. J. K. Li and C. Huang.)*

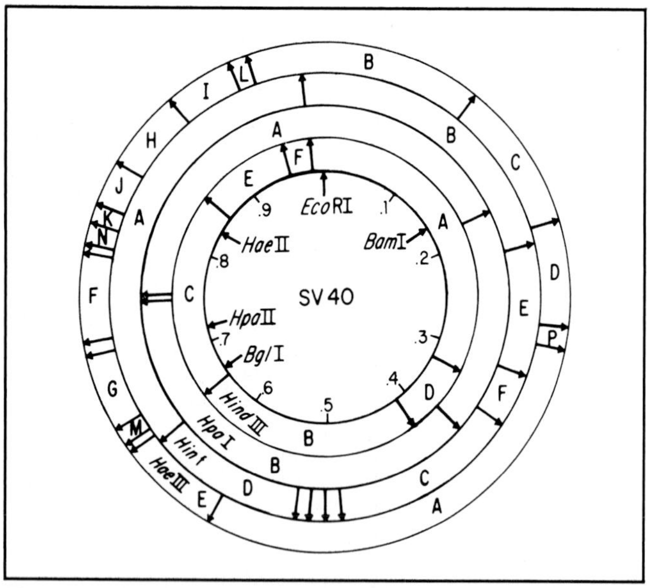

Fig. 55–7. Restriction endonuclease cleavage maps of SV40 DNA, using *Hin*dIII, *Hpa*I, *Hin*f, and *Hae*III. *Eco*RI, *Bam*I, *Bgl*I, *Hpa*II, and *Hae*II cleave only once. The origin of DNA replication is at a palindromic sequence, part of which forms the recognition sequence for *Bgl*I.

mutations into any desired location in a viral genome. This has, in turn, opened the way to identifying and defining not only the functions of virus-specified proteins but also the mechanisms by which the expression of the genes that encode them is regulated.

Multiplication Cycles of Double-stranded DNA-containing Viruses

Papovaviruses

Papovaviruses are among the smallest double-stranded DNA-containing viruses. They can infect cells both by the lytic virus-cell interaction, during which they initiate productive infection, multiply, and lyse their hosts, and by the transforming virus-cell interaction during which their genome is integrated into that of the host cell, thereby creating new, genetically different cells, namely, transformed cells, which can form benign or malignant tumors in animals. In general, the more permissive cells are, that is, the more readily they support productive infection, the less likely are they to become transformed. The transforming papovavirus-host cell interaction is discussed in Chapter 59. Here, we are concerned with the nature of their lytic multiplication cycles.

The multiplication cycle of polyomaviruses, such as polyoma virus, SV40, and BK virus, can be divided into well-defined early and late periods. During each period, different portions of the viral genome are transcribed into messenger RNAs, which are then processed and translated into proteins by the cellular protein-synthesizing system. We describe the nature of the functions that regulate the multiplication of SV40, the simplest papovavirus, in some detail because the principles on which they are based are applicable not only to the other papovaviruses, such as polyoma virus and the human papillomaviruses, which are of rapidly increasing medical importance, but also to the other dsDNA-containing viruses, namely, the adenoviruses, the herpesviruses, and the poxviruses.

Early Period

The genome of SV40 is a circular molecule about 5230 bp long, which has been completely sequenced. Its multiplication cycle is best understood by reference to the genetic and transcription maps of its genome (Fig. 55–8). During the early phase, which lasts a surprisingly long time (14–18 hours), about 50% of the viral DNA, namely, the region that extends from map position 0.65 (relative to the *Eco*RI restriction endonuclease cleavage site) to map position 0.17, is transcribed into RNA. The transcripts of this region are processed not into one but into two species of messenger RNA. The first is about 2230 nucleotides long and is composed of two parts that map to positions 0.65 to 0.60 and 0.54 to 0.17, respectively. RNA corresponding to the DNA between map positions 0.60 and 0.54 is not present in this messenger RNA because it is spliced out. The second messenger RNA also is composed of two exons, which correspond to map positions 0.65 to 0.55 and 0.54 to 0.17, respectively.

These two messenger RNAs encode two proteins. The 2230 nucleotide-long messenger RNA is translated into the large T antigen, a 708 amino acid–long nonstructural DNA-binding phosphoprotein with both ATPase and DNA helicase (DNA unwinding) activity, which has a variety of extremely important regulatory functions. First, it is essential for the initiation of DNA replication and regulates the SV40 transcription program by binding to several sites on SV40 DNA near map position 0.65, which is where the origin of DNA replication is located and where both early and late transcription begin. Second, it activates the transcription of several cellular genes involved in cellular DNA replication and cell cycle control by being a transactive transcriptional activator. As a result, it stimulates G0 arrested cells to enter S phase and divide. This is of little consequence for SV40 lytic infection but increases the likelihood that the viral genome will be integrated into that of the cell. Third, the large T antigen binds to at least two cellular proteins. One is p53, a nuclear protein implicated in the regulation of the cell division cycle. The other is the retinoblastoma susceptibility protein, $p110^{Rb}$, an antioncogene whose inactivation triggers the formation of retinoblastomas and osteosarcomas (Chap. 59). By binding these two proteins with growth suppressor functions, the large T antigen further stimulates uncontrolled cell multiplication. Fourth, although most large T antigen is located in the nucleus, about 5% of it is embedded in the plasma membrane where, in transformed cells, it serves as the tumor-specific transplantation antigen (TSTA). Fifth, the large T antigen can be modified in numerous ways: it can be phosphorylated, glycosylated, ADP-ribosylated, palmitylated, and *N*-acetylated, and it can exist in cells in the monomeric as well as in oligomeric forms. No doubt these modifications affect the manner in which it functions. For example, phosphorylation decreases its ability to bind DNA. Finally, as a result of exercising all these as well as perhaps additional functions, the large T antigen establishes and maintains cell transformation; it is, therefore, the SV40 oncogene.

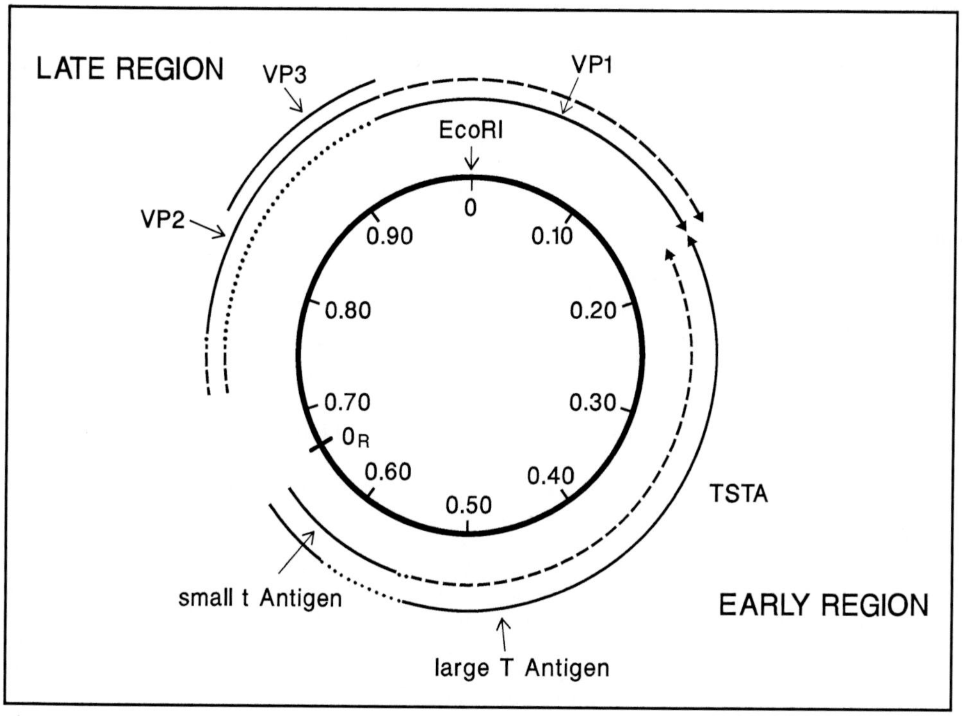

Fig. 55–8. The genetic and transcription map of SV40 DNA. It is drawn so that the restriction endonuclease *Eco*RI cleavage site is at the 12 o'clock position. O_R is the origin of replication of SV40 DNA. The coding sequences of messenger RNAs are indicated by solid lines, noncoding sequences by dashed ones. Sequences spliced out during the processing of transcripts to messenger RNAs are indicated by dotted lines. Note that the messenger RNAs for small t antigen, VP2, and VP3 are translated for only part of their length because of early occurring termination codons. The coding region for VP3 overlaps entirely with that of VP2 in the same reading frame; translation of both is terminated at the same termination codon. Furthermore, the initiation signal for VP1 lies about 120 nucleotides upstream of the VP2/VP3 termination codon, and VP1 is read in a different reading frame from VP2 and VP3.

The second species of early messenger RNA encodes a 174 amino acid–long protein known as the small t antigen. Whereas the large T antigen is encoded by the sequences that extend from map positions 0.65 to 0.60 and from 0.54 to 0.17, small t antigen is encoded by the sequence that extends from 0.65 to 0.55, where stop codons occur that are spliced out of the messenger RNA for large T antigen. Large T antigen and small t antigen, therefore, share their first 82 amino acids. As a result, they cross-react immunologically. Small t antigen is not required for SV40 multiplication, but together with large T antigen, it plays an essential role in cell transformation (Chap. 59).

In cells infected with polyoma virus, which is about 40% related to SV40, there is yet a third protein, middle T antigen (mol wt 57 kDa), which has the same amino terminal portion as large T and small t antigen and, therefore, shares antigenic determinants with both. In fact, the first 79 amino acids of all three polyoma T antigens are the same, and then the next 112 amino acids of small t and middle T antigen are the same. But then the messenger RNA for middle T antigen is spliced so that the termination codon that terminates small t antigen translation is removed, and translation continues for another 350 or so codons in a reading frame that is different from that used for large T antigen translation.

Polyoma middle T antigen is a phosphoprotein that is embedded in the plasma membrane via a hydrophobic region near its carboxy-terminus. It binds to several cellular proteins, one of which is the cellular protooncogene product $pp60^{c\text{-}src}$, a tyrosine kinase (Chap. 59), whose activity it enhances. Like large T and small t antigen, middle T antigen functions to maintain the transformed state.

Late Period

During the late period the early region continues to be transcribed to a decreasing extent as large T antigen accumulates, and the remainder of the SV40 genome begins to be transcribed. This region possesses three open reading frames (ORFs) that overlap, as shown in Figure 55–8. It is transcribed in the opposite direction, that is, from the opposite strand, as the early region. Late region transcripts are processed into two messenger RNAs that correspond to map positions 0.76 to 0.17 and 0.95 to 0.17, respectively. In addition, both possess leader sequences from the region around map position 0.74, which is about 250 nucleotides long for the latter but very much shorter for the former. The smaller mRNA is translated efficiently into the major capsid protein VP1 (362 amino acids) as well as very small 61 amino acid–long very basic nonstructural proteins of unknown function (the agnoprotein). The larger mRNA is translated inefficiently into the two minor structural proteins VP2 and VP3, whose reading frames overlap entirely.

Control of the SV40 Transcription Program

Early and late transcription are controlled largely by a remarkable region of the SV40 genome located at and near the origin of SV40 DNA replication (Fig. 55–8; it is enlarged in Fig. 55–9). It contains the following sequence elements.

1. A 27 bp sequence that is a near perfect GC-rich palindrome
2. A 17 bp sequence that is composed entirely of AT base pairs
3. A 21 bp sequence repeated tandemly (head-to-tail) three times
4. A 72 bp sequence repeated tandemly twice

The 72 bp repeats act as an enhancer for early transcription. Enhancers potentiate, activate, and generally enhance transcription even when located thousands of base pairs away in either direction. They probably serve as entry sites for RNA-dependent RNA polymerase II, which then moves along the DNA, searching for the first suitable promoter element.

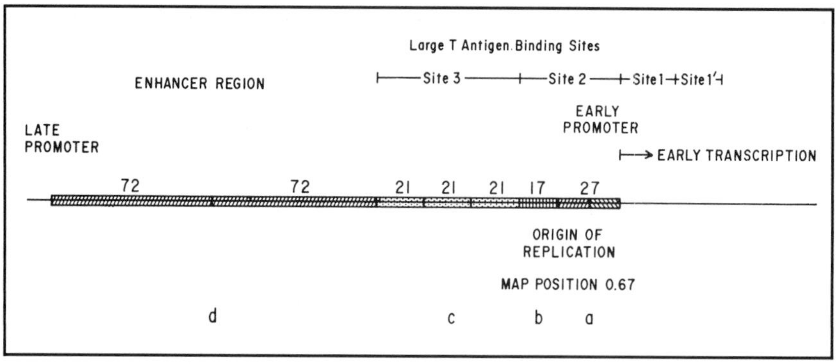

Fig. 55–9. The sequence elements that control the SV40 transcription program and contain the origin of replication. The strongest large T antigen binding site is site 1, followed by site 2 and site 3/site 1′. The late transcription start site is about 300 bp upstream of the 72 bp repeats.

The recognition, identification, and characterization of such transcriptional superpromoters, which also exist in eucaryotic genomes including the human genome, are important byproducts of molecular virology.

The promoters for the early messenger RNAs are located at or very near the 27 bp palindromic sequence; those for the late messenger RNAs are in a broad region centered just to the left of the second 72 bp segment. The significant fact is that the large T antigen plays a crucial role in controlling the extent of both early and late transcription. Large T antigen binds to four sequence elements in this region (Fig. 55–9), and the effect of such binding is to reduce early transcription and to increase late transcription. This is a progressive effect as more and more large T antigen is synthesized. It permits the early transcription program to be active early and the late transcription program to predominate at late stages of the multiplication cycle without totally arresting the early program.

Replication of SV40 DNA

The replication of SV40 DNA starts at map position 0.67, the origin of replication, in the region that encompasses the AT-rich sequences, the 27 bp palindrome, and the site where early transcription starts. This is also the region that contains the strongest large T antigen binding site; binding of large T antigen is essential for the initiation of each round of replication. The binding of large T antigen to this region (more precisely, to site 2, Fig. 55–9) is stimulated greatly by ATP, which causes it to bind in the form of a presumably bilobal double hexamer. This complex untwists and unwinds the DNA by virtue of its helicase activity, which permits DNA replication to commence. Once replication has initiated, it proceeds bidirectionally until the two forks meet again, one DNA strand being synthesized in a continuous manner and the other in the form of Okazaki fragments that are then joined. Newly replicated SV40 DNA does not exist in free form within infected cells but is complexed with histones into a chromatinlike structure. This structure differs from that of the minichromosomes present in SV40 particles (Chap. 53) in being more condensed. The reason for this is that the intracellular SV40 chromatin also contains histone H1 (in addition to histones H3, H4, H2A, and H2B), which causes the intranucleosomal distance to be reduced. H1 is removed before SV40 DNA is encapsidated.

General Observations on the Strategy of Papovavirus Gene Expression

The preceding discussion highlights the remarkable strategy according to which papovaviruses express the information encoded in their genomes. There are two promoters, one used early, the other late, the former controlling the expression of regulatory, the latter of structural proteins; transcripts are spliced according to multiple patterns to yield multiple messenger RNA species; there are multiple, often overlapping open reading frames; multifunctional proteins are transactive transcriptional regulators that also regulate their own expression. Complex DNA sequences feature palindromes, direct and inverse repeats, and atypical base composition segments (AT or GC rich) that specify protein binding sites. Multifunctional proteins initiate DNA replication by unwinding the double helix. Functional control is mediated by protein modifications, such as phosphorylation. All these features are also present in the multiplication cycles of the more complex double-stranded DNA-containing viruses.

Adenoviruses

The multiplication cycle of adenoviruses (Table 55–3, Fig. 55–10), whose 36,000 bp–long genome is almost seven times the size of that of SV40 or polyoma virus, lasts about 36 to 48 hours. It can be divided into an early period of about 8 hours, during which about 30% of the viral genome is transcribed, and a late period, during which the rest of the information that it encodes is expressed. Host macromolecular

TABLE 55–3. STRUCTURAL PROTEINS OF ADENOVIRUS (SEROTYPE 2)

Protein	Designation	Number per Virus Particle	Size (Mol Wt kDa)
Hexon	II	720 (3 per hexon)	120
Penton	III	60 (5 per penton)	85
Fiber	IV	36 (3 per fiber)	62
Major core protein	VII	1000	18
Minor core protein	V	200	48
Hexon-associated	VI	450	24
Hexon-associated	VIII	?	13
Hexon-associated (peripentonal)	IIIa	?	66
Hexon-associated	IX	?	12

Additional structural proteins, IVa1, IVa2, X, XI, and XII (mol wt 60, 56, 6.5, 6, and 5, kDa respectively), have been described.

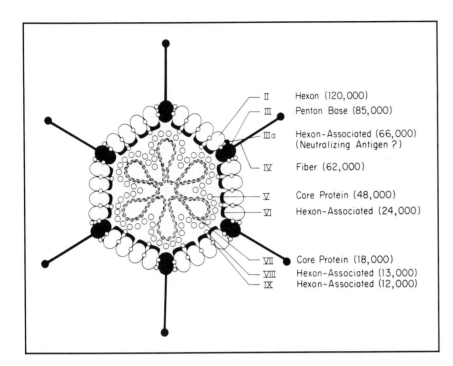

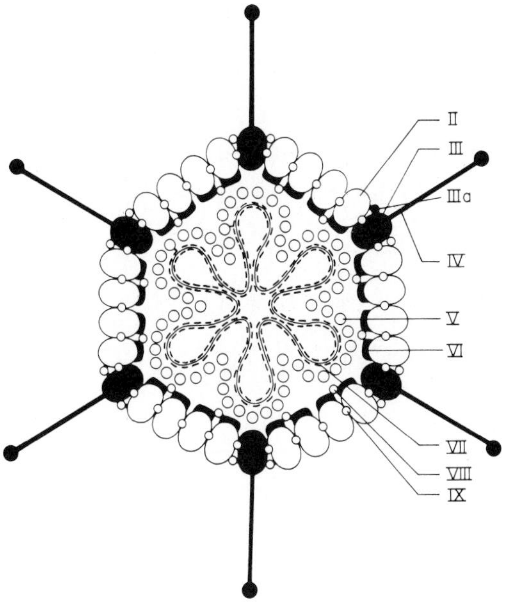

Fig. 55–10. Model of adenovirus showing the inner DNA protein core and the outer icosahedral capsid, as well as the location and sizes of the various structural proteins. The fiber is the viral cell-attachment protein, as well as the hemagglutinin. Proteins VI, VII, and VIII are synthesized in the form of precursors that are cleaved to the actual virus particle components. *(Adapted from Brown et al: J Virol 16:366, 1975.)*

biosynthesis (synthesis of host protein, RNA, and DNA) is not shut off until the late period has commenced. Late proteins are often synthesized in very large amounts, greatly in excess over what is assembled into progeny virus particles. Much of this protein often appears in infected cells in the form of quasi-crystalline arrays (see below).

Nature of Adenovirus Transcripts and Messenger RNAs

The location of many adenovirus genes has been determined by a variety of techniques, all of which take advantage of the fact that detailed restriction endonuclease cleavage maps are available for the DNAs of adenovirus strains of several serotypes. The location of important adenovirus genes is shown in Figure 55–13 (see below).

Just as in the case of SV40 described above, the primary adenovirus genome transcripts are not messenger RNAs; rather they must be processed to messenger RNAs. Processing involves three major modifications. First, the 5′-termini of transcripts must be capped (which involves guanylylation and methylation). Second, the 3′-termini of transcripts must be polyadenylated, and, third, the transcripts must be spliced. The purpose of capping is to provide strong ribosome binding sites to ensure efficient translation (although some messenger RNAs are known that are translated very efficiently, yet are not capped, and vice versa). The purpose of polyadenylation is not known; again, some messenger RNAs are known that are translated very efficiently yet are not polyadenylated. As for splicing, the discovery of spliced adenovirus RNAs in the spring of 1977, and the demonstration shortly thereafter that splicing is a general phenomenon that applies not only to viral but also to most eucaryotic cellular messenger RNAs, was one of the major discoveries in biology in recent times—one that changed fundamentally our ideas and concepts concerning the nature and arrangement of eucaryotic genetic material.

The basic discovery was that late adenovirus messenger RNA species hybridize to and, therefore, are transcribed from several widely separated regions of the viral genome. One of the techniques for showing this was the R-loop heteroduplex technique in which adenovirus DNA and RNA transcripts are mixed and partially melted; the DNA-DNA strands dissociate, and more stable RNA-DNA hybrids are formed instead. When these hybrids are examined with the electron microscope, the regions where RNA and DNA have hybridized are seen as loops (R loops), one arm of which is seen to be single stranded (one of the DNA strands), the other double stranded (the RNA-DNA hybrid) (Fig. 55–11). This technique is extremely powerful for defining the precise locations of transcribed regions because not only the lengths of R loops but also their positions (distance from the ends of DNA molecules) can be measured very precisely. Using this technique, it was shown that most late adenovirus messenger RNA molecules begin with a leader sequence that is derived from three locations at map positions 16.7, 19.7, and 26.7, the combined length of which is about 200 nucleotides (Fig. 55–12). The original transcripts encompass not only the leader sequences and the coding sequences but also the intervening sequences, the introns, which are spliced out as part of processing.

Adenovirus Transcription Program

For the purposes of expression/transcription, the adenovirus genome is organized functionally into five transcription units, each of which encompasses several genes (Fig. 55–13). Each unit uses its own set of promoters and leaders and is transcribed into one or several transcripts that are processed into messenger RNA species from which the individual proteins are translated, often from overlapping coding sequences read in the same or in different reading frames. Four of these units are expressed during the early phase of the multiplication cycle, in cascade-like fashion, transcription of the first unit being essential for transcription of the second, and so on, and one very large unit is expressed during the late period.

The first early transcription unit encompasses two genes, *E1A* and *E1B*, each of which encodes several proteins trans-

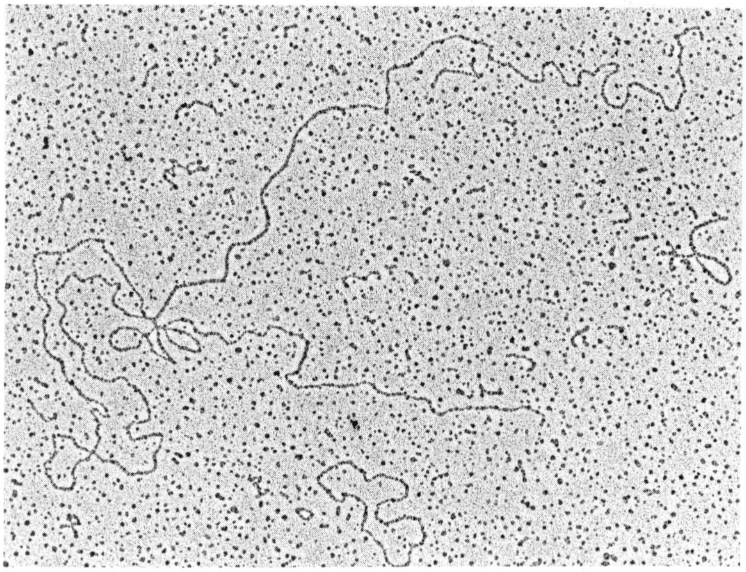

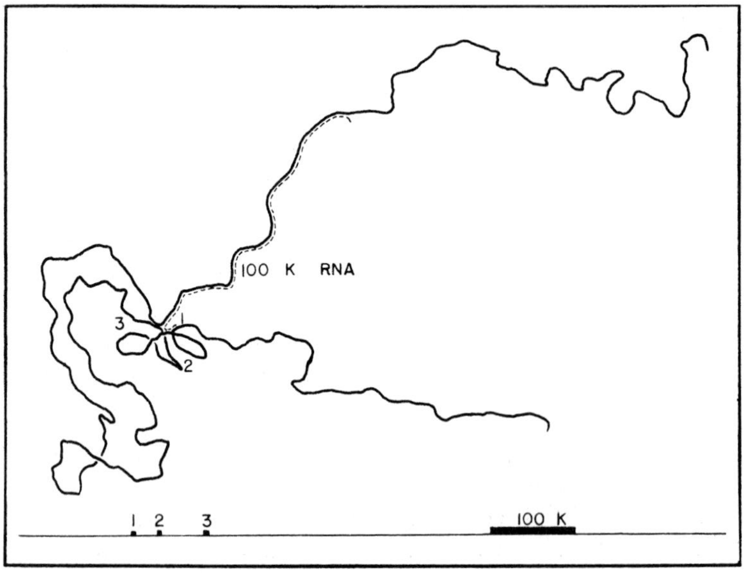

Fig. 55–11. R loops. An electron micrograph of a heteroduplex of human adenovirus serotype 2 (Ad2) RNA and DNA. The RNA was extracted from HeLa cells at a late time after infection. The DNA is constrained into a series of deletion loops corresponding to the intervening sequences removed from the spliced RNA. The first, second, and third leader segments and the main coding body of the messenger RNA are all clearly visible. *(From Chow and Broker: Cell 15:497, 1978.)*

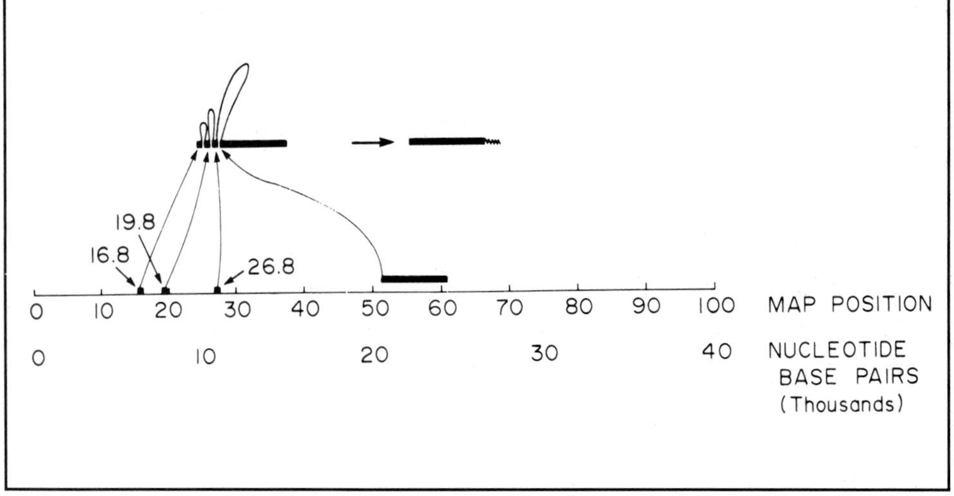

Fig. 55–12. Structure of the adenovirus hexon messenger RNA. It consists of five portions: (1) a leader sequence about 50 nucleotides long transcribed at map position 16.7, (2) a leader sequence about 80 nucleotides long transcribed at map position 19.7, (3) a leader sequence about 75 nucleotides long transcribed at map position 26.7, (4) a coding sequence about 3800 nucleotides long transcribed from a genome sequence beginning at map position 51.7, and (5) a poly(A) sequence about 200 nucleotides long. The intervening sequences between map position 16.7 and 19.7, 19.7 and 26.7, and 26.7 and 51.7, which are present in the primary transcript, are spliced out.

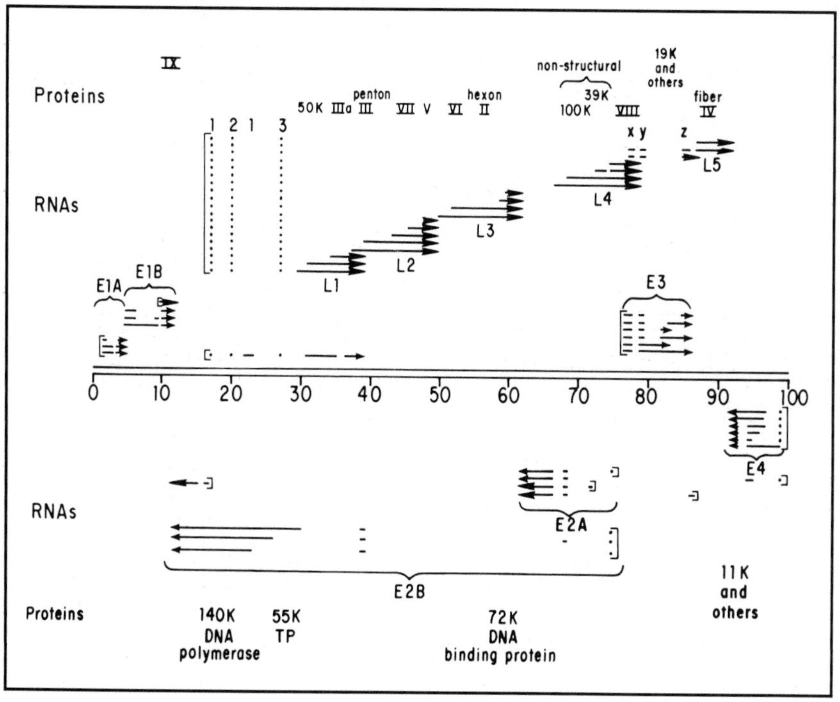

Fig. 55–13. The adenovirus transcription map. There are five major promoters, four early ones and one late one. The locations of the promoters ([or]), of the exons, and of the coding sequences of the most important proteins are indicated.

lated from differently spliced messenger RNAs, some of which are powerful *trans*-active transcription and replication cofactors that can turn on the transcription of heterologous genes or the replication of heterologous replicons. In particular, two E1A phosphoproteins activate the transcription of all other early adenovirus genes by either activating the transcription of or activating posttranscriptionally a series of cellular proteins that bind to the promoters of the E2, E3, and E4 transcription units and activate their transcription. They are also the major effectors of adenovirus-induced cell transformation (Chap. 59) and induce cellular DNA synthesis in G0-arrested cells. The proteins encoded by the *E1B* gene act similarly and reinforce and complement the functions of the E1A proteins. In essence, the E1A and E1B proteins are the counterparts of the SV40 T antigens.

The second region, E2, the transcription of which is activated by the E1A-induced cellular transcriptional activator E2F, encodes three proteins that are essential for adenovirus DNA replication: the adenovirus DNA polymerase and the terminal protein (TP) that is linked covalently to the 5′-termini of adenovirus DNA, both of which are made in small amounts only, and the heavily phosphorylated 72kDa DNA-binding protein (DBP), which is made in large amounts (see below).

The proteins encoded by early regions E3 and E4 are not as well characterized. The major E3 protein is a 19 kDa (159 amino acids) glycoprotein that possesses sequence similarity to a conserved domain in all major human histocompatibility complex (MHC) antigens, β_2-microglobulin and immunoglobulins. It binds to the α_1 and α_2 domains of class I antigens of the MHC (HLA antigens) in the endoplasmic reticulum and prevents their transport to the cell surface by interfering with their terminal glycosylation. As a result of this downregulation, cells infected with adenovirus are not recognized by cytotoxic T lymphocytes and escape immune surveillance. This permits them to set up persistent infections (Chap. 56) or, if transformed by adenovirus, to form tumors. Another E3 open reading frame encodes a 14.7 kDa protein that prevents lysis of adenovirus-infected cells by tumor necrosis factor (TNF), and a third encodes a 10.7 kDa protein that binds to the epidermal growth factor (EGF) receptor. As for region E4, it encodes several proteins that are required for efficient adenovirus DNA replication, late gene expression, and shutoff of host macromolecular biosynthesis; more specifically, one cooperates with E1A to activate E2F (see above), while another cooperates with E1B to activate late gene expression. Interestingly, region E3 and at least part of region E4 are not essential for adenovirus multiplication in cultured cells. In particular, the region from map units 79 to 86 is not required and can be both deleted and substituted by other DNA sequences (Chap. 57).

Adenovirus late proteins are translated from about 20 messenger RNAs that are all processed from a 25,000 nucleotide–long transcript that covers the entire region between map positions 30 and 100; all of them possess the same tripartite leader transcribed from short sequences at map positions 16, 19, and 27 (see above). They fall into five groups that share common 3′-termini at map positions 39, 49, 61, 78, or 91 (Fig. 55–13). Presumably, the nature of the splicing and of the polyadenylation signals controls both where, as well as how efficiently, splicing and polyadenylation occur, and no doubt this determines how many messenger RNA molecules of each type are made.

The proteins encoded by these messenger RNAs are of two types. First, there are the structural proteins, the most important of which are the 120 kDa hexon protein (II) and three hexon-associated proteins, namely, proteins VI (24 kDa), VIII (13 kDa), and IX (12 kDa); the penton base protein (protein III, 85 kDa), the fiber protein (protein IV, 62 kDa), and a protein associated with peripentonal hexons, protein IIIa (66 kDa); and the core proteins, protein V (48 kDa) and VII (19 kDa), both of which are rich in arginine. Some of these proteins, like the hexon protein (720 copies per virus particle), are required in large amounts. Others, like the fiber protein, are required in small amounts only (36 copies per virus particle). Second, there are some nonstructural late proteins that function during morphogenesis. For example, there is a 100 kDa late protein that is necessary as a *scaffold* for the assembly of the hexon trimers (each hexon consists of three protein II molecules). Scaffold proteins are defined as proteins that are necessary during the formation of assembled structures but that are absent from the final products. Two other scaffold proteins, 50 and 39 kDa, also function during the formation of capsids.

Like many other viral proteins, some adenovirus proteins, like the terminal protein (TP) and several of the structural proteins, are synthesized in the form of precursors that are cleaved more or less rapidly to the actual functional proteins. This is an expensive mechanism because precursor cleavage usually requires highly specific virus-encoded proteases. However, it can probably not be avoided, because structural proteins cannot be transported easily because they are very insoluble and possess high affinity for each other and because the conversion of precursors to products often serves to lock structural proteins into place irreversibly.

In summary, in the adenovirus genome, many genes overlap, both on the same strand and on the complementary strand. The adenovirus transcription program provides an extremely sophisticated system for regulating both when each gene is transcribed and the extent to which it is transcribed. The controlling features of this system are the use of common promoters for initiating transcription and the transcript processing mechanism, which provides the means, through splicing and polyadenylation, for specifying which transcript regions are to be translated. This system permits any given region of DNA to be used over and over again, given the fact that there are three reading frames and multiple splice donor and acceptor sites.

Virus-associated (VA) RNAs

Adenovirus DNA encodes two closely related small (155 nucleotide long) RNA species, VA RNA_I and VA RNA_{II}, which are transcribed in large amounts late in infection by cellular DNA-dependent RNA polymerase III (rather than polymerase II, which transcribes all other sequences). These two RNA species, particularly VA RNA_I, play a critical role in adenovirus multiplication. Apparently adenovirus infection activates a latent cellular protein kinase that phosphorylates the α subunit of protein synthesis initiation factor eIF-2, thereby inactivating it. As a result, the initiation of translation is prevented; for the phosphorylated form of eIF-2α sequesters the guanine nucleotide exchange factor, eIF-2B, which recycles GDP/GTP, in a tight complex, thereby preventing the formation of the ternary complex (met-$tRNA_{met}$:GTP:eIF2), which initiates translation. Translation initiation is, therefore, controlled by the phosphorylation state of eIF-2*. Now, the kinase(s) that phosphorylate(s) eIF-2α (a 68 kDa and perhaps also a 90 kDa protein) is/are activated by double-stranded (ds) RNA that is formed in adenovirus-infected cells as a result of symmetrical transcription (i.e., transcription of the same DNA sequence in both directions) late in infection. Therefore, translation of late messenger RNA is progressively inhibited. VA RNA_I, however, possesses a partially duplex structure and, by competing with the dsRNA, prevents activation of the

* Phosphorylation, and therefore inactivation, of eIF-2α is also postulated to be one of the mechanisms by which interferon inhibits viral messenger RNA translation (Chap. 58).

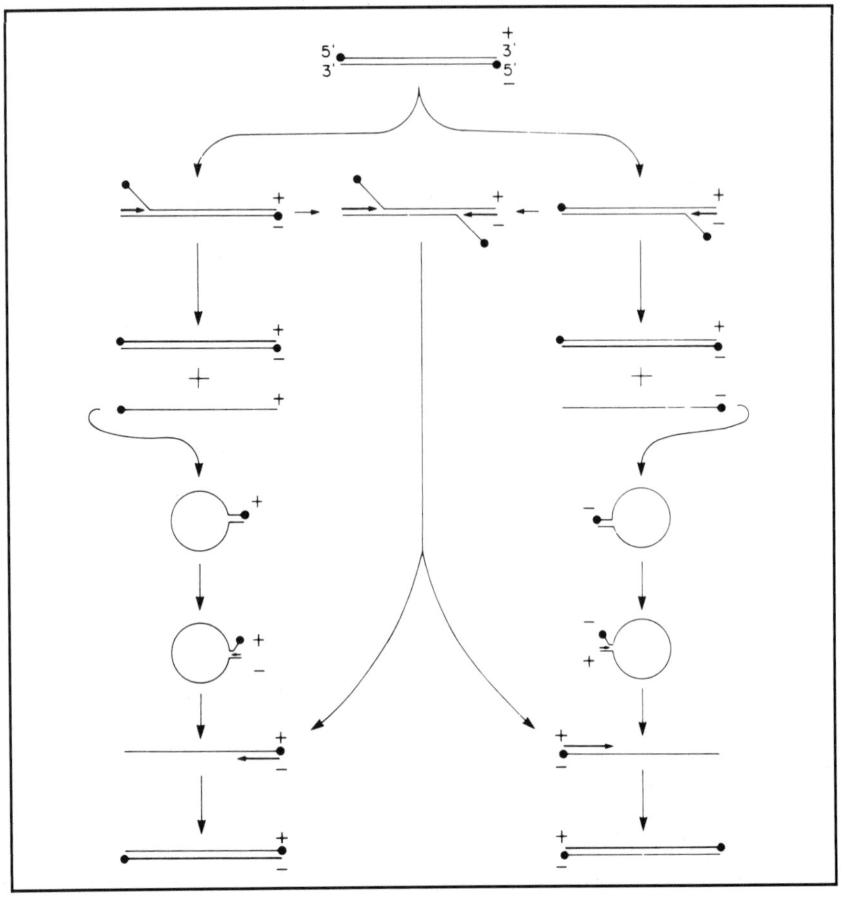

Fig. 55–14. Proposed model for adenovirus DNA replication. Replication commences at either end and causes the displacement of either the plus or the minus strand. The resulting single strands then cyclize via their inverted terminally repeated (ITR) sequences (Chap. 53) and are transcribed again, yielding double-stranded molecules. Occasionally, replication starts simultaneously at both ends, which would yield replication intermediates of the type indicated. ●, termination protein (TP), which is linked covalently to the 5′-termini of both DNA strands. *(Adapted from Lechner and Kelly: Cell 12:1007, 1977.)*

inactivating kinase. The ability of VA RNA_I to fulfill its vital function thus depends not on its sequence but on its secondary structure. This explains why the closely related VA RNA_{II} is far less effective, whereas two unrelated small RNA species encoded by the Epstein-Barr virus, a herpesvirus, are very active.

Adenovirus DNA Replication

Adenovirus DNA replication is unique because it uses protein for priming. It is the only eucaryotic or viral DNA whose replication can be initiated in vitro. The essential features of this mechanism, which is illustrated in Figure 55–14, are as follows. Initiation of replication requires newly synthesized terminal protein (TP), DBP (see above), the adenovirus DNA polymerase, and a cellular nuclear factor. The TP reacts with dCTP to form a TP-dCMP complex, which is the primer for transcription of the minus strand from its 3′-end, displacing the plus strand. The displaced plus strand can cyclize by virtue of possessing inverted terminal repeats (ITRs), forming a structure the panhandle ends of which are exactly the same as the ends of duplex (double-stranded) molecules. Thus, single strands can be replicated in exactly the same way as duplex molecules. Replication thus proceeds alternately by type I replication of duplex strands or by type II replication of the plus-stranded and minus-stranded single-stranded DNA molecules. Both processes are continuous elongation reactions, without Okazaki fragment formation.

Adenovirus Morphogenesis

The morphogenesis of adenovirus proceeds via intermediates that are intimately associated with the nuclear matrix. Several of the assembly-intermediate particles contain virus-encoded proteins that later are removed. These are the scaffold proteins referred to previously. Little is known of their specific functions. Cleavage of structural protein precursors by presumably highly specific proteases is also an essential feature of adenovirus morphogenesis. Little is known concerning the process of DNA encapsidation. Naked DNA is postulated to enter one of the immature capsid particles through an opening at one of the vertices. At the end of the multiplication cycle, infected cells often contain in the nucleus paracrystalline arrays of mature virus particles, of incomplete empty particles, and even of structural proteins that are often synthesized in great excess (Fig. 55–15).

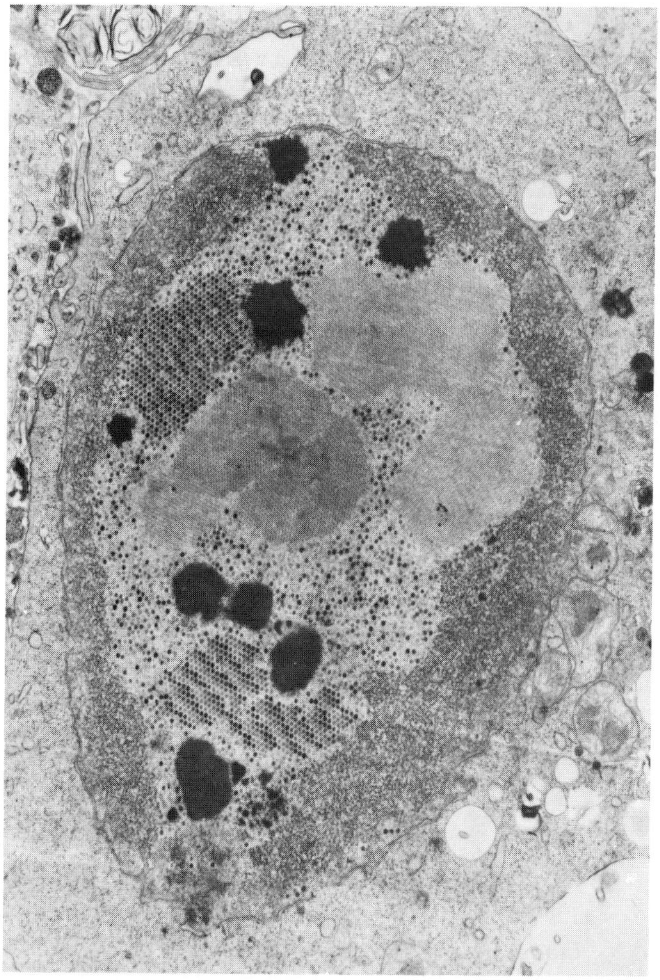

Fig. 55–15. The nucleus of a Vero African green monkey kidney cell 70 hours after infection with adenovirus type 2. Paracrystalline arrays of virus particles, crystals of core proteins, and intranuclear inclusions (the densely staining masses) are visible. × 10,000. *(From Henry et al: Virology 44:215, 1972.)*

Herpesviruses

Herpesvirus particles contain at least 33 proteins, six of which are present in the nucleocapsid and eight of which are glycoproteins located on the outer surface of the envelope.

The DNA of the prototype herpesvirus, herpes simplex virus type 1, is about 150,000 bp long (mol wt 96 × 10^6 Da). This is 30 times the size of SV40 and polyoma virus DNA and 4 times that of adenovirus DNA. The DNA of human cytomegalovirus (HCMV) (230 kbp) is half as large again. The DNA of HSV-1 consists of two regions, L and S, which account for 82% and 18% of the viral DNA, respectively. Each component consists of largely unique sequences, U_L and U_S, bracketed by inverted repeated sequences (Fig. 55–16). HSV-1 DNA extracted from virus particles consists of four isomers in which the orientations of the L and S components are inverted relative to each other. It therefore exists in four configurations. The mechanism that causes this state of affairs is intramolecular recombination within one of the direct repeats, DR4, in the terminally reiterated *a* sequences (Fig. 55–16). It is the result of generalized recombination mediated by the replication complex. The significance of this extraordinary anatomy of herpes simplex virus DNA is not clear because it is modified or even absent in other herpesviruses. Thus, in the genome of pseudorabies virus, a porcine herpesvirus, only the S segment is flanked by inverted repeated sequences and only the S segment inverts relative to the L segment, so that there are only two sequence isomers; and the genomes of Epstein-Barr virus and several other herpesviruses exist in only one configuration. Also, herpes simplex virus containing DNA with altered *a* sequences, so that it can exist in only one configuration, is infectious.

Herpesvirus Multiplication Cycle

The manner in which herpesvirus particles penetrate into cells is still a matter for debate. The evidence favors fusion of the

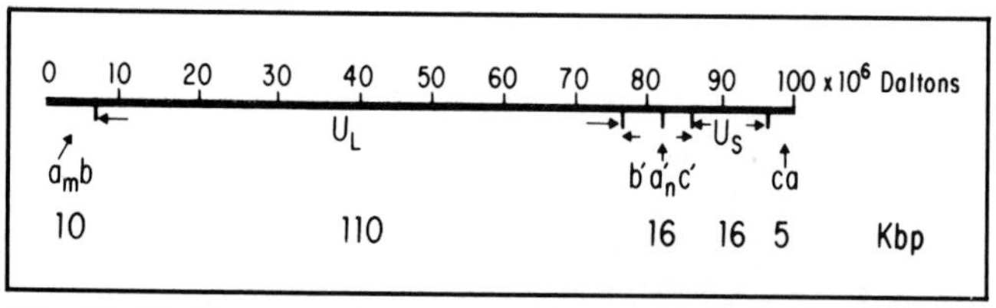

Fig. 55–16. The sequence arrangements in herpes simplex virus DNA. U_L and U_S are unique regions flanked by inverted repeats. Regions *a* and *a'*, etc, are inverted forms of the same sequence. U_L is flanked by *b* sequences (about 8000 base pairs) and a variable number of *a* sequences (about 400 base pairs). U_S is flanked by *c* sequences (about 5000 base pairs) and *a* sequences. The *a* sequence is itself composed of five smaller sequence elements (from 12 to 64 base pairs long), two of which are unique, while the others are present in 2, 2 to 3, and 19 to 22 copies, respectively. Note that the *a* sequence is present in the same orientation at the ends of the molecule and in the inverted orientation at the L–S junction (*a'*). During the course of infection, the L and S components invert relative to each other such that the progeny DNA consists of equimolar amounts of four isomers that differ from each other solely in the relative orientations of the two components. The signal that directs the inversion of L and S components relative to each other is contained solely in the *a* sequence; in fact, insertion of *a* sequences into the U_L region causes additional inversion to occur. As a rule, the segment that inverts is flanked by *a'* sequences; segments that are flanked by *a* sequences do not invert. The inversion itself results from intramolecular recombination between terminal and inverted *a* sequences.

viral membrane with the plasma cell membrane and liberation of naked nucleocapsids into the cytoplasm. Of the eight virion glycoproteins, three (gB, gD, and gH) are indispensable for viral entry into cells under laboratory conditions. The major glycoprotein gB possesses the fusion function. The other five glycoproteins no doubt have specialized cell-specific functions in infections of animals or humans.

Herpesvirus DNA is uncoated at nuclear pores, where the empty capsids remain while the DNA is released into the nucleoplasm. It begins to replicate after about 4 hours; the peak rate of herpesvirus DNA replication occurs at 6 to 8 hours, but it continues to replicate at a gradually diminishing rate until the end of the multiplication cycle at about 36 hours. Herpesvirus DNA replication is mediated by a virus-encoded DNA polymerase and probably proceeds via a rolling circle type mechanism that generates head-to-tail concatemers that are cleaved to generate unit length genomes bounded by terminally reiterated *a* sequences.

Herpesvirus Transcription Program

The herpesvirus transcription program has been investigated intensively by the techniques described for SV40 and adenovirus. Like the transcription programs of these viruses, it can be divided into an early and a late period, and within each period, several sets of genes are transcribed according to a precisely regulated program, that is, in cascade fashion, caused by the fact that in each set some genes encode proteins that are transactive transcription cofactors for turning on the next set of promoters (Fig. 55–17). The herpesvirus genome, by the way, is transcribed by the cellular DNA-dependent RNA

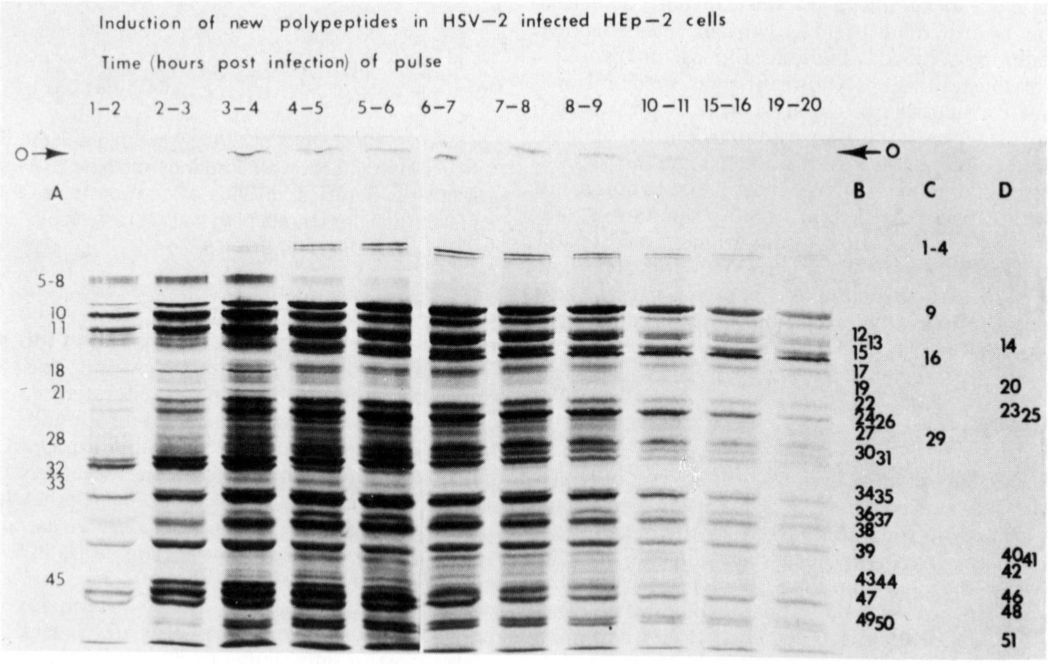

Fig. 55–17. Autoradiogram of a polyacrylamide gel in which the proteins synthesized at various stages of the herpesvirus infection cycle (i.e., pulse labeled with ^{35}S-methionine from 1–2 hours, 2–3 hours, 3–4 hours, and so on) had been electrophoresed. The direction of electrophoresis was from O (origin) downward. A, B, C, and D refer to kinetic groups to which the individual numbered proteins can be assigned, and which correspond roughly to the products of alpha, beta, and gamma genes. *(Courtesy of Dr. Richard J. Courtney.)*

polymerase II. Only few herpesvirus messenger RNAs are spliced, and only a few share 5′ or 3′ termini.

The first set of genes to be expressed are the alpha genes. Their transcription is turned on by a virus particle component, the α-transinduction factor (α-TIF), 500 to 1000 molecules of which are present in virus particles, acting in concert with several host proteins. Alpha genes, five of which are known, are widely dispersed in the viral genome; in fact, several are located in the *b* and *c* sequences, so that they are present as two copies each. Alpha genes encode phosphoproteins; four of them are transactive transcriptional activators of the next two sets of genes, the beta 1 and beta 2 genes. Among the beta gene products are a DNA-binding protein, as well as various enzymes, such as a DNA polymerase, a deoxypyrimidine kinase, and a component of a ribonucleotide reductase. The synthesis of these enzymes signals the onset of DNA replication. As for the gamma genes, their transcription is turned on after DNA replication has started. Most of them encode structural virus particle components.

Herpesvirus Morphogenesis and Release

Herpesvirus morphogenesis proceeds in the nucleus. Capsids are formed first, and newly formed viral DNA is then inserted into them. This DNA is in the form of head-to-tail concatemers; cleavage to unit length genomes and packaging appear to proceed hand-in-hand. It is clear that *a* sequences play a crucial role in this process, and inversion of L and S components may occur at this time. The DNA-containing capsids then attach to patches of modified inner lamella of the nuclear membrane and become enveloped in the process. The enveloped virus particles are then transported through the cytoplasm by an as yet unidentified mechanism and released either by reverse phagocytosis or via the Golgi apparatus following a pathway similar to that taken by secreted soluble proteins.

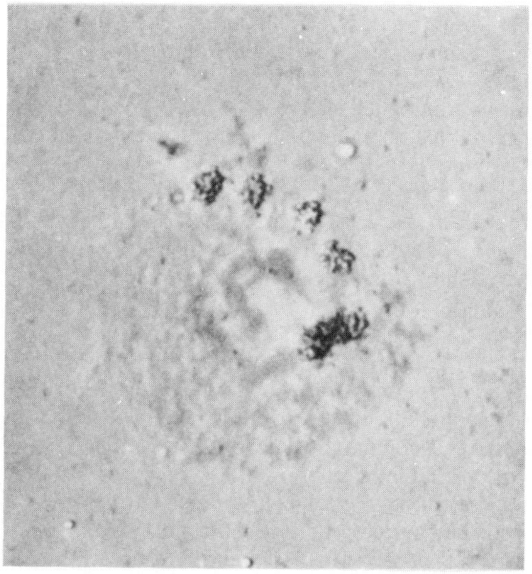

Fig. 55–18. Vaccinia virus factories in the cytoplasm of a HeLa cell. Cells growing on a coverslip were infected at a multiplicity of 6 plaque-forming units (PFU) per cell. At 6 hours after infection, tritiated thymidine was added, and at 7 hours, the cells were fixed. Autoradiographic stripping film was then applied, and the slide was stored for 2 weeks. On developing, the picture shown here was obtained. There are no grains (indicative of thymidine incorporation and, therefore, DNA replication) over the nucleus, but there are in the cytoplasm five labeled areas, or factories (one is actually composed of two coalesced areas)—this is where viral DNA is being synthesized. This cell had been stained with antibody to vaccinia virus coupled to fluorescein before autoradiography, and it was thereby demonstrated that the only areas in the cell that contained appreciable amounts of vaccinia virus antigens were the factories. Both viral DNA replication and viral morphogenesis, therefore, proceed within the factories. *(From Cairns: Virology 11:603, 1960.)*

Poxviruses

Poxviruses present at least three unique features. First, they are by far the most structurally complex of all viruses, with large cores, lateral bodies, outer coats, envelopes, and fibrils on the particle surface arranged in intricate patterns. There are more than 100 different protein species in poxvirus particles. Second, they are DNA-containing viruses that multiply in the cytoplasm. Therefore, they contain a complete transcription enzyme system, including a DNA-dependent RNA polymerase that consists of at least seven subunit species, a 5′-terminus capping system and a poly(A) polymerase. They also contain other enzymes that apparently function in DNA replication and DNA processing or modification, such as a topoisomerase, a deoxyribonuclease that also possesses DNA ligase activity and may function in the formation of the hairpin loops of vaccinia virus DNA, two DNA-dependent ATPases, and others (Chap. 53). Third, they are unique in that they require a newly synthesized protein for uncoating. Vaccinia virus particles are taken up into cells via phagocytic vesicles (coated vesicles; see above) from which they are liberated into the cytoplasm in the form of cores. In the presence of inhibitors of protein synthesis, these cores are not uncoated. Uncoating of cores requires the formation of a protein that is encoded by the DNA that they contain and that is transcribed by the RNA polymerase that is present within them.

Soon after infection, inclusions, known as B-type inclusions, are formed in the cytoplasm, within which uncoated DNA is transcribed further, replicates, and is encapsidated into progeny virions; they are "factories" for virus multiplication. These factories, which are easily visible by light microscopy, are composed of fibrillar material and may be located anywhere in the cytoplasm. Their number per cell is proportional to the multiplicity of infection, which suggests that each infecting virus particle initiates its own factory (Fig. 55–18).

Vaccinia Virus DNA Replication

The essential features of the structure of vaccinia virus DNA are illustrated in Figure 55–19. Vaccinia virus DNA replication begins very early, at about 1.5 hours after infection and is complete by about 5 hours (Fig. 55–20). During this brief period, up to 10,000 genomes are synthesized. This corresponds to about a quarter of the cellular genome, and this amount of DNA is formed during a period that is equivalent to about one third of the S-phase. Thus the rate of vaccinia virus DNA synthesis is extremely rapid. It proceeds at about the same rate as host cell DNA synthesis. Vaccinia virus DNA is synthesized in excess; usually only about one third of newly formed vaccinia virus DNA molecules are encapsidated into progeny virus particles.

As for the mechanism of vaccinia virus DNA replication,

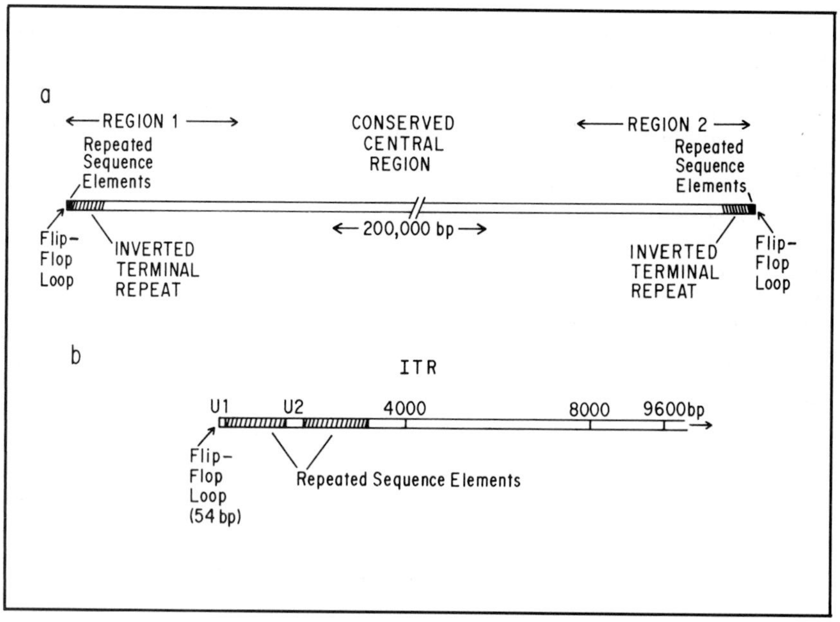

Fig. 55–19. Essential features of the structure of the poxvirus (vaccinia virus) genome. The typical DNA molecule is about 200,000 bp long. It possesses inverted terminal repeats (ITRs) at each end that are about 10 kbp long. Its two ends are in the form of the *flip-flop loops* shown in Figure 53–27. Just inside these terminal regions are two sets of repeated sequence elements; each of these sets, which are about 1000 bp long, is made up of a small number (two to six) of 30 to 40 bp long sequences that are related to each other and that are repeated 5 to 20 times. Since they are highly conserved, they probably serve some essential function, probably during replication. The central 60% of the poxvirus genome is conserved and contains the genes essential for replication. Regions 1 and 2 are less conserved and contain most of the type-specific information that relates to the interaction of the poxvirus particle with its environment (such as host range, tissue tropism, and pathogenicity). **a.** The structure of the orthopoxvirus genome. **b.** The structure of a typical ITR.

it is likely that it proceeds as illustrated in Figure 55–21. Either one (or perhaps both) of the strands appear to be nicked by a site-specific nuclease at the ends of the "flip-flop" loops, so that the free 3′ end(s) so created serve(s) as the primer(s) for DNA replication, displacing the other strand. This leads to the formation of concatameric forms of poxvirus DNA that accumulate in infected cells if late protein formation is prevented. These concatamers then resolve into linear molecules with complementary loops after nicking at their ends and rejoining parental to progeny strands.

Vaccinia Virus Transcription Program

The total number of proteins encoded by the vaccinia virus genome is large. Over 200 new proteins have been detected in extracts of infected cells by two-dimensional polyacrylamide gel electrophoresis.

Transcription of early genes starts as soon as cores are

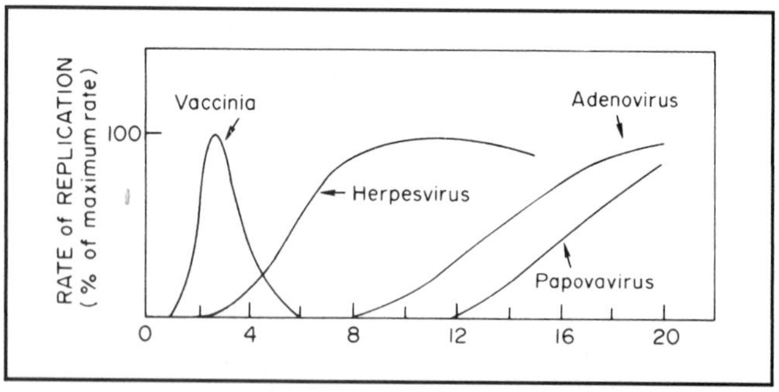

Fig. 55–20. The replication of vaccinia virus, herpesvirus, adenovirus, and papovavirus DNA. Vaccinia virus DNA is atypical in replicating only during a brief period of time early in the multiplication cycle. Progeny DNA molecules always form a pool from which individual molecules are selected at random for incorporation into progeny virus particles.

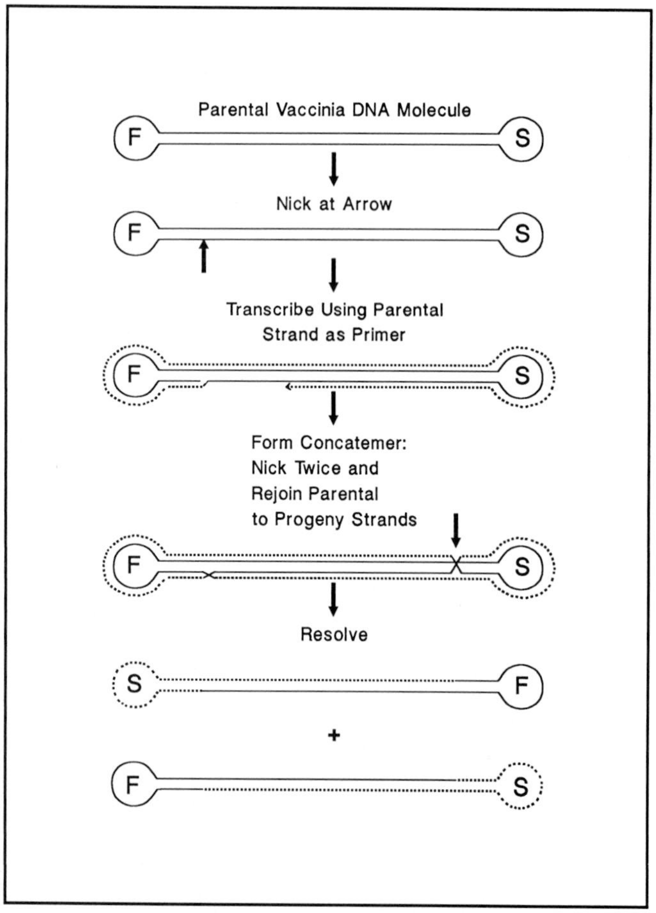

Fig. 55–21. Model for the replication of vaccinia virus DNA. Note that the F and S loops are complementary to each other (see Fig. 53–27) and are, therefore, transcribed into each other.

liberated into the cytoplasm. Transcription is initiated by a vaccinia virus early transcription factor (VETF), which possesses DNA-dependent ATPase activity and is present in cores. About 20 early promoters have been examined so far, and all are similar in structure: they possess a highly AT-rich 15 bp critical region, a rather less critical 11 bp spacer region, and then, at position −1 to +6, the consensus sequence TAAAAG. At their other end, all early genes possess the signal sequence TTTTNT about 50 nucleotides upstream of the site where transcription terminates. All vaccinia messenger RNAs are polyadenylated, but they are not spliced, presumably because they are synthesized in the cytoplasm.

During the early period, before the onset of viral DNA replication, about one half of the vaccinia virus genome is transcribed. Many of the approximately 100 early genes have been mapped on the viral genome, and many of the proteins that they encode have been identified (Table 55–4). Most early poxvirus proteins are nonstructural proteins. Some modify normal cell functions and, therefore, contribute to cellular and organismal pathogenicity. Others are enzymes involved in replication and the transcription of the viral DNA in the cytoplasm. These enzymes reveal fascinating patterns of relatedness with corresponding enzymes from other sources. For example, the vaccinia virus thymidine kinase is closely related (about 65%) to the human enzyme but unrelated to the herpesvirus enzyme, and its ribonucleotide reductase possesses about 75% identity to the mammalian enzyme but much less similarity to the herpesvirus or procaryotic enzymes. However, the vaccinia virus DNA polymerase possesses very significant sequence similarity to the herpesvirus and adenovirus DNA polymerases, its topoisomerase possesses a region of homology with the yeast enzyme, and one of the subunits of the vaccinia virus DNA-dependent RNA polymerase possesses extensive similarity to one of the yeast and *Drosophila* RNA polymerase subunits and less similarity to the second largest subunit of the *Escherichia coli* enzyme. Interestingly, one of the vaccinia virus RNA polymerase subunits may be a subunit of the host cell enzyme, a subunit that is translocated from the nucleus to the cytoplasm on infection and is packaged into mature virus particles as part of the viral enzyme.

TABLE 55–4. TRANSCRIPTION-TRANSLATION MAP OF THE VACCINIA VIRUS GENOME

***Hind*III Fragment**		**C**		**N + M + K**	**F**	**E**	**O + I**	**G**	**L + J**	**H**	**D**	**A**	**B**	**Total**
Size (mol wt × 10^{-6})	**5.9**	**4.4**	**3.8**	**5.3**	**8.9**	**9.9**	**5.3**	**6.0**	**5.8**	**5.6**	**10.3**	**30**	**19**	
Early proteins (mol wt × 10^{-3})	42	60	38	54	68	95	80	54	41	40	86	58	42	
	19	21	32	53	62	67	79		21	39	84	45	35	
	8	19	21	46	59	64	33		17	14	79	41	35	
		13	15	40	54	62	32			11	52	40	31	
		6	14	30	45	55	25				34	39	27	
			12	23	39	36					28	37	19	
				20	35	34					27	35	8	
				16	33	32					24	31		
				11	27	30					17	27		
				9	17	26					14	24		
					16	22					12	23		
					16	17						20		
					10	15						18		
												16		
Medium-early proteins			23					33	110					
								30						
Late proteins	—	22	40	—	52	12	46	65	44	55	70	96		
					40		35	44	37	46	35	84		
					15		11	33	36	36	17	45		
								30	33	30	14	22		
								14	30	28				
								12	28	18				
								9	28	17				
									19	16				
									19	13				
									18					
									14					

Adapted from Isle et al: Virology 112:306, 1981.

Extracts were prepared of HeLa cells infected with vaccinia virus under three sets of conditions: (1) in the presence of cycloheximide, an inhibitor of protein synthesis, when vaccinia virus cores are not uncoated and only *early* messenger RNA is made, (2) in the presence of cytosine arabinoside, an inhibitor of DNA replication, when both early and medium-early messenger RNAs are made, and (3) during the late period of the multiplication cycle, when some early and medium-early but also all late messenger RNAs are made. The viral messenger RNAs in these extracts were hybridized to cloned *Hind*III restriction endonuclease fragments of vaccinia virus DNA, and those that hybridized were translated in a cell-free protein synthesizing system prepared from reticulocytes in order to determine which proteins they encode. The *Hind*III C fragment was further divided into its *Eco*RI fragments, A, B, C and D. Because they are small, C and D are combined in this map. For the same reason, *Hind*III fragments N, M, and K, O and I, and L and J also are combined. *Hind*III fragments A and B are too large to be cloned readily and were used in uncloned form. Note the sizes of the proteins that were obtained, which range from over 100 to less than 10 kDa, and the fact that the early and late proteins are clustered on the vaccinia virus genome, late proteins being encoded primarily in the regions defined by *Hind*III fragments G, L, J, and H.

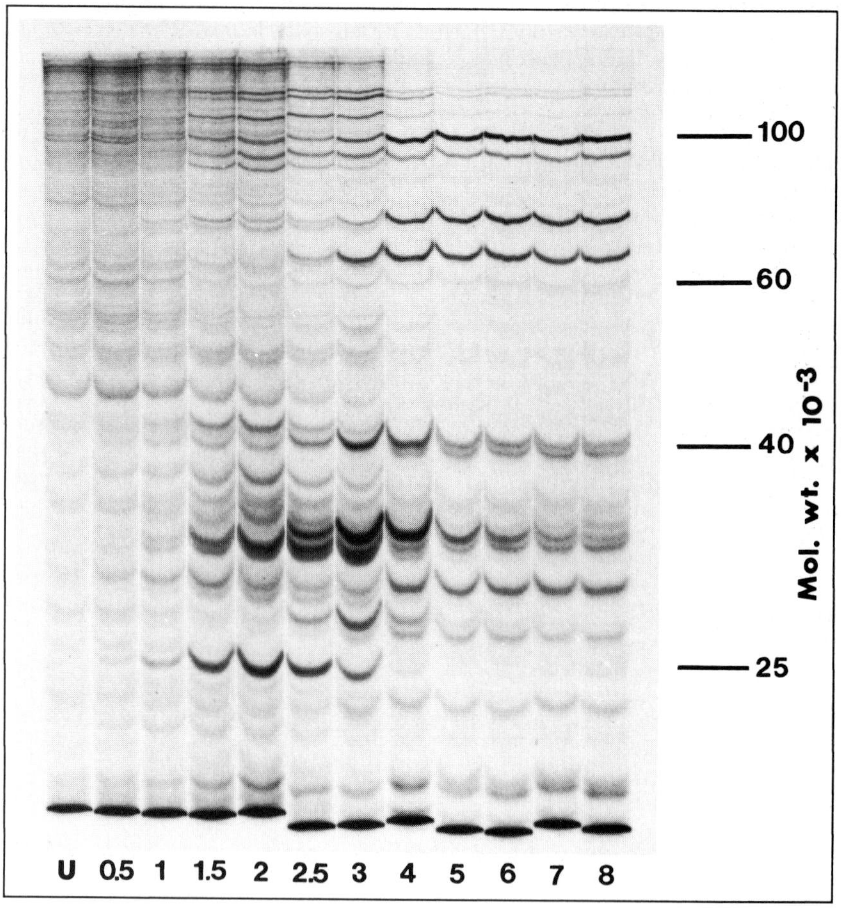

Fig. 55–22. Autoradiogram of a 9% polyacrylamide slab gel into which the proteins synthesized at various stages of the vaccinia virus multiplication cycle had been electrophoresed. At the times indicated (hours after infection), the cells were labeled for 15 minutes with ^{14}C-protein hydrolysate. At the right is a molecular weight scale as determined by electrophoresing proteins of known size under identical conditions. *(Courtesy of Dr. T. H. Pennington.)*

Whereas parental viral genomes serve as templates for RNA polymerase and early promoter-specific transcription factors, only naked newly replicated DNA is accessible to intermediate and late promoter-specific transactivators. As a result, intermediate genes are transcribed immediately after the onset of replication, whereas late genes, of which there are many more, are transcribed somewhat later. Like early promoters, late promoters share extensive sequence similarity. In particular, they all possess the sequence TAAAT in positions −1 to +4, the AT being the first two residues of the translation initiation codon. Remarkably, when the RNA polymerase transcribes this sequence, it tends to slip, which leads to reiterative transcription and causes late poxvirus messenger RNAs to possess 5′-poly(A) leaders from 5 to 40 residues long.

Although most early proteins are no longer synthesized after DNA replication, most of the viral genome continues to be transcribed. The reason is that late vaccinia messenger RNA molecules do not have defined 3′-ends. Transcription of late genes simply continues, through and even beyond adjacent early or late genes.

When one examines the nature of the proteins formed at the various stages of the vaccinia virus multiplication cycle, data are obtained such as are illustrated in Figure 55–22. Clearly, the viral proteins fall into several classes (Fig. 55–23). There are early proteins whose synthesis is switched off early, early proteins that continue to be synthesized throughout the

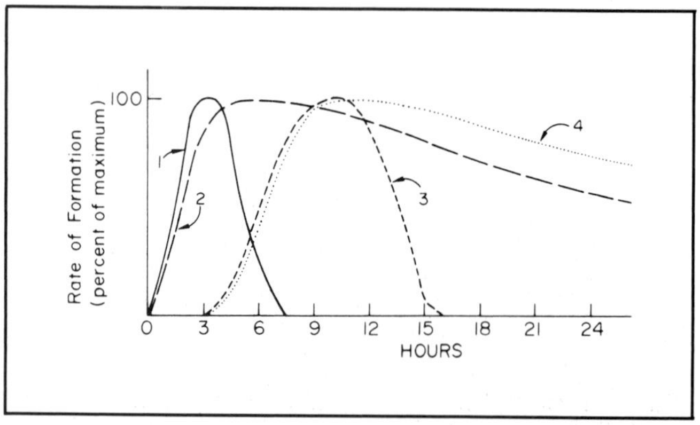

Fig. 55–23. The synthesis of four classes of vaccinia-specified proteins. First, there are some early proteins whose synthesis is switched off when DNA replication commences. Early enzymes and some nonstructural vaccinia virus proteins belong to this class. Second, there are early proteins whose synthesis continues throughout the multiplication cycle. One of the major components of immature virus particles belongs to this class. Third, there are late proteins that are synthesized for some time after the onset of DNA replication and that are then switched off. Finally, there are late proteins that are synthesized throughout the entire late period of the multiplication cycle. Most structural vaccinia virus proteins belong to this class. *(Adapted from Holowczak and Joklik: Virology 33:726, 1967.)*

multiplication cycle, late proteins that are synthesized until the end of the multiplication cycle, and late proteins whose synthesis is switched off soon after it has started. Clearly, there are at least four classes of vaccinia virus protein translation patterns, and there may be many more. About 40 late proteins have been mapped so far on the vaccinia virus genome by cell-free translation of late messenger RNAs selected by hybridization to restriction endonuclease fragments. Most of them are structural proteins and enzymes that are present in virus particles. In addition, there are the following: (1) the vaccinia virus hemagglutinin, a nonstructural glycoprotein that is a member of the immunoglobulin superfamily, possesses affinity for a protein on the surface of vaccinia virus particles and facilitates adsorption and penetration; (2) a protein that often forms large inclusions (A-type inclusions) in the cytoplasm and is formed in very large amounts late during the multiplication cycle; and (3) one or more proteins that inhibit the induction of the inflammatory response. One of these proteins possesses some sequence similarity to the superfamily of *serpins*, many (but not all) of which are serine protease inhibitors. One hypothesis of how this protein might function is that it may inhibit the protease that generates IL-1, one of the principal mediators of the inflammatory response, from its precursor. Finally, there is also a 19 kDa protein that shares sequence similarity and functional properties with epithelial growth factor (EGF) and T cell growth factor (TGF-α). It is a membrane protein but in cleaved form is secreted into the medium. It is not essential for virus multiplication, but by binding to the EGF receptor and causing it to be tyrosine-phosphorylated, it stimulates mitogenic activity and induces the hyperplastic response often elicited by poxviruses. It is a strong mediator of poxvirus virulence. Virus strains that lack it are markedly less virulent than strains that possess it.

The Switch-off Phenomenon

The fact that the synthesis of some vaccinia virus proteins ceases at a time when other viral proteins are being made at a rapid rate suggests the existence of a mechanism that controls the translation of various viral messenger RNAs, and indeed such a mechanism exists. This is the so-called switch-off mechanism (Fig. 55–24). It has been investigated particularly in relation to the switch-off of the synthesis of early enzymes, such as thymidine kinase and DNA polymerase. In essence, cessation of the synthesis of these early enzymes is not due to inhibition of the transcription of their genes, to instability of their messenger RNA species, or to instability of the enzymes themselves. Rather it is due to a suddenly developing inability of the messenger RNA species that encode them to be translated. If viral DNA replication and protein synthesis are inhibited, this inability does not develop. One of the first late proteins to be synthesized may, therefore, specifically prevent the translation of the messenger RNA molecules that encode certain early enzymes. This mechanism of controlling protein synthesis is obviously highly selective because many other viral messenger RNA molecules continue to be translated rapidly. It is of potential significance for antiviral chemotherapy because it implies the existence of a chemical difference between those messenger RNA molecules that continue to be translated and those that are switched off. It may prove possible to exploit this difference (Chap. 58).

Poxvirus Morphogenesis

Progeny genomes of DNA-containing viruses generally replicate faster than they are incorporated into virus particles. Thus they accumulate to form pools from which individual genomes are withdrawn at random for encapsidation; whereas some DNA molecules may be withdrawn very soon after they are formed, others remain naked for long periods of time. This is true particularly for vaccinia virus, the replication of whose genome ceases at about 5 hours after infection, whereas viral morphogenesis continues for about 25 hours. The time necessary for a complete virus particle to be assembled around a vaccinia DNA molecule is about 1 hour.

The morphogenesis of vaccinia virus particles proceeds in the cytoplasm via a series of intermediates, only some of which have been characterized (Fig. 55–25). Progeny virus particles are released by two distinct mechanisms. Most virus particles are released only when infected cells disintegrate. However, from 1% to 30% of particles, depending on virus strain and cell type, are released by a special mechanism that involves passage of particles through the Golgi apparatus, where they are enveloped in a double membrane, followed by transport to specialized microvilli from the tips of which they are released by fusion of one of the membranes surrounding them with the plasma membrane, which results in the liberation of particles surrounded by one layer of Golgi

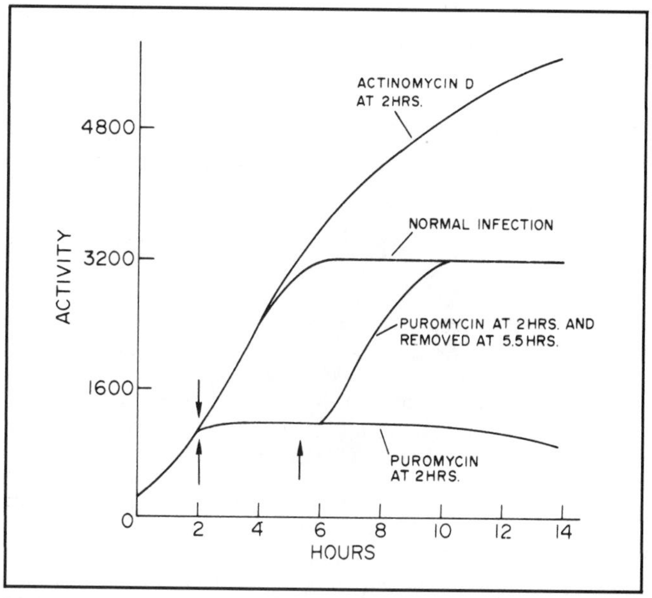

Fig. 55–24. The switch-off phenomenon. This graph depicts the synthesis of early enzymes, such as thymidine kinase and DNA polymerase, during vaccinia virus infection. Under normal conditions, these enzymes begin to be formed soon after infection, and their synthesis is "switched-off" at about 4 hours. If actinomycin D, which inhibits messenger RNA formation, is added at 2 hours, switch-off does not occur. This demonstrates (1) that the messenger RNAs from which these enzymes are translated are stable, and (2) that switch-off itself requires the synthesis of some other messenger RNA. If protein synthesis is inhibited with puromycin at 2 hours, enzyme synthesis ceases immediately; if puromycin is removed at 5.5 hours, enzyme synthesis resumes and is again switched off after a time interval equivalent to that between the addition of puromycin and the onset of normal switch-off. This indicates that switch-off is due to the accumulation of a certain amount of some specific protein. *(Adapted from McAuslan: Virology 21:383, 1963.)*

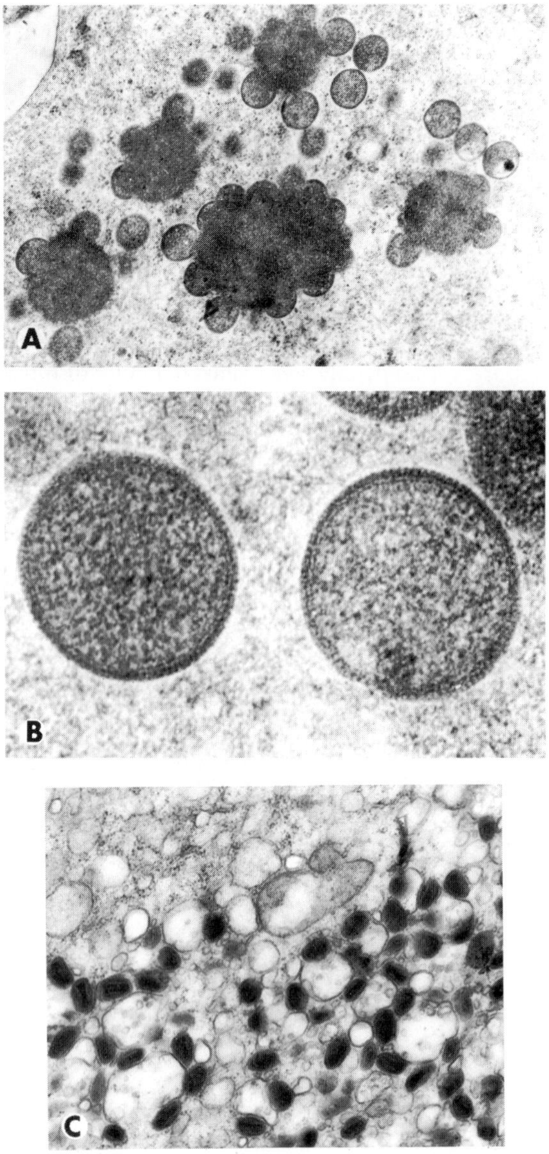

Fig. 55–25. Vaccinia virus particles in the cytoplasm of infected cells. **A.** Immature virus particles developing from intracytoplasmic inclusions 1 hour after reversal of vaccinia virus morphogenesis arrest by rifampin (Chap. 58). × 9000. **B.** Characteristic structure of immature vaccinia virus particles. × 48,000. **C.** Mature vaccinia virus particles in the cytoplasm of infected cells. × 12,000. (**A, B** *courtesy of Dr. T. H. Pennington;* **C** *from Dales and Siminovitch: J Biochem Biophys Cytol 10:475, 1961.*)

membranes (Fig. 55–26). These particles are not neutralized by antisera prepared against virus released by cell disruption. Their envelopes contain several cellular glycoproteins that are not components of normal vaccinia virus particles. The biologic significance of these enveloped virus particles is not known, but their specific infectivity is high, and their presence must be taken into account when planning vaccination programs.

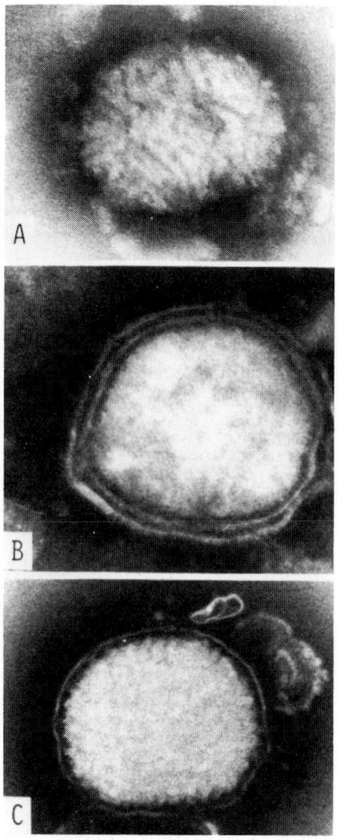

Fig. 55–26. Various forms of mature vaccinia virus particles. **A.** Naked virus particle such as are formed in large numbers in infected cells and are released when cells disintegrate. **B.** Intracellular virus particle enwrapped in intracytoplasmic membranes (intracellular double-membraned virus particle). Such virus particles migrate to the cell surface, where their outer membrane fuses with the plasma membrane as they are released. **C.** Released extracellular virus particle now surrounded by only a single membrane. *(From Payne and Kristenson: J Virol 32:614, 1979.)*

Multiplication Cycles of Retroviruses and Hepadnaviruses

Retroviruses

Retroviruses contain RNA, which they transcribe into double-stranded DNA with an enzyme that they encode and that they contain, namely, the reverse transcriptase. The double-stranded DNA form of their genome is then integrated into that of the host cell. Although not all retroviruses cause tumors, many of them do so. A major reason why they continue to create a great deal of interest is that their study provides the best hope, at this time, for discovering the nature of the reactions that transform normal cells into cancer cells. Their multiplication cycle is discussed in Chapter 59.

Hepadnaviruses

Hepadnaviruses employ a unique strategy of gene expression/replication, a strategy that also appears to include the reverse transcription of RNA into DNA. Although their multiplication cycles and that of retroviruses share some common elements, it is convenient to discuss them here, together with the other double-stranded DNA-containing viruses.

Hepatitis B virus (HBV) particles (Fig. 53–19) contain a double-stranded DNA genome with a minus strand that is 3200 nucleotides long and an incomplete plus strand that is

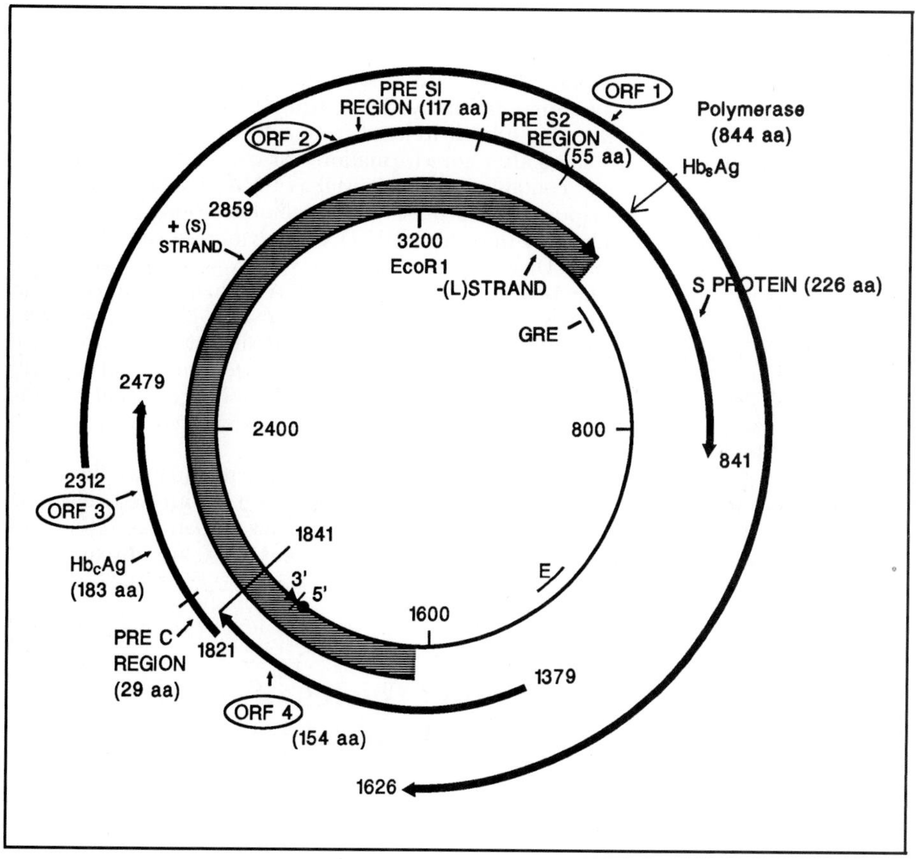

Fig. 55–27. The HBV genome. The minus strand is complete; the plus strand is incomplete in virus particles (broken line). The 5′-end of the minus strand is covalently linked to a protein (●). ORF 1, which completely overlaps ORF 2, may encode the DNA polymerase; ORF 2 encodes the HBsAg, ORF 3 encodes the HBcAg, and it is not clear yet which protein is encoded by ORF 4. ORF 2 actually encodes three proteins: P24 (S protein, 226 amino acids), P30 (pre-S-2 protein, 55 amino acids longer at the N-terminus), and P39 (pre-S-1 protein, 119 acids longer still at the N-terminus), which, collectively, are known as the HBsAg. P24 is always the major component. ORF 3 encodes two forms of HBcAg, one 183 amino acids long, and the other 29 amino acids longer at the N-terminus. Both possess c as well as e epitopes. Like the pre-S regions, the 29 amino acid long pre-c region appears to function in morphogenesis (by acting as a signal for cell membrane attachment). The HBV genome contains an enhancer (E) between nucleotides 1080 and 1234 that is tissue-specific, that is, is active only in human liver cells, and a glucocorticoid (steroid) responsive element (GRE).

anywhere from 1700 to 2600 nucleotides long. All plus strands possess the same 5′-end (Fig. 55–27). Since the 5′-ends of the plus and minus strands of this genome are separated by about 225 nucleotides, it is circular—not because the single strands themselves are covalent circles but because the sequences between the 5′-ends of the two strands are complementary to each other.

HBV particles consist of a core composed of the core antigen protein, HBcAg, surrounded by an envelopelike structure that contains about 30% lipid and is made up of three forms (see below) of a single protein or glycoprotein, the HBV surface antigen HBsAg. This protein possesses at least three epitopes; one, termed *a*, is common to all strains of HBV, whereas the other two are present in either one form or the other, that is, they are allelic. Thus there are HBsAg molecules that are a, d or y, and w or r. Several other minor epitopes behave similarly. The predominant forms of HBsAg present in Europe and North America are adw and ayw. In addition, HBV particles contain one molecule of DNA polymerase that is attached covalently to the 5′-end of the DNA minus strand.

The HBV genome contains four genes that overlap extensively (Fig. 55–27). They are as follows.

The first is the *S* gene, which encodes the HBV surface antigen, or HBsAg. Its reading frame is 400 codons long, but two internal AUG codons are also used to initiate protein synthesis, so that this gene encodes three HBsAg proteins 400, 281, and 226 amino acids long, all with the same C-terminus, which are known as the pre-S1, pre-S2, and S HBsAg, respectively. All three occur both in nonglycosylated and glycosylated form, and all three also occur as lipoprotein because of the presence of very hydrophobic domains. The S form of the HBsAg aggregates extremely readily to form 20 nm spherical particles of which it is the sole constituent, as well as filamentous particles (Fig. 53–19), of which it is the major and the pre-S2 form is a minor constituent. In the 42 nm Dane particles, which are the complete virus particles and which are often outnumbered by the 20 nm particles by a factor of more than 10,000 in the sera of infected individuals, all three forms of the HBsAg occur in roughly equal amounts.

Another gene is the *C* gene, which encodes the HBV core antigen, or HBcAg. This gene is 214 codons long, but the first AUG is not used efficiently. Most translation initiation events occur at an AUG some 30 codons downstream to provide a protein that is the actual HBcAg. The major function of the infrequently translated pre-C HBcAg appears to be to promote secretion of the HBcAg in a truncated form from which the C-terminal 34 amino acids are missing. This truncated protein readily associates with several serum proteins that mask its HBcAg epitope and cause it to display a new epitope, HBeAg, which is also unmasked when core particles are disrupted.

The third gene is the *X* gene, which encodes a 154 amino acid–long nonstructural protein, protein X, the precise function of which is not known. It acts as a transactive transcriptional activator. Among the sequences it activates is a *k*B-like enhancer in the LTR region of the human immunodeficiency virus (HIV) and the β-interferon gene. Finally, almost three quarters of the HBV genome is taken up, again in a different reading frame, by the *P* gene, which encodes the 845 amino acid long HBV polymerase, which can transcribe both RNA and DNA. It occurs in HBV particles covalently bound to the 5′-end of the minus strand.

The promoters of these four genes are controlled by an enhancer (E) (Fig. 55–27) that is tissue-specific (being most active in liver cells) and responsive to glucocorticoids (the glucocorticoid receptor binds to a specific sequence (GRE) on HBV DNA, which increases the activity of the enhancer five times).

HBV Replication

The replication of HBV is accomplished via a remarkable strategy (Fig. 55–28). It appears that parental HBV cores migrate to the nucleus and that the DNA polymerase first completes synthesis of the plus strand. The completely double-stranded DNA molecule is then transcribed into the various messenger RNAs and into a complete plus-stranded RNA strand. This RNA strand is encapsidated into cores, within which it is transcribed into minus-stranded DNA, with concomitant degradation of the template RNA strand. The cores are then assembled into complete virus particles by the addition of the HBsAg- and lipid-containing surface layer, and at the same time, the minus DNA strand is transcribed partially into the plus strand. Release from cells can apparently occur at any stage after core formation, for core particles and virus particles containing RNA as well as DNA at various stages of transcription are all present in the bloodstream.

The fact that the HBV DNA polymerase can transcribe RNA into DNA suggests that it may share structural similarity with the reverse transcriptases of retroviruses. Indeed, the HBV DNA polymerase and the retrovirus reverse transcriptase share very significant sequence similarity, as do other regions of the HBV and retrovirus genomes (particularly those of murine leukemia viruses). This suggests that hepadnaviruses and murine leukemia viruses evolved from a common ancestor.

HBV exhibits a marked tendency to integrate its DNA into that of host cells. This occurs both in infected cells that are not transformed and in primary hepatoma cells. The patterns of integration are complex and are discussed in Chapter 59.

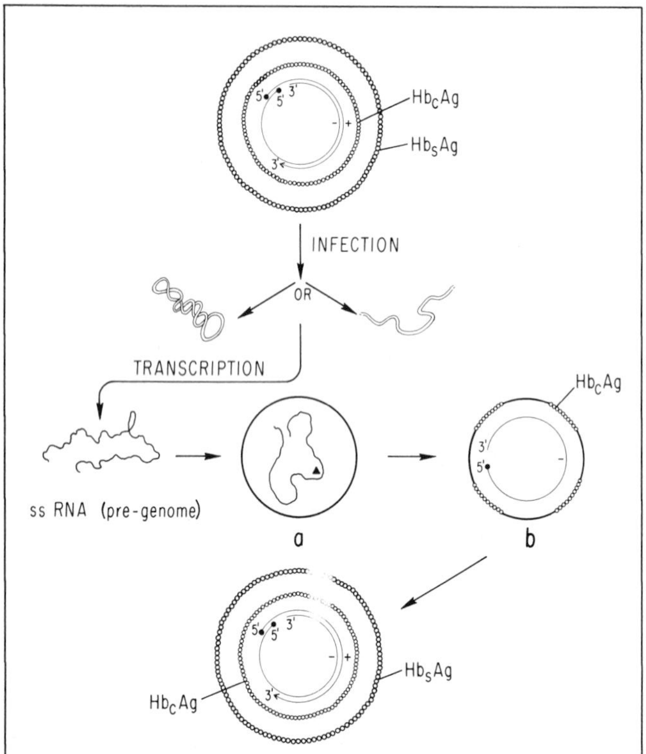

Fig. 55–28. The multiplication cycle of HBV. Concomitant with infection, transcription of the plus genome strand is completed, and intact double-stranded DNA is uncoated, presumably in circular (but not covalently circular) form. The viral DNA is then transcribed into plus-stranded RNA—the pre-genome. Some pre-genomes are translated, others are encapsidated into immature cores (a) that also contain the polymerase (▲). The pre-genome is then transcribed into negative-stranded DNA while the pre-genome is degraded (b). The outer coat consisting of HBsAg is then added, the minus DNA strand is partially transcribed into a plus strand, and the virus is liberated.

Multiplication Cycles of Single-stranded DNA-containing Viruses

Parvoviruses

Only one parvovirus, B19, is a human pathogen. It is the causative agent of transient aplastic crisis of hemolytic disease, the common childhood exanthem known as fifth disease, and a polyarthralgia syndrome in adults. In addition, antibodies against AAV serotypes 1, 2, 3, and 5, all of which are nonpathogenic, are widespread in human populations. Parvoviruses are generally thought of as being the simplest DNA-containing viruses, but their genomes, which are only slightly smaller than that of SV40, are surprisingly complex.

There are three genera in the family Parvoviridae: *Parvovirus* and *Densovirus*, members of which are known as the autonomous parvoviruses, and *Dependovirus*, members of which require a helper function for multiplication (see below). The following description concerns primarily dependoviruses, such as AAV, but also applies in all significant aspects to autonomous parvoviruses.

Parvovirus particles consist of three species of protein, a major species, VP3 (about 60 kDa), and two minor species, VP1 (about 85 kDa) and VP2 (about 70 kDa). The amino acid sequences of these three proteins are very closely related because VP3 is a cleavage product of VP1, and the coding sequences of VP1 and VP2 overlap extensively.

The organization of the Parvovirus genome is shown in Figure 55–29. It encodes two nonstructural proteins in the 3′-terminal portion of its negative-stranded (predominantly encapsidated) form and the three structural proteins in its 5′-terminal portion. There are three promoters, at map positions 5, 19, and 40, and at least six species of messenger RNA have been identified in both unspliced and spliced form. All are polyadenylated at their 3′-ends, which are the same for all, at about map position 96. The smallest of these messenger RNAs is translated into all three capsid proteins; the functions of

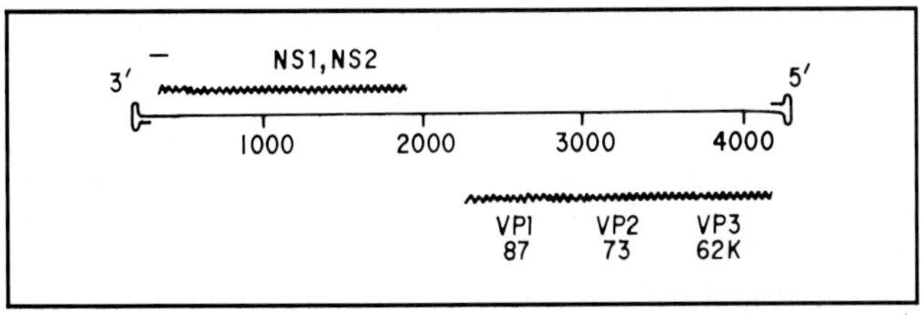

Fig. 55–29. Parvovirus genome organization. There are two long nonoverlapping reading frames, one encoding two nonstructural proteins, the other the three structural proteins. The coding sequences of the latter overlap extensively (see text). All messenger RNAs are spliced transcripts: the region from nucleotides 1907 to 2227 is missing from all.

the others are difficult to determine because they overlap extensively. One of the nonstructural proteins, rep 68, is an ATP-dependent site-specific endonuclease with DNA helicase activity and undoubtedly functions in viral DNA replication. Another is covalently attached to the 5′-termini of replicative form DNA and progeny single strands and may also be a transactive transcriptional activator.

Parvovirus genomes possess long palindromes at both ends that can, therefore, assume hairpin configurations. Like the flip-flop loops of orthopoxviruses (Fig. 53–27), these palindromes of parvoviruses, but not of dependoviruses, exist in two forms that are inverted complementary repeats of each other (Fig. 55–30). The replication of parvovirus DNA, which takes place in the nucleus, appears to proceed like that of vaccinia virus DNA (see p. 805): the palindromic hairpin ends serve as primers for transcription via a rolling hairpin type mechanism, with subsequent site-specific nicking generating unit length genomes from double or even quadruple size intermediates.

The multiplication of parvoviruses requires a helper function. For members of the genus *Parvovirus*, this function is supplied by multiplying, but not by resting, host cells. For members of the genus *Dependovirus*, it is usually supplied by replicating adenoviruses, herpesviruses, or poxviruses. In the case of adenoviruses, the helper function is supplied by E1A or most other early functions. It is likely, therefore, that the required function is a transactive transcription factor. This would fit with the finding that in cells infected with AAV in the absence of helper virus, the AAV genome is not transcribed. Recently, AAV replication has been demonstrated even in cells not infected with a helper virus but synchronized by treatment with hydroxyurea, cycloheximide, chemical carcinogens or UV irradiation. In the absence of a helper function, AAV particles can penetrate to the nucleus, where the AAV genome is integrated into the cell genome to establish a latent infection from which it can be recovered by subsequent helper virus infection. Integration appears to be fairly site-specific, at a site located on chromosome 19.

Multiplication Cycles of Single-stranded RNA-containing Viruses

The principles involved in the multiplication of single-stranded RNA-containing viruses differ in several respects from those described for the double-stranded DNA-containing viruses. Most importantly, their multiplication cycles cannot be divided into clearly defined early and late periods. Brief descriptions of the multiplication cycles of several families of single-stranded RNA-containing viruses follow.

Multiplication Cycles of Plus-stranded RNA-containing Viruses

Picornaviruses

The most intensively investigated picornavirus is poliovirus, the study of which has provided many breakthroughs. It was the first virus to be grown in cultured cells; in fact, attempts to propagate it in vitro provided the primary impetus for the development of tissue culture. The discoveries of the poliovirus RNA-dependent RNA polymerase and of the polyprotein as the primary product of gene expression were also of fundamental significance; both were the first of their kind to be characterized. Recently, the three-dimensional atomic structure of five picornaviruses, namely, poliovirus, rhinovirus types 14 and 1A, mengovirus, and foot-and-mouth disease virus (FMDV), has been established using x-ray diffraction analysis (Fig. 55–31). This provides an unparalleled opportunity for defining in molecular terms their interactions with their host cells and with the immune system.

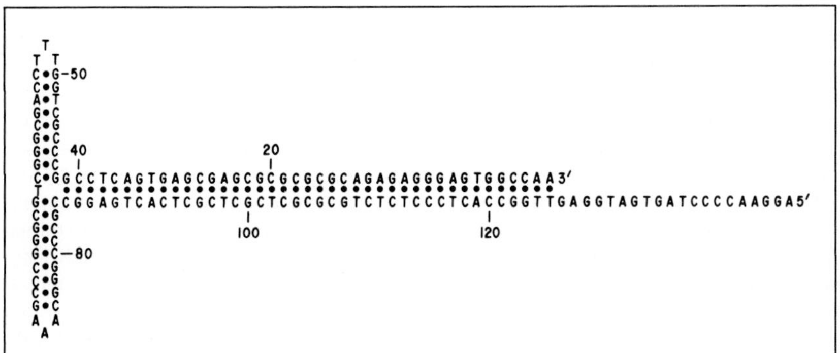

Fig. 55–30. Parvovirus genome organization. This is the 3′-end of the AAV genome, which comprises two internal palindromes (nucleotides 42–84) flanked by a more extensive palindrome (nucleotides 1–41 and 85–125). The 145 nucleotides at the 5′-end are an inverted repetition of the 3′-end. Each end can exist in two configurations, which are inversions of the terminal 125 nucleotide. For autonomous parvoviruses, including the human pathogen B19, the two ends of the genome are unrelated, but both are also palindromic. During replication, the 5′-terminal hairpin provides the primer for initiating DNA synthesis.

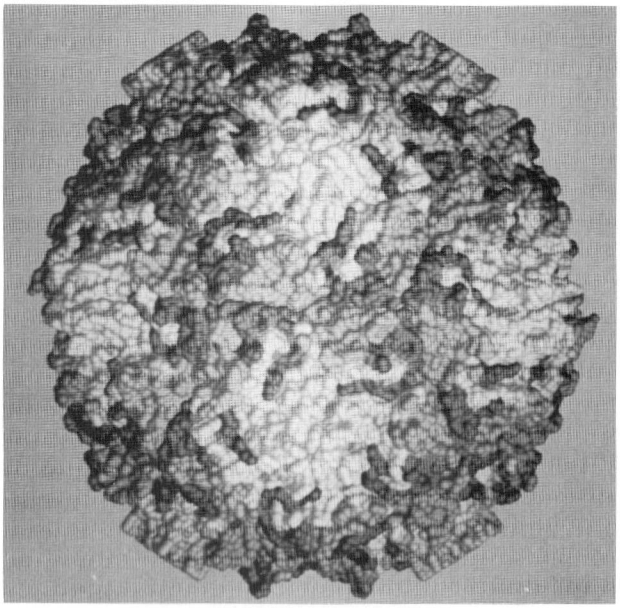

Fig. 55–31. The three-dimensional structure of poliovirus (From Hogle, Chow, and Filman: Science 229:1358, 1985. Photograph by David J. Filman and Arthur J. Olson.)

The poliovirus capsid is composed of 60 "protomers," each of which is made up of a 100 kDa protein that is cleaved during morphogenesis into four proteins, VP1, VP2, and VP3, which are roughly equal in size, and VP4, the molecular weight of which is about 7 kDa. These protomers are assembled into pentamers, 12 of which form the capsid shell. All major poliovirus epitopes are located on VP1.

The RNA of many picornaviruses has been sequenced. That of poliovirus is about 7400 nucleotides long, that is, about 40% larger than SV40 DNA. It is linked covalently at its 5′-end to a 22 amino acid–long protein, VPg.

The Poliovirus Multiplication Cycle

Poliovirus adsorbs to specific cellular receptors. This is readily apparent because poliovirus infects only humans and only very few types of human cells at that (cells of the nasopharynx, cells lining the intestinal tract, and anterior horn cells of the spinal cord). Receptors for poliovirus are not expressed on human kidney and amnion cells but are formed when these cells are cultured in vitro. Recently, the poliovirus receptor has been characterized as a new member of the immunoglobulin superfamily. The poliovirus cell attachment protein is VP1. Poliovirus is taken up by receptor-mediated endocytosis, and free RNA is released into the cytoplasm from endosomes via a pH-dependent process (i.e., a pH of between 5 and 6 is required).

The strategy of the poliovirus multiplication cycle is summarized in Figure 55–32. Once uncoated, poliovirus RNA acts as a messenger RNA and is translated into one large protein, the polyprotein, which is about 2200 amino acids long (Fig. 55–33). Since the poliovirus genome is about 7400 nucleotides long, this means that about 800 nucleotides must be in the terminal noncoding regions. In fact, about 750 of them are at the 5′-end. This noncoding region has important regulatory functions. Cellular proteins bind to multiple sites in it, and point mutations in them can affect the efficiency of viral protein synthesis, tissue tropism, virulence including neurovirulence, and cause temperature-sensitive phenotypes that are reversed by further nearby point mutations, which suggests that the basis of all these effects lies in three-dimensional structures recognized by cellular proteins.

The polyprotein is processed via a highly specific cleavage program effected by several virus-encoded proteases (Fig. 55–33). The P1 capsid precursor is released from the nascent polyprotein by protease 2A cleaving at its amino terminus. All other cleavages are effected by the 3C protease (or its precursor 3 CD) except that of VP0 to yield VP4 and VP2, which occurs as the last stage of morphogenesis and which is catalyzed by the M (or maturation) protease, which is probably VP0 itself, possibly in conjunction with bases in the RNA. Other viruses also encode highly specific proteases that cleave viral precursor proteins. Examples are the capsid protein C of togaviruses and the retrovirus protease (Chap. 59).

Whereas translation of the poliovirus genome into a single precursor protein has many advantages, there are also potential disadvantages. In particular, this strategy implies that all portions of the viral genome will be expressed with equal

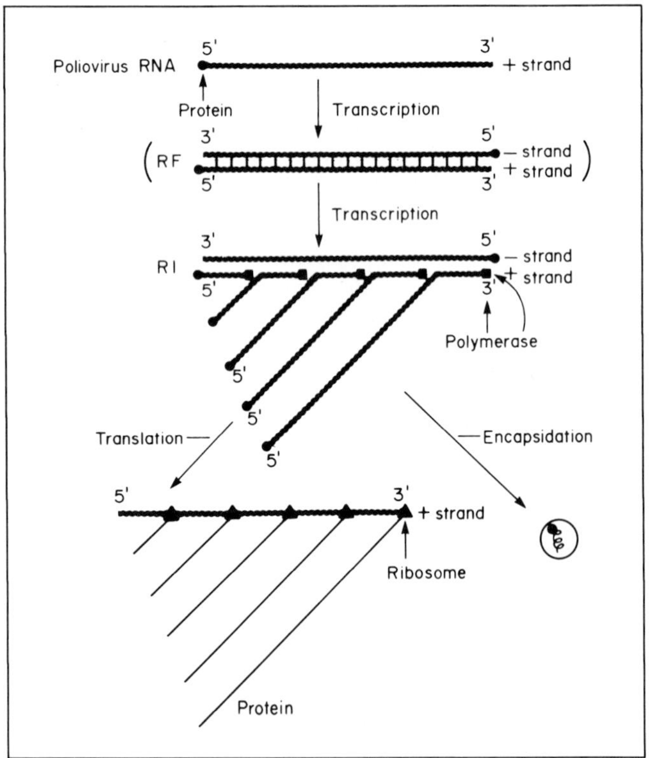

Fig. 55–32. The strategy of the poliovirus multiplication cycle. Parental RNA strands are translated into the polyprotein, and the polymerase derived from it then transcribes them into strands of minus polarity. Progeny plus strands are then transcribed repeatedly from the minus-strand templates. The structures consisting of minus-stranded templates and several plus-stranded transcripts at various stages of completion are known as replicative intermediates (RI). Progeny plus strands are either translated or encapsidated.

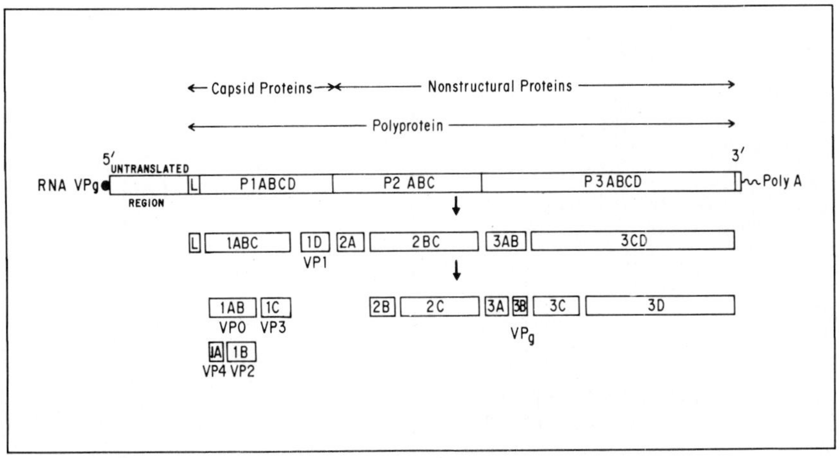

Fig. 55–33. The strategy of poliovirus RNA expression. The polyprotein is first cleaved into proteins L (a small *leader* protein of unknown function that is thought to possess proteolytic activity), P1, P2, and P3. P1 is cleaved sequentially into VP1, VP3, and VP0, which is cleaved into VP4 and VP2 as the final stage of morphogenesis (see below). 2A is the protease that effects the P1–P2 cleavage, 2B is thought to be a host range determinant, and 2C appears to be involved in the initiation of RNA synthesis, since it contains the guanidine resistance marker (Chap. 58). Finally, protein 3B is VPg, 3C is the protease that cleaves glutamine-glycine bonds and effects all cleavages except the initial autolytic cleavage of P1 from P23 and the VP4-VP2 cleavage, and 3D is the poliovirus RNA polymerase. Interestingly, protease 2A is also the enzyme that cleaves the 220K component of the host cell cap-binding complex eIF-4F (see p. 837). This cleavage is responsible for most (but not all) inhibition of host protein synthesis in poliovirus-infected cells.

frequency. This would be very wasteful because many more capsid protein molecules are required than, for example, polymerase molecules. In fact, the various processed poliovirus-specified proteins are not formed in equimolar amounts, especially during the later stages of the multiplication cycle. The mechanism by which such translational control is achieved is by premature termination of translation; that is, ribosomes *fall off* the poliovirus RNA as they translate it. Clearly, such a process would favor the formation of capsid proteins over that of nonstructural proteins because the latter are encoded in the 3′-terminal portion of the RNA.

Poliovirus RNA Replication

Poliovirus RNA replication (Fig. 55–32) starts within an hour or so of infection and occurs in association with smooth cytoplasmic membranes. It is catalyzed by the poliovirus RNA polymerase 3D in concert with a cellular 67K protein with UMP transferase activity. This enzyme is thought to add U residues to the 3′-poly(A)-containing ends of poliovirus RNA; the oligo U track is then postulated to fold back onto the poly(A) sequence, thereby forming a hairpin structure that can be used as a primer (like that described above for vaccinia virus and parvovirus DNA) for transcribing the plus strands into minus strands. Presumably, a specific nuclease then cleaves the dimers that result. Each minus strand is then transcribed repeatedly into plus strands via multistranded (since several rounds of transcription can be initiated before the first is completed), partially double-stranded complexes, known as replicative intermediates (RIs). Some progeny plus strands are also again transcribed into minus strands, but this is not a common occurrence. The total number of minus strands in infected cells probably does not exceed 10,000, whereas up to 500,000 plus strands may be formed.

There is evidence that proteins from the P2 region, that is, 2C or its precursor 2 BC, play a role in the structural organization of poliovirus RNA replication. This is also suggested by the fact that guanidine-resistant and guanidine-dependent mutants, in which RNA synthesis is affected, are 2C mutants.

Poliovirus Morphogenesis

Poliovirus capsids are built up from protomers that consist of VP1, VP3, and VP0 (VP4 plus VP2), which polymerize into pentamers, or *platelets*. These platelets then condense into capsids. It is not clear whether RNA becomes encapsidated as the capsid is being formed or whether the RNA is introduced into capsid precursors, termed *procapsids*. The particles become infectious when VP0 is cleaved to VP2 and VP4. Encapsidated RNA contains VPg, but plus strands that act as messenger RNA do not. Thus, VPg may serve as an encapsidation signal.

As is the case for other icosahedral viruses, poliovirus progeny particles often accumulate in the form of large, intracytoplasmic, paracrystalline arrays (Fig. 55–34). There appears to be no special mechanism for releasing poliovirus particles. Being small, they leak out of cells as cells break up.

Togaviruses

Togavirus particles, as exemplified by the alphavirus Semliki Forest virus (SFV), consist of an icosahedral nucleocapsid made up of 180 molecules of a single protein, the C protein, surrounded by an envelope composed of a lipid bilayer into which 80 spikes are inserted (Fig. 55–35). Each spike is a trimer of a glycoprotein that itself consists of three components (Fig. 55–36): glycoprotein E1, the hemagglutinin and therefore probably the cell attachment protein; glycoprotein E2, which contains the epitopes against which neutralizing anti-

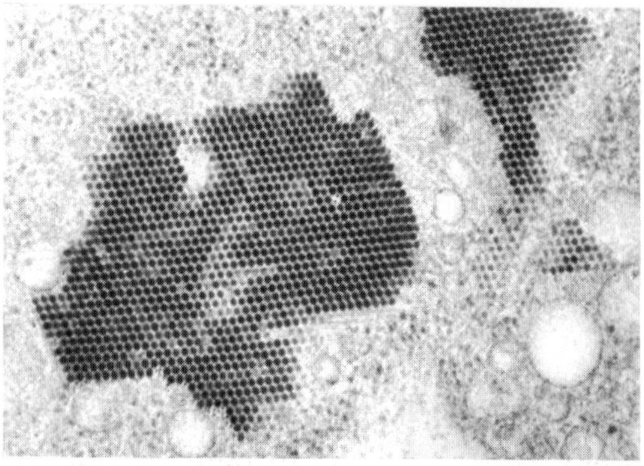

Fig. 55–34. A large crystal of progeny poliovirus particles in the cytoplasm of a HeLa cell infected for 7 hours. × 50,000. *(From Dales et al: Virology 26:379, 1965.)*

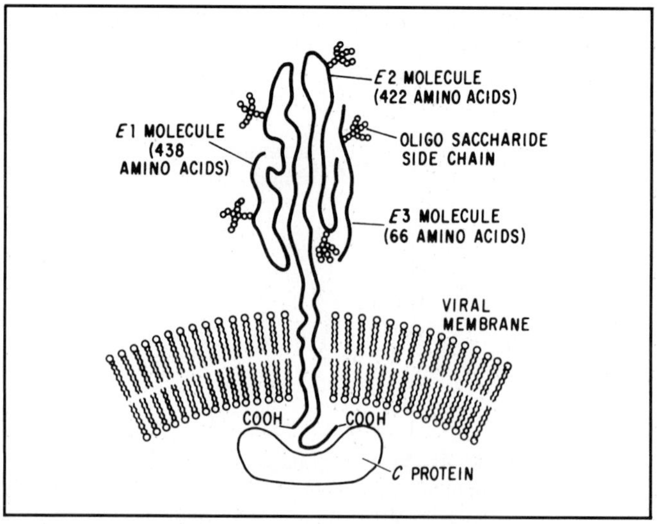

Fig. 55–36. The togavirus spike. Each spike consists of three glycoproteins, E1 (envelope protein 1) (mol wt 48 kDa), E2 (mol wt 46 kDa), and E3 (mol wt 7 kDa). E1 and E2 possess two carbohydrate chains, and E3 possesses only 1. The two large glycoproteins are anchored in the lipid bilayer; thirty-one amino acids of E2 and two amino acids of E1 penetrate through it into the interior of the particle, where they may make contact with C protein molecules. *(Adapted from Simons et al: Sci Am 246:58, 1982.)*

bodies are directed; and the small (65 amino acids) glycoprotein E3, which is cleaved from E2 after its insertion into the envelope. This cleavage is essential for virus release from the cell. In the closely related Sindbis virus, E3 is lost in the process. Interestingly, proteins E1 and E2 are not only glycosylated but also acylated; their *N*-termini are acetylated, and near their *C*-terminal membrane-spanning domains, several of their cysteine residues are linked to long-chain fatty acids, such as palmitic acid, via thioester bonds. Such acylation is a common modification of viral membrane proteins in general.

Togaviruses are taken up into cells via the normal endosome-mediated pathway that results in their genomes being released into the cytoplasm as a result of viral envelope–endosome membrane fusion effected by low pH activation of the viral spike glycoproteins. The uncoated nucleic acid, a plus-stranded RNA molecule about 11,700 nucleotides long (mol wt 4.3×10^6 Da, sedimentation coefficient 49S) then acts as messenger RNA; however not all of it is translated, but only its 5′-terminal two thirds (about 2300 codons) (Fig. 55–37). This portion of it is translated into a 270 kDa polyprotein, which is cleaved progressively, by nsP2, a both *cis*- and *trans*-acting protease, into four nonstructural proteins, about the functions of which little is known: nsP1 may be associated with methyltransferase activity, nsP3 is a phosphoprotein, and nsP4 is the RNA polymerase.

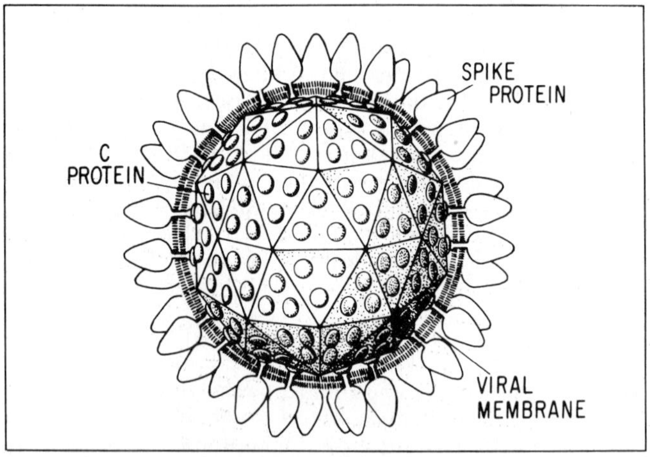

Fig. 55–35. Structure of the alphavirus Semliki Forest virus. One hundred eighty molecules of the C protein (mol wt 30 kDa) form the icosahedral nucleocapsid, and 80 spikes are inserted into the lipid bilayer of the envelope, where they are distributed in a regular icosahedral T=4 surface lattice (Fig. 53–16). *(Adapted from Simons et al: Sci Am 246:38, 1982.)*

The alphavirus RNA transcription and replication program proceeds as follows (Fig. 55–37). First, the parental genome is transcribed into a minus strand, which then acts as the template for plus-strand synthesis. The crucial point here is that two types of plus strands are transcribed: (1) full-length 49S plus strands, which, like the progeny plus strands of poliovirus RNA, either can function as messenger RNAs for more p270, act as template for the synthesis of additional minus strands, or become encapsidated into progeny virus particles, and (2) strands that are only about one third as long (about 3900 nucleotides, 26S). These RNA molecules represent the 3′-terminal one third of the 49S viral genome. Their transcription is initiated at a conserved (among various alphaviruses) 21-base sequence known as the junction sequence, which is located just upstream of the p270 stop codon. This 26S RNA encodes the four structural alphavirus proteins. It is translated first into a 130K precursor polyprotein (about 1250 amino acids), which is cleaved into its components, the C protein, gp62 (the E2 + E3 precursor), and the E1 protein, as it is being synthesized. The protease that effects the protein C-gp62 and the gp62-E1 cleavages is protein C. The cleavage that generates E2 and E3, as pointed out above, occurs only after gp62 has been inserted into the envelope and is essential for release of virus from the cell.

In essence, then, the alphavirus genome expresses itself via two messenger RNAs instead of only one. The 26S subgenomic messenger RNA is transcribed about three times

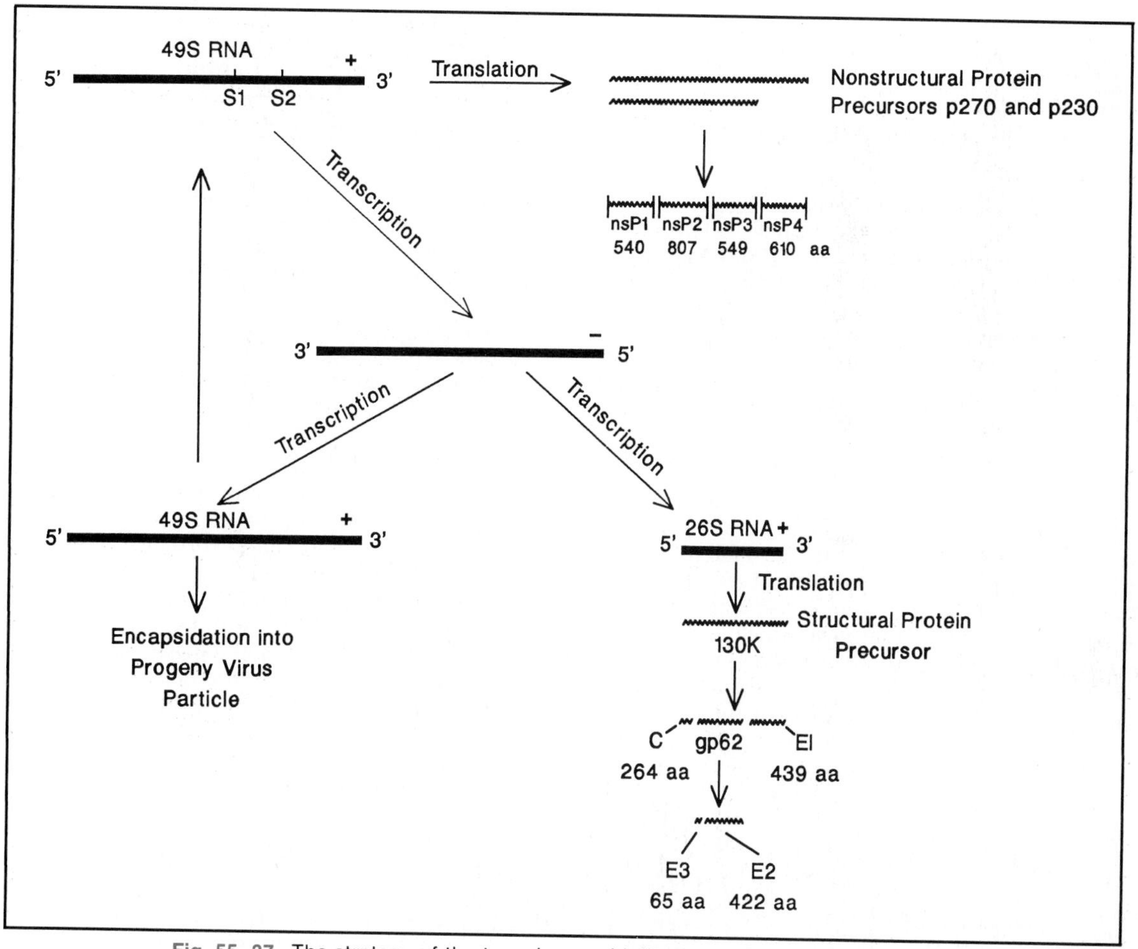

Fig. 55–37. The strategy of the togavirus multiplication cycle. For details, see text.

more frequently than the 49S RNA, which acts as the messenger RNA only for the nonstructural protein precursor. Their relative transcription frequencies are controlled by at least two proteins, namely, one of the nonstructural proteins, which promotes transcription of 26S RNA, and the C protein, which represses it.

The morphogenesis of alphaviruses involves the formation of cores or nucleocapsids that consist of 49S plus-stranded RNA and C protein and the budding of these cores through patches of the plasma cell membrane into which the glycosylated envelope proteins have been inserted. This process is discussed in more detail later (see p. 821).

Flaviviruses

Flavivirus particles are smaller than togaviruses (diameter 45 to 50 nm rather than 60 to 65 nm). They consist of a nucleic acid–containing core or nucleocapsid that is composed of a single protein species, surrounded by an envelope that consists of a lipid bilayer and the membrane (M) protein, to which are attached E glycoprotein spikes. Interestingly, flaviviruses gain access to cells not only by interacting with their (as yet unidentified) receptors but also by using an accessory receptor: when combined with nonneutralizing antibody molecules, they can bind to Fc receptors that are present on certain types of cells. The subsequent entry pathway appears to be normal, as far as one can tell. Why complexes with these particular antibody molecules should be processed normally is not known. The net effect of this mode of entry, known as antibody-modified enhancement of flavivirus replication, is to increase flavivirus yields because more receptors are used. The clinical consequences of such enhancement can be serious, since it causes infections to be more serious in individuals who possess antibodies than in those who do not (Chap. 54).

The flavivirus genome (Fig. 55–38), which is about 11 kb long, possesses a single open reading frame (ORF) flanked by 5′- and 3′-untranslated regions of 118 and 511 nucleotides, respectively. As in the case of picornaviruses, this ORF is translated into a single polyprotein that is 3411 amino acids long. This polyprotein is then cleaved into its component proteins; since pulse-chase experiments fail to detect cleavage intermediates, cleavage is assumed to be very rapid, perhaps cotranslational. Again, as in the case of picornaviruses, structural proteins are located in the N-terminal, nonstructural proteins in the C-terminal portion of the polyprotein. Cleavage of the bonds between the structural proteins is apparently effected by endoplasmic reticulum signalases; little is known

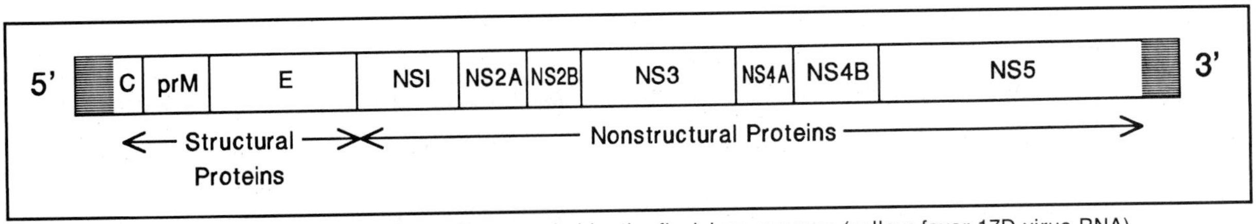

Fig. 55–38. The genetic information encoded by the flavivirus genome (yellow fever 17D virus RNA). The genome, which is about 11,000 nucleotides long, contains one long open reading frame that is 10,233 nucleotides (3411 aa) long. Just under a quarter of it encodes three structural proteins: the C or core protein (123 aa), the M or membrane protein (75 aa), which is synthesized in the form of a precursor, prM, which is cleaved as virus particles are liberated, and the E protein (about 480 aa) which is the spike glycoprotein. The remainder of the genome encodes six or seven nonstructural proteins, two of which, NS3 and NS5, are synthesized in readily detectable amounts. There is some evidence that they may function in RNA replication.

of the enzymes that effect the cleavages between the nonstructural proteins except that several specificities are involved. As for the proteins themselves, the C protein is small (about 110 amino acids), very basic, and not well conserved among the various flaviviruses, and the M protein is very small (about 75 amino acids), and its cleavage from prM, which is a glycoprotein (M is not glycosylated), is thought to occur in the Golgi apparatus concomitantly with virus release (see below). Little is known of the functions of the nonstructural proteins. Proteins NS3 and NS5 are highly conserved among flaviviruses. NS5 contains regions of similarity with those of the picornavirus and togavirus RNA polymerases.

The mode of flavivirus RNA replication is the same in principle as that of picornavirus and togavirus RNA.

Flaviviruses differ from togaviruses in the manner in which they are liberated. Togaviruses bud directly through the plasma cell membrane. Flaviviruses, on the other hand, bud from membranes of the endoplasmic reticulum and the Golgi apparatus into cytoplasmic vacuoles that are liberated by exocytosis and cell lysis (see p. 821).

Coronaviruses

Coronavirus particles possess a helical nucleocapsid that consists of a plus-stranded RNA molecule more than 27,000 nucleotides long—by far the longest RNA molecule known—tightly associated with a basic phosphoprotein, the N or nucleocapsid protein (about 520 amino acids). This nucleocapsid is enclosed within an envelope that consists of a lipid bilayer with which three proteins are associated: the E1 or M protein (220 amino acids), which is the matrix protein, the E2 or S protein, a large glycoprotein (about 1150 amino acids), dimers or trimers of which form the large coronavirus spikes, also known as peplomers, and the E3 or HE protein, a 550 amino acid–long glycoprotein that is the coronavirus hemagglutinin, binds to 9-0-acetylneuraminic acid (9-0-acNA) residues on cell membranes and, like an enzyme on the spikes of influenza C virus particles, is an acetylesterase that cleaves the acetyl group from 9-0-acNA and thus acts as a receptor-destroying enzyme. This protein is not present on all coronavirus strains. The S glycoprotein, which exists in the virus in cleaved form (near the middle), causes cell fusion, possesses the epitopes against which neutralizing antibodies are directed, and is also a coronavirus cell-attachment protein. It also binds the Fc fragment of immunoglobulin, and monoclonal antibodies against the Fc receptor precipitate it. Since the S glycoprotein is present on the surface of infected cells, this molecular mimicry may allow coronavirus-infected cells to escape destruction by the immune system.

Coronaviruses enter cells via the normal clathrin-coated vesicle-endosome mediated pathway, which results in the viral RNA being released into the cytoplasm. Coronavirus genome replication-expression then proceeds via a remarkable and unique mechanism (Fig. 55–39). The first step is the translation of the huge *L* gene into an RNA polymerase using the entire coronavirus RNA molecule as the template. The *L* gene, which represents the 5′-terminal three quarters of the molecule (more than 20,000 nucleotides long), contains two huge ORFs, each between 3000 and 4000 codons long, which overlap by 42 nucleotides, the second being in the −1 frame with respect to the first. These two ORFs are translated into one protein as a result of efficient ribosomal frame-shifting that suppresses the termination codon of the first ORF by virtue of the presence of the sequence UUUAAAC, which in concert with an adjacent system of stem-loop structures that fold into a pseudoknot, causes ribosomal slippage. (A similar mechanism operates at the junction of the *gag* and *pol* gene reading frames in retrovirus RNA [Chap. 59]). The huge protein that would then be formed has not yet been isolated, but there is no doubt that at least a part of it is the coronavirus RNA polymerase.

Once formed, this polymerase then transcribes the entire coronavirus genome into a minus strand. This minus strand is transcribed into full-length plus strands and into six or seven messenger RNAs (depending on the strain), which form a *nested* set. They possess identical polyadenylated 3′-ends (which are the same as that of genomic RNA), they possess different 5′-ends, and their coding sequences are located in their 5′-proximal regions. The proteins encoded by these messenger RNAs are, in order, a 30 kDa nonstructural protein of unknown function, the HE or E3 protein (if present), the E2 or S (spike) glycoprotein, 14, 13, and 10 kDa nonstructural proteins of unknown function, the E1 or M protein, and the N or nucleocapsid protein.

The mechanism by which these messenger RNAs are synthesized is remarkable. It turns out that the first 70 nucleotides of transcripts of the minus strand (which correspond to the 5′-terminal 70 nucleotides of the coronavirus genome) constitute a *leader sequence*, which has an independent existence. This leader sequence is synthesized in large amounts and serves as the primer for the transcription of each of the

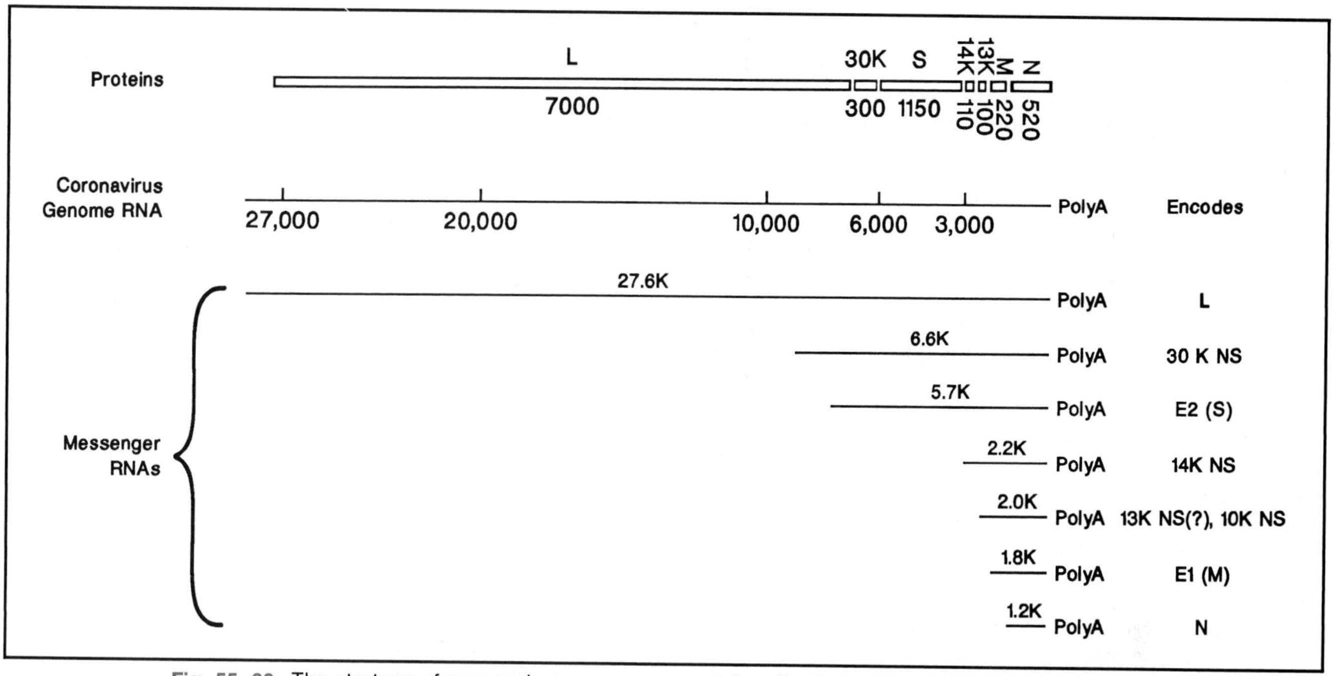

Fig. 55–39. The strategy of coronavirus genome expression. The L protein (the RNA polymerase) is translated from the entire viral genome acting as messenger RNA, and each of the other six proteins is translated from the 5′-proximal portion of its particular messenger RNA. The *L* gene contains a termination codon near its middle that is not observed owing to a −1 frameshift (see text). The leader sequences at the 5′-ends of messenger RNAs are not shown (see text). The numbers below the gene designations (**top**) are the sizes of the proteins that they encode (number of amino acids). The numbers above the messenger RNAs are their lengths (nucleotides).

six messenger RNA species by virtue of the existence at each of the six transcription start sites of short nonidentical but similar sequences with which the 3′-terminal portion of the leader sequence can base pair and which it therefore recognizes and to which it binds. In effect, the leader is the primer for messenger RNA transcription, and all messenger RNAs possess the leader sequence at their 5′-ends. Coronavirus messenger RNA transcription is thus "leader-primed." Furthermore, it seems that the relative frequency of transcription of each of the six messenger RNA species—for they are not transcribed in equimolar amounts—is a function of how efficiently the leader binds to each transcription start site.

Another remarkable feature of coronavirus replication is the manner in which the minus strand is transcribed into genomic plus strands. It appears that during transcription, the polymerase, with the portion of the transcript that it has just transcribed attached to it, can dissociate from the template and reinitiate transcription, at the correct site, on another minus strand. The effect of this is that in cells infected with two strains or variants of coronavirus, recombinants are formed very readily. There are only two other single-stranded RNA viruses that exhibit similar behavior, namely, poliovirus and foot-and-mouth disease virus (FMDV). However, for both, the frequency of template switching is far lower than for coronavirus.

Coronavirus particles mature like flaviviruses (see p. 818), that is, by budding into smooth-walled vesicles at membranes of the rough endoplasmic reticulum and in the Golgi apparatus, but they do not bud at the plasma membrane. The virus particle–containing vesicles are released either by fusion with the plasma membrane or by cell lysis. The budding-maturation process is described in detail below (see p. 821).

Multiplication Cycles of Negative-stranded RNA-containing Viruses

These viruses contain RNA with the polarity opposite to that of messenger RNAs. Since their RNAs cannot be translated, the first step of their multiplication cycles is their transcription into plus strands. Since cells cannot transcribe RNA from RNA, all negative-stranded RNA-containing viruses contain RNA-dependent RNA polymerases encoded by themselves.

The best way of viewing plus-, negative-, and double-stranded RNA-containing viruses is to consider them as virus particles that encapsidate, respectively, the messenger-sense form, the messenger-template form, and the replicative form of their genomes. The basic principle is the same for all: all RNA genomes must have a form that can be translated and a form that is the template for making the form that can be translated, and they must have a replicative form or intermediate. Any one of these can be encapsidated, depending on the nature of the virus.

Rhabdoviruses

The most important human pathogen in the Rhabdovirus family is rabies virus, infection with which without vaccination is invariably fatal. The most intensively studied rhabdovirus is vesicular stomatitis virus (VSV). It has a broad host range, its multiplication cycle is rapid, and the cytopathic effects that it causes are severe.

VSV particles, like all rhabdoviruses, are uniquely bullet-shaped (Fig. 53–5). They consist of two components. The first is the helical nucleocapsid, which consists of an approximately 11,000 nucleotide–long negative-stranded RNA molecule associated with about 1250 molecules of the N protein (422 amino acids). Each N protein molecule, therefore, covers about nine nucleotides. This nucleocapsid is associated with two proteins that transcribe and replicate the RNA: there are about 50 molecules of the very large L protein (about 2100 amino acids) and about 460 molecules of the NS protein, a phosphoprotein about 220 amino acids long. This ribonucleoprotein (RNP) core is surrounded by an envelope that consists of a lipid bilayer lined on its inner surface by the peripheral matrix or M protein (about 1800 molecules, about 230 amino acids long)—a basic protein that contacts both the acidic phospholipid head groups of the lipid bilayer and the nucleocapsid, thereby serving as a glue between them—and to the outer surface of which are attached the glycoprotein spikes that are composed of trimers of the G protein (about 1200 molecules, 500 amino acids long). These 400 spikes contain the epitopes that elicit the formation of neutralizing antibodies and are the viral cell attachment organs.

VSV enters the cell via invagination into clathrin-coated vesicles in which its envelope is removed and from which the RNP core is liberated into the cytoplasm. Removal of the envelope activates the transcription complex, of which the N protein, the L protein, and the fully phosphorylated form of the NS protein are all essential components and which transcribes the five VSV genes into messenger RNA molecules via a unique mechanism (primary transcription). The nature of the VSV genome is shown in Figure 55–40. It encodes, in order from the 3′-end, the *N*, *NS*, *M*, *G*, and *L* genes, each separated from the next by the dinucleotide sequence GA. During transcription into messenger RNA, the *N* gene is transcribed first (however, see below). The polymerase then encounters the sequence AUACUUUUUUU, which is a polyadenylation signal. It pauses there and copies the run of Us over and over until about 250 A residues have been added. The enzyme then starts transcription of the *NS* gene, at the end of which it encounters exactly the same 11-nucleotide polyadenylation signal—and so on, for all five genes.

The five VSV proteins are synthesized in about the same molar ratios as those in which they exist in virus particles. For example, about 25 times as many N as L protein molecules are synthesized. These ratios appear to be controlled at the level of transcription rather than translation. This presents a paradox, for the manner in which VSV RNA is transcribed implies that equal numbers of all five species of messenger RNA molecules should be formed. It seems, however, that there is a polarity effect (attenuation); that is, as the polymerase transcribes the RNA, it tends to detach so that the farther a gene is situated from the origin of transcription, the less likely is it to be transcribed. Indeed, the gene order 3′-N-NS-M-G-L-5′ in the VSV RNA minus strand parallels the frequency of transcription, in a decreasing sense, of each gene into messenger RNA.

In addition to the five species of messenger RNA, there is a sixth transcript: the extreme 3′-terminal region of VSV RNA, that which precedes gene *N*, is transcribed into a 48 nucleotide–long RNA, the so-called *leader* RNA. After transcribing the leader RNA, the polymerase often reinitiates at the beginning of the RNA rather than at the beginning of the *N* gene, so that leader RNA is synthesized in molar excess. Its function is not known with certainty. It has been suggested that it may shut down host DNA and RNA synthesis because is is transported rapidly into the nucleus. However, it is also known that leader RNA binds N protein strongly. Therefore it probably contains the encapsidation start site, that is, the site where N protein starts to bind to the *minus* RNA strands on the way to forming nucleocapsids; it should be noted that the sequence of the 5′-end of the (plus-stranded) leader RNA is very similar to that of the 5′-end of the (negative-stranded) virion RNA (see legend to Fig. 55–40). The reason for the separate existence of the leader RNA may, therefore, be a consequence of its containing the encapsidation start site, for if leader RNA were not a separate molecule, the messenger RNA for the *N* gene would also be encapsidated.

The replication of the VSV genome proceeds via the same mechanism by which all viral single-stranded RNA genomes replicate, that is, transcription into an RNA strand of opposite polarity, in this case, one of plus polarity, and then repeated transcription of that strand into progeny strands. The major problem here is: What causes minus strands to be transcribed into intact plus strands (to serve as templates for the transcription of progeny minus strands) rather than into messenger RNA molecules? The answer seems

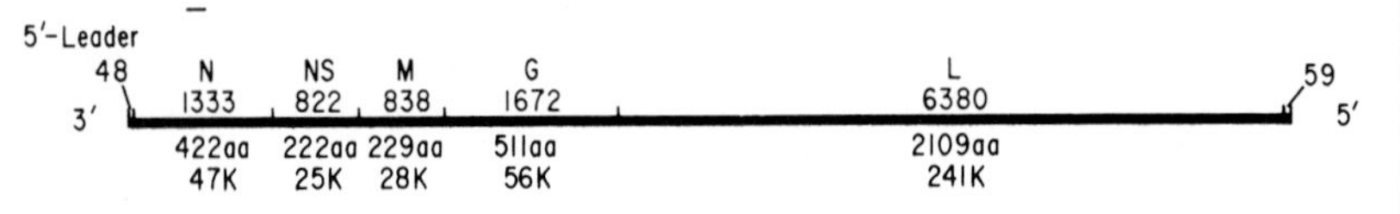

Fig. 55–40. The nature of the VSV genome. The genome is a negative-stranded RNA molecule. At its 3′-end, there is a 48 nucleotide–long noncoding sequence that is transcribed into the 5′-leader RNA; at its 5′-end, the noncoding sequence is 59 nucleotides long. Fifteen to twenty nucleotides at its two ends are almost perfect inverted complementary repeats (i.e., 3′UGCUUC .... GAAGCA5′). At the 5′-end of each gene there is an 11 nucleotide–long polyadenylation signal followed by the dinucleotide GA. The length of each gene is indicated, as are the length of each protein and its approximate molecular weight.

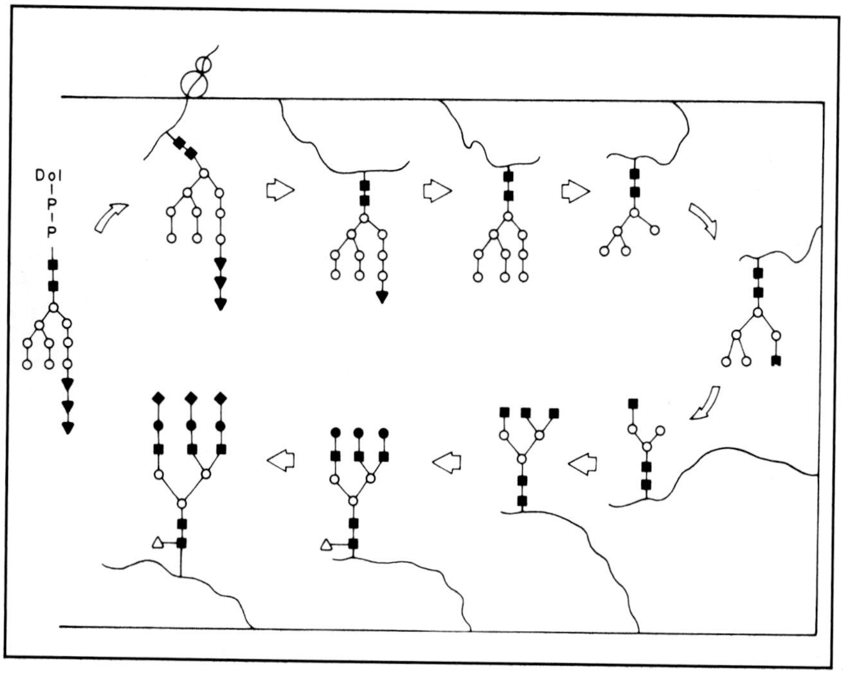

Fig. 55–41. Proposed sequence of reactions for the synthesis of the oligosaccharide subunit of the G spike protein of vesicular stomatitis virus. The first step is the transfer of a mannose-rich precursor from dolichol pyrophosphate to an asparagine residue of the G protein. This precursor is then processed to yield the final oligosaccharide unit. Dol, dolichol; ■, *N*-acetylglucosamine; ○, mannose; ▲, glucose; ●, galactose; ◆ sialic acid (*N*-acetylneuraminic acid); △, fucose. *(From Kornfeld et al: J Biol Chem 253:7771, 1978.)*

to be the formation of N protein. Transcription of messenger RNA does not require concomitant protein synthesis, but transcription of intact plus strands does. The protein that is primarily required is the N protein. Apparently, as progressively larger amounts of N protein are made, it complexes more and more extensively with the minus-stranded RNA template, covering up the termination signals at the 5′-ends of the leader sequence and of the various genes and thereby permitting uninterrupted transcription of intact plus strands.

Formation of Mature VSV Particles: Budding

Like other enveloped viruses, VSV has a special mechanism for being liberated from cells, namely, budding. G glycoprotein is synthesized on membrane-associated ribosomes and is transported to the Golgi apparatus, where it is inserted into membranes and glycosylated. Like other proteins that must pass through membranes, it possesses a hydrophobic leader sequence 16 amino acids long at its N-terminus that is cleaved off as soon as it has penetrated the lipid bilayer and led the rest of the protein chain through it. Membrane glycoproteins are usually, but not always, anchored in the lipid bilayer of the membrane by a strongly hydrophobic sequence close to their C-terminus. As a result, a short stretch of such proteins remains on the internal side of the membrane.

Glycosylation of glycoproteins proceeds in several stages, the first of which is the transfer of a mannose-rich precursor oligosaccharide from dolichol pryrophosphate to specific asparagine residues. These precursors are then processed in the Golgi apparatus to the final prosthetic groups via a series of reactions depicted in Figure 55–41. As discussed in Chapter 53, the precise composition of the oligosaccharide is determined in part by the nature and relative amounts of the various cellular glycosyl transferases and, in part, particularly beyond the mannose fork, by the nature of the protein that is being glycosylated. While glycosylation proceeds, the glycoproteins are transported through the cell membrane system to patches either on the plasma membrane or on membranes lining intracytoplasmic vacuoles, depending on the nature of the virus strain and of the cell type, where they replace host-specified membrane proteins. Ribonucleoprotein cores then migrate to these modified areas, which they recognize with great specificity, align themselves with them, and bud through them, becoming coated with them in the process (Figs. 55–42 and 55–43). The M protein appears to be incorporated into virus particles just before budding; it acts both as a nucleating agent for budding and as the agent that selects negative-stranded RNA rather than plus-stranded RNA containing RNP cores for budding. Interestingly, treatment of cells with cytochalasin B, a drug that disrupts actin-containing microfilaments, inhibits the release of enveloped viruses. This suggests

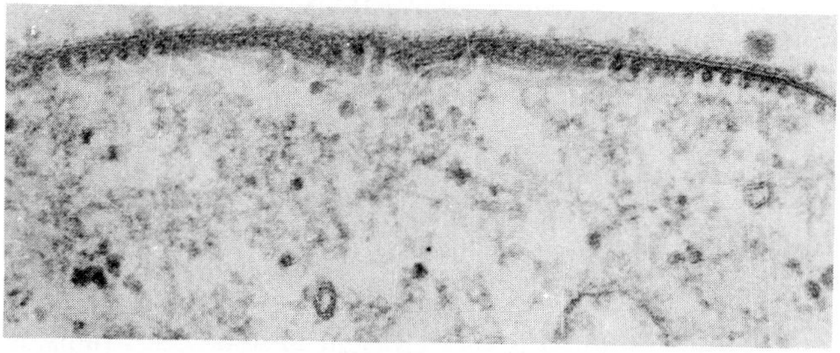

Fig. 55–42. Modification of the plasma membrane of a monkey kidney cell infected with the paramyxovirus SV5. A layer of dense material representing the spikes on viral envelopes is present on the outer surface of the membrane. Nucleocapsids, many seen in cross-section, are aligned immediately beneath the modified patches of cell membrane. In due course, they will bud through these patches and become enveloped by them in the process. × 76,000. *(From Compans et al: Virology 30:411, 1966.)*

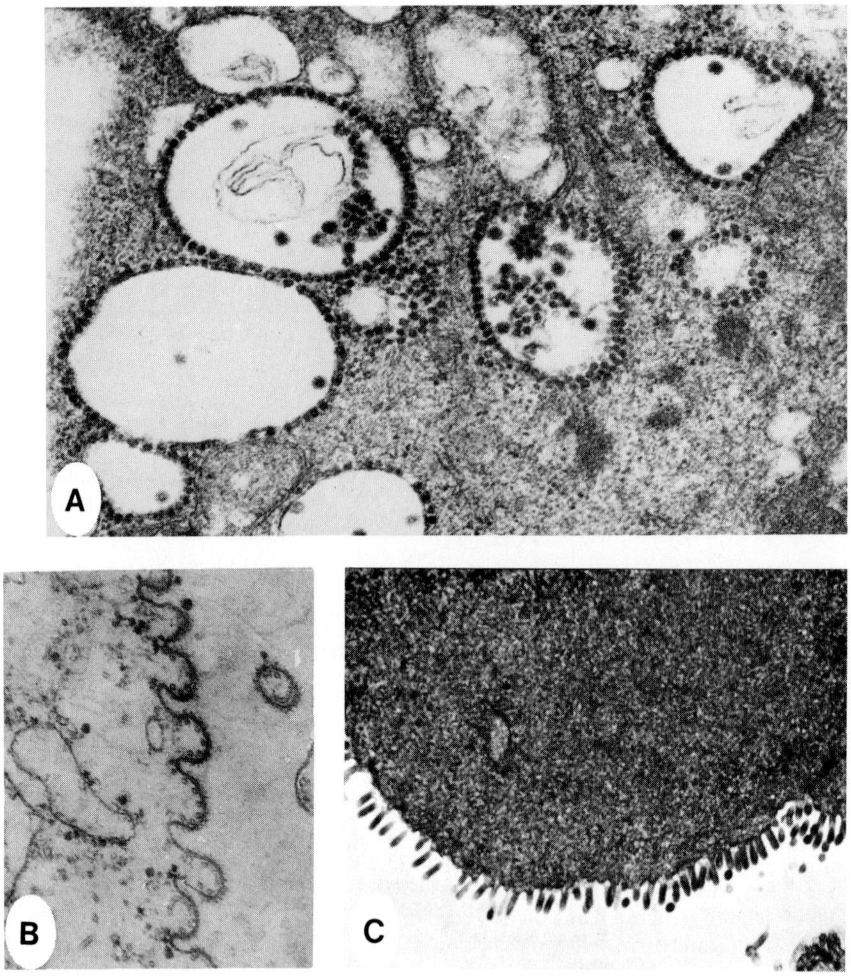

Fig. 55–43. Budding of enveloped viruses. **A.** A chick embryo cell infected with the togavirus Semliki Forest virus (SFV). Numerous nucleocapsids lining cytoplasmic vacuoles before budding into them can be seen. The virus-containing vacuoles will be liberated by exocytosis (transport to and fusion with the plasma membrane) or cell lysis. × 22,000. **B.** A row of SV5 particles budding from the plasma membrane of a monkey kidney cell, showing many nucleocapsids in cross-section. **C.** Vesicular stomatitis virus (VSV) budding from the plasma membrane of a mouse L cell. In L cells, the majority of VSV particles bud from the plasma membrane. In other cells, such as chick embryo fibroblasts and pig kidney cells, VSV buds mostly into cytoplasmic vacuoles. × 21,500. (**A** *from Grimley et al: J Virol 2:1326, 1968;* **B** *from Compans et al: Virology 30:411, 1966;* **C** *from Zee et al: J Gen Virol 7:95, 1970.)*

that such microfilaments play a role in the budding process, which can actually be demonstrated (Fig. 55–44).

The location where enveloped viruses bud is predicated both by the virus and by the cell. Togaviruses and rhabdoviruses usually bud through plasma membranes but may bud into cytoplasmic vesicles or vacuoles (Fig. 55–43). Flaviviruses and coronaviruses almost always bud into cytoplasmic vesicles or vacuoles, bunyaviruses bud into the Golgi apparatus, and paramyxoviruses, orthomyxoviruses, and arenaviruses almost always bud through plasma membranes. Further, some viruses, such as influenza virus, bud through apical plasma membranes of polarized cells, and others, such as VSV, bud through basolateral ones. The information that specifies budding targets is located in the amino acid sequence of the spike glycoproteins.

Whereas budding is very efficient in some cell strains, it is very inefficient in others. This sometimes leads to the accumulation in the cytoplasm of very large numbers of nucleocapsids (Fig. 55–45).

The budding process itself does not harm the host cell significantly. Many cells persistently infected with enveloped viruses (Chap. 56) remain normal in appearance and continue to multiply for many generations while viruses bud from their surfaces. This is not to say that enveloped viruses cannot be cytopathic; it merely says that budding per se is not a factor in cytopathogenicity.

Paramyxoviruses

Paramyxoviruses provide an interesting problem for classification. On the one hand, they share many properties with the Orthomyxoviruses (influenza viruses): like them, they possess proteins with hemagglutinin and neuraminidase activity, share a predilection for sialic acid–containing cell receptors, and exhibit marked respiratory pathogenesis. On the other hand, in the structure of their genomes, including gene order and nature of regulatory sequences such as gene-terminating and intergenic sequences, nature of the proteins that they encode, and strategy of their multiplication cycles, they resemble the rhabdoviruses much more closely. The conclusion is inescapable that rhabdoviruses, paramyxoviruses, and orthomyxoviruses share a common ancestor.

The multiplication cycles of several paramyxoviruses have been investigated extensively, particularly those of parainfluenza viruses, such as Sendai virus (murine parainfluenza virus type 1), SV5 (canine parainfluenza virus type 2), and

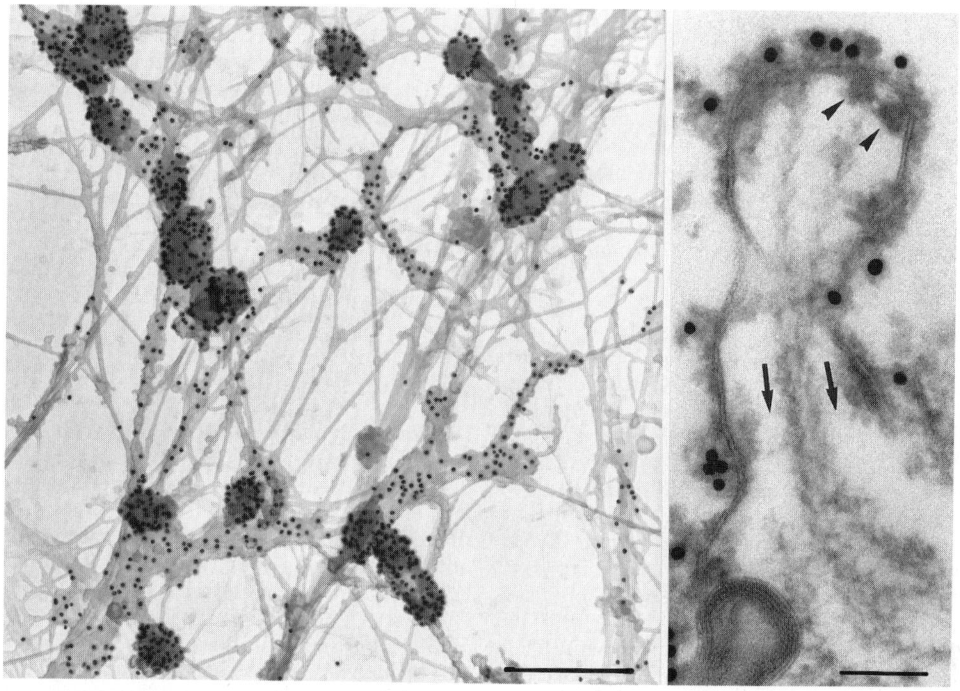

Fig. 55–44. Demonstration of the involvement of cytoskeleton actin filaments in the budding process. **Left.** Transmission electron micrograph of cytoskeleton protruding from HeLa cells infected with measles virus. Bar, 0.5 μm. Virus particles identified by immunogold-labeling with antibodies against the hemagglutinin are associated with the actin filaments. Budding commences with the gradual elevation of such filaments from the plasma membrane, which leads to the formation of stublike protrusions that then vesiculate and form spherical virus particles. This indicates that actin cables control the movement of viral structures at the plasma membrane, the M protein serving as the recognition site for actin. **Right.** Ultrathin section of a measles virus particle budding from the plasma membrane of a HeLa cell. The virus particle is identified as at **left**; actin was decorated with heavy meromyosin (HMM). The HMM arrowheads (→) indicate that the actin filaments terminate with their barbed ends on section profiles of measles virus nucleocapsid cores (▶). Bars, 0.1 μm. *(From Bohn et al: Virology 149:91, 1986.)*

some human parainfluenza viruses, mumps virus, Newcastle disease virus (NDV), measles virus, and respiratory syncytial virus (RSV). We will consider primarily Sendai virus and RSV, which are members of different genera and, therefore, differ in some significant aspects.

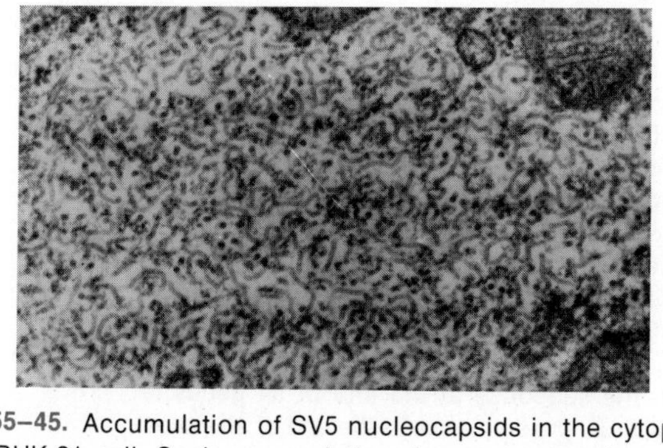

Fig. 55–45. Accumulation of SV5 nucleocapsids in the cytoplasm of a BHK-21 cell. Such accumulation does not occur in monkey kidney cells, from which nucleocapsids bud as rapidly as they are synthesized. × 34,000. *(From Compans et al: Virology 30:411, 1966.)*

Paramyxovirus Particles

Like rhabdoviruses, paramyxoviruses are RNP complexes that consist of a helical nucleocapsid composed of the RNA and the NP protein and associated transcription/replication complex proteins, including the very large L protein and the P (polymerase-associated) protein (the counterpart of the rhabdovirus NS protein), surrounded by a lipid bilayer membrane that is associated on its inner surface with the M (or membrane) protein, while two types of glycoprotein spikes are attached to its outer surface. For the paramyxoviruses (parainfluenza viruses, mumps virus, and Newcastle disease virus), these are composed of dimers of the F_0 protein, which possesses membrane fusion and therefore hemolytic activity, and dimers of the HN protein, which is the hemagglutinin and the neuraminidase. The situation is similar for the morbilliviruses, such as measles virus, except that their second type of spike glycoprotein (the H protein) lacks neuraminidase activity. In the pneumoviruses, such as RSV, the second type of glycoprotein (the G protein) lacks both neuraminidase and hemagglutinin activity, although it is still the cell attachment protein and possesses the epitopes that elicit the formation of neutralizing antibodies.

Paramyxovirus spike glycoproteins, particularly the F_0

protein, must be cleaved once in order for virus particles to be infectious. The fragments that result, F_1 and F_2, remain covalently bonded to each other via —SS— bonds. The reason why cleavage is essential for infectivity is that it generates a very hydrophobic F1 N-terminal sequence that is capable of inserting into membranes, thereby promoting membrane fusion even at neutral pH. Fusion between the viral envelope membrane and cellular plasma membranes is the mechanism by which paramyxovirus nucleocapsids gain entry into cells.

The Paramyxovirus Genome

Paramyxovirus genomes are somewhat larger than those of rhabdoviruses (about 15,000 nucleotides), but structurally they are very similar (Fig. 55–46). The paramyxovirus and measles virus genomes comprise six genes that encode the three ribonucleoprotein complex (*NP, P*, and *L*) and the three envelope proteins [*M*, F_O, and *HN(H)*]. In addition, the genomes of some paramyxoviruses also possess a small gene that encodes a small hydrophobic (SH) membrane protein (about 50 amino acids) between the F_O and the *HN(H)* genes. Further, the *P* genes often encode not only the P proteins but also additional proteins that tend to be membrane proteins. The additional proteins are translated either from the same or a different reading frame, or they are translated from second messenger RNAs into which one or two untemplated Gs are introduced into runs of G during transcription by a stuttering mechanism, thereby generating novel ORFs. Finally, the genome of RSV is somewhat more complex, since it also possesses two genes that encode small (about 130 amino acids) nonstructural proteins of unknown function, as well as a gene that encodes a 22K very basic envelope protein. In addition, there is also the *1A* gene that encodes the counterpart of the SH protein.

The cleavage of paramyxovirus spike proteins is accomplished by an endoprotease in conjunction with a carboxypeptidase that clips several amino acids from the fragment that is anchored in the envelope. Both are cellular enzymes. The efficiency of cleavage is a function both of cell type (some cells contain more of the endoprotease than others) and of the amino acid sequence at the cleavage site (some sequences, particularly basic ones, are more cleavable than others). Since cleavage may be inefficient, an excess of noninfectious virus is often produced. Noninfectious virus can be activated by treatment with proteases in vitro.

Strategy of Paramyxovirus Transcription/ Replication Program

The strategy of the paramyxovirus multiplication cycle closely resembles that of rhabdoviruses.

Orthomyxoviruses—Influenza Virus

Like other negative-stranded RNA-containing viruses, influenza viruses are enveloped helical RNP complexes. Their distinctive feature is that their genome is segmented. That of influenza A and B virus strains consists of eight segments, that of influenza C strains of only seven (because they possess only one type of glycoprotein spike). Table 55–5 summarizes information concerning the eight genome segments of influenza virus and the proteins encoded by them, and Figure 55–47 shows electropherograms of the genome segments of two influenza virus A strains.

The influenza virus envelope contains a typical transmembrane protein, M1, which is located mostly on its inner surface. It is encoded by the 5′-terminal three quarters of the plus-stranded form of the *M* gene. There is a second protein, M2, which is also encoded by the *M* gene, via a spliced messenger RNA. It is encoded predominantly by the 3′-terminal quarter of the plus-stranded form of the gene (Fig. 55–48). Proteins M1 and M2 share their first nine amino acids; after that, their reading frames overlap by 51 nucleotides, but in different reading frames. Protein M2 is also present in the viral envelope, but in very small amounts only. It clearly plays an essential role because antibodies against it strongly inhibit virus multiplication. It apparently exists as tetramers that form proton translocation channels capable of regulating the pH of vesicles in the trans-Golgi network that promote the correct maturation of the HA glycoprotein. Interestingly, M2 is the

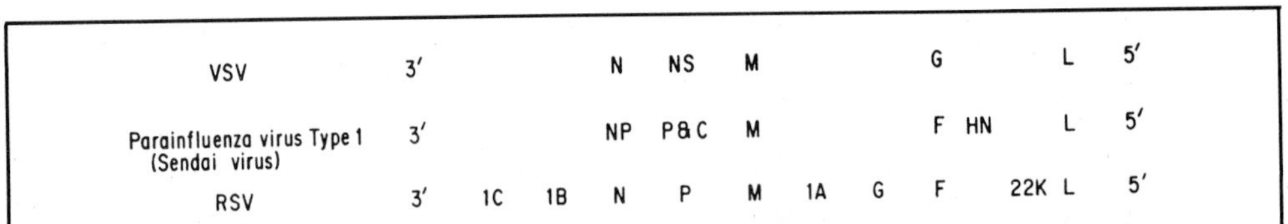
VSV
3′
N
NS
M
G
L
5′
Parainfluenza virus Type 1
(Sendai virus)
3′
NP
P&C
M
F
HN
L
5′
RSV
3′
1C
1B
N
P
M
1A
G
F
22K
L
5′

Fig. 55–46. Arrangement of genes in the genomes of the rhabdovirus VSV and two paramyxoviruses, parainfluenzavirus type 1 (Sendai virus), a member of the genus *Paramyxovirus*, and respiratory syncytial virus (RSV), a member of the genus *Pneumovirus.* Note the conserved functions of most of the proteins. Thus, N, NP, and N proteins are the nucleocapsid proteins; NS, P, and P are nucleocapsid-associated phosphoproteins that probably function in concert with the L proteins, the RNA polymerase proteins; all the M proteins are membrane or matrix proteins, as is the RSV 22 kDa protein; and G, F and HN, and G and F are spike glycoproteins. The C protein of parainfluenza viruses and 1A, 1B, and 1C of RSV are small nonstructural proteins, the function of which is not known. The nature of the paramyxovirus intergenic regions is of interest. For VSV, the sequence at the end of all genes is AUACUUUUUUU, followed by the intergenic GA. For Sendai virus, the sequence at the end of all genes is UNAUUCUUUUU, followed by an intergenic GAA. For RSV, the sequence at the end of all genes is $UCAAUN_{(1-4)}U_{(4-6)}$, followed by intergenic sequences that are all different and from 1 to 52 nucleotides long; but all RSV genes start with the sequence CCCGUUUA.

TABLE 55–5. THE EIGHT INFLUENZA VIRUS GENOME SEGMENTS AND THE PROTEINS THAT THEY ENCODE [INFLUENZA VIRUS STRAIN PR8 (HINI)]

Genome Segment Size (Nucleotides)	Protein	Size of Protein (Mol Wt kDa)	Approx. No. of Protein Molecules per Virus Particle	Approx. % of Virus Particle Protein	Function of Protein
2341	PB1	86.5	16	1	Initiation of transcription
2341	PB2	84	16	1	Cap-binding protein
2233	PA	82.5	16	1	Elongation of transcription
1778	HA HA1	36	500	17	Hemagglutinin spike. The sizes of the carbohydrate groups on HA1 and HA2 are 11,500 and 1,400 Da, respectively
	HA2	27	500		
1565	NP	56	1,000	31	Structural protein of the helical nucleocapsids
1413	NA	50	100	3	Neuraminidase
1027	M1	28	3,000	47	Matrix protein
	M2	11	?	?	Minor envelope component
890	NS1	27	0		Nonstructural protein of unknown function
	NS2	14	0		Nonstructural protein of unknown function

protein with which the anti-influenza A agent amantadine reacts (Chap. 58).

Influenza virus possesses two types of spikes. One is composed of the hemagglutinin (HA) protein, which is the cell attachment protein and the hemagglutinin, possesses the epitopes that elicit the formation of neutralizing antibodies, and effects the membrane fusion that is essential for liberating viral nucleocapsids into the cell cytoplasm. The cell receptor is provided by neuraminic acid containing oligosaccharides of cell surface glycoproteins. Each HA spike, of which there are about 170 per virus particle, is composed of a trimer of two —SS— linked proteins, HA1 and HA2, which are formed by cleavage of the HA protein by the same mechanism as was described for paramyxoviruses. This cleavage is essential for infectivity because it enables the highly hydrophobic N-terminus of the HA2 protein to exercise its membrane fusion function.

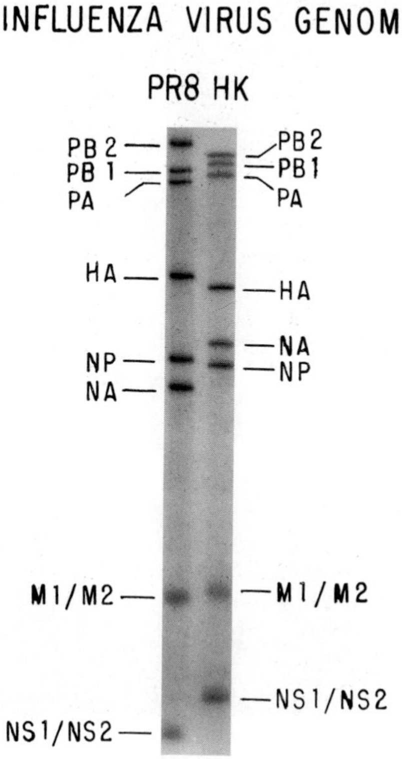

Fig. 55–47. Polyacrylamide gel electropherograms of the eight genome segments of influenza A virus strains PR8 and HK. The proteins encoded by each genome segments are indicated. For their functions, see Table 55–5 and text. *(Adapted Ritchey et al: J Virol 20:307, 1976.)*

The influenza virus hemagglutinin has, in recent years, become one of the most extensively studied proteins. Its three-dimensional structure has been established as a result of x-ray crystallographic analysis, the first membrane protein to be so studied. A large number of variants of it have been sequenced, and changes in amino acid sequence have been correlated with structure and function; and the nature of the epitopes of many variants has been correlated with sequence on the one hand and ability to react with a wide variety of monoclonal antibodies on the other (Fig. 55–49). As a result, structure-function studies for the influenza virus HA protein are as far advanced as those for any other protein.

The second type of spike is the neuraminidase (the NA spike). There are about 25 of these per virus particle, each made up of a tetramer of the NA protein. It is anchored in the lipid bilayer not by its C-terminus, like the HA, but by its N-terminus. Interestingly, whereas the distribution of the HA is uniform on the influenza particle surface, the NA tends to be localized in that region of the envelope where the budding virus particle separated from the cell membrane. It seems that concentration of the NA in that region facilitates release of newly formed virus particles from host cells.

The distribution of the cell attachment-hemagglutinin (HA), membrane fusion (F), and neuraminidase (NA) functions among the orthomyxovirus and paramyxovirus glycoprotein spikes is interesting (Table 55–6).

The three largest and the smallest influenza virus genome segments encode nonstructural proteins. The former encode

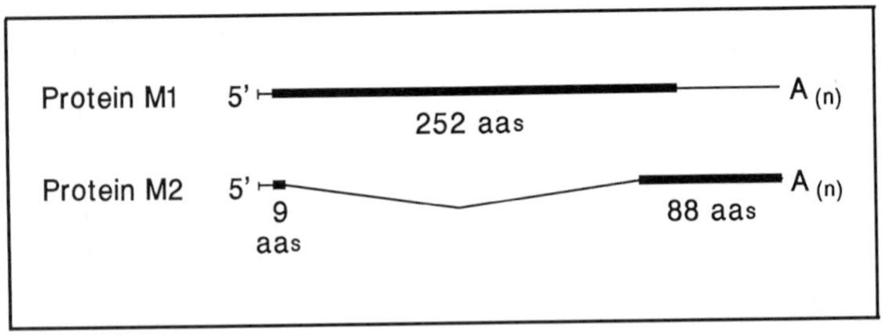

Fig. 55–48. Mode of translation of the influenza A M1 and M2 proteins. The M1 protein is translated from the unspliced plus-stranded transcript of the M genome segment until a termination codon is encountered. The M2 protein is translated from a messenger RNA from which almost three quarters of the sequence has been spliced out. The M1 and M2 proteins share the first nine amino acids; the other 86 amino acids of the M2 protein are translated from a reading frame that is different from that which encodes protein M1. The NS1/NS2 proteins are translated in similar fashion.

TABLE 55–6. FUNCTIONS OF PARAMYXOVIRUS AND ORTHOMYXOVIRUS GLYCOPROTEIN SPIKES

Virus	Functions[a]	
Parainfluenza viruses	HA/NA	F
Morbilliviruses (measles)	HA	F
Pneumoviruses (RSV)	Cell attachment	F
Influenza A and B	HA/F	NA
Influenza C	HA/Ac-Esterase/F	

[a] The HA also possesses the cell attachment function.

proteins that function in transcription/replication (see below); the latter encodes two nonstructural proteins, NS1 and NS2, which, like the two proteins encoded by the *M* gene, are also translated from a nonspliced and a spliced messenger RNA, respectively. NS1 is encoded by the 5′-terminal 80% of the plus-stranded form of the gene, NS2 by its 3′-terminal 40% portion. There is extensive overlap, in different reading frames, of their coding sequences. Both NS proteins are located in the nucleus.

Influenza viruses are classified into three types, A, B, and C, based on antigenic differences between their NP and M proteins. Type A influenza virus strains are subdivided into subtypes based on the antigenic characteristics of their surface

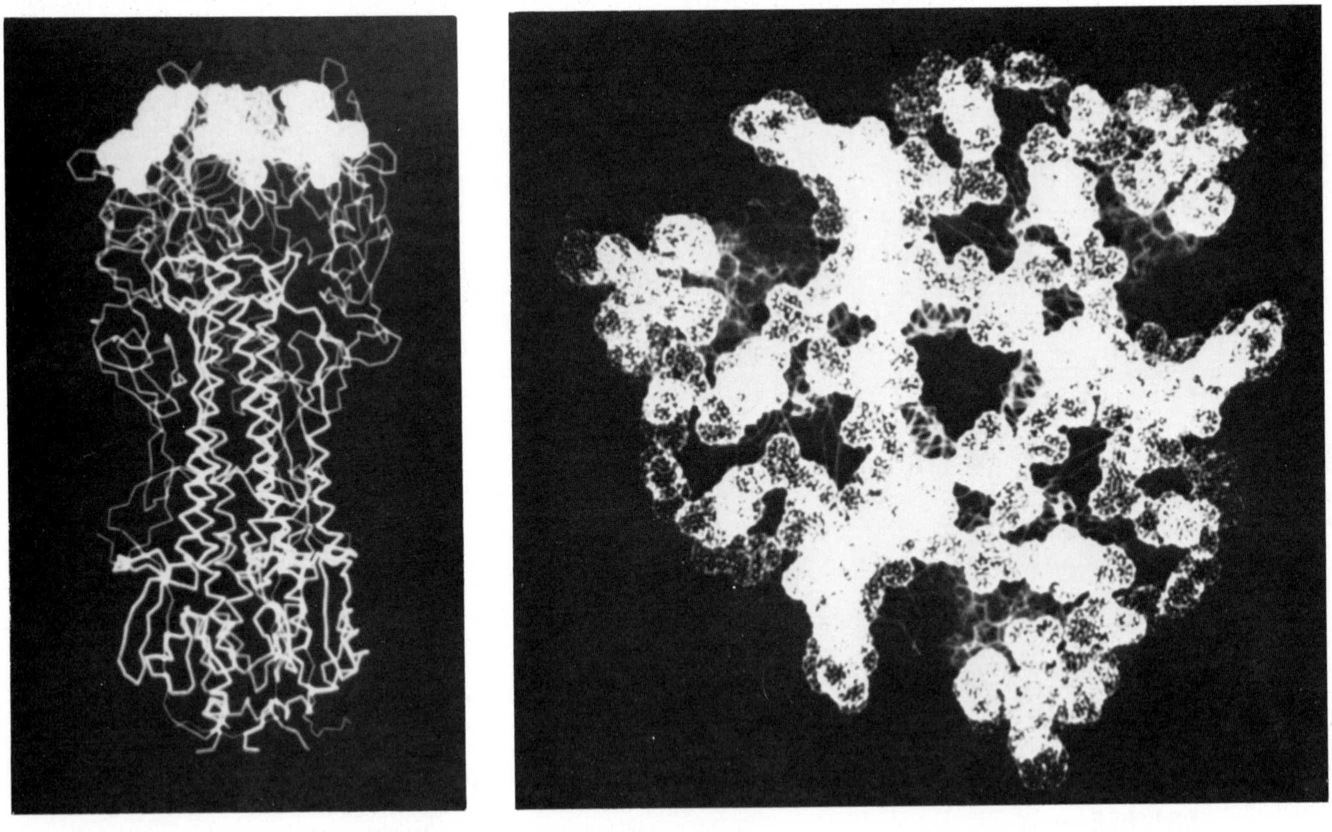

A B

Fig. 55–49. The structure of the influenza virus hemagglutinin as determined by x-ray crystallography. **A.** The hemagglutinin spike is a trimer of HA1 (thin lines) and HA2 (thick lines) polypeptide chains. The membrane anchoring sites are at the bottom, the receptor binding sites at the top. **B.** View of the hemagglutinin spike from the top, that is, looking at the receptor binding sites. Their trimeric arrangement is clearly visible. *(Courtesy of Dr. J. J. Skehel.)*

antigens, namely, the HA and NA proteins. Thirteen distinct HA subtypes and nine NA subtypes are currently recognized. Since human influenza viruses were first isolated (1933), human influenza A strains have contained HAs of three subtypes (H1, H2, and H3) and NAs of two subtypes (N1 and N2). The other HA and NA subtypes are present in influenza virus strains of other animal species (e.g., horses, swine, birds). The nature of the extensive antigenic variations that cause the emergence of the influenza virus strains responsible for successive human pandemics is discussed in Chapter 58.

Influenza Virus Multiplication Cycle

Influenza virus is transported into cells via the normal clathrin-coated vesicle/endosome-mediated pathway. Within the vesicle, low pH causes a conformational change in the HA spike, as a result of which the hydrophobic N-terminus of protein HA2 is exposed. This is then inserted into the vesicle membrane and causes fusion of the viral membrane with the vesicle membrane. As a result, the RNP complexes are released into the cytoplasm. Virus particles that contain HA that has not been cleaved adsorb to cells but are not internalized.

The released parental RNP complexes do not remain in the cytoplasm but migrate to the nucleus; influenza virus is the only RNA-containing virus that replicates in the nucleus. The reason is that the influenza virus RNA polymerase cannot initiate transcription of the negative-stranded RNA genome segments into messenger RNAs without a primer; it therefore uses for this purpose the 5′-terminal regions of cellular messenger RNAs, and all cellular messenger RNAs are synthesized in the nucleus. The mechanism of transcription initiation is outlined in Figure 55–50. Messenger RNA transcription does not proceed to the end of the negative RNA strands but stops about 20 nucleotides short of the end because polyadenylation signals are located there on all genome segments. Thus influenza virus messenger RNAs possess heterogeneous 5′-terminal 10 to 13 nucleotide long sequences pirated from host cell messenger RNAs and are about 20 nucleotides shorter at their 3′-ends than their negative-stranded templates [not counting their poly(A) tails].

In contrast to the transcription of messenger RNA molecules, transcription of plus strands, which are required as the templates for progeny minus-strand synthesis, proceeds without difficulty, that is, without the need for primers, from one end of each minus strand to the other. Thus, influenza RNA is replicated by the same mechanism as all other viral RNAs. Presumably a major factor that determines whether negative strands are transcribed into messenger RNAs or into intact plus-stranded antigenomes is the availability of NP protein; for intact RNA strands, both plus- and negative-stranded, are always encapsidated, messenger RNAs are always free. There is some evidence that the encapsidated nucleocapsids might be circular because the 15 or so nucleotides at each of their ends are complementary and could form double-stranded panhandles.

Influenza Virus Morphogenesis

The morphogenesis of influenza virus proceeds as described for VSV, but there are some unique features. One is that in order for influenza virus progeny to be infectious, the HA must be cleaved into two proteins HA1 and HA2, as described

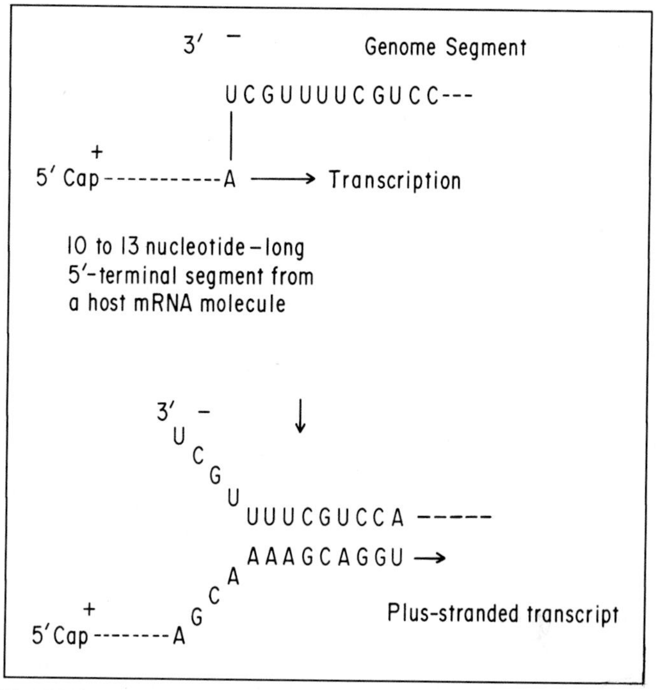

Fig. 55–50. Initiation of transcription of an influenza virus genome segment. The first step is cleavage of a capped cellular RNA molecule (the donor) 10 to 13 nucleotides from its 5′-end by an endonuclease activity that is probably located on protein PB2. The preferred cleavage site is on the 3′-side of an A residue; the product possesses a free 3′-OH group, as is required of primers for RNA transcription. All influenza virus RNA segments possess the same 12 nucleotide long 3′-terminal sequence, which starts with U. The A on the primer probably pairs with this U, thus positioning primer and template for transcription. PB1 then catalyzes the extension of the primer, adding first a G and using the negative-stranded genome segment as the template. The exact function of the PA protein is not known, but the three P proteins are thought to move along the template as a complex.

for the paramyxovirus HN and F proteins; another concerns the function of the influenza virus neuraminidase. It seems that the primary function of this enzyme is to remove neuraminic acid residues from the oligosaccharide moieties of the HA protein. If this is prevented (either by the addition of inhibitors or by the use of appropriate mutants), the newly formed virus either aggregates or readsorbs to cells; also, the HA protein cannot be cleaved unless neuraminic acid is first removed from its oligosaccharides.

Finally, the influenza virus genome segment assortment process poses a fascinating problem. How do the genome segments assort with each other into sets of eight unique segments if their sequences are masked by association with NP protein? One explanation that has been advanced is that there is in fact no specific assortment mechanism but that influenza virus particles contain more than eight randomly assorted segments. It can be shown that if each influenza virus particle contains no more than 10 random segments, about 1 in every 35 particles on average will contain one of each of the eight genome segments and, therefore, be viable.

TABLE 55–7. BUNYAVIRUS GENOME SEGMENTS AND THE PROTEINS THAT THEY ENCODE

Genome Segment	Size (Nucleotides)	Protein	Size (Amino Acids)	Function
L	6000–9000	L	2000	RNA polymerase
M	4000–6000	G	1300	Spike glycoproteins G1 (1000 aa) and G2 (300 aa)
		NS_M	150	Nonstructural protein
S	1000–2000	N	200–250	Nucleocapsid protein
		NS_S	150	Nonstructural protein

Bunyaviruses and Arenaviruses

Both the bunyaviruses and the arenaviruses include some very important human pathogens, but less work has been carried out on them than on viruses in other families. They are considered together here because they share several basic characteristics and because the strategies of their multiplication cycles are similar.

Bunyaviruses

Bunyaviruses, like orthomyxoviruses, possess segmented negative-stranded RNA genomes; they possess three genome segments termed L, M, and S (Table 55–7). Bunyavirus RNPs appear to be circular. The reason is probably that their RNAs possess about 50 nucleotide–long complementary inverted terminal repeats, that is, of the type A, B, C, D . . . D′, C′, B′, A′, which can base pair with each other, thereby forming double-stranded *panhandles*. Like all other negative-stranded RNA genomes or genome segments, bunyavirus RNA molecules are associated with many nucleocapsid (N) protein molecules and with a few molecules of a very large protein, the L protein, which is probably the RNA polymerase. The bunyavirus envelope is remarkable for not containing an M protein, but it possesses two glycoproteins, G1 and G2, that are cleaved from a common precursor, the G protein. The L protein is encoded by the L RNA segment, the glycoprotein precursor by the M RNA segment, and the N protein by the S RNA segment.

Some bunyaviruses, particularly members of the *Phlebovirus* and *Bunyavirus* genera, also encode two nonstructural proteins of unknown function. One is the NS_M protein encoded by the M genome segment; the other is the NS_S protein, which is encoded by the S genome segment. The NS_M protein is encoded by its own ORF, but the situation is different for the NS_S protein. The bunyavirus NS_S protein is translated from the same messenger RNA as the N protein but from a different overlapping reading frame. The messenger RNA of the phlebovirus NS_S proteins, however, is the product of a remarkable *ambisense* coding strategy (Fig. 55–51). Here the N protein is translated from a subgenomic messenger RNA that is transcribed from the negative, that is, the genome

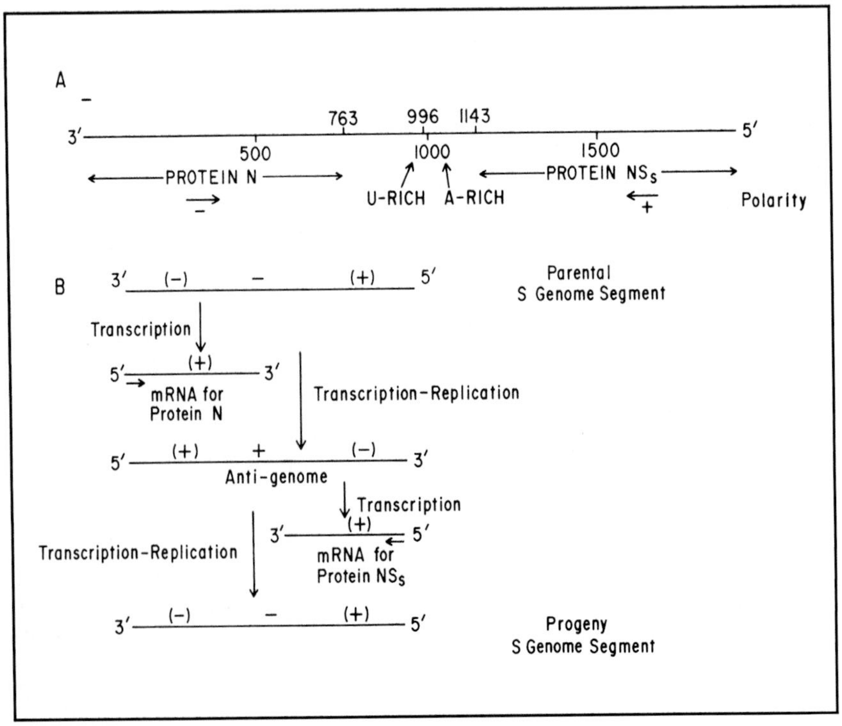

Fig. 55–51. **A.** The structure of the *Phlebovirus* S genome RNA segment. The coding information for protein N is in the left half, that for protein NS_S in the right half. The central portion of the RNA molecule contains a 206 nucleotide–long palindrome centered around nucleotide 996, the left side of which is very rich in U, the right side very rich in A residues. This palindrome is capable of forming a long hairpin structure that could be a major factor in mRNA transcription termination. **B.** A model for the transcription and replication of this genome segment. The N protein is postulated to be translated from a subgenomic messenger RNA that is transcribed from the left portion of the genome segment, the NS_S protein from a messenger RNA that is transcribed from the right portion of the antigenome segment. This could only occur after genome segment replication has commenced. Thus the function of the NS_S protein must be required only during the later stages of the multiplication cycle. Ambisense genome segments are thought to have been generated through a replication mistake that occurred when a polymerase that started transcription of a plus strand detached from the template and reinitiated transcription on a minus strand.

sense, strand, whereas the NS_S protein is translated from a subgenomic messenger RNA that is transcribed from the plus, that is, the antigenome sense, strand. Thus, one half (the left half) of the S genome segments of these viruses is minus stranded, and the other half is plus stranded—that is, the S genome segments are ambisense.

Bunyavirus messenger RNAs, like orthomyxovirus messenger RNAs, possess heterogeneous primer sequences about 14 nucleotides long at their 5′-termini that are derived from host cell messenger RNAs. Interestingly, however, bunyavirus messenger RNA transcription is not sensitive to the transcription inhibitor actinomycin D. Further, the bunyavirus transcription apparatus, which consists of only one protein, the L protein, is far simpler than that of orthomyxoviruses.

The bunyavirus replication cycle is similar in principle to that of other negative-stranded RNA viruses. Bunyaviruses bud into the cisternae of the Golgi apparatus, from which they are released in individual small vesicles, analogous to secretory granules. However, some bunyaviruses, like Rift Valley fever virus, can also bud from plasma membranes. It is not clear how the RNP complexes recognize the areas through which to bud, since bunyaviruses do not possess an M protein.

Arenaviruses

Like bunyavirus particles, arenavirus particles consist of four proteins, the N protein (about 550 amino acids), which is the structural nucleocapsid protein, the L protein (more than 7200 amino acids), which is the polymerase, and two glycoproteins, G1 and G2, which are derived from an approximately 500 amino acid–long precursor, designated GPC. Again, there is no M protein. A remarkable feature of arenavirus particles is that each contains several ribosomes, but this appears to be fortuitous because they perform no function relevant to arenavirus multiplication.

Arenaviruses possess negative-stranded RNA genomes. There are two genome segments, designated L (about 7000 nucleotides) and S (about 3000 nucleotides). They appear to be circular for the same reason, presumably, that bunyavirus RNPs are circular. The L genome segment encodes the polymerase and perhaps also, via ambisense strategy, an 11K protein of unknown function that contains a Zn finger domain. The S genome segment definitely is ambisense: it encodes both the N protein and the GPC protein, the former being encoded by its 3′-terminal sequences and translated from a messenger RNA transcribed from the negative (genome-sense) strand, the latter by its 5′-terminal sequences, translated from a messenger transcribed from the antigenome strand. Just as for the phlebovirus S genome segments, the two ORFs do not overlap but are separated by a very stable hairpin structure that serves as a transcription terminator. It should be noted that, like orthomyxovirus and bunyavirus messenger RNAs, arenavirus messenger RNAs possess heterogeneous 5′-termini pirated from nonviral messenger RNAs.

The strategy of the arenavirus multiplication cycle parallels that of bunyaviruses. In distinction to bunyaviruses, arenaviruses bud from plasma membranes.

Hepatitis Delta Virus (HDV)

Hepatitis delta virus is an important human pathogen discovered in 1977 in HBV patients experiencing unexpectedly severe liver disease. It either coinfects with HBV, which results in fulminant hepatitis, or it superinfects chronic HBV carriers, in which case chronic hepatitis and liver cirrhosis result. It is endemic in many parts of the world, often in intravenous drug users, who frequently are HBV carriers.

HDV is an incomplete virus that requires HBV as helper. It is a 36 nm particle that contains, within an HBsAg-containing outer coat, a very small (about 1700 nucleotide–long) single-stranded (ss), circular, viroidlike RNA molecule associated with the delta antigen, HDA, which consists of two RNA-binding phosphoproteins, $p24^{\delta}$ and $p27^{\delta}$. Interestingly, these two proteins are translated from two cytoplasmic polyadenylated messenger RNAs that are about 800 nucleotides long, possess the opposite polarity from HDV RNA (that is, HDV is a negative-stranded RNA virus), and differ from each other in a *single* nucleotide that changes the UAG termination codon at the end of the reading frame for the smaller protein to UCG, which extends the reading frame for another 19 codons. The sequences of $p24^{\delta}$ and $p27^{\delta}$ are therefore identical except that $p27^{\delta}$ is 19 amino acids longer. The two messenger RNAs are about 500 times less abundant than HDV RNA itself, which replicates in the nucleus via a unique mechanism. It appears that transcription is probably effected via a rolling circle-type mechanism by redirected host DNA-dependent RNA polymerase, that the HDA plays an as yet undetermined role in this process, and that both self-cleavage and self-ligation by HDA itself are involved.

The reason why HDV causes severe disease is also very interesting. It turns out that there is extensive sequence complementarity between HDV RNA and 7S RNA, a small cytoplasmic RNA that is a component of the signal recognition particle, the structure involved in the translocation of secretory and membrane-associated proteins. HDV RNA apparently either sequesters 7S RNA, thereby preventing it from functioning or, since it possesses ribozyme-like catalytic properties, cleaves it.

HDV is clearly a completely novel type of virus, which employs unique strategies for replicating and expressing its genome. It is being investigated intensively in order to determine what other surprises it holds and whether other similar agents are human pathogens.

Multiplication Cycle of Double-stranded RNA-containing Viruses

Finally, we come to a family of viruses the genome of which is double-stranded RNA. In essence, as will be seen, double-stranded RNA-containing viruses encapsidate the replicative forms of their genomes.

The important human pathogens in the reovirus family are the rotaviruses, which cause infantile gastroenteritis, the primary cause of death among infants in Third World countries. Human rotaviruses are difficult to grow in cultured cells. It is very likely that their multiplication cycle proceeds like that of reovirus, one of the most intensively studied of all viruses, which is described here.

The reovirus particle consists of about eight structural proteins, three in the outer capsid shell and five in the core (Table 55–8). The cell attachment protein, hemagglutinin and antigen that elicits the formation of the major neutralizing

TABLE 55–8. REOVIRUS GENOME (REOVIRUS SEROTYPE 3, STRAIN DEARING)

Genome Segment	Length		Protein	% in Virions	Location/Function
	Nucleotides	Codons			
L1	3860	1278	λ3	<2	Transcriptase
L2	3914	1289	λ2	12	Projections or spikes; guanylyltransferase
L3	3896	1233	λ1	12	Major core component
M1	2304	736	μ2	<2	Minor core component
M2	2203	708	μ1	35	Major outer capsid shell component; myristoylated at its N-terminus; mostly cleaved to μ1C (666 aas); possesses a protease motif
M3	2235	719	μNS	0	Nonstructural protein; binds ssRNA
S1	1416	455	σ1	2	Outer shell component; cell attachment protein; hemagglutinin; elicits formation of neutralizing antibodies
S2	1331	418	σ2	8	Major core component
S3	1198	366	σNS	0	Nonstructural protein; binds ssRNA
S4	1196	365	σ3	28	Major outer capsid shell component; binds dsRNA

antibodies and interacts primarily with cells of the immune system, is a protein, σ1, which is present on the virus particle surface in the form of 12 trimers inserted into the icosahedrally distributed projections or spikes (Fig. 53–14).

The reovirus genome consists of 10 segments of double-stranded RNA that range in size from about 1200 to 3800 bp (Table 55–8). The plus strands of all 10 genome segments terminate in 5′-GCUA- and -UCAUC-3′. The total length of the reovirus genome is about 23 kbp, which places reoviruses among the most complex of RNA containing viruses. Each RNA segment encodes one major primary protein; one also encodes a second, small protein (σ1S) in a different reading frame, and another encodes another protein (μNSC) in the major ORF by using an internal initiation codon. Two of the primary reovirus proteins (μNS and σNS) are nonstructural proteins that function during morphogenesis.

The double-stranded reovirus genome cannot express itself in cells. It must first be transcribed into plus-stranded RNA, which can then be translated. The enzymes that transcribe the double-stranded genome segments into messenger RNA are present in reovirus particles, more precisely, in reovirus cores. They include not only the transcriptase, that is, the double-stranded RNA-dependent RNA polymerase, but also the enzyme system that caps the 5′-termini of the messenger RNA molecules (Table 55–8).

When reovirus particles infect cells, their outer capsid shells are partially degraded within endosomes fused with lysosomes, and particles known as subviral particles (SVP) are released into the cytoplasm (Fig. 55–52). The partial disruption of the outer capsid shell activates the transcription of the 10 genome segments by permitting movement of polymerase relative to template, which is not possible in intact virus

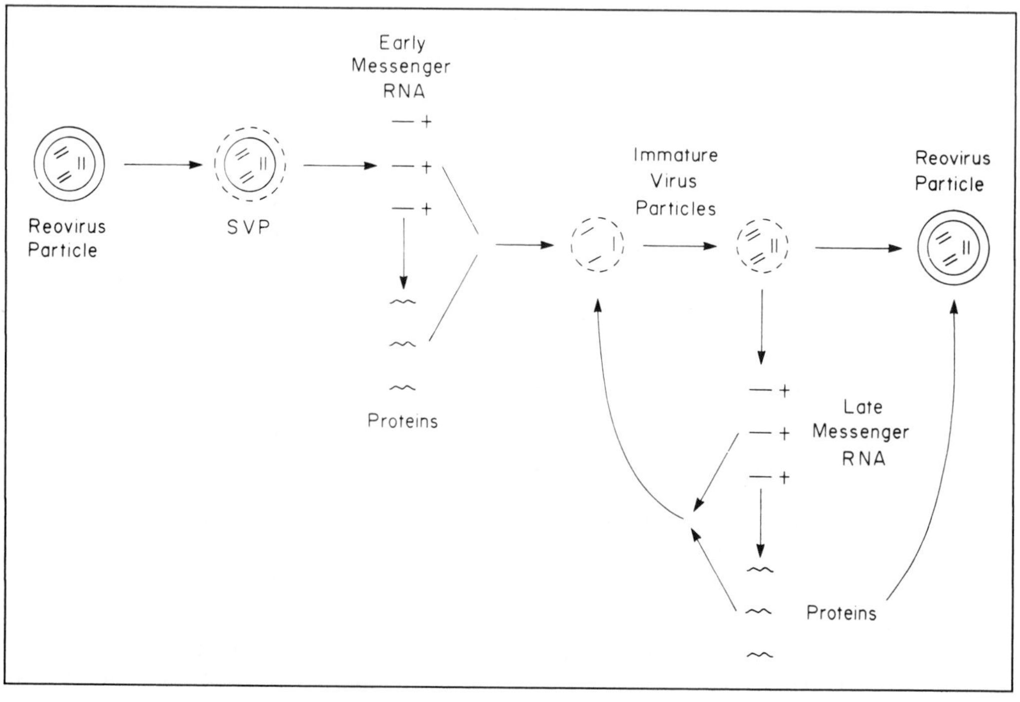

Fig. 55–52. The reovirus multiplication cycle. For details see text. The activation of transcription during the initial phase of the multiplication cycle involves the removal of two of the three proteins of the outer capsid shell as well as of a portion of the third. Activation of transcription does not involve activation of the transcriptase but removal of constraints that cause transcription in intact virus particles to abort when the nascent transcripts are no more than four nucleotides long.

particles (thereby causing reiterative abortive transcription of oligonucleotides no longer than four to six nucleotides long, many of which are trapped in reovirus particles). The products of transcription are capped but unspliced and not polyadenylated, plus-stranded RNA molecules. The parental double-stranded RNA genome segments never escape from the SVP, which persist in infected cells throughout the multiplication cycle.

The early phase of the reovirus multiplication cycle lasts for about 3 hours. At that time, the first plus-stranded RNA molecules, most of which are associated with the two nonstructural proteins μNS and σNS, begin to be transcribed once—and once only—into minus strands with which they remain associated, thereby giving rise to double-stranded (ds) RNA molecules, the progeny genome segments. Interestingly, although the existence of complexes that contain one of each of the ten plus strands cannot be demonstrated, the complexes that contain newly formed dsRNA molecules do contain them in equimolar amounts. Assortment of the 10 genome segments into units that contain one of each of them and dsRNA formation thus appear to be tightly linked; but the nature of the obviously highly specific RNA-RNA, RNA-protein, and protein-protein interactions that must be involved is not known. The immature progeny virus particles that contain the newly formed dsRNA molecules then transcribe more plus-stranded RNA molecules, which are translated into more proteins, thereby repeating the sequence of reactions. This is the *multiplication* step of the reovirus growth cycle. At the same time, these immature particles begin to shed the nonstructural proteins and associate first with core proteins and then with outer capsid shell proteins, which leads in stepwise fashion to the formation of mature virus particles.

One of the consequences of the type of genome segment assortment mechanism exhibited by reovirus is that genetic recombination through genome segment *reassortment* is highly efficient in cells simultaneously infected with different strains of reovirus. The same applies also to the other viruses with segmented genomes, that is, the orthomyxoviruses, the bunyaviruses, and the arenaviruses. This is discussed further in Chapter 57.

FURTHER READING

Books and Reviews

GENERAL

Challberg MD, Kelly TJ: Animal virus DNA replication. Annu Rev Biochem 58:671, 1958

Kelly TJ, Wold MS, Li J: Initiation of viral DNA replication. Adv Virus Res 34:1, 1988

Kielian M, Jungerwirth S: Mechanisms of enveloped virus entry into cells. Mol Biol Med 7:17, 1990

Krausslich H-G, Wimmer E: Viral proteinases. Annu Rev Biochem 57:701, 1988

Marsh M, Helenius A: Virus entry into animal cells. Adv Virus Res 37:107, 1989

Nevins JR: Mechanisms of viral-mediated trans-activation of transcription. Adv Virus Res 37:35, 1989

Pearse BMF: Clathrin and coated vesicles. EMBO J 6:2507, 1987

Stephens EB, Compans RW: Assembly of animal viruses at cellular membranes. Annu Rev Microbiol 42:489, 1988

White JM, Littman DR: Viral receptors of the immunoglobulin superfamily. Cell 56:725, 1989

PAPOVAVIRUSES

Borowiec JA, Dean FB, Bullock PA, Hurwitz J: Binding and unwinding—How T antigen engages the SV40 origin of DNA replication. Cell 60:181, 1990

Kelly TJ: SV40 DNA replication. J Biol Chem 263:17889, 1988

Lambert PF, Baker CC, Howley PM: The genetics of bovine papillomavirus type I. Annu Rev Genetics 22:235, 1988

Prives C: The replication functions of SV40 T antigen are regulated by phosphorylation. Cell 61:735, 1990

ADENOVIRUSES

Flint J, Shenk T: Adenovirus E1A protein: Paradigm viral transactivator. Annu Rev Genetics 23:141, 1989

Moran E, Mathews MB: Multiple functional domains in the adenovirus E1A gene. Cell 48:177, 1987

Nevins JR: Regulation of early adenovirus gene expression. Microbiol Rev 51:419, 1987

HERPESVIRUSES

Benson JD, Huang E-S: Recent progress in cytomegalovirus research. Virus Genes 303:263, 1990

Goding CR, O'Hare P: Herpes simplex virus Vmw65-octamer binding protein interaction: A paradigm for combinatorial control of transcription. Virology 173:363, 1989

Grose C: Glycoproteins encoded by varicella-zoster virus: Biosynthesis, phosphorylation and intracellular trafficking. Annu Rev Microbiol 44:59, 1990

Hammerschmidt W, Sugden B: DNA replication of herpesviruses during the lytic phase of their life cycles. Mol Biol Med 7:45, 1990

Knipe DM: The role of viral and cellular nucleoproteins in herpes simplex virus replication. Adv Virus Res 37:85, 1989

Mach M, Stamminger T, Jahn G: Human cytomegalovirus: Recent aspects from molecular biology. J Gen Virol 70:3117, 1989

McDougall JK (ed): Cytomegaloviruses. Curr Topics Microbiol Immunol, vol 154, 1990

Michael N, Spector D, Mavromara-Nazos P, et al: The DNA-binding properties of the major regulatory protein α4 of herpes simplex viruses. Science 239:1531, 1988

Ostrove JM: Molecular biology of varicella zoster. Adv Virus Res 38:45, 1990

Roizman B, Kenkins FJ, Kristie TM: Herpesviruses: Biology, gene regulation, latency, and genetic engineering. In Bercoff RP (eds): The Molecular Basis of Viral Replication. New York, Plenum, 1987

POXVIRUSES

Moss B: Regulation of vaccinia virus transcription. Annu Rev Biochem 59:661, 1990

Traktman P: The enzymology of poxvirus replication. Curr Topics Microbiol Immunol 163:93, 1990

Turner PC, Moyer RW: The molecular pathogenesis of poxviruses. Curr Topics Microbiol Immunol 163:125, 1990

HEPADNAVIRUSES

Howard CR: The biology of hepadnaviruses. J Gen Virol 67:1215, 1986

Neurath AR, Kent SB: The pre-S region of hepadnavirus envelope proteins. Adv Virus Res 34:65, 1988

PARVOVIRUSES

Berns KI: Parvovirus replication. Microbiol Rev 54:316, 1990

Berns KI, Labow MA: Parvovirus gene regulation. J Gen Virol 68:601, 1987

PICORNAVIRUSES

Jackson RJ, Howell MT, Kaminski A: The novel mechanism of initiation of picornavirus RNA translation. TIBS 15:477, 1990

Palmenberg AC: Proteolytic processing of picornaviral polyprotein. Annu Rev Microbiol 44:603, 1990

Racaniello VR: Poliovirus neurovirulence. Adv Virus Res 34:217, 1988

Stanway G: Structure, function and evolution of picornaviruses. J Gen Virol 71:2483, 1990

Tyrrell DAJ: Hot news on the common cold. Annu Rev Microbiol 42:35, 1988

TOGAVIRUSES

Vaux DJT, Helenius A, Mellman I: Spike-nucleocapsid interaction in Semliki Forest virus reconstructed using network antibodies. Nature 336:36, 1988

Wengler G: The mode of assembly of alphavirus cores implies a mechanism for the disassembly of the cores in the early stages of infection. Arch Virol 94:1, 1987

FLAVIVIRUSES

Hahn CS, Galler R, Rice CC: Flavivirus genome organization, expression, and replication. Annu Rev Microbiol 44:649, 1990

CORONAVIRUSES

Lai MM-C: Coronavirus. Organization, replication and expression of genome. Annu Rev Microbiol 44:303, 1990

Spaan W, Cavanagh D, Horzinek MC: Coronaviruses: Structure and genome expression. J Gen Virol 69:2939, 1988

RHABDOVIRUSES

Banerjee AK: Transcription and replication of rhabdoviruses. Microbiol Rev 51:66, 1987

Banerjee AK: The transcription complex of vesicular stomatitis virus. Cell 48:363, 1987

Banejee AK, Chattopadhyay D: Structure and function of the RNA polymerase of vesicular stomatitis virus. Adv Virus Res 38:99, 1990

PARAMYXOVIRUSES

Morrison TG: Structure, function, and intracellular processing of paramyxovirus membrane proteins. Virus Res 10:113, 1988

Vainionpää R, Marusyk R, Salmi A: The paramyxoviridae: Aspects of molecular structure, pathogenesis, and immunity. Adv Virus Res 37:211, 1989

ORTHOMYXOVIRUSES

Klenk H-D, Rott R: The molecular biology of influenza virus pathogenicity. Adv Virus Res 34:247, 1988

Nayak DP, Jabbar MA: Structural domains and organizational conformation involved in the sorting and transport of influenza virus transmembrane proteins. Annu Rev Microbiol 43:465, 1989

BUNYAVIRUSES

Elliott RM: Molecular biology of the Bunyaviridae. J Gen Virol 71:501, 1990

ARENAVIRUSES

Bishop DHL: Ambisense RNA genomes of arenaviruses and phleboviruses. Adv Virus Res 31:1, 1986

REOVIRUSES

Bellany AR, Both GW: Molecular biology of rotaviruses. Adv Virus Res 38:1, 1990

Emmons RW: Ecology of Colorado tick fever. Annu Rev Microbiol 42:49, 1988

Estes MK, Cohen J: Rotavirus gene structure and function. Microbiol Rev 53:410, 1989

HEPATITIS DELTA VIRUS

Taylor JM: Hepatitis delta virus: *cis* and *trans* functions required for replication. Cell 61:371, 1990

Selected Papers

GENERAL

Doxsey SJ, Brodsky FM, Blank GS, Helenius A: Inhibition of endocytosis by anti-clathrin antibodies. Cell 50:453, 1987

PAPOVAVIRUSES

Borowiec JA, Hurwitz J: Localized melting and structural changes in the SV40 origin of replication induced by T-antigen. EMBO J 7:3149, 1988

DeLucia AL, Deb S, Partin K, Tegtmeyer P: Functional interactions of the simian virus 40 core origin of replication with flanking regulatory sequences. J Virol 57:138, 1986

Mastrangelo IA, Hough PVC, Wall JS, et al: ATP-dependent assembly of double hexamers of SV40 T antigen at the viral origin of DNA replication. Nature 338:658, 1989

Pallas DC, Morgan W, Roberts TM: The cellular proteins which can associate specifically with polyomavirus middle T antigen in human 293 cells include the major human 70-kilodalton heat shock proteins. J Virol 63:4533, 1989

Scheffner M, Knippers R, Stahl H: RNA unwinding activity of SV40 large T antigen. Cell 57:955, 1989

ADENOVIRUSES

Gooding LR, Elmore LW, Tollefson AE, et al: A 14,700 MW protein from the E3 region of adenovirus inhibits cytolysis by tumor necrosis factor. Cell 53:341, 1988

Jefferies WA, Burgert H-G: E3/19K from adenovirus 2 is an immunosubversive protein that binds to a structural motif regulating the intracellular transport of major histocompatibility complex class I proteins. J Exp Med 172:1653, 1990

Katze MG, DeCorato D, Safer B, et al: Adenovirus VAI RNA complexes with the 68,000 M_r protein kinase to regulate its autophosphorylation and activity. EMBO J 6:689, 1987

Kenny MK, Hurwitz J: Initiation of adenovirus DNA replication: Structural requirements using synthetic oligonucleotide adenovirus templates. J Biol Chem 263:9809, 1988

Mak I, Mak S: Separate regions of an adenovirus E1B protein critical for different biological functions. Virology 176:553, 1990

Maran A, Mathews MB: Characterization of the double-stranded RNA implicated in the inhibition of protein synthesis in cells infected with a mutant adenovirus defective for VA RNA_I. Virology 164:106, 1988

Mellits KH, Kostura M, Mathews MB: Interaction of adenovirus VA RNA_I with the protein kinase DAI: Nonequivalence of binding and function. Cell 61:843, 1990

Neill SD, Hemstrom C, Virtanen A, Nevins JR: An adenovirus E4 gene product trans-activates *E2* transcription and stimulates stable E2F binding through a direct association with E2F. Proc Natl Acad Sci USA 87:2008, 1990

Svensson C, Akusjärvi G: A novel effect of adenovirus VA RNA_I on cytoplasmic mRNA abundance. Virology 174:613, 1990

Webster A, Russell WC, Kemp GD: Characterization of the adenovirus proteinase: Development and use of a specific peptide assay. J Gen Virol 70:3215, 1989

Zhang X, Bellett AJ, Hla RT, et al: Adneovirus type 5 E3 gene products interfere with the expression of the cytolytic T cell immunodominant E1a antigen. Virology 179:199, 1990

HERPESVIRUSES

Barker DE, Roizman B: Identification of three genes nonessential for growth in cell culture near the right terminus of the unique sequences of long component of herpes simplex virus 1. Virology 177:684, 1990

Cai W, Gu B, Person S: Role of glycoprotein B of herpes simplex virus type 1 in viral entry and cell fusion. J Virol 62:2596, 1988

Crute JJ, Tsurumi T, Zhu L, et al: Herpes simplex virus 1 helicase-primase: A complex of three herpes-encoded gene products. Proc Natl Acad Sci USA 86:2186, 1989

Kaner RJ, Baird A, Mansukhani A, et al: Fibroblast growth factor receptor is a portal of cellular entry for herpes simplex virus type 1. Science 248:1410, 1990

Mavromara-Nazos P, Roizman B: Delineation of regulatory domains of early (β) and late (γ2) genes by construction of chimeric genes expressed in herpes simplex virus 1 genomes. Proc Natl Acad Sci USA 86:4071, 1989

McKnight JLC, Kristie TM, Roizman B: Binding of the virion protein mediating α gene induction in herpes simplex virus 1-infected cells to its *cis* site requires cellular proteins. Proc Natl Acad Sci USA 84:7061, 1987

Mettenleiter TC, Kern H, Rauh I: Isolation of a viable herpesvirus (pseudorabies virus) mutant specifically lacking all four known nonessential glycoproteins. Virology 179:498, 1990

Rice RE, Knipe DM: Genetic evidence for two distinct transactivation functions of the herpes simplex virus α protein ICP27. J Virol 64:1704, 1990

Sekulovich RE, Leary K, Sandri-Goldin RM: The herpes simplex virus type 1 α protein ICP27 can act as a *trans*-repressor or a *trans*-activator in combination with ICP4 and ICP0. J Virol 62:4510, 1988

Weber PC, Levine M, Glorioso JC: Rapid identification of nonessential genes of herpes simplex virus type 1 by Tn5 mutagenesis. Science 236:576, 1987

CYTOMEGALOVIRUSES (CMV)

Adlish JD, Lahijani RS, St Jeor SC: Identification of a putative cell receptor for human cytomegalovirus. Virology 176:337, 1990

Pari GS, St Jeor SC: Human cytomegalovirus major immediate early gene product can induce SV40 DNA replication in human embryonic lung cells. Virology 179:785, 1990

HUMAN HERPESVIRUS 6 (HSV 6)

Di Luca D, Katsafanas G, Schirmer E, et al: The replication of viral and cellular DNA in human herpesvirus 6-infected cells. Virology 175:199, 1990

Ensoli B, Lusso P, Schachter F, et al: Human herpes virus-6 increases HIV-1 expression in co-infected T cells via nuclear factors binding to the HIV-1 enhancer. EMBO J 8:3019, 1989

Lawrence GL, Chee M, Craxton MA, et al: Human herpesvirus 6 is closely related to human cytomegalovirus. J Virol 64:287, 1990

Lusso P, Markham PD, Tschachler E, et al: In vitro cellular tropism of human B-lymphotropic virus (human herpesvirus-6). J Exp Med 167:1659, 1988

EPSTEIN-BARR VIRUS (EBV)

Fingeroth JD, Clabby ML, Strominger JD: Characterization of a T-lymphocyte Epstein-Barr virus/C3d receptor (CD21). J Virol 62:1442, 1988

VARICELLA-ZOSTER VIRUS (VZV)

Davison AJ, Taylor P: Genetic relations between varicella-zoster virus and Epstein-Barr virus. J Gen Virol 68:1067, 1987

Vafai A, Murray RS, Wellish M, et al: Expression of varicella-zoster virus and herpes simplex virus in normal human trigeminal ganglia. Proc Natl Acad Sci USA 85:2362, 1988

POXVIRUSES

Baroudy BM, Venkatesan S, Moss, B: Incompletely base-paired flip-flop terminal loops link the two DNA strands of the vaccinia virus genome into one uninterrupted polynucleotide chain. Cell 28:315, 1982

Buller RML, Chakrabarti S, Cooper JA, et al: Deletion of the vaccinia virus growth factor gene reduces virus virulence. J Virol 62:866, 1988

Howard ST, Chan YS, Smith GL: Vaccinia virus homologues of the Shope fibroma virus inverted terminal repeat proteins and a discontinuous ORF related to the tumor necrosis factor receptor family. Virology 180:633, 1991

Jin D, Li Z, Jin Q, et al: Vaccinia virus hemagglutinin: A novel member of the immunoglobulin superfamily. J Exp Med 170:571, 1989

Keck JG, Baldick CJ Jr, Moss B: Role of DNA replication in vaccinia virus gene expression: A naked template is required for transcription of three late *trans*-activator genes. Cell 61:801, 1990

Merchlinsky M: Resolution of poxvirus telomeres: Processing of vaccinia virus concatemer junctions by conservative strand exchange. J Virol 64:3437, 1990

Palumbo GJ, Pickup DJ, Fredrickson TN, et al: Inhibition of an inflammatory response is mediated by a 38-kDa protein of cowpox virus. Virology 172:262, 1989

Patel DD, Pickup DJ: Messenger RNAs of a strongly expressed late gene of cowpox virus contain 5′-terminal poly(A) sequences. EMBO J 6:3787, 1987

Perkus ME, Goebel SJ, Davis SW, et al: Deletion of 55 open reading frames from the termini of vaccinia virus. Virology 180:106, 1991

Perkus ME, Goebel S, Davis S, et al: Vaccinia virus host range genes. Virology 179:276, 1990

Pickup DJ, Ink BS, Hu W, et al: Hemorrhage in lesions caused by cowpox virus is induced by a viral protein that is related to plasma protein inhibitors of serine proteases. Proc Natl Acad Sci USA 83:7698, 1986

Pickup DJ, Ink BS, Parsons BL, et al: Spontaneous deletions and duplications of sequences in the genome of cowpox virus. Proc Natl Acad Sci USA 81:6817, 1984

HEPADNAVIRUSES

Levrero M, Balsano C, Natoli G, et al: Hepatitis B virus X protein transactivates the long terminal repeats of human immunodeficiency virus types 1 and 2. J Virol 64:3082, 1990

Miller RH: Close evolutionary relatedness of the hepatitis B virus and murine leukemia virus polymerase gene sequences. Virology 164:147, 1988

Salfeld J, Pfaff E, Noah M, Schaller H: Antigenic determinants and functional domains in core antigen and e antigen from hepatitis B virus. J Virol 63:798, 1989

Tokino T, Fukushige S, Nakamura T, et al: Chromosomal translocation and inverted duplication associated with integrated hepatitis B virus in hepatocellular carcinomas. J Virol 61:3848, 1987

Tur-Kaspa R, Shaul Y, Moore DD, et al: The glucocorticoid receptor recognizes a specific nucleotide sequence in hepatitis B virus DNA causing increased activity of the HBV enhancer. Virology 167:630, 1988

Yokosuka O, Omata M, Ito Y: Expression of pre-S1, pre-S2 and C proteins in duck hepatitis B virus infection. Virology 167:82, 1988

PARVOVIRUSES

Kotin RM, Berns KI: Organization of adeno-associated virus DNA in latently infected Detroit 6 cells. Virology 170:460, 1989

Kotin RM, Siniscalco M, Samulski RJ, et al: Site-specific integration by adeno-associated virus. Proc Natl Acad Sci USA 87:2211, 1990

Schlehofer JR, Ehrbar M, Zur Hausen H: Vaccinia virus, herpes simplex virus, and carcinogens induce DNA amplification in a human cell line and support replication of a helpervirus-dependent parvovirus. Virology 152:110, 1986

Yakobson B, Koch T, Winocour E: Replication of adeno-associated virus in synchronized cells without the addition of a helper virus. J Virol 61:972, 1987

PICORNAVIRUSES

Greve JM, Davis G, Meyer AM, et al: The major human rhinovirus receptor is ICAM-1. Cell 56:839, 1989

Mendelsohn CL, Wimmer E, Racaniello VR: Cellular receptor for poliovirus: Molecular cloning, nucleotide sequence, and expression of a new member of the immunoglobulin superfamily. Cell 56:855, 1989

Nicklin MJH, Kräusslich HG, Toyoda H, et al: Poliovirus polypeptide precursors: Expression in vitro and processing by exogenous 3C and 2A proteinases. Proc Natl Acad Sci USA 84:4002, 1987

Pilipenko EV, Blinov VM, Romanova LI, et al: Conserved structural domains in the 5′-untranslated region of picornaviral genomes: An analysis of the segment controlling translation and neurovirulency. Virology 168:201, 1989

Skinner MA, Racaniello VR, Dunn G, et al: New model for the secondary structure of the 5′ non-coding RNA of poliovirus is supported by biochemical and genetic data that also show that RNA secondary structure is important in neurovirulence. J Mol Biol 207:379, 1989

Tobin GJ, Young DC, Flanegan JB: Self-catalyzed linkage of poliovirus terminal protein VPg to poliovirus RNA. Cell 59:511, 1989

Ypma-Wong MF, Dewalt PG, Johnson VH, et al: Protein 3CD is the major poliovirus proteinase responsible for cleavage of the P1 capsid precursor. Virology 165:265, 1988

TOGAVIRUSES

Ding M, Schlesinger MJ: Evidence that Sindbis virus NSP2 is an autoprotease which processes the virus nonstructural polyprotein. Virology 171:280, 1989

Hardy WR, Strauss JH: Processing the nonstructural polyproteins of Sindbis virus: Study of the kinetics in vivo by using monospecific antibodies. J Virol 62:998, 1988

Lobigs M, Garoff H: Fusion function of the Semliki Forest virus spike is activated by proteolytic cleavage of the envelope glycoprotein precursor p62. J Virol 64:1233, 1990

Mi S, Durbin R, Huang HV, et al: Association of the Sindbis virus RNA methyltransferase activity with the nonstructural protein nsP1. Virology 170:385, 1989

Peränen J, Takkinen K, Kalkkinen N, Kääriäinen. Semliki Forest virus–specific non-structural protein nsP3 is a phosphoprotein. J Gen Virol 69:2165, 1988

Shirako Y, Strauss JH: Cleavage between nsP1 and nsP2 initiates the processing pathway of Sindbis virus nonstructural polyprotein P123. Virology 177:54, 1990

FLAVIVIRUSES

Chambers TJ, McCourt DW, Rice CM: Production of yellow fever virus proteins in infected cells: Identification of discrete polyprotein species and analysis of cleavage kinetics using region-specific polyclonal antisera. Virology 177:159, 1990

Chambers TJ, Weir RC, Grakoui A, et al: Evidence that the N-terminal domain of nonstructural protein NS3 from yellow fever virus is a serine protease responsible for site-specific cleavages in the viral polyprotein. Proc Natl Acad Sci USA 87:8898, 1990

Hase T, Summers PL, Eckels KH, Baze WB: An electron and immunoelectron microscopic study of dengue-2 virus infection of cultured mosquito cells: Maturation events. Arch Virol 92:273, 1987

Nowak T, Färber PM, Wengler G, Wengler G: Analyses of the terminal sequences of West Nile virus structural proteins and of the in vitro translation of these proteins allow the proposal of a complete scheme of the proteolytic cleavages involved in their synthesis. Virology 169:365, 1989

Rico-Hesse R: Molecular evolution and distribution of dengue viruses type 1 and 2 in nature. Virology 174:479, 1990

CORONAVIRUSES

Brierley I, Digard P, Inglis SC: Characterization of an efficient coronavirus ribosomal frameshifting signal: Requirement for an RNA pseudoknot. Cell 57:537, 1989

Lee H-J, Shieh C-K, Gorbalenya AE, et al: The complete sequence (22 kilobases) of murine coronavirus gene 1 encoding the putative proteases and RNA polymerase. Virology 180:567, 1991

Makino S, Stohlman SA, Lai MMC: Leader sequences of murine coronavirus mRNAs can be freely reassorted: Evidence for the role of free leader RNA in transcription. Proc Natl Acad Sci USA 83:4204, 1986

Schultze B, Wahn K, Klenk H-D, Herrler G: Isolated he-protein from hemagglutinating encephalomyelitis virus and bovine coronavirus has receptor-destroying and receptor-binding activity. Virology 180:221, 1991

RHABDOVIRUSES

Chattopadhyay D, Banerjee AK: Phosphorylation within a specific domain of the phosphoprotein of vesicular stomatitis virus regulates transcription in vitro. Cell 49:407, 1987

Hercyk N, Horikami SM, Moyer SA: The vesicular stomatitis virus L protein possesses the mRNA methyltransferase activities. Virology 163:222, 1988

Howard M, Wertz G: Vesicular stomatitis virus RNA replication: A role for the NS protein. J Gen Virol 70:2683, 1989

Yazaki K, Sano T, Okamoto T, et al: Intracellular vesicular stomatitis virus nucleocapsids and virions visualized by surface spreading. J Virol Methods 23:1, 1989

PARAMYXOVIRUSES

Blumberg BM, Crowley JC, Silverman JI, et al: Measles virus L protein evidences elements of ancestral RNA polymerase. Virology 164:487, 1988

Bohn W, Rutter G, Hohenberg H, et al: Involvement of actin filaments in budding of measles virus: Studies on cytoskeletons of infected cells. Virology 149:91, 1986

Curran J, Kolakofsky D: Ribosomal initiation from an ACG codon in the Sendai virus P/C mRNA. EMBO J 7:245, 1988

Hsu M-C, Scheid A, Choppin PW: Protease activation mutants of Sendai virus: Sequence analysis of the mRNA of the fusion protein (F) gene and direct identification of the cleavage-activation site. Virology 156:84, 1987

Kawano M, Bando H, Yuasa T, et al: Sequence determination of the hemagglutinin-neuraminidase (HN) gene of human parainfluenza type 2 virus and the construction of a phylogenetic tree for HN proteins of all the paramyxoviruses that are infectious to humans. Virology 174:308, 1990

Ryan KW, Morgan EM, Portner A: Two noncontinguous regions of Sendai virus P protein combine to form a single nucleocapsid binding domain. Virology 180:126, 1991

Vidal S, Kolakofsky D: Modified model for the switch from Sendai virus transcription to replication. J Virol 63:1951, 1989

Vidal S, Curran J, Kolakofsky D: A stuttering model for paramyxovirus P mRNA editing. EMBO J 9:2017, 1990

ORTHOMYXOVIRUSES

Copeland CS, Zimmer K-P, Wagner KR, et al: Folding, trimerization, and transport are sequential events in the biogenesis of influenza virus hemagglutinin. Cell 53:197, 1988

Hsu M-T, Parvin JD, Gupta S, et al: Genomic RNAs of influenza viruses are held in a circular conformation in virions and in infected cells by a terminal panhandle. Proc Natl Acad Sci USA 84:8140, 1987

Katze MG, Tomita J, Black T, et al: Influenza virus regulates protein synthesis during infection by repressing autophosphorylation and

activity of the cellular 68,000-M_r protein kinase. J Virol 62:3710, 1988
Kida H, Shortridge KF, Webster RG: Origin of the hemagglutinin gene of H3N2 influenza viruses from pigs in China. Virology 161:160, 1987
Raymond FL, Caton AJ, Cox NJ, et al: The antigenicity and evolution of influenza H1 hemagglutinin, from 1950–1957 and 1977–1983: Two pathways from one gene. Virology 148:275, 1986
Skorko R, Summers DF, Galarza JM: Influenza A virus in vitro transcription: Roles of NS_1 and NP proteins in regulating RNA synthesis. Virology 180:668, 1991
Sugrue RJ, Hay AJ: Structural characteristics of the M2 protein of influenza A viruses: Evidence that it forms a tetrameric channel. Virology 180:617, 1991
Weis W, Brown JH, Cusack S, et al: Structure of the influenza virus haemagglutinin complexed with its receptor, sialic acid. Nature 333:426, 1988
Yamashita M, Krystal M, Palese P: Comparison of the three large polymerase proteins of influenza A, B, and C viruses. Virology 171:458, 1989

BUNYAVIRUSES

Anderson GW Jr, Smith JF: Immunoelectron microscopy of Rift Valley fever viral morphogenesis in primary rat hepatocytes. Virology 161:91, 1987
Giorgi C, Accardi L, Nicoletti L, et al: Sequences and coding strategies of the S RNAs of Toscana and Rift Valley fever viruses compared to those of Punta Toro, Sicilian sandfly fever, and Uukuniemi viruses. Virology 180:738, 1991
Raju R, Kolakofsky D: The ends of La Crosse virus geome and antigenome RNAs within nucleocapsids are base paired. J Virol 63:122, 1989
Suzich JA, Kakach LT, Collett MS: Expression strategy of a phlebovirus: Biogenesis of proteins from the Rift Valley fever virus M segment. J Virol 64:1549, 1990

HEPATITIS DELTA VIRUS (HDV)

Chang M-F, Baker SC, Soe LH, et al: Human hepatitis delta antigen is a nuclear phosphoprotein with RNA-binding activity. J Virol 62:2403, 1988
Hsieh S-Y, Chao M, Coates L, Taylor J: Hepatitis delta virus genome replication: A polyadenylated mRNA for delta antigen. J Virol 64:3192, 1990
Kuo MY-P, Chao M, Taylor J: Initiation of replication of the human hepatitis delta virus genome from cloned DNA: Role of delta antigen. J Virol 63:1945, 1989
Luo G, Chao M, Hsieh S-Y, et al: A specific base transition occurs on replicating hepatitis delta virus RNA. J Virol 64:1021, 1990
Perrotta AT, Been MD: The self-cleaving domain from the genomic RNA of hepatitis delta virus: Sequence requirements and the effects of denaturant. Nucleic Acids Res 18:6821, 1990
Sharmeen L, Kuo MY-P, Taylor J: Self-ligating RNA sequences on the antigenome of human hepatitis delta virus. J Virol 63:1428, 1989
Weiner AJ, Choo Q-L, Wang K-S, et al: A single antigenomic open reading frame of the hepatitis delta virus encodes the epitope(s) of both hepatitis delta antigen polypeptides p24δ and p27δ. J Virol 62:594, 1988
Xia Y-P, Chang M-F, Wei D, et al: Heterogeneity of hepatitis delta antigen. Virology 178:331, 1990

HEPATITIS C VIRUS

Weiner AJ, Brauer MJ, Rosenblatt J, et al: Variable and hypervariable domains are found in the regions of HCV corresponding to the flavivirus envelope and NS1 proteins and the pestivirus envelope glycoproteins. Virology 180:842, 1991

REOVIRUS

Banerjea AC, Brechling KA, Ray CA, et al: High-level synthesis of biologically active reovirus protein σ1 in a mammalian expression vector system. Virology 167:601, 1988
Choi AHC, Paul RW, Lee PWK: Reovirus binds to multiple plasma membrane proteins of mouse L fibroblasts. Virology 178:316, 1990
Fraser RDB, Furlong DB, Trus BL, et al: Molecular structure of the cell-attachment protein of reovirus: correlation of computer-processed electron micrographs with sequence-based predictions. J Virol 64:2990, 1990
Furlong DB, Nibert ML, Fields BN: Sigma 1 protein of mammalian reoviruses extends from the surfaces of viral particles. J Virol 62:246, 1988
Nibert ML, Schiff LA, Fields BN: Mammalian reoviruses contain a myristoylated structural protein. J Virol 65:1960, 1991
Paul RW, Choi AHC, Lee PWK: The α-anomeric form of sialic acid is the minimal receptor determinant recognized by reovirus. Virology 172:382, 1989
Roner MR, Sutphin LA, Joklik WK: Reovirus RNA is infectious. Virology 179:845, 1990
Samal SK, El-Hussein A, Holbrook FR, et al: Mixed infection of *Culicoides variipennis* with bluetongue virus serotypes 10 and 17: Evidence for high frequency reassortment in the vector. J Gen Virol 68:2319, 1987
Wiener JR, Bartlett JA, Joklik WK: The sequences of reovirus serotype 3 genome segments M1 and M3 encoding the minor protein μ2 and the major nonstructural protein μNS, respectively. Virology 169:293, 1989

CHAPTER 56

Effect of Virus Infection on the Host Cell

The effect of viral infection on host cells is far more difficult to study in molecular terms than is the process of virus multiplication. Study of the multiplication process requires merely the ability to recognize and measure virus-specified macromolecules; study of the effect on host cells requires a detailed knowledge of the functioning of the normal cell. In fact, studies that have focused attention on the effect of viral infection on host cells have broadened our knowledge of the functioning of uninfected cells, and the acquisition of such knowledge has been one of the important spin-offs of the study of virus-cell interactions.

Whatever the reason that lytic viruses destroy their host cells, several causes can be ruled out. One is that virus synthesis creates an excessive demand for protein and nucleic acid precursors, so that competition causes a shortage of building blocks that prevents synthesis of host cell macromolecules. This is unlikely, because the amount of viral material that is synthesized rarely exceeds 10% of total host cell material and usually is less than 1%. Considerations of this nature also rule out the necessity for breakdown of host cell material in order to provide precursors for the synthesis of viral macromolecules.

Inasmuch as both nucleic acid and protein synthesis are absolutely dependent on the supply of energy, the largest virus yields would be expected in cells that are damaged least for the longest periods of time. Many highly lytic viruses, however, are very successful. This is because they take over the host cell's synthetic apparatus rapidly and multiply extensively in the brief period of time for which the apparatus continues to function.

Cytopathic Effects

The most easily detected effects of infection with lytic viruses are the cytopathic effects, which can be observed both macroscopically and microscopically. Plaque formation is caused by the cytopathic effect of viruses; viruses kill the cells in which they multiply, and plaques are the areas of killed cells. Both the light microscope and the electron microscope often reveal changes in a variety of cell organelles soon after infection. Frequently the nucleus is affected first, with pyknosis, changes in nucleolar structure, and margination of the chromatin. Changes in the cell membrane usually follow; cells gradually lose their ability to adhere to supporting surfaces and therefore round up and sometimes develop a strong tendency to fuse with one another (see below). Disruption of the cytoskeleton also often occurs, caused by depolymerization of one or more cytoskeletal fiber system(s). This is then often followed by the appearance, either in the nucleus or in the cytoplasm, of distinct spreading foci that generally are composed of fibrillar material. These are the classic inclusion bodies that have long been described by cytologists, and they represent the sites of virus-directed biosynthesis and morphogenesis. Finally, at about the time when structural viral protein synthesis proceeds at its maximum rate, necrotic and grossly degradative changes become noticeable. They may be attributed to at least three causes. First, by this time interference with host cell macromolecular biosynthesis generally is severe (see below). It is known that all host cell macromolecules turn over to a greater or lesser extent—that is, they are continually broken down and resynthesized by mechanisms that operate whether or not cells grow. Inhibition of resynthesis in the face of continuing breakdown clearly could lead to structural and functional failure. Second, plasma membrane function declines, probably because cell protein and lipid synthesis ceases and because patches of cell membrane proteins are replaced by virus-encoded ones. Certainly, permeability increases soon after infection, and before long loss of plasma membrane function results in failure to maintain the proper intracellular ionic environment and in diminished transport of essential nutrients into cells and of waste products out of them. Third, the membranes that line lysosomes also begin to fail, and as a result the degradative hydrolytic enzymes they contain begin to leak out into the cytoplasm, thereby exacerbating the effects caused by the other mechanisms.

The net result of cell necrosis is the release of those viruses that do not bud from the cell membrane. In general, the smaller the virus, the more readily is it released. Large viruses, such as poxviruses, often are retained in the ghosts of infected cells for considerable periods of time. In the body the situation may be different because damaged cells may become phagocytosed, thereby providing an additional mechanism for the dissemination of viral progeny.

In addition to these degenerative and necrotic changes that develop as virus multiplication progresses, some viruses cause cytopathic or cytotoxic changes very soon after infection. Most likely these early effects are caused by the structural viral proteins that are responsible for uncoating. These proteins are fusogenic and cause lysis of the clathrin-coated vesicles within which virus particles are transported into cells (Chap. 55); but they are also cytotoxic owing to their ability to fuse membranes. Examples of such proteins are the adenovirus penton/fiber protein, the surface tubule protein of vaccinia virus, and many glycoproteins of enveloped viruses, such as the G glycoprotein of vesicular stomatitis virus.

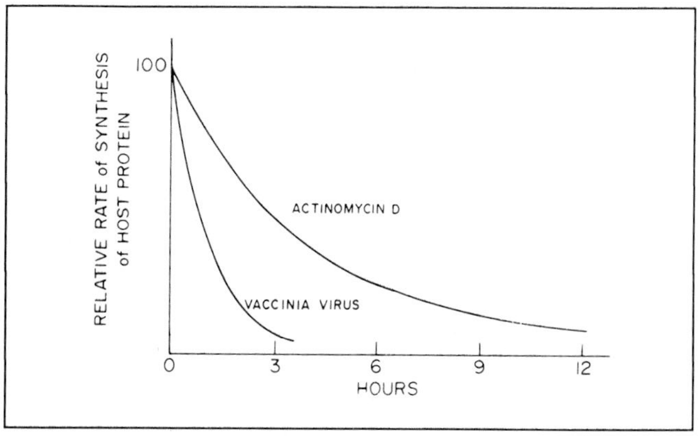

Fig. 56–1. Effect of infection with vaccinia virus, as well as of actinomycin D, on cellular protein synthesis in mouse L fibroblasts. Actinomycin D inhibits RNA transcription; therefore the decrease in the rate of protein synthesis in its presence reflects the stability of cellular messenger RNAs, whose average half-life is about 3 hours. Infection with vaccinia virus inhibits host protein synthesis much more rapidly. Presumably the infection either causes host messenger RNA to be inactivated, or it actively prevents host messenger RNA from being translated.

Inhibition of Host Macromolecular Biosynthesis

The induction of cytopathic effects early after infection may be intimately related to the more or less rapidly developing inhibition of host protein, DNA and RNA synthesis, which is a fundamentally important factor in the lytic virus-cell interaction.

Host protein synthesis is inhibited first. This effect is often missed if only the overall rate of protein synthesis is measured, because viral protein synthesis generally takes over as host protein synthesis declines. Inhibition of host protein synthesis then quickly causes inhibition of host DNA replication, which is known to depend on the activity of short-lived proteins. Host RNA synthesis also soon ceases, often not as a result of any direct effect on DNA-dependent RNA polymerases, RNA processing (splicing) or RNA transport—all of which could be, and indeed sometimes *are* targets where viral infection might inhibit—but because of changes in the physical state of the DNA (margination of chromatin, changes in nucleolar structure; see above) that prevent it from acting as a template for transcription. As a result, not only progressively less and less host cell messenger RNA is synthesized, but also the supply of new ribosomes is quickly interrupted. In fact, the only ribosomes that are usually available for protein synthesis during the virus multiplication cycle are those that are present in the cytoplasm at the time of infection.

The reasons why infection with viruses inhibits host protein synthesis have been studied extensively but are not well understood. Sometimes the reason may be that less and less host cell messenger RNA reaches the cytoplasm. It is clear, however, that in many viral infections the rate of host protein synthesis decreases far more rapidly than would be expected on the basis of messenger RNA present in the cytoplasm at the time of infection decaying at the normal rate; for example, infection with high multiplicities of vaccinia virus inhibits host protein synthesis by well over 90% within 2 hours (Fig. 56–1). This is not a *general* toxic effect on host cells, because viral proteins continue to be synthesized rapidly at the same time.

Different viruses employ different mechanisms for inhibiting host protein synthesis. Poxviruses and herpesviruses can cause this effect in the absence of new protein synthesis; that is, components of infecting virus particles must be responsible. It seems that this effect is caused primarily by increases in the rate of cellular messenger RNA degradation. More commonly, however, this is not the mechanism, because the continued existence of undiminished amounts of fully functional messenger RNA can often be demonstrated by its continuing ability to be translated efficiently in in vitro protein-synthesizing systems prepared from uninfected cells. In other words, shortly after infection mechanisms develop that actively prevent cellular messenger RNAs present in the cytoplasm at the time of infection from being translated. Among these mechanisms are the following. First, there is interference with the initiation of protein synthesis. For example, poliovirus infection causes cleavage of the 220 kDa component of the messenger RNA cap-binding complex (CBC or eIF-4F), which plays an essential role in the initiation of translation (Fig. 55–33); because poliovirus RNA is not capped and translation of it is initiated internally, its ability to be translated remains unaffected. Further, viral infection often activates a protein kinase that phosphorylates the α subunit of the protein synthesis initiation factor eIF2, thereby inactivating it and inhibiting the translation of host cell messenger RNAs, which is very dependent on the presence of eIF2.

Second, as pointed out above, the plasma cell membrane is often damaged soon after infection, and as a result the Na^+-K^+ gradient collapses, which causes the Na^+ concentration to rise and the K^+ concentration to fall. There is evidence that these changes inhibit the translation of host cell messenger RNAs more than that of viral messenger RNAs. Third, it has been suggested that viral messenger RNAs may, in general, be more efficient messenger RNAs than are host cell messenger RNAs; thus in vitro protein-synthesizing systems presented with mixtures of host and viral messenger RNAs often translate the latter preferentially. Finally, viral messenger RNAs are often translated almost exclusively simply because they soon outnumber host cell messenger RNA molecules; even if they were not translated preferentially, simple competition would cause host protein synthesis to be reduced.

Not only do viruses often inhibit host protein synthesis, but some viruses also actively degrade host proteins. Infection with poliovirus, for example, causes degradation not only of eIF-4F (see above) but also of several other proteins, including that of a transcription factor that is essential for ribosomal RNA synthesis, which ceases almost completely soon after infection with poliovirus.

Although the hypothesis that inhibition of host DNA and RNA synthesis is secondary to inhibition of host protein synthesis is probably correct for most virus infections, several exceptions have been reported. For example, there is some evidence that the vesicular stomatitis virus (VSV) leader RNA (p. 820) inhibits transcription by both RNA polymerase II and III, possibly in conjunction with a newly synthesized protein. Also, a component of parental poxvirus particles has been reported to inhibit host DNA synthesis; this appears to be a DNase specific for single-stranded DNA.

Changes in Regulation of Gene Expression

Viral infection may also affect the regulation of host genome expression. For example, the activity of several enzymes on the pathway of nucleic acid biosynthesis increases after infection with papovaviruses; infection with almost all viruses induces the synthesis of a new protein, interferon (Chap. 58). Thus cellular genes may be expressed in infected cells that are not expressed in uninfected cells.

The mechanisms responsible for this situation, insofar as they do not involve nonspecific effects attributable to gross cell damage, depend on whether expression of the genes that are turned on is regulated positively or negatively. If regulation is positive, the gene is under the control of a promoter to which transcription factors must be bound if it is to be expressed. Such factors may be limiting in uninfected cells. Several virus-encoded proteins, however, are transactive transcriptional activators of a variety of promoters, including cellular ones, and they may initiate or activate the expression of cellular genes. Examples of such proteins are the large T antigen of papovaviruses and the adenovirus E1A protein. If regulation of gene expression is negative, the promoter in question is active unless it is bound by a repressor, usually a protein. Inasmuch as most repressors are unstable (which is desirable because it permits rapid switching from the inactive to the active state), any interference with repressor protein synthesis, which may be a consequence of viral infection, could cause genes that are not expressed in uninfected cells to become expressed after infection. An example of this type of promoter is the interferon promoter.

Appearance of New Antigenic Determinants on the Cell Surface

Sooner or later after infection the outer cell membrane is modified. This manifests itself in a variety of ways; for example, cellular morphology changes, cells become more agglutinable by the lectin concanavalin A (Chap. 59), cell membrane permeability increases, and new antigenic determinants appear on the cell surface. When the infecting virus is an enveloped virus, these new determinants are likely to be viral envelope proteins that become incorporated into the cell membrane; however, new antigenic determinants also appear on the surfaces of cells that are infected with nonenveloped viruses. The presence of these determinants serves to alert the immune mechanism to the fact that the cells are infected and should be eliminated (Fig. 56–2).

Cell Fusion

Several viruses, particularly paramyxoviruses and herpesviruses, cause cells to fuse with one another, which results in the formation of giant syncytia, masses of cytoplasm bounded by one membrane and containing hundreds and even thousands of nuclei. Fusion seems to be caused by changes induced

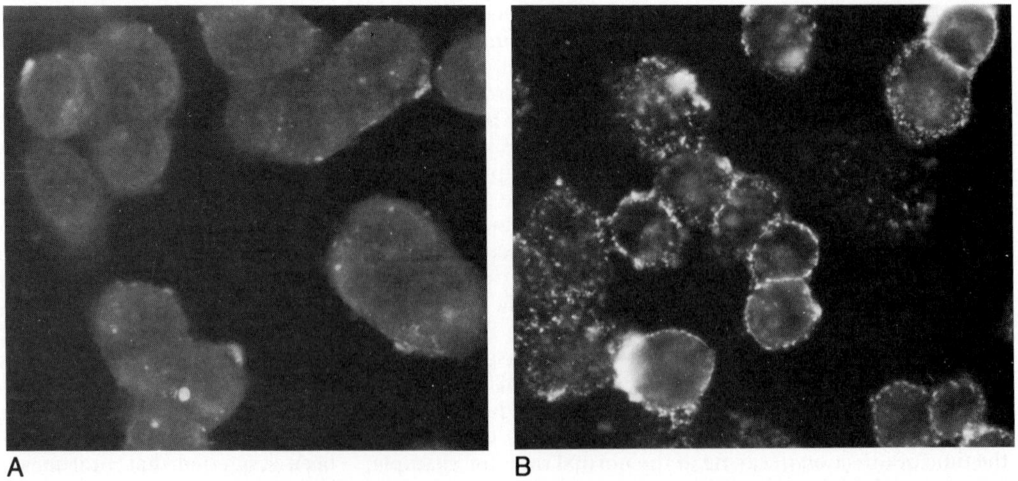

Fig. 56–2. Virus-specified surface antigen on HeLa cells infected with vaccinia virus. **A.** Uninfected cells. **B.** Cells infected for 8 hours. The cells were stained with rabbit antiserum to rabbit cells infected with vaccinia virus. *(Courtesy of Dr. Yoshiaki Ueda.)*

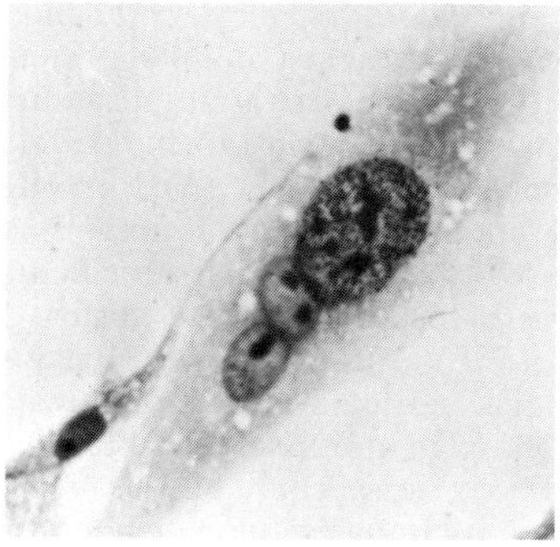

Fig. 56–3. Cell fusion induced by UV-inactivated Sendai virus. Three chick embryo fibroblasts have fused to yield the heterokaryon shown here, which contains three nuclei. The two small ones are normal chick nuclei; the large one is from a chick transformed with Rous sarcoma virus. × 400. *(From Svoboda and Dourmashkin: J Gen Virol 4:523, 1969.)*

in cell membranes by certain glycoproteins in viral envelopes (glycoproteins gB and gD in herpesvirus envelopes and the F spike glycoprotein of paramyxoviruses [p. 823]). Fusion can be induced not only among identical but also among different cells. The products of fusion are either heterokaryons—cells that contain several nuclei of different types (Fig. 56–3)—or hybrid cells that contain the fused nuclei of the parents. Hybrid cells are frequently viable and have become valuable tools for studies in somatic cell genetics. They are produced by fusing mixtures of the cells to be hybridized with inactivated Sendai virus or by treating them with polyethylene glycol and then cloning them. Hybrid cells are particularly useful for determining the chromosomal location of specific genes because as they multiply, they lose chromosomes, and one can correlate the loss of a particular gene function with the loss of a specific chromosome. In recent years many human genes have been assigned to chromosomes in this manner, using human-mouse hybrid cells that lose human chromosomes. The genetic factors that control susceptibility to viral infection and the expression of tumorigenicity can also be studied with the aid of somatic cell hybrids. In addition, the technique has become important in immunology for the production of hybridomas that produce monoclonal antibodies.

The Concept of Permissiveness

Viruses do not grow equally well in all cells of the body. In fact, any particular virus usually can grow in only very few types of cells, which is fortunate, because otherwise viral infections would have disastrous consequences. For example, influenza viruses grow only in cells lining the respiratory tract, rotaviruses in cells lining the intestinal tract, and so on. Cells in which a particular virus can multiply to high titer are said to be permissive for that virus; cells in which it cannot grow are said to be nonpermissive. In between there is a spectrum of degrees of permissiveness. In the extreme case, in which no virus is formed, the result is abortive infection (see below); if some virus is formed but the yields are low, persistent infections may result (see below).

There are many reasons why viruses can multiply to high titer in some cells and only minimally or not at all in others. Often, no doubt, the reason for nonpermissiveness is the fact that the cells in question lack the particular virus receptor on their surface; however, there are also other reasons that are not as well understood. The important points to remember are, first, the fact that cellular permissiveness can be altered, examples of which are discussed below, and, second, the fact that cellular permissiveness is not correlated with the severity of cytopathic effects; for viral infections may cause marked cytopathic effects, but virus ability to multiply may be limited, and virus may be able to grow to high titer while causing minimal cytopathic effects.

Abortive Infections

Most of the changes described so far relate to the lytic multiplication cycle under conditions of productive infection, that is, when a virus multiplies to high titer in permissive cells. Viruses, however, can also infect cells that are not fully permissive and even cells that are nonpermissive. Often, in such cells, viruses cannot multiply because some essential step of the multiplication cycle cannot proceed. Examples of this type are the abortive infection of HeLa cells by influenza virus, of dog kidney cells by herpes simplex virus, of pig kidney cells by certain mutants of rabbitpox virus, of monkey cells by human adenovirus, and many others. The infection of permissive cells in the presence of antiviral agents (Chap. 58) is also abortive. In such cases the viral genome usually begins to express itself, the alterations in host cells that were described above are likely to occur, and the cells die.

Persistent Infections

As a rule the infection of permissive cells with lytic viruses leads to productive infection and cell death. Occasionally, however, cell cultures are observed that, while multiplying more or less normally, nevertheless contain and release significant amounts of virus. Such cultures are said to be persistently infected. Stable relationships between cell growth and virus multiplication, which occur not only in vitro but also in vivo, are of two kinds.

The first involves infection by viruses that cause a minimum of the type of cell damage discussed above. A good example is provided by the paramyxovirus SV5. This virus interacts with many cells by means of a lytic, cytocidal interaction. When it infects monkey kidney cells, however, it causes practically no cell damage and permits the infected cells to grow freely while multiplying itself. In such cultures, all cells multiply, all cells are infected, and all cells produce virus. Infection of new cells plays no role in this situation; consequently, this type of infection cannot be cured by the addition of neutralizing antibody.

The second situation is quite different. Here the virus-cell interaction is lytic—that is, the cells that are infected die—but the extent of virus multiplication is limited, so that the yield is small. In addition, several factors reduce the probability of reinfection, so that the proportion of infected cells in the cell population is kept small and constant. The factors that induce and maintain this type of persistent infection are as follows. First, this type of infection occurs most readily in cells that are almost, but not quite, nonpermissive and that, therefore, produce only small amounts of virus. Second, it occurs in situations in which factors in the medium, such as antibody or interferon, prevent the major portion of released progeny virus from infecting new cells. The role of small amounts of interferon is sometimes not readily apparent but becomes obvious if antibody against interferon is added, when persistent infections become lytic infections. Third, many of the virus strains that have been isolated from persistently infected cells and animals are less virulent, less cytopathic, and interestingly, temperature-sensitive with respect to their ability to multiply. This has been found for foot-and-mouth disease virus, coxsackievirus, Sindbis virus and western equine encephalomyelitis (WEE) virus, influenza virus, Newcastle disease virus, Sendai virus, mumps and measles virus, VSV and herpesvirus, and others.

The fact that virus strains recovered from persistently infected cells are frequently temperature sensitive has aroused considerable interest, and, indeed, persistent virus infection can be established readily by infecting cells with temperature-sensitive mutants. The important fact, however, is not that virus strains present in persistently infected cells are temperature sensitive but rather that (1) they are less cytopathic and infectious than wild-type virus because they synthesize less messenger RNA and protein and sometimes possess a lower affinity for cell receptors and that (2) they interfere with the growth of wild-type virus at permissive, as well as at nonpermissive, temperatures by a mechanism that appears to involve competition between mutant and wild-type viral proteins.

Finally, persistently infected cells often contain not only infectious virus but also deletion mutants, that is, virus particles that lack a portion of their genome (Chap. 57). These virus particles, which are incapable of multiplying on their own, are nevertheless capable of interfering with the multiplication of infectious virus and are therefore known as defective interfering (DI) particles. Their presence dampens the effect of viral infection; that is, it reduces both cell damage and the amount of infectious virus that is produced. Their role in initiating and maintaining persistent infection is readily demonstrated by inoculating them into animals together with wild-type virus, when an otherwise severe disease is often converted to a slowly progressing persistent infection. Similarly, if cultured cells are infected with wild-type virus together with DI particles, persistent infections are readily established. The role of DI particles in persistent and chronic infections has now been demonstrated for influenza virus, Sendai virus, Newcastle disease virus (NDV), and measles, lymphocytic choriomeningitis virus, Sindbis virus, Semliki Forest virus, WEE and rubella, as well as vesicular stomatitis virus. The nature of the deletions in the DI particles of various viruses and the nature of the mechanisms that cause such particles to inhibit the multiplication of wild-type virus are discussed in Chapter 57.

In summary, the replacement of virulent by less virulent virus strains and the inhibition of virus multiplication by DI particles are major factors in the establishment and maintenance of persistent virus infection. Persistent infections of this type are important in the intact organism, where the presence of antiviral antibody and interferon in amounts too low to eliminate virus may provide conditions favorable for low-level persistent infections. It should be noted that this kind of persistent infection can be cured by the addition of large amounts of neutralizing antibody.

Latency

We have so far considered only persistently infected cells in which some infectious virus is formed. There are, however, persistently infected cells in which no infectious virus is formed because in them the multiplication cycle is completely arrested at some stage. In some cases, such arrest is permanent; but in others it is not, because under the influence of appropriate and as yet poorly understood stimuli, the virus multiplication cycle may be resumed after a period that may last from several weeks to many years, and infectious virus may then be formed and released. This is the phenomenon of latency, which is a central feature of infection by several herpesviruses, particularly HSV types 1 and 2, varicella-zoster virus, and Epstein-Barr virus (EBV). In the case of HSV, infecting virus quickly enters neurones of sensory ganglia, particularly the trigeminal ganglia, as well as sympathetic ganglia, and multiplies briefly; and then latency develops. The precise state of the viral genome in latently infected cells is not known; there is evidence that it is in the form of about 20 extrachromosomal plasmidlike circular viral genomes per cell. A great deal of work has been done to determine whether these genomes express themselves. Several species of latency-associated transcripts are usually detected, but the significance of their presence for the establishment or maintenance of the latent state has not been established. Under certain poorly defined conditions, transcription can be reactivated, virus, or some subviral form of it, is formed, and the virus then spreads to the epithelium where additional virus replication occurs and the virus is shed. These areas in humans are, most commonly, the lip (fever blisters) for HSV-1 and the genitalia for HSV-2. Other examples of latent infections are those by varicella-zoster virus (sensory ganglia), cytomegalovirus (CMV) (mononuclear cells), and EBV (B lymphocytes and nasopharyngeal cells). Adeno-associated virus can also enter a latent stage by integrating its DNA into that of host cells (which herpesviruses do not do).

Inapparent Infections

Whereas persistent infections of the type described above can usually be recognized because infectious virus *is* produced, there are indications that viruses often initiate infections in which multiplication and gene expression occur at so low a level that their presence can only be detected by very special measures. For example, the papovavirus BKV infects most individuals by adolescence and sets up minute and inapparent foci of infection in kidneys and in cells lining the urinary tract; infection only becomes apparent if the individual becomes immunocompromised, when the BKV begins to multiply and is shed. Other examples are provided by adenovirus, which can often be isolated from apparently normal adenoviral tissue, and the activation of viruses that cause the common cold syndrome in persons after exposure to cold temperatures. In fact, it is thought by some that the reason why resistance to viruses that cause diseases during childhood is retained throughout life is that the viruses persist in inapparent foci of infection where they constantly shed minute amounts of antigen.

Not surprisingly, latent and apparent or inapparent persistent infections may cause chronic and sometimes also progressive disease. Examples of the latter are subacute sclerosing panencephalitis (SSPE), an infection of the central nervous system caused by measles virus, and progressive multifocal leukoencephalopathy (PML), caused by the papovaviruses JCV and, more rarely, SV40. Both are slow degenerative diseases of the central nervous system caused by viral infections that persist but yield essentially no infectious virus. The reason, in the case of SSPE, is interesting. SSPE is one of the most thoroughly studied persistent infections of the human central nervous system. It develops 5 to 10 years after acute measles virus infections and invariably leads to death after months or years, and it is accompanied by a hyperimmune response in the absence of infectious virus production. The reason is hypermutation in the three measles virus envelope genes, particularly the M gene, which results in the formation of prematurely terminated, unstable, nonfunctional proteins. By contrast, the L, N, and P genes are not affected, and therefore large amounts of nucleocapsids accumulate in infected cells. The reason for the striking hypermutation of the M, H, and F genes, which over limited sequence segments is "biased"—that is, up to one quarter of the Us or As are converted to Cs or Gs, respectively—is not known.

Modification of Cellular Permissiveness

Cellular permissiveness is not invariate, but it can be modified. For example, the ability of HSV to grow in neuroblastoma cells is increased more than 1000-fold if the cells are treated with sodium butyrate. No doubt other substances that may be produced in the body could have a similar effect. Occasionally infection with one virus alters to an amazing extent the ability of other, unrelated, viruses to multiply. For example, adeno-associated virus (AAV) can multiply only in cells infected with adenovirus; SV40 enables human adenovirus to grow in monkey cells; and poxviruses, such as vaccinia and fibroma virus, enable VSV to multiply in rabbit cells. The helper function usually appears to involve translation of messenger RNA, that is, protein synthesis. For example, in rabbit cornea cells infected with VSV, viral messenger RNA is made and forms polyribosomes, but no VSV proteins are synthesized because VSV protein synthesis is inhibited at the stage of elongation. If such cells are also infected with vaccinia virus, VSV multiplies normally. Apparently vaccinia virus modifies the protein-synthesizing mechanism in such a way that VSV messenger RNA can be translated normally. The ability of SV40 to correct the inability of human adenoviruses to multiply in monkey cells appears to have a similar basis. Other mechanisms, however, may also be involved. For example, the reason why VSV cannot multiply in rabbit kidney cells appears to be the fact that it is not adsorbed; that is, the cells do not possess VSV receptors. If such cells are first infected with Shope fibroma virus, the plasma membrane is modified and VSV receptors appear; VSV can then adsorb and replicate.

FURTHER READING

Books and Reviews

PERSISTENT INFECTIONS

Dales S: Reciprocity in the interaction between the poxviruses and their host cells. Ann Rev Microbiol 44:173, 1990

Oldstone MBA: Viral persistence. Cell 56:517, 1989

Whitaker-Dowling P, Youngner JS: Viral interference-dominance of mutant viruses over wild-type virus in mixed infections. Microbiol Rev 51:179, 1987

LATENCY

Baichwal VR, Sugden B: Latency comes of age for herpesviruses. Cell 52:787, 1988

Roizman B, Sears AE: An inquiry into the mechanisms of herpes simplex virus latency. Annu Rev Microbiol 41:543, 1987

Stevens JG: Human herpesviruses: A consideration of the latent state. Microbiol Rev 53:318, 1989

Klein G: Viral latency and transformation: The strategy of Epstein-Barr virus. Cell 58:5, 1989

Sugden B: An intricate route to immortality. Cell 57:5, 1989

Selected Papers

INHIBITION OF HOST MACROMOLECULAR BIOSYNTHESIS

Blondel D, Harmison GG, Schubert M: Role of matrix protein in cytopathogenesis of vesicular stomatitis virus. J Virol 64:1716, 1990

Elgizoli M, Dai Y, Kempf C, et al: Semliki Forest virus capsid protein acts as a pleiotropic regulator of host cellular protein synthesis. J Virol 63:2921, 1989

Katze MG, DeCorato D, Krug RM: Cellular mRNA translation is blocked at both initiation and elongation after infection by influenza virus or adenovirus. J Virol 60:1027, 1986

Kwong AD, Frenkel N: The herpes simplex virus virion host shutoff function. J Virol 63:4834, 1989

Meyers G, Tautz N, Dubovi EJ, Thiel H-J: Viral cytopathogenicity correlated with integration of ubiquitin-coding sequences. Virology 180:602, 1991

O'Malley RP, Duncan RF, Hershey JWB, Mathews MB: Modification of protein synthesis initiation factors and the shut-off of host protein synthesis in adenovirus-infected cells. Virology 168:112, 1989

Simon KO, Whitaker-Dowling PA, Youngner JS, Widnell CC: Sequential disassembly of the cytoskeleton in BHK_{21} cells infected with vesicular stomatitis virus. Virology 177:289, 1990

Stein RW, Ziff EB: Repression of insulin gene expression by adenovirus type 5 Ela proteins. Mol Cell Biol 7:1164, 1987

Wyckoff EE, Hershey JWB, Ehrenfeld E: Eukaryotic initiation factor 3 is required for poliovirus 2A protease-induced cleavage of the p220 component of eukaryotic initiation factor 4F. Proc Natl Acad Sci USA 87:9529, 1990

PERSISTENT INFECTIONS

Cattaneo R, Schmid A, Spielhofer P, et al: Mutated and hypermutated genes of persistent measles viruses which caused lethal human brain diseases. Virology 173:415, 1989

Jordan JA, Youngner JS: Dominance of temperature-sensitive phenotypes. Dominance of temperature-sensitive phenotypes. II. Vesicular stomatitis virus mutants from a persistent infection interfere with shut-off of host protein synthesis by wild-type virus. Virology 158:407, 1987

Perlman S, Jacobsen G, Olson AL, Afifi A: Identification of the spinal cord as a major site of persistence during chronic infection with a murine coronavirus. Virology 175:418, 1990

Rosenthal KL, Zinkernagel RM, Hengartner H, et al: Persistence of vesicular stomatitis virus in cloned interleukin-2-dependent natural killer cell lines. J Virol 60:539, 1986

LATENCY

Block TM, Spivack JG, Steiner I: A herpes simplex virus type 1 latency-associated transcript mutant reactivates with normal kinetics from latent infection. J Virol 64:3417, 1990

Burke RL, Hartog K, Croen KD, Ostrove JM: Detection and characterization of latent HSV RNA by in situ and Northern blot hybridization in guinea pigs. Virology 181:793, 1991

Coen DM, Kosz-Vnenchak M, Jacobson JG, et al: Thymidine kinase-negative herpes simplex virus mutants establish latency in mouse trigeminal ganglia but do not reactivate. Proc Natl Acad Sci USA 86:4736, 1989

Kosz-Vnenchak M, Coen DM, Knipe DM: Restricted expression of herpes simplex virus lytic genes during establishment of latent

infection by thymidine-kinase-negative mutant viruses. J Virol 64:5396, 1990
Mellerick DM, Fraser NW: Physical state of the latent herpes simplex virus genome in a mouse model system: Evidence suggesting an episomal state. Virology 158:265, 1987
Sample J, Kieff E: Transcription of the Epstein-Barr virus genome during latency in growth-transformed lymphocytes. J Virol 64:1667, 1990

OTHER EFFECTS
Ash RJ: Butyrate-induced reversal of herpes simplex virus restriction in neuroblastoma cells. Virology 155:584, 1986
Hwang CBC, Shillitoe EJ: Analysis of complex mutations induced in cells by herpes simplex virus type-1. Virology 181:620, 1991
Remenick J, Kenny MK, McGowan JJ: Inhibition of adenovirus DNA replication by vesicular stomatitis virus leader RNA. J Virol 62:1286, 1988

CHAPTER 57

The Genetics of Animal Viruses

The genetic approach to studying virus multiplication and virus-host interaction is very powerful. The principal techniques of viral genetics are the isolation of mutants in the various viral genes, identification of their phenotype, and the structural and functional characterization of the proteins that they encode. These techniques permit dissection of the complex series of interactions that is initiated when viruses infect cells into its individual components.

Types of Virus Mutants

Viruses are encapsidated segments of genetic material, and like other genetic systems, viral genomes are not invariate but are subject to change by mutation. Spontaneous mutations occur constantly in the course of virus multiplication, and while many mutations are lethal, others are not. Thus virus populations may be regarded as genetically heterogeneous, because they are likely to contain mutants at each locus.

Mutant virus strains can also be generated in the laboratory as a result of mutagenesis, and it is from mutagenized virus populations that mutant isolation is usually undertaken. Among the procedures used for mutagenizing RNA-containing viruses are treatment of virus particles with nitrous acid, hydroxylamine, *N*-methyl-*N*-nitro-*N*-nitrosoguanidine (NTG), or ethane methane sulfonic acid, and propagation in the presence of 5-fluorouracil, 5-azacytidine, or proflavine (for the double-stranded RNA-containing reovirus). For DNA-containing viruses, treatment of virus particles with nitrous acid, hydroxylamine or ultraviolet irradiation, and growth in the presence of 5-bromodeoxyuridine, NTG, or proflavine are used most commonly.

All these procedures yield random mutations, that is mutations in any part of the viral genome. Such mutations must be sequenced for precise characterization. It is also possible to construct site-specific mutations in any desired region of the genome by the use of recombinant DNA technology.

There are two principal types of virus mutants: point mutants, in which there is a change in a single nucleotide base, and deletion mutants, in which a whole sequence or region of nucleic acid has been deleted. Deletion mutants will be considered below in the discussion of defective virus particles. The most important point mutants are the conditional lethal mutants.

Conditional Lethal Mutants

Conditional lethal mutants, as the name implies, can multiply under some conditions, but not under others. There are two classes of such mutants. The first comprises mutants that are temperature-sensitive (ts) with respect to their ability to multiply. Wild-type animal viruses generally can multiply over a temperature range that extends from a lower limit of 20C to 24C to an upper limit of about 39.5C for mammalian viruses and 40C to 41C for avian ones. In temperature-sensitive mutants there is a nucleic acid base substitution that causes an amino acid replacement in some virus-encoded protein, as a result of which it cannot assume or maintain the structural conformation necessary for activity at elevated or nonpermissive (restrictive) temperatures, although it still is able to do so at lower or permissive temperatures. Thus the typical temperature-sensitive mutation causes the formation of some enzyme or structural protein that cannot function above 36C.

In the second class of conditional lethal mutants are the host-dependent mutants, which have been very useful in bacterium/bacteriophage systems (Chap. 8). In these mutants, the codon for some amino acid is changed to a termination codon (UAG, UAA, or UGA), and, as a result, proteins are formed that are shorter than those specified by wild-type virus and that therefore cannot function. However, mutant bacterial strains exist that contain mutated transfer RNA (tRNA) molecules that recognize these termination codons as the codon for some amino acid (generally different from the original one), which is therefore inserted into the amino acid sequence, thereby again permitting a full-length protein to be formed. If the amino acid change is such that the altered protein can still function, the effect of the original nonsense mutation will therefore be suppressed. The mutated tRNA molecules are known as suppressor tRNAs and the mutant bacterial strains as suppressor strains. The mutations that give rise to UAG, UAA, and UGA are known as *amber*, *ochre*, and *opal*, respectively. Recent work has shown that this type of mutation also exists in mammalian cells and viruses.

The reason that conditional lethal mutants are so important in studies seeking to define the reactions essential for virus multiplication is that they permit study of the virus multiplication cycle with one, and only one, reaction unable to proceed. Use of such mutants permits both the assessment of the role of any particular known reaction during the course of virus multiplication and also the detection of hitherto unknown functions.

Mutants with Other Commonly Observed Phenotypes

In addition to temperature-sensitive and host-dependent mutants, several other mutant phenotypes are often observed, mostly because selection for them is easy and they are therefore readily observed and isolated.

Plaque-size Mutants

Many virus strains give rise to spontaneous mutants that form smaller plaques than wild-type virus because their adsorption is inhibited by sulfated polysaccharides present in agar (Fig. 57–1). Large-plaque mutants are also known, and in this case the ability of wild-type virus to adsorb is inhibited by the polysaccharides, whereas that of the mutants is not. In either case the site of the mutation is in the capsid protein that functions in adsorption.

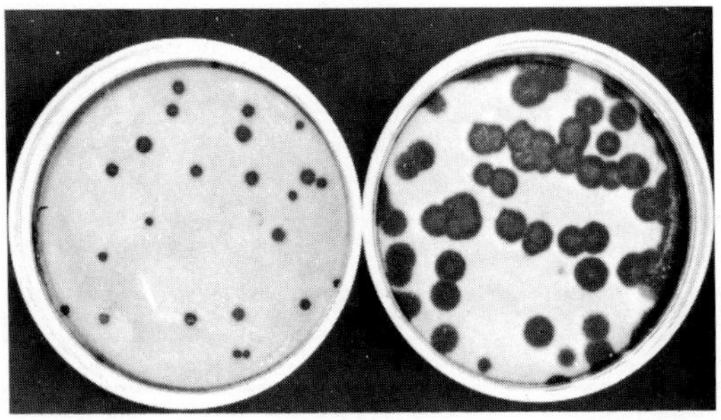

Fig. 57–1. Comparative sizes of two Mengovirus plaque-size variants, S-Mengo (left) and L-Mengo (right). The plaques are 49 hours old. The L mutant is more virulent in animals and more cytopathic in cell cultures. *(From Amako and Dales: Virology 32:184, 1967.)*

Host Range Mutants

Host range mutants are of two types: mutants in cell attachment protein genes and mutants in genes that encode regulatory proteins that interact with cellular proteins and that therefore control the ability of viruses to multiply in specific types of cells.

Drug-resistant Mutants

Drugs capable of inhibiting the multiplication of certain viruses are known (Chap. 58), and mutants exist that are resistant to such drugs. Examples are poliovirus mutants resistant to guanidine, herpesvirus mutants resistant to phosphonoacetic acid, and vaccinia virus mutants resistant to rifampin and isatin-β-thiosemicarbazone (IBT). Poliovirus mutants dependent on guanidine and vaccinia virus mutants dependent on IBT also exist.

Enzyme-deficient Mutants

Viruses encode several enzymes essential for virus multiplication, and mutations that destroy this ability are obviously lethal. Some viruses also encode enzymes that are not essential, and mutants that lack the ability to encode these are viable. For example, poxviruses and herpesviruses encode enzymes that phosphorylate thymidine (thymidine kinases). Virus mutants that are deficient in the ability to induce the synthesis of thymidine kinases are known; they multiply well, which suggests that the survival advantage conferred by the ability to encode them is small, at least in the laboratory cell strains generally used to study them.

Neutralization Escape Mutants

Mutations at or very close to antigenic sites or epitopes often result in the formation of mutants that are able to grow in the presence of antibodies that prevent the growth of the original wild-type virus. Such mutations are of obvious medical importance. They are particularly prevalent in enveloped viruses in which they occur in the spike glycoproteins. Neutralization escape mutants have been studied extensively, particularly in influenza virus, where they are responsible for the "antigenic drift" that causes the emergence of new antigenic variants in response to continual antigenic pressure. Neutralization escape mutants are widely used to locate and characterize the epitopes that elicit the formation of neutralizing antibodies.

Mutations in Noncoding Regions of Viral Genomes

The mutations considered so far have been tacitly assumed to be in genome sequences that encode proteins. Mutations however, also can occur in noncoding regions of viral genomes, and some have surprising phenotypes. For example, a single base change deep in the long-untranslated 5′-region of poliovirus RNA drastically alters neurovirulence, and deletion of one nucleotide close to the 5′-terminus of poliovirus RNA—hundreds of nucleotides removed from a protein-coding sequence—causes the virus to become temperature-sensitive, a defect that is reversed by changing a nearby G to U. The latter effect is thought to be due to the fact that the deletion alters local secondary structure by reducing the likelihood of hairpin formation, which changing G to U restores. Recently, the advent of two new and powerful technologies has greatly increased our ability to study the structure-function relationships of viral genomes. First, the advent of recombinant DNA technology has made possible the incorporation of any desired nucleotide substitution, insertion, or deletion into viral genomes; second, computer formulations in conjunction with chemical cross-linking studies are beginning to provide an insight into the three-dimensional structures of viral genomes that consist of single-stranded RNA. Used in concert, these two approaches should provide explanations of why mutations in noncoding regions can drastically alter viral phenotypes.

Physical and Functional Mapping of Viral Genomes

Physical maps of genomes are generated by restriction endonuclease analysis, followed by sequencing, which provides the ultimate physical genome maps. Physical maps can then be correlated with functional maps such as transcription maps, that is, maps that identify genes that are transcribed under various sets of conditions. For RNA-containing viruses, translational maps have proved valuable. Take, for example, the case of poliovirus, the genome of which is translated into the polyprotein, which is then cleaved into its various functional constituents. Here the pactamycin mapping technique established the gene order. The polyprotein was translated in the presence of pactamycin which inhibits initiation of protein synthesis while permitting the continued translation of already initiated protein molecules. If a radioactive amino acid label is added at the same time as pactamycin, most label will be incorporated into the sequences at the C-terminal end of the polyprotein, thereby ordering the various polyprotein components relative to the ends of the poliovirus genome.

Genetic Interactions Among Viruses

Under conditions of multiple infection, cells may become infected with two or more virus particles with different genomes. If they are sufficiently closely related—that is, if they belong to the same genus—they can interact genetically. There are several types of such interactions.

Recombination

The detection of recombination between two virus strains depends on the availability of techniques that permit recombinants to be detected in the presence of a large excess of the two parents. If the two parents are single-step mutants of some wild-type strain, each differing from it in some recognizable manner, some of the recombinants will have the wild-type genotype and phenotype and be easily detectable.

Viruses differ greatly in the ease with which they undergo recombination, the principal relevant factor being the nature of their genomes. Viral genomes that consist of double-stranded DNA recombine efficiently, probably by a mechanism that is analogous to that by which segments of cellular genomes recombine. By contrast, with two exceptions, viral genomes that consist of single-stranded RNA do not recombine; the exceptions are coronaviruses and several picornaviruses such as poliovirus and foot-and-mouth disease virus. The mechanism of recombination here is not breakage and reunion of RNA molecules but rather copy choice during the transcription of plus strands into minus strands, the polymerase switching template in the process of synthesizing a minus strand. It is of interest that template switching does not occur randomly throughout the genome but at preferred sites, with the potential for forming secondary structure elements capable of bringing together homologous regions of the two recombining genomes by means of the formation of intermolecular complexes. The nascent 3′-end of the strand being synthesized would then detach from a "parting" site on the first template and reattach to an identical or a closely related "anchoring" site on the second template.

The important point here is that viruses must be reasonably closely related for recombination to occur; only viruses within the same genus recombine, and ability to recombine is now recognized as being a useful taxonomic criterion. It should be noted, however, that very rarely totally unrelated viral genomes can recombine, such as those of SV40 and adenovirus (see below) or AAV and adenovirus.

Two-Factor and Three-Factor Crosses

Because recombination can occur at any nucleotide residue, the frequency of recombination between two markers is directly proportional to the distance between them. Measuring recombination frequencies in simple two-factor crosses therefore is an excellent way of genetically mapping mutations. Recombination frequencies, however, are not always additive, particularly for pairs of mutants that are either very close or very far apart. In such cases three-factor crosses can be used. Here the two mutations under investigation are used in conjunction with a third, say A, the location of which is known and which is not selected for or against while recombinants are selected for the other two. The A^+/A^- segregation pattern of the recombinants is then determined. If A lies outside the two mutations, either A^+ or A^- will predominate, the extent of the inequality depending on the distance of A to the nearest mutant locus. If the cross is then repeated with another nonselected marker, B, the position of which relative to A is known, the reciprocal locations of the two mutations under investigation can be unambiguously determined.

Genome Segment Reassortment

The most efficiently recombining viruses are those whose genomes are segmented. In such cases recombination proceeds not by classic recombination involving breakage and reformation of covalent bonds but by simple reassortment of segments into new genomic sets (Fig. 57–2). Both single-stranded and double-stranded RNA segments participate in this type of recombination, as shown by the fact that pairs of reovirus, influenza virus, bunyavirus, and arenavirus mutants with mutations in different genome segments generate wild-type virus with high frequency. In particular, genome segment reassortment is an important mechanism for generating new influenza virus strains; it is the cause of the major antigenic shifts that have occurred in human influenza virus during the last half century. The influenza viruses that exist in nature each possess one of 13 different kinds (subtypes) of hemagglutinin (H1 to H13) and one of 9 different subtypes of neuraminidase (N1 to N9). The proteins specified by these different subtypes differ markedly in amino acid sequence and possess quite different antigenic determinants. Before 1957 the influenza virus strains that circulated in humans had the constitution H1N1; in 1957 they were replaced by Asian influenza, which is H2N2; in 1968 the Hong Kong virus appeared, which is H3N2 and is still circulating. The mechanism responsible for the appearance of these new strains of influenza virus is the introduction, by genome segment reassortment, of new genome segments from some animal influenza viruses, most probably avian ones, into influenza virus strains circulating in and pathogenic for human populations.

Multiplicity Reactivation

Viruses that contain double-stranded DNA frequently exhibit multiplicity reactivation after being subjected to UV radiation. UV radiation damages nucleic acids in several ways. The most important are, first, the formation of covalent bonds between adjacent pyrimidines, thereby giving rise to cyclobutane derivatives. In DNA, the most commonly formed pyrimidine dimers are those between adjacent thymine rings; in RNA, dimers are formed between adjacent uracil and cytosine rings. Dimer formation inactivates viral genomes by preventing replication and probably also transcription and translation. Second, UV radiation causes the addition of water molecules across the C5–C6 double bond of pyrimidines in both DNA and RNA, which results in the formation of photohydrates (6-hydroxy-5,6-dihydro derivatives). These photohydrates represent a major portion of the lethal damage caused by UV light in many RNA-containing viruses.

The most radiation-sensitive property of a virus is its infectivity. The reason is that infectivity requires expression of the genome's entire information content and thus presents the largest target. Sometimes virus particles that have lost their ability to reproduce can still express some special function or group of functions that originate from genes that have not sustained radiation damage. Examples of such functions are the ability to synthesize early enzymes and the ability to transform cells.

Multiplicity reactivation is recognized by the fact that the frequency of viral survivors increases sharply with multiplicities of infection above 1. This effect is caused by cooperation between viral genomes that have been damaged by radiation and that can, therefore, no longer multiply on their own. The nature of the cooperation is recombination; that is, the damaged genomes recombine until an intact genome arises, which can then replicate and form progeny.

Complementation

Viral genomes can also interact indirectly by means of complementation. A typical example of this type of interaction is provided by infection of cells at restrictive temperatures with two virus mutants that bear temperature-sensitive mutations

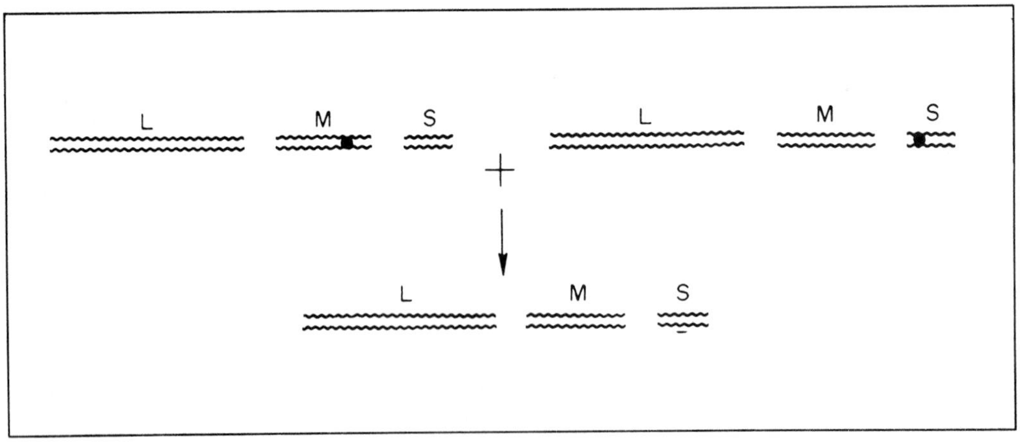

Fig. 57–2. Generation of wild-type genomes by reassortment of damaged genome segments. Two genomes, each consisting of three segments of double-stranded nucleic acid, are shown. One carries a mutation in an M segment, the other in an S segment. When they are introduced into the same cell, sets of undamaged segments are generated by reassortment. This type of mechanism can account for the generation of new genotypes among reoviruses, influenza viruses, bunyaviruses, and arenaviruses.

in different genes and neither of which can multiply alone. If complementation occurs, progeny comprising both mutants is produced. The explanation of this phenomenon is that each mutant produces functional trans-active gene products corresponding to all genes except the gene bearing the temperature-sensitive mutation, so that in cells infected with both mutants all gene products necessary for virus multiplication are formed, and both mutants can therefore multiply. Complementation plays a major role in permitting the survival of viruses with genomes that contain damaged or nonfunctional genes.

Phenotypic Mixing and Phenotypic Masking

The dual phenomena of phenotypic mixing and phenotypic masking represent a special case of complementation. When two closely related viruses, for example, poliovirus type 1 and poliovirus type 3, infect the same cell, the two types of progeny genomes may become encapsidated not only by their own capsids but also by hybrid capsids—that is, capsids composed of proteins encoded by both genomes (phenotypic mixing)—or even by capsids specified entirely by the other genome (phenotypic masking or transcapsidation) (Fig. 57–3). This situation is most readily detected by antigenic analysis. The former class of virus particles is neutralized by antiserum against either parent, whereas virus particles of the latter class are neutralized by antiserum against one of the parents, while their progeny is neutralized by antiserum against the other.

A similar phenomenon occurs among enveloped viruses, but here it involves not only viruses that are related but also viruses that are completely unrelated. In particular, the nucleocapsid of the rhabdovirus vesicular stomatitis virus (VSV) possesses the remarkable ability to become encapsidated in envelopes that are only partially, or not at all, specified by it. For example, among the yield from cells simultaneously infected with both VSV and the paramyxovirus SV5, there are bullet-shaped particles that contain VSV nucleocapsids encased in envelopes that bear not only VSV-specified glycoprotein spikes but also both types of SV5-specified spikes. Another example is provided by VSV nucleocapsids completely encased in RNA tumor virus envelopes. Inasmuch as such particles are easily and rapidly quantitated (because VSV causes plaques rapidly in cell monolayers), they are useful for studies on RNA tumor virus host range (which is specified by the envelope). Finally, VSV nucleocapsids can even be encased in herpesvirus envelopes. Nucleocapsids of one virus enclosed in envelopes specified by another are known as *pseudotypes*. Viruses differ in their propensity to form pseudotypes; those that do so most readily are VSV and RNA tumor viruses.

Suppression

Reversal of mutant phenotypes can occur by several mechanisms. The most obvious is simple reversion, that is, back mutation at the nucleotide of the original mutation. Reversal, however, also can occur as a result of additional mutations that reverse the effect of the original mutation. Several such mechanisms are known. One is suppression of chain-terminating mutations by host-encoded tRNAs; this is informational suppression which occurs primarily in procaryotes (see Chap. 8). Another is by means of mutations in the same gene (intragenic suppression), which typically causes frame-shift mutations that restore the original reading frame. A third is mediated by mutations in genes different from those that contain the original mutation (extragenic suppression). This mechanism operates through physical interaction between two mutated proteins; whereas interaction between a mutant protein with some wild-type protein would be nonproductive, interaction with a mutated version of this protein would be as productive as that between the two wild-type proteins. Extragenic suppression is most readily observed in viruses with segmented genomes because there intragenic suppression is not detectable. For example, reovirus exhibits a high frequency of reversions of temperature-sensitive (ts) mutations; however, the phenotypically wild-type revertant viruses still possess the original ts mutation, as well as an additional mutation that enables the ts mutant to grow at nonpermissive (for itself) temperatures. Extragenic suppression may be of considerable advantage to RNA viruses that cannot reverse the effects of deleterious mutations by recombination.

Defective Virus Particles

Several types of virus particles cannot multiply on their own but can multiply in cells simultaneously infected with infectious "helper" virus. They can be subdivided into two classes: those

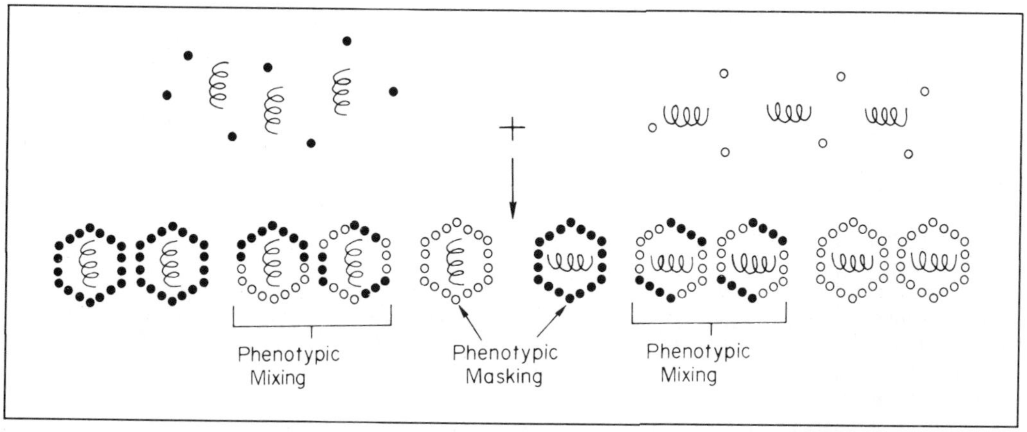

Fig. 57–3. Phenotypic mixing and phenotypic masking. Simultaneous infection with two related viruses is illustrated. Either genome can be encapsidated in capsids that are composed exclusively of homologous capsomers or mixed capsomers (phenotypic mixing) or exclusively of heterologous capsomers (phenotypic masking). The methods for detecting the latter two classes of particles are described in the text.

that interfere extensively with the multiplication of their helper virus and those that do not.

Defective Interfering (DI) Virus Particles

When viruses are passaged repeatedly at high multiplicity, the progeny frequently includes, in addition to mature virus particles, defective virus particles that are capable of interfering with the multiplication of homologous wild-type virus. Such virus particles have the following properties: (1) they contain the normal structural capsid proteins; (2) they contain only a part of the viral genome—that is, they are deletion mutants; (3) they can reproduce only in cells infected with homologous virus, which acts as helper virus; (4) although unable to reproduce on their own, they nevertheless can express a variety of functions in the absence of helper virus, such as inhibition of host cell biosynthesis, cell transformation, and protein synthesis; and (5) they interfere specifically with the multiplication of homologous virus.

The following are examples of defective interfering (DI) virus particles that have been characterized in some detail.

Defective Interfering Influenza Virus Particles

Under conditions of repeated passaging at high multiplicity, the infectivity of successive yields of influenza virus gradually decreases a millionfold or even more, although the total number of virus particles that is produced remains roughly the same. In other words, noninfectious, defective virus particles gradually replace virions in the yields. This phenomenon was first described in 1952 by von Magnus and bears his name. Defective particles are not formed if influenza virus is passaged at low multiplicity, and they are readily eliminated from virus stocks by passaging them at a multiplicity of less than 1, which shows that defective particles cannot multiply on their own. The ability of the defective particles to inhibit the multiplication of infectious virus is demonstrated by the fact that the addition of defective particles to inocula of influenza virus preparations free of them reduces the yield of infectious virus in most types of cells.

The essential difference between infectious and defective influenza virus particles is that the latter have lost most of their three large RNA segments (Chap. 55) and acquired instead several new RNA segments that are smaller than the smallest segment of wild-type virus and that are derived from the three largest segments. The loss of infectivity is a consequence of the deletions from the large segments; the ability to interfere with the multiplication of wild-type virus is due to the presence of the new small segments. The mechanism of formation and nature of several small influenza interfering RNA species is shown in Figure 57–4. The mechanism of the interference and the reason why these deletion mutants compete successfully with wild-type virus are discussed below.

Defective Interfering Particles of Other Viruses

DI particles of rhabdoviruses such as VSV contain RNA that is about one third as long as genome RNA. As a result, they are about one third as long as infectious virus particles, which makes them approximately spherical (Fig. 57–5). The interfering RNA molecules are, like those of influenza virus, the result of aberrant transcription. For reasons that are poorly understood, the VSV RNA polymerase suddenly switches transcription from one template sequence to another, causing (1) deletions if reinitiation occurs downstream on the same template or (2) the synthesis of sequences complementary to portions of the strand being synthesized if reinitiation occurs on itself (Fig. 57–6). As a result, interfering VSV RNA molecules possess either both ends of normal viral RNA or complementary copies of one end. Small interfering RNA

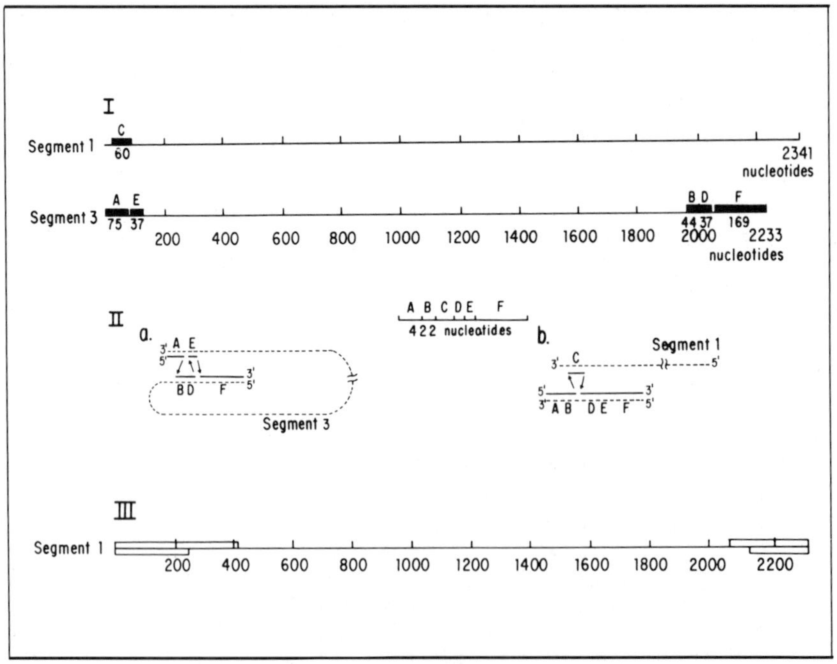

Fig. 57–4. **I.** Origin of one of the small interfering RNA molecules of influenza virus strain A/NT/60/68. It is 422 nucleotides long, a little less than one half as long as the smallest influenza virus gene (see Table 55–5). It is derived from five separate regions, four on genome RNA segment 1, including both ends, and one on genome RNA segment 3. The size of each region is indicated. **II. a** and **b.** Models for the origin of this small interfering RNA molecule. Template switching occurs when the RNA polymerase pauses at U-rich sequences and reinitiates synthesis at another site. **III.** The A/WSN/33 strain of influenza virus gives rise to two different interfering RNA molecules; each is derived from genome RNA segment 1 via a single large deletion. The larger and smaller RNA species (composed of the two terminal sequences indicated above and below the gene, respectively) are 683 and 441 nucleotides long, respectively. Note that all small interfering influenza RNA molecules contain both ends of influenza virus genes. *(From Fields and Winter: Cell 28:303, 1982; Nayak et al: Proc Natl Acad Sci USA 79:2216, 1982.)*

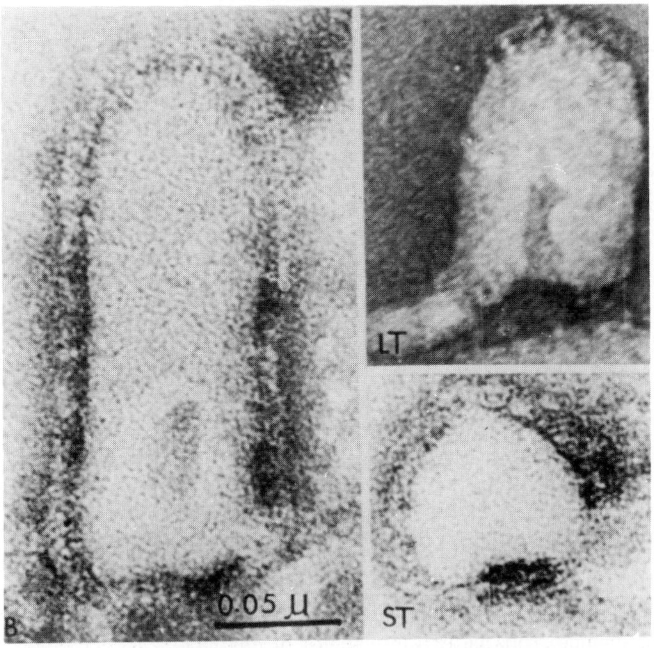

Fig. 57–5. Defective interfering particles of VSV. B, a bullet-shaped normal virus particle; LT, a long truncated particle; ST, a short truncated particle. LT particles are about one half as long as normal virus particles; ST particles, which are round, are about one third as long. The defective particles contain RNA molecules that are correspondingly shorter than the RNA molecules in normal virus particles. *(Courtesy of Dr. C. Y. Kang.)*

molecules of paramyxoviruses such as Sendai virus are quite similar.

DI particles of togaviruses such as Semliki Forest virus and Sindbis virus, contain small interfering RNA molecules one sixth to one half as long as full-length RNA. They are generated by a mechanism in which template switching is carried to the nth degree. They tend to comprise a short region derived from one end of the genome, two or three tandemly arranged copies of diverse regions 500 to 800 nucleotides long—regions that may themselves be repeated—and a short sequence derived from the other end of the viral genome. All sequences from the 3′-terminal one third of the viral genome, which comprises the structural togavirus genes (Chap. 55), usually are completely deleted. The generation of these molecules requires extensive template switching, with the RNA polymerase disengaging from the template it is transcribing and, although remaining attached to the transcript it is in the process of synthesizing, reinitiating transcription elsewhere on the same strand, either upstream or downstream or on a different strand, which may be the transcript to which it is attached.

DI particles also occur in high passage yields of polioviruses, reoviruses, bunyaviruses, coronaviruses, herpesviruses such as pseudorabies virus, and probably most other viruses. All are deletion mutants that require the presence of wild-type virus as helpers but outgrow them quickly. DI polioviruses tend to be simple deletion mutants, the deletions being only 4% to 15% of the genome, and DI mutants of reovirus simply lack one or two genome segments.

Molecular Basis of Interfering Function of DI Particles

DI particles interfere successfully with the multiplication of wild-type virus and outgrow it quickly. How do they accomplish this? Let us consider first DI particles of RNA-containing viruses. The small interfering RNA molecules that are their genomes may lack a wide variety of genes, but they all possess two regions: RNA polymerase recognition site(s) and encapsidation signals. Because these sites and signals are located near the termini of viral RNAs, all small interfering RNAs contain at least one end of intact RNA. All available evidence indicates that small interfering RNAs are encapsidated and serve as templates for RNA polymerase at least as efficiently as intact RNA. In addition, because they are smaller, they are formed much more rapidly than intact RNA molecules are; thus very soon most RNA polymerase recognition sites and encapsidation recognition signals are located on small interfering RNA molecules, not on intact ones. As a result, the multiplication of wild-type virus is severely inhibited. As for the DI particles of DNA-containing viruses, the arguments are similar except that here the genomes of all DI particles must contain an origin of replication, as well as the encapsidation signals.

Effect of Host Cells on Generation of DI Particles

Interestingly, the host cell can influence profoundly both the extent to which DI particles are formed and their nature. Thus a single clonal isolate of influenza virus or VSV will produce different types of small interfering RNA molecules in different cells and will produce DI particles in different cells with different efficiencies. Sometimes DI particles are not formed at all; for example, VSV will not form DI particles in cells treated with actinomycin D, which inhibits host DNA transcription, or in cells simultaneously infected with fibroma virus. All this evidence suggests that host factors are required for the generation of DI particles, but whether they function in the generation of small interfering RNAs (by decreasing the fidelity of transcription or by promoting template switching, or by both) or prevent their encapsidation is not known.

Role of DI Particles in Persistent Infections

DI particles play a role in the establishment and maintenance of persistent infections in nature. There is no question that persistent infections can be established readily in animals by infecting them with mixtures of infectious and DI particles and that DI particles often are present in persistently infected cells. What is the origin of these DI particles? It appears that persistent infections usually are associated with viral variants that are less cytopathic than wild-type virus (Chap. 56), and that these variants often generate DI particles at enormous rates, more than a million times faster than do wild-type virus. Perhaps the generation of DI particles is a mechanism for ensuring the survival of viruses by establishing and maintaining persistent infections. If this is true, DI RNA not only should be smaller than wild-type RNA, possess higher affinity for RNA polymerase, and replicate more rapidly but also should not encode structural viral proteins (so as to minimize cytopathic effects). The genomes of DI particles fulfill all these criteria.

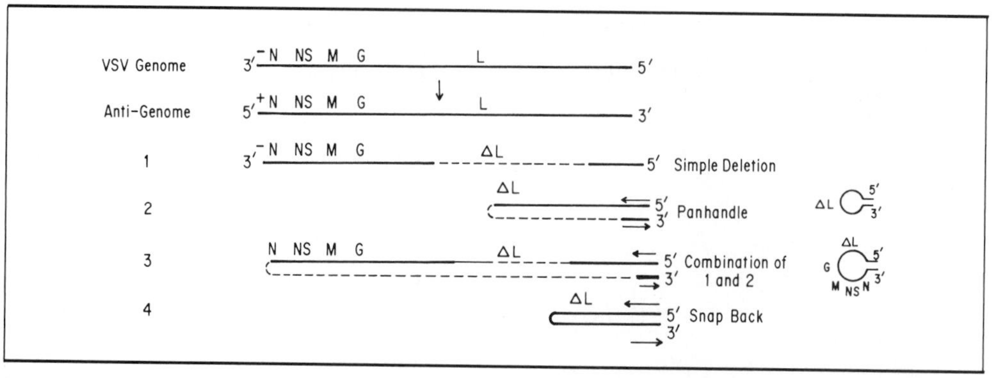

Fig. 57–6. The nature of four types of small interfering RNAs of VSV. The structures of intact VSV RNA and of its plus-stranded transcript (the antigenome) are shown at the top; N, NS, M, G, and L refer to the five VSV genes. The first small interfering RNA is a simple deletion mutant, with most of the L gene (ΔL) deleted; the complete RNA molecule consists of the heavy-lined sequences joined together. To generate the second small interfering RNA, the RNA polymerase transcribes part of the L gene, then stops, reinitiates on the transcript that it is in the process of synthesizing about 45 nucleotides from the end, and transcribes it back to the end. Many panhandle molecules of this type are generated in which the lengths of the L gene sequences that are transcribed are different, but the polymerase always starts transcribing backward at the same position, 43 to 48 nucleotides from the end, where there is a sequence, UUCUGG, that is also present in the opposite orientation near the end, at position 4 to 9, which probably is an RNA polymerase recognition sequence. Thus all RNA molecules of this type possess identical panhandles 43 to 48 base pairs long and varying lengths of L gene sequences. The third type of small interfering RNA is a combination of the first and the second, whereas in the fourth the polymerase transcribes the L gene for a certain distance and then immediately transcribes the sequence that it has just transcribed backward, probably using as template not the strand it has just synthesized but the strand that is being transcribed by the polymerase molecule immediately in front of it (note that one antigenome can be transcribed by several RNA polymerase molecules at the same time). *(From Schubert et al: Cell 18:749, 1979; Lazzarini et al: Cell 26:145, 1981.)*

Adenovirus and Papovavirus Deletion Mutants

When passaged repeatedly at high multiplicity, adenoviruses and papovaviruses give rise to a variety of interesting deletion mutants. For example, there are viable adenovirus deletion mutants. It turns out that a sizable region of the adenovirus genome centered around map position 83 is not essential for the ability to replicate. Mutants that lack more than 2200 base pairs in this region have been isolated and are viable. There are also nonviable adenovirus and papovavirus *evolutionary variants*, so named because they evolve over the course of repeated passaging from simple deletions or substitutions to more complex rearrangements. These particles contain DNA molecules that are almost the same size as the viral genomes but that comprise only a small fraction of them, the remainder being cell DNA. Usually they acquire a selective growth advantage (but do not interfere significantly with the multiplication of wild-type virus) and become a significant fraction of the virus yield; of course, they require infectious virus as helper. Like the genomes of DI particles, their DNAs must contain recognition sites for the initiation of viral DNA replication and encapsidation. Two extreme examples of adenovirus evolutionary variants are (1) a variant that contains only the leftmost 3% of the viral DNA and host DNA corresponding to 93% of the viral DNA and (2) a variant that contains about 6% of each end of viral DNA and host DNA corresponding to 80% of the viral DNA. Among extreme SV40 evolutionary variants is one with a DNA molecule that comprises three copies of a sequence of about 150 base pairs that includes the SV40 origin of replication linked to about 1500 base pairs of host cell DNA.

Adenovirus-SV40 Hybrid Particles

Human adenoviruses multiply poorly in monkey cells but will do so in the presence of the simian papovavirus SV40. The exact nature of the helper function provided by SV40 is not known; there is some evidence that the large T antigen transactivates the transcription of the functional forms of certain late adenovirus transcripts in much smaller amounts in monkey cells than in human cells. The progeny of such mixed infections sometimes includes particles that contain, within an adenovirus capsid, hybrid DNA molecules that contain portions of both adenovirus and SV40 DNA. One example of this type is the $E46^+$ strain of adenovirus serotype 7, which was generated during attempts to adapt human adenovirus to grow in monkey kidney cells for vaccine production. It turned out that the monkey kidney cells contained SV40, the DNA of which recombined with adenovirus DNA to produce molecules that lacked the adenovirus DNA sequences between map positions 5 and 21 and that contained instead two SV40 DNA sequences joined end to end—namely,

TABLE 57–1. NONDEFECTIVE ADENOVIRUS TYPE 2–SV40 HYBRIDS

	Portion of Adenovirus DNA Deleted		Portion of SV40 DNA Inserted	
Hybrid	Map Position[a]	Mol Wt	Map Position	Mol Wt
$Ad2^+ND_1$	80.6–86.0	1.24×10^6	0.29–0.11	0.58×10^6
$Ad2^+ND_2$	79.9–86.0	1.40×10^6	0.43–0.11	1.02×10^6
$Ad2^+ND_3$	80.7–86.0	1.22×10^6	0.18–0.11	0.22×10^6
$Ad2^+ND_4$	81.5–86.0	1.04×10^6	0.54–0.11	1.38×10^6
$Ad2^+ND_5$	78.9–86.0	1.63×10^6	0.39–0.11	0.90×10^6

[a] According to convention, the adenovirus and SV40 maps are referred to as being 100 and 1.00 map units long, respectively. Note that all adenovirus DNA deletions end at map position 86.0 and that all SV40 DNA inserted segments, which comprise from 7% to 43% of the viral genome, end at map position 0.11.

those between map positions 0.50 and 0.71 and between 0.11 and 0.66 (Fig. 55–8). These particles cannot multiply on their own because they contain neither a complete adenovirus genome nor a complete SV40 genome, but they can perform that function that enables human adenoviruses to multiply in monkey cells. They are therefore called *PARA* (particles aiding the replication of adenovirus). Further, they themselves can multiply in the presence of human adenovirus, which supplies the functions encoded by that region of adenovirus DNA that is missing in their own DNA. Thus here are two types of virus particles, human adenovirus and the hybrid PARA particle, neither of which can multiply in monkey cells by itself but both of which can multiply if they infect monkey cells simultaneously. The significance of this system is that viruses that can multiply only in cells also harboring other viruses may be of great importance in causing human diseases of still undefined etiology. These situations are difficult to detect and characterize, but detailed studies such as that described above can provide valuable clues for the search for others of clinical relevance.

Another interesting class of adenovirus-SV40 hybrids is represented by *infectious* adenovirus type 2–SV40 hybrids, five of which have been characterized in some detail (Table 57–1). In these hybrids a portion of the adenovirus genome is deleted from the region that is not essential for virus multiplication and is replaced by a portion of SV40 DNA. The largest of these pieces expresses all early SV40 functions, whereas the smallest encodes no more than 10 to 15 kDa of protein. Yet this is sufficient to endow even this hybrid with the ability to multiply in monkey cells.

Interference Between Viruses

It has been known for a long time that when two different viruses infect the same cell, they may interfere with each other and diminish each other's yield. There are two primary causes of interference. First, the first virus may inhibit the ability of the second virus to adsorb, either by blocking its receptors (certain pairs of enteroviruses) or by destroying its receptors (certain pairs of myxoviruses). Second, one virus may prevent the messenger RNAs of the second virus from being translated. Thus, just as poliovirus inhibits the translation of host-cell messenger RNA by inactivating the cap-dependent messenger RNA recognition mechanism (Chap. 56), so does it inhibit the translation of VSV messenger RNAs and thereby interferes with the ability of VSV to multiply. Similarly, the translation of vaccinia virus messenger RNA is prevented in cells infected with adenoviruses. The ability of Sindbis virus to interfere with the multiplication of VSV and Newcastle disease virus (NDV) and of rubella virus to interfere with the multiplication of NDV also may be due to interference with the ability of viral messenger RNAs to be translated. This mechanism of interference would account for the marked specificity of such inhibitory effects; for example, whereas cells infected with rubella virus become resistant to NDV, they remain susceptible to a variety of other viruses.

Yet another mechanism may operate in cells infected with VSV and herpesvirus. VSV inhibits host protein synthesis by inhibiting transcription; herpesvirus inhibits host protein synthesis by preventing the formation of polyribosomes (an effect of a capsid protein) and causing host messenger RNA to be degraded (a function of an early herpesvirus protein). In cells infected with both these viruses, VSV is dominant, because it inhibits herpesvirus transcription. In cells infected with both herpesvirus and adenovirus, however, transcription of adenovirus messenger RNAs is inhibited, a function, apparently, of yet another early herpesvirus protein.

Viruses as Vectors of Genetic Information

The genomes of many viruses contain genes that are not essential for multiplication under standard conditions. Therefore it is possible to clone foreign genes into them and place them under the control of powerful promoters; the viruses most commonly used for this purpose are vaccinia virus and baculovirus, an insect virus. The levels to which foreign genes can be expressed in cells infected with such hybrid genome–containing viruses can be very high; such expression vector systems are increasingly being used to produce large amounts of a variety of cellular and viral proteins.

Two other applications of viral vectors are also being developed actively. First, the genes of several important human viral pathogens that encode the proteins that elicit the formation of neutralizing antibodies are being inserted into the vaccinia virus genome. When the resulting hybrid vaccinia viruses are inoculated into animals, antibodies are formed not only against vaccinia virus but also against the viral pathogen whose genes they contain, thereby providing protective immunity against them (Chap. 58). The second application is in the area of gene replacement therapy, that is, for the purpose of introducing functioning genes into the genomes of individuals who possess genes with deleterious mutations such as the cystic fibrosis or the sickle cell anemia genes. The carriers of choice here are retroviruses, because the foreign gene must be introduced into the cell genome.

Evolution of Viruses

The development of efficient nucleic acid sequencing techniques has yielded a rapidly increasing body of information concerning the genetic relationships between viruses. Viral genomes clearly are genetic systems capable of rapid genetic change. What are the pressures and mechanisms that cause viruses to evolve on the one hand and to maintain their identity on the other?

The major factor that causes short-term genetic changes in viruses is undoubtedly mutation. In fact, mutants like neutralization escape mutants (see above) arise so rapidly for some enveloped viruses such as influenza virus (corresponding to mutation rates at the nucleotide level of about 1% per year, which is about a million times the rate for the human genome) that it is difficult to see how genetic stability can be maintained at all. Because these mutations occur much more frequently in influenza virus than in other enveloped viruses, is the influenza virus RNA polymerase inherently more error prone than are other viral RNA polymerases? This has been tested and the answer is no; the influenza virus RNA polymerase is not more error prone than, for example, the VSV or parainfluenza virus RNA polymerases, and the excess accumulation of influenza virus variants in vivo therefore must reflect specific selective pressures. The influenza RNA polymerase, however, is 10 times more error prone than is the poliovirus RNA polymerase, which in turn is more error prone than the polymerases of DNA-containing viruses (which possess a proofreading function that the polymerases of RNA-containing viruses lack). Thus short-term genetic diversity of viruses undoubtedly is caused by the lack of fidelity of viral nucleic acid polymerases.

Error-prone polymerases per se, however, do not spell long-term genetic instability. Viruses do not leave fossil records, but historic evidence concerning viral diseases in humans goes back a long time. There is, for example, an almost 4000-year-old rock carving of a Pharaoh with symptoms of poliomyelitis similar to those caused by poliovirus today; there is evidence from ancient Chinese manuscripts that smallpox many centuries ago behaved similarly to smallpox in this century before its eradication. Thus, irrespective of the different fidelities of poliovirus and smallpox virus nucleic acid polymerases, and in spite of their proneness to error, poliovirus and smallpox virus changed little in 4000 years despite causing innumerable epidemics. Clearly there must be factors that stabilize viral genomes. The two most important are as follows. First, mutations must be "acceptable" to the proteins in which they occur; that is, they must not cause loss of protein function. Proteins will differ in this regard; for example, spike glycoproteins, which have no nearest neighbors and therefore no structural constraints dictated by their environment, are likely to accept higher proportions of amino acid changes than are nucleocapsid proteins, such as the adenovirus hexon, which are intimately associated with their neighbors. The second factor is the nature of the selection process. It turns out that while some selective mechanisms—for example, those for neutralization escape mutants and drug-resistance mutants—are very strong, most others that operate on viruses are weak. In fact, positive selection resulting in long-term increased survival and therefore emergence as dominant population components is most probably difficult to achieve *in the same host.* Even the epitope changes discussed above provide only short-term advantages, because they are likely to be cyclical; that is, there are only a finite number of permitted alterations that can recur. The overall conclusion is that although viral genomes are relatively unstable genetic systems, the selective pressures to which they are subject in the *same* host *stabilize* them, at least over periods of time measured in thousands of years.

There are, however, factors other than mutations that cause viruses to "evolve"; and these are much more important. There are two such factors. The first is the acquisition of new genetic information by recombination or genome segment reassortment. Examples of such acquisitions are possession of a unique acetyl esterase by both influenza C viruses and coronaviruses and the fact that western equine encephalitis virus is a recombinant between New World and Old World togaviruses. The second factor is expansion of the host range, that is, ability to infect new hosts, which can be acquired either through the acquisition of new genetic information or as a result of mutation (e.g., cell attachment protein genes). New hosts are important because they provide *new* selective pressures that favor "fixing" permanently newly acquired functions. Examples of viral evolution involving the acquisition of new hosts are the existence of poxviruses, picornaviruses, togaviruses, reoviruses, rhabdoviruses, and influenza viruses, with not only vertebrate but also invertebrate and plant hosts, and the fact that picornavirus capsid proteins, togavirus nucleocapsid proteins, and yeast double-stranded RNA-containing virus capsid proteins are significantly related.

In summary, extensive virus evolution has taken place in the past. The mechanisms responsible have involved major acquisitions of new genetic material, selective pressures resulting from the acquisition of new hosts, and fine tuning by mutation for the selection of dominant population components.

FURTHER READING

Books and Reviews

Calisher CH: Evolutionary significance of the taxonomic data regarding bunyaviruses of the family Bunyaviridae. Intervirology 29:268, 1988

Cockley KD, Rapp F: Complementation for replication by unrelated animal viruses containing DNA genomes. Microbiol Rev 51:431, 1987

Gammelin M, Altmüller A, Reinhardt U, et al: Phylogenetic analysis of nucleoproteins suggests that human influenza A viruses emerged from a 19th-century avian ancestor. Mol Biol Evol 7:194, 1990

Goldbach R, Wellink J: Evolution of plus-strand RNA viruses. Intervirology 29:260, 1988

Smith DB, Inglis SC: The mutation rate and variability of eukaryotic viruses: An analytical review. J Gen Virol 68:2729, 1987

Strauss JH, Strauss EG: Evolution of RNA viruses. Annu Rev Microbiol 42:657, 1988

Selected Papers

RECOMBINATION IN RNA VIRUSES

Keck JG, Stohlman SA, Soe LH, et al: Multiple recombination sites at the 5′-end of murine coronavirus RNA. Virology 156:331, 1987

Kirkegaard K, Baltimore D: The mechanism of RNA recombination in poliovirus. Cell 47:433, 1986

Tolskaya EA, Romanova LI, Blinov VM, et al: Studies on the recombination between RNA genomes of poliovirus: The primary structure and nonrandom distribution of crossover regions in the genomes of intertypic poliovirus recombinants. Virology 160:54, 1987

DEFECTIVE INTERFERING VIRUSES

Bangham CRM, Kirkwood TBL: Defective interfering particles: Effects in modulating virus growth and persistence. Virology 179:821, 1990

Makino S, Shieh C-K, Soe LH, et al: Primary structure and translation of a defective interfering RNA of murine coronavirus. Virology 166:550, 1988

DePolo NJ, Giachetti C, Holland JJ: Continuing coevolution of virus and defective interfering particles and of viral genome sequences during undiluted passages: Virus mutants exhibiting nearly complete resistance to formerly dominant defective interfering particles. J Virol 61:454, 1987

VIRUS EVOLUTION

Air GM, Gibbs AJ, Laver G, Webster RG: Evolutionary changes in influenza B are not primarily governed by antibody selection. Proc Natl Acad Sci USA 87:3884, 1990

Air GM, Laver WG: The molecular basis of antigenic variation in influenza virus. Adv Virus Res 31:53, 1986

Buonagurio DA, Nakada S, Fitch WM, Palese P: Epidemiology of influenza C virus in man: Multiple evolutionary lineages and low rate of change. Virology 153:12, 1986

Bruenn JA, Diamond ME, Dowhanick JJ: Similarity between the picornavirus VP3 capsid polypeptide and the *Saccharomyces cerevisiae* virus capsid polypeptide. Nucleic Acids Res 17:7487, 1989

Domier LL, Shaw JG, Rhoads RE: Potyviral proteins share amino acid sequence homology with picorna-, como-, and caulimoviral proteins. Virology 158:20, 1987

Dominguez G, Wang C-Y, Frey TK: Sequence of the genome RNA of rubella virus: Evidence for genetic rearrangement during togavirus evolution. Virology 177:225, 1990

Fuller SD, Argos P: Is Sindbis a simple picornavirus with an envelope? EMBO J 6:1099, 1987

Hahn CS, Lustig S, Strauss EG, Strauss JH: Western equine encephalitis virus is a recombinant virus. Proc Natl Acad Sci USA 85:5997, 1988

Luytjes W, Bredenbeek PJ, Noten AFH, et al: Sequence of mouse hepatitis virus A59 mRNA 2: Indications for RNA recombination between coronaviruses and influenza C virus. Virology 166:415, 1988

Okazaki K, Kawaoka Y, Webster RG: Evolutionary pathways of the PA genes of influenza A viruses. Virology 172:601, 1989

Parvin JD, Moscona A, Pan WT, et al: Measurement of the mutation rates of animal viruses: Influenza V virus and poliovirus type 1. J Virol 59:377, 1986

Steinhauer DA, de la Torre JC, Holland JJ: Nigh nucleotide substitution error frequencies in clonal pools of vesicular stomatitis virus. J Virol 63:2063, 1989

MISCELLANEOUS

Kuge S, Nomoto A: Construction of viable deletion and insertion mutants of the Sabin strain of type 1 poliovirus: Function of the 5′-noncoding sequence in viral replication. J Virol 61:1478, 1987

Racaniello VR, Meriam C: Poliovirus temperature-sensitive mutant containing a single nucleotide deletion in the 5′-noncoding region of the viral RNA. Virology 155:498, 1986

Silverman L, Klessig DF: Characterization of the translational defect to fiber synthesis in monkey cells abortively infected with human adenovirus: Role of ancillary leaders. J Virol 63:4376, 1989

CHAPTER 58

Antiviral Chemotherapy, Interferon, and Vaccines

This chapter deals with the control and prevention of diseases caused by viruses. The purpose of antiviral chemotherapy and interferon is to control viral diseases by arresting and curing infections once they have started, whereas the purpose of vaccines is to prevent viral infections and therefore the onset of viral diseases.

Important Human Viral Diseases

Although the incidence of many severe, virus-caused diseases such as smallpox, poliomyelitis, yellow fever, and measles has

TABLE 58–1. IMPORTANT HUMAN VIRUS-CAUSED DISEASES

Virus	Comments
Human immunodeficiency virus (HIV)	Causes the acquired immunodeficiency syndrome (AIDS); by far the most important human viral pathogen at this time. More than 1 million Americans may by now be infected with this virus, and current evidence suggests that a high proportion of them will become immunodeficient. In Africa the number of infected persons appears to be at least 10 times higher
Hepatitis B virus (HBV)	The primary cause of acute and chronic liver disease and of primary liver cancer; at least 100 million humans are infected with this virus
Influenza virus	Causes widespread disease; life threatening in elderly persons. New pandemic strains possess the potential for killing millions
Herpes simplex virus	Widespread disease
Viruses that cause respiratory and diarrheal disease: coronaviruses, respiratory syncytial virus, parainfluenza viruses, and rotaviruses	Major causes of morbidity and mortality in children worldwide
Cytomegalovirus	Most common cause of congenital viral infection; feared pathogen in recipients of bone marrow transplantation; frequently fatal
Hemorrhagic fever viruses: dengue, Crimean-Congo hemorrhagic fever, Korean hemorrhagic fever (Hantaan), Lassa fever, Rift Valley fever, Argentinian (Junin) and Bolivian (Machupo) hemorrhagic fever	Frequently fatal
Encephalitis viruses: Japanese encephalitis and others	Frequently fatal

declined dramatically in recent decades owing to the success of widely used highly effective vaccines, other virus-caused diseases still present grave problems. The most important human viral pathogens are listed in Table 58–1. It is important to note that many of these viruses (e.g., the rotaviruses) present much greater problems in Third World countries than in developed countries. Further, several viruses that are under control in developed countries, such as poliomyelitis, measles, mumps, and rubella, are still major problems in Third World countries.

In addition to these viruses that cause acute, persistent, or latent disease, several viruses, either directly or by acting as cofactors, cause a variety of human malignancies. They are Epstein-Barr virus (Burkitt's lymphoma and nasopharyngeal carcinoma), hepatitis B virus (primary hepatoma), human papillomaviruses (cervical carcinoma), and human T cell leukemia virus (adult T cell leukemia).

Rational Approach to Antiviral Chemotherapy

A rational approach to antiviral chemotherapy includes an examination of where virus multiplication cycles can best be interrupted without detriment to the host. The following is a brief relevant analysis.

Adsorption, Penetration, and Uncoating

Until recently, inhibition of processes at the beginning of the multiplication cycle was not attempted seriously because not enough was known about the specific individual reactions involved. The only clinically important drug that inhibits penetration and uncoating is amantadine and the closely related rimantadine, which specifically inhibit the multiplication of influenza A viruses. During the last several years, however, the receptors for several viruses such as human immunodeficiency virus (HIV), human rhinovirus, and Epstein-Barr virus (EBV) (Chap. 55) have been identified, and as a result, efforts are being made to down-regulate their synthesis and to block specifically the interaction between them and viral cell-attachment proteins.

Replication of Viral Nucleic Acids

The replication of the nucleic acids of many viruses is catalyzed by enzymes that do not exist in uninfected cells. This is true for all RNA-containing viruses, as well as for poxviruses, herpesviruses, and adenoviruses. It is possible to isolate and characterize these enzymes and to design specific inhibitors against them.

Integration of Viral Genomes into Cellular Genomes

The genomes of several types of viruses are inserted into cellular DNA either as an essential part of their multiplication cycle (retroviruses) or as the first step in transforming normal cells into tumor cells (papovaviruses, herpesviruses, and hepatitis B virus) (Chap. 59). Some viruses use host cell enzymes for this purpose, but others, such as the retroviruses, encode their own integrases, which provide promising targets for antiviral chemotherapy.

Synthesis of Viral Messenger RNAs

Many viral messenger RNAs are synthesized by virus-encoded RNA polymerases; they are excellent targets for antiviral chemotherapy. Further, some viral messenger RNAs are capped at their 5′-ends by virus-encoded capping enzymes. Although these enzymes are analogous to corresponding host cell enzymes, they are different proteins and therefore also represent targets for intervention.

Synthesis of Viral Proteins

Several lines of evidence suggest that the translation of viral messenger RNAs differs from host cell messenger RNAs; in particular, translation of host cell messenger RNAs often diminishes greatly several hours after infection, at a time when translation of viral messenger RNAs proceeds rapidly. This suggests that viral messenger RNAs differ in some recognizable manner from host cell messenger RNAs, and this difference should be exploitable. A promising avenue of approach, therefore, is analysis of the features in which viral messenger RNAs differ from host cell messenger RNAs.

Viral Morphogenesis

Many viral capsid proteins are synthesized in the form of precursors that are cleaved to furnish the actual proteins used for the formation of virus particles. The proteases that cleave these precursors are virus-encoded. Several of these proteases are now being characterized, and inhibitors are being designed against them. Further, analogues of amino acid sequences cleaved by them possess antiviral activity.

Mode of Action of Certain Antiviral Agents

Many compounds inhibit virus multiplication effectively in cultured cells and have no adverse effect on the growth of uninfected cells. Unfortunately, many of them either inhibit virus multiplication in the body much less efficiently or have unacceptable toxic side effects. They are therefore not suitable for antiviral chemotherapy in humans. Clinical trials, however, have revealed a number of compounds with great promise. Most of them act by means of one of the mechanisms discussed above.

Analogues of Ribonucleosides and Deoxyribonucleosides

Analogue of ribonucleosides and deoxyribonucleosides are highly promising antiviral agents by virtue of their ability to inhibit RNA or DNA synthesis. They consist of nucleic acid bases or derivatives of them, linked either to ribose or deoxyribose or to analogues of ribose or deoxyribose. All must be phosphorylated to their triphosphate forms, which are then recognized as nucleic acid building blocks by nucleic acid polymerases. They inhibit viral RNA or DNA synthesis by two distinct mechanisms: (1) Those that contain nucleic acid base analogues are incorporated into nucleic acids, usually DNA, less commonly RNA; once incorporated, they interfere with the ability of the nucleic acid to function correctly. For example, 5′-iododeoxyuridine (idoxuridine, IDU) (Fig. 58–1) is an analogue of thymidine and is incorporated into DNA.

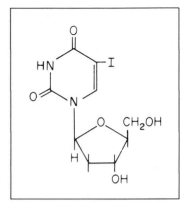

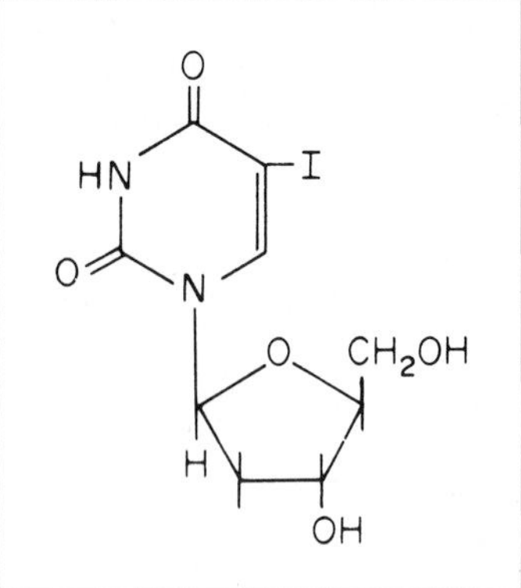

FIG. 58–1. 5′-Iododeoxyuridine (idoxuridine, or IDU). In trifluorothymidine (F_3T), I is replaced by CF_3.

Because iodouracil does not base-pair with adenine as faithfully as does thymidine, mismatching occurs during both the replication and the transcription of the substituted DNA. (2) Compounds containing analogues of ribose or deoxyribose that lack a 3′-OH group arrest nucleic acid synthesis by acting as chain terminators. Neither of these two mechanisms accounts for the selective inhibition of viral vis-à-vis cellular nucleic acid synthesis. Selectivity is, in fact, provided by two mechanisms. First, viral DNA polymerases often possess higher binding affinities for the analogue triphosphates than do the cellular enzymes, sometimes by as much as 100-fold. This means that analogue triphosphate concentrations that have little or no effect on host cell DNA replication inhibit viral DNA replication. Second, many analogues also tend to inhibit competitively cellular enzymes on the biosynthetic pathways that lead to the formation of RNA and DNA, including kinases that form monophosphates, diphosphates, and triphosphates, as well as enzymes that synthesize and interconvert purine and pyrimidine nucleotides. As a result, reduced amounts of the regular ribonucleoside or deoxyribonucleoside triphosphates are formed, thereby exacerbating the effects of the analogue triphosphates, which the viral nucleic polymerases often prefer in any case.

A discussion of the most important analogues of this type follows.

Idoxuridine and Trifluorothymidine

Idoxuridine and trifluorothymidine (F_3T) are analogues of thymidine (Fig. 58–1). IDU was the first active and effective deoxyribonucleoside analog tested. Both inhibit the multiplication of herpesviruses. Both are licensed by the Food and Drug Administration for the topical treatment of epithelial herpes simplex keratitis; they are too toxic for systemic use.

Vidarabine

Vidarabine (adenosine arabinoside, ara-A) inhibits the multiplication of herpes simplex virus (HSV) and varicella-zoster (VZ); cytomegalovirus and EBV are less sensitive. Vidarabine possesses good in vitro activity; it inhibits the viral DNA polymerases more than cellular DNA polymerases. Because it is phosphorylated by cellular kinases, it is active against thymidine kinase–deficient (TK^-) mutants of HSV (mutants resistant to it map to the pol gene). Unfortunately it is rapidly deaminated to the less active hypoxanthine arabinoside. Vidarabine is licensed by the FDA for topical use against herpes simplex keratitis and for intravenous use against herpes simplex encephalitis and neonatal herpes simplex.

Acyclovir

Acyclovir (9-[2-hydroxyethoxymethyl]guanine) consists of guanine linked to an open ring analogue of ribose or deoxyribose (Fig. 58–2). It is phosphorylated by the HSV and VZ thymidine kinases (TKs), which have a wider substrate specificity than the cellular TK, which only phosphorylates thymidine; thus it is phosphorylated only in herpesvirus infected cells (the target cells). Once converted to the triphosphate, it is incorporated into DNA by the viral DNA polymerases, which have a much higher affinity for it than cellular DNA polymerases. Because it has only one −OH group, it acts as a chain terminator, and because it cannot be excised by the polymerase-associated 3′-exonuclease, the DNA polymerase binds irreversibly to the acyclovir-terminated DNA and is inactivated. Mutants resistant to acyclovir are mutants either in the TK or in the DNA polymerase. It is much less active against CMV and EBV, which do not encode their own TKs. It is thus an extraordinarily specific anti-HSV and anti-VZ agent and, surprisingly, in view of its mode of action, is remarkably nontoxic.

Ganciclovir

Ganciclovir (9-[1,3-dihydroxy-2-propoxymethyl]guanine, or DHPG) is a close relative of acyclovir (Fig. 58–2). It is an even better substrate for HSV TK than is acyclovir and is a powerful inhibitor of HSV multiplication. It also is a much better inhibitor of CMV infections than is acyclovir; it is the best inhibitor of CMV infections currently in use. It is not known how it is phosphorylated; CMV does not encode a TK, yet more triphosphate is found in infected cells than in uninfected cells. Ganciclovir's mode of action is the same as that of acyclovir although it is probably not a strict chain terminator because it possesses 2′-OH groups.

Zidovudine

Zidovudine (azidothymidine, also known as retrovir or AZT) (Fig. 58–2) is an inhibitor of retrovirus reverse transcriptases for which its triphosphate has 100-fold greater affinity than for cellular DNA polymerases. Because it does not possess a 3′-OH group, it is a chain terminator. It is the only drug with demonstrated clinical efficacy in HIV infections.

Ribavirin

Ribavirin (virazole) (Fig. 58–2) is an analogue of the purine precursor 5′-aminoimidazole-4-carboxamide. It has a wide antiviral spectrum, including both RNA- and DNA-containing viruses. Its targets are virus-encoded nucleic acid polymerases: ribavirin triphosphate is a powerful noncompetitive inhibitor of transcription, primarily affecting elongation and to a lesser extent initiation. It is licensed by the FDA for the treatment in aerosol form of severe respiratory syncytial virus infections in children. Oral and intravenous ribavirin also reduce mortality in patients with Lassa fever.

Other Agents

Several other analogs of ribonucleosides and deoxyribonucleosides strongly inhibit herpesvirus DNA polymerases but not cellular DNA polymerases, possess low cytotoxicity, and are undergoing clinical trials. Among them are analogues of thymidine, exemplified by BVdU, and an analogue of cytosine, FIAC (Fig. 58–3).

Recently, 2′,3′-dideoxynucleosides have been found to inhibit strongly the multiplication of many retroviruses, including HIV. Although they are much more effective in some cells than in others, preliminary results against HIV are so promising that they are already undergoing clinical trials. Presumably they act primarily as chain terminators.

Finally, phosphonoformic acid (foscarnet) and the closely related phosphonoacetic acid (PAA) are potent, highly specific inhibitors of herpesvirus DNA polymerases (Fig. 58–4). Unfortunately, they are toxic because they accumulate in bones (because they act as phosphate analogues in bone metabolism)

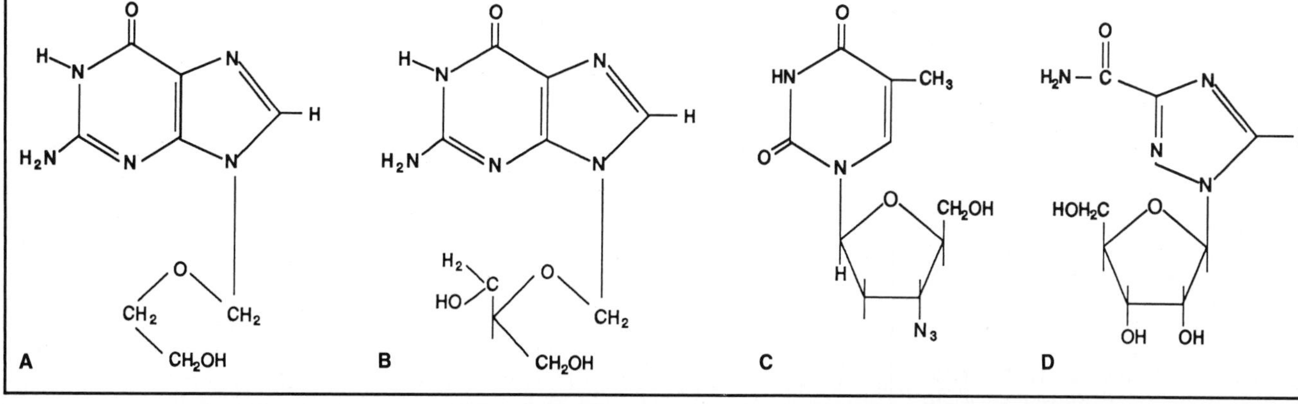

Fig. 58–2. **A.** Acyclovir (9-[2-hydroxyethoxymethyl]guanine, or acycloguanosine). **B.** Gancyclovir (9-[1,3-dihydroxy-2-propoxymethyl]guanine, or DHPG). **C.** Zidovudine ([3′-azido-3′-deoxy] thymidine, or azidothymidine, or retrovir, or AZT). **D.** Ribavirin (1-β-D-ribofuranosyl-1,2,4-triazole-3-carboxamide, or virazole).

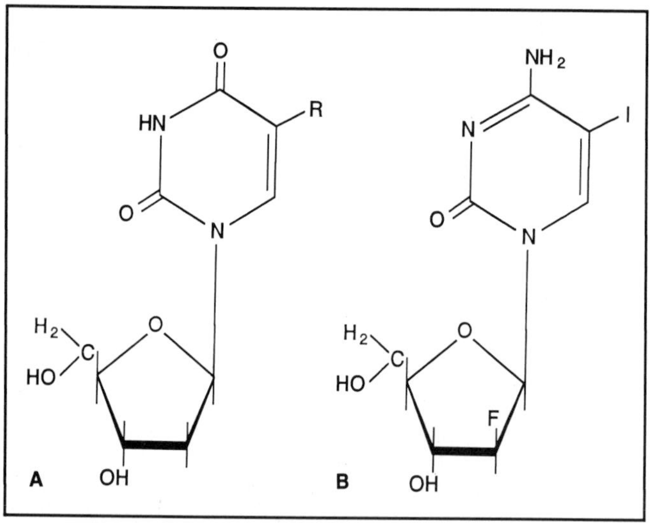

Fig. 58–3. A. R = CH=CH$_2$, 5-vinyl-2′-deoxyuridine; R = CH=CHBr, (E)-5-(2-bromovinyl)-2′-deoxyuridine (BvdU); R = CH=CHI, (E)-5-(2-iodovinyl)-2′-deoxyuridine (IVdU). **B.** FIAC (1-[2′-deoxy-2′-F-β-D-arabinofuranosyl]-5-iodocytosine).

and also cause nephrotoxicity, and mutants resistant to them emerge rapidly. In spite of these drawbacks foscarnet is undergoing clinical trials in immunosuppressed patients infected with CMV. Recently another methyl phosphonate derivative, (s)-HPMPA (Fig. 58–4), has been found to be a highly potent and selective inhibitor of a wide spectrum of DNA-containing viruses, including herpesviruses, poxviruses, and adenoviruses, as well as retroviruses. Further, another compound of this type, PMEA (Fig. 58–4), is a strong inhibitor of retrovirus multiplication and suppressor of tumor formation; it is also a potent and selective inhibitor of the replication of HIV in human T lymphocytes. In fact, its anti-HIV activity exceeds that of zidovudine.

Amantadine and Rimantadine

These two closely related compounds, which possess a remarkably rigid structure comprising three fused saturated six-membered rings (Fig. 58–5), are effective inhibitors of influenza A virus multiplication. They appear to interfere with the earliest stages of the multiplication cycle, namely penetration and uncoating; recent evidence, however, suggests that they may also inhibit budding/virus particle release. Mutants resistant to these two compounds map to the M2 ORF, which encodes a small protein that may form tetrameric channels in vesicles of the trans-Golgi network that are important for the proper formation of the HA glycoprotein spike (Chap. 55). Both have been licensed by the FDA for the prophylaxis and treatment of influenza A infections. There are some central nervous system side effects, which are less serious for rimantadine than for amantadine. Rimantadine is used extensively in the Soviet Union but not in the United States because it seems impractical to use chemoprophylaxis for control of a disease that is generally mild and that the individual patient has a good chance of avoiding. Either compound provides an excellent alternative to vaccination for protecting individuals at high risk in whom the disease may be serious, such as persons who are elderly or immunocompromised or who have allergies, as well as for epidemics in which the causative virus strain is significantly different from the vaccine strain.

Other Antiviral Agents

Many other compounds inhibit virus multiplication without significant effect on host cells. Some of these compounds have been used in humans, others in animals; many are of interest because they identify and illustrate targets for antiviral chemotherapy in virus multiplication cycles. A discussion of some of these compounds follows.

Isatin-β-thiosemicarbazone

Isatin-β-thiosemicarbazone (IBT) is a potent inhibitor of poxvirus multiplication (Fig. 58–6). In the presence of IBT, the

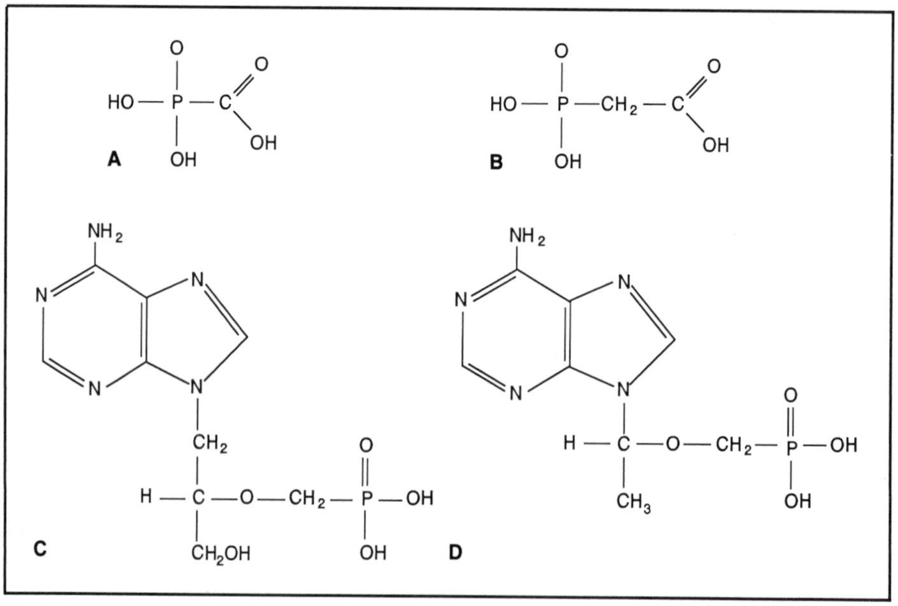

Fig. 58–4. A. Foscarnet (phosphonoformic acid, or PFA). **B.** Phosphonoacetic acid (PAA). **C.** (s)-9-(3-hydroxy-2-phosphonyl-methoxypropyl)adenine, or (s)-HPMPA. **D.** 9-(2-phosphonylmethoxyethyl)adenine, or PMEA.

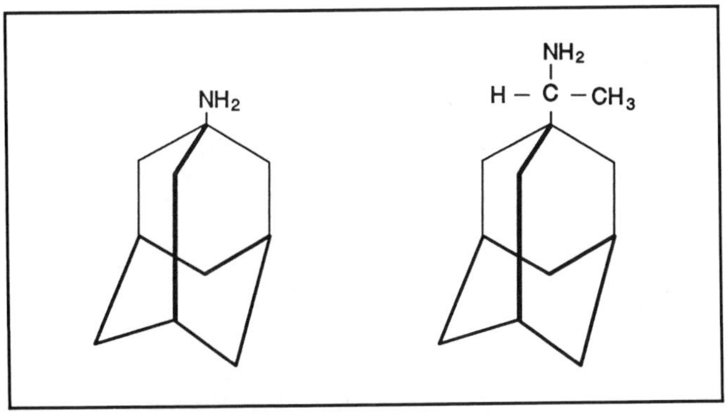

Fig. 58–5. Left, amantadine. **Right**, rimantadine.

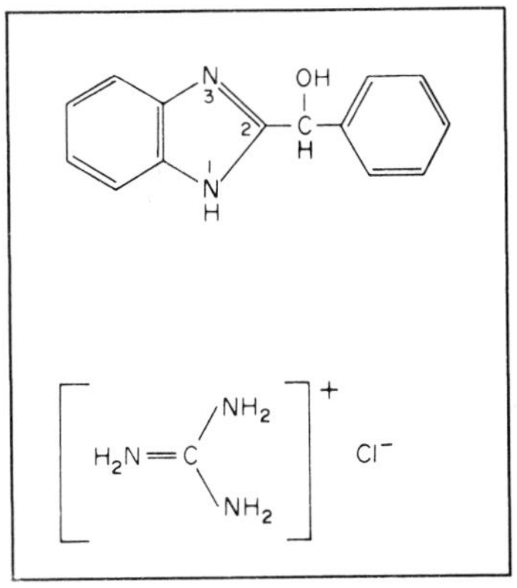

Fig. 58–7. 2-Hydroxybenzylbenzimidazole (HBB) and guanidine hydrochloride.

early period of the poxvirus multiplication cycle, viral DNA replication, and transcription of late messenger RNA (mRNA) all proceed normally, but late mRNA (as well as cellular RNA) is rapidly broken down so that the synthesis of late proteins, which include most of the viral capsid proteins, is prevented, and no progeny virus particles are formed. Recent evidence suggests that resistance or susceptibility to IBT is controlled by an early viral gene, but its function is not known.

A derivative of IBT, *N*-methyl-IBT (Marburan), was administered by mouth to known smallpox contacts in field trials in India and Pakistan during the smallpox eradication campaign, and beneficial results of this prophylactic treatment were observed.

2-Hydroxylbenzylbenzimidazole and Guanidine

The two reagents 2-hydroxylbenzylbenzimidazole (HBB) and guanidine (Fig. 58–7) inhibit the multiplication of many picornaviruses including poliovirus, echoviruses, Coxsackie viruses, and foot-and-mouth disease virus. They are examples of reagents that interfere with the replication of viral RNA; they prevent the initiation of the synthesis of progeny plus strands by interfering with the function of protein 2C (p. 815), a nonstructural protein that plays an essential but undefined role in picornavirus RNA replication. Although both drug-resistant and drug-dependent virus mutants emerge quickly, HBB has been used with some success in controlling enterovirus infections in animals.

Rifampin

Rifampin and related rifamycin derivatives bind to bacterial RNA polymerases, thereby preventing the initiation of transcription. Rifampin (see Fig. 9–21) does not bind to animal RNA polymerases, but it does inhibit the multiplication of poxviruses and adenoviruses. The mechanism by which it acts has been studied most intensively in vaccinia virus–infected cells. Inhibition of viral RNA polymerase is not involved, inasmuch as both early and late mRNAs are transcribed normally. Rather, the mechanism involves some event in viral morphogenesis, because in the presence of the drug immature virus particles that lack the normal dense spicule layer (Fig. 55–25) accumulate. Mutations to resistance to rifampin map to a gene that encodes a 65 kDa virion component, which in the presence of rifampin fails to associate with progeny virus particles.

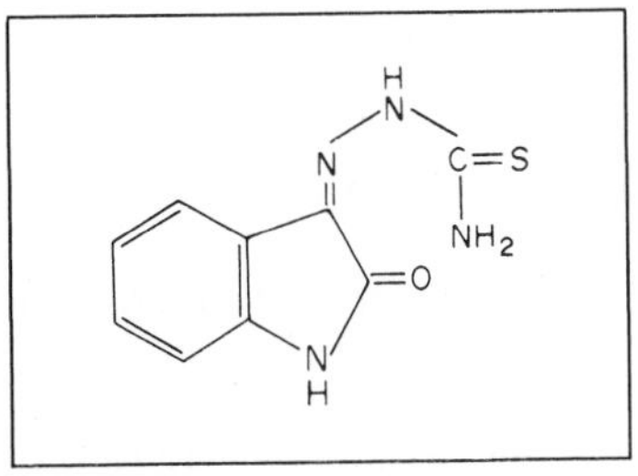

Fig. 58–6. Isatin-β-thiosemicarbazone (IBT).

Arildone, Rhodanine, and WIN 51711

Arildone, rhodanine, and WIN 51711 (disoxaril) (Fig. 58–8) are members of a group of compounds that inhibit the uncoating of picornaviruses such as poliovirus, echovirus, and rhinovirus. Although they do not affect adsorption or penetration, they prevent the pH-dependent uncoating events that take place in acidic endosomes. They do so by increasing the stability of these viruses to such an extent that active unde-

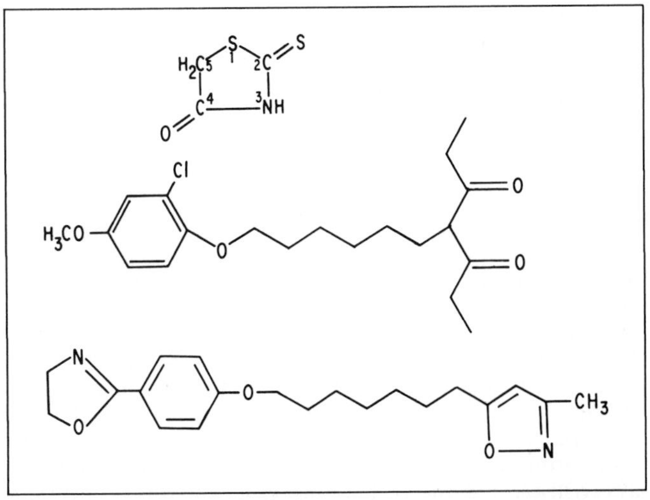

Fig. 58–8. Top, rhodanine (2-thio-4-oxothiazolidine). **Middle,** arildone (4-[6-(2-chloro-4-methoxyphenoxyl)hexyl]-3,5-heptanedione). **Bottom,** WIN 51711 (disoxaril).

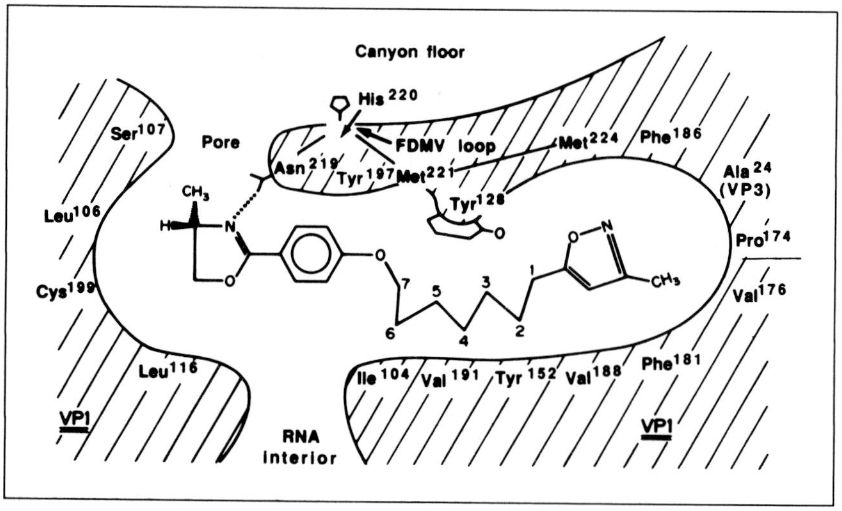

Fig. 58–9. Diagrammatic representation of the binding site of WIN 52084, a methyl derivative of WIN 51711, in the capsid of human rhinovirus 14. *(From Smith et al: Science 233:1286, 1986.)*

graded virus can be recovered from cells as long as 4 hours after infection with treated virus. How these compounds function at the molecular level has been elucidated for disoxaril by x-ray diffraction analysis. It appears that the 3′-methylisoxazole group of this compound (right-hand end) inserts itself into a hydrophobic pocket formed by capsid protein VP1 and that its other end covers the entrance to an ion channel also formed by VP1 (Fig. 58–9). Viral disassembly may be inhibited either by preventing the collapse of the hydrophobic pocket or by blocking the flow of ions into the virus interior. Arildone and rhodanine may act by analogous mechanisms.

Promising New Approaches

The search for new antiviral agents has been enormously stimulated by the AIDS epidemic, and many new approaches are now being tested in efforts to arrest its replication and spread within the body.

Inhibitors of Proteases

Many viral proteins are synthesized in the form of precursors that must be cleaved in order to yield the functional proteins required. Often, such as in the case of the picornaviruses, the togaviruses, and the retroviruses, these cleavages are effected by highly specific virus-encoded proteases that are prime targets for interference with virus multiplication. In particular, the three-dimensional structure of the HIV protease, which cleaves both the *gag* and *env* protein precursors (p. 899), has been solved at the atomic level by x-ray crystallographic analysis; strenuous efforts are now being made, with the use of computer modeling, to design inhibitors of it. This approach is also promising for viruses like the coronaviruses, the paramyxoviruses, and the orthomyxoviruses, in which envelope glycoproteins such as the fusion proteins and the hemagglutinins must be cleaved to permit these viruses to infect cells effectively. These cleavages, which occur in basic amino acid sequences, are carried out by host proteases that are often referred to as *trypsin-like*. In the case of influenza virus it has been shown that peptidyl chloroalkyl ketones (which bind covalently to the substrate-binding sites of proteolytic enzymes) strongly inhibit virus multiplication when they contain a palmityl residue, as well as at least two adjacent amino acids (e.g., palmityl-fluorophenylalanine-alanine-lysine-arginine-chlorethylketone).

Inhibition of Adsorption

The identification of an increasing number of viral receptors has stimulated attempts to interfere with the process of virus adsorption. In the case of HIV, its primary cellular receptor is the CD4 T cell antigen to which gp120, its spike glycoprotein, binds. Two strategies for inhibiting this interaction are as follows. First, soluble derivatives of CD4 are being prepared; they interact with the virus and thereby prevent it from binding to T cells. Because soluble CD4 is rapidly cleaved from the bloodstream, the CD4 is coupled to immunoglobulin to generate "immunoadhesins," which have a greatly increased half-life in the blood and which also target the virus for elimination by the immune system. Such complexes are already undergoing clinical trials. It should also be possible to prepare soluble derivatives of or analogues to gp120 that should attach to cell-associated CD4, thereby preventing HIV from attaching to cells.

Recently sulfated polysaccharides such as dextran sulfate and heparin have been found to inhibit HIV adsorption to target cells. Although their action appears to be nonspecific, they are highly active at nontoxic concentrations and are undergoing clinical trials.

Targeted Introduction of Toxins into Infected Cells

Targeted introduction of toxins into infected cells is another variant of the strategy employing the recognition event between virus and host cell receptors as a target for antiviral chemotherapy; that is, it is another "target cell approach" directed solely against *infected* cells, rather than against *all* cells in infected hosts. This approach is based on coupling toxins such as ricin or the *Pseudomonas* exotoxin (PE)—very few molecules of which kill cells—to CD4, which will then attach to gp120 present on the surface of infected cells and be internalized, thereby introducing the toxin into the infected cells. In another approach the toxin is coupled to a monoclonal antibody directed against gp41, which is the stalk component of HIV glycoprotein spikes. Preliminary experiments with the use of CD4 and antibody molecules as homing devices are promising. Similar approaches are being followed for other viruses, such as rhinoviruses and EBV, for which the receptors are known.

Introduction into Cells of Specific Anti-Sense RNA Sequences

As in many other areas, recombinant DNA technology has suggested new approaches to antiviral chemotherapy. One such approach takes advantage of the fact that many mRNA splice junctions have now been sequenced. It is possible to synthesize oligonucleotides capable of base-pairing with these splice junctions and to render them capable of entering cells by using their methylphosphonate derivates. It may be possible in this way to prevent viral splice junctions from being recognized by the splicing mechanism. The same approach should be applicable to the functional inactivation of mRNA translation initiation sequences and of regulatory nucleic acid sequences.

Preventing Interactions Among Protein Molecules

Another approach is to prevent the interactions among proteins or protein subunits by adding an excess of oligopeptides with the same sequence as the interacting sequence on one of the interacting partners. This approach has been found to inhibit the formation of herpesvirus ribonucleotide reductase, which consists of two subunits that must combine to form the active enzyme. Clearly, this approach is capable of wide applicability. For example, it is conceivable that the formation or association of capsomers, and therefore viral morphogenesis, could be inhibited in this way.

Interferons

An antiviral agent onto which a great deal of attention is being focused is one that is elaborated by living cells themselves. Virus-infected cells often produce a protein that protects uninfected cells against infection or, more precisely, greatly decreases the chance that virus infection will be able to initiate a productive multiplication cycle in them. This protein is called *interferon.* Interferon provides the first line of defense against virus infections: in animals treated with antiserum to interferon, virus infections progress much more rapidly and cause much more severe disease than in untreated animals.

Interferons are cellular proteins. Normal cells do not contain detectable amounts of interferon; the formation of interferons must be induced (see below). Interferons are host cell species–specific because they interact with cells via specific receptors; biologic activity is usually proportional to binding affinity. Target cell specificities are sometimes unexpectedly narrow and peculiar. For example, chick and duck interferons—like mouse and rat interferons—exhibit little if any cross-protective activity, but many human interferons protect bovine cells even better than does bovine interferon. Further, not all viruses are equally susceptible to interferons. Adenoviruses, for example, are rather resistant, as are poxviruses like vaccinia virus, in certain types of cells only, whereas orthomyxoviruses and rhabdoviruses are among the most susceptible.

Nature of Interferons

Human interferons are proteins that are about 145 amino acids long (mol wt about 17,000). There are three types of human interferon (IFN): IFN-α and IFN-β, produced predominantly by leukocytes and fibroblasts, respectively, in response to virus infection or to a variety of inducing agents (type 1 interferons), and IFN-γ, formerly called *immune* or type 2 interferon, which is produced by unsensitized lymphoid cells in response to mitogens and by sensitized lymphocytes when stimulated with specific antigens (Table 58–2).

IFN-β and IFN-γ are glycoproteins, but their oligosaccharide chains are not essential for antiviral activity; the IFN-α species are not glycoproteins. The type 1 interferons, but not IFN-γ, are remarkably resistant to low pH—they are quite stable at pH 2 at 4C—and retain activity in the presence of sodium dodecyl sulfate, an unusual property that is very useful in the final stages of their purification.

The separation of interferons into three classes is based primarily on antigenicity. The three classes of interferon are immunologically distinct; that is, antisera raised against any one class do not inactivate interferons in the other two classes.

There is evidence for two highly conserved domains in interferon molecules. One, in the aminoterminal half of the molecule, appears to contain the cell surface receptor binding site; the other, in the other half of the molecule, appears to modulate such binding and mediate other biologic functions.

Finally, interferons possess two types of biologic activity: antiviral and cell-regulatory. Interferons not only inhibit virus multiplication, which function was discovered first, but are also cytokines and lymphokines. The antiviral activity of all three classes of interferon is comparable, but the cell-regulatory activity of IFN-γ greatly exceeds that of type 1 interferons.

Assay of Interferons

The antiviral activity of interferons is usually assayed by exposing cells to serially diluted interferon preparations for about 12 hours and then infecting them with a standard amount of virus (usually vesicular stomatitis virus [VSV]) known to produce a certain number of plaques. The titer of an interferon preparation is the reciprocal of that dilution that reduces this number by 50%. The specific activity of pure interferons is 5 to 10 × 10^8 PRD_{50} (50% plaque reduction doses) per milligram. This astonishingly high biologic activity means that in some sensitive cell-virus systems interferon is detectable at concentrations as low as 10^{-14} M.

TABLE 58–2. CHARACTERISTICS OF HUMAN INTERFERONS

Type	Alpha (Leukocyte)	Beta (Fibroblast)	Gamma (Immune or Class 2)
Produced by	Peripheral leukocytes	Fibroblasts	Lymphocytes
Inducing agent	Virus infection dsRNA	Virus infection dsRNA	Mitogens Specific antigens
Number of genes	≥15	1	1
Presence of introns	No	No	Yes
Chromosomal location	9	9	12
Size of primary protein (number of amino acids)	166	166	166
Length of signal sequence (number of amino acids)	23	21	20
Size of actual protein (number of amino acids)	143	145	146
Molecular weight (kDa)	~17	~17	~17
Glycoprotein	No	Yes	Yes
Stability at pH 2	Yes	Yes	No
Activity in the presence of sodium dodecyl sulfate	Yes	Yes	No

Nature of Interferon Genes

There are at least 15 different human IFN-α genes, one IFN-β gene, and one IFN-γ gene (Table 58–2). All these genes encode proteins that are exactly the same length, namely, 166 amino acids long, 20 to 23 of which are *N*-terminal signal sequences that are cleaved off as the interferons are secreted. The various IFN-α genes are 80% to 90% related to each other. The coding sequences of the IFN-α genes and the IFN-β gene are about 30% related, which indicates that they diverged about 500 million years ago, before the emergence of vertebrates. The IFN-γ gene exhibits essentially no homology to the other interferon genes but clearly derives from a common ancestor, because it encodes a similar-sized protein in which several amino acids occupy the same positions as in IFN-α and IFN-β.

Most if not all IFN-α genes are arranged tandemly, or close to each other, on chromosome 9; the IFN-β gene is also located on chromosome 9; and the IFN-γ gene is located on chromosome 12. The latter is the only interferon gene that possesses introns.

In addition to these functional genes, the human genome also contains at least nine IFN-α pseudogenes whose sequences contain mutations or deletions that prevent the expression of full-length interferon proteins.

All human interferon genes have been sequenced. They have also been cloned into both procaryotic and eucaryotic expression vectors, which has greatly facilitated their production. The significance of this accomplishment is that cultured human cells can be induced to produce only small amounts of interferons (typically 0.1 mg/10^9 cells) before they die. By means of expression vectors, interferons can now be produced in very much larger amounts in either procaryotic or eucaryotic cells.

Another avenue that has been opened by the cloning of interferon genes is the possibility of constructing hybrid genes, that is, comprising different portions of two or more interferon genes, so as to encode interferons with more desirable biologic and pharmacologic properties, or with particular applicability in specific situations in the antiviral or in the cell regulatory (cancer, see below) area.

Induction of Interferons

Normal cells as a rule do not contain or synthesize interferons; all available evidence indicates that this is because interferon genes are not transcribed to any significant extent. Interferon formation, can however, be induced by a variety of inducers that include virus infection, double-stranded RNA (dsRNA), and various metabolic activators and inhibitors.

To understand how these disparate inducers activate the transcription of interferon genes, it is necessary to understand the nature of the regulatory sequences upstream of the interferon coding regions. Let us take, for example, the nature of the controls that regulate the expression of the IFN-β gene. The sequence crucial to transcription control is located between residues −77 and −37 upstream of the cap site, termed the *interferon gene regulatory element* (IRE). The IRE comprises three functional components: a negative regulatory domain (NRD I) and two positive regulatory domains (PRD I and PRD II). These three regulatory elements interact with several proteins. One is a repressor that normally binds to NRD I and blocks the binding of transcription factors to the positive regulatory domains. This is the normal state of affairs. Upon induction, the repressor is removed and two proteins, PRD I-BF_c and PRD II-BF, are modified, possibly by phosphorylation, and then bind to PRD I and PRD II, respectively, thereby activating transcription. Removal of the repressor is postulated to result from either direct inactivation or displacement by the two modified positive transcription factors.

The mechanism of induction of interferons by the various inducers can be explained as follows in the light of this model. It should be noted that most interferon inducers fall into the class of "noxious" stimuli; that is, they tend to be cytotoxic and inhibitors of protein synthesis.

Induction of Interferon by Viral Infection

The most important interferon inducer is infection with viruses. In general, RNA-containing viruses are good interferon inducers whereas DNA-containing viruses, with the exception of poxviruses, are rather poor interferon inducers. The kinetics of interferon production tend to be the same for most virus infections: interferon production begins about 4 hours after infection, reaches a peak when viral protein synthesis is proceeding at its maximal rate, and then declines.

Viruses most probably induce interferon because infection usually inhibits host protein synthesis. Because interferon repressors are labile proteins, even a moderate reduction of the rate at which they are replaced may be sufficient to deplete them sufficiently to permit the two transcriptional activators to bind to PRD I and PRD II.

Induction by Double-stranded RNA

Another important interferon inducer is dsRNA. All naturally occurring dsRNAs are interferon inducers, including the dsRNAs of reoviruses, as well as synthetic double-stranded polyribonucleotides such as poly-rI:poly-rC (usually abbreviated to poly-IC). Neither single-stranded RNA (ssRNA) or DNA nor dsDNA or RNA-DNA hybrid molecules are interferon inducers. Resistance to ribonuclease greatly augments interferon-inducing ability; for example, the ribonuclease-resistant thiophosphate derivative of poly-AU is a much more effective interferon inducer than is poly-AU, and the activity of poly-IC is greatly enhanced if it is complexed with polycations such as diethylaminoethyl dextran (DEAE), methylated albumin, protamine, polylysine, or histone.

Inducibility by poly-IC is governed by the same sequence between positions −77 and −37 as inducibility by virus infection. In particular, the PRD I element responds to dsRNA, and dsRNA also markedly increases the levels of the cellular transcription factor NF-κB, possibly by releasing it from combination with an inhibitory factor, which then binds to and activates the PRD II element. It is of interest that PRD I is activated by interferon itself, which may be the basis of "priming"; that is, treatment of cells with very low amounts of interferon greatly increases interferon production when they are subsequently exposed to inducing agents (see below).

Induction by Metabolic Activators and Inhibitors

Yet another important group of interferon inducers comprises metabolic activators and inhibitors. In the former class are the substances that induce the formation of IFN-γ, namely, mitogens and lymphokines such as IL-2 for uncommitted lymphocytes. Another class of metabolic activators capable of inducing all classes of interferons in different cells are tumor promoters, in particular, tetradecanoyl phorbol acetate (TPA); other compounds in this class are butyrate, bromodeoxyuridine, dexamethasone, and dimethylsulfoxide.

Metabolic inhibitors such as inhibitors of mRNA formation and of protein synthesis also induce the formation of interferon. It was, in fact, the realization that induction of interferon synthesis does not require de novo protein synthesis that provided the first indication that the interferon gene normally is repressed by a labile repressor.

Other Interferon Inducers

There are numerous other substances that induce interferons, generally in small amounts relative to those induced by viral infection. Among them are bacterial endotoxin and bacteria such as *Brucella abortus* and *Listeria monocytogenes*, trachoma-inclusion conjunctivitis agents, mycoplasmas, protozoa, and rickettsiae; synthetic polymers such as pyran, polyacrylic acid, maleic anhydride-divinyl ether copolymer, and polyvinyl sulfate; and polysaccharides such as mannans, dextran sulfate, sulfated polysaccharides from seaweed, and phosphomannan. The feature common to all these compounds is that they are cytotoxic and inhibit protein synthesis more or less severely.

Differential Synthesis of Different Interferon Species

Since the regions flanking the various interferon genes are different and since interferon gene expression is controlled by cellular factors—the relative amounts of which differ in different cells—it is not surprising that the formation of the various interferon species, even individual species of IFN-α, is induced to markedly different levels by different inducers in different cells. Specific examples are lymphoblastoid cells, which may produce IFN-α or IFN-γ constitutively (see below) but also form IFN-β when induced; human fibroblasts, which produce IFN-α and IFN-β in response to virus infections but only IFN-β when induced with poly-IC; and L cells in which IFN-β is formed when they are treated with poly-IC but in which IFN-α is produced when they are infected with Newcastle disease virus (NDV).

It is worth noting in this connection that interferons are not the only proteins whose synthesis is induced by "interferon inducers." In fact, the synthesis of more than 20 other proteins has also been found to be induced. It is likely that these are all proteins whose synthesis is also more or less repressed in normal cells by labile repressors encoded by short-lived mRNAs.

Spontaneously Interferon-producing Cells

Normal cells, as a rule, do not contain or synthesize interferon. Interferon genes, however, are transcribed constitutively in some cells, particularly in T lymphoblastoid cell lines (51). Some produce IFN-γ, but most produce IFN-α in amounts that range from 100 to 1000 U/mL.

The molecular basis of spontaneous interferon formation appears to be a modified NRD I region (see above) to which repressor binds less strongly, or the synthesis of insufficient amounts of repressor, or the synthesis of defective repressor.

Antiviral Activity of Interferons

Interferons interfere with virus multiplication; this is the property for which they are named.

The nature of the mechanism by which interferons inhibit viral protein synthesis has been investigated intensively. Interferons themselves are not the proteins that actually inhibit virus multiplication; rather they induce the synthesis of proteins that are the actual effectors of the antiviral state. The antiviral state usually lasts for several days and then decays. After a further period of several days the antiviral state can then once again be induced.

In many systems interferon-induced inhibition of virus multiplication involves interference with the ability of parental or early viral mRNA molecules to be translated. As a result, no virus-specified proteins are synthesized, no progeny viral genomes are formed, and infection is aborted.

This effect of interferon is remarkably specific: cellular protein synthesis is unaffected, and viral protein synthesis is inhibited. The mechanism can even discriminate between simian virus 40 (SV40) mRNAs transcribed from free viral genomes that are not translated and SV40 mRNAs transcribed from SV40 DNA integrated into the host cell genome in transformed cells, the translation of which is not inhibited. This discrimination can even be achieved in the same cell. Any mechanism of interferon-induced viral protein synthesis inhibition must be able to account for the ability to discriminate between viral and cellular mRNAs.

In the mid-1970s two observations were made that provided explanations in molecular terms of how interferon might inhibit or prevent viral mRNA translation. One was the demonstration by Kerr and associates of an inhibitor of translation in extracts of interferon-treated cells and its identification as 2′,5′-oligoA; the other was the demonstration that at least two new proteins are phosphorylated in interferon-treated infected cells. In both cases interferon proved to trigger the synthesis of enzymes that were essentially absent in untreated cells (Fig. 58–10).

The 2′,5′-oligo(A) System

Exposure to interferon induces the synthesis of an enzyme, 2′,5′-oligo(A) synthetase, which, in the presence of dsRNA, converts ATP to 2′-5′-linked oligo(A) molecules up to 15 residues long, the trimer being the most abundant. This 2′,5′-oligo(A) then activates an endoribonuclease, RNase L, which is present in normal cells in a latent inactive state, and then apparently hydrolyzes viral mRNAs, thereby inhibiting viral protein synthesis.

Many aspects of the molecular biology of this 2′-5′-oligo(A) system are well established. For example, the location of the interferon-responsive element in the promoter of the 2′,5′-oligo(A) synthetase gene is known, as is the fact that it contains three protein-binding segments, including a constitutive enhancer, an interferon-activated enhancer, and a region that binds a putative repressor. Significantly, the various classes of interferon differ in their ability to induce the synthetase in different cells; in particular, type 1 interferons often induce higher levels of it than does IFN-γ. As for RNase L, it appears that it occurs in some cells in much higher amounts than in others, and in some cells interferon increases its level by as much as twentyfold. It is not specific for viral mRNA; in fact, in many interferon-treated infected cells ribosomal RNA is broken down extensively.

Two aspects of the 2′,5′-oligo(A) system that are still unexplained are the source of the dsRNA that activates the synthetase and the feature of it that enables it to discriminate between viral and cellular mRNAs (which RNase L cannot). With respect to the former, it is hypothesized that naked replicative intermediates of RNA-containing viruses, as well as complementary regions of opposite sense transcripts of adjacent genes in the genomes of dsDNA-containing viruses, might be responsible. With respect to the latter, it has been suggested that 2′,5′-oligo(A) formation may be highly localized, so that newly formed 2′,5′-oligo(A) would immediately be bound by and activate RNase L in its immediate vicinity.

The P1/eIF-2α Protein Kinase

Interferon also often induces the synthesis of a 68 kDa protein kinase (P68 or p68 kinase), which autophosphorylates in the presence of dsRNA and then phosphorylates the small subunit of protein synthesis initiation factor eIF-2 (eIF-2α) (Fig. 58–10), which prevents initiation of protein synthesis by the same series of reactions as were described on page 802. The problems with this explanation of how interferon inhibits viral protein synthesis are similar to those enumerated above; in particular, it is not known how this mechanism discriminates between host cell mRNA translation, which is not inhibited, and viral mRNA translation, which is inhibited. It is interesting in this regard that several viruses encode inhibitors of the 68 kDa protein kinase and therefore are resistant to interferon. One such inhibitor is a small RNA encoded by adenoviruses, VA_I RNA, which can assume a dsRNA-like structure and binds to the protein kinase, thereby preventing its activation by dsRNAs. As a result, adenovirus is resistant to interferon (but a deletion mutant of it that lacks the VA_I gene is sensitive). Vaccinia virus also encodes an inhibitor of the protein kinase, as well as of the 2′,5′-oligo(A) synthetase, which is thought to be a dsRNA-binding protein. Vaccinia

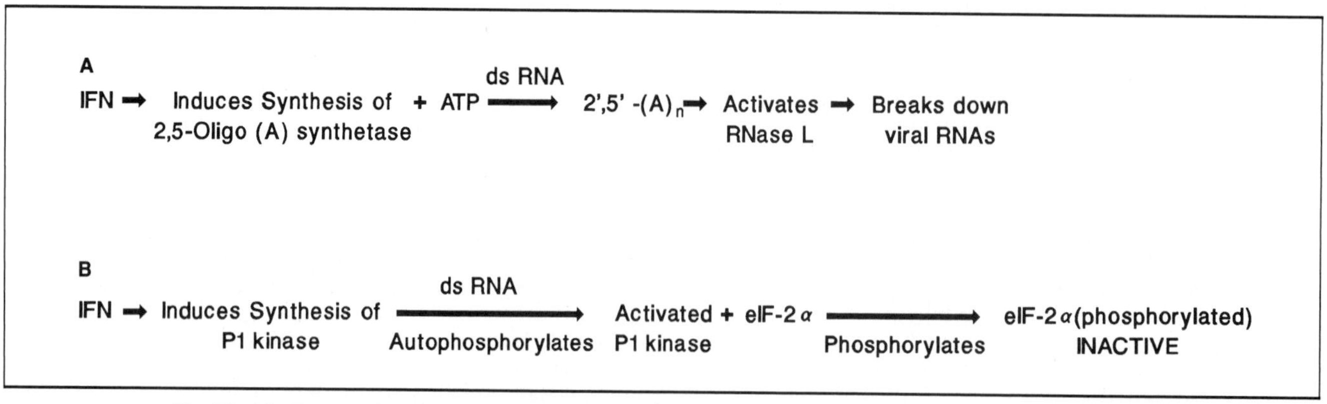

Fig. 58–10. Proposed mechanisms of action of interferon. **A.** The 2′,5′-oligo(A) system. **B.** The P1/eIF-2α protein kinase system. For details, see text.

virus, however, is sensitive to interferon in many types of cells. Influenza virus also regulates protein synthesis by inhibiting the protein kinase.

The Mx Protein

Mice possess an interferon-inducible gene, the Mx gene, which encodes a protein that prevents the multiplication of influenza viruses (and also of rhabdoviruses). In humans this gene, located on chromosome 21, encodes a homologous 76 kDa guanosine triphosphate (GTP)–binding protein. The precise function of the Mx proteins is not known. It is interesting, however, that a related G protein exists in yeast in which it functions during the sorting of proteins during secretion. G proteins are known to be involved in the secretory pathway.

Interferons as Cytokines and Lymphokines

Interferons were discovered and at first studied as antiviral agents. It then became clear, however, that they also affect and regulate a wide variety of cellular functions.

Interferons share the ability to induce, stimulate, and repress the expression of a bewilderingly wide variety of cellular genes with other members of a recently recognized family of small proteins known as *cytokines*. Cytokines mediate cell-cell communication. They are produced in one type of cell under the influence of a variety of stimuli that often include induction by other cytokines, are secreted, and then interact with receptors on other cells, regulating their proliferation and differentiation. Cytokines that are produced by cells of the immune system and affect immunomodulation are known as *lymphokines*. Cytokines and lymphokines often have antagonistic biologic effects; in fact, cellular homeostasis probably represents a balance between the effects caused by a variety of cytokines that together constitute what is known as the cytokine network.

The effects of interferons are exerted at plasma cell membranes by combination with specific glycoprotein receptors. There are two interferon receptors, one for type 1 interferons, the gene for which is located on chromosome 21, and the other for IFN-γ, the gene for which is located on chromosome 6. Interferons are rapidly internalized by receptor-mediated endocytosis and are rapidly transported to the nucleus. Genes whose transcription is turned on by interferons (interferon-stimulated genes, or ISGs) possess interferon-stimulated response elements (ISREs) in their promoters, the central regions of which are homologous to the PRD 1 element. Type 1 interferons activate ISREs by the induction of two proteins. One, interferon-stimulated gene factor 3 (ISGF-3), exists in normal cells in the form of two subunits, one of which is activated by interferon and thereby enabled to associate with the other. The synthesis of the other, ISGF-2, is induced by interferon. ISGF-3 rapidly activates the ISRE; ISGF-2 down-regulates it after several hours. IFN-γ acts like type 1 interferons in some cells—that is, rapidly and via ISGF-3—but in others acts more slowly, possibly by inducing the formation of one of the two components of ISGF-3, as well as of an additional protein, particularly in lymphocytes. IFN-γ does not induce the synthesis of ISGF-2, and therefore its antiviral effect is much longer lasting than that of type 1 interferons.

Interferons induce the expression of a large and seemingly disparate group of genes, all of which presumably possess ISREs in their promoters. They include not only the 2′,5′-oligo(A) synthetase, the P1/eIF-2α protein kinase, and the Mx protein, but also class I major histocompatibility complex (MHC) antigens, β_2-microglobulin, class II MHC antigens and Fc receptor, Ly-6 antigens, B cell and endothelial cell differentiation antigens, and many others of unknown function. Interferons also down-regulate many genes, probably by inducing the synthesis of transcriptional repressors or of proteins acting either posttranscriptionally or posttranslationally. Among such genes are various oncogenes, genes that encode various receptors, and genes that promote cell proliferation. Interferons therefore possess cell multiplication inhibitory activity.

Interferons, as components of the cytokine network, interact with many other cytokines and lymphokines. In IFN-β the cytokine characteristics predominate. For example, the antiviral effect of tumor necrosis factor (TNF) is due to its induction of IFN-β, and IFN-β plays a major role in the TNF-α–mediated increase of MHC class I antigens on cell surfaces; further, IFN-β is one of the agents capable of inducing the synthesis of IL-6, which was first designated IFN-β2. In IFN-α the lymphokine characteristics, not surprisingly, are expressed more strongly than in IFN-β, and IFN-γ is a powerful and versatile lymphokine. It possesses significant sequence homology with IL-2, is a macrophage activating factor (MAF), and as such enhances the synthesis of IL-1 and TNF-α, acts as a B cell maturation factor, activates natural killer (NK) cells, and functions in regulating antigen presentation. Because of its activation and mobilization of the immune system, IFN-γ is a major mediator of resistance to nonviral infectious agents such as *Toxoplasma gondii*, *Mycoplasma*, and even bacteria.

Prospects for Clinical Use

Many attempts have been made to exploit the powerful antiviral and cell regulatory properties of interferons in clinical situations. Although intranasal administration of type 1 interferons reduces the incidence of illness and infection after natural exposure to a variety of respiratory viruses, particularly rhinoviruses, it appears unlikely that interferons will find extensive use as antiviral agents in common non-life-threatening viral infections. Interferons, however, may be useful in life-threatening infections such as rabies, hemorrhagic fevers, and encephalitic infections, and they may also ameliorate or even eliminate persistent infections of hepatitis B virus, herpesvirus zoster, human papillomaviruses, and cytomegalovirus.

Intensive efforts have also been made to exploit the antiproliferative and immunomodulatory activities of interferons to treat human cancers. Table 58–3 lists the efficacies of interferon therapy for a variety of human tumors. The most sensitive tumor is hairy-cell leukemia (HCL), a rare B cell tumor, for which treatment with recombinant human IFN-α has been approved worldwide. Other interferon-sensitive tumors are chronic myelogenous leukemia (CML), cutaneous T cell lymphoma, Kaposi's sarcoma, and endocrine pancreatic neoplasms. Four aspects of the activity of interferons as anticancer agents are of particular interest. First, and most surprisingly, by far the most active type interferon is not IFN-γ but IFN-α. All the activities listed in Table 58–3 are those of IFN-α species. IFN-γ, a much more powerful lymphokine, is often highly effective in vitro, but, for reasons

TABLE 58–3. ANTITUMOR ACTIVITY OF α-INTERFERONS

Tumor	Percent Complete/ Partial Remissions
Hairy cell leukemia	90
Chronic myelocytic leukemia	90
T cell lymphoma	53
Kaposi's sarcoma	42
Endocrine pancreatic neoplasms	30
Non-Hodgkin's lymphomas	25–35
Renal carcinoma	10–25
Multiple myeloma	10–25
Breast carcinoma	0–25
Melanoma	3–20
Colon carcinoma	5
Bronchogenic carcinoma	0–2

From Quesada and Gutterman: J Int Res 7:575, 1987.

that are not clear, is rather ineffective clinically. Second, the interferon levels required are high (daily doses of 3 to 10 million units) and must be maintained for long periods of time. This used to be a problem but is no longer, because interferons can now be produced in large amounts through the use of highly efficient expression vectors (see above). Third, inasmuch as they are highly reactive molecules, interferons have undesirable side effects in humans, including uncontrollable nausea, anorexia, fatigue and malaise, myalgias, central nervous tissue toxicity, leukopenia, and renal and cardiac toxicity. Indeed, it has been suggested that many of the symptoms of influenza virus infections may be caused by interferon toxicity. Finally, because interferons are part of the cytokine network, the use of combination therapies involving interferons and other biologic response modifiers such as interleukins, TNF, and the like, may be a very promising avenue for future exploration.

Vaccines

The only currently feasible means of preventing diseases caused by viruses is through mobilization of the immune mechanism by means of vaccines. There are three types of antiviral vaccines: inactivated virus vaccines, attenuated active virus vaccines, and subunit vaccines.

Inactivated Virus Vaccines

The primary requirements for effective vaccines of this type are complete inactivation of infectivity coupled with minimum loss of antigenicity. These requirements are not easily met simultaneously because few reagents are available that inactive viral genomes—the source of infectivity—without also affecting viral proteins, the source of antigenicity. UV irradiation could accomplish this best but is inapplicable because virus inactivated in this manner is capable not only of expressing the functions of those genes that have not received lethal hits but also of undergoing multiplicity reactivation (Chap. 57). Photodynamic inactivation—in which virus is treated with dyes, such as neutral red, that are capable of intercalating between adjacent nucleic acid base pairs and is then irradiated with white light—inactivates viral nucleic acids efficiently and irreversibly without damaging viral proteins but suffers from similar drawbacks in that genes that have not received hits remain potentially functional. Beta-propiolactone is a potentially useful nucleic acid–inactivating agent but is a potent carcinogen. The best reagent for inactivating viral nucleic acids without compromising antigenicity is formaldehyde, which destroys infectivity by reacting with those amino groups of adenine, guanine, and cytosine that are not involved in base-pairing. Viruses that contain single-stranded nucleic acid are therefore inactivated readily, whereas those that contain double-stranded nucleic acid are not. At higher concentrations formaldehyde also reacts with amino groups in proteins, forming addition compounds of the Schiff's base type and cross-linking polypeptide chains. Reactions of this type are probably responsible for the occasional generation of formaldehyde-resistant infectious virus fractions. Careful control of reaction conditions and rigorous checks for residual infectious virus are mandatory for the preparation of formaldehyde-inactivated virus vaccines. The influenza virus vaccine currently in use is a vaccine of this type.

Attenuated Active Virus Vaccines

The second method of immunizing against viral pathogens is by administering attenuated virus strains, antibody against which neutralizes the pathogen. This is the principle on which Jenner's vaccination procedure against smallpox in 1798 was based; he inoculated with the relatively avirulent cowpox virus in order to induce antibodies against the highly virulent smallpox virus. Since then many attenuated virus vaccine strains have been developed, among them Theiler's yellow fever virus vaccine strain, the attenuated Sabin poliovirus vaccine strains, and attenuated measles, mumps, rubella, and adenovirus virus strains. The most commonly used method for isolating attenuated virus strains is by repeated passage of human pathogens in other host species, which results in the selection of multistep variants with drastically reduced virulence for humans.

Attenuated virus vaccines are effective in very small amounts, because the attenuated virus can multiply. This provides a powerful amplification effect: the viral progeny, rather than the virus in the inoculum, acts as the antigen. The attenuated vaccines also possess the advantage of stimulating the formation of all the correct types of antibody molecules (i.e., IgA and IgG).

Recombinant DNA technology has provided a powerful tool for improving attenuated virus vaccine strains. The genomes of many viruses have now been cloned, and many viral genes have been mapped. These include the genes responsible for specifying host range, tissue tropism, ability to spread and route of spread, efficiency of shedding, virulence, nature of cytopathic effects, capacity to establish latent or persistent infections, and immunogenicity. A wide variety of genetic techniques is now available for identifying and inactivating such genes. With their use, it should be possible to provide a new generation of safe and efficient active virus vaccines.

Subunit Vaccines

In recent years many of the viral proteins that elicit the formation of neutralizing antibodies have been identified and attempts have been made to use them as subunit vaccines. Such proteins are often very good antigens, but they do not, of course, elicit the formation of the same range of antibodies (such as secretory IgA and IgM) that infection with virus itself elicits. Still, they often provide very good protection. Here also the application of recombinant DNA technology is proving valuable. The genes of many of these proteins have now been cloned into expression vectors so that it is now much easier to isolate large amounts of these proteins than when they had to be isolated by dissociating virus particles or from infected cells.

Viral Vectors

The genes for many of the aforementioned proteins can be inserted into avirulent viral vectors such as vaccinia virus (Chap. 57). When these vectors are used to infect hosts, the inserted foreign genes are expressed without causing disease and the host develops antibodies to and immunity against the virus from which they were derived. The genes for many proteins that elicit the formation of neutralizing antibodies—from the HA gene of influenza virus to the glycoprotein B gene of herpesvirus and the surface antigen of HBV—have now been inserted into the thymidine kinase gene of vaccinia virus (which vaccinia virus does not need in order to multiply). In all cases, neutralizing antibodies against such viruses as influenza virus are formed when the recombinant vaccinia virus is used to infect animals. The major concern regarding this highly promising approach to inducing immunity against a wide variety of pathogenic viruses is the residual pathogenicity of vaccinia virus itself, which is not negligible in immunocompromised hosts and if the pathogenic agent whose gene it contains is not life threatening. It should not be impossible, however, to effect a substantial reduction of the pathogenicity of vaccinia virus. Inactivation of the thymidine kinase gene (into which the foreign gene is inserted) already reduces vaccinia virus pathogenicity markedly; inactivation of the vaccinia growth factor gene (p. 809) reduces it still further. In addition, genes such as those that encode IL-2 can also be cloned into vaccinia virus, which would greatly reduce the complications that arise in patients with an impaired immune system. Still further reductions of vaccinia virus pathogenicity along these lines are currently being explored.

FURTHER READING

Books and Reviews

ANTIVIRAL AGENTS

De Clercq ED: New acquisitions in the development of anti-HIV agents. Antiviral Res 12:1, 1989

Lentz TL: The recognition event between virus and host cell receptor: A target for antiviral agents. J Gen Virol 71:751, 1990

Montgomery JA: Approaches to antiviral chemotherapy. Antiviral Res 12:113, 1989

Rossmann MG: The structure of antiviral agents that inhibit uncoating when complexed with viral capsids. Antiviral Res 11:3, 1989

INTERFERON

Arnheiter H, Meier E: Mx proteins: Antiviral proteins by chance or by necessity? New Biologist 2:851, 1990

Billiau A: Redefining interferon: The interferon-like antiviral effects of certain cytokines (interleukin-1, interferon-β_2, interferon-γ) may be indirect or side effects. Antiviral Res 8:55, 1987

Levy D, Darnell JE Jr: Interferon-dependent transcriptional activation: Signal transduction without second messenger involvement? New Biologist 2:923, 1990

Samuel CE: Mechanisms of the antiviral action of interferons. Prog Nucleic Acid Res Mol Biol 35:29, 1988

Staeheli P: Interferon-induced proteins and the antiviral state. Adv Virus Res 38:147, 1990

Taylor JL, Grossberg SE: Recent progress in interferon research: Molecular mechanisms of regulation, action, and virus circumvention. Virus Res 15:1, 1990

VACCINES AND VECTORS

Piccini A, Paoletti E: Vaccinia: Virus, vector, vaccine. Adv Virus Res 34:43, 1988

Selected Papers

ANTIVIRAL AGENTS

Badger J, Krishnaswamy S, Kremer MJ, et al: Three-dimensional structures of drug-resistant mutants of human rhinovirus 14. J Mol Biol 207:163, 1989

Baltera RF Jr, Tershak DR: Guanidine-resistant mutants of poliovirus have distinct mutations in peptide 2C. J Virol 63:4441, 1989

Balzarini J, Naesens L, Herdewijn P, et al: Marked in vivo antiretrovirus activity of 9-(2-phosphonylmethoxyethyl)adenine, a selective anti-human immunodeficiency virus agent. Proc Natl Acad Sci USA 86:332, 1989

DeClercq E, Holy A, Rosenberg I: A novel selective broad-spectrum anti-DNA virus agent. Nature 323:464, 1986

Dubreuil M, Sportza L, D'Addario M, et al: Inhibition of HIV-1 transmission by interferon and 3′-azido-3′-deoxythymidine during de novo infection of promonocytic cells. Virology 179:388, 1990

Freitas VR, Fraser-Smith EB, Matthews TR: Increased efficacy of ganciclovir in combination with foscarnet against cytomegalovirus and herpes simplex virus type 2 in vitro and in vivo. Antiviral Res 12:205, 1989

Mul YM, van Miltenburg RT, De Clercq E, van der Vliet PC: Mechanism of inhibition of adenovirus DNA replication by the acyclic nucleoside triphosphate analogue (S)-HPMPApp: Influence of the adenovirus DNA binding protein. Nucleic Acids Res 17:8917, 1989

Neyts J, Snoeck R, Schols D, et al: Selective inhibition of human cytomegalovirus DNA synthesis by (S)-1-(3-hydroxy-2-phosphonylmethoxypropyl)cytosine [(S)-HPMPC] and 9-(1,3-dihydroxy-2-propoxymethyl)guanine (DHPG). Virology 178:41, 1990

Rankin JT Jr, Eppes SB, Antczak JB, Joklik WK: Studies on the mechanism of the antiviral activity of ribavirin against reovirus. Virology 168:147, 1989

Schols D, Pauwels R, Desmyter J, De Clercq E: Dextran sulfate and other polyanionic anti-HIV compounds specifically interact with the viral gp120 glycoprotein expressed by T-cells persistently infected with HIV-1. Virology 175:556, 1990

Shirasaka T, Murakami K, Ford H Jr, et al: Lipophilic halogenated congeners of 2′,3′-dideoxypurine nucleosides active against human immunodeficiency virus in vitro. Proc Natl Acad Sci USA 87:9426, 1990

Wray SK, Smith RHA, Gilbert BE, Knight V: Effects of selenazofurin and ribavirin and their 5′-triphosphates on replicative functions of influenza A and B viruses. Antimicrob Agents Chemother 29:67, 1986

Zeichhardt H, Otto MJ, McKinlay MA, et al: Inhibition of poliovirus uncoating by disoxaril (WIN 51711). Virology 160:281, 1987

NEW APPROACHES

Brücher KH, Garten W, Klenk HD, et al: Inhibition of endoproteolytic cleavage of cytomegalovirus (HCMV) glycoprotein B by palmitoyl-peptidyl-chloromethyl ketone. Virology 178:617, 1990

Garten W, Stieneke A, Shaw E, et al: Inhibition of proteolytic activation of influenza virus hemagglutinin by specific peptidyl chloroalkyl ketones. Virology 172:25, 1989

Kulka M, Smith CC, Aurelian L, et al: Site specificity of the inhibitory effects of oligo(nucleoside methylphosphonate)s complementary to the acceptor splice junction of herpes simplex virus type 1 immediate early mRNA 4. Proc Natl Acad Sci USA 86:6868, 1989

McClements W, Yamanaka G, Garsky V, et al: Oligopeptides inhibit the ribonucleotide reductase of herpes simplex virus by causing subunit separation. Virology 162:270, 1988

Till MA, Ghetie V, Gregory T, et al: HIV-infected cells are killed by rCD4-ricin A chain. Science 242:1166, 1988

INTERFERONS

Bischoff JR, Samuel CE: Mechanism of interferon action: Activation of the human P1/eIF-2α protein kinase by individual reovirus s-class mRNAs. s1 mRNA is a potent activator relative to s4 mRNA. Virology 172:106, 1989

Coccia EM, Romeo G, Nissim A, et al: A full-length murine 2-5A synthetase cDNA transfected in NIH-3T3 cells impairs EMCV but not VSV replication. Virology 179:228, 1990

Driggers PH, Ennist DL, Gleason SL, et al: An interferon γ-regulated protein that binds the interferon-inducible enhancer element of major histocompatibility complex class I genes. Proc Natl Acad Sci USA 87:3743, 1990

Dron M, Lacasa M, Tovey MG: Priming affects the activity of a specific region of the promoter of the human beta interferon gene. Mol Cell Biol 10:854, 1990

Fan C-M, Maniatis T: Two different virus-inducible elements are required for human β-interferon gene regulation. EMBO J 8:101, 1989

Fu X-Y, Kessler DS, Veals SA, et al: ISGF3, the transcriptional activator induced by interferon α, consists of multiple interacting polypeptide chains. Proc Natl Acad Sci USA 87:8555, 1990

Horisberger MA, McMaster GK, Zeller H, et al: Cloning and sequence analyses of cDNAs for interferon- and virus-induced human Mx proteins reveal that they contain putative guanine nucleotide-binding sites: Functional study of the corresponding gene promoter. J Virol 64:1171, 1990

Kitajewski J, Schneider RJ, Safer B, et al: Adenovirus VA1 RNA antagonizes the antiviral action of interferon by preventing activation of the interferon-induced eIF-2α kinase. Cell 45:195, 1986

Levy DE, Lew DJ, Decker T, et al: Synergistic interaction between interferon-α and interferon-γ through induced synthesis of one subunit of the transcription factor ISGF3. EMBO J 9:1105, 1990

Lew DJ, Decker T, Darnell JE Jr: Alpha interferon and gamma interferon stimulate transcription of a single gene through different signal transduction pathways. Mol Cell Biol 9:5404, 1989

Pavlovic J, Zürcher T, Haller O, Staeheli P: Resistance to influenza virus and vesicular stomatitis virus conferred by expression of human MxA protein. J Virol 64:3370, 1990

Pine R, Decker T, Kessler DS, et al: Purification and cloning of interferon-stimulated gene factor 2 (ISGF2): ISGF2 (IRF-1) can bind to the promoters of both beta interferon- and interferon-stimulated genes but is not a primary transcriptional activator of either. Mol Cell Biol 10:2448, 1990

Rothman JH, Raymond CK, Gilbert T, et al: A putative GTP binding protein homologous to interferon-inducible Mx proteins performs an essential function in yeast protein sorting. Cell 61:1063, 1990

Shan B, Vazquez E, Lewis JA: Interferon selectively inhibits the expression of mitochondrial genes: A novel pathway for interferon-mediated responses. EMBO J 9:4307, 1990

Visvanathan KV, Goodbourn S: Double-stranded RNA activates binding of NF-κB to an inducible element in the human β-interferon promoter. EMBO J 8:1129, 1989

VACCINES AND VECTORS

Bolognesi DP: Immunobiology of the human immunodeficiency virus envelope and its relationship to vaccine strategies. Mol Biol Med 7:1, 1990

Chambers TM, Kawaoka Y, Webster RG: Protection of chickens from lethal influenza infection by vaccinia-expressed hemagglutinin. Virology 167:414, 1988

Esposito JJ, Knight JC, Shaddock JH, et al: Successful oral rabies vaccination of raccoons with raccoon poxvirus recombinants expressing rabies virus glycoprotein. Virology 165:313, 1988

Flexner C, Hügin A, Moss B: Prevention of vaccinia virus infection in immunodeficient mice by vector-directed IL-2 expression. Nature 330:259, 1987

Mason PW, Pincus S, Fournier MJ, et al: Japanese encephalitis virus—vaccinia recombinants produce particulate forms of the structural membrane proteins and induce high levels of protection against lethal JEV infection. Virology 180:294, 1991

Morrison HG, Bauer SP, Lange JV, et al: Protection of guinea pigs from Lassa fever by vaccinia virus recombinants expressing the nucleoprotein or the envelope glycoproteins of Lassa virus. Virology 171:179, 1989

Murphy BR, Prince GA, Collins PL, et al: Current approaches to the development of vaccines effective against parainfluenza and respiratory syncytial viruses. Virus Res 11:1, 1988

CHAPTER 59

Tumor Viruses

Origins of Tumor Virology

Characteristics of Virus-transformed Cells

- **Possession of Viral Genome**
- **Tumorigenicity**
- **Morphology**
- **Changes in Growth Patterns**
- **Ability to Form Colonies in Soft Agar**
- **Changes in Membrane Transport Properties**
- **Acquisition of New Surface Antigens**
- **Increased Agglutinability by Lectins**
- **Changes in Chemical Composition of Plasma Cell Membrane Components**
- **Decreased Levels of Cyclic AMP**
- **Increased Secretion of Plasminogen Activator**
- **Chromosomal Changes**

DNA Tumor Viruses

Papillomaviruses

Polyomaviruses

- **Transformation by Polyomaviruses**
- **Function of Polyomavirus Tumor Antigens**
- **Rescue of Integrated Polyomavirus Genomes**
- **Revertants of Transformed Cells**

Adenoviruses

Herpesviruses

Epstein-Barr Virus

- **EBV as Human Tumor Virus: Its Role in Etiology of Burkitt's Lymphoma and Nasopharyngeal Carcinoma**

Herpes Simplex Virus Type 2 and Human Cytomegalovirus

Poxviruses

Hepatitis B Virus

Retroviruses

Nature of Retrovirus Particles

Retrovirus Genome

Molecular Biology of Retroviruses

- **Formation and Integration of Proviral DNA**
- **Transcription of Integrated Proviral DNA**

Biology of Retroviruses

Host Range

- **Interference**

Transmission

Endogenous Retroviruses

Basis of Tumorigenicity of Retroviruses

Sarcoma–Acute Leukemia Viruses

Transforming Genes: Oncogenes

Proto-Oncogenes

Nature and Functions of Proteins Encoded by *onc* Genes

Growth Factors

Transmembrane Growth Factor Receptors with Tyrosine-specific Protein Kinase Activity

Membrane-bound Tyrosine-specific Protein Kinases

Membrane-bound G Proteins

Cytoplasmic Serine-Threonine-specific Protein Kinases

Nuclear Factors Involved in Regulating Gene Expression, DNA Replication, or Cell Division

Oncogenes with Miscellaneous Functions

Antioncogenes

- **Interactions Between Antioncogenes and "Oncogenes" of DNA-containing Viruses**

Cooperation Between Oncogenes and Antioncogenes in Multistep Progression Toward Tumorigenesis

How Do Retroviruses that Lack Oncogenes Cause Cancer?

Proviral Insertion

Recombination with Endogenous Viral Genomes: MCF Viruses

Mechanisms Causing Overexpression of Proto-Oncogenes

- **Chromosomal Translocation**
- **Oncogenes in Amplified DNA**

Mouse Mammary Tumor Virus

Human Retroviruses

Human T Cell Leukemia Virus Types I and II

Human Immunodeficiency Viruses

- **Replication of HIV**
- **Genome of HIV**
- **Role of Other Viral Infections in HIV Infections**
- **Prospects for Prevention and Control of HIV Infections**

Human Endogenous Retroviruses

Nature and Function of Retroposons

Intracisternal A-type Particles

VL30 Elements

Retroposons in *Drosophila*

Ty Elements of Yeast

Viruses are at the forefront of a large effort that is being devoted to discovering how normal cells are transformed into cancer cells; they are at the cutting edge of studies of the mechanisms of tumorigenesis. There are two reasons for this. First, infection with tumor viruses is capable of transforming *all* cells in a population into potential tumor cells; with all other agents the frequency of transformation is far lower. As a result, virus-induced transformation can be studied at the biochemical and molecular level, but transformation caused by other agents cannot. Second, mutants of tumor viruses exist that cannot transform or maintain the transformed state at nonpermissive temperatures (typically at 38C and above) but can do both at permissive temperatures (typically at 35C and below). Cell transformation is therefore a function of a *single viral gene*. Clearly it should be possible to identify such genes and the proteins that they encode, determine their functions, identify their targets, and thereby gain insight into the basic reactions that cause normal cells to be converted to tumor cells. Such studies are impossible with any other carcinogenic agent.

Both RNA-containing and DNA-containing viruses can cause various types of neoplasms in animals and in humans. Awareness of the principles of tumor virology is therefore very important for the medical practitioner.

Origins of Tumor Virology

The concept that infectious agents may be involved etiologically in the cancer process was advanced as early as 1908 by Ellerman and Bang, who observed that the mode of transmission of leukemia in the fowl was similar to that of an infectious disease. Shortly thereafter Rous demonstrated that the infectious agent in avian sarcomas could pass through filters that would not permit passage of bacteria. For many years this discovery remained an isolated finding until in 1932 Shope discovered in wild cottontail rabbits a viral agent that transmitted a wartlike growth not only to cottontail but also to domestic rabbits. Although most warts in cottontails remain benign or regress, those in domestic rabbits sometimes develop into highly malignant carcinomas. Then in 1938 Bittner discovered in mammary gland tumors of mice the mammary tumor virus, or milk factor, a virus that is passed from mother to offspring through suckling. The finding that, more than any other, elicited the upsurge of interest in viruses as carcinogenic agents was the discovery by Gross in 1951 of a virus that induces leukemia in mice, a disease that is remarkably similar to leukemia in humans. Efforts to develop animal models applicable to the human disease have resulted in the isolation of a large number of viruses that cause many kinds of cancers in every major group of animals.

Characteristics of Virus-transformed Cells

Discussion of the virus-cell interaction up to this point has focused on the lytic interaction, which involves multiplication of the virus and destruction of the host cell. However, certain DNA viruses can interact with cells not only by means of the lytic interaction, but also by means of an interaction in which virus multiplication is repressed and the host cell is not destroyed. In this type of interaction the viral DNA either is integrated into the genome of the host cell or replicates as a plasmid. In either case a new entity, the transformed or tumor cell, is created that can multiply indefinitely.

In addition, a family of RNA-containing viruses, the retroviruses, can also transform cells and cause tumors. At first, the problem of how viral RNA could be integrated into the host genome presented a major conceptual hurdle. This was overcome by the discovery in retroviruses of a DNA polymerase that transcribes their RNA into DNA; this is the so-called reverse transcriptase. It is the DNA transcribed from viral RNA by this enzyme that is integrated into the cellular genome.

Transformed or tumor cells differ from normal cells in several important respects; since these changes are at the genetic level, they are passed on to the cells' descendants. Discussion of the principal properties in which virus-transformed cells differ from normal ones follows.

Possession of Viral Genome

Transformed cells contain either the whole or a part of the genome of the virus that causes the transformation. More often than not, this genome is integrated into the cell DNA, but in the nuclei of some transformed cells it may exist as a free plasmidlike entity. The extent to which viral genetic information is expressed in transformed cells varies widely, from full expression, with resultant formation of progeny virus particles, to complete silence, as judged by the absence of messenger RNA transcribed from it or proteins encoded by it.

Tumorigenicity

Transformed cells generally give rise to tumors when injected into animals, particularly immunosuppressed or immunologically deficient animals such as athymic nude mice. Like naturally occurring tumors, the various lines of virus-transformed cells exhibit wide variations in invasiveness. Even large numbers of some types of transformed cells produce only benign tumors at the site of infection; but even small numbers of others give rise to highly invasive cancers.

Morphology

Normal and transformed cells differ in morphology. There are two major differences. First, transformed cells are usually more rounded and refractile than normal cells; second, normal and transformed cells differ in the orientation of cells relative to each other. Normal cells usually arrange themselves in regular patterns, but transformed cells tend to orient themselves randomly (Fig. 59–1; see also Fig. 52–5).

Changes in Growth Patterns

Most types of untransformed cells grow in vitro to a certain cell density; cell division ceases (or almost ceases) when a monolayer of uniformly spread cells has formed. Under the same conditions, transformed cells continue to divide so that very much higher cell densities are attained. This alteration of growth patterns is due primarily to two factors: loss of contact inhibition and reduction in the requirement for serum.

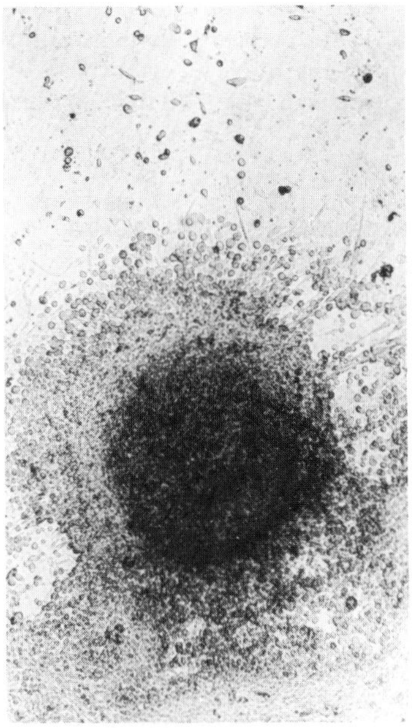

Fig. 59–1. Focus of chick embryo fibroblasts transformed with Rous sarcoma virus. Note drastically altered morphology and growth pattern of the transformed cells, which are densely piled on top of one another in the center of the focus. (*Courtesy of Dr. P.K. Vogt.*)

LOSS OF CONTACT INHIBITION. When an untransformed cell comes into contact with another cell, the rapid movement of pseudopodia (ruffles) that are constantly extended and retracted ceases, and forward movement is arrested. At the same time the cell stops dividing. This dual phenomenon is known as contact inhibition. The ability to respond to contact with other cells ensures that any given cell grows only in its appropriate location within the organism and does not proliferate unless it receives a signal that more of its kind are needed for the organism's orderly growth or maintenance.

Transformed cells are always much less susceptible to contact inhibition than their untransformed counterparts. Loss of contact inhibition represents release from normal controls over multiplication; it accounts in part for unregulated cell growth in the organism. Some transformed cells, such as the cells of benign tumors, have lost only the ability to respond to contact with each other but are still inhibited by contact with other cell types; others, such as those of metastasizing tumors, respond to contact neither with each other nor with other types of cells.

REDUCTION IN REQUIREMENT FOR SERUM. Contact inhibition is not the only factor that limits cell growth. The addition of serum to nondividing, contact-inhibited monolayers of untransformed cells often results in further rounds of division so that cells may actually pile up on top of one another. Virus transformation markedly reduces cellular serum dependence; transformed cells require much less serum to initiate division than do untransformed cells. For example, NIH 3T3 cells, a line of mouse fibroblasts, will not grow optimally unless the serum concentration is greater than 5%. By contrast, NIH 3T3 cells transformed with simian virus 40 (SV40) can divide to a small but significant extent in serum concentrations as low as 0.5%. The nature of the serum factors required by cells and how these factors act are not known. It is hoped that studying them will hasten the deciphering of the signals that guide cells through their growth cycles.

Ability to Form Colonies in Soft Agar

Untransformed cells of fibroblast origin must attach to a solid surface before they can divide; this requirement is known as *anchorage dependence of multiplication*. By contrast, transformed cells will divide in suspension culture. In particular, the ability to grow and form colonies when suspended in soft (0.5%) agar (Fig. 59–2) provides not only a very useful test for the stably transformed state, but also the basis for a selective procedure that permits the isolation of transformed cells from populations of predominantly untransformed ones.

Changes in Membrane Transport Properties

Simple sugars and other nutrients are transported several times more rapidly across the plasma membrane of trans-

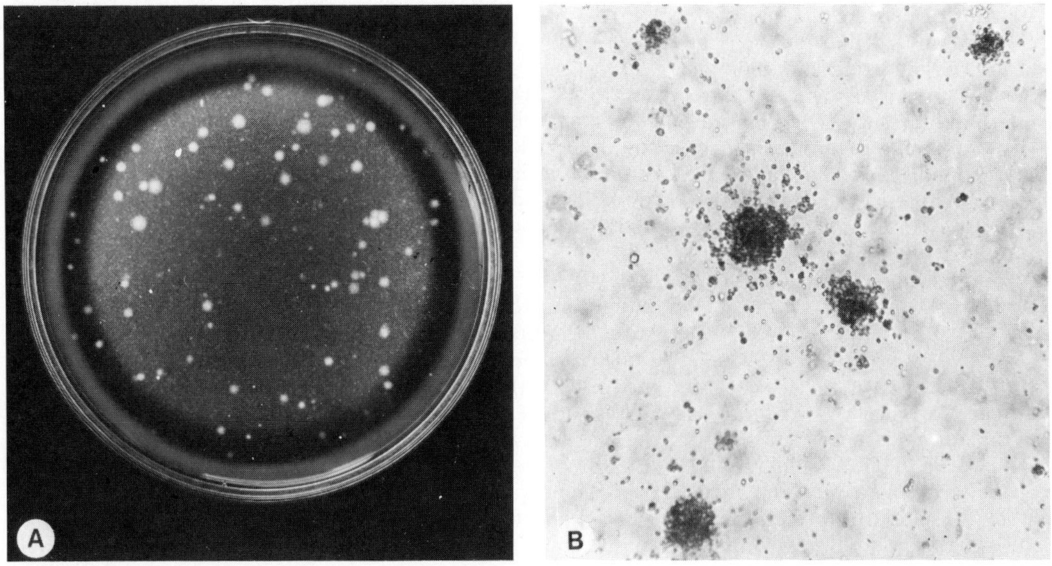

Fig. 59–2. Suspension colonies in soft agar of chick embryo fibroblasts transformed with Rous sarcoma virus. **A.** Numerous colonies 14 days after infection and plating. **B.** Enlargement of several colonies (8 days after infection and plating). (*Courtesy of Dr. Thomas Graf.*)

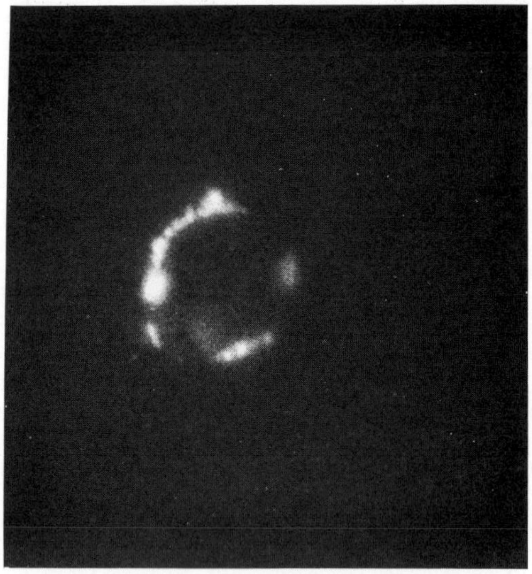

Fig. 59–3. Demonstration, by means of immunofluorescence, of the tumor-specific transplantation antigen (TSTA) on a cell derived from a tumor induced in hamsters with adenovirus type 12. The cell was treated first with a hamster antiserum to such cells and then with rabbit anti-hamster immunoglobulin conjugated with fluorescein isothiocyanate. The hamster antiserum was prepared by repeated injection of adenovirus type 12, followed by one injection of tumor cells. Note the annular pattern of specific fluorescence on the cell membrane. TSTA on cells transformed with papovaviruses can be demonstrated by analogous procedures. (*From Vascencelos-Costa: J Gen Virol 8:69, 1970.*)

formed than of untransformed cells. This is generally the earliest observable change after transformation. It is conceivable that increased sugar transport into transformed cells is responsible, at least in part, for the increased rate of glycolysis that is generally observed in transformed cells.

Acquisition of New Surface Antigens

The surfaces of virus-transformed cells possess antigenic determinants not present on untransformed cells. These new surface antigens can be detected by immunofluorescence (Fig. 59–3) or by tests for cytotoxic and cell-mediated immunologic responses. Indeed, their presence causes transformed cells to be recognized as foreign and therefore subject to immune surveillance. Most of these new antigenic determinants are virus specified; some may be encoded by the host genome. Among the mechanisms that may cause new host-specified antigens to manifest themselves after transformation are derepression of genes that do not normally express themselves and unmasking or exposure of determinants that are not normally apparent.

Increased Agglutinability by Lectins

Many animal cells are agglutinated by certain glycoproteins and proteins that are present in plant seeds, snails, crabs, and some fish and that possess affinity for sugars in general and glycoproteins in particular; they are collectively known as *lectins* (or *agglutinins*). Some of these lectins preferentially agglutinate tumor cells. The two lectins that best discriminate between normal and transformed cells are the jack bean agglutinin concanavalin A (Con A) and wheat germ agglutinin (WGA). They agglutinate tumor cells more efficiently than normal cells because their receptors are dispersed in the latter but clustered in the former.

Changes in Chemical Composition of Plasma Cell Membrane Components

Whereas the protein composition of plasma membranes appears to be fairly constant, their lipid, glycolipid, and glycoprotein carbohydrate components are notoriously variable; they are exquisitely sensitive to changes in the medium, changes in the cell growth rate, and changes in growth conditions in general. It is difficult, therefore, to pick out changes attributable to transformation, but the following appear to be significant:

1. When untransformed cells become density (contact) inhibited, their glycolipids become larger and more complex. Transformed cells do not exhibit this cell density–dependent glycolipid extension response. Fucose-, galactose-, and *N*-acetyl neuraminic acid (NANA)–containing glycolipids are present in transformed cells in smaller amounts than in untransformed cells and are smaller in size.
2. Changes of a similar but opposite nature occur in the oligosaccharides of glycoproteins; in transformed cells these groups are larger than in untransformed cells, and they contain more NANA (which always occupies a terminal position).
3. One of the major components of plasma membranes of normal cells is fibronectin, a large polymorphic glycoprotein (subunit mol wt 200 to 250 kDa). Fibronectin possesses affinity for collagen, fibrin, heparin, and cell surfaces. Transformed cells usually, but not always, lack this protein, which is also known as LETS (large external transformation-sensitive) protein. Its absence may decrease cell-cell and cell-tissue matrix interactions; its absence may also increase membrane fluidity, thereby facilitating access to nutrients (thus lowering the requirement for serum) and lateral movement of membrane components (which would explain the increased agglutinability by lectins).

Decreased Levels of Cyclic AMP

In normal cells the level of cyclic AMP increases as they reach confluence; lowering the concentration of serum in the medium has a similar effect. Transformed cells generally possess lower levels of cyclic AMP than normal ones, and lowering the serum concentration fails to elevate these levels.

Increased Secretion of Plasminogen Activator

Most cells produce small amounts of a protease, known as *plasminogen activator*, which converts plasminogen to plasmin, the protease that digests fibrin. Many, but not all, transformed cells produce very much more plasminogen activator than their normal counterparts. The significance of this increased level of protease production is not clear. Since normal cells produce less plasminogen activator when contact inhibited than when growing and since tumor cells are less subject to contact inhibition than normal cells, production of high levels of plasminogen activator may play a role in cell growth stimulation.

Chromosomal Changes

Transformation generally results in changes in karyotype. Among the most common changes are deletion of portions of some chromosomes, duplication or amplification of portions of others, translocation of material from one chromosome to another, and duplication of entire chromosomes.

Members of six virus families are known to be tumorigenic and capable of transforming cultured cells. The manner in which transformation by these viruses is established, maintained, transmitted, and detected will now be described.

DNA Tumor Viruses

Papillomaviruses

Papillomaviruses cause both benign and malignant tumors in a wide variety of animals. For example, the Shope papilloma virus induces skin warts in rabbits that transform into squamous cell carcinomas; and in cattle, bovine papilloma viruses induce upper alimentary tract papillomas that convert to carcinomas, adenomas and adenocarcinomas of the intestine, urinary bladder tumors, meningiomas, fibropapillomas, penile and esophageal papillomas, and urinary bladder papillomas.

To date, more than 50 types of human papillomavirus (HPV) have been isolated (see Table 53–4). They are classified by degree of genetic relatedness: If the DNAs of two isolates hybridize to less than 50% under standard conditions, they are regarded as different types. Based on sequence comparison, the degree of relatedness of HPVs ranges from more than 95% to less than 20%.

The capsid of HPVs consists of several proteins, one of which (mol wt 57 kDa) accounts for 80% of the total viral protein and possesses genus-specific epitopes. Several smaller proteins are also present, which may contain the species-specific epitopes that are located on the virion surface.

The various HPV serotypes cause a variety of lesions (Table 59–1). Many form benign warts, but some give rise to transformed cells that eventually progress to malignant carcinomas. The HPV-associated human malignancy on which most attention is focused at this time is cervical intraepithelial neoplasia (CIN), which can progress to carcinoma of the cervix. Worldwide, where it is the most frequent female malignancy (24% of all cancers), about 500,000 new cases of invasive cancer of the cervix occur annually; in the United States it accounts for 7% of all female cancers (4800 deaths annually).

Elucidation of the mechanism by which HPVs cause cancers is made more difficult by the fact that they do not grow in cultured cells. The HPV genome is about 7900 base pairs long and, like that of all papovaviruses, circular. At least 9 have been sequenced so far, and although the organization of their genomes is similar, the exact locations and lengths of the various open reading frames (ORFs) are different for each. The genome organization of HPV-16, the HPV most commonly associated with cervical carcinoma, is shown in Figure 59–4. It is remarkably complex. There are at least eight ORFs, all on the same strand but in different reading frames and overlapping extensively; they are transcribed, using at least six promoters, into transcripts that are extensively spliced. Six of these ORFs, E1 to E7 (there is no E3), encode regulatory proteins; two, L1 and L2, encode structural proteins. Only the former are transcribed in transformed cells. The protein encoded by E1 is a DNA-binding protein; the E2 protein is an enhancer-binding protein; E4 may encode a later nonstructural cytoplasmic protein; and the E6 and E7 proteins, which are 158 and 98 amino acids long, respectively, together constitute the papillomavirus "oncogene." The evidence for this is that the E6 protein in conjunction with the E7 protein (which is also a transactive transcriptional activator) transforms cells such as human foreskin keratinocytes. The mechanisms by which these two proteins achieve this is that they bind to two cellular proteins, the p53 protein (E6) and the retinoblastoma (Rb) gene product $p110^{Rb}$ (E7). These two proteins suppress cell division and proliferation, presumably by controlling the expression of certain critical genes; when they are removed, uncontrolled growth results. The genes that encode

TABLE 59–1. LESIONS IN HUMANS CAUSED BY HPVs

Lesions	HPV Type	Comment
Plantar warts	1	
Common warts	2, 27, 29, 54; 4	
Flat warts	3, 10, 28, 41	
Butcher's warts	7, 40	Common warts on the hands of butchers
Reddish brown (macular) plaques of epidermodysplasia verruciformis	5, 8, 12, 14, 19–23, 25, 36, 46, 47, 49; 9, 15, 17; 37, 38; 24	May become malignant in light-exposed areas
Anogenital warts (condyloma); laryngeal papillomas	6, 11	Anogenital warts (vagina, vulva, rarely the cervix, penis, anus, perineum) are a commonly transmitted disease; respiratory papillomatosis, with malignant transformation, is a rare disease probably acquired at birth
Cervical intraepithelial neoplasia (CIN) and cervical cancer		Lower genital tract cancers
Strong association	16; 18	
Moderate association	31, 33, 35, 45, 51, 52, 56	

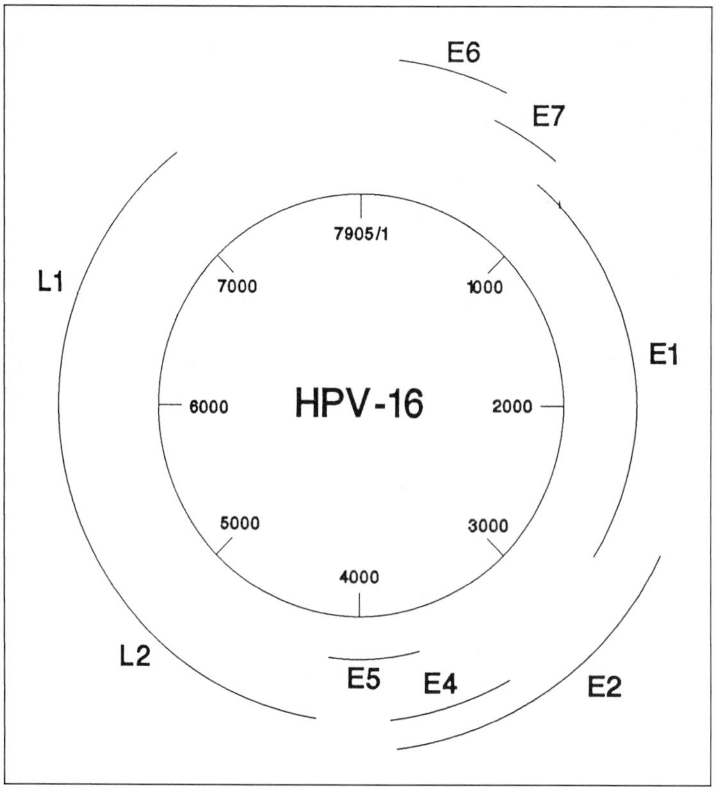

Fig. 59–4. Genetic and transcription map of HPV 16.

p53 and p110^{Rb} are therefore known as *growth* or *tumor suppressor genes* or *antioncogenes* (see p. 892).

Although E6 together with E7 ORF expression is capable of transforming cultured cells, it is not clear whether HPVs *alone* are capable of causing tumors or whether and to what extent cofactors are involved. Both episomal and integrated forms of HPV-16 DNA are associated with invasive cervical carcinomas, whatever the clinical tumor stage. Both forms are amplified by treating cells with the mutagen *N*-methyl-*N′*-nitroso-*N*-nitrosoguanidine (MNNG), irradiating them with ultraviolet light, or infecting them with herpes simplex virus type 1, all of which can thus be regarded as tumor formation cofactors. Significantly, the ability of the HPV-16 E6 plus E7 proteins to transform cells is also increased by cofactors, specifically the presence of the *ras* oncogene (see p. 893). Thus although almost 100% of cervical biopsies that contain precancerous changes contain HPV DNA, the question of whether HPVs themselves cause cancer or whether they do so in conjunction with cofactors—chemical, physical, or viral—remains open.

Polyomaviruses

Polyoma virus, isolated from mice, only rarely causes tumors in nature. When injected into newborn mice or hamsters, it produces a wide variety of histologically distinguishable tumors, hence its name.

SV40 was first isolated from apparently normal cultures of monkey kidney cells. The only host in which it causes tumors (lymphocytic leukemia, lymphosarcoma, reticulum cell sarcoma, and osteogenic sarcoma) is the baby hamster.

There are also two human polyomaviruses: BK virus and JC virus (*BK* and *JC* are the initials of the individuals from whom they were isolated in 1971). BKV was isolated from the urine of an immunosuppressed renal transplant patient, whereas JCV was isolated from the brain of a patient with progressive multifocal leukoencephalopathy (PML). They are quite distinct from each other; both are related more closely to SV40 than to polyoma virus. Both viruses are very widespread in humans; infection occurs in childhood, and most adults have antibodies to them. Apparently primary infections are asymptomatic and are followed by low-grade lifelong persistent infections that are activated when the immune system is compromised. The viruses then establish silent foci of infection in the urinary tract, which causes them to be excreted in the urine; and in a very few individuals JCV reaches oligodendrocytes in the brain and causes PML, a chronic, fatal demyelinating disease. Interestingly, a very similar disease occurs in rhesus monkeys, the natural host of SV40; and two human PML cases have yielded SV40 rather than JCV.

Both BKV and JCV possess oncogenic potential; both transform cultured cells and cause tumors in a variety of animals. Both are markedly neurotropic; thus JCV induces brain tumors in owl monkeys, and most of the tumors caused by BKV in Syrian hamsters are ependymomas, whereas JCV shows a predeliction for neuroectodermal cells. However, neither virus is associated with any form of cancer in humans.

Transformation by Polyomaviruses

Polyomaviruses not only interact with cells by means of the lytic pathway (Chap. 55) but also transform cells. Cells are transformed if they are nonpermissive; or if they are permissive, they can be transformed if they are infected with defective virus particles such as the deletion mutants that arise with repeated passage at high multiplicity (Chap. 57) or if they are infected with inactivated virus particles (e.g., by photodynamic inactivation). In other words, if a polyomavirus can multiply in a cell, that cell will in general not be transformed; if it cannot multiply, the cell may be transformed. The establishment of the transforming papovavirus–cell interaction requires high multiplicities of infection (10^6 to 10^7 particles per cell). There is evidence that the frequency of transformation is enhanced, by some as yet unknown mechanism, by treating cells with chemical carcinogens such as 4-nitroquinoline-1-oxide. The essential feature of the transforming polyomavirus-cell interaction is that viral DNA becomes stably integrated into the DNA of the host cell. As a result, it cannot multiply except as a cellular gene, and no progeny virus is produced.

Polyomavirus DNA can integrate at many sites in the cellular genome. The number of integrated viral genomes generally varies from one to three but can be as high as 20 to 50. Integration of the genome of one polyomavirus does not preclude integration of the genome of another or of genomes of unrelated viruses. Thus double transformants of SV40 and polyoma, of SV40 and adenovirus, and of SV40 and various retroviruses have been isolated and studied.

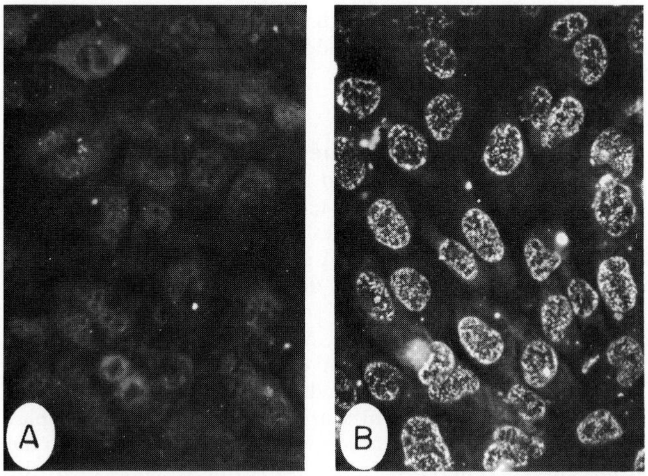

Fig. 59–5. Demonstration of the SV40 large T antigen by means of immunofluorescence. Cells from a tumor induced by SV40 in a hamster were exposed to fluorescein-conjugated serum from a non-tumor-bearing hamster, **A**, and a tumor-bearing hamster, **B**. ×280. *(From Rapp, Butel, Melnick: Proc Soc Exp Biol Med 116:1131, 1964.)*

Function of Polyomavirus Tumor Antigens

Although viral DNA in transformed cells does not replicate except as part of the host genome, it does express itself. However, not the entire viral genome is transcribed but only that portion of it that encodes the early functions, that is, the various tumor antigens (large T and small t in the case of SV40 and large T, middle T, and small t antigens in the case of polyoma virus [Chap. 55]). These proteins are responsible for the induction and maintenance of the transformed state, and much work has been carried out to define their functions; clearly, knowledge of these functions could provide fundamentally important clues concerning the mechanisms by which normal cells are transformed into cancer cells. This work has permitted the following conclusions:

1. Three functions contribute to the cell-transforming activity of large T antigen. First, large T antigen (Fig. 59–5) stimulates host cell DNA synthesis, a function that can be separated from its ability to initiate viral DNA replication. Second, it is a transactive transcriptional activator capable of initiating the transcription of inappropriate cellular genes. Third, large T antigen binds to the two cellular antioncogene proteins, p53 and $p110^{Rb}$ (see above), which inactivates their growth suppressor function (see above).
2. Small t antigen complements the functions of large T antigen. It causes loss of contact inhibition, ability to produce increased amounts of plasminogen activator (see p. 872), and dissolution of the intracellular actin cable network, absence of which is a hallmark of fully transformed cells.
3. In cells infected with polyoma virus, middle T antigen plays a vital role in enhancing full expression of the transformed phenotype; in fact, expression of middle T antigen alone causes transformation to highly tumorigenic cells. Since polyoma middle T antigen by itself is capable of fully transforming cells, it is what is known as an *acute transforming gene* product (see below, p. 886). Middle T antigen is located in cytoplasmic membranes, including the plasma membrane. It occurs in transformed cells complexed with several cellular proteins, particularly the proto-oncogene products $pp60^{c\text{-}src}$ and $p62^{c\text{-}yes}$ (see p. 888), both of which are tyrosine-specific protein kinases, and with phosphatidylinositol 3-kinase and protein phosphatase 2A. Association with middle T antigen stimulates the activity of the kinases, and it is itself phosphorylated by them; in addition, middle T antigen independently causes the phosphorylation of the ribosomal protein S6. Middle T antigen thus appears to regulate the phosphorylation of cellular proteins. It should be noted that phosphorylation of tyrosine residues in proteins also occurs in cells transformed with retroviruses (see below), and a great deal of research is currently directed at determining the significance of tyrosine phosphorylation in the cancer process. The reason for the excitement is that most phosphoproteins in normal cells are phosphorylated on serine and threonine, not on tyrosine residues.

Rescue of Integrated Polyomavirus Genomes

Whereas polyomavirus DNA in transformed cells never expresses itself in its entirety, it is nevertheless the entire viral DNA that is integrated, not portions or segments of it, as can be proved by several types of experiments. For example, the genome of SV40 can be rescued from transformed cells by fusing them (using inactivated Sendai virus [Chap. 56]) with uninfected permissive cells, which induces a normal lytic multiplication cycle; alternatively, transformed cells can be shown to harbor the entire SV40 genome because infectious SV40 DNA can be extracted from them. It should be noted, however, that it is by no means essential for the *entire* viral genome to be integrated into the cellular genome in order for transformation to occur; portions of the viral genome that encode the capsid proteins are clearly not necessary, and it has already been pointed out that cells are transformed if the polyoma virus gene that encodes middle T antigen alone is introduced into them.

Revertants of Transformed Cells

Numerous attempts have been made to isolate revertants of transformed cells. Among the techniques that have led to the selection of revertant cell lines that exhibit growth control comparable to that of normal cells are selection for serum dependence, passage at high dilution, resistance to nucleic acid-base analogues at high cell density (i.e., inability to multiply at high cell density), and resistance to con A. All these methods yield cells that display contact inhibition of growth and resemble normal cells morphologically. However, almost always they still synthesize the tumor antigens, display unaltered virus-specific transcription patterns, and contain the viral genome. Therefore reversion is due to changes in the cellular, rather than loss of the viral, genome. In fact, revertant cell lines often contain more chromosomes than their transformed antecedents. This has suggested a hypothesis that the cell phenotype is modified as a result of changes in the relative numbers of chromosomes with genes that promote and genes that prevent transformation.

Adenoviruses

Human adenoviruses can be divided into three groups on the basis of their oncogenicity. Serotypes 12, 18, and 31 are highly oncogenic; when injected into newborn hamsters, they cause tumors rapidly and with high frequency. Serotypes 3, 7, 14, 16, and 21 are weakly oncogenic; they produce tumors in newborn hamsters with low frequency and after a long latent period. Most of the remaining serotypes, exemplified by serotypes 2 and 5, are nononcogenic, but even they can transform rodent cells in culture.

Adenovirus-transformed cells display many of the properties described above for cells transformed by polyomaviruses, but there are also important differences. For example, in contrast to integrated SV40 and polyomavirus DNA, adenovirus DNA integrated into the genomes of transformed cells cannot be rescued by fusion with permissive cells. This suggests either that only a portion of adenovirus DNA is integrated or that it is integrated in the form of fragments. Analysis of the nature of viral DNA sequences present in a variety of cells transformed by several adenoviruses has shown that (1) none of them contain the complete adenovirus genome, (2) some contain most of the viral genome but in fragmented form, and (3) all contain at least the left-hand 8% of the viral genome where the E1A and E1B genes, which together comprise the adenovirus-transforming region, are located. The transcripts of these two regions are processed through differential splicing into messenger RNAs that are translated into several proteins that are modified extensively posttranslationally and associated with several cellular nuclear proteins; in particular, the E1A protein(s) binds to $p110^{Rb}$, and the E1B protein(s) binds to p53 (see above). Further, like papovaviruses, adenoviruses require the functions of *two* proteins for complete transformation; E1A expression immortalizes cells, but complete transformation requires the additional expression of the E1B region, whose function can also be supplied by the H-*ras* or the *myc* oncogene (see below).

Whereas E1A and E1B gene expression transforms cells cultured in vitro, the survival and growth of transformed cells in animals (i.e., tumor progression) require an additional E1A function. The E1A proteins of highly oncogenic adenoviruses, but not of weakly oncogenic or nononcogenic adenoviruses, down-regulate major histocompatibility complex (MHC) class I gene expression by repressing their promoters. As a result, cells transformed by these viruses evade immune surveillance even more efficiently than through the mechanism mediated by the E3/19K protein and are thereby able to establish progressive tumors.

Herpesviruses

Numerous herpesviruses are either oncogenic, are associated with tumors, or can transform cells in vitro (Table 59–2); they include herpesviruses of primates and other mammals, birds, and amphibians. In humans no fewer than three herpesviruses may be involved in tumorigenesis: (1) Epstein-Barr virus, the genome of which is often present in cultured Burkitt lymphoma and nasopharyngeal carcinoma cells and which can transform human B lymphocytes; (2) herpes simplex virus type 2 (HSV 2), which, seroepidemiologic evidence suggests, may be associated with carcinoma of the cervix and which can transform a variety of cells, especially when inactivated with ultraviolet irradiation to preclude the productive or lytic virus-cell interaction; and (3) human cytomegalovirus (HCMV), which may also be implicated in the etiology of cervical carcinoma and perhaps also of Kaposi's sarcoma and which can also transform cultured cells after exposure to ultraviolet irradiation.

Epstein-Barr Virus

Burkitt's lymphoma is a tumor that is relatively common in East Africa and New Guinea, but rare in other parts of the

TABLE 59–2. ONCOGENIC HERPESVIRUSES

	Host	Host Cell	Malignancy
Epstein-Barr virus	Humans	B lymphocyte	Burkitt's lymphoma, nasopharyngeal carcinoma
Herpesvirus pan	Chimpanzee	B lymphocyte	Lymphoma
Herpesirus papio	Baboon	B lymphocyte	Lymphoma
Marek's disease virus	Chicken	T lymphocyte	Lymphoma
Herpesvirus saimiri	Squirrel monkey	T lymphocyte	Lymphoma
Herpesvirus ateles	Spider monkey	T lymphocyte	Lymphoma
Herpesvirus sylvilagus	Rabbit	B lymphocyte	Lymphoma
Lucké frog herpesvirus	Frogs		Adenocarcinoma of the kidney

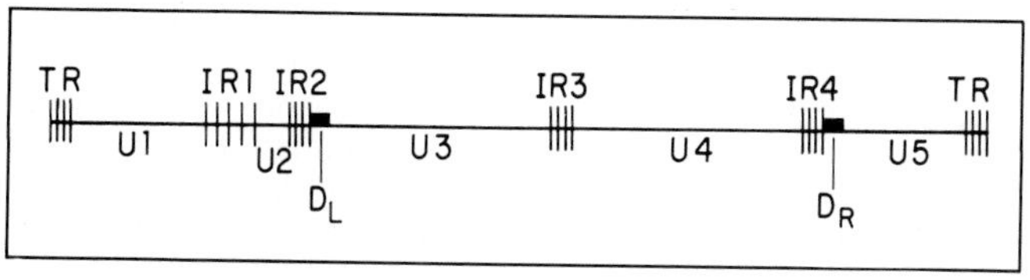

Fig. 59–6. Schematic representation of the DNA of the Epstein-Barr virus (EBV). Its size is similar to that of herpes simplex virus (about 110×10^6 or 175,000 base pairs [bp]). The various regions are not drawn strictly to scale. About three quarters of the sequences of EBV DNA are distributed in five unique regions, whereas about one quarter are present in the form of repeated sequence elements. IR1 is transcribed very extensively into messenger RNA, but the proteins that it encodes have not yet been identified. IR2 appears to contain the origin of replication. IR3 is also transcribed very actively and encodes the EBV nuclear antigen, EBNA (mol wt, 78 kDa), a protein with a remarkable composition: more than two thirds of its amino acids are alanine and glycine. TR, terminal repeat, about 500 bp, repeated 6 to 12 times; IR1, internal repeat 1, about 3000 bp, repeated 6 to 12 times; IR2, internal repeat 2, about 123 bp, repeated 8 to 12 times; IR3, internal repeat 3, about 123 bp, repeated about 7 times; IR4, internal repeat 4, about 103 bp, repeated 6 to 12 times; D_L and D_R, partially homologous regions about 2000 bp long.

world; it occurs primarily in children 5 to 12 years of age. The tumor cells contain no infectious virus, but a small proportion of lymphoblastoid cells established in vitro from tumor tissue produce a herpesvirus that is known as Epstein-Barr virus (EBV) after its discoverers. EBV is also present in the cells of patients with nasopharyngeal (postnasal) carcinoma (NPC), which occurs with rather high frequency in southern Chinese and, to a lesser extent, in northern native American populations.

EBV is widely distributed: 80% of adults worldwide possess antibodies against it. Conversion from the seronegative to the seropositive state occurs during the acute phase of infectious mononucleosis; thus EBV is the etiologic agent of infectious mononucleosis. Presumably, most infections with EBV are subclinical; some cause overt infectious mononucleosis; and rarely in most populations but more frequently in others in which special factors may be operative, Burkitt's lymphoma or NPC ensues.

EBV is one of three tumorigenic B-lymphotropic herpesviruses of humans and primates, with the others being herpesvirus papio (baboons) and herpesvirus pan (chimpanzees), the genomes of which share approximately 40% sequence homology. All cause lymphoproliferative disease. Their host range is narrow; only B lymphocytes possess receptors for them, which is the C2 complement receptor C021.

Infection of B lymphocytes with EBV transforms them into immortalized lymphoblastoid cells, that is, into tumor cells with an infinite life span. In these cells EBV DNA (Fig. 59–6) exists in the form of 2 to more than 200 episomal closed circles. Productive virus multiplication occurs in only a small proportion of such cells. This proportion can be increased by arginine deprivation or treatment with bromodeoxyuridine, TPA (12-*O*-tetradecanoylphorbol-13-acetate, a tumor promoter), 5-azacytidine, or dimethyl sulfoxide.

Immortalization and transformation of B lymphocytes are the functions of two sets of early proteins: the Epstein-Barr nuclear antigen (EBNA) proteins, of which EBNA-1 is essential for EBV DNA persistence as an episome, EBNA-2 is a transcriptional transactivator, and EBNA-LP regulates a cell growth factor or growth factor receptor important in the establishment of primary B lymphocyte growth transformation; and the LMP membrane proteins, whose synthesis is induced by EBNA-2. LMP1 is the primary effector of lymphocyte transformation, that is, is the EBV oncogene, whereas LMP2A and LMP2B are mediators of tyrosine-specific plasma membrane protein phosphorylation and are transformation cofactors.

EBV as Human Tumor Virus: Its Role in Etiology of Burkitt's Lymphoma and Nasopharyngeal Carcinoma

EBV is the only oncogenic human herpesvirus; in some genetically predisposed or severely immunodeficient humans EBV infection can evolve into rapidly fatal lymphoproliferative disease. EBV also causes papillomatous proliferation of epithelial cells in acquired immunodeficiency disease syndrome (AIDS) patients (oral hairy leukoplakia).

As for the involvement of EBV in the etiology of Burkitt's lymphoma (BL) and NPC, the fact that it plays some role is undoubted; but tumors develop only in patients with these diseases long after primary EBV infection, and it is therefore thought that EBV probably is a cofactor of malignancy rather than its primary cause. The arguments concerning BL are as follows. First, although EBV infections are common throughout the world, BL occurs with high frequency in only two areas: tropical Africa and New Guinea, areas where malaria is hyperendemic. Second, all BL tumor cell lines contain a reciprocal exchange between the terminal portions of chromosomes 8 and 14 or, less frequently, between chromosome 8 and chromosomes 2 or 22. The portion of chromosome 8 that is translocated contains the proto-oncogene c-*myc* (see below), and in being translocated, its expression is activated by the IgH, Ig-κ, or Ig-λ enhancers, respectively. Thus BL tumor cells contain greatly elevated levels of the c-*myc* protein, which stimulates cell proliferation (see below). The most likely scenario for the etiology of BL is therefore that EBV performs the essential function of initiating the replication of B cells, that malaria suppresses the immune response, and that sooner or later a chromosomal translocation occurs that activates the c-*myc* proto-oncogene, which causes the actual malignant transformation.

Herpes Simplex Virus Type 2 and Human Cytomegalovirus

Numerous reports during the last two decades have suggested an association between genital infections with HSV 2 and, more recently, with HCMV and uterine cervical carcinoma. The evidence is primarily epidemiologic: women with genital herpetic infections have a higher-than-average incidence of cervical carcinoma, and women with cervical carcinoma have a higher-than-average incidence of antibodies against HSV 2. Further, HSV 2 DNA is present in some, although not all, tumor cells. In summary, HSV 2 and HMCV are candidates for the induction of premalignant or malignant disease, but there is so far no evidence for a viral oncogene. The most persuasive roles for HSV 2 and HCMV in human tumorigenesis are as activators of the transcription of normally not expressed genes or as mutagens (by causing chromosomal translocations [see above]).

Poxviruses

Two types of poxviruses are tumorigenic: fibroma viruses, including the classic rabbit Shope fibroma virus, as well as several closely related viruses pathogenic for deer, squirrels, and hares; and Yaba monkey tumor virus, which is pathogenic for several species of monkeys and for humans. Both produce benign tumors that soon regress. In immunosuppressed rabbits fibroma virus produces invasive fibrosarcomas.

The interest in poxvirus tumorigenicity derives from the fact that poxviruses are DNA-containing viruses that have always been thought to multiply exclusively in the cytoplasm. There have been several reports of the presence of poxvirus DNA in the nuclei of infected cells, but none have been substantiated; the finding that the nucleus must be present during the early part of the poxvirus multiplication cycle if infection is to be productive has now been traced to the fact that one of the subunits of the complex poxvirus DNA-dependent RNA polymerase is of host origin (Chap. 55). When fibroma virus transforms cells, host DNA replication is first arrested, and viral DNA replication is initiated. However, viral DNA replication quickly ceases, host DNA replication recommences, and the cells become transformed. They then multiply more rapidly than before, exhibit an altered morphology, are less sensitive to contact inhibition, and display new antigens on their surface. Recently, the region of the fibroma virus genome responsible for transforming cells has been located within its inverted terminal repeats. When it is introduced into a myxoma virus, the resulting hybrid virus produces invasive tumors. Apparently the tumors produced by the fibroma virus soon regress because they cannot evade immune surveillance; presumably the tumors produced by the hybrid virus can do so. The situation may be analogous to that for cells transformed by adenovirus (see above).

Hepatitis B Virus

The only known host of hepatitis B virus (HBV) is humans. About 200 million people are currently infected with this virus, which causes hepatitis B or serum hepatitis. Many of them are carriers in whom the virus establishes a chronic or persistent infection manifested by the circulation of high concentrations of HBsAg particles and small amounts of infectious virus in the bloodstream for months or years. In other individuals the virus establishes a highly virulent, often fatal disease; and in others still it causes, or is a major factor in causing, the most common fatal cancer in humans—primary hepatic carcinoma. The most compelling evidence for this view is the fact that most (75% to 85%), but not all, hepatoma cells contain integrated HBV DNA, often in the form of multiple copies. There is no preferred site of integration into cellular DNA. The integrated HBV genomes are generally fragmented; their sequences are rearranged by duplication and transposition, and major portions of them are deleted.

How HBV causes cell transformation is not known. It does not possess an oncogene, nor does it integrate near known oncogenes or cause oncogene activation by inducing specific chromosomal translocations like EBV does. Instead, it probably acts as a direct mutagen through an as-yet unidentified mechanism such as postintegration DNA rearrangement or as an indirect mutagen owing to the generation of oxidants (such as active oxygen radicals and peroxides) by phagocytic cells during the chronic inflammation of cirrhosis. Such oxidants can cause single-strand DNA breaks and are strong tumor promoters in some systems.

Retroviruses

Retroviruses are the most intensively studied of all tumor viruses. Their study has led to several important discoveries such as the demonstration that RNA can be transcribed into DNA and the identification of oncogenes. Both discoveries are of fundamental importance for an understanding of differentiation and development on the one hand and of carcinogenesis on the other. In fact, study of the functions of oncogenes incorporated into retrovirus genomes provides the best hope for understanding how normal cells are transformed into cancer cells.

The above refers only to the Oncovirinae ("Oncovirus") subfamily of the Retroviridae. There are two other subfamilies. The Spumavirinae are known as contaminants of primary cultured cells in which they cause a "foamy" degeneration (*spuma*, foam). They have not been studied extensively. The other subfamily, the Lentivirinae, includes the visna and maedi viruses that cause, in sheep, progressive neurologic damage and chronic pneumonia, respectively, after long latent periods. Interest in this little-studied group of viruses has increased enormously in recent years with the realization that the human AIDS virus is a lentivirus.

Most of the discussion in this chapter is devoted to the oncoviruses. Because they are by far the largest and best studied of the retrovirus subfamilies, they are referred to in this text by the more commonly used name of *retroviruses*.

Nature of Retrovirus Particles

Retrovirus particles possess an electron-dense nucleoid or core surrounded by two shells (Figs. 59–7 and 59–8), an inner nucleocapsid shell that appears to possess icosahedral symmetry, and an outer shell that consists of a lipid bilayer membrane to which glycoprotein spikes are attached.

There are three morphologic types of retrovirus particles: (1) C-type particles (most leukemia and sarcoma viruses); (2) B-type particles (mammary tumor viruses), which differ from C-type particles in the eccentric rather than central location of their nucleocapsid in thin sections, their more prominent glycoprotein spikes, and in the fact that their nucleoids can often be seen in the cytoplasm of infected cells (these are the so-called *intracytoplasmic* A-type particles); and (3) D-type particles (viruses isolated from a variety of primates), the morphology of which is intermediate between those of C-type and B-type retrovirus particles.

Retrovirus particles comprise six structural and two nonstructural proteins (Tables 59–3 and 59–4). Two are -SS-linked glycoproteins, and trimers of them comprise the envelope spikes—the larger forming the knob, the smaller, the stalk. They are encoded by the *env* gene. The other structural proteins are nucleocapsid components that are derived by cleavage of a precursor that is the primary protein product

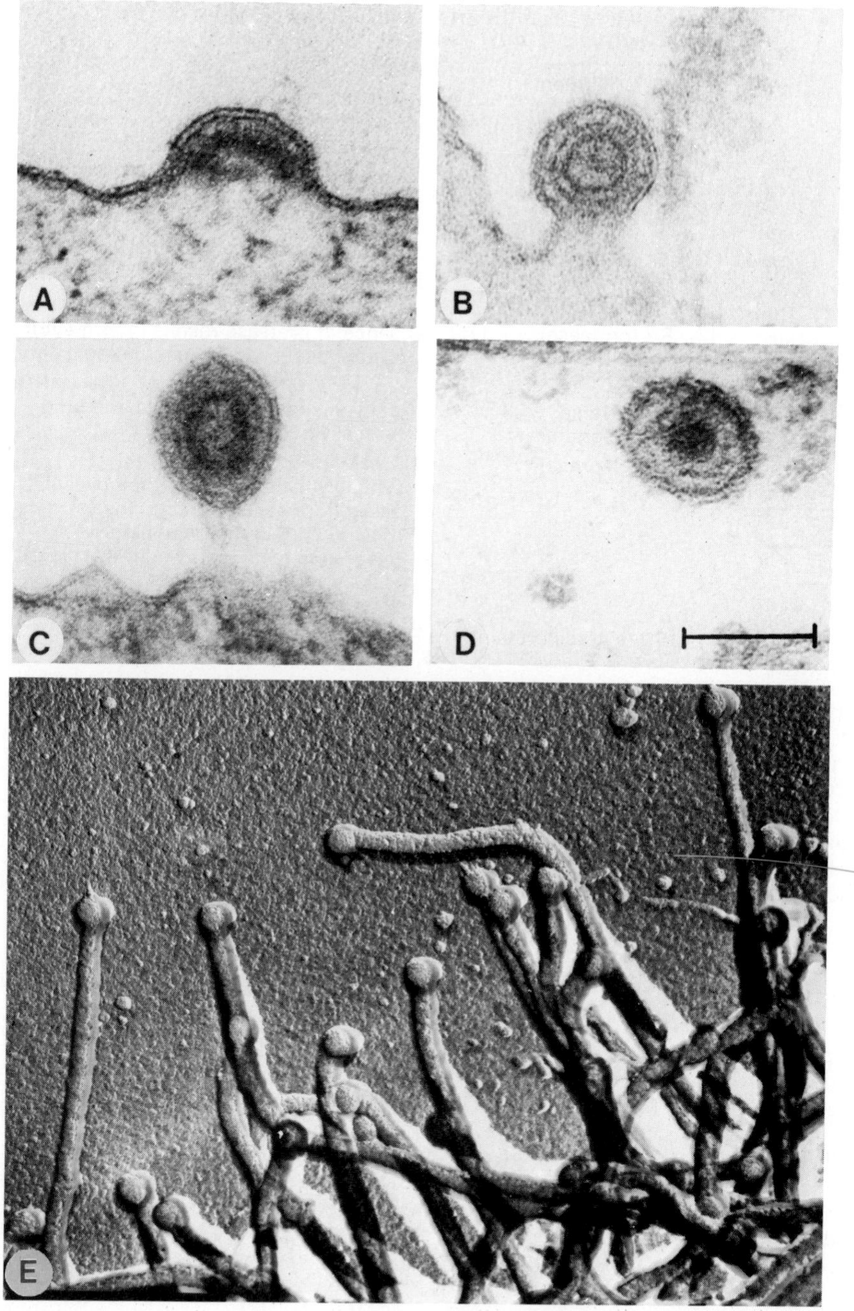

Fig. 59–7. Morphogenesis and structure of retroviruses. **A–D**. Four stages in the budding of a C-type avian retrovirus. Note the electron-lucent center or core in immature particles (**B** and **C**) and the electron-dense core in mature particles (**D**). **E**. Micrograph of a surface replica of a GR cell that is producing murine mammary tumor virus particles (B-type retrovirus). The micrograph shows the cell margin with microvilli, from the tips of which the virus buds. (*Panels **A** to **D**, courtesy of Dr. Heinz Bauer; panel **E**, courtesy of Dr. J. B. Sheffield.*)

of another retrovirus gene, the so-called *gag* protein gene (see below). The enzyme that effects this cleavage, encoded by the *pro* gene, is synthesized as part of a fusion protein with the *gag* or *pol* or both gene products (see below); it is a dimeric aspartic proteinase that cleaves itself autocatalytically out of the *gag* precursor polyprotein (like the poliovirus proteinase [see p. 815]) at the time of, or shortly after, budding and then cleaves the polyprotein further to the various nucleocapsid proteins listed in Table 59–3. This results in an obvious morphologic conversion (see Fig. 59–7) to the mature particle configuration. Because of its key role in this process, the protease is a prime target for antiviral chemotherapy. Several retrovirus proteases, including that of human immunodeficiency virus (HIV), have been crystallized, and their three-dimensional atomic structure has been determined, clearing the way for the design of specific inhibitors.

Retrovirus particles also contain several molecules of each of two proteins encoded by the *pol* gene. Like the *gag* gene, the *pol* gene is translated into a precursor, which is then cleaved into two enzymes by the protease. One is the so-called reverse transcriptase (RT), which actually possesses two enzymic activities, namely, a DNA polymerase activity capable of transcribing either RNA or DNA into DNA and a ribonuclease activity known as RNase H (for hybrid), which breaks

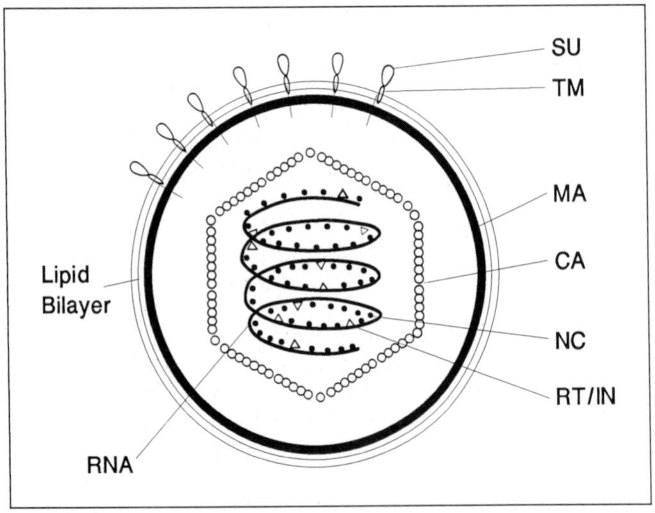

Fig. 59–8. Model of a retrovirus particle. For further details, see text and Tables 59–3 and 59–4.

down RNA as soon as it is transcribed. RT activity is readily detectable in disrupted virus particles; used with the synthetic primer-template poly(rC)·oligo(dG), assaying its presence provides a sensitive and simple technique for detecting retroviruses.

The second protein encoded by the *pol* gene is the IN protein or integrase. It is a double-stranded (ds) DNA-binding protein with endonuclease activity. The evidence for its role in integration is primarily genetic.

TABLE 59–3. PROPERTIES AND FUNCTIONS OF RETROVIRUS PROTEINS

Protein	Properties and Function
MA (matrix protein)	In most retrovirus groups the *N*-terminal domain is myristylated, which is essential for membrane association and budding
CA (capsid protein)	Forms the core shell, which is clearly visible in electron micrographs
NC (nucleic acid binding protein)	Basic protein with affinity for RNA; required for RNA encapsidation
PR (protease)	Absence of protease results in formation of noninfectious and immunologically immature particles
RT (reverse transcriptase)	Mutants lacking RT assemble and bind normally but are noninfectious
IN (integrase)	A DNA-binding endonuclease that is probably the enzyme that removes 2 bases from each 3′-end of linear proviral DNA at the beginning of integration (see Fig. 59–13); its role in nicking host cell DNA has not yet been demonstrated
SU (surface protein)	Required for receptor binding, adsorption, and entry; contains the major epitope against which neutralizing antibodies are synthesized; usually heavily glycosylated; linked by —SS—bonds to TM
TM (transmembrane protein)	Anchors the SU protein to the envelope; is generally less heavily glycosylated than the SU protein; cytoplasmic domain is generally short (20–30 amino acids)

Retrovirus Genome

The retrovirus genome consists of two identical plus-stranded RNA molecules that are 3500 to 9000 nucleotides long (mol wt 1 to 3 × 10^6). They are thought to be hydrogen-bonded to each other through palindromic sequences approximately 40 nucleotides long that are centered about 80 nucleotides from their 5′-ends (Fig. 59–9).

The essential features of the basic retrovirus genome, that is, the genome of nondefective avian and mammalian (particularly murine) leukosis and leukemia viruses (ALV and MLV), are shown in Figure 59–10. It possesses four genes, namely the *gag* gene, which encodes the nucleocapsid proteins; the *pro* gene, which encodes the protease; the *pol* gene, which encodes the RT and IN proteins; and the *env* gene, which encodes the glycoprotein spike components (the SU and the TM proteins). The manner in which the proteins encoded by these three genes are expressed is discussed below (see Fig. 59–15).

These four genes are flanked by two regions with regu-

TABLE 59–4. SIZES OF VARIOUS PROTEINS SPECIFIED BY THE MAJOR GROUPS OF RETROVIRUSES

Gene	gag				pro	pol		env	
Protein[a]	MA	?[b]	CA	NC	PR	RT	IN	SU	TM
Avian sarcoma–leukemia virus	p19	p10	p27	p12	p15	p68	p32	gp85	gp37
Mammalian C-type viruses	p15	p12	p30	p10	p14	p80	p46	gp70	gp15E
HTLV	p19		p24	p15	p14	?	?	gp46	gp21
Lentiviruses (HIV)	p17		p25	p7	p12	p66	p32	gp120	gp41

[a] The reading frame order of these proteins is 5′ to 3′ from left to right.

[b] Function is unknown; therefore it is as yet unnamed.

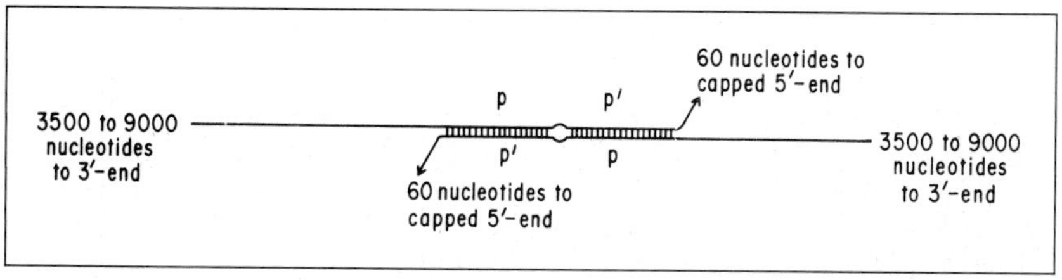

Fig. 59–9. Retrovirus genome. Its two subunits are thought to be held together by base-pairing between the palindromic sequences p and p′ near their 5′-ends. (*Adapted from Haseltine et al: Proc Natl Acad Sci USA 74:989, 1977.*)

latory functions. At the outer end of each region there is an identical region that may be as short as 12 (murine mammary tumor virus, MMTV) and as long as 235 (bovine leukemia virus, BLV) nucleotides and that is termed the *R region* because it represents a direct repeat. It effects the template switch during the transcription of viral RNA into dsDNA (see below). An 80 to 120 nucleotide long unique region termed *U5* is at the 5′-end, and a unique region that varies greatly in length (200 to 1200 residues) termed *U3* is at the 3′ end of the molecule. Both contain numerous functional/regulatory/signal elements. Further, just inside the U5 region is a 16- to 19-nucleotide-long binding site for transfer RNA molecules that serve as primers for the transcription of the RNA into negative-stranded DNA (primer binding, PB); and just inside the U3 region is a 10 to 20 nucleotide long purine-rich sequence that is the initiation site for the synthesis of plus-stranded DNA (polypurine, PP) (see below). Finally, there are relatively long 5′-untranslated leader sequences between the PB site and the 5′-end of the *gag* reading frame that contain splice donor sites (for the generation of the *env* and other messenger RNAs [see below]) and the packaging signals for incorporating viral RNA into virus particles; and there are relatively short untranslated regions downstream of the *env* reading frame and upstream of the U3 region.

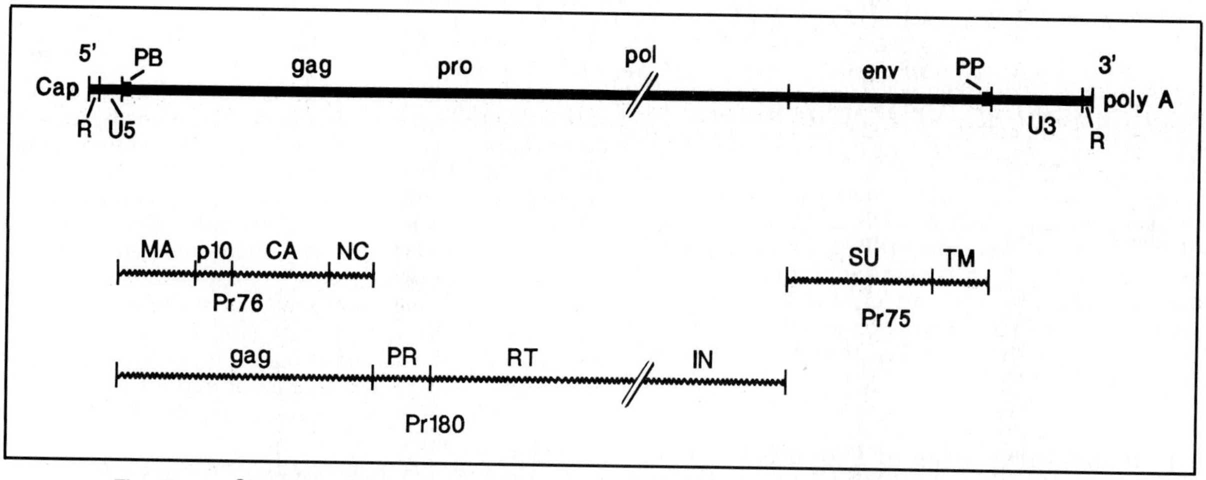

Fig. 59–10. Structure of the basic retrovirus genome: the genome of nondefective avian or murine leukemia/leukosis viruses. Note that the RNA is capped at its 5′-terminus and polyadenylated at its 3′-terminus.

R: 30–60 nucleotides repeated at both ends.

U5: 80–120 nucleotide unique sequence.

PB: a sequence complementary to the 16–19 5′-terminal residues of $tRNA^{trp}$, $tRNA^{pro}$, $tRNA^{glu}$, or $tRNA^{lys}$ in avian leukosis viruses (ALVs), murine leukemia viruses (MLVs), endogenous murine retroviruses, and murine mammary tumor viruses (MMTVs), respectively. The tRNAs bind to these sites to serve as primers for the transcription of the RNA into complementary DNA (cDNA).

gag, *pro*, *pol*, and *env*: genes that encode the nucleocapsid (*gag*) proteins, the *pro*tease, the RT and IN enzymes, and the *env*elope proteins (SU and TM).

Pr76: precursor of the ALV *gag* proteins (the precursor of MLV *gag* proteins is a Pr65).

Pr180: infrequently formed read-through product of the *gag*, *pro*, and *pol* genes, cleavage of which provides the RT and IN enzymes.

Pr57: precursor of gp85 and gp37, the knob and stalk proteins of the spikes of ALVs. The corresponding MLV precursor protein is a Pr80.

PP: a short highly conserved purine-rich sequence that serves as the primer for *positive* strand DNA synthesis.

U3: a unique region 200 to 1000 nucleotides long. It contains a powerful transcriptional promoter.

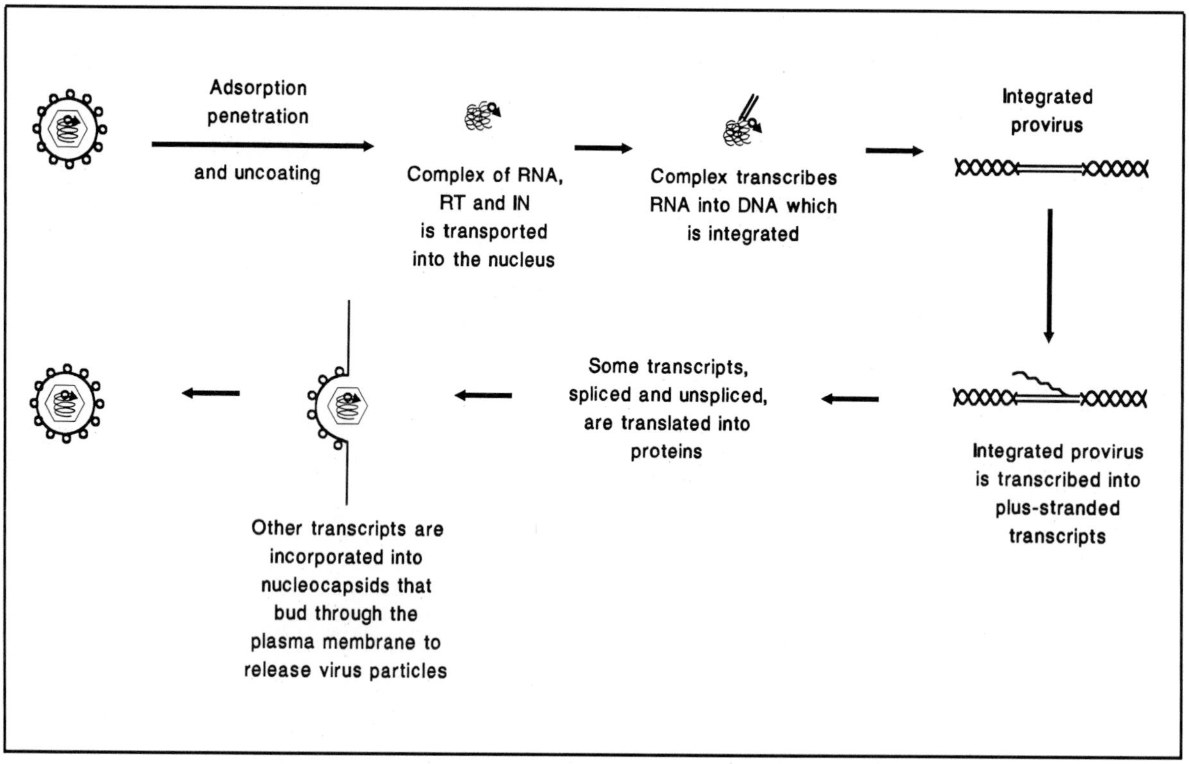

Fig. 59–11. Strategy of the retrovirus multiplication cycle.

Molecular Biology of Retroviruses

The unique feature of retrovirus molecular biology is the reverse transcription of RNA into DNA, independently discovered by Temin and Baltimore in 1970. First believed to be confined to retrovirology, it is now known to be utilized by hepadnaviruses and a wide variety of transposable elements that may have evolved from a common ancestor.

The strategy of the retrovirus multiplication cycle is illustrated in Figure 59–11.

Formation and Integration of Proviral DNA

After adsorption and penetration into the cell via the receptor-mediated endocytosis mechanism typical of enveloped viruses (Chap. 55), the RNA in parental nucleocapsids is transcribed by the reverse transcriptase into linear ds DNA by a fascinating series of reactions depicted in Figure 59–12. The linear proviral DNA then moves to the nucleus and is integrated into the genome of the host cell. Little is known concerning the enzymology of this process, which includes the loss of 2 base pairs from each end of the viral genome and duplication of a 4- to 6-base pair–long sequence of cellular DNA at the integration site in such a way that one copy of it is at one end of the integrated provirus and the other is at the other end (Fig. 59–13). Retroviral proviral insertion is highly efficient; almost all reverse-transcribed molecules are integrated.

Proviral insertion into cellular DNA does not occur randomly but rather into a limited number of strongly preferred sites. Analysis of flanking sequences of randomly picked proviral integration sites has indicated that there are 500 to 1000 highly preferred sites in transcriptionally active regions of the cell genome into which about 20% of proviral insertions occur and which are used about 1 million times more frequently than would be expected if integration occurred randomly. In fact, about one in 5000 integrations occurs into the *same* preferred insertion site where integration often occurs at precisely the same nucleotide base pair.

It should be pointed out that the reverse transcriptase makes errors at a high rate ($1{\cdot}4 \times 10^{-4}$ mutations per nucleotide per replication cycle). Therefore, although able to integrate, many proviruses cannot express themselves in the form of infectious virus particles because they contain inactivating point mutations.

The structure of integrated proviruses is shown in Figure 59–14. As a consequence of the transcription and integration processes described in Figures 59–12 and 59–13, their coding sequences are flanked by two identical long terminal repeats (LTRs) composed of the U3, R, and U5 regions. In addition, integrated proviruses are *always* flanked by 4- to 6-base pair–long direct repeats (DR) of host origin that result from the integration process and that are the invariate hallmarks of transposons. The mechanism of provirus integration is thus formally analogous to the often observed insertion of transposable elements into the genomes of bacteria, yeasts, *Drosophila,* and higher organisms.

Once integrated, proviruses are stable genetic elements. There appears to be no limit on the number of different types of proviral genomes in any given cellular genome; mouse cells are known to contain more than 10 different kinds of proviruses, each present in the form of multiple copies.

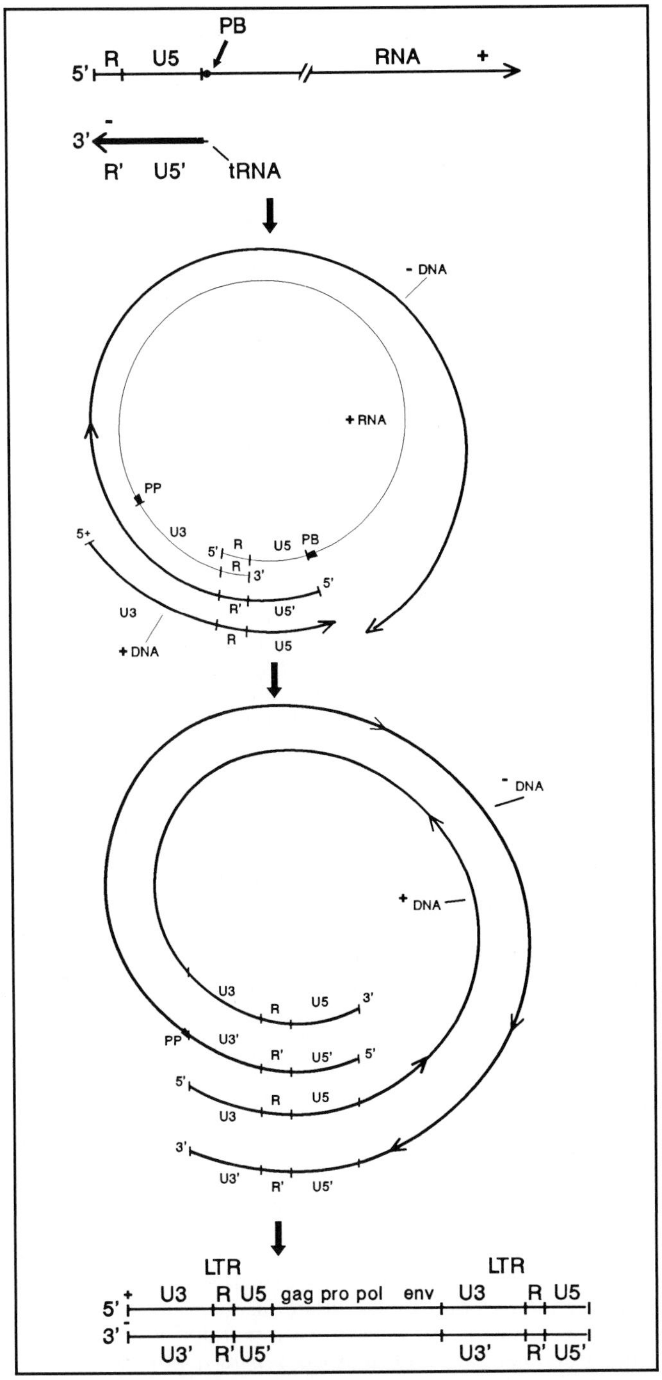

Fig. 59–12. Scheme for the transcription of retrovirus RNA into double-stranded DNA. Step 1: Using tRNA as primer, the approximately 150 nucleotides of the U5 and R regions are transcribed. Step 2: Transcription continues after degradation of the R RNA region by the RNase H activity of the RT and template switching to the R region at the other end of the same molecule or of the other RNA molecule. As transcription of the ⁻DNA strand continues, transcription of the ⁺DNA strand commences at the PP site. Step 3: Transcription of both strands continues. As the RNA is progressively degraded, the DNA strands themselves serve as templates. Step 4: The final product is a double-stranded DNA molecule flanked by the long terminal repeats (LTRs; the U3-R-U5 regions).

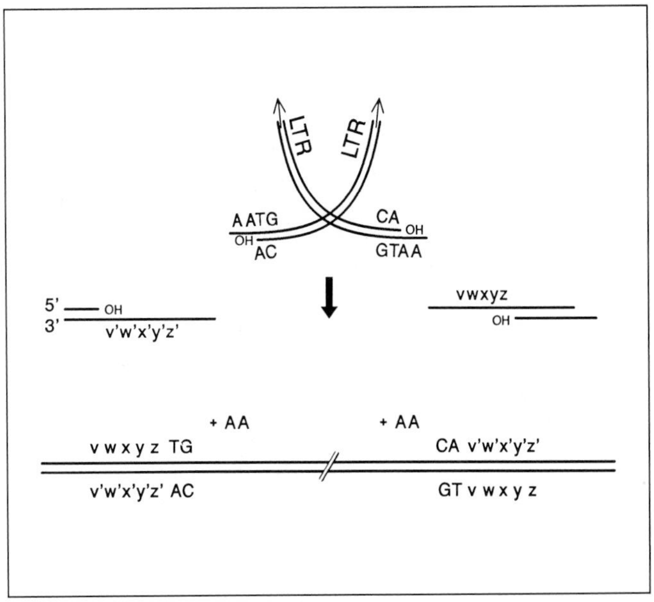

Fig. 59–13. Scheme for the integration of proviral DNA into cellular DNA. As proviral DNA approaches the site where it will integrate, enzymes (perhaps IN) remove two bases from each 3′-end of the provirus, cleave the cellular DNA, and remove four to six nucleotides from each 3′-end. Ligation and repair follow. Presumably this is all a concerted reaction. The result is loss of 2 bps from each end of the provirus and duplication at each end of the provirus of the cellular DNA sequence into which it integrated.

Transcription of Integrated Proviral DNA

Integrated proviral DNA is transcribed by cellular RNA polymerase II into transcripts that are capped at their 5′-ends and polyadenylated at their 3′-ends. These transcripts are used in one of three ways. First, they may be translated either into the *gag* gene product, a polyprotein that is cleaved by the protease into the several *gag* proteins, or, infrequently, into the *gag-pro-pol* polyprotein, which is then cleaved to the *pro* and *pol* gene products and to the *gag* proteins (Fig. 59–15). This mode of synthesizing the *pol* gene products (i.e., without a messenger RNA of their own and by infrequent read-through or frameshift of a messenger originating in the upstream gene) provides a mechanism for ensuring that they will not be synthesized in excessive amounts (clearly far more *gag* gene products are required for viral morphogenesis than *pol* gene products).

Second, provirus transcripts may have the *gag*, *pro*, and *pol* gene sequences spliced out, thereby providing messenger RNA molecules that are translated into the *env* gene products. The splice donor site is located in the *gag* gene 5′-untranslated region; the splice acceptor site is generally close to the *pol* termination codon. If a transforming gene is also present in the provirus (see below), the same 5′-splice signal is observed.

Third, provirus transcripts may be encapsidated, pairwise, into progeny virus particles.

The extent to which proviral genomes are expressed depends on the nature of the LTRs that contain signals

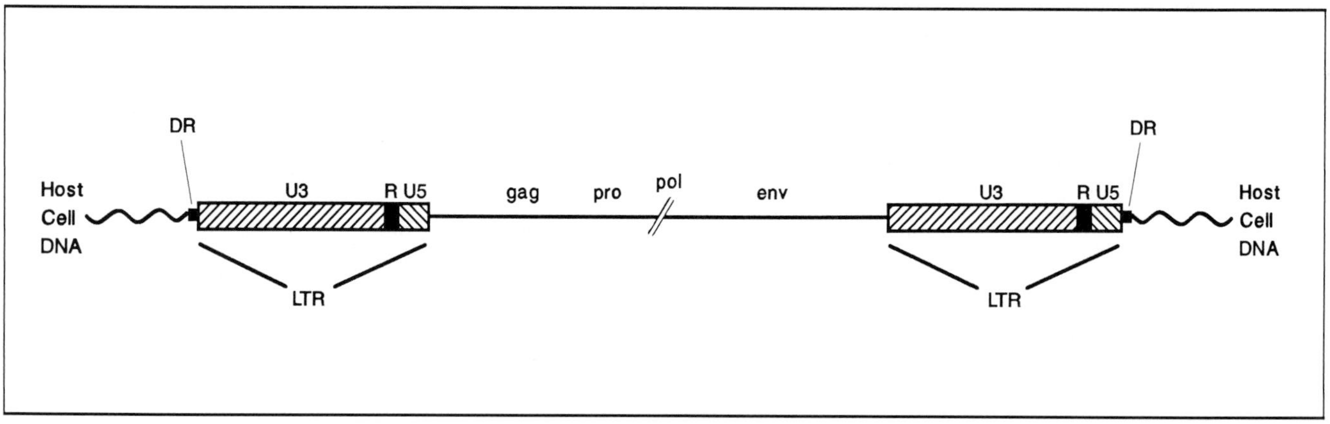

Fig. 59–14. Structure of the integrated provirus. The coding sequences of the *gag*, *pro*, *pol*, and *env* genes are flanked by long terminal repeats (LTRs) from 250 to 1200 bp long, depending on the virus, each composed of the U3, R, and U5 regions. The entire provirus is flanked by direct repeats (DR) 4 to 6 bp long that are of host cell origin.

recognized by the cellular transcription apparatus. Included are signals for the initiation of transcription (at the U3-R junction) and polyadenylation (at the end of the R region) and an enhancer (in the U3 region) capable of binding and responding to factors with a wide range of cell- and differentiation state–specificity. These factors, which are present or active in some cells and absent or inactive in others, with a wide spectrum between, control target cell specificity, pathogenesis, and the ability to form tumors. Thus any provirus can be expressed, depending on the cell type.

Biology of Retroviruses

Retroviruses are very widely distributed in nature. They have been found in most vertebrates, and retrovirus-like sequences occur even in invertebrates such as *Drosophila*. Under normal conditions, most retroviruses are restricted to a single animal species. The most intensively studied retroviruses are the avian ones, which are often grouped together as the avian sarcoma/avian leukosis viruses (ASV/ALV), and the corresponding murine viruses (MSV/MLV); other well-studied groups are the feline, bovine, and primate retroviruses and recently the human retroviruses.

Host Range

Retrovirus host range is specified primarily by the presence or absence of receptors on cell surfaces. Usually the host range is narrow; murine retroviruses infect only mouse cells, feline retroviruses, cat cells, and so on. Some animal species possess multiple nonallelic retrovirus receptors, the expression of which is genetically controlled. For example, chickens possess five different types of glycoprotein retrovirus receptors known as *A* through *E*. Thus there are five groups of ASV/ALV, each of which adsorbs to and infects the cells that express its particular receptor. In the mouse the situation is different. Here there are retroviruses, the *ecotropic* viruses, that use a receptor present only on mouse cells; retroviruses that use receptors present in cells of many nonmouse species but not in mouse cells are the *xenotropic* viruses; and retroviruses present on both mouse cells and cells of other species are the *amphotropic* and *polytropic* viruses.

Interference

Cells productively infected with one type of retrovirus are resistant to superinfection by retroviruses that use the *same* receptor. The reason for this interference phenomenon is that retroviral glycoprotein SU formed in these cells saturates all receptor molecules, thus preventing potentially superinfecting virus from adsorbing. Measurement of viral interference is a convenient and widely used method for identifying and classifying retroviral glycoproteins and therefore retrovirus strains.

Transmission

Most retroviruses are transmitted exogenously, like other viruses. However, retroviruses integrate their genomes into those of host cells, and the proviruses of some retroviruses have, during the course of evolution, inserted themselves into the genomes of germ cells. Such proviruses are transmitted vertically as heritable genetic material, like any other gene. Retroviruses whose proviruses are integrated into germ-line cellular genomes are known as *endogenous* retroviruses.

Endogenous Retroviruses

The genomes of most if not all vertebrate animal species contain retroviral proviruses. Many endogenous retroviral genomes are defective and cannot yield an infectious virus; this is the case, for example, for all human endogenous retroviral proviruses (see p. 900). The reasons for defectiveness range all the way from the accumulation, during the course of evolution, of mutations that result in premature termination codons, to deletion of major portions of proviral

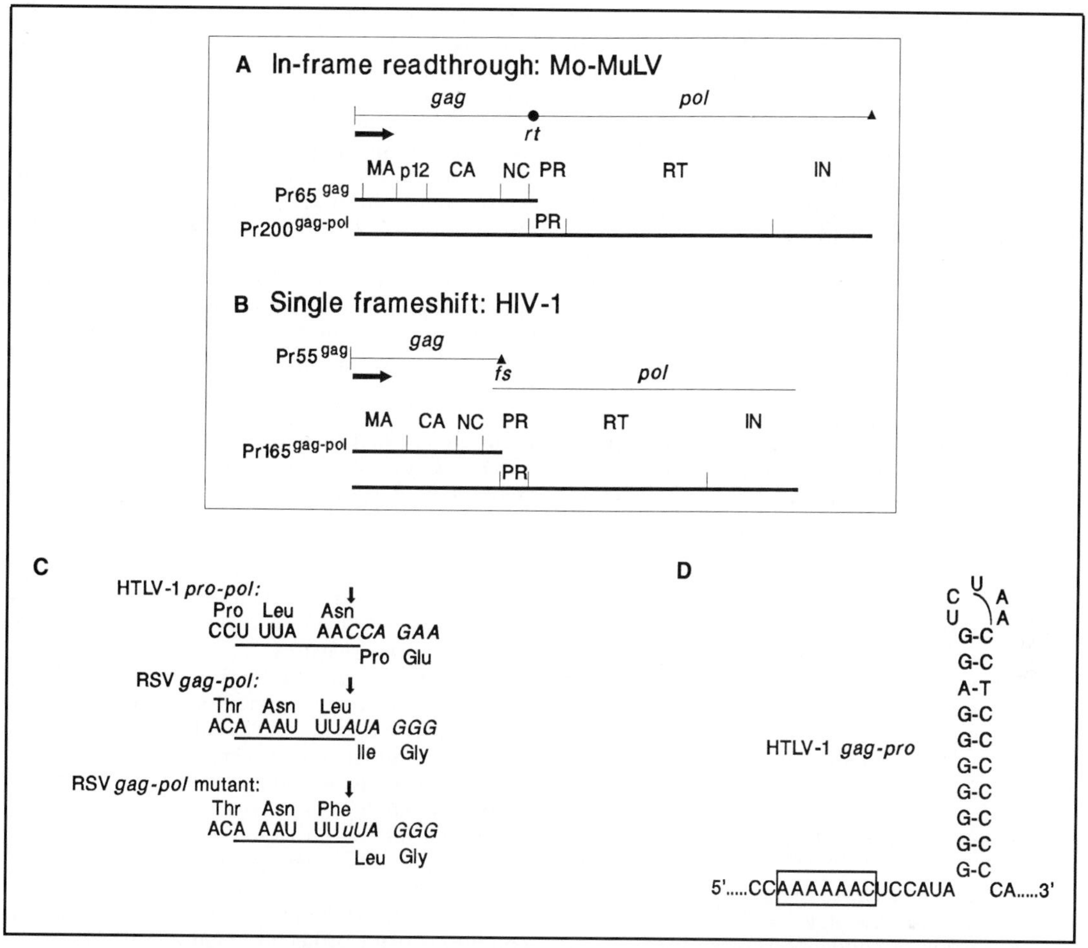

Fig. 59–15. Expression of the proteins encoded by the *gag*, *pro*, *pol*, and *env* genes. Expression of the *gag* and *env* genes is unremarkable: the *gag* gene is translated from the full-length RNA into a polyprotein, whereas the *env* gene is translated from transcripts of the integrated provirus from which the *gag*, *pro*, and *pol* reading frames have been spliced out. Expression of the *pro* and *pol* genes, however, is very interesting. In some viruses such as the mammalian type C viruses, **A**, the *gag* and *pro* genes are separated by a single termination codon, the amber codon UAG (at rt). Here the UAG is read as glutamine about 1 time out of 20, which results in the formation of a read-through *gag-pro-pol* polyprotein that is cleaved into its constituent seven components by the protease. Thus only about one twentieth as much of the RT and IN proteins, which are enzymes, is made as of the structural *gag* proteins.

In other viruses such as Rous sarcoma virus (RSV), HTLV-I, and HIV, **B**, the *gag* and *pro* reading frames overlap by as little as 13 or as much as 178 nucleotides. Here also both reading frames are translated into a single *gag-pol* polyprotein because a frameshift (fs) of −1 occurs somewhere in the overlap, again with a frequency of about 5%. In the frameshift, it is thought that both the peptidyl-tRNA and the aminoacyl-tRNA slip simultaneously by one base in the 5′ direction, causing the ribosome to read the −1 frame and then continue translating it to the termination codon at the end of the *pol* gene. Two types of signal are required for the frameshift to occur. One is provided by one of three sequences, A AAC, U UUA, or U UUU, in which asparagine (AAC), leucine (UUA), and phenylalanine (UUU) are read in the 0 reading frame, and C, A, and U are the first codon positions of the first codon to be read in the −1 frame, **C**. The second signal is the presence of a stem-loop structure, **D**, which may also exist as a pseudoknot, immediately downstream of the frameshift signal sequence.

In some viruses, such as murine mammary tumor viruses, two frameshifts are required to enable synthesis of the *gag-pro-pol* polyprotein because not only do the *gag* and *pro* reading frames overlap, but also the *pro* and *pol* reading frames. (Adapted from Hatfield and Oroszlan: TIBS 15:186, 1990.)

genomes including one or more of their genes. In fact, several types of repeated sequence elements in vertebrate genomes are clearly amplified, highly degenerate endogenous retroviral genomes (see below).

However, the genomes of some animals also contain intact retroviral proviruses capable of generating infectious virus particles. For example, chickens contain at least 16 different functional proviruses, and mice harbor at least 10 different complete proviruses, each present to the extent of about 10 copies. Some fascinating evolutionary relationships have emerged now that many retrovirus genomes have been sequenced. For example, the cat endogenous xenotropic virus RD114 was acquired in the Pliocene from a monkey; and the two exogenous primate retroviruses, simian sarcoma virus and gibbon ape leukemia virus, are derived from an endogenous murine xenotropic virus. Although the acquisition of endogenous retroviral sequences is clearly a rare event, it can be observed experimentally; highly inbred strains of mice such as the high-incidence-of-leukemia AKR strain (see below) integrate new proviral genomes into the genomes of their germ cells at the rate of 1 per 40 to 50 generations. The effective rate of such acquisition in feral populations under natural conditions is many orders of magnitude lower.

Some endogenous proviruses are under very tight cellular control. Such proviruses never express themselves under natural conditions but can be induced to express themselves by treatment with a variety of substances, including inhibitors of protein synthesis, inhibitors of nucleic acid synthesis such as halogenated deoxyribonucleosides, inhibitors of glycosylation, and B lymphocyte mitogens. Different inducers induce different endogenous retroviruses, indicating that the nature of the cellular controls that regulate their ability to express themselves is diverse.

Other endogenous proviruses express themselves to varying degrees, depending on the age of the host. In feral populations the expression of endogenous proviruses as virus particles is greatly repressed; but breeding programs for mice and chickens, in particular, have produced many strains of inbred animals in which the mechanisms that control endogenous provirus expression have been dissociated from the proviruses themselves, with the result that in these animals retroviruses are produced continuously and often throughout the animals' life. For example, mice such as the albino AK and the C58BL strains have large numbers of leukemia virus particles in their bloodstream and develop leukemia at 6 to 12 months of age with high frequency; these mice are high-incidence-of-leukemia mouse strains. In other strains of mice, such as BALB/c and DBA, endogenous proviruses express themselves during embryonic life, even to the extent of virus particle formation, but then become repressed so that the virus is generally undetectable in young adults. Later in life, however, these proviruses again express themselves, and leukemia may result, albeit with low frequency. Mice that harbor such endogenous proviruses are known as low-incidence-of-leukemia mouse strains. Finally, some mice such as NIH Swiss and NZB mice do not develop leukemia at all because the endogenous proviruses capable of producing spontaneous leukemia have been bred out of them.

Although endogenous retroviruses usually do not express themselves to the extent of virus particle formation, they do sometimes express their *env* genes. For example, a strain of Rous sarcoma virus (RSV) whose RNA contains a deletion in the *env* gene (the Bryan strain) is incapable of growing in some chick cells but is capable of growing in others, which are therefore said to possess a "chick-helper-factor" (chf). This factor is the spontaneously expressed *env* glycoprotein of an endogenous chick retrovirus known as RAV-0, which the Bryan strain can use to form virus particles.

Another example is found in the mouse. A differentiation alloantigen designated G_{IX} (since it appears to be specified by a gene in linkage group IX) is present in the thymocytes of certain mouse strains. It is also present in the serum of some mouse strains (particularly strain 12A), in epithelia associated with the digestive tract, and in the epithelial lining of the male reproductive tract and therefore in seminal fluid. This G_{IX} antigen represents the gp70 glycoprotein specified by the *env* gene of an endogenous provirus, which expresses itself irrespective of *gag* and *pol* gene expression, just like chf mentioned previously.

Not only can portions of endogenous proviruses express themselves, but proviruses can also recombine with the genomes of superinfecting retroviruses. For example, the development of spontaneous leukemia tends to be associated with the generation of a new class of retroviruses that are amphotropic and induce focal morphologic alterations in a mink lung cell line; therefore they are often referred to as mink cell focus (MCF)–incuding viruses. They are recombinants between exogenous retroviruses and the *env* genes of endogenous retroviruses.

Finally, the question arises as to whether endogenous retroviruses serve an essential normal function; for example, do they play a role in cellular differentiation? This is unlikely; not only is endogenous provirus gene expression idiosyncratic with respect to tissue and age in different mouse strains, which is not compatible with provirus expression playing an essential functional role in ontogeny, but healthy chickens that do not contain any endogenous provirus have also been bred. However, it is conceivable that possession of endogenous proviruses may confer some form of survival advantage under natural conditions (e.g., protection against infectious exogenous retrovirus particles; see above).

Basis of Tumorigenicity of Retroviruses

C-type retroviruses can be divided into two groups. Most of them possess the four genes, *gag*, *pro*, *pol*, and *env*, which are essential for multiplication; they are *replication competent*. They do not transform cells in vitro; thus they are said to be transformation defective. Although they are widely distributed and the animals they infect are generally viremic throughout life, they cause tumors (lymphocytic, myeloid, and erythroblastic leukemias, osteopetrosis, nephroblastoma, and thymic and generalized lymphosarcomas) only late in life; and when injected in large amounts into animals, they cause neoplasms only after long latent periods. These are the viruses commonly known as the *leukemia viruses* (but some of them also cause nonneoplastic diseases such as wasting diseases and neurologic disorders).

Sarcoma–Acute Leukemia Viruses

The second group of C-type viruses possess high oncogenic potential; they are *transformation competent*. They transform

TABLE 59–5. SOME WELL-KNOWN SARCOMA-ACUTE LEUKEMIA VIRUSES (TRANSFORMATION COMPETENT–REPLICATION DEFECTIVE) AND THEIR ONCOGENES

Virus	Type of Tumor	Animal	Oncogene	Protein Product
Rous sarcoma virus (RSV)[a]	Sarcoma	Chicken	v-*src*	$pp60^{v\text{-}src}$
Fujinami sarcoma virus (FSV)	Sarcoma	Chicken	v-*fps*	$pp140^{v\text{-}gag\text{-}fps}$
Avian myeloblastosis virus (AMV)	Leukemia	Chicken	v-*myb*	$P48^{v\text{-}myb}$
Avian myelocytomatosis virus (MC29)	Carcinoma, sarcoma, leukemia	Chicken	v-*myc*	$P110^{v\text{-}gag\text{-}myc}$
			v-*erb* A	$p75^{v\text{-}gag\text{-}erb\ A}$
Avian erythroblastosis virus (AEV)	Leukemia and sarcoma	Chicken	v-*erb* B	$p140^{v\text{-}gag\text{-}erb\ B}$
Moloney murine sarcoma virus (Mo-MSV)	Sarcoma	Mouse	v-*mos*	$P37^{v\text{-}mos}$
Kirsten murine sarcoma virus		Rat		
Harvey murine sarcoma virus	Sarcoma and leukemia	Rat	v-*ras*	$p21^{v\text{-}ras}$
FBJ murine sarcoma virus	Sarcoma	Mouse	v-*fos*	$p55^{v\text{-}fos}$
Abelson murine leukemia virus	Leukemia	Mouse	v-*abl*	$p160^{v\text{-}gag\text{-}abl}$
			v-*fes*	$p140^{v\text{-}gag\text{-}fes}$
			v-*fms*	$gp180^{v\text{-}gag\text{-}fms}$
			v-*kit*	$p80^{v\text{-}gag\text{-}kit}$
Feline sarcoma virus (FeSV) (various strains)	Sarcoma and leukemia	Cat	v-*fgr*	$p70^{v\text{-}gag\text{-}actin\text{-}fgr}$
Simian sarcoma virus	Sarcoma	Woolly monkey	v-*sis*	$P28^{v\text{-}sis}$

[a] Replication competent.

fibroblasts and hematopoietic cells in vitro and rapidly cause a wide variety of tumors of the hematopoietic system as well as sarcomas, endotheliomas, neurolymphamatosis, and splenomegaly. The reason for this is that their genomes contain an additional gene, a transforming gene or oncogene, which encodes a protein that triggers the transformation of normal cells into cancer cells. They are thus said to be v-*onc*$^+$, as opposed to the leukemia viruses, which are v-*onc*$^-$. The first virus of this group to be discovered and studied was the avian sarcoma virus, Rous sarcoma virus. This virus possesses five genes: *gag*, *pro*, *pol*, *env*, and a gene denoted *src* (for sarcoma), which encodes $pp60^{src}$, a phosphoprotein that possesses tyrosine-specific protein kinase activity. The *src* gene is a transforming gene: mutants with temperature-sensitive lesions in it are temperature sensitive with respect to ability to transform or maintain transformation. Thus RSV is both *transformation competent and replication competent* since it possesses all genes necessary for multiplication.

However, RSV is the only transformation-competent virus that is replication competent; all other v-*onc*$^+$ viruses are replication defective because in these viruses—the so-called sarcoma-acute leukemia viruses—the v-*onc* gene is inserted into their genome in such a way that either one or more of the genes essential for replication are either wholly or partially deleted. Usually the amount of deleted genetic material exceeds that which replaces it, so the genomes of the replication-defective sarcoma/acute leukemia viruses are generally smaller than, and sometimes no more than one half the size of, standard leukemia virus genomes. Therefore they can multiply only in the presence of a helper virus, typically a leukemia virus, which encodes the missing nucleocapsid, polymerase, or envelope proteins. Strains of these viruses consist of two types of particles, the helper virus particles and particles that are composed of proteins specified by the helper virus and contain the genome of the defective sarcoma/acute leukemia virus. These particles are known as *pseudotype* particles and are denoted as follows: Mo-MSV (Mo-MLV) for Moloney murine sarcoma virus, with the virus in parentheses denoting the helper virus, which is generally present in large excess. Usually any one of numerous leukemia viruses can serve as the helper.

Some well-known transformation-competent retroviruses are listed in Table 59–5. They include avian sarcoma viruses such as RSV and the Fujinami sarcoma virus; avian acute leukemia viruses such as avian myeloblastosis virus (AMV), avian myelocytomatosis virus (MC29), and avian erythroblastosis virus (AEV); murine sarcoma viruses such as the Moloney, Kirsten, and Harvey murine sarcoma viruses; murine acute leukemia viruses such as the Abelson murine leukemia virus; feline sarcoma viruses; and simian sarcoma virus.

Transforming Genes: Oncogenes

The reason sarcoma/acute leukemia viruses transform cells readily in vitro and rapidly induce cancer in animals is that they possess special genes, the transforming genes or oncogenes. More than 30 such genes have been discovered so far on the basis of the presence in retroviral genomes of specific nucleic acid sequences and the detection in cells transformed by them of proteins encoded by them. Many of these oncogenes are identified in Table 59–6, and the physical maps of the proviruses that contain some of them are depicted in Figure 59–16.

Proto-Oncogenes

The transforming genes present in retroviral genomes are closely related to certain cellular genes; in fact, each viral oncogene, v-*onc*, has a cellular counterpart or homologue, c-*onc*. Virtually all c-*onc* genes, which are generally termed *proto-oncogenes*, encode components of the signal transduction pathway that is activated when cells are stimulated to divide and proliferate by growth factors produced by other cells (i.e., cytokines or lymphokines) binding to receptors on their sur-

TABLE 59–6. SOME ONCOGENES AND THEIR FUNCTIONS

Oncogene	Virus	NIH/3T3 Transfection Assay	Function
Growth Factor Analogues			
v-*sis*	SiSV		Analogue of B chain of PDGF
fgf		+ (Kaposi's sarcoma)	Member of FGF family
int-2[a]			Member of FGF family
Transmembrane Glycoprotein Growth Factor Receptors with Tyrosine-specific Protein Kinase Activity			
erb B	AEV		Very similar to or identical with EGF receptor
erb B2 *HER2*(human) *neu*(mouse)		+	Closely related to EGF receptor; ligand unknown
fms	Susan-McDonough FeSV		Macrophage colony-stimulating factor (M-CGF or CMS-1) receptor
kit	Hardy-Zuckerman FeSV		Related to CMS-1 and PDGF receptors
mas		+ (epidermoid carcinoma)	Related to or identical with angiotensin receptor
met		+ (carcinogen-induced osteogenic sarcoma)	Ligand unknown
mpl	Myeloproliferative leukemia virus (MPLV)		Related to hematopoietic cytokine receptors; ligand unknown
ros	UR2-ASV		Closely related to insulin receptor
sea	AEV-913		Member of insulin receptor family
tcr	Defective FeLV		β-chain of T cell antigen receptor
trk-2		+ (breast cancer)	Ligand unknown
Membrane-associated Tyrosine-specific Protein Kinases			
abl	Abelson murine leukemia virus		Not known
fes	Gardner-Arnstein and Snyder-Theiler FeSV		Not known
fps	Fujinami avian sarcoma virus		Not known
src	RSV		Not known; association with polyoma middle T antigen increases its tyrosine-specific protein k nase activity
fgr	Gardner-Rasheed FeSV		Member of *src* family
yes	ASV-Y73		Member of *src* family
blk, fyn, hck, lck, and *lyn*			Members of *src* family identified by transfection assay or by probing gene libraries
Membrane-bound Guanine Nucleotide–binding Proteins: G Proteins			
ras (Ha-*ras*, Ki-*ras*, N-*ras*)	Harvey and Kirsten murine sarcoma viruses		Not known; cooperates with c-*fos* and c-*jun* in inducing site-specific DNA binding
Cytoplasmic Serine- and Threonine-specific Protein Kinases			
mil	MH2-ASV		Not known
raf-1	MuSV-3611		Murine version of *mil*
mos	Moloney-MuSV	+	Cytostatic factor (CSF)
pim-1[b]			Not known
Nuclear Factors Involved in Regulation of Gene Expression, DNA Replication, or Cell Division			
cbl	CasNS-1 murine retrovirus		Binds to T cell receptor–α enhancer; related to GCN4
ets	AEV E26		Related to Pu.1, a macrophage-specific transcription factor
fos	FBJ-MuSV		Associates with c-*jun* to form an enhancer-binding complex

(*continued*)

TABLE 59–6. SOME ONCOGENES AND THEIR FUNCTIONS (*continued*)

Oncogene	Virus	NIH/3T3 Transfection Assay	Function
jun	ASV17		In conjunction with c-*fos* is AP-1, an enhancer-binding protein that stimulates gene expression in response to growth factors and phorbol esters
maf	Avian musculo-aponeuritic fibroma virus U2 (AS 42)		Not known
myb	AMV; ASV E26		Sequence-specific DNA-binding protein
myc	Avian myelocytomatosis MC29; CM11; OK10		Sequence-specific DNA-binding protein; activates expression of G0/G1 transition genes
ski	Sloan-Kettering ASV		Distantly related to *myc*
Oncogenes with Miscellaneous Functions			
crk	ASV-CT10		Structure similar to group C oncogenes but possesses no protein kinase activity
erb A	AEV		c-*erb A* is the thyroid receptor; v-*erb A* is a thyroid hormone receptor antagonist
int-1[a]			Is secreted and becomes associated with the cell surface; may determine fate of surrounding cells
rel	Avian reticuloendotheliosis (REV-T)		c-*rel* binds to the κB enhancer; v-*rel* inhibits the function of NF-κB

SISV, simian sarcoma virus; AEV, avian erythroblastosis viruses; AMV, avian myeloblastosis virus; ASV, avian sarcoma virus; FeSV, feline sarcoma virus; FeLV, feline leukemia virus; FGF, fibroblast growth factor; MuLV, murine leukemia virus; MuSV, murine sarcoma virus; PDGF, platelet-derived growth factor; RSV, Rous sarcoma virus; EGF, epidermal growth factor.
[a] Identified in breast carcinomas induced by MMTV.
[b] Identified in MuLV-induced T cell lymphomas.

faces. Interaction with their ligands activates these receptors and initiates a cascade of events in which each activated protein activates some other protein, the overall result being the transmission of signals from the outer surface of the plasma cell membrane to the nucleus in which novel sets of transcriptional activators initiate the transcription of genes, the function of which is to promote cell proliferation. The key to the correct functioning of such cascadelike signal transduction pathways is that activation of each component, that is, their existence in the "on" state, must be limited to the period for which the stimulating signal is present; that is, when the supply of growth factor ceases, all pathway components must return rapidly to their inactive "off" state, and cell proliferation must cease.

Proto-oncogenes become incorporated into retroviral genomes with surprising ease. When mutants of RSV with large deletions in their *src* genes are injected into chickens, viruses can soon be recovered that can again cause tumors. The reason is that in the newly transformation-competent viruses, the deleted v-*src* gene has been replaced by the chicken c-*src* gene, which has in effect been "pirated" by the viral genome. Exactly how proto-oncogenes are incorporated into retroviral genomes is not known. Presumably the proto-oncogene first recombines with and is inserted into the provirus, and its introns are lost when the transcript of this new recombinant provirus is spliced to yield the genome of the new transforming virus. Such insertion of cellular material into the retroviral genome apparently provides the opportunity for further recombination with homologous regions within the host cell genome because sequencing studies have shown that viral oncogenes such as the v-*ras* gene are flanked by several sets of sequences derived from cellular DNA and are generated through numerous recombination events.

Not all known oncogenes have yet been found in such essentially "cloned" form in retroviral genomes. About 10 years ago Weinberg found that when the DNA of certain human tumors is transfected into cultured mouse NIH–3T3 cells, foci of transformed cells result. Approximately 5% to 10% of human tumors react positively in this transfection assay. Most of them are members of an oncogene family, the *ras* gene family, members of which are also incorporated into retroviral genomes (Fig. 59–16 and Tables 59–5 and 59–6); thus the "activated" form (see below) of the c-Ha-*ras*-1 gene is present primarily in human bladder carcinomas and urinary tract tumors, lung carcinoma, melanoma, and chemically induced tumors, whereas that of the c-Ki-*ras*-2 gene is present primarily in human lung, colon, pancreatic, gallbladder, and primary ovarian carcinomas as well as in adult lymphocytic leukemia and rhabdomyosarcoma. A third member of this family, the N-*ras* gene, which has not yet been found integrated into any retroviral genome, is also reactivated in a wide variety of human tumors.

In addition to the *ras* genes, several other oncogenes have been identified by the cell transfection assay technique. Some, like *ras*, were also later found to be v-*onc* genes (e.g., *mos*); others, also listed in Table 59–6, have not yet been found integrated into any retroviral provirus. In addition, several oncogenes have been identified because they are overexpressed as the result of the activity of an enhancer in a nearby provirus (*int*-1, *int*-2, *met*, and *pim*-1; [Table 59–6]), and several

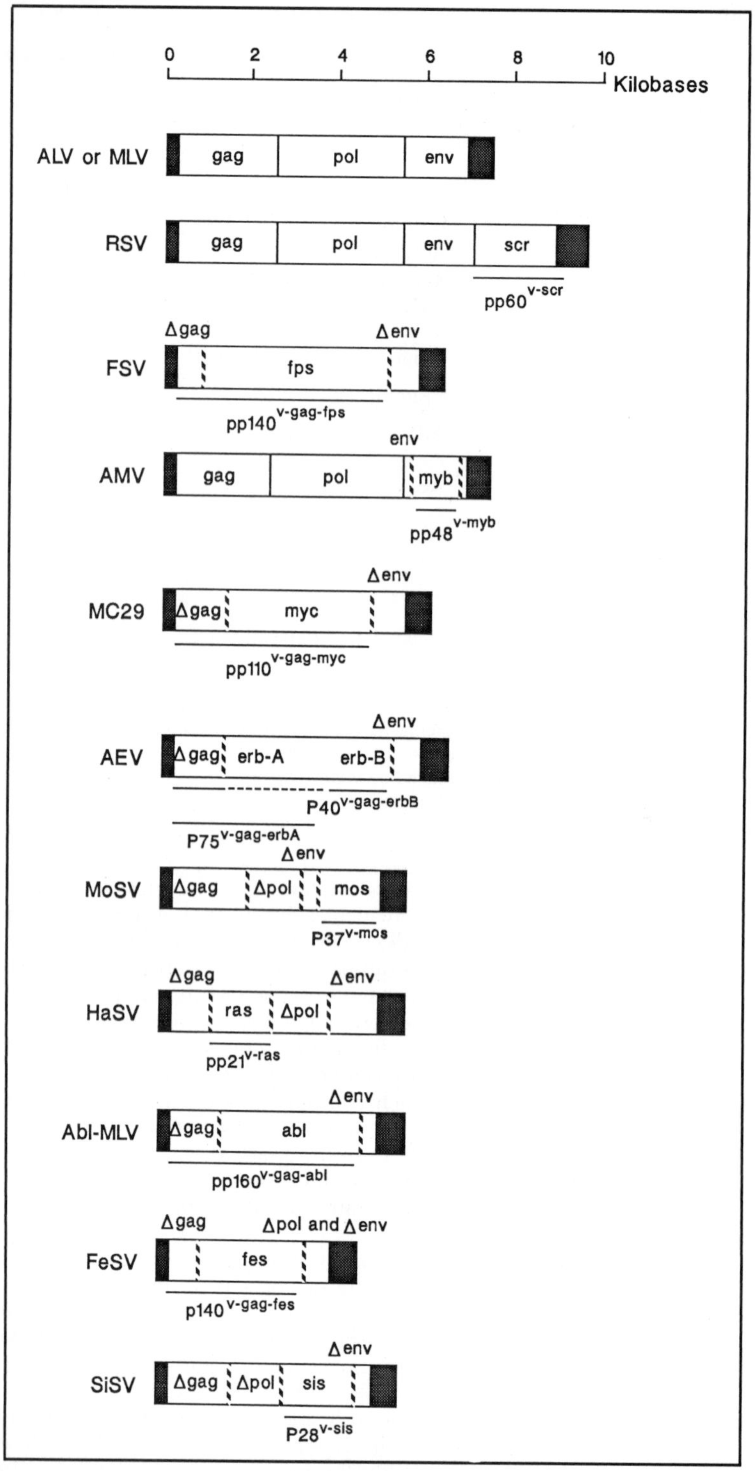

Fig. 59–16. Genomes, transforming genes, and transforming gene products of acute leukemia/sarcoma viruses. The genomes of avian and murine leukemia viruses and of Rous sarcoma virus, which are nondefective, are shown for comparison. The transforming proteins are indicated beneath the RNA sequences that encode them. Phosphoproteins are denoted by the prefix pp, other proteins by the prefix P. Note that some transforming proteins are fusion proteins in which their *N*-terminal portions are the *N*-terminal portions of the *gag*-encoded protein, while the remainder is encoded by the specific oncogene (the v-*myc*, v-*fps*, v-*abl*, and v-*fes* gene products), and others (v-*src*, v-*myb*, v-*mos*, v-*ras*, and v-*sis* gene products) are specified entirely by the oncogene. Note that in all cases except RSV the transforming gene replaces a very substantial portion of the normal retrovirus genome, leaving partially deleted genes (*gag*, *pol*, and *env*), which are not large enough to encode functional proteins/enzymes. ALV and MLV, avian and murine leukemia virus, respectively; RSV, Rous sarcoma virus; FSV, Fujinami sarcoma virus; AMV, avian myeloblastosis virus; MC29, a strain of avian myelocytomatosis virus; AEV, avian erythroblastosis virus; MoSV, Moloney murine sarcoma virus; HaSV, Harvey murine sarcoma virus; Abl-MLV Abelson murine leukemia virus; FeSV, feline sarcoma virus; SiSV, simian sarcoma virus.

oncogenes have been identified in and isolated from gene libraries through the use of probes comprising sequences of known oncogenes.

Under normal conditions the proteins encoded by proto-oncogenes do *not* transform cells. By contrast, proteins encoded by oncogenes do; and they do so because they are locked permanently into the activated, or "on," mode. The most common reason for this is loss or functional inactivation of regulatory domains that are usually located in their C-terminal regions, as illustrated for the c-*src* gene in Figure 59–17. The regulatory domain is either deleted or modified by several mutations, probably at the time when proto-onco-

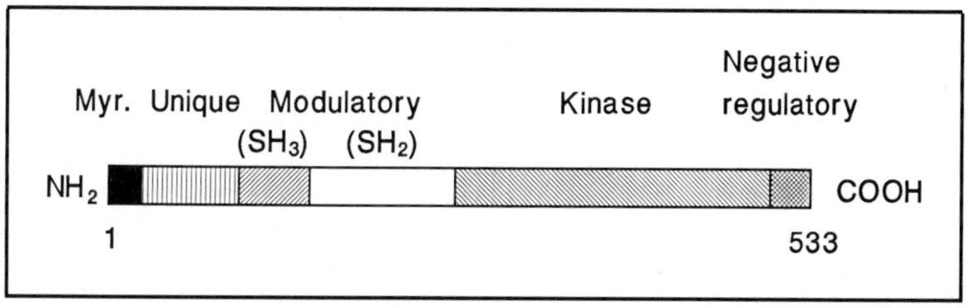

Fig. 59–17. Functional map of pp60$^{c\text{-}src}$, a typical membrane-associated, tyrosine-specific protein kinase–containing signal transduction pathway component. The protein is anchored in membranes via a myristylated site near its *N*-terminus. Next there is a unique region that may be responsible for substrate specificity, followed by two regions, SH_2 and SH_3 (for *src h*omology), that modulate the protein's activity. These two regions, which are also present in other components of the signal transduction pathway such as GTPase activator protein (GAP) and phospholipase $C\gamma 1$, possess high affinity for activated growth factor receptors; they provide a mechanism by which diverse regulatory proteins can associate physically with activated receptors and thereby couple growth factor stimulation to intracellular signal transduction pathways in a cell-specific manner. There follows a tyrosine-specific protein kinase domain and finally a regulatory domain in the C-terminal region, loss or functional modification of which activates these proteins irreversibly and converts them to oncogenes. These proteins also possess several transmembrane domains that could target them to distinctive subcellular locations and may endow them with diverse biologic functions. For example, pp60$^{c\text{-}src}$ is associated with plasma membranes, perinuclear membranes, secretory organelles, and growth cones in developing neurons.

genes are integrated into proviruses. Another way in which regulatory domains may be lost is by fusion with genes normally far removed (through translocation or rearrangement of genetic material). Interestingly, in the case of the *ras* proteins, permanent conversion to the "on" mode is caused by a *single* mutation, usually in position 12 or in position 61.

Although under normal conditions proteins encoded by proto-oncogenes do not transform cells, some do so if they are overexpressed. This happens when proto-oncogenes are brought under the control of powerful constitutive enhancers, again through the rearrangement of genetic material such as may be caused by chromosomal translocations.

The net result of all these changes is that signal transduction pathways are switched permanently to the "on" mode; thus cells are permanently stimulated to proliferate, that is, are transformed into tumor cells. Since in all these situations the modified or overexpressed proto-oncogene products exert a positive effect, these genes are *dominant* oncogenes. As is shown below, examples are also known of *recessive* oncogenes.

Nature and Functions of Proteins Encoded by *onc* Genes

As may be expected, signal transduction pathways are multiple, varied, and complex. They comprise several families of proteins, each composed of proteins that are related and that exercise similar type functions but that differ in specificity, that is, with respect to the nature of the proteins that activate them and the proteins that they activate. Since these genes are essential to correct cellular functioning, they are highly conserved during evolution; many are present not only in all vertebrate, but probably in all metazoan genomes. For example, *src*-, *myc*-, and *ras*-related genes are present in *Drosophila*; an *abl*-related gene is present in nematodes; and *ras*-related genes are present and expressed in amebae and in yeast.

The functions of the families of signal transduction pathway components of which oncogenes are permanently activated members follow (see also Table 59–6).

Growth Factors. The v-*sis* oncogene encodes an altered version of the β-chain of the platelet-derived growth factor (PDGF), and the *int*-2 and K-*fgf* gene products are related to the fibroblast growth factor.

Transmembrane Growth Factor Receptors with Tyrosine-specific Protein Kinase Activity. These are glycoproteins that possess large *N*-terminal extracellular regions, a transmembrane spanning region, and an intracellular portion that possesses tyrosine-specific protein kinase activity. The oncogenes in this family are permanently activated (i.e., possessing high kinase activity in the absence of ligand) versions of the epidermal growth factor (EGF), colony-stimulating factor (CSF1), thyroid hormones, angiotension receptors, the β-chain of the T cell receptor, and possibly the insulin or insulin-like factor receptors.

Membrane-bound Tyrosine-specific Protein Kinases. Many oncogenes are permanently activated versions of genes that encode membrane-bound tyrosine-specific protein kinases. Some of these kinases phosphorylate many proteins, others only a few. Among their substrates are lipid kinases that phosphorylate phosphoinositol, which, when cleaved by phospholipase C, yields secondary messengers such as inositol triphosphate (which releases calcium from intracellular stores, which in turn activates a variety of calcium-dependent functions), and diacylglycerol (DAG), which, together with calcium, activates protein kinase C. Other substrates may be cytoplasmic serine-threonine kinases involved in transmitting signals to the nucleus. The nature of these protein kinases, particularly those of the *src*-like family (*src*, *blk*, *fgr*, *fyn*, *hck*, *lck*, *lyn*, and *yes*) is shown in Figure 59–17.

Membrane-bound G Proteins. Another group of proteins involved in signal transduction are the membrane-bound G proteins, proteins that bind GTP/GDP. When activated, they exchange guanosine diphosphate (GDP) for guanosine triphosphate (GTP) and then activate either adenylate cyclase, with resultant increases in the concentration of cyclic AMP (the prototype of second messengers) or ion channels, or phospholipase C, which then generates DAG and inositol triphosphate as described above. One of the most intensively investigated oncogenes, the *ras* oncogene, is a G protein. G proteins that are oncogenes have lost their intrinsic capacity to hydrolyze GTP and therefore permanently transduce their signal, which results in unregulated cell growth.

Cytoplasmic Serine-Threonine-specific Protein Kinases. These kinases appear to belong to the protein kinase C family. In response to mitogenic signals they are recruited to the membrane, where they are activated by becoming phosphorylated on tyrosine residues, causing them to autophosphorylate serine or threonine residue, which "turns on" their regulatory domains. Once activated, they migrate to the nucleus; thus they are thought to provide a link in the signal transduction pathway between external signals generated at the membrane and nuclear proteins that regulate gene expression and cell division. Oncogene-encoded versions of these enzymes have lost their C-terminal regulatory domains.

Nuclear Factors Involved in Regulating Gene Expression, DNA Replication, or Cell Division. These proteins are sequence-specific DNA-binding proteins and/or transactive transcriptional activators. Several oncogenes encode proteins that are, or possess sequence similarity to, more-or-less well-characterized members of this family of nuclear factors.

Oncogenes with Miscellaneous Functions. In addition to the oncogenes that are analogues of components of the signal transduction pathway, there are several with miscellaneous functions. One oncogene, *int*-1, acts at the cell membrane and may function in cell-to-cell signaling; another, *erb A*, is a nuclear thyroid hormone receptor antagonist; and others are cytoplasmic proteins with functions reminiscent of, but not identical with, those of the oncogenes discussed previously.

Antioncogenes

Several years ago a study of the rare hereditary disease retinoblastoma led to the discovery of a fundamentally different class of cancer genes—a class of genes that function in normal cells not to promote cell proliferation but to suppress it.

There are two forms of retinoblastoma: a sporadic form seen in children who have no family history of the disease, which usually affects only one eye, and a familial form that occurs in children whose parents also suffer from the disease, which usually affects both eyes. In 1971 Knudson proposed that both forms involve two genetic inactivating lesions (through mutation or deletion); in the former both lesions were postulated to occur somatically in an embryonic cell in the retinal lineage, whereas in the familial form of the disease one lesion was thought to be already present in the fertilized egg and only the second occurred somatically. The targets of these inactivating lesions were the two copies of a gene located on chromosome 13, termed the *Rb gene*. Both copies of this gene were subsequently indeed found to be functionally inactive, not only in all cases of retinoblastoma, but also in many cases of bladder cancer, breast cancer, osteosarcoma, and small cell lung carcinoma.

Since it is the absence of a functional Rb protein that causes malignancy, the gene has been referred to as a *recessive* oncogene, a tumor or growth suppressor gene, or simply as an antioncogene.

At the same time it was recognized that p53, a cellular protein that had been studied extensively in cells infected with DNA-containing tumor viruses (adenoviruses, SV40, and papillomaviruses), was present in many tumors in abnormal form. Functionally inactivated versions of this protein, encoded by a gene on chromosome 17 in a region subject to frequent translocations, have been found in about one half of human malignancies: in chronic myelocytic and myelogenous leukemia, hepatocellular carcinoma, osteogenic sarcoma, colon, colorectal, and esophageal cancer, breast cancer, lung cancer, and malignant neurofibrosarcomas in von Recklinghausen's neurofibromatosis. In many of these malignancies at least one p53 allele has suffered a mutation, deletion, or rearrangement that results in the formation of nonfunctional p53 protein; but it is not necessary that *both* alleles be inactivated since the functional form of p53 is a homooligomeric complex so that inactive p53 can exert a transdominant inactivating effect. Further, as for the Rb gene, inactivated forms of the p53 gene can exist in germ line cells, thereby predisposing to tumorigenesis, as is the case in the rare dominantly inherited Li-Fraumeni syndrome of breast cancer and other malignancies. Finally, p53 exists in functionally inactive form in many cultured cell lines, which may conceivably contribute to their immortalization. Cell lines in which both p53 genes have been inactivated exist and are viable (e.g., HL60 human promyelocytic leukemia cells).

The Rb (mol wt 105 kDa) and p53 proteins have similar functions. Both are expressed in all cells, especially during embyrogenesis. Both are nuclear proteins subject to cell cycle phase-specific phosphorylation: they are not phosphorylated in the G0/G1 phases and exist in the form of multiple phosphorylated species thereafter. The cdc protein kinase and a DNA-activated protein kinase are among the enzymes that phosphorylate them. It is not known exactly how they suppress cell division/proliferation; it is thought that they control the expression of genes that are critical for entry into the cell cycle. If they are inactivated, the result is uncontrolled cell growth.

It is unlikely the Rb and p53 genes are the only antioncogenes. Indeed, about 12 other chromosomal regions contain genes that act in a tissue-specific manner to regulate cell proliferation because each contributes to tumorigenesis when both functional alleles are lost.

Interaction Between Antioncogenes and "Oncogenes" of DNA-containing Viruses

All available evidence indicates that absence of functional Rb and p53 proteins leads to uncontrolled cell proliferation. Such absence may be caused not only by sequence modifications that result in the formation of inactive protein species but also by the binding of Rb and p53 proteins by other proteins to form functionally inactive complexes. Several such proteins have been identified; interestingly, they are the E1A and E1B proteins of adenovirus, the SV40 large T antigen, and the E6 and E7 proteins of papillomaviruses, proteins that have long been considered the oncogenes of these DNA-containing

TABLE 59–7. INTERACTIONS OF "ONCOGENES" OF DNA TUMOR VIRUSES WITH ANTIONCOGENE PROTEINS p53 AND $p110^{Rb}$

Virus	Protein	Function	Antioncogene Protein Bound
SV40	Large T antigen (domain 1–120 aas)	Immortalizes primary cells Transcriptional transactivator	$p110^{Rb}$
SV40	Large T antigen (domain 272–625)	Transforms some cells Helicase Binds to DNA polymerase	p53
Adenovirus	E1A proteins	Immortalize cultured cells Transcriptional transactivators	$p110^{Rb}$
	E1B proteins	Transforms cells	p53
HPV 16	E7	Transforms cells with E6 Transcriptional transactivator	$p110^{Rb}$
	E6	Transforms cells with E7	p53

viruses (see p. 873). These proteins express several functions that together are required for tumor formation: immortalizing cells, transforming cells, transcriptional trans-activating activity, and miscellaneous ancillary functions. The domains that express these functions and that are located on either a single protein or on two separate proteins possess affinity for either the Rb protein or for p53 (Table 59–7): the domains with transcriptional transactivating activity bind to the Rb protein, and domains with cell-transforming activity bind p53. In both cases the complexes that are formed are inactive with respect to the tumor suppressor function of the two antioncogenes. In fact, recent evidence indicates that combination of p53 with the E6 protein stimulates its degradation by the ubiquitin-dependent protease system.

The affinity of the E1A and E1B proteins of adenoviruses, the large T antigen of SV40, and the E6 and E7 proteins of papillomaviruses for the Rb and p53 proteins raises questions concerning (1) their own oncogenicity and (2) the significance of these interactions during their lytic multiplication cycles. Regarding the first question, there is no doubt that the ability of the viral oncogenes to inactivate the antiproliferative effects of the Rb and p53 proteins is a major factor in the oncogenicity of adenoviruses and papovaviruses; but the ability of the E1A protein, the SV40 large T antigen, and the papillomavirus E7 protein to activate the transcription of genes with cell proliferation promoting functions is undoubtedly also functionally very important. With respect to the second question, adenoviruses, SV40, HPV16, and HPV18 have most probably evolved the ability to inactivate the antiproliferative Rb and p53 genes so as to stimulate cell division/proliferation because they themselves multiply best in replicating cells. Alternatively, if they infect nonpermissive cells, they integrate their genomes into cellular genomes and then still express the E1A/E1B, large T antigen and E6/E7 proteins, which again antagonize the antioncogenes, thereby again stimulating the multiplication of the cells that now contain their genomes.

Cooperation Between Oncogenes and Antioncogenes in Multistep Progression Toward Tumorigenesis

Although cell transformation from the normal state to a form capable of unrestricted growth in vitro and in vivo can be elicited by single oncogenes, tumorigenesis itself, (i.e., the establishment of cancer cells with metastatic potential) is a complex multistep process. Unfortunately, there are few, if any, model systems in which the progression that this process involves can be studied in molecular terms. One of the major difficulties is that the mechanisms underlying tumorigenesis differ widely with the nature of the malignancy; another is that, although it is often possible to establish the nature of the oncogene that *initiates* tumorigenesis, the *subsequent* interactions are exceedingly complex. However, it is becoming increasingly apparent that the two basic mechanisms involved are interactions among and between oncogenes and antioncogenes on the one hand and selection of cells optimally transformed for the particular stage of progression attained on the other. The two systems that have yielded the most insight are cultured cells and certain malignancies that exhibit clearly identifiable stages. For example, primary rat embryo fibroblasts cannot be transformed by an activated *ras* oncogene alone. They can be *immortalized* after transfection of the *myc* oncogene, the adenovirus E1A gene, or a mutant p53 antioncogene; but production of *transformed* cells requires the introduction of *two* oncogenes such as *ras* plus E1A, *ras* plus mutant p53, or *ras* plus *myc*. As for an example of the development of malignancies in hosts, progression through the clinical stages of colorectal cancer is characterized first by *ras* activation, followed in sequential fashion by the functional inactivation of p53 and of at least two other unidentified genes at specific chromosomal locations. There is evidence that the complete development of malignancies may involve more than 10 genetic alterations, which suggests that most "oncogenes" involved in human neoplasia have not yet been identified. In particular, more than 24 chromosomal translocations in various groups of lymphoid tumors have not yet been characterized with respect to what genes are being inactivated, modified/caused to be overexpressed, and there may be many more. Finally, it is becoming increasingly apparent that the more c-*onc* proteins are examined in tumors, the more are found to possess abnormal structure or function. For example, in a significant proportion of bronchiogenic carcinomas, the *myc*, *ras*, *raf*, *jun*, and *erb* B2 (*neu*) protooncogenes have been altered, as well as one or both of the Rb and p53 antioncogenes.

How Do Retroviruses that Lack Oncogenes Cause Cancer?

Retroviruses that lack oncogenes also cause cancer, but they usually do so infrequently, after long latent periods, and generally late in life. Two mechanisms are primarily involved in this process.

Proviral Insertion

The first mechanism is proviral insertion, also often termed *insertional activation* or *promoter insertion*. Its basis is that much of the proviral insertion into cellular DNA does not occur randomly but rather into strongly preferred target sites (see p. 882). Since the long terminal repeats (LTRs) of proviruses contain signals specifying activation of transcription (promoters and enhancers), the expression of genes flanking integrated proviruses is greatly increased. This becomes crucial if these genes are proto-oncogenes, particularly if they are mutated by the genetic disturbance caused by the proviral integration event and if this results in loss of a regulatory domain, so that what is overexpressed is not the normal proto-oncogene protein but rather a mutated proto-oncogene protein in the "on" mode (see above). Examples of insertional activation are B cell lymphomas caused, after latent periods of 6 months or more, by an avian leukosis virus (ALV) in chickens, which express *myc*; erythroleukemias caused similarly in chickens by an ALV in which the provirus has invariably inserted within the c-*erb* B locus, which results in the expression of a truncated growth factor receptor that has lost its ligand-binding domain and is thus permanently in the "on" position; and several genes, expression of which is activated by insertion of MMTV proviruses, including *int*-1 and *int*-2 (see Table 59–6). *Pim*-1, a cytoplasmic protein with serine-threonine-specific protein kinase activity, *ras* and *mos*, *fms*, which encodes either the CSF-1 receptor or a close homologue of it, and *lck*, a cytoplasmic tyrosine-specific protein kinase–containing signal transduction pathway component, are also activated by proviral insertion.

Proviral insertion may also disrupt the coding regions of cellular genes. The resultant damage, however, is usually not apparent because cellular genomes are diploid. Nevertheless, there is one consequence of this type of disruptive proviral insertion that *is* noticeable and that occurs when there is insertion into antioncogenes. This is the case in tumors induced by the Friend murine leukemia virus, which often involves proviral insertion into both alleles of the p53 gene.

Recombination with Endogenous Viral Genomes: MCF Viruses

The development of leukemia in mice is often preceded by the generation of a novel class of retroviruses, the so-called MCF viruses (because they form foci in [i.e., transform] cultured mink cells). MCF viruses are recombinants between proviruses of murine leukemia viruses and *env* genes of endogenous viruses. The significance of their generation lies in the fact that retrovirus host range and ability to interact with host cell genomes is controlled by *env* genes and proviral LTRs, respectively; generation of MCF viruses thus creates new virus strains, with new target cells and with additional opportunities for transforming cells by insertional mutagenesis.

The generation of MCF viruses highlights a unique property of retroviruses, namely, their extraordinarily high rate of recombination, not only between infecting exogenous viruses but also, as demonstrated here, between exogenous and endogenous viruses. Oncogene capture is another expression of this phenomenon; the sequences in regions flanking captured oncogenes often bear witness to multiple recombinational events. A clue to the nature of the mechanisms involved in the generation of recombinants is provided by the fact that recombinants are not produced in cells infected with two *different* retroviruses; recombination requires infection with *heterozygous* virions (i.e., virus particles containing two *different* RNA strands). The mechanism involved in the generation of recombinants is often referred to as *forced copy choice*, the basis of which is the fact that retroviral RNA strands often contain breaks; when the reverse transcriptase encounters a break, it switches template to the homologous sequence on the other strand. This mechanism may be crucial for retrovirus survival.

Mechanisms Causing Overexpression of Proto-Oncogenes

There are two major mechanisms that cause proto-oncogenes to be overexpressed and transform cells.

Chromosomal Translocation

Many types of cancer cells display chromosomal abnormalities caused by translocations in which portions of two chromosomes exchange positions. Some of these translocations occur repeatedly in certain types of tumors; and in them proto-oncogenes are relocated so that they are brought under the control of strong promoters or enhancers, thus causing their expression to be activated or increased and tumors to form. There are many examples of this type. One is the human c-*myc* gene, which in Burkitt lymphoma cell lines is translocated from its normal location on chromosome 8 to chromosome 14, 2, or 22, where it is activated by IgH, Igκ, or Igλ enhancers, respectively. Another example is provided by c-*abl*, which is translocated from chromosome 9 to chromosome 22 in human chronic myelogenous leukemia cells. In the resultant chromosome, the Philadelphia (Ph) chromosome, the c-*abl* gene is fused to the bcr (breakpoint cluster region) in such a way that instead of the normal $pp145^{c\text{-}abl}$, the abnormal $pp210^{bcr\text{-}abl}$ is formed, which possesses a more active tyrosine-specific protein kinase activity than the normal protein and has lost its regulatory domain. A similar translocation occurs in acute lymphoblastic leukemia cells. Other oncogenes activated by chromosomal translocation are *met*, *ret*, *trk*-1, and *trk*-2 (in which cellular tyrosine-specific protein kinases are activated by fusion to a tropomyosin gene and a ribosomal protein gene, respectively), *bcl*-2 (which is activated in human B cell lymphomas by a [18:14] translocation that places c-*bcl*-2 under the control of the IgH enhancer), *ets* (lymphocytic and myelogenous leukemia), and *dbl*.

Oncogenes in Amplified DNA

Tumor cells often contain regions of DNA that, for reasons not well understood, are amplified. The degree of amplification may be only fivefold to fiftyfold, but it may also reach 1000-fold or more; at such levels the amplified DNA can be detected by karyologic techniques as double-minute chromosomes or homogeneously staining regions (HSRs). Several proto-oncogenes are located in the amplified DNA, and their

TABLE 59–8. PROTO-ONCOGENES IN AMPLIFIED REGIONS OF TUMOR CELL DNA

Proto-Oncogene	Tumor
c-*myc*	Promyelocytic leukemia Small-cell lung carcinoma Bursal lymphoma
N-*myc*	Neuroblastoma Retinoblastoma Small-cell lung carcinoma
c-*abl*	Chronic myeloid leukemia Acute lymphoblastic leukemia
c-*myb*	Colon carcinoma Acute myeloid leukemia
c-*erb B*	Epidermoid carcinoma
c-Ki-*ras*-2	Primary lung, colon, bladder, and rectal carcinomas
N-*ras*	Mammary carcinoma
c-*ets*	Acute myelomonocytic leukemia Small lymphocytic cell lymphoma

presence is always correlated with increased levels of RNA transcribed from them. Examples of proto-oncogenes in amplified human tumor cell DNA are listed in Table 59–8.

Mouse Mammary Tumor Virus

Mouse mammary tumor virus (MMTV), the prototype of B-type retroviruses, can be transmitted both vertically and horizontally. The genome of mice contains about 15 different MMTV proviruses that were probably acquired as a result of germ line infection events and that behave like cellular genes. Some are silent because they are in transcriptionally inactive chromatin regions; others are defective. However, two encode infectious MMTV particles that can be transmitted horizontally. They are the Mtv-1 provirus which encodes the MMTV strain known as the Bittner milk factor which is present in large amounts in lactating mammary tissue and therefore in milk; as a result, it is passed on readily to young animals in which it induces mammary adenocarcinomas with high frequency early in life. In animals reared by foster mothers whose milk contains no MMTV, it causes mammary tumors at an incidence of 20% to 50% at 1½ to 2 years of age. The other complete provirus is Mtv-2, which causes mammary tumors at high incidence (90%) at an early age and is also present in milk.

The extent to which MMTV proviruses are expressed in various tissues varies greatly; in virus-producing tumors and lactating mammary tissue there are more than 1000 genome equivalents of MMTV RNA per cell, but in most other tissues there are essentially none. The reason is that MMTV LTRs, which are very long (more than 1300 base pairs), possess a steroid hormone (glucocorticoid, estrogen)-responsive enhancer.

MMTV does not possess an oncogene; it causes tumors by proviral insertion. The most commonly activated proto-oncogenes are *int*-1 and *int*-2 (see Table 59–6).

Sequences closely related to MMTV proviruses and to *int*-1 and *int*-2 are present in the human genome.

Human Retroviruses

Human retrovirology is a relatively young field; although virologists have searched for human retroviral pathogens since the beginning of the century, it has been only 10 years since the first human retrovirus was isolated.

Human T Cell Leukemia Virus Types I and II

There are two human exogenous C-type retroviruses that are specific for T cells and transform them into cells capable of growing in the absence of exogenous T cell growth factor (IL-2). Human T cell leukemia virus type I (HTLV-I) was first identified in a T-lymphoblastoid cell line established from a patient diagnosed with cutaneous T cell lymphoma; more likely the patient had adult T cell leukemia (ATL), a disease first described in certain regions of southern Japan where there are about 1 million infected individuals (about 10% of the population in Kyushu), and 300 to 500 cases of ATL are diagnosed annually. HTLV-I is also endemic in other regions of the Orient, the Caribbean basin, northeastern South America, and Central Africa. The incidence of HTLV infection is increasing in Europe and in the United States, primarily among intravenous drug abusers and homosexuals. In addition to causing ATL, it is also the cause of the neurologic disorder known as *tropical spastic paraparesis* (HTLV-I-associated myelopathy).

Human T cell leukemia virus type II (HTLV-II) is far less common. It was first identified in a T cell line established from a patient with hairy-cell leukemia. However, it has been isolated only a very few times, and a definite etiologic role for it in the epidemiology of human malignancy has not yet been established.

HTLV-I and HTLV-II are most closely related to bovine leukemia virus (BLV) and simian T cell leukemia virus (STLV). Like them, they are oncogenic but do not possess an oncogene. Their most remarkable feature is possession of at least two regulatory genes that control their replication. They therefore form a distinctive subfamily among the C-type oncornaviruses.

The organization of the HTLV genome is shown in Figure 59–18. It resembles that of other type C retroviruses: it possesses the U3-R-U5-containing LTRs, a *gag* gene, a *pol* gene, and an *env* gene. It also possesses a region that encodes, in different reading frames, two proteins with regulatory functions. The *tax* protein is a *trans*-active transcriptional activator that increases the rate of transcription initiation from the promoter in the 5′-LTR; it is also capable of *trans*-activating heterologous promoters such as the adenovirus E3, the IL-2, the IL-3, and the GM-CSF promoters. Its mechanism of action is indirect. It is not a DNA-binding protein but either interacts with, modifies, or activates one or more cellular transcription factors that bind to a variety of regulatory sequences at or near the transcription initiation site at the U3-R junction of the 5′-LTR.

The *rex* gene encodes two proteins of 27K and 21K that share C-termini. They control the differential posttranscriptional expression of viral proteins by controlling whether doubly spliced (for the *tax* and *rex* proteins) or unspliced and singly spliced mRNAs (for *gag*, *pol*, and *env* proteins, respectively) are transported to the cytoplasm.

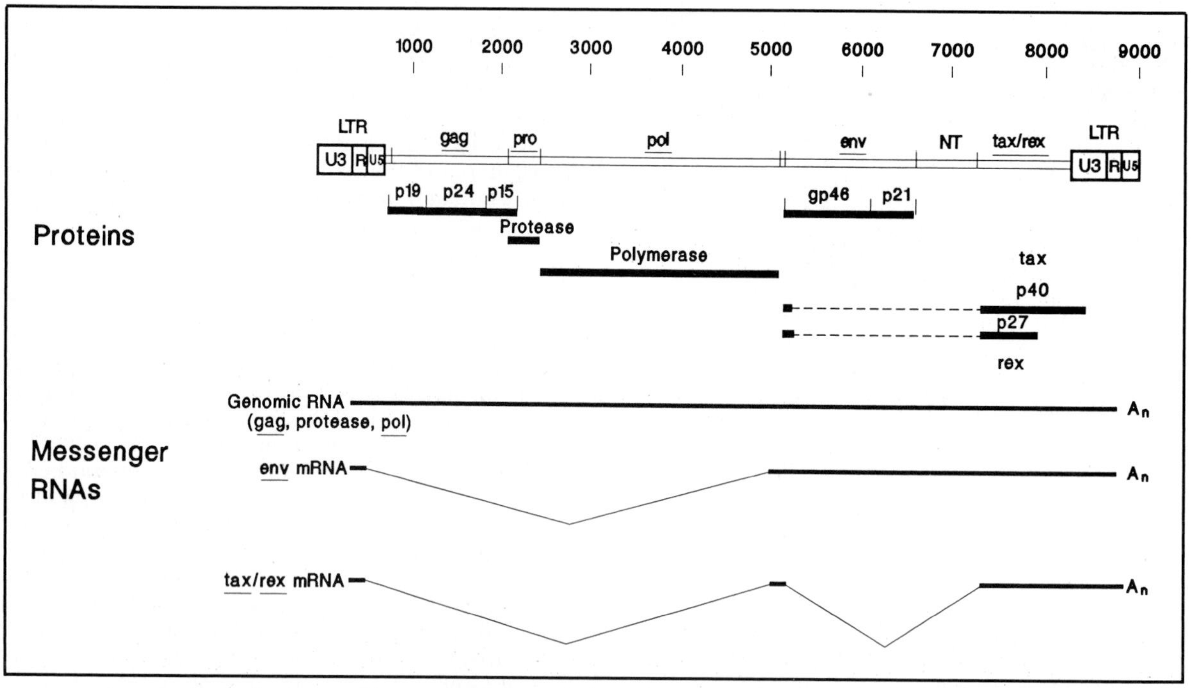

Fig. 59–18. The HTLV-I genome: structure and expression strategy. Note the overlapping *gag*, *pro*, and *pol* gene reading frames; the *pro* gene overlaps both the 3′-end of the *gag* gene and the 5′-end of the *pol* gene. Synthesis of the respective proteins is probably achieved by two ribosomal frameshifts (see Fig. 59–15). The 3′-end of the *pol* gene overlaps slightly, in a different reading frame, that of the *env* gene, which encodes the 46K SU protein and the 21 kDa TM protein. The *env* open reading frame (ORF) is followed by a large (about 600 nucleotides long) untranslated region of unknown function and then by the *tax* and *rex* genes. The *tax* and *rex* proteins are both translated from a single messenger RNA that consists of two minor exons and one major exon; large portions of the ORFs of the *tax* and *rex* genes overlap entirely in different reading frames.

The molecular mechanism by which HTLV transforms cells is not clear. It does not possess an oncogene, nor is there a common integration site in different tissues; thus proviral insertion also is not operative. Conceivably it is the inappropriate transcriptional activation of T cell proliferation genes by the *tax* protein that results in uncontrolled cell proliferation.

Human Immunodeficiency Viruses

The primary etiologic agent of the human acquired immunodeficiency syndrome (AIDS) is human immunodeficiency virus (HIV), a retrovirus (Fig. 59–19). HIV is not, however, a member of the subfamily Oncovirinae but belongs to the subfamily Lentivirinae (see Table 53–4), viruses whose most striking characteristic is their ability to initiate persistent chronic infections that result in debilitating progressive diseases both of the nervous system and of other organs. They do so using several strategies for evading immune surveillance; in particular, they can reside in cells in latent form, which they can do because they encode a variety of proteins designed to regulate various phases of their multiplication cycle. HIV is not a tumor virus; it does not transform cells but destroys them. However, it is considered here because it is by now the most intensively studied retrovirus because of its great clinical importance.

HIV was identified as the etiologic agent of epidemic AIDS in 1983. Epidemiologic evidence indicates that it arose in Central Africa. There are actually two forms of HIV: HIV-I, which is the predominant form not only in Africa, but worldwide; and HIV-II, which is endemic in West Africa. The two human HIVs are 50% to 60% related to each other and to several immunodeficiency viruses that have been isolated from several species of monkeys and primates (Fig. 59–20), but HIV-I is about 85% related to an immunodeficiency virus isolated from chimpanzees, and HIV-II is equally closely related to an immunodeficiency virus isolated from sooty mangabeys and to another isolated from macaques. Whether HIV-I and HIV-II evolved from simian immunodeficiency viruses, acquiring the ability to infect humans in the process, or are the products of recombination among simian immunodeficiency viruses is not known.

The major biologic and genetic features of HIV-I and HIV-II are very similar. Since HIV-I causes many more human infections and is also somewhat more virulent, most of the discussion that follows focuses on it.

The most significant feature of the spectrum of diseases caused by HIV is the fact that the HIV receptor is the CD4 T lymphocyte antigen. Thus the multiplication of the virus is

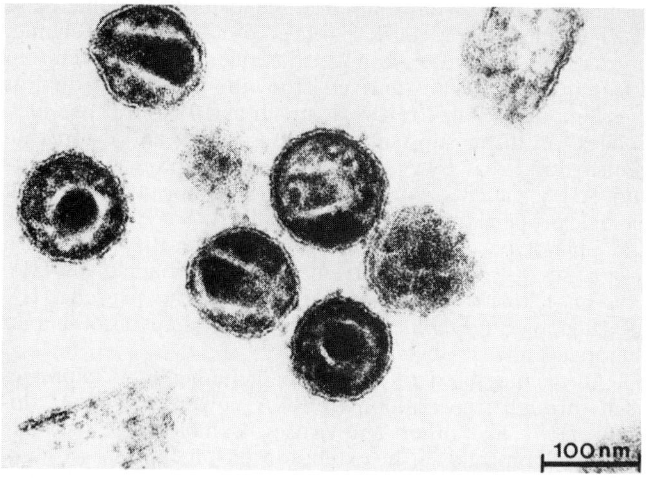

A

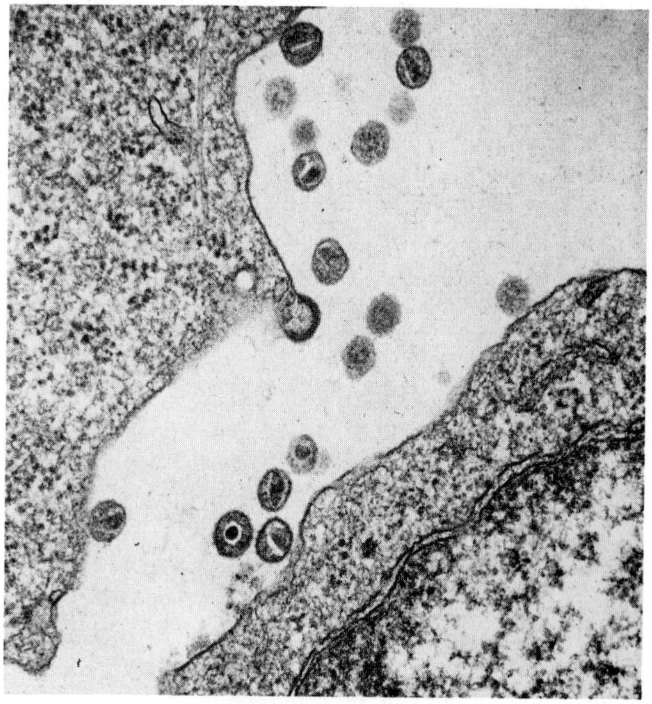

B

Fig. 59–19. **A.** Electronmicrographs of HIV-I, showing the highly characteristic arrangement of the core, which is wedge-shaped or circular depending on the angle of view. **B.** HIV-II particles, the morphology of which is indistinguishable from that of HIV-I. One particle is shown in the process of budding. (*Courtesy of Dr. Reinhard Kurth*).

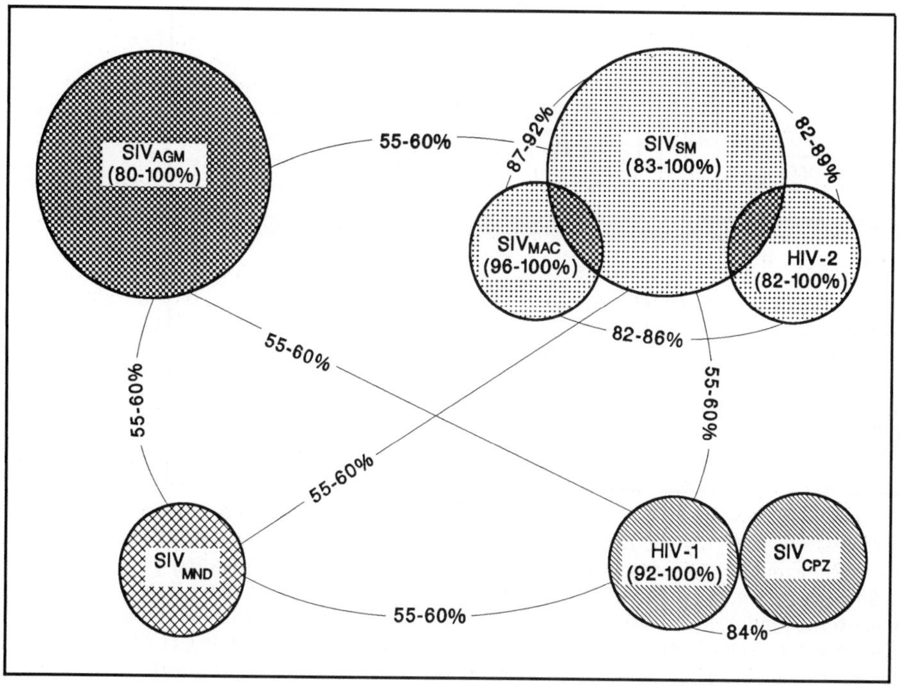

Fig. 59–20. Genetic relatedness patterns among primate immunodeficiency viruses. Percentages in the lines are amino acid identities in *pol* gene products; those in parentheses are the ranges of *pol* gene product identities in different isolates of each virus. SIV, simian immunodeficiency virus; AGM, African green monkey; MND, mandrill; MAC, macaque; SM, sooty mangabey; CPZ, chimpanzee. (*From Desrosiers: Nature 345:288, 1990.*)

restricted to cells that display it, primarily helper/inducer T lymphocytes, monocytes and macrophages, as well as astrocytes and microglia. Progressive, lethal immunodeficiency disease is the result of the total destruction of helper/inducer T lymphocytes and the progressive central nervous system degeneration caused by this virus. However, HIV has also been linked to a broader array of pathologic processes, including Kaposi's sarcoma and aggressive nonHodgkin's B cell lymphoma, in which its involvement may be stimulation of the production of a variety of lymphokines by cells infected by it, for another fundamental feature of HIV is its ability, referred to previously, to initiate and maintain persistent latent infections by virtue of the various regulatory proteins that it encodes.

Replication of HIV

The primary targets for HIV in the human body are cells that express the CD4 antigen on their surfaces, primarily T lymphocytes and glial cells in the central nervous system. Interestingly, entry of HIV into cells does not proceed via receptor-mediated endocytosis or pH-dependent entry via endosomes but via fusion of the viral envelope with the cell membrane, like that of paramyxoviruses. Once inside the cell, HIV RNA is transcribed into double-stranded DNA, which is integrated into randomly, as far as one can tell, located sites in the genome of the cell. An important point here is that the HIV reverse transcriptase is extremely error prone. Its error rate is about one in 2000 nucleotides; since HIV RNA is about 9000 nucleotides long, this means that there are up to five errors in every DNA minus strand that must serve as the template for the synthesis of progeny RNA (which is performed by the far more accurate cellular RNA polymerase II). The consequences of this large error rate are far-reaching. It turns out that the amino acid sequences of proteins in different HIV isolates derived from the same individual at the same time can differ by as much as 10%, and that such isolates can differ substantially in host range and cytopathogenicity; and that HIVs isolated from asymptomatic carriers and AIDS patients can also possess significantly different biologic properties. Indeed, it is very likely that HIV genotype and phenotype change progressively as the disease pattern progresses. Clearly, the extreme genetic variability of HIV presents a formidable obstacle to attempts to prevent HIV infection by immunologic means (and perhaps also chemotherapeutically [see below]).

Once integrated into the host genome, HIV expresses itself through transcription by RNA polymerase II. At this point HIV, like other lentiviruses, exhibits a remarkable degree of control over the extent to which it expresses itself—from complete silence to very active synthesis of structural proteins. This is achieved by the interplay of two mechanisms: control of transcription and posttranscriptional transcript processing. Transcription is controlled by a multiplicity of cellular transcription factors and one that is encoded by HIV itself. At least six cellular factors have been identified as binding upstream of the transcription start site, and four downstream (Fig. 59–21); their relative abundance is of primary importance in specifying the frequency of HIV provirus transcription. For example, the synthesis of NF-κB is induced in T lymphocytes after mitogenic stimulation, so that HIV gene expression is initiated when T cells are activated. As for the viral transcriptional activator, it binds to a sequence downstream of the transcription start site, and its availability is

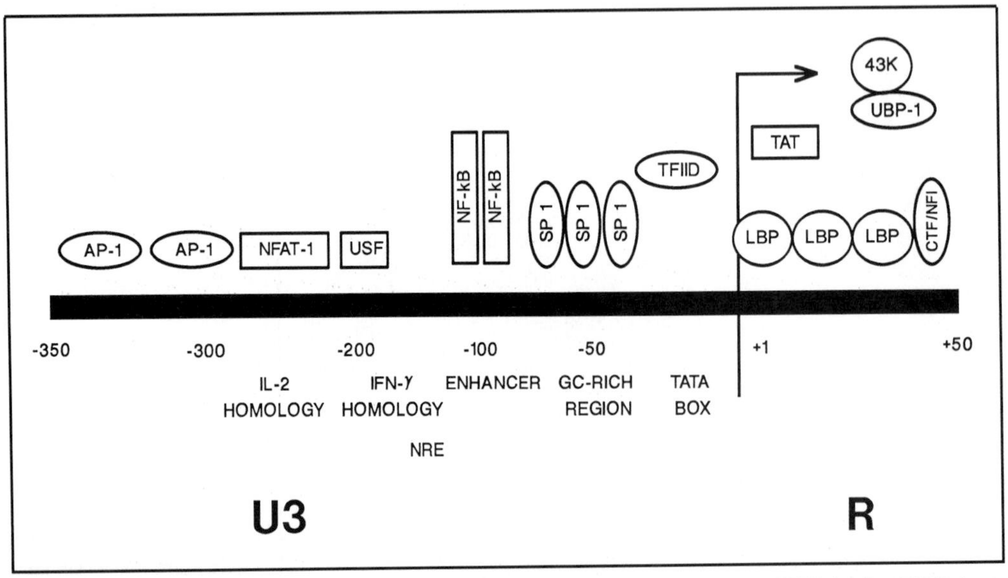

Fig. 59–21. *Cis*-acting regulatory elements in the HIV long terminal repeat. TFIID is the TATA box binding protein; SP1 binds to the three GC-rich sequences; the inducible transcription factor NFκB expressed in immunoglobulin-producing B cells binds to the enhancer, as does the enhancer-binding protein EBP-1 (not shown); and the upstream binding factor (USF), the nuclear factor of activated T cells (NFAT-1), and the cellular transcription factor (AP-1) bind to regions upstream of the enhancer, which also contain a negative regulatory element (NRE). Several factors also bind to the 5′-untranslated leader region. They include the leader-binding protein (LBP), CTF/NF1, and the TAT protein. (*From Steffy and Wong-Staal: Microbiol Rev 55:193, 1991.*)

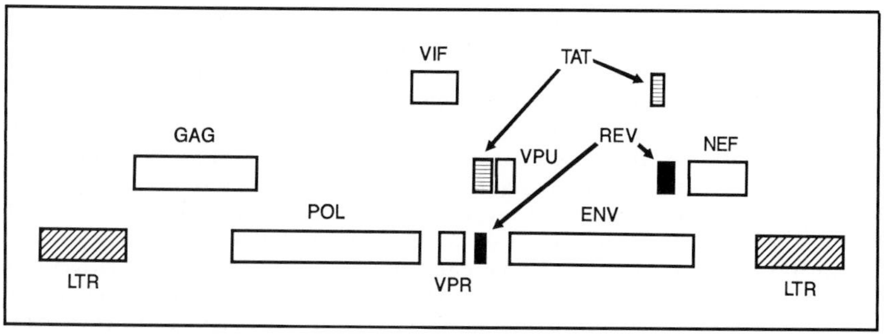

Fig. 59–22. Genomic structure of the HIV genome. In addition to the *gag*, *pro* (not shown, at *gag-pol* interface), *pol*, and *env* genes, there are six genes that encode regulatory proteins. Like their counterparts in the HTLV-I genome, the *tat* and *rev* genes each possess two exons. The *env* gene is translated from a singly spliced mRNA and most of the regulatory genes from multiply spliced mRNAs. (*Adapted from Steffy and Wong-Staal; Microbiol Rev 55:193, 1991.*)

controlled by another regulatory protein encoded by the virus itself (see below).

Genome of HIV

The genome of HIV is surprisingly complex—even more so than that of HTLV-I and HTLV-II and much more so than that of oncornaviruses (Fig. 59–22). It contains the four genes present in all retroviruses; *gag*, *pol*, *pro*, and *env*. As for all other retroviruses, the *gag* polyprotein is translated from the unspliced proviral transcript, the *gag-pro-pol* precursor from the unspliced transcript via a −1 ribosomal frameshift, and the *env* proteins from a singly spliced transcript from which the *gag-pro-pol* sequences have been removed. The *env* polyprotein is cleaved and processed to the gp120 (SU) and the gp41 (TM) glycoproteins, which constitute the HIV glycoprotein spikes that have such high affinity for the CD4 receptor.

In addition, however, the HIV genome contains at least six additional genes that encode proteins with regulatory functions, that is, functions that affect the extent to which the HIV genome expresses itself and the nature of the virus particles that are produced (Table 59–9). These proteins are translated from a series of multiply spliced messenger RNAs formed by using at least four splice-donor and six splice-acceptor sites. The two proteins whose function has been studied most intensively are *tat* and *rev* The *tat* (*trans*-activator) protein (86 amino acids long) binds to an RNA sequence, the TAR (*trans*-activation response) element, that is located between positions plus 19 and plus 42 in the viral RNA (see Fig. 59–21) and possesses a highly characteristic stem-loop secondary structure. The *tat* protein binds to this sequence immediately it is transcribed, together with LBP (leader binding protein) and nuclear factor-1 (NF-1); by binding to this sequence, it increases the amount of complete HIV transcripts that are formed by about 100-fold. There is some evidence that it may act as an antiterminator (i.e., prevent transcription termination within the first 60 nucleotides).

The *rev* protein (116 amino acids long) is, like the *tat* protein, essential for viral replication. It binds to another sequence in HIV transcripts, the *rev* response element (RRE), which is located in the *env* gene. It is about 230 nucleotides long and contains a 66-nucleotide-long stem-loop subdomain that is absolutely essential for *rev* binding. By binding to HIV transcripts, *rev* antagonizes splicing and promotes the transport of species that contain *gag* and *env* sequences (unspliced and singly spliced species) to the cytoplasm. Thus early during HIV transcription, little *rev* is available, and most HIV transcripts are multiply spliced to form the messengers that encode *tat*, *rev*, and the other regulatory proteins; as transcription continues, these proteins accumulate, and the increased amounts of *rev* promote the transport to the cytoplasm of increasing amounts of those messenger RNA species that encode the structural proteins of HIV.

The functions of the other regulatory proteins are less clear and are also summarized in Table 59–9. In distinction to *tat* and *rev*, both of which are *essential* for HIV replication, mutants lacking them do form some progeny HIV.

TABLE 59–9. FUNCTIONS OF REGULATORY HIV PROTEINS

Protein	Size	Function
tat	p14	Transactivator of transcription
rev	p19	Regulates transport to the cytoplasm of unspliced and singly spliced transcripts
nef	p27	Precise function unknown; binds GTP; possesses GTPase activity: there are unconfirmed reports it downregulates HIV transcription
vpr	p18	Precise function unknown; present in virus particles; may facilitate an early stage of infection; weak transactivating activity
vif	p23	Precise function unknown; required for viral infectivity; may function in morphogenesis
vpu	p15	Precise function unknown; associated with cytoplasmic membranes; may function in budding

Role of Other Viral Infections in HIV Infections

Infections with HIV are frequently accompanied by infections with other viruses. The question arises as to whether the presence of such viruses can affect the course of HIV-caused disease. For at least two viruses this appears to be at least theoretically possible. First, HIV infections are to an increasing extent accompanied by HTLV-I infections; and the HTLV-I *tax* protein can transactivate, through an inducible cellular factor that interacts with the NF-κB binding site, transcription of the HIV provirus. Second, a human herpesvirus, HHV-6, has recently been identified that also uses the CD4 antigen as its receptor. This virus contributes to HIV infections in two ways: it *trans*-activates HIV transcription, and it contributes to the destruction of $CD4^+$ cells, thereby exacerbating the extent of immune deficiency.

Prospects for Prevention and Control of HIV Infections

HIV poses a public health problem of international proportions. More than 1 million individuals are infected with HIV-I in the United States alone, where more than 160,000 AIDS cases have been reported and more than 100,000 have died so far. Tens of millions are infected worldwide, most of them in Africa. Prevention and control of HIV infections is therefore a top priority research goal. The following approaches are currently being investigated most intensively.

DEVELOPMENT OF A VACCINE. Epitopes eliciting the formation of neutralizing antibodies are located on the gp120 spike glycoprotein. This approach is fraught with difficulties because of the genetic instability of HIV (see above).

PREVENTION OF ADSORPTION OF HIV PARTICLES TO CD4 PROTEIN ON T LYMPHOCYTES. Two approaches appear promising. First, adsorption can be inhibited by nonspecific inhibitors such as dextran sulfate, which are highly effective in vitro but much less so in the body. Second, soluble forms of the CD4 antigen, modified to prevent its rapid clearance from the bloodstream, are being used to saturate HIV particles, thereby preventing their adsorbing to CD4 on T lymphocytes.

DESIGN OF INHIBITORS OF REVERSE TRANSCRIPTASE AND PROTEASE. Both proteins have been crystallized. Determination of their atomic structure should provide clues for the design of highly specific and effective inhibitors.

DEVELOPMENT OF TRANSDOMINANT VARIANTS OF *TAT* AND *REV* PROTEINS. The *tat* and *rev* proteins are essential for HIV replication. Truncated forms of these proteins have been identified that bind to the same RNA response elements as the wild-type proteins but do not exercise the functions of the wild-type proteins. Attempts are underway to introduce genes encoding such transdominant variant proteins into cellular genomes to render the cells resistant to HIV infection.

USE OF GP41-RICIN AND CD4-RICIN TO KILL HIV-INFECTED CELLS. Cells infected with HIV display patches of its *env* proteins on their surface; from such areas progeny virus particles bud. These *env* proteins serve as receptors for two types of molecules: antibodies and CD4 antigen. When such antibodies, for example, monoclonal antibodies against gp41 or CD4, are coupled to the A chain of the powerful plant toxin ricin, the AB-ricin^A and CD4-ricin^A complexes adsorb to infected cells and are internalized, thereby introducing into cells the toxin, which is an *N*-glycosidase that removes one specific adenine residue from 28S ribosomal RNA, thereby inactivating ribosomes, completely inhibiting protein synthesis, and causing cell death. *Pseudomonas* exotoxin is another toxin being examined in this regard (Chap. 58).

Human Endogenous Retroviruses

The human genome, like that of other animals, contains multiple copies of numerous retroviral proviruses that are the products of germ line cell infections at some time in the past; in fact, about 0.1% of the human genome consists of retroviral elements. However, in distinction to the endogenous retroviral proviruses of most other animal species, all such proviruses so far encountered in the human genome are defective: they possess either variously truncated LTRs, minor or major deletions in the *gag*, *pro*, *pol*, and *env* genes, termination codons in these genes, or any combination of these.

There are several types of human endogenous proviral elements, and they can be grouped according to several criteria. Some are related to the human exogenous retroviruses HTLV-I and HTLV-II and no doubt evolved from them; others are related more or less closely to simian retroviruses. These proviruses are present in the form of a single copy only in the haploid genome. There are also two groups of proviruses, each of which comprises many members, more or less closely related, each present in the form of up to 1000 copies per haploid genome, and many present not only in the form of the provirus itself but also in the form of very large numbers (more than 1000) of solitary LTRs (LTR-ISs). These groups can be classified further according to the tRNA that they use as primer for DNA synthesis; some use *glu*-, *his*-, or *pro*-tRNAs and are related to C-type retroviruses, plus others use *lys*-tRNA and are related to B- (MMTV), D-, and A-type retroviruses.

No function has yet been associated with any of these proviruses. Although most are in transcriptionally silent regions of the genome, many are transcribed into a variety of messenger RNAs, both in normal tissues such as placental and fetal tissues and in various tumors and tumor cell lines. Further, their transcription can be activated because some possess steroid-response elements in their LTRs or by azacytidine, an inhibitor of DNA methyltransferases, which reverses the effect of hypermethylation in silencing transcription. The major question is whether these messenger RNAs are translated into proteins. There are some reports of the synthesis of *gag*, *pol*, and *env* proteins encoded by human endogenous retroviruses (HERVs); but are the particles resembling retroviruses that are often observed in human reproductive and embyronic tissues the products of provirus expression? The difficulty has been that these particles are produced only in small amounts, and so far, it has been impossible to isolate and sequence them.

However that may be, the presence or expression of endogenous proviruses in the human genome has not so far been linked with any human disease, but such a link cannot be ruled out. The particles that are seen are certainly noninfectious; and no case of proviral insertional activation of any inappropriate human gene has yet been found, although there is no question that their LTRs do contain both *cis*- and *trans*-active enhancer and promoter sequences.

Nature and Function of Retroposons

Retroposons, also called *retrotransposons* or *retroelements*, are sequences whose generation and propagation depend on reverse transcription. They are found in various kingdoms of the living world, ranging from bacteria to humans; they include retroviral proviruses and proviruslike elements in vertebrates, retrotransposable elements in insects and nematodes, and retrotransposons in yeasts and plants. Clearly all have evolved from an extremely ancient common precursor;

increasingly, it is being realized that reverse transcription may be a strong driving force in evolution. As much as 10% of the human genome is thought to have arisen by reverse transcription-mediated processes.

The various retroposons listed above share two basic characteristics: all encode a reverse transcriptase that transcribes their transcripts into DNA, and they integrate this DNA into cellular DNA through the same unique set of reactions by which retroviral DNA is integrated (see Fig. 59–13). Most retroposons transcribe their RNA and integrate the transcribed DNA into some other site of the genome in the *same* cell; retroviruses are a special type of retroposon because they also encode *env* genes, which, by permitting them to form virus particles, provide them with an extracellular phase and enable them to integrate into the genomes of new cells. The overall importance of retroposons in evolutionary processes derives from the fact that the insertions of mobile elements results in the activation/inactivation of cellular genes (see below).

The characteristics of four families of retroposons follow.

Intracisternal A-type Particles

Intracisternal A-type particles (IAPs), which have been studied primarily in mice and hamsters, are defective retroviruses (Fig. 59–23). There are two types of IAPs: type I IAPs whose genomes are organized like those of C-type retroviruses, with LTRs and functional *gag* and *pol* genes but lacking *env* genes; and type II IAPs that lack varying amounts of the sequences normally between the two LTRs and possess instead characteristic short (270 base pair–long) insertions called AIIins. Type II IAPs are often extensively amplified in myeloma cells (more than 1000 IAP proviruses per haploid genome). Since IAPs lack functional *env* genes, they have no extracellular phase; but IAP RNA *can* be encapsidated into C-type retrovirus particles and thus spread to other cells.

The two major questions concerning IAP proviruses are how extensively they express themselves and what the effect of their presence is on cells. IAPs are abundant in fetal tissue and the thymus and in many tumors, including embryonal carcinomas, hybridomas, plasmacytomas, and B cell lymphomas, during the differentiation of which their number increases approximately fourfold. They bud abundantly into the cisternae of the rough endoplasmic reticulum (RER). Usually they remain attached to the RER membrane, but in many myelomas they are released in extracellular form (but are not infectious). Although their expression in the form of particles has no apparent consequences for the producing cells, the integration of IAP proviruses into new locations can have important physiologic effects. Among observed effects are the constitutive activation of the c-*mos* gene, the IL-3 gene, the GM-CSF gene, and the homeobox-2,4 gene; inactivation of the κ light chain gene; and replacement of internal IAP sequences by the IL-6 receptor gene or the immunoglobulin E binding factor gene, with resultant elevated expression of these genes.

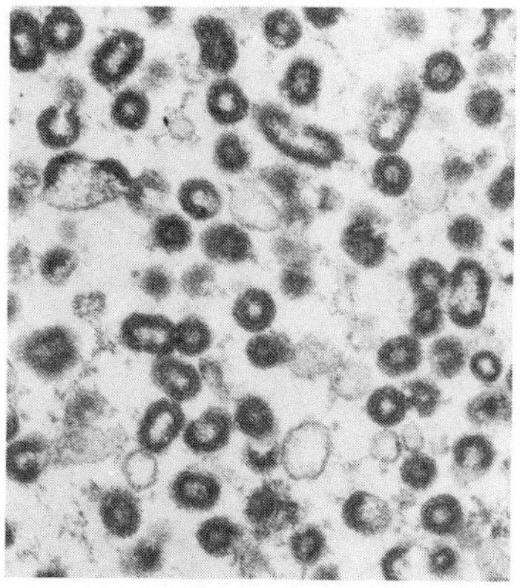

Fig. 59–23. Intracisternal A-type particles (IAP) extracted from the mouse plasma cell tumor MOPC 104E and partially purified by sucrose density gradient centrifugation. × 70,000. (*Courtesy of Dr. N.A. Wivell.*)

VL30 Elements*

The genomes of many mammalian species contain about 200 VL30 elements that are 5000 to 6000 bp long and possess either no or only very slight sequence similarity to retroviruses. However, they retain many of the structural hallmarks of retroviral proviruses: LTRs that contain enhancers and promoters, priming sites that permit reverse transcription of their transcripts into DNA, and encapsidation signals that permit encapsidation of their transcripts, in diploid form, into pseudovirions supplied by endogenous or exogenous C-type retroviruses. This provides them with the means to retrotranspose into other cells. However, the 4000 to 5000 bp long sequences between their LTRs possess no open reading frames; no VL30-encoded proteins have yet been identified.

VL30s are a very heterogeneous family. Some are expressed in adult tissue, others in transformed cells, and others still in cells stimulated to divide by treatment with serum, EGF, or activators of protein kinase C such as tissue plasminogen activator (TPA).

Like IAPs and other proviral elements, VL30 elements may function as insertional mutagens to activate the transcription of cellular genes, including proto-oncogenes. The ability of VL30 elements to recombine with retroviral proviruses may also be of significance; for example, the genome of Harvey murine sarcoma virus contains VL30-specific sequences.

Retroposons in *Drosophila*

The genomes of insects such as *Drosophila* contains at least 40 families of retroelements that comprise approximately 10% of it. One of these families is composed of retrovirus-like elements, the best known of which are the copia and gypsy/17.6 subfamilies. The copialike elements possess LTRs and a functional *pol* gene; gypsy/17.6-like elements possess LTRs and three open reading frames, one of which encodes a *pol*, *pro*, and endonuclease containing polyprotein that possesses extensive sequence similarity to corresponding retroviral proteins. RNA-containing particles resembling retrovirus cores occur in the cytoplasm of *Drosophila* cells.

Transposition of these retroelements is associated with spontaneous mutations resulting from insertional activation/inactivation. They can be grouped according to when during development they are transcribed and transposed. Some, such as 17.6, are transcribed mainly during the early larval and pupal stages of development; others are more active during

* So-called because they are *virus*like and the diploid form of their RNA transcripts has a sedimentation coefficient of 30 S.

the larval than the pupal stages, and the transcripts of still others such as copia are present as maternal messengers in unfertilized embryos. Thus different regulatory sequences, presumably under the control of different cellular genes, regulate the expression of these elements. It is interesting in this regard that the LTRs of some of these elements possess multiple ecdysteroid receptor binding sites that presumably function as regulatory sequence elements.

Ty Elements of Yeast

The genome of *Saccharomyces cerevisiae* contains at least three families of retrotransposons, Ty1, Ty2, and Ty3. Approximately 35 copies of these elements are present in each haploid genome. They are about 6 kbp long and possess LTRs known as delta sequences and two genes, TYA and TYB, that correspond to and share sequence similarity with retroviral *gag* and *pro-pol* genes. The extent of sequence similarity between the Ty genes and those of other retrovirus-like retroelements is variable among Ty subfamilies but is often remarkable; for example, 43% of the amino acids of the *pro-pol* proteins of the Ty3 transposon and the *Drosophila* 17.6 element are identical.

Together, the TYA and TYB proteins form RNA-containing particles in the cytoplasm that resemble retrovirus cores and presumably function in the integration events that constitute transposition. In all major respects the Ty elements function in a manner analogous to endogenous retroviral proviruses.

The existence of genetic elements that transpose through reverse transcription in life forms as low as yeast focuses attention on the question of their biologic role, which is surely fundamentally important in view of the extraordinary extent to which they have been conserved during evolution. It is likely that Ty, with its two genes, represents the basic functional retroelement: one gene encodes the proteins that package the RNA; the other encodes the enzymes necessary for processing the polyproteins, reverse transcription, and integration. Presumably retroviruses then evolved from these elements by acquiring *env* genes that endowed them with an extracellular phase and a correspondingly expanded transposition potential. The raison d'être for the continued existence of retroelements may be their ability to generate that most essential prerequisite for evolution—genetic diversity.

FURTHER READING

Books and Reviews

DNA TUMOR VIRUSES

Galloway DA, McDougall JK: Human papillomaviruses and carcinomas. Adv Virus Res 37:126, 1989

Kaplan DR, Pallas DC, Morgan W, et al: Mechanisms of transformation by polyoma virus middle T antigen. Biochim Biophys Acta 948:345, 1988

Kieff E, Wang F, Birkenbach M, et al: Molecular biology of lymphocyte transformation by Epstein-Barr virus. In Origins of Human Cancer. New York, Cold Spring Harbor Press, 1991

Knippers R, Levine AJ (eds): Transforming proteins of DNA tumor viruses. Curr Top Microbiol Immunol 144:1, 1989

Macnab JCM: Herpes simplex virus and human cytomegalovirus: Their role in morphological transformation and genital cancers. J Gen Virol 68:2525, 1987

Schröder CH, Zentgraf H: Hepatitis B virus related hepatocellular carcinoma: Chronicity of infection—The opening to different pathways of malignant transformation? Biochim Biophys Acta 1032:137, 1990

Sousa R, Dostatni N, Yaniv M: Control of papillomavirus gene expression. Biochim Biophys Acta 1032:19, 1990

SARCOMA/LEUKEMIA VIRUSES

Gallo RC, Wong-Staal F (eds): Retrovirus Biology and Human Disease. New York, Marcel Dekker, 1990

Grandgenett DP, Mumm SR: Unraveling retrovirus integration. Cell 60:3, 1990

Hatfield D, Oroszlan S: The *where, what* and *how* of ribosomal frameshifting in retroviral protein synthesis. Trends Biomed Sci 15:186, 1990

Katz RA, Skalka AM: Generation of diversity in retroviruses. Ann Rev Genet 24:409, 1990

Mason WS, Taylor JM, Hull R: Retroid virus genome replication. Adv Virus Res 32:35, 1987

Schuepba CH: Human retrovirology: Facts and concepts. Curr Top Microbiol Immunol 142:1, 1989

Skalka AM: Retroviral proteases: First glimpses at the anatomy of a processing machine. Cell 56:911, 1989

Stoltzfus CM: Synthesis and processing of avian sarcoma retrovirus RNA. Adv Virus Res 35:1, 1988

Swanstrom R, Vogt PK (eds): Retroviruses: Strategies of replication. Curr Top Microbiol Immunol vol 157, 1990

Varmus H: Retroviruses. Science 240:1427, 1988

ONCOGENES

General

Bourne HR, Sanders DA, McCormick F: The GTPase superfamily: Conserved structure and molecular mechanism. Nature 349:117, 1991

Bruker BJ, Mamon JH, Roberts TM: Oncogenes, growth factors, and signal transduction. N Engl J Med 321:1383, 1989

Casey PJ, Gilman AG: G protein involvement in receptor-effector coupling. J Biol Chem 263:2577, 1988

Cosman D, Lyman SD, Idzerda RL, et al: A new cytokine receptor superfamily TIBS 15:265, 1990

Perlmutter RM, Marth JD, Ziegler SF, et al: Specialized protein tyrosine kinase proto-oncogenes in hematopoietic cells. Biochim Biophys Acta 948:245, 1988

Pierce JH: Oncogenes, growth factors and hematopoietic cell transformation. Biochim Biophys Acta 989:179, 1989

Pimentel E: Oncogenes. Boca Raton, Fla, CRC Press, 1986

Rivera VM, Greenberg ME: Growth factor–induced gene expression: The ups and downs of *c-fos* regulation. New Biologist 2:751, 1990

Stroms RW, Bose HR Jr: Oncogenes, proto-oncogenes, and signal transduction: Toward a unified theory? Adv Virus Res 37:1, 1989

Ullrich A, Schlessinger J: Signal transduction by receptors with tyrosine kinase activity. Cell 61:203, 1990

Vogt PK (ed): Oncogenes: Selected reviews. Curr Top Microbiol Immunol vol 147, 1989

Vogt PK (ed): Oncogenes and retroviruses: Selected reviews. Curr Top Microbiol Immunol vol 148, 1989

SPECIFIC ONCOGENES

Curran T, Franza BR Jr: Fos and jun: The AP-1 connection. Cell 55:395, 1988

Damm K, Thompson CC, Evans RM: Protein encoded by v-*erbA* functions as a thyroid-hormone receptor antagonist. Nature 339:593, 1989

Gibbs JB, Marshall MS: The *ras*-oncogene—An important regulatory element in lower eucaryotic organisms. Microbiol Rev 53:171, 1989

Hall A: *ras* and GAP—Who's controlling whom? Cell 61:921, 1990

Hannink M, Donoghue DJ: Structure and function of platelet-derived growth factor (PDGF) and related proteins. Biochim Biophys Acta 989:1, 1989

Maihle NJ, Kung H-J: C-*erbB* and the epidermal growth-factor receptor: A molecule with dual identity. Biochim Biophys Acta 948:287, 1988

McCormick F: *ras* GTPase activating protein: Signal transmitter and signal terminator. Cell 56:5, 1989

Milburn MV, Tong L, deVos AM, et al: Molecular switch for signal transduction: Structural differences between active and inactive forms of protooncogenic *ras* proteins. Science 247:939, 1990

Ramakrishnan L, Rosenberg N: *abl* genes. Biochim Biophys Acta 989:209, 1989

Ransone LJ, Verma IM: Nuclear proto-oncogenes FOS and JUM. Ann Rev Cell Biol 6:539, 1990

Rosenberg N, Witte ON: The viral and cellular forms of the Abelson (*abl*) oncogene. Adv Virus Res 35:40, 1988

Shen-Ong GLC: The *myb* oncogene. Biochim Biophys Acta 1032:39, 1990

Sherr CJ: The *fms* oncogene. Biochim Biophys Acta 948:225, 1988

Williams LT: Signal transduction by the platelet-derived growth factor receptor. Science 243:1564, 1989

ANTIONCOGENES

Cooper JA, Whyte P: RB and the cell cycle: Entrance or exit? Cell 58:1009, 1989

Green MR: When the products of oncogenes and anti-oncogenes meet. Cell 56:1, 1989

Levine AJ: The p53 protein and its interactions with the oncogene products of the small DNA tumor viruses. Virology 177:419, 1990

Levine AJ, Momand J: Tumor suppressor genes: The p53 and retinoblastoma sensitivity genes and gene products. Biochim Biophys Acta 1032:119, 1990

Stanbridge E: Human tumor suppressive genes. Ann Rev Genet 24:615, 1990

Stanbridge EJ, Nowell PC: Origins of human cancer revisited. Cell 63:867, 1990

MOUSE MAMMARY TUMOR VIRUS

Salmons B, Günzburg WH: Current perspectives in the biology of mouse mammary tumour virus. Virus Res 8:81, 1987

HUMAN T-CELL LEUKEMIA VIRUSES

Blattner WA (ed): Human Retrovirology: HTLV. New York, Raven Press, 1990

HUMAN IMMUNODEFICIENCY VIRUS (HIV)

Braun MM, Heyward WL, Curran JW: The global epidemiology of HIV infection and AIDS. Ann Rev Microbiol 44:555, 1990

Chang DD, Sharp PA: Messenger RNA transport and HIV *rev* regulation. Science 249:614, 1990

Cullen BR: The HIV-1 tat protein: An RNA sequence-specific processivity factor? Cell 63:655, 1990

Cullen BR, Green WC: Regulatory pathways governing HIV-1 replication. Cell 58:423, 1989

Cullen BR, Greene WC: Functions of the auxiliary gene products of the human immunodeficiency virus type 1. Virology 178:1, 1990

Desrosiers RC: Simian immunodeficiency viruses. Ann Rev Microbiol 42:607, 1988

Evans LA, Levy JA: Characteristics of HIV infection and pathogenesis. Biochim Biophys Acta 989:237, 1989

Gelderblom HR, Özel M, Pauli G: Morphogenesis and morphology of HIV structure-function relations. Arch Virol 106:1, 1989

Greene WC: Regulation of HIV-1 gene expression. Annu Rev Immunol 8:453, 1990

Hammarskjöld M-L, Rekosh D: The molecular biology of the human immunodeficiency virus. Biochim Biophys Acta 989:269, 1989

Kieber-Emmons T, Jameson BA, Morrow WJW: The gp120-CD4 interface: Structural, immunological and pathological considerations. Biochim Biophys Acta 989:281, 1989

Pavlakis GN, Felber BK: Regulation of expression of human immunodeficiency virus. New Biologist 2:20, 1990

Robey E, Axel R: CD4: Collaborator in immune recognition and HIV infection. Cell 60:697, 1990

Sattentau QJ: HIV infection and the immune system. Biochim Biophys Acta 989:255, 1989

Steffy K, Wong-Staal F: Genetic regulation of HIV. Microbiol Rev vol 55, 193, 1991

Volberding PA, McCutchan JA: The HIV epidemic: Medical and social challenges. Biochim Biophys Acta 989:227, 1989

Zack JA, Arrigo SJ, Chen ISY: Control of expression and cell tropism of human immunodeficiency virus type I. Adv Virus Res 38:125, 1990

RETROELEMENTS

Berg DE, Howe MH: On the impossibility of knowing more. Cell 60:703, 1990

Boeke JD, Corces VG: Transcription and reverse transcription of retrotransposons. Ann Rev Microbiol 43:403, 1989

Kingsman AJ, Kingsman SM: Ty: A retroelement moving forward. Cell 53:333, 1988

Larsson E, Kato N, Cohen M: Human endogenous proviruses. Curr Top Microbiol Immunol 148:115, 1989

Levy SB, Miller RV: Migrant DNA in the bacterial world. Cell 60:7, 1990

Sandmeyer SB, Hansen LJ, Chalker DL: Integration specificity of retrotransposons and retroviruses. Ann Rev Genet 24:491, 1990

Will H, Hull R: Molecular biology of retroelements. Virus Genes 4:93, 1990

Selected Papers

DNA TUMOR VIRUSES

Bedrosian CL, Bastia D: The DNA-binding domain of HPV-16 E2 protein interaction with the viral enhancer: Protein-induced DNA bending and role of the nonconserved core sequence in binding site affinity. Virology 174:557, 1990

Cohen JI, Wang F, Mannick J, Kieff E: Epstein-Barr virus nuclear protein 2 is a key determinant of lymphocyte transformation. Proc Natl Acad Sci USA 86:9558, 1989

Hawley-Nelson P, Vousden KH, Hubbert NL, et al: HPV16 E6 and E7 proteins cooperate to immortalize human foreskin keratinocytes. EMBO J 8:3905, 1989

Manservigi R, Cassai E, Deiss LP, et al: Sequences homologous to two separate transforming regions of herpes simplex virus DNA are linked in two human genital tumors. Virology 155:192, 1986

Matsukura T, Koi S, Sugase M: Both episomal and integrated forms of human papillomavirus type 16 are involved in invasive cervical cancers. Virology 172:63, 1989

Phelps WC, Yee CL, Münger K, Howley PM: The human papillomavirus type 16 E7 gene encodes transactivation and transformation functions similar to those of adenovirus E1A. Cell 53:539, 1988

Talmage DA, Freund R, Young AT, et al: Phosphorylation of middle T by pp60$^{c\text{-}src}$: A switch for binding of phosphatidylinositol 3-kinase and optimal tumorigenesis. Cell 59:55, 1989

SARCOMA/LEUKEMIA VIRUSES

Dai HY, Etzerodt M, Baekgaard AJ, et al: Multiple sequence elements in the U3 region of the leukemogenic murine retrovirus SL3-2 contribute to cell-dependent gene expression. Virology 175:581, 1990

Hoatlin ME, Kozak SL, Lilly F: Activation of erythropoietin receptors by Friend viral gp55 and by erythropoietin and down-modulation by the murine *Fv-2*ʳ resistance gene. Proc Natl Acad Sci USA 87:9985, 1990

Ishimoto LK, Halperin M, Champoux JJ: Moloney murine leukemia virus IN protein from disrupted virions binds and specifically cleaves its target sequence *in vitro*. Virology 180:527, 1991

Jacks T, Madhani HD, Masiarz FR, Varmus HE: Signals for ribosomal frameshifting in the Rous sarcoma virus *gag-pol* region. Cell 55:447, 1988

Martinelli SC, Goff SP: Rapid reversion of a deletion mutation in Moloney murine leukemia virus by recombination with a closely related endogenous provirus. Virology 174:135, 1990

Shih C-C, Stoye JP, Coffin JM: Highly preferred targets for retrovirus integration. Cell 53:531, 1988

Sitbon M, Ellerbrok H, Pozo F, et al: Sequences in the U5-*gag-pol* region influence early and late pathogenic effects of Friend and Moloney murine leukemia viruses. J Virol 64:2135, 1990

ONCOGENES

Anderson D, Koch CA, Grey L, et al: Binding of SH2 domains of phospholipase Cγ1, GAP, and Src to activated growth factor receptors. Science 250:979, 1990

Ballard DW, Walker WH, Doerre S, et al: The v-*rel* oncogene encodes a κB enhancer binding protein that inhibits NF-κB function. Cell 63:803, 1990

Bos TJ, Bohmann D, Tsuchie H, et al: v-*jun* encodes a nuclear protein with enhancer binding properties of AP-1. Cell 52:705, 1988

Cartwright CA, Simantov R, Cowan WM, et al: $pp60^{c\text{-}src}$ expression in the developing rat brain. Proc Natl Acad Sci USA 85:3348, 1988

Chen-Levy Z, Nourse J, Cleary ML: The *bcl*-2 candidate proto-oncogene product is a 24-kilodalton integral-membrane protein highly expressed in lymphoid cell lines and lymphomas carrying the t (14;18) translocation. Mol Cell Biol 9:701, 1989

Di Fiore PP, Pierce JH, Fleming TP, et al: Overexpression of the human EGF receptor confers an EGF-dependent transformed phenotype to NIH 3T3 cells. Cell 51:1063, 1987

Eva A, Vecchio G, Rao CD, et al: The predicted *DBL* oncogene product defines a distinct class of transforming proteins. Proc Natl Acad Sci USA 85:2061, 1988

Hirai H, Varmus HE: Mutations in *src* homology regions 2 and 3 of activated chicken c-*src* that result in preferential transformation of mouse or chicken cells. Proc Natl Acad USA 87:8592, 1990

Kaplan JM, Varmus HE, Bishop JM: The *src* protein contains multiple domains for specific attachment to membranes. Mol Cell Biol 10:1000, 1990

Langdon WY, Hyland CD, Grumont RJ, Morse HC: The c-*cbl* proto-oncogene is preferentially expressed in thymus and testis tissue and encodes a nuclear protein. J Virol 63:5420, 1989

Lonardo F, Di Marco E, King CR: The normal *erb*B-2 product is an atypical receptor-like tyrosine kinase with constitutive activity in the absence of ligand. New Biologist 2:992, 1990

Lugo TG, Witte ON: The *BCR-ABL* oncogene transforms *rat*-1 cells and cooperates with v-*myc*. Mol Cell Biol 9:1263, 1989

Meijlink F, Curran T, Miller AD, Verma IM: Removal of a 67-base-pair sequence in the noncoding region of protooncogene *fos* converts it to a transforming gene. Proc Natl Acad Sci USA 82:4987, 1985

Miller AD, Curran T, Verma IM: c-*fos* protein can induce cellular transformation: A novel mechanism of activation of a cellular oncogene. Cell 36:51, 1984

Moran MF, Koch CA, Anderson D, et al: Src homology region 2 domains direct protein-protein interactions in signal transduction. Proc Natl Acad Sci USA 87:8622, 1990

Ness SA, Marknell A, Graf T: The v-*myb* oncogene product binds to and activates the promyelocyte-specific *mim*-1 gene. Cell 59:1115, 1989

Privalsky ML, Sharif M, Yamamoto KR: The viral *erbA* oncogene protein, a constitutive repressor in animal cells, is a hormone-regulated activator in yeast. Cell 63:1277, 1990

Roussel MF, Downing JR, Rettenmier CW, Sherr CJ: A point mutation in the extracellular domain of the human CSF-1 receptor (c-*fms* proto-oncogene product) activates its transforming potential. Cell 55:979, 1988

Sagata N, Watanabe N, Vande Woude GF, Ikawa Y: The c-*mos* proto-oncogene product is a cytostatic factor responsible for meiotic arrest in vertebrate eggs. Nature 342:512, 1989

Stahl ML, Ferenz CR, Kelleher KL, et al: Sequence similarity of phospholipase C with the non-catalytic region of *src*. Nature 332:269, 1988

Thompson TC, Southgate J, Kitchener G, Land H: Multistage carcinogenesis induced by *ras* and *myc* oncogenes in a reconstituted organ. Cell 56:917, 1989

Tsujimoto Y: Overexpression of the human *BCL*-2 gene product results in growth enhancement of Epstein-Barr virus–immortalized B cells. Proc Natl Acad Sci USA 86:1958, 1989

Tsukamoto AS, Grosschedl R, Guzman RC, et al: Expression of the *nt*-1 gene in transgenic mice is associated with mammary gland hyperplasia and adenocarcinomas in male and female mice. Cell 55:619, 1988

Turner R, Tjian R: Leucine repeats and an adjacent DNA binding domain mediate the formation of functional c*Fos*-c*Jun* heterodimers. Science 243:1689, 1989

Zenke M, Muñoz A, Sap J, et al: v-*erbA* oncogene activation entails the loss of hormone-dependent regulator activity of c-*erbA*. Cell 61:1035, 1990

Zhou H, Duesberg PH: A retroviral promoter is sufficient to convert proto-*src* to a transforming gene that is distinct from the *src* gene of Rous sarcoma virus. Proc Natl Acad Sci USA 87:9128, 1990

ANTIONCOGENES

Bressac B, Galvin KM, Liang TJ, et al: Abnormal structure and expression of p53 gene in human hepatocellular carcinoma. Proc Natl Acad Sci USA 87:1973, 1990

Hollstein MC, Metcalf RA, Welsh JA, et al: Frequent mutation of the p53 gene in human esophageal cancer. Proc Natl Acad Sci USA 87:9958, 1990

Scheffner M, Werness BA, Huibregtse JM, et al: The E6 oncoprotein encoded by human papillomarvirus types 16 and 18 promotes the degradation of p53. Cell 63:1129, 1990

Takahashi T, Nau MM, Chiba I, et al: p53: A frequent target for genetic abnormalities in lung cancer. Science 246:491, 1989

T'Ang A, Varley JM, Chakraborty S, et al: Structural rearrangement of the retinoblastoma gene in human breast carcinoma. Science 242:263, 1988

HUMAN IMMUNODEFICIENCY VIRUS (HIV)

Balachandran R, Thampatty P, Enrico A, et al: Human immunodeficiency virus isolates from asymptomatic homosexual men and from AIDS patients have distinct biologic and genetic properties. Virology 180:229, 1991

Berkhout B, Silverman RH, Jeang K-T: Tat *trans*-activates the human immunodeficiency virus through a nascent RNA target. Cell 59:273, 1989

Byrn RA, Sekigawa I, Chamow SM, et al: Characterization of in vitro inhibition of human immunodeficiency virus by purified recombinant CD4. J Virol 63:4370, 1989

Chaudhary VK, Mizukami T, Fuerst TR: Selective killing of HIV-infected cells by recombinant human CD4-*Pseudomonas* exotoxin hybrid protein. Nature 335:369, 1988

Dubreuil M, Sportza L, D-Addario M, et al: Inhibition of HIV-1 transmission by interferon and 3′-azido-3′-deoxythymidine during de novo infection of promonocytic cells. Virology 179:388, 1990

Egberink H, Borst M, Niphuis H, et al: Suppression of feline immunodeficiency virus infection *in vivo* by 9-(2-phosphonomethoxyethyl) adenine. Proc Natl Acad Sci USA 87:3087, 1990

Gojobori T, Moriyama EN, Ina Y, et al: Evolutionary origin of human and simian immunodeficiency viruses. Proc Natl Acad Sci USA 87:4108, 1990

Maddon PJ, McDougal JS, Clapham PR, et al: HIV infection does not require endocytosis of its receptor, CD4. Cell 54:865, 1988

Malim MH, Tiley LS, McCarn DF: HIV-1 structural gene expression requires binding of the Rev *trans*-activator to its RNA target sequence. Cell 60:675, 1990

Rando RF, Srinivasan A, Feingold J, et al: Characterization of multiple molecular interactions between human cytomegalovirus (HCMV) and human immunodeficiency virus type 1 (HIV-1). Virology 175:87, 1990

Watkins BA, Dorn HH, Kelly WB, et al: Specific tropism of HIV-1 for microglial cells in primary human brain cultures. Science 245:549, 1990

Weber J Clapham P, McKeating J, et al: J Gen Virol 70:2653, 1989

RETROELEMENTS

Adams SE, Mellor J, Gull K, et al: The functions and relationships of Ty-VLP proteins in yeast reflect those of mammalian retroviral proteins. Cell 49:111, 1987

Dührsen U, Stahl J, Gough NM: *In vivo* transformation of factor-dependent hemopoietic cells: Role of intracisternal A-particle transposition for growth factor gene activation. EMBO J 9:1087, 1990

Heidmann, O, Heidmann T: Retrotransposition of a mouse IAP sequence tagged with an indicator gene. Cell 64:159, 1991

Kröger B, Horak I: Isolation of novel human retrovirus-related sequences by hybridization to synthetic oligonucleotides complementary to the $tRNA^{Pro}$ primer-binding site. J Virol 61:2071, 1987

Lankenau D-H, Huijser P, Jansen E, et al: Micropia: A retrotransposon of *Drosophila* combining structural features of DNA viruses, retroviruses and non-viral transposable elements. J Mol Biol 204:233, 1988

Mariani-Costantini R, Horn TM, Callahan R: Ancestry of a human endogenous retrovirus family. J Virol 63:4982, 1989

Mietz JA, Grossman Z, Leuders KK, Kuff EL: Nucleotide sequence of a complete mouse intracisternal A-particle genome: Relationship to known aspects of particle assembly and function. J Virol 61:3020, 1987

CHAPTER 60

Bacteriophage

In 1915, Twort published a note describing the infectious destruction of micrococcal colonies by an agent that seemed to be viral because it passed through bacteria-proof filters, was inactivated by heating to 60C for 1 hour, and could not grow autonomously. d'Herelle, who discovered this phenomenon independently, soon demonstrated the particulate nature of what he called *bacteriophage*. The viral nature of bacteriophage was confirmed by the elegant work of Burnet and of Schlesinger in the 1930s.

Bacteriophage and Development of Molecular Biology

Early hopes of using bacteriophage as a means of preventing and treating infectious diseases were not fulfilled. However, Delbrück and a group of investigators in the 1940s realized that the availability of viruses multiplying in clonal populations of rapidly growing host cells provided an ideal tool for gaining insight into basic biologic mechanisms. Their expectation has been amply borne out. Bacteriophage systems are highly amenable to experimentation, and intensive investigations over the last four decades have provided many of the fundamental concepts concerning molecular genetics, nucleic acid replication, and the transcription and translation of genetic information. Bacteriophage systems continue to provide some of the most advanced model systems for studying problems of basic biologic importance.

Measurement of Bacteriophage

A rapid and reliable method for measuring bacterial virus stocks was developed more than 50 years ago, initiating a quantitative approach toward understanding the virus life cycle. In this *plaque assay*, a moderate number of bacteriophage particles are mixed with a suspension of bacterial host cells and a small amount of molten agar, and the mixture is then spread over a Petri plate containing nutrient agar. The molten agar quickly solidifies, and, during an overnight incubation, the bacterial host grows into a confluent lawn. The lawn is interrupted, however, by a number of holes called *plaques*, each plaque originating from a single virus particle in the initial mixture. Each single phage particle first infects one bacterium and undergoes an infective cycle, killing the host cell and releasing many progeny phage a short time later. The progeny phage particles then diffuse until they find additional hosts, and the process repeats itself. Several cycles of phage infection thereby lead to a plaque containing numerous phage, all of which are the direct descendants of the same single phage particle from the initial mixture. The plaque is visible as a hole in the bacterial lawn because phage propagation has killed most or all bacterial cells within that area.

The plaque assay generally is conducted by performing serial dilutions of a phage stock and testing the diluted samples for the number of plaque-forming units (PFU), thus establishing the titer of PFU/mL in the original phage stock. Importantly, for many bacteriophage, the titer of PFU/mL is equal to the titer of virus particles visible in the electron microscope. Thus, essentially every virus particle is infective and the efficiency of plating (EOP, infective particles per total particles) is 1.0. This remarkable efficiency implies that all steps critical to a productive bacteriophage infection occur essentially without fail and that defective phage particles are not produced in significant numbers. As described previously (Chaps. 52 and 55), the EOP of many animal viruses is far less than 1, presumably because of the more complex steps involved in the animal virus infective cycle.

Classic Experiments

An important advance in understanding viral infective cycles was the development of synchronous infections in *one-step growth* experiments designed by Ellis, Delbrück, and Doermann in the 1940s. To this day the analysis of synchronous infections is central to almost every dissection of bacteriophage and animal virus multiplication cycles (Chap. 55). To conduct a one-step growth experiment, a concentrated stock of bacteriophage first is added to a suspension of bacterial hosts, generally at a multiplicity of infection (MOI) of several phage per cell. Most of the phage particles successfully infect a host cell within a short period (e.g., 2 minutes). To ensure synchrony in the infective cycle, any phage particles that have not infected a cell within that time period are inactivated, for example, by adding antiserum directed against the phage or by extreme dilution. As a function of time after infection, the titer of PFU is measured by plaque assay with appropriate dilutions.

If the infection is allowed to proceed unperturbed, the number of PFU per infected cell is initially equal to 1 and remains at this level for a period of time, called the *latent period* (Fig. 60–1, circles). During this time the plaque assay is detecting the infected cells rather than free phage particles. The latent period is the time during which the viral life cycle is progressing in an orderly fashion; each bacteriophage studied has a characteristic latent period, usually in the range of 15 to 30 minutes. Upon completion of the latent period, the bacterial hosts lyse and many progeny phage are released into the medium during the *rise period*. The average burst size (number of progeny phage produced per infected cell) for most bacteriophage is in the range of 50 to 500.

Two important facets of the viral life cycle are revealed if the infected bacteria are prematurely lysed by the addition of chloroform just before plaque assay (Fig. 60–1, triangles). First, the infected cells during the early part of the latent period contain no infective phage particles, even though they can produce many such phage if allowed to proceed without chloroform addition. Because infective phage disappear when assayed with premature lysis, this is called the *eclipse period*. Evidently, the complete virus particle dissociates into noninfectious subunits during the eclipse period. Viral growth was thereby shown to follow a completely different strategy than does cell multiplication. The second facet is that the rise in PFU occurs significantly sooner if the infected cells are prematurely lysed with chloroform during the latter part of the

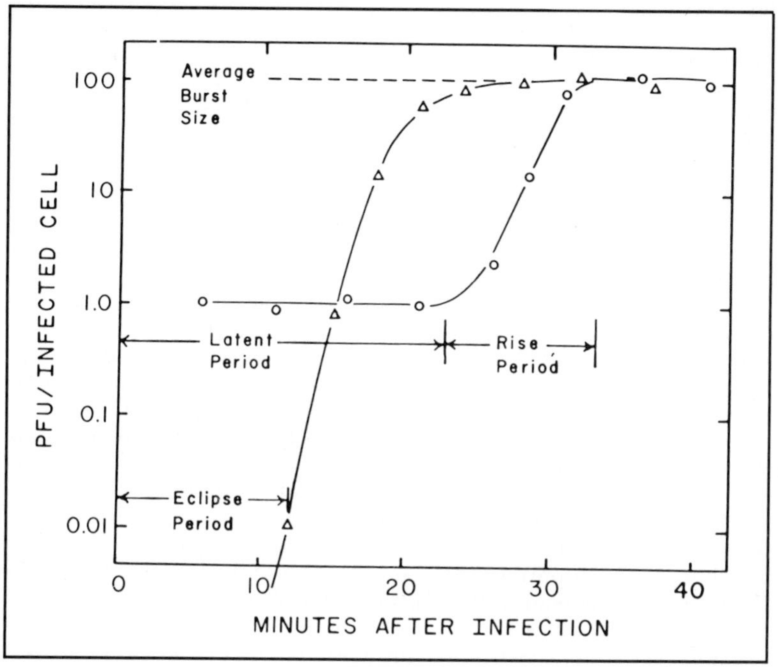

Fig. 60–1. One-step growth of phage T4. Samples were harvested as a function of time after the synchronized infection. The open circles are the results obtained when the samples were tested for plaque-forming units (PFU) directly, whereas the open triangles are those obtained when the samples were first treated with chloroform to induce premature lysis. *(From Mathews: Bacteriophage Biochemistry. Van Nostrand Reinhold Co, 1971.)*

latent period (Fig. 60–1; compare circles and triangles). This result implies that, in the absence of chloroform treatment, fully infectious progeny phage particles accumulate within the infected cells before the bacteriophage-directed lysis of the host cell.

By about 1950 it was clear that bacteriophage generally contain both protein and DNA, but the relative importance of each was uncertain. At that time, the central role of DNA as genetic material was not uniformly accepted, and the Watson-Crick model for DNA structure had not been formulated. In one of the milestones of virology, Hershey and Chase demonstrated that the nucleic acid of bacteriophage contains all the information necessary for phage multiplication, whereas the proteins of the parental virus particle are discarded during the infective cycle. They infected bacteria with a phage called T2, labeled in its protein with radioisotope ^{35}S. After an incubation period of several minutes, the phage particles and bacteria were separated by shearing in a Waring blender. Very little of the radioactive label was associated with the bacteria, even though the cells could go on to produce a normal burst of phage progeny. When the experiment was repeated with phage in which the DNA had been labeled with the radioisotope ^{32}P, the radioactive label was found associated with the cells. Thus the viral DNA had passed into the interior of the cell, whereas the protein coat of the virus had remained attached to the outer cell surface from which it could be dislodged by shearing forces. The inescapable conclusion is that the viral DNA constitutes the genetic material of the phage and is fully capable of directing a productive phage multiplication cycle once inside a cell. The protein coat has since been shown to be a complex structure that protects the DNA, recognizes appropriate hosts, and allows delivery of DNA into the cell interior. The separation of the genetic material from the delivery system explains the eclipse period described above.

Numerous fundamental aspects of molecular biology have emerged from bacteriophage systems—a few of these will now be summarized. One of the most important is the discovery of messenger RNA (mRNA), first detected in 1956 when Volkin and Astrachan noted that the base composition of newly synthesized RNA in T2-infected cells resembled that of T2 DNA rather than that of the host. In 1961, Brenner, Jacob, and Meselson firmly established the concept of mRNA by showing that this RNA combines with ribosomes and is responsible for phage protein synthesis. Another key landmark in the development of molecular biology was the elucidation of the nature of the genetic code. Crick and colleagues determined that the code must be triplet by combining various frameshift mutations in a gene of phage T4 (a close relative of T2). Certain combinations, such as three one-base deletions, restored functionality to the gene product. Evidently, the triple-mutant protein was functional because the correct reading frame was restored downstream from the three mutations (Chap. 7). Finally, it is worth noting that all the current genetic engineering approaches trace their origins to phage biology. Many bacteria were found to encode restriction systems that blocked the growth of certain bacteriophage (see below), and these restriction systems later were shown to encode restriction enzymes, the most important tool in the genetic engineering arsenal. Many other important enzymes used in genetic engineering are encoded by bacteriophage, and phage themselves often serve as the vector for recombinant DNA experiments.

Bacteriophage Genetics

The very rapid growth of bacteriophage quickly results in enormous numbers of clonally identical phage in a stock, a situation that is ideal for genetic investigations. Consider a typical phage that produces an average burst of about 300 in 20 minutes. With the availability of sufficient host cells, a single such phage particle would produce more than 10^{12} progeny in less than 2 hours. Even considering the very low frequency of spontaneous mutation (Chap. 8), this number of progeny phage is sufficient to contain interesting mutants of virtually every kind. The isolation of clonally pure phage stocks is critical for genetic analyses and can be easily accomplished by seeding a bacterial culture with a single plaque from an overnight lawn.

Early genetic analyses of bacteriophage centered on mutants that could easily be recognized. For example, a variety of bacteriophage mutants produce an altered plaque morphology that can be visually identified. Mutants of bacteriophage T4 that lyse the host cell more *r*apidly (*r*I, *r*IIA, *r*IIB, and *r*III mutants) produce larger plaques because of the more rapid diffusion of phage particles in the development of the plaque on the bacterial lawn.

A second category of phage mutants have an altered range of permissive hosts and are thereby called *host-range* mutants. The most common type of host-range mutants affect the adsorption process by which the phage particle binds to the envelope of the bacterial cell (see below). Host-range mutants were the first category for which the great power of genetic selection could be utilized. With the appropriate combination of (initially) nonpermissive host and phage strains, an enormous number of phage particles (e.g., 10^9) can be mixed with bacteria and spread on an agar plate. The parental (wild-type) phage cannot attach to the host and therefore do not form plaques. Rare host-range mutants with an altered attachment organ, however, can attach to the host bacteria and thereby form plaques. Thus host-range mutants can be readily isolated even if they occur at frequencies in the range of 10^{-9}.

The foundation for all bacteriophage genetics was established with just these few categories of mutants. Mixed infections of two different mutants were found to produce two types of recombinant phage, one that carried both mutations and the other that carried neither. Thus the existence of genetic recombination between phage genomes was established. By comparing the frequency of recombination between various pairs of mutants, rudimentary genetic maps also were established.

Only a very limited number of genes can, in the mutant form, cause altered plaque morphology or host range. The great potential of the genetic approach in bacteriophage biology therefore was not realized until collections of *conditional lethal* mutants were isolated in the 1960s. As described earlier (Chaps. 7, 8, and 57), conditional lethal mutants are those that are unable to propagate under some restrictive condition but that are viable under an alternative permissive condition. Thus *temperature-sensitive* mutants can grow only at low temperatures, and *nonsense* mutants require the presence of a suppressor transfer RNA (tRNA) to propagate. The critical point is that such mutations, in principle, can occur in any essential gene of an organism. A large collection of conditional lethal mutants therefore defines most or all essential genes, regardless of whether the corresponding gene products are involved in transcription, DNA replication, or phage particle morphogenesis.

The isolation of conditional lethal mutants greatly accelerated the molecular dissection of the phage life cycle. Every conditional lethal mutant can readily be propagated under permissive conditions, allowing the production of mutant phage stocks. The normal function of the mutant gene then can be assessed by examining the result of an infection under restrictive conditions. Among the first set of conditional lethal T4 mutants, mutations in 10 genes resulted in defective DNA replication, 7 in defective head assembly, and 11 in defective tail assembly. The class of nonsense mutants also can be exploited to identify the protein product of a mutant gene. Virus-encoded proteins can be labeled with radioisotope ^{35}S and separated by means of gel electrophoresis. The product of a particular gene can be identified in these gels because a nonsense mutation in the gene results in a truncated protein in nonsuppressing bacterial hosts but in a normal protein in suppressing hosts. In this way, most of the essential proteins of the commonly studied bacteriophage have been identified.

The process of *complementation* can be used to decide whether any two mutations are located in the same gene. If two conditional lethal mutants coinfect a restrictive host, a productive infection can result when the two mutations are in different genes (e.g., genes *A* and *B*). Complementation occurs because the A^- mutant phage provides functional B^+ product, whereas the B^- mutant phage provides A^+ product. When the two mutations are in the same gene, neither phage produces a functional product for that gene. Therefore the infection is nonproductive, except for the small number of wild-type recombinants that might be produced (see below).

Recombination studies of bacteriophage advanced rapidly once numerous mutants were available. Any two nonoverlapping mutations in the genomes of coinfecting bacteriophage can interact to produce recombinants, even when the two mutations are within the same gene. Studies of bacteriophage recombination have shed important light on diverse recombination mechanisms and also have been useful in deducing the genome structure of various bacteriophage. With some exceptions, the frequency of recombination is a direct function of the distance between two mutations, and thus recombination frequencies can be used to generate genomic maps. Physical studies of phage genomes complemented the genetic approach, culminating in determination of the complete nucleotide sequence of bacteriophage genomes as large as that of phage λ (48,502 base pairs).

Structure of Bacteriophage

There are bacteriophage for essentially every bacterial species that has been studied. Very few have been investigated in detail, but intense concentration on a small number of them has permitted rapid progress. Many of the well-studied phage are active on *Escherichia coli* or on *Bacillus* or *Pseudomonas* species (Table 60–1).

Phage Capsids

The structure of bacteriophage capsids is governed by the same principles described for animal viruses in Chapter 53. Among the smallest phage, some have icosahedral capsids (e.g., ϕX174 and MS2), whereas others are filamentous with capsids that display helical symmetry (e.g., fl) (Figs. 60–2 and 60–3, respectively). Consistent with their small genome sizes, these phage specify very simple capsids composed of only three to five distinct protein species. The *Pseudomonas* phage PM2 uses a somewhat more complex icosahedral capsid and a lipid envelope (Fig. 60–4).

The larger bacteriophage that have been analyzed have considerably more complex capsids. These phage generally consist of a head structure that contains the phage genome and a tail that serves both as a cell attachment organ and as a tube through which the DNA passes into the host cell. The phage head structures are icosahedral in design, with some being elongated and some symmetrical. The heads are produced by complex assembly pathways (see below) and can consist of more than 10 different protein species. For certain bacteriophage, particular proteins are found attached to the outside of the capsid (decoration proteins) and others are found within the capsid, often complexed with the nucleic acid (internal proteins). Remarkably, some of these internal proteins enter a newly infected cell along with the DNA, presumably by traversing the tail tube. One vertex of each phage head has a unique protein structure and is the site at which the tail is attached.

Bacteriophage tails vary greatly in composition and complexity, with three basic morphologic patterns. The first pattern consists of a very short tail containing only a few protein species, as found in coliphage T3 and T7 (Fig. 60–5). The second pattern consists of a very long but relatively simple tail, such as those of coliphage T1 and λ. The phage λ tail is a noncontractile flexible tube composed, on average, of 32 stacked disks, with a fine fiber protruding from the distal end (Fig. 60–6). The third morphologic pattern, exhibited by coliphage T2, T4, and T6 (the so-called T-even phage) is much more complex (Fig. 60–7). These large tails are composed of more than 20 different protein species and undergo complex structural rearrangements that allow injection of viral DNA through the cell envelope into the cytoplasm of the infected cell. The hollow core of the tail is covered with a sheath structure composed of 24 annuli. The sheath is assembled in a high-energy extended state and collapses into

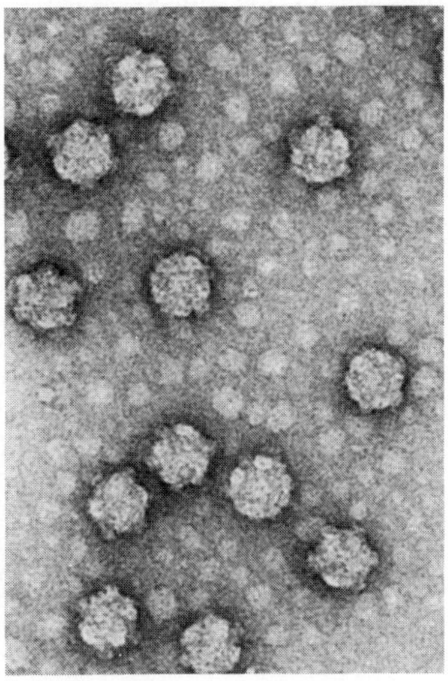

Fig. 60–2. Bacteriophage ϕX174. × 225,000. *(Electron micrograph by Dr. R. B. Luftig.)*

TABLE 60–1. CHARACTERISTICS OF SOME WELL-STUDIED BACTERIOPHAGE

Phage	Common Host	Particle Dimensions (nm) Head	Tail Length	Structure	Nucleic Acid Type	Mol Wt × 10^6	Structure
T1	*E. coli*	50	150	Icosahedral, simple tail	dsDNA	27	Linear, terminally redundant
T2, T4, T6	*E. coli*	85 × 110	110	Prolate icosahedral head, complex tail with fibers	dsDNA	110	Linear, circularly permuted, terminally redundant, contains glucosylated 5-hydroxy-methylcytosine
T3, T7	*E. coli*	60	15	Icosahedral, short tail	dsDNA	25	Linear, terminally redundant
T5	*E. coli*	65	170	Icosahedral, simple tail	dsDNA	80	Linear, terminally redundant
N4	*E. coli*	70	15	Icosahedral, short tail	dsDNA	40	Linear, terminally redundant
λ	*E. coli*	64	140	Icosahedral, simple tail	dsDNA	32	Linear, cohesive ends
P22	*S. typhimurium*	61	20	Icosahedral, complex tail	dsDNA	29	Linear, circularly permuted, terminally redundant
SP01, SP82	*Bacillus subtilis*	90	200	Icosahedral, complex tail	dsDNA	85	Linear, terminally redundant, contains 5-hydroxymethyluracil
φ29	*B. amyloliquefaciens*	30 × 40	30	Prolate icosahedral head with attached fibers, complex tail	dsDNA	12	Linear, covalently attached terminal protein
PM2	*Pseudomonas Bal-31*	60	None	Icosahedral, envelope contains lipid	dsDNA	6	Circular
φX174, S13, M12, G4	*E. coli*	27	None	Icosahedral	ssDNA	1.7	Circular
fl, fd, M13	*E. coli*	7 × 900	None	Filamentous	ssDNA	2.1	Circular
φ6	*Pseudomonas phaseolica*	65	None	Icosahedral, envelope contains lipid	dsRNA	9.5	3 linear segments (2.2, 2.8, and 4.5 × 10^6)
MS2, f2, fr, Qβ	*E. coli*	24	None	Icosahedral	ssRNA	1.2	Linear

a more compact structure to drive the hollow tube covered by the sheath through the cell envelope (Fig. 60–8). Many of the complex tails possess multiple tail fibers at their ends; these fibers serve to recognize specific binding sites on the host cell and thereby initiate the attachment of the phage particle to its host.

Phage Nucleic Acids

Genome Structure. A variety of different forms have been found for the genomes of various bacteriophage (Table 60–1). The smallest phage genomes are either single-stranded DNA circles (e.g., φX174, M13) or single-stranded RNA

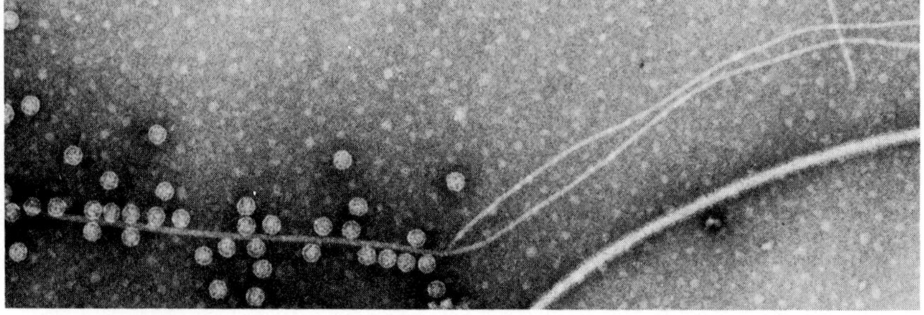

Fig. 60–3. An F-pilus with two types of male-specific phage attached: icosahedral RNA-containing MS2 and filamentous DNA-containing fl. The former are attached along the entire length of the F pilus; the latter are adsorbed by their ends to the tip of the pilus. *(From Caro and Schnos: Proc Natl Acad Sci USA 56:128, 1968.)*

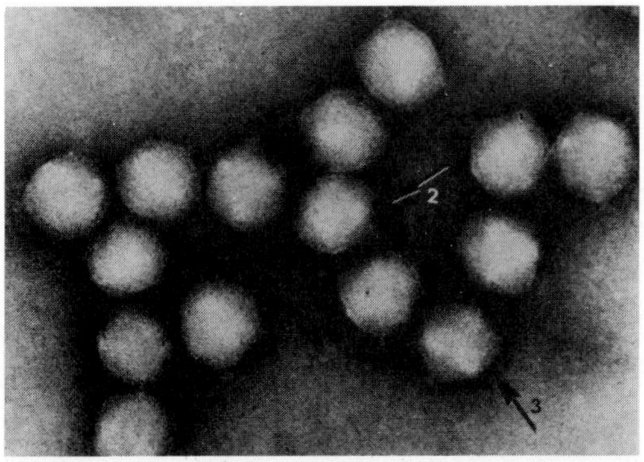

Fig. 60–4. The enveloped phage PM2 fixed with glutaraldehyde and negatively stained with phosphotungstate. The numbered arrows indicate axes of twofold and threefold symmetry. × 120,000. *(From Silbert et al: Virology 39:666, 1969.)*

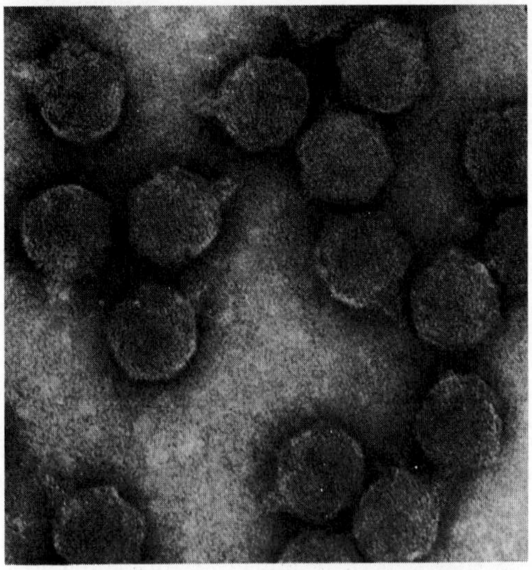

Fig. 60–5. Bacteriophage T7. × 225,000. *(Electron micrograph by Dr. R. B. Luftig.)*

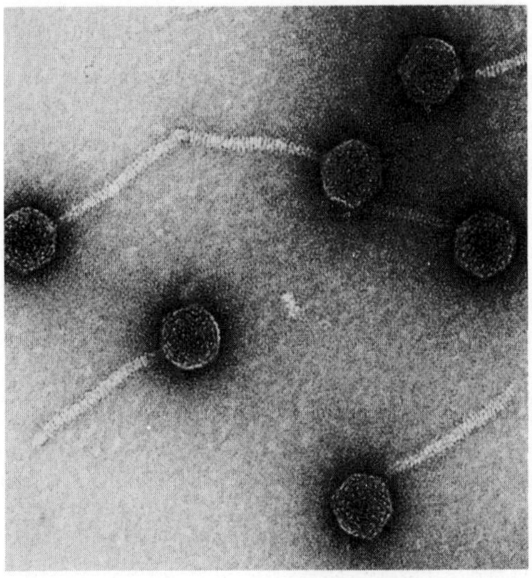

Fig. 60–6. Bacteriophage λ. × 135,000. *(Electron micrograph by Dr. R. B. Luftig.)*

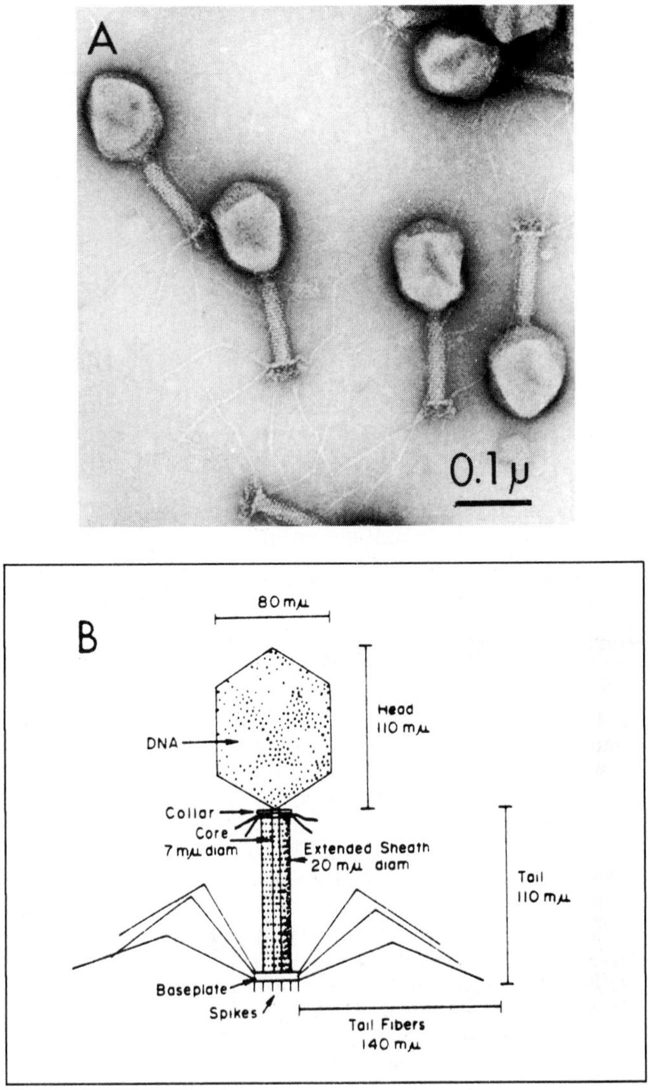

Fig. 60–7. **A.** Bacteriophage T4. × 100,000. **B.** Model of phage T4. *(Electron micrograph by Dr. R. B. Luftig.)*

linears (e.g., MS2, Qβ). In both classes the single strand packaged in the phage particle is of the same polarity as the mRNA of the bacteriophage, and the viral genome therefore is considered to be of positive polarity. Phage φ6, which infects *Pseudomonas phaseolica*, has an unusual bacteriophage genome consisting of duplex RNA. Like the duplex RNA genomes of animal viruses, the φ6 genome is segmented, with three unique chromosomes that must each be present in the virion.

The larger, more complex bacteriophage generally contain single, duplex DNA chromosomes that vary in length from about 10 to 300 kilobase pairs. A few of these bacteriophage, such as PM2, contain a circular genome, but the majority use linear duplex DNA. Any linear duplex chromosome poses a major problem for replication, and this *end problem* must be appreciated to understand the structures of bacteriophage genomes. DNA polymerases can synthesize product only in the 5′ to 3′ direction, and generally they use RNA primers to initiate each newly synthesized DNA fragment

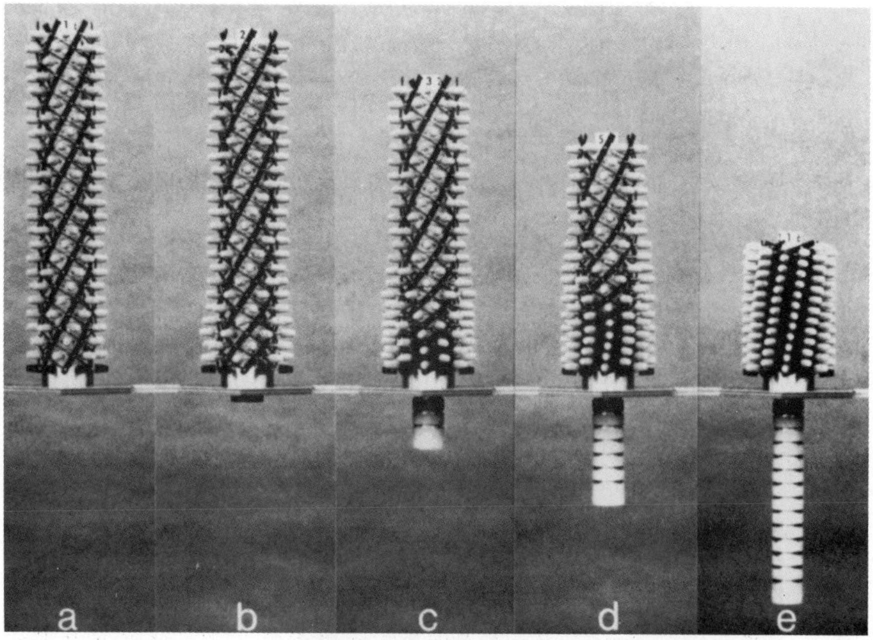

Fig. 60–8. A mechanical model for the contraction of the phage T4 tail. Panels a through e show steps in the progressive collapse of the extended sheath. In this model, extended springs, rather than protein conformational changes, provide the driving force for collapse of the sheath. Note that the rigid central tail tube is driven down through the surface as a result of sheath collapse. *(From Caspar: Biophys J 32:103, 1980.)*

(Chap. 7). Even if an RNA primer is situated at the extreme 3′ terminus of a linear DNA template to begin daughter strand replication, the RNA segment subsequently would be excised. Thus the daughter strand would be at least several bases shorter than the parental strand after one round of replication. The problem is even worse, because RNA primers can be synthesized only at certain sequences. These sequences cannot always be present precisely at the 3′ terminus when that terminus is becoming shorter during every round of replication. Without some mechanism to solve this problem, a linear chromosome would become shorter and shorter with every replication cycle. Bacteriophage with linear genomes demonstrate several different strategies to bypass this difficulty, and all the strategies are reflected in the genome structure.

The phage ϕ29 uses a terminal protein that directs priming at the ends of the genome, so that a DNA base is inserted opposite the extreme 3′-terminal residue of the parental strand. Like the adenovirus terminal protein, the ϕ29 terminal protein is covalently linked to each 5′ end of the DNA. Other bacteriophage, such as λ, possess complementary single-stranded regions at the two ends of the genome. These *cohesive ends* anneal to each other immediately after the DNA enters the cell, converting the genome into a circular form. Thus, phage λ solves the end problem by using a circular replicative intermediate without ends.

Two additional strategies to solve the end problem involve *terminally redundant* DNA. The first strategy, used by phage such as T3 and T7, involves the generation of identical viral genomes, all containing the same terminal redundancy. For example, the viral DNA of coliphage T7 contains a perfectly repeated sequence of 160 base pairs at its left and right ends. During an infection the processes of replication and recombination convert the viral DNA into long concatemers in which many genomes are covalently linked end-to-end, with only one copy of the terminal repeat between each pair of genomes (Fig. 60–9A). Late in infection, each single copy of the terminal repeat is duplicated during the maturation of the DNA. Presumably, staggered single-strand cleavages are introduced at the two ends of the 160–base pair terminal repeat, providing 3′ termini that are used by DNA polymerase to initiate replication of the terminal repeats (Fig. 60–9B). Replication of the repeats would convert the concatemeric intracellular form of T7 DNA into monomeric forms, complete with both copies of the 160–base pair repeat, suitable for packaging into phage particles.

The second strategy, used by phage such as T4, involves viral DNA that is both terminally redundant and *circularly permuted* (Fig. 60–10). In addition to having direct repeats at the two ends, the repeated ends of any one T4 DNA molecule are different from those of another molecule. Considering a simple alphabetic genome, the sequence of some molecules is ABCDE . . . XYZAB; of others, BCDEF . . . YZABC; and so on. In phage T4, it appears that any one base position out of the entire 170-kilobase genome is the terminal base in some viral DNA molecules (i.e., the ends are completely random). This kind of genome structure is generated in two steps. First, the infecting phage DNA is replicated and recombined into long concatemers, as in the case of phage T7 (Fig. 60–9A). These concatemers are then a substrate in the second step, the packaging of DNA into phage heads during viral assembly (Fig. 60–10). DNA is packaged into a preexisting phage head until the head is full. Because a full phage head contains slightly more DNA than is required for the complete genetic content of the phage, *headful packaging* results directly in the observed terminal redundancy. Further, because excess DNA is packaged into each phage head, successive packaging events from the same concatemeric DNA precursor result in the circular permutation of terminal sequences.

Phage nucleic acids can be infectious, just as are the nucleic acids of animal viruses. Naked phage DNA, however, can penetrate only a bacterial cell that is competent for DNA

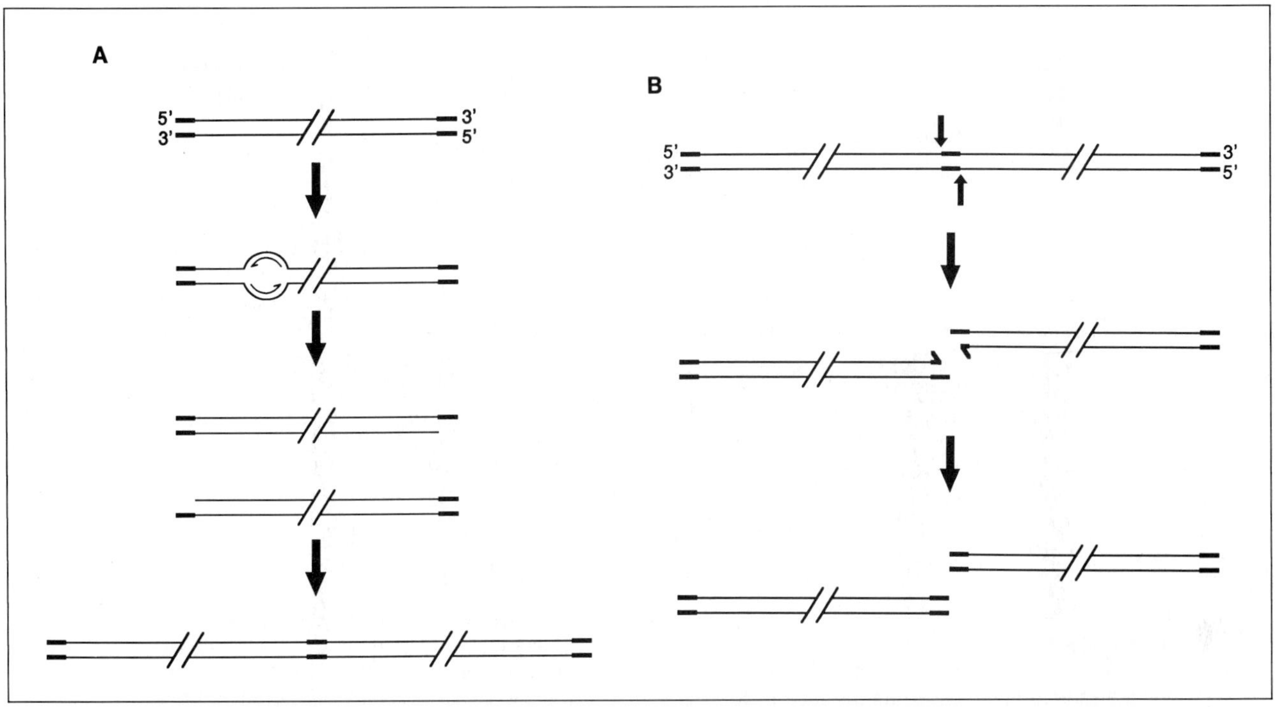

Fig. 60–9. Model for phage T7 DNA metabolism. **A.** The monomeric infecting DNA is converted into concatemeric DNA. Replication from an internal origin leads to single-stranded regions in the terminal repeats (bold lines) at each 3′ end of the parental DNA. Because the two single-stranded regions are complementary, recombination can join the two products into a concatemeric structure. Multiple rounds of replication and recombination produce concatemers with many genomes linked end-to-end. **B.** Concatemeric DNA is the substrate for a specific cleavage event that nicks on both sides of the terminal repeat sequence. Subsequent DNA replication converts the two single-stranded repeats into the duplex form. *(Adapted from Watson: Nature New Biol 239:197, 1972.)*

uptake (see the discussion of transformation in Chap. 8). Thus, competent *Bacillus subtilis* can be *transfected* with naked phage DNA, as can artificially induced (e.g., Ca^{++}-treated) competent cells of *E. coli.*

Unusual Nucleic Acid Bases. The genomes of several bacteriophage contain unusual nucleic acid bases. For example, the T-even coliphage DNAs contain 5-hydroxymethylcytosine in place of cytosine, and the majority of the hydroxymethylcytosine residues in these DNAs also are glucosylated. The DNA of certain *B. subtilis* phage show a remarkable diversity of thymine replacements, including uracil, 5-hydroxymethyluracil, glycosylated and phosphorylated 5-(4′,5′-dihydroxypentyl) uracil, and α-glutamyl thymine.

These various base substitutions confer an important advantage on infecting phage genomes—namely, they render the DNA resistant to degradation by host restriction systems. As described in Chapter 8, many bacterial cells produce restriction enzymes that degrade foreign DNA, and nearly all restriction enzymes are inactive against these substituted phage DNAs. A second advantage of the substituted bases is that the infecting phage is able to specifically degrade the host DNA (containing normal bases), thereby generating a large pool of nucleotide precursors for its own replication. Each bacteriophage with unusual bases simply induces nucleases that degrade only DNA with normal bases, providing the necessary specificity to prevent degradation of phage DNA.

A second class of unusual bases often is found in the DNA of both bacteriophage and bacterial cells and results from the action of specific methylation systems. Many bacterial cells contain specific restriction-modification systems that act at particular nucleotide sequences in DNA (Chap. 8). For example, bacteria with the *Eco*RI system produce both a restriction enzyme and a DNA adenine methylase, each of which recognizes the sequence 5′-GAATTC-3′. The methylase normally methylates the second A residue in that particular sequence, rendering the DNA resistant to cleavage by the *Eco*RI restriction endonuclease. Bacteriophage DNA that has been produced in the presence of a particular restriction-modification system also will contain the methyl groups at the same characteristic sequence. Thus, phage produced in a cell with the *Eco*RI system will be protected from *Eco*RI digestion in a subsequent infection of a cell with the *Eco*RI system. Conversely, if the same phage infects a cell with a different restriction system, the phage DNA may be destroyed by that restriction system unless it has some protection (e.g., by the unusual bases described above). As described in Chapter 8, the restriction systems do not operate with 100% efficiency; thus a small number of phage particles can survive destruction and produce progeny. The progeny of such surviving phage will contain the modifications specified by the host and thereby

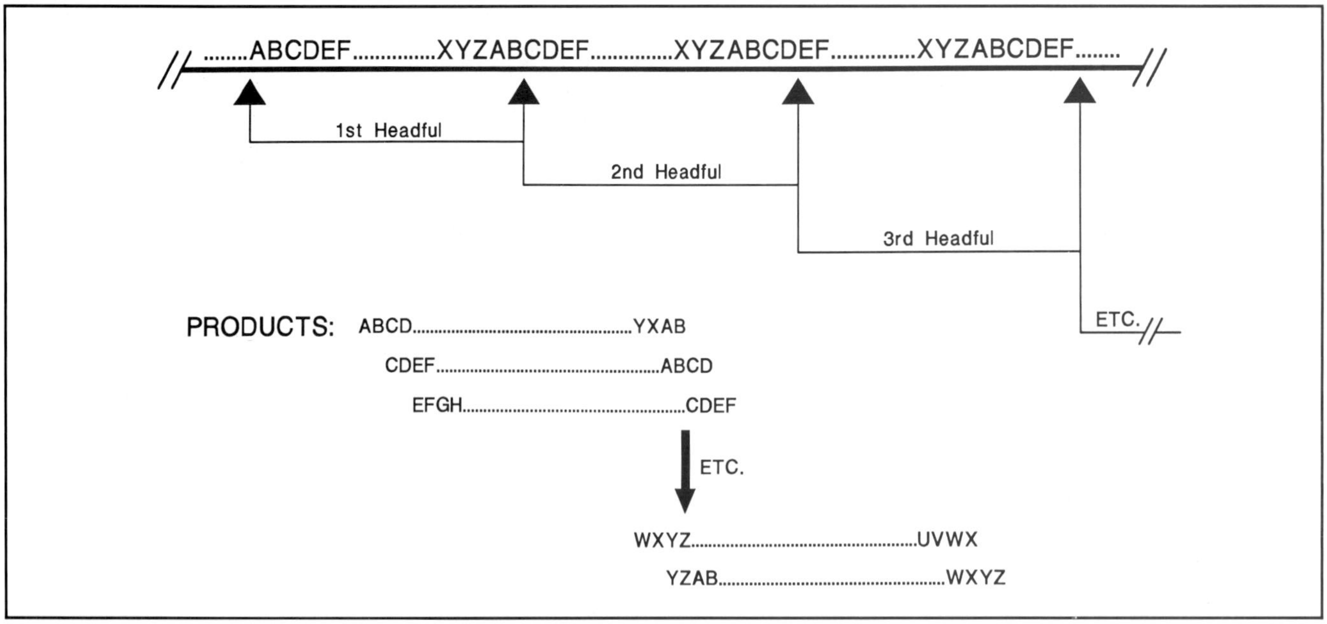

Fig. 60–10. Headful packaging of phage T4 DNA. A concatemeric intermediate is generated during phage T4 infections by mechanisms similar to those described for phage T7 (Fig. 60–9A). The concatemer is then a substrate for headful packaging, which generates the circularly permuted and terminally redundant genomes found in the virion.

break the restriction barrier. Because these methylation systems depend on the genotype of the bacterial host, they are referred to as *host-induced modifications*.

Virulent Bacteriophage

Some bacteriophage always lyse their hosts, and these are known as the *virulent* phage. The multiplication cycle of virulent phage is formally analogous to that of animal viruses (Chap. 55) but proceeds much more rapidly. The length of the latent period is at least 4 hours for poliovirus and 12 hours for vaccinia virus, but it is only about 13 minutes for phage T1, T7, and ϕX174 and about 20 to 25 minutes for the T-even phage and MS2. The life cycle of duplex DNA bacteriophage is illustrated here by focusing mostly on that of the well-studied phage T4. Figure 60–11 presents the T4 genetic map, along with the function of many T4 gene products. Important aspects of other virulent phage life cycles also are mentioned where appropriate.

A second class of bacteriophage either can undergo a lytic cycle much like that of the virulent phage or, alternatively, can enter into a dormant state in which they are passively maintained by an otherwise normal bacterial cell. These so-called temperate or lysogenic phage form a relationship with their host that is similar to that of the animal tumor viruses described in Chapter 59. The life cycle of lysogenic bacteriophage is considered in detail below. However, because the lytic phase of the lysogenic life cycle is exactly analogous to that of the virulent phage being discussed in this section, the lytic multiplication of lysogenic bacteriophage also is considered in this section.

Life Cycle of Duplex DNA Phage

Attachment and DNA Entry. The initial step in a phage infective cycle is the attachment of the phage particle to virus-specific receptors on the host cell surface. Phage receptors vary considerably, with some composed of lipopolysaccharide, others of lipoprotein, and still others of a specific protein or protein complex.

Most bacteriophage are highly specific for a limited number of bacterial hosts, and this specificity resides primarily in the attachment step. Conversely, bacteria capable of adsorbing the same phage often are antigenically related. This observation has found application in the practice of phage typing. In this method, the sensitivity and resistance patterns of bacterial strains to a series of known bacteriophage are determined. Because these patterns are both readily determined and highly characteristic, they can be useful for bacterial strain identification in diagnosis and epidemiology.

Bacteriophage T4 first contacts the outer surface of its bacterial host by means of its multiple tail fibers. Depending on the bacterial host, the fibers bind either to lipopolysaccharide or to a specific cell surface protein encoded by the *ompC* gene. This stage of binding is reversible and may allow the phage a chance to wander around the cell surface until it finds an appropriate location to inject its DNA into the cell. The transition from reversible to irreversible binding of the phage to the cell is coincident with the association of the base of the tail to special sites on the cell surface. These sites appear to be the locations where the inner and outer membranes of

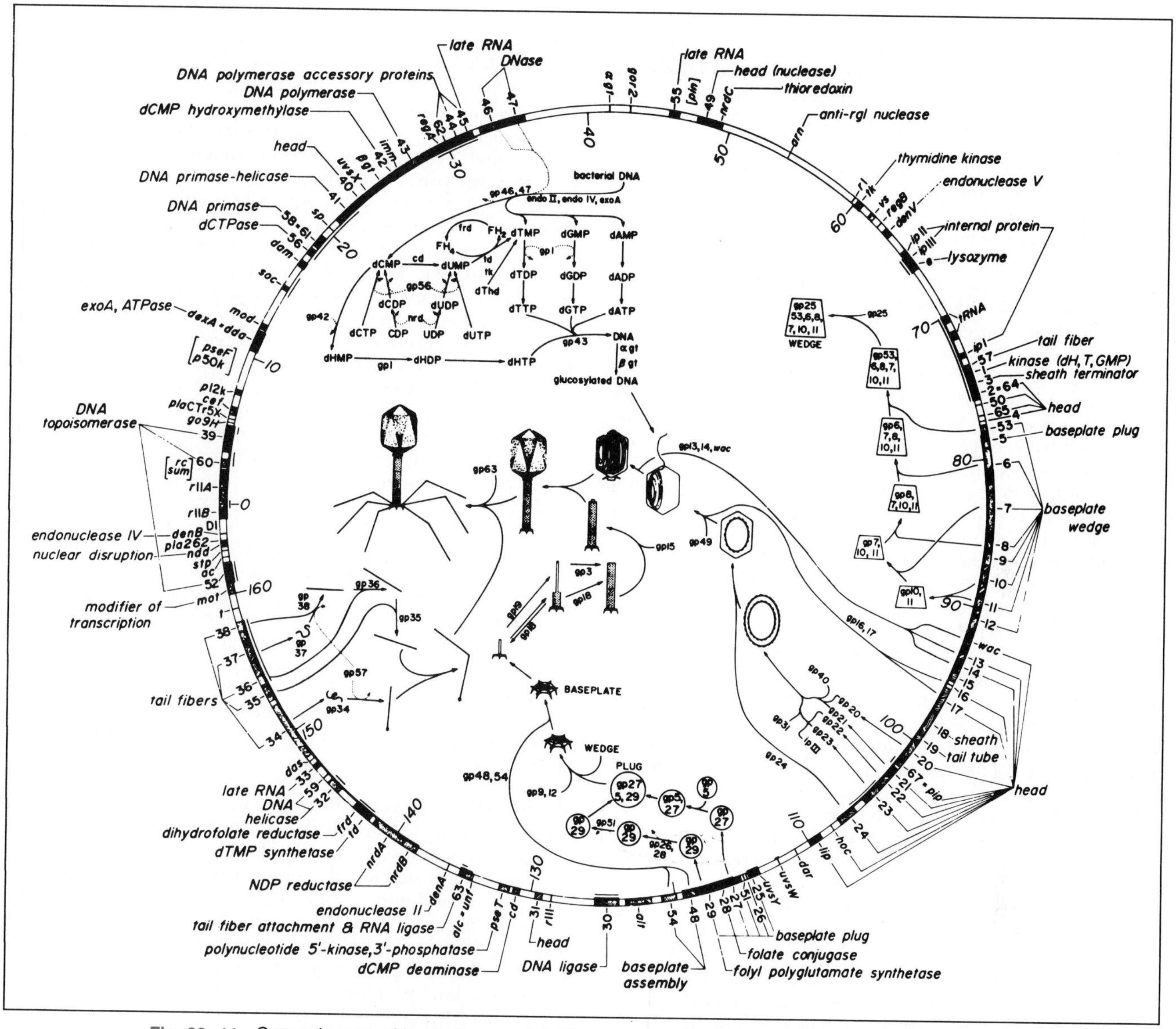

Fig. 60–11. Genomic map of bacteriophage T4. The map coordinates just inside the circle are in kilobase pairs, increasing clockwise from the junction of genes *r*IIA and *r*IIB. The functions of many of the gene products are indicated next to the gene designations, and simplified pathways for nucleotide and DNA synthesis and for phage assembly are depicted within the circle. *(Courtesy of Dr. E. Kutter and Dr. B. Guttman.)*

the cell contact each other (adhesion zones). The adhesion zones presumably are used as sites of DNA injection because the entering DNA would thereby avoid the periplasm of the cell, which contains numerous hydrolytic enzymes, including nucleases (Chap. 3). Once the phage is bound irreversibly, the tail structure undergoes a complex series of structural transitions. As described above (Fig. 60–8), the tail sheath contracts, driving the tail tube into the bacterial cell. The actual transport of DNA from the phage head, through the tail tube, and into the interior of the cell is a poorly understood process.

Regulation of Gene Expression. During the phage multiplication cycle, the genetic information encoded in the viral genome expresses itself according to an exquisitely refined regulatory program, exerted mostly at the level of transcription. One important class of regulatory events modulates the quantities of particular gene products synthesized. Some proteins are needed in large amounts, some in very small amounts, and the requirement for others may depend on the exact growth conditions. A second important class of events regulates the time course of synthesis of various gene products. The utility of temporal regulation is obvious: for example, enzymes that replicate phage DNA need to be made early in infection, whereas enzymes that break down the cell envelope need to be made very late in infection to avoid premature lysis.

The temporal programs used by bacteriophage have been extensively studied by hybridizing phage RNA produced at various times after infection to restriction fragments and to separated strands of the viral genome. All the duplex DNA bacteriophage were found to produce, in sequence, several classes of mRNA. Within any one temporal class, the transcribed phage genes tend to be organized within the phage genome, generally being transcribed from the same strand of DNA and often from one or a few contiguous regions. Often, genes of related function are transcribed into polycistronic mRNA species, allowing coordinate regulation of several genes from a single promoter region.

Because the first transcripts synthesized during a phage infection precede any phage-directed protein synthesis, T4 and almost every other bacteriophage depend on the host RNA polymerase for transcription of *early* genes. Early promoters in phage DNA generally are indistinguishable from host promoters, containing the same consensus sequences in the −10 and −35 regions (Chap. 7). The only clear exception to this pattern is provided by a coliphage, N4, which injects its own RNA polymerase (synthesized in the previous infection cycle) along with viral DNA to transcribe early genes. In a bizarre twist, phage N4 uses the host RNA polymerase for transcription of its late genes.

Among the early transcripts directed by various bacteriophage are those encoding proteins that change the transcriptional apparatus, sometimes in very complex manners. Phage T4 changes the transcriptional specificity of the host RNA polymerase by inducing a positive transcriptional activator, which is the product of an early gene called *motA* (*mo*dulator *of t*ranscription). The *motA* protein binds to *middle* promoters in the phage genome; these promoters apparently are transcribed by the host RNA polymerase only when the *motA* protein is bound. The process of transcription termination also is modified relatively early in phage T4 infection, increasing transcription of certain genes located downstream of transcription terminator sequences. Regulation of gene expression at the level of transcription termination, which also is used extensively by the temperate phage lambda, is discussed in the context of the lysogenic state later in this chapter.

A second major switch in the T4 transcriptional program involves the replacement of the normal σ subunit of the host RNA polymerase. The phage gene *55* specifies a new σ subunit that redirects the host RNA polymerase to the *late* T4 promoters. Several important bacterial regulatory circuits, including those involved in the heat shock response, sporulation, and nitrogen metabolism, also use a σ subunit replacement strategy (Chap. 7). The overall strategy used by phage T4 to direct a temporal program of gene expression therefore involves modifying the host RNA polymerase so that it sequentially recognizes three classes of promoters. In addition, phage T4 also specifies numerous other modifications of the host enzyme, including both covalent modifications (adenosine diphosphate [ADP] ribosylation and phosphorylation) and the addition of several new subunits. The precise role (or roles) of these other changes in the T4 transcriptional program currently are unclear.

Alteration of the host RNA polymerase is not the only strategy used by bacteriophage to program transcription. Phage T7 and its relatives utilize the host RNA polymerase only for early gene expression. The product of the early gene *1* is a phage-encoded RNA polymerase, which then goes on to transcribe all later genes. Because it is a fairly simple and efficient enzyme, the T7-encoded (and related phage SP6-encoded) RNA polymerase currently is being used extensively in recombinant DNA procedures.

Although bacteriophage gene expression is regulated predominantly by alterations in transcription, control at the translational level also has been documented. During phage T4 infections, translation of the single strand binding protein (the gene *32* protein) is autogenously regulated. The protein serves as a translational repressor by binding to the translational initiation region of its own mRNA and blocking ribosome attachment. This repression fixes the free pool of the single strand binding protein at a level that is optimal for replication, recombination, and other metabolic processes. Phage T4 also encodes a more global regulator of translation, the product of the *regA* gene. This protein represses synthesis of a variety of proteins involved in DNA synthesis and thereby may regulate the overall extent of phage DNA replication.

Perhaps the most entertaining method of temporal regulation has been demonstrated for phage T5. Only about 15% of the phage T5 genome enters the infected cell during the initial attachment, and this segment contains all the early genes. The late genes are present in the remaining 85% of the phage DNA, which lingers for several minutes in the phage capsid outside the cell! The early genes in the first segment of DNA have a variety of functions, including, for example, the arrest of host transcription. Two early gene products are required to bring the remainder of the phage DNA into the cell. Late promoters in this segment then are recognized by the host RNA polymerase to complete the regulatory program. Phage T5 thereby regulates expression simply by transporting the early versus late genes into the cell at different times.

Phage DNA Replication. As in transcription, bacteriophage use a variety of strategies to replicate their DNA. Some phage rely extensively on the host replication machinery, whereas others replace the host system with phage-encoded enzymes. In addition, a wide variety of mechanisms are used to initiate bacteriophage DNA replication. In general, various bacteriophage have provided critical model systems for studying mechanistic aspects of DNA replication, and even the *E. coli* replication machinery was first uncovered by studying replication of phage that utilize the host enzymes.

The total amount of DNA that needs to be synthesized during a phage infection often exceeds the amount made in uninfected cells. For example, 500 copies of T4 DNA, which can be synthesized during the 20- to 30-minute infective cycle, is equivalent in mass to about 20 copies of the *E. coli* genome. Before infection, the bacterial cell does not contain sufficient nucleotide precursors to synthesize this much DNA. Many bacteriophage therefore must augment the supply of nucleotide precursors to achieve a high synthetic rate. In addition, the use of unusual DNA bases by certain bacteriophage necessitates the production of novel nucleotide synthesizing enzymes.

One source of nucleotide precursors used by many phage is the DNA of the bacterial host. In the case of phage T4, the bacterial DNA is broken down into constituent deoxynucleoside monophosphates by a combination of phage-encoded endonucleases and exonucleases. After conversion to the appropriate deoxynucleoside triphosphates, this process provides a significant (although nonessential) source of DNA precursors. The degradation of the host genome also contributes to the phage-induced arrest of host transcription, translation, and replication.

T4 and many other phage encode enzymes that function in the synthesis of nucleotide precursors for replication. Because T4 DNA contains glucosylated 5-hydroxymethylcytosine instead of cytosine, the following enzymes generally are important for growth: (1) an enzyme that destroys deoxycytosine triphosphate (to prevent incorporation of the unmodified base into phage DNA), (2) an enzyme that hydroxymethylates deoxycytosine monophosphate, and (3) two enzymes that glucosylate 5-hydroxymethylcytosine residues in polymerized DNA. Several other enzymes specified by T4 function in the synthesis of the other three deoxyribonucleoside triphosphates; these generally are not essential for phage growth, because similar host enzymes can partially substitute for their function. The cumulative effect of these various enzymes is a drastic alteration in the nucleotide pools after T4 infection. Many of the simpler phage do not induce enzymes to alter the nucleotide pools but, rather, use only precursors synthesized by the host nucleotide-metabolizing machinery.

Several bacteriophage DNA replication reactions have been reproduced in vitro and thus have contributed significantly to our understanding of DNA synthesis. The events that occur at a replication fork are essentially the same in various bacteriophage systems and in the host (Chap. 7), although in each case a somewhat different number and variety of proteins may be involved. In vitro replication in the T4 system requires the phage-encoded DNA polymerase and DNA polymerase accessory proteins (encoded by genes *43* and *44*, *45*, and *62*, respectively), which together constitute the polymerase holoenzyme complex (Chap. 7). In addition, the single-strand binding protein (gene *32* protein) interacts with the polymerase complex and stabilizes single-stranded regions at the replication fork. Finally, a complex of two proteins (the genes *41* and *61* proteins) assists in replication by providing helicase activity to unwind the parental DNA and primase activity to initiate Okazaki fragment synthesis. In addition to these, phage T4 induces its own DNA ligase, type II DNA topoisomerase, and other proteins that are required for optimal replication of phage DNA.

Bacteriophage use diverse mechanisms to initiate their DNA replication. The replication of T4 DNA occurs by two very different processes, depending on the time of infection. At early times, several replication origins located throughout the genome are active. Each origin analyzed to date contains either early or middle promoters for transcription. The function of RNA polymerase may be to provide the first primer for replication of the leading strand at the origin, although other possibilities have not been ruled out. Surprisingly, T4 replication does not require replication origin sequences at late times of infection. Rather, a set of proteins involved in genetic recombination is required to initiate replication, and replication apparently starts at any location in the genome. The simplest model is that recombination intermediates are converted into replication forks. This and other examples illustrate the very intimate connections between the processes of replication and recombination during bacteriophage infections. As discussed above, T4 and other phage synthesize concatemeric DNA intermediates as an obligatory intermediate in their life cycles; the precise roles of replication and recombination in the generation of concatemeric DNA remain to be determined.

The replication scheme of phage ϕ29 DNA is much like

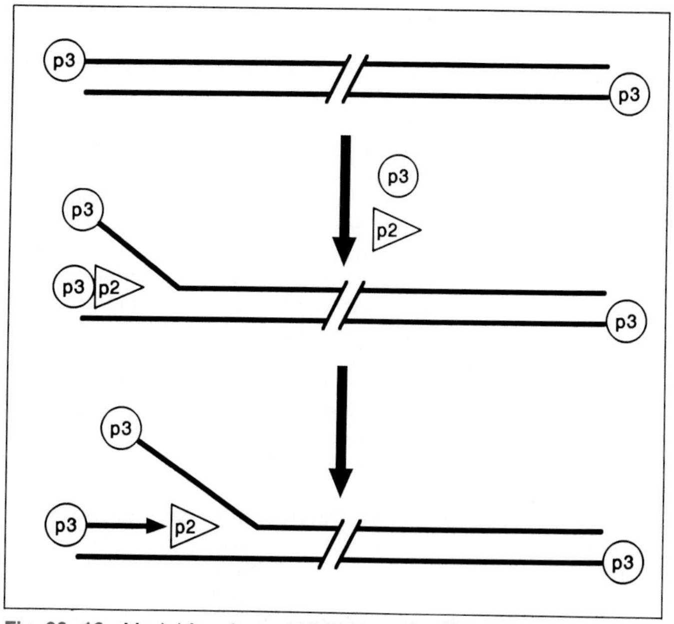

Fig. 60–12. Model for phage ϕ29 DNA replication. The ϕ29 genome has terminal protein (p3) covalently attached to each 5′ end. Initiation of replication involves the association of free p3 protein with one terminus. Replication by the DNA polymerase (p2) begins with the use of the p3 as a protein primer. *(Adapted from Salas: In Calendar (ed): The Bacteriophages, vol 1. Plenum Press, 1988.)*

that of the adenovirus genome (Chap. 55). ϕ29 contains a linear duplex genome with a terminal protein, p3, covalently attached to each 5′ terminus (Fig. 60–12). As discussed above, replication initiating from the terminal protein allows complete replication of the linear genome. Initiation of ϕ29 DNA replication involves first the formation of a phosphodiester bond between deoxyadenosine monophosphate (dAMP) and the hydroxyl group of a serine residue in a free molecule of p3. Formation of the bond requires the ϕ29 DNA polymerase (p2 protein). The p3-dAMP complex associates with one of the p3 molecules covalently attached to a 5′ terminus of the parental DNA. The 3′-hydroxyl group provided by the dAMP residue is then used as the primer to initiate replication, with the parental 5′ terminus–p3 complex being displaced as the daughter molecule is synthesized by the ϕ29 DNA polymerase (Fig. 60–12). Initiation of replication at both ends of the parental DNA leads to a complete duplication of the phage genome.

The initiation of phage λ DNA replication during the lytic phase of its life cycle has been studied in great detail. The strategy adopted by λ is to appropriate the host replication machinery rather than to replace it with a phage-encoded system. Phage λ encodes two key replication proteins, the products of genes *O* and *P*. The *O* protein specifically recognizes four adjacent 19–base pair repeats within the λ origin of replication, which is itself located within the *O* gene. The *P* protein serves as the bridge between the λ and host components, binding both to the *O* protein at the origin and to the host *dnaB* protein (Chap. 7). The loading of the host *dnaB* protein onto λ DNA at the origin allows localized DNA unwinding, utilizing the helicase activity of the *dnaB* protein. After DNA unwinding, RNA priming by the host *dnaG* primase and subsequent elongation by the DNA polymerase III holoenzyme complex creates a functional replication fork.

Finally, the lytic replication of temperate phage Mu DNA is remarkable and important because it occurs solely by a replicative transposition mechanism (Chap. 8). Most transposable elements transpose at a very low frequency, typically 10^{-5} per cell generation or less. During a lytic infection by phage Mu, however, several hundred replicative transposition events occur in a similar time span. This extremely high frequency of phage Mu transposition led to the first in vitro reconstitution of transposition and thereby contributed greatly to our understanding of this important genetic process. Mu encodes two proteins that are directly involved in transposition. These proteins recognize the ends of phage Mu DNA and catalyze the strand exchange reaction critical for transposition (Chap. 8). During a lytic infection, the host replication machinery is then recruited to complete the replicative transposition process.

Morphogenesis of Phage Particles. Because of the excellent genetic and biochemical approaches available, phage particle morphogenesis provides an unparalleled system for answering important questions concerning biologic form determination. Morphogenesis has been investigated most intensively for coliphage T4, T7 and λ, and for the *Salmonella* phage P22. For each, two distinct classes of proteins have been found to be involved in assembly. In addition to the structural proteins found in the mature phage particle, several other proteins act as catalysts during the assembly pathways. The proteins involved in particle morphogenesis generally are of the late class, being synthesized only after the intracellular pool of phage DNA has increased dramatically as the result of DNA replication. An interesting exception is the early production of two T4 proteins (products of genes *31* and *40*) involved in head assembly. Both proteins are necessary for the initiation of the head assembly process, presumably explaining why they are synthesized before all the other proteins involved in morphogenesis.

The structural proteins that become part of the mature phage particle generally are synthesized in large amounts, because most of these proteins are required in many copies per mature virion and because each infected cell produces hundreds of progeny phage. In contrast, many of the proteins that play a catalytic role in phage assembly are produced in only very small amounts. The number of different gene products involved in phage assembly can be quite high. Phage T4 has more than 30 different structural protein species, and about 20 other proteins are required for the assembly pathways. Even the simpler phage, such as T7 and λ, contain on the order of 10 to 15 different structural proteins.

An invaluable approach for deciphering phage assembly has been to study the products of infection of each of a large number of conditional lethal mutants that are defective in morphogenesis. Cells infected under restrictive condition accumulate not mature phage particles but, rather, normal or abnormal phage components, such as one or another form of prohead, mature heads, tail fibers, tail cores, and/or other partially completed tail structures. This analysis allowed the grouping of phage genes into those involved in the assembly of the individual parts of the phage and demonstrated that phage assembly involves several distinct pathways that could be separated.

These assembly pathways have been further dissected by their reconstruction in vitro. When extracts of cells infected with two different assembly mutants are mixed, the complete assembly of mature, infectious virus can proceed. This *in vitro complementation* approach has allowed the purification of many important assembly proteins. Imagine that a mix of a gene A^- mutant extract and a gene B^- extract allows assembly of infectious phage in vitro. The product of the wild-type *A* gene can now be purified without any further information about its precise function. The gene B^- extract is fractionated by biochemical techniques (e.g., one or another type of column chromatography), and every fraction is assayed for the ability to complement the gene A^- extract in the production of infectious phage. The only component missing from that extract is the gene *A* protein itself; thus the assay is completely specific for that protein. By repeating this procedure with many different mutants of a variety of phage, the products of many genes involved in phage particle morphogenesis have been purified and characterized.

The in vitro reconstitution of assembly also has provided a very detailed picture of the precise sequence of events in each of the assembly pathways. A somewhat simplified scheme for the assembly of phage T4 is shown in Figure 60–13. As is obvious from inspection of that figure, heads, tails, and tail fibers are assembled independently of each other and then combine to form complete phage particles. Heads begin as complex core-containing immature proheads that are assembled on the cytoplasmic membrane of the bacterial cell. They are then processed to mature proheads, which are released from the membrane and filled with DNA. The packaging of DNA into the minuscule volume of a phage head is a remarkable process that can proceed at rates well in excess of 100,000 base pairs per minute. Independent pathways result in the synthesis of the tail structure and the tail fibers, so that three distinct pathways contribute to the final assembly of a T4 phage particle. On the basis of examples provided by phage systems, complex biologic structures generally may be constructed by the independent assembly of several component parts.

The stepwise assembly of proteins in phage morphogenesis reveals another general principle of biologic structure assembly—namely, that the addition of one protein species to a growing structure can facilitate the subsequent addition of another protein. Apparently, the conformational changes induced in a protein by assembly onto a growing structure can generate the reactive site(s) necessary for addition of the subsequent protein, and these reactive sites are not present in the free (unassembled) proteins. This orderly assembly of proteins has at least two important benefits. First, the assembly process can be readily controlled at any one single point, and second, a huge variety of useless subassemblies and dead-end structures are avoided.

Several other principles can be gleaned from the results of phage morphogenesis experiments. First, phage morphogenesis often involves the processing of capsid proteins by means of proteolytic cleavage, for example, in the assembly of T4 heads and λ tails. In the case of T4 head assembly, the major protease apparently is assembled as an inactive zymogen. Upon correct assembly, the zymogen is itself activated by proteolytic cleavage and is then competent to cleave about 10 different head proteins. Specific proteolysis reactions may serve to make the overall assembly pathway irreversible. Proteolysis within the growing phage particle also may generate reactive sites for binding of the next protein species, thereby assisting the stepwise assembly of proteins discussed above.

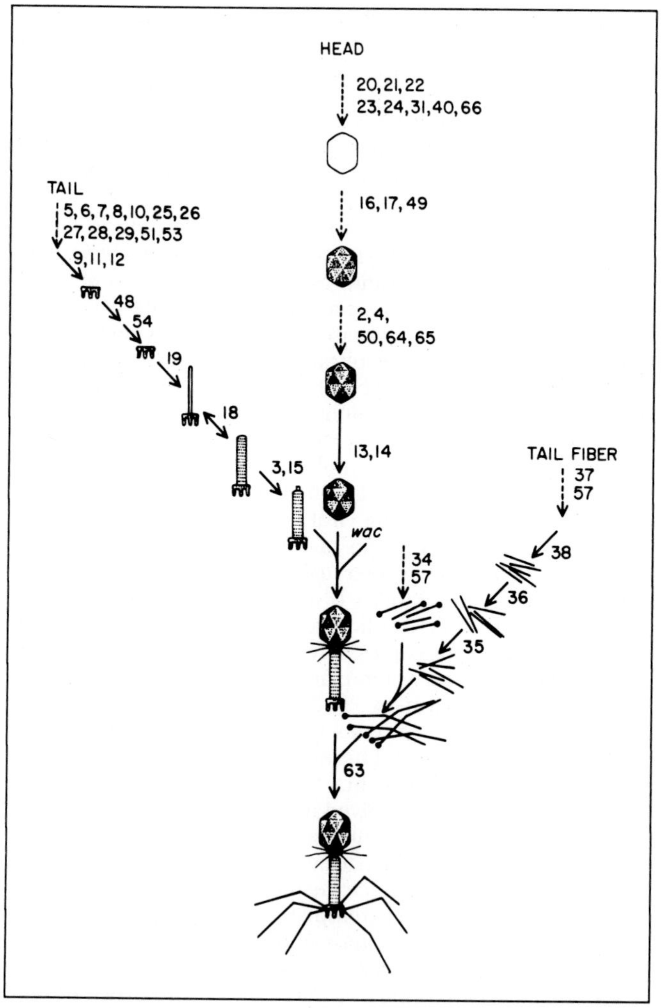

Fig. 60–13. The morphogenetic pathway of phage T4. There are three principal branches leading independently to the formation of heads, tails, and tail fibers. The numbers refer to the gene products involved in each step. Also see Figure 60–11. *(From Wood and Crowther: In Mathews et al (eds): Bacteriophage T4. American Society for Microbiology, 1983.).*

A second principle from phage morphogenesis is the use of a *scaffolding* protein that is central for assembly but completely eliminated from the mature phage particle. Phage P22 assembles a prohead structure with several hundred molecules of such a scaffolding protein. The protein components of the mature head are assembled around this scaffolding protein, which subsequently exits the prohead as phage DNA is inserted. The scaffolding protein plays a role in the determination of the shape of the head. In addition, the exit of the scaffolding protein may expose charged sites in the interior of the head, allowing DNA to collapse into the requisite compact structure.

The mechanisms used to precisely determine biologic forms also have been illuminated by viral assembly reactions. The assembly of proteins into icosahedral shells has already been discussed extensively in the context of animal viruses (Chap. 53). In the simplest case, capsid assembly occurs by self-association of many copies of a major capsid protein. A related issue deals with the mechanism of length determination. How can a particular biologic structure, such as a bacteriophage tail, always assume exactly the same length? In the case of phage λ and probably others, a protein ruler is used to gauge the correct length. A central component of the λ tail is the product of gene *H*, present in six copies per tail. Tails formed in the absence of this protein are called *polytubes* and are indefinitely long. More important, deletion of a number of amino acids from the gene *H* protein results in a proportional shortening in the length of the tail. Therefore, this protein, presumably extending the full length of the tail, acts as a ruler to measure out the correct length during tail assembly.

Lysis and Release of Progeny Phage. Most bacteriophage are liberated from their hosts after lytic growth by a mechanism that differs fundamentally from any employed by animal viruses (Chap. 55); the bacterial cell suddenly lyses, thereby liberating the entire progeny. In the case of phage T4, cell lysis is the result of the function of at least two late phage-encoded enzymes. One is a well-characterized lysozyme that hydrolyzes the cell wall, and the other is reported to be a lipase that attacks the cell membrane.

Life Cycle of Single-stranded DNA Phage

Two large groups of bacteriophage contain a circular single-stranded DNA genome. As their names imply, the icosahedral group package the genome in a simple icosahedral shell, whereas the filamentous phage utilize a long protein tube that contains the genome in an extended configuration. Both groups have a small genome consisting of only about 6000 nucleotide residues. This small size severely limits the range of proteins that can be encoded, forcing extensive use of host proteins in all phases of the life cycle. In addition, the regulatory capabilities of the phage are limited. None of the single-stranded DNA phage appear to regulate transcription in a temporal fashion, and the infective cycle therefore is considerably simpler than that of the duplex DNA phage discussed above. Nonetheless, many features of the infective cycle are similar in broad outline to those of the duplex DNA phage life cycle and therefore will not be belabored here.

The best studied member of the icosahedral group is φX174, whose genome is a plus-stranded circle of 5386 nucleotides. The φX174 genome contains 11 genes, 9 of which are essential for phage growth. The φX174 genome was the first shown to contain overlapping genes, both in the same and different reading frames (Fig. 60–14). The various roles of the 11 gene products encoded by the phage are listed in Table 60–2 and include six involved in morphogenesis.

A major problem posed by the discovery of this class of bacteriophage relates to the nature of their genome. How does a single-stranded genome allow replication and transcription while still obeying the rules of base pairing? This question was answered when it was found that upon entering the host cell, the single-stranded DNA is rapidly converted into a duplex replicative form.

The single-stranded DNA bacteriophage have provided ideal model systems for studying DNA synthesis, and their mechanisms of replication are known in intimate detail. Each of the phage depends on particular combinations of host proteins for its replication, and so these viruses also have

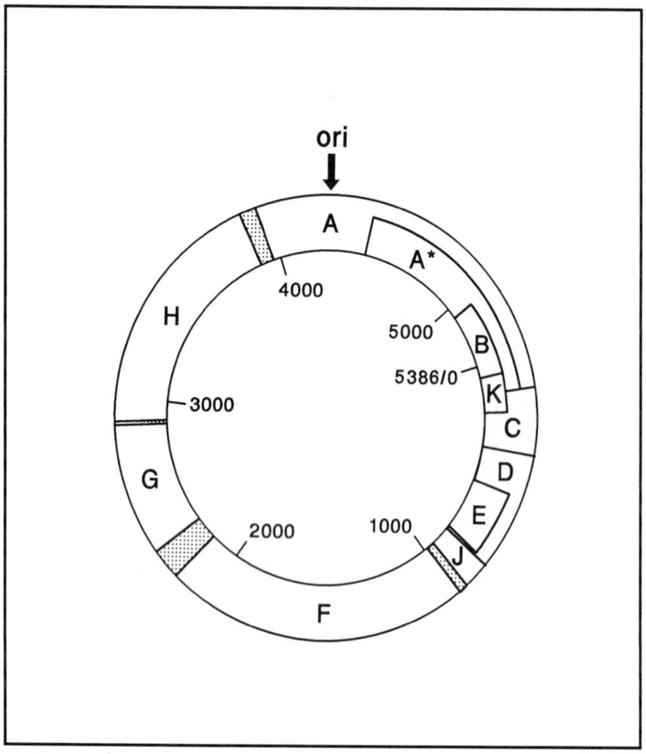

Fig. 60–14. Genomic map of phage φX174. The locations of φX174 genes, intergenic regions (stippled), and origin of viral strand replication (ori) are shown. *(Adapted from Kornberg: Supplement to DNA Replication. W. H. Freeman, 1982.)*

TABLE 60–2. GENES AND GENE FUNCTIONS OF THE SINGLE-STRANDED DNA-CONTAINING BACTERIOPHAGE φX174

Gene Designation	Mol Wt of Protein Product	Function
A	56,000	DNA synthesis
*A**	37,000	Shut off host DNA synthesis?
B	13,800	Morphogenesis
K	6,400	Unknown
C	7,000	DNA maturation
D	16,800	Morphogenesis
E	9,900	Host cell lysis
J	4,000	Morphogenesis
F	48,400	Major capsid protein
G	19,000	Spike (vertex) protein
H	35,800	Spike (vertex) protein

Adapted from Kornberg: Supplement to DNA Replication. W. H. Freeman, 1982.

The coding regions for the *A** and *A* proteins overlap in the same reading frame, with the coding region of *A** being the rightward (C-terminal) three fifths of that of *A*. The coding region for the *B* protein is entirely within that of the *A/A** proteins but in a different reading frame. The coding region for the *K* protein overlaps the adjacent *A/A** and *C* coding regions. The coding region for the *E* protein overlaps that of the *D* protein in a different reading frame. With the overlaps noted above, the gene order is as listed in the table from top to bottom, corresponding to the clockwise direction around the genetic map.

provided an important window through which cellular DNA replication can be viewed. In fact, many host replication proteins were first identified and purified by use of these bacteriophage replication reactions. The φX174 genome encodes only one protein that is directly involved in replication, the product of the *A* gene. Several other phage-encoded proteins are required to couple the processes of DNA replication and DNA packaging (see below).

The overall scheme of φX174 DNA replication is shown schematically in Figure 60–15. The first stage is conversion of the infecting single strand (SS) into a duplex replicative form (RF). This involves a specific RNA priming event that is catalyzed by the host primase in concert with seven other host proteins, followed by replication by the host DNA polymerase III holoenzyme (Chap. 7). The RF product from the first stage is competent as a substrate for the second stage of DNA replication. This stage occurs by the rolling-circle mechanism, with a single template molecule producing many copies of product successively (Fig. 60–15). The second stage is initiated by the action of the viral *A* protein, which recognizes and cleaves the φX174 origin of replication. The site-specific cleavage provides the primer used in stage two replication, and the gene *A* protein also is involved in terminating each cycle of rolling-circle replication. Second-stage replication results in roughly 60 copies of duplex product per infected cell, and these then act as templates for extensive transcription and subsequent replication. The third stage of replication is similar to the second but does not include any minus strand synthesis (Fig. 60–15). Therefore the product is single-stranded progeny DNA rather than duplex replicative form. Several phage proteins involved in particle morphogenesis are required for stage-three synthesis, indicating that replication is tightly coupled to DNA packaging. Third-stage replication also occurs by the rolling-circle mechanism initiated by the viral *A* protein, and each template molecule therefore produces many viral single strands in a continuous reaction.

The multiplication cycles of the filamentous phage (e.g., f1, fd, and M13) are similar to that of φX174 in broad outline but differ in several important details. First, the filamentous phage utilize the conjugative pili (e.g., F pili) for attachment to their hosts. The phage apparently bind to the tips of the pili and subsequently are brought to the cell surface by means of pilus retraction (Chap. 8). Second, as mentioned above, a somewhat different repertoire of host replication proteins are involved in the first stage of replication; notably, phage M13 uses host RNA polymerase rather than primase to provide the RNA primer for conversion of SS to RF. Third, the filamentous phage produce single-stranded progeny DNA in a reaction that is not directly coupled to DNA packaging. The SS progeny DNA is first found complexed with a phage-encoded single-strand binding protein and subsequently is encapsidated at the cell membrane. Fourth, unlike virtually every other bacteriophage, the filamentous phage do not lyse their host cells. Instead, intact progeny virus are continually extruded through the cell membrane in a process that is somewhat analogous to that by which the enveloped animal viruses are released from their hosts. Phage extrusion apparently occurs at the adhesion zones where inner and outer bacterial membranes are fused. As in the case of the duplex DNA phage injection discussed above, the adhesion zones probably are used for filamentous phage extrusion to avoid the periplasmic space. Remarkably, bacterial cells infected with filamentous phage are not killed. Cell viability is maintained through unlimited cell generations, and large numbers

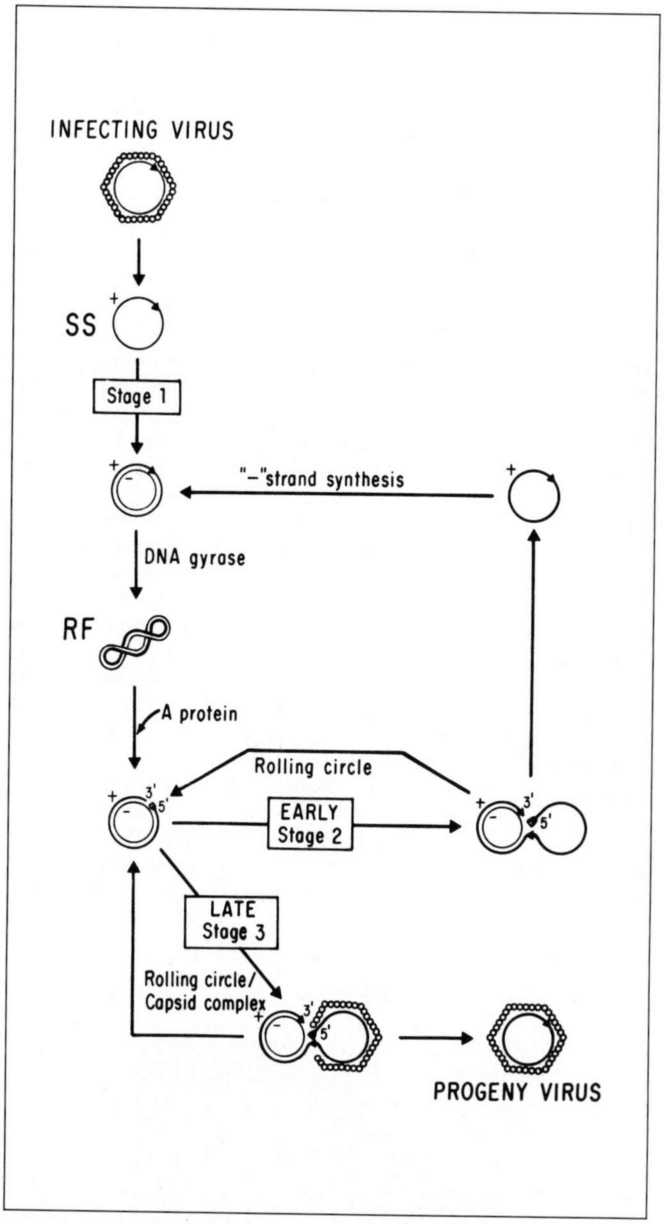

Fig. 60–15. The mechanism of replication of phage ϕX174 DNA. In stage 1, the infecting single strand (SS, + polarity) is converted into a duplex replicative form (RF) by complementary strand (– polarity) synthesis followed by DNA gyrase action. Both stages 2 and 3 depend on the viral gene *A* protein, which cleaves RF DNA at a specific internucleotide linkage on the plus strand (see text). This cleavage provides a primer for rolling-circle replication, in which many copies of the plus strand are synthesized sequentially by the same replication complex. The gene *A* protein also is required to linearize and then circularize the plus strand products, thereby freeing them from the replication complex. During stage 2, the resultant circular plus strands are converted into duplex RF by complementary strand synthesis, increasing the number of RF molecules. Stage 3 is coupled to DNA packaging, and therefore, the plus strand products are not converted to duplex form but instead are packaged in the single-stranded form. *(Adapted from Dressler et al: In Denhardt et al (eds): The Single-Stranded DNA Phages. Cold Spring Harbor Laboratory, 1978.)*

of progeny phage are continually produced and extruded into the medium during this time.

Life Cycle of Single-stranded RNA Phage

Single-stranded RNA phage are small icosahedral viruses that resemble the picornaviruses. The capsids of the RNA phage are quite simple, consisting mainly of 180 identical coat protein molecules. In addition, each capsid contains one molecule of the maturation protein, which is required both for proper assembly and for ability to adsorb to the host. The linear genomes of RNA phage are very small; for example, the MS2 genome consists of 3569 bases that encode only four proteins (Fig. 60–16, map of MS2 genome).

Most of the well-studied RNA phage are coliphage. MS2, f2, R17, and others form one closely related serologic group, whereas Qβ belongs to another. In spite of the fact that Qβ is serologically distinct from the others and has a genome some 15% larger, its genome organization and protein products are quite similar to the MS2 group, implying a common evolutionary origin. Like the filamentous phage discussed above, the RNA phage depend on conjugative pili for attachment to their host cell. Unlike the filamentous phage, however, the RNA phage bind to the sides of the pilus in a reaction that requires the single molecule of maturation protein.

The relative simplicity of a small RNA genome has made the RNA phage fascinating objects for the elucidation of fundamental biologic processes. In spite of this simplicity, the RNA phage are among the most prolific viruses known: a single MS2-infected *E. coli* cell can produce on the order of 20,000 progeny phage. In addition, studies of the multiplication cycle of RNA phage continue to provide important clues for investigations of animal viruses that contain RNA.

Beginning at the 5′ terminus, the four genes of the MS2 genome encode the maturation protein, the coat protein, the lysis protein, and the RNA replicase (Fig. 60–16). The latter protein actually is only one of four subunits that together constitute the functional replicase, the others being three bacterial proteins involved in protein synthesis (elongation factors Tu and Ts and ribosomal protein S1).

Replication of RNA Genome. The replication of the RNA phage genome is certain to be interesting for several reasons. Bacterial cells do not generally replicate RNA, and the single infecting RNA phage genome must be recognized for duplication among a vast excess of assorted cellular RNAs. In addition, bacterial cells such as *E. coli* contain an enzyme, ribonuclease III, that destroys duplex RNA, which would be expected as an intermediate in replication of the RNA genome.

The involvement of both phage- and host-encoded proteins in formation of the RNA replicase probably relates to the first two points raised above. There is no evidence for a host RNA replicase; thus the phage presumably would need to encode the catalytic subunit of the enzyme. The three bacterial proteins appear to play an important role in the initiation of replication, probably in the recognition of the RNA template. In the uninfected cell, these three proteins are involved in translation. Perhaps recognition of the RNA phage genome by one or more of these proteins somehow mimics the recognition of a cellular RNA during translation.

The RNA replicase must use the rules of base pairing to correctly duplicate the genome, implying that duplex RNA must exist at least transiently at the site of replication. The

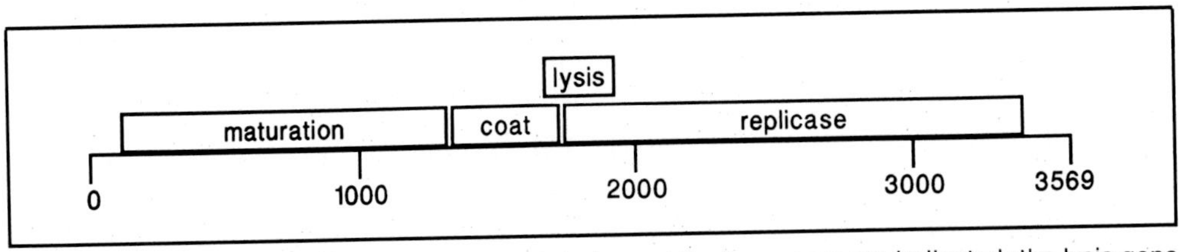

Fig. 60–16. Genomic map of phage MS2. The locations of the four genes are indicated; the lysis gene overlaps both the coat and replicase genes. *(Adapted from van Duin: In Calendar (ed): The Bacteriophages, vol 1. Plenum Press, 1988.)*

replicase, however, denatures the template and nascent progeny strands as it synthesizes, preventing formation of extensive regions of template-progeny duplex. This active denaturation presumably prevents attack by the host ribonuclease III.

Another interesting feature of RNA replication relates to the fidelity of synthesis. Replicative DNA polymerases generally contain a proofreading capability that excises incorrectly incorporated bases, thereby reducing the mutation rate during replication by several orders of magnitude (Chap. 8). The RNA replicase, however, has no proofreading ability and therefore produces mutations during replication at frequencies between 10^{-3} and 10^{-4} per base replicated. This is thought to limit the genome to its very small size; if an RNA phage had a genome of 10,000 bases, most progeny molecules would acquire one or more new mutations in every round of replication. Even with the small genome size of the well-studied RNA phage, every stock contains numerous mutants.

Regulation of RNA Phage Gene Expression. The genomes of the RNA phage possess plus polarity and start functioning as mRNA very soon after they enter cells. After effecting the translation of the RNA replicase, the infecting strand then serves as a template for the synthesis of complementary minus strands, which in turn are used in the synthesis of progeny plus strands. The two proteins necessary for capsid formation (coat and maturation proteins) are then produced. As soon as their concentrations are sufficiently high, encapsidation of RNA commences and mature progeny phage accumulate (Fig. 60–17).

The infective cycle of RNA phage, like that of many other viruses, is carefully programmed to produce optimal levels of each protein in an appropriate temporal sequence. Yet the genome of an RNA phage is too small to encode proteins with a purely regulatory function. How then does it happen that coat protein, which is present in virus particles in 180-fold excess over maturation protein, is in fact synthesized in vastly greater amounts than is maturation protein? What mechanism causes the RNA replicase to be synthesized early in the infective cycle, when it is needed, and not at late times in the cycle? Further, because parental RNA genomes must be both translated and replicated, what mechanism prevents collisions between ribosomes, which traverse mRNA in the 5′ to 3′ direction, and replicase, which traverses its template in the opposite direction?

The answers to these questions reveal a most elegant program for controlled gene expression, involving both multifunctional proteins and the secondary structure of the RNA genome. As the genome is itself the mRNA, all control mechanisms must operate at the translational level. The infecting plus strand is a polycistronic message with three distinct ribosome binding sites, each possessing unique properties. Like other RNAs, the genomes of RNA phage possess extensive secondary structure that is specified by base pairing between complementary stretches of nucleotide sequence. These regions of duplex RNA are presumably too short to be recognized by ribonuclease III. Because of the secondary structure, however, there is a marked difference in the accessibility of the ribosome binding sites at the 5′ termini of the various genes. In normal phage RNA, the only accessible site for initiation of translation is at the beginning of the coat gene. Therefore a small amount of coat protein is produced early in infection, even though the protein itself is not needed at that time. Translation of the coat gene at early times is important, however, because it triggers translation of the replicase gene. The ribosome binding site for the replicase gene normally is embedded in secondary structure, but the translation of the coat gene destroys the base pairing required for that secondary structure. Therefore translation of the coat gene activates translation of the replicase gene. Once replicase protein increases to a sufficient concentration, the replicase acts as a translational repressor of coat protein synthesis by binding to the translational initiation site of the coat protein

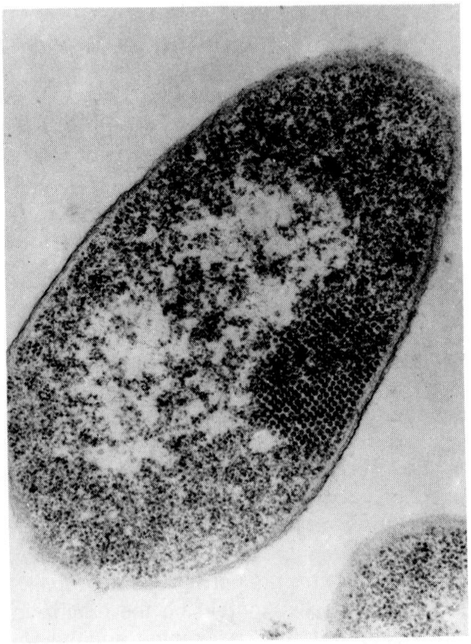

Fig. 60–17. An *E. coli* cell 50 minutes after infection with MS2. Note the paracrystalline virus particle array. The virus is slightly larger than the ribosomes that are present throughout the cell. This cell is about to lyse. × 37,500. *(Courtesy of Dr. M. Van Montagu.)*

gene. Because translation of the coat protein gene is required for translation of the replicase gene (see above), the critical concentration of replicase protein blocks all translation of the infecting genome. The translational repression by replicase thereby solves the potential problem of the replicase colliding with an opposing ribosome: by the time RNA replication commences, all translation has been shut off by the repressor action of replicase.

Once this initial burst of protein synthesis is complete, the RNA replicase proceeds to synthesize minus, and then plus, progeny strands. As a result of this replication, the concentration of replicase complex per plus strand decreases dramatically, and therefore, translational repression of the coat protein is ineffective. As there are now many copies of the coat protein mRNA (i.e., plus strand progeny), extensive synthesis of coat protein ensues. When coat protein increases to a sufficiently high concentration, it now acts as a translational repressor of replicase synthesis by binding to the replicase gene translational initiation region. The concentration of coat protein necessary for repression is achieved only at late times of the infective cycle, when many copies of plus strand are actively synthesizing coat protein. Therefore, at late times, a large concentration of coat protein but very little replicase is synthesized. To summarize the interactions between coat protein and replicase: (1) translation of the coat protein gene activates replicase synthesis, but coat protein itself later represses translation of replicase; (2) replicase protein acts as a translational repressor of the coat protein gene and yet induces the synthesis of large amounts of coat protein by increasing the copy number of the genome as the infection progresses. It is quite remarkable that these two proteins engage in such sophisticated control, particularly as the primary functions of the coat and replicase proteins have nothing to do with translational regulation.

The maturation protein is the minor capsid protein required for assembly and adsorption, and its translation also is carefully programmed. The ribosome binding site of the maturation protein gene, like that of the replicase gene, is embedded in secondary structure. Ribosomes apparently bind to the beginning of this gene only during the period during which the plus strand RNA is in the process of being synthesized, limiting synthesis of maturation protein to very small amounts. The fourth RNA phage-encoded protein, the lysis protein, is required in small amounts and must be produced only late in infection. Translation of the lysis protein also appears to be regulated by a mechanism involving genome secondary structure, but the molecular details currently are unknown.

It is clear therefore that the RNA phage genome regulates a very sophisticated replication and translation program. The salient features of this regulation are the use of multifunctional proteins and genome secondary structure. Both of these features presumably are caused by the constraints inherent in a very small genome size. The economy in genome size also is evidenced in the use of overlapping genes (Fig. 60–16) and the utilization of host proteins Tu, Ts, and S1 as subunits of the functional replicase complex.

The Lysogenic Bacteriophage

Not all phage infections result in immediate progeny production and lysis of the host cell. There are many phage that, upon entering a sensitive cell, either undergo a lytic cycle such as those described above or, alternatively, enter into a benign relationship with their hosts. While in this benign state, only one or a few viral genes are expressed, and the viral genome exists either inserted into the host chromosome or as a free plasmid form in the bacterial cell. The phage genome in this state, called the *prophage*, replicates along with the bacterial chromosome whether the viral DNA is integrated or in plasmid form. It is important to realize that this is a legitimate means of reproduction for a bacteriophage; the prophage is multiplying just as rapidly as the cell in which it resides. The bacterial cell with a resident prophage appears perfectly normal, with only one or a very few altered properties (see below). Occasionally, however, the integrated prophage is excised from bacterial DNA, and phage multiplication and subsequent cell lysis ensue. This phenomenon therefore was named *lysogeny*; bacteria that harbor prophage are called *lysogens*, and phage capable of eliciting this response are called *lysogenic*, or *temperate*, bacteriophage.

When it was discovered that certain animal viruses could enter into similar relationships with their hosts (Chap. 59), the analogy between them and lysogenic phage was quickly recognized. Although there are, of course, differences in the manner in which tumor viruses and lysogenic phage interact with their respective hosts, the concepts that evolved from studies of the lysogenic phage have profoundly influenced our approaches to tumor viruses.

Nature of Prophage

As mentioned above, various lysogenic bacteriophage either integrate into the host genome or exist as free plasmids in the bacterial cell. Of the first class, most phage integrate into unique sites of the chromosome, called *attachment sites*. The attachment site for coliphage λ is between the *gal* and *bio* operons of the *E. coli* genome, but other phage use sites elsewhere in the genome. In addition to these phage that integrate into unique sites on the chromosome, phage Mu has no specific integration site. During lysogenization, Mu integrates in an essentially random fashion anywhere in the bacterial genome. As discussed above, phage Mu is a large transposable element that also uses transposition as its replicative mechanism during lytic growth. Some lysogenic bacteriophage, such as P1, lysogenize by forming a stable plasmid that replicates autonomously. Like many other plasmids (Chap. 8), the P1 prophage plasmid employs special mechanisms to ensure efficient segregation—the plasmid is lost only about once in every 10^6 cell divisions.

Regardless of the location of the prophage DNA, all lysogenic phage maintain most of their genes in a repressed state during lysogeny. All the promoters for genes involved in the lytic growth cycle are stringently controlled so as not to have any detrimental effect on the host cell. The repressor responsible for this control is encoded by the prophage genome and is one of the very few proteins synthesized from the phage genome during lysogeny. The existence of repressor in the lysogen has a very important consequence: the cell becomes immune to superinfection by another member of the same phage family. The repressor produced from the endogenous prophage genome is just as active on the superinfecting phage DNA as on its own and blocks the transcription necessary for lytic growth. The stability of the prophage state discussed above is not absolute. A resident prophage can

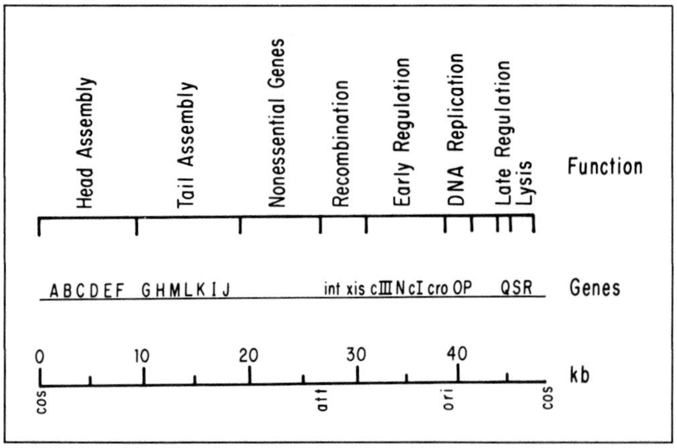

Fig. 60–18. A simplified genetic map of bacteriophage λ. The scale at the bottom is in kilobase pairs of DNA and shows the location of the two cohesive ends (cos), the attachment side (att) used for integration into the host chromosome, and the origin of replication (ori). A number of important genes are shown in the middle, and the function of the corresponding gene products are shown at the top. *(Adapted from Daniels et al: In Hendrix et al (eds): Lambda II. Cold Spring Harbor Laboratory, 1983.)*

suddenly terminate the lysogenic relationship and undergo a normal lytic cycle, producing many progeny viruses and lysing the host cell. Normally, this prophage *induction* occurs with a very low frequency, on the order of 10^{-5} per cell generation. Various noxious physiologic conditions, however, can result in quantitative prophage induction (see below). This response can be viewed as an attempt by the prophage to escape from a cell that has been seriously, or perhaps terminally, damaged.

Bacteriophage λ

The best known of the many lysogenic bacteriophage is the coliphage λ, probably the most intensively studied of all viruses. The exquisite and intricate mechanisms that control its interactions with the host and its multiplication represent the paramount system with which to study biologic control. Therefore this discussion focuses on the mechanisms that operate in lysogeny in terms of the λ system. A simplified genetic map of the λ genome is shown in Figure 60–18; the genome has been sequenced in its entirety and is composed of 48,502 base pairs.

When λ DNA enters a cell, it is converted into covalently closed circles by the host enzyme DNA ligase acting at the complementary cohesive ends described earlier in this chapter. The circular intermediate is then rapidly converted into a superhelical form by the host enzyme DNA gyrase (Chap. 7). Within a brief critical time, the decision is made as to whether a lytic multiplication cycle is to be initiated or whether the phage genome is to be repressed to form a lysogen. As described below, the decision is a logical one based on important parameters, namely the physiology of the host cell and the multiplicity of infection.

Genetic Identification of Regulatory Components. The elucidation of the regulatory mechanisms that guide the lysis-lysogeny decision depended critically on exhaustive genetic analyses of the phage. Essentially all the important genes and DNA sites involved in the λ life cycle have been defined by finding mutants in which the gene or site is inactive. The genes essential for λ lytic growth were identified by isolation of conditional lethal mutants. These essential genes were named with capital letters according to map order, *A* through *R* from left to right on the map (Fig. 60–18).

Most of the genes whose products are involved in the lysis-lysogeny decision are not essential for lytic growth and therefore were not identified by means of conditional lethal mutants. Instead, these genes were identified by finding mutations that affect the lysis-lysogeny decision, for example, those that abolish the lysogenic response. The simplest method to find such mutants involves the plaque morphology of phage λ. Wild-type phage form turbid plaques as a result of the growth of lysogenic cells within the plaque itself. Recall that lysogens are immune to superinfection, and therefore a lysogenic bacterial cell can survive and propagate within the plaque. Mutants of λ that cannot lysogenize are readily identified as those with *c*lear plaques, and these define three genes, *c*I, *c*II and *c*III. Mutations in another important regulatory gene (*cro*, signifying *c*ontrol of *r*epressor and *o*ther genes) result in a strong bias in favor of lysogeny during the lysis-lysogeny decision. Finally, mutants that fail to *int*egrate the viral DNA defined the *int* gene, and mutants that fail to *ex*c*is*e prophage DNA upon induction defined the *xis* gene. The regulatory sites in the λ genome, many of which were identified by genetic analysis, also have been given sensible names. The critical promoters are called p_L (*l*eftward *p*romoter), p_R (*r*ightward *p*romoter), p_{RE} (*p*romoter for *r*epressor *e*stablishment), p_{RM} (*p*romoter for *r*epressor *m*aintenance), and p_I (*p*romoter for *i*nt gene). Likewise, the two most important operator regions, in which the regulatory proteins modulate transcription, are called o_L and o_R (*l*eftward and *r*ightward *o*perator, respectively).

Competition Between *cro* and *c*I Proteins. The crucial regulatory genes and control regions in λ DNA are illustrated in Figure 60–19, which presents an enlargement of one portion of the λ genetic map. The critical regulatory region to focus on contains two oppositely oriented promoters, p_R and p_{RM}. Transcription from these promoters is modulated by the binding of the *c*I and *cro* proteins to the overlapping operator o_R, which actually consists of three tandem sites. The binding of *c*I and *cro* proteins to this operator are the most intensively studied and best understood interactions between protein and DNA. Recent advances, including x-ray crystallographic analyses, have provided a detailed three-dimensional picture of these binding events.

We will now trace the molecular events that occur during the lysis-lysogeny decision, focusing first on the events at the critical regulatory region mentioned above. Ultimately, the lysis-lysogeny decision rests on whether the activity of the *c*I protein or the *cro* protein dominates at this region. Domination by *c*I protein leads to the lysogenic response, whereas domination by *cro* protein results in a lytic infection. It is important to realize that the two divergent promoters, p_R and p_{RM}, direct transcription of the *cro* and *c*I genes, respectively (Fig. 60–19). As is discussed in detail below, this fact results in an amplification of the difference between *c*I and *cro* protein concentrations and also allows autoregulation by both proteins.

The two possible outcomes of the lysis-lysogeny decision cannot be understood without appreciating the alternative physiologic states of the critical regulatory region (Fig. 60–20).

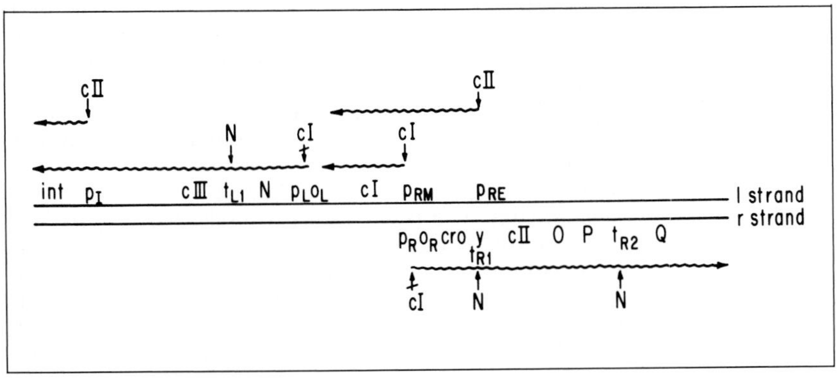

Fig. 60–19. A map of the regulatory elements of phage λ. Wavy lines indicate the location of various transcripts, with arrowheads showing the direction of transcription. Vertical arrows without slashes at the start of a transcript indicate that the gene product activates transcription at that particular promoter; vertical arrows with slashes denote repression of that promoter. Vertical arrows in the middle of transcripts show the sites where the *N* gene product prevents transcription termination from occurring. *(From Wulff and Rosenberg: In Hendrix et al (eds): Lambda II. Cold Spring Harbor Laboratory, 1983.)*

In the absence of any regulatory proteins, the rightward promoter p_R is active but the leftward p_{RM} is inactive (Fig. 60–20A), resulting in the synthesis of *cro* protein. This would correspond to the state of λ DNA immediately after infection, because no λ regulatory proteins would be present. The modulation of transcription by the regulatory proteins depends on an inverse preference for the three binding sites within o_R. The *c*I protein binds preferentially to o_R1, and repressor bound to o_R1 greatly facilitates binding to o_R2; the o_R3 site is bound weakly, that is, only at high *c*I concentrations. The preferences of *cro* protein are essentially the opposite; that is, o_R3 is bound much more strongly than is o_R1 or o_R2. When modest concentrations of *c*I protein are present, the protein binds cooperatively to o_R1 and o_R2 (Fig. 60–20B). The first important consequence is that transcription from p_R is blocked by repression, preventing synthesis of *cro* protein. Second, transcription from p_{RM} is activated by the presence of *c*I protein at o_R2, resulting in the further synthesis of *c*I protein. Depending on where it binds, the *c*I protein can therefore act as either a transcriptional repressor or a transcriptional activator. When the concentration of *c*I protein increases to a very high level, the protein binds to all three

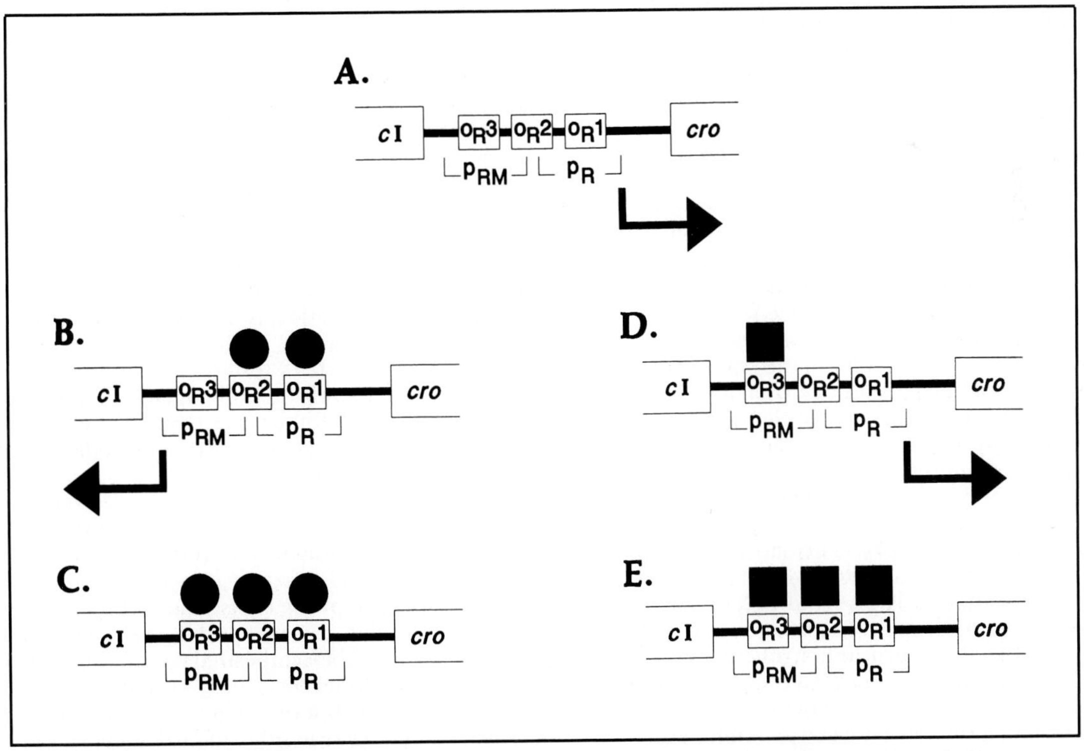

Fig. 60–20. Transcription control by λ *cI* and *cro* proteins. The central regulatory region of phage λ consists of two divergent promoters, p_{RM} and p_R. **A.** The activity of p_R but not p_{RM} in the absence of regulatory proteins. The effect of *cI* protein (spheres) binding to the operator sites is indicated in **B** and **C**, whereas the effect of *cro* protein (squares) binding is shown in **D** and **E**. See text for detailed descriptions. *(Adapted from Herskowitz and Hagen: Annu Rev Genet 14:399, 1980.)*

sites and thereby represses transcription from both p_R and p_{RM} (Fig. 60–20C). The binding of *cro* protein to o_R can have two important effects. When *cro* protein is present in modest amounts, it preferentially binds to o_R3 and blocks any possible transcription from p_{RM} (Fig. 60–20D). Finally, when the concentration of *cro* protein is high, all three operator sites are bound and transcription from both promoters is blocked (Fig. 60–20E).

As indicated above, when the activity of the *c*I protein exceeds that of *cro* protein, the infecting phage is destined to take the lysogenic pathway. The binding of *c*I protein to o_R blocks further transcription from p_R, preventing synthesis of *cro* and other proteins involved in the lytic infective cycle. Furthermore, the binding of *c*I activates transcription of additional *c*I protein from p_{RM}. These two effects combine to amplify the dominance of *c*I over *cro* protein and to establish the lysogenic state. The *c*I protein then serves as the repressor that maintains λ in the lysogenic state, preventing expression of lytic genes from the prophage. In this state the *c*I protein autoregulates its own synthesis by stimulating transcription from p_{RM} when the protein concentration falls (Fig. 60–20B) and by inhibiting its own synthesis when the concentration rises (Fig. 60–20C). In the lysogenic state, transcription from a second lytic promoter, p_L, also is repressed by means of the *c*I protein binding to the overlapping o_L operator.

On the other hand, when the activity of *cro* protein dominates over that of *c*I protein, the infecting λ is destined to undergo the lytic infective cycle. The binding of *cro* protein to o_R blocks transcription from p_{RM}. Therefore, further synthesis of the key *c*I repressor protein is prevented. The net effect is to maintain the activity of the p_R promoter, thereby allowing a continued increase in the concentration of *cro* protein. Once again, the regulatory switch is amplified, this time in favor of the *cro* protein and the lytic response. As the lytic infection proceeds, *cro* protein has a second role. As the concentration of the protein increases, it eventually reaches a level that is sufficient to completely block transcription from p_R and the other early promoter, p_L. The *cro* protein therefore assists in the switch from early to late gene expression during the lytic cycle.

Importance of *c*II Protein Concentration. If the relative levels of *c*I and *cro* proteins determine the fate of an infecting λ genome, what then modulates the balance of these two proteins? Moving one step backward in the regulatory cascade, we encounter two more phage-encoded proteins, the products of the *c*II and *c*III genes. The concentration of the *c*II protein is the key modulator in the lysis-lysogeny decision. As described above, the *c*I repressor is necessary for the lysogenic pathway, and *c*I repressor can induce its own synthesis from the promoter p_{RM}. In the absence of *c*I protein, however, no transcription is possible from p_{RM}. The only promoter capable of directing transcription of a message for the *c*I repressor in the absence of that protein is p_{RE}, and p_{RE} is active only in the presence of the λ *c*II protein. Therefore, upon λ infection, *c*II protein is required to begin the synthesis of *c*I protein; without *c*II protein, the infecting phage cannot traverse the lysogenic pathway. As described above, once *c*I protein is synthesized, it can amplify its levels by activating p_{RM}.

The concentration of *c*II protein varies widely during infection under different conditions. The *c*II protein is degraded by a specific host protease, but this protease is neutralized by the λ *c*III protein. The degradation of *c*II protein by the host protease explains how an infecting phage genome can sense the physiologic state of the cell, because the host protease is negatively controlled by the catabolite activation system (Chap. 7). The net effect is that starved cells have low levels of protease, and therefore *c*II protein is stable. As described above, this in turn results in production of *c*I protein and thereby favors the lysogenic response. This complex regulatory circuit makes good sense, because a lytic infection would proceed very poorly in starved cells. When the host is not able to support a productive lytic cycle, phage λ prefers to enter into the lysogenic relationship. Conversely, the lytic response is favored in cells growing rapidly in rich medium. Again because of the catabolite activation system, such cells have high levels of the protease, which in turn results in decreased levels of *c*II protein and a consequent preference for the lytic cycle.

The fact that *c*III protein neutralizes the specific host protease also allows λ to sense the relative number of infecting phage genomes. When the multiplicity of infection of a particular cell is high, λ preferentially enters the lysogenic state. This also is a sensible decision, because a high multiplicity of infection implies that available (i.e., uninfected) hosts must be in short supply. The preference for the lysogenic state is a direct consequence of the fact that *c*III protein synthesis is proportional to the number of infecting λ genomes, whereas the level of the host protease is not affected by multiplicity. When many λ genomes infect the same cell, the high level of *c*III protein neutralizes the host protease, resulting in stabilization of *c*II protein and subsequent synthesis of the *c*I repressor.

Regulation by Transcriptional Antitermination. Another early regulatory protein of phage λ is a transcriptional antiterminator, the product of the essential gene *N*. In the absence of *N* protein, the host RNA polymerase terminates λ transcription at a series of specific sequences (terminators; see Chap. 7) and does not produce transcripts for the majority of the λ genome. The *N* protein allows RNA polymerase to ignore these sequences and thereby is required for the synthesis of all subsequent λ proteins (Fig. 60–19). The mechanism of antitermination is exceedingly complex and involves several host proteins and a specific binding site that is distinct from the terminator sequence described above. *N* protein–directed antitermination is important for both the lysogenic and the lytic pathways. Without *N* protein, the *c*II protein cannot be synthesized, resulting in no synthesis of the *c*I repressor and, therefore, no lysogeny. In addition, *N* protein action is required for transcription of genes involved in λ replication and late gene expression, both important events in the λ lytic cycle.

A second case of antitermination plays an important role in the switch from early to late gene expression. Like the *N* protein, the λ *Q* protein is a transcriptional antiterminator. However, *Q* protein acts at completely different sites than does *N* protein, allowing transcriptional read-through into the genes responsible for λ capsid formation. Although the *Q* protein begins to be synthesized soon after *N* protein directs antitermination (Fig. 60–19), *Q* protein is active only after it accumulates to high levels. Thus antitermination by *Q* protein is delayed until later in infection when the capsid proteins are needed.

Integrative Recombination. In cases in which *c*I repressor activity has dominated and the infecting genome chooses the lysogenic pathway, the genome of λ becomes integrated into

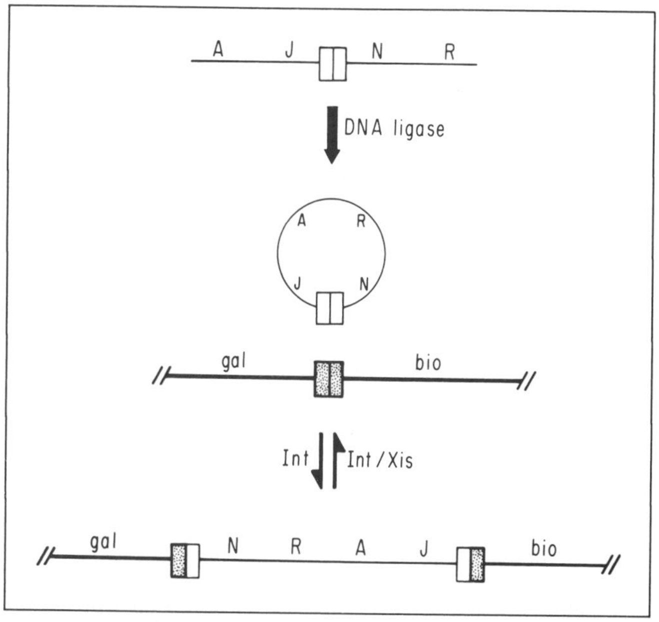

Fig. 60–21. Integration and excision of the lambda genome. The infecting viral DNA is shown at the top, with four representative genes shown for orientation (*A, J, N,* and *R*). DNA ligase action at the two cohesive ends results in a circular genome (first step), and the circular DNA is then converted into a supercoiled form by the action of DNA gyrase (not shown). Site-specific recombination occurs between the attachment site in the phage DNA (indicated by two open boxes) and a related site in the bacterial chromosome (indicated by two filled boxes). Integration requires the phage-encoded *int* protein, whereas excision requires *int* and *xis*; both reactions also require host proteins (see text).

the bacterial chromosome at the specific attachment site mentioned above. This integration reaction is an example of a site-specific recombination reaction (Chap. 8) occurring by the cleavage, exchange, and resealing of phosphodiester bonds (Fig. 60–21). This integrative recombination has been duplicated in vitro and studied in great detail, to the point where the exact nucleotide linkages involved are known. The reaction is catalyzed by the phage *int* protein, with the assistance of several host proteins.

As would be expected, synthesis of *int* protein is coupled to the decision to undergo the lysogenic response. Transcription of the *int* gene is positively activated by the action of *c*II protein at the promoter p_I; *c*II protein is thus a transcriptional activator for both the *c*I and *int* genes.

Induction of Prophage. The termination of the lysogenic state, or induction, requires both release from repression and excision of the phage DNA from the host chromosome. As mentioned above, although induction occurs spontaneously at a low frequency, it occurs in nearly every lysogenic cell when the bacterial SOS pathway becomes activated. A variety of conditions that damage DNA or block host DNA replication activate the protease activity of the host *recA* protein to induce the SOS pathway (Chap. 8). The *recA* protease, in addition to cleaving the host *lexA* repressor, also cleaves the λ *c*I protein, and a lytic cycle ensues. Two of the first proteins synthesized from the λ genome are the products of genes *int* and *xis*. As described above, the *int* protein is required for integrative recombination during the establishment of lysogeny. The combination of *int* and *xis* proteins allows the reverse reaction, excisive recombination (Fig. 60–21). Excision results in the restoration of the free circular form of λ DNA, which then undergoes the events characteristic of a normal lytic infective cycle.

Medical Significance of Lysogeny: Lysogenic Phage Conversion

The lysogenic potential of the temperate bacteriophage has important ramifications. It allows the process of specialized transduction and thereby increases the exchange of genetic information between bacterial cells (Chap. 8). In addition, lysogenic phage can endow bacterial cells with novel properties. This is of widespread importance because every bacterial cell may well possess one or more prophage. In addition to normal lysogenic phage such as λ, there are numerous defective prophage that lack the complete set of information necessary for phage multiplication. Such defective phage can nonetheless confer novel properties to their host cells.

One property conferred by prophage upon bacterial cells is the immunity to superinfecting phage described above. With some lysogenic phage, important properties other than phage immunity also are conferred, and these are referred to as cases of lysogenic phage conversion. Several examples of conversion have great medical importance.

The first involves the phage-mediated conversion of somatic O antigen, an important virulence determinant in *Salmonella* (Chap. 35). This antigen forms part of the lipopolysaccharide structure of the cell wall and is composed of highly esterified lipid (lipid A) linked to a polysaccharide core; side chains consisting of repeating sequences of a variety of sugars are attached to the polysaccharide core (Chap. 6). The antigenic specificity resides in the sugars and can be modified by altering their nature. A wide variety of lysogenic *Salmonella* phage can modify the antigenic properties of the somatic O antigen—for example, by the addition of a D-glucosyl residue. The chemical alterations in *Salmonella* polysaccharides are clearly phage induced inasmuch as phage genes have been shown to encode the appropriate enzymes involved in generating the sugar linkages. These converting functions are not essential for growth of the phage. The alterations in the somatic O antigen, however, do affect adsorption of related phage to the lysogenic cell. The advantage of this type of lysogenic conversion to the phage therefore may involve an augmented immunity to superinfecting phage that are not sensitive to the repressor of the prophage.

Some of the most potent toxins known to medical science are encoded by bacteriophage. Toxigenic strains of the gram-positive *Corynebacterium diphtheriae* carry the corynephage β in the prophage state, and nontoxigenic strains can be made toxigenic by lysogenization with β. In general details, corynephage β is similar to the various coliphage discussed in this chapter. β has an icosahedral head connected to a long, noncontractile tail, as well as a duplex DNA genome of about 35 kilobase pairs. In addition, like phage λ, β integrates into bacterial DNA by site-specific recombination and is inducible by conditions that damage the host DNA. Clearly, the structural gene for diptheria toxin is located within the phage genome, because phage mutants coding for defective toxin have been isolated. It is not clear, however, what advantage the phage gains by coding for a protein with the remarkable biologic and enzymatic properties of the toxin (Chap. 30).

Several other important toxins also are induced by bacteriophage. For example, the pyrogenic exotoxins produced by *Streptococcus pyogenes*, which cause scarlet fever, are encoded by a family of lysogenic bacteriophage. Likewise, the most common enterotoxin involved in *Staphylococcus aureus* food poisoning is encoded within the genome of a lysogenic phage. Of interest is that the structural genes that encode all three of the above-mentioned toxins are located directly adjacent to the attachment sites within the phage genomes, where recombination with the host chromosomes occur. These and other findings argue that the toxin genes were perhaps gained from some bacterial host in the evolution of the toxin-producing bacteriophage.

A final example involves *Clostridium botulinum* types C and D, which produce toxin only when demonstrably infected with certain bacteriophage. The relationship between host cell and phage, however, may be more similar to an ongoing lytic infection than to true lysogeny, because infected *C. botulinum* becomes nontoxigenic when treated with antiserum to phage.

These simple cases of potent phage-encoded toxins represent some of the best-studied determinants of bacterial virulence. As additional virulence determinants are studied in molecular detail, it would not be surprising to find many others that are encoded by bacteriophage. Indeed, even phage λ, the prototype for lysogenic phage, has recently been shown to encode two proteins that are apparently involved in bacterial virulence.

FURTHER READING

Books and Review

DOUBLE-STRANDED DNA PHAGE

Anderson TF: Reflections on phage genetics. Annu Rev Genet 15:405, 1981

Cairns J, Stent GS, Watson JD: Phage and the Origins of Molecular Biology. Cold Spring Harbor, NY, Cold Spring Harbor Laboratory, 1966

Calendar R: The Bacteriophages, vols 1 and 2. New York, Plenum, 1988

Casjens S, King J: Virus assembly. Annu Rev Biochem 44:555, 1975

Chamberlin M, Ryan T: Bacteriophage DNA-dependent RNA polymerases. In Boyer PD (ed): The Enzymes, vol 15. New York, Academic Press, 1982, p 87

Earnshaw WC, Casjens SR: DNA packaging by the double-stranded DNA bacteriophages. Cell 21:319, 1980

Koerner JF, Snustad DP: Shutoff of host macromolecular synthesis after T-even bacteriophage infection. Microbiol Rev 43:199, 1979

Kruger DH, Schroeder C: Bacteriophage T3 and bacteriophage T7 virus-host cell interactions. Microbiol Rev 45:9, 1981

Mathews CK: Bacteriophage Biochemistry. New York, Van Nostrand Reinhold, 1971

Mathews CK, Kutter EM, Mosig G, et al (eds): Bacteriophage T4. Washington, DC, American Society for Microbiology, 1983

Murialdo H, Becker A: Head morphogenesis of complex double-stranded deoxyribonucleic acid bacteriophages. Microbiol Rev 42:529, 1978

Schmidt FJ: RNA splicing in prokaryotes: Bacteriophage T4 leads the way. Cell 41:339, 1985

Warren RAJ: Modified bases in bacteriophage DNAs. Annu Rev Microbiol 34:137, 1980

Watson JD: Origin of concatemeric T7 DNA. Nature New Biology 239:197, 1972

PHAGE λ: LYSOGENY

Calendar R, Geisseloder J, Sunshine MG, et al: The P2-P4 transactivation system. In Fraenkel-Conrat H, Wagner RR (eds): Comprehensive Virology, vol 8. New York, Plenum, 1977, p 329

Gottesman S: Lambda site-specific recombination: The *att* site. Cell 25:585, 1981

Greenblatt J: Regulation of transcription termination by the *N* gene protein of bacteriophage lambda. Cell 24:8, 1981

Hendrix RW, Roberts JW, Stahl FW, et al (eds): Lambda II. Cold Spring Harbor, NY, Cold Spring Harbor Laboratory, 1983

Hershey AD (ed): The Bacteriophage Lambda. Cold Spring Harbor, NY, Cold Spring Harbor Laboratory, 1971

Herskowitz I, Hagen D: The lysis-lysogeny decision of lambda: Explicit programming and responsiveness. Annu Rev Genet 14:399, 1980

Nash HA: Integration and excision of bacteriophage lambda: The mechanism of conservative site-specific recombination. Annu Rev Genet 15:143, 1981

Ptashne M: A Genetic Switch. Gene Control and Phage Lambda. Palo Alto, Calif, Blackwell, 1986

Shimatake H, Rosenberg M: Purified lambda regulatory protein *c*II positively activates promoters for lysogenic development. Nature 292:128, 1981

Ward DF, Gottesman ME: Suppression of transcription termination by phage lambda. Science 216:946, 1982

SINGLE-STRANDED NUCLEIC ACID PHAGE

Baas PD: DNA replication of single-stranded *Escherichia coli* DNA phages. Biochim Biophys Acta 825:111, 1985

Blumenthal T, Carmichael GG: RNA replication: Function and structure of Qβ-replicase. Annu Rev Biochem 48:525, 1979

Denhardt DT, Dressler D, Ray DS (eds): The Single-Stranded DNA Phages. Cold Spring Harbor, NY, Cold Spring Harbor Laboratory, 1978

Fiers W: Structure and function of RNA bacteriophages. In Fraenkel-Conrat H, Wagner RR (eds): Comprehensive Virology, vol 13. New York, Plenum, 1979, p 69

Kornberg A, Baker TA: DNA Replication, ed 2. New York, W. H. Freeman & Co, 1992

Ray DS: Replication of filamentous bacteriophages. In Fraenkel-Conrat H, Wagner RR (eds): Comprehensive Virology, vol 8. New York, Plenum, 1977, p 105

Zinder ND: Portraits of viruses: RNA phage. Intervirology 13:257, 1980

Selected Papers

THE LYTIC PHAGE MULTIPLICATION CYCLE

Black LW, Silverman DJ: Model for DNA packaging into bacteriophage T4 heads. J Virol 28:643, 1978

Blanco L, Salas M: Replication of phage ϕ29 DNA with purified terminal protein and DNA polymerase: Synthesis of full-length ϕ29 DNA. Proc Natl Acad Sci USA 82:6404, 1985

Brennan SM, Chelm BK, Romeo JM, et al: A transcriptional map of the bacteriophage SPO1 genome. II. The major early transcription units. Virology 111:604, 1981

Brenner S, Jacob F, Meselson M: An unstable intermediate carrying information from genes to ribosomes for protein synthesis. Nature 190:576, 1961

Caspar DLD: Movement and self-control in protein assemblies. Biophys J 32:103, 1980

Coombs DH, Eiserling FA: Studies on the structure, protein composition and assembly of the neck of bacteriophage T4. J Mol Biol 116:375, 1977

Crick FHC, Barnett L, Brenner S, et al: General nature of the genetic code for proteins. Nature 192:1227, 1961

Crowther RA, Lenk EV, Kikuchi Y, et al: Molecular reorganization in the hexagon to star transition of the base plate of T4. J Mol Biol 116:489, 1977

Dodson M, Roberts J, McMacken R, et al: Specialized nucleoprotein structures at the origin of replication of bacteriophage λ: Complexes with λO protein and with λO, λP, and *Escherichia coli* DnaB proteins. Proc Natl Acad Sci USA 82:4678, 1985

Doermann AH: The intracellular growth of bacteriophages. I. Liberation of intracellular phage T4 by premature lysis with another phage or with cyanide. J Gen Physiol 35:645, 1951

Edgar RS, Wood WB: Morphogenesis of bacteriophage T4 in extracts of mutant-infected cells. Proc Natl Acad Sci USA 55:498, 1966

Ellis EL, Delbrück M: The growth of bacteriophage. J Gen Physiol 22:365, 1939

Epstein RH, Bolle A, Steinberg CM, et al: Physiological studies of conditional lethal mutants of bacteriophage T4D. Cold Spring Harbor Symp Quant Biol 28:375, 1963

Formosa T, Burke RL, Alberts BM: Affinity purification of bacteriophage T4 proteins essential for DNA replication and recombination. Proc Natl Acad Sci USA 80:2442, 1983

Fuller MT, King J: Purification of the coat and scaffolding proteins from procapsids of bacteriophage P22. Virology 112:529, 1981

Hersey AD, Chase M: Independent functions of viral protein and nucleic acid in growth of bacteriophage. J Gen Physiol 36:39, 1952

Kassavetis GA, Geiduschek EP: Defining a bacteriophage T4 late promoter: Bacteriophage T4 gene 55 protein suffices for directing late promoter recognition. Proc Natl Acad Sci USA 81:5101, 1984

Katsura I, Hendrix RW: Length determination in bacteriophage lambda tails. Cell 39:691, 1984

Lemair G, Gold L, Yarus M: Autogenous translational regulation of bacteriophage T4 gene 32 expression in vitro. J Mol Biol 126:73, 1978

McCorquodale DJ, Chen CW, Joseph MK, et al: Modification of RNA polymerase from *Escherichia coli* by pre-early gene products of bacteriophage T5. J Virol 40:958, 1981

Mizuuchi K: In vitro transposition of bacteriophage Mu: A biochemical approach to a novel replication reaction. Cell 35:785, 1983

Nordstrom B, Randahl H, Slaby I, et al: Characterization of bacteriophage T7 DNA polymerase purified to homogeneity by antithioredoxin immunoadsorbent chromatography. J Biol Chem 256:3112, 1981

Volkin E, Astrachan L: Phosphorus incorporation in *Escherichia coli* RNA after infection with bacteriophage T2. Virology 2:149, 1956

von Gabain A, Bujard H: Interaction of *Escherichia coli* RNA polymerase with promoters of several coliphage and plasmid DNAs. Proc Natl Acad Sci USA 76:189, 1979

PHAGE λ: LYSOGENY

Barondess JJ, Beckwith J: A bacterial virulence determinant encoded by lysogenic coliphage λ. Nature 346:871, 1990

Ho Y-S, Lewis M, Rosenberg M: Purification and properties of a transcriptional activator: The *c*II protein of phage lambda. J Biol Chem 257:9128, 1982

Hochschild A, Douhan J, Ptashne M: How λ repressor and λ Cro distinguish between o_R1 and o_R3. Cell 47:807, 1986

Hochschild A, Irwin N, Ptashne M: Repressor structure and the mechanism of positive control. Cell 32:319, 1983

Hoyt MA, Knight DM, Das A, et al: Control of phage lambda development by stability and synthesis of *c*II protein: Role of the viral *c*III and host *hflA, himA* and *himD* genes. Cell 31:565, 1982

Pabo CO, Krovatin W, Jeffrey A, et al: The N-terminal arms of λ repressor wrap around the operator DNA. Nature 298:441, 1982

Sanger F, Coulson AR, Hong GF, et al: Nucleotide sequence of bacteriophage lambda DNA. J Mol Biol 162:729, 1982

Sauer RT, Ross MJ, Ptashne M: Cleavage of the lambda and P22 repressors by *recA* protein. J Biol Chem 257:4458, 1982

Sauer RT, Yocum RR, Doolittle RF, et al: Homology among DNA-binding proteins suggests use of a conserved super-secondary structure. Nature 298:447, 1982

Shimatake H, Rosenberg M: Purified lambda regulatory protein *c*II positively activates promoters for lysogenic development. Nature 292:128, 1981

Takeda Y, Folkmanis A, Echols H: Cro regulatory protein specified by bacteriophage lambda: Structure, DNA-binding and repression of RNA synthesis. J Biol Chem 252:6177, 1977

SINGLE-STRANDED NUCLEIC ACID PHAGE

Arai K-I, Kornberg A: Mechanism of *dnaB* protein action. IV. General priming of DNA replication by *dnaB* protein and primase compared with RNA polymerase. J Biol Chem 256:5267, 1981

Beremand MN, Blumenthal T: Overlapping genes in RNA phage: A new protein implicated in lysis. Cell 18:257, 1979

Berkhout B, Van Duin J: Mechanism of translational coupling between coat protein and replicase genes of RNA bacteriophage MS2. Nucl Acid Res 13:6955, 1985

Fiers W, Contreras R, Duerinck F, et al: Complete nucleotide sequence of bacteriophage MS2-RNA: Primary and secondary structure of the replicase gene. Nature 260:500, 1976

Grant RA, Lin T-C, Konigsberg W, et al: Structure of the filamentous bacteriophage f1. J Biol Chem 256:539, 1981

Meyer TF, Geider K: Enzymatic synthesis of bacteriophage fd viral DNA. Nature 296:828, 1982

Sanger F, Coulson AR, Friedmann T, et al: The nucleotide sequence of bacteriophage ϕX174. J Mol Biol 125:225, 1978

Shlomai J, Polder L, Arai K-I, et al: Replication of ϕX174 DNA with purified enzymes. I. Conversion of viral DNA to a supercoiled, biologically active duplex. J Biol Chem 256:5233, 1981

DIPHTHERIA TOXIN PRODUCTION

Uchida T, Kanei C, Yoneda M: Mutations in corynephage ϕ that affect the yield of diphtheria toxin. Virology 77:876, 1977

SECTION V

CLINICAL VIROLOGY

CHAPTER 61

Pathogenesis of Viral Infections

As knowledge concerning the nature of viruses and the strategies according to which their genomes express the functions that they encode has expanded, our understanding of virus infections in humans has become increasingly detailed. The chapters that follow focus on the clinical manifestations of viral infections and on the management of virus-caused disease. The purpose of this chapter is to summarize current knowledge of host-virus interactions in terms of the rapidly emerging field of molecular pathogenesis. This is a field of vital importance, particularly for the young clinician, because here we focus on the nature of the problems concerning viral infections of humans that are now becoming susceptible to experimental investigation; that is, these are the areas in which major advances may be expected during the next several decades, and these are the areas in which new insights will have the greatest impact on the management of virus-caused disease.

Host-virus interaction can be viewed from two perspectives. The first is in terms of the successive stages of pathogenesis; the second is in terms of the type of host-virus interactions that result. Superimposed on these two perspectives are considerations concerning the nature of the host and the route of infection.

Nature of Host

The nature of the host is one of the most critical factors that govern the outcome of virus-host interactions. The age of the host is clearly of primary importance. For example, in the case of herpes simplex virus, an overwhelming disseminated infection may occur in the newborn infant who acquires infection during delivery. In the absence of immunocompromise, this is an almost unheard of event in older individuals. In contrast, in the case of rotaviruses, infection of the newborn is almost always asymptomatic; but rotaviruses are the leading cause of diarrhea in infants between the ages of 6 months and 18 months. Further, although hepatitis B virus can infect and ultimately cause serious disease in an individual of any age, it is far more likely to become established as a persistently infecting agent if an infant acquires this virus; more than 90% of infants who become infected with this virus in the perinatal period become chronic carriers of hepatitis B virus (HBV). This is clearly not the case in older children or adults. Adenoviruses can cause severe and overwhelming pneumonia in infants, but this is very unusual in older persons unless immunosuppression or immunodeficiency exists. Finally, many of the normal childhood diseases like measles, mumps, and chickenpox are far less serious in children than in adolescents or adults. The differential susceptibility to viral infections of persons of different ages probably reflects the balance of several competing factors, such as the ability of cells to support virus multiplication, which is proportionately higher in the younger person; the ability to withstand loss of cells, which is likely to be greater in the young than in the old, owing to their greater capacity for tissue regeneration; and the ability to mount an effective immune response, which is highest in children, adolescents, and young adults.

Another important factor is the nutritional state of the host. Again there are competing factors. Viruses tend to multiply less well in nutritionally deficient hosts for a variety of reasons, including the presence of fewer receptors and the reduced capacity to sustain macromolecular biosynthesis, but the ability to replace infected cells and to mount an adequate immune defense is likely to be compromised to an even greater extent. As a result, the severity of viral infections is usually enhanced by malnutrition.

Finally, genetic factors are of major importance in regulating susceptibility and resistance to viral infection. A well-known example is the Mx gene of mice. This gene controls the susceptibility to infection with influenza virus; allele Mx^+ encodes a nuclear protein that is induced by interferon α or β and that confers resistance to influenza virus (see p. 865). Humans possess an analogous gene. The existence of several other situations of this general type—that is, genetic predisposition or resistance to viral infection—is suggested by epidemiologic observations. For example, southern Chinese and Algerians are much more likely than other populations to contract nasopharyngeal carcinoma; the incidence of Burkitt's lymphoma is much higher in Central Africa than in other parts of the world, and an X-linked inability to limit Epstein-Barr virus (EBV) replication has been defined and is known as Duncan's syndrome. In view of observations of this type and the suspected but as yet unproved role of MHC gene polymorphism in influencing susceptibility to viral infections, further genetic studies in this area should yield very interesting and valuable results.

Mode of Viral Entry into Host

The virus must first gain access to the host. Most commonly this occurs via the mucous membranes of the respiratory, gastrointestinal, or genitourinary tracts. Aerosolization of virus affords entry into the respiratory tract, whereas direct inoculation of virus occurs with fecal-oral spread and sexual transmission. Virus may also gain entry through the skin or by direct introduction into the bloodstream, such as occurs with insect vectors or transplacental transmission of viruses. Each portal of infection poses problems for virus entry. For example, in the case of mucous membranes, cell surfaces are bathed in an array of secretions that contain nonspecific as well as specific defenses against invasion by viral pathogens, like sialic acid–containing mucoproteins capable of interacting with viruses of the orthomyxovirus and paramyxovirus families. Competition between such mucoproteins and the glycoproteins that are the viral receptors on cell surfaces is, for such viruses, a factor that diminishes infectivity. As for viruses that multiply in cells lining the gastrointestinal tract or that gain access to the body through the gastrointestinal tract, such viruses must be able to survive the acid environment of the stomach, as well as the protease-rich environment of the small intestine. These viruses, like the enteroviruses, rotaviruses, and certain adenoviruses, possess capsids that resist acid pH and protease digestion. For example, reovirus serotype 3, but not reovirus serotype 1, is inactivated by treatment with proteolytic enzymes. As a consequence, reovirus serotype 3 cannot replicate in the gastrointestinal tract (of newborn mice), whereas reovirus serotype 1 can replicate there. Thus the M2 gene, which encodes the protein (μ1C) that is cleaved, controls the efficiency with which reovirus establishes infection in and gains access to the body across the gastrointestinal tract.

Primary Replication

Invading virus particles infect and multiply in the first susceptible cells that they encounter. Susceptible cells must possess two characteristics: they must display receptors for the virus in question, and they must be permissive; that is, they must be capable of supporting replication of the virus. Clearly, only a minority of cells in the body possess receptors and are permissive for any particular virus; if the situation were otherwise, viral infections would commonly be much more generalized than they are. Expression of the viral receptor is a simple plus/minus situation. Permissiveness is much more complex and involves functions relevant to viral uptake and uncoating, initiation of viral RNA transcription, viral messenger RNA translation, viral genome replication, morphogenesis, and other functions.

Some viruses replicate extensively at the primary site of entry because that is where they encounter the cells that are their primary targets and in which they multiply most extensively. Examples of such viruses are viruses that infect the respiratory tract (e.g., the orthomyxoviruses, paramyxoviruses, and coronaviruses) and viruses that cause gastrointestinal infections (e.g., the rotaviruses and various types of adenoviruses). However, many other viruses multiply only minimally at the primary site of entry and spread from there to the organs in which they subsequently replicate extensively and cause disease. For example, mousepox virus (ectromelia) replicates in the skin at the site of inoculation and then in the regional lymph nodes before systemic spread via the bloodstream; in enterovirus infections, primary replication occurs in epithelial cells and lymphoid follicles around the nasopharynx, which is followed by viremia and replication in other tissues such as those of the central nervous system.

Viral Spread

Viruses that cause systemic disease set up major foci of infection in parts of the body other than those where primary infection occurs. The ability of viruses to spread and the manner in which they spread are, therefore, vital factors in determining the outcome and severity of viral diseases. Viruses spread via a variety of pathways, depending on the specific entry point and the targets involved. Some viruses spread via the extracellular environment, that is, the bloodstream or the lymphatic system. Examples of viruses that spread via the bloodstream are the enteroviruses, which spread in free form, and rubella virus, cytomegalovirus (CMV), and lymphocytic choriomeningitis (LCM) virus, which circulate primarily within cells. An example of a virus that spreads via the lymphatic system is reovirus, which spreads from Peyer's patches via the lymphatic system. Spread via the extracellular environment in free form is subject to inhibition by the various humoral elements of the immune system, such as antibodies. Other viruses, such as the paramyxoviruses, can spread directly from cell to cell by fusion of the membranes of adjacent cells; in this case prevention of viral spread requires the destruction of infected cells by the cell-mediated factors of the defense system. Still other viruses, such as rabies virus, spread via neuronal pathways.

All viruses display tissue tropism, that is, a marked preference for multiplying in some particular tissue or organ where the cells are both susceptible and permissive. Susceptible cells must display the appropriate virus receptors, the presence of which can be tested experimentally by in vitro binding assays. The receptor for human immunodeficiency virus (HIV), for example, is the CD4 glycoprotein that is present on T4 lymphocytes, astrocytes, and microglia, as well as on certain other cells; the receptor for poliovirus is present on cells lining the respiratory tract and the gastrointestinal tract, as well as on anterior horn cells of the central nervous system; and the receptor for EBV is present on B lymphocytes and on epithelial cells in the respiratory tract and in the cervix. It should be noted, however, that although cells cannot be infected if they do not possess receptors on their surfaces, not all cells that possess such receptors are permissive; indeed, many cells can be infected, but virus cannot multiply in them because some reaction essential for the formation of virus progeny fails to proceed. Such cells are infected abortively. The factors involved in permissiveness were discussed in

Chapter 56. A special case of permissiveness, specifically for orthomyxoviruses and paramyxoviruses, is possession of a proteolytic enzyme capable of cleaving their HA or F protein, thereby providing the hydrophobic N-termini required for uncoating their nucleocapsids (Chap. 55). As a result, cells that possess the appropriate receptor but lack the requisite protease cannot be infected by orthomyxoviruses and paramyxoviruses that contain uncleaved HA or F proteins.

Most cells in the body can probably be infected by some virus or other. Among them are skin and subcutaneous tissue, muscle tissue, mucosal membranes lining the respiratory and the gastrointestinal tracts, cells of the immune system such as lymphocytes, monocytes, and macrophages, cells lining the blood vessels, cells of the various organs including liver, spleen, and kidney, and cells of the nervous system. Centers of viral infection are identified most readily by staining sections of suspected target organs with fluorescein-labeled antibody against the virus in question (Chap. 54) or by in situ hybridization with probes amplified by polymerase chain reaction (PCR) technology.

Host Response to Viral Infection

The host response to viral infection takes numerous forms. Some responses are mounted against viral infections in general and affect most if not all viruses; others are specific for specific viruses.

A very important general antiviral response mechanism is the formation of interferon. Interferon is formed in the body as soon as virus multiplication begins at the primary site of infection. The first response is the formation of type I interferon (IFN-α and β), which inhibits virus multiplication by the mechanisms outlined in Chapter 58. Somewhat later proliferating lymphocytes begin to synthesize type 2 interferon, or IFN-γ, which strongly influences the nature of the immune response. The importance of the interferon system in reducing the extent of early virus multiplication is readily demonstrable by infecting animals with virus in the presence of antibody against IFN-α and β, when the severity of the disease is much greater than when such antibody is absent. It should be noted, however, that not all viruses induce the formation of interferon efficiently, nor is the multiplication of all viruses inhibited equally (Chap. 58).

The immune response to viral infection is complex. In essence, viral proteins, either as part of virus particles or expressed on the surfaces of infected cells (Chap. 54), interact with macrophages that bear type II histocompatibility antigens (Ia antigens) on their surfaces, thereby initiating a cascade that results in the development of both cellular and humoral immunity (Chap. 17). The primary humoral response is the formation of antibodies, including immunoglobulins G, M, and A. Antibodies with many specificities are made against virus particles; most viruses display several proteins on their surfaces, each with several epitopes distributed in several functional domains, and as a result the spectrum of antibodies formed against any particular virus particle is highly complex. The formation of neutralizing antibodies is generally elicited by only one or two viral surface proteins, but nonneutralizing antibodies may also play a role in specifying the immune response to viral infection (Chap. 54).

The cellular limb of the immune system is also activated during viral infection. Its salient features, within the present context, include activation of cytotoxic T lymphocytes (CTLs), natural killer (NK) cells, and macrophages (Chap. 17). It should be noted that macrophages and NK cells may lyse infected cells by antibody-dependent cellular cytotoxicity (ADCC) and that both NK cells and macrophages are activated by IFN-γ (Chaps. 17 and 54).

The complement system may also play a role in the pathogenesis of viral infection. For example, the alternate complement pathway is activated by alphavirus spike glycoproteins, the extent of complement activation being regulated by their sialic acid content (decreasing amounts of sialic acid correlating with increased complement activation and more rapid bloodstream clearance). Complement may initiate lysis of free virus and of virus-infected cells in the presence of antibody (Chap. 54).

The formation of various types of antibodies and the development of mechanisms for lysing and destroying infected cells are general defensive mechanisms that are activated in response to infection with most, although not all, viruses, but the exact nature of the immune response mounted varies for each particular virus. Delineating specific features is aided by studying situations in which the immune status of the host has been compromised, as in immunodeficient or in immunosuppressed patients. For example, children with combined humoral and cellular immune deficiencies have chronic pulmonary infections with respiratory syncytial and parainfluenza viruses because they are unable to eradicate them from their respiratory tract. The deficient cellular immunity seems more important, because children with only humoral immune deficiency do not have such chronic infections. Individuals lacking normal cellular immunity may have gastrointestinal disease for prolonged periods of time due to noncultivatable adenoviruses and rotaviruses, as well as fatal infections with varicella virus and measles virus, but individuals with only humoral antibody deficiency are able to cope normally with many common viral infections, such as those caused by varicella, measles, influenza, respiratory syncytial virus (RSV), herpes simplex, and CMV viruses. However, inability to limit the replication of poliovirus and other enteroviruses in the central nervous system is now recognized as being a consequence of humoral antibody deficiency, and patients with this condition sustain persistent and chronic infections with these viruses in this sequestered location.

Immunosuppression

Viral infection itself may alter the host's ability to respond to infection. For example, the cellular receptor for HIV is the CD4 antigen, which is expressed on only a few types of cells in the body, in particular T4 lymphocytes. These cells are therefore the primary hosts for this virus and, as they play a key role in the normal immune response, their destruction triggers the collapse of the entire immune system (Chaps. 59 and 77). Several other viruses also multiply in cells of the immune system. For example, EBV multiplies in B lymphocytes; measles virus infects lymphocytes and decreases their ability to begin replication and differentiation; and influenza virus and RSV diminish the oxidative burst in stimulated neutrophils (but this may not require virus multiplication in host cells). In addition, many structural viral proteins are cytotoxic (Chap. 56) and may affect the functioning of cells of the immune system with consequent immunosuppressive effects. Indeed, one of the major considerations in designing subunit vaccines is ruling out the possibility that the candidate proteins that are intended to induce the formation of neutralizing antibodies do not themselves cause immunosuppression.

Adverse Consequences of Immune Response

Whereas the immune response is absolutely essential for protection against viral infections, its efficient functioning sometimes has adverse results. Two such effects have already been described elsewhere. One is the effect of the cellular response during LCM infection (Chap. 54); the other is the effect of the antibody-complement interaction in the hemorrhagic shock syndrome elicited by a flavivirus, dengue virus, as well as by certain arenaviruses such as Junin virus (Argentinean hemorrhagic fever) (Chap. 54). In both cases an efficiently operating immune response leads to disaster for the host. Another example of this type is the problem of immune complex formation. Whereas immune complexes are normally not formed in excessive amounts and are readily eliminated, they are sometimes formed in very large amounts and cannot then be dealt with adequately. In such cases virus-antibody complexes may damage the host. For example, infants congenitally infected with CMV have circulating complexes of virus and antibody that are deposited in the kidney, and patients with HBV infection have circulating immune complexes and resultant pathology, such as arthritis and glomerulonephritis. An animal model of this condition that has been investigated extensively is that of LCM. In utero and in neonates, infection of mice with this virus produces an initially asymptomatic infection; persistent lifelong viremia is established, and the blood contains virus-antibody complexes. Although antibody to each of the viral proteins is present, virus is not cleared from the animal; in fact, the infectious virus that circulates is protected by being bound to antibody. These complexes may lead to glomerulonephritis, choroiditis, and vasculitis, with virus subsequently multiplying in the tissues where the complexes are deposited. It is not clear in this animal model why cytotoxic T cells are not detectable. Initially viral antigens are expressed on the surface of infected cells as well as in the cytoplasm; subsequently, the surface antigen diminishes, which may be related to capping and subsequent stripping of the antigen from the cell surface by antibody. The viral nucleoprotein in the cytoplasm persists, but the cell is then no longer susceptible to specific lysis, as there are no expressed viral antigens on its surface. The concept that these persistently infected cells manage to survive despite intracellular virus replication is important. There are no hallmarks of tissue destruction or inflammation in this setting, and by light microscopy the tissue morphology appears normal. With the use of appropriate antisera, however, viral nucleoprotein can be demonstrated within the cytoplasm of the cells. This infection would go undetected without knowledge of the infectious agent and the use of specific antisera.

Another complication is the generation of autoantibodies directed against normal tissues that have not themselves been infected by the virus. For example, newborn mice infected with reovirus serotype 1 develop a polyendocrinopathy, with antibodies directed against antigens in pancreatic islets, the anterior pituitary, and the gastric mucosa. Immunosuppression with antilymphocyte serum prevents the development of polyendocrine disease. Further, anti-idiotypic antibodies may be produced as part of the immune response against viruses, and some experimentally produced anti-idiotypic antibodies have been shown to bind to specific viral cell surface receptors in a fashion similar to that of virus itself. It is conceivable that tissues not actually infected with virus may be injured or have their functions altered or impaired by attachment of such anti-idiotypic antibodies.

Finally, adverse consequences may result from interactions between the host and altered or modified virus particles. Atypical measles is an example. The atypical measles syndrome occurs in persons who receive inactivated measles virus vaccine and are infected months to years later with active measles virus. In the inactivated measles vaccine the F protein (Chap. 55) is altered by the formalin used to inactivate the virus. Therefore, vaccine recipients do not form antibody against the F protein but do form antibodies against the HN and other proteins. Introduction of infectious virus into such hosts elicits an anamnestic antibody response with respect to the HN protein and a cell-mediated immune response against the other viral proteins, but virus replication and cell-to-cell spread are not prevented until antibody against F protein is formed. In the meantime infected cells express viral antigens on their surface, exhibit capping, and liberate antigen-antibody complexes. The clinical manifestations of measles virus infection in these individuals are very unusual: they include prominent pulmonary disease, a vasculitic-type rash, arthritis, and hepatic dysfunction. Similar considerations—that is, the possible results of viral infection after immunization with incomplete antigen—must be taken into account whenever the use of subunit vaccines is contemplated.

Viral Virulence Genes

Recombinant DNA technology has placed within our grasp the means to identify the viral genes that are responsible for specific aspects of virus-host interactions. As described in the preceding chapters, it is now possible to identify, by the use of both naturally occurring and engineered mutants and variants, the functions of many of the proteins encoded by viral genes. Many aspects of molecular pathogenesis have, therefore, become amenable to experimentation. This problem can be approached most directly with the viruses that possess segmented genomes, such as reovirus and influenza virus. For example, there are three serotypes of mammalian reovirus—serotypes 1, 2, and 3—that differ in their ability to arrest host cell DNA, RNA, and protein synthesis, in the nature of their cytopathic effects on host cells, and in the nature of the disease that they produce in experimental animals. By using reassortants that possess certain genome segments of one serotype and others of another serotype, it is possible to assign phenotypic behavior to individual genome segments and therefore to specific proteins. For example, this type of reassortant analysis has shown that genome segment S4, which encodes the outer capsid shell protein $\sigma 3$, inhibits host RNA and protein synthesis and that the S1 gene product $\sigma 1$, is (1) the cell attachment protein and, therefore, the hemagglutinin; (2) the protein against which the serotype-specific neutralizing antibodies, serotype-specific cytotoxic T lymphocytes, and delayed-type hypersensitivity are directed; (3) the protein that induces the formation of autoantibodies, controls virus spread across the gastrointestinal tract wall to mesenteric lymph nodes and the spleen, and controls neural cell tropism by the presence of specific receptors; and (4) the protein that shuts off host DNA replication. Furthermore, the M2 gene product, μ1C, the major component of the reovirus outer capsid shell (1), determines virulence by regulating virus survival in the gastrointestinal tract, (2) induces the formation of suppressor T lymphocytes, and (3) modulates neurovirulence by regulating the extent of virus replication in cells of the CNS. Finally, the L2 gene product, λ2, which is a core component but penetrates through the outer capsid to the virus particle surface, determines virus shedding and transmission between hosts.

In the case of viruses that do not possess segmented genomes, this type of analysis is more difficult; however, the following insights have been obtained.

1. Cowpox virus (CPV) produces lesions that are hemorrhagic as a result of the lack of the normal inflammatory responses to infection. It appears that CPV genes encode proteins that can inhibit inflammatory responses. Several viral genes are probably required to effect this inhibition because host inflammatory responses can be activated by any one of several different mechanisms. One CPV gene that is required for this inhibition has been identified; several candidate inflammation-inhibitory genes are under investigation. The virulence of the virus is directly related to the products of these genes because their primary function is to inhibit host defenses against viral infection.
2. Vaccinia virus encodes a protein that is similar to the epithelial growth factor (EGF) and transforming growth factor α (TGFα). The vaccinia virus growth factor (VGF) binds to the EGF receptor and activates the signal transduction pathway (Chap. 59) by stimulating it to autophosphorylate. This suggests that VGF may enable the vaccinia virus to subvert EGF receptor-dependent functions. For example, VGF is mitogenic; it induces localized hyperplasia at the site of infection. Other members of the poxvirus family, such as Shope fibroma virus, Yaba monkey tumor virus, and molluscum contagiosum virus, also induce pathogenic proliferation effects, and these effects may be caused by similar VGF-like proteins specified by these viruses.
3. Recent evidence suggests that postinfectious demyelinating encephalomyelitis and neuritis may be due to immunologic cross-reactions evoked by specific viral antigenic determinants homologous to regions in target myelins of the central and peripheral nervous systems. Computer searches have revealed regions of similarity in several human myelin basic proteins and proteins encoded by several viruses including vaccinia virus, measles virus, EBV, influenza virus A and B, and several others that cause upper respiratory infections.
4. Recently a vaccinia virus gene has been identified that is required for multiplication in human cells. The function of the protein that it encodes is currently under intensive investigation.
5. A discovery that has created a great deal of interest is that variants of herpesvirus and vaccinia virus that lack thymidine kinase are less virulent than wild-type virus. For example, normal herpes simplex virus type 2 replicates to high titer in the guinea pig vagina and spinal cord, and infected animals develop severe clinical disease. Infection with variants lacking the TK gene results in similar vaginal virus titers, but little or no clinical illness results. TK^- mutants establish latency in trigeminal ganglia but do not reactivate. Vaccinia virus TK^- mutants are also much less virulent than wild-type virus and possess dramatically reduced neurovirulence, which is of great interest vis-á-vis attempts to use vaccinia virus as a carrier for genes of other viruses that encode the proteins that possess epitopes eliciting the synthesis of neutralizing antibodies (Chap. 58).
6. The reassortant analysis technique for assessing virulence has been applied to a bunyavirus, LaCrosse virus. The neurovirulence determinants were found to be complex. For example, when two LaCrosse virus strains were examined that differed in virulence by a factor of 30,000 (that is, 30,000 times more of one virus was required to cause the same clinical symptoms than of the other virus), it was found that the M RNA segment was the major determinant of neurovirulence but that the other two genome segments, S and L, modulated the virulence of the nonneuroinvasive virus strain. Elaboration of this approach should yield data concerning specific neurovirulence determinants. A start has been made by determining that a spike glycoprotein variant with altered fusion function—it requires a lower pH for activation of fusion and also fuses cells less efficiently—exhibits diminished neuroinvasiveness.
7. Another type of virulence factor was demonstrated in a study that analyzed the difference in sensitivity to interferon among mouse hepatitis viruses with high and low virulence for mice. Growth of less virulent viruses was more suppressed in interferon-treated cells than growth of more virulent viruses. The difference was at the level of viral messenger RNA and protein synthesis.
8. Just as the S1 gene of reovirus directs the spread of virus from the primary focus of infection, so has a herpes simplex virus type 1 gene been identified that directs the spread of virus from the cornea to the central nervous system. More specifically, the sequences in the herpesvirus genome that lie between map positions 0.31 and 0.44 direct this spread. Clearly, this region contains many genes, but work currently under way should soon identify the actual gene that is responsible for facilitating this spread.
9. Neurovirulence determinants are also being investigated for vesicular stomatitis virus (VSV), Semliki Forest virus, and mumps virus. In all cases the spike glycoproteins (G, E2, and HN, respectively) control ability to infect the CNS.
10. One of the most interesting investigations in this regard is the characterization of poliovirus neurovirulence determinants. Such determinants are spread over several areas of the poliovirus genome; unexpectedly, some are located in its 5′-noncoding region. The fact that neurovirulence is controlled by viral proteins is not unexpected, but the fact that neurovirulence determinants are also located in a genome region that does not encode protein is surprising. A possibly related finding is that the genomes of attenuated and virulent poliovirus strains (that is, without

and with neurovirulence) differ in the relative efficiencies with which they are translated; neurovirulent strains are translated more efficiently than nonneurovirulent ones. Thus the situation here parallels that which occurs with other viruses, where neurovirulence is also controlled by the extent of virus multiplication in the CNS.

11. Efforts have been made to identify the virulence genes of influenza viruses. Influenza pathogenicity has a complex basis; reassortant analysis indicates that several genes contribute to the overall pathogenic profile. There is no question, however, that the predominant determinant of pathogenicity here is the hemagglutinin. Influenza virus acquires virulence suddenly; a single critical point mutation in the HA gene of avirulent forms of the virus is all that is required to produce highly virulent virus. In other words, in such cases the virus already possesses the other genes necessary for virulence and it is the extra change in the HA gene that converts a relatively avirulent strain to a highly virulent one. As for the factors that determine whether a given HA protein specifies high virulence or low virulence, the most important is susceptibility to the proteolytic enzymes present in the various types of cells in the body. The reason for this is that only cleaved HA (or F protein in the case of paramyxoviruses) possesses the latent hydrophobic HA2 N-termini that fuse viral envelopes and endosomal vesicle membranes and thereby permit the liberation of free nucleocapsids into the cytoplasm (Chap. 55). Although other factors are presumably also involved, pathogenesis of influenza viruses is determined primarily by cleavability of their HAs.
12. Measles virus virulence is associated with suppression of immune function. The virus infects T lymphocytes, B lymphocytes, and monocytes, but does not produce cytolysis. One consequence of infection is the failure of T and B lymphocyte mixtures to cooperate in secreting immunoglobulins. This defect resides in the infected B lymphocytes. Measles virus appears to suppress B cell development at the activation or proliferation stage but does not affect terminal differentiation into immunoglobulin-secreting cells.
13. A key factor in eradicating viral infections is the generation of cytotoxic T lymphocytes (CTLs). There are two classes of such CTLs. The first are directed against the neutralizing type- or strain-specific epitopes located on viral antigens such as the spike glycoproteins of enveloped viruses, the $\sigma 1$ protein of reoviruses, the VP1 of poliovirus, the fiber protein of adenoviruses, and so on (Chaps. 54 and 55). These are the strain-specific CTLs. The other CTLs are the cross-reactive CTLs. They are directed against either nonstructural virus-encoded proteins or internal structural viral components. Among such are the proteins encoded by certain immediate early (IE) herpesvirus genes, genes that are expressed immediately after infection and encode proteins that regulate viral genome expression; the large T antigen of papovaviruses (Chap. 55); and the influenza virus NP, PB1, and PB2 proteins, all nucleocapsid components, as well as the nonstructural protein NS1. All these proteins are located both in the nucleus and in the cytoplasm of infected cells. How they function in CTL recognition of infected cells is not known. Recent evidence indicates that the ability to recognize them cosegregates with MHC haplotype.
14. It has been suspected for some time that viruses can cause insulin-dependent (type 1) diabetes mellitus (IDDM) via an anti-self immune response. Recently it has been shown, in a mouse transgenic model, that a viral gene introduced into the germ line and expressed in islet of Langerhans cells does *not* produce tolerance when the host is exposed to the virus later in life; rather, the induced anti-self (viral) CTL response then causes selective and progressive damage to β cells, resulting in IDDM.

In summary, techniques are now becoming available for identifying the functional roles of many viral proteins in pathogenesis. As more and more viral virulence determinants are being identified, techniques are being devised to inactivate them so as to provide harmless vaccine strains. This is easier for DNA- than for RNA-containing viruses. In the case of DNA-containing viruses, all that is necessary is to identify the genes responsible for some aspect of pathogenicity and to clone nonspecific segments of DNA into them. This effectively and permanently inactivates them as virulence determinants. Efforts are being made to inactivate virulence determinants of RNA viruses also, but this is proving to be more difficult because many of their virulence determinants are structural viral proteins. However, it should be possible to introduce appropriate multiple mutations into these proteins and thereby construct engineered viral strains that are avirulent but still possess the epitopes that elicit the formation of neutralizing antibodies.

Identifying and modifying viral genes that control virulence is a most exciting area of research in clinical virology at this time.

Types of Viral Infections

The final factor to be considered in patterns of host-virus interactions is the type of infection that results.

1. The type of illness that is thought of as the standard viral infection is acute and self-limited (e.g., respiratory tract and gastrointestinal infections).
2. Damage due to acute infection may have other consequences (e.g., congenital malformations). Viruses such as rubella and CMV are well appreciated causes of intrauterine infections. The consequences of such infections depend on such factors as the time of infection, the agent causing the infection, and the response of the host. For example, rubella virus causes alterations in organogenesis, whereas CMV causes destruction of poorly differentiated tissue. Because the immature fetus does not mount an adult-type immune response to infection, viruses such as rubella may replicate and be present for months.
3. Many human viruses can cause persistent infections. A well-known example is HBV, which may persist in carriers in large amounts for years. The results of this persistent infection can be asymptomatic infection or symptomatic liver disease, with cirrhosis and hepatocellular carcinoma as possible outcomes. Central nervous system infection by enteroviruses in patients

with agammaglobulinemia is another example of persistent infection but one that is dependent on an abnormal host response. Virus may be detectable for years in the central nervous system, with progressive and ultimately fatal disease. Furthermore, serologic studies indicate that human papovaviruses (BKV and JCV) asymptomatically infect the majority of persons by adulthood; yet disease becomes apparent only with immunosuppression. Finally, subacute sclerosing panencephalitis (SSPE) is the result of measles infection proceeding in an incomplete manner over a period of many years.

4. A special example of persistent infection is latency (Chap. 56). The herpes group of viruses elicit a type of virus-host interaction in which initial infection is followed by a variable period of time when no demonstrable signs of infection are present. Subsequently, recurrent active infection occurs. For example, herpes simplex virus is notorious for its ability to cause intermittent overt infection; it is latent in neural tissue. CMV infection also cannot be eliminated because the virus becomes latent, always with the capacity to reactivate. CMV may be intermittently excreted by infected individuals; when appropriate studies are done, such as restriction endonuclease analysis, only the originally infecting virus is found to be involved. Similarly, varicella virus infection induces a primary generalized illness and in subsequent years a localized infection in the form of zoster, and EBV, the etiologic agent of infectious mononucleosis, causes latent infection of circulating lymphocytes and perhaps of other cells.
5. The final example of this spectrum of viral illness is oncogenesis. It now seems quite certain that several human viruses either cause or are cofactors in carcinogenesis. HBV is associated with hepatocellular carcinoma; EBV is a cofactor in Burkitt's lymphoma and a polyclonal malignant lymphoma, as well as in nasopharyngeal carcinoma; the recently recognized human T cell leukemia viruses—HTLV-1 and HTLV-2—cause human leukemias; and several types of human papillomavirus causes or are cofactors in cervical carcinoma. Thus our appreciation of the virus-host interaction extends across the spectrum from acute, temporally limited illness through teratogenesis and persistent infection, latency and recurrent infection, to oncogenesis.

In summary, virology is at a fascinating stage because recombinant DNA technology is now providing us with the tools not only for defining which viral genes and proteins are determinants of pathogenicity in acute infections but also for identifying the viral genes and proteins that specify virus-host interactions in terms of persistent infection, latency, and oncogenesis.

FURTHER READING

Books and Reviews

Ada GL, Jones PD: The immune response to influenza infection. Curr Top Microbiol Immunol 128:1, 1986

Albert MJ: Enteric adenoviruses. Arch Virol 88:1, 1986

Berns KI, Labow MA: Parvovirus immune regulation. J Gen Virol 68:601, 1987

Buller RML, Palumbo GJ: Poxvirus pathogenesis. Microbiol Rev 55:80, 1991

Fan HY, Chen ISY, Rosenberg N, Sugden W (eds): Viruses that affect the immune system. Washington, American Society for Microbiology, 1991

Friedmann A, Lorch Y: Theiler's virus infection: A model for multiple sclerosis. Progr Med Virol 31:43, 1985

Haase AT: The pathogenesis of slow virus infections: Molecular analyses. J Infect Dis 153:441, 1986

Haase AT: Pathogenesis of lentivirus infections. Nature 322:130, 1986

Herberman RB, Ortaldo JR: Natural killer cells: Their role in defenses against disease. Science 214:24, 1981

Kirchner H: Immunobiology of human papillomavirus infections. Progr Med Virol 33:1, 1986

Macnab JCM: Herpes simplex virus and human cytomegalovirus: Their role in morphological transformation and genital cancers. J Gen Virol 68:2525, 1987

Morrison LA, Fields BN: Parallel mechanisms in neuropathogenesis of enteric virus infections. J Virol 65:2767, 1991

Parsonson IM, McPhee DA: Bunyavirus pathogenesis. Adv Virus Res 30:279, 1986

Raccah B: Nonpersistent viruses: Epidemiology and control. Adv Virus Res 31:387, 1986

Rosen L: The natural history of Japanese encephalitis virus. Ann Rev Microbiol 40:395, 1986

Sharpe AH, Fields BN: Pathogenesis of reovirus infection. In Joklik WK (ed): The Reoviridae. New York, Plenum Press, 1983, pp 229–286.

Zinkernagel RM, Doherty PC: MHC-restricted cytotoxic T cells: Studies on the biologic role of polymorphic major transplantation antigens determining T-cell restriction-specificity, function and responsiveness. Adv Immunol 27:51, 1979

Selected Papers

Beattie E, Tartaglia J, Paoletti E: Vaccinia virus-encoded eIF-2α homolog abrogates the antiviral effect of interferon. Virology 183:419, 1991

Bloom DC, Edwards KM, Hager C, Moyer RW: Identification and characterization of two nonessential regions of the rabbitpox virus genome involved in virulence. J Virol 65:1530, 1991

Buller RML, Chakrabarti S, Cooper JA, Twardzik DR, Moss B: Deletion of the vaccinia virus growth factor gene reduces virus virulence. J Virol 62:866, 1988

Buller RML, Smith GL, Cremer K, et al: Decreased virulence of recombinant vaccinia virus expression vectors is associated with a thymidine kinase-negative phenotype. Nature 317:813, 1985

Coen DM, Kosz-Vnenchak M, Jacobson JG, et al: Thymidine kinase-negative herpes simplex virus mutants establish latency in mouse trigeminal ganglia but do not reactivate. Proc Natl Acad Sci USA 86:4736–4740, 1989

Dietzschold B, Wunner WH, Wiktor TJ, et al: Characterization of an antigenic determinant of the glycoprotein that correlates with pathogenicity of rabies virus. Proc Natl Acad Sci USA 80:70, 1983

Finberg R, Spriggs DR, Fields BN: Host immune response to reovirus: CTL recognize the major neutralization domain of the viral hemagglutinin. J Immunol 129:2235, 1982

Finberg R, Weiner HL, Fields BN, et al: Generation of cytolytic T lymphocytes after reovirus infection: Role of S1 gene. Proc Natl Acad Sci USA 76:442, 1979

Gillard S, Spehner D, Drillien R, et al: Localization and sequence of a vaccinia virus gene required for multiplication in human cells. Proc Natl Acad Sci USA 83:5573, 1986

Gonzalez-Scarano F, Janssen RS, Najjar JA, et al: An avirulent G1

glycoprotein variant of LaCrosse bunyavirus with defective fusion function. J Virol 54:757, 1985
Gresser I, Tovey MC, Bandu MT, et al: Role of interferon in the pathogenesis of virus diseases in mice as demonstrated by the use of anti-interferon serum. II. Studies with herpes simplex virus, Moloney, sarcoma virus, Newcastle disease virus and influenza virus. J Exp Med 144:1316, 1976
Graham S, Green CP, Mason PD, Borysiewicz LK: Human cytotoxic T cell responses to vaccinia virus vaccination. J Gen Virol 72:1183, 1991
Halstead SB, O'Rourke EJ: Dengue viruses and mononuclear phagocytes. I. Infection enhancement by non-neutralizing antibody. J Exp Med 146:201, 1977
Herrler G, Klenk H: The surface receptor is a major determinant of the cell tropism of influenza C virus. Virology 159:102, 1987
Hinrichs SH, Nerenberg M, Reynolds RK, et al: A transgenic mouse model for human neurofibromatosis. Science 237:1340, 1987
Hirsch RL, Griffin DE, Winkelstein JA: Host modification of Sindbis virus sialic acid content influences alternative complement pathway activation and virus clearance. J Immunol 127:1740, 1981
Howard ST, Chan YS, Smith GL: Vaccinia virus homologues of the Shope fibroma virus inverted terminal repeat proteins and a discontinuous ORF related to the tumor necrosis factor receptor family. Virology 180:631, 1991
Hrdy DB, Rubin DH, Fields BN: Molecular basis of reovirus neurovirulence: Role of the M2 gene in avirulence. Proc Natl Acad Sci USA 79:1298, 1982
Janssen RS, Nathanson N, Endres MJ, et al: Virulence of LaCrosse virus is under polygenic control. J Virol 59:1, 1986
Javier RT, Thompson RL, Stevens JG: Genetic and biological analyses of a herpes simplex virus intertypic recombinant reduced specifically for neurovirulence. J Virol 61:1978, 1991
Kauffman RS, Wolf JL, Finbert R, et al: The §1 protein determines the extent of spread of reovirus from the gastrointestinal tract of mice. Virology 124:403, 1983
Löve A, Rydbeck R, Christensson K, et al: Hemagglutinin-neuraminidase glycoprotein as a determinant of pathogenicity in mumps virus hamster encephalitis: Analysis of mutants selected with monoclonal antibodies. Virol 53:67, 1985
McChesney MB, Fujinami RS, Lampert PW, et al: Viruses disrupt functions of human lymphocytes. II. Measles virus suppresses antibody production by acting on B lymphocytes. J Exp Med 163:1331, 1986
Meyer H, Sutter G, Mayr A: Mapping of deletions in the genome of the highly attenuated vaccinia virus MVA and their influence on virulence. J Gen Virol 72:1031, 1991
Morrison LA, Sidman RL, Fields BN: Direct spread of reovirus from the intestinal lumen to the central nervous system through vagal autonomic nerve fibers. Proc Natl Acad Sci USA 88:3852, 1991
Oakes JE, Gray WL, Lausch RN: Herpes simplex virus type 1 DNA sequences which direct the spread of virus from cornea to central nervous system. Virology 150:513, 1986
Ohashi PS, Oehen S, Buerki K, et al: Ablation of "tolerance" and induction of diabetes by virus infection in viral antigen transgenic mice. Cell 65:305, 1991
Oldstone MBA, Nerenberg M, Southern P, et al: Virus infection triggers insulin-dependent diabetes mellitus in a transgenic model: Role of anti-self (virus) immune response. Cell 65:319, 1991
Palumbo GJ, Pickup DJ, Fredrickson TN, et al: Inhibition of an inflammatory response is mediated by a 38-kDa protein of cowpox virus. Virology 172:262, 1989
Perkus ME, Goebel S, Davis S, et al: Vaccinia virus host range genes. Virology 179:276, 1990
Perkus ME, Goebel SJ, Davis SW, et al: Deletion of 55 open reading frames from the termini of vaccinia virus. Virology 180:406, 1991
Pilipenko EV, Blinov VM, Romanova LI, et al: Conserved structural domains in the 5'-untranslated region of picornaviral genomes: An analysis of the segment controlling translation and neurovirulency. Virology 168:201, 1989
Reddehase MJ, Fibi MR, Keil GM, et al: Late-phase expression of a murine cytomegalovirus immediate-early antigen recognized by cytolytic T lymphocytes. J Virol 60:1125, 1986
Rubin DH, Fields BN: The molecular basis of reovirus virulence: The role of the M2 gene. J Exp Med 152:853, 1980
Sarnow P, Bernstein HD, Baltimore D: A poliovirus temperature-sensitive RNA synthesis mutant located in a noncoding region of the genome. Proc Natl Acad Sci USA 83:571, 1986
Simmons A, Nash AA: Role of antibody in primary and recurrent herpes simplex virus infection. J Virol 53:944, 1985
Smith GL, Chan YS: Two vaccinia virus proteins structurally related to the interleukin-1 receptor and the immunoglobulin superfamily. J Gen Virol 72:511, 1991
Stanberry LR, Kit S, Myers MG: Thymidine kinase-deficient herpes simplex virus type 2 genital infection in guinea pigs. J Virol 55:322, 1985
Svitkin YV, Maslova SV, Agol VI: The genomes of attenuated and virulent poliovirus strains differ in their *in vitro* translation efficiencies. Virology 147:243, 1985
Taguchi F, Siddell SG: Difference in sensitivity to interferon among mouse hepatitis viruses with high and low virulence for mice. Virology 147:41, 1985
Tardieu M, Boespflug O, Barbé T: Selective tropism of a neurotropic coronavirus for ependymal cells, neurons, and meningeal cells. J Virol 60:574, 1986
Taylor G, Stott EJ, Wertz G, Ball A: Comparison of the virulence of wild-type thymidine kinase (tk)-deficient and tk^+ phenotypes of vaccinia virus recombinants after intranasal inoculation of mice. J Gen Virol 72:125, 1991
Twardzik DR, Brown JP, Ranchalis JE, et al: Vaccinia virus-infected cells release a novel polypeptide functionally related to transforming and epidermal growth factors. Proc Natl Acad Sci USA 82:5300, 1985
Tyler KL, McPhee DA, Fields BN: Distinct pathways of a viral spread in the host determined by reovirus S1 gene segment. Science 233:770, 1986
Yahnke U, Fischer EH, Alvord EC Jr: Sequence homology between certain viral proteins and proteins related to encephalomyelitis and neuritis. Science 229:282, 1985

CHAPTER 62

Rapid Viral Diagnosis

The direction in diagnostic virology today is to employ the evolving technologies of antigen detection and molecular biology to achieve a more rapid viral diagnosis. Antiviral chemotherapy is largely responsible for this impetus and makes a rapid, sensitive, specific viral identification a necessity. The advent of monoclonal antibodies coupled with immunofluorescent antibody (FA) and enzyme immunoassay (EIA) techniques, DNA hybridization, and polymerase chain reaction (PCR) technology make rapid diagnosis possible and practical for the laboratory.

In this chapter, the standard techniques of viral diagnosis will be described, as well as rapid methodologies being used and developed for the laboratory.

Laboratory Diagnosis

Laboratory diagnosis of a viral infection requires (1) the detection of the virus itself, (2) components of the virus, or (3) an immune response to the virus. Detecting the virus itself or components of the virus (Table 62–1) determines whether the patient is currently infected with a given virus. Viruses are detected by various culture methods or, in some instances, by electron microscopy. Assays for viral components may be done by a number of techniques, including FA, EIA, and DNA hybridization. Serum antibody assessment determines whether the person has ever experienced infection with the agent in question. In specific circumstances, it is possible to determine when the infection occurred, for example, with a seroconversion occurring in a defined time period. A number of techniques are used to determine antibody in serum including complement fixation (CF), FA, radioimmunoassay (RIA), and EIA.

Specimen Collection, Treatment of Specimens

The crucial element to making the laboratory diagnosis of a virus, regardless of the method employed, is the acquisition and processing of the appropriate clinical specimen(s). A clinical diagnosis will direct the laboratory toward the appropriate test to be performed. Attempts at virus isolation, EIA, or nucleic acid detection techniques will not be successful unless the correct specimen is collected properly. In addition, the best specimens are usually collected early in the illness when virus is being excreted at relatively high levels and has not yet been bound by antibody. Specimens obtained within the first 72 hours of an illness are more likely to yield infectious virus than specimens obtained later in the course of illness. After 7 days, it is usually not worthwhile to obtain viral cultures in immunocompetent hosts. In unusually slow or chronic viral infections, however, especially in immunocompromised hosts, virus may be present for long periods of time.

Specimens should be obtained aseptically if virus isolation is to be attempted. The volume of the sample should be sufficient to permit direct testing as well as virus isolation when possible. Storage of some of the specimen for retesting in additional tests, for example PCR, may also be necessary. Inoculation of specimens into tissue culture within 2 to 4 hours is best for virus isolation. Many viruses tend to be unstable at an acid pH or at temperatures above 40C. Specimens should be kept at 4C or on crushed ice until inoculated. If more prolonged transport is required, most specimens can be preserved at −70C, although some viruses, such as respiratory syncytial virus (RSV), may not survive the freeze-thawing process. As a general rule, however, delay of more than 4 days until inoculation requires freezing of the specimens at −70C for optimal preservation of infectious virus.

TABLE 62–1. SUGGESTED SPECIMENS TO BE SUBMITTED FOR VIRAL DIAGNOSIS

Specimen	Cell Culture	Direct Examination
Respiratory		Immunostaining
Nasopharyngeal secretions	Yes	Respiratory syncytial virus
Endotracheal secretions	Yes	Adenoviruses
		Parainfluenza, influenza
Bronchoalveolar lavage	Yes	Measles
Lung biopsy	Yes	
Throat swab	Only method available	
Gastrointestinal		Electron microscopy
Diarrhea only		Rotaviruses
Stool	Not helpful	Adenoviruses
		Coronaviruses
		Norwalk-like viruses
		Astroviruses
		Caliciviruses
		Enzyme immunoassay and latex agglutination for rotaviruses only
Systemic illness (more symptoms than diarrhea)	Preferred method	
Stool (preferred)		
Rectal swab (less optimal)		
Skin		Immunostaining
Vesicles	Yes	HSV
Pustules	Yes	VZV
Biopsy	Yes	Vaccinia
Eye		Immunostaining
Tears	Yes	HSV
Tissue	Yes	VZV
		Adenoviruses
Blood		Experimental use of in situ nucleic acid hybridization for CMV, EBV, and antigen detection for HIV
Anticoagulated with citrate	Only method for most viruses	
Genitourinary		Experimental use of in situ nucleic acid hybridization for CMV
Urine	Yes	
Cervical/vaginal/urethral secretions	Yes	Immunoasays for HSV
Central Nervous System	Yes	Experimental antigen detection for HSV, cDNA/RNA hybridization for enteroviruses
CSF		
Brain tissue	Essential; animal inoculation may be essential for coxsackie A, LCM, and some arboviruses	Immunostaining for HSV or rabies

HSV, herpes simplex virus; VZV, varicella-zoster virus; CMV, cytomegalovirus; EBV, Epstein-Barr virus; HIV, human immunodeficiency virus; LCM, lymphocytic chorlomeningitis virus.

Typical sources for viral culture include nasopharynx, urine, stool, blood, cerebrospinal fluid, specific tissue (brain, lung, liver, spleen, kidney), and skin vesicles. In addition, pleural fluid, pericardial fluid, bone marrow, and skin scrapings can all be used for viral culture. Tissue specimens from biopsies or postmortem examination are suitable for attempted virus isolation if fresh or frozen but not in formalin or other fixative.

A clinical diagnosis will direct the laboratory toward the rapid appropriate test(s) to be performed and help determine the appropriate cell lines on which the specimen should be inoculated. Commonly needed information, in addition to the clinical diagnosis, includes patient identification, age, source of specimen(s), and the date the specimen(s) were obtained. It is often helpful to know whether the patient has recently received viral vaccines or antiviral therapy. Because viral agents are not affected by antimicrobial agents, cultures may be obtained even if therapy for potential pathogens has been previously initiated. Such materials are obtained from the same site(s) as specimens for bacterial culture. In addition, many viruses do not withstand drying. Swabs of mucosal surfaces, skin scrapings, and tissues should be placed in a transport medium that provides stability with an essential protein source free of antibodies that may neutralize or inhibit the virus. Albumin, gelatin, or antibody-free serum and a buffered salt solution are commonly used to preserve infective virus. All of these media have antibiotics added to prevent overgrowth by resident host bacterial and fungal flora and to decrease exogenous contamination of the specimen.

Virus Isolation

The foundation of diagnostic virology is the detection of the virus or its components. The standard by which all other tests are measured in diagnostic virology is isolation of the virus itself, usually in cell culture and, to a much lesser degree, in organ culture, eggs, or animals.

Virus isolation is unequaled in sensitivity and also has extremely high specificity. A positive culture may be obtained with a single infectious virion. Because only the virus is amplified, sensitivity is increased without loss of specificity. In addition, virus isolation can permit the identification of the etiologic agent as well as its recovery and preservation.

However, there are several disadvantages to virus isolation. First, the process is often slow, requiring days to weeks for identification. Therefore virus identifications may not be available in time to affect patient care. It is also labor intensive, expensive, and requires technical expertise and experience. In addition, it requires the use of appropriate culture systems. For example, four or five cell lines or types are needed for optimal detection of respiratory viruses. Furthermore, cell culture methods for a number of viruses, such as the agents that cause gastroenteritis (e.g., rotaviruses, Norwalk agents, and enteric adenoviruses), are not readily available. Finally, it must be remembered that isolation of a virus, especially from a mucosal surface, does not always prove it is the etiologic agent.

Evidence of host cell infection and damage is called cytopathic effects (CPEs). By killing cells in which they multiply, newly formed virions spread to involve more and more cells in the culture. Viruses are detected and often identified by the particular cytopathic effects produced over time in a particular cell culture. Most CPEs can be readily observed in unfixed, unstained cell cultures under low power of the light microscope. The characteristics of the CPEs, as well as the length of time after inoculation at which cytopathic changes first become detectable, provide good presumptive identification of a particular virus. A trained virologist can distinguish several types of CPE on unstained living cultures. However, fixation and staining of the cell monolayer are necessary to visualize such details as inclusion bodies and syncytia.

The cell tropism of the virus and the specific morphologic alterations provide enough information for the preliminary identification of many viruses. Enteroviruses, for example, which grow rapidly, often show detectable CPEs after 24 to 48 hours, destroying the monolayer completely by 3 days. On the other hand, some of the more slowly growing viruses, such as cytomegalovirus (CMV), may not produce detectable CPEs for weeks, during which time the general condition of the inoculated monolayers and even uninfected control monolayers may deteriorate unless fresh medium is maintained.

Direct Examination

Tissue Pathology

For some viruses, direct histopathology can provide a presumptive diagnosis. Most of the procedures are dependent on a typical histopathologic appearance of the virus that is present during active infection. The viruses most likely to be detected are herpes simplex and herpes zoster viruses and CMV. Cutaneous lesions, such as vesicles, macules, or pustules, may also be examined for the presence of multinucleated giant cells and inclusion-bearing cells. Materials obtained from such lesions can be examined easily and quickly. The vesicle is sponged with alcohol (if no virus cultures are to be taken from the lesion), and the roof of the vesicle is reflected. The fluid is blotted and the base of the lesion is scraped, with gross bleeding avoided when possible. A scraping of cells at the base of a young vesicle suspected of containing herpes simplex or varicella zoster virus can be spread onto a slide, fixed with methyl alcohol, and stained with hematoxylin-eosin, Wright's, or freshly made Giemsa stains. On direct light microscopy, multinucleated giant cells, intranuclear inclusions, or both in a lesion would indicate an infection with either herpes simplex or herpes (varicella) zoster. These stains cannot, however, differentiate between these two herpesviruses. The sensitivity of these staining methods depends heavily on the skill with which the specimen is prepared, stained, and examined, but in experienced hands this method, originally described by Tzanck, is useful in guiding therapy and prognosis. Similarly, herpes simplex infection of the female genital tract can be diagnosed by obtaining a swab of the cervix and examining it by Papanicolaou stain for giant cells and intranuclear inclusions. Another similar direct procedure examines urine samples for cytomegalic cells. Although only 25% to 50% of urine from infants with cytomegalic inclusion disease (CID) will have these large cells with intranuclear inclusions, they are diagnostic of congenital CMV infection except in rare cases of neonatal herpes simplex virus infection. Beyond the neonatal period, however, this test is of no value in diagnosing acute CMV infection. Similar samples and staining methods have been used to diagnose measles by scraping of Koplik spots.

Tissue specimens can be examined for the presence of multinucleated giant cells containing intranuclear inclusions, which is strong evidence for the presence of either herpes simplex virus or varicella zoster virus. In addition, tissue samples can be examined for cytomegalovirus. The presence of large 25 to 40 μm cells with 8 to 10 μm intranuclear inclusions that stain eosinophilic with hematoxylin-eosin stain are typical of CMV infection. However, CMV can invade tissues without producing morphologic changes. Therefore failure to find cytomegalic cells does not exclude CMV infection. Virologic or serologic confirmation of histologic findings is necessary for definitive diagnosis.

Electron Microscopy

Direct and rapid diagnosis of viral infections can be accomplished by ultrastructural study in limited clinical situations. Negative staining with heavy metal salts allows electron microscopic visualization and morphologic characterization of the virus group. For electron microscopy (EM) to be useful, large numbers of morphologically distinct virus particles must be present in the clinical sample and the particles must be sufficiently free of background debris to permit recognition of viral morphology. An electron microscope scans a field of approximately 1 millionth of a milliliter; therefore the specimen must contain at least 1 million viruses per milliliter for detection to be made. Such levels of excretion are normally present only during the first 48 hours of viral diarrhea.

The sensitivity of direct visualization by electron microscopy can be increased with use of the pseudoreplica technique, in which the specimen is added to an agarose surface and the virus is subsequently collected onto a form or film. This serves to concentrate the virus in the specimen as the fluid and interfixing substance such as salts are absorbed into the agarose. This technique may permit detection of human CMV in urine specimens with a particle concentration as low as 1×10^4/mL. Sensitivity of EM for virus detection has also been increased with the use of high-speed centrifugation to pellet virus directly onto the specimen grid. Also, the use of specific antisera causes adherence of virions to antibody and results in clumping of virus particles. This clumping permits detection of virus present in smaller quantities, 10^4 particles. Electron microscopy particularly is useful for detecting viruses that will not readily grow in cell culture or are difficult to grow, such as the agents of gastroenteritis, Norwalk agent, astroviruses, caliciviruses, rotaviruses, minirotaviruses, and adenovirus types 40 and 41. Historically, discovery of the etiologic agent of hepatitis B was accomplished by ultrastructural visualization of the virus. Electron microscopy (EM) of vesicular lesion fluid distinguishes members of the herpes virus group from members of the poxvirus group. Unfortunately, most clinical specimens, including tissue samples, have too few virus particles for the viruses to be visualized directly by electron microscopy. Stool is an ideal specimen for electron microscopy, however, since many noncultivable viruses are found in large numbers in the stool. Rotavirus, for example, has a distinctive double-wheel shape and distinct size, 70 nm in diameter, and is found in quantities up to 10^{11} virus particles per gram of feces.

Antigen Detection

Immunofluorescence

One of the oldest and most widely used techniques in the clinical laboratory is immunofluorescence microscopy. This procedure is technically simple, and it is probably the most broadly applicable rapid technique practiced in diagnostic laboratories today. The immunofluorescence staining protocol may be direct or indirect. The direct procedure uses a fluorescence-labeled specific antibody; for the indirect procedure, a fluorescence-labeled antiglobulin is used to detect the unlabeled specific antibody. Meticulous preparation of materials is required, and antisera must be both sensitive and specific. The advent of specific monoclonal antibodies for use as antisera has increased the specificity and in some cases the sensitivity of these assays. Immunofluorescent staining may be used for rapid virus identification on the direct specimen, or the technique may be used for confirmation of CPE seen in cell culture. However, the technique is somewhat time consuming and highly dependent on the quality of reagents, and of course it requires a fluorescence microscope. There is no objective end point; a conclusion or laboratory diagnosis is based mainly on experience and judgment. Other potential difficulties include the collection and preparation of a suitable specimen, autofluorescence, and nonspecific binding of antibody molecules.

Even so, immunofluorescence microscopy by an experienced person is useful for rapid identification of certain viruses, such as respiratory viruses. Respiratory epithelial cells obtained by elution of cells from a nasal washing or a nasopharyngeal swab or by aspiration of endotracheal secretions may be examined with the use of monoclonal antibodies directed against many of the common respiratory viruses (RSV, parainfluenza 1, 2, 3, influenza A and B, and adenovirus). The method provides an etiologic diagnosis within one working day. Also, with the use of monoclonal antibody specific for CMV immediate early antigens (IEA), the presence of CMV in cell culture can be determined in some cases days before cytopathic effects are recognized. Monoclonal antibodies conjugated to fluorescence isothionate (FITC) can be used to subtype viral species, such as herpes simplex virus (HSV) type 1 and type 2.

Immunoperoxidase staining is similar to immunofluorescence staining and is the preferred technique in some laboratories. The procedure entails a few additional steps; however, it requires only a light microscope. It permits antigen-specific staining on a background of standard staining, can be performed on paraffin-embedded tissue, and results in permanent slides. In addition to eluted cells from clinical specimens, immunofluorescence or immunoperoxidase staining may be used on tissue touch preparations or on frozen tissue sections fixed in acetone. Although immunofluorescence and immunoperoxidase techniques are now widely used in diagnostic laboratories, reagents are available for only a limited number of clinically important viruses and testing of patient samples requires multiple antisera.

Solid-phase Immunoassays

All solid-phase immunoassays depend on the immobilization of either antigen or antibody on a surface, followed by a series of interactions with antibody or antigen. These end either with visible particle agglutination or in RIAs and EIAs in the attachment of a marked molecule, which is quantitated as a measure of the amount of antigen or antibody bound at some earlier step.

If the surface is a particle, agglutination can occur in the presence of antigen and antibody. Agglutination tests depend on the initial attachment of specific antiviral antibodies to erythrocytes or latex particles. This reagent is then incubated with the clinical sample in which antigen is sought, and the particles agglutinate if adequate antigen is present. These tests are generally supplemented or confirmed by other tests because of a high percentage of nonspecific reactions.

Since the first use of RIA methods for the detection of insulin in human plasma in 1959, there has been a tremendous growth in the use of immunologically labeled reagents for detecting infectious diseases. Identification of hepatitis B virus (HBV) in human sera made it essential that a means of antigen detection be developed to screen donor blood. Solid-phase immunoassays have progressed to the currently used RIAs and EIAs.

RIA procedures are rapid and sensitive, have an objective end point, and can be automated. RIAs that use ^{125}I or ^{131}I can detect either antigens or antibodies. Either the antigen or the antibody is labeled with isotope and processed by standard procedures. The test is extremely sensitive and can detect substances present in nanogram- or picogram-per-milliliter quantities, such as the hepatitis B surface antigen in serum. However, the use of EIAs with their longer reagent shelf life, relative low cost, and lack of radioactivity, have supplanted RIA procedures in most instances of viral antigen detection. EIA is essentially similar to solid-phase RIA and has similar sensitivity. These assays are capable of measuring nanogram quantities of protein and have an objective end point. Frequently this equates with 10^3 to 10^4 infectious virus particles. The specificity is often much less in clinical specimens than in cell cultures because of contaminants in the specimen, such as bacteria. EIAs can be applied to a large volume of samples and can also be automated. They are stable and do not carry the potential hazards of radioisotopes. However, the disadvantages of EIAs include the carcinogenicity of some reagents, the expense of the automated equipment used, and insufficient sensitivity.

EIAs for antigen detection most often are based on a capture antibody bound to a solid phase, usually a microtiter well or a plastic bead. A viral antigen present in a clinical specimen binds to the antibody bound to the solid phase. The bound viral antigen is then detected with another antibody, which is conjugated to an enzyme either directly or by means of an indirect sandwich technique. The bound enzyme is then detected and quantitated by the development of color or fluorescence when an appropriate substrate is added. These assays can be performed with automated equipment, the results can be read in seconds by specially designed spectrophotometers, and the data can be promptly collated and analyzed by computer. Some EIA assays are Food and Drug Administration (FDA) approved for visual reading of the color reaction, therefore eliminating the use of a spectrophotometer. Such assays can detect various viral pathogens, such as rotavirus, Norwalk agent, adenovirus, and RSV, but in many infections insufficient virus is present for successful detection of the pathogen.

For routine diagnostic virology, immunoenzymatic methods are of value in the direct detection of some viral antigens in selected clinical samples, detection and identification of viral antigen in cell culture, rapid typing of viruses isolated in cell culture, and serologic study. As mentioned before, EIAs are capable of detecting virus to a limit of 10^3 to 10^4 infectious virus particles. Therefore, relatively large amounts of antigen must be present in clinical samples to be measurable by these methods. The specificity is often much less in clinical specimens than in cell cultures because of contaminants in the specimen, such as bacteria.

Ideally, a rapid technique would be at least as sensitive as virus isolation, but available assays currently fall short of this goal. Even the introduction of monoclonal antibodies has not improved the sensitivity of these assays to that of virus isolation. Specificity, however, has been improved since the advent of monoclonal antibodies. There are two reasons why the sensitivity of rapid antigen tests have reached the maximum level of sensitivity achievable by these tests and not significantly improved beyond that point. First, solid-phase assays require multiple washes, and a certain number of specific antigen-antibody complexes are also removed. Moreover, monoclonal antibodies often have low-affinity constants, and they make poor candidates for use in immunoassays that require high-affinity antibodies. Therefore specific binding is less than optimal.

Further advances in EIA protocols have led to the enzyme immunofiltration staining assay in which cells and cell debris from clinical specimens are nonspecifically captured and immobilized on the solid phase, which consists of glass fiber filters contained in a specially designed filtration manifold. This technique differs from other methods that capture soluble viral antigens with the use of agent-specific capture antibodies.

The problem of low-affinity constant monoclonal antibodies is overcome by use of the avidin-biotin complex. Avidin and biotin have a very strong affinity for each other. Viral antigens first bind biotinylated monoclonal antibodies, which then bind streptavidin conjugated to horseradish peroxidase. Each IgG molecule of the specific monoclonal may bind four biotin molecules, which in turn will bind the streptavidin–horseradish peroxidase complex. An insoluble red reaction product forms on the infected cells after the enzyme substrate, 3-amino-9-ethyl carbazole (AEC) is added. Therefore the test reaction is amplified without altering sensitivity or specificity. The immunofiltration method is rapid, inexpensive, and technically easy to perform, does not require complicated equipment, and is applicable to multiple viral agents.

From a practical point of view, in addition to being limited by insufficient amounts of viral antigens in certain infections and certain specimens, diagnostic laboratories are limited by commercial availability of reagents, especially specific monoclonal antibodies, so that experience with immunoassays for some viruses has been limited to a few research laboratories.

Nucleic Acid Hybridization

DNA in its natural state is composed of two complementary strands of deoxyribonucleotide polymers joined in an antiparallel arrangement to form a stable double helix. The linkage between the double strands is through hydrogen bonds formed between the complementary bases. The double-stranded helix can be "denatured" into single strands by breaking the hydrogen bonds by heat or alkali. On cooling, the single strands will reanneal or hybridize to re-form double-stranded DNA.

With the use of molecular cloning procedures, large quantities of specific nucleic acids can be generated for use as probes in hybridization assays for clinical diagnosis. A probe for specific viral nucleic acid is produced by cloning a DNA fragment that represents a subfragment or the entire genome of an organism to screen for the presence of the organism. The discovery of restriction endonucleases has made it possible to excise selected nucleotide sequences from nucleic acids. These extracted sequences, called restriction fragments, can then be labeled, denatured, and used as probes to detect the presence of specific genes unique to a particular virus.

There are myriad hybridization protocols described in the literature. In addition to DNA-DNA hybridization, RNA-RNA and RNA-DNA hybridizations have been described. Each hybridization protocol falls into one of three categories: solid support hybridization, solution hybridization, or in situ hybridization. Most protocols for detecting viral nucleic acid use solid support hybridization. Target or probe nucleic acids may be immobilized on solid supports (dual-phase hybridizations) or in solution (single-phase hybridization). Nevertheless, all hybridization protocols share four phases: (1) preparation of the sample or target nucleic acids, (2) preparation of the reference probe, (3) the hybridization reaction, and (4) the detection of hybrid formation.

Solid-support hybridization involves the dotting of sample nucleic acid onto nitrocellulose filters. Single-stranded DNA or RNA is immobilized directly onto a filter and then hybridized with the desired single-stranded specific radiolabeled probe. However, a major problem with nucleic acid hybridization done on solid supports is that less than 10% of sample DNA is available for hybridization. Hybridization performed in solution alleviates this problem by making the entire specimen accessible to the probe. In situ hybridization employs a thin section of tissue to which a desired probe is directly hybridized. In situ hybridization is particularly useful for identifying the specific cells infected by an infectious agent or the number of copies of the organism infecting a given cell.

The polymerase chain reaction (PCR) is an ingenious tool

of molecular biology that is so sensitive that a single DNA molecule can be amplified, and single-copy genes are routinely extracted out of complex mixtures of genomic sequences and visualized as distinct bands on agarose gels. There are many diverse PCR applications throughout scientific and medical research. The DNA sample that one wishes to copy can be pure, or it can be a minute part of an extremely complex mixture of biologic materials. The natural function of DNA polymerase is to repair and replicate DNA. These enzymes can lengthen a short oligonucleotide "primer" by attaching an additional nucleotide to its 3′ end, but only if the primer is hybridized, or bound, to a complementary strand called a template. For the reaction to occur, the surrounding solution must also contain nucleotide triphosphate molecules as building blocks. The nucleotide to which the polymerase attaches will be complementary to the base in the corresponding position on the template strand. By repeating this process over and over, the polymerase can extend the 3′ end of the primer all the way to the 5′ terminus of the template. The fragment of specific viral DNA can be amplified through PCR to a level at which the viral DNA can be detected by standard hybridization procedures.

In principle, nucleic acid hybridization techniques can be applied to detect any microorganism, and these techniques have been applied to a wide range of DNA and RNA viruses. Some viruses for which cloned probes are currently being developed and tested include adenovirus, CMV, Epstein-Barr virus (EBV), enterovirus, HSV-1 and HSV-2, HBV, influenza virus, parainfluenza virus, RSV, and rotavirus.

At present, however, none of these tests is routinely available to the clinical diagnostic virology laboratory, and nucleic acid probes are still reserved for the most part for a small but growing number of research laboratories. Several advances in technology are required before such detection systems can be used regularly by clinical laboratories. Simplification of hybridization procedures, the development of sensitive and inexpensive nonisotopic detection systems, standardization of the techniques, and the availability of specific probes will be necessary and no doubt will come about in the near future. With the specificity of these hybridization techniques coupled with the extreme sensitivity of PCR, clinical relevance of the viral nucleic acid detected in patient specimens may become the major issue in interpretation of laboratory results, particularly for viruses known to remain latent in the human host after primary infection.

Despite these obstacles, nucleic acid hybridization has a great potential to influence how we diagnose viral infections, especially since the advent of the PCR technology.

Antibody Measurement

Most acute primary viral infections induce an increase in serum antibody that can be used for diagnosis. Exceptions involve infections in immunoincompetent hosts, including certain young infants, and acute infections acquired in the presence of passively transferred antibody, such as perinatally acquired CMV, HSV, and human immunodeficiency virus (HIV) infections. Although serodiagnosis is useful in clinical virology, it usually cannot provide a definitive diagnosis during the acute phase of an illness because sera from both acute and convalescent phases are required. A single serum can tell only whether the person has ever been infected with virus.

Standard Serologic Procedures

The conventional methods for serodiagnosis of viral infections include complement fixation (CF), neutralization, hemagglutination inhibition (HI), and in certain infections passive hemagglutination (PHA). Each of these procedures has its advantages and limitations, and none is uniformly applicable to all of the common viral infections of humans.

The CF test has been the most widely used in vitro method for serodiagnosis of viral infections because of its versatility, broad reactivity, and effectiveness in detecting rises in antibody titer. It is a functional antibody assay that is used to assess many antigen-antibody systems, but it is also independent of specific antiviral functions. However, its disadvantage is that it is relatively insensitive, particularly for detecting antibody of long duration, and the test requires high concentrations of antigen. Reliable CF antigens are not available for all the important human viruses. Also, valid results cannot be obtained on anticomplementary sera or those containing antibodies against host components.

However, CF offers a relatively rapid, efficient way of screening sera for a number of viral antibodies. It is particularly useful in determining that recent infection has occurred. As a general rule, the antibodies detected are virus group–specific and not type-specific. For example, adenovirus antibody to type 1 adenovirus can be distinguished from poliovirus antibody, but antibody to type 1 adenovirus cannot be distinguished from any other adenovirus CF antibody. CF antibodies usually decline more rapidly than do specific neutralizing antibodies. Therefore their absence does not necessarily eliminate suspicion of the virus in question.

The neutralization test is based on the reaction of antibody with virus to render it noninfectious for a susceptible host. One of the major limitations of the procedure is that it depends on cell culture, which is time-consuming, to obtain results. The major advantage of neutralization is its specificity. Neutralizing antibody is of long duration, and in many cases its presence is associated with host immunity.

The HI test is based on the property that some viruses can agglutinate erythrocytes of certain species; however, combination of the virus with specific antibody will prevent this reaction. Therefore this test will assess the ability of antibody to block a specific viral infection. Viral antibody can be assayed by demonstrating ability of the test serum to inhibit agglutination of red blood cells (RBCs) by a standard dose of viral antigen. The HI tests are limited (1) by the fact that nonantibody serum components may inhibit hemagglutination, which must be removed or inactivated before a valid antibody assay can be performed, and (2) by the fact that not all viruses have a hemagglutinin. The advantages of the HI test are that it is inexpensive, that it is easy to perform an in vitro system, that it yields results in 24 hours while maintaining sensitivity, and that its specificity is similar to that of the neutralization test.

Other tests, such as indirect immunofluorescence (IF) or immunoperoxidase (IP) techniques, are more cumbersome than other in vitro viral antibody assays since they require microscopic reading and are therefore generally reserved for those infections for which other adequately sensitive and specific in vitro tests are not available, such as EBV infections and arenavirus infections. Improved technology has led the way for solid-phase indirect EIA systems that use instrument readings for viral antibody assays.

PHA tests are useful in vitro systems for viruses that do not hemagglutinate RBCs directly (e.g., human herpesviruses and HBV). The tests are simple and relatively sensitive and can detect viral antibody of the IgM class. Improved methods for stabilization and storage of antigen-coated RBCs have made the procedures more practical for routine use. Disadvantages are the requirement for purified antigens in some cases and occasional nonspecific agglutination of RBCs by the test sera. Erythrocytes can be made to absorb viral antigens to their surface by treatment with tannic acid, glutaraldehyde, or chromic chloride, and these can be used in PHA tests for assay of viral antibodies.

In interpreting any of these traditional test procedures, the commonly accepted serologic confirmation of acute infection is a fourfold or greater rise in antibody titer when serial twofold dilutions of serum are employed.

Newer Methods for Assay of Viral Antibodies

In recent years, newer methods have been developed for detection of viral antibodies and have proved to be improvements over conventional tests in many cases in terms of economy, sensitivity, specificity, or rapidity. These assays do not measure the function of antibody.

Solid-phase indirect RIAs, in which antigen in the form of virus-infected cells, lysates of infected cells, or purified virus is immobilized on plastic microtiter plates or beads, have shown high sensitivity for detection of viral antibody. Although efforts generally have been made to substitute EIA procedures for RIA in viral antibody assays, the high sensitivity of RIA may make this a (more) satisfactory approach for detecting low levels of viral antibody in fluids such as cerebrospinal fluid. RIA is also useful for detecting viral antibodies in eluates from virus-infected tissues and can be a useful tool for indirectly identifying the presence of virus in tissues from certain chronic diseases.

Solid-phase indirect EIAs, commonly referred to as ELISA, have been widely applied in recent years to the assay of viral antibodies. They have become standard and routine serologic procedures for detection of antibodies against many viral agents. Viral antigens are immobilized on a solid phase (bead, microtiter cup, or plastic paddle); test sera are added; incubation is followed by thorough washings; and antibodies coupled with the test antigen are detected through addition of an enzyme-labeled antispecies immune globulin, followed by the appropriate substrate. Results can be read with a spectrophotometer or fluorimeter and in some cases visually. This system is most suitable for assay of viral antibodies of the IgG class.

RIAs, EIAs, and quantitative immunofluorescence report numerical values that have no obvious correlation with traditional results given as the reciprocal of twofold serum dilutions. To interpret each test, a new set of values must be compared to the accepted standards. There is no major guideline interpretation of the newer tests corresponding to a fourfold rise in titer that can be applied to such tests as CF, HI, and neutralization. Each method requires individual interpretation. Currently such serologic procedures are coming into general use.

The EIA systems for assay of viral antibodies are now becoming available from commercial sources. In evaluating these kits, researchers have found that results have generally been in agreement with those of standard assay procedures, but some problems have been encountered in obtaining reproducible results on sera containing low levels of antibody. This has resulted in setting higher levels for positive readings and in establishing an equivocal range of results, which requires the performance of another type of backup antibody assay. It has also become apparent that results obtained from EIA systems are not linearly proportional to antibody titers and that the antibody in a test serum cannot be accurately quantitated from results on a single concentration of the serum. This is related to variations in specificities, affinities, and immunoglobulin classes in the antibody responses of different individuals to a viral infection. Many laboratories are dependent on the manufacturers' standards and are not aware of the limitations of the prelicensure testing or of the variability of tests.

Advantages of these EIA tests include versatility, sensitivity, objectivity when read by instrument, adaptability of automation, lack of interference by nonspecific inhibitors in test sera, stability, and safety of the labeled antibodies. In practice, they have shown greater ability than conventional serologic procedures to demonstrate seroconversion. The use of purified viral subunit antigens can increase the specificity and diagnostic value of EIAs, for example, to detect subtype-specific antibody titer elevations to H2 or H3 hemagglutinin of influenza A viruses or type-specific antibody responses to HSV. EIA is also a useful test for the measurement of antibodies to human retroviruses.

Other Newer Methods for Assay of Viral Antibodies

Latex Agglutination Tests

A test using latex particles coated with rubella antigen has been developed in recent years to test for rubella antibody. A drop of test serum is mixed with a drop of the antigen preparation, and a positive agglutination reaction is demonstrable within a few minutes. For the most part, this test has shown a sensitivity for rubella antibody detection or for demonstration of seroconversion similar to those of HI and neutralization. Sera with high levels of rubella antibody may give a prozone reaction when tested undiluted, and for this reason it may be desirable to examine diluted as well as undiluted sera. Preliminary evidence suggests that it may be able to detect IgM as well as IgG viral antibody. Because of its simplicity, rapidity, and economy, this test system probably will be extended for assay of antibodies to a wider range of viral agents.

Significance of Antibody Measurement to Rapid Viral Diagnosis

The antibody response in the human host is polyclonal, and it is frequently useful to dissect the temporal pattern of antibody formation against a specific viral antigen. For example, antibodies against virus capsid antigen (VCA) of EBV appear earlier than antibodies against Epstein-Barr nuclear antigen (EBNA); the sequential samples that document the appearance of EBNA antibodies provide evidence of recent infection. Similarly, detection of antibody against hepatitis B surface antigen (HBsAg) signifies infection with this virus at some time in the past and rules out the possibility of chronic carriage. Antibody to hepatitis B core antigen does not rule out the possibility of chronic HBV carriage, and an HBsAg determination has to be made if that information is relevant.

Difficulties in the use of antibody measurement are encountered often. There are immune-deficient persons who cannot form antibody and for whom antibody is therefore not a reliable measure. The newborn infant who has passively acquired maternal antibodies will transiently have antibody, regardless of whether he or she is infected. The presence of maternal antibody against CMV will temporarily obscure development of antibody by the baby if he or she should become infected.

In some instances the speed of specificity of viral serodiagnosis may be improved by the assay of viral antibodies in specific classes of immunoglobulins, particularly IgM. The postnatal viral infections IgM antibodies characteristically appear within 7 to 10 days after infection and generally persist at detectable levels for between 3 and 6 months. Thus the presence of viral IgM antibody implies a current or recent infection with the agent, and this offers the possibility of making a rapid diagnosis by demonstrating viral IgM in a single, acute-phase serum specimen, for example, for hepatitis A infection. Since maternal IgM antibody does not cross the placenta, virus-specific IgM in the newborn can be assumed to be a result of congenital infection, and viral IgM assays can provide a more rapid diagnosis than can be achieved by demonstrating persistence of antibody in a later specimen taken from the infant at a time when maternal antibody would have disappeared. Rubella-specific IgM antibody in a newborn infant is diagnostic of intrauterine infection. There continue to be technical problems with many IgM assays, including rheumatoid factor, which needs to be absorbed from serum. Unfortunately, IgM responses against other viruses in older children and adults are variable. The antibodies may last for months and may reappear with reactivation or reinfection, making the diagnosis of acute infection unreliable.

FURTHER READING

Books and Reviews

Hsiung GD: Diagnostic Virology, ed 3. New Haven, Yale University Press, 1982

Innis MA, Gelfand DH, Sninsky JJ, White TJ (eds): PCR Protocols: A Guide to Methods and Applications. San Diego, Academic Press, Inc, 1990

Lennette EH, Schmidt NJ (eds): Diagnostic Procedures for Viral, Rickettsial and Chlamydial Infections, ed 5. Washington, DC, American Public Health Association, 1979

McIntosh K: Diagnostic Virology. In Fields BN, Knipe DM, Chanock RM, et al (eds): Virology, ed 2. New York, Raven Press, 1990

Spector SA, Dankner WM: Rapid Viral Diagnostic Techniques. In Aronoff SC, Hughes WT, Kohl S, et al (eds): Advances in Pediatric Infectious Diseases, vol 1. Chicago, Year Book Medical Publishers, 1986

Viral agents of gastroenteritis: Public health importance and outbreak management. MMWR vol 39, April 27, 1990

Yolken RH: Laboratory diagnosis of viral infections. In Galasso GJ, Whitley RJ, Merigan TC (eds): Antiviral Agents and Viral Diseases of Man, ed 3. New York, Raven Press, Ltd., 1990

Selected Papers

Cleveland PH, Richman DD: Enzyme immunofiltration staining assay for immediate diagnosis of herpes simplex virus and varicella zoster virus directly from clinical specimens. J Clin Microbiol 25:416, 1987

Eisenstein BI: The polymerase chain reaction: A new method of using molecular genetics for medical diagnosis. N Engl J Med 322:178, 1990

Meegan JM, Evans B, Horstmann DM: Comparison of the latex agglutination test with the hemagglutination inhibition test, enzyme-linked immunosorbent assay, and neutralization test for detection of antibodies to rubella virus. J Clin Microbiol 16:644, 1982

Mullis KB: The unusual origin of the polymerase chain reaction. Sci Am 56:262, April 1990

Richmond DD, et al: Rapid viral diagnosis. J Infect Dis 149:298, 1984

Sever JL, Tzan NR, Schekrachi IC, Madden DL: Rapid latex agglutination test for rubella antibody. J Clin Microbiol 17:52, 1983

CHAPTER 63

Poxviruses

Poxviruses causing disease in vertebrates are divided into eight established genera (Table 53–4). Of these, only four genera (*Orthopoxvirus, Parapoxvirus, Molluscipoxvirus*, and *Yatapoxvirus*) contain viruses that can cause human disease. Historically, the most important of these is the genus *Orthopoxvirus*, which includes smallpox (variola), vaccinia, monkeypox, cowpox, and camelpox viruses, raccoon poxvirus, tatera poxvirus, vole poxvirus, Uasin Gishu poxvirus, and mousepox (ectromelia) virus (Table 63–1). Smallpox was a major worldwide health problem until its global eradication in 1979. A resurgence of interest in poxviridae has occurred because one of the family members, vaccinia, may be useful as a vaccine vector for the prevention of a number of other infectious diseases.

Smallpox

History

For more than 3000 years, smallpox was an extremely important infectious and communicable disease worldwide. Now the disease is of primarily historical significance. Smallpox is the only infectious disease that has been eradicated through the conscious and intensive efforts of man.

Pharaoh Ramses V is considered the earliest known victim of smallpox. His mummified remains from 1157 BC have lesions suggesting smallpox. Early epidemics were apparently confined to the Orient, the Middle East, and Africa until Arab expeditions carried the disease into Europe during the sixth century. The term *smallpox* distinguished the disease from great pox (syphilis) until AD 570, when Bishop Marius of Avenches used the term *variola* to describe an epidemic in Italy and France. The disease was devastating, with high mortality rates. In 1707, 18,000 of Iceland's 50,000 people died of smallpox. Fourteen years later, 5889 of Boston's 12,000 inhabitants were infected with smallpox, with a fatality rate of 15%.

The first attempt at preventing smallpox was variolation, or the inoculation of smallpox from a nonfatal case. The fatality rate was 2% with this practice, a marked improvement over naturally acquired disease. Intradermal inoculation rather than acquisition of virus by inhalation may have been important in diminishing the severity of infection. By 1792, when another outbreak arrived in Boston, 97% of the population had been inoculated. Edward Jenner's first vaccinations were given in 1796, but it took more than 100 years before epidemics were eliminated from the United States and Europe.

The World Health Organization started its eradication program in 1966, and the last naturally occurring case of smallpox was detected in Merka, Somalia, in October 1977. The last two cases of smallpox were in 1978 and were associated with a laboratory exposure. Since 1984 the only known reservoirs of the virus have been the Centers for Disease Control in Atlanta and the Research Institute for Viral Preparations in Moscow.

Epidemiology

Man is the only natural host for smallpox, a fact that was crucial to the eradication of the disease. Primates have been infected in the laboratory but did not acquire natural disease when smallpox was endemic. Another factor important to the eradication program was that asymptomatic infection did not occur or occurred rarely. Persons were infected and communicable before the disease was recognized, but asymptomatic carriage was unknown. Transmission was from one person to another, primarily by respiratory tract secretions. Virus has

TABLE 63–1. SPECIES OF THE GENUS *ORTHOPOXVIRUS*

Species	Natural Infection of Man	Natural Animal Host
Camelpox virus	N	Camel
Cowpox virus	Y	Cow, elephant, gerbil, rat, carnivores
Ectromelia virus	N	Mouse, ?vole
Monkeypox virus	Y	Monkey, great ape, squirrel, anteater
Raccoon poxvirus	N	Raccoon
Tatera poxvirus	N	Gerbil
Uasin Gishu poxvirus	N	Horse
Vaccinia virus	Y	Buffalo, cow, pig, rabbit
Variola virus	Y	None
Vole poxvirus	N	Vole

been recovered from sloughed scabs long after the illness, although this was a minor mode of transmission. Once the virus was introduced into a community, it could be passed to those individuals who had never been infected with smallpox or immunized with vaccinia virus. It was originally thought that smallpox was a highly contagious disease, similar to varicella. Careful epidemiologic studies during the eradication program showed that it was a more slowly moving disease with secondary attack rates of 26% to 44%.

Clinical Features

Figure 63–1 illustrates the typical course of infection with smallpox. After an incubation period of 7 to 17 days, there was an acute onset of high fever, headache, chills, back pain, and prostration lasting 2 to 4 days. The temperature dropped as the rash started, initially with maculopapules on the face or hands and forearms, and then on the trunk and legs. The lesions became vesicular within 24 to 48 hours and often umbilicated. By the seventh to the ninth day, they were frank pustules. The pustules dried, and scabbing began with crusts separating about the twelfth or thirteenth day. A secondary fever was common at about this time as part of the disease and was not necessarily due to secondary bacterial infection. The mortality rate was 30% among unvaccinated persons, but only 3% among those who had been previously vaccinated.

The spectrum of illness included patients with flat lesions, where the pocks were soft and velvety with little if any projection above the surrounding skin. Mortality from this form was 94% in unvaccinated individuals. The most severe illness was described as hemorrhagic because extensive bleeding appeared during the prodrome, with death occurring during the first week of illness. The overall mortality was 95% to 100%.

Modified illness occurred primarily in individuals who had been previously vaccinated. The prodrome was often severe, but few lesions developed and they were completely crusted within 10 days. There was no associated mortality.

The above descriptions and mortality figures refer to classic smallpox or variola major. Variola minor (alastrim) and intermediate strains produced the same four clinical pictures, but there was a marked shift toward the modified form. Variola minor had a case-fatality rate of 1% to 1.5%.

The most common complications were secondary bacterial infections of the skin and respiratory tract. In addition, keratitis with corneal damage, encephalitis, and peripheral neuritis were seen. Treatment consisted of supportive therapy and appropriate management of any secondary complications. *N*-methylisatin-β-thiosemicarbazone (methisazone) had very little benefit in established cases.

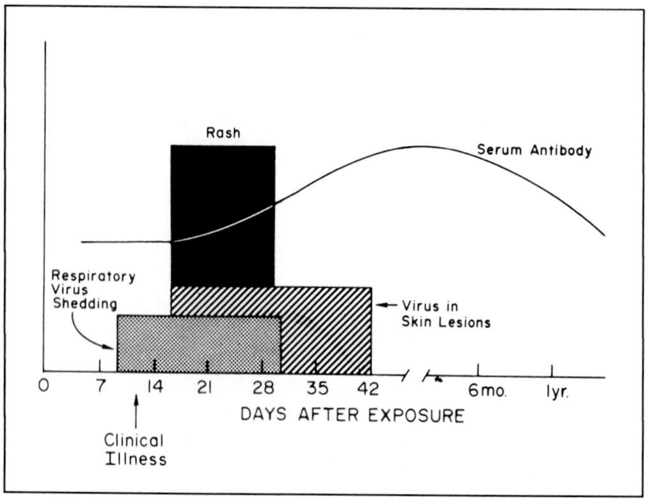

Fig. 63–1. The course of infection with smallpox.

Pathology and Pathogenesis

The virus entered by way of the respiratory tract and spread to regional lymph nodes. A primary viremia led to dissemination to liver, spleen, bone marrow, lymph nodes, and lung. After additional replication, there was a secondary viremia and spread to the skin and mucous membranes. The skin lesions showed swollen epithelial cells with cytoplasmic inclusions (Guarnieri bodies) before vesicle formation.

Diagnosis

Originally, the clinical diagnosis of smallpox was based on the course of the disease, contact, and susceptibility. Laboratory diagnosis is now essential for any suspected cases. Rapid diagnosis is possible with direct visualization of a poxvirus under the electron microscope or agar gel precipitation for viral antigens. At the time smallpox was eradicated, the optimal method for differentiating between poxviruses was to characterize the DNA after digestion by restriction endonucleases. Fluorescent antibody and complement fixation techniques have been used to detect antigens. Identification is also possible by isolation of the virus on the chorioallantoic membrane of fertilized eggs, where characteristic pocks will form. A retrospective diagnosis can be made with a variety of serologic methods.

Prevention

Smallpox has been eradicated through the use of vaccination. Inoculation with vaccinia confers protective immunity for a period of 3 to 20 years. Protection is longer after natural infection with smallpox. Vaccination is now recommended only for those laboratory workers directly involved with the use of poxviruses. Methisazone was effective in decreasing the secondary spread among susceptible individuals. Vaccinia-immune globulin has also been used to provide transient protection.

Vaccinia

In 1757 Edward Jenner at 8 years of age, underwent the customary treatment—being bled, purged, and dieted—and then was inoculated with smallpox. Jenner continued this practice after he became a country physician in England. However, he noticed that variolation did not succeed among persons who gave a history of having acquired lesions on their hands after contact with pox lesions on cows. In 1796 he took pus from a lesion on the hand of a milkmaid and inoculated it superficially into the arm of an 8-year-old boy. There was a local reaction only, and 7 weeks later the boy was inoculated with material from a smallpox pustule. There was no disease. After repeating these experiments, Jenner published his findings in 1798.

It is not possible to establish with any certainty what virus Jenner actually used, or what happened to it over nearly two centuries of passage through animal and man. Jenner believed his virus actually came from horsepox that had been passed in cows before transfer to man. Over the years, Jenner's virus has been passaged in humans, cattle, and sheep. In some places, it has even been mixed with smallpox. DNA analysis shows distinct differences between vaccinia, cowpox, and smallpox. It is not clear whether vaccinia represents genetic recombination, a new species of smallpox or cowpox virus derived by serial passage, or a species that no longer exists in nature.

Vaccinia is administered intradermally by puncture or scarification or by air jet. There are three basic responses that can be seen. The vaccinia or primary response occurs if there is no existing immunity. A papule appears at the site of inoculation by the third or fourth day. This progresses to become a pustule by the eighth to tenth day and then crusts over. The scab falls off after about 3 weeks, leaving a typical pockmark.

A vaccinoid or accelerated response may be seen in people with partial immunity. The lesion progresses through the same stages as in the vaccinia response but more rapidly and with less intensity. The severity of the reaction corresponds with the level of immunity.

The immediate or "allergic" reaction that has been described is actually a delayed hypersensitivity reaction. It is a response to the viral protein, and thus viral replication is not required. This reaction does not correlate with the presence of protective immunity.

Universal vaccination was not without its complications. One of the more serious risks was progressive vaccinia. The initial lesion failed to heal, with the appearance of secondary lesions elsewhere. The lesions progressed, leading to death in more than 50% of these individuals 2 to 5 months after vaccination. This rare complication occurred only among individuals with a deficient cell-mediated immune system. Treatment with vaccinia-immune globulin or methisazone was rarely effective.

Eczema vaccinatum was much more common. It occurred among those individuals with eczema who were vaccinated or who came in contact with recently vaccinated individuals. Eczema was a contraindication to vaccination in many countries. The mortality rate was 30% to 40% but could be reduced to 7% if vaccinia-immune globulin was used for treatment.

Generalized vaccinia occurred when there was hematogenous spread from the inoculation site. Lesions could appear at multiple distant sites, but each lesion went through the same progression as the primary one. There was no associated immune deficiency. The mortality rate was about 10%. Vaccinia-immune globulin was effective in hastening the resolution of lesions.

Central nervous systems (CNS) disease was the most serious complication of vaccination, with a 25% to 50% mortality rate. Its occurrence was unpredictable and did not depend on an underlying immune defect or skin disorder. The association was proved only by the isolation of vaccinia in rare cases, but the temporal relationship of the clinical course implicated the vaccine. Autopsies on children under 2 years of age usually showed an encephalopathy with histologic findings of brain edema and hyperemia. Older individuals had an encephalitis with demyelinization similar to that seen in other postinfectious encephalitides.

Other less serious complications included secondary bacterial skin infections and autoinoculation, especially to the eye or perineum. Contacts of vaccinated individuals were also at risk of acquiring the virus. Recent complications have been seen in children with underlying diseases who have been exposed to a family member in the military who has received the vaccine. There has also been a case of disseminated vaccinia in a military recruit in whom AIDS was subsequently diagnosed.

The incidence of complications is hard to evaluate. There were many different strains of vaccinia used around the world. The vaccine used in Holland had a high incidence of CNS effects, estimated at 1 in 4000 doses, whereas the vaccine in the United States caused encephalitis in only 2.3 to 2.9 per million vaccinees. Table 63–2 shows the incidence of complications of primary vaccination in a national survey in the United States in 1968. There were six vaccinia-related deaths in that study, or about one death per million doses of vaccine. The number of complications after revaccination was about one-tenth that after primary vaccination, although there were still two vaccinia-related deaths in this group of 8.5 million revaccinations.

The complications of vaccinia eventually outweighed the risk of acquiring smallpox, and routine vaccination of all children was stopped after 1971–1972. Vaccination was continued among hospital personnel until 1976. The eradication of smallpox finally led to the cessation of vaccination and the abolishment of required vaccination for international travel. The resulting savings, including the costs of vaccinations, port health inspections, and the medical treatment required for complications of smallpox vaccination, have been estimated to be about $1 billion annually.

Administration of vaccinia virus has no role in the treatment of any disease. For a short time, vaccinia was administered by some individuals to prevent or treat herpes simplex virus infections. Rather than hasten improvement in these patients, it often caused more severe disease, especially in patients in whom compromised immune systems had not been

TABLE 63–2. COMPLICATION RATES OF PRIMARY SMALLPOX VACCINATION IN UNITED STATES, 1968

		Cases per Million				
Age (y)	No. of Immunizations	Postvaccinia Encephalitis	Progressive Vaccinia	Eczema Vaccinatum	Generalized Vaccinia	Accidental Infection, Other
<1	614,000	6.5	—	8.1	70.0	27.7
1–4	2,733,000	2.2	0.4[a]	11.3	17.2	47.9
5–9	1,533,000	3.2	0.6[a]	7.1	12.9	25.8
10–19	406,000	—	2.5[a]	7.4	12.3	9.9
>19	288,000	3.5[a]	6.9[a]	24.3	45.1	41.3
Total	5,594,000	2.9	0.9	10.4	23.4	37.2

From Lane et al: N Engl J Med 281:1201, 1969.
[a] Based on three or fewer cases.

recognized. The only individuals who should be immunized are laboratory workers involved in poxvirus research.

A newer use for vaccinia is its role as a vector for the expression of other genes. Recombinant DNA techniques have allowed investigators to insert foreign genes into vaccinia. As the vaccinia replicates, these genes are expressed. At least 25 kilobases of foreign DNA can be inserted into the vaccinia virus genome. If a gene that can provoke a protective immune response is used, an effective vaccine can be produced. Several of these vaccines have been tried in animal systems with the production of antibodies and protection when challenged with the pathogen of interest. It is also possible to have a recombinant vaccinia virus that will express multiple foreign genes, raising the possibility that a single inoculation could protect against several different infections. A recombinant vaccinia virus containing genes from herpes simplex virus, hepatitis B, and influenza A has been tried in animals, and antibodies were made to all three antigens. Other poxviruses that have been used as vectors include cowpox virus, raccoon poxvirus, and fowlpox virus.

This work is progressing along several paths. The first is the identification of specific genes that can invoke protection against an infectious agent. Increased expression of these genes with the use of appropriate promoters, as well as the ease of construction of the vector must be considered. Enhancement of the immunologic response is being studied. Equally important are the studies of vaccinia itself aimed at decreasing the pathogenicity of the virus. Several genes that have roles as virulence factors have been identified. In addition, the host range can be narrowed through appropriate mutations. It is clear that recombinant vaccinia vaccines will be useful only where the potential benefit of protection against an agent outweighs the risk of the complications from vaccinia itself.

Monkeypox

Human monkeypox occurs sporadically in the tropical rain forests of west and central Africa, primarily Zaire. The virus was first recovered in 1958 from monkeys that had become ill while in captivity. At least four species of monkey are infected in nature, and there is evidence of infection in chimpanzees. In addition, monkeypox-specific antibodies have been found is several species of squirrel.

The World Health Organization has conducted extensive surveillance of human monkeypox infections. In Zaire there were only 52 cases identified between 1970 and 1981. Surveillance was intensified, and a total of 338 cases were identified in a population of 5 million from 1981 to 1986.

The disease is clinically indistinguishable from smallpox except for the presence of cervical and frequently inguinal lymphadenopathy in monkeypox infections. Infection may be subclinical or may cause an extensive rash. The disease usually lasts 2 to 4 weeks. Prior vaccination against smallpox is at least partially protective. In a study of 250 unvaccinated and 32 vaccinated patients with monkeypox, there were 27 deaths. All were in the unvaccinated group. The case fatality rate was about 11% in this group and was highest among the youngest patients.

Secondary cases occur about 7 to 24 days after contact with a primary case. The attack rate for household contacts is about 11% if there is no prior history of vaccination, compared to about 1.7% if a vaccination scar is present. This low transmission rate makes it unlikely that monkeypox can be sustained in humans alone. The longest reported chain of human-to-human transmission is only five generations. However, monkeypox is endemic in an area where the majority of people have been immunized against smallpox. As the population changes to include more unvaccinated individuals, monkeypox transmission may become more significant.

Cowpox

For years, it has been assumed that all human cases of cowpox were acquired by direct contact with cows. Other data now suggest that rodents are the true natural reservoir of cowpox. Cows, cats, and possibly humans are infected by these rodents. A wide range of zoo and circus animals with cowpox have also been reported. Cowpox is a European disease, with no reports of the virus isolated elsewhere in the world in recent years.

The disease in man is usually found on the hands after contact with an infected animal. It can be spread to other parts of the body, frequently the eye, through autoinoculation. The lesions are similar to those of primary vaccination with vaccinia, with vesicle and pustule formation before scabbing. Local findings, including edema, lymphangitis, and lymphadenitis, may be greater than those that follow vaccination. Fever may persist for a few days. Cowpox in children may be a severe illness.

Diagnosis of cowpox depends on a high index of suspicion. The classic history of milking cows no longer applies. Contact with appropriate animals, consistent skin lesions, and residence in an endemic area should prompt the performance of appropriate cultures and electron microscopy. The disease is self-limited, and only symptomatic care is needed.

Orf

Orf is caused by a member of the genus *Parapoxvirus*. Also known as ecthyma contagiosum, contagious pustular dermatitis, and scabby mouth, it is primarily a disease of young sheep and goats. The virus is found worldwide. Human infection is acquired through direct contact with an infected animal but can also be spread through fomites. The incubation period is about 3 to 6 days, with symptoms lasting from 3 to 24 weeks. The initial lesions are macular at the site of contact but become papular. They then develop a red center with a white ring, surrounded by red, inflamed skin. Central umbilication is seen, followed by a papillomatous stage. Unlike most other poxvirus lesions, these are painful. They may be accompanied by low-grade fever and regional lymphadenopathy.

The diagnosis can be made on a clinical basis. The virus can be cultured, and it has a characteristic appearance on electron microscopy. Lesions require no treatment, and there has been no documented transmission from human to human.

Milker's Nodule Virus

Also known as pseudocowpox or paravaccinia, milker's nodule is caused by another member of the genus *Parapoxvirus*. It is characteristically a disease of cows and is found in all parts of the world. Jenner recognized that there was more than one disease causing vesicular lesions on the teats of cows, not all of which were protective against smallpox. Human infection is acquired through skin abrasions by direct contact with an infected animal. Lesions usually appear 5 to 7 days after contact. The initial lesions are red papules. These enlarge, forming smooth, firm, purple nodules up to 2 cm in diameter. The lesions are painless but may itch. They gradually resolve over 4 to 8 weeks.

Infection with paravaccinia does not confer immunity to cowpox or vaccinia. Immunity to paravaccinia does not last long, and reinfection can occur.

Tanapox

On the basis of morphologic, serologic, and restriction endonuclease analyses, it has been proposed that tanapox virus and the related Yaba monkey tumor virus be placed into a new genus, *Yatapoxvirus*. Tanapox virus was first isolated in 1962 after it caused epidemics in 1957 and 1962 among populations living on the flood plains of the Tana River in Kenya.

Tanapox affects both sexes and all age groups. Prior vaccination against smallpox is not protective. The virus is found in monkeys, but the reservoir host has not been identified. The mode of transmission from animal to man is not known. It has been suggested that there may be an arthropod vector. The skin lesions usually appear on exposed parts of the body and about three fourths of the patients only have a single lesion. There is also a seasonal increase in the incidence of tanapox, coinciding with the period in which mosquitoes and other blood-sucking insects are active.

There are two phases to the disease. The first, preeruptive stage is characterized by fever in most patients. Severe headache and backache may also be present. The first skin symptom is itching at the site of inoculation. A macule appears and becomes papular. This may become umbilicated. It then progresses to form a nodule 10 to 15 mm in diameter, surrounded by a large erythematous areola and edematous skin. Regional lymphadenopathy is usually present at this stage and may be painful. The lesion then ulcerates and heals, leaving a scar about 6 weeks into the illness. Even the most severely affected patients recover without complications.

The clinical diagnosis is made on the basis of a characteristic skin lesion in an endemic area. However, it can be confused with monkeypox. Electron microscopy reveals that tanapox is usually enveloped. Unlike monkeypox, tanapox will not grow on the chorioallantoic membrane of a developing chick embryo.

Yaba Monkey Tumor Virus

Yaba monkey tumor virus was first isolated in 1958 during an outbreak in a colony of rhesus monkeys in Yaba, Nigeria. The virus produces histiocytomas in monkeys and humans. Natural infection of humans has not been seen, but experimental and accidental cases have been reported. The incubation period is not known. Following one accidental exposure, no tumor appeared at the site of inoculation until 4 months had elapsed. The lesions, usually on the heads or limbs of animals, swell up to 40 mm in diameter. The tissue mass eventually sloughs off and healing occurs in 6 to 12 weeks.

Molluscum Contagiosum

Molluscum contagiosum is a benign, self-limited skin disease that occurs primarily in children and young adults. The virus is considered to be a member of the poxvirus group based on its morphology since it does not replicate serially in any current in vitro tissue culture system. Unlike other poxviruses, it cannot be grown on the chorioallantoic membrane of the developing chicken embryo.

The virus affects only humans and has low infectivity, although epidemics can occur. Transmission can be either direct personal contact or indirect contact with towels or washcloths, although the source of the infection is frequently unknown. The incubation period varies widely, from 14 to 50 days. There have been reports suggesting that molluscum contagiosum can act as an opportunistic pathogen in patients with AIDS.

These asymptomatic lesions are recognized by their umbilication caused by central degeneration and by the formation of satellite nodules at the periphery of the parent lesion. Each lesion is usually 2 to 5 mm long, although giant molluscum lesions may be greater than 15 mm in diameter. The lesions are characteristically discrete, dome-shaped, waxy papules that vary in color from white to pink to yellow. The number of lesions varies from 1 to 20 but may be much higher. In children the trunk, face, extremities, and occasionally the conjunctivae are the usual sites of involvement. Genital lesions are much more common in adults, probably due to sexual transmission.

Pathologic examination shows a mass of hypertrophied and hyperplastic epidermis up to 6 times the normal width. The epidermidis projects into the dermis but does not cross the basement membrane. The umbilication near the center of the lesion contains a mass of epidermal cells filled with virus. Large, acidophilic, intracytoplasmic inclusions (molluscum or Henderson-Patterson bodies) can be found in the epidermis.

The disease is benign and self-limited. Resolution of lesions may take months to years, although an inflammatory response following trauma or secondary bacterial infection may shorten the course. Removal of the lesions is recommended to prevent transmission to other body sites or to other people. Successful physical removal methods include surgery, cautery, and cryotherapy.

REFERENCES

Baxby D: Human poxvirus infection after the eradication of smallpox. Epidemiol Infect 100:321, 1988

Behbehani AM: The smallpox story: In words and pictures. Kansas City, University of Kansas Medical Center, 1988

Benenson AS: Smallpox. In Evans AS, ed: Viral Infections of Humans. New York, Plenum Publishing Co, 1989, p 633

Fenner F, Henderson DA, Arita I, et al: Smallpox and its eradication. Geneva, World Health Organization, 1988

Fenner F, Wittek R, Dumbell KR: The Orthopoxviruses. San Diego, Academic Press, 1989

Fine PE, Jezek Z, Grab B, Dixon H: The transmission potential of monkeypox virus in human populations. Int J Epidemiol 17:643, 1988

Gill MJ, Arlette J, Buchan KA, Barker K: Human orf: A diagnostic consideration? Arch Dermatol 126:356, 1990

Jezek Z, Arita I, Szczeniowski M, et al: Human tanapox in Zaire: Clinical and epidemiological observations on cases confirmed by laboratory studies. Bull World Health Organ 63:1027, 1985

Jezek Z, Marennikova SS, Mutombo M, et al: Human monkeypox: A study of 2510 contacts of 214 patients. J Infect Dis 154:551, 1986

Jezek Z, Szczeniowski M, Paluku KM, Mutombo M: Human monkeypox: Clinical features of 282 patients. J Infect Dis 156:293, 1987

Katzman M, Carey JT, Elmets CA, et al: Molluscum contagiosum and the acquired immunodeficiency syndrome: Clinical and immunological details of two cases. Br J Dermatol 116:131, 1987

Knight JC, Novembre FJ, Brown DR, et al: Studies on Tanapox virus. Virology 172:116, 1989

Porter CD, Muhlemann MF, Cream JJ, Archard LC: Molluscum contagiosum: Characterization of viral DNA and clinical features. Epidemiol Infect 99:563, 1987

Quinnan GV Jr (ed.): Vaccinia viruses as vectors for vaccine antigens. New York, Elsevier Science Publishing Co., Inc., 1985

Spencer AJ: Diagnostic exercise: Subcutaneous nodules in rhesus monkeys. Lab Anim Sci 35:79, 1985

Tartaglia J, Pincus S, Paoletti E. Poxvirus-based vectors as vaccine candidates. Crit Rev Immunol 10:13, 1990

Walker DH, Voelker FA, McKee AE Jr, Nakano JH: Diagnostic exercise: Tumors in a baboon. Lab Anim Sci 35:627, 1985

CHAPTER 64

Herpesviruses

Of more than 50 herpesviruses in the animal world, only eight are associated with infection in humans. The human herpesviruses are a family of seven viruses encompassing a broad spectrum of clinical illness. The group includes herpes simplex virus types 1 and 2, varicella-zoster virus, Epstein-Barr virus, cytomegalovirus, human herpesvirus 6, and human herpesvirus 7. A simian virus, herpes B virus, is a rare cause of serious infection in monkey handlers.

The common feature of these large enveloped DNA viruses is the ability to establish latency in the body after primary infection, despite the presence of antibodies. Reactivation of virus occurs at variable rates. Infections range in severity from asymptomatic to fatal; however, the majority of clinical episodes are uncomplicated and self-limited. Herpes infections are of particular importance in immunocompromised patients, who are susceptible to prolonged or severe infections and sequelae.

Herpes Simplex Virus (HSV)

Although herpes infections have become more prevalent in the last two decades, they have been described throughout history. The term *herpes* is believed to have been coined around AD 100 (Greek *herpein:* to creep) with reference to the spreading nature of herpes labialis. Genital herpes was first described in the eighteenth century. Changes in the natural history of herpes are occurring in the wake of changes in both immunosuppressive therapy and sexual mores.

Epidemiology

HSV may be found worldwide. The virus is spread by direct contact with infected secretions. Lesions are highly infectious to susceptible individuals. Auto-inoculation of multiple sites (e.g., eyes or fingers) may occur by touching a lesion. Good handwashing and protective barriers reduce the risk of transmission. Asymptomatic excretion of virus appears to result in less efficient transmission, but it provides an important reservoir for the continued spread of herpes. The risk of fomite transmission is negligible, since herpesviruses are unable to survive for long outside the body. Infants may be infected during delivery by exposure to the virus in the birth canal.

Serologic studies show that HSV-1 is acquired in early childhood. Seroprevalence rates range from 30% to 100% according to the socioeconomic status of the population surveyed. The presence of HSV-2 antibodies generally correlates with the onset of puberty and peaks in the early years of sexual activity.

Antibodies to herpes are not protective against subsequent outbreaks. Recurrences are common and represent reactivation of latent virus, although exogenous reinfection has also been described. After the onset of primary infection, neutralizing antibodies and antibody-dependent cellular cytotoxic antibodies appear within 2 to 6 weeks. Subsequent exposure to the heterologous virus type generally results in milder symptoms. The first episode of genital herpes in a patient with a history of herpes labialis would be referred to as initial nonprimary infection.

Herpes simplex types 1 and 2 share many common antigens. Most commonly available serologic tests cannot distinguish between the two types. This often results in confusion if serologic testing is used for diagnosis of recurrent disease. Type-specific tests available in some research settings measure responses to glycoproteins gG-1 and gG-2 and identify antibodies to HSV-1 and HSV-2, respectively.

Pathogenesis

After contact with a mucous membrane or a break in the skin, HSV undergoes initial replication in the parabasal and intermediate epithelial cells, which lyse and invoke an inflammatory response. The characteristic changes of herpes infection include the formation of multinucleated giant cells, ballooning degeneration, edema, and intranuclear inclusion bodies of Cowdry type A. Lysis of the cell results in the formation of a vesicle, a clear fluid-filled space teeming with virus between the dermis and epidermis. As white cells respond, the lesion becomes pustular and forms a scab. Little or no virus can be recovered from scabbed lesions.

After initial replication on the skin, the virus migrates to the dorsal root ganglion and establishes lifelong latency. If stimulated, HSV returns to the skin along sensory nerves and causes a recurrent infection. The characteristic vesicle is rarely observed on mucous membranes. Here the epithelium is so thin that lesions ulcerate rapidly.

If viral replication continues unchecked, then viremia and visceral dissemination ensue. Infected organs exhibit hemorrhagic necrosis.

Clinical Manifestations

Oropharynx

Primary infection with HSV-1 usually occurs in preschool children. Most cases are asymptomatic; however, symptomatic cases appear as gingivostomatitis. After an incubation period of 2 to 12 days, infection is manifest as fever, drooling, and pain in the mouth. Pharyngeal erythema and edema are followed by transient vesicles on the pharynx, buccal mucosa, and gingiva. The vesicles rapidly become shallow ulcers. The lesions are accompanied by cervical and submandibular adenopathy. Oral pain may be severe enough to impair intake and lead to dehydration. Healing occurs in 1 or 2 weeks. Herpes gingivostomatitis must be differentiated from herpangina, which is caused by Coxsackie A virus and is usually limited to the posterior pharynx, and from trench mouth, which is associated with anaerobic infection of the gingiva.

Young adults may have primary involvement of the tonsils with primary HSV-1 infection. This must be distinguished from streptococcal pharyngitis and infectious mononucleosis. Pharyngitis has also been observed in approximately 10% of patients with primary genital herpes.

Oral herpes infection recurs as herpes labialis, commonly known as a cold sore or fever blister. Approximately one fourth of the U.S. population has herpes labialis. It may be reactivated by stress, menses, trauma, or exposure to ultraviolet light. Recurrences typically occur at the vermilion border of the lip, in the same location each time. Many persons experience a prodrome of pain, tingling, or itching before the appearance of the lesions. Erythema and edema progress to a papule and a vesicle with 24 hours. The vesicle ulcerates and then heals within 10 days.

Genitalia

Primary genital herpes may range from asymptomatic or unnoticed to severely debilitating. The course of the infection may be moderated in individuals with prior exposure to HSV-1. After an incubation period of 2 to 7 days, patients develop multiple painful vesicles and ulcers with a vaginal or urethral discharge. Primary genital herpes heals in 3 weeks. Systemic symptoms include fever, regional adenopathy, malaise, myalgia, and headache. Involvement of the urethra may result in dysuria and urinary retention. Some patients have sacral autonomic dysfunction and rarely radiculomyelitis. Viral meningitis occurs in approximately 5% of cases as a result of viremic spread and may be diagnosed by mild cerebral spinal fluid (CSF) pleocytosis and isolation of HSV. In contrast, virus isolation from CSF is unusual in herpes encephalitis.

Recurrent genital herpes is a milder illness. Lesions are limited to a smaller area. A prodrome of pain or tingling often precedes the development of a small cluster of vesicles or shallow ulcers. Pain may last for 4 days, and lesions usually heal within 10 days. Constitutional symptoms are uncommon. The average number of recurrences is five to eight per year. The annual rate of recurrences may decrease over time. Asymptomatic shedding of virus from the cervix and urethra occurs to an unknown extent. The frequency and severity of recurrences correlate with the serotype of the initial genital infection. HSV-1 infection of the genitalia is milder and less frequent than HSV-2 genital infection.

Genital herpes need not be confined to the perineal area. Many recurrences go undiagnosed on the buttocks or in the perianal area. Perirectal herpes or herpetic proctitis is being recognized increasingly, particularly in homosexual men. Severe ulcerative perirectal lesions are often seen in patients with acquired immunodeficiency syndrome (AIDS), and their presence fulfills one of the major diagnostic criteria for AIDS.

Although recurrent genital herpes resolves spontaneously, it may have a profound life-disrupting effect on some patients. The emotional stress of carrying a chronic, sexually transmissible disease may be overwhelming. Pregnant women may transmit infection to their infants. Infected patients need counseling and screening for other sexually transmitted diseases. In addition, there are theories about the potential role of HSV in altering the course of human immunodeficiency virus (HIV) infection, either by facilitating transmission of HIV through genital ulcers or by stimulating HIV replication. The potential role of HSV in oncogenesis is controversial. HSV-2 has been associated with carcinoma of the cervix on the basis of detection of herpes DNA in some cancer cells. More recent studies implicate papillomaviruses as a more likely co-factor.

Skin

Intact dry skin is the best host defense against herpes simplex. Herpetic whitlow represents inoculation of the finger. A pustule is often mistaken for a paronychia, but incision and drainage only exacerbate the infection. The lesion may be accompanied by marked neuralgia and axillary adenopathy. Whitlow is an occupational hazard for medical and dental personnel, because of chronic exposure to saliva of infected patients. The risk should be lessened with the increasing use of gloves and universal precautions for contact with all secretions.

Superficial abrasions may become infected with HSV. This is known as herpes gladiatorum in wrestlers and as scrumpox in rugby players.

More widely damaged areas of skin provide access for cutaneous dissemination of HSV. Patients with eczema may develop a potentially fatal form of infection known as eczema herpeticum (formerly called Kaposi's varicelliform eruption). Burn patients are susceptible to herpes infection of eschar or denuded skin.

Brain

Although rare, herpes simplex encephalitis is the most common cause of fatal sporadic encephalitis in the U.S. (approximately 2000 cases per year). The mortality rare is 70% in untreated cases.

Except in infancy, when central nervous system infection occurs after exposure to an infected birth canal, herpes encephalitis is usually caused by HSV-1. The mechanism of involvement of the brain is not understood. Encephalitis may occur with primary or recurrent infection. Few patients have had cold sores at the onset of encephalitis, so there is no evidence that it represents dissemination.

The onset may be sudden or gradual, with nonspecific flulike symptoms. Fever, headache, stiff neck, and behavioral changes are common. Focal neurologic signs can be demonstrated. Examination of the spinal fluid reveals elevated protein, pleocytosis, and erythrocytosis. Temporal lobe localization is characteristic, but other areas of the brain may be involved.

Brain biopsy is generally recommended for histologic diagnosis and virus isolation. Antiviral therapy may begin while the patient awaits surgery, since a favorable outcome depends on early intervention. Noninvasive diagnostic techniques are less reliable than biopsy, especially in the early stages of infection. Although some authors believe that the safety of antiviral agents is adequate to justify empiric therapy, a large clinical study showed that one third of the patients with a characteristic clinical diagnosis of herpes encephalitis had other treatable illnesses diagnosed by biopsy.

The course of untreated infection is rapid progression to coma and death from progressive hemorrhagic necrosis of the brain. The survivors suffer severe neurologic sequelae. Treatment with acyclovir or vidarabine has been shown to decrease mortality and is discussed below.

Eye

Herpes infections of the eye are usually caused by HSV-1. This is the most common infectious cause of corneal blindness in the United States. Primary infection results in an acute follicular keratoconjunctivitis, with or without vesicles on the periocular skin, accompanied by regional adenopathy. Coarse punctate opacities may be observed with fluorescein staining. In some patients dendrites develop. The lesions heal spontaneously within 3 weeks. If the cornea is involved, wiping debridement is performed with a cotton applicator to remove loose epithelial cells. Antiviral therapy is recommended.

Neonates

Potentially fatal infections are seen in neonates. Neonates have the highest rate of dissemination and mortality of any population studied. A small number of infants have congenital infection acquired in the second half of pregnancy. Most infected infants have had contact with herpesvirus during delivery. Infants become ill within 1 month of age. About 70% of neonatal disease is caused by HSV-2. HSV-1 may be acquired from infected family members or hospital staff shortly after delivery. Despite improved prenatal screening procedures, most cases of neonatal herpes occur in children of mothers with no known history of herpes. Routine culturing of all mothers for HSV is not a cost-effective means of prevention. Instead, the presence of lesions on the vulva or cervix and the length of time from rupture of membranes are the major determinants of the need for abdominal delivery.

Congenital infection is manifest shortly after birth by seizures, irritability, jaundice, hepatosplenomegaly, bleeding, chorioretinitis, pneumonitis, and skin vesicles. Rapid respiratory and cardiac deterioration follow.

Infection acquired during delivery is usually diagnosed between 10 and 21 days of life. Skin vesicles alone have been observed in 70% of infants at presentation, but involvement of other sites occurred in 70%. For infants in whom vesicles never develop, surveillance cultures of eyes, throat, and rectum must be relied upon for diagnosis. A high level of suspicion is necessary since early symptoms may be nonspecific.

Involvement of the central nervous system or disseminated infection result in 50% and 80% mortality, respectively. Disease limited to the skin, eyes, or mouth has a better prognosis, with a mortality of 30%. Antiviral therapy has decreased mortality from 65% to 25%. Recurrences after treatment may lead to long-term neurologic complications or developmental delays. Improved diagnostic methods and treatment regimens are currently under intense investigation.

Immunocompromised Host

Reactivation of herpes simplex is affected by the immune status of the patient. The risk of severity of infection correlates directly with the degree of immune suppression of cell-mediated immunity. Patients who are seropositive for HSV before bone marrow, cardiac, liver, or renal transplantation reactivate virus at rates of 35% to 85% within 1 month of the transplant. Some reactivation consists of asymptomatic viral shedding, but most cases are associated with morbidity. In some cases, fatal dissemination occurs.

Infection in patients with congenital or acquired deficiencies of cell-mediated immunity (e.g., severe combined immunodeficiency syndrome [SCIDS] or AIDS) have more severe and persistent infections. Viral shedding persists for 3 weeks, as opposed to 4 days in immunocompetent patients. Healing may take 4 weeks. The characteristic appearance of lesions may not be present. Mucositis may mimic inflammation caused by chemotherapy or radiation or may be masked by fungal superinfection. Perirectal ulcers may be mistaken for pressure sores. A high index of suspicion is necessary for therapeutic intervention.

Diagnosis

Diagnosis of herpes infection may be made on clinical grounds. Patients with fever, vesicles, or ulcers of the mucous membranes and with constitutional symptoms should be considered to have HSV infection. A history of similar episodes strongly suggests recurrent herpes. Many patients without a history of herpes recall past outbreaks when they are shown photographs of lesions. Asymptomatic infection in many instances may simply be unrecognized infection. Since results of therapy are dependent on early initiation, treatment should not be delayed pending the outcome of viral cultures, particularly for patients with severe or life-threatening infections.

Virus isolation is the most reliable method for confirmation of the clinical diagnosis. HSV grows rapidly, so characteristic cytopathic effects are observed in 24 to 48 hours if an adequate specimen is obtained. Vesicular fluid contains the highest titer of virus. Virus is rarely obtained from crusted lesions. Specimens should be placed in viral transport media and inoculated into tissue culture as soon as possible. Specimens should be refrigerated (up to 24 hours) until they are inoculated. If there is a longer delay, then specimens in transport media should be frozen at −70C. Storage at −20C in a standard freezer compartment results in significant loss of virus.

Several methods have been developed for rapid diagnosis of HSV. Accelerated viral cultures combine virus-specific monoclonal antibodies or DNA hybridization techniques with colorimetric, fluorescent, or radioactive indicators. The Tzanck preparation or Papanicolaou stain shows cytologic changes in scrapings from the base of a vesicle or mucous membranes. The stains cannot differentiate between herpes simplex and varicella-zoster infections.

Serologic testing may be useful in primary infection to show a rise in neutralizing antibodies. In the transplant setting, the presence of antibodies before transplantation is a useful indicator to identify patients at risk of virus reactivation. Serologic testing is unreliable for diagnosis of recurrent genital diseases because of the high rate of cross-reactivity with HSV-1.

Treatment

The recent development of antiviral therapy for herpes infections is a major milestone in virology. Many nucleoside analogues interrupt virus replication in vitro. However, some are too toxic for systemic use. None of the antiviral agents eradicates latent virus.

Vidarabine, a purine analogue, is phosphorylated within the cell. Vidarabine triphosphate preferentially inhibits viral DNA polymerase over cellular DNA polymerase. In its intravenous form, vidarabine was the first antiviral agent effective against serious herpes infections. Multicenter studies demonstrated that it reduced mortality from herpes encephalitis or neonatal herpes. It is widely used in topical form against herpes keratitis.

Acyclovir is noteworthy as the first antiviral agent with selective toxicity. By targeting HSV-infected cells and viral DNA polymerase, acyclovir has a low potential for toxicity in uninfected host cells.

Acyclovir is phosphorylated by HSV-encoded thymidine kinase to the monophosphate. Acyclovir monophosphate is further converted to the triphosphate by cellular enzymes. Acyclovir triphosphate is incorporated into growing chains of viral DNA by viral DNA polymerase and acts as a chain terminator, preventing further virus replication. The triphosphate also inhibits HSV DNA polymerase to a much greater extent than cellular DNA polymerases.

Acyclovir is available in several formulations for intravenous, oral, or topical administration. An ophthalmic preparation is not available in the United States. For serious infections, parenteral administration is preferred. Intravenous acyclovir is effective for treatment of mucocutaneous infections in immunocompromised patients by inhibiting viral shedding, limiting progression of the infected area, and reducing pain. Recurrences in immunocompromised patients at risk of reactivation have been suppressed by daily treatment with acyclovir throughout the periods of highest risk. For treatment of herpes encephalitis or neonatal herpes, multicenter studies comparing acyclovir and vidarabine have favored acyclovir for efficacy or ease of administration. In patients with biopsy-proven herpes encephalitis, mortality was 28% for patients treated with acyclovir compared with 54% for vidarabine. In neonatal infections, the mortality rates after acyclovir were similar to those after vidarabine at the doses studied. Intravenous acyclovir is also recommended for treatment of severe initial genital herpes.

The predominant use of oral acyclovir is for treatment of genital herpes. Acyclovir is the only available antiviral drug effective against initial and recurrent genital herpes. Controlled clinical trials demonstrated that treatment with acyclovir reduced the duration of viral shedding, promoted healing, and reduced pain in comparison with placebo. Chronic suppression of recurrences is warranted for patients troubled by frequent recurrences. In one study patients have been treated daily for more than 5 years to reduce the frequency of their recurrences. The optimal duration of suppressive treatment is not known, since the frequency of recurrences may decrease over the years.

The use of acyclovir for treatment of herpes labialis is less clearly defined. Preventive use has been shown to be effective in one study of patients known to reactivate cold sores after prolonged exposure to sunshine.

Idoxuridine and trifluridine, deoxythymidine analogues, are effective topical agents for treatment of herpes keratitis. Idoxuridine inhibits thymidine kinase and is incorporated into both viral and cellular DNA. Trifluridine is believed to be incorporated directly into viral DNA. Myelosuppression after systemic administration limits the usefulness of both to topical preparations. Trifluridine is more effective for stromal keratitis and may be used in patients intolerant of or resistant to idoxuridine or vidarabine.

A growing number of compounds are being investigated for potential antiherpes activity by virtue of antiviral or immune modulating effects. Isoprinosine (inosine pranobex) has been studied in a comparative trial with acyclovir in patients with genital herpes and was not shown to be effective. Foscarnet (phosphonoformate) is a derivative of phosphonoacetic acid, which is active in vitro against HSV but too toxic for development. Foscarnet is principally for treatment of cytomegalovirus infections, but it may play a role in treatment of some infections that are resistant to acyclovir in patients with HIV disease.

Prevention

Currently there is no effective therapy to prevent infection with HSV. Avoidance of direct contact with lesions or infected secretions is the primary means of prophylaxis. Young children should not be kissed by an individual with herpes labialis. Patients with genital herpes should be advised to abstain from intimate contact while lesions or prodromal symptoms are present and to use condoms at other times.

No studies have demonstrated effective postexposure prophylaxis of antiviral therapy. Prophylactic antiviral treatment of mothers and infants for neonatal herpes has not been evaluated. Although chronic suppression of recurrent genital herpes with acyclovir decreases the frequency of outbreaks, sporadic viral shedding occurs. Consequently, there is no clinical evidence that acyclovir can block transmission of herpes.

Vaccination for herpes would be the ideal preventive measure. Vaccine development for HSV is fraught with theoretical and practical difficulties. Prevention of a disease that reactivates in the presence of antibodies has been a major hurdle. Development strategies have focused on demonstrating immunogenicity of harvested or recombinant DNA envelope glycoproteins. Concerns about potential oncogenicity, teratogenicity, or latency hamper development of live-virus vaccines.

Varicella-Zoster Virus (VZV)

VZV infection is a common childhood infection in temperate parts of the world. In the United States, more than 90% of the population is infected by adulthood. Primary infection with the virus causes varicella (chickenpox). Reactivation of the virus in later life or in response to immune suppression results in herpes zoster (shingles). Studies by Weller in 1958 confirmed that these two clinical entities are caused by the same virus.

Epidemiology

Chickenpox occurs worldwide, with a seasonal distribution in the winter and early spring. Transmission occurs by close contact, but indirect evidence strongly supports respiratory transmission of aerosolized virus. Epidemiologic studies document transmission rates that could be achieved only by aerosolization. Transmission may occur before the rash appears. Vesicular fluid contains high titers of virus. The risk of transmission is low when all lesions have crusted.

Varicella may be acquired in utero. If a pregnant woman has chickenpox during the first trimester, the chance of infecting the fetus with resultant congenital varicella syndrome is about 2% (3/131) with a range of 0.5% to 6.5%. Infection as late as 28 weeks into pregnancy has resulted in congenital varicella. Infection in late pregnancy may result in healthy infants in whom the first manifestation of infection is shingles.

Herpes zoster occurs without seasonal variation. Patients of all ages who have had chickenpox are affected with increasing frequency in older decades. By the age of 85 years, 50% of the population should have experienced herpes zoster. Alterations in cell-mediated immunity also result in increased risk of reactivation. Epidemics of zoster have been described in older literature, but recombinant DNA technology has shown that apparent outbreaks were caused by different viruses.

Pathogenesis

There is no adequate animal model of VZV infection. Hope-Simpson, in 1965, outlined a working hypothesis based on clinical observation, which holds to this day. After initial contact with the virus via the respiratory route, the virus undergoes limited replication, enters the bloodstream, and is borne to the skin. From small blood vessels in the corium, virus is spread to adjacent cells to form characteristic multinucleated giant cells. The fluid accumulating under the epidermis accounts for vesicle formation. Polymorphonuclear leukocytes invade the vesicle, which becomes cloudy and pustular. The fluid resorbs, leaving a crust which subsequently sloughs.

The events leading to latency are poorly understood. Presumably, during the viremic phase the virus migrates to the ganglion associated with the area of the body with the highest viral load. Virus particles have been demonstrated in ganglia and perineural cells. Reactivation depends on the integrity of cellular immune responses. After reactivation, the virus travels along sensory nerves to the skin. Lesions resembling vesicles of chickenpox are usually confined to one dermatome and may coalesce. The involved nerve may show intense inflammation, loss of large fibers, and hemorrhagic necrosis of nerve cells. In rare cases, patients may experience dermatomal neuralgia without lesions (zoster sine herpete).

Clinical Manifestations

Varicella

Chickenpox is considered the last major viral exanthem in children. After an incubation of 10 to 23 days, the rash characteristically begins on the scalp and trunk and spreads to the extremities. A vesicular lesion on an erythematous base is the hallmark. Macules evolve in 2 to 3 mm vesicles, which evolve in successive crops. Lesions on mucous membranes are easily traumatized and may appear as ulcers. Lesions appear in the mouth, conjunctivae, rectum, and vagina. The average number of lesions is 200 but varies from a few to several hundred confluent lesions. Children may have a mild to moderate (38C to 39C) fever for 2 days. Constitutional symptoms include headache, sore throat, loss of appetite, irritability, and pruritus. The differential diagnosis formerly included smallpox, which has been completely eradicated.

Varicella is more severe in older children and adults. The rash is more extensive, and a larger proportion of patients have fever. Varicella pneumonia had been observed in 14% of military recruits. Mortality is higher than in children.

Complications in healthy children are uncommon but may be sufficient to necessitate hospitalization. Cerebellar ataxia is the most common neurologic complication and appears late in the course of the illness. Fulminant encephalitis may occur with the onset of lesions in fewer than 1 per 1000 cases. Some of these cases may represent Reyes syndrome, which has been linked epidemiologically to use of aspirin during chickenpox. Rare neurologic complications include aseptic meningitis, Guillian-Barré syndrome, and transverse myelitis.

Thrombocytopenia and hepatitis have been observed. The most common complication is bacterial superinfection of the skin.

Immunosuppressed patients may have a prolonged course. Lesions may continue to form for 2 to 3 weeks. Temperatures may be elevated to 41C. Lesions may become deeply ulcerated. Visceral dissemination may result in pneumonitis, hepatitis, or meningitis. The mortality from disseminated infection may approach 20%, in contrast to 7% in those with cutaneous dissemination.

Congenital and Neonatal Varicella

Infection in the first trimester of pregnancy may result in congenital varicella syndrome. A wide variety of manifestations include cicatricial lesions of a limb in a dermatomal distribution, microphthalmia, cataracts, chorioretinitis, deafness, or cortical atrophy of the brain.

If the mother develops varicella within 5 days before or after delivery, the infant does not receive tranplacental antibody and the attack rate in the newborn is 20%. The mortality rate is 35%, presumably because the cellular immune response to VZV is immature. Treatment with varicella-zoster immune globulin for the mother before term and for the infant at delivery is recommended to prevent or modify neonatal varicella. Treatment of neonatal varicella with acyclovir may reduce mortality, but this has not been studied. Most neonates have maternal IgG antibody transmitted across the placenta and are protected from severe disease.

Herpes Zoster

Reactivation of VZV is heralded by radicular pain. The vesicular rash appears in a unilateral dermatomal distribution. New lesions appear for 3 to 4 days, occasionally involving adjacent dermatomes. Satellite lesions (fewer than 25) may appear in a remote dermatome and are not cause for alarm. Thoracic involvement is the most common, followed by involvement of the ophthalmic division of the trigeminal nerve. Vesicles evolve like those of chickenpox, and healing of the skin is complete within 2 weeks. There is no correlation between the extent of the rash and the severity of the symptoms.

The most common complication of zoster is postherpetic neuralgia (PHN). Pain in the affected dermatome may persist for months or years after the rash has healed. Because of the lack of standard definition, the true incidence of postherpeutic neuralgia is not known. PHN occurs more commonly in elderly patients. Pain may be characterized by burning, itching, or tingling sensations and may be severe enough to interrupt sleep or daily activities. Hyperesthesia is a common component of PHN. Other neurologic complications include encephalitis or myelitis. Ipsilateral cerebral ischemia is an infrequent inflammatory response occasionally manifest days to months after ophthalmic zoster. Ophthalmic complications are frequent and include keratitis, iritis, uveitis, conjunctivitis, scleritis, or ophthalmoplegia. Complications of infection of cranial nerves VII and VIII include Bell's palsy and Ramsay-Hunt syndrome.

Patients with altered cell-mediated immunity have a higher rate of zoster and its attendant complications. Patients receiving radiation therapy or transplants, or those with hematologic malignancy have the highest incidence of reactivation. Although studies associate a high risk of reactivation in patients with lymphoreticular malignancies, there is no reason to suspect cancer in a young patient with zoster. Zoster may be an early indicator of HIV infection. In a young patient at risk for HIV, the appearance of zoster is an indication for evaluation of the possibility of HIV infection.

In immunocompromised patients, there is an increased risk of cutaneous and visceral dissemination of VZV. Dissemination will occur in approximately 25% of immunosuppressed patents. Multidermatomal zoster is common in patients with advanced HIV infection. The course of infection is prolonged. New lesions appear for 3 weeks, and healing may occur for a month. A chronic, verrucous form of zoster has been observed recently in patients with AIDS.

Diagnosis

The characteristic appearance of chickenpox and zoster enables most cases to be diagnosed on clinical grounds. A history of exposure to chickenpox can usually be elicited in children, but many elderly patients will be unable to recall their primary infection.

Culture of the vesicular fluid for virus is the definitive diagnostic test. It will distinguish HSV from VZV when the appearance is similar; however, culture of VZV is not easily accomplished. Fluid must be obtained from a fresh vesicle and transported promptly to the laboratory at 4C or inoculated directly onto tissue culture at the bedside. Antigen-detection tests for rapid diagnosis are becoming increasingly available.

If confirmation is necessary, acute and convalescent serum will show a rise in titer of antibody to VZV by ELISA (enzyme-linked immunosorbent assay), which is the most practical test today. For determination of susceptibility, the most sensitive assays are necessary, such as FAMA (fluorescent antibody to membrane antigen), anti-complementary CF, and RIA (radioimmunoassay), which are not commercially available. The ELISA has become widely available but is somewhat less sensitive.

Treatment

Uncomplicated varicella is usually treated only with supportive measures. Antihistamines such as diphenhydramine may be used for pruritus. Aspirin should be avoided because of the possible association with Reye's syndrome. Drying agents, such as calamine or colloidal oatmeal baths, are soothing and help prevent secondary bacterial infections.

Antiviral therapy is investigational. Most clinical experience involves immunosuppressed children. High-dose interferon decreased new lesion formation and dissemination when compared with placebo in a study of varicella in children with cancer. Vidarabine has also been shown to decrease new lesion formation and duration of fever and to prevent visceral dissemination. Acyclovir has also been shown to prevent visceral dissemination in immunosuppressed children. In healthy children, one study showed that treatment with acyclovir reduced duration of fever and the number of lesions. Multicenter studies in children and adolescents confirmed that prompt treatment resulted in fewer lesions, more rapid healing, and more rapid resolution of constitutional symptoms.

Treatment of zoster in immunocompromised patients is undertaken to limit dissemination. Both vidarabine and acyclovir are licensed for treatment of zoster in immunocompromised patients. In one comparative study of acyclovir and vidarabine in recipients of bone marrow transplants, acyclovir was superior in the rate of healing and the number of treatment failures.

In immunocompetent patients, the primary objective of treatment is to alleviate pain. Oral acyclovir in multicenter studies reduced the duration of formation of new lesions, shortened time to healing, and reduced the duration of pain and dysesthesia by a mean of 5 weeks.

Prevention

The major efforts at prevention are targeted at immunocompromised patients at risk of substantial morbidity and mortality. Patients with chickenpox or shingles require respiratory and contact isolation, respectively, to prevent transmission to susceptible immunosuppressed patients. Seronegative health care workers must refrain from patient contact during the latter part of the incubation period if they are exposed to VZV.

Varicella-zoster immune globulin (VZIG) is available for passive immunization of high-risk patients. Derived from high-titer normal donor plasma, VZIG modifies or prevents illness if administered within 72 hours of exposure.

The availability of live-attenuated vaccine is imminent. It is immunogenic and prevents or limits the infection in both immunosuppressed and healthy children. The duration of the protection is unknown, but protective antibody titers and protective immunity were measured after 10 years in normal children in Japan. Whether booster doses will be needed is not known. Reinfection is common, but symptoms have been mild when present.

Cytomegalovirus (CMV)

Cytomegalovirus infection is ubiquitous and results in a wide spectrum of illness, ranging from asymptomatic infection to severe life-threatening disease, which clearly establishes CMV as a significant pathogen. Cytomegaloviruses as a group are widely distributed among several animal species, but there remains a high degree of species specificity.

In vivo and in vitro infection of cells with CMV produces cell enlargement. These cytomegalic cells were first described in 1904 on the basis of histopathologic findings in the kidneys and parotid glands of infants studied at autopsy. In 1956, Smith first isolated "human salivary gland virus" from infants dying of cytomegalic inclusion disease. Weller subsequently defined the term *cytomegalovirus* to reflect the morphologic change in virus-infected cells.

Since that time the development of serologic tests has enabled investigators to define the epidemiology and clinical manifestations of human CMV infection. Infection in normal children and adults usually causes no symptoms and is detected only through viral shedding, seroconversion, or both, although in immunocompromised hosts, CMV may cause severe opportunistic infections with high morbidity and mortality. The past decade has witnessed advances mainly in the treatment and prevention of CMV disease in the increasing numbers of immunocompromised patients. This patient population is expanding because of the increased use of transplantation and more aggressive cancer chemotherapy regimens, in addition to the epidemic of AIDS.

Epidemiology

CMV infection is endemic rather than epidemic; there is no seasonal variation. The virus is transmitted by close or intimate person-to-person contact. In general, the prevalence of CMV infection is related to the socioeconomic status of a population and, to a certain extent, to geographic location. Infection rates increase in early childhood and peak at 1 to 2 years of age. There is a slow increase in primary infection rates in adolescents and adults. The prevalence of CMV infection in the adult population ranges from 40% in Europe to almost 100% in Africa and the Far East.

Potential sources of virus include saliva, urine, semen, breast milk, cervical and vaginal secretions, blood, and transplanted donor organs. Maternal infections play an important role in transmission of CMV to neonates, whereas sexual transmission becomes a predominant mode of acquisition in adult life. CMV can be reactivated during gestation, and the virus may be transmitted to the fetus in utero despite circulating maternal antibody. Approximately 1% of infants are found to be congenitally infected, as shown by viruria detectable at birth. Congenital infections may follow primary, recurrent (exogenous reinfection), or reactivated maternal infections. After primary maternal infection, CMV transmission occurs in 40% to 50% of the cases and 5% to 10% of these congenitally infected infants will have symptoms. In contrast, babies born to mothers who have reactivation infection are much less likely to have symptoms, which suggest that preexisting maternal immunity reduces the severity of the infant's infection. There is increased cervical CMV excretion during the last trimester, which increases the risk of neonatal acquisition during birth. Seropositive mothers excreting CMV in their breast milk may also transmit virus to their breast-fed infants.

Viral transmission by exposure to oral secretions among preschool children in day care centers is extremely high, and infection rates subsequently increase rapidly at the age of entry into school. By puberty, generally 40% to 80% of all youths have been infected with CMV. In lower socioeconomic areas, 90% to 100% of the population may acquire primary CMV infection during childhood.

Sexual transmission is a significant mode of spread for CMV. Approximately 8% to 10% of women shed CMV from the cervix, and approximately 30% of symptom-free homosexual men have CMV in their semen. In adults the type of sexual activity and the number of sexual partners are stronger predictors of the prevalence of CMV infection than race, age, or socioeconomic status. Approximately 100% of male homosexuals or bisexuals with human immunodeficiency virus (HIV) infection also have CMV infection, whereas the rate of CMV infection among other HIV-infected patient groups, such as persons with hemophilia, is similar to populations without HIV.

Primary or recurrent CMV infection occasionally follows blood transfusion or organ transplantation. Susceptible infants of low birth weight who receive blood from seropositive donors are at significant risk of severe CMV infection. This has led to the use of screened CMV seronegative blood products in these patients. In older patients, posttransfusion CMV infection is most often asymptomatic, but a mild hepatitis or mononucleosis-like syndrome may develop. The risk of acquiring CMV is about 3% per unit of blood transfused. For either transfusion- or transplant-acquired CMV, the risk is greatest if donors are seropositive and recipients are seronegative. In renal transplant recipients, an average of 53% of seronegative patients acquire primary CMV infections, and 85% of seropositive subjects develop recurrent CMV infections. High rates of CMV infection also occur in recipients of solid organ and bone marrow transplants. In general, 70% to 85% of the transplant recipients have symptoms with primary infection, while only 20% to 40% develop symptoms with recurrent infections. This indicates that preexisting immunity offers some protection against developing symptomatic illness after rechallenge. The mortality rate of CMV pneumonia in transplant patients with primary CMV infection is higher than in those individuals with recurrent infection. Patients with cancer in whom immunosuppression develops during chemotherapy are also at risk of symptomatic CMV infection.

Clinical Manifestations

Congenital and Perinatal Infection

Congenital CMV infection may be asymptomatic or may result in severe disease with hepatosplenomegaly, jaundice, chorioretinitis, petechiae, respiratory distress, and neurologic abnormalities such as microcephaly and focal calcifications in the brain. Although most congenitally infected infants (≥90%) are asymptomatic at birth, 5% to 20% of these infants may develop late manifestations of CMV infection, such as hearing loss and poor intellectual performance. Transfusion-acquired CMV, especially in low-birth-weight neonates, can be serious and sometimes fatal. Congenital or perinatal CMV infections usually result in persistent chronic viral excretion over months or years.

Infection in Normal Hosts

Primary CMV infections in normal children and adults are usually asymptomatic but may result in a mononucleosis-like illness with fever, lethargy, myalgias, headache, and mild hepatitis. A similar illness, the "postperfusion syndrome," may develop after transfusion of large amounts of blood, such as commonly occurs during cardiopulmonary bypass surgery. CMV causes only 8% of all infectious mononucleosis syndromes, and EBV causes the majority of cases. CMV mononucleosis generally resembles the mononucleosis caused by Epstein-Barr virus (EBV), but certain clinical features differ. CMV-infected patients are older, with a mean age of 28 years, compared with EBV-infected patients, who have a mean age of 19 years. With CMV mononucleosis, the duration of fever is longer (mean duration, 18 days) than in patients with EBV mononucleosis (mean duration 10 days). Pharyngitis, tonsillitis, lymphadenopathy, and lymphocytosis with atypical lymphocytes are more commonly associated with EBV than with CMV. Another cause of a mononucleosis-like syndrome that must be considered in sexually active adults is HIV (Chap. 77). Other complications of CMV infections in normal hosts are rare but include rash, granulomatous hepatitis, Guillain-Barré syndrome, meningoencephalitis, myocarditis, pneumonia, hemolytic anemia, and thrombocytopenia.

Infection in Immunocompromised Hosts

In immunocompromised patients, CMV infection may be asymptomatic, or it may be a serious opportunistic infection with high morbidity and mortality. CMV infection may result in severe prolonged mononucleosis-like syndromes, leukopenia, pneumonitis, retinitis, cholecystitis, and colitis. CMV infection itself is immunosuppressive, and complications include bacterial, fungal, or parasitic superinfections and possibly an increased risk of allograft rejection, although the latter remains speculative. The high incidence of CMV infection after transplantation may be attributed to reactivation of latent virus by immunosuppressive drugs, as well as transmission of virus by latently infected donor tissues or blood. It is important to determine whether infection occurring after transplantation is primary, reactivated, or due to exogenous reinfection, as primary infections more frequently result in more serious disease.

In patients with AIDS, CMV causes variable clinical manifestations similar to those that follow transplantation. In addition to disseminated infection, patients with AIDS commonly develop localized infections, such as chorioretinitis, erosive CMV esophagitis, colitis, pneumonitis, adrenalitis, or meningoencephalitis.

Laboratory Diagnosis

A laboratory diagnosis of suspected CMV infection may be confirmed by several methods, including viral isolation, serologic study, electron microscopy, histologic evaluation, immunohistochemical staining of tissues, and nucleic acid hybridization techniques. Histopathologic detection in biopsy or autopsy material involves demonstration of the characteristic large cells with intranuclear and occasional cytoplasmic inclusions. The presence of these cytomegalic cells suggests CMV infection, but virologic or serologic confirmation is desirable.

A serologic diagnosis may be made by comparing antibody titers present in acute-phase sera with those in convalescent-phase sera obtained 2 to 3 weeks later. A seroconversion or fourfold or greater rise in titer is diagnostic of recent infection. If congenital infection is suspected, both maternal and infant sera should be examined. The presence of IgG class CMV antibodies alone in the infant's serum indicates passive acquisition of maternal antibodies, whereas the detection of CMV IgM antibodies usually indicates actual congenital infection. Common serologic methods include the complement fixation (CF) test, the indirect immunofluorescent antibody (IFA) test, and the anticomplement immunofluorescent (ACIF) test, the latter two being more sensitive than CF. Enzyme-linked immunosorbent assays (ELISA) are also available for CMV serologic testing.

Isolation of CMV is the most specific diagnostic test. CMV may be cultured from throat washings, urine, cervical swabs, blood (buffy coat), or biopsy specimens. In immunosuppressed patients, buffy coat cultures are better indicators of symptomatic infection or disease than positive CMV cultures from urine or throat washings. Positive urine isolates must be interpreted cautiously, since shedding may persist up to 2 years after initial infection. Human fibroblast cultures are routinely used for viral diagnostic purposes, with the time required for virus isolation dependent on the virus titer present. Cultures may be positive within 2 to 10 days, or they may take up to 6 weeks to show cytopathic effects. Recently described is a centrifugation culture technique that allows for a more rapid diagnosis. This involves centrifugation of the specimen onto monolayer cell cultures and the subsequent immunoassay for CMV antigens expressed early during the viral replication cycle. More recently, the sensitive polymerase chain reaction (PCR) method with CMV-specific synthetic oligonucleotide primers has been used to detect viral DNA in clinical specimens.

Treatment

The most promising drugs for the treatment of CMV disease include the antiviral agents ganciclovir (DHPG, 9-[1,3-dihydroxy-2-propoxymethyl] guanine) and phosphonoformate (PFA, foscarnet sodium). Patients with CMV retinitis usually stabilize or improve on therapy with either of these antiviral agents, but patients with CMV pneumonia or colitis often respond poorly. If treatment is terminated, most AIDS patients with these manifestations of CMV disease relapse; therefore maintenance therapy in this particular patient population is necessary. Recent studies in bone marrow transplant recipients with CMV pneumonia demonstrate greater efficacy of ganciclovir in combination with immunoglobulin with high anti-CMV titers. Interferon, transfer factor, adenine arabinoside, acyclovir, and combinations of these agents have been tried without success for treatment of patients with severe CMV disease.

Prevention

Approaches to prevent CMV disease studied thus far include passive and active immunization as well as antiviral agents. Although cell-mediated immunity is important, circulating antibody has some value in preventing CMV disease. Studies in patients with bone marrow and renal transplants reveal that intravenous hyperimmune globulin results in less severe CMV disease. This is especially important in seronegative recipients of transplants from seropositive donors or when the use of seronegative blood products cannot be guaranteed.

Two live attenuated CMV vaccines (AD 169 and Towne 125) have been shown to be safe and immunogenic. Vaccination has been shown to offer partial protection from severe CMV disease after renal transplantation, but immunity wanes rapidly after immunization. Several laboratories are presently developing inactivated subunit vaccines.

Acyclovir (acycloguanosine) is an antiviral agent with selective anti-HSV and anti-VZV activity but limited in vitro anti-CMV activity. In trials involving its use for prophylaxis, acyclovir has been shown to modify the severity of CMV disease after renal transplantation. Similar studies are ongoing in patients with progressive HIV disease to determine whether acyclovir prevents CMV infection and disease in patients with AIDS.

Epstein-Barr Virus

The Epstein-Barr virus (EBV) is ubiquitous and causes a spectrum of diseases, most commonly a self-limited mild illness in adolescents and young adults. Various severe diseases induced by EBV have been described in patients with either inherited, iatrogenically induced or acquired immunodeficiency disorders. The virus is associated with several malignancies of B cell or epithelial cell origin: Burkitt's lymphoma, nasopharyngeal carcinoma, and lymphoma in immunocompromised hosts. These tumors are associated with the presence of EBV genome and antigens in tumor tissue. Like other herpesviruses, EBV establishes latent infection, primarily in the B lymphocyte.

In 1964, Epstein, Achong, and Barr first discovered the virus in persistently infected lymphoblastoid cell lines derived from Burkitt's lymphoma (BL) tissue. The Henles developed serologic methods to diagnose EBV infections which led to their discovery of the association of acute EBV infection with an infectious mononucleosis syndrome when one of their laboratory technicians became ill and EBV seroconversion was demonstrated.

Epidemiology

Infection is ubiquitous and seropositivity to EBV is associated with socioeconomic status. Developing countries have a higher seroprevalence in a younger age group compared with the developed world, where acquisition of EBV infection is often delayed until adolescence or early adulthood. In U.S. college populations, 35% to 80% of the students have EBV antibodies at entry, and 10% to 15% of those without antibody become infected each year they are in college. EBV seropositivity occurs in 90% to 95% of most adult populations.

Pathogenesis

EBV requires close person-to-person contact for transmission. The virus is excreted in saliva, and epithelial cells of the oropharynx are the primary site for viral attachment and productive infection. B lymphocytes are also very important target cells; a complement (C3d) receptor on the lymphocyte also has EBV receptor function. EBV develops latent infection in the throat, lymphoid tissue, and blood. Transmission by transfusion and bone marrow transplantation can occur, but this is less frequent than with CMV. Infection of B lymphocytes induces polyclonal proliferation and EBV antigen expression, and a subset of these cells becomes permanently infected. The normal host immune response will control EBV replication. Intermittent viral reactivation can occur, but it is generally subclinical unless the host is immunosuppressed. It has recently been demonstrated that higher levels of EBV excretion occur with advanced HIV disease than in less advanced HIV infection or normal hosts with infectious mononucleosis.

Clinical Manifestations

Asymptomatic primary infection is the most frequent, and viral shedding in the saliva occurs intermittently at low titer for years. Symptomatic illness usually occurs 4 to 7 weeks after infection and most commonly results in an infectious mononucleosis syndrome with fever, tonsillitis, lymphadenopathy, hepatosplenomegaly, and occasionally hepatitis. The fever may last from 1 to 3 weeks. Approximately 50% of patients develop splenomegaly. Lymphadenopathy may be generalized or localized only to cervical lymph nodes. Occasional patients develop a mild skin rash or one that is extensive and maculopapular in nature. A majority of patients with EBV-induced infectious mononucleosis will develop a skin rash if they are given ampicillin or related drugs.

A majority of patients have recovered completely in 1 to 4 weeks. Younger patients typically have mild symptoms and a short duration of illness, whereas older patients have more prolonged illness. Primary EBV infections in infants and young children are frequently asymptomatic. When symptoms occur in childhood, a variety of disorders have been observed, including otitis media, diarrhea, upper respiratory tract infection, and abdominal complaints.

Although fatal cases are unusual in otherwise normal hosts, the major causes of death associated with EBV infection include neurologic complications (Guillain-Barré syndrome, meningitis, encephalitis, myelitis), splenic rupture, and secondary infections. Splenic rupture may occur secondary to trauma or rarely after deep palpation of the spleen during physical examination. Autoimmune hemolytic anemia, aplastic anemia, agranulocytosis, and thrombocytopenia are also complications of EBV-induced infectious mononucleosis. On rare occasions, some of the symptoms of acute infectious mononucleosis may become chronic and an ill-defined chronic EBV syndrome ensues. The frequency and even the existence of this chronic EBV syndrome as it may or may not relate to the recently described chronic fatigue syndrome is questioned by some and remains to be better defined.

The presence of EBV DNA and antigens has recently been demonstrated in oral hairy leukoplakia (OHL) lesions, which are oral manifestations specifically associated with the development of advanced HIV disease. OHL is believed to be the result of permissive infection of EBV in epithelial cells of the tongue and oral mucosa.

In severe immunodeficiency states when cellular immunity is depressed, EBV may reactivate and cause uncontrolled viral replication. This may result in a severe mononucleosis-like syndrome with fever, leukopenia, and intensified immunosuppression or widespread lymphoproliferation, and lymphomas can develop. The rate of EBV reactivation is augmented by the degree of immunosuppression with some examples of regression of lymphomas after discontinuation of immunosuppressive therapy, such as has been reported in renal transplant patients.

EBV is associated with several lymphoproliferative diseases of B cell origin, including Burkitt's lymphoma and lymphoma of immunocompromised hosts. In addition, this virus has recently been associated with Hodgkin's lymphoma, non-Hodgkin's lymphoma in homosexual men, and lymphoid interstitial pneumonitis in children with AIDS.

Evidence of the association of EBV with Burkitt's lymphoma includes several findings: viral DNA or antigens in tumor tissue, transformation of cultured B lymphocytes by EBV in vitro, induction of lymphomas by EBV in nonhuman primates, significantly higher EBV antibody titers in patients with Burkitt's lymphoma than in control populations as well as a correlation between EBV antibody patterns and prognosis. Cultures from BL tissue explants are monoclonal, and these cells contained distinctive chromosomal translocation from the No. 8 chromosome to No. 14, which involves activation of the c-*myc* oncogene. This chromosomal aberration is not present in EBV-infected cells from patients with infectious mononucleosis. Burkitt's lymphoma is epidemic in regions of equatorial Africa, with only a sporadic occurrence in the United States and western Europe. In the past decade a relatively high frequency of BL has been described in persons with AIDS.

Nasopharyngeal carcinoma (NPC) is a malignant tumor of the epithelial lining behind the nose. There is a high prevalence of NPC in southern China, east Africa, Alaska, and Tunisia. All biopsy tissues of NPC have EBV DNA, which is lacking in tissues examined from other cancers of the head and neck. Specific EBV antibody patterns and titers correlate with the course of tumor progression or regression during treatment.

Diagnosis

Lymphocytosis with many atypical lymphocytes is present during acute infectious mononucleosis. A decreased T helper (CD4+)/T suppressor (CD8+) ratio due to increased CD8+ cells is also seen. A positive heterophile antibody titer is found on laboratory examination. Most patients develop positive heterophile antibodies, which are named for their ability to cross-react with unrelated antigens from different animal species.

Immunologic responses to EBV are complex. In persons with negative tests for heterophile antibodies, tests for specific EBV antibodies should be performed. Specific antibodies to EBV antigens that have been studied thoroughly and found to be of diagnostic importance include those to viral capsid antigen (VCA), early antigens (EA), and Epstein-Barr nuclear antigen (EBNA). With acute infection, IgM to VCA develops first, with IgG developing later. IgM antibodies are transient and disappear after a few weeks or months. Also, antibody to EA develops acutely and disappears after a few weeks or months. Antibodies to the nuclear antigen (EBNA) are the last to appear and detectable EBNA titers are not usually found until 1 to 2 months after acute infection. In persons with past infection, IgG antibodies to VCA and EBNA antibodies are detectable, without VCA-IgM or EA antibodies. Thus, in acute or recent primary EBV infection, one or more of the following serologic responses occur: the presence of VCA-specific IgM antibodies, high titers of VCA-specific IgG antibodies (>1:320), detection of anti-EA (>1:20), and the absence of anti-EBNA. In young infants, however, VCA-IgM and EA antibody responses are detectable in only 50% to 60% of the cases during acute EBV infection.

Treatment

EBV infections are usually self-limited. Treatment for patients with infectious mononucleosis is supportive, with bed rest and symptomatic therapy for fever and sore throat with antipyretics, analgesics, and so on. Severe manifestations, such as tonsillitis with potential airway obstruction and hematologic and neurologic complications, can be treated with coricosteroids.

EBV is inhibited in vitro by vidarabine, acyclovir, and zidovudine. Clinical trials of oral acyclovir for use in the treatment of infectious mononucleosis showed no significant response.

Human Herpesvirus 6 (HHV-6)

In 1986, a novel virus, human herpesvirus 6 (HHV-6), was isolated from six patients with lymphoproliferative disorders. HHV-6 has been found in vitro to infect T and B lymphocytes, monocyte-macrophage cell lines, and megakaryocyte and glioblastoma cells. It has recently been shown in vitro that HHV-6 and HIV can productively coinfect T helper (CD4+) lymphocytes, resulting in accelerated HIV expression and cell death. Whether coinfection with HHV-6 and HIV in vivo results in a course of more progressive HIV disease remains to be determined.

Seroepidemiologic studies indicate that HHV-6 infection is widespread, like other herpesvirus infections, with 60% to 90% of the general population shown to be infected with HHV-6. There appears to be an age-related decline in HHV-6 seroprevalence, which might indicate waning immunity. Higher infection rates have been reported in patients with HIV, lymphoma, and the ill-defined chronic fatigue syndrome. HHV-6 has been associated with the development of roseola (exanthem subitum), a benign rash illness of infants and young children. This illness is characterized by 3 to 5 days of fever and occasionally cervical lymphadenopathy and upper respiratory infection symptoms. Within 48 hours after defervescence, a maculopapular rash on the trunk and neck appears. Primary HHV-6 infection in adults has been associated with a mild mononucleosis-like syndrome. Simultaneous acquisition of HHV-6 and CMV has been reported in transplant recipients. Studies are under way to determine whether HHV-6 is an opportunistic pathogen in the setting of the immunocompromised state.

Diagnosis and Treatment

Serologic testing for HHV-6 is not widely available. Virus isolation is labor intensive, is not well-standardized, and requires cord blood. Thus an efficient culture system has yet to be developed. Foscarnet, acyclovir, and ganciclovir have been found to have antiviral activity. If HHV-6 is found to be a significant pathogen, these antiviral agents may be studied in clinical trials to determine whether they are useful.

Human Herpesvirus 7 (HHV-7)

A new virus, human herpesvirus 7 (HHV-7), described in 1990, was isolated from CD4+ T lymphocytes from healthy individuals. The epidemiology of HHV-7 and its association with any infectious syndrome remain to be determined.

Herpes B Virus

Herpesvirus simiae (B virus) is a close relative of herpes simplex that is enzootic in Old World monkeys. A recent cluster of cases in humans established the importance of B virus as a pathogen.

Epidemiology

Monkeys, particularly macaques, are the reservoir for B virus. In its natural milieu, infection is self-limited and may recur. Little is known about infection in humans, but the natural history is much more severe. The disease has occurred in isolated cases from handling infected monkeys. One case of human-to-human transmission by direct contact has been described.

Of 18 well-detailed cases reviewed, 13 were fatal and three of the five remaining cases resulted in serious neurologic sequelae. A cluster of four cases was reported in Florida in 1987. Three cases resulted from penetrating injuries while monkeys were being handled. The fourth was the spouse of one of the index patients. Two of the Florida cases were identified late, and the patients died of encephalitis despite attempted treatment with acyclovir or ganciclovir. Two patients with localized infection were given long-term treatment with acyclovir. As a result of this outbreak, the Centers for Disease Control and the National Institutes of Health issued recommendations for appropriate care of persons exposed to the virus. The role of antiviral therapy has not been defined. Treatment with acyclovir or ganciclovir has been attempted because of the high risk of mortality and the in vitro susceptibility of herpes B virus to both agents.

FURTHER READING

HERPES SIMPLEX VIRUS

Corey L, Spear PG: Infections with herpes simplex viruses. N Engl J Med 314:686, 749, 1986

Straus SE: Herpes simplex virus infection: Biology, treatment and prevention. Ann Intern Med 103:404, 1985

Johnson RE, et al: A seroepidemiologic survey of the prevalence of herpes simplex virus type 2 infection in the United States. N Engl J Med 321:7, 1989

Spruance SL, et al: The natural history of recurrent herpes simplex labialis. N Engl J Med 297:69, 1977

Corey L, et al: Genital herpes simplex virus infections: Clinical manifestations, course, and complications. Ann Intern Med 98:958, 1983

Corey L, et al: Genital herpes simplex virus infections: Current concepts in diagnosis, therapy, and prevention. Ann Intern Med 98:973, 1983

Koutsky LA: The frequency of unrecognized type 2 herpes simplex virus infection among women: Implications for the control of genital herpes. Sex Transm Dis 17:90, 1989.

Siegal FP, et al: Severe acquired immunodeficiency in male homosexuals, manifested by chronic perianal ulcerative herpes simplex lesions. N Engl J Med 305:1439, 1981

Stamm WE, et al: The association between genital ulcer disease and acquisition of HIV infection in homosexual men. JAMA 260:1429, 1988

Laurence J: Molecular interactions among herpesviruses and human immunodeficiency viruses. J Infect Dis 162:338, 1990

Rawls WE, et al: Serological and epidemiological considerations of the role of herpes simplex virus type 2 in cervical cancer. Cancer Res 36:829, 1976

Galloway DA, McDougall JK: The oncogenic potential of herpes simplex viruses: Evidence for a "hit-and-run" mechanism. Nature 302:21, 1983

Gill MJ, et al: Herpes simplex virus infection of the hand. J Am Acad Dermatol 22:111, 1990

Selling B, Kibrick S: An outbreak of herpes simplex among wrestlers (herpes gladiatorum). N Engl J Med 270:979, 1964

Bork K, Brauninger W: Increasing incidence of eczema herpeticum: Analysis of seventy-five cases. J Am Acad Dermatol 19:1024, 1988

Whitley RJ, et al: Herpes simplex encephalitis: Vidarabine therapy and diagnostic problems. N Engl J Med 304:313, 1981

Whitley RJ, et al: Vidarabine versus acyclovir therapy in herpes simplex encephalitis. N Engl J Med 314:144, 1986

Whitley RJ, et al: Diseases that mimic herpes simplex encephalitis: Diagnosis, presentation and outcome. JAMA 262:234, 1989

Liesegang TJ: Ocular herpes simplex infection: Pathogenesis and current therapy. Mayo Clin Proc 63:1092, 1988

Whitley RJ, et al: Predictors of morbidity and mortality in neonates with herpes simplex virus infections. N Engl J Med 324:450, 1991

Arvin AM, et al: Failure of antepartum maternal cultures to predict the infant's risk of exposure to herpes simplex at delivery. N Engl J Med 315:796, 1986

Hirsch MS: Herpes group virus infections in the compromised host. In Rubin RH, Young LS (eds): Clinical Approach to Infection in the Compromised Host. New York, Plenum, 1988

Corey L: Laboratory diagnosis of herpes simplex virus infections: Principles guiding the development of rapid diagnostic tests. Diagn Microbiol Infect Dis 4:111S, 1986

Mindel A. Treatment, prevention and control. In Herpes Simplex Virus. London, Springer-Verlag, 1989

Dorsky DI, Crumpacker CS: Drugs five years later: acyclovir. Ann Intern Med 107:859, 1987

Whitley RJ, et al: A controlled trial comparing vidarabine with acyclovir in neonatal herpes simplex virus infection. N Engl J Med 324:444, 1991

Kurtz T, et al: Safety and efficacy of long-term suppressive Zovirax treatment of frequently recurring genital herpes: Year 5 results (Abstr. 1107). In 30th Interscience Conference on Antimicrobial Agents and Chemotherapy, 1990.

Erlich KS, et al: Foscarnet therapy for severe acyclovir-resistant herpes simplex virus type-2 infections in patients with the acquired immunodeficiency syndrome. Ann Intern Med 110:710, 1989

Mertz GJ, et al: Double-blind, placebo-controlled trial of a herpes simplex virus type 2 glycoprotein vaccine in persons at high risk for genital herpes infection. J Infect Dis 161:653, 1990

VARICELLA ZOSTER VIRUS

Straus SE: Varicella-zoster infections: Biology, natural history, treatment, and prevention. Ann Intern Med 108:221, 1988

Hyman RW: Natural History of Varicella-Zoster Virus. Boca Raton, Fla., CRC Press, 1987

Weller TH: Varicella and herpes zoster: Changing concepts of the natural history, control and importance of a not-so-benign virus. N Engl J Med 309:1362, 1434, 1983

Hope-Simpson RE: The nature of herpes zoster: A long-term study and a new hypothesis. Proc R Soc Med 58:9, 1965

Croen KD, et al: Patterns of gene expression and sites of latency in human nerve ganglia are different for varicella-zoster and herpes simplex viruses. Proc Natl Acad Sci USA 85:9773, 1988

Dolin R: Herpes zoster-varicella infections in immunosuppressed patients. Ann Intern Med 89:375, 1978

Preblud SR: Varicella: Complications and costs. Pediatrics 78(Suppl):728, 1986

Brunell PA: Varicella in the womb and beyond. Pediatr Infect Dis J 9:770, 1990

Burgoon CF, et al: The natural history of herpes zoster. JAMA 164:265, 1957

Ragozzino MW, et al: Population-based study of herpes zoster and its sequelae. Medicine 61:310, 1982

DeMoragas JM, Kierland RB: The outcome of patients with herpes zoster. Arch Dermatol 75:193, 1957

Hope-Simpson RE: Postherpetic neuralgia. J R Coll Gen Pract 25:572, 1975

Loeser JD: Herpes zoster and postherpetic neuralgia. Pain 25:149, 1986

Hoppenjans WB, et al: Prolonged cutaneous herpes zoster in acquired immunodeficiency syndrome. Arch Dermatol 126:1048, 1990

Prober CG, et al: Acyclovir therapy of chickenpox in immunosuppressed children: A collaborative study. J Pediatr 101:622, 1982

Balfour HH, et al: Acyclovir treatment of varicella in otherwise healthy children. J Pediatr 116:633, 1990

Arvin A, et al: A double-blind placebo controlled trial of acyclovir (ACV) treatment of chickenpox in healthy children. Abstr. 725. In 30th Interscience Conference on Antimicrobial Agents and Chemotherapy, 1990.

Whitley RJ et al: Early vidarabine therapy to control the complications of herpes zoster in immunosuppressed patients. N Engl J Med 307:971, 1982

Balfour HH, et al: Acyclovir halts progression of herpes zoster in immunocompromised patients. N Engl J Med 308:1448, 1983

Shepp DH, et al: Treatment of varicella-zoster virus infection in severely immunocompromised patients: A randomized comparison of acyclovir and vidarabine. N Engl J Med 314:208, 1986

Huff JC, et al: Therapy of herpes zoster with oral acyclovir. Am J Med 85(Suppl 2A):84, 1988

Morton P, Thomson AN: Oral acyclovir in the treatment of herpes zoster in general practice. N Z Med J 102:93, 1989

Williams WW: CDC guideline for infection control in hospital personnel. Infect Control 4:326, 1983

Centers for Disease Control: Varicella-zoster immune globulin for the prevention of chickenpox. Ann Intern Med 100:859, 1984

Gershon AA: Live attenuated varicella vaccine. Ann Rev Med 38:41, 1987

CYTOMEGALOVIRUS

Weller TH: The cytomegalovirus: Ubiquitous agents with protean clinical manifestations. N Engl J Med 285:203, 1971

Ho M: Cytomegalovirus, Biology and Infection. New York, Plenum, 1982

Huang ES, et al: Molecular epidemiology and oncogenicity of human cytomegalovirus. In Harris CC (ed): Biochemical and Molecular Biology of Cancer. UCLA Symposium on Molecular and Cell Biology New Series 40:323, 1986

Hanshaw JB: Congenital cytomegalovirus infection: A fifteen year perspective. J Infect Dis 123:555, 1971

Stagno S, et al: Congenital cytomegalovirus infection: Occurrence in an immune population. N Engl J Med 296:1254, 1977

Stagno S, et al: Congenital cytomegalovirus infection: The relative importance of primary and recurrent maternal infection. N Engl J Med 306:945, 1982

Stagno S et al: Primary cytomegalovirus infection in pregnancy: Incidence, transmission to fetus, and clinical outcome. JAMA 256:1904, 1986

Handsfield HH, et al: Cytomegalovirus infection in sexual partners: Evidence for sexual transmission. J Infect Dis 151:344, 1985

Reynolds DW, et al: Inapparent congenital cytomegalovirus infection with elevated cord IgM levels: Casual relationship with auditory and mental deficiency. N Engl J Med 290:291, 1974

Kumar ML et al: Congenital and postnatally acquired cytomegalovirus infections: Long-term follow-up. J Pediatr 104:674, 1984

Chatterjee SN, Jordan GW: Perspective study of the prevalence and symptomatology of cytomegalovirus infection in renal transplant recipients. Transplantation 28:457, 1979

Smiley ML, et al: The role of pretransplant immunity in protection from cytomegalovirus disease following renal transplantation. Transplantation 40:157, 1985

Klemola E, et al: Cytomegalovirus mononucleosis in previously healthy individuals. Ann Intern Med 71:11, 1969

Gleaves CA, et al: Rapid detection of cytomegalovirus in MRC-5 cells inoculated with urine specimens by using low-speed centrifugation and monoclonal antibody to early antigen. J Clin Microbiol 19:917, 1984

Shepp DH, et al: Activity of 9-[hydroxy-1-(hydroxymethyl)ethoxymethyl] guanine in the treatment of cytomegalovirus pneumonia. Ann Intern Med 103:368, 1985

Laskin OL, et al: Use of gancyclovir to treat serious cytomegalovirus infections in patients with AIDS. J Infect Dis 155:323, 1987

Collaborative DHPG Treatment Study Group: Treatment of serious cytomegalovirus infections with 9-(1,3-dihydroxy-2-propoxymethyl) guanine in patients with AIDS and other immunodeficiencies. N Engl J Med 314:801, 1986

Yeager AS et al: Prevention of transfusion-acquired cytomegalovirus infections in newborn infants. J Pediatr 98:281, 1981

Snydman DR, et al: Use of cytomegalovirus immune globulin to prevent cytomegalovirus diseases in renal-transplant recipients. N Engl J Med 317:1049, 1987

Plotkin SA, et al: Clinical trials of immunization with the Towne 125 strain of human cytomegalovirus. J Infect Dis 134:470, 1976

EPSTEIN-BARR VIRUS

Cheeseman SH: Infectious mononucleosis. Semin Hematol 25:261, 1988

Epstein MA, Achong BG (ed): The Epstein-Barr Virus, New York, Springer-Verlag, 1979

Fleisher GR, Pasquariello PS, Warren WS, et al: Infrafamilial transmission of Epstein-Barr virus infections. J Pediatr 98:16, 1981

Kieff E, Dambaugh T, Heller M, et al: The biology and chemistry of Epstein-Barr virus. J Infect Dis 146:506, 1982

Miller G: Epstein-Barr virus: Biology, pathogenesis and medical aspects. In Fields BN, Knipe DM (eds): Fields Virology, ed 2, vol 2. New York, Raven Press, 1990

Purtilo DT, Tatsumi E, Manolov G, et al: Epstein-Barr virus as an etiological agent in the pathogenesis of lymphoproliferative and aproliferative diseases in immune deficient patients. Int Rev Exp Pathol 27:113, 1985

Robinson J, Brown N, Andiman W, et al: Diffuse polyclonal B cell lymphoma during primary infection with Epstein-Barr virus. N Engl J Med 302:1293, 1980

Sayer RN, Evans AS, Niederman JC, et al: Prospective studies of a group of Yale University freshmen. I. Occurrence of infectious mononucleosis. J Infect Dis 123:263, 1971

Stagno S, Whitley RJ: Herpesvirus infections of pregnancy. I. Cytomegalovirus and Epstein-Barr virus infections. N Engl J Med 313:1270, 1985

Tosato G, Blaese RM: Epstein-Barr virus infection and immunoregulation in man. Adv Immunol 37:99, 1985

Straus SE: The chronic mononucleosis syndrome. J Infect Dis 157:405, 1988

Sullivan JL: Epstein-Barr virus and lymphoproliferative disorders. Semin Hematol 25:269, 1988

Thorley-Lawson DA: Basic virological aspects of Epstein-Barr virus infection. Semin Hematol 25:247, 1988

HUMAN HERPESVIRUSES 6 AND 7

Frenkel N, et al: Isolation of a new herpesvirus from human CD4+ T cells. Proc Natl Acad Sci USA 87:748, 1990

Irving WL, Cunningham AL: Serological diagnosis of infection with human herpesvirus type 6. Br Med J 300:156, 1990

Lopez C, Pellett P, Stewart J, et al: Characteristics of human herpesvirus-6. J Infect Dis 157:1271, 1988

Niederman JC, Liu C-R, Kaplan MH, Brown NA: Clinical and serological features of human herpesvirus-6 infection in three adults. Lancet 2:817, 1988

Okuno T, Takahashi K, Balachandra K, et al: Seroepidemiology of human herpesvirus 6 infection in normal children and adults. J Clin Microbiol 27:651, 1989

Russler SK, et al: Susceptibility of human herpesvirus 6 to acyclovir and ganciclovir. Lancet II:817, 1989

Salahudden SZ, Ablashi DV, Markham PD, et al: Isolation of a new virus, HBLV, in patients with lymphoproliferative disorders. Science 234:596, 1986

Spira TJ, Bozeman LH, Sanderlin KC, et al: Lack of correlation between human herpesvirus-6 infection and the course of human immunodeficiency virus infection. J Infect Dis 161:567, 1990

Yamanishi K, Okuno T, Shiraki K, et al: Identification of human herpesvirus-6 as a causal agent for exanthem subitum. Lancet 1:1065, 1988

HERPES B VIRUS

Centers for Disease Control: Guidelines for prevention of herpesvirus simiae (B virus) infection in monkey handlers. MMWR 36:41, 1987

Holmes GH, et al: B virus (Herpesvirus simiae) infection in humans: Epidemiologic investigation of a cluster. Ann Intern Med 112:833, 1990

CHAPTER 65

Adenoviruses and Adeno-associated Viruses

Adenoviruses

Human adenoviruses are medium-sized DNA viruses that belong to the family of Adenoviridae, genus of *Mastadenovirus*. These agents were first isolated in the early 1950s by two independent groups of researchers. In 1953, while working with epithelial cell lines derived from adenoid tissue, Rowe and collaborators isolated an agent capable of producing cytopathic effects. Almost simultaneously, an agent causing acute respiratory distress (ARD) in military recruits was found. Further studies with these new viruses determined that they produced similar cytopathologic changes and were antigenically related. In 1956 Enders and coworkers gave the name *adenovirus* to these agents as a reminder of the source of the original prototype strain and also to designate the prominent involvement of lymphoid tissue that occurs during these infections.

Adenoviruses have been recognized mainly as pathogens of the eye and respiratory tract. Since their initial recovery, however, they have been isolated from individuals with diseases affecting most other organ systems. In more recent years, the ability of these agents to produce disseminated disease in the immunocompromised host has become evident. Of the 41 serotypes now identified, some have been related to specific disease entities.

These viruses were the first human DNA viruses with a demonstrable oncogenic potential in animals. This feature, added to their ability to produce persistent infections, encouraged studies directed to an understanding of the mechanisms governing virus replication and cell transformation. Results of these studies have given insight into basic mechanisms of cellular biology. For example, the process of messenger RNA splicing was originally described in adenoviruses. The genome of some of these agents has been structurally and functionally mapped, and the techniques originally applied to these efforts are now used to study other viral agents.

Classification

There are at present 41 recognized serotypes of human adenoviruses. The 41 human adenoviruses are subdivided by their biophysical, biochemical, biologic, and immunologic characteristics into seven subgroups (A through G), as indicated in Table 53–4. The biophysical and biologic characterizations of these viruses and the clinical syndromes caused by the subgroups are remarkably parallel. Subgroup A adenoviruses (types 12, 18, and 31) are regularly isolated from the feces of apparently healthy humans, and the incidence of antibody to them is high. This group of adenoviruses is associated with the induction of tumors in hamsters. Subgroup B adenoviruses (types 3, 7, 11, 14, 16, 21, 34, and 35) are most frequently isolated from the throat washings of patients during epidemics of acute respiratory illness and may be associated with severe pneumonia. This group of adenoviruses is not associated with latency. Subgroup C adenoviruses (types 1, 2, 5, and 6) are most commonly isolated from the respiratory and gastrointestinal tracts of children with mild upper respiratory tract infections; they are also isolated from long-term cultures of adenoid or tonsillar tissue. Apparently, subgroup C adenoviruses are able to establish latent infections in lymphoid tissue, which persist for extended periods of time. Subgroup D adenoviruses (types 8 to 10, 13, 15, 17 to 20, 22 to 30, 32, 33, and 36 to 39) are most often associated with the clinical entities of conjunctivitis and pharyngoconjunctival fever. They are not usually associated with the development of latent infections. Antibodies to these serotypes are also less commonly detected in seroepidemiologic surveys of the population. The only subgroup E adenovirus is adenovirus type 4, which has been associated with severe respiratory disease in both sporadic and epidemic forms and with pharyngoconjunctival fever. Adenovirus type 40 constitutes subgroup F, and adenovirus type 41 is the only virus of subgroup G. Adenoviruses 40 and 41 are characterized as fastidious enteric adenoviruses.

Pathogenesis and Pathology

Adenoviruses are capable of establishing productive infections of the respiratory, conjunctival, and gastrointestinal mucosal lining cells. From these primary sites of infection, newly replicated virus may enter the bloodstream and establish infection in other body tissues; subsequent events depend on the complex interplay of host and viral factors. The various adenoviral serotypes have unique tissue tropisms. Most cases of severe lower respiratory tract and disseminated infections have involved adenoviruses 1 to 5, 7, and 21. Ocular infections are usually due to adenoviruses 3, 4, 7, 11, and 37; more severe ocular infections occur with adenoviruses 8 and 19. Occasionally, adenovirus 7 has been implicated in infections of the central nervous system.

So far there are no satisfactory animal models in which to study the pathological effects of adenovirus infections. Therefore the pathology of these infections has been studied in tissues obtained from fatal cases of disseminated disease or severe pneumonia. In the respiratory tract, these infections cause extensive necrosis of the bronchial epithelium and bronchial glands. The alveolar spaces are distended by an eosinophilic exudate, and the interstitial tissue is infiltrated by mononuclear cells. As with other viral infections, intranuclear inclusions are frequently present. Initially, these are basophilic intranuclear deposits, and amphophilic or eosinophilic intranuclear inclusions appear later. Electron microscopic visualization of these inclusion bodies shows that they are made of typical paracrystalline arrays of virus particles. In acutely infected livers, tissue necrosis, mononuclear infiltration, and basophilic or amphophilic inclusions are also seen.

The pathologic changes described are thought to be due to direct tissue damage determined by the virus replication process within susceptible cells. Tissue injury may also occur through immunopathologic mechanisms. For example, the chronic inflammatory sequelae of adenoviral keratitis evolves in the absence of recoverable virus. It is thought that persistent antigen-antibody complexes elicit an inflammatory response that determines continued injury to the cornea.

Immunologic clearance of infective virus requires the successful interaction of macrophages, lymphocytes, natural killer cells, and humoral factors, including antibody, complement, interferon, and lymphokines. Although there is some evidence that humoral responses can modify adenoviral infections, cell-mediated immune mechanisms are responsible for the containment and eventual resolution of these infections. Most cases of severe or disseminated adenovirus infections have been documented in patients in whom cellular immunity is abnormal or absent. Susceptible individuals include neonates, immunosuppressed cancer or transplant patients, children with congenital thymic aplasia or other T-cell disorders, and HIV-infected individuals.

A possible outcome of an adenoviral infection is the establishment of persistent infections despite adequate function of the immune system. These infections are accompanied by asymptomatic chronic shedding of viable viral particles, indicating a failure of immune clearance. The mechanisms by which these agents are able to persist in an organism with an intact immunologic system have not been elucidated but are the subject of intense research.

Clinical Associations

Adenoviruses show a predilection for infections of conjunctival, respiratory, and intestinal epithelium, in addition to regional lymphoid tissue. Incubation periods have been 1 to 2 weeks where discernible. Latent infections, clinically asymptomatic infections, and prolonged viral shedding after clinical illness (particularly in the intestine) have all been described.

Respiratory Infections

Adenoviruses are able to replicate in all areas of the respiratory tract, producing acute upper and lower respiratory tract infections. The potential to produce latent infections with prolonged colonization of the upper respiratory tract and adjacent lymphoid tissues is evidenced by the frequent isolation of these agents from respiratory secretions or stool specimens of asymptomatic individuals. Serologic surveys have estimated that 5% to 10% of all respiratory infections in children under 5 years of age are due to adenoviruses. They are the third most common viral respiratory pathogen in children, after respiratory syncytial virus and parainfluenza virus. Serotypes of groups B and C are the usual isolates that cause respiratory infections.

The most common respiratory illnesses caused by these agents are pharyngitis, tonsillitis, and nasopharyngitis. Adenoviruses are rarely associated with the common cold syndrome. Sore throat with redness, tonsillar exudates, and cervical adenopathy are the common clinical symptoms, lasting 5 to 7 days. One fourth of the cases of exudative pharyngitis in children of preschool age are due to adenoviruses. They are also an important cause of nonstreptococcal pharyngitis in military recruits. Most upper respiratory infections are mild and are followed by complete resolution.

Sporadic mild cases of croup (acute laryngotracheitis) caused by adenoviruses type 1, 2, 3, 5, 6, and 7 have been reported in young children. However, other viruses are more important causes of this syndrome.

It is estimated that 5% of acute bronchiolitis is due to adenoviruses. The disease is usually mild and sporadic, with clinical symptoms similar to those in cases caused by other viral pathogens. Rarely, severe cases with residual lung damage or death have resulted from infections with these agents. Usual serotypes involved in bronchiolitis have been types 3, 7, and 21.

Childhood pneumonias due to adenoviruses are less frequent than those caused by respiratory syncytial virus and parainfluenza. However, adenoviruses cause more severe disease and appear to be more frequently associated with fatalities. Severe pneumonia usually occurs in infants 3 to 18 months of age. High fever, cough, respiratory distress, rales, vomiting, and lethargy are frequent. In severe cases, dissemination of infection with the involvement of central nervous system, liver, skin, myocardium, and kidneys has been described. Recovery with residual lung damage is not unusual after severe pneumonia. Some patients develop bronchiolitis obliterans and have a waxing and waning course with wheezing, respiratory distress, cough, fever, and pneumonia. Unilateral hyperlucent lung syndrome may also be the result of a severe infection. The syndrome is caused by a reduction in the number and size of pulmonary vessels with the resultant hypoperfusion, decrease in lung size, and poor aeration of all or part of a lung field. Adenoviruses 7 and 21 have been associated with this complication.

Types 3 and 7 have been described as causing pneumonia in healthy adults. Death secondary to adenoviral pneumonias usually occur in young infants and in children with underlying diseases, malnutrition, and crowding, and it may follow previous viral infections such as measles.

A pertussislike syndrome in children less than 3 years of age has been described. Progressive cough develops over 1 or 2 weeks and becomes paroxysmal in nature. Approximately half the children have the typical whoop. Leukocytosis with lymphocytosis and elevated platelet counts are usual.

Military recruits constitute a population group that is very susceptible to infections by these agents. Acute respiratory disease (ARD) is an influenza-like syndrome that affects recruits in early stages of their training. Adenoviruses 4, 7, and 21 are the typical isolated serotypes. Crowding and fatigue appear to be important predisposing factors. Initial studies of this disease reported a hospitalization rate of approximately 20%. The disease occurs in epidemics with a higher incidence during winter months. Affected individuals present with pharyngitis, cervical adenitis, fever, cough, chest pain, myalgias, diarrhea, and rales. X-ray films of the chest may show bilateral mottled infiltrates. Occasional fatalities have been reported in persons infected with serotypes 4 and 7.

Ocular Infections

Ocular infections caused by adenoviruses can be grouped into three distinct clinical entities: acute follicular conjunctivitis, pharyngoconjunctival fever, and epidemic keratoconjunctivitis.

The first of these entities is the most common eye infection produced by adenoviruses. It is a benign unilateral follicular conjunctivitis with no extraocular manifestations. After an incubation period of 5 to 7 days, the conjunctiva becomes hyperemic; there is increased lacrimation, and clear eye drainage with a sensation of a foreign body develops. The condition is self-limited and resolves completely in 10 to 14 days. Various adenoviral types have been recovered from conjunctival scrapings. Most cases occur sporadically and are most likely transmitted by direct contact.

Pharyngoconjunctival fever (PCF) was recognized as a distinct entity in the nineteenth century, when it was thought to be caused by *Chlamydia trachomatis.* In 1955, a few years after the initial isolation of adenoviruses, the association between these agents and PCF was made. The most frequent serotypes involved are types 3 and 7; other serotypes implicated at times are 1, 4, and 14. Although sporadic cases of the disease occur, the typical scenario is that of a focal outbreak or epidemic centered around a recreational swimming facility or a summer camp. Usually children or young adults are affected. Secondary spread to siblings, parents, or close contacts occurs frequently. In some outbreaks the virus has been recovered from contaminated water. In episodes that occur around a swimming pool, poor chlorination of the water has been demonstrated and implicated as the cause of the outbreak.

Transmission occurs by direct contact of contaminated water or respiratory secretions with the conjunctival mucosa. Direct inoculation into the conjunctival sac appears to be necessary for disease production with subsequent spread to the upper respiratory tract or by autoinoculation with respiratory secretions. The incubation period is usually 6 to 9 days, but it may be shorter.

The onset of disease is abrupt, with sore throat, fever, and conjunctivitis. The pharynx appears red, the tonsils are frequently enlarged and may have exudates, and postnasal drainage and coryza are common. Most patients have a high fever for 3 to 4 days. In 10% of the patients the febrile illness continues for 7 to 10 days.

The eyes are hyperemic, with increased tearing and crusts; the palpebral conjunctiva appears granular, and small bulbar hemorrhages may be present. Associated symptoms such as headache, malaise, vomiting, and diarrhea are common, especially in young children. Adults appear to have a milder condition, mainly limited to ocular involvement. This may be due to partial immunity acquired from previous exposures. The disease gradually subsides after 2 weeks, with complete resolution. Adenoviruses may be recovered from the conjunctiva, throat, and stool of infected persons.

The most serious ocular infection caused by these agents is epidemic keratoconjunctivitis (EKC), a condition that also has been retrospectively recognized from reports of epidemics occurring in the early twentieth century. The association of disease with adenoviral infection was established in 1955 with the isolation of adenovirus 8 from affected individuals. Subsequently, other serotypes have been isolated in cases of EKC. Severe cases are associated with types 5, 8, and 19. In recent epidemics type 37 has been the most frequent isolate in Europe and the United States.

The disease occurs sporadically or in epidemics affecting mainly adults. Early on, it was described in industrial workers. During World War II it was common in shipyards, where it was known as "shipyard eye." Apparently, the disease spread from Hawaii to the West Coast of the United States and has gradually extended to the East Coast. More recently it has been the cause of epidemics in Vietnamese refugee camps and in large ophthalmology centers. Transmission occurs by direct contact from person to person through contaminated hands or ophthalmologic instruments.

Adenovirus 8 is widely distributed in Southeast Asia, where it is endemic. In this area 40% to 60% of school-aged children have demonstrable antibody titers against this viral type. In contrast, school-aged children in the United States are seronegative for this type.

The disease is characterized by a follicular conjunctivitis with palpebral edema, pain, and photophobia accompanied by preauricular adenopathy; sore throat and coryza are usual. As the conjunctival involvement begins to resolve, corneal erosions develop. Initially these are superficial and centrally located; later they become subepithelial and heal gradually, leaving corneal opacities that may impair vision and persist for months.

In Japan an infantile form of this disease has been recognized. It takes the form of a conjunctivitis with systemic symptoms and no corneal involvement. The disease follows an incubation period of 5 to 7 days and may begin with unilateral eye involvement, only to spread to the unaffected eye 2 to 7 days later.

The diagnosis may be suggested by the clinical presentation and epidemiologic characteristics of the disease. Rapid diagnostic tests are helpful and detect the presence of viral antigens in the clinical specimen. The virus can be recovered from the conjunctiva or throat. Later the agent may be isolated in the stool. One study indicated that immunofiltration can detect antigen in the conjunctiva of patients with symptomatic disease for 7 days after the onset of symptoms. Chronic cases with prolonged viral shedding have been reported. Giemsa stains can be positive for the presence of viral inclusion bodies.

Infections of Genitourinary Tract

Acute hemorrhagic cystitis (AHC) is a unique adenoviral infection of the urinary tract. It was first described in Japan in 1968. Typically, this disease affects young males, who develop sudden onset dysuria, gross hematuria, and suprapubic pain. The lack of associated hypertension and abnormal renal function tests help differentiate this condition from glomerulonephritis. The disease usually lasts 5 days, resolving spontaneously without residual dysfunction. Adenoviruses 11 and 21 are the usual serotypes isolated in these cases and can be recovered from urine. Immunofluorescence of exfoliated bladder cells is positive in some cases and can assist with the diagnosis.

Renal involvement has occasionally accompanied severe adenoviral pulmonary infections; red blood cell casts and proteinuria have been described. In renal transplant patients adenoviruses 34 and 35 have been recovered in the urine and may persist for prolonged periods of time. HIV-infected individuals have also had prolonged viruria with adenovirus type 35.

Adenoviruses 19 and 37 have been isolated from the genitourinary tract of males and females attending a sexually transmitted diseases clinic. Cervicitis by adenoviruses has been described and occasionally may accompany herpetic infections. Oculogenital involvement has been reported with adenovirus type 19.

Gastrointestinal Infections

Although adenoviruses were frequently isolated from stool specimens, their role in the production of disease localized to the gastrointestinal tract was unclear. Patients who have experienced infections caused by these agents frequently shed viruses in their stools long after symptoms have resolved. Many clinicians believed that these agents were important causes of infantile diarrhea, but isolation of these agents in symptom-free patients obscured their real significance. During electron microscopic screenings of stools of children with a diarrheal illness adenovirus-like particles were visualized. Initial attempts to culture these agents were not successful. Subsequently, it was shown that these adenoviruses were defective viruses that required human embryonic kidney (HEK) cells modified by adenovirus 5 to replicate and produce cytopathic effects. The fastidious or enteric adenoviruses are serotypes 40 and 41.

These adenoviruses cause diarrhea in young children. The disease can be prolonged and accompanied by respiratory symptoms. It is estimated that 5% to 12% of cases of infantile diarrhea are produced by enteric adenoviruses 40 and 41. The disease may occur in epidemics, and nosocomial transmission has been documented. In some populations, 50% of the children develop antibodies to these serotypes by the time they are 4 years of age.

Hepatic involvement, with elevated liver function tests, hepatomegaly, and jaundice, is described in cases of disseminated disease affecting the young infant or the immunocompromised patient. Recently outbreaks of adenoviral hepatitis in American Indians have been reported with the isolation of adenoviruses types 1, 2, and 3. Adenovirus 5 has been implicated in sporadic cases of uncomplicated hepatitis.

Other gastrointestinal diseases in which the isolation of adenoviruses has been reported include intussusception, mesenteric adenitis, and appendicitis. However, many patients with these illnesses have no evidence of an adenoviral infection. It is possible that their illnesses are the result of multiple possible etiologic factors. Recently some investigators have tried to establish a relationship between adenoviral infections and celiac disease. It appears that an early viral protein product of adenovirus 12 has similar amino acid sequences to α-gliadin, a major component of gluten. One study reported that patients with celiac disease were more likely than healthy controls to have antibodies to adenovirus 12. This has not been confirmed by other reports.

Other Clinical Adenovirus Infections

Several other syndromes and illnesses have rarely been associated with adenovirus infection. Among them are myocarditis, arthritis, acute and subacute meningoencephalitis, and general exanthems. Many of the higher adenovirus serotypes have been recovered from persons with inapparent infections, and their significance in disease is uncertain. Adenovirus 35 has been isolated from immunosuppressed patients, particularly those with AIDS and AIDS-related complex (ARC), and may cause life-threatening infections, primarily interstitial pneumonitis. Adenoviruses 11, 34, and 35 have been reported to cause serious and at times life-threatening illnesses in patients with bone marrow transplants. These infections may represent reactivation of latent virus in a manner analogous to cytomegalovirus infections in this population.

Epidemiology and Transmission

Adenoviruses are ubiquitous agents that infect humans of all ages, races, and nationalities. All the known human adenoviruses have been recovered from patients with a wide range of epidemic or sporadic illnesses. For clinical purposes, adenoviruses can be divided into three overlapping groups: (1) adenoviruses that are endemic in early childhood; (2) those that determine epidemics; (3) and those that are predominantly sporadic. The lower-numbered adenoviral serotypes (adenoviruses 1, 2, 5, and 6) appear to be endemic in many areas of the world. In western Europe and the United States between one third and one half of the children under the age of 1 year have acquired antibodies to one or more of the adenovirus types. Adenoviruses 3, 4, 7, 8, and occasionally 11, 14, 19, and 21 tend to be implicated in epidemic infections. Adenoviruses 3, 4, and 7 are commonly associated with epidemics of PCF. Adenoviruses 4 and 7 and less often 11, 14, and 21 are associated with ARD in military recruits. Adenoviruses 8 and 19 are associated with EKC. Outbreaks of gastroenteritis have been attributed to the fastidious enteric adenoviruses 40 and 41.

Adenoviral infections have been documented in tropical

and temperate climates and occur throughout the year. Seasonal differences in infection rates are not as marked in the tropical settings as they are the temperate zones, where a midwinter and a midsummer peak of adenoviral respiratory illness are seen. ARD in military recruits is largely confined to the cooler months of the year.

The major means of transmission, at least in childhood, is the fecal-oral route. Adenoviruses continue to be excreted from the feces for months or years after an initial infection. Although chronic viral shedding from the respiratory tract occurs, fecal shedding appears to be more intense and prolonged. ARD can be transmitted experimentally by oral inoculation of infective respiratory secretions to healthy volunteers. PCF is thought to be transmitted through direct contact of contaminated swimming pool water or other infected materials with the nose or eyes.

The incubation period for the various clinical presentations of adenoviruses varies from 4 to 10 days. PCF usually is preceded by 5 to 10 days' incubation, with a mean of 7 days, whereas the incubation period for EKC is usually 7 to 10 days. Outbreaks of ARD have an incubation period of 7 to 10 days.

Laboratory Diagnosis

Although the diagnosis of an adenoviral infection can be entertained on the basis of epidemiologic and clinical information, the isolation of the agent from the clinical specimen or the demonstration of viral antigens in the specimen is required to establish the diagnosis with certainty.

Adenoviruses have been isolated from the respiratory, genital, and gastrointestinal tracts, from the conjunctival mucosa, and occasionally from the central nervous system. Body fluids and secretions, including those from the throat, nasopharynx, bronchoalveolar lavage, urine, stool, blood, biopsy, or autopsy tissues, are cultured in the laboratory.

Because of the special tropism of adenoviruses for epithelial cells, these agents are best recovered when inoculated onto epithelial cell lines and grow less well when human diploid fibroblast lines are used. Primary HEK cells and monkey kidney cells are the epithelial cell lines frequently used for virus isolation. Some continuous malignant cell lines such as Hep-2, KB, or HeLa may also be used to isolate adenovirus.

The fastidious enteric adenoviruses fail to produce visible cytopathic effects in human kidney cells and human diploid fibroblasts. These adenoviruses, serotypes 40 and 41, may be isolated with some difficulty in the Chang conjunctival cell line, primary cynomolgus monkey kidney, or in Graham 293 cells. The 292 cell line was derived by transforming HEK cells with adenovirus 5.

Cell lines permissive to infection with adenovirus typically show cytopathic effects in 3 to 5 days. However, some specimens may require several weeks to grow, depending on the specific adenoviral type involved and the amount of viable virus present in the sample. Infected cells typically become swollen, rounded, and refractile; many have large intracytoplasmic vacuoles. Certain adenoviral subtypes will determine grapelike clustering of infected cells in the tissue culture monolayer.

Newly formed adenoviruses are "cell associated," and few free virus particles can be demonstrated in the tissue culture media. Harvesting cells after the disruption of an inoculated monolayer by freeze/thawing increases the viral titer by freeing viable virus particles. This procedure should be used when a clinical specimen in a highly suspicious case remains negative despite the use of adequate cell lines and specimens.

Indirect immunofluorescence using a monoclonal antibody to the cross-reactive hexon antigen can be used for rapid viral diagnosis by demonstrating common adenoviral antigens in cells from the respiratory tract, including the throat, nasopharynx, and bronchoalveolar lavage, or from the conjunctiva or cornea, or the urine. Enzyme immunoassays (EIA) can also be employed to detect soluble viral antigen in feces or nasopharyngeal secretions. These rapid methods can be used in specimens obtained directly from the patient, or they may be used for confirmation of an isolate obtained in tissue culture. The noncultivable enteric adenoviruses can be identified from fecal specimens by these methods or by immunoelectron microscopy after the detection of an adenovirus by electron microscopy. Adenoviruses have a distinct morphology and size that can be readily identified by electron microscopy.

Neutralization assays using antisera to the 41 adenoviral subtypes permit further identification of a clinical isolate. However, these assays are cumbersome, time-consuming, and expensive. Therefore neutralization assays with intersecting pools of antisera are used to avoid these disadvantages. With information obtained from the intersecting pools, a neutralization assay using two of three individual antisera may be done to complete the identification of the isolate.

Restriction endonuclease mapping and hybridization of isolated adenoviral DNA are research tools that are being used to characterize possible new species. These techniques are not practical for identifying isolates in the diagnostic laboratory at the present time.

Serology is rarely used to diagnose an ongoing infection. For epidemiologic surveys, however, evidence of past infection can be detected with EIAs that use the cross-reactive hexon antigen. Further subtyping of specific antibodies can be done by hemagglutination inhibition assays using rat or rhesus monkey erythrocytes.

Interpretation of the significance of an isolate depends on the origin of the specimen. Recovery of the adenovirus from the eye, genital tract, lung, or brain is diagnostic; from the throat of a patient with respiratory disease, suggestive; and from feces, ambiguous. This is because adenoviruses are shed in large numbers and for long periods of time in the feces, particularly in children with persistent infections of tonsils and adenoids. Furthermore, recrudescent shedding may be precipitated by infection with another agent or immunocompromise of the host.

Treatment

As with other viral infections, there is no specific treatment for adenoviral infections. Although bacterial superinfection is rare, antibiotic therapy is helpful to reduce further organ or tissue damage. Although immunoglobulins, interferon, and at times steroids have all been used in the treatment of occasional patients with adenovirus infections, their role has not been clearly defined.

Prevention

The development of vaccines for the prevention of adenovirus infections was stimulated because of the severity of respiratory disease in restricted population groups (i.e., military recruits). Enteric coated orally administered vaccines for adenoviruses 4 and 7 have been developed. These vaccines contain live non-attenuated virus and produce an asymptomatic infection of the gastrointestinal tract with the development of a systemic immune response. The use of the vaccine has been generally restricted to military populations, where it appears to have produced a decrease in the incidence of ARD by types 4 and 7. The virus is excreted in stools for weeks.

More recent efforts to develop vaccines are concentrating on the use of antigenic viral subunits. This concept is attractive because these agents have the potential to produce persistent infections.

Adeno-associated Viruses

The adeno-associated viruses (AAVs) are small DNA viruses of the parvovirus family. AAVs were first observed on electron microscopy as small particles in adenovirus preparations. They were thought to represent either precursor or breakdown products of the adenovirus virions. It was later determined that they represented a second virus that was biologically and structurally different from adenovirus. Five serotypes of AAV have been identified. Since the initial demonstration of AAV, serotypes of bovine, avian, equine, and canine origin have been discovered. The host range of AAVs is not as limited as that of their helper adenoviruses: avian AAVs can productively infect humans using a human adenovirus helper, and herpes simplex viruses type 1 and 2 can provide the necessary helper functions for AAV replication.

Several epidemiologic studies have shown that AAV infection is common in the general population. Antibodies are generally acquired between the ages of 6 months and 2 years, and 50% to 80% of persons tested can be shown to have serologic evidence of AAV infection. AAV cryptically infects human and primate cells in vivo, and latent infection of human cells with AAV has been documented. No overt clinical syndromes have been associated with the AAV infection.

Coinfection or previous infection of cells with AAV may modify the ability of some DNA viruses to transform those cells or induce tumor formation in animal models. The ability of adenovirus 12 to induce tumors in hamsters is decreased from 44% to 18% by AAV infection. Perinatal transplacental infection of mice with AAV protects these mice against a lethal postnatal adenovirus infection. In a study of patients with either cervical carcinoma or carcinoma of the prostate, neoplasms for which an etiologic role of herpes simplex virus has been discussed, the incidence of antibodies to AAV 2 and AAV 3 was lower than in a comparable group of patients without carcinoma who were matched for sex and age. Similar low antibody titers in patients with cervical adenocarcinoma have been seen for AAV 5. The suggestion implicit in these studies is that patients with AAV infection may be at decreased risk of either cervical or prostatic carcinomas when later exposed to herpes simplex virus. These data are provocative and not proven. Any role of AAV in human disease remains to be established.

FURTHER READING

Books and Reviews

ADENOVIRUSES

Baum SG: Adenovirus. In Mandell GL, Douglas RG, Bennett JE (eds): Principles and Practice of Infectious Diseases, ed 3. New York, John Wiley & Sons, 1990

Berns KI: Parvoviridae and their replication. In Fields BN, Knipe DM, et al (eds): Fundamental Virology, ed 2. Raven Press, Ltd., New York, 1991

Horowitz AS: Adenoviridae and their replication. In Fields BN, Knipe DM, et al (eds): Fundamental Virology, ed 2. New York, Raven Press, 1991

Spencer MJ, Cherry JD: Adenoviral infections. In Feigin RD, Cherry JD (eds): Textbook of Pediatric Infectious Diseases, ed 2. Philadelphia, WB Saunders, 1987

ADENO-ASSOCIATED VIRUSES

Berns KI, Hauswirth WW: Adeno-associated viruses. Adv Virus Res 25:407, 1979

Berns KI, Bohenzky RA: Adeno-associated viruses: An update. Adv Virus Res 32:243, 1987

Selected Papers

ADENOVIRUSES

Baraff LJ, Wilkins J, Wehrie PF: The role of antibiotics, immunizations, and adenoviruses in pertussis. Pediatrics 61:224, 1978

Enders JF, Bell JA, Dingle JH, et al: Adenoviruses: Group name proposed for new respiratory-tract viruses. Science 124:119, 1956

Fox JP, Hall CE, Cooney MK: The Seattle virus watch. Am J Epidemiol 105:362, 1977

Ginsberg HS, Lundholm-Beauchamp U, Horswood RL, et al: Role of early region 3 (E3) in pathogenesis of adenovirus disease. Proc Natl Acad Sci USA 86:3823, 1989

Ginsberg HS, Valdesuso J, Horswood RL, et al: Adenovirus gene products affecting pathogenesis. In Chanock RM, Lerner RA, Brown F, Ginsberg H (eds): Vaccines '87 Modern Approaches to New Vaccines: Prevention of AIDS and other Viral, Bacterial, and Parasitic Diseases. Cold Spring Harbor, Cold Spring Harbor Laboratory, 1987

Gooding LR, Wold WSM: Molecular mechanisms by which adenoviruses counteract antiviral immune defenses. Immunology 10:53, 1990

Griffiths PD, Ellis DS, Zuckerman AJ: Other common types of viral hepatitis and exotic infections. Br Med Bull 46 (2):512, 1990

Hilleman MR, Werner JH: Recovery of a new agent from patients with acute respiratory illness. Proc Soc Med Exptl Biol 85:183, 1954

Howdle PD, Zaidel B, Smart LK, et al: Lack of a serologic response to an E1B protein of adenovirus 12 in coeliac disease. Scand J Gastroenterol 24:282, 1989

Jones LF: Latent or persistent infection with adenovirus. Rev Respir Dis 139:1327, 1989

Kagnoff MF: Celiac disease: Adenovirus and alpha gliadin. Micro and Immuno 145:67, 1989

Kotloff KL, Losonsky GA, Morris JG, et al: Enteric adenovirus infection and childhood diarrhea: An epidemiologic study in three clinical settings. Pediatrics 84:219, 1989

Levine AJ: The adenovirus early proteins. Microbiol Immunol 110:143, 1984

Nelson KE, Gavitt F, Batt MD, et al: The role of adenoviruses in the pertussis syndrome. J Pediatr 86:335, 1975

Paabo S, Severinsson L, Anderson M, et al: Adenovirus proteins and MHC expression. Adv Cancer Res 52:151, 1989

Pacini DL, Collier AM, Henderson FW: Adenovirus infections and respiratory illnesses in children in group day care. J Infect Dis 156:920, 1987

Routes JM, Coor JL: Resistance of human cells to the adenovirus E3 effect on Class I MHC antigen expression. J Immunol 114:2763, 1990

Rowe WP, Huebner RJ, Gilmore LK, et al: Isolation of a cytopathogenic agent from human adenoids undergoing spontaneous degeneration in tissue culture. Proc Soc Exp Biol Med 84:570, 1953

Schmitz H, Wigand R, Heinrich W: Worldwide epidemiology of human adenovirus infections. Am J Epidemiol 117:455, 1983

Yolken RH, Lawrence F, et al: Gastroenteritis associated with enteric type adenovirus in hospitalized infants. J Pediatr 101:21, 1982

ADENO-ASSOCIATED VIRUSES

Blacklow NR, Hoggan MD, Kapikian AZ, et al: Epidemiology of adenovirus-associated virus infection in a nursery population, Am J Epidemiol 88:368, 1986

Buller RML, Janik JE, Sebring ED, et al: Herpes simplex virus type 1 and 2 completely help adenovirus-associated virus replication. J Virol 40:241, 1981

George-Fries B, Biederlack S, Wolf J, et al: Analysis of proteins, helper dependence and seroepidemiology of a new human parvovirus. Virology 134:64, 1984

Lipps BV, Mayor HD: Defective parvoviruses acquired via the transplacental route protect mice against lethal adenovirus infection. Infect Immun 37:200, 1982

Maza M, Carter BJ: Inhibition of adenovirus oncogenicity in hamster by adeno-associated virus DNA. J Natl Cancer Inst 67:1323, 1981

Rosembaum MJ, Edwards EA, Pierce WE, et al: Serologic surveillance for adenovirus-associated satellite virus antibody in military recruits. J Immunol 106:711, 1971

CHAPTER 66

Human Papovaviruses

Papillomaviruses and polyomaviruses have been grouped together as the *Papovaviridae* family (see Table 53–4). The members of this family of viruses share the following properties: they are nonenveloped, they have a double-stranded circular DNA genome, which is small (5000 to 8000 bp), and they have an icosahedral capsid. Current understanding of the differences among these viruses indicates that papillomaviruses and polyomaviruses have distinctive characteristics and should be classified as subfamilies of papovaviruses. Major differences include smaller genome size (5000 bp for polyomaviruses compared with 8000 bp for papillomaviruses) and antigenic characteristics that are shared within the subfamilies but not among them.

Papillomaviruses

Papillomaviruses are the etiologic agents that cause warts in humans and papillomas in many mammals and birds. The inability to propagate human papillomaviruses in cell culture systems has impeded their classification and characterization on the basis of biologic properties. Papillomaviruses have now been assigned to several different groups in terms of patterns of restriction endonuclease digestion of their DNA, DNA homology, and serologic cross-reactivity. A classification of human papillomaviruses is provided in Table 53–4. By 1989 more than 60 types had been described in the literature.

Biologic Characteristics

Papillomaviruses are both species specific and have pronounced tropism for squamous epithelial cells. The infected cells show a relative failure of terminal differentiation, leading to increased numbers of cells in the intermediate epidermal layers, hyperkeratosis. Intranuclear inclusions and intracytoplasmic distortions may be seen on routine histologic examination of some infected tissue. Cells that are permissive for the production of infective virions commonly display a ballooned cytoplasmic vacuole that lies against the darkened nucleus and is termed *koilocytosis.*

Virus replication, including the production of viral capsid proteins and assembly of infectious virions, occurs in the terminally differentiated layer of squamous epithelium, whereas viral DNA and RNA transcripts for early gene expression are found in the basal layer. This linkage between virus replication and progressive cellular differentiation may account for the failure to achieve growth of human papillomaviruses (HPVs) in in vitro cell culture systems.

The genomes of the various types resemble each other in containing about 8000 bp and having similar genomic organizations. There are nine designated open reading frames (ORFs) that encode seven early and two late functions. The late functions are expressed in productively infected cells, and many human infections are characterized by the production of little or no infectious virus but abundant DNA production. There is also a long control region in which there are no ORFs. All ORFs and the long control region occur on one strand of the viral DNA, which serves as the template for DNA transcription.

The recognized functions of the early and late ORFs are listed in Table 66–1. (See a fine summary by Howley [1991] for further information on this burgeoning field of investigation.)

Epidemiology and Clinical Associations

The human diseases associated with papillomavirus infection are summarized in Table 66–2. The papillomaviruses associated with common warts (common, plantar, or flat warts) are usually found in children and young adults. Natural transmission of these viruses is presumed to be through contact

TABLE 66–1. GENETICALLY ASSIGNED FUNCTIONS OF HUMAN PAPILLOMAVIRUS GENES

No.	Portion	Function
E1	5′ portion	Replication repression
	3′ portion	Replication
E2	Full length	Transcriptional transactivation (HPV types 6, 11, 16)
	3′ portion	Transcriptional repression; binds to long control region
E3		No known product or function
E4		Cytoplasmic phosphoprotein in warts (HPV-1)
E5		Transformation (HPV-6)
E6		Transformation in cooperation with E7 (HPV types 16, 18); complexes with p53 (HPV types 16, 18)
E7		Transcriptional transactivation (HPV-16); complexes with p105-RB (HPV types 6, 16); co-operates with ras oncoprotein (HPV-16); domain for casein kinase II
L1		Major capsid protein
L2		Minor capsid protein (HPV-1)

and minor abrasions. There are no specific predisposing factors for the development of common warts, although more extensive warty disease may be seen in individuals with primary immunodeficiencies and in patients treated with immunosuppressive therapy. Dermal warts usually are caused by HPV types 1 through 4. HPV types 1 through 3 are commonly isolated from warts of patients aged 5 to 15 years, whereas HPV-4 warts occur predominantly in patients between the ages of 20 to 25 years. HPV-7 infection is also associated with the development of common hand warts in meat handlers. The natural resolution of these lesions is spontaneous regression.

TABLE 66–2. DISEASE IN WHICH HUMAN PAPILLOMAVIRUSES HAVE BEEN IMPLICATED

Anogenital condyloma acuminatum
Cervical dysplasia
Cervical carcinoma of the cervix
Multiple juvenile laryngeal papillomatosis
Conjunctival papillomatosis
Corneal keratosis
Squamous cell carcinoma of sinuses
Squamous cell carcinoma of lung
Carcinoma of anus
Carcinoma of penis
Carcinoma and keratosis in epidermodysplasia verruciformis
Carcinoma of periungual areas
Common skin warts (verruca vulgaris)
Malignant transformation of venereal and skin warts in immunocompromised patients, including those with acquired immunodeficiency virus (AIDS)
Chronic renal failure
Bone marrow transplantation
Wiskott-Aldrich syndrome

The warts and macular lesions associated with epidermodysplasia verruciformis may be seen throughout the lifetime of infected individuals. The natural route of transmission for the HPV serotypes associated with these lesions (HPV types 5, 8, 9, 12, 14, 15, 17, and 19 to 25) is not known. Epidermodysplasia verruciformis is a familial disease that may be linked to an autosomal recessive gene. It is usually associated with depressed cell-mediated immunity, which may contribute to the lifetime persistence of disseminated wart lesions. Malignant conversion of some of the warty lesions, particularly those associated with HPV-5, is observed in approximately 25% of the affected patients. Those warts that undergo malignant transformation usually occur in sun-exposed areas.

Condylomata acuminata are genital warts caused primarily by HPV type 6 or 11. They generally occur in young adults, and their transmission is mainly venereal. Sexual promiscuity and changes in hormone balance (e.g., in pregnancy) may be predisposing factors for their development. Condylomata acuminata may regress spontaneously but are subject to recurrence and may give rise to extensive lesions. Malignant conversion of these anogenital warts has been observed in rare instances in lesions of the vulva, penis, and anus. In adults, condyloma acuminatum is a sexually transmitted disease, and some studies show that lesions will develop in up to 75% of persons after unprotected intercourse with an infected partner. In children, anogenital condyloma acuminatum is primarily a sexually transmitted disease and highly associated with sexual abuse, although perinatal transmission with lesions in early infancy may also occur.

Highly sensitive methods for assaying specimens for HPV have recently been developed. These techniques amplify the HPV DNA that is present in the specimen using the polymerase chain reaction (PCR). The amplified DNA may then be characterized with hybridization methods. By means of DNA amplification techniques, various populations have been assessed for the prevalence of genital HPVs. The results have shown that many populations of men and women who have no evidence of clinically diagnosable HPV-associated disease nevertheless show a high incidence of HPV DNA. An interpretation of these findings is that many types of HPVs are highly prevalent in a subclinical form and that other factors are necessary for the development of the overt diseases of genital warts or cervical dysplasias. The trauma of sexual activity and smoking are two probable cofactors in the development of disease.

Recurrent respiratory papillomas form another group of HPV-caused lesions. The juvenile type of laryngeal papillomatosis is generally found in children younger than 5 years of age. HPV type 6 or 11 genomes have been demonstrated in some of these lesions, which suggests that the development of these papillomas follows transmission of virus at birth from mothers with condylomata acuminata to their children. Recurrent respiratory papillomas are also seen in adults, and a small percentage of these lesions can be shown to contain HPV genomes. These papillomas show frequent and rapid recurrence after excision, but their malignant conversion is only rarely observed. Reported transformation has usually been seen after radiation therapy of the lesions. In the absence of radiation therapy, malignant transformation may be associated with heavy smoking.

Epidermal infection with human papillomaviruses is associated with the development of serotype-specific antibodies and cell-mediated immunity. Both IgM and IgG humoral antibodies appear in patients with warts. Detection of IgG antibodies and cell-mediated immunity correlate with resolution of the warts.

Treatment

Therapy for warts is generally directed toward removal of the lesion rather than treatment of the papillomavirus infection. Topical application of caustic agents, such as podophyllin, has been the treatment of choice for genital warts for many years. Cryosurgery is used for removal of common warts. Laser therapy may be employed for refractory genital or respiratory lesions. Recently successful therapy has been reported using more specific antiviral or immunodulating therapy. Both systemic and intralesional alpha-interferon have been used to treat extensive refractory genital and respiratory papillomatosis. Topical idoxuridine has been used with some success in patients with extensive genital warts. Systemic cytotoxic chemotherapy also has been tried in some cases. The use of hypnosis and suggestion as a means of eradicating hand warts has been studied and is highly effective.

Human Papillomaviruses in Cancer

Most HPVs, including the etiologic agents of common, plantar, and flat warts, are entirely benign and are not associated with subsequent development of carcinomas. As indicated previously, however, several HPVs have recently been implicated in the malignant transformation of special groups of warty lesions to squamous cell carcinomas. HPV-6 is related to juvenile laryngeal papillomatosis and the malignant transformation of condyloma acuminatum. HPV-5-specific and less commonly HPV-8– and HPV-14-specific nucleotide sequences have been identified in the squamous carcinomas evolving from the chronic wart disease epidermodysplasia verruciformis. In one such patient, HPV-5 DNA was present both in the warty lesions and in a subcutaneous metastatic tumor.

Cervical Neoplasia

Evidence is rapidly accumulating to implicate HPV as a primary factor in the development of premalignant and malignant lesions of the uterine cervix, vagina, and vulva. Many cervical intraepithelial neoplasia (CIN) lesions are found to be associated with HPV infection, most commonly HPV-16 and less often HPV types 18, 33, and 35 or other less common types. HPV-16 genome can be demonstrated in approximately 25% of grade III CIN lesions; 33% to 70% of patients with invasive cervical carcinoma have evidence of HPV-16 infection in their malignant lesions. In a pathologic study of precancerous cervical lesions, biopsy specimens from 22 to 23 women (95%) contained DNA sequences that were specific for HPV types 6, 11, 16, or 18. A prospective study of women with cytologic evidence of HPV infection showed that there was a fifteen-fold increased risk of subsequent development of cervical malignant disorders in these infected women.

Several points can be made regarding the relationship between papillomaviruses and carcinomas. The oncogenic potential of any given papillomavirus type is unique. HPV-16 and HPV-18 are clearly related to cervical neoplasia and malignant change. The role of cocarcinogens may be crucial to potentiating papillomavirus-induced malignant transformation. This is particularly evident in epidermodysplasia verruciformis, in which malignant transformation of warty lesions occurs only in those areas exposed to UV light. In women with cervical HPV-associated lesions, smoking appears to be a powerful contributor to malignant progression. In addition, the malignant transformation associated with HPV-6 in laryngeal papillomatosis appears to occur only after radiation therapy of the lesions. The immunocompetence of the host also affects the transformation of viral papillomas. Defects in immunity in patients with epidermodysplasia verruciformis or immunosuppression (such as in patients receiving renal transplants) are associated with both an increased number of warts and an increased incidence of cutaneous carcinomas.

Polyomaviruses

In 1971 two human papillomaviruses were isolated. Each was designated by the initials of the person from whom it was obtained. BK virus (BKV) was isolated by Gardner and associates from the urine of a patient receiving immunosuppressive therapy after kidney transplantation. This urine contained transitional epithelial cells with enlarged inclusion-bearing nuclei. Electronmicroscopic examination of the exfoliated cells showed structures typical of polyomaviruses. The virus causes hemagglutination of human type O and guinea pig red blood cells. In serologic tests, BKV reacts slightly with antisera specific for SV40 but not with antisera against polyoma virus or human papillomaviruses. JC virus (SCV) was isolated by Padgett and associates from brain tissue obtained at autopsy from a person with progressive multifocal leukoencephalopathy. JCV also hemagglutinates human and guinea pig erythrocytes. Weak reactions are detected between JCV and antisera against SV40.

Other viruses serologically indistinguishable from BKV and JCV have been recovered from a wide variety of patients. Although these viruses are isolated with the highest frequency from patients immunocompromised either by virtue of inherent defects in immunity or by immunosuppression due to pregnancy or suppressive medication, they can also be isolated at a low frequency from apparently normal individuals. In addition, recent studies have demonstrated that continuous shedding of JCV occurs in a large proportion of nonimmunosuppressed, well older persons. All JCV-related viruses tested appear to be identical to prototype JCV. Most BKV-related viruses are similar to the prototype BKV, although some differences may be seen with DNA reassociation techniques and restriction endonuclease mapping.

Epidemiology

Several epidemiologic studies of human polymavirus have shown that these infections are widespread in many parts of the world. Infection with these viruses is a common occurrence during childhood, with BKV and JCV infections occurring independently. Approximately 80% of children aged 5 to 9 years can be found to have antibodies to BKV present in their serum. Antibody to JCV may be acquired somewhat later in life. Padgett and Walker found that 65% of children in Wisconsin were JCV-seropositive by 10 to 14 years of age. In another study, 50% of the children had antibodies to JCV by the age of 3 years. Seventy to one hundred percent of adults are seropositive for antibodies to both JCV and BKV. There is probably no animal reservoir for these viruses.

The high incidence of infection with these viruses implies that they are transmitted easily. However, almost nothing is known about the route of transmission. The viruses, with rare exception, have been recovered only from the urine. It may be, however, that a respiratory route of viral transmission is the source of most primary BKV and JCV in infections.

Several recent studies have addressed the possibilities of congenital infections with human polyomaviruses. For example, in a serologic study of pregnant women in the United States, fourfold or greater polyomavirus antibody rises during pregnancy occurred. These antibody titer changes were all consistent with virus reactivation. Virus-specific IgM was detected in the serum of mothers after BKV reactivation but not after JCV reactivation. No evidence of congenital transmission of either JCV or BKV has been found in either English or American studies, although some Japanese studies have shown some positive evidence.

A high percentage of adults have antibodies to BKV and JCV that are detectable decades after their primary childhood infection. Many patients have significant levels of antibody against BKV before immunosuppression and nevertheless show fourfold or greater rises of titer thereafter. In some persons this increase has been correlated with the appearance of IgM antibodies in the serum. These data suggest that there is lifelong persistence of virus with reactivation of virus subsequent to immunosuppression and the aging process.

Primary Infection

A mild respiratory illness has been recorded in children at the time of appearance of antibodies against BKV. Goudsmit and associates retrospectively investigated sera from 177 children admitted to hospital for acute respiratory disease. Sera from seven of these children showed seroconversion suggestive of primary infection with BKV. All children with BKV infection had upper respiratory tract infections, and BKV was associated with 8% of all upper respiratory tract infections in this series. Tonsillar tissue from children with recurrent attacks of acute respiratory disease has been found to contain BKV DNA by hybridization with cloned genomic DNA of prototype BKV, but no infectious virus could be isolated from these tonsils.

Primary infection with JCV has not been documented. The lack of data regarding primary JCV infections may be related to difficulty in obtaining primary fetal glial cells for virus isolation. In addition, the slightly older age children when infected may make primary JCV disease less severe and may preclude patients from seeking medical attention.

Urinary Tract Infection

BKV was first isolated from the urine of an immunosuppressed patient who had received a kidney and ureter graft 3 months previously. Virus-containing cells were shed from the lumen of a stenosed donor ureter. Subsequently, Coleman and associates documented the excretion of large quantities of polyomavirus-infected cells in the urine of renal transplant patients who had been given large doses of corticosteroids for possible rejection episodes. The transplanted ureters of these patients proved to be stenosed and ulcerated, and the urothelium contained cells with large inclusion bodies that contained polyomavirus particles. Hogan and associates studied infection of JCV and BKV in 61 immunosuppressed renal transplant patients. Polyomavirus excretion was detected in the urine of 12 of 61 patients (20%), 11 of whom excreted JCV, and 9 excreted BKV. Serologic data suggested that most JCV infections were primary, whereas most BKV infections resulted from virus reactivation. Urinary tract excretion of polyomavirus is associated with drug-dependent diabetes mellitus, arterial occlusive disease, and urethral stricture with loss of renal function.

Progressive Multifocal Leukoencephalopathy

The one disease closely linked to human polyomaviruses is progressive multifocal leukoencephalopathy (PML). PML is an uncommon, generally fatal, demyelinating disease that occurs in patients with altered immunocompetence. It recently has been reported in 2% to 4% of patients with neurologic complications of acquired immunodeficiency syndrome (AIDS). It also occurs frequently as a complication in patients with chronic lymphocytic leukemia or Hodgkin's disease and may be seen in patients who are immunosuppressed after renal transplantation or with inherited immunodeficiency syndromes.

PML is caused by infection of oligodendrocytes by polyomavirus (most commonly JCV). Several cases of PML have been associated with an SV40-like virus designated as SV40-PML. Pathologic lesions of PML occur in both the gray and the white matter and may be distributed throughout the neuraxis. These lesions are classically small, discrete areas of demyelination that may become confluent. The outstanding cytologic features are unusual astrocytes with bizarre chromatin patterns and atypical oligodendroglia with enlarged, ill-defined inclusions. As a result of the infection of the oligodendrocytes, demyelination occurs. Presumably, this oligodendroglial degeneration is secondary to activation of previously latent JCV by immunosuppression.

Subacute encephalitis with severe dementia occurs in approximately 20% of adults with AIDS, and several studies have attempted to identify the factors leading to this complication. PML has been found at biopsy of some of these patients. A notable finding on the biopsies has been the histologic association between areas of oligodendroglial and astrocytic disease, which are characteristic of PML and the close spatial localization of macrophages that produce human immunodeficiency virus (HIV). The two diseases may potentiate the severity of each component, and further understanding of the disease process is needed.

Although PML is now recognized as a viral disease, diagnosis of this illness still rests on finding the characteristically altered oligodendroglia in biopsied brain tissue. Studies of serum antibody levels are not helpful because of the high background level of antibody in the general population and because affected patients often have impaired immune responses. Neither specific JCV antibodies nor other proteins characteristic of demyelinating disease have been found in the cerebrospinal fluid. In a reported case of PML in a male homosexual with T cell insufficiency, oligoclonal bands were documented.

There is no known treatment for PML. Human leukocyte interferon has been used successfully for prophylaxis of BKV and JCV infections in renal transplant patients.

Oncogenicity of Human Polyomaviruses

The human polyomaviruses BKV and JCV are oncogenic in neonatal hamsters. Malignant, histologically distinct brain tumors developed in two of four adult owl monkeys inoculated with JCV intercerebrally, subcutaneously, and intravenously simultaneously. Four owl monkeys inoculated similarly with BKV and four inoculated with SV40 did not develop tumors after 3 years.

Attempts have been made to associate BKV and JCV infection with human tumors, using both serologic and DNA hybridization techniques on hundreds of patients and tumors. All results have been uniformly negative. No data, therefore, exist linking BKV or JCV to human carcinomas.

SV40 is tumorigenic in laboratory animals. It produces subclinical infections indicated by serum antibody prevalence and virus isolation in humans. SV40-contaminated poliovirus vaccine was administered to millions of people in the early 1960s. Although it has been reported that SV40-like antigens are present in the tumors of patients with meningiomas and other brain tumors, there is no evidence that cancer trends have been affected by poliovirus vaccine containing SV40. Mortimer and associates reported on the 17- to 19-year follow-up of newborns exposed to SV40-contaminated poliovirus vaccine in the first 3 days of life and found no excess risk of cancer of any sort.

FURTHER READING

Selected Papers

PAPILLOMAVIRUSES

Herman-Giddens M, Gutman LT, Berson NL: Association of coexisting vaginal infections and multiple abusers in female children with genital warts. Sex Transm Dis 15:63, 1988

Howley PM: Papillomavirinae and their replication. In Fields BN, Knipe DM, et al (eds): Fundamental Virology, ed 2. New York, Raven Press, 1991

Howley PM, Munger K, Werness BA, et al: Molecular mechanisms of transformation by the human papillomaviruses. In Knudson AG Jr, et al (eds): Genetic Basis for Carcinogenesis: Tumor Suppressor Genes and Oncogenes. Tokyo Japan Science Press, 1990

Kadish AS, Burk RD, Kress Y, et al: Human papillomaviruses of different types in precancerous lesions of the uterine cervix: Histologic, immunocytochemical and ultrastructural studies. Hum Pathol 17:384, 1986

Kataja V, Syrjanen K, Syrjanen S, et al: Prospective follow-up of genial HPV infections: Survival analysis of the HPV typing data. Eur J Epidemiol 6:9, 1990

Kiviat NB, Koutsky LA, Paavonen JA, et al: Prevalence of genital papillomavirus infection among women attending college student health clinic or a sexually transmitted disease clinic. J Infect Dis 159:293, 1989

Macnab JCM, Walkinshaw SA, Cordiner JW, et al: Human papillomavirus in clinically and histologically normal tissue of patients with genital cancer. N Engl J Med 315:1052, 1986

Mounts P, Shah KV, Kashima H: Viral etiology of juvenile- and adult-onset squamous papilloma of the larynx. Proc Natl Acad Sci USA 79:5425, 1982

Ostrow RS, Bender M, Niimura M, et al: Human papillomavirus DNA in cutaneous primary metastasized squamous cell carcinomas from patients with epidermodysplasia verruciformis. Proc Natl Acad Sci USA 70:1634, 1982

Reeves WC, Rawls WE, Brinton LA: Epidemiology of genital papillomaviruses and cervical cancer. Rev Infect Dis 11:426, 1989

Syrjanen KJ, Syrjanen SM: Human papillomavirus (HPV) infections related to cervical intraepithelial neoplasia (CIN) and squamous cell carcinoma of the uterine cervix. Ann Clin Res 17:45, 1985

POLYOMAVIRUSES

Arthur RR, Shah KV: Occurrence and significance of papovaviruses BK and JC in the urine. Prog Med Virol 36:42, 1989

Coleman DV, et al: A prospective study of human polyomavirus infection in pregnancy. J Infect Dis 142:1, 1980

Daniel R, Shah K, Madden D, et al: Serological investigation of the possibility of congenital transmission of papovavirus JC. Infect Immun 33:319, 1981

Dei R, Marmo F, Corte D, et al: Age-related changes in the prevalence of precipitating antibodies of BK virus in infants and children. J Med Microbiol 15:285, 1982

Goudsmit J, Wertheim–van Dillen P, van Strien A, et al: The role of BK virus in acute respiratory disease and the presence of BKV DNA in tonsils. J Med Virol 10:91, 1982

Grossi MP, Moneguzzi G, Chenciner N, et al: Lack of association between BK virus and ependymomas, malignant tumors of pancreatic islets, osteosarcomas and other human tumors. Intervirology 15:10, 1981

Hogan TF, Borden EC, McBain JA, et al: Human polyomavirus infections with JC virus and BK virus in renal transplant patients. Ann Intern Med 92:373, 1980

Houff SA, Major EO, Katz DA, et al: Involvement of JC virus–infected mononuclear cells from the bone-marrow and spleen in the pathogenesis of progressive multifocal leukoencephalopathy. N Engl J Med 318:301, 1988

Kitamura T, Aso Y, Kuniyoshi N, et al: High incidence of urinary JC virus excretion in nonimmunosuppressed older patients. J Infect Dis 161:1128, 1990

Mortimer EA, Lepow ML, Gold E, et al: Long-term follow-up of persons inadvertently inoculated with SV40 as neonates. Med Intell 305:1517, 1981

Padgett BL, Walker DL, ZuRhein GM, et al: Cultivation of papovalike virus from human brain with progressive multifocal leucoencephalopathy. Lancet 1:1257, 1971

Rochford R, Villareal LP: Polymavirus DNA replication in the pancreas in a transformal pancreas cell line has distinct enhancer requirements. J Virol 65:2108, 1991

Stoner GL, Ryschkewitsch CF, Walker DL, et al: JC papovirus large tumor (T) antigen expression in brain tissue of acquired immune deficiency syndrome (AIDS) and non-AIDS patients with progressive multifocal leukoenceophalopathy. Proc Natl Acad Sci USA 83:2271, 1986

Vazeux R, Cumont M, Girard PM, et al: Severe encephalitis resulting from coinfections with HIV and JC virus. Neurology 40:914, 1990

Walker DL, Padgett BL: The epidemiology of human polyomaviruses. In Sever J, Madden D (eds): Polyomaviruses and Human Neurological Diseases. New York, Liss, 1983, p 99

Yogo Y, Kitamura T, Sugimoto C, et al: Sequence rearrangement in JC virus DNAs molecularly cloned from immunosuppressed renal transplant patients. J Virol 65:2422, 1991

CHAPTER 67

The Enteroviruses

The genus *Enterovirus* of the family Picornaviridae contains many significant human pathogens. Polioviruses, hepatitis A virus, the Coxsackie viruses, and the echoviruses are all enteroviruses. These agents are classified together on the basis of their morphology and behavior in cell culture and animal model systems. The notoriety of these agents, as well as the ease with which they can be grown in tissue culture, has meant that the enteroviruses have been among the most intensively studied of all human pathogens. The war on poliomyelitis led by the National Foundation for Infantile Paralysis (the March of Dimes) produced many breakthroughs in the science of virology, most notably the nonneural growth and neutralization of the polioviruses by Enders, Robbins, and Weller, work for which they received the Nobel prize. Other major advances tied to research on the enteroviruses have included important discoveries in the replication of RNA viruses and the x-ray crystallographic characterization of this group of viruses. In addition, combining information gathered by crystallography with data on neutralization of the viruses by monoclonal antibodies and genetic sequencing has allowed an exquisite mapping of the surface of these agents, information that will be vitally useful in the exploration of viral pathogenesis.

Classification

The enteroviruses are small, nonenveloped, and have a single positive-sense RNA strand. The viral particles are 27 to 30 nm spheres, with a capsid made up of 60 copies each of four proteins, VP1, VP2, VP3, and VP4. There may also be a few copies of VP0, the uncleaved precursor of VP2 and VP4. The intricate interweaving of these proteins has been characterized using x-ray crystallography (Chap. 55).

Because the enteroviruses have no lipids in their capsid, they are stable against treatment with ether, ethanol, and various detergents. They are acid stable and can remain viable for hours on laboratory surfaces if left slightly moist. The enteroviruses can be inactivated by ultraviolet light, by formalin, and by chlorine (or sodium hypochlorite bleach).

The enteroviruses are assigned species names by their reactions with specific antisera and by their behavior in cell culture and animal model studies. The three serotypes of poliovirus, for example, are defined as a group by their growth in cell culture and their propensity to cause paralytic disease in primates. The other human enteroviruses include the echoviruses, Coxsackie A and B viruses, and the more recently categorized species that have been labeled only by a serotype number. The full categorization of the genus *Enterovirus* of the family Picornaviridae is shown in Table 67-1. Echoviruses can be grown fairly easily in cell culture, but they rarely multiply to any significant extent in mice. Although many Coxsackie A viruses can be grown in cell culture, it is difficult to isolate them in vitro with routine methods. They grow in suckling mice, an animal in which they cause a clinically and pathologically apparent myositis. The Coxsackie B viruses are similar to the Coxsackie A viruses in that they cause disease in mice, but the illness tends to be more diffuse than myositis alone and often includes encephalitis, pancreatitis, and myocarditis. The Coxsackie B viruses are generally more easily grown in cell culture systems that are the Coxsackie A viruses.

Beginning in 1970, new species of enteroviruses have been labeled by serotype number. The first new serotype was designated enterovirus type 68, and the most recently categorized serotype is enterovirus type 72, also known as hepatitis A virus. Hepatitis A virus is unique among the enteroviruses in many ways, including the fact that it grows quite well in cultured cells without producing any recognizable cytopathic effects.

Epidemiology

The enteroviruses are spread from person to person by the fecal-oral route. Once the viral particles are swallowed, they

TABLE 67–1. THE HUMAN ENTEROVIRUSES

Polioviruses	Serotypes 1, 2, and 3
Echoviruses	Serotypes 1–9, 11–27, 29–34[a]
Coxsackie A viruses	Serotypes 1–22, 24[b]
Coxsackie B viruses	Serotypes 1–6
Enteroviruses	Serotypes 68–71
Hepatitis A virus	(Enterovirus 72)

[a] Echovirus 10 is now classified as reovirus type 1, whereas echovirus 28 is classified as human rhinovirus 1A.
[b] Coxsackie A 23 is now classified as echovirus 9.

either can adsorb to the mucosal cells of the oropharynx or can pass into the gastrointestinal tract. The protein capsid of the virus is stable in acid conditions; therefore the virus particles are able to traverse the stomach intact and pass into the small intestine. Once the intestines are reached, the virus adsorbs and replicates. Gastrointestinal replication can continue for weeks, even months, during the primary infection with most of the enteroviruses. Virus particles are shed, often in large numbers, into the feces while the gastrointestinal tract replication proceeds. In countries with sophisticated sewage disposal and good hygiene, the feces are flushed down the toilet and treated; thus the viruses tend to spread in the community fairly slowly. In areas where sewage disposal is less advanced, the virus can remain stable in the environment for fairly long periods of time. It can be spread to people on unwashed foods, particularly in areas where fecal material is used as fertilizer, or it may be transmitted on the feet of vectors such as houseflies. Infants, with their feces contained in diapers, are also a major route of enteroviral dissemination, particularly in day-care settings.

An individual who has been infected by a serotype of enterovirus thereafter is immune to symptomatic reinfection with that same serotype. If reexposed to a serotype by the fecal-oral route, many persons shed the virus transiently in their feces, which implies the presence of gastrointestinal virus replication, but the fecal shedding will be brief, and invasive viral disease almost never occurs. It is assumed that serum antibodies and memory B cells generated by the primary infection protect against invasion by the virus, even though they may not completely eradicate gastrointestinal replication.

The best studied example of enteroviral epidemiology is poliovirus. Until the 1955 introduction of the inactivated (Salk) polio vaccine, poliomyelitis was an epidemic disease throughout most of the developed world. Even now, more than 30 years after the introduction of vaccine, there are still thousands of cases of poliomyelitis each year in the Third World. The Sabin attenuated vaccine was licensed in 1961, further decreasing the number of cases in those countries in which it was used.

Within temperate climates, most major epidemics of enteroviral disease, including poliomyelitis, occur during the late summer months. The season during which enteroviruses are active generally lasts from May through late October. The reason for this seasonality is unknown, but temperature and relative humidity may play a role. Epidemics in those parts of the United States that have shorter summers and more variation among seasons, such as New England, tend to be of shorter duration and more intense than in the Southeast. The tropics have almost no seasonal variation in poliovirus incidence, and disease occurs throughout the year. Within the United States the highest number of recognized cases of paralytic poliomyelitis occurred in 1952, when 21,269 cases were reported. The inactivated vaccine reduced the number to 988 cases in 1961, whereas the oral attenuated vaccine has further decreased the incidence of paralytic disease in the United States to roughly 10 cases per year. Most of these cases are caused by the vaccine virus, rather than by wild-type virus strains. Since 1986 there has been virtually no detectable circulation of virulent poliovirus within the confines of the United States.

Other features of enteroviral epidemiology were clarified by the intense work on poliomyelitis: (1) There are many more infections with an enterovirus than there are symptomatic cases. For poliovirus, although the paralytic case-to-infection ratio varied in different studies, the average probably was one paralytic case for every 100 to 150 infections. (2) Most of the human enteroviruses are species-specific. Their life cycles do not include major animal reservoirs.

The role of age in determining the paralytic case–to-infection ratio in poliomyelitis is controversial. Traditional thinking has been that after the neonatal period (when protective maternal antibodies are circulating), the susceptibility to paralysis increases with age. Thus young children were more often infected but not as frequently paralyzed as were older individuals. This hypothesis has been invoked as an explanation for the observation that paralytic poliomyelitis became an epidemic disease only after good sanitary practices became extant in a region. Improved sanitation delayed the age at which primary infection occurred, increasing the incidence of paralytic disease. Fortunately, the decline in the frequency of poliovirus infection makes it unlikely that the relationship of age and rates of paralytic disease will ever be clearly resolved.

Table 67–2 shows the pattern of nonpolio enteroviral isolates within the United States during the period from 1970 to 1983. The large year-to-year variations are perhaps related to the immunity generated against an epidemic strain, decreasing its incidence in subsequent years. One factor affecting the results of surveys such as that in Table 67–2 is the ease with which a given serotype is isolated. The Coxsackie A viruses, for example, probably cause more disease than the table would suggest inasmuch as they are relatively difficult to isolate using routine methods.

Some of the enteroviral serotypes tend to circulate with greater regularity than others. The Coxsackie B viruses have a periodicity of about 2 to 5 years. As a consequence the adult population in the United States has a high level of antibody seropositivity against all six Coxsackie B virus serotypes.

Pathogenesis

The basic pathogenesis of most of the human enteroviral infections is the same. They enter the body through the mucosa of the oropharynx and upper respiratory tract, then begin to multiply in the tissues around the oropharynx. The exact cells in which the virus multiplies are not known, although there is some reason to suspect the reticuloendothelial system. The virus is shed back into the oral secretions, whence it is swallowed. Because the enteroviruses are stable in acidic conditions, they are able to pass through the stomach into the intestines, where they undergo further rounds of replication. Roughly at the same time as it reaches the intestine, the virus begins to spill into the systemic circulation. This

TABLE 67–2. THE 15 MOST COMMON TYPES OF NONPOLIO ENTEROVIRUSES REPORTED ISOLATED IN THE UNITED STATES FROM 1970 to 1983

	Percentage of Total Isolates by Year														
NPEV Type[a]	1970–1983	1970	1971	1972	1973	1974	1975	1976	1977	1978	1979	1980	1981	1982	1983
E11	12.2	2.8	3.5	8.2	6.4	8.7	7.5	1.6	1.0	4.5	36.2	19.9	8.2	20.2	8.3
E9	11.3	11.5	29.0	6.8	7.1	9.3	37.0	2.4	6.6	30.0	2.1	3.9	13.1	6.1	3.8
CB5	8.7	0.4	0.4	40.0	21.3	0.2	0.1	0.6	5.9	4.9	1.7	3.0	3.6	5.1	20.2
E30	6.8	1.2	1.1	0.5	1.2	1.0	1.1	4.7	2.8	6.0	7.8	8.7	19.9	16.9	9.6
E4	6.3	12.5	31.0	6.9	4.5	12.3	6.4	7.4	1.8	10.2	2.4	1.5	2.4	1.3	0.5
E6	5.5	13.1	3.3	7.5	7.1	9.0	4.4	8.8	23.0	4.2	1.8	3.4	1.3	2.2	4.2
CB2	4.8	2.7	5.6	4.1	5.3	10.3	3.9	15.8	2.9	2.0	6.7	6.9	1.0	4.0	3.3
CB4	4.6	3.3	3.3	3.6	6.9	4.1	5.5	13.8	1.7	5.1	4.9	3.7	6.1	5.1	1.4
CB3	4.5	1.6	1.9	2.7	5.5	6.3	2.2	11.3	7.6	2.1	1.1	18.1	1.6	2.3	3.1
CA9	4.5	2.5	1.1	4.0	11.6	0.6	5.5	8.1	6.4	6.7	1.4	4.6	7.3	2.0	3.8
E3	3.2	33.4	4.4	0.9	0.6	0.0	0.1	0.2	4.9	0.2	0.2	0.7	7.9	1.1	0.7
E7	3.0	0.3	0.9	1.2	1.9	0.4	0.4	0.9	1.0	3.1	15.5	1.0	0.7	0.9	1.4
E5	2.0	0.4	0.4	0.3	0.7	1.8	1.3	0.6	0.5	1.1	0.6	1.5	7.5	6.4	2.5
E24	1.8	0.0	0.1	0.0	0.1	0.1	0.1	0.1	0.0	0.4	3.0	2.8	0.9	2.1	8.4
CB1	1.6	0.9	1.4	1.8	0.7	0.5	0.1	2.1	8.7	0.4	0.7	2.6	1.6	1.2	1.6
Other	19.1	13.5	12.5	11.2	19.1	35.5	24.2	21.5	25.2	19.2	13.8	17.8	17.1	23.1	27.5
Total No. of isolates	23,481	1100	1589	2062	1376	829	1355	850	1172	1782	3088	2204	2130	1518	2426

From Strikos RA, Anderson LJ, Parker RA: J Infect Dis 153:346, 1986.
[a] E. echovirus; CB, coxsackievirus group B; CA, coxsackievirus group A; other, all other types of NPEV (nonpolio enteroviruses).

early (primary) viremic phase usually is asymptomatic and involves fairly low titers of virus in the blood. During the primary viremia, tissues are seeded according to the tropism of the virus (those tissues for which it does or does not have an affinity). In the case of the polioviruses the tissues infected include neurons, especially the anterior horn cells of the spinal cord. However, for reasons that are not clear, seeding of the central nervous system does not occur in all persons infected with poliovirus. After the primary viremia, the virus replicates in susceptible tissues and symptomatic manifestations of the disease begin to occur. There is often fever, malaise, and symptoms of other organ involvement, such as aseptic meningitis and myocarditis. In many instances during this symptomatic phase there is a secondary viremia that can be detected by culturing the blood for virus.

The immune response to an enteroviral infection begins with the initial penetration of mucosal tissues. As the virus spreads into tissues, the immune system recognizes the presence of foreign antigens and produces antibodies and specific T cells. Antibodies can be detected in the circulation by the seventh to tenth day after exposure, roughly the same time as the symptomatic disease and secondary viremia occur. With the exception of the gastrointestinal tract, the viral replication in tissues soon slows to a halt. In contrast, gastrointestinal tract viral multiplication and fecal shedding can continue for weeks after the development of high neutralizing antibody titers. The cellular location for this replication is not clear, nor is the reason the infection can persist in the face of neutralizing antibodies known.

The varied manifestations of the different serotypes of the enteroviruses probably reflect diversity in the tropism of the virus. In some cases there are also clearly different cell-virus interactions. The best example of an atypical cell-virus interaction is that of hepatitis A virus, which does not directly lyse infected cells. The virus persistently infects those cells in which it is replicating, apparently without destroying them. One corollary to this pattern is that the virus must also have an unusual, nonlytic, egress route from the cell. The mechanism used by hepatitis A virus to exit from the cytoplasm has not yet been determined.

Viral tropism appears to be determined by cellular receptor molecules. Each enterovirus group has certain cellular proteins to which it attaches in order to enter the cell. For example, all three poliovirus serotypes bind to a protein encoded by human chromosome 19. Using monoclonal antibodies against the cellular poliovirus receptors, researchers have been able to simultaneously neutralize infections by all three poliovirus serotypes. The antibody does not react with the virus at all; instead neutralization occurs because the virus is unable to bind to its target cell. This mechanism of neutralization works for the enteroviruses because they have a mandatory extracellular phase. If the viruses were able to move through intercellular bridges from cytoplasm to cytoplasm, by-passing the membrane attachment step, surface binding antibody would have little effect. In contrast to the ability to generate antireceptor antibodies, production of antibodies able to neutralize all three poliovirus serotypes by binding to the viral capsid has not been possible.

The role of cell-mediated immunity in enteroviral infections is not clear, although there are examples in which a role for the cellular immune system in enteroviral pathogenesis seems probable. The best studied example is Coxsackie B virus–produced myocarditis, at least in murine model systems. In that model, lytic T cells contribute to cell damage yet do not appear to be critical for virus elimination. Mice depleted of T cells do not have myocarditis as severely as mice with normal T cell function; yet both groups eradicate the virus at essentially the same rate. Another aspect of Coxackie virus–induced myocarditis is the apparent role of antibody-mediated cytotoxicity. In some mouse strains, autoantibodies generated against cardiac myocytes seem to be the mediator for tissue damage. Whether T lymphocyte–mediated or antibody-induced cell damage is more important in human myocarditis has not been resolved.

Cellular immunity seems to be an important aspect in the production of disease by hepatitis A virus. Virus replication appears to slow just before symptomatic disease begins. In addition, specific in vitro recognition of hepatitis A–infected cells by lytic T cells and natural killer cells has been demonstrated.

A major recent advance in enteroviral research has been the visualization of viral structure using x-ray crystallography. This technique is possible because the icosahedral symmetry of the picornaviruses is regular enough to allow the generation of virus crystals. Combining structural information from crystallography with knowledge about the nucleic acid and peptide sequences has helped solve several important riddles in enteroviral pathogenesis.

Virologists have long puzzled over why the enteroviruses form groups (such as the polioviruses, echoviruses, and Coxsackie viruses), which share a common cellular receptor and thus probably a common viral attachment protein locus, yet against which group-specific antibodies have been difficult to generate. The reason for this discrepancy appears to be that the viral attachment protein site is located in canyons on the surface of the virus. These canyons are large enough to allow the receptor molecule to enter but too narrow for antibody-binding sites.

Another stride made possible by the combination of sequence data and crystallography has been clarification of the virus neutralization sites. It was first recognized that there are areas in the enteroviral genome critical for the generation of mutations that can escape from neutralization by monoclonal antibodies. In many cases altering even one peptide in these critical regions is enough to prevent neutralization by a given monoclonal antibody. Crystallography demonstrates that these critical protein sequences are largely on the surface of the viral capsid, forming small loops that are exposed and thus available for antibody binding.

The combination of crystallographic and sequence data holds great potential to clarify many important points in enteroviral pathogenesis. The fine geography of the antigen-antibody complex can be analyzed at a molecular level. The interaction of the cellular receptor and viral attachment protein should also become clear at a molecular level, perhaps allowing interventional schemes to be developed to prevent virus binding. Further, data regarding capsid structure already have been used to clarify the mechanism of action of antienteroviral drugs that operate to prevent viral uncoating and the release of RNA.

Clinical Manifestations

The enteroviruses cause a variety of clinical syndromes, with a great deal of overlap among the different serotypes. A brief discussion of the diseases most closely associated with the enteroviruses follows.

Poliomyelitis

The polioviruses are the cause of most paralytic disease caused by the enteroviruses, although both the Coxsackie A and B viruses can occasionally cause paralysis or muscle weakness. Poliomyelitis is typically a biphasic disease. The first manifestations, termed the *minor illness,* come within a few days after exposure and include fever, malaise, headache, sore throat, and vomiting. The *major illness* follows 3 or 4 days after the end of the minor illness. The symptoms are those of aseptic meningitis (fever, headache, stiff neck, vomiting), with or without paralysis. Paralytic disease begins with muscle stiffness, proceeds to hyperactivity of deep muscle reflexes and fasciculations in the muscles that will be involved with the paralysis, and evolves to severe weakness. The type of poliomyelitis can be categorized as *spinal,* if the muscle groups involved are supplied by nerves emanating from the spinal cord, or *bulbar,* if the major involvement is in the distribution of the cranial nerves. Characteristic of the spinal form is asymmetric involvement of the limbs. Bulbar poliomyelitis can affect the respiratory centers in the medulla, as well as the muscles in the pharynx, soft palate, and vocal cords. Involvement of the respiratory system is perhaps the worst element of poliomyelitis and may require prolonged ventilatory support.

Nonspecific Febrile Illness

Most patients with enteroviral infections are asymptomatic. Among those with clinical manifestations of infection, the most common pattern is a nonspecific febrile illness. This disease is generally of little consequence except in children in the first few months of life. Because serious bacterial infections can present as no more than a fever in young children, patients with enteroviral fevers are often admitted to the hospital to "rule out" bacterial sepsis. Enterovirally produced fevers are probably among the commonest causes of hospital admission of small children, especially during the late summer and early fall, although the infection itself generally has a benign prognosis.

Perinatal Infections

The enteroviruses can cause severe disease in some newborns. The virus can be acquired either across the placenta (most often immediately before delivery) or by ingestion of contaminated materials during the birth process. The serotypes most frequently implicated as the cause of severe neonatal disease include the Coxsackie B viruses and some of the echoviruses, particularly type 11. The disease is generally multisystem, with manifestations that include fever, meningitis, myocarditis, hepatitis, and adrenal cortical involvement. It appears that maternal antibody is protective for the infant; therefore the most serious disease occurs in babies whose mothers acquire virus in the few days before delivery (so that there is insufficient time to develop and deliver protective antibodies) or in babies who are infected shortly after delivery. Many well-documented nursery outbreaks have been described. The stability of the enteroviruses to soaps and other disinfecting agents makes nosocomial spread particularly difficult to stop.

Febrile Diseases With Rashes

Many of the enteroviruses have been associated with outbreaks of febrile illnesses with rashes. Both exanthems (skin rashes) and enanthems (lesions on mucosal surfaces) occur, with widely varied appearances. Most of the exanthems are maculopapular, sometimes with petechiae. Vesicular lesions may be seen, particularly with the hand-foot-and-mouth syndrome caused by various Coxsackie A virus serotypes. The Coxsackie A viruses are also frequently associated with enanthems. Herpangina is a particularly notable example. This disease causes vesicular and ulcerative lesions on the soft palate and throat and may be extremely painful.

Viral Meningitis and Meningoencephalitis

The enteroviruses are the commonest cause of viral meningitis, a generally benign illness that is often mistaken for bacterial meningitis. Viral meningitis presents with fever, headache, stiff neck, and malaise. Patients with an element of encephalitis can also manifest changes in their mental status. The laboratory findings in enteroviral meningitis include a cerebrospinal fluid (CSF) pleocytosis, which can initially have a high percentage of polymorphonuclear cells and then evolve rapidly to a lymphocyte predominance. The CSF protein concentration will be mildly elevated or normal, and the CSF glucose levels will be normal. Most patients with enteroviral central nervous system infections (other than polio) will have nearly complete recovery. Longitudinal studies on young children who had recovered from viral meningitis have suggested mild neurologic defects, particularly in receptive language function. Prospective studies are being conducted to delineate the frequency and nature of sequelae.

Myocarditis

The Coxsackie B viruses are strongly associated with myocarditis, although the echoviruses and Coxsackie A viruses can also cause the disease, particularly in younger children. The clinical illness presents with chest pains, fever, fatigue, cardiac arrhythmias, and sometimes with evidence of cardiac failure. Electrocardiographic changes are also generally present. Myocarditis can be fatal or lead to a persistent deficit in cardiac performance.

Hepatitis

Hepatitis A virus (HAV) is a major cause of viral hepatitis. The symptoms include fever, malaise, increased liver size, and jaundice. The illness is less severe than hepatitis B disease, has a shorter incubation period (2 to 7 weeks), and is much more contagious. Unlike hepatitis B, HAV does not cause chronic liver disease. The illness generally lasts less than 3 to 4 weeks, although liver function tests (aspartate aminotransferase, alanine aminotransferase) may take 2 to 3 months to return to normal. Virus is shed in the feces before and during the earliest symptomatic stages but is rarely detected after the onset of jaundice. Hepatitis A is discussed further in Chapter 76.

Respiratory Disease and Pleurodynia

The enteroviruses can cause an upper respiratory infection clinically indistinguishable from other etiologies of the common cold. These viruses can also cause pneumonia, usually mild, particularly in newborns.

Pleurodynia, also known as Bornholm disease or "the devil's grippe," is another disease caused by an enterovirus, usually one of the Coxsackie A viruses. The symptoms of pleurodynia include fever and sharp episodic pains in the side of the chest. The disease actually involves the intercostal

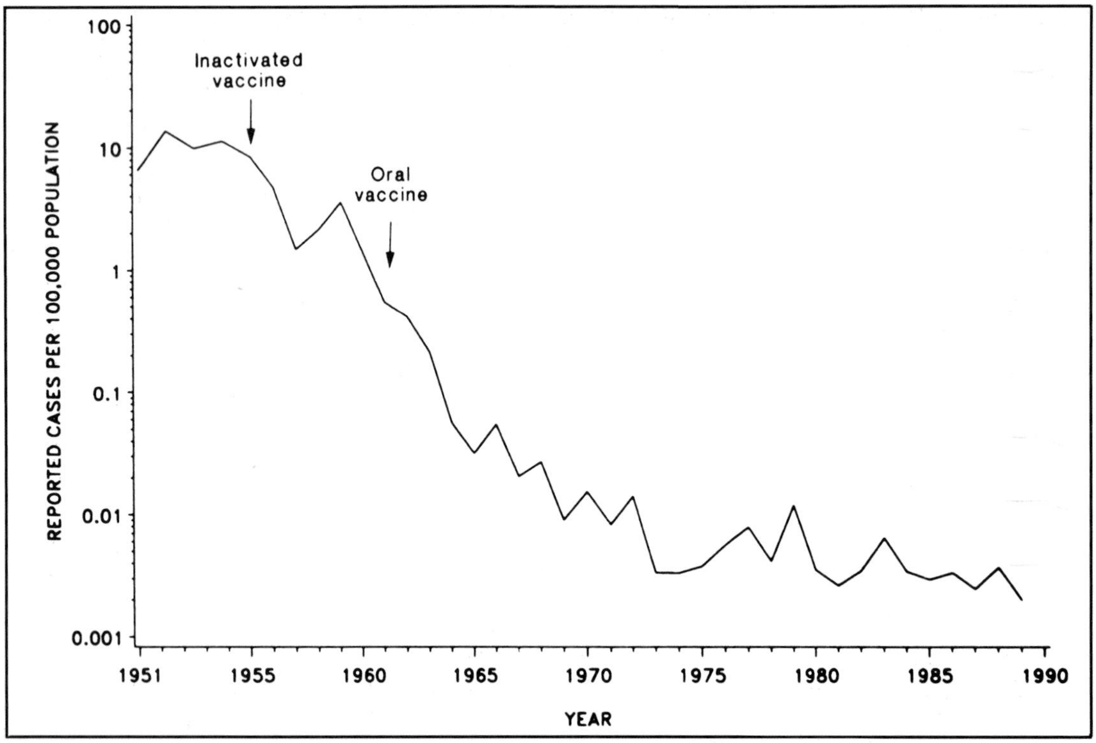

Fig. 67–1. Poliovirus incidence. Reported cases of paralytic poliomyelitis per 100,000 population per year in the United States, 1951–1989. *(From Summary of Notifiable Diseases, United States, 1989. MMWR 38(54), 1989.)*

muscles to a greater degree than the pleura and has a duration of several weeks.

Treatment and Prevention

The conquest of epidemic poliomyelitis has been one of the public health landmarks of the twentieth century. Thousands of lives have been saved, millions have been spared the pain and anxiety of paralytic disease, and many millions of dollars have been saved by the use of polio vaccine. This last point is an especially crucial one: prevention of a disease is much cheaper than treatment, and in most cases the price of research to develop a vaccine is cheaper than the cost of caring for all the patients with an epidemic disease.

The first attempts at an inactivated poliovirus vaccine were made in the early twentieth century, but these pioneering efforts failed, in part because of the lack of appreciation that there were three serotypes of poliovirus. The first successful inactivated trivalent polio vaccine was developed by Salk and was field tested in 1954 (Fig. 67-1). The licensure of Salk's vaccine in the following year led to an immediate and dramatic reduction in the number of poliomyelitis cases.

Even after the inactivated vaccine came into use, efforts were made to perfect an attenuated vaccine, and after a fiercely competitive process the strains of poliovirus attenuated by Albert Sabin were accepted as the standards for vaccine use and licensed in 1961. The orally administered live attenuated vaccine has several advantages, including the production of mucosal immunity and lower cost. The attenuated virus is transmissible and therefore may infect persons who have not been given vaccine. This increases the number of immune persons but carries the risk of inadvertent paralytic disease in a vaccine contact. People immune to poliovirus can be reinfected, as defined by the intestinal excretion of virus, but the period of fecal shedding tends to be shorter and the quantity of virus smaller than in nonimmune individuals. In addition, the excretion of attenuated viruses repetitively exposes the population to polio, although the overall contribution of circulating virus to maintenance of protective immunity is unknown.

Inactivated vaccine also dramatically decreases the occurrence of paralytic illness. Mucosal immunity, however, is not present, and when wild-type virus is reintroduced into the population, it replicates in the gastrointestinal tract, is excreted in large quantities, and is transmitted rapidly throughout the population. As a result of this community-wide dissemination, persons who lack immunity may be few in number but still at risk of acquiring virus and disease. A question has been raised concerning susceptibility of persons previously immunized with unactivated vaccine whose serum antibodies have waned. In a recent Scandinavian outbreak paralytic disease occurred in 10 persons, most of whom were immunized. Thus it may be possible that gastrointestinal replication occurs with viremia before an anamnestic humoral response is generated.

The issue of whether the United States should change from the predominant use of live attenuated vaccine to inactivated vaccine remains controversial. The relative merits of the attenuated vaccine's ability to produce mucosal immunity versus the inactivated vaccine's superior safety have been argued for decades, and it is quite likely that in the future a regimen combining both vaccines will prevail.

FURTHER READING

Hogle JM, Chow M, Filman DJ: Three-dimensional structure of poliovirus at 2.9 Å resolution. Science 229:1358, 1985

Hughes JR, Wilfert CM, Moore M: Echovirus 14 associated with fatal neonatal hepatic necrosis. Am J Dis Child 123:61, 1972

Huovilainen A, Hovi T, Kinnunen L, et al: Evolution of poliovirus during an outbreak: Sequential type 3 poliovirus isolates from several persons show shifts of neutralization determinants. J Gen Virol 68:1373, 1987

Melnick JL: Portraits of viruses: The picornaviruses. Intervirology 20:61, 1983

Modlin JF: Fatal echovirus 11 disease in premature neonates. Pediatrics 66:775, 1980

Modlin JF, Polk BF, Horton P, et al: Perinatal echovirus infection: Risk of transmission during a community outbreak. N Engl J Med 305:368, 1981

Nathanson N, Langmuir AD: The Cutter incident, I, II, III. Am J Hyg 78:16, 1963

Paul JR: A History of Poliomyelitis. New Haven, Yale University Press, 1971

Rossmann MG: The canyon hypothesis. Viral Immunol 2:143, 1989

Rotbart HA, Kinsella JP, Wasserman RL: Persistent enterovirus infection in culture-negative meningoencephalitis: Demonstration by enzymatic RNA amplification. J Infect Dis 161:787, 1990

Zhaori G, Sun M, Faden HS, Ogra PL: Nasopharyngeal secretory antibody response to poliovirus type 3 virion proteins exhibit different specificities after immunization with live or inactivated poliovirus vaccines. J Infect Dis 159:1018, 1989

CHAPTER 68

Viruses in Gastrointestinal Tract Infections

Acute infectious diarrheal illness is recognized as one of the leading causes of morbidity and mortality in developing nations. Even in developed countries, infectious gastroenteritis is cited as second only to respiratory infections as a cause of morbidity in childhood. Viral agents recognized during the past decade have been shown to be responsible for a large proportion of the diarrhea for which an etiologic agent can be defined. Acute viral gastroenteritis affects all age-groups of people and may occur in either sporadic or epidemic form. Most such illnesses are self-limited, and in normal hosts recovery is complete. If severe dehydration occurs, morbidity and even mortality may be substantial.

Infection of the gastrointestinal tract with agents such as the enteroviruses is usually asymptomatic. The initial virus replication, however, may be followed by viremia, with spread of virus to other target organs and symptoms related to the infection of the additional tissues. Contrary to early suggestions, enteroviruses do not appear to be responsible for any significant proportion of gastrointestinal tract disease. It is also necessary to note briefly that several nondiarrheal diseases of the gastrointestinal tract have a postulated viral etiology. Intussusception occurs most commonly in children younger than 2 years of age, and mesenteric lymph node enlargement in the area of the terminal ileum has been observed at the time of surgery. Because lymphoid hyperplasia may occur in association with viral infection and adenoviruses have been isolated from children with intussusception, they are among the etiologic agents suggested for this entity. Coxsackie B viruses have been epidemiologically associated with diabetes mellitus, and several case reports have associated Coxsackie B4 with the development of diabetes mellitus. Experimentally, other viruses have been shown to infect pancreatic beta cells, and reovirus type 3 and murine encephalomyocarditis virus can produce a diabetes-like syndrome in inbred strains of mice. It must be emphasized that intussusception and diabetes mellitus have not been proved to have a viral etiology. It may be that virus infection represents only one of several factors contributing to the development of subsequent disease.

The viral agents discussed in detail in this chapter are those that seem to be associated with clinical symptoms related to virus replication within the gastrointestinal tract.

Rotaviruses

In 1943 an outbreak of diarrhea in infants was reported by Light and Hodes, who isolated from stool specimens a filterable agent that caused diarrhea in calves. They established the incubation period and reproduced diarrhea with serial passage of the agent. The pathology of the bowel, the development of immunity to the agent, and passive protection by the administration of immune serum were described. At the time there was no confirmation of a viral etiology of the diarrhea inasmuch as no agent could be detected in available cell culture systems. It was not until 1973 when virus particles were visualized in a duodenal biopsy by electron microscopy that the etiologic agent was finally defined as a rotavirus. In the past decade, rotaviruses have come to be appreciated as the single most common agents causing epidemic diarrhea in infants from 6 to 24 months of age. Rotaviruses are known to cause diarrhea in foals, lambs, piglets, rabbits, deer, monkeys, and other species. Experimental infection of animals other than the species of origin occurs with most rotaviruses.

Rotaviruses constitute one genus of the family Reoviridae. The rotavirus genome consists of 11 segments of double-stranded RNA, each coding for a virus protein, and rotavirus particles possess a double shell of outer and inner capsids (Fig 68-1A). The internal core contains VP1, VP2, and VP3; the inner capsid contains VP6; and the outer capsid contains VP4 and VP7. At least 3 of the 11 rotavirus genes contribute to antigenic diversity. Gene 8 or 9 codes for VP7, which induces neutralizing antibody responsible for serotype specificity. Gene 6 codes for a common group antigen and a subgroup specific antigen. Gene 4 codes for an outer capsid protein (VP 3), which is the hemagglutinin and also induces neutralizing antibody contributing to serotype specificity. It is the fourth gene that restricts ability of human rotaviruses to grow in cell culture. If this gene is supplied by a bovine rotavirus (all animal rotaviruses can grow in cultured cells), the reassortant is able to grow. Rotavirus groups A through F have been described, but only groups A, B, and C have been identified in humans. Group A viruses are common causes of gastroenteritis in children. There are 11 serotypes (determined by VP7) of group A viruses, and types 1 through 4 are the major causes of human disease.

Epidemiology and Clinical Illness

Sporadic diarrhea occurring predominantly in infants and young children is a significant illness of worldwide importance. In the United States, rotaviruses are the etiologic agents for at least 35% to 50% of the cases of infantile diarrhea that require hospitalization. It has been estimated that hospitalization due to rotavirus occurs with an incidence of 3.67/1000 in the first year of life in children cared for by a health maintenance organization. In developing nations the problem is of greater magnitude as it is estimated that 10% of episodes of diarrhea per child from 6 to 11 months of age are due to rotaviruses; 90% of children will have rotavirus antibody by 24 months of age. Peak prevalence of rotavirus infection occurs during the cooler months of the year in temperate climates, but in tropical areas cases are identified throughout

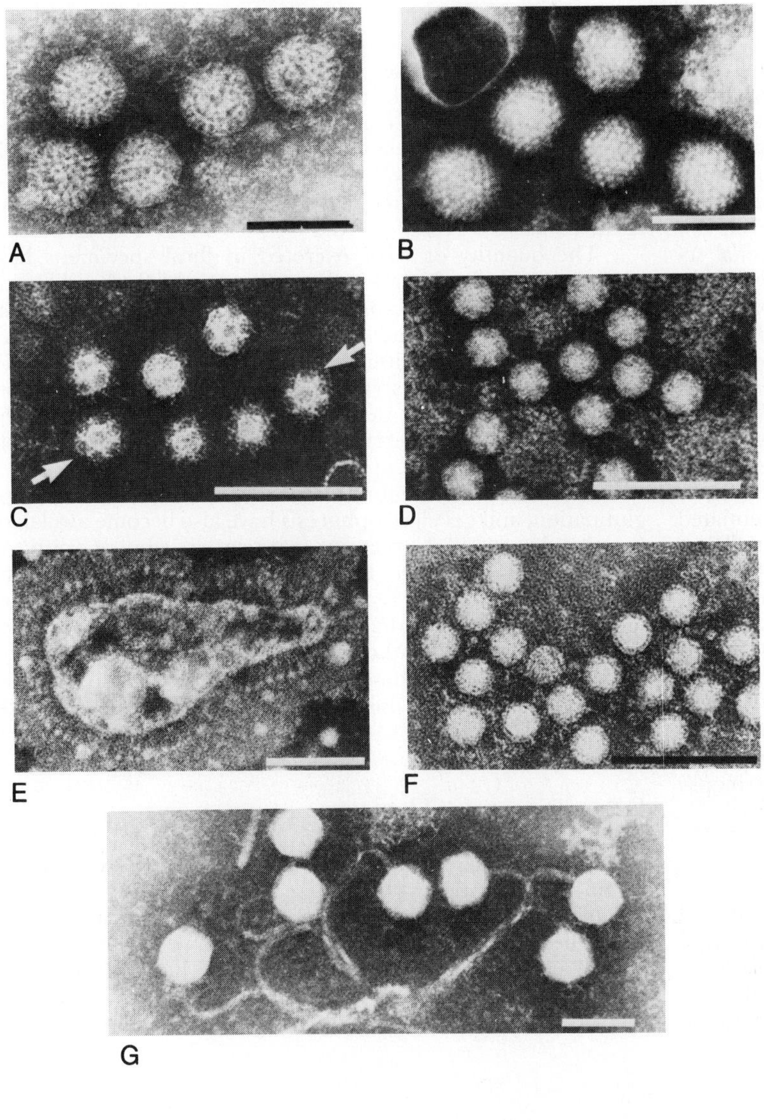

Fig. 68–1. Viruses found in feces from patients with gastroenteritis, showing a negative stain reaction with 2% potassium phosphotungstate at pH 6.5. Bars represent 100 nm. **A.** Rotaviruses. **B.** Adenoviruses: the icosahedral morphology is evident. **C.** Caliciviruses: two particles (arrowed) clearly exhibit the characteristic six-pointed star morphology. **D.** Astroviruses: some particles show a five- or six-pointed star on the surface. **E.** Coronavirus: pleomorphic particle with surface projections above 20 nm long. **F.** Small round viruses (SRV): particles with no obvious morphology and a diameter of 27 to 30 nm. **G.** Bacteriophages: these particles have hexagonal heads with long flexible tails, and are attached to pieces of bacterial debris. *(Courtesy of Dr. H. A. Davies.)*

the year. Serotypes 1 and 3 are the most frequent in the United States.

Virus is excreted in feces from approximately 2 days before to 10 days after onset of symptoms and in large amounts, with as many as 10^{11} virus particles per gram of feces. Virus does not seem to be commonly shed from the respiratory tract, but aerosolization of fecally contaminated material may result in inhalation or ingestion of infectious virus. Rotavirus transmission occurs from person to person by the fecal to oral route. Experimental human infection can be accomplished either by oral or by enteric administration of virus, and the incubation period is 2 to 5 days. Children from 6 months to 2 years of age most often show symptoms of the infection. Newborn infants are infected and excrete virus, but only an estimated 8% to 28% are symptomatic suggesting important age-related differences in the immature host. Furthermore, infants who are infected in the newborn period have fewer episodes of subsequent diarrheal illness with rotavirus. Adults become infected but frequently are without symptoms. Asymptomatic infections occur in up to 50% of children in day care. Thus infection is transmissible from symptom-free persons transiently infected with virus. Recurrent infections are common in day care and other settings in which exposure is frequent.

Acute infection due to rotaviruses is characterized by the rather abrupt onset of severe diarrhea that is not characteristically associated with blood or mucus in the stool. Fecal leukocytes are seen in a minority of patients. Fever and vomiting are often present at the onset of illness. Those most severely infected and affected are between the ages of 6 and 24 months. The mean duration of illness in normal hosts is 5 to 7 days. Dehydration and metabolic acidosis are observed in children ill enough to be hospitalized with this infection.

Rotavirus particles have been visualized by electron microscope in intestinal epithelial cells, aspirated duodenal secretions, and feces of infected persons. Morphologically, shortening and blunting of the villi of the duodenum and small intestine occur early and can be seen within 30 minutes of experimentally induced infection. Virus particles are visualized in the cytoplasm and bud into the cisternae of the endoplasmic reticulum of the enterocytes. Immunofluorescence studies have demonstrated rotavirus antigens in the cytoplasm of the villus epithelial cells but not in the cells of the crypts or lamina propria. This suggests that the specificity of the virus particle is for the mature or differentiated enterocytes located in the mid and upper villus epithelium. The destruction of mature enterocytes is associated with a decrease in the surface areas of the intestine and decreased production of one or more mucosal disaccharidases. The destroyed infected cells are replaced by immature cells, which results in a deficit in glucose-facilitated sodium transport. Diarrhea then results from decreased absorption secondary to the altered ion transport in immature cells. In contrast to the toxin-mediated diarrheas, there is no increase in intestinal secretion. Complete recovery has been documented by biopsy as early as 4 weeks after the episode of diarrhea.

Host Response

Specific antibody has been demonstrable in the stool and serum. Primary infection produces an initial serum IgM response, followed by an IgG and an IgA response. Secretory IgA is formed in the gastrointestinal tract. Adults with rotavirus infection manifest an anamnestic response with elevation of IgG antibodies. Persons may experience more than one infection with rotaviruses, and the role of serum homotypic and heterotypic humoral antibodies and secretory antibodies is under study. It is likely that protective immunity is attributable to VP7 or VP4, or both.

Specific antibody has been demonstrated in colostrum and milk for as long as 9 months of lactation. In nurseries in which rotavirus infection has been endemic, breast-fed infants seem to acquire infection less often than do formula-fed infants. Those who are infected excrete less virus and have fewer symptoms. Antibodies in human colostrum and milk are capable of neutralizing rotavirus in vitro, and experimental feeding of human IgG with rotavirus antibody diminished virus excretion and illness in infants in an endemically infected nursery. Weaning from breast milk in developing nations is temporally associated with the onset of a diarrhea-malnutrition cycle. The humoral response in infants may be homotypic but becomes heterotypic as they become older and sustain second or third infections. Despite the fact that breast milk has been shown to have preventive activity against undifferentiated infantile diarrhea and, even more specifically, has been shown to contain antibodies against some of the causative agents, breastfeeding is declining in popularity in many parts of the world with the greatest incidence of diarrheal disease.

Diagnosis

Human rotaviruses are extremely fastidious, but recent progress has been made in the cell culture propagation of these agents. Human rotavirus strains have now been efficiently propagated directly from clinical specimens into cell cultures. In particular MA 104 cells, which are a line derived from embryonic rhesus monkey kidney, have been successfully used.

The quantity of virus excreted in fecal specimens has enabled various antigen detection systems to identify virus in the stool. Electron microscopic (EM) examination of fecal extracts obtained during the acute stage of gastroenteritis, particularly when specific antiserum (immune electron microscopy [IEM]) is used to agglutinate virus particles, is almost invariably positive. EM detects other viruses associated with gastroenteritis and therefore where available is the most efficient diagnostic test.

Enzyme-linked immunosorbent assay (ELISA), latex agglutination, and gel electrophoresis have also become available for the detection of rotavirus particles in stool. Group A rotaviruses are detected by ELISA and latex agglutination assays. Electrophoretic typing is a useful epidemiologic tool but is not practical for diagnosis. ELISA is as sensitive as EM for group A viruses, and commercially marketed reagent kits are now available for detection of rotavirus in stool. Oligonucleotide probes and polymerase chain reaction (PCR) tests are being evaluated.

Prevention and Therapy

Therapy of viral gastroenteritis is limited to supportive measures, since there are no effective antiviral agents available for specific treatment.

There can be no doubt that prevention of rotavirus illness would be a major contribution to reduction of morbidity from gastroenteritis. For immunization to be effective, immunity within the gastrointestinal tract is probably a necessity. Various approaches to immunization are being considered. Reassortant rotavirus viruses containing the VP7 gene from human rotavirus and the remaining 10 genes from an animal rotavirus are being studied. Oral vaccines of rhesus monkey and bovine origin show promise inasmuch as they are immunogenic, have an acceptably low occurrence of fever or diarrhea, and are not transmissible to contacts. Further clinical studies are needed to determine if morbidity due to rota viruses can be decreased by administration of vaccine.

Norwalk-like Group of Viruses

Epidemic gastroenteritis occurs in a form that produces an explosive, self-limited disease lasting for 24 to 48 hours, that may be community-wide, and that affects school-aged children, family contacts, and adults. Such an outbreak of gastroenteritis occurred in Norwalk, Ohio, in 1969. Within a matter of 48 hours gastrointestinal illness developed in half the students and teachers in an elementary school, with the secondary symptomatic attack rate affecting approximately one third of family contacts. A bacteria-free filtrate from a stool specimen produced gastroenteritis in several volunteers, and stools from the infected individuals could be serially passaged in additional volunteers, but no agent could be isolated in the usual cell culture systems. In 1972, immune electron microscopy (IEM) with serum from a patient with symptomatic disease demonstrated small, nonenveloped 27-nm diameter particles in an infectious stool filtrate. Norwalk agent particles contain single-stranded RNA of about 8 kb in length and only a single protein species with a molecular weight of 59,000. Several morphologically similar but antigenically different viruses are identified from outbreaks of illness. The inability to propagate these viruses in cell culture has hindered studies.

Epidemiology and Clinical Infection

Roughly one third of outbreaks of gastroenteritis can be attributed to a Norwalk-like agent. This is a surprisingly high number and suggests that the antigenically unique viruses of this group may be limited in number. Thus far, five serotypes of these 27 nm particles have been identified. The settings in which such outbreaks have occurred include schools, recreational camps, cruise ships, and nursing homes. Ingestion of contaminated water and food (shellfish, salads, cake frosting) and person-to-person spread transmit infection. Outbreaks have occurred at all times of the year, and antibody surveys document that the agent or agents occur worldwide. In most undeveloped nations, infection occurs at an early age. In the United States, antibody is uncommon during childhood and approximately one half of persons in the fifth decade of life have antibodies. Although respiratory symptoms are unusual, the rapidity of spread suggests that some aerosolization of virus may occur either from fecal contamination of the environment or from vomitus that has been shown to contain virus.

Infection with these agents results in delayed gastric emptying although the gastric mucosa is morphologically normal. Microscopic broadening and blunting of the villi in the jejunum are apparent. The mucosa remains histologically intact, but there is mononuclear cell infiltration of the lamina propria. Virus has not yet been detected in involved mucosal cells by electron microscopy but shortening of the microvilli and dilatation of the endoplasmic reticulum are seen.

The majority of patients who sustain these infections have nausea, vomiting, and abdominal cramps, and about one half of them have associated diarrhea. Some have fever and chills. The symptoms last from 12 to 24 hours, and the incubation period appears to be around 48 hours. Usually the stools are not bloody and do not contain mucus or leukocytes. A transient lymphopenia has been observed in volunteers challenged with these agents.

Host Response

Immunity to these viruses is a puzzling feature of the infections that they cause. Challenge of volunteers produces disease in some persons and not in others. Repeat challenge with homologous virus within several months of the original infection will not produce clinical illness. Subsequent challenge 2 to 4½ years later produces disease in the same volunteers who had symptomatic illness with the first contact with the virus. Those individuals who were symptom-free and did not acquire infection with the first contact do not do so with subsequent challenge. Those individuals who acquire clinical infection have demonstrable antibody within 72 hours after onset of illness. Antibody wanes and then has an anamnestic boost with a subsequent challenge. Volunteers in whom illness fails to develop have no demonstrable antibody. Measurement of intestinal antibody also showed that those individuals in whom illness developed have higher mean antibody titers in jejunal fluid than do those in whom illness failed to develop. Neither serum nor local intestinal antibody correlates with resistance to a Norwalk challenge. Thus individuals who have demonstrable serum antibody are those who are at risk for symptoms induced by infection. These findings are not understood. It is possible that some individuals are not susceptible to these viruses by reason of genetically determined factors such as the absence of appropriate intestinal receptors.

Diagnosis and Therapy

IEM and radioimmunoassay are the best available procedures for identifying members of this group of agents. The radioimmunoassay and ELISA are more efficient than IEM because they are able to detect soluble as well as particulate antigens. These tests, however, are not commercially available and depend on the availability of appropriate high-titered serum. In research laboratories, radioimmunoassay, immune adherence hemagglutination, and immune electron microscopy have also been used to assess serum antibody status.

The illnesses associated with the Norwalk group of agents are generally self-limited and mild. No specific therapy is available. Replacement fluid therapy is essential in the management of such patients. The rather simplistic approach of good hand-washing and effective hygiene is the best we have to offer to prevent the spread of these viruses.

Coronaviruses

The Coronaviridae are pleomorphic, enveloped, single-stranded RNA-containing viruses with widely spaced 20 nm club-shaped surface projections (Fig. 68–1E). This family of viruses has been well identified as an etiologic agent of respiratory and intestinal disease in animals. In 1960 the first of these agents was isolated from a human with a cold. It grew in human tracheal organ culture and was morphologically similar to infectious bronchitis virus, an avian coronavirus. A second isolate, now the prototype strain of human coronavirus (229E), was isolated in human kidney cell culture in 1962.

Human coronaviruses were first etiologically associated with upper respiratory tract disease in adults and with lower respiratory tract disease in hospitalized children. Coronaviruses may be responsible for an exacerbation of the respiratory symptoms in children hospitalized because of asthma. Coronavirus infections tend to occur in small outbreaks that take place during the late winter and early spring but sporadically occur in other seasons. A specific serotype may recur in the community in cycles of 2 to 3 years. Reinfection with coronaviruses is a frequent event, as shown by the presence of infection in persons with preexisting neutralizing antibodies.

It was predicted in the mid-1970s that an association of coronaviruses with enteric disease of humans would be identified because of the known involvement of these agents with enteric disease in animals. Electron microscopic examination of stools then revealed coronavirus-like particles in human feces. In fecal specimens it has been estimated that there are as many as 10^8 coronavirus particles per gram. Many of these particles are defective, which suggests that maturation may be faulty within the gastrointestinal tract.

Of interest is an apparent difference in the epidemiology of these viruses. They seem to be less likely to be responsible for diarrhea within the first year of life and are more commonly visualized in the diarrheal stools of older children and young adults. Enteric coronaviruses can be excreted for as long as 18 months, and in some cases of persistent excretion, chronic gastroenteritis is present. Prolonged viral excretion complicates conclusions concerning the epidemiology, because symptom-free individuals can be excreting virus. It has been documented that endemic diarrheal disease occurs in situations in which poor hygiene exists, and acquisition of virus does coincide with development of gastroenteritis.

Work with the coronaviruses isolated from humans has been difficult because they grow best in organ cultures, and those from the respiratory tract appear to require the use of ciliated epithelium. There are at least two antigenic groups of mammalian coronaviruses, and the successful cultivation in vitro of several human strains is beginning to advance our knowledge of these viruses. Human coronaviruses possess four major structural proteins; the surface projections that are responsible for hemagglutination and complement fixation consist of two large glycoproteins. These coronaviruses do not appear to bud from the plasma membrane of infected cells but bud into the cisternae of the endoplasmic reticulum and are found in large intracytoplasmic vesicles. Postmortem examination of the small intestine of an infant with diarrhea and newborns with necrotizing enterocolitis showed coronavirus particles within cytoplasmic vesicles of epithelial cells and in the lumen of the intestine.

Fastidious (Enteric) Adenoviruses

The fastidious adenoviruses were first described by Flewett in 1975. Adenoviruses of a variety of serotypes are often present in stool and can be isolated in cell culture. Fastidious (enteric) adenoviruses, however, which do not grow easily in cell culture but are visualized by EM, seem to be causally associated with enteric illness. These agents have been established as a significant pathogen of diarrheal illness in children and are second to rotaviruses in frequency. Preliminary characterization of agents isolated from geographically distinct outbreaks indicates that they are all representatives of serogroup F and comprise only serotypes 40 and 41 (Fig. 68–1B). These agents did not grow in the usual cell culture systems, and successful in vitro cultivation depended on the use of 293 Graham cells, a human embryonic kidney cell line containing some of the genome of adenovirus type 5. In these cells the cytopathic effects produced are typical of adenoviruses. Subsequently these viruses have also been propagated successfully in HeLa, HEp-2, Ch'ang conjunctiva, and cynomolgus monkey kidney cells.

These agents most often appear to be responsible for acute diarrhea in infants younger than 1 year of age. After an incubation period of 3 to 10 days the onset of illness manifests with diarrhea, and the young child may also have respiratory symptoms, including cough, rhinorrhea, or wheezing. Pneumonia and conjunctivitis have also been seen in association with adenovirus gastroenteritis. The illness is usually mild to moderate in severity, lasting 6 to 9 days, and may occur in any month of the year. The viruses can be visualized in the feces of patients for a period of 4 days to 2 weeks. There is a suggestion that more prolonged symptomatic illness of 8 to 12 days may also occur.

The estimated frequency of adenoviruses as a cause of diarrhea varies. If the study period is selected when rotavirus disease is not occurring, adenoviruses are responsible for a larger proportion of illness, recorded to be as high as 50%. When prospective study is extended over a several-year period, 4% to 8% of all the diarrhea observed may be associated with these fastidious adenoviruses. Serologic studies suggest that approximately one half of children have antibodies by 3 to 4 years of age.

The diagnosis of these agents depends on demonstration of the virus particles or antigen in stool. Visible adenoviruses that do not grow in cell culture are almost all enteric serotypes. Initial recognition by electron microscopy has been followed by the development of an ELISA that employs monoclonal antibodies. Serologic assessment is also available in research laboratories, as is serotyping of enteric adenoviruses and restriction enzyme analysis.

Astroviruses

Astroviruses were described in 1975 after they were visualized in the stool of newborn infants. They are 28 to 30 nm particles and are shed in the stool in very large numbers. The RNA genome encodes four structural proteins, and there are currently five known antigenic types of these viruses. They are present in the stools of infants both with and without acute gastroenteritis. The five- to six-pointed-star shape designates the agents as astrovirus particles (Fig 68–1D). Similar morphologic structures have been identified in feces from both adults and children and in diarrheal feces from lambs and calves. These agents infect monolayers of human embryonic kidney cells without producing cytopathic effects. EM, IEM, and immunofluorescence of cell cultures will detect virus. Monoclonal antibodies have made the development of an ELISA possible.

Early serologic studies have demonstrated seroconversion in association with demonstrable infection and fecal excretion. Yet feeding of these agents to adult volunteers resulted in poor transmission of disease but antibody rises in the majority of volunteers. More than 80% of adults, however, have previously met the agents and have antibody. Therefore they may be protected against disease. These viruses have been associated with disease in many countries. Outbreaks in pediatric wards, schools, and nursing homes have been associated with these agents. Illness includes malaise, low-grade fever, and watery diarrhea lasting about 3 days. The incubation period is 1 to 4 days, and residual lactose intolerance may follow acute illness.

In lambs, these agents infect the epithelial cells and the subepithelial macrophages of the villi of the small intestine. Atrophy of the villi is demonstrable.

Caliciviruses

Calicivirus particles are 35 to 39 nm in diameter with a star of David appearance (Fig 68–1C). Five antigenic types of virus are known, and almost all children have antibodies by 5 years of age. Diarrheal illness and symptom-free infection have been documented. The illness is similar to rotavirus diarrhea. Fecal-to-oral spread occurs, and these agents may be involved in food-borne outbreaks of gastroenteritis. EM will detect virus in stool, and on a research basis, IEM assay and ELISA have been developed.

Other Viruses

The interest in examining feces by electron microscopy has resulted in the description of numerous virus species. Some of them are clearly defined as etiologic agents of gastroenteritis, and others have yet to be assigned a definitive etiologic role. The relationship to each other or other morphologic species also remains to be determined. These unidentified and unclassified types of particles are discussed below.

Small, Round Viruses (Picorna-Parvovirus-like)

This heterogeneous collection of small round viruses is visualized in stools. The particles, 27 to 30 nm in diameter, have no detectable surface structure and do not grow in vitro in routine cell culture systems (Fig. 68–1F). They have been seen in stools of patients with diarrhea and of patients with no clinical symptoms.

Minireovirus and Minirotaviruses

These agents are 30 nm particles with a double capsid and with no serologic relationship to rotaviruses or reoviruses. They have been visualized in stools of children with diarrhea and in infants who have acquired diarrhea within hospital settings.

Pestiviruses are 40 to 60 nm in diameter as visualized by EM and have been identified in stools.

An agent resembling Breda virus of calf diarrhea (torovirus) has been detected in children's diarrheal stools. These agents are elongated with rounded ends and are 40 by 100 nm.

Additional information is needed to establish the role of these viruses as etiologic agents in gastroenteritis.

FURTHER READING

General

Barnett BB: Other viruses with etiologic roles in childhood gastroenteritis. Pediatr Infect Dis J 5:575, 1986

Tyrrell DAJ, Kapikian AZ (eds): Virus Infections of the Gastrointestinal Tract. New York, Marcel Dekker, 1982

Rotavirus

Dennehy PH, Gauntlett DR, Tente WE: Comparison of nine commercial immunoassays for the detection of rotavirus in fecal specimens. J Clin Microbiol 26:1630, 1988

Estes MK, Cohen J: Rotavirus gene structure and function. Microbiol Rev 53:410, 1989

Flores J, Nakagomi O, Nakagomi T, et al: The role of rotaviruses in pediatric diarrhea. Pediatr Infect Dis J 5:S53, 1986.

Green KY, Tamguchi K, Mackow ER, et al: Homotypic and heterotypic epitope specific antibody responses in adult and infant rotavirus vaccinees: Implications for vaccine development. J Infect Dis 161:664, 1990

Kapikian AZ, Flores J, Hoshino Y, et al: Rotavirus: The major etiologic agent of severe infantile diarrhea may be controllable by a "Jennerian" approach to vaccination. J Infect Dis 153:815, 1986

Losonsky GA, Rennels MB, Kapikian AZ, et al: Safety, infectivity, transmissibility, and immunogenicity of rhesus rotavirus vaccine (MMU 18006) in infants. Pediatr Infect Dis J 5:25, 1986

Prasad BVV, Burno JW, Mariette K, et al: Localization of VP4 neutralization sites in rotavirus by three dimensional cryoelectron microscopy. Nature 343:476, 1990

Rotbart HA, Yolken RH, Nelson WL, et al: Confirmatory testing of rotazyme results in neonates. J Pediatr 107:289, 1985

Vesikari T, Isolauri E, Delem A, et al: Clinical efficacy of the RIT 4237 live attenuated bovine rotavirus vaccine in infants vaccinated before a rotavirus epidemic. J Pediatr 107:189, 1985

Vesikari T, Kapikian AZ, Delem A, et al: A comparative trial of rheusus monkey (RRV-1) and bovine (RIT 4237) oral rotavirus vaccines in young children. J Infect Dis 153:832, 1986

Yolken, RH, Miotti P, Viseidi R: Immunoassays for the diagnosis and study of viral gastroenteritis. Pediatr Infect Dis J 5:46, 1986

Norwalk-like Agents

Adler I, Vicki R: Winter vomiting disease. J Infect Dis 119:668, 1969

Agus SG, Dolin R, Wyatt RG, et al: Acute infectious nonbacterial gastroenteritis: Intestinal histopathology. Histologic and enzymatic alterations during illness produced by the Norwalk agent in man. Ann Intern Med 79:18, 1973

Morse DL, Guzewich JJ, Hannahan JP, et al: Widespread outbreaks of clam- and oyster-associated gastroenteritis: Role of Norwalk virus. N Engl J Med 314:678, 1986

Nakata, S, Chiba S, Terashima, H: Humoral immunity in infants with gastroenteritis caused by human calicivirus. J Infect Dis 152:274, 1985

Ryder RW, Singh N, Reeves WC, et al: Evidence of immunity induced by naturally acquired rotavirus and Norwalk virus infection on two remote Panamanian islands. J Infect Dis 151:99, 1985

Other Viruses

Battaglia M, Passarani N, DiMatteo A, et al: Human enteric coronaviruses: Further characterization and immunoblotting of viral proteins. J Infect Dis 155:140, 1987

Brandt CD, Kim HW, Rodriguez WJ, et al: Adenoviruses and pediatric gastroenteritis. J Infect Dis 151:437, 1985

Gerna G, Passarani N, Battaglia M, et al: Human enteric coronaviruses: Antigenic relatedness to human coronavirus OC43 and possible etiologic role in viral gastroenteritis. J Infect Dis 151:796, 1985

Hertman JE, Novod NA, Perron-Henry DM, et al: Diagnosis of astrovirus gastroenteritis by antigen detection with monoclonal antibodies. J Infect Dis 161:226, 1990

Kotloff KC, Lasonsky GA, Morris JG, et al: Enteric adenovirus infection and childhood diarrhea: An epidemiologic study in three clinical settings. Pediatrics 84:219, 1989

Madeley CR: The emerging role of adenoviruses as inducers of gastroenteritis. Pediatr Infect Dis J 5:63, 1986

Matson DO, Este MK, Tanaka T, et al: Asymptomatic human calicivirus infection in a daycare center. Pediatr Infect Dis J 9:180, 1990

Mortensen ML, Ray CG, Payne CM, et al: Coronaviruslike particles in human gastrointestinal disease: Epidemiologic, clinical, and laboratory observations. Am J Dis Child 139:928, 1985

Rettig PJ, Altshuler GP: Fatal gastroenteritis associated with coronaviruslike particles. Am J Dis Child 139:245, 1985

Rodriguez WJ, Kim HW, Brandt CD, et al: Fecal adenoviruses from a longitudinal study of families in metropolitan Washington, D.C.: Laboratory, clinical, and epidemiologic observations. J Pediatr 107:514, 1985

Yolken RH, Franklin CC: Gastrointestinal adenovirus: An important cause of morbidity in patients with necrotizing enterocolitis and gastrointestinal surgery. Pediatr Infect Dis J 4:42, 1985

CHAPTER 69

Influenza Viruses

Outbreaks of influenza virus infection of varying severity occur annually, typically in the colder months of the year in temperate climates. The question is not whether influenza virus infections will occur but when, with what strains, and how severe in terms of clinical illness and numbers of persons affected. Epidemics in which more than 10% of the local population become infected will cause increases in school and industrial absenteeism, physician visits, hospitalizations, and deaths. Most infections occur in children and young adults, but the increases in hospitalizations and deaths occur primarily among older adults, especially those who have chronic heart or lung disease or reside in a nursing home. The use of current influenza control measures—vaccine and an antiviral agent—is aimed at reducing the severe morbidity and mortality among the latter population.

Clinical Features

Influenza is a highly contagious infection that can spread by aerosol or by person-to-person contact. The incubation period for influenza is 1 to 4 days. Primary target cells for the virus are those of the respiratory epithelium from the upper respiratory tract down to the alveoli. Infected cells will slough, allowing extravasation of fluid and secondary submucosal inflammation; alveolar collapse secondary to loss of surfactant and hemorrhagic viral pneumonia can occur. Influenza viruses are rarely detected outside the respiratory tract, and it is thought that most of the prominent generalized symptoms of influenza may result from release of cellular toxins such as tumor necrosis factor and interleukin-1. Secondary bacterial infections, including otitis media, sinusitis, pharyngitis, bronchitis, and pneumonia, contribute in a major way to the morbidity and mortality incurred in influenza epidemics. Among the effects of the influenza virus infection that may facilitate these secondary infections are impaired mucociliary clearance, extravasated fluid that serves as a good culture medium, impaired function of both phagocytic cells and lymphocytes, and enhanced adherence of bacteria to altered epithelial cells.

The typical influenza syndrome in previously healthy older children and adults consists of the rather sudden onset of fever and tracheobronchitis with a dry cough that causes substernal discomfort. Systemic symptoms, including myalgia, headache, generalized aches, malaise, and lethargy, often are prominent. Upper respiratory symptoms such as nasal obstruction and a scratchy throat may be present but are often overshadowed by the systemic symptoms and tracheobronchitis. Physical examination usually reveals only an uncomfortable, febrile, coughing patient with flushed skin and mucosal injection. The white blood cell count and differential may be within normal limits or may reveal neutropenia, a potential help in distinguishing effects of the virus from those of secondary bacterial infection. Pulmonary function studies commonly yield evidence of impaired gas exchange and increased peripheral airway resistance, even in uncomplicated influenza, and these effects may take several weeks to clear. Bronchial hyperreactivity also occurs as a result of the infection and can precipitate asthmatic attacks in patients with preexisting reactive airways disease. Uncomplicated influenza illness typically lasts 3 to 6 days, but cough and lassitude may persist for several additional days or weeks.

Findings during influenza virus infections in infants and young children differ for several reasons. These individuals will likely lack cross-reactive immunity generated by prior influenza virus infections and will exhibit both larger amounts of virus in respiratory secretions and a longer duration of shedding than do their older siblings and parents. Moreover, their airways are of relatively small caliber, which increases the likelihood of obstruction by the inflammatory response to infection. Also, they will be unable or less able to describe their symptoms. Fever, cough, and rhinorrhea are common findings, and bacterial otitis media is a frequent complication. Vomiting and diarrhea may occur, although the pathogenesis is unclear. Frequent diagnoses for children admitted to the hospital with what is later proved to be influenza virus infection are viral and/or bacterial pneumonia, laryngeotracheobronchitis (croup), and unexplained fever. The occurrence of febrile convulsions, vomiting, and irritability in such patients may suggest meningitis. Recovery from the more severe manifestations of the infection usually occurs in 3 to 6 days, but rhinorrhea and cough may persist for several more days or weeks.

The clinical diagnosis of influenza in elderly individuals can also be difficult. Some of the patients may not complain of typical symptoms because of mental impairment. Increased lassitude, confusion, anorexia, or unexplained fever may be the primary findings of uncomplicated disease in such patients. Moreover, complications of influenza virus infection are more frequent in the elderly (see below), and symptoms and signs of the complicating illness may overshadow those of the initial virus infection.

The most frequently recognized severe complication of influenza is pneumonia. The virus infection can cause scattered rales that are heard on auscultation of the chest and increased interstitial markings on chest radiographs, with a good prognosis for full recovery. Much more ominous is primary influenzal pneumonia with diffuse pulmonary infiltrates and acute respiratory failure. This illness carries a high mortality rate, and diffuse pulmonary fibrosis has been observed among some of those that survive. Primary influenzal pneumonia is uncommon and occurs primarily during major influenza A virus epidemics. Occasionally, combined viral and bacterial pneumonia will occur as a progression of the initial illness and, like primary influenzal pneumonia, carries a high mortality rate.

The much more frequent type of pneumonia complicating influenza virus infection is secondary bacterial pneumonia signified by a recurrence of fever, along with cough productive of purulent sputum when the patient seemed to be recovering from the initial influenzal illness. These pneumonias occur 5 to 10 days after onset of the viral illness. A variety of bacteria can be involved, but the most frequent are pneumococci. This type of pneumonia typically responds well to appropriate antimicrobial therapy. *Staphylococcus aureus* pneumonia occurs more frequently during influenza epidemics than at other times and tends to be associated with a higher mortality rate than that due to other organisms.

A sustained increase in the number of deaths due to pneumonia and influenza over the expected number is a traditional marker of influenza epidemics. Total excess mortality exceeded 10,000 persons in 19 different epidemics during the 30-year period of 1957 through 1986 and has exceeded 40,000 during several recent epidemics. It should be noted that deaths attributed to ischemic heart disease also increase during influenza epidemics; these deaths are usually about twice as numerous as those attributed to pneumonia and influenza and are likely a result of complications of the infection, such as congestive heart failure. Infrequent complications of influenza virus infections include myositis, myocarditis, pericarditis, encephalopathy, transverse myelitis, and Goodpasture's syndrome (pulmonary hemorrhage and nephritis due to an autoantibody). Guillain-Barré syndrome (GBS), an ascending paralytic illness that can persist for months, has been observed after both influenza virus infection and vaccination but, with the exception of influenza A/New Jersey/76 (H1N1) vaccine (see below), neither appears to be an important trigger for the illness. Reye's syndrome, characterized by vomiting, lethargy, and progressive mental deterioration, occurs infrequently in children after a variety of viral illnesses, including influenza; occurrence of this syndrome is associated with ingestion of salicylates during the antecedent illness, and such medication should be avoided in children with influenza.

An important contributing factor to the development of severe influenzal disease and complications, including death, is the presence of certain underlying chronic diseases. Among children these include congenital cardiovascular disease, bronchopulmonary dysplasia, cystic fibrosis, asthma, sickle cell disease, and a variety of neurologic, metabolic, and renal disorders. Most prominent among adults are chronic diseases of the heart or lungs, which, individually, increase the risk of death due to pneumonia or influenza more than 100-fold during epidemics and, together, increase the risk some 800-fold. Metabolic diseases such as diabetes mellitus, renal dysfunction, anemia, and immunosuppression also contribute to the risk. Increasing age in the absence of one of these high-risk conditions is associated with only a modest increase in the frequency of complications during influenza virus infection. Nevertheless, healthy persons older than 65 years of age are considered to be at increased risk, in part because some will have covert underlying diseases that only become apparent with the stress of infection.

Epidemiology

Influenza viruses are classified as types A, B, and C on the basis of the antigenicity of their nucleoproteins and matrix proteins that rarely varies. Epidemic influenza disease is caused by types A or B, or both. Type C influenza virus differs from types A and B genetically and epidemiologically, causing widespread but milder and more sporadic infections; it will not be considered further. Antigenically stable internal proteins of influenza viruses are important targets for cytotoxic T cells that can speed recovery from infection, but protection against infection is mediated primarily by antibody directed against the hemagglutinin (H), one of the two glycoproteins projecting from the virus envelope. Antibody directed against the second surface glycoprotein, neuraminidase (N), does not prevent infection but can impair spread of the virus and thus make illness less severe. The H and N glycoproteins of both types A and B influenza viruses exhibit frequent minor antigenic variations because of genetic mutations that result in change of one or more amino acids. This antigenic drift reduces the effectiveness of antibodies induced by prior strains and thus allows the viruses to cause repeated outbreaks of infection. Influenza A strains predominate most frequently, with B strains predominating at 2 to 4 year intervals.

Type A influenza viruses can also exhibit major shifts in their H and N glycoproteins, creating new subtypes. The mechanism by which this occurs appears to involve reassortment of the eight RNA segments of the viral genome when individuals become dually infected with a human strain to which they are partially immune and an animal strain possessing different surface glycoproteins. Type A (but not B) influenza viruses can infect many animal species, which serves to maintain several distinct H and N glycoproteins in nature. Virus strains adapted to growth in animals do not usually cause significant infection in humans because their genes that control replication do not function well in human cells, but they can donate their distinctive glycoproteins to create "new" human subtypes if the necessary dual infection occurs. The host's antibodies will be ineffective against these new influenza A virus subtypes, thus permitting more severe infections that may then be transmitted to other persons. Because of the lack of significant immunity in the population, such new influenza A virus subtypes can spread extensively, causing worldwide pandemics and displacing the preceding subtype. The Far East appears to be a fertile area for the generation of new influenza A subtypes, perhaps because the density of human and swine or duck populations increases the likelihood of dual infections of persons with both human and animal strains. Influenza A virus subtypes that have caused pandemics are A/H1N1 in 1918, A/H2N2 in 1957, and A/H3N2 in 1968. An unusual situation arose with the return of A/H1N1 influenza in 1977 after a 20-year absence; persons older than 25 years of age were largely immune because of prior infection, and A/H3N2 and A/H1N1 subtypes have circulated simultaneously since then.

Outbreaks of influenza virus infection occur annually over a 6- to 10-week period, predominantly during the winter months in temperate climates. A partial explanation for the winter occurrence may be the increased stability of influenza viruses at low humidity, which would favor transmission during cooler periods, but epidemics can also occur during the rainy season in the tropics. Congregation of people in close quarters may be a more important factor in influenza virus transmission and the generation of epidemics. Despite searches, influenza viruses cannot be found in a given population during large parts of the year; the viruses appear to be reintroduced into a population annually in the course of their travel from person to person around the globe.

Effects of influenza outbreaks in the community tend to follow a typical pattern. Increases in school and industrial absenteeism, emergency room visits for respiratory illness, hospital admissions for pneumonia, and an excessive number of deaths attributable to pneumonia or influenza, or both, usually are detectable when the cumulative influenza attack rate is at least 10% and always are noted with more severe epidemics that have attack rates of 20% or more. The highest attack rate of influenza illness in any segment of the population early during an epidemic is usually among schoolchildren, who appear to play an important role in propagation of epidemics by carrying the virus home to younger siblings and parents. Preschoolers may ultimately have equally as high or higher attack rates, whereas those for parents tend to be lower because of partial immunity from prior infection with related viruses, especially so in the case of influenza A/H1N1 and B viruses. Older adults tend to have the lowest overall attack rates, in part because of the additional factor of less frequent exposure to schoolchildren.

Age-related patterns for hospitalization and mortality rates during influenza epidemics are very different from that for the illness attack rate and from each other. Opposite ends of the age spectrum—infants and adults 65 years of age or older—consistently have the highest hospitalization rates. Hospitalization because of pneumonia or other complications occurs in about 1/25 to 50 infants and 1/10 or fewer elderly adults with influenza illness but in less than 1/100 older children and young adults. As to mortality, 80% to 90% of the deaths during influenza epidemics in excess of the expected number occur in elderly adults. Among persons hospitalized with complications of influenza, death occurs in only 1% to 2% of those younger than the age of 45 years but in 10% to 15% of those 65 years of age or older. Thus, even though elderly individuals are less likely to acquire influenza virus infection than are younger persons, they are much more likely to develop complications of the infection that require hospitalization and lead to death. As described earlier, a major contributing factor to this severe morbidity and mortality because of influenza virus infection is the presence of underlying chronic disease, particularly of the heart or lungs.

Explosive outbreaks of influenza and other infections that are spread by the respiratory route can occur in residential communities. Congregation of people in close quarters such as barracks, classrooms, or communal recreation and dining areas facilitates transmission of these infections. Agents with a relatively low potential for spread in the open population can be involved; for example, the influenza A/New Jersey/76 (H1N1) outbreak that precipitated a national "swine" influenza vaccine campaign ultimately proved to be limited to military personnel at Fort Dix. Occurrence of an influenza outbreak in a nursing home occupied by elderly individuals, many of whom have underlying diseases, can be devastating; influenza illness attack rates approximating 60% are well described, and complications leading to hospitalization or death may occur in as many as 40% of those affected. The decline in T cell function that occurs with increasing age may contribute to the severity of influenza outbreaks among nursing home residents and may also impede efforts at prophylaxis with vaccine. Nevertheless, control of influenza in nursing homes with combined use of vaccine and an antiviral effective against influenza A viruses is feasible and has a high priority.

Diagnosis

The clinical diagnosis of influenza virus infection cannot be accomplished in the absence of an epidemic, because many different infections can produce similar clinical findings. However, in the midst of an influenza epidemic confirmed by laboratory studies on a portion of the patients, the likelihood that an influenza-like illness is due to infection with the virus is high inasmuch as other respiratory viruses are displaced during epidemics.

The most commonly employed method for laboratory diagnosis is recovery of the virus from specimens containing respiratory secretions, such as a nasal wash, nose and throat swab, or sputum. Virus titers in respiratory secretions will be highest early in the illness, and positive cultures longer than 5 days after onset are infrequent except in young children. Carrier medium for the specimen must contain protein and be kept cold to stabilize the virus. Attempts at virus culture should be initiated as soon as possible because a gradual loss of viability will occur, but influenza virus can still be recovered after several days of refrigeration in an appropriate carrier medium. The specimen should be frozen at −70C for prolonged storage.

Virus isolation can be accomplished by inoculation of the allantoic and amniotic sacs of 10-day-old embryonated chicken eggs or by inoculation of one of several types of tissue culture. One of the more convenient and effective tissue cultures for recovery of influenza viruses consists of continuous Madin-Darby canine kidney (MDCK) cells supplemented with trypsin (the viral hemagglutinin must be proteolytically cleaved in order for the virus to be infectious). The virus induces few or only nonspecific cytopathic effects and must be detected by hemagglutination, hemadsorption, or immunofluorescence. Specific identity of the virus may be accomplished employing hemagglutination inhibition (HI) assays with specific antisera.

Rapid diagnosis of influenza virus infection can be achieved by immunofluorescent detection of the virus in respiratory epithelial cells, by detection of virus in secretions using an enzyme immunoassay, or by fluorometric detection of neuraminidase in secretions, but these methods are not as sensitive as virus isolation and are not generally available.

Serologic diagnosis of influenza virus infection is primarily of use for epidemiologic purposes or for attempting to confirm the viral etiology of some unusual or severe disease manifestation. It can be accomplished most precisely by demonstrating a significant increase in antibody to the virus in convalescent-serum specimens collected 2 to 4 weeks after illness onset as compared with that in acute-phase serum. Assays for neutralizing antibody titers of the sera with demonstration of a four-fold or greater rise in titer are sensitive for this purpose but are cumbersome and expensive. HI assays are about equally as sensitive and considerably less cumbersome and expensive. Sera frequently contain nonspecific inhibitors of influenza virus hemagglutination that sometimes will themselves agglutinate the commonly employed chicken erythrocytes, but after the sera are treated to remove these interfering factors, HI assays can detect long-lived (years), strain-specific antibody whose titer correlates well with that of neutralizing antibody. Complement fixation (CF) assays can detect short-lived (3 to 6 months) antibodies to internal proteins of influenza viruses, as well as the longer-lived antibodies to the surface glycoproteins if a test virus homologous to that which caused the infection is used. If a test virus with irrelevant glycoproteins is employed, then an elevated CF titer (e.g., ≥1:32) on a single convalescent serum suggests recent infection with an influenza virus of the same type as the test virus, although this cannot be considered absolutely diagnostic. Alternative antibody assays such as enzyme immunoassays that employ isolated viral proteins are being used in some centers to investigate immune responses to influenza viruses and may offer improvements in the ability to diagnose these infections.

Treatment

Rest is an important component of the management of acute influenza virus illness and also serves to reduce dissemination of the virus in the community. Increasing fluid intake above normal will help overcome increased losses due to fever. Adequate hydration is important to maintain the flow of respiratory secretions, which may reduce the likelihood of secondary bacterial infections, and a decongestant such as pseudoephedrine should be used as necessary to promote this flow. Use of antihistamines may be indicated for excessive secretions that interfere with rest. Antipyretic analgesics such as acetominophen, ibuprofen, or aspirin may be administered to adults as necessary to promote comfort and rest; acetominophen should be used for this purpose in children because of its documented safety and the association of aspirin with Reye's syndrome.

An additional therapeutic measure to be considered for influenza-like illness during a type A epidemic is use of an antiviral medication. Two orally administered medications, amantadine and its congener, rimantadine, can inhibit an early step in intracellular replication of influenza A viruses, but not influenza B or other viruses, in clinically achievable concentrations. Only amantadine is presently available commercially. Amantadine is well absorbed after oral administration and is excreted renally without being metabolized. Central nervous system side effects such as insomnia, nervousness, dizziness, fatigue, and difficulty concentrating occur in up to one third of healthy young adults taking the recommended dose of amantadine for prophylaxis against influenza (see below). These side effects are usually mild, always disappear when the medication is discontinued, and may abate even when the medication is continued at the same dose. Their frequency increases with higher blood levels and may be reduced by splitting the daily dose into two equal portions or reducing it by half, although halving the recommended dose of amantadine for a person with normal renal function may approach the limit of therapeutic and prophylactic efficacy. The dosage of amantadine must be reduced in patients with impaired renal function to avoid accumulating toxic blood levels, and an automatic halving of the dose is recommended for persons 65 years of age or older because of the natural decline in renal function with increasing age. Amantadine has increased seizure activity in persons with an underlying seizure disorder, and its dose should always be reduced by half in such persons. High doses of amantadine are teratogenic in rats, and it should not be used during pregnancy except for life-threatening situations.

Treatment of presumptive influenza A virus illness with amantadine begun within 48 hours of onset when virus titers are highest and continued for 5 days has been shown repeatedly to reduce the duration of fever and symptoms by 1 to 2 days. It can also hasten resolution of the increase in peripheral airway resistance that occurs with influenza virus infection. The side effects of amantadine described above are usually obscured by those of the illness during therapy. A risk of using amantadine therapeutically is the development of drug-resistant virus that can spread to contacts even if the latter are receiving amantadine prophylaxis. Thus it may be better to reserve amantadine therapy for high risk patients in whom it is hoped that complications of the infection can be averted. No evidence exists for a therapeutic benefit of orally administered amantadine when it is delayed until complications of influenza A virus infection have occurred. Administration of amantadine, rimantadine, or another antiviral, ribavirin, by small-particle aerosol appears in mouse-model studies to offer therapeutic benefits later in the course of influenza A virus pneumonia than enterally administered medication, and ribavirin also is active against influenza B and other viruses (e.g., see respiratory syncytial virus); however, the usefulness and practicality of aerosol therapy for influenza virus disease requires further study.

Prevention

Two means are presently available for attempting to prevent influenza virus infection, killed virus vaccine and amantadine. Their practical usefulness is not in controlling influenza epidemics but in reducing the associated severe morbidity and mortality in high risk individuals. Influenza virus vaccine is the primary means of prevention.

Currently available influenza vaccines are prepared from virus grown in embryonated chicken eggs and rendered noninfectious by treatment with formalin. The vaccines are reformulated each spring to contain antigens of the most current influenza viruses. They are presently trivalent and contain 15 μg of hemagglutinin each from representative A/H1N1, A/H3N2, and type B strains. Whole-virus vaccine consists of a suspension of purified virus particles, whereas subvirion vaccine contains partially purified surface glycoproteins derived after chemical disruption of the virus particles. Only subvirion vaccine should be used in children under 13 years of age, because whole-virus vaccine is significantly more reactogenic in this age range, but older individuals respond similarly to each type of vaccine.

Vaccination should be performed during the fall months, optimally in November so that antibody titers will be at their peak when influenza outbreaks usually start in December or January. The vaccine should be administered intramuscularly in the deltoid muscle or, for infants and young children, in the anterolateral aspect of the thigh. Local tenderness lasting 1 to 2 days will occur in up to one third of vaccinees, and occasional individuals will develop local erythema and/or induration lasting a few days. Systemic symptoms such as malaise and myalgia may occur in 5% to 10% of vaccines, and fever in a smaller portion; these usually begin within a few hours of vaccination and last 1 to 2 days. Immediate allergic reactions such as anaphylaxis are extremely rare and presumably are due to traces of egg protein remaining in the vaccine; persons who cannot eat eggs because of allergic reactions should not receive influenza vaccine. GBS occurred within a few weeks of receipt of "swine" influenza vaccine in about 1/100,000 recipients in 1976-1977, but no association of this syndrome with subsequent influenza vaccines has been found and it is not considered at present to be a risk of the vaccine.

Influenza vaccines have been shown to reduce attack rates of influenza illness by 70% to 90% during epidemics among military personnel when a good match existed between vaccine and epidemic strains. If vaccine was similarly efficacious in schoolchildren, it might have the benefit of actually reducing the severity of influenza epidemics. Attempts to do this in Japan, however, have yielded no direct evidence that annual vaccination of 50% to 60% of the schoolchildren affected the incidence of influenza in the community. Studies with influenza vaccines in an English boarding school for boys found that the cumulative attack rate for influenza among those who received annual vaccinations was similar over three A/H3N2 epidemics to that of boys who received no vaccine. Vaccine appeared less effective when given to boys who had received one or more prior vaccinations, but once influenza illness had occurred, protection was nearly absolute against subsequent A/H3N2 illness. These and similar studies suggest that rather than receiving annual vaccinations, healthy individuals at low risk for severe influenza disease may be better served by being allowed to acquire influenza virus infection and develop the stronger, more durable immunity that follows.

Influenza vaccines are not as effective against influenza virus illness in elderly individuals as they are in military personnel, but their efficacy against the more severe consequences of influenza such as hospitalization and death are equally as high. Protection begins as early as 2 weeks after vaccination. It does not appear, however, to persist as long as 1 year in elderly individuals; thus annual vaccinations are indicated even if the vaccine composition remains unchanged. Evidence for vaccine-induced "herd immunity" has been found in studies of nursing homes. If more than 70% to 80% of the residents are vaccinated, the likelihood of an influenza outbreak in the nursing home is significantly reduced. Thus the available data indicate that currently formulated influenza virus vaccines can reduce the severe consequences of influenza if they are administered annually to a significant proportion of high risk individuals. It is also important to vaccinate care giver and housemates of high risk individuals in an attempt to reduce transmission of influenza viruses.

The alternative to vaccine for prophylaxis against influenza is amantadine (see discussion of clinical pharmacology and side effects under Treatment). This medication has an efficacy for the prevention of influenza A virus infections that approximates that of vaccine. Among its advantages are protection against all influenza A strains rather than being limited to strains closely related to those in the vaccine, as well as onset of protection within a day of starting the medication as opposed to 2 weeks for vaccine. Disadvantages of amantadine are that protection lasts only as long as it is taken regularly, it lacks activity against influenza B viruses, bothersome side effects may occur, and costs will exceed those of vaccination if it is used for longer than approximately 2 weeks. Rimantadine exhibits similar or greater activity against influenza A viruses, with fewer side effects, and may displace amantadine for prophylaxis when and if it becomes available.

One of the uses of amantadine is to provide protection to individuals at high risk for the 2 weeks required for vaccine to induce protection when vaccination has been delayed until after onset of an influenza A epidemic; amantadine will not interfere with the antibody response to vaccine. Amantadine can also serve as the primary means of protection for high risk individuals who cannot take vaccine because of allergy or prior severe reactions or when vaccine and epidemic influenza A virus strains are known to differ. In these situations, amantadine prophylaxis will need to be continued for the duration of significant influenza activity in the community. It appears that the protective effects of antibody and amantadine are at least additive; thus high risk individuals who received appropriate vaccination may also benefit from supplemental amantadine prophylaxis during an influenza A epidemic, particularly if exposure is likely or known to have occurred. An important aspect of the latter use is that amantadine prophylaxis can actually help abort influenza A outbreaks in institutionalized populations such as nursing home residents. The first objective of an influenza control program for such institutions is to achieve a vaccination level of 80% or more in the hope of averting an outbreak by means of herd immunity. If, however, a cluster of residents with influenza-like illness is identified when influenza A viruses are known to be active in the surrounding community, amantadine prophylaxis should be initiated for all residents regardless of their vaccination status. Rapid action is necessary because of the frequently explosive nature of influenza A outbreaks in residential institutions. It should be noted that a portion of the residents already may be infected when the administration of amantadine is begun in the latter setting (i.e., they will be receiving treatment rather than prophylaxis). Thus, to minimize the risk of spread of drug-resistant virus if it should develop, any ill residents should be isolated while they have symptoms.

It would be desirable to have more effective control measures for influenza, perhaps even methods that could prevent epidemics rather than merely reduce the severe consequences. Studies are proceeding with various means to enhance immune responses to killed virus vaccine, including increasing the antigenic content, combining topical and parenteral routes of administration, and using adjuvants and other immune stimulators. Investigations of live attenuated influenza virus vaccines administered intranasally are also proceeding. Candidate live attenuated vaccine strains can be rapidly prepared by reassortment to contain six "internal" genes from an attenuated, cold-adapted strain and genes for the two surface glycoproteins from a new wild-type strain. These cold-reassortant vaccines may offer the best possibility for effective immunization of children, although their replication in older adults may be insufficient to provide significant benefit. Antiviral drugs having greater effectiveness, broader antiviral spectrum, and no bothersome side effects are also needed. Much developmental work remains to be done, but, for the present, more effective use can be made of the influenza control measures currently available.

FURTHER READING

Symposia and Books

Douglas RG Jr (ed): Prevention, management and control of influenza. A mandate for the 1980's. Am J Med 82(6A):1, 1987

Kendal AP, Patriarca PA (eds). Options for the Control of Influenza. New York, Alan R Liss, 1986

Kilbourne ED: Influenza. New York, Plenum, 1987

Schild GC (ed): Influenza. Br Med Bull 35:1, 1979

Stuart-Harris CH, Potter CW: The Molecular Virology and Epidemiology of Influenza. New York, Academic Press, 1984

Stuart-Harris CH, Schild GC, Oxford JS: Influenza. The Viruses and the Disease. Baltimore, Edward Arnold, 1985

Selected Papers

Arden NH, Patriarca PA, Fasano MB, et al: The roles of vaccination and amantadine prophylaxis in controlling an outbreak of influenza A (H3N2) in a nursing home. Arch Intern Med 148:865, 1988

Barker WH, Mullooly JP: Pneumonia and influenza deaths during epidemics. Implications for prevention. Arch Intern Med 142:85, 1982

Belse RB, Burk B, Newman F, et al: Resistance of influenza A virus to amantadine and rimantadine: Results of one decade of surveillance. J Infect Dis 159:430, 1989

Budnick LD, Stricof RL, Ellis F: An outbreak of influenza A in a nursing home, 1982. NY State J Med 84:235, 1984

Current status of amantadine and rimantadine as anti-influenza-A agents: Memorandum from a WHO meeting. Bull WHO 63:51, 1985

Douglas RG Jr: Prophylaxis and treatment of influenza. N Engl J Med 322:443, 1990

Glezen WP: Serious morbidity and mortality associated with influenza epidemics. Epidemiol Rev 4:25, 1982

Glezen WP, Couch RB: Interpandemic influenza in the Houston area, 1974–76. N Engl J Med 298:587, 1978

Glezen WP, Payne AA, Snyder DN, Downs TD: Mortality and influenza. J Infect Dis 146:313, 1982

Hoskins TW, Davies JR, Smith AJ, et al: Assessment of inactivated influenza A vaccine after three outbreaks of influenza A at Christ's Hospital. Lancet 1:33, 1979

Immunization Practics Advisory Committee: Prevention and control of influenza. I. Vaccines. MMWR 38:297, 1989

Johnson PR, Feldman S, Thompson JM, et al: Immunity to influenza A virus infection in young children: A comparison of natural infection, live cold-adapted vaccine and inactivated vaccine. J Infect Dis 154:121, 1986

Levine M, Beattie BL, McLean DM, Corman D: Characterization of the immune response to trivalent influenza vaccine in elderly man. J Am Geriatrics Soc 35:609, 1987

Meiklejohn G, Hoffman R, Graves P: Effectiveness of influenza vaccine when given during an outbreak of influenza A/H3N2 in a nursing home. J Am Geriatr Soc 37:407, 1989

Moser MR, Bender TR, Margolis HS, et al: An outbreak of influenza A aboard a commercial airliner. Am J Epidemiol 110:1, 1979

Patriarca PA, Weber JA, Parker RA, et al: Efficacy of influenza vaccine in nursing homes. Reduction in illness and complications during an influenza A (H3N2) epidemic. JAMA 253:1136, 1985

Patriarca PA, Weber JA, Parker RA, et al: Risk factors for outbreaks of influenza in nursing homes. A case-controlled study. Am J Epidemiol 124:114, 1986

Perrotta DM, Decker M, Glezen WP: Acute respiratory disease hospitalizations as a measure of impact of epidemic influenza. Am J Epidemiol 122:468, 1985

Powers DC, Spears SD, Murphy BR, et al: Systemic and local antibody responses in elderly subjects given live or inactivated influenza A virus vaccines. J Clin Microbiol 27:2666, 1989

Schonberger LB, Hurwitz ES, Katona P, et al: Guillaine-Barré syndrome: Its epidemiology and associations with influenza vaccine. Ann Neurol 9(suppl):31, 1981

CHAPTER 70

Paramyxoviruses

The paramyxoviruses are enveloped viruses with a helical nucleocapsid and a nonsegmented single-stranded RNA genome. Viruses belonging to the family Paramyxoviridae measure roughly 150 nm in diameter. Members of this family of viruses cause a wide spectrum of disease in humans, ranging from bronchiolitis, pneumonia, and croup to measles and mumps. Since the introduction of both the measles and the mumps vaccines, the number of measles and mumps cases have been dramatically reduced in the United States. Vaccines to prevent illness secondary to respiratory syncytial virus and the parainfluenza viruses are not presently available. Therefore RSV remains the most significant cause of lower respiratory tract disease in infants in developed countries, and the PIVs remain the second leading cause of lower respiratory infections in young children. Like other viral agents associated with respiratory tract infection, RSV and PIV can be associated with each of the respiratory syndromes. RSV, however, is most frequently the cause of bronchiolitis and viral pneumonia in young children whereas PIVs are most commonly the cause of viral croup.

Respiratory Syncytial Virus

Respiratory syncytial virus (RSV) is primarily a respiratory tract pathogen that causes both upper and lower respiratory tract infections. It is the only human pathogen in the genus *Pneumovirus*. The RNA genome encodes for 10 virus-specific messenger RNAs (mRNAs), which in turn encode for 10 unique viral proteins that are expressed in infected cells. Three major transmembrane glycoproteins of RSV (F, G, and SH) are expressed on the surface of virions and infected cells. The attachment (G) glycoprotein mediates attachment of the virus to the plasma membrane of target host cells. The fusion (F) glycoprotein facilitates the spread of infection in the host by cell-to-cell fusion and induces the cytologic hallmark of infection in these cells—syncytium formation. The carbohydrate side chains of the F and G glycoproteins appear to be essential for infectivity because treatment of the virus with specific endoglycosidase, or inhibition of glycosylation, alters viral infectivity. RSV possesses no neuraminidase or hemagglutinin activity.

Natural infection with RSV appears to be limited to humans and chimpanzees. Closely related bovine strains of RSV have also been recovered during winter epidemics of bronchiolitis and pneumonia in cattle. On the basis of reactivity to monoclonal antibodies two major strains of RSV are recognized: strain Long (subgroup A or 1) and strain 18537 (subgroup B or 2). These two strains can circulate in parallel. The Long strain has been shown to predominate. The relative epidemiologic importance of these strain differences has yet to be determined.

Clinical Illness

Infection with RSV usually starts as an upper respiratory infection with profuse rhinorrhea, nasal congestion, pharyngitis, cough, and fever. Infection in adults is typically contained to the upper respiratory tract. In infants 6 weeks to 6 months of age who are encountering RSV for the first time there appears to be a 25% to 40% chance of developing a lower respiratory tract infection, most often manifesting as bronchiolitis and pneumonia. Laryngotracheobronchitis (croup) and bronchitis are less frequently encountered syndromes associated with RSV infection in children. Repeat infection with RSV is the expected occurrence and is usually less severe than the first infection. After 3 years of age, repeated infections most commonly manifest as upper respiratory tract illness or tracheobronchitis.

Hospitalization is reported to occur from 1/50 to 1/1000 infections with RSV in children. It is estimated that 40% of children hospitalized with bronchiolitis and 25% of children hospitalized with pneumonia are admitted because of RSV. RSV bronchiolitis is an infection of the smaller bronchi and bronchioles, characterized by labored and rapid respirations with a prolonged expiration. Wheezes, ronchi, and rales can be auscultated on examination of the chest. Chest radiographs reveal hyperaeration with air trapping and may reveal infiltrates secondary to subsegmental atelectasis. RSV pneumonia is an infection of smaller airways and alveoli characterized by rales or evidence of pulmonary consolidation on physical examination or radiograph. Most infants requiring hospitalization have hypoxemia due to ventilation perfusion mismatching in the lungs.

Children usually recover from RSV infection within 6 to 10 days, but involvement of the lungs with RSV infection may be severe enough to require assisted ventilation. The mortality rate in normal infants hospitalized with RSV is less than 1%. In infants with underlying diseases the mortality and morbidity associated with RSV is markedly higher. Conditions that place a child at risk of severe or fatal RSV infection include bronchopulmonary dysplasia, cystic fibrosis, prematurity, congenital heart disease, immunodeficiency disease, or therapy causing immunosuppression.

Nonobstructive apnea may occur as a complication of RSV infection. Predisposing factors that correlate with apnea in association with RSV infection include premature birth and young chronologic age at the time of infection. Other syndromes associated with RSV infection of the upper respiratory tract include both otitis media and conjunctivitis. Infection with RSV is a predisposing factor for the development of acute otitis media. Both bacteria and RSV have been recovered from the middle ear effusions of children with RSV. Bacterial pneumonia can also complicate the course of RSV lower respiratory tract disease.

Studies have raised the possibility that RSV infections in infancy may result in persistent abnormalities in lung function in later life. Low oxyhemoglobin levels and peripheral airway obstruction may be detected sequentially through the first 8 years of life in children who were hospitalized during infancy with acute lower respiratory tract illness due to RSV. Whether RSV infection in infancy is related to chronic obstructive airway disease in the adult remains unclear.

Pathogenesis and Pathology

RSV initially comes in contact with the mucosal surface of the eyes and nose. The incubation period ranges from 2 to 8 days, with 4 to 6 days being most common. Virus replication occurs in mucosal epithelial cells and macrophages. In infants RSV achieves an average titer of 10^4 to 10^6 median tissue culture infective dose ($TCID_{50}$) per milliliter of nasal wash specimen. Infection can spread to the lower respiratory tract and generally remains confined to the respiratory system. Virus-induced cytopathologic effects and the inflammatory response to RSV are most prominent in the smaller airways. Although viral antigen has been detected in peripheral blood leukocytes, the clinical significance has not been determined.

Bronchiolitis is characterized by peribronchial lymphocytic infiltration and edema. In the bronchiole lumen there is proliferation and necrosis of the bronchiolar epithelium and hypersecretion of mucus. Mucous plugs containing cellular debris and fibrin lead to small airway obstruction, with air trapping distal to the obstruction. Young infants are particularly vulnerable because they have small airways with a high resistance to airflow, a relative deficiency in lung elastin, soft bronchial cartilage, and relatively increased compliance of the thoracic cage.

Infants with RSV pneumonia have mononuclear cell infiltrates in interstitial tissues, alveoli, small bronchioles, and alveolar ducts. There may be syncytia formation and intracytoplasmic inclusions consistent with but not pathognomonic of RSV infection. Necrosis and edema can lead to alveolar filling. Many children with RSV lower respiratory tract infection have findings consistent with both bronchiolitis and pneumonia.

Host Response

In general both serum and secretory antibody responses to RSV are brisk and short-lived. This may be the reason reinfection is the rule with RSV. The IgM serum antibody response appears a few days after the initial illness and lasts from 2 to 10 weeks. During primary infection serum IgA and IgG antibodies are detectable at the tenth day of illness, and peak titers occur after 3 or 4 weeks of illness but persist for less than 6 months. RSV-specific secretory IgA, as well as IgG and IgM, appear in respiratory tract secretions within 3 days and reach peak titers 8 to 13 days after the onset of illness. Antibody is detectable for less than 6 months. The secretory IgA antibody response is typically greater in children older than 6 months of age. With repeat infection by the virus an anamnestic response is seen. Enhanced and more persistent antibody responses occur in both serum and secretions with reinfection.

RSV envelope glycoproteins F and G are the major determinants for antibodies that neutralize viral infectivity in vitro. Antibodies to the F surface glycoprotein inhibit syncytia formation and are broadly reactive against the two major RSV subgroups. Antibodies to the G surface glycoprotein are subgroup specific. Neutralizing antibodies can distinguish the two virus subgroups. The role that antigenic differences between the two virus subgroups plays in reinfection of infants and children is unclear. Antibody directing antibody-dependent cell-mediated cytotoxicity (ADCC) against cells infected with RSV has been demonstrated to be present in serum, colostrum, and respiratory secretions. The potential role of ADCC in the eradication of RSV infection remains unclear.

The search for an effective vaccine against RSV has led to a significant body of knowledge about both the humoral and the cellular immune responses to RSV infection. The host response is not completely protective, and there has been concern that illness was enhanced by the host response. Epidemiologically, the peak incidence of disease occurs in infants younger than 6 months of age, when levels of passively acquired maternal antibody are the highest. Several lines of evidence now suggest that RSV-specific antibody is beneficial. The severity of illness caused by RSV is inversely related to the level of passively acquired maternal neutralizing antibody in the neonate. Animal model studies have demonstrated protection against viral replication in the lungs when animals are given high-titered antibody directed against RSV. Infants with RSV bronchiolitis or pneumonia who have been treated with human immune serum globulin containing high-titered RSV-neutralizing antibody have experienced more rapid improvements in their oxygenation and a more rapid diminution in the amount of virus shed. Last, epidemiologic studies suggest that breast feeding may provide some protection against RSV infection. RSV-specific IgA can be found in the colostrum of the majority of breast-feeding women, but the IgA titers in the breast milk decline over the course of lactation.

Further evidence suggesting that host response plays a role in disease pathogenesis is the observation that RSV-specific IgE and histamine have been demonstrated to appear more frequently and in higher titers in patients with wheezing due to RSV infection than in patients infected with RSV who do not have wheezing. High levels of RSV-IgE and histamine also correlate significantly with hypoxia, and it is likely that other mediators of airway obstruction play a role in the severity of illness as well. Leukotriene CP_4 has recently been shown to be higher in the respiratory secretions of wheezing patients. A high RSV-IgE response at the time of RSV bronchiolitis may also be predictive of subsequent wheezing episodes.

The cellular component of the immune response appears to be critical to the containment of viral infection in the respiratory tract. This conclusion is supported by the fact that children with compromised immune function are at risk from persistent and severe or fatal infection with RSV. These children also tend to shed virus for significantly prolonged periods, 6 weeks or longer. Cell-mediated immune responses to viral antigen appear to be greatest in patients with lower respiratory tract involvement at the time of infection. Some further evidence suggests that the cell-mediated responsiveness seen in bronchiolitis may in fact be related to suppressor cell dysfunction. Cytotoxic lymphocytes (CTLs) appear to be primarily directed against F protein determinants but also against nucleocapsid protein.

Epidemiology

RSV occurs worldwide and in temperate climates causes yearly epidemics of respiratory illness that alternate from mid-winter to late spring in occurrence. Outbreaks of RSV disease appear to interfere with outbreaks of influenza or parainfluenza so that these viruses tend not to reach concurrent epidemic peaks. When RSV epidemics are at their peak, there is a large increase in the number of hospitalizations because of bronchiolitis and pneumonia, especially among children younger than 6 months of age. RSV outbreaks have also been linked to winter peaks of deaths from lower respiratory illness in infants younger than 1 year of age. An attack rate of 50% is estimated for exposed infants during the first year of life, and virtually all infants have been infected by 2 years of age. About 50% of children have experienced two episodes of infection by 2 years of age. RSV is generally introduced into a family by an older, school-aged sibling. Attack rates are high among all the family members. The severity of illness among family members is age related, with younger members having the most severe manifestations of disease. Attack rates for RSV are also high among day-care attendees.

Transmission of RSV is by direct or close contact. Direct inoculation of large droplets or self-inoculation by touching contaminated surfaces may occur. Once infants are infected, virus can be shed from their respiratory tracts for up to 21 days. Excreted virus may persist on environmental surfaces for several hours and on human skin for 30 minutes or longer.

Nosocomial spread of RSV infection among hospitalized infants is a major problem. Up to 45% of children admitted to the pediatric ward of a hospital during RSV season may acquire RSV nosocomially. The infants most at risk of suffering severe nosocomially acquired RSV infection are those infants with cardiopulmonary disease. During outbreaks, rates of infection among hospital staff members are also as high as 60%. Hospital personnel play a crucial role in the nosocomial spread of the virus. The most effective means of preventing transmission of virus is consistent hand washing. The use of masks plus goggles by hospital staff has also been demonstrated to decrease nosocomial spread of RSV. Outbreaks of RSV have occurred in nursing homes among elderly residents.

Diagnosis

During epidemics of RSV infection, infants presenting with the clinical syndromes of bronchiolitis or pneumonia can usually be assumed to have infection with RSV. Infection can be confirmed by virus culture, antigen detection, or serologic means. RSV detection depends on obtaining an appropriate respiratory specimen. The virus can be recovered from a throat or nasal swab, but the preferred specimen is a nasal wash. Once the specimen is obtained, it should be transported promptly to the laboratory for culture because RSV is a relatively labile virus. RSV is usually cultivated on a continuous human epithelial cell line. In cell culture the virus induces a typical cytopathic effect with syncytia formation. This usually occurs within 5 days of inoculation of the culture.

With the availability of antiviral agents to treat RSV infection, the need to diagnose RSV infection reliably and expediently has become more essential. Most diagnostic laboratories are utilizing antigen detection as a means for confirming RSV infection. Antigen detection requires only several hours to perform and may be more sensitive than is culture. Viral antigen can often be detected late in the course of infection despite the presence of antibody that may neutralize the infective virus in secretions. Techniques widely used for antigen detection are the indirect immunofluorescent method and the enzyme-linked immunosorbent assay (ELISA). For antigen detection by immunofluorescence the rapidity with which the clinical specimen is processed is still critical because the integrity of infected cells must be preserved for accurate interpretation of the results. The indirect immunofluorescence method uses mouse anti-RSV monoclonal antibodies and a fluorescein-conjugated goat antimouse IgG. The indirect immunofluorescence test is qualitative and is somewhat more sensitive than the ELISA in the detection of RSV antigen. The accuracy depends on the experience and judgment of the person performing the test. The ELISA does not require a fluorescent microscope and, when automated, can produce an objective endpoint.

Serologic diagnosis of RSV can be accomplished by a complement fixation (CF) assay, a neutralization assay, a plaque reduction assay, or an ELISA. To demonstrate infection both an acute and a convalescent serum specimen are needed. A fourfold rise in antibody indicates recent infection. CF often fails to detect antibodies in the sera of young infants recovering from RSV infection. Both the plaque reduction assay and the ELISA are more sensitive at detecting infection in the young infant.

Therapy

Therapy for RSV infection depends on the clinical status of the patient and is principally supportive. Moderately or severely ill children should be admitted to the hospital. Children with hypoxemia should receive humidified oxygen. The severely ill child may require intubation and assisted ventilation. Ribavirin administered as an aerosol is a specific therapeutic agent available for the treatment of RSV infections. It is a synthetic nucleoside analogue that appears to interfere with the expression of mRNA and to inhibit viral protein synthesis. Ribavirin should be considered for use in selected groups of infants hospitalized with lower respiratory tract disease caused by RSV. Selected infants include those at high risk for severe or complicated RSV infection, especially children with cardiopulmonary disease, immunodeficiency disease, or prematurity, as well as severely ill infants. Preliminary studies indicate that therapy with intravenous immunoglobulin may be of some benefit in the treatment of RSV infection. Further studies are required.

Prevention

Attempts to decrease the morbidity and mortality associated with RSV infection have focused on the development of a vaccine. Particular problems associated with development of an RSV vaccine include the young age at which children are infected and the lack of complete immunity after natural infection. In the 1960s an alum-precipitated, formalin-inactivated RSV vaccine failed to offer protection to vaccinated children despite the fact that the vaccine induced both neutralizing and CF antibodies. When these children encountered naturally occurring infection, pneumonia developed more often in vacinees than in a control (unimmunized) population, suggesting that the immune response was detrimental. Subsequent studies suggest that the formalin inactivation may have altered the fusion protein so that antibodies produced did not hinder cell fusion. The vacinees then sustained virus replication and had worse illness because the host response to viral proteins could not stop viral infectivity. Because of the adverse side effect encountered, the development of the inactivated vaccine was abandoned.

Subsequent research was directed toward the development of a live virus vaccine. Temperature-sensitive mutants of RSV that could be administered intranasally and induce local immunity were given to both adults and children. Theoretically, at the lower temperatures encountered in the upper respiratory tract, the live, temperature-sensitive mutant virus could propagate and induce an immune response while at core body temperatures encountered in the lower respiratory, the mutant virus could not replicate and therefore could not cause a lower respiratory infection. Mutant viruses tested were not genetically stable, did not provide protection from subsequent infection, or were poorly infectious. When given intramuscularly, live virus vaccine was not efficacious.

Currently, efforts in RSV vaccine research are being directed toward the development of purified G or F protein as immunogens. Complete pulmonary resistance developed in cotton rats immunized with G or F protein when they were challenged with RSV. Because the F protein appears to be highly immunogenic, inducing both a humoral and a cellular response, and because antibodies to the F protein are broadly reactive against both strains of RSV, the F protein appears to be a logical choice as an immunogen. Thus an RSV subunit vaccine containing purified F protein is now being tested in humans. Other strategies for the development of a potential RSV vaccine include the insertion of the cloned genes for F and G protein into vectors expressed in vaccinia virus and administration of a vaccinia-RSV recombinant. Cotton rats and nonhuman primates immunized with vaccinia-RSV recombinants also have demonstrated pulmonary resistance to challenge with RSV.

One other potential strategy for the prevention of RSV infection is the prophylactic administration of intravenous immunoglobulin to infants at high risk during epidemics of RSV. Current animal data suggest that if high enough levels of neutralizing antibody are achieved in the circulation, RSV replication can be reduced in the lower respiratory tract. Therefore prophylactic administration of immunoglobulin to infants at high risk may decrease the severity of lower respiratory tract infection. Further investigation of the role of immunoglobulin prophylaxis for RSV infection is required before a recommendation for routine use is made.

Parainfluenza Viruses

The parainfluenza viruses (PIVs) are primarily respiratory tract pathogens and are important causes of both upper and lower respiratory tract infections. PIVs are members of the Paramyxovirus family and belong to the genus *Paramyxovirus*. There are four serotypes of the human PIVs (types 1, 2, 3, and 4). The serotypes vary in their epidemiologic and clinical manifestations. Among the PIVs the structure of PIV type 3 has been studied the most extensively. The genome of PIV type 3 encodes for six structural proteins. Two of the structural proteins, the hemaglutinin-neuraminidase (HN) protein and the fusion (F) protein, are glycoprotein spikes contained on the surface of the viral envelope.

The HN surface glycoprotein mediates attachment of the virus to the plasma membranes of target cells, as well as hemagglutination and neuraminidase activities. The HN glycoprotein attaches to host-cell sialic acid moieties and initiates infection. The F protein mediates viral envelope fusion to the target cell membrane, as well as viral penetration into the host cell. F protein activity also results in fusion of infected cells with neighboring uninfected cells and facilitates the cell-to-cell spread of infection. As a consequence of fusion activity, cells may form syncytia. The F glycoprotein mediates red blood cell hemolysis as well. Proteolytic cleavage of the F glycoprotein by a trypsinlike host enzyme is required for activation of infectivity. This process is an important determinant of virus tissue tropism and therefore pathogenesis.

Clinical Illness

Like other viruses that are respiratory tract pathogens, the PIVs can involve the respiratory tract in different ways. Illness may range from a mild upper respiratory tract illness to a more severe lower respiratory tract infection. Primary infection with PIV is usually symptomatic and often results in lower respiratory tract disease in the young child. PIVs are the largest cause of viral laryngotracheobronchitis or croup, leading to more than 40% of the cases. Types, 1, 2 and 3 PIV all manifest most often as croup but may also present clinically as pneumonia, bronchiolitis, and bronchitis. PIV type 1 is the most common cause of viral croup. PIV type 2 typically causes milder lower respiratory tract disease. PIV type 3 is second to RSV as the most frequent cause of pneumonia and bronchiolitis in children younger than 6 months of age. PIV type 4 is infrequently isolated and tends to cause only mild upper respiratory illness. With increasing age, primary infection with one of the PIVs is less likely to cause severe lower respiratory tract disease. Reinfection with PIV is common throughout life. Repeat infections are less likely to result in significant lower respiratory tract disease. Illness in adults usually but not always is confined to the upper respiratory tract.

The symptoms of infection with PIV are often indistinguishable from those of a cold, with cough, sore throat, and rhinorrhea. Fever is frequently present. After 24 to 48 hours a hoarse voice and a brassy cough will develop in a child whose infection progresses to a crouplike illness. The cough is often described as sounding like a barking seal. Signs of upper airway obstruction may become apparent, including stridor, a prolonged inspiratory phase, an increased respiratory rate, and increased work of breathing. A radiograph of the neck shows subglottic narrowing. Fever may persist for up to 4 days. Most children have a mild course, and symptoms last from 3 to 7 days. Rarely, hypoxemia and cyanosis secondary to severe airway obstruction may occur. In these cases the duration of illness tends to be longer.

PIV can cause both prolonged respiratory infection and more severe infection in children with immunodeficiency. PIV has been isolated from extrapulmonary sites in several immunocompromised patients, suggesting that dissemination can occur with altered host defenses.

Pathogenesis and Pathology

The PIVs initially infect the epithelium of the pharyngeal and nasal mucosa. Spread of the virus occurs by cell-to-cell transfer of the virus. There have also been several reports of viremia occurring after both primary and secondary infection. The incubation period ranges from 2 to 6 days. Symptomatic results of infection of the upper airway are nasal congestion and pharyngeal irritation. The mean titer of virus isolated from children with PIV infection has been demonstrated to be 10^3 $TCID_{50}$ per milliliter of nasal wash specimen. Higher titers of virus tend to be shed in younger children and in children with laryngitis, pharyngitis, or fever.

The PIVs can subsequently spread from the upper respiratory tract to the epithelium of the larynx and trachea. Inflammation of the glottic and tracheal surfaces result in narrowing of the subglottic area and causes the symptoms of croup. Histologically, edema and cellular infiltration occur in the lamina propria, submucosa, and adventitia of the larynx and trachea.

The pneumonia associated with PIV infection is characterized by a peribronchial lymphocytic infiltration, plugging of the bronchioles with mucus and cellular debris, and necrosis of the bronchiolar epithelium. Lymphocytic infiltration of the alveolar walls and interstitial lung tissue also may occur.

In vitro, tracheal ring cultures have been used to describe the sequential morphologic events attendant on PIV. Examination by means of immunofluorescence demonstrates viral antigens in the cytoplasm of epithelial cells within 24 hours after infection. Ciliary motion is lost, and the pseudostratified columnar organization of the epithelial layer disappears as some ciliated cells are lost and others fuse to form multinucleate giant cells. Such fusion is also seen in the lamina propria and in the cartilage. Budding virus particles from these cells are visible by electron microscopic examination.

Studies with closely related avian paramyxoviruses indicate that cleavage of the F glycoprotein by host cell proteases must occur for the virus to be infectious. Viral pathogenesis is related to both susceptibility of the F glycoprotein to cleavage and to the activity of the host cell protease. The tissue tropism of the paramyxoviruses has been related to the ability of the cells in the target tissue to cleave the F glycoprotein.

Host Response

Infection with PIV does not confer immunity to infection or symptomatic illness. Consequently, reinfection with both homotypic and heterotypic virus is common throughout life. Infection causes the host to produce humoral antibody as measured by hemagglutination inhibition, neutralization, and complement fixation. Antibodies to the HN protein can be measured by hemagglutination inhibition, neuraminidase inhibition, neutralization of infectivity, or inhibition of hemadsorption. Antibodies to the F protein neutralize virus infectivity and inhibit syncytia formation. The antibody response to the HN protein is greater in primary PIV infection than is the antibody response to F protein. It is likely that both antibody specificities are important in preventing clinical infection.

The PIVs share no single common antigen but remain antigenically related. The primary response to PIV is usually fairly specific for the infecting serotype. Primary infection has been shown to induce protection from subsequent lower respiratory tract involvement with a homotypic strain but not a heterotypic strain. Reinfection stimulates an anamnestic response with heterotypic antibodies to other serotypes. Studies with PIVs types 1 and 2 have shown that immunity is better correlated with secretory IgA than with the level of circulating antibody. Patients show homologous IgA antibody formation in nasal secretions, usually within 7 to 10 days after the onset of symptoms, reaching maximum titers in 2 weeks. Virus-neutralization activity is also demonstrable but does not correlate with IgA.

Animal studies suggest that passively administered antibody is protective against infection with PIV type 3. Levels of neutralizing antibody have been best correlated with protection. Infants born with high levels of passively acquired maternal neutralizing antibody to PIV type 3 are at lower risk of acquiring infection and serious illness with PIV type 3.

Levels of PIV-specific serum IgE and histamine in respiratory secretions have been shown to be higher in children with PIV-induced croup and wheezing than in children with PIV-associated upper respiratory symptoms alone. Thus the immune response may contribute to the pathogenesis of PIV-induced respiratory disease.

The importance of the cytotoxic T cell response to infection with PIV has not been well studied. Cellular host responses appear to play a role in the immune response and possible eradication of these viruses. Prolonged shedding of PIVs occurs in hosts with deficient cellular immunity. Systemic infection is well documented in children with severe combined immunodeficiency, but whether these are mutant viruses that have evolved in a defective host or whether this is due only to the host's deficits remains to be determined.

Epidemiology

PIVs are found throughout the world. Animals may be infected with antigenically related strains of paramyxoviruses, but there is little evidence to suggest that animals serve as a reservoir of infection for the human PIVs. Outbreaks of infection due to PIV types 1 and 2 occur as biannual epidemics in the autumn of the year. For several years outbreaks of PIV type 1 tended to alternate years with outbreaks of PIV type 2. In recent years outbreaks of both serotypes have occurred during the same season. The major increase in the number of croup cases in the fall of the year can usually be attributed to an outbreak of PIV type 1. Infection with PIV type 3 occurs endemically throughout the year. Springtime outbreaks of infection due to PIV type 3 have also been noted in recent years.

Illness associated with primary infection with PIV types 1 or 2 is more likely to occur in the child older than 2 years of age. Passively acquired maternal antibody appears to play a potentially protective role in the young infant exposed to PIV types 1 and 2. Severe lower respiratory tract disease is infrequent in children younger than 4 months of age who have infection caused by either PIV type 1 or 2. Almost three fourths of all children have demonstrable antibody to PIV type 1 by 5 years of age. More than half of all children have serum antibody to PIV type 2 by the same age. The majority of children appear to be infected with PIV type 3 during the first year of life, and more than 90% of children have demonstrable antibody to PIV type 3 by 2 years of age. Infection with PIV type 3 often occurs at a time when there is still circulating maternal antibody.

Although croup appears to be more common in boys than in girls, rates of infection with the PIVs appear to be similar for both sexes. The clinical manifestations of infection seem to be more severe in boys.

Transmission of the PIVs is by person-to-person contact or by spread of contaminated nasopharyngeal secretions. PIV type 1 is usually shed from the nasopharynx for 4 to 7 days, whereas PIV type 3 is shed over a period of 8 to 10 days and occasionally for up to a month. Nosocomial spread of the PIVs occurs readily in susceptible hospitalized infants. PIV type 3 appears to be the most efficient of the PIVs at person-to-person spread within a closed population.

Diagnosis

Infection secondary to PIV can be clinically suspected, depending on the clinical manifestations, the age of the patient, and the time of year. Because of the overlapping spectrum of respiratory disease caused by a number of viral respiratory pathogens, the etiologic agent may be defined only by identification of the responsible virus. Identification of the offending respiratory pathogen can be accomplished by viral antigen detection, tissue culture isolation of the virus, or by serologic means. For tissue culture isolation and viral protein or antigen detection, the preferred specimen from the patient is either a nasal wash specimen or a pharngeal swab. Because PIV is labile and infected cells are fragile, the respiratory specimen should be rapidly transported to the laboratory for culture or antigen detection.

Immunofluorescence allows the direct, rapid detection of PIV in infected respiratory epithelial cells. When obtained properly, the nasal wash specimen contains a large number of epithelial cells and therefore is the best specimen for antigen detection. An anti-PIV mouse monoclonal antibody can be applied to fixed epithelial cells and will bind viral antigen. After the addition of fluorescein isothiocyanate conjugated anti-mouse immunoglobulin, the specimen can be examined under a fluorescence microscope. The cytoplasm of epithelial cells infected with PIV will fluoresce green. Type-specific monoclonal antibodies can identify serotypes of PIV; however cross-reactions among the serotypes does occur. Other techniques for the rapid diagnosis of PIV infection include both the ELISA and immunoperoxidase staining for viral antigen detection, but these tests are not generally available.

Culture remains the standard method for confirmation of PIV infection. The viruses are best cultivated on primary monkey or human embryonic kidney cells. The PIVs may also be isolated on the continuous primate cell line LLC-MK2. Isolation and identification of the virus in culture may take up to 2 weeks. Cytopathic effects, including syncytia formation, may sometimes be observed in culture with PIV type 2 or 3. After every 5 days in culture, guinea pig red blood cells should be employed in order to detect a hemadsorbing agent, which may produce no evident cytopathic effect. Hemadsorption can presumptively confirm PIV infection. Specific identification of the PIV serotype depends on inhibition of hemadsorption by serotype-specific antisera. Immunofluorescence with monoclonal antibodies is an alternate, rapid method for tissue culture confirmation and serotype identification.

Serologic confirmation of PIV infection requires that an acute serum specimen be taken at the time of the diagnosis of infection and that a convalescent serum specimen be obtained 2 to 3 weeks later. A fourfold rise in antibody titer indicates infection. Serologic diagnosis can be made by complement fixation, hemagglutination inhibition, neutralization, or ELISA. The parainfluenza viruses do not always elicit an antibody response in young children. Serotype specificity is also a problem with all the serologic tests.

Therapy

There is currently no approved specific antiviral therapy for infection with PIV. Thus the therapy for respiratory infection associated with PIV is mainly supportive. It is agreed that hydration, maintenance of an adequate airway, and therapy for bacterial superinfection are important. Treatment of croup, however, remains controversial. Cool mist therapy is the cornerstone of management in the majority of cases. In more severe croup, oxygen is indicated, and an artificial airway may be necessary. The use of nebulized racemic epinephrine and steroids in the management of croup is still debated. There is some in vitro evidence to suggest that ribavirin has an antiviral effect. Ribavirin has been used to treat PIV infection in children with severe combined immunodeficiency, but its efficacy has not been proved.

Prevention

Vaccines for the PIVs are currently under development. Early trials with formalin-inactivated PIV vaccines failed to induce significant protection from naturally occurring infection. It subsequently has been shown that the formalin alters the F protein so that antibody produced to the formalin-inactivated material does not inhibit cell fusion. The goal of a potential vaccine candidate is to prevent serious lower respiratory tract infection secondary to PIV and to prevent morbidity associated with PIV infection. Because immunity to naturally occurring infection modifies illness but does not prevent reinfection, a vaccine may achieve comparable effects but not prevent infection. Furthermore, protection against serious PIV type 3 infection would require immunization during infancy, whereas protection against PIV types 1 and 2 would allow for immunization at a later time.

Live virus vaccine candidates include PIV type 3 cold-adapted, temperature-sensitive mutants, bovine PIV type 3 vaccine, which is antigenically related to PIV type 3, and PIV type 1 protease-activation mutants. The latter viruses have mutations that decrease host enzyme cleavage of the F protein and thus diminish viral infectivity. Recombinant vaccinia viruses containing the HN or F glycoprotein of PIV type 2 or 3 have been developed as well. All these vaccines have been shown in animal studies to be both attenuated and efficacious in restricting virus replication. Studies with vaccinia virus recombinants have demonstrated that HN appears to play a greater role in protective immunity than does the F protein.

The use of subunit vaccines that contain both the HN and the F glycoproteins of PIV type 3 or either purified F or HN glycoproteins is also being pursued. HN glycoprotein induces the hemagglutination inhibition and neutralizing antibodies, whereas F glycoprotein induces the production of fusion inhibition and neutralizing antibodies. It appears as if both determinants may be required for protection from PIV type 3. The HN gene from PIV type 3 has also been inserted into baculovirus vectors as a method of production of virus antigen for immunization.

With the current number of different strategies being employed in the development of vaccines against the PIVs, there is hope that in the future one or more of these promising candidate vaccines will be effective in preventing the serious sequelae of PIV infection.

Mumps Virus

Mumps virus is the etiologic agent associated with epidemic parotitis. Unlike RSV and the parainfluenza viruses it causes a disseminated generalized illness with frequent involvement of the central nervous system and certain glands. The mumps virus is a member of the Paramyxoviridae family and, along with the PIVs, is a member of the genus *Paramyxovirus*.

The mumps virion contains five major proteins, including two envelope glycoproteins, a nucleocapsid (NP)-associated protein also called the soluble antigen (S antigen), a polymerase, and a small, membrane-associated protein. The larger envelope glycoprotein contains the hemagglutinin-neuraminidase (HN) molecule (also called the V antigen), which mediates the adsorption of the mumps virus to host cells. Distinct sites responsible for either red blood cell adsorption or neutralization have been localized to domains on the HN molecule. The smaller glycoprotein is associated with fusion (F) activity and is required for penetration of the mumps virus nucleocapsid into the host cell. The hemolytic activity of the mumps virus has been localized to the F glycoprotein.

Mumps virus isolates differ in relation both to in vitro cytopathogenicity and to neurovirulence in a hamster animal model. It has been noted that neurovirulent virus isolates typically induce syncytia formation in vitro, whereas less virulent strains cause little cytopathicity. It was suggested that syncytia formation was regulated by neuraminidase activity, with a more active enzyme promoting rapid viral progeny release and not allowing time for cell fusion to occur. Subsequent observations suggest that both in vitro cytopathology and neuraminidase activity may not be reliable markers for animal neurovirulence. Strong evidence, however, exists to suggest that neurovirulence in hamsters is determined by the HN glycoprotein.

Clinical Illness

Illness associated with mumps virus is often preceded by several days of nonspecific symptoms, including fever, headache, malaise, and anorexia. The most classic and typically the first recognizable manifestation of mumps infection is parotid gland enlargement. Infection of the parotid gland or parotitis is accompanied by painful swelling of the parotid gland. Infection may also involve other salivary glands, including the submaxillary and, less commonly, the sublingual glands. The clinical manifestations associated with salivary gland involvement may be highly variable. Parotid gland involvement is typically bilateral but may be unilateral. There can also be involvement of the submaxillary and sublingual glands without involvement of the parotids. Fever typically lasts from 1 to 6 days, whereas salivary gland involvement lasts from 2 to 10 days. Involvement of the salivary glands occurs in about two thirds of cases. Mumps frequently is unrecognized as a clinical illness because symptoms may be totally inapparent in up to 30% of infected persons.

Central nervous system (CNS) manifestations of mumps virus infection are common. Cerebrospinal fluid (CSF) pleocytosis has been demonstrated in up to 60% of individuals hospitalized with mumps parotitis. Only half of these patients had CNS-related symptoms. Symptomatic CNS involvement or mumps meningoencephalitis has been estimated to occur in 1% to 10% of all mumps cases. CNS involvement is a more frequent complication of mumps infection among adults and also occurs more commonly in males with mumps. Mumps CNS disease is a result of either direct invasion of the CNS by the mumps virus or a postinfectious process with white matter demyelinization. Meningoencephalitis resulting from direct invasion of the CNS usually occurs 2 to 10 days after the onset of parotitis and may also occur in the absence of any parotid involvement. Postinfectious encephalitis usually occurs 10 to 14 days after the resolution of salivary gland involvement.

The term *mumps meningoencephalitis* is an inadequate term that reflects two quite distinct CNS manifestations of mumps virus infection. The first manifestation results in a clinical picture of mumps meningitis indistinguishable from other types of aseptic meningitis. Mumps meningitis results from meningeal invasion by the virus and represents the majority of mumps meningoencephalitis cases. The symptoms typically include fever, headache, vomiting, irritability, and nuchal rigidity. CSF findings in mumps meningitis are a pleocytosis with a lymphocytic predominance, a normal or low glucose concentration, and an elevated protein level. Mumps meningitis is typically self-limited and lasts only for 3 to 4 days. Before routine immunization, mumps was the most commonly identified cause of aseptic meningitis. The second manifestation of mumps-associated CNS infection resulting from either direct viral invasion or a postinfectious process is mumps encephalitis. Mumps encephalitis has been estimated to occur in only 0.2% of mumps cases. The encephalitis is a severe illness characterized by fever, impairment of locomotion, seizures, psychic disorders, and a depressed level of consciousness. It cannot be distinguished from mumps meningitis on the basis of CSF findings. The case fatality rate for mumps encephalitis has been reported to be 1.4%. Mumps encephalitis accounts for the majority of fatal mumps cases. Complications include both ataxia and behavioral disturbances. Aqueductal stenosis and hydrocephalus have also been demonstrated in rodent models after infection with the mumps virus, and the temporal association of hydrocephalus with mumps meningoencephalitis has been reported.

Orchitis or infection of the testes occurs as a manifestation of mumps infrequently in prepubescent males and in approximately 30% of postpubescent males who sustain mumps infection. Bilateral infection may occur in as many as 30% of patients with orchitis. In orchitis the testes become tender and swollen. The overlying scrotum is erythematous and edematous. Other systemic manifestations include fever, chills, nausea, headache, and abdominal pain. Orchitis usually occurs in the first week of infection and may occur without evidence of salivary gland infection. Orchitis generally resolves after 4 days. Mumps orchitis frequently leads to testicular atrophy of the involved testis. Infertility is infrequent but has been reported after cases with bilateral involvement. Epididimytis may occur in addition to orchitis or may occur alone without orchitis.

Mumps virus has a predilection to infect other glandular tissue in addition to the testes. Mastitis or infection of the breast tissue has been reported in up to 31% of women with mumps infection who are older than 15 years of age. Ovarian involvement or oophritis may also occur and is usually characterized by the development of lower abdominal pain or pelvic pain. Pancreatitis infrequently is associated with mumps infection. The clinical features of pancreatitis include epigastric abdominal pain, vomiting, and fever. The mumps virus has been shown to infect the beta cells of the endocrine pancreas, and temporally associated cases of diabetes mellitis have been reported after the onset of mumps. Although there is serologic evidence to suggest that infection with coxsackievirus may lead to the development of diabetes mellitis, it is unclear as to whether the relationships between infection with either mumps virus or coxsackievirus and diabetes are coincidental or causally related.

Mumps is rarely complicated by deafness. In most cases the loss of hearing secondary to mumps infection is unrelated to the occurrence of meningoencephalitis. The sensorineural hearing loss is caused by direct infection of the organ of Corti. Impaired hearing may occur suddenly during the parotid swelling and is often associated with vertigo, tinnitis, ataxia, and vomiting. In some cases the onset may be more gradual. The hearing loss is typically unilateral but in some cases may be bilateral. Permanent unilateral hearing loss has been reported in 1/20,000 cases of mumps. Transient high frequency hearing loss has also been reported to occur in up to 4% of patients with mumps.

Mumps myocarditis has been reported. It is usually self-limited but may be severe. Abnormal electrocardiographic findings are not uncommon during the course of mumps infection. Abnormal renal function is frequent in adults with mumps infection. Fatal nephritis has also been reported to occur in association with mumps infection. Rare complications of mumps that have been reported include arthritis, hepatitis, hemolytic anemia, and thrombocytopenia.

A higher occurrence of fetal death after mumps infection in the first trimester of pregnancy has been reported. Infection with the mumps virus during pregnancy, however, has not been linked to any pattern of mumps embryopathy. When attenuated mumps vaccine was given to women scheduled for therapeutic abortion, virus was recovered from the placenta but virus was not isolated from the fetal tissues. Case reports describing perinatally acquired mumps infection in infants suggest transplacental transmission of mumps virus. On the basis of skin test reactions to the mumps virus, there are some conflicting reports attempting to link the development of endocardial fibroelastosis to intrauterine mumps-virus infection. There is only one actual clinical case report of an infant with endocardial fibroelastosis born to a mother with mumps infection. Thus there is no confirmed evidence to support this proposed relationship.

Pathogenesis and Pathology

Mumps virus is transmitted by respiratory droplet spread. The incubation period is typically 16 to 18 days, with a range of 12 to 25 days. The virus initially comes in contact with the mucosa of the mouth and nose. The actual site of initial viral replication is unknown. The mumps virus could multiply in the mucosa of the upper respiratory tract, in the salivary glands, or in the regional lymph nodes and eventually enter the bloodstream, causing a transient viremia. The transient viremia allows for infection to develop in certain target organ systems, including the CNS and glandular tissues. Mumps virus can replicate in vitro in human lymphocyte culture and has been shown to preferentially infect T cell lines. In the face of a protective humoral immune response, circulating mumps-infected T lymphocytes can serve as an alternate means for dissemination of infection. Virus can be isolated from the saliva for 7 days before the onset of symptoms and for about 4 or 5 days after the onset of symptoms. During the acute illness, virus has also been isolated from blood, urine, and from CSF. The temporal relationships of virus excretion and communicability of the illness, along with the clinical symptoms and host antibody response, are shown in Fig. 70–1.

Parotitis is characterized histologically by periductal interstitial edema and a local inflammatory reaction composed mainly of mononuclear cells. The inflammatory reaction is confined largely to the interstitial stroma of the parotid gland, but occasionally the acini are involved. Degeneration of the

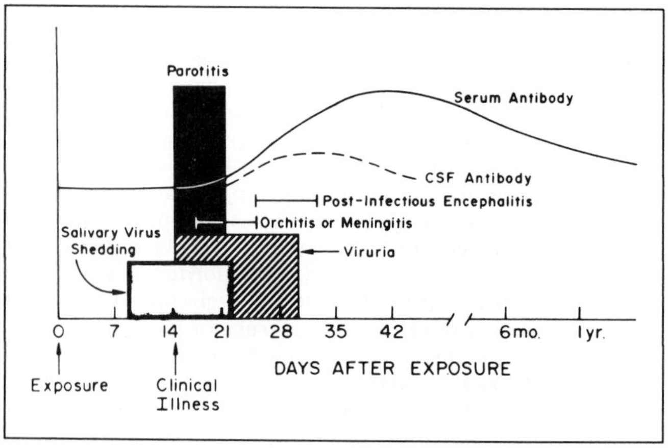

Fig. 70–1. The course of mumps virus infection.

cells of the ducts may occur, with an intraluminal accumulation of necrotic debris and polymorphonuclear leukocytes. The lesions in both the pancreas and the testes associated with mumps infection are similar. The testicular lesions associated with mumps orchitis are marked by diffuse interstitial edema with mononuclear cell infiltration and occasional scattered polymorphonuclear cells. Necrosis of the epithelium of the testicular tubules may occur, and the tubules may fill with necrotic debris. Hemorrhage into the interstitium may also occur. Because of the marked interstitial edema, the testicular blood supply may be compromised and microinfarctions may occur. Residual fibrosis and atrophy of the testicle result.

Infection of the CNS occurs by viral invasion across the choroid plexus. Infection is usually limited to the meninges. In the rarer cases in which the mumps infects the brain tissue, causing encephalitis, neuronolysis has been noted. The rare cases of postinfectious encephalitis are characterized by perivascular myelin loss and infiltration with mononuclear cells. CNS lesions associated with mumps virus cannot be distinguished pathologically from other viral causes of encephalitis.

Host Response

After infection with the mumps virus the immunity conferred is lifelong. The development of immunity does not depend on the particular clinical manifestations of the infection. Although occasional reports of reinfection do occur, it is likely that many of these reports actually represent misdiagnoses. If symptomatic reinfection occurs, it probably represents a small number of cases.

Mumps viremia is terminated at the time a humoral antibody response develops. The initial serologic antibody response to mumps virus infection is an IgM-specific antibody. A rise in serum IgM mumps-specific antibody can be noted as early as 3 days after the onset of symptoms and may persist for several months. Mumps-specific IgG is detectable within the first week of illness and persists for prolonged periods. Antibodies to different antigenic determinants of the mumps virus appear at different times in the course of the illness. Antibodies to the S or NP antigen are usually detectable during the first week of illness, peak at 10 days, and disappear in 8 to 9 months. Antibodies to the NP antigen are measurable by complement fixation and do not confer protective immunity. Antibodies to the V or HN antigen appear at about the tenth day of illness, peak at about 4 weeks, and persist for years. Antibodies to the HN antigen are measurable by complement fixation, neutralization of viral infectivity, or hemagglutination inhibition. Neutralizing antibodies and hemagglutination-inhibition antibodies to the HN antigen correlate with protection from disease. IgG mumps-specific antibodies cross the placenta and probably are responsible for the low incidence of mumps infection among infants younger than 1 year of age.

Virus-specific secretory IgA in the saliva generally appears 5 days after the onset of symptoms and coincides with the end of virus shedding in the saliva. Likewise both IgG and IgM mumps-specific antibody have been measured in the CSF of patients with mumps meningoencephalitis. The antibodies are synthesized in the CSF and appear during the first week of CNS symptoms. The IgG is oligoclonal and in some cases may persist for years.

The role of cell-mediated immunity in the recovery from infection is unclear. In vitro lymphocyte proliferative responses can be measured in seropositive individuals. Mumps-specific cytotoxic T lymphocytes can also be demonstrated after natural infection in humans. In addition, antibody-dependent cellular cytotoxicity has been demonstrated in vitro. There are no reported cases of severe mumps infection in compromised hosts.

Epidemiology

Naturally occurring infection with mumps virus is limited to humans. There are no known animal reservoirs or human carriers of the virus. Infection occurs throughout the world and may occur at any time during the year. In temperate climates the peak incidence of infection occurs during the winter and spring, with the majority of outbreaks taking place in March and April. Epidemics of infection have been reported recently in junior and senior high school students, in military populations before the availability of vaccine, and in other closed communities.

The source of mumps virus infection is infected saliva or other secretions that may contain virus. Infection is acquired when infected secretions come in contact with the oropharyngeal mucosa of a susceptible individual. Relative to measles and chickenpox, mumps virus appears to be less contagious. The period of communicability usually lasts about 7 to 10 days. Virus may be present in secretions for as long as 7 days but typically for 1 to 2 days before the onset of symptoms. The virus can persist in secretions for a period of 5 to 9 days after the onset of symptoms. In general it is not advised to quarantine ill individuals because there is a high rate of inapparent infection and because virus is shed before the onset of symptoms. Hospitalized patients with mumps should be isolated.

Mumps virus epidemiology has been significantly altered since the introduction of the mumps vaccine. The vaccine was licensed in 1967 and was recommended for routine use in 1977. The use of vaccine varied by community and state policy. In 1967 there were 185,691 cases of mumps reported in the United States. The majority of the clinically evident infections occurred in children between the ages of 5 and 10 years. Since that time the number of mumps cases per year in the United States steadily decreased and in 1985 reached an all-time low of 2982 cases reported. Cases of mumps encephalomyelitis, as well as the incidence of deaths from mumps, declined commensurately. A sizable increase in the number of mumps cases was noted in both 1986 and 1987. In 1987 the majority of mumps cases occurred in persons from 10 to 19 years of age. It is thought that the incremental introduction of the vaccine from 1967 up until 1977 left many young people both unimmunized and never exposed to natural infection. A cohort of unvaccinated young adults and adolescents was left susceptible to infection. As a result, outbreaks of mumps infection occurred in high schools, colleges, military populations, and the workplace.

Diagnosis

Before the routine use of mumps vaccine, the diagnosis of mumps could often be made on the basis of clinical findings alone. In the current era of vaccine use, confirmatory diagnostic testing should be performed on any person with clinically suspected mumps infection. Mumps should be considered in the differential diagnosis of any patient with parotitis. Mumps parotitis can often be confused with other disorders that cause swelling of the parotid glands or regional lymph nodes. Furthermore, acute parotitis can also be caused by infection with other viral agents, including coxsackievirus, parainfluenza virus, and influenza virus. In addition, parotitis is not an infrequent finding in patients with human immunodeficiency virus infection. Further, infection with mumps virus should be considered in any patient with either orchitis or aseptic meningitis. Confirmatory testing should be performed to make the definitive diagnosis. Laboratory confirmation is achieved by either virus isolation or serologic means.

Confirmatory diagnosis of mumps infection by virus isolation requires access to a diagnostic laboratory that is skilled at virus isolation. Laboratory personnel should also be alerted to the fact that mumps is a diagnostic consideration. Mumps virus can be cultured from the saliva, urine, CSF, or blood of infected individuals. Virus can be isolated from the saliva of patients in the first 2 to 3 days of illness. It can also be isolated from the CNS for up to 5 days after the onset of CNS symptoms and can usually be isolated in the urine for up to 2 weeks after the onset of illness. The virus is labile, and specimens should be transported promptly to the laboratory for inoculation into cell culture. The virus, which is best cultivated on either primary monkey kidney cells or on primary human embryonic kidney cells, causes a cytopathic effect in culture. The cells in the culture monolayer typically become rounded and fused and may form multinucleated giant cells. If infected by the mumps virus, the cell monolayer will hemadsorb guinea pig erythrocytes. Hemadsorption inhibition, immunofluorescence with a fluorescein-conjugated mumps antiserum, or neutralization can be used to confirm mumps infection of the culture.

Serologic tests for mumps are widely available and should be used to confirm all suspected cases. Mumps-specific antibody can be detected by hemagglutination inhibition, complement fixation, neutralization, and ELISA. Ideally a specimen should be obtained during the acute phase of illness and 3 weeks later during the convalescent phase. A fourfold increase in titer of antibody indicates acute infection. A rise in HN antibody occurs at about the tenth day of illness and persists for years. Serologic diagnosis of infection can also be made early in the course of infection, that is, before a convalescent-phase serum specimen is obtained. Antibody to the NP antigen appears during the first week of infection and disappears early. Antibodies to the NP antigen are detectable by the complement fixation assay and if present indicate an acute or a recent infection. Mumps-specific IgM can be detected by ELISA as early as 2 days after the onset of symptoms and also indicates acute infection. Neutralization assays and ELISA testing offer the advantage of being more sensitive than the other antibody tests. Because the ELISA is both sensitive and also relatively easy to perform, it is an effective test for determining immune status. This is particularly true in determining the immune status of vaccinated individuals in whom titers of mumps-specific antibody may not be high enough to detect by less sensitive methods.

Therapy

There is no specific antiviral therapy for mumps infection. There appears to be no role for therapy with immunoglobulin, and mumps-specific immunoglobulin is no longer available. Care of the patient with mumps infection is mainly supportive and consists of antipyretics for fever and analgesics for associated pain and discomfort.

Prevention

A live, attenuated mumps virus vaccine was licensed for use in 1966, and routine vaccination was recommended in 1977. The vaccine virus is the Jeryl-Lynn strain, named for the child from whom it was originally isolated. The live mumps virus vaccine is currently grown in chicken embryo cell cultures. Studies have shown that the vaccine is 95% effective in preventing disease, and immunity persists for as long as the 20 years it has been studied. The vaccine is effective in reducing disease morbidity, mortality, and the calculated cost of illness. Therefore it is recommended that the vaccine be administered to all susceptible children, adults, and adolescents. The vaccine may be given alone or in combination with the measles and rubella vaccines as a single injection. The combination vaccine should be administered routinely to all children after their first birthday. Mumps vaccine is not routinely advised for persons born before 1957 unless they are known to be seronegative. Most persons born before 1957 are likely to have had naturally occurring infection.

Mild parotitis and low-grade fever have been reported infrequently after immunization. More serious adverse reactions are rare. CNS complications after vaccination do not occur above the baseline incidence observed in an unvaccinated population. The vaccine should not be given to pregnant women or to women planning to conceive within the next 3 months because of the potential risk of fetal infection and the theoretic risk of harm with the vaccine virus. The mumps vaccine virus can infect the placenta. It has not been related to teratogenesis. Persons with a history of severe anaphylactic reaction to eggs should receive live mumps vaccine only with extreme caution. With one exception, patients with immunosuppressive disorders should not receive the vaccine. The vaccine has been demonstrated to be safe in children with immunodeficiency caused by human immunodeficiency virus and should be given to these children at 15 months of age. No immunocompetent host has had severe mumps due to either wild-type virus or vaccine virus. Passively acquired antibody may interfere with the immune response to the vaccine. Therefore vaccine should not be given within 3 months of the administration of either immunoglobulin or a blood transfusion.

In a susceptible person exposed to the naturally occurring virus, subsequent administration of the vaccine will not prevent infection from occurring. The short incubation period of the naturally occurring virus probably does not allow time for the development of a protective immune response to the vaccine virus. The vaccine can still be given in this situation inasmuch as it will cause no harm if the person does become infected and it will protect the person from future exposures if he or she does not become infected. Hyperimmunoglobulin has not been shown to be protective in the exposed individual and is no longer commercially available.

FURTHER READING

General

Denny FW, Clyde WA: Acute lower respiratory tract infections in nonhospitalized children. J Pediatr 108:635, 1986

Heilman CA: Respiratory syncytial and parainfluenza viruses. J Infect Dis 161:402, 1990

Henderson FW: Pulmonary infections with respiratory syncytial virus and the parainfluenza viruses. Semin Respir Infect 2:112, 1987

Murphy BR, Prince GA, Collins PL: Current approaches to the development of vaccines effective against parainfluenza and respiratory syncytial viruses. Virus Res 11:1, 1988

Tyeryar FJ: Report of a workshop on respiratory syncytial virus and parainfluenza viruses. J Infect Dis 148:588, 1983

Respiratory Syncytial Virus

Anderson LJ, Parker RA, Strikas RL: Association between respiratory syncytial virus outbreaks and lower respiratory tract deaths of infants and young children. J Infect Dis 161:640, 1990

Bruhn FW, Mokrohisky ST, McIntosh K: Apnea associated with respiratory syncytial virus infection in young infants. J Pediatr 90:382, 1977

Domurat F, Roberts NJ Jr, Walsh EE, et al: Respiratory syncytial virus infection of human mononuclear leukocytes in vitro and in vivo. J Infect Dis 152:895, 1985

Frank AL, Taber LH, Wells CR, et al: Patterns of shedding of myxoviruses and paramyxoviruses in children. J Infect Dis 144:433, 1981

Fulginetti VA, Eller JJ, Sieber F, et al: Respiratory virus immunizations. I. A field trial of two inactivated respiratory virus vaccines; An aqueous trivalent parainfluenza virus vaccine and an alum-precipitated respiratory syncytial virus vaccine. Am J Epidemiol 89:435, 1969

Glezen WP, Paredes AP, Allison JE: Risk of respiratory syncytial virus infection for infants from low-income families in relationship to age, sex, ethnic group, and maternal antibody level. J Pediatr 98:708, 1981

Graman PS, Hall CB: Nosocomial viral respiratory infections. Semin Respir Infect 4:253, 1989

Hall CB, Douglas RG, Geiman JM: Respiratory syncytial virus infections in infants: Quantitation and duration of shedding. J Pediatr 89:11, 1976

Hall CB, Douglas RG, Schnabel KC: Infectivity of respiratory syncytial virus by various routes of inoculation. Infect Immun 33:779, 1981

Hall CB, Hall WJ, Gala CL: Long-term prospective study in children after respiratory syncytial virus infection. J Pediatr 105:358, 1984

Hall CB, McBride JT, Walsh EE: Aerosolized ribavirin treatment of infants with respiratory syncytial viral infection. N Engl J Med 308:1443, 1983

Hall CB, Powell KR, MacDonald NE: Respiratory syncytial viral infection in children with compromised immune function. N Engl J Med 315:77, 1986

Hemming VG, Prince GA: Immunoprophylaxis of infections with respiratory syncytial virus: Observations and hypothesis. Rev Infect Dis 12:S470, 1990

Henderson FW, Collier AM, Clyde WA: Respiratory-syncytial-virus infections, reinfections and immunity—A prospective, longitudinal study in young children. N Engl J Med 300:530, 1979

Hendry RM, Burns JC, Walsh EE: Strain-specific serum antibody responses in infants undergoing primary infection with respiratory syncytial virus. J Infect Dis 157:640, 1988

Lamprecht CL, Krause HE, Mufson MA: Role of maternal antibody in pneumonia and bronchiolitis due to respiratory syncytial virus. J Infect Dis 134:211, 1976

MacDonald NE, Hall CB, Suffin SC: Respiratory syncytial viral infection in infants with congenital heart disease. N Engl J Med 307:397, 1982

McIntosh K: Respiratory syncytial virus infections in infants and children: Diagnosis and treatment. Pediatr Rev 9:191, 1987

Monto AS, Ohmit S: Respiratory syncytial virus in a community population: Circulation of subgroups A and B since 1965. J Infect Dis 161:781, 1990

Mufson MA, Belshe RB, Orvell C: Respiratory syncytial virus epidemics: Variable dominance of subgroups A and B strains among children, 1981–1986. J Infect Dis 157:143, 1988

Taber LH, Knight V, Gilbert BE: Ribavirin aerosol treatment of bronchiolitis associated with respiratory syncytial virus infection in infants. Pediatrics 72:613, 1983

Walsh EE, Schlesinger JJ, Brandriss MW: Protection from respiratory syncytial virus infection in cotton rats by passive transfer of monoclonal antibodies. Infect Immun 43:756, 1984

Welliver RC, Kaul A, Ogra PL: Cell-mediated immune response to respiratory syncytial virus infection: Relationship to the development of reactive airway disease. J Pediatr 94:370, 1979

Welliver RC, Sun M, Rinaldo D: Predictive value of respiratory syncytial virus-specific IgE responses for recurrent wheezing following bronchiolitis. J Pediatr 109:776, 1986

Welliver RC, Wong DT, Sun M: The development of respiratory syncytial virus-specific IgE and the release of histamine in nasopharyngeal secretions after infection. N Engl J Med 305:841, 1981

Parainfluenza Viruses

Chanock RM, Parrot RH, Cook MK: Newly recognized myxoviruses from children with respiratory disease. N Engl J Med 258:207, 1958

Choppin PW, Scheid A: The role of viral glycoproteins in absorption, penetration, and pathogenicity of viruses. Rev Infect Dis 2:40, 1980

Denny FW, Murphy TF, Clyde WA, et al: Croup: An 11-year study in a pediatric practice. Pediatrics 71:871, 1983

Glezen WP, Frank AL, Taber LH, et al: Parainfluenza virus type 3: Seasonality and risk of infection and reinfection in young children. J Infect Dis 150:851, 1984

Gross PA, Green RH, Curnen MG: Persistent infections with parainfluenza type 3 virus in man. Am Rev Respir Dis 108:894, 1973

Gross PA, Green RH, Lerner E: Immune response in persistent infection. Further studies on persistent respiratory infection in man with parainfluenza type 3 virus. Am Rev Respir Dis 110:676, 1974

Hall CB, Geiman JM, Breese BB: Parainfluenza viral infections in children: Correlation of shedding with clinical manifestations. J Pediatr 91:194, 1977

Klein JD, Collier AM: The pathogenesis of human parainfluenza type 3 virus infection in hamster tracheal organ culture. Infect Immun 10:883, 1974

McIntosh K, Kurachek SC, Cairns LM, et al: Treatment of respiratory viral infection in an immunodeficient infant with ribavirin aerosol. Am J Dis Child 138:305, 1984

Welliver RC, Wong DT, Middleton E: Role of parainfluenza virus-specific IgE in pathogenesis of croup and wheezing subsequent to infection. J Pediatr 101:889, 1982

Welliver RC, Wong DT, Tai-Soon C: Natural history of parainfluenza virus infection in childhood. J Pediatr 101:180, 1982

Yanagihara R, McIntosh K: Secretory immunological response in infants and children to parainfluenza virus type 1 and 2. Infect Immun 30:23, 1980

Mumps

Fleischer B, Kreth HW: Mumps virus replication in human lymphoid cell lines and in peripheral blood lymphocytes: Preference for T cells. Infect Immun 35:25, 1982

Hayden GF, Preblud SR, Orenstein WA: Current status of mumps and mumps vaccine in the United States. Pediatrics 62:965, 1978

Hilleman MR, Buynak EB, Weibel RE: Live, attenuated mumps-virus vaccine. N Engl J Med 278:227, 1968

Koplan JP, Preblud SR: A benefit-cost analysis of mumps vaccine. Am J Dis Child 136:362, 1982

Koskiniemi M, Donner M, Pettay O: Clinical appearance and outcome in mumps encephalitis in children. Acta Pediatr Scand 72:603, 1983
Love A, Rydbeck R, Kristensson K: Hemagglutinin-neuraminidase glycoprotein as a determinant of pathogenicity in mumps virus hamster encephalitis: Analysis of mutants selected with monoclonal antibodies. J Virol 53:67, 1985
McDonald JC, Moore DL, Quennec P: Clinical and epidemiologic features of mumps meningoencephalitis and possible vaccine-related disease. Pediatr Infect Dis J 8:751, 1989
Merz DC, Wolinsky JS: Biochemical features of mumps virus neuraminidases and their relationship with pathogenicity. Virology 114:218, 1981
Morbidity and Mortality Weekly Report. Mumps—United States, 1985–1988. 38:101, 1989
Siegel M: Congenital malformations following chickenpox, measles, mumps, and hepatitis. JAMA 226:1521, 1973
Wharton M, Cochi SL, Williams WW: Measles, mumps, and rubella vaccines. Infect Dis Clin North Am 4:47, 1990
Yamaugh T, Wilson C, St Geme JW: Transmission of live, attenuated mumps virus to the human placenta. N Engl J Med 290:710, 1974

CHAPTER 71

Measles and Subacute Sclerosing Panencephalitis

Measles (Rubeola)

Because of its distinctive clinical features, measles was recognized as a disease entity by seventh- and tenth-century Hebrew and Arabic physicians long before the demonstration of its viral etiology. Home, a Scottish physician, demonstrated in 1758 the transmissibility of the disease by scarification of susceptible individuals with blood taken from infected patients. Measles virus was first isolated successfully in tissue culture in 1954 by Enders and associates. This technique permitted investigations of the virus, studies of immunity, and the development and selection of variants for vaccine evaluation.

The use of live attenuated vaccines began in 1963 and has extended to many parts of the world, altering dramatically the incidence and epidemiology of the disease. Where infant measles immunization is widely practiced, the illness has become uncommon. In other lands, especially among economically disadvantaged nations, measles persists in epidemic fashion, responsible for the deaths of approximately 2 million infants and children each year. The World Health Organization, however, through its Expanded Program on Immunization has targeted measles for enhanced control efforts in the 1990s.

Pathogenesis and Pathology

Measles is acquired as an infection of the respiratory tract, with principal damage to surface mucosal lining cells. Secondary bacterial infections may be enhanced by diminished function of alveolar macrophages. The virus spreads to regional lymphoid cells and then, by an initial viremia, through the blood to the reticuloendothelial system. Continued virus replication then produces a more prolonged secondary viremia that distributes measles virus to lymphoid cells throughout the body. The large, inclusion-bearing, multinucleated giant cells found in reticuloendothelial and epithelial tissues are quite similar to those produced by measles virus when grown in vitro. Patients excrete large amounts of virus during the catarrhal phase. Virus can be recovered from the blood, particularly from the white cell fraction, for several days before rash appears but rarely thereafter. Viruria may persist up to 4 days after the onset of rash. The pathology of acute central nervous system (CNS) involvement includes edema, congestion, and scattered petechial hemorrhages, with perivascular demyelination in the later stages.

Measles viral antigens have been detected in mononuclear cells, macrophages, epithelial cells, and capillary endothelium of lymphoid organs and other tissues. Viral microtubular aggregates have been observed by electron microscopic examination of nuclei and cytoplasm of skin biopsy specimens. They are also found in the oral lesions (Koplik's spots). An important host mechanism for controlling the viral infection is the recognition and lysis of measles-infected cells by cytotoxic T lymphocytes. Rash reflects an intact component of the immune response as virus-infected cells in capillaries and small blood vessels are recognized by immune-reactive T cells. Malnourished, immunodeficient, or immunosuppressed children often undergo more severe measles illness, with prolonged virus replication, giant cell pneumonia, virus dissemination to many organs, and high case-fatality rates. Depressed T-cell function appears to be the liability shared by these patients. Further evidence of an interaction of measles infections and cellular immune mechanisms is the loss of delayed hypersensitivity to tuberculoprotein among tuberculin-positive patients with measles. This persists for weeks to months after acute infection. A worsening of underlying tuberculosis in children or adults who acquire measles infection has been reported.

Recent studies indicate that a selective deficiency of vitamin A in malnourished children is accentuated during measles by greatly increasing vitamin utilization at a time when dietary intake and intestinal absorption are reduced so that previously marginal hepatic stores are rapidly depleted. This deficiency predisposes to corneal xerophthalmia, corneal ulcers, and blindness as a result of measles. There is an additional epidemiologic suggestion that this vitamin A deficiency state is accompanied by a fourfold increase in the mortality rate of measles. The cause of such a rise in deaths is less clear, but even mild signs of vitamin A deficiency were associated with a striking increase in diarrhea and respiratory complications. In contrast to rubella, intrauterine measles is not teratogenic. However, it has resulted in stillbirth, premature delivery, and fatal congenital measles.

Clinical Course

Measles has an incubation period of 10 to 14 days (Fig. 71–1). A prodromal stage marked by catarrhal symptoms of cough, coryza, and conjunctivitis is accompanied by fever, which rises steadily until the appearance of rash 2 to 4 days after onset. Preceding the rash, the pathognomonic Koplik's spots appear. They are pinpoint and grayish white surrounded by bright red inflammation and found over the lateral buccal mucosa and the inner lips, occasionally involving the entire inner mouth. They may also be detected in the palpebral conjunctiva. The exanthem begins on the head, behind the ears, on the forehead, and on the neck. Discrete red macular and papular lesions progress downward to involve the trunk and upper extremities. Over a period of 3 days, the entire body becomes involved. When the lower extremities show discrete lesions, those on the head and the neck have begun to coalesce. With rash on the lower extremities, fever recedes dramatically. The bright red rash fades, to leave a brown discoloration that does not blanch with pressure.

The respiratory tract manifestations vary in severity but include laryngitis, tracheobronchitis, bronchiolitis, and interstitial pneumonitis from the viral damage of surface mucosal cells. With defervescence, there is improvement, but secondary bacterial infections of the respiratory tract may complicate the recovery phase in 5% to 10% of patients. These include otitis media, sinusitis, mastoiditis, and pneumonia. Acute encephalomyelitis occurs in approximately 0.1% of cases. This follows a 3- to 4-day period of recovery from the acute illness and is marked by a sudden onset, with seizures, confusion, and coma. The mortality rate of CNS involvement approaches 25%. Nearly half of those who survive are left with some sequelae involving impaired intellectual, motor, or emotional development. The responsibility of measles virus for later CNS complications has also been firmly established. Subacute sclerosing panencephalitis is an uncommon degenerative CNS disorder that does not manifest until 5 to 7 years after the initial measles virus infection. A third CNS complication of an intermediate type (progressive infectious measles encephalitis) has been observed among immunocompromised patients, with an incubation period ranging from 6 weeks to 6 months. SSPE occurs in 1 or 2/100,000 measles cases and is discussed in greater detail later in this chapter.

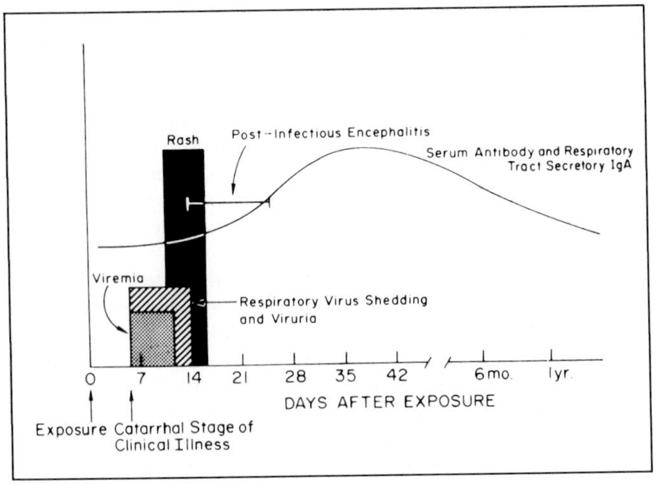

Fig. 71–1. The course of measles virus infection.

Epidemiology

Measles is one of the most highly communicable of all virus infections, so that nearly all susceptible children acquire the infection. In rural settings or among isolated communities, it has been possible for a population to reach adult life without exposure. Under such circumstances the introduction of measles virus produced devastating epidemics. Panum, a young Danish physician, in 1846 described such an outbreak in the Faroe Islands. He showed the persistence of lifelong immunity among individuals who had acquired the infection six and seven decades previously.

In the temperate zones, measles occurred in winter-spring epidemics in 2- or 3-year cycles, apparently related to the new groups of susceptible children born since the last outbreak. Because maternal immunoglobulin G (IgG) antibody is acquired transplacentally by the infant, infection in infants younger than 6 months of age is rare. As shown in Figure 71–1, the catarrhal stage of the illness is marked by extensive respiratory virus excretion, so that transmission most often is by large respiratory droplets in crowded settings such as day-care centers, classrooms, and homes. The virus can also persist for several hours in fine droplets, and airborne spread has been demonstrated in physicians' waiting rooms. A single attack confers lifelong immunity.

Although measles is a member of the genus *Morbillivirus*, which includes the agents of canine distemper, peste des petits ruminants, rinderpest of cattle, and a recently identified phocine distemper virus responsible for the deaths of many seals in the Baltic and North Seas, there is no evidence of natural spread among species. Except for minor variations, only one distinct serotype of measles virus has been identified. Infection sustained in any part of the world confers enduring, uniform geographic protection. With the striking decline of indigenous measles in the United States (Table 71–1) an increasing proportion of cases is the result of disease importations from other countries. A second change has been an upward shift in the age-specific incidence rate, with sporadic outbreaks in high schools and on college campuses. In 1989 and 1990, however, there were marked increases in measles cases predominantly among unimmunized, inner city, preschool infants and children. Outbreaks occurred in Los Angeles, Houston, Milwaukee, Dallas, Chicago, and San Diego. Case fatality rates were 3 to 5/1000 in contrast to <1/1000 in past years. Nearly 20% of the patients required hospitalization. Genomic analyses of current and past measles virus isolates

TABLE 71–1. REPORTED MEASLES CASES AND DEATHS IN THE UNITED STATES

Year	No. of Cases	No. of Deaths	Year	No. of Cases	No. of Deaths
1963	385,566	364	1977	57,345	15
1964	458,093	421	1978	26,871	11
1965	201,904	276	1979	13,597	6
1966	204,136	261	1980	13,506	11
1967	62,705	81	1981	3,032	2
1968	22,231	24	1982	1,697	2
1969	25,826	41	1983	1,497	4
1970	47,351	89	1984	2,587	1
1971	75,290	90	1985	2,822	4
1972	32,275	24	1986	6,273	2
1973	26,690	23	1987	3,588	2
1974	22,094	20	1988	2,933	N/A
1975	24,374	20	1989	16,236	41
1976	41,126	12	1990	26,520	97

N/A, not available.

revealed changes in only one to four nucleotides with no significant antigenic alterations. The important antigenic determinants were highly conserved.

Diagnosis

Diagnosis is clinically ascertained on the basis of the typical history and findings. Examination of the urinary sediment or nasal smears may reveal characteristic inclusion-bearing syncytia, and there is a peripheral leukopenia. Indirect immunofluorescence microscopy has been used to show measles antigen in nasopharyngeal cells. Although virus can be isolated from blood, respiratory tract secretions, conjunctival secretions, or urine, this is not ordinarily required or readily available.

A number of serologic tests use the antigens of the measles virion or its infectivity. These include virus neutralization, hemagglutination inhibition, complement fixation, enzyme-linked immunosorbent assay (ELISA), and immunofluroescence. Antibodies rise very rapidly after the appearance of rash and reach peak titers in the next 30 to 60 days. A pair of serum specimens, one obtained early in the course of illness and one 7 to 14 days thereafter, will show a marked rise in antibody titer by any of the methods described. Because of its relative simplicity, rapidity, and sensitivity, an ELISA is the method most commonly used to assay measles-specific antibodies.

Treatment and Prevention

The primary viral disease is not amenable to any current therapy. Supportive measures may be employed to reduce fever, ameliorate cough, and maintain hydration. Secondary bacterial complications are treated with antibiotics selected by culture of appropriate specimens. The treatment of encephalomyelitis is also based on symptoms, with careful attention to the maintenance of an airway, reduction of increased intracranial pressure, control of seizures, and provision of fluid, electrolyte, and caloric requirements. The administration of immunoglobulin (IG) early in the incubation period of measles may completely abort or modify the infection, depending on the amount employed. At a dose of 0.05 mL/kg body weight, IG will reliably modify measles so that a more benign course ensues, followed by lasting immunity. With use of a larger dose of 0.25 mL/kg body weight, it is possible to abort the infection completely, and the patient remains susceptible to future infection after catabolism of the exogenous globulin.

The prevention of measles by proper use of the available attenuated active virus vaccines offers the most reliable and enduring protection. Vaccines are recommended for all healthy children at or after 15 months of age. In developing nations where many cases of measles occur in infants younger than 1 year age, the EPI (Expanded Program of Immunization) of the World Health Organization administers the vaccine at age 9 months. Studies are under way to evaluate the efficacy of measles vaccine given as early as 4 to 6 months of age. The virus is propagated in chick embryo fibroblast or human diploid cell cultures. It is given parenterally, with successful infection in at least 95% of susceptible subjects. The attenuated infection is usually occult but may cause fever in 15% of recipients. Rarely, there is moderate, transient rash after the fever. This vaccine-induced attenuated infection is noncommunicable and results in antibody responses somewhat lower than those that follow natural measles. In patients studied to date, antibodies have persisted for more than 20 years after immunization. When exposed to natural infection, immunized children remain solidly protected.

From 1963 to 1967 an inactivated measles vaccine also was available. It has been abandoned because a severe, unusual illness followed the exposure of children to naturally occurring measles several years after the receipt of inactivated vaccine. Fever, pneumonitis, and an unusual centrifugal rash with petechiae developed, which seemed to represent a hypersensitivity reaction. The formalin or detergent treatment required to prepare the inactivated vaccine apparently degraded the F (fusion, hemolytic) protein of the outer viral envelope so that recipients lacked specific antibody to that antigen despite the presence of antibodies to the other five virion proteins. On exposure to natural measles, virus penetrated mucosal cells, with spread of newly synthesized virus by cell-to-cell fusion. These inactivated vaccines have been withdrawn from the market.

In the initial 5 years after the onset of vaccine use in the United States, reported cases of measles were reduced by 90%. Table 71–1 demonstrates the striking decline in reported cases of measles in the United States since vaccine licensure in 1963 and public health immunization programs began in 1966. A nadir was achieved in 1983 with fewer than 1500 reported cases, but the goal of measles elimination has proved to be elusive. Epidemiologic investigations disclosed two persisting foci of transmission. The major group was preschool, unimmunized, indigent, inner-city youngsters. Often these were the children of immigrants and illegal aliens who were not enrolled in health programs because of fear of contact with government agencies. A second, smaller focus was found among adolescents who constituted well-immunized groups where the presence of only a small number of susceptibles nevertheless supported an outbreak when exposed to a single case. These latter clusters have prompted the recommendation of a second dose of measles vaccine for all children to reduce even further that 5% in whom the primary vaccination failed, since apparently they are sufficient in numbers to support measles infection and spread when virus is introduced.

Recent public concerns about the hazards of immunization

TABLE 71–2. RATES OF COMPLICATIONS OF MEASLES AND MEASLES IMMUNIZATION

Adverse Reaction	Measles per 10^5	Vaccine per 10^5
Encephalomyelitis	50–400	0.1
SSPE	0.5–2.0	0.05–0.1
Pneumonia	3800–7300	—
Seizures	500–1000	0.02–19
Deaths	10–10,000	0.01

Adapted from reports of the Centers for Disease Control and World Health Organization.

have prompted the collection of data, such as those in Table 71–2, to permit a statistical comparison of the risks of the natural disease and of the attenuated vaccine. The higher rates of pneumonia and deaths represent figures collected in India, Nigeria, Gambia, Bangladesh, and other nations with developing health systems. Continued attention to immunization of all susceptible infants and children is needed to attain the goal of measles elimination.

Subacute Sclerosing Panencephalitis

Subacute sclerosing panencephalitis (SSPE), a degenerative disease of the brain, was first described in 1933 but was not attributed to measles infection until 1967. Since that time abundant laboratory data have confirmed the etiologic agent as measles virus (or a defective variant) that persists in the host's CNS after initial measles in infancy or early childhood.

Clinical Features

SSPE occurs almost exclusively in children and adolescents, usually between the ages of 5 to 10 years and predominantly in boys (3:1). Rarely, young infants are affected, and a very few cases have been reported in adults. The usual clinical course is outlined in Table 71–3. The progress of the disease sometimes may appear to be arrested for periods of years, usually when the patient is in coma, but almost invariably the patients die, often of inanition and intercurrent infection. A rare older patient with well-documented disease allegedly has recovered.

Epidemiology

Although the incidence of SSPE varies, it is estimated that one case follows each 100,000 cases of measles. The majority of patients give a history of uncomplicated natural measles at a younger-than-average age, and all remain well during the intervening 5 to 10 years until the onset of their CNS disease. Occasionally, no prior history of measles is elicited, or the only remembered exposure to measles virus has been vaccine. No consistent cellular or humoral immunologic defects have been demonstrated in patients with SSPE.

Past data have suggested that the disease may have been more common in the southeastern United States, that the primary measles infection occurred at a younger age in such patients, and that rural rather than urban residents were at greater risk. With the widespread use of vaccine and the resultant sharp decline of measles, SSPE has practically disappeared in the United States. Before measles vaccination programs, 20 to 40 cases of SSPE occurred annually; currently it is difficult to find a single new case. SSPE continues to appear, however, in nations where vaccine programs are nonexistent or poorly developed.

Diagnosis and Pathogenesis

SSPE diagnosis should be suspected on the basis of the history and the clinical findings of progressive personality changes, myoclonus, and variable focal neurologic deficits. A characteristic spike wave discharge is seen on the electroencephalogram, and the cerebrospinal fluid is usually normal except for the presence of oligoclonal measles antibodies produced locally in the CNS. The diagnosis is confirmed by the finding of measles antibodies in the cerebrospinal fluid and markedly elevated level of serum antibodies. Brain biopsy is not necessary for diagnosis, but should tissue become available, it may show perivascular round cell infiltration, neuronal degeneration, gliosis, and type A Cowdry intranuclear inclusion bodies when stained with hematoxylin and eosin and examined with the light microscope. With the electron microscope, these inclusion bodies contain microtubular filaments, corresponding in size and configuration to the nucleocapsids of measles virus. With appropriate fluorescent antibody staining, measles antigen can be demonstrated at these sites. Measles virus RNA can be detected by in situ hybridization. Finally, when brain tissue is cocultivated in the laboratory with permissive cells, complete infectious virus may be recovered.

Although measles virus infects CNS cells, there is no incorporation of the newly replicated components into cell membranes to form complete new infectious virus. Because of defects in expression of M, H, and F genes, the SSPE virus

TABLE 71–3. SUBACUTE SCLEROSING PANENCEPHALITIS

Clinical	Laboratory	
Personality change; declining school performance; intellectual deterioration often manifested by impaired memory, altered judgment, and inappropriate behavior; occasionally chorioretinitis; impaired motor activity, gait difficulty, speech difficulty; myoclonic jerks progressing to repetitive, often sound-sensitive myoclonic seizures; paralysis; gradual deterioration in consciousness; coma; death	EEG:	Paroxysmal, synchronous spike discharges with interim suppression of electrical activity
	CSF:	Usually acellular; normal total protein; increased gamma globulins (IgG); detectable measles antibody
	Blood:	Markedly elevated measles antibody
	Brain:	Specific immunofluorescence to measles antigen; microtubular filaments within nuclear inclusions on electron microscopy; SSPE virus recovered in tissue culture

EEG, electroencephalogram; CSF, cerebrospinal fluid.

is defective, with variable expression of the three gene product antigens at the cell surface. This explains the failure to recover infectious measles virus except by cocultivation with known permissive cells, antibodies in serum and cerebrospinal fluid to measles proteins, and the abortive persistent infection. The detection of measles virus RNA and antigens in SSPE brain tissue and spinal cord contrasts with acute measles encephalomyelitis, in which the absence of these findings has led to the hypothesis that the acute disorder may represent an autoimmune mechanism that does not require viral invasion of the CNS.

Treatment

Although numerous approaches to therapy for this condition have been attempted, all have failed. At present one can only offer general supportive care for the patient, attempt to control seizures, and try to provide early diagnosis and proper explanation.

FURTHER READING

Annunziato D, Kaplan MH, Hall WW, et al: Atypical measles syndrome: Pathologic and serologic findings. Pediatrics 70:203, 1982

Centers for Disease Control: Measles prevention: Recommendations of the immunization practices advisory committee (ACIP). MMWR 38:5, 1989

Fournier JG, Tardieu M, Lebon P, et al: Detection of measles virus RNA in lymphocytes from peripheral blood and brain perivascular infiltrates of patients with subacute sclerosing panencephalitis. N Engl J Med 313:910, 1985

Holt EA, Boulos R, Halsey NA, et al: Childhood survival in Haiti: Protective effect of measles vaccination. Pediatrics 85:188, 1990

Hussey GD, Klein M: A randomized controlled trial of vitamin A in children with severe measles. N Engl J Med 323:160, 1990

Istre GR, McKee PA, West GR, et al: Measles spread in medical settings: An important focus of disease transmission? Pediatrics 79:356, 1987

Katz SL: Measles in the United States: 1989 and 1990. In Aronoff SC (ed): Advances in Pediatric Infectious Diseases, vol 6. St Louis, Mosby–Year Book, 1991

Katz SL, Krugman S, Quinn TC: International symposium on measles immunization. Rev Infect Dis 5(suppl):389, 1983

CHAPTER 72

Rubella (German Measles)

On the basis of its molecular virology rubella virus has been classified as a positive-sense, single-stranded, enveloped RNA sole member of the *Rubivirus* genus of the family Togaviridae. Its replication is in the cytoplasm of infected cells, with assembly involving budding into intracellular organelles, and its biophysical structure and replicative functions are similar to those of the Alphaviridae. However, it has no interactions with arthropod vectors, does not replicate in insect cells, and is distinctive in its relations to humans, its only natural host. It is provocative to consider that other alphaviruses, transmitted by mosquitoes, can produce somewhat similar clinical syndromes characterized by fever, rash, and arthralgia or arthritis. These are Chikungunya, O'nyong-nyong, Sindbis, and Ross River viruses. Only a single serotype of rubella virus has been identified, coinciding with the clinical observation that a single infection generally confers lifelong immunity. Although rubella virus infection can be established in several laboratory animals (especially ferrets) and some primates, human beings are the only natural host.

From the mid-nineteenth century until 1941, rubella was regarded as a benign childhood rash disease. When the Australian ophthalmologist, Sir Norman Gregg, reported the association of intrauterine rubella infection with congenital cataracts, this attitude changed completely. Subsequently, deafness, congenital heart disease, and other malformations were found to result from maternal rubella during the first 4 months of pregnancy. The recovery in 1962 of rubella virus in cell culture systems led to the development and, in 1969, the licensure of attenuated active vaccines that have proved safe and effective. Congenital rubella has become rare in the United States and other nations where vaccine has been widely administered.

Clinical Features and Pathogenesis

Rubella postnatally is a mild rash disease that occurs principally in children but is seen at all ages. As shown in Figure 72–1, the incubation period is approximately 2 weeks, with minimal prodromal signs or symptoms. Most often, the first awareness of illness is mild fever and respiratory symptoms immediately preceding the onset of rash. The exanthem consists of pink macules and papules, at first on the face and then on the neck, trunk, and extremities, where they remain discrete and rarely coalesce. The rash has ordinarily disappeared by the third day. Preceding and accompanying the rash there is lymphadenopathy, which may involve the postauricular, suboccipital, and cervical nodes. Rash is observed commonly among children, but infection may be occult or only a febrile pharyngitis in as many as one third of adult patients. Little is known of the actual pathology of the postnatal disease because it is not a fatal one. Although major complications are rare (thrombocytopenic purpura and encephalitis), the incidence of transient arthralgia and/or arthritis is much greater than generally appreciated. The frequency of joint involvement is directly correlated with increasing age and appears also to be more common among women. In a few patients, persistence of rubella virus in synovial cells has been associated with polyarthritis and arthralgia of lengthy duration. Usually joint involvement is acute and short-lived without sequelae (Fig. 72–1). Whether rubella virus infection can be responsible for more chronic forms of arthritis (systemic juvenile arthritis, rheumatoid arthritis of pauciarticular and polyarticular forms, spondyloarthritis) is a topic of continuing investigation.

The route of infection is by the respiratory tract, with spread to regional lymphatics and then to the blood. Both viremia and respiratory tract shedding of virus may precede the rash by 1 week, and the latter may follow it for another several weeks. Because much virus excretion occurs before the recognition of illness, secondary infection of intimate contacts usually has transpired before the primary patient has been diagnosed.

The pathogenesis of congenital infection has been well studied during and since the 1964 pandemic. Maternal viremia is followed by infection of the placenta, which often leads to virus invasion of the fetus, especially in the first 16 weeks of pregnancy. Multiple tissues and organs support the replication of virus, which continues to multiply throughout the remainder of pregnancy and in the postnatal period. A large percentage of maternal infections that occur in the first 3 months of pregnancy result in fetal illness. There is a diminishing number in the fourth month, and it is controversial whether any fetal infections have resulted from maternal rubella in later pregnancy. Although the exact mechanism of damage to fetal organs is not clear, rubella infection of human embryonic cells in vitro is associated with both chromosomal breakage and inhibition of normal mitosis. Infants with congenital rubella suffer from intrauterine growth retardation and have a subnormal number of cells in some infected organs, suggesting that these same features have occurred in vivo.

Congenital rubella infection may result in a large variety of abnormalities, including deafness, congenital heart disease, eye defects (cataracts, glaucoma, retinitis, microphthalmia), growth retardation, thrombocytopenic purpura, osteitis, hepatitis, interstitial pneumonitis, encephalitis, and cerebral damage with mental retardation. In contrast to the postnatal infection, intrauterine disease is marked by a continued replication and excretion of virus, which may persist throughout the first year of life and has been demonstrated in selected tissues, such as the lens of the eye, as long as 3 or 4 years postnatally. In addition to those manifestations compatible with extrauterine life, intrauterine rubella infection may cause fetal death, abortion, or neonatal death. Although many of the acute neonatal manifestations resolve over the first months of life, long-term sequelae result in multiple developmental handicaps. Recent studies also indicate a significant increase in diabetes mellitus, chronic pneumonitis, thyroiditis, and late-onset degenerative encephalitis among the long-term survivors of intrauterine infection. One of the most interesting late manifestations of congenital rubella has been insulin-dependent diabetes mellitus. Of uncertain pathogenesis, it may represent persistent infection of islet cells or an autoimmune disorder with genetic predisposition. In favor of the latter hypothesis has been the detection of pancreatic islet cell antibodies and increased frequency of human leukocyte antigens (HLAs) DR3 and DR4 among the patients with diabetes. Vascular lesions involving renal, pulmonary, and coronary arteries result apparently from virus replication in endothelial cells, with eventual obstructive lesions such as renal artery stenosis and peripheral pulmonary artery and supravalvular aortic stenoses, as well as coronary artery intimal thickening.

The panencephalitis has temporal similarities to measles subacute sclerosing panencephalitis but only a dozen cases have been reported or studied. Onset of symptoms is delayed until the second decade, and the course is protracted, with degeneration over the subsequent 5 to 10 years. It too seems to be associated with a latent or persistent virus infection of the brain and with the replication of defective virus that stimulates rubella antibody production, with elevated cerebrospinal fluid levels.

The immunity that follows naturally acquired postnatal rubella is enduring. Only one serologic type of virus has been identified, and a single attack confers lifelong immunity. The immunologic events that accompany intrauterine infection differ strikingly. The antibody response in utero is principally one of IgM rather than IgG. Although IgG specific for rubella is found in fetal circulation, it is mainly of maternal origin and transplacentally acquired. Despite the presence of specific IgM and IgG in the fetal circulation, chronic infection of cells continues. Postnatally, the infected infant synthesizes rubella-specific IgG. Virus replication diminishes gradually over ensuing months. A small number of congenitally infected infants have developed unusual forms of hypogammaglobulinemia in the first year of life. Another group lost all detectable rubella antibody postnatally but nonetheless proved resistant to challenge with attenuated rubella viruses. The explanations for a number of these immunologic paradoxes are not yet known.

A recent review of the long-term effects among survivors of congenital rubella acquired in the 1964–1965 pandemic revealed that in their twenties approximately one third remain severely disabled and are institutionalized; one third are able to live independently and maintain normal lives; one third are at home but require substantial family support.

Epidemiology

In most urban communities, rubella infection was acquired during early childhood, principally in the school years. Because it is not as highly communicable as measles or varicella, 15% to 20% of women reached childbearing age without having acquired natural immunity. In the United States, large epidemics occurred at 6- to 8-year intervals, with smaller numbers of cases in the intervening years. This cycle was interrupted in 1969 by the introduction of rubella vaccine programs, and no large epidemic has developed in the United States in the 27 years since the 1964–1965 pandemic. The usual transmission is by the respiratory route, but the prolonged viruria of congenitally infected infants may be of importance in spread to close contacts. In situations in which adolescents and young adults have been placed in crowded living conditions, rubella outbreaks have been observed. Examples were regularly seen in the past among armed forces recruits, preparatory school and college groups, and summer camps. With widespread use of rubella vaccines, childhood outbreaks have disappeared, and only sporadic clusters of cases are reported now on college campuses and among other teen-age groups that have escaped both immunization and natural infection.

Since 1969, more than 140 million doses of rubella vaccine have been administered in the United States. After a 99% decline in rubella incidence from 1969 to 1988, the United States experienced a small increase in reported cases in 1990 (1093 total, with 11 cases of congenital rubella syndrome). Most patients resided in southern California and had no history of rubella immunization. Small clusters of cases occurred among adults in a variety of settings, including Amish communities, hospitals, college campuses, factories, and other workplaces and recreational settings. In contrast to the record in the United States, other countries that have not initiated aggressive rubella vaccine programs have continued to experience major outbreaks and to report the subsequent birth of infants with congenital rubella.

Diagnosis

Until 1962 the specific diagnosis of rubella was entirely a clinical one and quite unreliable because enteroviruses, adenoviruses, and other agents produced identical clinical syndromes. Currently, virus isolation techniques are not readily available. They involve the use of cell culture systems susceptible to the virus, with direct observation for cytopathic effect, or use of an interfering agent as an indicator of virus replication. Because these are time-consuming and technically demanding, serologic tests have been more commonly used. The antigens of rubella virus are responsible for the induction of a number of antibody types that can be assayed in serum. These include complement fixation (CF), virus-neutralizing, hemagglutination inhibition (HI), immunodiffusion, enzyme-linked immunosorbent assay (ELISA), and immunofluorescent antibodies. The HI test had been the most commonly employed. The rubella virus contains three structural proteins: E1 and E2, which are envelope glycoproteins, and NC, a nonglycosylated protein. E1 contains the principal hemagglutinin activity so that HI antibodies are directed against it; HI, however, does not detect the antibodies against the other proteins of rubella virus. For that reason, and for convenience of standardization, ELISA has replaced the HI test in most laboratories. Paired serum specimens obtained early in the course of illness and 10 to 20 days thereafter will demonstrate an antibody rise. The diagnosis of intrauterine rubella is more complicated but may be accomplished on a single serum specimen if neonatal blood is assayed for IgM antibodies specific to rubella virus. If an IgM technique is not available, it may be necessary to test paired specimens obtained over a period of several months to determine whether there is active postnatal antibody synthesis by the infant or merely a decline of transplacentally acquired IgG antibody.

Treatment and Prevention

There is no specific therapy for rubella virus infection. In the case of documented maternal infection during the first trimester of pregnancy, therapeutic abortion was commonly employed in the past. Even though rubella is confirmed virologically and/or serologically in the mother, it is not possible to be absolutely certain that fetal infection has occurred. Prospective studies showed that maternal rubella in the first 12 weeks of gestation carried a 90% incidence of fetal infection. After the third month this dropped to 25%, and little fetal damage was observed because organogenesis was complete. Amniocentesis has been employed in a few cases to examine cells and fluid for evidence of rubella virus infection, but there are insufficient data to evaluate the overall reliability of this method.

The use of immunoglobulin (IG) to prevent fetal rubella in an exposed pregnant woman has been ineffective and misleading. In most situations, it has been difficult to ascertain for how long a mother has been exposed to the virus. As depicted in Figure 72–1, she may have had a week's exposure

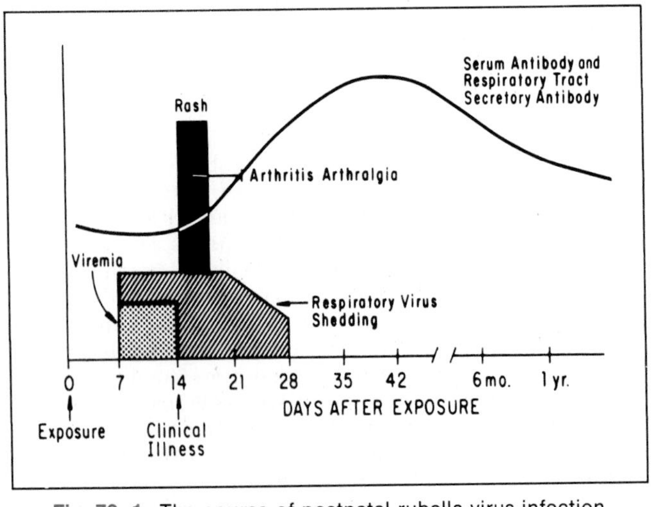

Fig. 72–1. The course of postnatal rubella virus infection.

to respiratory shedding from a contact by the time that individual contact develops rash disease.

Since 1969, attenuated active rubella virus vaccines have been used. These vaccines confer safe, lasting, effective immunity. They have been prepared in cell cultures of duck embryo, canine kidney, rabbit kidney, and a human diploid line (WI-38). In this country the diploid cell vaccine (RA27/3 strain) is the only one now used. Some respiratory shedding of the vaccine virus occurs for 7 to 28 days after vaccination. In contrast to that following natural infection, this is not transmissible. A serologically detectable antibody response is produced in more than 95% of susceptible vaccine recipients within 4 to 6 weeks of immunization. As with naturally acquired rubella, vaccination may be followed by joint complaints but in a far smaller percentage of recipients. Approximately 25% of adult female vaccinees 2 to 4 weeks after immunization experience arthralgia but only 1% true arthritis. Vaccine virus can cross the placenta to reach the products of conception, but no teratogenesis has been detected in 22 years' accumulated experience. Of more than 365 infants born to seronegative mothers who inadvertently received rubella vaccine in the early weeks of pregnancy, none has had a detectable congenital malformation. The use of vaccine in pregnant women remains nonetheless inadvisable.

Reinfection with wild rubella virus has been demonstrated to occur after either naturally acquired or vaccine-induced immunity. This usually happens in individuals whose antibody titers have fallen to low levels. The virologic events of such reinfections are markedly abbreviated. There is a rapid secondary type of antibody response with no overt illness. Continued study will be required to answer fully all the questions raised by the vaccines. In 22 years of utilization in the United States, they have produced a striking reduction in reported cases of both intrauterine and postnatal rubella. Prospective surveillance will continue to assess the long-range effects of these changes in population immunity and in the reduction of circulation of rubella virus.

FURTHER READING

Burke JP, Hinman AR, Krugman S: International symposium on prevention of congenital rubella infection. Rev Infect Dis 7(suppl 1): 1, 1985

Centers for Disease Control: Increase in rubella and congenital rubella syndrome—United States 1989–1990. MMWR 40:93, 1991

Centers for Disease Control: Rubella vaccination during pregnancy—United States 1971–1988. MMWR 38:289, 1989

Chu SY, Bernier RH, Stewart JA, et al: Rubella antibody persistence after immunization: Sixteen year follow-up in the Hawaiian Islands. JAMA 259:3133, 1988

Ginsberg-Fellner F, Witt ME, Fedun B, et al: Diabetes mellitus and autoimmunity in patients with congenital rubella syndrome. Rev Infect Dis 7(suppl):170, 1985

Gregg NM: Congenital cataract following German measles in the mother. Trans Ophthalmol Soc Aust 3:335, 1942

Munro ND, Sheppard S, Smithells RW, et al: Temporal relations between maternal rubella and congenital defects. Lancet 2:201, 1987

Smith CA, Petty RE, Tingle AJ: Rubella virus and arthritis. Rheum Dis Clin North Am 13:265, 1987

Waxham MN, Wolinsky JS: Rubella virus and its effects on the central nervous system. Neurol Clin 2:307, 1984

CHAPTER 73

Arboviruses

The past two or three decades have revealed many highly pathogenic viruses that were previously unknown. These viruses emerged not as a result of virus mutation from avirulence to virulence but rather because of dramatic changes in human living habits and practices (e.g., hemorrhagic fever viruses in Africa and human immunodeficiency virus [HIV] worldwide). The arboviruses, because of their widespread distribution and malleable genetic ecologic nature, have great potential for emerging in this way from previously undisturbed ecologic or genetic niches to produce significant human and animal disease. Among more than 500 recognized arboviruses about 100 are known to infect humans, and another 50 or so affect domestic and wild animals.

The term *arbovirus,* derived from arthropod-borne virus, was coined at a time when all the known viruses transmitted to humans by mosquitoes, ticks, flies, and other insects (arthropods) were grouped taxonomically under this heading. Modern studies of virus morphology and genetics have demonstrated that otherwise unrelated viruses are transmitted by arthropods, so that viruses from some several different virus families and genera are now included. On the other hand, some viruses that fall into the arbovirus classification because of their morphology and molecular organization, are now known to be spread to humans from animal reservoirs without intermediate arthropod vectors (e.g., Hantaan virus). (See specific reviews elsewhere for details of virus genetics and aspects of biochemistry, ecology, epidemiology, or disease associated with individual viruses.) The clinical syndromes caused by arboviruses are disparate. They cause mostly mild but acute, undifferentiated febrile illness, which, depending on the infecting virus, may be complicated by rash, hemorrhage, encephalitis, hepatitis, or renal failure. These more severe manifestations are not mutually exclusive, and some viruses are able to produce more than one syndrome (Fig. 73–1).

Arboviruses are found in ecologic niches virtually in every part of the world, including the Arctic. They have been responsible for some of the most devastating outbreaks of disease in humans and domestic animals over the centuries and thus have had a major impact on human history. Yellow fever is a prime example. That these outbreaks are not confined to past history is illustrated by the outbreak of Rift Valley fever in Egypt in the late 1970s, which affected more than 1 million people, and the outbreaks of yellow fever in West Africa from 1986 to 1991, which caused thousands of cases, many fatal. These human yellow fever infections in highly populated rural areas appear to a play a substantial role in continued virus transmission. Such situations may act as a precursor to outbreaks of urban yellow fever. Because the transmission of many of these diseases depends on basic human activities, such as water storage, travel, and raising domestic animals, their investigation and control has often required not only sound scientific principles but also some sense of adventure and not a little cultural and political diplomacy.

Virus Structure and Genetics

The Togaviridae, Flaviviridae, and Bunyaviridae families contain most of the arboviruses that cause serious human disease (see Chaps. 53 and 55). Togaviridae include four genera, of which only the arthropod-borne is genus *Alphavirus.* Members of the *Flavivirus* and *Alphavirus* genera have single-stranded genomes, approximately 4×10^6 in molecular weight, which are infectious (plus stranded) and which therefore act as the messenger RNA for translation of proteins and as the template for the transcription of negative sense RNA. The resultant product is then used to make more positive-sense RNA in the virus genomic replicative cycle. The alphaviruses are spherical, 60 to 70 nm in size, with three structural proteins—the capsid and the glycosylated E2 and E1 proteins—that compose the

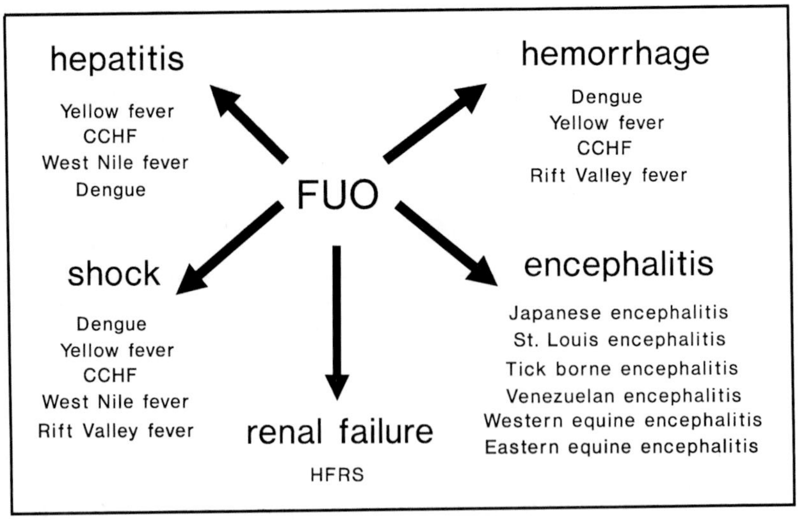

Fig. 73–1. Clinical syndromes associated with arbovirus diseases.

virion surface. The flaviviruses are smaller—40 to 50 nm in diameter—and have three structural proteins, a capsid, a glycosylated protein, and a small nonglycosylated protein that may be membrane associated. Both viruses encode several nonstructural proteins that appear to be important in the replicative cycle. Bunyaviridae of importance in human infections include members of the Bunyamwera virus, *Phlebovirus*, *Nairovirus*, and hantavirus genera. They are larger viruses ranging from 80 to 100 nm in diameter. They have a three-segment genome of negative-stranded RNA. The two glycosylated proteins are encoded in the M or middle RNA segment, the nucleocapsid is encoded by the S or small RNA segment, and the polymerase and perhaps other nonstructural proteins important in virus replication are encoded by the L or large RNA segment. Within each of the bunyavirus genera there is extensive antigenic cross-reactivity, especially with the nucleocapsid antigens. The alphaviruses, flaviviruses, and bunyaviruses are sensitive to lipid solvents and heat.

An important mechanism of survival for most viruses, especially arboviruses, is the ability to generate genetic diversity. This ability permits escape from host immune responses, adaptation to new hosts, or even the ability to alter replication patterns in an existing host (e.g., by altering the target organ or tissue). Arboviruses utilize several genetic processes to maintain their diversity. Those with segmented genomes undergo genetic drift as a result of deletions, mutations, and inversions and genetic shift through genome segment reassortment. The multigenomic arboviruses (bunyaviruses and orbiviruses) therefore demonstrate somewhat more genetic diversity than do the single genome viruses (alphavirus, flavivirus, rhabdovirus), which appear to depend on genetic drift alone. The genetic stability of these RNA viruses is substantially less than for DNA viruses because the DNA replication enzymes are less error prone in their transcription and the DNA viruses generally have enzymes that verify their DNA transcripts. An additional method of generating genetic diversity—recombination—used by some RNA viruses (e.g., poliovirus, influenza) remains unknown for arboviruses. These viral genetic mechanisms all occur in the context of diverse hosts (mostly avian and mammalian), vectors (such as mosquitoes, ticks, and flies), climate, and many other factors, all of which exert the selective pressures that mold the evolution and epidemic potential of arboviruses. The complexity of the interaction of the viruses with their vectors, hosts, and surrounding ecology are illustrated by the transmission cycles of St. Louis encephalitis virus in North America (Fig. 73–2) and yellow fever virus in Africa (Fig. 73–3). The significance of the transmission cycles in producing antigenic variety is illustrated by extensive antigenic cross-reactions among the arthropod-borne flaviviruses, whereas the nonarthropod ones, with fewer and less varied transmission cycles, are antigenically unique.

Diagnosis

Because of prior exposure to an antigenically related virus, specific serologic diagnosis of an acutely ill patient may be difficult in geographic areas containing several viruses of a genus that share antigenic circulation sites. Absolute antibody titers may be misleading because the highest titers in an acutely ill patient may result from an anamnestic response to a virus that the patient previously encountered rather than from the current related but biologically distinct infecting virus. In the future the use of virus-specific peptides may help to distinguish such infections, but their availability and use presently are limited. Virus-specific IgM antibody titers may be helpful in some cases. Also, the incubation period of many of these infections is short, so that a primary antibody response to the infecting virus may not yet have developed in the acutely ill patient.

The most accurate method of diagnosis is by isolation of virus from serum, and for many viruses the most sensitive method is intracerebral inoculation of suckling mice. For some viruses, however, specific continuous cell lines, such as mosquito cells, have been developed or adapted both for primary isolation from human, animal, or arthropod sources and for virus propagation in the laboratory. Virus isolation is not rapid enough to benefit the medical decisions required for care of the patient, but reagents for polymerase chain reaction have been developed for some viruses and may soon be available for rapid diagnosis. As more antiviral chemotherapy becomes available, such techniques will be essential for effective patient management.

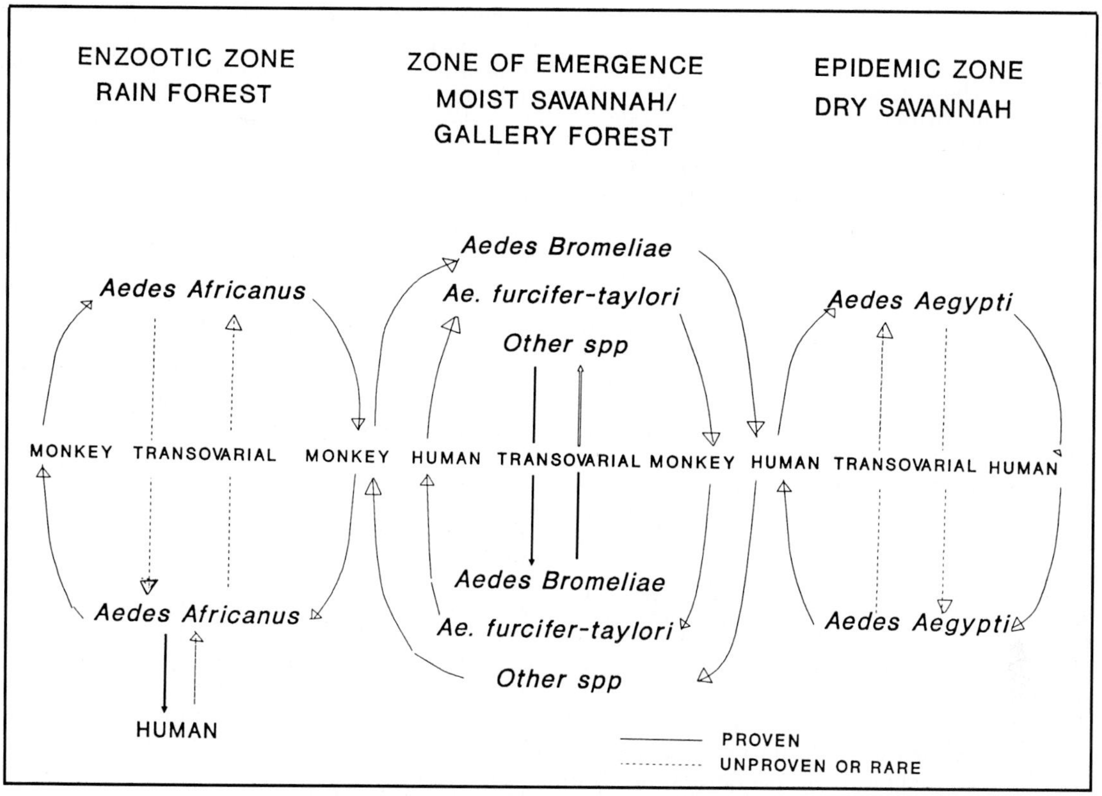

Fig. 73–2. Yellow fever virus transmission cycles in Africa.

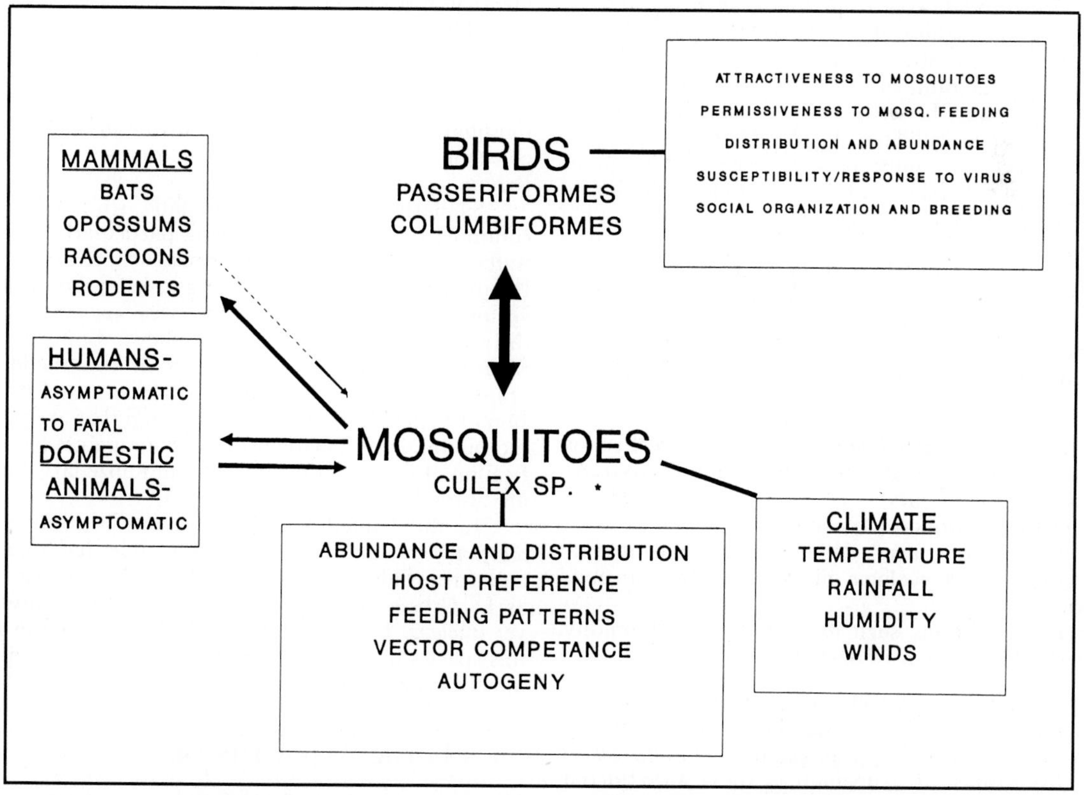

Fig. 73–3. Transmission of St. Louis encephalitis virus in North America. *Note large number of vectors (at least seven species of *Culex* involved) and multiple variables affecting host and vector ability to transmit virus.

Epidemiology

The epidemiology of arboviruses may be understood to some extent by grouping the viruses according to their mode of transmission. Thus mosquito-borne, tick-borne, phlebotomus (midge or mite)-borne, and "non-arthropod-borne" viruses are convenient categories. Despite its usefulness, this categorization hides an infinite complexity of epidemiologic ecosystems, many of which are unique to only one of the more than 500 known viruses. Many viruses have proved sufficiently versatile to be able to replicate in a number of hosts rather than in a single primary host (e.g., western equine encephalomyelitis, eastern equine encephalomyelitis, Japanese encephalitis, and Congo-Crimean hemorrhagic fever [CCHF] viruses). Humans are not normally primary hosts, and human infection is not an essential part of the natural history of most arboviruses, especially where fatal human disease is common—the death of the host normally not being to the advantage of the virus. The major exception is dengue, for which humans and perhaps monkeys are the only known nonarthropod hosts. For those viruses, however, in which humans can be a reservoir for transmission (e.g., yellow fever, Rift Valley fever, and CCHF), transmission to other humans may be greatly augmented by the presence of a number of highly viremic humans. Such transmission may occur by a vector intermediate (e.g., yellow fever) or by direct transmission (e.g., CCHF).

Several important concepts apply to the epidemiology of arboviruses regardless of their host or arthropod vector. Most viruses have amplifying vertebrate hosts that range from birds to equines (Table 73–1). Some of these amplifying hosts manifest illness (e.g., pigs and equines do so from Japanese encephalitis virus, and horses from Venezuelan equine encephalitis virus), but others do not (birds apparently are symptom-free). These hosts must have several characteristics in order to amplify the number of infected arthropods. Their degree of viremia must be sufficient (1 million to 1 billion infectious viruses per milliliter of blood) to easily infect arthropod vectors. They must be a favorite and frequent target for vector blood meals, and they must have a high rate of turnover to maintain a substantial population susceptible to infection. Nonamplifying (dead-end) hosts are those that do not reinfect the arthropod vector because of low levels of viremia, scarcity of the vertebrate, or infrequent feeding by the arthropod on the host.

Important determinants that directly affect the arthropods and therefore their efficiency in virus transmission include the following:

1. The ability of virus to traverse the gut of the arthropod and replicate in the salivary glands, from where transmission readily occurs
2. Size of the arthropod population
3. Biting habits (nocturnal, daytime) and flight ranges
4. Geographic and ecologic distribution of arthropod species
5. Climatic conditions such as temperature, humidity, rainfall, and number of daylight hours

Climatic conditions decisively affect the vector, the amplifying host, and the virus. In warm climates the arthropod and host are more affected by rainfall than by temperature variations. This is especially true in areas where wide fluctuations in rainfall are observed (the Savannah areas of Africa). In areas that normally experience several months of low rainfall each year, the virus often survives through transovarial transmission to the arthropod eggs, which may lie dormant for months before hatching but which will produce infectious adult arthropods on incubation. Thus the virus adapts to the life cycle of its arthropod vector, not only for transmission but also to evade adverse conditions. Rift Valley fever virus and yellow fever virus are believed to be two examples of this phenomenon in the tropics. Similarly, in temperate climates where transovarial transmission is also common, the virus must be able to survive the effects of low temperature.

Mosquito-borne Arbovirus Disease

Most mosquito-borne diseases are tropical in distribution and concentrated in areas of high mosquito population densities. Some are transmitted by sylvatic mosquitoes. In these circumstances infection of humans is an accidental event and thus not common. Problems for human populations occur when the virus brought in from the forest is able to adapt to peridomestic mosquitoes adept at breeding in urban communities, such as *Aedes aegypti* in water containers. This may result in explosive urban epidemics, prime examples being yellow and dengue fevers. In the tropical rain forests of Africa, yellow fever is maintained primarily in the mosquito *Aedes africanus* and monkey hosts (Fig. 73–2). The flexibility of the virus, however, allows it to adapt to many mosquitoes species. This is illustrated by its rapid establishment in America. After being brought over on the slave ships, probably both in humans and in the mosquitoes breeding in fresh water containers, yellow fever virus was able to adapt rapidly both to American mosquitoes and to South American jungle primates, in which, unlike the African monkeys, and like humans, it frequently causes fatal disease. The current West African epidemics are alarming in that adaptation to the rapidly increasing urban environments of the twentieth century may allow the virus to survive entirely in humans and peridomestic mosquitoes without the support of the jungle cycle. Thus the constant threat of yellow fever epidemics will remain in this region.

Similarly, Japanese encephalitis, spread by mosquitoes, continues to be a major problem, particularly with changes in water management, such as construction of new dams and flooding to enlarge rice farming areas. Like malaria control, vector control on a large scale, with present technology, is difficult if not impossible to achieve. Control therefore is focused on vaccination programs in conjunction with new approaches, such as breeding of larvivorous fish and dispersion of nematodes, bacteria, and fungi that are pathogens for mosquito larvae. Personal protection against bites and modification of irrigation practices to minimize larval proliferation are also important.

In the United States the recent introduction of *Aedes albopictus* in imported used tire casings has raised concerns about transmission of dengue, as well as native viruses such as La Crosse encephalitis. The long-term consequences are yet unclear, but it seems very possible that the potential of this species to transmit a number of pathological arboviruses may be realized in North America.

Tick-borne Arbovirus Disease

Members of at least three families of viruses cause human disease after transmission by ticks (ticks are arachnids with

TABLE 73–1. EPIDEMIOLOGIC SYNOPSIS OF MEDICALLY IMPORTANT ARBOVIRUSES

Virus	Family/Genus	Hosts: Invertebrate (vector)	Hosts: Vertebrate (amplifier)	Geographic Distribution	Clinical Manifestation	Comment
Mosquito-borne Viruses						
Dengue	Flavivirus	Aedes	Humans, monkeys	Worldwide especially tropics	Nonspecific fever, hemorrhage and shock	Water storage is important source for mosquito breeding
Yellow fever	Flavivirus	Aedes	Humans, monkeys	Africa South America	Hepatitis, hemorrhagic fever	Urban yellow fever depends on human reservoir
Japanese encephalitis	Flavivirus	Culex	Pigs, equines, birds	Asia	Encephalitis	Rural predominance Vaccine effective
West Nile	Flavivirus	Culex	Birds, equines?	Africa, Europe, Central Asia	Nonspecific fever, encephalitis, hepatitis	Mostly rural High prevalence
Murray Valley	Flavivirus	Culex	Birds	Australia		
St. Louis encephalitis	Flavivirus	Culex	Birds	North America	Encephalitis	Can produce large urban outbreaks
Rocio encephalitis	Flavivirus	Culex	?	South America	Encephalitis	Sporadic rural disease
Ilheus	Flavivirus	Psorophora, ? others	Birds, wild mammals, marsupials	South America	Encephalitis	—
Chikungunya	Alphavirus	Aedes	Wild mammals, humans	Africa, Asia	Nonspecific fever	Can cause large urban epidemics
O'Nyong-nyong	Alphavirus	Anopheles	Wild mammals, humans	Africa	Nonspecific fever	Similar to chikungunya
Ross River	Alphavirus	Culex, Aedes	Wild mammals	Australia, South Pacific islands	Nonspecific fever, polyarthritis	Similar to chikungunya
Venezuelan equine encephalitis	Alphavirus	Aedes, Culex, Mansonia, Psorophora	Equines, humans, marsupials	South and Central America	Severe encephalitis in humans and equines	Enzootic cycle in Culex Epidemic/ epizootic in Aedes, Mansonia, Psorophora Effective vaccine
Eastern equine encephalitis	Alphavirus	Aedes, Culiseta	Birds, equines	North America, South America, Caribbean	Encephalitis in humans and equines	Effective vaccine for equines
Western equine encephalitis	Alphavirus	Culex, Culiseta	Birds, equines	North America, (West) South America	Encephalitis in humans and equines	Effective vaccine for equines
Rift Valley fever	Bunyavirus Phlebovirus	? Culex	Wild mammals, domestic animals	Africa	Nonspecific fever, hemorrhage; hepatitis and encephalitis may occur	Severely affects domestic livestock
Bunyamwera	Bunyavirus Bunyamwera	Aedes, ? others	Wild mammals	Africa	Nonspecific fever Encephalitis	Origin of name Bunyavirus
California encephalitis	Bunyavirus	Aedes	Small mammals	North America	Usually mild fever in minority of infections	Endemic infection includes La Crosse, Jamestown Canyon Snow Shoe hare

(continued)

TABLE 73–1. EPIDEMIOLOGIC SYNOPSIS OF MEDICALLY IMPORTANT ARBOVIRUSES (*continued*)

Virus	Family/Genus	Hosts: Invertebrate (vector)	Hosts: Vertebrate (amplifier)	Geographic Distribution	Clinical Manifestation	Comment
Tick-borne Viruses						
Crimean-Congo hemorrhagic fever	Bunyavirus Nairovirus	Ixodid and Argasid (27 species)	Wild and domestic animals	Africa, Asia, Eastern Europe	Hemorrhagic disease, hepatitis	Endemic infection person to person transmission, nosocomial
Thogoto	Orthomyxovirus	Boophilus, ? other	Domestic and wild animals	Africa, Middle East	Encephalitis, optic neuritis	Appears to cause sporadic infections
Kyasanur forest	Flavivirus	Haemaphysalis	Monkeys, ? other	Asia (India)	Encephalitis	Sporadic outbreaks Multiple laboratory infections
Russian Spring-Summer	Flavivirus	Ixodes and Dermacentor	Birds	Russia	Encephalitis	Sporadic, severe disease
Tick-borne encephalitis	Flavivirus	Ixodes	Mammals	Europe, East Russia	Severe encephalitis	Includes Absetarov anzalova Hypr, and Kumlinge viruses
Langat	Flavivirus	Ixodes	Small mammals	Asia	Encephalitis but no natural infection known	Disease seen only in patients with tumors who were experimentally infected
Louping ill	Flavivirus	Ixodes	Birds, mammals	United Kingdom	Encephalitis	Restricted to Scotland
Powassan	Flavivirus	Ixodes	Small mammals	North America	Encephalitis	—
Colorado tick fever	Reovirus Orbivirus	Ixodid and Argasid	Small mammals	North America	Fever with meningo-encephalitis	Sporadic disease

fused head, thorax, and abdomen and with four pairs of legs). The diseases produced by tick-borne arboviruses include a complete clinical spectrum from nonspecific illness (e.g., Colorado tick fever and Dugbe infection) to hemorrhage and encephalitis (CCHF and tick-borne encephalitis). Much like the mosquito-borne arboviruses, the tick-borne viruses have intermediate vertebrate hosts. Furthermore, the viruses also replicate in their tick vectors, and many are passed both transovarially and transstadially. Tick vectors of arboviruses also represent a wide biologic range of ticks, including soft and hard ticks and those that require one, two, or three different hosts to complete their life cycle.

Unlike mosquito vectors, ticks move over small distances by themselves, but they are able to increase their range by attaching themselves to a vertebrate host. For example, because many ticks are parasites of birds, disease may be spread immense distances by ticks on migrating birds. Thus disease can be multifocal, and the viruses are often present on several continents. Like the factors that affect mosquito-borne viruses, diverse natural histories determine both the spread of virus to humans, as well as the maintenance of the virus in tick vectors or amplifying hosts. Many of the principles already cited that apply to mosquito-borne viruses may be applied to those borne by ticks. In any event, the risk to humans is less than for mosquito-borne diseases because it is easier to deliberately avoid tick contact. Persons at risk are usually farmers, veterinarians, or others with close contact with livestock or wild animals. Human infections consequently are most likely to be sporadic and endemic, rather than epidemic, and to reflect occupational risk factors and tick exposure.

Phlebotomus (midge or mite)-Borne Disease

Few diseases are known to be transmitted by midges (Table 73–1), but their distribution is wide. These small flies have a limited flight range but locally may be so plentiful that the entire human population will have acquired infection and thus antibody early in life. Observed outbreaks therefore are likely to be associated with movement of a large, susceptible adult population into an endemic area, as may occur in war or with development of tourism.

Non-Arthropod-borne Disease

The most important of the non-arthropod-borne viruses is the Hantaan virus, which is carried by rodents, particularly *Apodemus, Rattus,* and *Clethrionomys* species. Infections in humans are numerous, particularly in Asia, where the virus causes hemorrhagic fever with renal syndrome (HFRS). Although aerosol spread may occur, the main route of human infection appears to be direct contact with rodents or their excreta, most often in conditions of poor housing. Repeated attempts to identify an insect vector have been unsuccessful, and this is now thought to be an unlikely component in the spread of hantaviruses.

Clinical Features and Pathophysiology

Diseases caused by arboviruses are diverse and span the entire spectrum of clinical infectious disease. Although they cannot be fitted neatly into clinical pigeonholes, for the purposes of this discussion it is useful to group them by their involvement of main target organs (Fig. 73–1 & Table 73–1). Most infections, which produce a mild or even subclinical illness with fever and headache, are often the culprits in fevers of unknown origin. Some viruses, however, have the potential to involve the central nervous system, the liver, and the kidney or to produce fluid loss and hypotensive shock occasionally accompanied by a hemorrhagic diathesis.

Nonspecific Febrile Disease

All of the 70 or more known arboviruses that cause human illness can produce a febrile disease of varying severity, indistinguishable from many other infectious syndromes. Some of the most important in terms of the numbers of cases worldwide are West Nile fever, Chikungunya, Ross River fever, Phlebotomus (sandfly) fever, and dengue.

The shortness of the incubation period of these infections, 3 to 7 days, probably is related to their direct inoculation into the bloodstream by the vector, thus obviating the need for a primary epithelial site of replication. Nevertheless, some viruses are believed to replicate in the skin at the site of entry. Most of these fevers manifest with abrupt onset of fever, severe frontal headache—often with orbital pain—myalgia, backache, flushing of the skin or rash, conjunctivitis, and anorexia. This flulike syndrome suggests common fever inducers such as interferon and other lymphokines. Nausea and vomiting may occur with the more severe forms of some of the diseases, and leukopenia is often a feature; thus, as with many viral diseases, mild transient immunosuppression is likely to occur.

Most infections subside without development of localizing features and without complications, in most cases resulting in the development of neutralizing antibodies and lifelong immunity. This immunity, however, frequently is type-specific, and reinfections with closely related viruses occur. In these circumstances the clinical disease, with the notable exception of dengue (see below), is likely to be mild or asymptomatic. Most of the data on the immune response to these infections concern the humoral response and are virtually absent for the cellular immune response, which may be of importance both in virus clearance and protection against reinfection.

Nearly all these agents are capable of producing severe disease, and it is unclear whether host factors, virulence of the infecting virus, or the size or route of inoculum, or all these factors, determine illness severity. What is clear is that some agents are more likely to induce life-threatening disease than are others: mostly those that are frankly neurotropic or hepatotropic. Disease is often biphasic, the initial febrile stage being followed a few days later by a specific syndrome associated with a particular virus. In these circumstances the acute, mild, self-limiting disease can be considered an aborted form of the full syndrome, with virus replication in lymphatic tissue and subsequent viremia, but without significant involvement of target organs such as the brain or liver.

Central Nervous System Disease

Viral encephalitis may be caused by members of the alphaviruses, flaviviruses, and bunyaviruses (Table 73–1). These may cause a mild or inapparent disease, a moderate febrile illness, or severe encephalitis. The clinical manifestations include fever, headache, and somnolence, often followed by vomiting, tremors, confusion, and general seizures. Focal neurologic manifestations or paralysis are unusual. Equines may have fever, uncoordinated gait, tremors, convulsions, and in rare instances blindness. Among these viruses some warrant special mention either because of their high mortality rates—St. Louis encephalitis (8%), Venezuelan encephalitis (10%), and Japanese encephalitis (20% to 30%)—or the enormous number of affected individuals—Japanese encephalitis. It should be remembered, however, that high mortality rates in some outbreaks reflect identification of only the most severe cases; thus direct comparisons need cautious interpretation.

Hepatitis

Arboviruses can cause disease that clinically and pathologically has features in common with acute fulminant hepatitis B infection. In addition to yellow fever, it seems that CCHF and West Nile viruses may also be associated with severe fatal hepatitis, although the number of studies has been small and laboratory and histologic data limited. Yellow fever and CCHF begin abruptly with a high fever and headache, back pain, and severe myalgia. There is often flushing of the face and upper portion of the body. Gastrointestinal symptoms with anorexia are prominent, and severe thrombocytopenia may occur early, often with a frank hemorrhagic diathesis. Current evidence suggests this may involve a consumption coagulopathy with consequent thrombocytopenia. Studies of yellow fever in primates have shown that severe hepatitis is a significant cause of death, and in primates and patients during this period there is a high level of viremia. Although signs and symptoms of yellow fever, including fever, may remit for a few hours, the patient may subsequently worsen with more frequent vomiting, epigastric pain, the appearance of profound jaundice and more prominent and diffuse bleeding. Death is preceded by ever-increasing jaundice accompanied by high serum transaminase levels and acute renal failure, ending with hypothermia, encephalopathy, and coma. The clinical course of CCHF is often equally rapid. Severe jaundice is less common, but the patient's condition deteriorates equally rapidly, with onset of shock and uncontrollable bleeding.

Shock

Although shock may develop at any stage during infection by these viruses, there remains a distinct syndrome of clinical shock associated with volume depletion; extravasation of protein into the tissues; pericardial, pleural, and sometimes pericardial spaces; and proteinuria—all characteristic of the so-called viral hemorrhagic fevers. Five arbovirus diseases are classified as hemorrhagic fevers: dengue, HFRS, CCHF, yellow fever, and Kyasanur Forest disease, but other arboviruses may occasionally cause similar syndromes. Although the shock may be associated with a hemorrhagic diathesis, it is attributable not to the loss of blood but to selective fluid and macromolecular loss through a dysfunctional capillary endothelium. This appears, in most instances, to be due to reversible biochemical dysfunction of the endothelium rather than lytic destruction of the cells by viral, or vasculitic, processes. Patients become diaphoretic and restless, and their extremities become cold as blood and pulse pressures decrease. Respiration becomes shallow and rapid, and frank adult respiratory distress syndrome may ensue, with interstitial pneumonitis, mainly because of vascular leakage. Additional evidence of vascular leakage such as pericardial or pleural effusions, facial edema, and ascites is common. Intravenous fluid therapy can be lifesaving, but fluid balance is a delicate problem, with a high risk of patients dying of overhydration, especially those with dengue and HFRS. Hypoxia, hypothermia, delirium, and coma, often with hiccoughs, are associated with fatal disease.

Hemorrhage

As with the hemorrhagic fevers caused by Arenaviruses and Filoviruses (Lassa, Junín, Ebola), some arboviral infections, especially HFRS, dengue, yellow fever, and CCHF, may begin with evidence of disordered hemostasis. The usual initial manifestation is petechiae, especially in HFRS and dengue; frank hemorrhage, with either epistaxis or mucosal bleeding, may develop in only a few patients (<8%). Intractable bleeding, often with intracranial hemorrhage, remains the main cause of death in approximately 1% of patients with HFRS and dengue who do not survive. Other clinical signs of impaired hemostasis include bleeding from puncture sites and bruising. Bleeding in yellow fever may be severe, but CCHF is unique in that there are often characteristic and extensive ecchymoses. These are signs of a poor prognosis, and uncontrollable bleeding from the gastrointestinal tract is a common consequence.

The pathogenesis of dengue is distinct in that it may be immune mediated. Existing antibodies against dengue serotype 1, 3, or 4 early in life, or the possession by an infant of maternal antibodies—in both instances in low titer—may in fact enhance the infection by dengue 2 serotype. On the basis of in vitro experiments this appears to occur by attachment of infectious immune complexes of dengue type 2 virus to type II Fc receptors on macrophages and other cells of the immune system, presumably increasing the number of virus particles that infect cells of the reticuloendothelial system. Thus dengue type 2, which is normally a mild disease as a primary infection, may be made more virulent by immune-enhanced entry into macrophages and subsequent increase in virus replication. Such immune enhancement has been demonstrated in vitro for other flaviviruses, but its clinical significance is unknown for those other viruses. Nonetheless, direct evidence for dengue virus induction of the characteristic shock and hemorrhagic diathesis by this mechanism or, indeed, induction by immune complexes is at present lacking.

Acute Renal Failure

Although the severe systemic manifestations of the arboviral diseases may be associated with acute renal failure, especially yellow fever, acute renal failure is a major and unique component of HFRS. HFRS begins after 3 weeks or more of incubation, with the abrupt onset of fever, chills, and constitutional symptoms, among which headache and myalgia are particularly prominent. Abdominal pain occurs after 3 to 4 days, along with anorexia, nausea, and vomiting. Classic signs include flushing of the face, neck, and body; conjunctival injection; petechiae that are particularly prominent in the axillae, palate, and upper portion of the body; and tenderness in the renal angle. Proteinuria is copious and invariable. Hypotension with diminished pulse pressure develops after 3 to 4 days, followed rapidly by a phase of oliguria or anuria. Bleeding may occur at this stage or later in disease. A polyuric phase heralds a prolonged phase of convalescence. Permanent renal sequelae are not reported. As with dengue, circumstantial evidence suggests that immune complexes may underlie the pathology of this disease, but at present there is no direct proof of their role.

Treatment

There is no specific treatment for arbovirus infections. However, the broad-spectrum antiviral drug, ribavirin, which has activity against a wide range of RNA viruses, may be effective against the viruses of HFRS and CCHF. It is not effective against yellow fever virus. It may also be effective against encephalitis viruses, such as Japanese encephalitis, although effective therapy in central nervous system viral infections depends on good penetration of drug to the brain. Specific therapy with immune plasma from convalescent patients has been suggested for some diseases such as CCHF, but its benefits are uncertain, and the risk of using unscreened plasma has to be considered carefully.

It must be emphasized that specific therapy has to be instituted early for any hope of success because much of the pathology caused by these viruses is already well established early in infection, and by the time of hospitalization the disease may be much less reversible. Infections are self-limiting, however, and for those that require hospitalization good medical supportive care is often sufficient. Management of the fluid balance problems in those infections that induce hypovolemic shock can be difficult, and success depends on careful rehydration without risking fluid overload. Effusions usually clear without active management. Fulminant hepatitis and severe bleeding with or without hepatitis present the greatest difficulty, and until the processes underlying the bleeding become clearer, which may be difficult for each virus, recommendations are for replacement—again, with care to avoid overload. In the absence of evidence for a primary role for disseminated intravascular coagulation, heparin therapy is potentially dangerous.

Vaccination

The 17-D strain of yellow fever virus has been an effective and a safe vaccine since the 1940s. It has been widely used, is responsible for a great degree of the control of yellow fever, and has the enormous advantage of being highly effective, probably for life, after a single injection. The problem is now that it is not delivered to all or even to a significant portion of the population at risk. That outbreaks continue to occur is an indictment of the care systems that fail to deliver such an effective, inexpensive, and safe remedy to those who need it. Effective vaccines also exist for Japanese encephalitis and some tick-borne encephalitides. The Japanese encephalitis vaccine is a purified, inactivated mouse brain vaccine, and for reliable protection, three doses need to be administered. An attenuated live virus vaccine for Rift Valley fever virus, made by site-specific mutagenesis techniques, appears highly effective in animals, but it is not yet tested in humans. CCHF vaccines are reported to be used in Bulgaria and China, but data on efficacy and safety in clinical trials are not available. Vaccine candidates for dengue are being developed and evaluated, including a monovalent, live attenuated vaccine that has reached clinical trials. Concern about immune enhancement from prior exposure to dengue virus makes the development of a dengue vaccine a complex undertaking. To be effective, however, arbovirus vaccines need to be delivered early in life, preferably with the childhood vaccine programs. Because of the zoonotic reservoirs, eradication is presently impracticable, and indefinite surveillance will be needed to achieve control.

FURTHER READING

Books and Reviews

Calisher CH, Thompson WH: California serogroup viruses. Prog Clin Biol Res vol 123, 1983

The epidemiology of mosquito-borne virus encephalitides in the United States, 1943–1987. Am J Trop Med Hyg 37(suppl):1, 1987

Halstead SB: Dengue. Trop Geogr Med 72:675, 1990

Johnson RT: Arboviral encephalitis. Trop Geogr Med 74:691, 1990

McCormick JB, Fisher-Hoch SP: Viral hemorrhagic fevers. Trop Geogr Med 75:700, 1990

Monath TP (ed): The Arboviruses: Epidemiology and Ecology, vols I-V. Boca Raton, Fla, CRC Press, 1988

Schlesinger S, Schlesinger MJ (eds): The Togaviridae and Flaviviridae. New York, Plenum, 1986

Tesh RB: Undifferentiated arboviral fevers. Trop Geogr Med 73:685, 1990

Selected Papers

Brandt WE: From the World Health Organization. Development of dengue and Japanese encephalitis vaccines. J Infect Dis 162:577, 1990

Halstead SB, O'Rourke EJ: Dengue viruses and mononuclear phagocytes. I. Infection enhancement by non-neutralizing antibody. J Exp Med 146:201, 1977

Hoke Ch, Nisalak A, Sangawhipa N, et al: Protection against Japanese encephalitis by inactivated vaccines. N Engl J Med 319:608, 1988

Kliks SC, Nisalak A, Brandt WE, et al: Antibody-dependent enhancement of dengue virus growth in human monocytes as a risk factor for dengue hemorrhagic fever. Am J Trop Med Hyg 40:444, 1989

Littana R, Kurane O, Ennis FA: Human IgG Fc receptor II mediates antibody-dependent enhancement of dengue virus infection. J Immunol 144(8):3183, 1990.

Nasidi A, Monath TP, DeCock K, et al: Urban yellow fever epidemic in western Nigeria. Trans R Soc Trop Med Hyg 83:401, 1987

Reed W, Carroll J, Agramonte A, Lasear JW: Etiology of yellow fever: Preliminary note. Philadelphia Med J 6:790, 1900

Rosen L, Shroyer DA, Tesh RB, et al: Transovarial transmission of dengue viruses by mosquitoes *Aedes albopictus* and *Aedes aegypti*. Am J Trop Med Hyg 32:1108, 1983

Theiler M, Smith HH: Use of yellow fever virus modified by in vitro cultivation for human immunization. J Exp Med 65:787, 1937

CHAPTER 74

Rhabdoviruses and Filoviruses

Rhabdoviridae

Joseph Meister, a 9-year-old boy from Alsace, France, was bitten 14 times by a rabid dog on July 6, 1885. Sixty hours after the bites were inflicted, he was taken to Louis Pasteur in Paris. Pasteur had been working on a method of vaccinating dogs with desiccated spinal cords from rabbits that had been inoculated with fixed rabies virus. Despite "real and tormenting" doubts, Pasteur administered 13 subcutaneous inoculations of increasingly virulent spinal cord preparations to the boy over a period of 10 days. The boy survived, and in adulthood Meister became a concierge at the Pasteur Institute. This dramatic experiment more than 100 years ago was not only one of the earliest exercises in experimental medicine, but remains one of the most brilliant in demonstrating the etiology and at the same time effective prevention of what had hitherto been a uniformly fatal human disease. It is one of the most important early applications of basic science to the practice of medicine, one of many by Louis Pasteur. The understanding of rabies, initiated by Pasteur, has led to its eradication in some island nations and more recently by application of newly designed vaccines, to eradication from some sectors of wildlife. However, rabies continues to flourish in many parts of the world, especially in developing tropical countries where domestic dogs remain the primary source of human infection. Enzootic or epizootic cycles in wild vertebrates continue to play an important role in the maintenance of the disease. Other rhabdoviruses also cause disease in humans and animals, but rabies is the most important one.

Human Rabies

Human rabies and its association with dog bites were recognized in ancient Babylon and were dealt with by a wide variety of measures by virtually every recorded civilization since that time. The term *hydrophobia* was used to describe the disease by the Greeks. By the time of the European renaissance period, the clinical disease in humans was well described. Rabies in humans begins insidiously with malaise, chills and fever, headache, anorexia, myalgia, fatigue, and emotional lability. The progression of the disease may take two forms. The fulminant form (furious rabies) is classic rabies with hydrophobia, aerophagia, and extreme central nervous system (CNS) lability, with hallucinations and periods of aggressive behavior, often requiring restraint, alternated with episodes of complete lucidity. The hydrophobia is evoked by multiple stimuli, especially the sound, touch, smell, or even thought of water. It takes the form of a painful spasm of the inspiratory and laryngeal muscles, which can progress to seizures and cardiorespiratory arrest. Episodes of extreme bradycardia are characteristic of rabies; in fact, patients may die from cardiac arrhythmia. Paralytic or "dumb" rabies is recognized in less than 20% of infections. In this form the disease progresses through parasthesias and an ascending flaccid paralysis of the limbs to eventual fatal paralysis of the respiratory muscles. This form of disease may be much more common and may be misdiagnosed as postvaccinial or other encephalitis.

Pathogenesis

Rabies virus (Fig. 74–1) is contained in the saliva of infected animals and is inoculated into tissue at the time of a bite. It replicates in muscle fibers and possibly other cells and eventually reaches neuromuscular junctions. It then replicates in neuronal cells and is transmitted to the CNS through the axoplasm. Subsequently, it spreads to other nerves in the CNS and through those nerves infects other motor, sensory, and autonomic nerves, returning the virus to all of the peripheral organs. During this entire process the immune response to rabies is limited, perhaps because replicating virus is sequestered from those elements of the immune system required

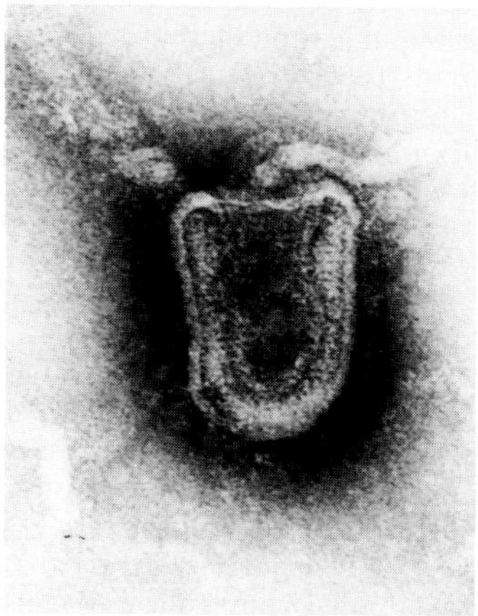

Fig. 74–1. Rabies virus, showing external membrane and internal nucleocapsid structure. × 226,500.

for virus clearance. Thus in natural infection, despite an often long incubation period, little or no neutralizing antibody and minimal inflammatory response are present at the onset of disease. As infection of the CNS progresses, the limbic system is particularly heavily affected, perhaps accounting for the aggressive behavior manifested in cases of classic rabies (especially in carnivores). This may be the key to the survival of rabies virus because this behavior drives the transmission of the virus by causing animals to bite. Large amounts of virus may be recovered from tissue with dense innervation such as exocrine tissues, especially salivary glands, from which the virus may then be transmitted to the next victim.

The mechanism of the virus's effect on nerve cells is not understood. In many instances there is little observable histologic damage to nerve cells, yet large quantities of viral antigen are present. Therefore the effects of the virus may be more on neurotransmitter receptors than on cell destruction, suggesting that some viral effects may be reversible. Most of these observations have been made in animal models of rabies and may or may not apply to the human condition about which only anecdotal data exist. These are important questions for future research on the pathogenesis of rabies.

Although the level of neutralizing antibody against rabies virus glycoprotein is clearly associated with protection against the rabies virus, there is also evidence of a cytotoxic T cell response. The role of the cell-mediated immune response in rabies pathogenesis and in the prevention of illness also is not yet understood. In vitro studies show that neutralizing antibodies prevent the spread of the virus from cell to cell. This may be one of the mechanisms by which the administration of postexposure immune globulin prevents rabies—by stopping the spread of the virus before it enters the CNS where it may be less accessable to antibodies. In vitro studies also suggest that a cell-mediated immune response may be responsible for eventual clearance of the virus from cells and that the presence of antibody may enhance the cell-mediated immune response. However, histologic evidence shows very little cellular (e.g., lymphocytic) response to rabies-infected cells in the CNS. Therefore it is not clear how virus clearance from neuronal cells of the CNS is accomplished, which may be how rabies evades the host immune response. Some evidence suggests that lymphocytes from acutely ill patients with rabies encephalitis proliferate in the presence of rabies antigen, suggesting that indeed a cellular immune response exists. However, patients with paralytic disease do not have such a proliferative response.

Recent advances in the molecular virology of the rabies virus have opened new avenues for understanding its morphology at the molecular level and for controlling its ability to multiply. The rabies virus genome, a single negative strand of nonsegmented RNA approximately 11,000 nucleotides long, has been cloned, and several of its genes have been sequenced, in particular, the G gene. It encodes the glycoprotein that comprises the spikes on the rabies virus surface, functions as the cell attachment protein (and therefore controls the tissue tropism of the virus), and is the antigen that elicits the formation of neutralizing antibodies. As a result, the virulence of the virus can be greatly attenuated by single amino acid changes in critical positions of the glycoprotein; the development of monoclonal antibodies against the glycoprotein that are capable of distinguishing between different strains of the virus has helped greatly to clarify the epidemiology of the virus, and several improved rabies virus vaccines have been developed—among them, an attenuated virus vaccine, a subunit vaccine, and a recombinant vaccinia virus vector vaccine. Many of these vaccines are currently under field trial in an effort to immunize wild animals.

Laboratory Diagnosis

Diagnosis can be made by immunofluorescence on impressions made from the brain, by identification of Negri bodies in the brain, or by mouse inoculation. The diagnosis in humans is best made by identification of antigen in a biopsy of the skin. The result from a brain biopsy, if available, is also reliable, but corneal impressions, although widely reported as useful in diagnosis, have proven difficult to obtain and unreliable for antigen detection. Virus may also be isolated occasionally during the first week of illness from selected sites such as saliva, cerebrospinal fluid (CSF), and sometimes urine, but can be isolated consistently only from brain. Primary isolation of the rabies virus is most readily accomplished in suckling mice, although it does replicate in some cell lines, especially BHK and CER cells. The identification of IgM antibody against rabies virus in CSF or blood is also a reliable indicator of acute infection. The use of the polymerase chain reaction (PCR), in those laboratories with such capability, may greatly improve the sensitivity, rapidity, and specificity of rabies diagnosis.

Prevention and Prophylaxis

The mammalian host range of rabies is so large that the virus can maintain itself by endemic transmission in virtually any area of the world. The areas free of rabies are primarily island nations such as Australia, Great Britain, and Guam, where eradication efforts, combined with strict quarantine measures, have eliminated the enzootic cycles. Rapid and simple transport of infected animals incubating disease may introduce it into an area of no or low infection or, more significantly, reintroduce it into areas with effective eradication programs. This transmission occurs slowly but persistently; therefore a vigorous ongoing program of animal vaccination and surveillance is required to prevent such reintroductions.

The vaccination of domestic dogs and cats is the cornerstone of human rabies prevention in most areas of the world, especially in urban areas where dogs and cats are the major reservoirs. Effective urban control of dog and cat populations is also critical, but often difficult, in densely populated cities. Dogs and cats should be vaccinated against rabies beginning at 3 months of age, followed by a vaccine of 3-year duration given 1 year after the initial dose of vaccine. Dogs or cats that are unvaccinated and exposed to a rabid animal should be destroyed immediately. Vaccinated animals should be revaccinated and kept under owner surveillance for 90 days. The development of genetically engineered vaccines in live virus vectors (such as poxviruses or adenoviruses) that can be placed in animal bait offers the possibility of programs to vaccinate selected wildlife populations as a means of control. Such a program has already had a significant effect on zoonotic rabies in Switzerland, France, and Germany.

When human exposure to rabies is believed to have occurred, prompt local wound treatment and appropriate passive and active immunization are necessary to prevent the spread of virus. The wound is carefully cleaned with soap and water and preferably is not sutured. Inactivated rabies virus grown in human diploid cell vaccine is given at days 0, 3, 7, 14, and 28 after exposure. Human rabies immune globulin (HRIG) is given immediately after exposure or as soon as it is available or any time up to 8 days after beginning the vaccine. Half is infiltrated into the wound area and the other half given at a site different from the initial vaccination site. Previously vaccinated individuals known to have antibody to rabies virus do not usually need HRIG but do require booster vaccinations.

Epidemiology

Rabies is spread to humans in more than 90% of instances by the bites of a domestic dog or, less often, a cat. Despite the availability of domestic animal vaccine programs, an average of more than 300 cats and dogs with rabies is reported each year in the United States. Half the animals are 1 year of age or less, and more than 80% are from rural areas. Dogs at highest risk for rabies are males kept as pets that have contact with wildlife. More than half the cats with rabies are not pets, and they represent more of a risk to humans and other animals, presumably because of more aggressive behavior from rabies. Because of the increased frequency of contact between children and dogs and cats in the United States, a disproportionately large number of cases are in children, although all age groups are equally susceptible. Only a few hundred cases of rabies are reported per year to the World Health Organization, although by all estimates the disease is largely underreported. Also, many cases of fatal encephalitis do not receive an etiologic diagnosis, especially in many of the developing countries. Although most cases of human rabies occur in association with bites of rabid animals, aerosol transmission has occurred in caves with large bat populations presumably heavily infected with rabies. Two laboratory infections have been associated with the generation of large aerosols.

Rabies virus is maintained in the wild by transmission, usually by bites, of the virus between animals, mostly carnivores. Each species of animal involved generally forms its own ecologic and epidemiologic niche. Different species are often the principal wild reservoir in different geographic areas (Fig. 74–2). Thus in the Caribbean, Central America, and parts of South America, vampire bats play an important role, especially in rabies in domestic cattle. In the western parts of the United States, skunks form an important reservoir, and in the eastern part of the United States foxes and racoons maintain an enzootic cycle (Fig. 74–2).

In Europe a slowly progressing epidemic of rabies in foxes is occurring. It is the interface between these wild animal reservoirs of rabies virus and domestic dogs or other animals that plays the principal role in introducing rabies into the human population. Rabies has also been associated with bats in Europe, where a virus closely related to Duvenhage currently is circulating in Denmark and Germany.

In recent years the use of molecular markers such as monoclonal antibodies specific for particular viral epitopes has supplied the tools to begin to understand the strain variation that occurs among rabies viruses. Strains vary both by geographic location and by animal species of origin. The biologic significance, if any, of these strain variations in terms of transmissibility or pathogenicity is not yet understood. Present evidence shows that the currently used and newer vaccines protect against all of the various strains identified by monoclonal antibodies.

Rabies-related Viruses

There are at least five rabies-related viruses, three of which have been isolated from vertebrates. Mokola virus was isolated

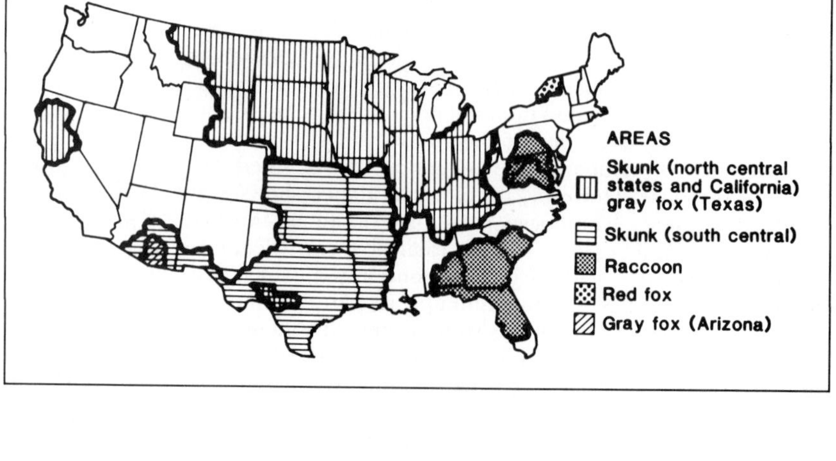

Fig. 74–2. Distribution of five antigenically distinct rabies virus strains and the predominant wildlife species affected—contiguous United States.

from shrews in the district of Mokola, Nigeria, in 1968. Subsequently, it has been isolated from Nigeria to South Africa from a number of humans, some of whom died of diseases similar to rabies and some of whom recovered after severe encephalitis. Lagos bat virus was originally isolated from fruit bats in Nigeria and later from bats in the Central African Republic and in South Africa. Duvenhage virus was first isolated from a man with a disease indistinguishable from rabies who had been bitten by a bat. It has since been isolated again in South Africa and more recently in Hamburg, West Germany, and Denmark, all from bats. Fatal rabies infection occurred in Denmark in an 11-year-old boy from whom a Duvenhage-related virus was isolated. Thus at least some of these viruses cause a fatal disease indistinguishable from that of classic rabies.

Vesicular Stomatitis Virus

Vesicular stomatitis virus (VSV) causes a vesicular lesion in domestic cattle and occasionally affects humans. There are seven related viruses, five of which occur in North America and two others in Asia and Africa. Circumstantial evidence suggests that they may be transmitted by arthropods such as sandflies, mites, blackflies, and mosquitoes. The disease occurs in domestic livestock and is generally benign, but it can emulate foot-and-mouth disease. Human disease is mild and consists of fever, malaise, headache, and myalgias, with occasional gastrointestinal symptoms and occasional vesicles in the mouth. The epidemiologic picture of VSV does not necessarily fit with purely arthropod transmission; more information is needed to understand the nature of the transmission of these viruses.

Filoviridae

Originally considered rhabdoviruses but now known not to be, the Filoviridae have been associated with dramatic and mysterious epidemic disease in humans as well as nonhuman primates. The first of these outbreaks occurred in persons exposed to tissues and blood from African Green monkeys imported into Germany and Yugoslavia from Uganda in 1967. There were 25 primary infections with seven deaths, and all five secondarily infected persons survived. Only people who had handled blood or tissues without protective gloves were infected. A novel virus was isolated and termed *Marburg virus* after the town in Germany where the outbreak was first recognized. Simultaneous epidemics of a fatal hemorrhagic disease occurred in 1976 in Northern Zaire and Southern Sudan. A new distinct virus was isolated. The virus was named Ebola after a river in Zaire. In 1989 macaques shipped from the Philippines were infected with a previously unrecognized filovirus, which appears endemic in Asia. It can cause severe illness in monkeys but seems to be of little or no pathogenecity for humans. Thus the geographic scope of the filoviruses is much greater than previously recognized. Despite many years of study and several outbreaks of human and now nonhuman primate filovirus infections, the natural reservoir of this virus remains one of the mysteries of virology. The filoviruses have a unique morphologic structure; they are the only filamentous mammalian viruses (Fig. 74–3).

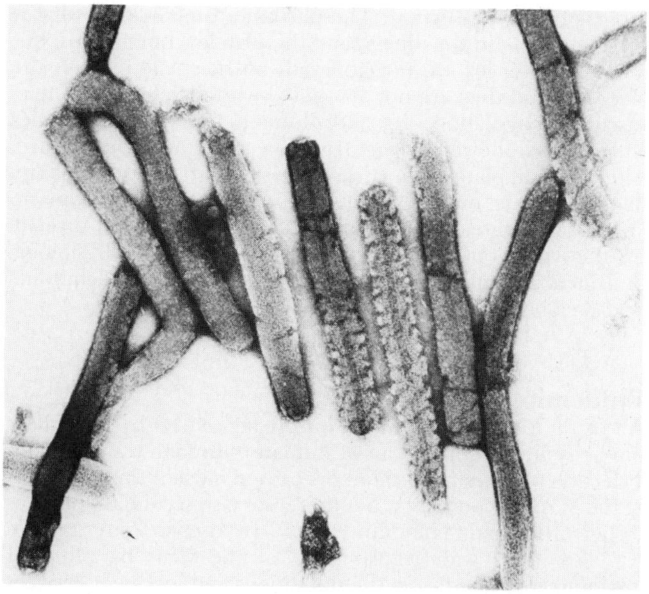

Fig. 74–3. Marburg virus, demonstrating its unique filamentous structure and internal nucleocapsid organization. It is from 900 to 1400 nm long and 80 nm wide. × 75,330.

Clinical Features

The illness is of sudden onset after 7 to 10 days incubation. It begins with fever, headache, weakness, myalgia, arthragia, and lethargy. Gastrointestinal symptoms develop in most patients on the second or third day of illness, with abdominal pain and cramping followed by diarrhea and vomiting. Sore throat is a common symptom, often associated with severe swelling and dysphagia. Bleeding is a hallmark of filovirus infections. The bleeding begins about the fifth day of illness and is most commonly gastrointestinal and mucosal. Death occurs in a large proportion of patients and is associated with hypovolemic shock and severe bleeding (290 deaths in 318 people with infections in Zaire in 1976). Most Ebola virus infections have occurred in areas with few medical resources. The case fatality rate might be substantially lower in areas where modern medical care is available. No antiviral therapy, including convalescent plasma, and no antiviral compounds have been shown effective against human Ebola virus infection.

Pathogenesis

Although Marburg and Ebola viruses cause fatal infections with bleeding and shock in a high proportion of affected patients, histopathologic changes are insufficient to explain the observed physiologic observations. Studies of primates infected by Ebola virus have demonstrated the early development of and progression to complete platelet dysfunction (despite adequate numbers of circulating platelets) and endothelial cell dysfunction. The partial thromboplastin time is prolonged late in the illness, and the platelet count drops, but these occurrences are not generally sufficient to explain the bleeding, and they are not associated with disseminated intravascular coagulation. In both human and animal studies leukopenia followed by neutrophilia is a consistent feature. Alterations in platelet function suggest that the platelets' ability to degranulate may be altered, and they therefore can no longer aggregate. Endothelial cells are not damaged directly by the virus but rather manifest a reversible physiologic dysfunction as measured by a marked decline in arachidonic acid metabolism.

Epidemiology

All of the recognized human outbreaks caused by filoviruses have resulted from a chain of human-to-human transmission. Infection of humans by monkeys caused most of the infections in the Marburg outbreak, but there was also secondary person-to-person spread. The outbreak of 318 cases in Zaire in 1976 was associated with transmission of the virus by reuse of contaminated needles in the outpatient and inpatient services of a hospital. Subsequently, dissemination of the disease into villages was followed by human-to-human transmission within the villages. The outbreaks in Sudan in 1976 (250 cases and 140 deaths) and 1979 (34 cases and 22 deaths) were caused by human-to-human transmissions in the hospital followed by similar transmission within families in villages. The spread of the Asian filovirus among macaques in animal quarantine facilities in the Philippines and the United States appeared to be animal to animal. How the virus was introduced into the animal population is unknown. The great secret remains the original source of the monkey and human infections. Outbreaks of human disease may be unusual because the primary infection from the natural reservoir to humans is apparently rare, or alternatively, it is possible that primary infections do not result in secondary transmission except in special circumstances such as existed in the hospitals involved in the original human outbreaks or in the crowded conditions associated with animal holding facilities in Asia. Thus far there have been few clues to the ecology of the Filoviridae. Searches for evidence of viral infection in many species of animals captured in central African countries have failed to provide any clues as to the possible reservoir. What is clear, however, is that transmission from person to person or animal to animal is a real hazard. The risk factors associated with human-to-human transmission are care of an infected individual, nosocomial infection from contaminated materials such as needles, contact with any secretions, preparation of a body for burial, or occasionally by sexual contact. Aerosol transmission has not been implicated.

Prevention and Control

There is no vaccine or other biologic method of preventing primary infections with filoviruses. However, because most infections result from nosocomial or person-to-person spread in families, the best methods of preventing infection are the early identification of infected patients, appropriate barrier nursing, and the use of isolation to prevent further transmission. Present progress in cloning and sequencing the various genes of Ebola virus will greatly assist in the construction of a genetically engineered vaccine, which would be applicable to hospital workers in endemic areas and to laboratorians.

FURTHER READING

Books and Reviews

Baer GM (ed): The Natural History of Rabies. New York, Academic Press, 1975

Kaplan C, Turner GS, Warrell DA: Rabies, The Facts. Oxford, Oxford University Press, 1986

Koprowski H, Plotkin SA (eds): Worlds Debt to Pasteur. New York, Liss, 1985

Martini GA, Siegert R (eds): Marburg Virus Disease. New York, Springer-Verlag, 1971

Murphy FA: The pathogenesis of rabies virus infection. In Koprowski H, Plotkin SA (eds): World's Debt to Pasteur. New York, Liss, 1985

Pattyn SR (ed): Ebola Virus Hemorrhagic Fever. Amsterdam, Elsevier/North Holland Biomedical Press, 1978

Smith JS: Rabies virus epitopic variation: Use in ecologic studies. Adv Virus Res 36:215, 1989

Wunner WH, Larson JK, Dietzschold B, Smith CL: The molecular biology of rabies viruses. Rev Infect Dis 10(s4):771, 1988

Selected Papers

ACIP: Rabies prevention United States, 1984. MMWR 33:393, 1984

Baron RC, McCormick JB, Zubier OA: Ebola virus disease in southern Sudan: Hospital dissemination and intrafamilial spread. Bull WHO 61:997, 1983

Cox NJ, McCormick JB, Johnson KM, Kiley MP: Evidence for two subtypes of Ebola virus based on oligonucleotide mapping of RNA. J Infect Dis 147:272, 1983

Eng T, Fishbein DB: Epidemiological factors, clinical findings, and vaccination status of rabies in cats and dogs in the United States in 1988. National Study Group on Rabies. J Am Vet Med Assoc 197(2):201, 1990

Fekadu M, Shaddock JH, Baer GM: Intermittent excretion of rabies virus in the saliva of a dog two and six months after it had recovered from experimental rabies. Am J Trop Med Hyg 30:1113, 1981

Fisher-Hoch SP, Platt GS, Neild GH, et al: Pathophysiology of shock and hemorrhage in a fulminating viral infection (Ebola). J Infect Dis 152:887, 1985

Johnson KM, Webb PA, Lange JV, et al: Isolation and partial characterization of a new virus causing acute haemorrhagic fever in Zaire. Lancet 1:569, 1977

Kiley MP, Cox N, Elliott LH, et al: Physiochemical properties of Marburg virus: Evidence for three distinct virus strains and their relationship to Ebola virus. J Gen Virol 69(8):1957, 1988

Kissling RE: Growth of rabies virus in non-nervous tissue culture. Proc Soc Trop Med Hyg 98:223, 1958

Koprowski H, Cox HR: Studies on chick embryo adapted rabies virus. I. Culture characteristics and pathogenicity. J Immunol 60:533, 1948

McCormick JB, Bauer SP, Elliott LH, et al: Biologic differences between strains of Evola virus from Zaire and Sudan. J Infect Dis 147:264, 1983

Murphy FA, Harrison AK, Winn WC, Bauer SP: Comparative pathogenesis of rabies and rabies-like viruses. Viral infection and transit from inoculation site to the central nervous system. Lab Invest 28:361, 1973

Pasteur L: Methode pour prevenir La Rage apres morsure. CR Acad Sci (Paris) 101:765, 1885

Pawan JL: The transmission of paralytic rabies in Trinidad by the vampire bat (*Desmodus rotundus murinus*). Ann Trop Med Parasitol 30:101, 1936

Sanchez A, Kiley MP: Identification and analysis of Ebola virus messenger RNA. Virology 157:414, 1986

Wandeler AI, Capt S, Kappeler A, Hauser R: Oral immunization of wildlife against rabies: Concept and first field experiments. Rev Infect Dis 10(4):649, 1988

Warrell DA, Davidson W, Pod HM, et al: Pathophysiological studies in human rabies. Am J Med 60:280, 1976

Wiktor TJ, Koprowski H: Antigenic variants of rabies virus. J Exp Med 159:99, 1980

World Health Organization: Ebola haemorrhagic fever in Sudan, 1976. Report of a WHO international commission. Bull WHO 56:247, 1978

World Health Organization: Ebola haemorrhagic fever in Zaire, 1976. Report of a WHO international commission. Bull WHO 56:271, 1978

CHAPTER 75

Arenaviruses

Arenaviruses are natural parasites of rodents (and in one instance of bats), in which they establish silent persistent infection throughout life. Thirteen different viruses from five different continents (Fig. 75–1) have been isolated, four of which are known to cause human disease. Lymphocytic choriomeningitis virus (LCMV), the geographically most widespread arenavirus, causes subclinical to severe infections, the latter being characterized by a rarely fatal meningoencephalitis. Junin and Machupo viruses from Argentina and Bolivia, respectively, are closely related and cause severe, often fatal hemorrhagic fever. Lassa virus in West Africa produces a similar disease. All of the human arenaviruses infect rodents either in utero or as suckling neonates, leading to persistent, lifetime infection of the animal and chronic viruria. Contact with rodent urine is considered the major source of human infection, although Lassa virus also is transmitted frequently from person to person.

Immunology

Classic central nervous system (CNS) disease induced by infecting older mice with LCMV is mediated by active cytotoxic T lymphocyte (CTL) response, with infiltration and destruction of nervous tissue. Conversely, immunosuppression of the infected adult mouse cell-mediated immune system results in persistent infection. Observations of persistent LCMV infections in newborn and adult mice have led to seminal ideas in immunology, including self-tolerance, virus-induced autoimmune disease, and CTL and major histocompatability complex (MHC) class restriction. Similarly, persistent infection can be induced in utero or in newborn mice with most arenaviruses. Infections are characterized by a lack of virus-specific MHC class I–restricted CTL activity and failure to clear the virus from infected tissues. The mechanism by which the CTL response to arenaviruses is either eliminated or prevented during infection of the unborn or newborn rodent is unclear. Transgenic adult mice expressing a T cell receptor of appropriate genetic background for LCMV are tolerant of LCMV infection. Such animals show a profound lack of CD+4CD+8 lymphocytes, which are precursors to CD+4CD8– or CD–4CD+8 lymphocytes, suggesting that the elimination of immature precursor lymphocytes may be important in the establishment of arenavirus tolerance in young rodents. An LCMV variant exists, which may or may not establish persistence in adult mice depending on the presence of phenylalanine in position 260 of the viral envelope glycoprotein (which eliminates persistence) or leucine in that position, which promotes persistence. The difference would appear to be the relative ability of the two viruses to replicate in macrophages and lymphocytes. The persistent variant is able to replicate efficiently in both of these cell types, whereas the nonpersistent type replicates poorly. The ability to replicate well in lymphocytes and macrophages may suppress the CTL response to these viruses and allow persistence. The CTL response to the nonpersistent virus is substantial.

A CTL immune response to natural infection by most arenaviruses in rodents is required to eliminate the virus. The CTL epitopes for LCMV for certain mouse MHC haplotypes have been identified on the NP and glycoprotein. Indeed, a vaccine in the form of a peptide replicating a known glycoprotein epitope has protected mice from lethal challenge.

The genome of arenaviruses consists of the large, or L, gene, which encodes the viral transcriptase and another nonstructural protein, and the small, or S gene, which encodes the envelope and nucleoproteins. Virulence of LCMV in guinea pigs maps at least in part to the L gene, whereas MHC-restricted CTL response maps to the S gene segment (Chap. 55). This suggests that the rate of virus replication is a key factor in virulence and that the efficiency of the immune response to viral structural proteins is critical in limiting virus production and reducing disease severity.

These viral elements are undoubtedly also key to human disease, but the complementary host factors related to virulence are not known. However, the nature of the human immune response to arenaviruses depends greatly on the virus. Neutralizing antibodies to Junin and Machupo viruses are sufficient, and probably necessary, for virus clearance and to convey immunity in humans and animals as shown by the successful treatment of acute Junin virus infection by immune plasma that contains an adequate virus neutralization titer.

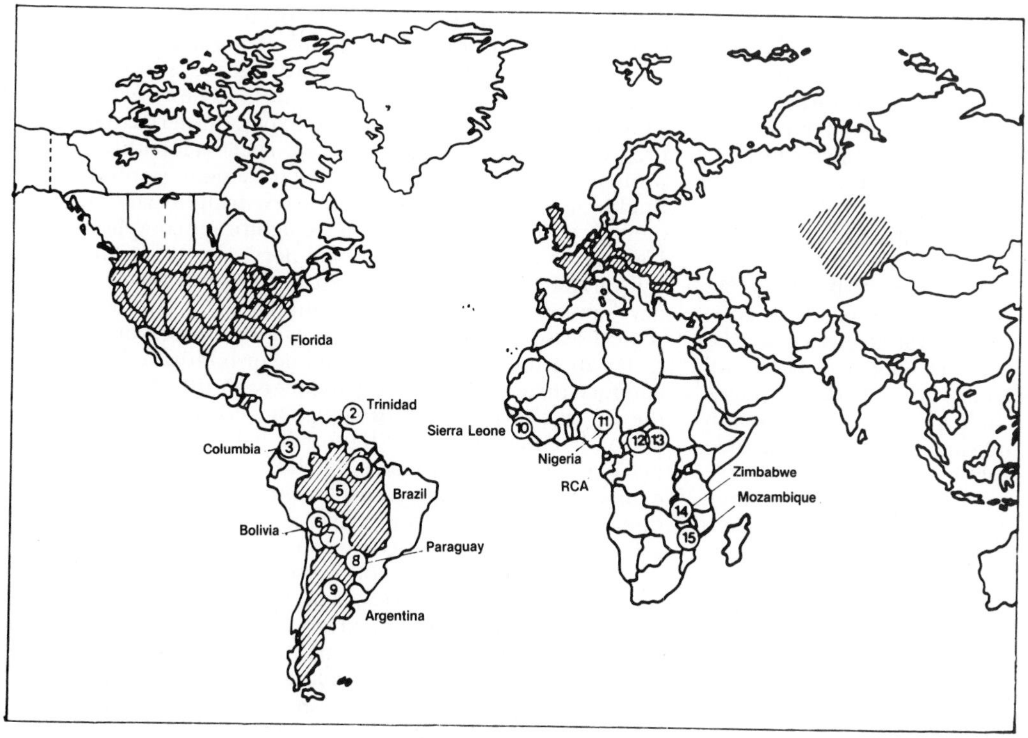

Fig. 75–1. Geographic distribution of arenaviruses. 1. Tamiami; 2. Tacaribe; 3. Pichinde; 4. Flexal; 5. Amapari; 6. Machupo; 7. Latino; 8. Parana; 9. Junin; 10,11. Lassa; 12. Mobala; 13. Ippy; 14,15. Mopeia. In gray, the geographic distribution of lymphocytic choriomeningitis virus.

Although a substantial cell-mediated immune response is also induced, whether it is sufficient or even necessary for virus clearance is uncertain. Presently, a live attenuated Junin virus vaccine against Argentinian hemorrhagic fever (AHF) is in a phase 3 trial in Argentina. All of the initial phases of the vaccine testing have been promising, but final proof of efficacy is another 1 to 2 years away.

In contrast, clearance of Lassa virus by infected humans is not related to the development of serum antibodies. Indeed, plasma from humans convalescent from Lassa fever rarely contains in vitro neutralizing antibodies, despite the fact that antibodies to all structural proteins are present. Furthermore, patients with Lassa fever continue to have high viremia well after the development of a brisk humoral immune response. Studies in one area of West Africa have shown that human Lassa fever does not respond to therapy with convalescent plasma.

Work with inactivated, recombinant, and live vaccines to Lassa virus suggest that a cell-mediated immune response to Lassa virus is both necessary and sufficient to protect monkeys from a lethal dose of Lassa virus. Killed vaccine induces a substantial immune response to structural proteins, but no neutralizing antibody is produced, no limitation of virus replication occurs, and, consequently, no protection from lethal challenge is afforded. Live recombinant vaccinia virus expressing the glycoprotein of Lassa virus induces little measurable antibody to the envelope protein, yet protection from lethal challenge is induced. The same is true for live virus vaccine. The human and experimental vaccine data taken together speak strongly for the importance of the cellular immune response to Lassa virus in protection and virus elimination.

Lassa Fever

Lassa virus causes Lassa fever, a disease found in West Africa from the northeastern plains of Nigeria to the forests of Guinea, an area encompassing nearly 100 million people. Human infection occurs primarily from contact with the commensal rodent *Mastomys natalensis,* ubiquitous in West Africa and the only known reservoir of Lassa virus. Human-to-human transmission also occurs. Human infection occurs year-round, with increases during the dry season. Transmission occurs primarily in houses in which *Mastomys* may comprise 50% or more of the rodents. Human infection appears to occur primarily through contact with rodent urine deposited on surfaces such as floors, tables, and beds in infested houses. Human-to-human transmission may account for 10% to 20% of cases. The disease is believed to be more common in rural areas, but the rapid urbanization of many areas of West Africa appears to have opened the door for *Mastomys* invasion of larger cities, as evidenced by cases occurring in these cities. The incidence of infection varies widely from village to village, ranging from less than 1/100 population per year in coastal areas where *Mastomys* are less abundant to as high as 15 to 20 infections per 100 population per year in the most active villages in the savannah and secondary forest areas where *Mastomys* proliferate. Large scale (>75%) reduction of rodent populations in high-incidence villages has a short-term effect on the incidence of disease.

Lassa fever begins with the gradual onset of fever, weakness, and malaise after 7 to 18 days of incubation. More than half the patients develop joint and lumbar pain and a nonproductive cough by the fourth day of illness. Severe frontal headache and a painful sore throat develop in 70% of patients by the fifth day of illness. Many also develop severe retrosternal chest pain, and about half will have vomiting or diarrhea and abdominal pain. Those developing more severe illness requiring hospitalization are usually admitted between the fourth and eighth illness day when a typical physical examination reveals fever and an elevated respiratory rate (22 to 25) and pulse (>100). The blood pressure may be low at admission. Seventy percent have pharyngitis, often exudative, and conjunctivitis occurs in about one third of patients. Respiratory signs often include fine diffuse rales suggesting pneumonitis, and pleural effusions are common (7% to 10%). Pericardial rubs are also common, with variable electrocardiographic changes, but usually they are not associated with clinical manifestations of myocarditis. A syndrome of polyserositis has been observed in some patients weeks or months after the acute episode. This syndrome may include effusions into the pleural, pericardial, and abdominal cavities, with fever and generalized edema. Lassa virus is not present in the fluids, but high titered antibodies to Lassa virus are present. Pericardial effusion with tamponade and resultant congestive heart failure may occasionally occur in the convalescent period.

The abdomen is tender in half of hospitalized patients. Edema of the face and neck is uncommon but is associated with poor prognosis, and it occurs in the absence of peripheral edema, indicating capillary leakage rather than cardiac dysfunction and impaired venous return. The severity of Lassa fever is highly associated with the level of viremia and ultimately with the rate of virus replication. This association is reflected in a more practical and useful prognostic measure, the level of serum aspartate aminotransferase (ASAT), which increases with severity. Viremia may persist for 4 to 5 weeks, even in the presence of a humoral immune response. Although viral excretion has been demonstrated in urine of humans infected with Lassa virus for up to 2 months, there is no evidence of a persistent infection such as that seen in rodents. Proteinuria is highly associated with Lassa fever, occurring in 80% of hospitalized patients. Although the mean white blood cell count in patients with Lassa fever on admission to hospital is 6×10^9 L, there is characteristically early lymphopenia, mild thrombocytopenia, and in severe cases later relative or absolute neutrophilia.

The pathologic changes observed in patients with fatal Lassa fever are few, with variable focal necrosis of the liver being the most substantial. The degree of liver damage is never sufficient to produce hepatic failure. Focal necrosis of other organs is minor. Bleeding is seen in only 15% to 20% of patients, limited primarily to the mucosal surfaces or occasionally to conjunctival hemorrhages or gastrointestinal or vaginal bleeding. However, bleeding is associated with a 50% case fatality rate. Since there is minimal disturbance of the intrinsic and almost none of the extrinsic coagulation system, and there is no increase in fibrinogen breakdown products, and platelet and fibrinogen turnover in experimental primate infections is normal, disseminated intravascular coagulation (DIC) is not a factor. Although platelet numbers are only moderately depressed, in severe disease their function is almost completely abolished by a circulating inhibitor of platelet function. The origin of this inhibitor appears to be the host, where it apparently exerts its effect by interference with cellular second-messenger systems. In the platelet it blocks dense granule and ATP release and thus abolishes the secondary wave of in vitro aggregation while sparing the arachidonic acid metabolite–dependent primary wave. The exact nature of this host-derived molecule is unknown.

Neurologic signs during acute disease are related to severity and may carry a poor prognosis. They usually begin with fine tremors, attributed to an hyperadrenergic state, and progress to confusion then to severe encephalopathy, with or without general seizures but without focal signs. Cerebrospinal fluid is usually normal but with a few lymphocytes and low titers of virus relative to serum. A significant complication of Lassa fever is acute eighth cranial nerve deafness. The onset is invariably during the convalescent phase of illness, and its development and severity are unrelated to severity of the acute disease. Nearly 30% of patients with Lassa fever infection suffer an acute loss of hearing in one or both ears. The mean auditory threshold of these patients is 55 dB. About half of the patients show a near or complete recovery over the 3 to 4 months after onset, but the other half continue with permanent, significant sensorineural deafness. Many patients also exhibit cerebellar signs during convalescence from severe disease, particularly tremors and ataxia, but this usually resolves over a period of weeks to months.

Lassa fever is a common cause of maternal mortality in many areas of West Africa, and there is a nearly twofold increase in the number of third-trimester Lassa virus infections requiring hospitalization, as compared to the first two trimesters, and a corresponding twofold to threefold greater risk of maternal death from infection in the third trimester. Very high levels of virus replication have been found in placental tissue in third-trimester patients. A fourfold reduction was noted in case fatality among women in all trimesters who spontaneously or were therapeutically aborted compared to those who were not (odds ratio for fatality with pregnancy intact is 5.47 compared to those with uterine evacuation). The excess mortality in the third trimester may be related to relative immunosuppression of pregnancy. Fetal or neonatal loss is 87%. Lassa virus is present in the breast milk of infected mothers; therefore neonates are at risk of congenital, intrapartal, and puerperal infection with Lassa virus.

Intravenous ribavirin is effective in treating Lassa fever. It reduces case fatality by fivefold to tenfold when administered during the first 6 days of illness and twofold to fourfold when given later in illness. Its effectiveness appears to be related to its ability to reduce or limit virus replication, and therefore it is even more effective in patients presenting with high viremias ($\geq 10^3$ pfu/mL). An accumulation of experience suggests that the severity of Lassa virus infection and perhaps the host response may vary in different regions of West Africa, although the clinical manifestations are the same. Thus disease in Nigeria may be more severe, with higher levels of viremia and a higher case fatality rate than that in Sierra Leone and surrounding countries. More research will be required to characterize these possible differences further, particularly as they relate to both vaccine development and antiviral therapy.

Lymphocytic Choriomeningitis Virus

LCMV was originally associated with sporadic transmission of the virus from feral rodents to humans, probably through direct contact with rodent urine containing the virus deposited in the home. Prevalence of antibody to LCMV in the general population is less than 0.1% in the United States. Case reports are few, and it is possible that the disease is commonly misdiagnosed. Areas of higher prevalence and therefore increased risk of LCMV infection may exist (e.g., in inner cities). LCMV occurs in Argentina, but there are no data from the rest of the Americas. In Europe infection has been found in Germany but not in Scandinavia. Beyond that little is known in Europe and virtually nothing in Asia. Studies in Africa have not found evidence of antibody to LCMV. The largest number of confirmed cases come from contact with infected laboratory or pet mice or hamsters. Since perinatally infected or immunoincompetent rodents such as nude mice may be silently, but heavily infected with virus, the source may often not be recognized until several cases occur. In this setting it may be that high doses in aerosol form are able to infect humans. There has never been a reported case of person-to-person transmission.

In the largest existing study of human LCMV infections, 33 of 94 (35%) were asymptomatic, 47 (50%) were mild-to-moderate febrile illnesses without significant CNS manifestations, and 14 (15%) were typical LCMV. Although rarely fatal, the disease can be severe, resulting in hospitalization and a prolonged convalescence. The typical disease in humans follows an incubation period of 1 to 3 weeks, with fever, malaise, weakness, anorexia, nausea, myalgia, and severe, often retro-orbital headache with photophobia. Fifty percent of patients have sore throat, vomiting, arthralgias, or all three, with chest pain and pneumonitis occurring less frequently. Alopecia, orchitis, and transient arthritis of the hands have been reported. Physical examination shows pharyngeal inflammation, usually without exudate. More severely ill patients have meningeal signs, including nuchal rigidity, about one third of whom will develop encephalopathy, whereas the rest will exhibit primarily aseptic meningitis. Convalescence is prolonged, with persistent fatigue, somnolence, and dizziness. Neurologic sequelae are unusual but have been reported, including a single reported case of permanent unilateral deafness similar to that with Lassa fever. The white blood cell count is often 3000/mm^3 or less, with mild thrombocytopenia; but a bleeding tendency has never been reported, and the major pathology apparently involves the leptomeninges. In one report of a fatal case with primarily neurologic manifestations there was evidence of perivascular infiltration of macrophages in multiple areas of the brain. Antigen was observed in the meninges and cortical cells by indirect fluorescent antibody (IFA), consistent with virus replication in the CNS. In animal studies the leptomeninges have been densely infiltrated with lymphocytic cells containing antigen, with little involvement of the brain parenchyma.

Junin Virus

Argentinian hemorrhagic fever (AHF), caused by Junin virus, was first recognized in the 1950s in northwestern Buenos Aires Province, Argentina, an area of very fertile farmland. More than 25,000 cases have been reported, with peak incidence in May. The disease has spread over the 30 years or so since its recognition from an area of 16,000 km^2 and a quarter of a million persons to an area greater than 120,000 km^2 containing a population of more than 1 million persons. AHF is predominant in adult males and has a seasonal peak in the harvest season of April and May when there is frequent contact with the major rodent hosts, *Calomys* sp., during the harvest of corn, sorghum, and sunflower fields.

The major route of human infection is through contact with virus-infected dust and grain products through cuts and abrasions on the skin or through airborne dust generated primarily by killing and scattering of rodents during mechanized farming. All ages and both sexes are susceptible, but most victims are male agricultural workers. Recent data from the endemic area show an overall antibody prevalence in humans of 12%, with typical predominance still in agriculture workers, and an illness to infection ratio of approximately 2:3. However, no data are available from this study on the size of the population actually at risk of infection based on their occupation.

The clinical aspects of AHF and Bolivian hemorrhagic fever (BHF) are similar, with insidious onset of malaise, fever, general myalgia, and anorexia. Lumbar, epigastric, and retro-orbital pain, often with photophobia, nausea, vomiting, and constipation, occur commonly. Unlike LCM and Lassa fever, respiratory symptoms and sore throat are infrequent in AHF and BHF. Conjunctivitis and erythema of the face, neck, and thorax are prominent, and petechiae may be observed in the axillae by the fourth or fifth day of the illness, with pharyngeal enanthem but no pharyngitis. The second stage of illness manifests as epistaxis or hematemesis or both, pulmonary edema, or acute neurologic disease. In contrast to patients with Lassa fever or LCM, bleeding is seen in nearly half of the patients, either from mucosal surfaces or into the skin. Up to 70% of patients with BHF and AHF experience hypotension, accounting for death in the majority of fatal cases. Fifty percent of AHF and BHF patients also have tremors of the hands and tongue, progressing in some patients to delirium, oculogyria, and strabismus.

Lymphopenia ($<1000/\text{mm}^3$) and thrombocytopenia ($<100{,}000/\text{mm}^3$) are invariable. Proteinuria is common, sometimes with microscopic hematuria. Alterations in clotting functions are minor, and DIC is not a significant part of the diseases. Liver and renal function test results are only mildly abnormal. As in patients with Lassa fever or LCM, convalescence is long (3 to 6 weeks) and is characterized by weakness, weight loss, autonomic instability, and occasionally allopecia.

Bolivian Hemorrhagic Fever

BHF was recognized in 1959, and by 1962 more than 1000 cases with a 22% case fatality rate had been identified in an area of two provinces in the Beni area of Bolivia, to which the human disease has always been confined. The cause, Machupo virus, was first isolated in 1964. The only known reservoir is *Calomys callosus*, a cricetid rodent found in highest density at the borders of tropical grassland and forest. The distribution of this rodent includes the eastern Bolivian plains, northern Paraguay, and adjacent areas of western Brazil. The largest known epidemic of BHF, involving several hundred cases, occurred in the town of San Joaquin in 1963 and 1964. This outbreak followed a marked increase in the *Calomys* population and their invasion of the town. They normally favor a rural habitat and avoid man. There has not been any increase in the geographic areas affected by BHF in the last decade, and virtually no cases have been reported.

AHF and BHF closely resemble each other, but their patients differ from those with Lassa fever by characteristically having a skin rash, petechiae, and bleeding. Bleeding is more pronounced with AHF and BHF than with Lassa fever, but it is not the cause of shock and death. There is mild edema of the vascular walls, with capillary swelling and perivascular hemorrhage and large areas of intraalveolar or bronchial hemorrhage without inflammation. Proteinuria frequently is present, and acute tubular necrosis occurs in about half the fatal cases. Capillary leakage is significant but with no evidence for disseminated intravascular coagulation (DIC). Although the petechiae suggest direct endothelial damage, no clear evidence of virus replication in and damage of endothelium has been demonstrated.

FURTHER READING

Books and Reviews

Ahmed R, Stevens JG: Viral persistence. In Fields BN (ed): Virology, ed 2. New York, Raven Press, 1990

Armstrong C, Lillie RD: Experimental lymphocytic choriomeningitis of monkeys and mice produced by a virus encountered in studies of the 1933 St. Louis encephalitis epidemic. Public Health Rep 49:1019, 1934

Buckley SM, Casals J, Downs WG: Isolation and antigenic characterization of Lassa virus. Nature 227:174, 1970

Cole GA, Nathansen N, Pendergast RA: Requirement for theta-bearing cells in lymphocytic choriomeningitis virus-induced central nervous system disease. Nature 238:335, 1972

Frame JD, Baldwin JM Jr, Gocke DJ, Troup JM: Lassa fever, a new virus disease of man from West Africa. I. Clinical description and pathological findings. Am J Trop Med Hyg 73:219, 1970

Jahrling PB, Hesse RA, Eddy GA, et al: Lassa virus infection of rhesus monkeys: Pathogenesis and treatment with ribavirin. J Infect Dis 141:580, 1980

McCormick JB: The arenaviruses. In Fields BN (ed): Virology, ed 2. New York, Raven Press, 1990

McCormick JB, Fisher-Hoch SP: Viral hemorrhagic fevers. In Mahmoud AF, Warren KS (eds): Tropical and Geographical Medicine, ed 2. New York, McGraw-Hill, 1989

Oldstone MBA (ed): Arenaviruses: Biology and Immunotherapy. New York, Springer-Verlag, 1987

Oldstone MBA (ed): Arenaviruses: Genes, Proteins and Expression. New York, Springer-Verlag, 1987

Selected Papers

Cummins D, McCormick JB, Bennett D, et al: Acute sensorineural deafness in Lassa fever. JAMA 16:2093, 1990

Fisher-Hoch SP, McCormick JB, Sasso D, Craven RB: Hematologic dysfunction in Lassa fever. J Med Virol 26:127, 1988

Fisher-Hoch SP, McCormick JB, Auperin D, et al: Protection of rhesus monkeys from fatal Lassa fever by vaccination with a recombinant vaccinia virus containing the Lassa virus glycoprotein gene. Proc Natl Acad Sci U S A 85:317, 1989

Fisher-Hoch SP, Mitchell SW, Sasso DR, et al: Physiologic and immunologic disturbances associated with shock in a primate model of Lassa fever. J Infect Dis 155(3):465, 1986

Holmes GP, McCormick JB, Trock SC, et al: Lassa fever in the United States: Investigation of a case and new guidelines for management. N Engl J Med 323:1120, 1990

Johnson KM: Epidemiology of Machupo virus infection. III. Significance of virological observations in man and animals. Am J Trop Med Hyg 14:816, 1965

Johnson KM, Mackenzie RB, Webb PA, Kuns ML: Chronic infection of rodents by Machupo virus. Science 150:1618, 1965

Klavinskis LS, Whitton JL, Oldstone MB: Molecularly engineered vaccine which expresses an immunodominant T-cell epitope induces cytotoxic T-lymphocytes that confer protection from lethal virus infection. J Virol 63:4311, 1989

MacKenzie RB: Epidemiology of Machupo virus infection. I. Pattern of human infection, San Joaquin, Bolivia, 1961–1964. Am J Trop Med Hyg 14:808, 1965

Maiztegui JI, Fernandez NJ, de Damilano AJ: Efficacy of immune plasma in treatment of Argentine haemorrhagic fever and association between treatment and a late neurological syndrome. Lancet 2:1216, 1979

Matloubian M, Somasundaram T, Kolhekar SR, et al: Genetic basis of viral persistence: Single amino acid change in the viral glycoprotein affects ability of lymphocytic choriomeningitis virus to persist in adult mice. J Exp Med 172:1043, 1990

McCormick JB, King IJ, Webb PA, et al: A case-control study of clinical diagnosis and course of Lassa fever. J Infect Dis 155:445, 1987

McCormick JB, Webb PA, Krebs JW, et al: A prospective study of the epidemiology and ecology of Lassa fever. J Infect Dis 155:437, 1986

McCormick JB, Webb PA, Scribner CL, et al: Lassa fever: Effective therapy with ribavirin. N Engl J Med 314:20, 1986

Monath TP, Newhouse VF, Kemp GE, et al: Lassa virus isolation from *Mastomys natalensis* rodents during an epidemic in Sierra Leone. Science 185:263, 1974

Oldstone MBA, Sinha YN, Blount P, et al: Virus induced alterations in homeostasis: Alterations in differentiated functions of infected cells in vivo. Science 218:1125, 1982

Parodi AA, Greenway JD, Rugiero HR, et al: Sobre la etiologia del brote epidemico de Junin. El Dia Medico 30:2300, 1958

Price ME, Fisher-Hoch SP, Craven RB, McCormick JB: Prospective study of maternal and fetal outcome in acute Lassa fever during pregnancy. Br Med J 297:584, 1988

Rivers TM, Scott TFM: Meningitis in man caused by a filterable virus. Science 81:439, 1935

Riviere Y, Southern PJ, Ahmsad R, Oldstone MC: Biology of cloned cytotoxic T lymphocytic specific for LCM virus. V. Recognition is restricted to gene producers encoded by the viral sRNA segment. J Immunol 136(1):304, 1986

Ruo SL, Mitchell SW, Kiley MP, et al: Antigenic relatedness between arenaviruses defined at epitopic level by monoclonal antibodies. J Gen Virol 1991 (in press)

Traub E: Factors influencing the persistence of choriomeningitis virus in the blood of mice after clinical recovery. J Exp Med 68:229, 1938

Weber EL, Buchmeier MJ: Fine mapping of a peptide sequence containing an antigenic site conserved among arenaviruses. Virology 164:30, 1988

Whitton JL, Tishon A, Lewicki H, et al: Molecular analyses of a five-amino-acid cytotoxic (CTL) epitope: An immunodominant region which induces nonreciprocal CTL cross-reactivity. J Virol 63:4304, 1989

Zinkernagel RM, Doherty PC: Restriction of in vitro T cell–mediated cytotoxicity in lymphocytic choriomeningitis within a syngeneic or semiallogeneic system. Nature 248:701, 1974

CHAPTER 76

Hepatitis Viruses

There has been a virtual explosion of information about viral hepatitis over the past 2 to 3 decades. Although clinically described for many years, the recognition of multiviral causation and distinctive epidemiologic features, the isolation and biochemical characterization of the viruses, and the development of effective control measures have occurred only in the past 30 years. This chapter summarizes the current state of knowledge about these hepatitis-related viruses and their associated diseases.

Characterization of Hepatitis Viruses

The hepatitis viruses consist of at least five human pathogens: hepatitis A (HAV), hepatitis B (HBV), hepatitis C (HCV) or parenterally transmitted non-A, non-B hepatitis, delta (δ)-associated hepatitis (HDV), and hepatitis E (HEV) or enterically transmitted non-A, non-B hepatitis. Table 76–1 summarizes some of their known characteristics, and Figure 76–1 shows the electron microscopic morphology of HAV, HBV, and HEV and a schematic diagram of HDV. These viruses share the propensity to cause liver diseases of various types, but in most other respects they are very different from each other.

Identification depends on the recognition of the virus-specific antigens and antibodies listed in Table 76–2. Although there is a simple interpretation for each marker, the sequence of emergence or loss of these markers is usually more informative in the definition of specific disease states. Commercially available reagents are available for most of these hepatitis virus markers, the currently preferred choices of methods being radioimmunoassay (RIA) and enzyme-linked immunosorbent assay (ELISA). There are no intervirus, cross-reactive antigens, nor are there intravirus group strains with unique virulence, disease predilection, sequelae, or complications. Within groups the number of strains is limited. HBV has one common subtype (a) and four allelic subtype determinants (d and y, r and w), but HAV, HCV, HDV, and HEV are all thought to be single strains.

Although the human viruses are very different in many fundamental respects, several have unique and distinctive features such as the synthesis of the DNA plus strand of HBV DNA on an RNA template by a reverse transcriptase mechanism such as that found in retroviruses. Another unique feature is the absolute dependence of the RNA-containing HDV on the coexistence of infection with HBV, the surface antigen (HBsAg) of which serves as the surrounding coat as noted in Figure 76–1D. Finally, the identification of at least one of the major immunoreactive peptides of HCV by primary cloning of a viral gene in a λgT11 expression vector constitutes the first use of this powerful technique to detect uncharacterized pathogens.

Pathogenesis and Pathology

Acute viral hepatitis associated with all classes of the virus consists of variable amounts of infiltration by inflammatory cells and parenchymal necrosis in the portal and periportal areas on examination by light microscopy. There are no reliable distinguishing pathologic features between the hepatitis viruses by light or electron microscopy, but the immunoperoxidase stains for viral antigens are specific when tissue is available. The intensity of the inflammatory reaction correlates only very roughly with the severity of the acute self-limited disease and does not accurately predict persistence of the viral infection with the development of chronic infection or the carrier state. Acute fulminant hepatitis may occur with any of the human virus infections, and pathologically the liver is small and devoid of recognizable liver architecture. Generally, other organs are not directly affected by the hepatitis viruses.

The mechanism of liver injury is incompletely understood. Although a direct cytopathic effect may contribute to the areas of necrosis, neither HBV nor HCV is known to be

TABLE 76–1. CHARACTERISTICS OF HEPATITIS VIRUSES

Virus	Virus Family	Virus Genus	Size (nm)	Nucleic Acid	Sequenced and/or Cloned	Grown in Tissue Culture	Identified by EM	Specific Serologic Tests	Infectious for Animals	Special Characteristics
HAV	Picornaviridae	*Enterovirus* 72	27	Single-stranded, positive sense RNA, 7.5 kbp	Yes	Yes	Yes	Yes	Yes	—
HBV	Hepadnaviridae	*Hepadnavirus* type 1	42; Dane particle 22; surface antigen	Primarily circular, double-stranded DNA, 3.2 kbp	Yes	Yes[a]	Yes	Yes	Yes	—
HCV	Togavirus-like		36–62	Positive strand RNA	Yes	No	No	Yes	Yes	—
HDV	Defective virus		35–37	Negative strand RNA 1.7 kbp	Yes	No	Yes	Yes	Yes	Requires HBV for replication
HEV	Calicivirus-like		32–34	RNA[b] positive strand 7.6 kbp	Yes	No	Yes	Yes[c]	Yes	Recognized only in developing countries

[a] Reported.
[b] Provisional.
[c] Immune electron microscopy.

directly cytopathic. Because only HAV has been cultivated successfully in vitro, it has been difficult to assess the isolated activity of the other viral classes on individual cells, but HAV does have a cytopathic effect. Other plausible mechanisms of liver cell injury include the participation of the humoral and cellular immune systems to mediate immunocytopathologic effects both in the liver and peripherally such as occurs with immune-complex deposition on articular surfaces. A variety of immunologic phenomena have been documented, but their importance has not been established.

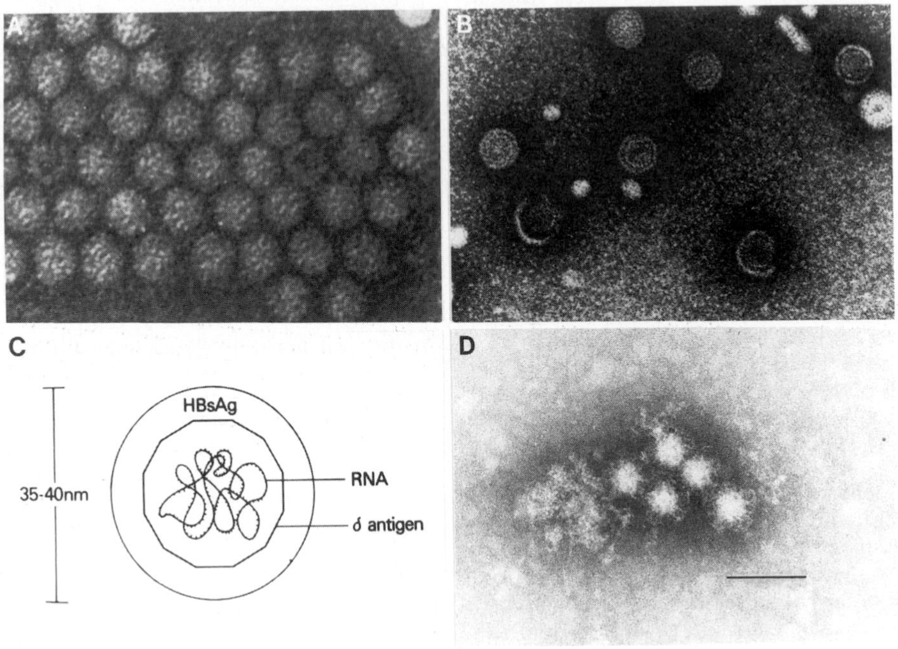

Fig. 76–1 A. Hepatitis A particles, 27 to 32 nm in diameter. **B.** Hepatitis B particles, 42 nm in diameter, with electron-dense core. **C.** Schematic diagram of delta (δ) agent. **D.** Hepatitis E virus (HEV) particles detected by immune electron microscopy. An immune complex of five typical HEV particles (electron-dense with possible surface indentations, diameter of approximately 29 nm) is coated with antibodies that have the staplelike morphology thought characteristic of IgM molecules. The bar at the bottom of the figure represents 100 nm. (**A** and **C** from Hollinger and **B** from Robinson. In Fields (ed): Virology. Raven, 1985. **D** courtesy of John Ticehurst, Walter Reed Army Institute of Research.)

TABLE 76–2. NOMENCLATURE OF THE HEPATITIS VIRUS ANTIGENS AND ANTIBODIES AND THEIR GENERAL INTERPRETATION

	Antigens		Antibodies	
Virus	Name	Interpretation	Name	Interpretation
Hepatitis A virus (HAV)	HA Ag (major antigen of HAV)[a]	Acute infection	Anti-HA	
			IgG	Immune to HAV
			IgM	Recurrent or current acute infection
Hepatitis B virus (HBV)	HBsAg (surface antigen of HBV)	Prior exposure to HBV	Anti-HBs	Immune to HBV
	Subtypes ayw, ayw2, ayw3, ayw4, ayr, adw2, adw4, and adr	Distinctive strains of HBV		
	HBcAg (core antigen of HBV)[a]	Infectivity: acute or chronic	Anti-HBc	Early or late convalescence or chronic hepatitis
	HBeAg (core-related antigen)	Infectivity: acute or chronic	Anti-HBe	Late convalescence
Posttransfusion non-A, non-B hepatitis virus (HCV)	Not available	Not available	Anti-HBc	Late convalescence or chronic hepatitis
Delta-associated agent (HDV)	Delta antigen[a]	Acute delta-associated hepatitis	Anti-Delta	Immune to delta-associated hepatitis (low titer) or chronic HDV
Enterically transmitted non-A, non-B hepatitis virus (HEV)	Viruslike particles by immune electron microscopy[a]	Acute infection	Anti-HEV[a]	Immune to HEV

[a] Research tool only.

Clinical Disease

The acute infection is commonly asymptomatic (30% to 70% of reported cases for each of the five human hepatitis viruses). When the acute illness does occur, it consists of a range of symptoms and signs, including lassitude, anorexia, weakness, nausea, vomiting, headache, chills, abdominal pain, fever, jaundice, and dark urine. Typically, laboratory studies reflect liver cell necrosis manifest most often by impressive elevations of aminotransferases and, less frequently and less impressively, alkaline phosphatase and bilirubin. The laboratory abnormalities precede and follow the clinical illness by 1 to 4 weeks, and the patient is very often ill for 2 to 4 weeks. There is considerable variation in the specific constellation of symptoms and signs in both the acute illness and the longer-term consequences of infection among patients. Exceptions to the typical course include the apparent immune-mediated phenomena (arthritis, arthralgia, glomerulopathy, polyarteritis) associated principally with HBV but also reported in HCV and HDV. Figure 76–2 summarizes, schematically, the clinical and laboratory chronology expected for each virus.

The majority of infections resolve spontaneously over a period of 1 to 6 months, although there may be a waxing and waning pattern to the clinical illness during that time period. Table 76–3 indicates the common and unique sequelae for each agent. The distinctive features follow.

Hepatitis A

Hepatitis A is characterized by an absence of many of the other features found in other forms of hepatitis. In particular, there are no extrahepatic manifestations of the acute infection, no chronic hepatitis, no long-term carrier state, and no recognized association with either cirrhosis or primary hepatocellular carcinoma. A fulminant form of acute hepatitis occurs in about 1% of patients as it does with the other viruses.

Hepatitis B

Hepatitis B differs from hepatitis A in a number of significant respects. First, there is a wide range of extrahepatic manifestations, including arthralgias, particularly of the small joints, and a variety of apparently immunologically mediated diseases such as arteritis, nephritis, and dermatitis.

Second, there are chronic forms of hepatitis B, defined as those illnesses with demonstrable liver injury lasting longer than 6 months. These fall into two general classifications: chronic persistent hepatitis and chronic aggressive hepatitis. Chronic persistent hepatitis is, generally, a benign illness in terms of the ultimate outcome. This form of hepatitis ordinarily is not symptomatic, but patients who are tested show abnormal findings on liver function tests and the persistence of many HBV markers, including HBsAg, HBeAg, and anti-HBc antibody. Liver biopsy findings further reveal the transient abnormalities associated with acute hepatitis and, most importantly, the absence of the more advanced pathology found in the more serious and second form of chronic hepatitis B, namely, chronic aggressive hepatitis.

In chronic aggressive hepatitis the patient is clinically indistinguishable from the one with chronic persistent hepatitis. However, the anti-HBc antibody may be present in very high titer, and the liver biopsy shows widespread lymphocyte infiltration of portal tracts and lobules, piecemeal necrosis, and bridging necrosis. This pathologic picture is a recognized precursor to cirrhosis and possibly to primary hepatocellular

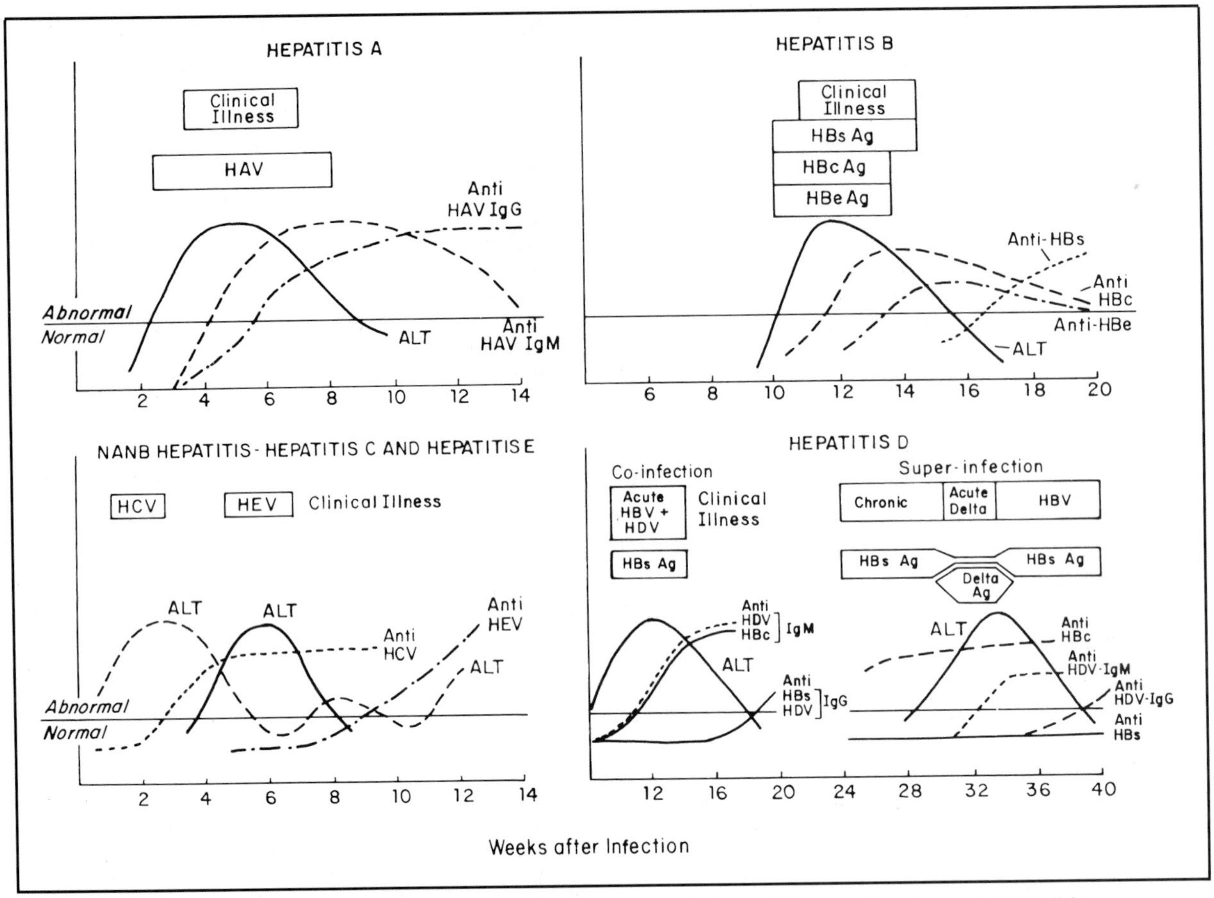

Fig. 76–2. Schematic diagram of the time relationships of clinical illness, laboratory abnormalities, and serologic responses to the hepatitis viruses.

carcinoma. As yet, it is not possible to predict the frequency with which this sequence of events occurs, but the cause-and-effect association seems secure. How long it takes to develop these very serious consequences also is not known. Once it has developed, however, most cases of chronic aggressive hepatitis seem to persist indefinitively. As desirable as the ability to predict which cases of acute hepatitis B will become chronic might be, no reliable markers have yet been identified to allow this prognostication. Risk factors for chronicity, however, include age (<1 year), sex (male), immune status (immunosuppression), and likely other cofactors (HDV).

Hepatitis B e antigen (HBeAg) was described by Magnius and Espmark in 1972. Distinct from either the 22 nm free HBsAg and the 42 nm Dane particle, this antigen is a soluble protein that correlates with HBcAg and DNA polymerase. It is a marker of infectivity, and its presence suggests continued activity of chronic hepatitis. In addition, HBeAg-IgG immune complexes are considered pathogenic in the induction of

TABLE 76–3. CLINICAL CHARACTERISTICS AND CONSEQUENCES OF VIRAL HEPATITIS

Virus	Asymptomatic (%)	Incubation Period (d)	Acute	Extrahepatic Manifestations	Fulminant/ Mortality (%)	Chronic Hepatitis: Persistent (%)	Chronic Hepatitis: Aggressive (%)	Chronic Hepatitis: Carrier (%)	Associated With Cirrhosis/ Hepatocellular Carcinoma
HAV	Children >80 Adults <20	25	+	–	+/1–4	–	–	–	–/–
HBV	>50	75	+	+	+/1–4	2–4	2–4	5	+/+
HCV	75	14–28	+	+	+/0.1	15	30	+/?	+/?
HDV	Unknown	28–90	+	+	+/+	2–4	2–4	5	+/–
HEV	Unknown[a]	22–60	+	–	+/[b]	–	–	–	–

[a] Usually recognized as part of epidemic.
[b] Pregnant women.

membranous glomerulonephritis. On the other hand, antibody to HBeAg correlates with the absence of HBcAg and DNA polymerase, much less infectivity, a better prognosis for chronic hepatitis, and possibly the omission of nephritis. Continued liver disease, however, may be observed independent of infectious virus, and immunopathologic mechanisms may continue to play a role in the pathogenesis.

Third among the differences, the patient with hepatitis B may be a carrier for long periods of time of either the whole, infectious virus or the HBsAg. Approximately 0.1% to 1% of the adult population are asymptomatic carriers, and approximately 5% of the recognized cases of acute HBV infection will become carriers of HBV. Some patients will spontaneously cease to be carriers, but most will persist beyond 6 months after the acute infection. The most likely to be long-term carriers are (1) nonCaucasians, (2) males, (3) infants infected in the newborn period, and (4) those who are immunosuppressed such as dialysis patients, patients who are receiving immunosuppressive drugs, and human immunodeficiency virus (HIV)-infected patients. The carrier may or may not be infectious. No currently available tests make this distinction, but again several types of patients seem more prone to being an infectious carrier: (1) those who have had a recent infection, (2) those who have a high titer of anti-HBc antibody, (3) those who have detectable HBeAg, and (4) those who are immunocompromised. In contrast, those with anti-HBs or anti-HBe antibodies are less likely to be infectious. Hoofnagle has proposed a system that combines clinical, laboratory, immunohistochemical, and nucleic acid hybridization studies to help distinguish the carrier from the patient with chronic hepatitis. From a practical point of view, all carriers of HBsAg should be considered potentially infectious.

Fourth, cirrhosis and primary hepatocellular carcinoma are probable sequelae of hepatitis B. The HBV genome is integrated into the DNA of tumor cells, and epidemiologic studies have confirmed a significant association of HBV infection and hepatocellular carcinoma.

Fifth, perinatal transmission of HBV is a very serious risk to the infants born to mothers who are HBeAg positive. Not only is the efficiency of transmission very high in this setting, but 90% of infants so infected develop chronic hepatitis B. Of all the recognized cases of HBV in the newborn, 95% are acquired at the time of delivery, whereas transplacental transmission occurs in less than 5%. Screening of all women who are pregnant has been recommended by the Advisory Committee on Immunization Practices (ACIP), the US Public Health Service.

Hepatitis C

Parenterally transmitted non-A, non-B (NANB) hepatitis, now known as hepatitis C (HCV), can be identified by a specific serologic test for anti-HCV antibodies. Previously this diagnosis could be made only after the exclusion of HAV (with an IgM anti-HAV antibody), HBV (with HBsAg and an IgM anti-HBc antibody), and a variety of other infectious and noninfectious diseases, such as infectious mononucleosis, cytomegalovirus, syphilis, measles, varicella, rubella, mumps, leptospirosis, bacterial sepsis, cholecystitis, ischemic necrosis, and Wilson's disease. Because the test for HCV measures antibody and because the presence of antibody may indicate only a prior infection or because the absence of antibody may be a reflection of inappropriate timing or immunosuppression, it is essential that other diagnostic possibilities be considered in the individual patient with liver disease.

In addition, it has been clear for some time that more than one virus causes NANB hepatitis. For one there is a wide range of incubation periods: one rather short incubation period (2 to 4 weeks) and the other rather long (16 to 24 weeks). For another, there are second episodes of NANB. Other evidence includes a different route of infection (enteric) and the cross-challenge experiments in chimpanzees, which demonstrated no cross-protection in challenge experiments using prototype viruses derived from human diseases associated with either parenteral transmission or enteric transmission. It is now evident that at least one of the parenterally transmitted forms of NANB hepatitis is HCV and that HEV is the major cause of enterically transmitted NANB hepatitis. Because HCV has not been demonstrated to account for all of the parenterally transmitted NANB hepatitis, others may be found as well.

HCV is the leading cause of posttransfusion hepatitis (PTH). Programs to screen blood for HCV antibody should improve the current screening method, which eliminates blood for transfusion that contains one or more of the NANB-associated surrogate markers (serum alanine aminotransferase [ALT] >75 IU/mL, HBsAG, HIV antibody, history of prior hepatitis or high-risk activities such as sex with a prostitute or another man). A test for HCV antigen, which is not presently available, could be very useful since the additional logistic and financial costs of both screening and donor exclusion are enormous. It is not yet clear what proportion of the NANB hepatitis in other groups such as hemodialysis patients and patients with hemophilia will be accounted for by HCV, although it is very unlikely to be all.

Both chronic, asymptomatic carriers and chronic hepatitis have been documented with HCV. The frequency of chronic hepatitis seems to be even greater with this virus than it is with HBV. Posttransfusion chronic hepatitis may occur in up to 54% of cases. Although the frequency of chronic HCV hepatitis is high, its course is thought to be less severe than that of HBV, with complete resolution common. In some groups with parenterally acquired disease (illicit drug use, immunosuppressed patients, hemodialysis, and HIV-infected patients) HCV replication is enhanced, and liver disease progresses variably—dependent, in part, on the competence of the immune system. Because the immune system seems to mediate the actual disease, it is not unusual for immunocompromised patients to have relatively little disease and modest abnormalities of tests for liver function and yet have chronic progressive histopathologic abnormalities that may be accentuated with improvement of the immune status.

Delta-associated Agent

Rizzetto and his colleagues described the delta/anti-delta antigen/antibody system in 1977. They detected delta (δ) antigen in the nuclei of liver cells of only HBsAg-positive patients with chronic liver disease. Antibody to delta antigen was later found to be associated with, but distinctive from, HBV (it was present in 19.1% of the patients with chronic hepatitis, in 2.6% of chronic carriers of HBsAg, and in low titers transiently in 4.8% of the patients with acute HBV infection), and it was not detected in the sera of HBsAg-negative controls. Patients who had been multiply transfused and were HBsAg-positive had a higher incidence of anti-delta antibody than nontransfused HBsAg carriers did. These data suggested that the delta-associated agent was transmitted both parenterally and nonparenterally by superinfection or coinfection of HBsAg carriers. Animal studies confirmed that it is transmissible and that it requires HBV as some sort of helper while it inhibits the replication of HBV. It has been further characterized biochemically and biophysically and consists of an RNA core surrounded by HBsAg in a particle 35 to 37 nm in diameter. Recent studies suggest that it may be a very important determinant in the development of the carrier state and chronic liver disease.

Hepatitis E

Now recognized as the enterically transmitted form of NANB hepatitis, HEV may be the major cause of hepatitis worldwide. Occurring as the cause of major epidemics in the Far East and little, if at all, in North America, less is known about this class of hepatitis viruses than others, principally because of the difficulty of diagnosis. The disease associated with HEV has been described as especially fulminant in pregnant women, but other distinctive characteristics have not been reported. Now that the virus has been cloned, more readily available diagnostic tools should improve the precision with which the acute and long-term consequences of HEV are understood.

Epidemiology

A consideration of the trends in occurrence, risk factors, and modes of transmission is extremely important for understanding viral hepatitis. During the 15 years from 1970 to 1984, the number of new reported cases of hepatitis of all types has decreased. This decrease is accounted for by a reduction in the rate (cases per 100,000) of hepatitis A from 27.87 in 1970 to 10.39 in 1987. Hepatitis B incidence increased from 4.08 to 10.65 over the same interval. Unspecified hepatitis decreased from 3.95 in 1974 to 1.27 in 1987. The Centers for Disease Control estimates 300,000 new cases of HBV each year, 1 million carriers, 4000 deaths due to cirrhosis, and 1000 deaths from hepatocellular carcinomas in the United States alone. Worldwide the problem is many times greater, especially in developing countries, where the incidence of HBV and chronic carriage is much higher.

Viral hepatitis is transmitted by a wide variety of routes. Table 76–4 summarizes these routes and their relative frequency. HAV is present in the feces of infected patients during the 2 weeks preceding and several weeks following the onset of clinical disease. It may be present in the blood and other body fluids for a short period of time, but fecal-oral transmission of HAV is by far the most prevalent route. The finding of an unexpectedly high incidence of HAV among male homosexuals suggests the possibility of sexual transmission, but more likely, this is due to fecal-oral transmission during oral-anal contact.

For HBV, HCV, and HDV, blood is the major vehicle, although other body fluids may possibly transmit the virus as well. This has been especially well documented for HBV. In contrast with HAV, feces is not infectious for HBV unless contaminated by blood. Not surprisingly then, the usual mode of transmission is by parenteral exposure to viral-contaminated blood or blood products. This mechanism is facilitated because HBV and HCV may persist in the serum of carriers. It is especially important to recognize that blood and blood products from different sources have different risks. Most whole blood and its derivatives, which are not prepared by the pooling of units, have a relatively smaller risk of inducing infection with HBV. This is due to the infrequency of HBV carriage in the normal adult population, the exclusion of potentially infected donors, and perhaps most importantly, the routine testing of donor blood for HBsAg, antibody to HCV, and other surrogate markers. Preparations generally considered safe are serum albumin, thrombin, profibrinolysin, fibrinolysin, immune serum globulin (ISG), and all hyperimmune globulins. At higher risk are blood and blood products derived from commercial (as opposed to volunteer) donors and those derived from pools of plasma and clotting factors I, II, VII, IX, and X. Washed and frozen human blood cells are not reliably virus free and should also be considered a risk. At present posttransfusion hepatitis is most often due to HCV. Hepatitis caused by either HBV or HCV may be acquired by other parenteral routes such as illicit drug use, accidental needlestick, or accidental injury such as might occur during surgery.

Nonparenteral routes of transmission have also been reported for HBV, HCV, and HDV. There is strong evidence that all these viruses, but particularly HBV, may be transmitted by close personal contact, including sexual contact. It is difficult to be certain however, which particular sexual activity constitutes the major risk factor.

Several of the classes of viral hepatitis are increasing in patients who are immunosuppressed such as hemodialysis, transplant, and oncology patients and now patients with HIV infection. This is true for HBV and HCV. In these two instances the immunosuppression appears to accentuate the

TABLE 76–4. EPIDEMIOLOGY OF VIRAL HEPATITIS TRANSMISSION

Virus	No. of Cases 1990[a]	Major Infectious Body Fluid	Route[b]				
			Transfusion/IV Drug Use	Fecal/Oral	Sexual	Vertical	Occupational
HAV	29,000	Feces	–	4+	1+	–	+/–
HBV	20,000	Blood and other body fluids	–/4+	+/–	3+	3+	3+
HCV	3,000	Blood	2+/4+	+/–	1+	+/–	2+
HDV	NR	Blood	–/4+	1+	3+	3+	+/–
HEV	NR	Feces	–	4+	Unknown	Unknown	Unknown

[a] Approximate number and exclusion of cases of "unspecified cause" ~ 2000.
[b] Estimates of relative frequency or efficiency.

TABLE 76–5. RECOMMENDATIONS FOR USE OF IMMUNE GLOBULINS

Virus Exposure	Time of Evaluation	Nature of Exposure	Immune Globulin Recommended	
			ISG[a]	HBIG[b]
HAV	Before exposure	Travel to endemic area	+	NA
	After exposure	Household or day-care center	+	NA
		School or work	−	NA
		Institution	+/−	NA
		Primate handler	+	NA
		Medical and paramedical personnel	−	NA
		Common-source epidemic	+	NA
HBV	Before exposure	Personnel or family members attending an infected patient	−	+
	After exposure	Parenteral transfusion of HBsAg-positive blood	−	+
		Accidental: needlestick, surgical injury, or blood on open wound or mucous membrane	−	+
		Nonparenteral: intimate contact	+	+ (optional)
		Postnatal	−	+
HCV	After exposure	Parenteral		
		Transfusion	+	NA
		Accidental	+	NA
HDV	—	—	−	NA
HEV	—	—	−	NA

[a] Immune serum globulin dose: 0.02 mL/kg body weight within 14 days of exposure if possible; 0.06 mL/kg every 5 months for prolonged travel.
[b] Hepatitis B immune globulin dose: 0.05–0.07 mL/kg within 7 days of exposure and repeated 1 month later.

likelihood of the increased exposure and acute infection to result in chronic infection. Paradoxically, the patients appear to have less attendant morbidity, and the viruses replicate unchallenged, both features presumably due to the compromised immune system. Restoration of the immune system has beneficial effects on the reduction of viral replication but may be accompanied by increased disease, reflecting the dual role of the immune system in the pathogenesis of viral hepatitis.

Prevention

The mainstays of viral hepatitis prevention are the correct diagnosis and reporting of new cases, the attention to standard principles of cleanliness and hygiene, and specific measures to eliminate the sources of infection. Because these methods are only partially successful, additional measures have been used. Passive immunity through the use of immune globulin is one such approach. Table 76–5 summarizes the current recommendations for the use of immune serum globulin or hyperimmune hepatitis B immune globulin. There is general, but not complete, agreement on these recommendations among authorities.

Active immunization is now a viable option for the prevention of HBV. The first licensed vaccine (Heptavax-B, Merck Sharp & Dohme) is a preparation of purified HBsAg derived from the plasma of known chronic carriers of HBV. In studies performed, beginning in 1978, on more than 20,000 recipients, the vaccine induced anti-HBs antibody in more than 95% of normal adult recipients. Since anti-HBs antibody is considered the immunologic defense that confers immunity, it is not surprising that it is 85% to 95% effective in the prevention of naturally acquired hepatitis B. In the same studies, minor self-limited side effects were observed at a rate equal to that of the placebo control, but no serious long-term side effects were observed in the period up to 7 years after

TABLE 76–6. HEPATITIS VACCINE RECOMMENDATIONS

	HBIG[a]	Vaccine
HBV Before Exposure		
Health care workers	−	+
Institutions for mentally retarded		
Staff	−	+
Clients	−	+
Hemodialysis patients	−	+
Homosexually active males	−	+
Users of illicit injectable drugs	−	+
Recipients of certain blood products	−	+
Household and sexual contacts of HBV carriers	−	+
Contacts of populations with high HBV endemicity	−	+
HBV After Exposure; Source HBsAg-Positive		
Perinatal	+	+
Sexual	+	+
Percutaneous		
Previously unvaccinated	+	+
Previously vaccinated with anti-HBs		
Responders (anti-HBs present)	−	−
Nonresponders or anti-HBs absent	+	+
Booster		
Normal hosts <7 years since complete immunization	NA	−
Hemodialysis patients; anti-HBs <10 mIU/mL	NA	+

[a] See Centers for Disease Control: MMWR 39:1, 1990, for recommended doses and schedules of hepatitis B immune globulin and vaccines.

immunization. This vaccine has been given to millions of individuals worldwide who are members of targeted risk groups. In addition, there currently are vaccines prepared by recombinant DNA technology (Recombivax HB, Merck Sharp & Dohme; Engerix-B, SmithKline Beecham) that also consist of purified HBsAg. Although relatively less is known about the efficacy of these preparations, both are licensed for use in the United States. Table 76–6 summarizes the recommendations of the U.S. Public Health Service for recipients of HBV vaccine. Special recommendations exist for the immune compromised patients because of their reduced ability to respond to standard regimens.

In addition, vaccines are being developed for HAV. The approaches include using live, attenuated virus, inactivated virus, and recombinant viral vaccines in selected populations.

Treatment

No specific form of therapy other than supportive care is available for patients with acute hepatitis due to any of the five classes of viral hepatitis. Various forms of treatment have been used in the treatment of chronic hepatitis, some more effective than others in selected patient subsets with HBV, HCV, and HDV. In a review of studies before 1986, no conclusively beneficial therapeutic regimen was found. Subsequently, trials of interferon with or without a prior tapered course of prednisone have demonstrated reduced liver function abnormalities and viral replication for up to 9 to 12 months in as many as 50% to 60% of patients with chronic hepatitis B. The addition of the prednisone taper appears beneficial. Although less well studied, benefits of these or similar regimens have been detected for chronic HCV and HDV. It is not yet clear, however, that these courses of therapy for any chronic form of hepatitis will be durably effective or practical in all patients.

FURTHER READING

Aach RD: The treatment of chronic type B viral hepatitis. Ann Intern Med 109:89, 1988

Alter HJ, Purcell RH, Shih JW, et al: Detection of antibody to hepatitis C virus in prospectively followed transfusion recipients with acute and chronic non-A non-B hepatitis. N Engl J Med 321:1494, 1989

Alter MJ: Non-A, non-B hepatitis: Sorting through a diagnosis of exclusion. Ann Intern Med 110:583, 1989

Beasley R, Hwang L-Y, Lin C-C, Chien C-S: Hepatocellular carcinoma and hepatitis B virus: A prospective study of 22,707 men in Taiwan. Lancet 2:1129, 1981

Blumberg BS, Gerstley BJS, Hungerford DA, et al: A serum antigen (Australia antigen) in Down's syndrome, leukemia and hepatitis. Ann Intern Med 66:924, 1967

Blumer G: Infectious jaundice in the United States. JAMA 81:353, 1923

Bonino F, Smedile A, Verme G: Hepatitis delta virus infection. Adv Intern Med 32:345, 1987

Burke CA: A statistical view of clinical trials in chronic hepatitis B. J Hepatol 3:S261, 1986

Centers for Disease Control: Hepatitis Surveillance. US Department of Health and Human Services. Public Health Services 52:1, 1989

Centers for Disease Control: Protection against viral hepatitis. MMWR 39:1, 1990

Centers for Disease Control: Update on hepatitis b prevention. Ann Intern Med 107:353, 1987

Choo QL, Kuo G, Weiner AJ, et al: Isolation of a cDNA clone derived from a blood-borne non-A, non-B viral hepatitis genome. Science 244:359, 1989

Davis G, Hoofnagle J: Interferon in viral hepatitis: Role in pathogenesis and treatment. Hepatology 6:1038, 1986

Dienstag JL: Viral hepatitis in the compromised host. In Rubin RH, Young LS (eds): Clinical Approach to Infection in the Compromised Host. New York, Plenum Medical Book Co, 1988

Feinstone SM, Kapikian AZ, Purcell RH: Hepatitis A: Detection by immune electron microscopy of a viruslike antigen associated with acute illness. Science 182:1026, 1973

Gerety R (ed): Non A Non B Hepatitis. New York, Academic Press, 1981

Grady G, Lee V, Prince A, et al: Hepatitis B immune globulin for accidental exposures among medical personnel: Final report of a multicenter controlled trial. J Infect Dis 138:625, 1978

Hadler SC, Judson FN, O'Malley PM, et al: The outcome of hepatitis B virus infection in homosexual men and its relationship to prior human immunodeficiency virus infection. J Infect Dis 163:454, 1991

Hollinger G, Dienstag J: Hepatitis viruses. In Lennette EH, Balows A, Hausler WJ Jr, Shadomy HJ, (eds): Manual of Clinical Microbiology. Washington DC, American Society for Microbiology, 1985

Hoofnagle JH: Antiviral treatment of chronic type B hepatitis. Ann Intern Med 107:414, 1987

Hoofnagle JH, Shafritz DA, Popper H: Chronic type B hepatitis and the "healthy" HBsAg carrier state. Hepatology 7:758, 1987

Ishak K: Light microscopic morphology of viral hepatitis. Am J Clin Pathol 65:787, 1976

Jacyna MR, Brooks MG, Loke RH, et al: Randomised controlled trial of interferon alfa (lymphoblastoid interferon) in chronic non-A, non-B hepatitis. Br Med J 298:80, 1989

Krugman S, Giles JP, Hammond J: Hepatitis virus: Effect of heat on the infectivity and antigenicity of the MS-1 and MS-2 strain. J Infect Dis 122:423, 1970

Krugman S, Giles JP, Hammond J: Infectious hepatitis: Evidence for two distinctive clinical epidemiological and immunological types of infection. JAMA 200:365, 1967

Kuo G, Choo QL, Alter HJ, et al: An assay for circulating antibodies to a major etiologic virus of human non-A, non-B hepatitis. Science 244:362, 1989

Lemon S: Type A viral hepatitis—New developments in an old disease. N Engl J Med 313:1059, 1985

Perrillo R, Campbell C, Strang S, et al: Immune globulin and hepatitis B: Immune globulin prophylactic measures for intimate contacts exposed to acute type B hepatitis. Arch Intern Med 144:81, 1984

Perillo RP, Regenstein FG, Peters MG, Al E: Prednisone withdrawal followed by recombinant alpha interferon in the treatment of chronic type B hepatitis: A randomized, controlled trial. Ann Intern Med 109:95, 1988

Perillo RP, Regenstein FG, Roodman ST: Chronic hepatitis B in asymptomatic homosexual men with antibody to the human immunodeficiency virus. Ann Intern Med 105:382, 1986

Provost P, Hilleman M: Propagation of human hepatitis A virus in cell culture in vitro. Proc Soc Exp Biol Med 160:213, 1979

Ratzan KR, Gregg MB, Hanson B: Transfusion-associated hepatitis in the United States: An epidemiologic analysis. Am J Epidemiol 94:425, 1971

Redeker AG, Mosley JW, Gocke DJ, et al: Hepatitis B immune globulin as a prophylactic measure for spouses exposed to acute type B hepatitis. N Engl J Med 293:1055, 1975

Reyes G, Purdy M, Kim J, et al: Isolation of a cDNA from the virus responsible for enterically transmitted non-A, non-B hepatitis. Science 247:1335, 1990

Rizzetto M: Biology and characterization of the delta antigen. In Szmuness W, Alter HJ, Maynard JE (eds): Viral Hepatitis—1981 International Symposium. Philadelphia, Franklin Institute Press, 1982

Rizzetto M, Canese MG, Arico S, et al: Immunofluorescence detection of a new antigen-antibody serum (delta/anti-delta) associated to hepatitis B virus in liver and in serum of HBsAg carriers. Gut 18:997, 1977

Rizzetto M, Hoyer B, Canese MG, et al: Delta agent: Association of delta antigen with hepatitis B surface antigen and RNA in serum of delta-infected chimpanzees. Proc Natl Acad Sci U S A 77:6124, 1980

Robinson WS, Marion PL, Feitelson M, Siddiqui A: The hepadna virus group: Hepatitis B and related viruses. In Szmuness W, Alter HJ, Maynard JW (eds): Viral Hepatitis—1981 International Symposium. Philadelphia, Franklin Institute Press, 1982

Rumi MG, Colombo M, Gringeri A, Mannucci PM: High prevalence of antibody to hepatitis C virus in multitransfused hemophiliacs with normal transaminase levels. Ann Intern Med 112(5):379, 1990

Summers J, Mason WS: Replication of the genome of a hepatitis B–like virus by reverse transcription of an RNA intermediate. Cell 29:403, 1982

Szmuness W, Stevens CE, Harley EJ, et al: Hepatitis B vaccine: Demonstration of efficacy in a controlled clinical trial in a high-risk population in the United States. N Engl J Med 303:833, 1980

Ticehurst J, Cohen JI, Feinstone SM, et al: Replication of hepatitis A virus: New ideas from studies with cloned cDNA. In Semler BL, Ehrenfeld E (eds): Molecular Aspects of Picornavirus Infection and Detection. Washington DC, American Society for Microbiology, 1989

Zeldis JB, Depner TA, Kuramoto IK, et al: The prevalence of hepatitis C virus antibodies among hemodialysis patients. Ann Intern Med 112(12):958, 1990

CHAPTER 77

Human Retroviruses

The discovery of the first exogenous pathogenic human retrovirus, the human T cell lymphotropic virus type I (HTLV-I) (Fig. 77–1) in 1980 opened a new era in the study of human disease. Not only did HTLV-I prove to be the causative agent of adult T cell leukemia, but the techniques first used to isolate and characterize HTLV-I were subsequently used to identify the causative agent of the acquired immunodeficiency syndrome (AIDS), the human immunodeficiency virus type 1 (HIV-1) (Fig. 77–2). More recently, these techniques have been used to identify primate variants of HTLV-I and HIV-1 and to identify and characterize two other human retroviruses, HTLV-II and human immunodeficiency virus type 2 (HIV-2).

Human T Cell Lymphotropic Virus Type I (HTLV-I)

Epidemiology

The original isolates of HTLV-I were made from leukemic cells of patients with aggressive forms of T cell malignancies from the southern United States, Japan, and the Caribbean basin. The clinical syndromes seen in patients with HTLV-I were identical to recently recognized T cell malignancies seen in Caribbean immigrants to London and identical to the clinical syndrome of adult T cell leukemia described in 1977 in Japan. Epidemiologic surveys of serum samples from patients with forms of T cell malignancies demonstrated the presence of HTLV-I antibodies in virtually all cases of Japanese T cell leukemia, in cases of T cell leukemias and lymphomas from the Caribbean, and in some cases of T cell malignancies from Blacks in the southern United States, Ethopian Jews in Israel, and Japanese immigrants to Hawaii. Virologic studies have confirmed the presence of HTLV-I in T cells from seropositive subjects. Comparison of HTLV-I isolates from the United States, Japan, the Caribbean, and Israel has demonstrated them to be the same based on nucleic acid homology. Comparison of a retrovirus isolated by Hinuma and coworkers, called *adult T cell leukemia virus* (*ATLV*), with HTLV-I isolates similarly demonstrated ATLV to be identical to HTLV-I. From studies of worldwide serum samples by Blattner and colleagues, endemic areas of HTLV-I infection have been identified in Asia, Africa, the Mideast, Europe, and the Western hemisphere (Table 77–1).

There is wide variation in the prevalence of HTLV-I seropositivity, depending on population, location, and age. Adjacent villages in Japan have been found with HTLV-I antibody prevalence rates of 0 and 12%. In Japan in subjects without malignancies, seropositivity to HTLV-I rises from approximately 2% at age 10 to 30% at age 60. HTLV-I is clearly an exogenous retrovirus that is transmitted horizontally. A role for sexual transmission of the virus has been suggested by (1) studies of husbands and wives showing that wives of HTLV-I-positive husbands are more likely to be HTLV-I positive than wives of HTLV-I-negative men; (2) antibody prevalance continues to increase in women after age 40 but remains constant in men after that age (suggesting predominantly male-to-female viral transmission); and (3)

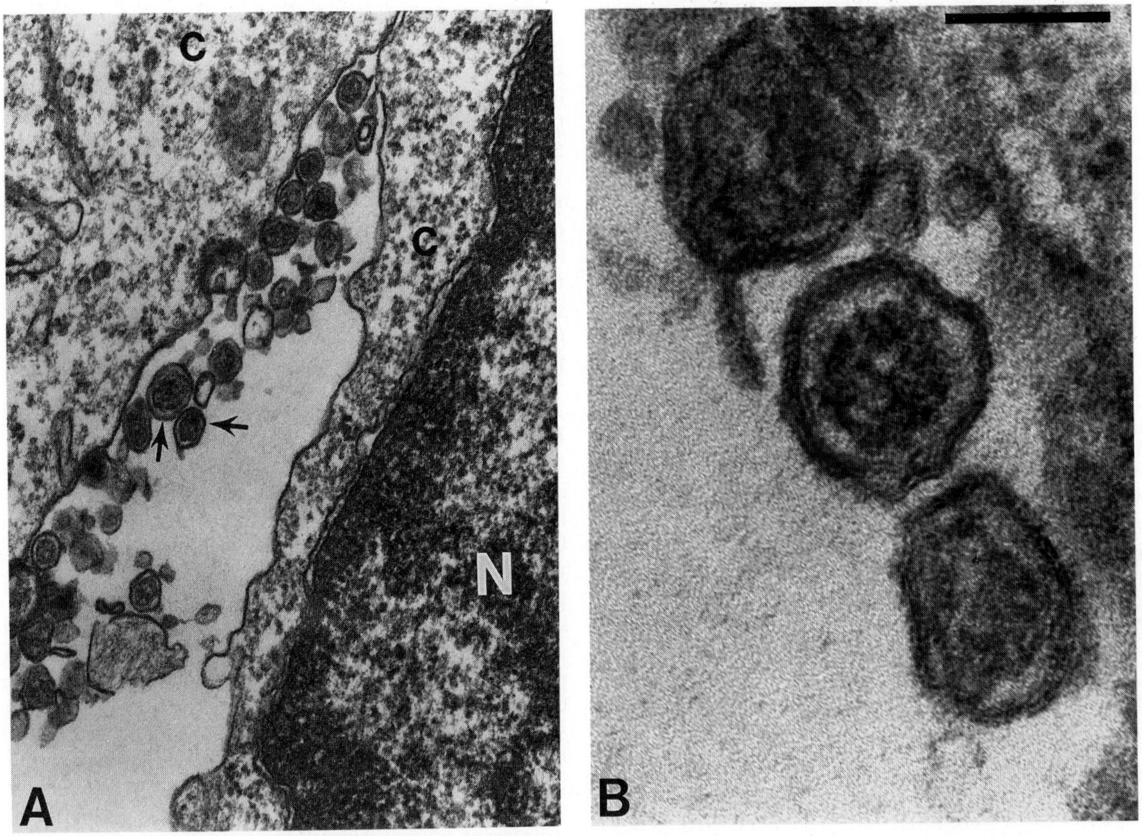

Fig. 77–1. Morphology of HTLV-I. **A.** The cytoplasm (C) of two adjacent T cells with mature extracellular HTLV-I virions (arrows) between the cells. N, nucleus of T cell on the right. **B.** High magnification of three extracellular HTLV-I mature virions. Bar, 0.1 μM. (**B** from Haynes; Proc Natl Acad Sci USA 229:675–679, 1985.)

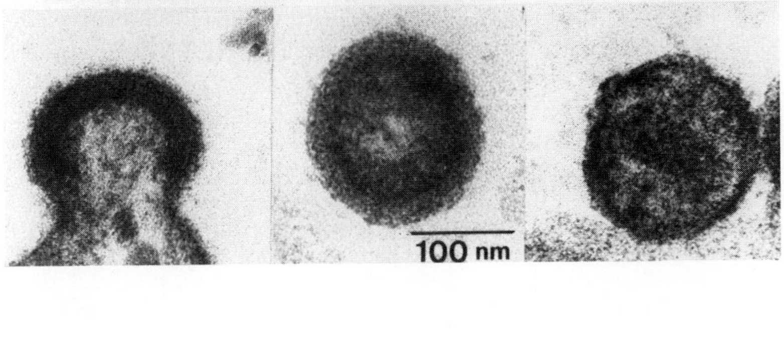

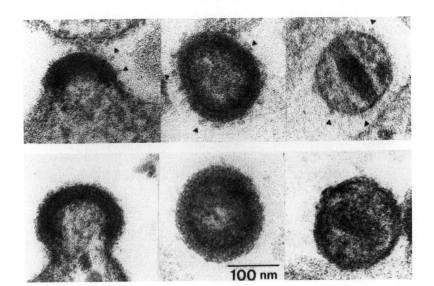

Fig. 77–2. Morphology of HIV-1 **(top row)** and HIV-2 **(bottom row).** Arrowheads indicate the presence of surface envelope spikes. Left panels show budding particles; center panels show immature particles; right panels show mature virions. (From Clavel et al: Science 233:343, 1986. Copyright 1986 by the American Association for the Advancement of Science.)

TABLE 77–1. ENDEMIC AREAS OF HTLV-I INFECTION

Asia	Western Hemisphere
Kyushu, Japan	Jamaica
Shikolu, Japan	Trinidad
Okinawa, Japan	Martinique
New Guinea	Guadeloupe
Africa and Mideast	Venezuela
Nigeria	Panama
Ghana	Columbia
Zaire	Guyana
Uganda	Southern United States (African-Americans)
Israel (Ethiopian Jews)	Hawaii (Japanese immigrants)
Europe	
England (Caribbean immigrants)	
Southern Italy	

Adapted from Clark, Blattner, Gallo; Harrison's Textbook of Medicine Update No. 8. New York, McGraw-Hill, 1985.

HTLV-I-positive lymphocytes in semen have been detected in seropositive men.

Family studies of HTLV-I-positive subjects have suggested that parent-to-child transmission can occur within the household setting since the prevalence of HTLV-I antibodies is higher in family members of HTLV-I-positive subjects than in the general population. Moreover, lymphocytes infected with HTLV-I have been found in the milk of antibody-positive mothers. HTLV-I-infected cells have also been detected in the cord blood of a child born to a seropositive mother, demonstrating that infection with HTLV-I can occur in utero. Finally, transmission of HTLV-I has also been shown to occur through parenteral administration of blood or blood products. This is evidenced by the documentation of transfusion-associated cases of HTLV-I infection and by the presence of HTLV-I antibodies in some intravenous (IV) drug users and patients with hemophilia. Thus the majority of HTLV-I infections occur later in life, possibly through a combination of sexual transmission and blood transfusion. The majority of individuals who are infected remain so for life, with the cumulative incidence of forms of adult T cell leukemia occurring in approximately 4% of those infected. The latency period for development of HTLV-I-induced adult T cell leukemia has been deduced from epidemiologic surveys to be between 10 and 30 years. The prevalence of seropositivity to HTLV-I or HTLV-II among blood donors in the United States has been estimated to be 0.025%.

Clinical Manifestations

Since the recognition that HTLV-I infection was associated with T cell leukemia in Japan and T cell malignancies elsewhere, it has become clear that HTLV-I infection is associated with a typical syndrome now termed *HTLV-I-associated adult T cell leukemia or lymphoma (ATL)*. The clinical features of HTLV-I-associated ATL include high peripheral white blood cell counts and frequent leukemic involvement of skin, often with lymphomatous vasculitic lesions (Fig. 77–3); enlargement of liver, spleen, and lymph nodes; involvement of the central nervous system, lungs, and gastrointestinal tract; a paraneoplastic syndrome characterized by increased bone resorption and hypercalcinemia; and a rapidly fatal clinical course. The malignant cells in ATL are mature T cells with pleomorphic irregular nuclei that express the helper T cell marker CD4 and lack the pan T cell CD7 (3A1) marker. Indeed, infection of $CD4^+$ T cells has emerged as a hallmark of all the human retroviruses.

Another clinical sequela of HTLV-I infection is a neurodegenerative syndrome called *tropical spastic paraparesis (TSP)* or *HTLV-I-associated myelopathy (HAM)*, characterized by a slowly progressing, indolent weakening of the legs, culminating in paraparesis or paraplegia. Associated neuropathologic findings include meningoencephalomyelitis, inflammatory changes at the spinal cord level, and foci of increased periventricular intensity on magnetic resonance imaging.

Diagnosis

Diagnosis of infection with HTLV-I can be made by serologic analysis or by isolation of the virus from lymphocytes grown in culture. For serologic analysis, enzyme-linked immunosorbent assay (ELISA) or radioimmunoassays (RIA) are used with whole disrupted viral proteins as antigen to detect the presence of HTLV-I-specific serum antibodies. Positive results in ELISA or RIA tests are confirmed using Western blot analysis to detect antibodies against gp46 *env*- and p19 and p24 *gag*-encoded core proteins. Food and Drug Administration (FDA)-approved test kits are available for testing human sera for reactivity to HTLV but cannot discriminate between human antibodies directed to HTLV-I or HTLV-II. Polymerase chain reaction (PCR) techniques are currently the most sensitive assays for detection of HTLV infection and can, with the use of appropriate oligonucleotide primers, discriminate between these two retroviruses.

To identify the presence of HTLV-I in culture, T cells are grown in the presence of a mitogen such as phytohemagglutinin (PHA) and the T cell growth factor IL-2 and are assayed for magnesium-dependent reverse transcriptase or for core proteins p19 and p24, using monoclonal antibodies and indirect immunofluorescence assays. Finally, a virus isolate of HTLV-I can be obtained by co-culture of irradiated patient leukemic cells with uninfected cord blood T cells, yielding an HTLV-I-transformed cord blood T cell line. PCR techniques for detection of HTLV-I or HTLV-II infection in vitro can also be used.

Treatment

To date there is no specific antivirus agent that can eliminate or control infection with HTLV-I. Those HTLV-I-positive subjects that go on to ATL can be treated with combination cytotoxic chemotherapeutic regimens with brief clinical remissions obtained. However, even with such treatment, the mean survival time of ATL patients in the United States is only 11 months. Recently, some success in treating HTLV-I-associated ATL has been achieved in Japan with deoxycoformycin and in the United States with radiolabeled monoclonal antibodies directed to the IL-2 receptor.

Prevention

Since HTLV-I is transmitted sexually and through blood products, the prevalence of seropositivity is gradually increasing in the United States, particularly in populations at risk for these modes of transmission such as hemophiliacs, IV

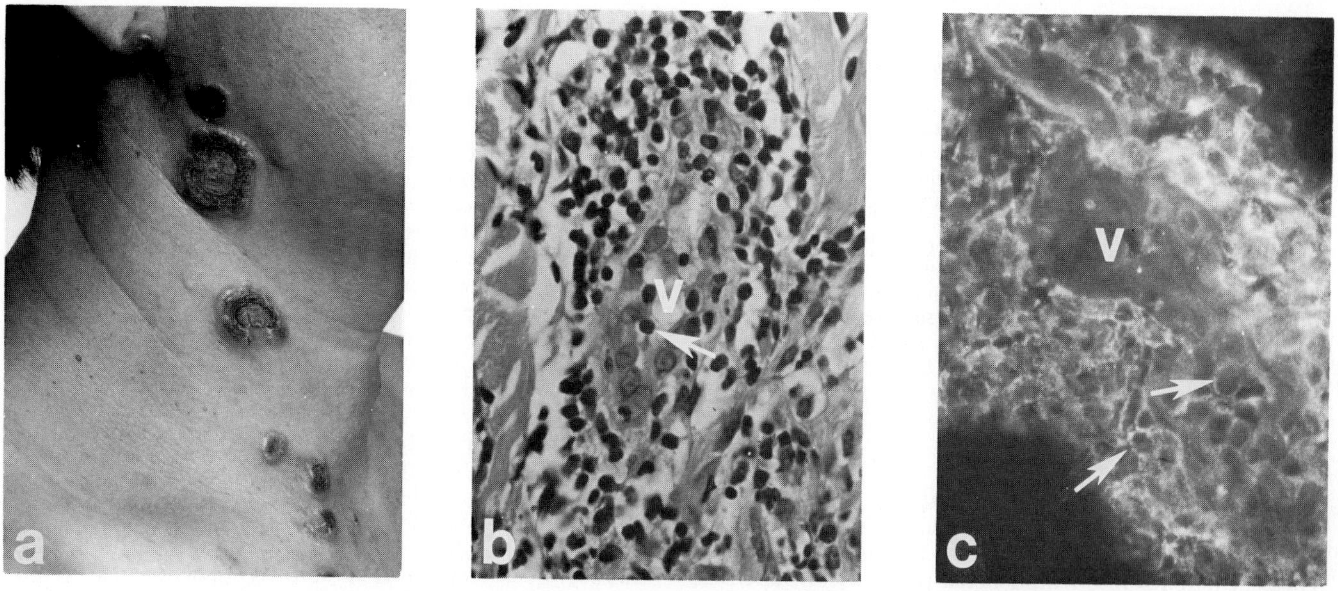

Fig. 77–3. HTLV-I–associated adult T cell lymphoma or leukemia (ATL). **A.** Typical ulcerating skin lesions on the neck of a patient with HTLV-I–associated ATL. **B.** Dermal infiltrating malignant T cells in the skin biopsy of the same patient as in **A**, with a vessel shown (V) with invading ATL cells (arrow). **C.** Indirect immunofluorescence of the skin lesion shown in **A** and **B**, demonstrating reactivity of the malignant cells with an antibody against the T cell receptor–associated CD3 (T3) antigens. V shows a vessel, and arrow points to malignant ATL cells in and around vessel wall. × 400. (**C** and **D** from Haynes BF et al: Proc Natl Acad Sci USA 229:675–679, 1985.)

drug users, and homosexuals. At present, the most effective measures for control of infection are adequate screening of blood and blood products for HTLV-I and education of populations at risk regarding mode of transmission.

Human Immunodeficiency Virus (HIV)

Introduction and Nomenclature

In 1983 and 1984 retrovirus isolates were described by Montagnier and colleagues from hemophiliac patients with lymphadenopathy (called *lymphadenopathy-associated virus* or *LAV-1*) and from patients with frank AIDS (called *immunodeficiency-associated virus* or *IDAV*). Also in 1984 Gallo and coworkers described numerous isolates of a retrovirus, HTLV-III, from homosexual and hemophiliac patients with AIDS and AIDS-related syndromes. Levy and colleagues in late 1984 reported the isolation and characterization of an AIDS-related retrovirus (ARV). Finally, in 1986 Montagnier and coworkers described a retroviral isolate called *LAV-2* from T cells of an African AIDS patient. Subsequent work by a number of investigators has demonstrated that LAV-1, HTLV-III, IDAV, and ARV are all isolates of the same virus, now called *human immunodeficiency virus type 1 (HIV-1)*. A more recent isolate, LAV-2, appears to be a virus distinct from HIV-1 and to be more closely related to the simian immunodeficiency viruses SIVsm and SIVmac. LAV-2 now appears to be a member of a distinct family of human lentiviruses called *human immunodeficiency virus type 2 (HIV-2)*.

Epidemiology

AIDS was first identified in 1981 and represents an unprecedented epidemic of immunologic deficiency with enormous implications for world health. First recognized in homosexual men and IV drug abusers, other risk groups have since been identified and include hemophiliacs receiving blood products, female and male sexual partners of persons with HIV infection, transfusion recipients, and infants and children of HIV-seropositive women.

HIV-1 has conclusively been shown to be the etiologic agent of AIDS based on demonstration of anti-HIV-1 antibodies and isolation of the HIV-1 virus from AIDS patients and patients with AIDS-related syndromes. In particular, studies in transfusion-associated AIDS cases have carefully documented the etiologic role of HIV-1 and have demonstrated an incubation period of 5 to 65 months for the development of AIDS after transfusion with HIV-1-positive blood. Unlike HTLV-I, which appears to have been endemic in populations for many years with a relatively low attack rate of clinical disease (3% to 5% lifetime risk), HIV-1 is a virus new to the populations at risk, with a high attack rate of clinical disease (approaching 100%). The distribution of HIV is worldwide, with large epidemics currently ongoing in the United States, the Caribbean, Europe, and Africa. Recent epidemiologic data suggest that unlike the U.S. epidemic that initially involved homosexual men and IV illicit drug users, the African AIDS epidemic primarily involves otherwise normal heterosexual men and women. Serologic studies of sera drawn from subjects in Uganda, Kenya, Tanzania, and the Ivory Coast in the early 1970s have shown 1% to 3% HIV-positivity—giving credence to the notion that the AIDS virus first caused disease in Africa. From Africa, HIV was presumably spread to the Caribbean and then into the U.S. homosexual population in 1978 and 1979. The documented modes of transmission of HIV are similar to those of HTLV-I: sexual contact, mother to child, and exposure to blood or blood products. HIV has been isolated from blood, semen, mother's milk, tears, cerebrospinal fluid, and saliva of infected patients. However, to date, transmission by fluids other than semen, blood, and human milk has not been reported.

As of December 1990, approximately 110,000 persons have been reported as having AIDS, with 55,00 cases reported in 1990. Seroepidemiologic data suggest that approximately 1 million people in the United States are infected with HIV-1, and based on current attack rates, by 1993 the cumulative total number of AIDS deaths in the United States will exceed 300,000.

Mechanisms of HIV Pathogenicity

Early in the study of AIDS, immunologic abnormalities were noted that provided important clues to the cause of the disease. These included severe lymphopenia primarily of the CD4+ T cell subset, decreased or absent delayed cutaneous hypersensitivity reactions, loss of cytotoxic natural killer cell function, abnormal monocyte function, and polyclonal hypergammaglobulinemia. That CD4+ lymphocytes were depleted selectively in AIDS patients gave rise to the observation that HIV selectively infected CD4+ T cells in vitro. Moreover, the CD4 molecule itself serves as the cellular receptor for HIV, resulting in HIV entering and infecting CD4+ T cells. In addition to infecting CD4+ T cells, HIV also has been shown to infect peripheral blood monocytes, monocytoid cell lines, and various forms of tissue macrophages such as follicular dendritic cells of lymph node germinal centers, skin, and thymus Langerhans cells, and microglial cells in brain—all cell types that recently have been shown to express the CD4 molecule. Thus in both T and monocyte lineage cells, HIV uses the CD4 molecule as a receptor for entering and infecting cells. Recent studies suggest T cell precursors in bone marrow and the thymus may become infected with HIV-1. Thus mechanisms of HIV-induced immunodeficiency include infection of peripheral T cells, infection of T cell precursors, and infection of tissue macrophages and dendritic cells. Infection of these cell types by HIV-1 suggests that HIV-1 can both decrease the functional capacity of existing peripheral T lymphocytes and antigen-presenting cells and inhibit the production and maturation of T cell precursors, thus preventing reconstitution of the peripheral T cell pool.

Once inside cells through receptor-mediated endocytosis, HIV undergoes a life cycle typical of lentiviruses (Chap. 59). Retroviruses of this subgroup cause slowly developing nontumorigenic diseases and replicate through complementary DNA (cDNA) intermediates that can be found either as unintegrated circular or linear double strands or as integrated cDNA in the host genome (provirus form). An important characteristic of HIV is that its replication in some cells in vivo appears restricted, resulting in maintenance of HIV in a latent form. Latent infection allows the HIV genome to be present in T cells and macrophages in the absence of expressed viral proteins, resulting in persistently infected cells that remain invisible to the host immune system.

Activation of latent HIV-infected cells both in vitro and in vivo can be induced by numerous immune cell cytokines, including tumor necrosis factor (TNF) and IL-6, and leads to several biologic effects of mature virus expression, including a cytopathic effect that leads to death of infected T cells and fusion of infected cells with uninfected cells to form multinucleated giant cells. Co-infection of HIV-1-infected cells with either HTLV-I or human herpes virus 6 (Chap. 59) enhances the expression of HIV-I in vitro. Lysed HIV-1-infected T cells release large numbers of infectious particles that rapidly adsorb to and infect nearby uninfected CD4+ cells. Cell-cell transmission of HIV also results from T cell fusion and giant cell formation. In addition to free virus released from lysed cells, soluble viral proteins are also released, including soluble external envelope protein capable of binding to the CD4 molecule. Soluble envelope molecules can coat uninfected CD4+ cells, making them vulnerable both to complement-mediated lysis and to antibody-dependent cellular cytotoxicity by Fc receptor bearing–cells.

Several important features of HIV make host-virus interactions extremely complex and make HIV a formidable infectious agent for the human immune system. That the CD4 molecule is a biologically relevant receptor for HIV infection is devastating to the normal host immune response. CD4+ cells are central regulatory and effector cells of the immune system. CD4+ macrophages and dendritic cells are essential for presenting antigen peptide fragments to T cells and for performing inductive functions essential for normal lymphopoiesis in the bone marrow and thymus. The CD4 molecule itself directly participates in stabilizing T cell–macrophage interactions and binds directly to macrophage major histocompatibility complex (MHC) class II molecules during antigen presentation to T cells. Therefore HIV-1 envelope protein binding to the CD4 molecule can potentially function as an off signal to T cell activation, thereby inhibiting anti-HIV-1 cellular and humoral responses.

Another important point regarding host-HIV-1 interactions involves cell-cell transmission of virus. Given that HIV infection is transmitted between people by transfer of allogeneic cells, the first cells to come in contact with infected cells are normal alloreactive T cells, which thus are likely the first host cells to become infected. Therefore noninfected host effector T cells responding to HIV-1-infected cells run the risk of being infected themselves during the mediation of normal anti-HIV-1 cellular immune responses.

Thus the pathogenicity of HIV-1 relates to its tropism for CD4+ cells and to complex host-virus interactions that lead to subversion of normal host immune responses, subsequently leading to destruction of host immunity and host death due to opportunistic infections.

Clinical Manifestations

Since the discovery of HIV-1 as the causative agent of AIDS, it has become clear that AIDS represents a broad spectrum of clinical conditions (Table 77–2). Figure 77–4 outlines the clinical stages of HIV infection correlated with HIV expression and anti-HIV serum antibody responses. The immunodeficiency of AIDS relates to a primary HIV-1-induced T cell deficiency, to a secondary dysfunction of B cells with polyclonal hypergammaglobulinemia and defective specific antibody responses, and to a defect in natural killer cell function.

A number of opportunistic infections routinely occur in AIDS patients. The most common organisms and their common clinical syndromes are *Pneumocystis carinii* (pneumonia), cytomegalovirus (disseminated, pneumonia, retinitis, encephalitis), atypical mycobacteria (disseminated), *Toxoplasma gondii*

TABLE 77–2. CLINICAL SPECTRUM OF HIV INFECTION IN MAN

Group I	Acute infection
Group II	Asymptomatic infection
Group III	Persistent generalized lymphadenopathy
Group IV	Other HIV-1–related syndromes
Subgroup A: Constitutional disease (fever, weight loss, diarrhea)	
Subgroup B: Neurologic disease (dementia, myelopathy, peripheral neuropathy)	
Subgroup C: Secondary infectious diseases	
Subgroup D: Secondary malignancies (Kaposi's sarcoma, nonHodgkin's lymphoma, primary lymphoma of the brain)	
Subgroup E: Other conditions attributed to HIV-1 infection (e.g., chronic lymphoid interstitial pneumonitis, autoimmune syndromes associated with HIV-1 infections, other nonclassified HIV-1–associated syndromes)	

Adapted from Centers For Disease Control Classification System for HIV-1 Infections: MMWR 35:334, 1986.

(encephalitis), *Candida albicans* (disseminated, esophagitis), herpes simplex (progressive infections), *Cryptococcus neoformans* (disseminated, meningitis), and *Cryptosporidium* (enteritis).

Malignancies develop in AIDS patients and are a hallmark of the syndrome. The most common is Kaposi's sarcoma, an otherwise rare tumor of vascular endothelium that occurs in approximately 40% of homosexual men with AIDS. Other malignancies associated with AIDS include non-Hodgkin's B cell lymphomas and carcinomas of the rectum and tongue.

An important component of the AIDS syndrome recognized recently is the occurrence of neurologic syndromes in approximately 40% of patients. These syndromes include encephalitis, progressive dementia, spinal cord degeneration, acute aseptic meningitis, chronic meningitis, and peripheral neuropathy. Studies in AIDS patients have demonstrated HIV in cells in cerebrospinal fluid and in microglial cells and multinucleated giant cells in brain. This is of particular interest since HIV is morphologically and genetically related to the visna virus that causes a chronic degenerative neurologic disease in sheep.

In addition to patients with typical AIDS, there are patients in all risk groups who have an AIDS-related complex (ARC), consisting of generalized lymphadenopathy or fever or both, malaise, fatigue, night sweats, weight loss, loss of appetite, diarrhea, or low platelet counts (Table 77–2). These features can all be part of the typical AIDS syndrome or may represent a prodrome for the development of AIDS.

With an increase in the number of women infected with HIV has come an increase in children with HIV infections. Eighty percent of all children with HIV infection acquire the disease perinatally, either just before or after delivery. Some children present with an HIV-induced wasting syndrome, including opportunistic infections and neurologic disease, early (4 to 8 months) after birth. Other children develop symptoms of HIV infection later in childhood, with lymphoid infiltration in the lung (lymphoid pneumonia) and recurrent bacterial infections.

Diagnosis

The diagnosis of HIV-1–related syndromes (Table 77–2) is made by the combination of the recognition of a clinical syndrome compatible with ARC or AIDS and the demonstration of serum anti-HIV antibodies by ELISA or RIA and Western blot assay. Although not routinely clinically available, HIV-1 can also readily be isolated by co-culture of patient T cells with leukemic CD4+ T cell lines that do not undergo cell lysis after infection with HIV-1, so that a viral isolate of HIV can be obtained. As with HTLV-I, anti-HIV monoclonal antibodies are available that identify HIV-infected cells in culture. Sensitive PCR techniques can also be used to detect proviral forms of HIV-1 in cells and tissues. Although 70% of children born to HIV-infected women are not infected with HIV, the diagnosis of HIV infection in infants is complicated by the presence of maternal antibody in the infant's blood. Thus in infants the diagnosis of HIV infection is more complicated than in adults and relies on HIV culture results, PCR analysis of infant DNA samples, and other clinical measurements.

Treatment

Currently there are no antivirus agents available that will eradicate or prevent HIV-1 infection. A number of agents

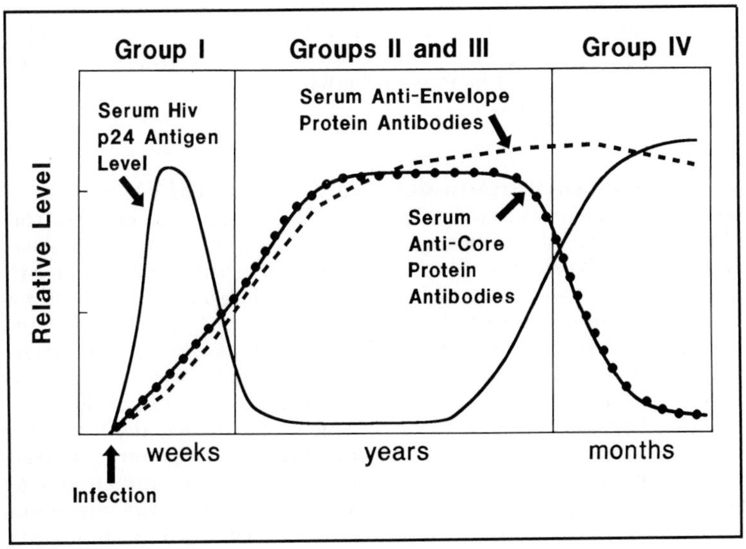

Fig. 77–4. Clinical stage of HIV infection in man correlated with HIV expression and anti-HIV antibody responses. HIV patient groups I through IV refer to groups in Table 77–2. Arrow labeled "infection" refers to the time point at which an individual initially becomes infected with HIV. During the initial acute stage of HIV infection (group I patients) HIV is expressed at a high level as measured by *gag* p24 protein levels in serum, and serum antibodies to core and envelope HIV proteins begin to rise. During the asymptomatic or lymphadenopathy phase of the infection (groups II and III) antibody levels to core and envelope proteins are high, and HIV expression (serum p24 levels) is low. This phase may last for many years and is probably maintained by successful host anti-HIV cellular and humoral immune responses. With the development of frank AIDS (group IV), antibodies to HIV envelope proteins are maintained, but anti-core antibody levels fall. HIV virus expression, as measured by serum p24 levels, again rises as AIDS progresses.

have demonstrated inhibitory activity of HIV-1 infectivity of T cells in vitro, including suramin, HPA-23, dideoxycytidine (ddC), dideoxyinosine (ddI), foscarnet, ribavirin, and 3′-azidothymidine (AZT). To date, only AZT has shown some degree of clinical efficacy in controlled trials in AIDS patients in vivo and is approved for use in adults and children. A metabolite of AZT acts as an irreversible inhibitor of DNA synthesis when incorporated into viral DNA and inhibits new infection of T cells by HIV in vitro. Other nucleosides are in trials, with approval pending results. Soluble CD4 has been tried in vivo and is without efficacy.

Prevention

The observation that HIV-1 infection can occur through transfusion has prompted a national program to screen all blood and blood products in the United States for HIV-1. In a remarkable effort beginning in 1984, screening assays for serum anti-HIV antibodies were licensed, resulting in screening of virtually the entire blood supply of the United States for HIV by 1986. However, since rare seronegative HIV-infected subjects can exist, screening blood and blood products has not completely eliminated the risk of transfusion-associated AIDS, although it has reduced the risk considerably.

More recently, all donors of organs such as hearts and kidneys and donors of semen for artificial insemination have been screened for anti-HIV serum antibodies, thus further reducing the risk of transmission of HIV. In spite of these efforts, HIV infection continues to spread within the United States, particularly in IV drug users and through heterosexual transmission. Continued intensive efforts are needed to control the spread of HIV-1 within populations at risk and to alert members of nonrisk populations to the dangers of risk-group contacts. Public health efforts at education, coupled with intensive research toward anti-HIV treatments and a protective vaccine, are necessary to ultimately control the AIDS epidemic.

Other Novel Human Retroviruses

Human T Cell Lymphotropic Virus Type II (HTLV-II)

HTLV-II is a novel human retrovirus isolated in 1982 from the Mo T cell line that was derived in 1976 from a patient with the T cell form of hairy cell leukemia. HTLV-II is similar in genomic organization, T cell transforming capability, and morphology (Fig. 77–1) to HTLV-I and has 60% nucleic acid homology to HTLV-I. Unlike HTLV-I, however, HTLV-II to date has been isolated only from a limited number of patients with the T cell form of hairy cell leukemia, AIDS, or hemophilia. Serologic surveys have demonstrated that HTLV-II infection occurs in select populations of IV drug users and hemophiliacs in the United States. Although the data are suggestive for an etiologic role of HTLV-II in T cell hairy cell leukemia, confirmation of this association awaits further studies.

Human Immunodeficiency Virus Type 2 (HIV-2)

In 1986 Montagnier and colleagues described the isolation of a new virus, LAV-2, from two patients with AIDS in West Africa. Although most cases of AIDS in Africa are caused by HIV-1, occasional African AIDS patients have been HIV-1 seronegative, and from two such cases LAV-2 was isolated. Based on antigenic cross-reactivity, it appears that LAV-2 (now called *HIV-2*) is more closely related to strains of simian immunodeficiency virus (SIV) (the etiologic agent of simian AIDS in captive macaques) than to HIV-1. However, the morphology of HIV-2 is similar to that of HIV-1 (Fig. 77–2), and HIV-2 is similarly tropic for CD4+ cells. HIV-2 has been most commonly found in Western Africa in 3% to 64% of female prostitutes and appears to be associated with a reduced pathogenicity relative to HIV-1. Genomic differences between HIV-1 and HIV-2/SIV include the presence of the *vpu* gene in HIV-1 only, whereas HIV-2/SIV contains the *vpx* gene, which HIV-1 lacks (Chap. 59). However, it is unclear whether these genomic distinctions are responsible for the reduced pathogenicity of HIV-2 in humans.

Simian Retroviruses Related to Human Retroviruses

Simian T Cell Lymphotropic Virus Type I (STLV-I)

Antibodies reactive with HTLV-I antigens have been found in several Old World monkey species, including Japanese and Chinese macaques, African green monkeys, and baboons. However, analysis of DNA from a T cell line established from a baboon that was seropositive for HTLV-I revealed viral sequences related to, but distinct from, HTLV-I and HTLV-II. This HTLV-I–related virus in baboons, called *simian T cell lymphotropic virus type I (STLV-I)*, may be involved in leukemogenesis in primates since STLV-I has been associated with the development of lymphomas in three species of macaques. Serologic surveys of primate species in Japan and Africa have documented the distribution of STLV-I is much wider than HTLV-I is in humans. These observations suggest this virus has been in primate and human populations for many years and that entry of STLV-I into primates and HTLV-I into man occurred independently many years ago rather than through present-day primate-to-man transmission. HTLV-I and STLV-I have greater nucleic acid sequence homology (90%) than HTLV-I and HTLV-II (60%), suggesting a close phylogenetic relationship between human and primate leukemia viruses.

Simian Immunodeficiency Virus (SIV)

SIVmac was first discovered in 1985 when it was isolated from captive rhesus macaques (*Macaca mulatta*), a species of Asian Old World primates. After this initial discovery, other SIV isolates were isolated from captive pigtailed (*Macaca nemestrina;* SIVmne), cynomolgus (*Macaca fascicularis;* SIVcyno), and stumptailed (*Macaca arctoides;* SIVstm) macaques. SIV isolates similar to SIVmac at the genomic level also were identified in healthy African sooty managabeys (SIVsm) and green monkeys (SIVagm). Subsequent seroepidemiologic and molecular studies revealed that SIVmac was not indigenous in Asian macaques but likely was inadvertently transmitted during captivity from African sooty mangabeys to Asian macaques. Moreover, certain strains of SIV derived from rhesus macaques and sooty mangabeys were closely related (80%) to HIV-2 at the genomic level and somewhat less related to HIV-1 (50%).

Serologic cross-reactivity between envelope glycoproteins of SIVmac, SIVsm, and HIV-2 provides further evidence that SIVmac, SIVsm, and HIV-2 are related members of a group of primate lentiviruses. Other primate lentiviruses representing an additional three distinct groups have been isolated from the African green monkey (SIVagm), mandrills (SIVmnd), and humans (HIV-1), all lentiviruses that may have been diverged from a common ancestor long before the spread of AIDS in humans.

From 20% to 50% of African green monkeys in Kenya, Ethiopia, and South Africa have antibodies to SIV and yet exhibit no apparent AIDS-like symptoms characteristic of SIV infection in Asian macaques. Similarly, African sooty mangabeys (*Cercocebus atys*) in their native habitat and in captivity are also SIV-infected and healthy, suggesting that SIV have been present in these two species for a long enough time to allow host adaptation to SIV infection through selective pressure. Infection of macaques with some strains of SIVmac and SIVsm results in a dramatically different outcome involving a fatal simian AIDS-like disease (SAIDS) that closely parallels the pathologic hallmarks of HIV-1 infection in humans. One of the earliest reports of an AIDS-like disease in primates observed in a colony of rhesus macaques describes SIV-infected animals dying of lymphoma or opportunistic infections, most commonly *P. carinii,* and displaying a wasting syndrome with decreased circulating CD4+ T cells and a primary encephalitis similar to that observed in some AIDS patients. Experimental inoculation of SIVmac isolates into rhesus monkeys at a number of primate centers confirmed the association of SIV infection with the AIDS-like syndrome. SIV is a lentivirus with genomic organization, cell tropism, receptor utilization, cytopathic effect, activation pathways, and pathology (in the appropriate host) similar to HIV-1 in humans. SIV-infected macaques are currently regarded by many as an excellent AIDS-like model system in which to study the pathology of primate lentivirus and to test therapeutic and interventive strategies, including vaccines.

FURTHER READING

GENERAL

Bartholomew C, Cleghorn F: Retroviruses in the Caribbean. Bull Pan Am Health Organ 23:76, 1989

Blattner WA: Human T-lymphotropic viruses and diseases of long latency. Ann Intern Med 111:4, 1989

Essex M, Kanki PJ: The origins of the AIDS virus. Sci Am 359:64, 1988

Gallo RC: Human retroviruses: Their role in neoplasia and immunodeficiency. Ann NY Acad Sci 567:82, 1989

Green Pl, Chen IS: Regulation of human T cell leukemia virus expression. FASEB J 4:169, 1990

McFarlin D, Koprowski H: Neurological disorders associated with HTLV-1. Curr Top Microbiol Immunol 160:100, 1990

Smith TF, Srinivasan A, Schochetman G, et al: The phylogenetic history of immunodeficiency viruses. Nature 333:573, 1988

Thomas BJ, Dalgleish AG: Human Retroviruses. Blood Rev 2:211, 1988

Wong-Staal F, Gallo RC: Human T-lymphotropic retroviruses. Nature 317:395, 1985

Yip MT, Chen IS: Modes of transformation by the human T cell leukemia viruses. Mol Biol Med 7:33, 1990

HTLV-I

Bunn PA, Schechter GP, Jaffe E, et al: Clinical course of retrovirus-associated adult T-cell lymphoma in the United States. N Engl J Med 309:257, 1983

Hanly SM, Rimsky LT, Malim MH, et al: Comparative analysis of the HTLV-I *rex* and HIV-1 *rev* trans-regulatory proteins and their RNA response elements. Genes Dev 3:1534, 1989

Liberski PP, Rodgers-Johnson P, Char G, et al: HTLV-I like viral particles in spinal cord cells in Jamaican tropical spastic paraparesis. Ann Neurol 23:5185, 1988

Palker TJ, Tanner ME, Scearce, et al: Mapping of immunogenic regions of human T-cell leukemia virus type I (HTLV-I) gp46 and gp21 envelope glycoproteins with *env*-encoded synthetic peptides and a monoclonal antibody to gp46. J Immunol 142:971, 1989

Ratner L, Vander Heyden N, Paine E, et al: Familial adult T cell leukemia/lymphoma. Am J Hematol 34:215, 1990

Shaw GM, Broder S, Essex M, Gallo RC: Human T cell leukemia virus: Its discovery and role in leukmogenesis and immunosuppression. Adv Intern Med 30:1, 1984

Waldmann TA: IL-2 receptor expression in the hematologic malignancies: A target for immunotherapy. Cancer Surv 8:891, 1989

Weinberg JB, Spiegel RA, Blazey DL, et al: Human T-cell lymphotropic virus I and adult T-cell leukemia: Report of a cluster in North Carolina. Am J Med 85:51, 1988

Williams AE, Fang CT, Slamon DT, et al: Seroprevalence and epidemiological correlates of HTLV-I infection in U.S. blood donors. Science 240:643, 1988

Yoshida M, Inoue J, Fijisawa, et al: Molecular mechanisms of regulation of HTLV-I gene expression and its association with leukemogenesis. Genome 31:662, 1989

HIV-1

Alizon M, Wain-Hobson S, Montagnier L, et al: Genetic variability of the AIDS virus: Nucleotide sequence analysis of two isolates from African patients. Cell 46:63, 1986

Barre-Sinoussi F, Chermann JC, Rey F, et al: Isolation of a T lymphotropic retrovirus from a patient at risk for the acquired immunodeficiency syndrome. Science 220:868, 1983

Berman PW, Gregory TJ, Riddle L, et al: Protection of chimpanzees from infection by HIV-1 after vaccination with recombination gp120 but not gp160. Nature 345:662, 1990

Broder S, Gallo RC: A pathogenic retrovirus (HTLV-III) linked to AIDS. N Engl J Med 311:1292, 1984

Broder S, Mitsuya H, Yarchoan R, et al: NIH conference. Antiretroviral therapy in AIDS. Ann Intern Med 113:604, 1990

Chin IM, Yaniv A, Dahlberg JE, et al: Nucleotide sequence evidence for relationship of AIDS retrovirus to lentiviruses. Nature 317:366, 1985

Ensoli B, Barillari G, Salahuddin SZ, et al: *Tat* protein stimulates growth of cells derived from Kaposi's sarcoma lesions in AIDS patients. Nature 345:84, 1990

Gallo RC, Salahuddin SZ, Popovic M, et al: Frequent detection and isolation of cytopathic retroviruses (HTLV-III) from patients with AIDS and at risk for AIDS. Science 224:500, 1984

Gottlieb US, Groopman JE, Weinstein W, et al: The acquired immunodeficiency syndrome. Ann Intern Med 99:208, 1983

Hart MK, Palker TJ, Matthews TJ, et al: Synthetic peptides containing T and B cell epitopes from human immunodeficiency virus envelope gp120 induce anti-HIV proliferative responses and high titers of neutralizing antibodies in rhesus monkeys. J Immunol 145:2677, 1990

Ho DD, Rota TR, Schooley RT, et al: Isolation of HTLV-III from cerebrospinal fluid and neural tissue of patients with neurologic syndromes related to the acquired immunodeficiency syndrome. N Engl J Med 313:1493, 1985

Koenig S, Fauci AS: Immunopathogenesis and immune response to the human immunodeficiency virus. In Devita VT, Hellman S, Rosenberg SA (eds): AIDS: Etiology, Diagnosis, Treatment and Prevention. New York, JB Lippincott, 1988

La Rosa G, Davide JP, Weinhold K, et al: Conserved sequence and structural elements in the HIV-1 principal neutralizing determinant. Science 249:932, 1990

Laspia MF, Rice AP, Matthews MB: HIV-1 *tat* protein increases transcriptional initiation and stabilizes elongation. Cell 59:283, 1989

Levy JA, Hoffman AD, Kramer SM, et al: Isolation of lymphocytopathic retroviruses from San Francisco patients with AIDS. Science 225:840, 1984

Palker TJ, Clark ME, Langlois AI, et al: Type-specific neutralization of the human immunodeficiency virus with antibodies to *env*-encoded synthetic peptides. Proc Natl Acad Sci USA 85:1932, 1988

Pizzo PA, Wilfert CM (eds): Pediatric AIDS. The Challenge of HIV Infection in Infants, Children and Adolescents. Baltimore, Williams & Williams, 1991

Rossi P, Moschese V, Broliden PA, et al: Presence of maternal antibodies to human immunodeficiency virus 1 envelope glycoprotein gp120 epitopes correlate with the uninfected status of children born to seropositive mothers. Proc Natl Acad Sci USA 86:8055, 1989

Schnittman S, Denning SM, Greenhouse JJ, et al: Evidence for susceptibility of intrathymic T-cell precursors and their progeny to human immunodeficiency virus infection: A mechanism for $CD4^+$ (T4) lymphocyte depletion. Proc Natl Acad Sci USA 87:7727, 1990

Wong-Staal F: HIV gene regulation and pathogenesis. Cancer Detect Prev 14:295, 1989

HTLV-II

Green WC, Leonard WJ, Wano Y, et al: Transactivator gene of HTLV-II induces IL-2 receptor and IL-2 cellular gene expression. Science 232:877, 1986

Hjelle B, Scalf R, Swenson S: High frequency of human T-cell leukemia/lymphoma virus type II infection in New Mexico blood donors: Determination by sequence specific oligonucleotide hybridization. Blood 76:450, 1990

Kalyanaraman US, Sarngadharan MG, Robert-Guroff M, et al: A new subtype of human T cell leukemia virus (HTLV-II) associated with atypical hairy cell leukemia. Science 218:571, 1982

Kwok S, Gallo D, Hanson C, et al: High prevalence of HTLV-II among intravenous drug abusers: PCR confirmation and typing. AIDS Res Hum Retroviruses 6:561, 1990

Lee TH, Coligan JE, Lane MF, et al: Serological cross-reactivity between envelope gene gradients of type I and type II human T cell leukemia virus. Proc Natl Acad Sci USA 81:7579, 1984

Rosenblatt JD, Chen IS, Colde DW: HTLV-II and human lymphoproliferative disorders. Clin Lab Med 8:85, 1988

Rosenblatt JD, Giorgi JV, Golde DW, et al: Integrated human T-cell leukemia virus II genome in $CD8^+$ T cells from a patient with "atypical" hairy cell leukemia: Evidence for distinct T and B cell lymphoproliferative disorders. Blood 71:363, 1988

Rosenblatt JD, Golde DW, Wachsman W, et al: A second isolate of HTLV-II associated with atypical hairy cell leukemia. N Engl J Med 315:372, 1986

HIV-2

Clavel F, Guetard D, Brun-Vezinet F, et al: Isolation of a new human retrovirus from West African Patients with AIDS. Science 233:343, 1986

De Cock KM, Brun-Vezinet F: Epidemiology of HIV-2 infection. AIDS 3:589, 1989

Homma T, Kanki PJ, King WW, et al: Lymphoma in macaques: Association with virus of human T lymphotropic family. Science 225:716, 1984

Kumar P, Hui HX, Kappes JC, et al: Molecular characterization of an attenuated human immunodeficiency virus type 2 isolate. J Virol 64:890, 1990

Lyons SF, Clausen L, Schoub BD: HIV-2–induced AIDS in southern Africa. AIDS 2:406, 1988

Romieu I, Marlink R, Kanki P, et al: HIV-2 link to AIDS in West Africa. J AIDS 3:220, 1990

Sattentau QJ, Clapham, PR, Weiss RA, et al: The human and simian immunodeficiency viruses HIV-1, HIV-2, and SIV interact with similar epitopes on their cellular receptor, the CD4 molecule. AIDS 2:101, 1988

Schultz TF, Whitby D, Hoad JG, et al: Biological and molecular variability of the human immunodeficiency virus type 2 isolates from Gambia. J Virol 64:5177, 1990

STLV-I

Ishikawa K, Fukasawa M, Tsujimoto H, et al: Serological survey and virus isolation of simian T-cell leukemia/T-lymphotropic virus type I (STLV-I) in non-human primates in their native countries. Int J Cancer 40:233, 1987

Watanabe T, Seiki M, Hirayama Y, et al: Human T-cell leukemia virus type I is a member of the African subtype of simian viruses (STLV). Virology 148:385, 1986

Watanabe T, Seiki M, Tsujimoto H, et al: Sequence homology of the simian retrovirus genome with human T cell leukemia virus type I. Virology 144:59, 1985

SIV

Allan JS, Kanda P, Kennedy RC, et al: Isolation and characterization of simian immunodeficiency viruses from two subspecies of African green monkeys. AIDS Res Hum Retroviruses 6:275, 1990

Daniel MD, Desrosiers RS: Use of simian immunodeficiency virus for evaluation of AIDS vaccine strategies. AIDS 3:5131, 1989

Daniel MD, Letvin WL, King NW, et al: Isolation of T cell tropic HTLV-III-like retrovirus from macaques. Science 228:1201, 1985

Desrosiers RC, Daniel MD, Li Y: HIV related lentiviruses of non-human primates. AIDS Res Hum Retroviruses 5:463, 1989

Gardner MD: SIV infection rhesus macaques: An AIDS model for immunoprevention and immunotherapy. Adv Exp Med Biol 251:279, 1989

Hirsch VM, Olmsted RA, Murphey-Corb M, et al: An african primate lentivirus (SIVsm) closely related to HIV-2. Nature 339:389, 1989

Kanki PJ, McLane MF, King NW, et al: Serologic identification and characterization of a macaque T-lymphotropic retrovirus closely related to HTLV-III. Science 228:1199, 1985

CHAPTER 78

Rhinoviruses, Reoviruses, and Parvoviruses

Rhinoviruses

More than 100 serotypes comprise the genus *Rhinovirus* of the Picornaviridae family. These 25 to 30 nm particles have a naked icosahedral nucleocapsid containing a single-stranded RNA genome. The first isolate in 1956 was initially classified as echovirus 28. Since then it has been learned that the rhinoviruses are acid labile and destroyed at a pH of less than 3. They have a buoyant density of 1.38 to 1.41 g/cm^2 in cesium chloride, which is higher than that of enteroviruses. All picornaviruses share the property of capsid assembly in the cytoplasm of infected cells, and mature virus particles contain four capsid proteins as a result of cleavage of a common precursor. Rhinoviruses (*rhino*, nose) are important causes of acute respiratory infections, with the predominant illness, the "common cold," occurring in the airway above the larynx. Roughly 30% of colds are produced by rhinovirus infections.

Clinical Illness

The usual symptoms of a rhinovirus infection are nasal obstruction and discharge, sneezing, scratchy throat, mild cough, and malaise. Virus replication is limited to the respiratory tract, and the incubation period to onset of virus shedding is 1 to 4 days. The titer of virus in nasal secretions reflects the extent of mucosal involvement and correlates with the severity of illness. Human epithelial cells containing rhinovirus antigens have been demonstrated in the nasal mucus of infected individuals, suggesting the virus multiples primarily in the epithelial surface of nasal mucosa. The amount of damage to the nasal epithelium appears to be minimal, with edema of subepithelial connective tissue and sparse infiltrates of inflammatory cells apparent. Experimental small-particle aerosol inoculation can produce tracheobronchitis. Severe tracheobronchitis and even atypical pneumonia occur rarely with natural infection in adults. Rhinovirus infection has been associated in a few studies with acute exacerbation of chronic obstructive pulmonary disease and with sinusitis. As with influenza and respiratory syncytial virus (RSV) infections, hyperreactive small airways have been demonstrated in adult volunteers with rhinovirus-caused illness, a problem that may manifest itself as an asthma attack. Fever and significant lower respiratory tract involvement in the form of bronchiolitis or pneumonia are more common with rhinovirus infection of children than adults. Although the rhinoviruses are common and a nuisance, as causes of respiratory disease they are not of the medical seriousness of RSV or the parainfluenza viruses.

Pathogenesis

The rhinoviruses replicate preferentially at 33C to 35C. The lack of viremia with the rhinoviruses and their predilection for infecting only the upper respiratory tract probably result from the higher temperatures present in blood and the lower respiratory tract. Virus yield in vitro may fall as much as 90% at the standard body temperature of 37C. The combination of stomach acidity and the rhinoviruses' acid lability also probably prevents gastrointestinal infection and excretion.

The symptomatic manifestations of a cold (swollen nasal membranes, increased mucus production, fever) are only to a small degree a product of tissue damage produced directly by these cytolytic viruses. Much more important are secreted vasoactive peptides (kinins), which are released in response to the infection. The kinins increase vascular permeability, allowing serum proteins such as albumin to escape from the mucosal capillaries, and accelerate a local inflammatory response. The number of polymorphonuclear leukocytes in the mucus increases, and as these cells degranulate, they produce further tissue irritation. The kinins may also be related to increased mucus secretion.

The immune response to rhinovirus infections includes serum neutralizing antibodies, mucosally secreted IgA antibodies, and a mild cellular response. Since rhinoviruses do not invade the circulation, it appears that the major function of the circulating neutralizing antibodies occurs when these proteins are included in the inflammatory transudates resulting from infection. The presence of detectable serum neutralizing antibodies against a given rhinovirus serotype generally indicates protection against reinfection by that serotype. However, the fact that there are more than 100 serotypes of rhinovirus limits the utility of these antibodies. In addition, antibody concentrations wane over a matter of years when there is no restimulation, so people can be infected either with one of the rhinovirus serotypes to which they have never been exposed or by a serotype with which they had been infected years before.

At a cellular level the receptor for more than 90% of rhinovirus serotypes is the intracellular adhesion molecule 1 (ICAM-1). ICAM-1 is a cell membrane protein used for intercellular binding and attachment in a number of cell-cell interactions. The levels of expressed ICAM-1 in membranes are normally fairly low, but inflammatory mediators (e.g., cytokines and leukotrienes) increase the expression of these proteins. Although it has not been confirmed experimentally, it seems reasonable to speculate that as a rhinovirus infection progresses, it creates a positive-feedback loop for itself. The virus produces inflammation, the inflammation up-regulates ICAM-1 expression on cell surfaces, and the increased levels of the ICAM-1 enhance the cellular attachment, entrance, and replication of the rhinoviruses. During the infection the process of making neutralizing antibodies is ongoing, and eventually the levels become sufficient to terminate viral replication. Serum IgG and IgM antibodies can be detected as early as 6 to 7 days in a primary (first) infection with a new rhinovirus serotype or after 3 to 4 days if the individual had been exposed previously to that serotype.

The structure of rhinovirus particles also contributes to their interaction with cells. The capsid proteins form a spherical particle with deep crypts, or canyons, on the virus surface. Within these canyons are the virus attachment sites that bind to ICAM-1. The canyons are too narrow for immunoglobulin molecules to penetrate, so neutralizing antibodies that could bind to more than one rhinovirus serotype at the attachment site are not generated.

Epidemiology

Rhinovirus infections have been documented in all populations studied. They occur throughout the year, but in a temperate climate there is some tendency for an increased frequency in early fall and late spring. Children frequently serve to introduce rhinoviruses into the family unit, with subsequent illnesses occurring usually after a 2- to 3-day incubation period in about 50% of contacts. Occasional epidemics with a single serotype have been described, but more often multiple serotypes appear to be circulating in the community at the same time. Some serotypes seem to be more easily transmissible, and a limited number of serotypes seem responsible for the majority of illness. Evidence suggests that antigenic variation of these viruses continues to occur and may contribute to the epidemiology. Human rhinoviruses are limited in their host range, and only the chimpanzee and gibbon have been shown to be susceptible experimentally.

Shedding of rhinoviruses in respiratory tract secretions has been amply documented. Experimental studies of transmission of these viruses have shown that transmission may occur by way of aerosols under intimate circumstances and by hand contact and self-inoculation of the mucous membranes of the eye or nasal mucosa. The importance of the hand contact and self-inoculation observed in experimental circumstances in which the variables are well controlled raises questions as to the main mode of transmission of infection in naturally occurring infection. Viral contamination of objects in the environment frequently occurs. Experimental studies tend to support the concept that rhinoviruses ordinarily are not transmitted in public gathering places or with relatively short exposure to friends or relatives with colds. Rather, transmission is more likely where hand contact with virus-containing secretions occurs. Finally, studies have successfully interrupted experimental rhinovirus transmission by the use of local application of aqueous iodine solution to the hands. Effectiveness of iodine in interrupting virus transmission in volunteers suggests that hand contamination and self-inoculation of the virus may provide the most important route by which these agents are transmitted.

Only 60% of rhinovirus infections produce symptoms; 40% are asymptomatic. The symptomatic infections produce higher concentrations of virus and are more contagious than asymptomatic cases.

Diagnosis

Acute upper respiratory symptoms can be caused by many different viruses. A tentative assignment of probable rhinovirus etiology can be made to illnesses occurring in the characteristic seasonal pattern and producing typical mild symptoms. To distinguish rhinovirus infection specifically from other etiologic agents requires virus isolation and demonstration of a rise in antibody titer between acute and convalescent sera. The assays for antibody must be done with neutralization tests against the specific rhinovirus causing the infection. This specific serologic identification of the agent requires multiple cross-neutralization tests and is impractical for general use.

Rhinoviruses are best recovered by inoculating a nasal specimen into human fibroblast cells or human embryonic kidney cell cultures. To obtain an optimal yield of these viruses, the culture should be incubated at 33C to 35C and at a neutral pH. The cytopathic effects usually become visible within the first week after inoculation, and infected cells are visible as a focus of oval or refractile cells. Cell lysis and a diminution in cell number occur. At the present time, detection of antigen by immunofluorescence of respiratory secretions is impractical because the large number of rhinovirus serotypes requires multiple antisera. No commercially available sources of hyperimmune sera exist. An isolate can be identified as a rhinovirus by its physicochemical properties, especially its acid lability, which distinguishes rhinoviruses from enteroviruses.

Treatment and Prevention

Treatment of rhinovirus infection is generally aimed at relief of symptoms. Providing hydration and preventing obstruction of the airways, paranasal sinuses, and eustachian tubes are the mainstays of therapy. Aspirin has been commonly prescribed, and although some diminution in symptoms may occur, increased virus shedding has been documented in persons receiving aspirin therapy, probably in part related to the reduction in body temperature (since higher temperatures suppress rhinovirus production).

Interferon alpha has been tested for effectiveness as prophylaxis against rhinovirus infections. When it was given as a nasal spray to household contacts, the total number of rhinovirus infections decreased. However, the drug had to be administered soon after exposure to the infected patient, it did not prevent the 70% of colds produced by other respiratory viruses, and the interferon produced a 10% rate of minor nasal bleeding. As of 1991, interferon prophylaxis is an interesting but impractical approach to preventing the common cold.

Several experimental antirhinoviral agents have been directed at the virus attachment site. A family of arylalkyl ketones, exemplified by disoxaril, have shown antivirus activity in vitro and in animal model systems. These agents fit into a canyon on the virus's surface (the area of the putative virus attachment protein) and stabilize the capsid, preventing it from releasing its RNA. Purified ICAM-1 also attaches to the virus, probably to the canyon region, and blocks access to cell-associated receptor molecules, thus decreasing viral replication. Neither of these families of agents have yet demonstrated efficacy in clinically relevant situations.

Resistance to reinfection with the same rhinovirus serotype can be shown after an initial infection, suggesting that a vaccine might be useful. The major obstacle to the development of vaccines is the more than 100 antigenically distinct serotypes of rhinoviruses. In addition, trials have suggested that production of materials of appropriate potency is difficult. At the present time, vaccination appears unlikely to be a successful method of prophylaxis against rhinovirus colds. Furthermore, vitamin C has not significantly decreased the number of colds in apparently well-designed studies.

Probably of greater importance than a vaccine is the possibility of diminishing the spread of infection. Recognition that contaminated hands play a role provides the opportunity to interrupt transmission with such basic measures as hand disinfection. One study has shown that antiviral tissues, virucidal for rhinoviruses, successfully diminished the incidence of respiratory illness in a closed setting. However, whether this type of approach will be useful outside a laboratory setting remains unanswered.

Reoviruses

Human reoviruses were first isolated in the early 1950s, but the name *reovirus* was not suggested until 1959. The name is derived from the isolation of virus from *r*espiratory and *e*nteric sources and the *o*rphan status (i.e., the lack of any associated human disease). A human isolate from 1953 was designated as echovirus 10 until it was reclassified as reovirus serotype 1, the Lang strain. Two other human strains, D5 Jones and Dearing, became the prototypes for serotypes 2 and 3, respectively.

Epidemiology

Reoviruses are ubiquitous in nature. Antibodies have been found in the sera of all mammals tested except whales. Orthoreoviruses have been isolated from many species of animals, including man, chimpanzees, calves, pigs, dogs, cats, mice, sheep, and birds. Newborn mice are particularly susceptible to experimental infection, which is frequently fatal.

Serologic surveys in different geographic and cultural areas have produced very similar results. The incidence of antibodies rises sharply in the first few years of life. Infections occur all year with no peak season. Virus can be cultured easily from water sources and sewage effluents, suggesting that they represent a potential source for human infection.

Pathogenesis

Mice have been used frequently in the study of reovirus infections. The segmented genome of reoviruses has facilitated their study because gene assortment occurs easily and is readily detected in recombinant progeny. A biologic difference can then be readily mapped to a single gene or group of genes. This has allowed the identification of some of the factors associated with virulence in the mouse system.

The first stage of viral pathogenesis is entry into the host, usually through the intestinal tract. Reovirus type 1, but not type 3, establishes infection in the mouse gut. This infection is associated with the activity of an outer capsid protein, μ1C, a cleavage product of protein μ1, which is encoded by genome segment M2. In reovirus serotype 1, μ1C confers resistance to the proteolytic enzymes in the gastrointestinal tract, allowing reovirus type 1 to penetrate through the intestinal epithelium and appear rapidly in Peyer's patches. Replication in lymphoid tissue occurs, followed by dissemination.

Another protein that is important in determining virulence is the σ1 protein, encoded by the S1 gene. Located on the outer capsid, this protein is responsible for the determination of cell and tissue tropism. Intracerebral inoculation of reovirus type 3 in newborn mice causes an acute, fatal encephalitis with massive neuronal involvement. Reovirus type 1, which has a different σ1 protein, produces a nonfatal infection of the ependymal cells with little or no effect on the neurons.

The σ1 protein is also responsible for the specificity of hemagglutination. Reovirus type 1 agglutinates human erythrocytes, whereas reovirus type 3 agglutinates bovine erythrocytes. Also identified as the viral protein responsible for the specific response to neutralizing antibody, σ1 determines type specificity. Therefore a reassortant virus that obtained the σ1 gene from reovirus type 1 but every other gene from reovirus type 3 would be identified as reovirus type 1.

Two other proteins, σ3 encoded by the S4 gene and λ2 encoded by the L2 gene, are capable of inducing neutralizing antibodies. However, unlike the antibodies to σ1, the antibodies to σ3 and λ2 can neutralize the infectivity of all three serotypes. The σ3 gene is responsible for inhibiting cellular RNA and protein synthesis. It is also a site of frequent mutations, which decrease the ability of the reovirus to lyse the host cells. Finally, it plays a role in the establishment of persistent infection.

Clearly, the mechanisms controlling virulence of the reoviruses involve several genes. As can be predicted from the information above, creating a recombinant virus with a serotype 1 M2 gene that produces a serotype 1 μ1C protein and a serotype 3 S1 gene that produces a serotype 3 σ1 protein yields a virus capable of infecting the mouse by the oral route, followed by dissemination and death from a fatal encephalitis.

Clinical Illness

The term *orphan* still applies to the reoviruses. Direct correlation between the reoviruses and disease has been difficult. Mammalian reoviruses are found primarily in the gastrointestinal tract but, in addition, have been isolated from respiratory tract secretions. They have been recovered from healthy humans and from individuals with a variety of minor gastrointestinal and respiratory illnesses. In infants, reovirus infection has been associated with a mild, febrile illness, diarrhea, and exanthem. Volunteers who were infected with reovirus remained asymptomatic or developed mild upper respiratory symptoms. The most characteristic pattern of adult infection, as judged by recovery of virus, is that of an afebrile coryzal illness occurring in the winter. Asymptomatic infections documented by virus isolation are common. The presence of neutralizing antibody in serum seems to be relatively protective against infection with the homologous serotype and may give some degree of protection against infection with heterologous types.

Reovirus serotype 3 infection in weanling mice produced a chronic obstructive jaundice associated with choledochal obliteration. The similarities between these pathologic changes and those seen in human congenital biliary atresia prompted further investigation. Some serologic studies have found a high percentage of infants with biliary atresia who were also seropositive to reovirus serotype 3. In an ultrastructural and immunocytochemical study, evidence of reovirus type 3 was found in the porta hepatis of an infant with extrahepatic biliary atresia. Other investigators, also using serologic techniques, found no association between reovirus type 3 antibodies and either biliary atresia or neonatal hepatitis. The data linking a role for reovirus in the pathogenesis of biliary atresia remain inconclusive.

All three serotypes have been isolated from sporadic cases of encephalitis, meningitis, pneumonia, and hepatitis that included rare fatalities. However, there has been no clearly defined role for reoviruses in these illnesses. Experimental infections have increased the number of possible diseases related to reoviruses. Infected animals have developed diabetes mellitus in mice; hydrocephalus in hamsters, ferrets, rats, and mice; encephalitis in mice; chronic infection with runting in mice; and lymphomas in mice with chronic infection.

Diagnosis

There are no specific clinical features of reovirus infections that allow their diagnosis without the aid of laboratory testing. Mammalian reoviruses replicate and produce visible cytopathic effects in a variety of tissue culture systems. Primary rhesus cell cultures have been used, but care must be taken in their interpretation since reoviruses can be contaminants of monkey tissue cultures. Primary human kidney cells have also been used successfully. Isolates have been obtained primarily from fecal specimens and, less often, from the respiratory tract. They have also been seen on occasion from other sources such as urine, cerebrospinal fluid, and various tissues obtained at autopsy.

Paired serum specimens can also be used to identify, retrospectively, an acute infection with reovirus. The antibody rise is measured by hemagglutination inhibition, neutralization, or indirect immunofluorescence. An enzyme-linked immunosorbent assay (ELISA) has been developed for the measurement of reovirus IgG, IgA, and IgM. The ELISA is not serotype specific, although this may become possible. Infection with one serotype causes a heterologous rise in antibodies to the other serotypes. This is explained primarily by the antibody to λ2, which is not serotype specific. Because there is such a high prevalence of antibodies to reovirus, paired sera demonstrating a rise in titer are necessary to make the serologic diagnosis of an acute reovirus infection.

Treatment and Prevention

Because of the lack of identifiable disease, no treatment is indicated for reovirus infections. However, ribavirin has been shown to inhibit reovirus replication in vitro. In addition, inactivated vaccines that induce high titer antibodies have been developed for animal use.

Parvoviruses

Two genera of the Parvoviridae family infect humans. The adeno-associated viruses (*Dependovirus*) are discussed in Chapter 65, and these defective agents require co-infection with an adenovirus for replication. The other genus of parvoviruses contains both agents that infect other vertebrate species and those that affect humans. The agents infecting humans require the special conditions found in the S phase of the cell cycle for replication. Thus these viruses have a propensity to infect rapidly dividing tissues. These agents are 18 to 26 nm in diameter, are nonenveloped, with icosahedral symmetry, and contain a linear single-stranded DNA molecule. Viral DNA replication occurs with the initial synthesis of the complementary strand to form monomer duplex DNA. Replication then proceeds, with formation of dimer duplex DNA from which the progeny DNA is made. The presence of both forms of DNA indicates replication is occurring. Plus and minus sense DNA are both encapsidated.

Serendipity led to the original identification of human parvoviruses in serum. In 1975, donor blood was being tested for the presence of hepatitis B surface antigen. Several units of donated blood gave a line of precipitate by counterimmunoelectrophoresis (CIE) with polyvalent human sera. These donor units were negative for hepatitis B surface antigen, and electron microscopy of the serum revealed a single species of virus particle with a mean diameter of 23 nm. One of these virus-containing units of blood has been designated *B19* and is frequently referred to in parvovirus studies. At the time of recognition of these viruses they were not associated with any known clinical entity. A review of the 11 viremic individuals identified by the blood screening procedures suggested a spectrum of vague symptoms was associated with the time when they were viremic. A pilot study was then performed in 1981, screening sera from children aged 2 to 12 years for parvovirus. Two children had parvovirus viremia, and review of their records revealed that they had sickle cell disease and had been admitted to the hospital because of an aplastic crisis. Thus the association with this entity was made for the first time. Subsequent investigation of other individuals with chronic hemolytic anemia and aplastic crises confirmed the association with parvovirus. The work on the agent and aplastic crises continued in Great Britain. Two children with a febrile illness and rash were observed in the family of a viremic donor. This raised the possibility that erythema infectiosum might be connected to these agents. Epidemiologic investigations have subsequently confirmed this association, and a second illness was attributable to parvoviruses. Subsequent clinical observations have also demonstrated that arthritis in adults and hydrops fetalis are associated with infections with these viruses.

Pathogenesis and Pathology

It seems probable that the respiratory tract is the usual portal of entry, although the parvoviruses can be transmitted by blood or blood products. Volunteer studies have used virus obtained from the original donor units of blood and inoculated the agent by intranasal instillation. Successful infection of antibody-negative volunteers occurs. In one individual viral DNA reappeared in nasal washings 10 days after inoculation, suggesting that local replication in the respiratory tract was occurring. In the volunteer studies seronegative individuals developed viremia as early as 6 days after inoculation, with peak titers as high as 10^5 for as long as 7 days. Viral excretion was detected in nasal washes and gargle specimens between days 7 and 11 from three of four volunteers. Virus was also demonstrable in urine specimens, but these specimens were contaminated with blood; therefore their source of virus is uncertain.

The volunteers experienced transient fever and nonspecific symptoms, including malaise, myalgia, headache, and itching, which was synchronous with the viremia. When rash was present, it appeared later than the viremia, as did arthritis and arthralgia. This biphasic illness suggests that the later manifestations may be attributable to secondary involvement of tissues or to the host response or both. The volunteers developed a temporary decrease in reticulocytes and a fall in hemoglobin of approximately 1 g/dL. These viruses replicate in erythroid precursors and are capable of inhibiting erythroid colony formation in vitro. These observations are consistent with a need for cell functions that are found in the late phases of mitosis; thus it appears the virus replicates in rapidly dividing erythroid precursors. It is likely that one infection protects against subsequent infection; therefore the patients with hemolytic anemia may be at risk for an aplastic crisis only on their first encounter with parvovirus. The ability to protect these vulnerable patients against aplastic red cell crisis would be desirable and may provide the impetus for development of a vaccine preventing this infection.

On the basis of the findings in volunteers, it seems plausible that these agents are in fact the etiologic cause of erythema infectiosum, although viremia is not detectable at the time of appearance of the rash. Inoculation of a small number of volunteers has demonstrated a spectrum of illness with nonspecific findings, fever, rash, arthritis, and demonstrable alterations in red cell production.

During an outbreak of erythema infectiosum six women were observed who had serologic evidence of human parvovirus infection during pregnancy. Two of these women had midtrimester abortions, and both of the fetuses were hydropic. Necrosis of individual hepatocytes with acidophilic inclusions and excessive iron pigment were observed. There was a simultaneous increase in the population of erythroid-myeloid precursor cells in the hepatic sinusoids. The nucleus of the erythroid cells also showed a homogeneous eosinophilic inclusion body. Other hematopoietic precursor cells in varying tissues showed similar nuclear changes. Parvoviruses were demonstrated in the placental and fetal tissues by using dot hybridization studies. The fetal infection with viral destruction of erythroid precursors results in hemolysis, anemia, and ultimately cardiac failure. Many aspects in the hydropic infants are the same as those caused by rhesus isoimmunization. Electron microscopic examination of the sections of fetal tissue did not reveal intact viral particles. Only examination of tissue homogenates has revealed viral particles.

Thus it is now apparent that parvoviruses may cause human illness by the respiratory route, by infusion of coagulation factor replacement, or alternatively by movement across the placenta from the maternal bloodstream to the fetus.

Epidemiology

Serologic studies show that antibody acquisition occurs most commonly between the ages of 4 and 10 years. In the United Kingdom where the majority of the serologic studies have been done, it has been demonstrated that 25% to 40% of individuals older than 16 years of age will have demonstrable parvovirus antibody. With more sensitive techniques, as many as 61% of a population of healthy blood donors in the United Kingdom were found to be seropositive. These serologic findings are consistent with the well-described epidemiology of erythema infectiosum and with the occurrence of aplastic crises in patients with hemolytic disease. Of particular interest is the seroprevalence that approaches 100% in children with hemophilia. These individuals have received large quantities of blood products for therapy of their disease, and it would appear that the clotting factor concentrates are more likely to contain virus than whole blood transfusions.

In 1985 and 1986 in the United Kingdom more than 2000 cases of B19 infection were diagnosed by detection of specific IgM antibodies or by detection of viral DNA. A spring and summer peak of infection has been described for school outbreaks of erythema infectiosum. Cases occurred in all months of the year, but the peaks were in the winter and spring. More than 80% of the illnesses resembled erythema infectiosum. Aplastic crisis in patients with chronic hemolytic anemias constituted a rather small percentage of the total cases, about 5%. There were individuals who were symptom free and were recognized as contacts of patients with clinical illness. The diagnosis of erythema infectiosum has been based on the appearance of a rash, but we now understand that infection with this virus does not always produce recognizable rash. Outbreaks of erythema infectiosum have been described as being confined to family, school, or other institutional groups and as being community wide. The disease has been recognized throughout the world, and clinical illness primarily occurs in children 2 to 12 years old.

Erythema infectiosum has not been considered a highly

communicable illness. A recent study following susceptible household contacts has estimated that the secondary attack rate is approximately 50%. The risk of infection in susceptible day-care personnel has been found to be 20% to 30%. Concurrent outbreaks of aplastic crisis and erythema infectiosum clearly demonstrate the association of each of these clinical entities with parvovirus B19 infection.

Clinical Illness

Parvoviruses cause a spectrum of clinical illness from nondescript febrile illness with vague headache and arthritis to defined clinical entities such as erythema infectiosum, hydrops fetalis, and aplastic crisis in the presence of hemolytic anemia. When a large number of infected persons are identified, approximately 30% of them will have rash and arthropathy. Another third will have either rash or arthropathy, and only 15% will have erythema infectiosum.

Erythema infectiosum is a well-described clinical entity characterized by a typical eruption. The rash appears first on the face and is described as "a slapped cheek" appearance. It may originate as a number of erythematous maculopapules that coalesce and develop into an erysipeloid confluent rash. The circumoral area has a contrasting pallor, and there may be scattered discreet lesions on the forehead and chin and behind the ears. The rash subsequently involves the upper and lower extremities and appears as small maculopapular red spots. Within several days the spots involve the flexor surfaces, the distal parts of the extremities, and the trunk. As the earlier lesions are fading, the rash develops its lacelike appearance. This rash may persist for several days. Precipitants such as trauma and sunlight and extremes such as hot and cold weather may cause the rash to reappear. Thus its appearance, distribution, evanescence, and tendency to recur are characteristic of this exanthem. It is well known that arthritis and arthralgia may occur during the course of the illness, and these manifestations are usually transient and self-limited and occur more commonly in adults than in children. This illness is usually mild, with minimal systemic or respiratory symptoms. Illness may last as long as 2 weeks.

Association of parvovirus with arthropathy in adults has been confirmed by studies initiated in a clinic taking care of patients with arthritis. Patients most often present with acute symmetric peripheral arthritis usually starting in the hands or knees. Within 48 hours other joints, including the wrists, ankles, feet, elbows, and shoulders, become involved. The pain, stiffness, and variable swelling are common but improve within 2 weeks. In several cases the symptoms were documented to have persisted for several months.

Aplastic crises associated with parvovirus infection are well described. It is probable that the increased number of erythroid progenitor cells in the bone marrow of the patients with hereditary hemolytic anemias facilitates virus replication because there are increased numbers of target cells for this agent. Furthermore, availability of susceptible cells may be the reason that such large quantities of virus are detectable in the blood. Patients with chronic hemolytic anemia who have a steady-state hemoglobin level of 7 to 9 g/dL and a red cell life span of 10 to 15 days will have a recognizable fall in hemoglobin level when the virus causes an arrest of erythropoiesis. The events are sufficiently rapid that viremia can be detected at the time of presentation of the patient with clinical symptoms. This is in marked contrast to normal individuals undergoing parvovirus infection in whom a red blood cell life span of 120 days and a hemoglobin level of 13 to 15 g/dL will obscure a transient decline in erythropoiesis. Thus viremia goes undetected, and it is usual for a characteristic rash to appear a week or more after the viremia has occurred.

Chronic or persistent infection has been documented in children with congenital immunodeficiency, patients receiving immunosuppressive therapy, and those infected with human immunodeficiency virus (HIV). They have erythroid hypoplasia, IgM antibodies but no IgG antibodies, and prolonged viremia. Intravenous immunoglobulin has been used with some success.

The risk of parvovirus infection in pregnancy is beginning to be defined. This virus can cross the placenta, infect the fetus, induce anemia, and ultimately induce hydrops fetalis. Too little experience is available to assess the degree of risk. Data suggest that a primary encounter with this virus is the only one placing the fetus at risk. The current information suggests that not all infections are transmitted to the fetus because six pregnant women with seroconversions were followed during an outbreak of parvovirus infection, and two of them delivered hydropic fetuses. The four healthy infants delivered to these women had no serologic incidence of infection. This information plus other case reports suggest that acquisition of virus by the fetus may induce fatal anemia resulting in hydrops, but no asymptomatic or less severely involved infant has yet been detected. Thus it remains possible that transplacental infection always results in fetal death or stillbirth. It is also possible that some infants have recovered from this infection, have lost their IgM antibody, and by the time of delivery have only IgG antibody and therefore cannot be determined to have been infected in utero. Estimates of risk to the fetus after exposure of pregnant women are low. An estimated 50% of adults are not susceptible because of prior experience with the virus. The maximal chance of maternal infection is 15% to 25%, and the risk of transplacental transmission is 33%, leaving an estimated risk of fetal death of less than 1.5% if a woman is exposed at a school or day care center and less than 2.5% if she is exposed at home to a household member. If exposure occurs to a susceptible woman, ultrasonoagraphy and α-fetoprotein measurements are used to monitor her pregnancy.

Host Response

Parvovirus infection elicits the appearance of IgM antibody and subsequently IgG antibodies. The IgM antibody reaches high titers during the second week of experimental inoculation, and IgG antibody can be detected at the end of the second or the beginning of the third week after experimental infection. An anamnestic response in antibody has been observed in a volunteer with preexisting IgG antibodies. Immune complexes have been detected during viremia but not during the later development of rash and arthralgia. Sequential observations of polymorphonuclear cells and lymphocytes during infection show transient but mild neutropenia developing approximately 1 week after infection and lasting a few days. Similarly, lymphocyte counts decreased approximately 1 week after infection and remained lower than their preinoculation counts for approximately 3 days.

Diagnosis

The human parvoviruses have been detected in serum by immune electron microscopy, counter immunoelectrophoresis, and radioimmunoassay. A more sensitive means of detecting virus is that of dot-blot hybridization using cloned viral DNA. A portion of the B19 genome has been cloned in pAT153 and used as a ^{32}P-labeled probe in the hybridization assay. The test is highly sensitive and detects virus in microliter volumes of serum. The sensitivity appears to be that of 0.5 pg of viral DNA, which is roughly equivalent to 10^4 virus particles. An advantage of the hybridization is that the presence of antibody does not interfere with detection of the virus. Most recently, polymerase chain reaction has been used to amplify and detect virus in peripheral blood. Unfortunately, the availability of these assays is limited.

Serologic diagnosis of parvovirus infection is most commonly approached by measuring parvovirus-specific IgM antibodies in the serum of the patient. Monoclonal antibodies to human parvovirus were developed and are used to develop a solid-phase-specific antibody-capture radioimmunoassay assay. The detection of IgM antibody or a fourfold rise in IgG antibodies can be used as presumptive evidence of parvovirus infection. The presence of IgM antibody clearly designates recent infection and is the test available through the Centers for Disease Control. The development of a cell line (Chinese hamster ovary) that expresses B19 structural proteins in the form of empty capsids will provide antigen for antibody assays and increase their availability.

Treatment and Prevention

There are no specific means of disease prevention or treatment. All the appropriate supportive measures are indicated for patients with chronic hemolytic disease and a red blood cell aplastic crisis. Fortunately, the majority of illness is sufficiently mild and self-limited that intervention is not necessary.

FURTHER READING

RHINOVIRUSES

Butler WT, Waldmann TA, Rossen RD, et al: Changes in IgA and IgG concentrations in nasal secretions prior to the appearance of antibody during viral respiratory infection in man. J Immunol 105:584, 1970

Cate TR, Roberts JJ, Russ MA, et al: Effects of common colds on pulmonary function. Am Rev Respir Dis 108:858, 1973

Dick CE, Jennings LC, Mink KA, et al: Aerosol transmission of rhinovirus colds. J Infect Dis 156:442, 1987

Douglas RM, Moore BW, Miles HB, et al: Prophylactic efficacy of intranasal alpha$_2$-interferon against rhinovirus infections in the family setting. N Engl J Med 314:65, 1986

Greve JM, Davis G, Meyer AM, et al: The major human rhinovirus receptor is ICAM-1. Cell 56:839, 1990

Gwaltney JM, Moskalski PB, Hendley JO: Hand-to-hand transmission of rhinovirus colds. Ann Intern Med 88:463, 1978

Gwaltney JM, Moskalski PB, Hendley JO: Interruption of experimental rhinovirus transmission. J Infect Dis 142:811, 1980

Hayden FG, Albrecht JK, Kaiser DL, et al: Prevention of natural colds by contact prophylaxis with intranasal alpha$_2$-interferon. N Engl J Med 314:71, 1986

Hsia J, Goldstein AL, Simon GL, et al: Peripheral blood mononuclear cell interleukin-2 and interferon-γ production, cytotoxicity, and antigen-stimulated blastogenesis during experimental rhinovirus infection. J Infect Dis 162:591, 1990

Marlin SD, Staunton DE, Springer TA, et al: A soluble form of intercellular adhesion molecule-1 inhibits rhinovirus infection. Nature 344:70, 1990

Naclerio RM, Proud D, Lichtenstein LM, et al: Kinins are generated during experimental rhinovirus colds. J Infect Dis 157:133, 1988

Smith TJ, Kremer MJ, Luo M, et al: The site of attachment in human rhinovirus 14 for antiviral agents that inhibit uncoating. Science 233:1286, 1986

REOVIRUSES

Brown WR, Sokol RJ, Levin MJ, et al: Lack of correlation between infection with reovirus 3 and extrahepatic biliary atresia or neonatal hepatitis. J Pediatr 113:670, 1988

Fields BN: Molecular basis of reovirus virulence. Brief review. Arch Virol 71:95, 1982

Jackson GG, Muldoon RL, Johnson GC, Dowling MF: Contributions of volunteers to studies on the common cold. Am Rev Respir Dis 88(Suppl):120, 1963

Joklik WK: The Reoviridae. New York, Plenum Press, 1983

Lerner AM, Cherry JD, Klein JO, Finland M: Infections with reoviruses. N Engl J Med 267:947, 1962

Morecki R, Glaser JH, Cho S, et al: Biliary atresia and reovirus 3 infection. N Engl J Med 307:481, 1982

Morecki R, Glaser JH, Johnson AB, Kress Y: Detection of reovirus type 3 in the porta hepatis of an infant with extrahepatic biliary atresia: Ultrastructural and immunocytochemical study. Hepatology 4:1137, 1984

Rankin JT Jr, Eppes SC, Antczak JB, Joklik WK: Studies on the mechanism of the antiviral activity of ribavirin against reovirus. Virology 168:147, 1989

Richardson SC, Bishop RF, Smith AL: Enzyme-linked immunosorbent assays for measurement of reovirus immunoglobulin G, A, and M levels in serum. J Clin Microbiol 26;1871, 1988

Sabin AB: Reoviruses. A new group of respiratory and enteric viruses formerly classified as ECHO type 10 is described. Science 130:1387, 1959

PARVOVIRUSES

Anand A, Gray ES, Brown T, et al: Human parvovirus infection in pregnancy and hydrops fetalis. N Engl J Med 316:183, 1987

Anderson MJ, Higgins PG, Davis LR, et al: Experimental parvoviral infection in humans. J Infect Dis 152:257, 1985

Anderson MJ, Jones SE, Minson AC: Diagnosis of human parvovirus infection by dot-blot hybridization using cloned viral DNA. J Med Virol 15:163, 1985

Anderson MJ: Human parvoviruses. J Infect Dis 161:603, 1990

Cartter MC, Farley TA, Rosengren S, et al: Occupational risk factors for infection with parvovirus B19 among pregnant women. J Infect Dis 163:282, 1991

Chorba T, Coccia P, Holman RC, et al: The role of parvovirus B19 in aplastic crisis and erythema infectiosum (fifth disease). J Infect Dis 154:383, 1986

Cohen BJ, Mortimer PP, Pereira MS: Diagnostic assays with monoclonal antibodies for the human serum parvovirus-like virus (SPLV). J Hyg (Camb) 91:113, 1983

Gillespie SM, Cartter ML, Asch S, et al: Occupational risk of human parvovirus B19 infection for school and day care personnel during an outbreak of erythema infectiosum. JAMA 263:2061, 1990

Plummer FA, Hammond GW, Forward K, et al: An erythema infectiosum-like illness caused by human parvovirus infection. N Engl J Med 313:74, 1985

Schwartz TF, Roggendorf M, Deinhardt F: Human parvovirus B19 infection in United Kingdom 1984–86. Lancet 2:738, 1987

White DG, Mortimer PP, Blake DR, et al: Human parvovirus arthropathy. Lancet 2:419, 1985

CHAPTER 79

Subacute Spongiform Encephalopathies and Unconventional Agents

The subacute spongiform encephalopathies (SSE) are slow infections of the central nervous system that produce progressive degeneration of the gray matter with characteristic histopathologic changes. The agents that cause the SSEs have not been fully characterized; they present unusual chemical and physical properties that suggest that they may be smaller and simpler than conventional viruses. In humans the recognized SSEs are kuru, Creutzfeldt-Jakob disease (CJD), and the Gertsmann-Sträussler syndrome. The animal diseases include scrapie, transmissible mink encephalopathy (TME), bovine spongiform encephalopathy (BSE), and chronic wasting disease of captive mule deer and elk. The histologic changes are typical and common to all the members of this group. They include (1) neuronal loss, (2) astrocytic proliferation and hypertrophy, (3) neuronal vacuolation, and (4) little inflammatory response. The presence of multiple small vacuoles in a brain specimen is termed *spongiform change*; the predominance of large vacuoles is classically named *status spongiosus*. The degree with which each of these histopathologic changes is present varies during the course of the disease and from disease to disease. Amyloid deposits also have been described in all these entities but are apparently not as uniformly present.

All the SSEs are transmissible conditions involving the central nervous system exclusively. They are characterized by a prolonged incubation period followed by a protracted but relentlessly progressive clinical course.

Another unique feature of these diseases is that their devastating effects progress in a state of "immunologic indifference." There is no inflammatory reaction in the tissues involved (central nervous system) and no measurable host cellular or humoral immunity to these agents. Infected hosts have no impairment of overall function of the immune system, and experimentally induced immunosuppression of infected hosts does not alter the course of these diseases.

The agents causing SSEs have been more difficult to characterize than the conventional viruses. Various studies of resistance and susceptibility of these agents to the effects of physical and chemical agents have given some insight regarding their possible nature. They generally are susceptible to agents that denature proteins but are resistant to those that modify nucleic acids, suggesting that proteins are important components of the infectious particle.

Although they are considered viruses by many investigators, no recognizable viral particles have been visualized by electron microscopy of infected cells or in highly infectious preparations concentrated by density gradient banding. No viral agents have been isolated using conventional culture procedures. Their resistance to physical and chemical treatments that normally inactivate viruses and the lack of any detectable immune response would appear to put these agents in a category apart from conventional viruses.

Distinctive fibrils are found in brains infected with these agents; these fibrils were described in 1981 by Merz and named *scrapie-associated fibrils (SAFs)*. Using elaborate purification procedures on scrapie-infected brain, other investigators isolated a unique 27 to 30 kDa protein and named it PrP27-30 (prion protein 27-30). PrP27-30 is a sialoglycoprotein associated with cellular membranes. It is resistant to proteinase K digestion and copurifies with infectivity in some experiments. The PrP27-30 protein is part of a larger molecule of 33 to 35 kDa (PrP33-35). These proteins polymerize into rodlike structures that have amyloid characteristics. Whether these rodlike structures are identical to the SAFs obtained by different techniques has been questioned by some investigators. However, SAFs appear to be composed of a protein of similar molecular weight to the PrP27-30 and react with monoclonal antibodies against PrP27-30. *N*-terminal amino acid sequencing of the SAF protein also suggests that it is very similar to PrP27-30.

Experimental data obtained from animal scrapie models have shown that there are different strains of the agent determining variability in incubation periods and susceptibility to infection. The presence of these strain variations argues in favor of the presence of a genome, although no agent-specific nucleic acids have been found. Also, these agents are unusually resistant to physical and chemical treatments that modify nucleic acids, suggesting that they lack nucleic acids or that their genome is very small and protected from the effects of these treatments, possibly by a protein envelope.

Some experiments have found that the PrP27-30 protein copurifies with infectivity. Prusiner and colleagues have proposed that this protein is a major component of the scrapie agent itself. They postulate that a proteinaceous pathogen resistant to procedures that modify nucleic acids is the causative agent of these diseases. These novel agents have received the designation of prions (proteinaceous infectious particle).

Other investigators propose that the agent may be a small nucleic acid surrounded by a coating of host-derived protein. The small size of the molecule and a thick protein envelope would be responsible for the resistance of these agents to substances capable of denaturing or modifying nucleic acids. They use the term *virino* to describe these unique pathogens.

Surprisingly, the gene encoding for PrP27-30 has been found both in scrapie-infected brains and in normal brains; however, the protein encoded for by the gene in normal brain does not polymerize into rodlike structures, and it is degraded by proteinase K. A posttranscriptional error may determine changes in the physicochemical properties of PrP27-30 that alter its processing within the affected cells.

Whether these agents are viruses, prions, or virinos remains to be determined and continues to be a subject of great controversy among researchers. The availability of monoclonal antibodies to PrP27-30 and the development of large scale purification techniques will help increase our understanding of these diseases.

Infections of Humans

Kuru

The Fore people of Papua, New Guinea's eastern highlands, used the word *kuru* to describe trembling from fear or cold. Kuru came to be the name of a disease characterized by tremors that was confined to this Melanesian tribe of 35,000 persons living in isolated Mesolithic villages. When the illness was first described by Gajdusek and Zigas in 1957, it was the most common cause of death among those people, and the death rate was as high as 1% annually.

Kuru was thought to be a genetically determined degenerative disease until 1959 when Hadlow noted the striking pathologic similarities between kuru and scrapie, an infectious disease of sheep. Gajdusek and coworkers were then prompted to test the transmission of kuru to animals. In 1966 primates inoculated intracerebrally with brain tissue of kuru patients developed a "kurulike" illness. Kuru became the first human SSE shown to be infectious.

Kuru is a distinctive neurologic syndrome of extraordinary uniformity in its clinical manifestations and course. Clinical disease is initially recognized by the development of clumsiness in walking or inability to maintain balance. These relatively minor changes in coordination may be associated with personality and mood alterations that persist for 12 to 18 months before more generalized disease becomes apparent. Once definite neurologic symptoms are recognized, the course of the disease is ordinarily fatal over the following 12 to 18 months. The clumsiness progresses so that the patient becomes unable to sit, stand, or perform any voluntary movement. At this stage, excessive contraction of synergistic muscles and associated movements in other limbs create exhausting ineffective muscular activity. Speech is slurred and becomes unintelligible, and chewing and swallowing are affected. The clinical examination of affected patients reveals signs of cerebellar dysfunction. Further changes in mood, emotional lability, depression, and episodes of confusion are common. Disability of memory and language functions is apparent. Unable to eat, aspirating secretions, and developing pneumonia and decubitus ulcers, the patients die.

Epidemiology

Kuru has only been found affecting members of the Fore linguistic group in New Guinea. The disease was unknown to tribal elders before the introduction of ritual cannibalism. Women and children of both sexes were commonly affected by the disease. They were directly involved in the preparation of the body and internal organs (including the brain) of the deceased for the ceremonial rituals. Although the adult men practiced cannibalism, they did not participate in the preparatory stages of the rituals, and they rarely contracted the disease. It is likely that the handling of the infected tissues allowed entry of the agent through breaks in the skin or mucosa, and the actual consumption of these tissues was less important in transmission of the disease. Pregnant women became infected, but no transplacental transmission of the disease occurred.

Pathology

The pathology of this disease is limited to the central nervous system, and it is as uniform as the clinical illness. Macroscopically, the cerebral hemispheres appear normal, and the cerebellum is atrophied. Microscopically, the most severe degeneration occurs in the cerebellum, where there is a loss of Purkinje and granule cells. Proliferation and hypertrophy of astrocytes occur throughout the brain. The spongiform changes of gray matter of the cerebral cortex and cord seem to be a result of coalescing vacuolation of neuronal processes, apparently intradendritic in origin. Accumulations of membranous material in these swellings are apparent. Microglial cells are seen in all stages of phagocytic activity. There is no evidence of inflammatory reaction or demyelination of white matter. In the majority of cases, birefringent amyloid-containing plaques are found. This amyloid material is composed of SAFs and their subunit (PrP27-30). Similar amyloid deposits are found in animals with scrapie and to a lesser degree also in patients with Creutzfeldt-Jakob disease. As observed by amino acid sequencing and immunoreactivity to anti-PrP antibody, the amyloid deposits appear to be of identical composition.

Kuru has been transmitted to experimental animals, and the pathology of nonhuman primates resembles that of humans. Infectivity is as high as 10^9 infectious units per gram of brain tissue, and animal inoculation studies have shown lower concentrations present in spleen, liver, or lymph nodes. Infectivity has not been found in blood, cerebrospinal fluid, urine, leukocytes, milk, amniotic fluid, or placenta. Intracerebral, intravenous, intramuscular, subcutaneous, and intraperitoneal injections transmit infection; and incubation periods range from 1 to 8½ years. A single experiment successfully transmitted infection orally to squirrel monkeys, whereas many other similar experiments have failed. These results suggest that penetration of the agent through skin or mucous membranes is a more likely avenue of infection for humans as well.

Creutzfeldt-Jakob Disease

Clinical and Epidemiologic Features

Creutzfeldt-Jakob disease (CJD) is a rare, progressive, and fatal disease of the human central nervous system that occurs in middle life and affects both sexes. It was originally described in the late 1920s as a form of presenile dementia. Vague prodromal symptoms are followed by dementia, with subsequent rapid progression to coma and death, occurring usually within 2 years after recognition of symptoms. The dementia can be accompanied by other neurologic manifestations. The association with myoclonus is characteristic and almost diagnostic. Signs of focal cortical degeneration, both upper and lower motor neuron involvement, extrapyramidal signs, cerebellar ataxia, and seizures also have been described and contribute to the variability in the clinical syndrome. During the course of their illness, approximately half the patients develop characteristic electroencephalographic changes, which, when present, are useful for diagnostic purposes.

The disease has worldwide distribution, with a prevalence rate estimated to be one or two cases per million population. Libyan Jews have a rate more than 30 times higher than the overall prevalence rate. A familial form of the disease has been recognized in 10% to 15% of patients, affecting members in several generations. Transmission of the infectious form of the disease is not highly efficient, since (1) only two cases of conjugal disease have been reported, and (2) people in closest contact with CJD patients do not appear to be at any higher risk of contracting infection than the general population.

The mechanisms involved in the natural transmission of the disease are not known. Transmission to humans has occurred after the use of contaminated neurosurgical and ophthalmologic equipment. Iatrogenic transmission of the disease to patients receiving corneal transplants, dura mater grafts, and human growth hormone derived from pituitary extracts have also been reported. Approximately 20 cases of CJD occurring in young adults have been attributed to the use of human growth hormone unknowingly contaminated with the infectious agent.

Concerns regarding the risk of occupational infection in those exposed to infected human tissues during surgery or postmortem examination have been raised by the occurrence of the disease in a neurosurgeon, two physicians, a dentist, and two of the dentist's patients. The incubation period in cases occurring after direct inoculation is estimated to be at least 15 to 20 months. The latency period in naturally occurring disease is probably much longer because of the absence of this disease in children or young adults.

The transmissible nature of CJD is well established. Gajdusek and associates reported the transmission of disease to nonhuman primates inoculated with 218 postmortem brain specimens obtained from patients with CJD. The results of additional inoculations are still pending. Brain tissue has been shown to contain at least 10^8 infectious units per gram. The agent has been found less regularly and at lower concentrations in lymph nodes, liver, kidney, spleen, lung, cornea, and cerebrospinal fluid; but it has not been isolated from body surfaces, secretions, or excretions. The natural acquisition of the disease may occur by tissue penetration as is the case with kuru.

Pathology

The diverse clinical manifestations of CJD are matched by the spectrum of the distribution and severity of the pathologic lesions. Brains may appear normal, or they may be small and atrophic. The microscopic changes always include neuronal loss, status spongiosus (less marked than in kuru), and proliferation of hypertrophic astrocytes. SAFs with PrP27-30 are present. Brain tissue of inoculated animals demonstrates status spongiosus as one of the major pathologic findings, together with neuronal loss, proliferation of astrocytes, and absence of inflammation.

Disinfection for Creutzfeldt-Jakob Disease Agent

No special ward isolation procedures are warranted. In fact, such procedures may be an inconvenience to both patient and personnel and, if specified, may prevent optimal care of the patient or admission to a long-term care facility. Exposure to breath, saliva, nasopharyngeal secretions, or urine of CJD patients should not cause special concern. Washing of hands or other exposed areas of the skin with appropriate detergent is recommended, as for contact with any patients with transmissible diseases. Although a patient's blood or cerebrospinal fluid could be infectious, simple washing should be sufficient to protect exposed persons. Caution must be taken to avoid accidental percutaneous exposure to blood, cerebrospinal fluid, or brain tissue. If puncture occurs, careful washing in iodine solution, phenolic antiseptic, 0.5% sodium hypochlorite solution, or with a 1 N sodium hydroxide solution is appropriate. Some of the physical and chemical properties of these agents are listed in Table 79–1. Surgical instruments, tonometers used on demented patients, and all instruments used in eye operations should be considered contaminated. The preferred method of disinfection of equipment is either by immersing it in a 1 N sodium hydroxide solution (three times for 30 minutes) or autoclaving it at 121C (15 psi for 4½ hours). The method of choice depends on the nature of the material being treated. Patients suffering a dementing illness should not be used as donors of blood, organs, or tissues for use in transplants or as the source of biologic products for human use.

TABLE 79–1. SOME PHYSICAL AND CHEMICAL PROPERTIES OF THE UNCONVENTIONAL AGENTS

Sensitive (loss of infectivity) to autoclaving (121C, 15 psi, 60 min), phenol, 1 N sodium hydroxide (three treatments of 30 minutes)—reduction of infectivity titers by 10^6 to 10^8

Moderately sensitive (decrease in titer by 10^2 to 10^4) to 0.5% sodium hypochlorite (decrease by 10^4), ether extraction (10^2)

Resistant to formaldehyde, β-propiolactone, ethylenediaminetetraacetic acid (EDTA), proteases (trypsin, pepsin, pronase, proteinase K), nucleases (DNase, micrococcal nuclease), phospholipases, nonionic or mildly ionic detergents (Triton, NP-40, sarkosyl, deoxycholate); ultraviolet radiation, ionizing radiation; 80C heat

Subacute Spongiform Encephalopathies in Animals

Scrapie

Scrapie has been known for some 200 years as a clinical entity in sheep in Europe. Also for more than 100 years, a chronic disease affecting the central nervous system of sheep was prevalent in a region of northern Iceland. The name of the disease in Icelandic, *rida*, means either ataxia or tremor. Rida is a progressive and fatal disease of adult sheep. The sheep fail to thrive; they become apprehensive and excitable; then tremor and uncoordinated movements of the head appear. The animals become clumsy, with initial involvement of the hind limbs. Finally, they become unable to walk and, despite remaining alert, are totally immobilized by tremors and spastic movements. This disease in Iceland is scrapie but without the characteristic pruritus seen in other geographic locations.

The pathogenesis of the pruritus with scrapie is unknown, but it can be severe enough to cause the affected animal to scratch incessantly against posts or trees. It is from this manifestation of the disease that the term *scrapie* is derived.

The transmissible nature of the disease was recognized by shepherds who found that sheep grazing in pastures previously occupied by infected flocks contracted the disease. Cuille and Chèlle experimentally confirmed the transmissibility of scrapie in 1936. As mentioned previously, the link between scrapie and kuru was suggested by Hadlow because of the similar central nervous system pathologic manifestations found in these entities.

Horizontal transmission is frequent in nature. Transmission of the disease from ewe to newborn lamb is usual, and placental tissues have been shown to be infectious. The time at which infection occurs, whether in utero or postpartum following contact with infected tissues or secretions, has not been identified.

Scrapie has been successfully adapted to laboratory animals, and much of what is known about the agents that cause these diseases stems from studies done in animals experimentally inoculated with the scrapie agent. Transmission of the agent to various laboratory animals is accomplished by parenteral inoculations. Sheep and mice also have been infected through the oral route.

The pathogenesis of scrapie has been studied in mice, and, although the route of infection influences the incubation period and ultimate outcome, several general features emerge. The inoculated agent can be almost completely recovered from spleen in the first week after infection. Infectivity is no longer detectable for the subsequent several weeks. Approximately 1 month after inoculation, replication becomes apparent, with initial reappearance of the agent in the spleen and lymph nodes and with subsequent spread to the central nervous system through peripheral nerves. Replication in lymphoid tissue does not appear to alter immune function or produce any pathology. Approximately 3 months after inoculation, infectivity is detectable in salivary glands, lung, intestine, and other tissues. The animals remain asymptomatic for a total of 4 to 5 months.

Transmissible Mink Encephalopathy

Transmissible mink encephalopathy (TME) is a rare sporadic disease of farm-raised mink. The first outbreak occurred in 1942 in two mink breeding farms in Wisconsin. Later outbreaks were reported in the 1960s and, more recently, in the 1980s. The disease exclusively affects the central nervous system, producing a chronic progressive illness that ends with death.

The pathologic changes are similar to those described with scrapie, varying only in the topographic location of the lesions in the brain. The first clinical manifestations of disease follow an incubation period of 8 to 9 months after oral inoculation; parenteral inoculation of the TME agent results in a shorter incubation period (approximately 5 or 6 months). Typically, behavioral manifestations mark the onset of disease; lack of grooming and decreased cleanliness are followed by excitability, eating difficulties, ataxia, somnolence, and increasing immobility.

Epidemiologic data suggest that the disease was introduced to the mink population accidentally by the use of infected tissues, possibly of ovine origin, as a dietary supplement. Disease transmission within the mink population is probably the result of inoculation of the agent through wounds inflicted by litter mates or through acts of cannibalism; vertical transmission does not occur. Mink are considered dead-end hosts.

Experimental transmission using other mink has successfully produced disease both by parenteral and oral routes. Sheep, goats, ferrets, and hamsters have also been infected after the parenteral inoculation of brain tissue of affected animals. In primates the disease is very similar to CJD. Transmission experiments, however, have been unsuccessful with mice. Chinese hamsters infected with the TME agent developed disease that suggested the presence of different strains of the agent; there were differences in the incubation period and topographic distribution of lesions in the central nervous system.

Bovine Spongiform Encephalopathy

Bovine spongiform encephalopathy (BSE) is the most recently recognized of the transmissible encephalopathies. Cases affecting cattle were first diagnosed in the United Kingdom between 1985 and 1986. Since then the disease has been diagnosed in thousands of animals. The clinical manifestations and remarkable pathology link it to scrapie and the other scrapielike illnesses of animals. The outbreak created great consternation because of concerns about the possibility of disease transmission to humans by the consumption of infected bovine products.

Changes in behavior, ataxia, excitability, and aggressiveness declare the onset of the disease. Subsequently, the animal shows signs of progressive wasting, its health deteriorates gradually over the ensuing 4 or 5 months, and the animal dies.

The incubation period appears to vary from 2½ to 8 years and would therefore place the introduction of the disease to cattle to the early 1980s. The source of infection is thought to be scrapie-infected sheep carcasses used in cattle feed. However, the use of ovine protein to supplement nutrition was not unusual before the beginning of the epidemic, and various hypotheses have been proposed to explain the abrupt outbreak. Changes in the procedures used during the processing of sheep carcasses used in animal feed took place in various rendering plants and may have exposed the bovine population to high titers of the infective agent. Mutational changes in the scrapie agent or immunologic changes in the host or both may have been important factors contributing to the expression of disease in cattle and leading to the outbreak.

There is no doubt that this disease is an SSE caused by a scrapielike agent. SAFs have been found in diseased cattle brain. PrP27-30 isolated from cattle is remarkably similar in its amino acid sequence to the scrapie PrP27-30 and differs in one amino acid from the mouse and CJD proteins. Also, this PrP protein cross-reacts with anti-PrP antibody of mouse origin and has similar lectin-binding abilities. The abnormal PrP27-30 protein found in affected cattle is not found in healthy cattle brain. Experimental transmission to mice using infected brain tissues by parenteral and oral routes emphasizes the similarities of BSE with the other entities considered in this chapter.

So far, there is no evidence of horizontal or vertical transmission of this disease within the bovine population; the infected animals are considered dead-end hosts. To prevent further extension of the epidemic, sheep protein has been banned from ruminant feed in the United Kingdom; infected animals and their offspring are sacrificed. With these measures, the epidemic should decrease considerably in the coming years.

There is no evidence that BSE can be transmitted to humans. However, surveillance programs designed to evaluate changes in the incidence of CJD have been instituted, and bovine tissues that may be potentially infectious (e.g., brain, spinal cord, and lymphoid tissues) have been removed from the food chain in the United Kingdom.

Transmissible Spongiform Encephalopathy of Mule Deer and Elk

This disease affects only animals in captivity. A chronic wasting disease of captive mule deer and elk with clinical and histopathologic similarities was described in 1978 and 1982, respectively. Experimental transmission of this disease has been accomplished, and SAFs have been found in brain tissue of diseased animals. It is thought that these diseases also represent the manifestation of scrapie in an accidental host.

FURTHER READING

Books and Reviews

Chesebro B: Spongiform encephalopathies: Transmissible agents. In Fields BN, Knipe DM, et al (eds): Virology, ed 2. New York, Raven Press, 1990

Gadjusek DC: Subacute spongiform encephalopathies: Transmissible cerebral amyloidoses caused by unconventional viruses. In Fields BN, Knipe DM, et al (eds): Virology, ed 2. New York, Raven Press, 1990

Lehrich JR, Tyler KL: Slow infections of the central nervous system. In Mandell GL, Douglas RG, Bennett JE (eds): Principles and Practice of Infectious Diseases, ed 3. New York, John Wiley & Sons, 1990

Prusiner SB, McKinley MD (eds): Prions: Novel Infectious Pathogens Causing Scrapie and Creutzfeldt-Jakob Disease. New York, Academic Press, 1987

Prusiner SB, Hsiao K, Kingsbury DT, et al: Human slow infections caused by prions. In Gilden DH, Lipson HL (eds): Clinical and Molecular Aspects of Neurotropic Virus Infection. Kluwer Academic Publishers, Norwell, Mass, 1989

Tyler KL: Prions. In Mandell GL, Douglas RG, Bennett JE (eds): Principles and Practice of Infectious Diseases, ed 3. New York, John Wiley & Sons, 1990

Selected Papers

Barry RA, Prusiner SB: Monoclonal antibodies to the cellular and scrapie prion proteins. J Infect Dis 154:518, 1986

Bendheim PE, Potempska A, Bolton DC, et al: Purification and partial characterization of the normal cellular homologue of the scrapie agent protein. J Infect Dis 158:1198, 1988

Brown P: Human growth hormone therapy and Creutzfeldt-Jakob disease: A drama in three acts. Pediatrics 81:85, 1988

Chesebro B, Race R, Haase A, et al: Identification of scrapie prion protein-specific mRNA in scrapie-infected and uninfected brain. Nature 315:331, 1985

Gadjusek DC, Gibbs CJ, Alpers MP: Experimental transmission of a kuru-like syndrome to chimpanzees. Nature 209:794, 1966

Gadjusek DC: Fantasy of a "virus" from the inorganic world: Pathogenesis of cerebral amyloidoses by polymer nucleating agents and/or "viruses." Hamatol Und Bluttransfusion 32:481, 1989

Gibbs CJ, Gadjusek DC, et al: Creutzfeldt-Jakob disease (spongiform encephalopathy): Transmission to the chimpanzee. Science 161:388, 1968

Hope J, Reekie LJD, Hunter N, et al: Fibrils from brains of cows with new cattle disease contain SAF protein. Nature 336:390, 1988

Hsiao K, Prusiner SB: Inherited human prion diseases. Neurology 40:1820, 1990

Kimberlin RH, Walker CA: Pathogenesis of mouse scrapie: Dynamics of agent replication in spleen, spinal cord, and brain after infection by different routes. J Comp Pathol 89:551, 1979

McKinley MP, Bolton DC, Prusiner SB: A protease-resistant protein is a structural component of the scrapie prion. Cell 35:57, 1983

Merz PA, et al: Scrapie-associated fibrils in Creutzfeldt-Jakob disease. Nature 306:474, 1983

Merz PA, Somerville RA, Iqbal K, et al: Abnormal fibrils from scrapie-infected brain. Acta Neuropathol 54:63, 1981

Piccardo P, Safar J, Gibbs CJ, et al: Immunohistochemical localization of prion protein in spongiform encephalopathies and normal brain tissue. Neurology 40:518, 1990

Prusiner SB: Scrapie prions. Ann Rev Microbiol 43:345, 1989

SECTION VI

MEDICAL MYCOLOGY

CHAPTER 80

General Characteristics of Fungi

The biological Kingdom of the fungi is composed of approximately 50,000 species characterized by pronounced differences in structure, physiology, and modes of reproduction. Fewer than 300 species of fungi have been implicated directly as agents of human or animal disease, and fewer than a dozen of these species cause about 90% of all fungous infections. However, infections caused by unusual fungi are often difficult to identify and manage. To understand how fungi develop, how some become pathogenic, and how they can be recognized as pathogens, it is necessary to have an understanding of the characteristics of fungi in general. The study of fungi is called mycology, which is derived from the Greek word *mykos*, meaning mushroom.

Since all fungi are eucaryotic organisms, each fungal cell has at least one nucleus, and nuclear membrane, endoplasmic reticulum, and mitochondria. Fungi synthesize lysine from α-aminoadipic acid. Fungous cells resemble those of higher plants and animals and are quite advanced microorganisms. Most fungous cells possess a rigid cell wall, and many species produce flagellated, motile cells. Some of the higher fungi display more than rudimentary differentiation into tissues and specialized structures. Unlike members of the plant kingdom, fungi lack the property of photosynthesis.

The natural habitats for most fungi are water, soil, and decaying organic debris. Most fungi are obligate or facultative aerobes. They are chemotrophic organisms and obtain their nutrients from chemicals found in nature. Fungi survive by secreting enzymes that degrade a wide variety of organic substrates into soluble nutrients, which are then passively absorbed or taken into the cell by active transport systems.

Morphology

Growth Forms

Yeasts

Fungi grow in two basic morphologic forms, as yeasts or molds. The yeast morphology reflects the unicellular growth of fungi. Yeast cells are usually spherical to ellipsoidal and vary in diameter from 3 to 15 μm. Although a few undergo division by binary fission, most yeasts reproduce by budding, which may also be referred to as the formation of blastoconidia (Fig. 80–1). The budding process is initiated by localized lysis of the cell wall at a specific point. The internal pressure on this area of weakened cell wall causes the wall to balloon outward. This swollen portion enlarges, the nucleus divides by mitosis, and a progeny nucleus migrates into the newly formed bud. The nascent bud may then continue to enlarge. The cell wall grows together at the constricted point of

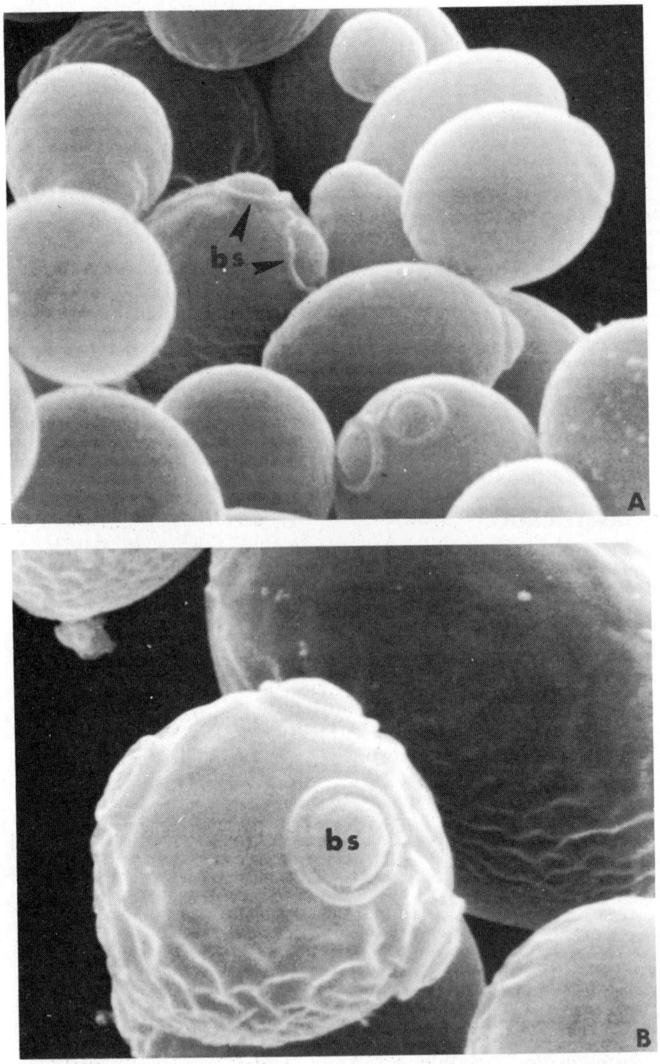

Fig. 80–1. *Saccharomyces cerevisiae.* **A.** Scanning electron photomicrograph of budding yeast cells. × 1800. **B.** Bud scars. × 9800. (*Courtesy of Dr. S. Miller.*)

attachment. Eventually, the bud breaks off from the parent cell, and the cycle of replication is complete and ready to be repeated. Yeasts retain a characteristic scar on their cell walls where a bud was once attached (Fig. 80–1B). Some species of yeasts typically produce multiple buds before detachment occurs. If single buds fail to separate, chains of spherical yeast cells are formed. Some species produce buds that characteristically fail to detach and become elongated; the continuation of the budding process then produces a chain of elongated yeast cells that resemble hyphae (see below) and are called *pseudohyphae.* The cells that compose a stretch of pseudohyphae are characteristically constricted where they are attached to each other (Chap. 85).

After growth on an agar medium for 1 to 3 days, yeasts produce colonies that are pasty and opaque and generally attain a diameter of 0.5 to 3.0 mm. A few species have characteristic pigments, but most are cream-colored. In microscopic and colonial morphology most yeast species differ very little, and physiologic tests are required for their speciation (Chap. 85).

Molds

The mold (or mould) form of growth refers to the production of multicellular, filamentous colonies. These colonies consist basically of branching cylindrical tubules varying in diameter from 2 to 10 μm and termed hyphae (singular, hypha). The hyphal width of a given species remains relatively constant during growth. Hyphal growth occurs by apical elongation (i.e., by extension in length from the tip of the filament or hypha). Hyphal tips contain densely packed, membrane-enclosed vesicles, many of which fuse with the cell membrane during active growth. The mass of intertwined hyphae that accumulates during active growth in the mold form is called a *mycelium* (plural, mycelia). Some hyphae are divided into cells by *septa* or crosswalls, which are typically formed at regular intervals during filamentous growth. Other species of molds are composed of nonseptate or sparsely septate hyphae. Since hyphal septa are perforated, cytoplasmic continuity is maintained in septate as well as nonseptate mycelia.

Molds tend to grow well on the surface of natural substrates or laboratory media. In such situations, hyphae that penetrate the supporting medium and absorb nutrients are termed vegetative or substrate hyphae. These hyphae also serve to anchor the mycelium to its natural substrate or to laboratory agar medium. Other hyphal filaments project above the surface of the mycelium into the air, and this aerial mycelium usually bears the reproductive structures of the fungus. Molds are generally identified by observation of their morphology. Macroscopic examination of a mold isolate should include notation of such characteristics as the rate of growth, topography (e.g., glabrous, verrucose), surface texture (e.g., velvety, cottony, powdery), and any pigmentation (surface, reverse, or diffusible into the medium). Microscopically, the types of spores or other reproductive structures (pigment, size, shape, mode of attachment) and their ontogeny are characteristic for each species.

Dimorphism

Most fungous species grow only as yeasts or molds, but some species are dimorphic and are capable of growing in more than one form under different environmental conditions. Some of the pathogenic fungi exhibit thermal dimorphism; they grow as yeasts at 37C and and in the mold form at lower temperatures, such as 25C or 30C. The morphogenesis of other dimorphic fungi is regulated by certain nutrients, carbon dioxide, cell density, age of the culture, or combinations of these factors.

Subcellular Structure

The fine structure of all fungi includes a unique cell wall, cell membrane, and cytoplasm containing an endoplasmic reticulum, nuclei, nucleoli, storage vacuoles, mitochondria, and other organelles (Fig. 80–2).

Capsule

Some fungi produce an external coating of slime or a more compact capsule. The capsule or slime layer is composed

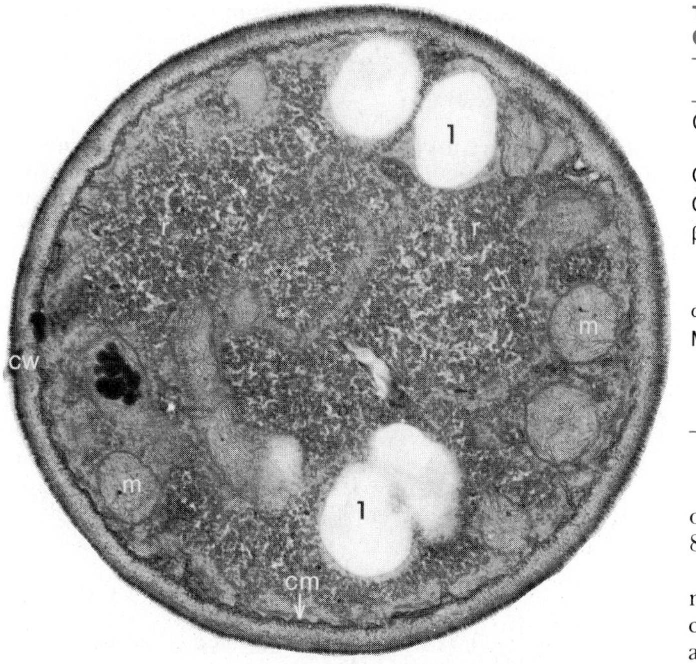

Fig. 80–2. *Candida albicans.* Transmission electron photomicrograph of yeast cell showing internal structure: cw, multilayered cell wall; cm, cell membrane; m, mitochondrium; l, lipid; r, ribosomes. × 20,000. (*Courtesy of Dr. S. Miller.*)

predominantly of amorphous polysaccharides that may be mucilaginous and cause the cells to adhere and clump together. The capsular polysaccharides of different species vary in quantity, chemical composition, antigenicity, and physical properties such as viscosity and solubility. The capsule does not appear to affect permeability or other functions of the cell wall and membrane. However, because of its gelatinous nature, the capsular material may influence the growth of the fungus by preventing the dissociation of buds from yeast cells or the dispersion of yeasts in air or water. The capsule of *Cryptococcus neoformans* has antiphagocytic properties and is associated with virulence (Chap. 85).

Cell Wall

The cell wall is an essential component and composes approximately 15% to 30% of the dry weight of a fungus. The cell wall provides rigidity and strength, and it protects the cell membrane from osmotic shock. As the wall determines the shape of any fungus, the process of fungal morphogenesis (e.g., sporulation or yeast-mold dimorphism) involves changes in the cell wall. The cell wall is generally thicker in yeasts (200 to 300 nm) than in molds (200 nm), but in both cases it is a multilayered structure that appears highly refractile under light microscopy.

Composition. Eighty percent or more of the cell wall is carbohydrate. Actually, a relatively small number of major polysaccharides are usually found in the walls of a wide variety of species of fungi, albeit in different quantities and in combination with varying amounts of other polysaccharide components that may be less common or even unique. Some of the more prevalent polysaccharides are listed in Table 80–1.

TABLE 80–1. MAJOR POLYSACCHARIDES OF FUNGAL CELL WALLS

Polymer	Monomer	Linkage and Structure
Chitin	*N*-acetylglucosamine	β-1,4-long, unbranched polymer
Chitosan	D-glucosamine	β-1,4-
Cellulose	D-glucose	β-1,4-
β-Glucan	D-glucose	β-1,3-linked backbone with β-1,6-linkages at branchpoints
α-Glucan	D-glucose	α-1,3 and α-1,4-
Mannan	D-mannose	α-1,6-linked backbone with frequent α-1,2- and α-1,3-linked branches of one to five residues each

As a result of the similarity among these polysaccharides, many fungi share surface antigens. However, because the side chains of glucans vary considerably in the number, length, and linkage of their residues, many unique antigenic determinants can also be found. Therefore, some cell wall antigens are widespread among fungi, whereas others are found only within certain taxa or even individual species. This concept is illustrated in Table 80–2, which indicates the association of certain polysaccharides with broad taxonomic groups. Antigenic analysis of cell walls is a powerful tool for the study of classification and phylogeny among fungi. The detection of water-soluble, species-specific surface antigens has provided a rapid method for the identification of slow-growing and/or poorly sporulating pathogenic fungi (Chaps. 81 and 82). Some species can be identified with monoclonal antibodies to cell wall antigens (Chap. 85).

Perhaps 10% of the composition of fungal cell walls consists of protein and glycoprotein. These proteins include enzymes involved in wall growth, certain extracellular enzymes, and structural proteins that cross-link the polysaccharide chains. The concentration of wall protein is higher near the cell membrane. Wall proteins have large amounts of sulfur-containing amino acids and disulfide bonds. Disulfide bonds are more prevalent in hyphal walls than in yeast walls, and in some species (*Candida albicans, Histoplasma capsulatum,* and *Paracoccidiodes brasiliensis*) the reduction of these disulfide bonds is associated with transformation from the mycelial to the yeast form of growth.

TABLE 80–2. DISTRIBUTION OF MAJOR CELL WALL POLYSACCHARIDES

Fungous Group	Predominant Cell Wall Polysaccharides
Lower aquatic fungi	Cellulose
Class Zygomycetes	Chitin, chitosan
Ascomycetous yeasts	β-glucans, mannans
Basidiomycetous yeasts	Chitin, mannans
Fungi with septate hyphae	Chitin, β-glucans

From Bartnicki-Garcia: Ann Rev Microbial 22:87, 1968

Ultrastructure. Cell wall polysaccharides are fibrillar in structure and multilayered. The polysaccharides appear as long microfibrils (Fig. 80–2). Four to eight distinct layers are usually observed, but the degree of organization, whether a linear alignment or a cross-hatched pattern, varies considerably. Generally, the most compact layer is nearest the cell membrane, and the external layer(s) tend to be more amorphous, less organized, and less compact. Some fungal cell walls contain tightly interwoven microfibrils embedded in an amorphous, polysaccharide matrix.

Methods of Study. Fungal cell walls may be studied in situ by several techniques, which are often coupled with light or electron microscopy. Some routine approaches to analysis of fungal cell walls are listed below:

1. Lectin-binding (e.g., concanavalin A)
2. Chemical stains (e.g., periodic acid–thiocarbohydrazide–silver, calcofluor white)
3. Selective enzymatic digestion of exposed surface components
4. Susceptibility to selective chemical degradation (e.g., solubility in hot acid or alkali)
5. Immunologic analysis of cell wall antigens (e.g., fluorescent antibody, agglutination, colloidal gold, or ferritin labels)
6. Incorporation and localization of radiolabeled cell wall precursors (cell-associated label, autoradiography).

A more precise compositional analysis can be made by studying the isolated cell walls. As a first step in the preparation of cell walls, fungal cells can be disrupted by physical means, during which the cytoplasmic contents are released. Cell walls vary in toughness, and a number of methods differing in harshness have been used. They include the following:

1. Grinding fungal suspensions with mortar and pestle to break the cells
2. Sonification
3. Shredding the cells in a blender
4. Use of high pressure to crack the cells (e.g., French press, Ribi press)
5. Violent mixing with sand, glass beads, or steel pellets.

With all these procedures, certain precautions should be observed, such as preventing the system from overheating and buffering with inhibitors of degradative enzymes (proteinases, nucleases) to minimize autodigestion of macromolecules. After the cells are broken, the walls can be separated from intact cells and cytoplasmic contents by differential filtration or centrifugation and extensive washing. Purified cell walls are essentially membrane-free on examination by electron microscopy.

Biochemistry. Isolated cell walls can be subjected to routine techniques of carbohydrate biochemistry. After removal by hot alkali or acid, polysaccharides can be purified by chromatographic or electrophoretic techniques. Once purified, a polysaccharide can then be hydrolyzed and its component sugar(s) identified. If more than one sugar is present, the relative proportion of each may be determined. The linkage of an intact polysaccharide can be studied by optical rotation, x-ray crystallography, or nuclear magnetic resonance spectrometry. The specific structure can be analyzed by determination of reducing sugars and susceptibility to specific enzymes (e.g., β-glucosidase and endo-β-1,3-gluconase). Acetylation and methylation analyses can be used to identify exposed hydroxyl groups. These and other methods have been combined to determine the size, composition, and linkage of several cell wall polysaccharides.

Polysaccharide Biosynthesis. Chitin is a major component of the cell walls of many fungi. Chitin is a homopolymer of *N*-acetylgucosamine (GlcNAc) and, like cellulose, which it structurally resembles, it is insoluble in water and forms crystalline arrays of parallel chains.

Polymerization of chitin is catalyzed by the enzyme chitin synthase, which is located in the cell membrane. The amino sugar donor, uridine-diphospho-*N*-acetyl-glucosamine (UDP-GlcNAc), is derived de novo from fructose-6-phosphate and glutamine. In the following general type of reaction, the enzyme is allosterically activated on complexing with UDP-GlcNAc, and the preexisting chitin polymer is extended in length by one monomeric unit as an aminosugar is added.

$$\text{UDP-GlcNAc} + \underset{\substack{\text{Preexisting}\\ \text{chitin}\\ \text{chain}}}{(\text{GlcNAc})_n} \xrightarrow[\text{synthase, Mg}^{++}]{\text{chitin}} \underset{\substack{\text{Lengthened}\\ \text{chitin}\\ \text{chain}}}{(\text{GlcNAc})_{n+1}} + \text{UDP}$$

Chitin synthase exists in a latent (zymogen) state and is activated by partial proteolysis.

Glucans are synthesized by similar reactions. The enzyme glucan synthase is involved, Mg^{++} is required, and UDP serves as carrier for the D-glucose monomer. In the synthesis of mannan, guanosine-diphosphomannose is produced in the cytoplasm and transferred to a lipid carrier, polyprenolmannose phosphate. Mannan biosynthesis probably occurs on the endoplasmic reticulum with the monomeric units being transported to the cell wall by the lipid intermediate. In the cell wall, two mannan chains are linked to a peptide. Mannan synthase requires Mn^{++}.

Cell Wall Biosynthesis. Fungal cell wall polysaccharides are synthesized in situ between the membrane and the existing wall. With hyphal growth, the apical vesicles contain the components of the synthetic machinery, the wall precursor material, biosynthetic enzymes, lytic enzymes, and cofactors. Lytic enzymes are believed to be transported to the site of new wall growth, where they cleave glycosidic bonds of polysaccharides. The biosynthesis of yeast cell walls involves similar components and mechanisms.

A unified theory has been advanced by Bartnicki-Garcia to explain the events involved in wall biosynthesis. The steps may occur in sequence or simultaneously. During growth, vesicles migrate to the site of wall growth, fuse with the cell membrane, and empty their contents into the space between the membrane and wall. These vesicles contain lytic enzymes that cleave the polysaccharide fibrils, the ends of which may serve as biosynthetic primers for further elongation of polymer. This cleavage weakens the wall, and the internal pressure causes it to stretch and increase in surface area. Activating factors, such as proteases and UDP-sugar carriers, are also carried in vesicles and deposited in this space. Wall growth occurs as synthases construct new polysaccharide to lengthen broken fibrils and strengthen the wall. This filling-in of the increased surface area caused by the pressure-stretched wall produces growth.

This concept leaves a number of fundamental questions unanswered. What governs the spatial orientation of newly formed polysaccharide? After focal disruption and biosynthesis, the integrity of the wall and arrangement of the microfibrils is somehow preserved. What controls the balance between wall lysis and synthesis? The process of wall biosynthesis is probably similar in both yeast and molds. If so, the difference in shape between yeasts and molds may reflect the result of diffuse versus localized (apical) wall growth, respectively; indeed, dimorphism in fungi involves regulation of cell wall growth. These and a number of other questions (e.g., the molecular basis of bud formation, sporulation, and germination) are currently under active investigation. These areas of research have obvious relevance to morphogenesis, regulation of the cell cycle, and eucaryotic cell transformation, and fungi provide excellent models for study. Practical benefits may also emerge as results are applied to medically important fungi. As more becomes known about how fungal growth is controlled, it may be possible to devise ways to perturb the growth of fungi. For example, a natural inhibitor of chitin synthase has been isolated. If this or a similar inhibitor were effective against pathogenic fungi, transported into fungi, stable and nontoxic for human tissue, it would have excellent promise as an antibiotic.

Medical Importance of Fungous Cell Walls. During exposure or infection, the host is initially confronted by the fungous cell surface. Mounting evidence suggests that the cell wall is not only essential for growth and survival but also governs fungous pathogenicity. The cell walls of the major pathogenic fungi have been shown to possess components that mediate attachment to host cells (Chap. 81), including phagocytes, epithelial cells, and endothelial cells. Cell surface ligands, receptors, and other components promote colonization and invasion, as well as evasion and subversion of host defenses. For example, strains of *C. albicans* have a cell wall protein that mimics the mammalian CR3 receptor for iC3b (Chaps. 15 and 85); other lectin like proteins recognize fucose and glucosamine residues on epithelial cell membranes, and portions of the wall mannan may mediate adherence to ligands, such as fibrinogen, fibronectin, and laminin.

Strains of *C. albicans* and other fungi also differ in cell surface hydrophobicity, and hydrophobic cells appear to be more virulent. Since the surface of both fungi and mammalian cells generally have negative charges, their contact may be facilitated by surface hydrophobic forces.

Fungous cell walls are potent antigens. Humans and animals develop specific immune responses to a number of wall determinants, some of which can be identified as specific oligosaccharides. Through normal environmental exposure, most adults have become immunized to the more prevalent mannans and glucans. In fact, exposure to some fungal antigens (*Candida*, dermatophytin) is so widespread that reactivity to them confirms a normal immunologic status. Atopic persons may develop severe hypersensitivity reactions to specific cell wall determinants (Chap. 81, 82, and 85). It is not clear in all cases whether the wall immunogen is purely carbohydrate or how much, if any, protein must be present. Many wall extracts lose their immunogenicity on fractionation into polysaccharide, protein, and glycoprotein components.

Mammalian tissues lack the enzymes to degrade many wall polysaccharides, and, as a result, fungal walls are cleared from the body very slowly. The retention of wall material may contribute to the pathogenesis of fungal infection. Specific examples of this are cited in subsequent chapters.

Staining Properties. The cell wall polysaccharides have unique staining properties that can be exploited for histopathologic observation. Fungi are often poorly stained or too sparse to be detected by the routine hematoxylin and eosin preparation. Two very helpful fungal wall stains are the periodic acid–Schiff reagent and the methenamine silver stain. These are true wall stains; neither the internal contents nor the capsular material is stained by them. Calcofluor white is a highly sensitive fluorescent stain that binds cellulose and chitin. Fungi can be easily recognized in specimens of tissue or fluids. The Gram stain is usually not applied to fungi because it does not help in their identification and may obscure internal structures. However, the Gram stain is useful for the examination of smears for both *Candida* and bacteria.

Cell Membrane

Fungi have a bilayered membrane similar in structure and composition to the cell membranes of higher eucaryotes. The cell membrane protects the cytoplasm, regulates the intake and secretion of solutes, and facilitates the synthesis of the cell wall and capsular material. The membrane contains several phospholipids, and their relative amounts vary with different species. Most prevalent are phosphatidylcholine and phosphatidylethanolamine, with smaller amounts of phosphatidylserine, phosphatidylinositol, and phosphatidylglycerol; there are other phospholipids in the cell membranes of some species. The phospholipid content varies not only among species but also within strains of a species and within a given strain, depending on the conditions of growth.

Unlike bacteria (except the mycoplasmas) but similar to other eucaryotes, fungal membranes contain sterols. Sterols are essential for viability of nearly all fungi. The principle fungal sterols are ergosterol and zymosterol; mammalian cell membranes contain cholesterol. This difference has been exploited in the successful use of the polyene antibiotics, which complex with sterols both in solution and in membranes. Their effect is to perforate intact membranes (Chaps. 7 and 81). The major antifungal antibiotic, amphotericin B, is a polyene that has greater affinity for ergosterol than cholesterol. The interaction of this antibiotic with sterols probably explains both its effectiveness against fungi and its toxicity for humans.

The triazole and imidazole antifungals interfere with the synthesis of ergosterol. These drugs block the cytochrome P-450–dependent 14 α-demethylation of lanosterol, which is a precursor of ergosterol in fungi and cholesterol in mammalian cells. However, the fungal cytochrome P-450s are approximately 100 to 1000 times more sensitive to the azoles than mammalian systems.

Cytoplasmic Content

Fungous cells, both yeasts and molds, often contain several nuclei. All hyphae can be considered multinuclear, as cytoplasmic continuity is maintained. Hyphal filaments with crosswalls or septa have pores, which can be simple perforations or complex devices. The septal pores of higher fungi are capable of opening and closing to permit the streaming of cytoplasmic contents through the hypha and the regulated migration of organelles, including nuclei, between cells.

The mitochondria of fungi resemble those of plant and animal cells. The number of mitochondria per cell varies considerably and correlates with the level of respiratory activity. For example, the sporulation process demands a large expense of energy, and is followed by a reduction in respiration, number of mitochondria, and overall metabolic activity. Profound but transient reductions in respiration and protein synthesis also accompany the mold-to-yeast morphogenesis in *Histoplasma capsulatum* (Chap. 82). In tissue, fungi may also have fewer mitochondria. Spore germination is accompanied by an increase in respiratory activity. In several species, germination has been correlated with increased energy consumption, increased numbers of mitochondria, and higher ratios of mitochondrial DNA to cellular DNA. Although increased respiration seems to be required for spore germination, it is not certain that other observed changes, such as synthesis of mitochondrial DNA, are actually necessary.

The cells of many fungal species have characteristic vacuoles (Fig. 80–2), which are complex organelles. Vacuoles may contain a variety of hydrolytic enzymes. They also serve to store ions and metabolites, such as amino acids, polyphosphates, and other compounds. The secretory apparatus and transport mechanisms of yeast cells have been well characterized. Fungous plasmids, viruses, which are mainly double-stranded RNA viruses, and other extrachromosomal genetic systems also have been described.

Several strains of *Saccharomyces cerevisiae, Candida, Cryptococcus,* and other yeasts have been shown to produce killer toxins. Killer strains secrete a toxin to which they are immune but which is lethal to sensitive yeasts. In most cases, the toxin is produced by a dsRNA mycovirus; a second dsRNA virus makes capsid proteins for both mycoviruses. The major toxins that have been studied have a narrow pH range, are proteins or glycoproteins, require binding to the cell wall of the target yeast, and probably involve a second receptor at the cell membrane. Although these toxins have a limited spectrum of activity, they may be exploited for the identification of isolates. Therapeutic applications are currently impractical.

Some fungi elaborate characteristic secondary metabolites. These are usually small compounds that are not essential for viability and that have no obvious function or survival value. Secondary metabolites include a number of compounds with diverse and pronounced biologic effects, such as carcinogens (e.g., aflatoxin), toxins (e.g., amanitin), antibiotics, anticancer substances, and pharmacologically active compounds (e.g., ergotamine).

A discussion of the genetics of fungi is beyond the scope of this chapter, but several reviews are listed at the end. Fungi such as the yeast *Saccharomyces cerevisiae* and the mold *Neurospora crassa,* as well as others, have become classic models for the investigation of eucaryotic molecular genetics.

Reproduction

Asexual Reproduction

Fungi reproduce by asexual, sexual, or parasexual processes. Asexual reproduction can occur simply as vegetative growth and expansion of a mold or yeast colony as the cells replicate. When a few yeast cells or fragments of hyphae are transferred to a fresh substrate, as is routinely done in the laboratory when fungi are transplanted from one culture to another, the transferred portion grows to produce a new colony. However, asexual reproduction usually refers to the production of spores or propagules, which are generally more resistant to adverse environmental conditions. The properties of spores that facilitate their dispersion are often essential for the dissemination and propagation of the fungus in nature. For example, spores are usually dry and easily airborne. Some spores are equipped with rough surfaces for adherence to fomites or animals that might transport them to another location.

Conidia are the major asexual propagules or spores. *Conidia* are produced by specialized structures, conidiogenous cells, and classified according to their developmental process. Although the method of conidial formation is often not discernible with routine light microscopy, the conidia of many fungi are distinctive and can be easily identified. Two basic types of conidial ontogeny are thallic and blastic. These terms, and others applicable to medically important fungi, are described below. They represent only a portion of the diversity of conidiogenesis among the fungi.

Thallic conidia are derived from cells of the thallus or body of the fungus. That is, a hyphal cell becomes delineated by a septum and is transformed into a conidium. One example is the chlamydospore, which is a large, spherical, thick-walled, unicellular structure formed by enlargement of a hyphal cell. *Chlamydospores* (chlamydoconida) may be produced in a lateral, intercalary, or terminal position on a hypha (Fig. 80–3B). An *arthroconidium* is a unicellular, thallic conidium produced by condensation of the cytoplasm and thickening of the wall of a hyphal cell. Usually adjacent cells, or alternative cells, as in the case of *Coccidioides immitis,* undergo this transformation into small, dense conidia to produce a chain of rectangular arthroconidia from a hypha. With maturation, the arthroconidia become desiccated and fragment to form an easily aerosolized batch of conidia, quite uniform in size (Fig. 80–3C). The dermatophytic mold species (Chap. 84) also develop thallic conidia, usually from terminal hyphal cells; they may be unicellular (microconidia) or multicellular (macroconidia). A fungus species may characteristically produce either or both microconidia and macroconidia (Fig. 80–4). The production of arthroconidia, chlamydospores, and other thalloconidia is not specific for any single species; a given fungus may produce none or one or more than one type of thallic conidia.

In the formation of *blastic* conidia, only a portion of the conidiogenous cell contributes to the development of the conidium, and conidium formation is initiated before the conidium becomes delimited by a septum. Two major types of blastic conidia are recognized—holoblastic and enteroblastic. In *holoblastic* conidiogenesis, all of the cell wall layers of

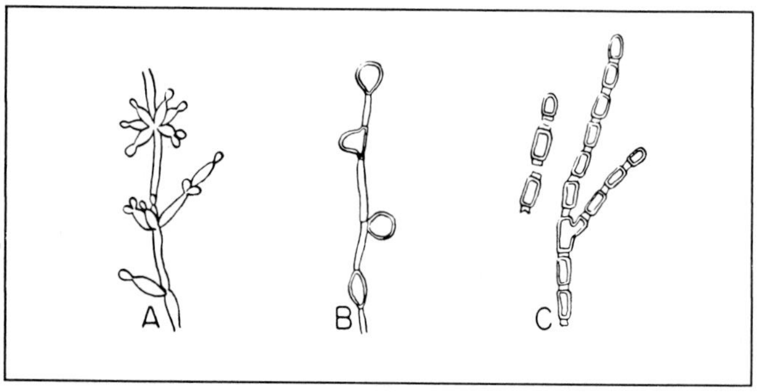

Fig. 80–3. Various types of asexual spores. **A.** Blastoconidia and pseudohyphae. **B.** Chlamydospores. **C.** Arthroconidia. (*From Conant et al: Manual of Clinical Mycology, ed 3. Saunders, 1971.*)

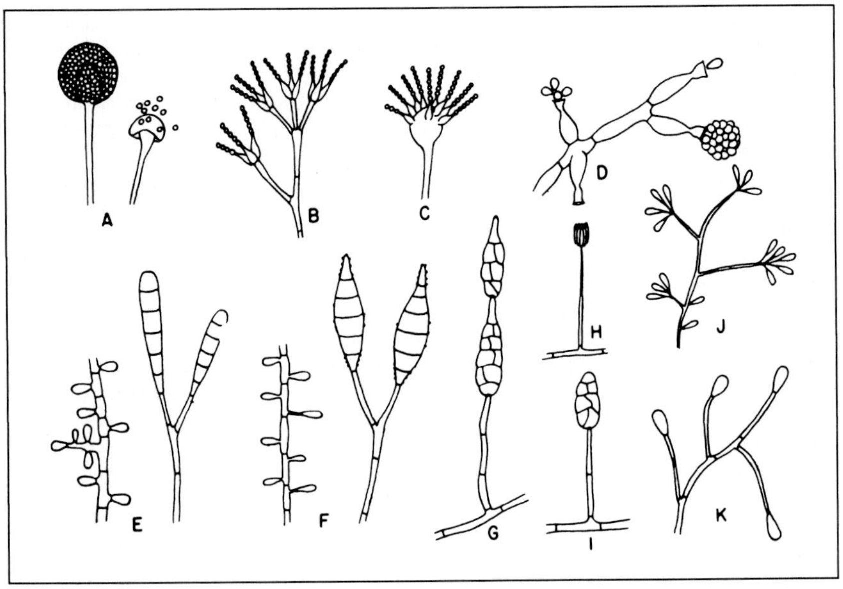

Fig. 80–4. Various types of asexual spores. **A.** Sporangia and sporangiospores. **B, C, D.** Phialoconidia, *Penicillium* **(B)**, *Aspergillus* **(C)**, *Phialophora* **(D)**. **E, F.** Thallic microconidia and macroconidia, *Trichophyton* **(E)**, *Microsporum* **(F)**. **G.** Tretic macroconidia, *Alternaria*. **H–K.** Other types of conidia and conidiophores. (*From Conant et al: Manual of Clinical Mycology, ed 3. Saunders, 1971.*)

the conidiogenous cell participate in conidium development. The buds formed by most species of yeasts, including pseudohyphae, are examples of holoblastic conidia, or blastoconidia (Fig. 80–3A). The mold genus *Cladosporium* produces chains of holoblastic conidia.

With *enteroblastic* conidia, only the inner cell wall layer(s) or no portion of the cell wall of the conidiogenous cell contributes to the development of the conidium. Several of the varieties or subtypes of enteroblastic conidiogenesis are important in medical mycology. *Tretic* conidia develop through a channel or pore in the outer wall of the conidiogenous cell, and the inner wall layer(s) participates in formation of the conidium. *Phialides* are flask-shaped conidiogenous cells that produce conidia through a distal opening in the cell wall, but no portion of the phialide cell wall contributes to the cell walls of the conidia (phialoconidia). Several familiar genera including *Aspergillus*, *Penicillium*, and *Phialophora*, produce phialoconidia. An *annellide* is another blastic conidiogenous cell; it elongates with the production of each conidium and acquires ring-shaped scars or annellations at the point of conidial production. Annelloconidia are produced by *Scopulariopsis*, *Exophiala*, and other genera. (Phialoconidia and annelloconidia are discussed further in Chapter 83.)

Conidia that are not released during their production (some are forcibly discharged) are usually liberated by physical dislodgment or by the disintegration of adjacent cells. A specialized hypha that bears the conidia or conidiogenous cells is called a *conidiophore*. A conidiophore may be a simple and undistinguished hyphal stalk to which the conidium is attached; other conidiophores are branched, complexly modified, or uniquely shaped. For example, *Aspergillus* species produce at the end of the conidiophore a swollen vesicle from which short phialides project, and these in turn produce radiating chains of globose, unicellular, often pigmented phialoconidia (Fig. 80–4C). This type of conidial formation is *basipetal*, as the conidia are extruded from the attached end of the chain. The newest and youngest conidium is the one nearest the point of attachment of the chain to the phialide. With other fungi (e.g., *Cladosporium*), conidial chains are formed in an *acropetal* manner, whereby chains of blastoconidia are produced by a budding process from the youngest conidium at the distal end.

The asexual structures of many of the lower fungi are produced in a saclike structure termed a *sporangium* (Fig. 80–4A). The sporangium develops at the tip of a *sporangiophore*, and the spores formed within it are called *sporangiospores*. On maturation, the sporangial wall or membrane ruptures to release its spores.

Sexual Reproduction

Sexual reproduction in fungi follows the same pattern as in higher eucaryotes. The process is initiated by plasmogamy, whereby two compatible, haploid nuclei are brought together in the same cell. Karyogamy is the fusion of these two nuclei to form a diploid nucleus. Karyogamy may immediately follow plasmogamy, or it may be delayed, as in some higher fungi, with the development of a mycelium consisting of binucleate cells. Sooner or later meiosis occurs, resulting in genetic exchange, reduction, and then division to yield four haploid progeny nuclei. This sequence occurs in all the fungi for which a sexual cycle has been discovered, but many variations exist among the different kinds of fungi. Some fungi produce distinct sex organs and gametes. In others, the somatic nuclei perform the sexual function. In some species, nuclei within a single thallus are capable of fusion, and in others, sexual compatibility is genetically determined, and compatible thalli are required for mating. Nuclei from two compatible thalli may be brought together by specialized gametangia or by anastomosis of their hyphae and exchange of nuclei by migration from the hypha of one to the other. Hyphal fusion and migration of nuclei and cytoplasmic contents from one hypha to another are a common phenomenon among the same species of fungi.

Because the sequence of plasmogamy, karyogamy, and meiosis is not a single continuous event for many fungi, it is helpful to describe the life cycle of a fungus as consisting of (1) a *haplophase*, during which the uninuclear or multinuclear thallus contains only haploid nuclei, (2) a *dikaryophase*, in which two genetically distinct haploid nuclei occupy each cell of the thallus, and (3) a *diplophase*, which refers to the diploid nucleus formed as a result of karyogamy. Most of the lower fungi lack a distinct dikaryophase, and the haplophase is the predominant state. In the more complex higher fungi, the dikaryophase assumes greater prominence. With mushrooms, for example, the binucleate mycelium of the dikaryophase constitutes most of the macroscopic structures. In some species both the haplophase and the dikaryophase occupy significant portions of the life cycle, and asexual sporulation may serve to propagate either phase.

After meiosis, the progeny nuclei develop into sexual spores. The basic type of sexual spore that is formed and the supporting tissue, if any, that is produced are the features that define the major taxonomic groups of fungi.

Parasexual Reproduction

Parasexuality refers to a sequence of events that culminates in genetic exchange by mitotic recombination. First described by Pontecorvo, parasexual reproduction has become a laboratory tool for the genetic analysis of many imperfect fungi. It has also been shown to occur in several species of ascomycetes, basidiomycetes, and deuteromycetes (see following classification scheme).

Parasexuality is initiated by the formation of a heterokaryon, a thallus that contains haploid nuclei of two different genotypes. Heterokaryons are most commonly formed by hyphal anastomosis and nuclear exchange between genetically different strains of the same species. Rarely, nuclear fusion will occur with the formation of a stable diploid heterozygote that multiplies along with the two haploid nuclei. During mitosis of the diploid nuclei, homologous chromosomes may pair up and permit somatic recombination to occur. The cycle is completed when the diploid undergoes haploidization to the original chromosome number and the haploid recombinant is isolated.

The parasexual process, or mitotic recombination, provides a natural mechanism for genetic exchange among imperfect fungi. It also provides a model for genetic manipulation in other somatic systems, such as mammalian tissue cultures.

Classification

Fungous taxonomy is a dynamic area of investigation that undergoes constant refinement and revision. The criteria by which various taxa, including species, are defined continue to change as new information becomes available about the significance of differences in selected properties. The bases for establishing phylogenetic relationships among groups and species of fungi are frequently challenged and reviewed. The product of sexual reproduction, such as zygospores, ascospores, or basidiospores, has been used to separate very large groups of fungi, such as the zygomycetes, ascomycetes, and basidiomycetes, respectively. At the species level, sexual compatibility can be used to confirm species identity. However, many fungi lack a sexual reproductive cycle, and they must be classified on the basis of vegetative and asexual morphology, physiology, and similar characters. There are few reliable criteria for separating many genera and families, and any given character, such as the production of pseudohyphae, may have major or minor significance in different taxa. Recently, comparisons of DNA (guanosine and cytosine content or sequence homology) have clarified several relationships.

Growth as a yeast or mold does not constitute a major taxonomic separation. Indeed, subgroupings of each major taxon contain species of yeasts and dimorphic fungi.

The following is an abridged list of taxonomic groups of special interest in medical mycology. Classification into the major groups within the fungous kingdom depends primarily on the type of spore that is formed after sexual reproduction (i.e., the "perfect" or *teleomorphic* state). Fungi that do not reproduce sexually (or for which a sexual reproductive cycle has not been discovered) are termed imperfect, or *anamorphic*, and may be classified within the subdivision of deuteromycetes based on the morphology of their asexual reproductive structures.

Sometimes a given fungus has more than one name and placement in the classification scheme. For example, a fungus, typically in its haplophase, may be identified on the basis of its characteristic asexual reproductive structures as a specific anamorphic species in the subdivision Deuteromycotina, but during sexual reproduction, the same fungus is recognized by its sexual spores as a teleomorphic species with another name. In many cases, both names must be retained because a sexually reproducing (teleomorphic) species may produce more than one corresponding anamorphic form during asexual reproduction. Conversely, an anamorphic species may actually represent the mating type of more than one teleomorphic species; that is, two or more teleomorphic (sexual) species may reproduce asexually to form the same, indistinguishable anamorph.

Class Myxomycetes

The myxomycetes, or slime molds, are fungi whose vegetative form is an aseptate mass of protoplasm called a plasmodium, which contains many diploid nuclei. *Dictyostelium* is a myxomycete genus.

Class Zygomycetes

These fungi include water molds, arthropod parasites, and various types of motile, flagellated fungi. In most cases the mycelium of the zygomycetes lacks crosswalls or is sparsely septated. The class Zygomycetes contains molds that reproduce sexually by the fusion of two compatible gametes or hyphae to form a *zygospore* and asexually by the production of conidia or sporangiospores. The zygomycetes and several smaller classes of fungi were once called phycomycetes, a term that is no longer taxonomically legitimate.

Order Mucorales. Asexual reproduction occurs by the production of sporangia. This order includes the genera *Absidia, Cunninghamella, Mortierella, Mucor, Phycomyces, Pilobolus, Rhizomucor, Rhizopus,* and *Saksenaea*, among others (Chap. 85).

Order Entomophthorales. Asexual reproduction occurs by conidia that are forcibly discharged. Some genera are *Basidiobolus, Condidiobolus,* and *Entomophthora* (Chap. 83).

Subdivision Ascomycotina

Sexual reproduction involves a saclike structure, an *ascus*, that contains the spores produced after karyogamy and meiosis. The yeast *Saccharomyces cerevisiae* is an ascomycete; after sexual reproduction, the ascospores develop within the ascus that was formed by the fusion of two sexually compatible yeast cells. In the mold *Neurospora crassa*, each ascus contains a row of eight ascospores.

Order Eurotiales. In the order Eurotiales the asci are produced within a *cleistothecium*, a closed structure composed of compact specialized hyphae. Many of the medically important, imperfect fungi for which sexual phases have been discovered have now been reclassified into this order (Chaps. 82–84).

FAMILY GYMNOASCACEAE. Members of the family Gymnoascaceae produces spherical cleistothecia with unorganized peridial hyphae. Genera include *Arthroderma*, which represents the teleomorphic states of species of the anamorphic genera *Trichophyton* and *Microsporum*, and *Ajellomyces*, the teleomorph for *Blastomyces* and *Histoplasma*.

FAMILY EUROTIACEAE. With molds of the family Eurotiaceae the peridial hyphae around the cleisotothecium are more compact and tissuelike. This group contains *Pseudallescheria boydii* and many of the teleomorphs of *Aspergillus* species (e.g., *Emericella, Eurotium, Sartorya*) and of *Penicillium* species (e.g., *Carpenteles, Talaromyces*).

Subdivision Basidiomycotina

Sexual reproduction results in progeny spores produced on a special structure called a *basidium*. The basidiomycetes are a large and complex group of fungi, some of whose members show a high degree of differentiation. The basidiomycetes include many plant and insect pathogens, the smuts and rusts, puffballs, bracket fungi, and mushrooms, as well as *Filobasidiella neoformans*, which is represented in its dominant haplophase by the important pathogenic yeast, *Cryptococcus neoformans* (Chap. 85).

Subdivision Deuteromycotina (Fungi Imperfecti)

The Deuteromycotina group contains all the fungi for which a sexual reproductive cycle has not been discovered. The anamorphic states are characterized by asexual reproduction. The taxa within this group do not reflect phylogenetic relationships (Chaps. 82–85).

Class Blastomycetes. The class Blastomycetes contains the imperfect (asexual) yeasts, some of which may produce pseudohyphae or true hyphae. The genera include *Candida, Cryptococcus, Malassezia, Rhodotorula, Torulopsis*, and *Trichosporon*.

Class Hyphomycetes. Fungi of the class Hyphomycetes produce septate mycelia and reproduce asexually by conidia that are not borne on a highly specialized tissue stroma. Most of the pathogenic fungi belong here. Some of the genera are *Alternaria, Aspergillus, Blastomyces, Epidermophyton, Geotrichum, Histoplasma, Microsporum, Penicillium*, and *Trichophyton*. Cell walls of the hyphae, conidia, or both, of *dematiaceous* molds contain melanins and are typically darkly pigmented. This large group includes the genera *Alternaria, Cladosporium, Exophiala*, and *Phialophora*.

FURTHER READING

Books and Reviews

Ainsworth GC, Sussman AS (eds): The Fungi: An Advanced Treatise. Vol I: The Fungal Cell. Vol II: The Fungal Organism. Vol III: The Fungal Population. London, Academic Press, 1965, 1966, 1968

Ainsworth GC, Sparrow FK, Sussman AS (eds): The Fungi: An Advanced Treatise. Vol IVA: Ascomycetes and Fungi Imperfecti. Vol IVB: A Taxonomic Review with Keys: Basidiomycetes and Lower Fungi. London, Academic Press, 1973

Alexopoulos CJ, Mims CW: Introductory Mycology, ed 3. New York, John Wiley & Sons, 1979

Bartnicki-Barcia: Cell wall chemistry, morphogenesis, and taxonomy of fungi. Annu Rev Microbiol 22:87, 1968

Bennett JW, Lasure LL (eds): Gene Manipulations in Fungi. Orlando, Academic Press, 1985

Burnett JH: Fundamentals of Mycology, ed 2. London, Arnold Ltd, 1976

Carmichael JW, Kendrick WB, Conners IL, et al: Genera of Hyphomycetes, Edmonton, Alberta University Press, 1980

Cole GT, Kendrick WB (eds): Biology of Conidial Fungi. vols. 1 and 2. New York, Academic Press, 1981

Deadon JW: Introduction to Modern Mycology. New York, John Wiley & Sons, 1980

Farkas V: Biosynthesis of cell walls of fungi. Microbiol Rev 43:117, 1979

Garraway MD. Evans RC: Fungal Nutrition and Physiology. New York, John Wiley & Sons, 1984

Hudson HJ: Fungal Biology. Arnold Ltd, 1986

Kendrick WB: The Fifth Kingdom. Waterloo, Ontario, Mycologue, 1985

Nickerson WJ: Symposium on the biochemical basis of morphogenesis in fungi. IV. Molecular basis of form in yeast. Bacteriol Rev 27:3305, 1963

Pontecorvo G: The parasexual cycle in fungi. Annu Rev Microbiol 10:393, 1956

Prescott DM: Methods in Cell Biology. Vol XI-XII: Yeast Cells. New York, Academic Press, 1975

Rose AH, Harrison JS (eds): The Yeasts. ed 2. Vol I: Biology of Yeasts. Vol II: Yeasts and the Environment. London, Academic Press, 1987

Ross IK: Biology of the Fungi. New York, McGraw-Hill, 1979

Smith JE, Berry DR: An Introduction to Biochemistry of Fungal Development. London, Academic Press, 1974

Smith JE, Berry DR (eds): The Filamentous Fungi. Vol II: Biosynthesis and Metabolism. Vol III: Developmental Mycology. London, Arnold Ltd, 1975, 1978

Sypherd PS, Borgia PT, Paznokas JL: Biochemistry of dimorphism in the fungus *Mucor*. Adv Microb Physiol 18:67, 1978

Szaniszlo PJ, Harrison JS (eds): Fungal Dimorphism—with Emphasis on Fungi Pathogenic for Humans. New York, Plenum Press, 1985

Webster J: Introduction to Fungi; ed 2, Cambridge, Cambridge University Press, 1980

Seleted Papers

Barkai-Golan R, Sharon N: Lectins as a tool for the study of yeast cell walls. Exp Mycol 2:110, 1978

Cabib E, Farkas V: The control of morphogenesis: An enzymatic mechanism for the initiation of septum formation in yeast. Proc Natl Acad Sci USA 68:2052, 1971

Calderone RA, Braun PC: Adherence and receptor relationships of *Canidia albicans*. Microbiol Rev 55:1, 1991

Domer JE: *Candida* cell wall mannan: A polysaccharide with diverse immunologic properties. Crit Rev Microbiol 17:33, 1989

Elmer GW, Nickerson WJ: Nutritional requirements for growth and yeastlike development of *Mucor rouxii* under carbon dioxide. J Bacteriol 101:595, 1970

Klionsky DJ, Herman PK, Emr SD: The fungal vacuole: composition, function, and biogenesis. Microbiol Rev 54:266, 1990

Lopez-Romero E, Ruiz-Herrera J, Bartnicki-Garcia S: Purification and properties of an inhibitory protein of chitin synthetase from *Mucor rouxii*. Biochem Biophys Acta 525:338, 1978

Novick P, Ferro S, Schekman R: Order of events in the yeast secretory pathway. Cell 25:461, 1981

Orlowski M, Ross JF: Relationship of internal cyclic AMP levels, rates of protein synthesis and *Mucor* dimorphism. Arch Microbiol 129:353, 1981

Prasad R: Nutrient transport in *Candida albicans*, a pathogenic yeast. Yeast 3:209, 1987

Ruiz-Herrera J, Lopez-Romero E, Bartnicki-Garcia S: Properties of chitin synthetase in isolated chitosomes from yeast cells of *Mucor rouxii*. J Biol Chem 252:3338, 1977

Shepherd MG: Cell envelope of *Candida albicans*. CRC Crit Rev Microbiol 15:7, 1987

Ulane RE, Cabib E: The activating system of chitin synthetase from *Saccharomyces cerevisiae*. J Biol Chem 251:3367, 1976

CHAPTER 81

Principles of Fungous Diseases

Species of fungi can be isolated globally from soil, air, and water. These ubiquitous microorganisms constitute an essential, unique, and fascinating biologic domain. As a group, the fungi exert profound effects, both beneficial and detrimental, on all forms of life. The collective degradative enzymes produced by saprophytic fungi in soil are essential for the biologic recycling of organic matter. Cellulolytic fungi decompose vegetative debris into humus. Fungi also serve humankind quite directly. Species of yeasts are necessary for the preparation of certain foods, such as beer, cheese, bread, and wine. Higher fungi, mostly basidiomycetes, may be eaten directly as mushrooms. Other fungi are phytopathogens and have a tremendous economic impact on the agricultural industry and the annual food supply by causing plant diseases.

For many years, scientists have employed fungous models to explore such fundamental areas as genetic regulation, the cytoplasmic transmission of sensory stimuli, and the control of morphogenesis. In medicine, fungi are an important source of biologically active compounds, including hallucinogens, adrenergic alkaloids, vitamins, mutagens, carcinogens, antibiotics, immunosuppressive agents, and potential anticancer substances. Recent investigations have focused on the ability of several fungous components to function as powerful immunomodulators.

Types of Fungous Diseases

Fungi are able to cause human disease in three generalized ways:

1. Allergies may follow sensitization to specific fungous antigens.
2. Fungi may elaborate or indirectly generate toxic substances.
3. Some fungi are able to cause infection and grow actively on an animal host.

Fungous Allergies

The respiratory tracts of all animals, including humans, are constantly exposed to the aerosolized conidia and spores of many saprophytic fungi. These spores, or other fungous components, may contain potent allergens to which certain individuals may respond with a strong hypersensitivity reaction. The manifestation of these allergies does not require growth or even viability of the inducing fungus, although in some cases both infection and allergy may occur simultaneously.

The fungous spore census in outdoor air varies considerably with geographic location, season, time of day, and weather conditions. The average spore concentration in normal outdoor air is approximately 10^5 spores per cubic meter. In enclosed areas with growth conditions suitable for the proliferation of fungous contaminants, such as farm buildings, the spore counts may exceed 10^9 spores per cubic meter. Persons exposed to such heavy doses of fungous aerosols are likely to become sensitized to the fungous (and actinomycetous) antigens, which may lead to allergic reactions on subsequent exposure.

Depending on the site of deposition of these allergens, patients may exhibit rhinitis, bronchial asthma, alveolitis, or generalized pneumonitis. Atopic persons are more susceptible. Table 81–1 lists some of these well-characterized syndromes. Farmer's lung is a classic example of extrinsic allergic alveolitis. In general, the clinical manifestations are determined by the immune responses of the host and the nature of the fungous challenge—namely, particle size, antigenicity, and amount of inoculum. The clinical description, mechanisms of immuno-

TABLE 81–1. RESPIRATORY ALLERGIES (RHINITIS, BRONCHIAL ASTHMA, ALVEOLITIS) CAUSED BY FUNGI AND ACTINOMYCETES

Allergy	Source	Etiology
Cheese washer's lung	Cheese	*Penicillium casei*
Maltster's lung	Barley malt	*Aspergillus clavatus*
Maple-bark stripper's lung	Maple tree bark	*Cryptostroma corticale*
Sequoiosis	Redwood sawdust	*Aureobasidium pullulans, Graphium*
Suberosis	Cork	*Penicillium frequentans*
Wood-pulp worker's disease	Wood pulp	*Alternaria*
Farmer's lung	Stored hay	*Faenia rectivirgula, Thermoactinomyces vulgaris*
Bagassosis	Sugar cane	*Thermoactinomyces saccharii*
Humidifier lung	Humidifiers, air conditioners	*Thermoactinomyces vulgaris, Thermoactinomyces candidus*

pathology, and management of these hypersensitivity diseases are covered in Chapter 19. These factors are also discussed in Chapter 85 in reference to one of the more ubiquitous genera, *Aspergillus*. In addition to specific medical treatment, these allergies may also be controlled by eliminating the environmental hazard or otherwise removing the patient from the allergen.

Mycotoxicoses

Fungi can generate substances with direct toxicity for humans and animals. Such toxins are secondary metabolites (Chap. 80) that are synthesized and secreted directly into the environment. They include a variety of mycotoxins elaborated by mushrooms. Exposure to these toxins after their inadvertent ingestion results in a disease termed *mycetismus*, whose severity depends on the amount and type of mycotoxin ingested. A recent history of mycophagy precedes the manifestation of symptoms by several hours. Heating of mycotoxins has little effect on reducing the toxicity. Table 81–2 summarizes the common clinical forms of mycetismus.

Amatoxins and Phallotoxins. The amatoxins and phallotoxins represent two important families of mycotoxins. The amatoxins are among the most potent. The phallotoxins, which are not absorbed by the gastrointestinal tract and are not a cause of mycetismus, have been studied in animals after injection. Both toxins are produced by poisonous mushrooms, such as *Amanita*, which may yield several toxins, including phalloidin, phalloin, and α-, β, and γ-amanitin. The amatoxins are cyclic octapeptides, and the phallotoxins are cyclic heptapeptides. The liver is a target organ for both families of toxins. α-Amanitin binds to a subunit of RNA polymerase II and consequently interferes with mRNA and protein synthesis.

TABLE 81–2. SUMMARY OF HUMAN MYCETISMUS (ABRIDGED)

Site of Involvement	Latent Period	Duration	Etiology	Mycotoxin	Mechanism of Action	Symptoms	Prognosis and Treatment
Gastrointestinal tract	Minute to hours	36–72 h	*Boletus satanas, Lactarius torminosus, Lepiota morgani, Russula emetica,* and others	Unidentified		Nausea and diarrhea; mild to severe	Spontaneous recovery
Gastrointestinal tract (cholera-type and parasympathetic nervous system)	6–24 h		*Amanita phalloides, Amanita virosa*	Amatoxin(s) (phallotoxins)	Cholinergic effect on smooth muscles and exocrine glands	Diphasic (1) violent vomiting, diarrhea, dehydration, muscle cramps, (2) renal and hepatic failure, confusion, perspiration, lacrimation, salivation, twitching, jaundice, coma	Second phase treated with atropine; often fatal; thioctic acid
		15–30 min	*Clitocybe* species, *Inocybe* species	Muscarine	Same	Violent gastrointestinal upset, perspiration, salivation; central nervous system symptoms: delirium, hallucination, or coma; high doses cause cardiac and/or respiratory failure	Same
		6–8 h	*Helvella esculenta*	Gyromitrin (volatilized with heating)	Gastrointestinal toxicity, hemolysis	Nausea, vomiting, diarrhea; hemoglobinuria, jaundice	Usually self-limiting
Central nervous system	30–60 min	5–10 h	*Psilocybe cubensis, Psilocybe* species	Psilocybin		Hallucination	Spontaneous recovery

From Becker et al: West J Med 125:100, 1976

Phalloidin binds to actin in cell membranes. Globular actin (G-actin), after binding adenosine triphosphate (ATP) and Ca^{2+}, is converted to the fibrous form (F-actin). Phalloidin binds to and stabilizes F-actin, causing vacuolization, membrane leakage, and disruption of the endoplasmic reticulum.

Treatment for mushroom poisoning is largely supportive, as specific antidotes are not available. The basis for the efficacy of thioctic acid in some patients is not apparent. In addition to these and other direct toxins, fungous contamination and breakdown of grains and other foods may result in degradative by-products that are toxic on ingestion.

Aflatoxins and Other Tumorigenic Mycotoxins. Other fungi elaborate a variety of mutagens and carcinogens; their production is not essential for survival of the fungus. Although these toxins can be lethal or tumorigenic for animals, no direct evidence has yet linked any of the carcinogenic mycotoxins with human disease. The most potent and best characterized example is *aflatoxin*, of which eight varieties are produced by certain strains of *Aspergillus flavus* and other molds. The name *aflatoxin* is derived from *A. flavus* toxin.

The structures of the two most potent aflatoxins, B_1 and G_1, are shown in Figure 81–1. Aflatoxins are converted in the host (e.g., by liver microsomal enzymes) into active, unstable compounds that bind to DNA, prevent base-pairing, and induce frameshift mutations. Aflatoxin B_1, the most potent liver carcinogen, also induces many other molecular changes. Birds are extremely sensitive to aflatoxin, and the seminal investigation of aflatoxicosis was stimulated by a lethal outbreak in Great Britain that was called turkey X disease until the mechanism of disease was traced to aflatoxin contamination of the African groundnuts in feed. Sublethal amounts of aflatoxin in the avian diet may cause a multitude of dose-related effects, including fatty liver changes, reduced liver enzymes, anemia, decreased leukocyte chemotaxis and phagocytosis, and increased susceptibility to infection. Since the pathologic condition also includes a reduction in growth and in egg production, aflatoxicosis has had a devastating effect on the poultry industry.

Other mycotoxins with proven carcinogenicity for experimental animals include ochratoxin, sporidesmin, zearalenone, and sterigmatocystin. They are produced by species of *Aspergillus*, *Penicillium*, *Helminthosporium*, and other ubiquitous saprophytic fungi. As mentioned, there is no direct evidence to implicate mycotoxins in human disease, but some provocative epidemiologic investigations have correlated liver damage in certain tribal populations with dietary exposure to aflatoxin. There is regular monitoring of levels of aflatoxins and other mycotoxins in grains, corn, peanuts, and other foods frequently contaminated with the toxin-producing fungi.

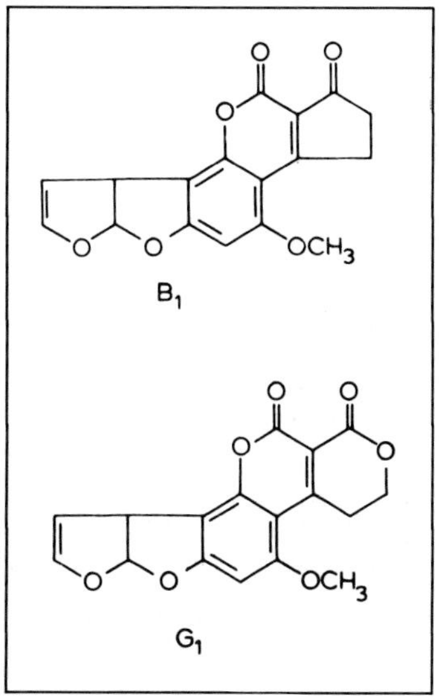

Fig. 81–1. Structures of aflatoxins B_1 and G_1. *(From Fishbein & Falk: Chromatog Rev 12:42, 1970.)*

Mycoses

The most common form of mycotic disease is infection, which refers to the actual growth of a fungus on a human or animal host. The term *mycosis* refers to an infection caused by a fungus. The names of many fungous infections are formed by coupling *mycosis* as a suffix to another word that designates the etiologic agent (e.g., coccidioidomycosis) or the site of involvement (e.g., otomycosis). Several other mycoses are named by adding the suffix *-sis* denoting "state or condition" to the etiologic designation, such as aspergillosis or candidiasis.

In general, the establishment of a mycosis depends on the state of the host defenses, or lack thereof, the route of exposure, the size of the inoculum, and the virulence of the fungus. Chapters 82 through 85 cover the ecology, mycology, pathogenesis, and immunology of the more prevalent infectious fungi and the epidemiology, clinical symptoms, diagnosis, and treatment indicated for the respective mycoses. The remainder of this chapter develops some general principles of the host-fungus interaction that pertain to exposure, pathogenesis, diagnosis, and treatment.

Mycosis

Incidence

Since the mycoses are not reportable diseases, their prevalence is unknown. An accurate report of the incidence cannot be obtained either by the Centers for Disease Control in the United States or by the World Health Organization. However, it is apparent that dermatophytoses and pityriasis versicolor are among the most common infectious diseases in the world. Furthermore, they have always been prevalent; the lesions are superficial, and historical descriptions of ringworm date from antiquity. Other historical accounts are compatible with many of the systemic mycoses. For example, there is compelling evidence that the curse of Tutankhamen's tomb was actually residual conidia of *Aspergillus*.

Several mycologists have attempted to estimate the incidence of systemic mycoses. Through 1983 the Centers for Disease Control recorded the annual deaths that were voluntarily reported; Table 81–3 indicates these deaths for selected years, adjusted for the total number of annual deaths. These figures represent a gross underestimation of the prevalence of the infections. Not all deaths due to fungous infection are reported, since reporting is not required by law. Many mycotic deaths are undiagnosed, misdiagnosed, or unspecified because they are secondary to some preexistent malady.

Despite the lack of more reliable data, it is apparent from Table 81–3 that in recent years there has been a steady increase in the overall prevalence and mortality from the

TABLE 81–3. MORTALITY RATES DUE TO MYCOSES FOR SELECTED YEARS, BASED ON VOLUNTARY REPORTS TO CDC[a]

Mycosis	1955	1960	1965	1970	1975	1980	1983
Aspergillosis	NR[b]	NR	NR	2.0	3.3	4.0	6.8
Blastomycosis	1.2	0.9	1.6	0.2	0.1	1.3	0.8
Candidiasis	NR	6.3	5.1	8.0	11.4	11.7	21.1
Coccidioidomycosis	4.1	3.2	2.8	2.2	3.2	3.0	2.8
Cryptococcosis	4.8	4.2	3.4	5.8	6.9	5.6	8.3
Histoplasmosis	3.5	4.7	4.1	2.9	3.1	2.6	2.3

[a] Number of mycotic deaths per 100,000 adult deaths. Calculated from *Morbidity and Mortality Weekly Reports,* Annual Summary and Vital Statistics Reports, Vols 7–33, U.S. Department of Health and Human Services.
[b] NR, Mycotic deaths not recorded by Centers for Disease Control (CDC).

opportunistic mycoses, aspergillosis, candidiasis, and cryptococcosis. Conversely, the attack rates of the primary pathogens have remained stable or declined. However, since 1983, the AIDS epidemic has dramatically increased the incidence of opportunistic candidiasis, cryptococcosis, histoplasmosis and coccidioidomycosis.

The incidence of mycotic disease is not geographically uniform. Most mycoses are caused by fungi that reside saprophytically in nature, but their distribution varies considerably. For this reason, the attack rates and incidence of specific mycoses vary widely in different areas. Because the mortality rate for primary systemic infection with any of the three dimorphic fungi endemic to this country (blastomycosis, coccidioidomycosis, and histoplasmosis) is clearly less than 5%, the number of patients with active clinical diseases in any year is at least 20 times greater than the number of deaths. Many fungous infections are chronic; the management and care of individual patients may extend for years.

To estimate the incidence of mycoses requiring hospitalization, Hammerman et al. examined data from the Commission of Professional and Hospital Activities, which consisted of vital statistics and discharge diagnoses from more than 10 million hospital records of participating acute-care hospitals during the year 1970. From these data, regional and national projections of incidence and mortality were made for specific diseases. For histoplasmosis and coccidioidomycosis, the prevalence of skin test reactivity in the population was used for extrapolation. The projected number of hospitalized cases of histoplasmosis per 100,000 population was between 2.2 and 3.2 in the endemic area. Coccidioidomycosis is largely confined to the southwestern states, and the projected number of hospitalized cases per 100,000 population in these states varied from 1.2 to 24.7. Overall incidence of other mycoses (as the primary diagnosis) requiring hospitalization was estimated at between 0.02 and 0.09 per 100,000 Table 81–4 shows the actual number of cases reported, the case fatality rate, and the projected number of mycoses that would require hospitalization throughout the United States in 1970. These estimates on incidence are conservative, as patients not requiring hospitalization have been excluded, and none of the Veterans Administration or other federal hospitals contributed to the data base. It is apparent from Table 81–4 that certain mycotic agents, such as *Coccidioides immitis* and *Blastomyces dermatitidis*, occur more often as primary pathogens, whereas others, such as *Candida*, are encountered predominantly as opportunists. In all cases, the mortality rates are double for secondary or opportunistic fungous infection in a previously compromised patient; as reflected in Table 81–3, these mycoses are on the rise. The study also reported that the average time of hospitalization varied from 11 days for patients with acute histoplasmosis to 30 days for those with aspergillosis.

Portal of Entry

To establish an infection, a potential fungal pathogen must first enter the body. This can occur in only a limited number of ways. The skin presents a strong barrier to fungal penetration. Most fungi lack the enzymes or other invasive properties that would permit them to penetrate intact skin; however, if the skin surface has been abraded, burned, or macerated or

TABLE 81–4. INCIDENCE OF HOSPITALIZED CASES OF SYSTEMIC MYCOTIC INFECTIONS[a]

	Fungal Disease as Primary Diagnosis			Fungal Disease as Secondary Diagnosis		
Infection	Cases Reported	Case Fatality Rate (%)	Cases Projected	Cases Reported	Case Fatality Rate (%)	Cases Projected
Aspergillosis	42	7.1	144	53	22.6	235
Blastomycosis	39	7.7	145	14	14.3	35
Candidiasis (systemic)	31	6.5	88	76	13.2	250
Coccidioidomycosis	270	1.5	1389	146	4.1	695
Cryptococcosis	39	18.0	139	38	36.8	121
Histoplasmosis	449	1.6	1462	855	2.6	2544

From Hammeramn et al: Sabouraudia 12:33, 1974
[a] Number of cases and percentage of fatalities reported to Commission of Professional and Hospital Activities and projected number of hospitalized cases for the United States during 1970.

its integrity has otherwise been compromised, fungi and other microorganisms are able to gain access to the cutaneous and subcutaneous tissue, and the opportunity for infection vastly increases. Several studies have shown that the chances of establishing an experimental cutaneous mycosis with *Candida albicans* or the dermatophytes are greatly enhanced by abrading the skin before challenge. Although the protective defenses of the skin have not been completely defined, both anatomic and physiologic factors are involved. For example, dermatophytes are fungi that preferentially infect the skin, hair, or nails (Chap. 84). Certain chemicals that are often present on the skin surface (amino acids, fatty acids) and lipids found in sebum inhibit the growth or conidial germination of some dermatophytes. Although lysozyme is not a potent antifungal agent, the dermatophytes may be actively deterred by other factors, such as hormone-induced changes in the skin or hair chemistry, salinity, pH, and the secretion of specific growth inhibitors.

Inhalation is the most important method of initiating a fungous infection. Throughout life the respiratory tract is exposed to a barrage of airborne fungi; yet the incidence of respiratory mycoses is relatively low. A natural barrier is the anatomy of the respiratory tract, which determines the depth to which particles can be inhaled. The size of the inhaled fungal cells or conidia will delimit the extent of penetration. Particles of 10 μm or larger may be deposited on the tracheal or nasal epithelium, where they are usually retained and then expelled from this area. Particles 5 to 10 μm in diameter may penetrate the bronchioli, but they are usually removed by bronchial secretions and the ciliated epithelial lining of the respiratory tract. Therefore, fungal inocula greater than 5 μm in diameter usually are limited to local colonization of the nasal sinuses or bronchial tree. Fungous surface antigens may induce a local allergic response; this reaction is also associated with inert allergens, such as pollen and dust particles. Yeast cells, conidia, or other fungous cells less than 5 μm in diameter may be inhaled to the alveoli.

In the alveolus, the fungous cell is confronted by surfactant, humoral serum components, alveolar macrophages, and a subsequent inflammatory response. The host response may culminate in either inactivation of the fungus, after which it will be cleared slowly from the host, or protracted interaction between the fungus and the host. This transient episode is characterized by a mild or asymptomatic lung infection, pulmonary infiltration, sensitization of the host to fungous antigens, and, eventually, a stabilized or arrested lesion (usually granulomatous) that becomes sealed off for an indefinite period. Alternatively, the host defenses may be inadequate to quell the fungous challenge, and a progressive infection ensues. Symptoms vary considerably. The developing mycosis may be acute, subacute, or chronic; the fungus may remain localized in the lung, or it may metastasize. Whether the fungal challenge is successfully contained or results in clinical disease depends on the dynamic interaction of three determinants—integrity of the host defenses (both immunologic and nonspecific), the pathogenic potential of the fungus, and the extent of exposure.

In addition to the skin and respiratory tract, the other two epithelial surfaces infrequently serve as portals of entry for fungous infection. The urogenital tract is occasionally bridged by endogenous fungi such as *C. albicans* when their growth is enhanced by physiologic changes in the local mucosa. Similarly, the gastrointestinal tract may become a source of fungous infection after changes induced by age, trauma, neoplasm, certain drugs, or an imbalance in the normal flora. As discussed in Chapter 85, yeasts, such as *C. albicans*, have cell wall determinants that mediate their specific attachment to receptors on the membrane of mucosal, epithelial, and other cells.

Iatrogenic inoculation—through contaminated indwelling catheters, during surgery, after antibacterial or immunosuppressive chemotherapy, administration of steroids, or radiation treatment—has dramatically increased the incidence of opportunistic mycoses in recent years. Under these conditions, either fungi are introduced into the host directly, often bypassing natural defense mechanisms, or the host defenses are sufficiently suppressed to permit enhanced fungous invasion (Chap. 85).

Classification

No clinical classification of mycoses is entirely adequate. Fungous infections are usually organized on the basis of the general body area predominantly involved. This classification, presented in Table 81–5, reflects both the portal of entry and the major site of involvement. For example, most primary systemic mycoses are initially pulmonary whereas subcutaneous mycoses follow traumatic inoculation of the skin. Exceptions are common, however, as systemic or deep mycotic agents can produce cutaneous and subcutaneous lesions after dissemination from the lung as well as from primary cutaneous inoculation. Similarly, many subcutaneous mycoses may have systemic manifestations.

The term *opportunistic mycoses* is not precise. It generally refers to fungous infections in patients whose host defenses have been somehow compromised. However, under the appropriate circumstances, any pathogenic fungus may be opportunistic. Furthermore, the fungi generally regarded as opportunistic may also cause primary disease. Because the range of host-compromising conditions has not been fully defined, it may be that many more mycoses are opportunistic than are recognized as such. Opportunism is a frequently and loosely used term, and it is probably best applied functionally and not confined to specific pathogens.

Pathogenesis

Fungous Determinants. For a mycotic infection to develop, contact between the host and the fungal pathogen must be established. Most fungi that can produce disease exist saprophytically in a natural reservoir and are acquired through exogenous contact. Some fungi (e.g., *C. immitis*) are confined to specific geographic regions, whereas others (e.g., *A. fumigatus*) are ubiquitous. The conditions of exposure (inoculum size, route, host immunity) will determine whether infection ensues. A few common pathogens are endogenous and either are part of the human flora (*Candida* species) or have adapted for persistent infection (certain dermatophytes).

Another important determinant of whether infection follows contact is the inherent virulence of the fungus. Experimental infections have shown wide differences in indices of pathogenicity (e.g., mortality, fungal census in target organs) among various fungous species or strains of a single species. In many cases, the bases of these differences in virulence are poorly understood. Tissue-reactive enzymes, irritants, attachment to host cells, antiphagocytic properties, and inflammatory components have been described for many

TABLE 81–5. CLINICAL CLASSIFICATION OF MYCOTIC INFECTIONS (ABRIDGED)

Area of Predominant Involvement	Mycosis	Etiology
Superficial	Pityriasis versicolor	*Malassezia furfur*
	Tinea nigra	*Phaeoannellomyces werneckii*
	White piedra	*Trichosporon beigelii*
	Black piedra	*Piedraia hortae*
Cutaneous	Dermatophytosis	*Microsporum* species, *Trichophyton* species, and *Epidermophyton floccosum*
	Candidiasis of skin, mucosa, or nails	*Candida albicans*, other *Candida* species
Subcutaneous	Sporotrichosis	*Sporothrix schenckii*
	Chromomycosis	*Philaphora verrucosa, Fonsecaea pedrosoi*, and others
	Mycetoma	*Pseudallescheria boydii, Madurella mycetomatis,* and others
	Rhinosporidiosis	*Rhinosporidium seeberi*
	Lobomycosis	*Loboa loboi*
	Subcutaneous phycomycosis	*Basidiobolus haptosporus*
	Rhinoentomophthoromycosis	*Conidiobolus coronatus*
Systemic	Primary mycoses	
	Coccidioidomycosis	*Coccidioides immitis*
	Histoplasmosis	*Histoplasma capsulatum*
	Blastomycosis	*Blastomyces dermatitidis*
	Paracoccidioidomycosis	*Paracoccidioides brasiliensis*
	Opportunistic mycoses	
	Candidiasis, systemic	*Candida albicans*, other *Candida* species
	Cryptococcosis	*Cryptococcus neoformans*
	Aspergillis	*Aspergillus fumigatus*, other *Aspergillus* species
	Mucormycosis	Species of *Rizopus, Absidia, Mucor*, and others

infectious fungi. (Virulence factors as unambiguous and potent as bacterial exotoxins are not produced.) Some of the properties correlated with virulence or shown to affect pathogenicity are presented in Table 81–6. Most of the potential fungous determinants of pathogenicity are complex factors that are variably expressed and strongly effected by the host milieu. For example, most of the systemic pathogens have been shown to release cell wall and other components that produce direct or indirect immunomodulatory effects. Details and more specific information are included in the subsequent chapters.

In vivo morphology is a fundamental determinant. Fungi may produce hyphae, spherical structures (yeasts, sporangia, sclerotic cells), or both, and this morphology influences pathogenesis. Anatomically, hyphae tend to penetrate the lumina of vessels and lymphatics. Yeasts are less confined and can be transported through the circulation to virtually any part of the body and therefore, in theory, their pathogenic potential is unlimited.

Another crucial factor is attachment of the fungus to host tissue. *C. albicans* and other fungi have surface ligands and receptors that facilitate attachment and binding to host cells and products. Some of these components and processes have been clearly associated with pathogenicity, as will be discussed in Chapters 82 and 85.

The concept of infection and disease must be clearly understood. Some fungi are completely superficial; they grow on the host without invasion and cause minimal irritation. Two examples are piedra (the formation of nodules on hair), and the colonization of the external ear or nasal sinuses by *Aspergillus* species. *Aspergillus* can also colonize the bronchial tree and the pulmonary cavity. However, some colonizing fungi such as *Aspergillus* have the potential to cause more serious disease. In other situations, fungi involve tissue and elicit inflammation but produce only asymptomatic infection. Fungous disease is usually a symptomatic infection and is generally associated with more extensive damage to host tissue.

Many fungous pathogens closely resemble each other in morphology, taxonomic relationship, antigenic determinants, cell wall composition, growth requirements, and physiologic properties. These similarities are relevant to the diagnosis and treatment of specific fungal infections. Cross-reactive antigens may preclude the development of a specific and diagnostic serologic test.

Host Factors. Considering the high prevalence of fungi in the environment and the low incidence of mycotic disease, it is apparent that most humans are highly resistant to fungous invasion. During infection both humoral and cellular immune responses are stimulated. In general, the antibodies that form are not protective, although they may be useful in establishing a diagnosis and evaluating prognosis. Resistance to several mycoses (e.g., disseminated coccidioidomycosis, chronic mucocutaneous candidiasis) is clearly associated with the thymus-dependent immune system. Furthermore, patients are predisposed to the opportunistic mycoses by a cellular immunodeficiency resulting from various sarcomas (and their treatments), steroids, or immunosuppressive therapy after organ transplantation. The importance of the host immune response in controlling mycotic infections, where understood, is discussed more fully under the individual mycoses. Adequate neutrophils are essential for optimal defense against systemic candidiasis and invasive aspergillosis.

Other host factors that have been shown to influence susceptibility to fungal infection in specific instances include age, sex, race, heredity, and physiologic condition. Table 81–7

TABLE 81–6. EXAMPLES OF POSSIBLE DETERMINANTS OF FUNGOUS PATHOGENICITY (ABRIDGED)

Feature	Examples, Responsible Factor or Mechanism
Morphology	Yeast cells are more easily transported and disseminated Hyphal invasion is anatomically restricted Expression of *C. albicans* surface antigens, receptors and binding components differs between yeast cells and germ tubes or hyphae
Attachment	*C. albicans* surface components bind to receptors on phagocytes, epithelial cells and endothelial cells
Growth requirement	*S. schenckii* and dermatophytes exhibit restricted growth at 37C.
Enzymes	*C. neoformans*, phenoloxidase *C. albicans*, proteinases *A. fumigatus*, elastase Dermatophytes, keratinases
Toxins, irritants	*C. albicans*, shock-producing toxin *A. fumigatus*, gliotoxin *B. dermatitidis*, cell walls induce granulomata Dermatophytes induce inflammation
Antigens	*C. immitis*, immune complexes may induce suppression of cell-mediated immunity *C. albicans* may induce autoimmunity *A. fumigatus* and other fungi, allergens
Interference with nonspecific host defenses	*A. fumigatus* inhibits activation of the alternative complement pathway *C. neoformans*, capsule inhibits phagocytosis *C. immitis*, inhibition of phagolysosomal fusion *C. albicans*, CR-3-like and other surface receptors
Immunosuppression or modulation	*C. albicans*, cell wall mannoproteins, glycoproteins *C. neoformans*, mannoprotein induces suppressor cells *C. immitis*, induction of tumor necrosis factor

presents some of the associations of certain mycoses with abnormal or impaired host defenses. Obviously there is considerable overlap, and many patients with severe diseases, such as leukemia or transplantation, experience multiple risk factors.

Dynamics of Host-Fungus Interactions. Except for fungi that may be confined to the skin because of restricted growth at higher temperatures, the pathogenesis of fungous infections is determined by the interplay of host defenses with the invading fungus. After a fungous cell has bridged one of the body surfaces, it confronts numerous nonspecific, immunologic, humoral, and cellular host defenses.

The nonspecific humoral defenses include inhibitors of fungous growth in serum (e.g., transferrin), hormones that may inhibit growth or regulate phagocytosis, serum substances that clump yeast cells, and opsonins. Both neutrophils and macrophages are able to phagocytize most pathogenic yeasts, but the extent of phagocytosis is inversely related to the size of the yeast cells. The ability to kill ingested yeasts, though inefficient, may be adequate to ensure resistance to infection. Activated macrophages are more phagocytic, but the killing ability of macrophages from different sources varies considerably. The antifungal activity of murine natural killer cells has been described. Specific antibodies do not appear to be directly injurious to most pathogenic fungi; however, antibodies can serve as opsonins to enhance phagocytosis, and they participate in antibody-dependent cellular cytotoxicity against fungi. Lymphocytes from sensitive persons may serve a protective function directly or through the mobilization of macrophages or modulation of other immunologic components.

Blocking factors, immune complexes, and suppressor lymphocytes have also been implicated as possible mechanisms to enhance fungous disease. Subsequent chapters will present summaries of the available information regarding the pathogenesis of each mycosis. Information about the host risk factors and fungous determinants of pathogenic potential are becoming increasingly relevant to the diagnosis and management of mycoses.

Diagnosis

Three diagnostic approaches are routinely applied in clinical mycology—direct examination, culture, and serology. The direct microscopic examination of specimens can often establish a diagnosis or narrow the etiologic possibilities. Pathogenic fungi are large enough to be observed in skin scrapings, tissue biopsy material, or body fluids digested with 10% potassium hydroxide. The method of choice for fresh preparations is calcofluor white, a nonspecific fluorescent stain for fungous cell walls. Fungous cells may be seen in histologic sections that are stained with hematoxylin and eosin. If few organisms are present, material can be concentrated or stained with calcofluor white, fluorescent antibody reagents, or histochemical stains (periodic acid–Schiff, methenamine silver) for fungous cell wall material.

Regardless of the results of a direct examination, specimens are cultured for pathogenic fungi. Nonsterile specimens (e.g., skin scrapings, sputa) are planted on media containing antibiotics to inhibit bacteria and nonpathogenic fungous contaminants. The routine fungous culture medium is Sabouraud's agar, consisting of 2% or 4% glucose, 1% neopeptone, and 2% agar. Many laboratories obtain improved recovery of fungi with Inhibitory Mold Agar, which is a complex medium containing chloramphenicol and gentamicin to inhibit bacteria. Rich media, such as brain-heart infusion agar with sheep blood, are used for the isolation of fungi from normally sterile specimens and when certain fungi, such as *H. capsulatum*, are suspected. Routine cultures are incubated at 25C to 30C and must be retained for several weeks before they are reported as negative. Fungous isolates are identified by appropriate morphologic, physiologic, or antigenic properties.

Serology is the third laboratory tool with established diagnostic and prognostic value for certain mycotic infections. The value, limitations, specificity, sensitivity, and predictive value of the available serologic tests are described in the following chapters under specific mycoses. Mycoserologic techniques include the measurement of specific antibodies, antigens, and delayed and immediate hypersensitivity. Complete immunologic evaluation of patients, both in vivo and in vitro, including enumeration and functional capacity of T cell subpopulations, immunoglobulin classes, and lymphokine pro-

TABLE 81–7. EXAMPLES OF HOST FACTORS THAT MAY PREDISPOSE TO MYCOTIC INFECTION

Host Condition	Examples or Mechanisms	Associated Mycoses
Impaired cell-mediated immunity	Inherent cellular immunodeficiency; AIDS; hematologic malignancies; treatment with steroids, immunosuppressive, or cytotoxic drugs associated with transplantation or anticancer therapy	Chronic mucocutaneous candidiasis Superficial candidiasis Secondary (disseminated) coccidioidomycosis Disseminated histoplasmosis Cryptococcosis Paracoccidioidomycosis
Neutropenia or impaired neutrophils	Chronic granulomatous disease; hematologic malignancy; treatment with steroids, immunosuppressive or cytotoxic drugs associated with transplantation or anticancer therapy	Systemic candidiasis Invasive aspergillosis Mucormycosis
Atopy	Hereditary predisposition to develop immediate hypersensitivity	Allergic bronchopulmonary aspergillosis
Iatrogenic	Surgery, antibacterial antibiotics, indwelling catheters, hyperalimentation	Systemic candidiasis Fungemia due to species of *Candida, Trichosporon, Malassezia furfur*
Impaired epithelium	Burns, trauma, maceration	Mucormycosis Superficial candidiasis
Abnormal pulmonary space	Cavity formed by previous disease (e.g., tuberculosis, sarcoid); emphysema	Aspergilloma Cavity histoplasmosis

duction, yields information of prognostic value in several mycoses.

In the near future, the polymerase chain reaction will be used for the direct and rapid amplification of fungous DNA in clinical specimens to effect an immediate diagnosis. DNA probes, analysis with restriction endonucleases, and other methods are currently being used to biotype or fingerprint strains of pathogenic fungi, including *C. albicans*, *C. neoformans*, and *A. fumigatus*, that differ in virulence, epidemiology, resistance to antifungal drugs or other properties.

With some mycoses, additional diagnostic methods (e.g., radiology, clinical chemistry) can be helpful.

Therapy

Each of the limited number of antibiotics that is used currently to treat fungous infections has one or more drawbacks, such as profound side effects, a narrow antifungal spectrum, poor penetration of certain tissues, or selection of resistant organisms. However, research to develop new antifungal drugs has never been more intense, and treatment breakthroughs may soon be forthcoming. Among the current drugs are the polyenes (Chap. 7), flucytosine (5-fluorocytosine), and the azoles (imidazoles and triazoles).

The mechanism of action of the polyenes involves the formation of complexes with ergosterol in fungous cell membranes. The major systemic antifungal, amphotericin B, has greater affinity for ergosterol than cholesterol, the predominant sterol in mammalian cell membranes. Packaging of amphotericin B in liposomes has shown greater experimental efficacy. The azoles interfere with the synthesis of ergosterol. They block the cytochrome P-450-dependent 14 α-demethylation of lanosterol, which is a precursor of ergosterol in fungi and cholesterol in mammalian cells. However, the fungous cytochrome P450s are approximately 100 to 1000 times more sensitive to the azoles than mammalian systems. Flucytosine is converted by fungous cytosine deaminase to 5-fluorouracil and incorporated into 5-fluorodexoyuridylic acid monophosphate, which perturbs thymidylate synthetase and DNA synthesis. The current applications of the available antifungal drugs are summarized in Table 81–8. More specific information on treatment of specific mycoses is discussed in the following chapters.

In many systemic mycoses, cell-mediated immunity is transiently suppressed during active infection, and after chemotherapy, as the fungous antigen burden is reduced, the cell-mediated immune responses of the host are restored. However, with profound depression of underlying cellular immunity, as in patients with chronic mucocutaneous candidiasis or cryptococcal meningitis and AIDS, the relapse rate is very high, which has led to the concept and practice of maintenance or suppression therapy. Patients receive low-dose treatment for long periods to control the mycotic disease. Suppression therapy has been prescribed with ketoconazole, oral nystatin, or low-dose amphotericin B.

Several clinical trials have evaluated antifungal prophylaxis in high risk patients, such as those with transplants or hematologic malignancies, whose management often includes corticosteroids, cytotoxic drugs, and antibacterial antibiotics. Although promising results have been achieved with ketoconazole, oral nystatin, and low-dose amphotericin B, often in combination or with other drugs, a standard regimen has not been adopted. The usual criteria for prophylaxis include persistent neutropenia and fever that does not respond to antibacterial antibiotics, administration of corticosteroids, or unexplained progressive pulmonary infiltrates, debilitation, or major organ failure.

In addition to antibiotics, other therapeutic approaches have been applied to certain mycoses; these include topical chemical preparations, heat, surgery, hyperbaric oxygen, and administration of transfer factor, cytokines, or immunomodulators.

TABLE 81–8. SUMMARY OF ANTIFUNGAL ANTIBIOTICS

Drug	Indications	Adult Dosage	Side Effects	Comments
Nystatin	Oral thrush	Solution of 1–2 × 10^5 units, PO, daily for 1–2 wk	Rarely diarrhea, nausea	
	Cutaneous candidiasis	Topical ointment of 10^5 units, 2–3 times daily	Rarely hypersensitivity	
Amphotericin B (AMB)	Systemic mycoses	1–5 mg/d IV, increased to 0.3–0.6 mg/kg/d in 5% glucose with mannitol; total dose 1–3 g	Manifold; especially renal toxicity; thrombophlebitis, hypokalemia, anemia, chills, fever, headache, nausea, anorexia	Monitor BUN and creatine levels; intrathecal administration for some meningitis cases
Flucytosine (5FC)	Candidiasis Cryptococcosis Aspergillosis Chromomycosis	150 mg/kg/d PO in 4 doses for 4 or 6 wk	Skin rash, diarrhea, nausea, hematopoietic (aplastic anemia, granulocytopenia) and hepatic toxicities	Resistant organisms emerge; check WBC and liver function weekly; patients with impaired renal function may accumulate toxic levels
Amphotericin B and flucytosine	Cryptococcosis Systemic candidiasis		Reduced toxicity due to lower dose of AMB	See above
Griseofulvin	Dermatophytosis	0.5–1.0 g PO daily after fatty meal	Some GI distress; rarely neurologic symptoms	
Tolnaftate	Dermatophytosis of skin	Topical; 1% solution in cream base		Not effective against hair or nail infections
Miconazole nitrate	Dermatophytosis of skin	Topical; 2% in cream base		
Miconazole	Systemic mycoses	0.2–1.2 mg IV q 8 h for 3–6 wk	Phlebitis, nausea, anemia, hyponatremia, pruritus, rash, cardiac arrhythmia; rarely marrow, liver toxicity	May administer intrathecally
Ketoconazole	Chronic mucocutaneous candidiasis Superficial candidiasis Dermatophytosis Systemic mycoses, especially paracoccidioido-mycosis	200–1200 mg PO in multiple daily doses for 1–6 mo or more	Nausea, vomiting, rash; rarely liver toxicity, gynecomastia, endocrine dysfunction, pruritus	Monitor liver function
Itraconazole	Aspergillosis Sporotrichosis Chromomycosis Systemic and cutaneous mycoses	50–200 mg PO daily	Nausea, headache, pyrosis	Monitor liver function
Fluconazole	Superficial candidiasis Cryptococcal meningitis in AIDS patients Coccidioidal meningitis	50–400 mg PO daily	Nausea, vomiting; rarely liver toxicity	May administer IV

IV, intravenous administration; PO, oral administration; BUN, blood urea nitrogen; GI, gastrointestinal; WBC, white blood cell count.

FURTHER READING

Books and Reviews

Abramovici A: Mycotoxins and abnormal fetal development. Contrib Microbiol Immunol 3:81, 1977

Ajello L: Comparative ecology of respiratory mycotic disease agents. Bacteriol Rev 31:6, 1967

Al-Doory Y (ed): The Epidemiology of Human Mycotic Disease. Springfield, Ill, Charles C Thomas, 1975

Al-Doory Y, Domson JF (eds): Mould Allergy. Philadelphia, Lea & Febiger, 1984

Al-Doory Y, Wagner GE (eds): Aspergillosis. Springfield, Ill, Charles C Thomas, 1985

Becker CE, Tong TG, Buerner U, et al: Diagnosis and treatment of

Amanita phalloides-type mushroom poisoning: Use of thioctic acid. West J Med 125:100, 1976
Beneke ES, Rogers A: Medical Mycology Manual, ed 4. Minneapolis, Burgess, 1980
Bode FR, Pare JAP, Fraser RG: Pulmonary diseases in the compromised host. Medicine 53:255, 1974
Bodey GP, Fainstein V (eds): Candidiasis. New York, Raven Press, 1985
Borgers M, Vanden Bossche H, Cauwenbergh G: The pharmacology of agents used in the treatment of pulmonary mycoses. Clin Chest Med 7:439, 1986
Chandler FW, Kaplan W, Ajello L: Color Atlas and Text of the Histopathology of Mycotic Diseases. Chicago, Year Book, 1980
Conant NF, Smith DT, Baker RD, et al: Manual of Clinical Mycology, ed 3. Philadelphia, WB Saunders, 1971
Cox RA (ed): Immunology of the Fungal Diseases. Boca Raton, Fla, CRC Press, 1989
Davies SF, Sarosi GA: Role of serodiagnostic tests and skin tests in the diagnosis of fungal disease. Clin Chest Med 8:135, 1987
DiSalvo AF (ed): Occupational Mycoses. Philadelphia, Lea & Febiger, 1983
Emmons CW, Binford CH, Utz JP, et al: Medical Mycology, ed 3. Philadelphia, Lea & Febiger, 1977
Fromtling RA: Fungi. In Balows A, Hausler WJ, Herrmann KL, et al (eds): Manual of Clinical Microbiology, ed 5. Washington, DC, American Society for Microbiology, 1991, p 579
Galgiani JN: Fluconazole, a new antifungal agent. Ann Intern Med 113:177, 1990
Hay RJ, Dupont B, Graybill JR (eds): First international symposium on itraconazole. Rev Infect Dis 9:51, 1987
Howard DH (ed): Fungi Pathogenic for Humans and Animals. Part A. Biology. Part B. Pathogenicity and Detection: I and II. New York, Marcel Dekker, 1983 (A and BI) and 1985 (BII)
Kaufman L, Reiss E: Serodiagnosis of fungal diseases. In Rose NR, Friedman H, Fahey JL: Manual of Clinical Immunology, ed 3. Washington DC, American Society for Microbiology, 1986, p 446
Kerridge D: Mode of action of clinically important antifungal drugs. Adv Microbiol Physiol 27:1, 1986
Kobayashi GS, Medoff G: Antifungal agents: Recent developments. Annu Rev Microbiol 31:291, 1977
Koneman EW, Roberts GD, Wright SF: Practical Laboratory Mycology, ed 3. Baltimore, Williams & Wilkins, 1985
Krustak E (ed): Immunology of Fungal Diseases. New York, Marcel Dekker, 1989
Lincoff G, Mitchel DJ: Toxic and Hallucinogenic Mushroom Poisoning. New York, Van Nostrand Reinhold, 1977
Litten W: The most poisonous mushrooms. Sci Am 232:90, 1975
McGinnis MR: Laboratory Handbook of Medical Mycology. New York, Academic Press, 1980
McGinnis MR, D'Amato RF, Land GF: Pictorial Handbook of Medically Important Fungi and Aerobic Actinomycetes. New York, Praeger, 1982
McGinnis MR, Schell WA: Classifying the medically important fungi. Diagn Med p 30, March 1985
Moore GS, Jaciow DM: Mycology for the Clinical Laboratory. Reston, Va, Reston Publishing Co, 1979
Odds FC: Candida and Candidosis, ed 2. London, Bailliere Tindall, 1988
Palmer DF, Kaufman L, Kaplan W, et al: Serodiagnosis of Mycotic Diseases, Springfield, Ill, Charles C Thomas, 1977
Polak A: 5-Fluorocytosine. Contrib Microbiol Immunol 4:158, 1977
Reiss E: Molecular Immunology of Mycotic and Actinomycotic Infections. New York, Elsevier, 1986
Rippon JW: Medical Mycology, ed 3. Philadelphia, WB Saunders, 1988
Rumack BH, Salzman E: Mushroom Poisoning: Diagnosis and Treatment. Boca Raton, Fla, CRC Press, 1978
San-Blas G: The cell wall of fungal human pathogens: Its possible role in host-parasite relationships; a review. Mycopathologia 79:159, 1982
Smith JE, Moss MO: Mycotoxins. Formation, Analysis and Significance. Chichester, John Wiley & Sons, 1985
Smith JMB: Opportunistic Mycoses of Man and Other Animals. Oxon, UK, CAB Internatl Mycological Institute, 1989
Speller DCE: Antifungal Chemotherapy. Chichester, UK, John Wiley & Sons, 1980
Vanden Bossche H: Biochemical targets for antifungal azole derivatives: Hypothesis on mode of action. Curr Top Med Mycol 1:313, 1985
Vanden Bossche H, Mackenzie DWR, Cauwenbergh G, et al (eds): Mycoses in AIDS Patients. New York, Plenum Press, 1990
Warnock DW, Richardson MD (eds): Fungal infection in the Compromised Patient. Chichester, UK, John Wiley & Sons, 1982
Wentworth BB (ed): Diagnostic Procedures for Mycotic and Parasitic Infections, ed 7. Washington, DC, American Public Health Association, 1988, Chap. 1–11
Weiland T, Faulstich H: Amatoxins, phallotoxins, phallolysin, and antamanide: The biologically active components of poisonous *Amanita* mushrooms. Crit Rev Bicohem 5:185, 1978
Wogan GN: Mycotoxins. Annu Rev Pharmacol 15:437, 1975
Wright DE: Toxins produced by fungi. Annu Rev Microbiol 22:269, 1967

Selected Papers

Fraser DW, Ward JI, Ajello L, et al: Aspergillosis and other systemic mycoses: The growing problem. JAMA 242:1631, 1979
Haley LD, Trandel J, Coyle MB: Practical Methods for the Culture and Identification of Fungi in the Clinical Microbiology Laboratory. Cumitech 11. Washington, DC, American Society for Microbiology, 1980
Hammerman KJ, Powell KE, Tosh FE: The incidence of hospitalized cases of systemic mycotic infections. Sabouraudia 12:33, 1974
McCormick DJ, Arbel AJ, Gibbons RB: Nonlethal mushroom poisoning. Annu Intern Med 90:332, 1979
Mote RF, Muhm RL, Gigstad DC: A staining method using acridine orange and auramine O for fungi and mycobacteria in bovine tissue. Stain Technol 50:5, 1975
Polak A: Melanin as a virulence factor in pathogenic fungi. Mycoses 33:215, 1989
Schlueter DP, Fink NJ, Hensley GT: Wood-pulp workers' disease: A hypersensitivity pneumonitis caused by *Alternaria*. Ann Intern Med 77:907, 1972
Stobo JD, Paul S, Van Scoy RE, Hermans PE: Suppressor thymus-derived lymphocytes in fungal infection. J Clin Invest 57:319, 1976
Stoddert RW, Herbertson BM: The use of lectins in the detection and identification of human fungal pathogens. Biochem Soc Trans 5:233, 1977

CHAPTER 82

Systemic Mycoses

Each of the four major, primary systemic mycoses—coccidioidomycosis, histoplasmosis, blastomycosis, and paracoccidioidomycosis—is caused by a thermally dimorphic fungus. The fungi that cause coccidioidomycosis and histoplasmosis exist in nature normally in dry soil or in soil mixed with guano, respectively. The agents of blastomycosis and paracoccidioidomycosis are presumed to exist in nature, but their habitats have not been clearly defined. The prevalence and geographic distribution of these mycoses are delimited. Inhalation of any one of these fungous cells can lead to pulmonary infection, which may or may not be symptomatic. Dissemination to other parts of the body may occur. Except for a few extremely rare cases, there is no evidence of transmission among humans or animals. Table 82–1 compares some of the mycologic, ecologic, and epidemiologic features of these four, usually primary, systemic mycoses due to exogenous, dimorphic fungi.

Although most symptomatic cases of coccidioidomycosis, histoplasmosis, and paracoccidioidomycosis occur in patients without significant preexisting and predisposing disease, persons with defects of cell-mediated immunity have long been recognized to be at risk for these mycoses in the appropriate endemic areas. The incidence of each of these three mycoses as opportunistic mycoses in patients with AIDS has sharply increased in recent years.

Coccidioidomycosis

Coccidioidomycosis is caused by *Coccidioides immitis*, a dimorphic fungus that normally lives in soil in a highly restricted geographic area. Both the fungus and the infection it causes are almost entirely limited to this endemic area. The organism was discovered in 1892 in tissue from a fatal case and was named *Coccidioides* (i.e., *Coccidia*-like) because the tissue forms (spherules) resemble *Coccidia*; the species name, *immitis*, means not mild. Most early cases were diagnosed at autopsy, and until 1930 the disease was erroneously thought to be invariably severe and disseminated. It was recognized quite early that coccidioidomycosis is confined to the southwestern United States, contiguous regions of northern Mexico, and specific areas of Central and South America. The more common primary form is a mild, respiratory ailment, also called valley fever or San Joaquin Valley fever.

Much of the early knowledge of coccidioidomycosis was provided by Dr. Charles E. Smith and his associates at Stanford University. The ecology of *C. immitis* and the epidemiology of coccidioidomycosis were elucidated by Smith in a series of pioneering investigations that began in the 1930s and inspired many subsequent mycologic studies. Smith discovered the natural reservoir of *C. immitis* by isolating it from soil samples collected throughout the Southwest, and he determined the environmental conditions under which the organism was propagated. From mycelial culture filtrates, he developed coccidioidin, the skin test antigen used to detect exposure to *C. immitis*, and conducted population studies of skin reactivity. His contributions extended beyond the accumulation of information about coccidioidomycosis to the establishment of fundamental concepts of mycotic infection.

Morphologic and Cultural Characteristics

Dimorphism. As depicted in Figure 82–1, the life cycle of *C. immitis* encompasses at least four distinct morphologic structures that are produced under different conditions. In nature and in the laboratory, *C. immitis* grows as a mold (Fig. 82–1, A–E). It produces hyaline, branching, septate hyphae, and as the culture ages, characteristic arthroconidia are produced, usually but not invariably in alternate hyphal cells (Figs. 82–1E and 82–2). In older cultures, the arthroconidium-forming hypha fragments and readily releases unicellular, barrel-shaped arthroconidia, the ends of which often retain appendage-like remnants of wall material from adjacent cells. Arthroconidia are approximately 3 by 6 μm in size, are easily airborne, and are small enough to be inhaled into the alveoli. They are highly resistant to desiccation, temperature extremes, and deprivation of nutrients, and they may remain viable for years. Under appropriate growth conditions, the arthroconidia will germinate to recycle the saphrophytic mycelial phase (Fig. 82–1B).

After their inhalation, the arthroconidia become spherical (Fig. 82–1A, F, and G). In the infected host, *C. immitis* exists as spherules—spherical thick-walled structures 15 to 80 μm in diameter—that are filled with a few to several hundred endospores. As a spherule enlarges (Fig. 82–1H to S), the nuclei undergo mitosis, the cytoplasm condenses around these nuclei, and a cell wall forms around each developing endospore. At maturation, the spherule ruptures to release its endospores. The endospores are 2 to 5 μm in size and may, in turn, enlarge to form mature spherules (Fig. 82–1H to S). Hyphae as well as spherules may form in the tissues and appear in sputum of patients with coccidioidal cavities of the lungs.

TABLE 82-1. SUMMARY OF EPIDEMIOLOGIC FEATURES OF PRIMARY SYSTEMIC MYCOSES

Feature	Coccidioiodomycosis	Histoplasmosis	Blastomycosis	Paracoccidioiomycosis
Saprophytic form (<35C): hyaline, septate hyphae	Yes	Yes	Yes	Yes
Tissue form	Spherules	Yeasts	Yeasts	Yeasts
High infection rate in endemic areas	Yes	Yes	?	Yes
≥90% of infections are initiated by inhalation	Yes	Yes	Yes	Yes
≥90% of infections are asymptomatic	Yes	Yes	?	Yes
≥90% of infections are self-limited	Yes	Yes	?	Yes
≥90% of infections involve immunocompetent patients	Yes	Yes	Yes	Yes
Approximate percentage of males among patients with disease	75%–90%	80%–90%	50%–90%	95%

From Walsh TJ, Mitchell TG: In Balows et al (eds): Manual of Clinical Microbiology, ed 5. Washington DC, American Society for Microbiology, 1991, p 630

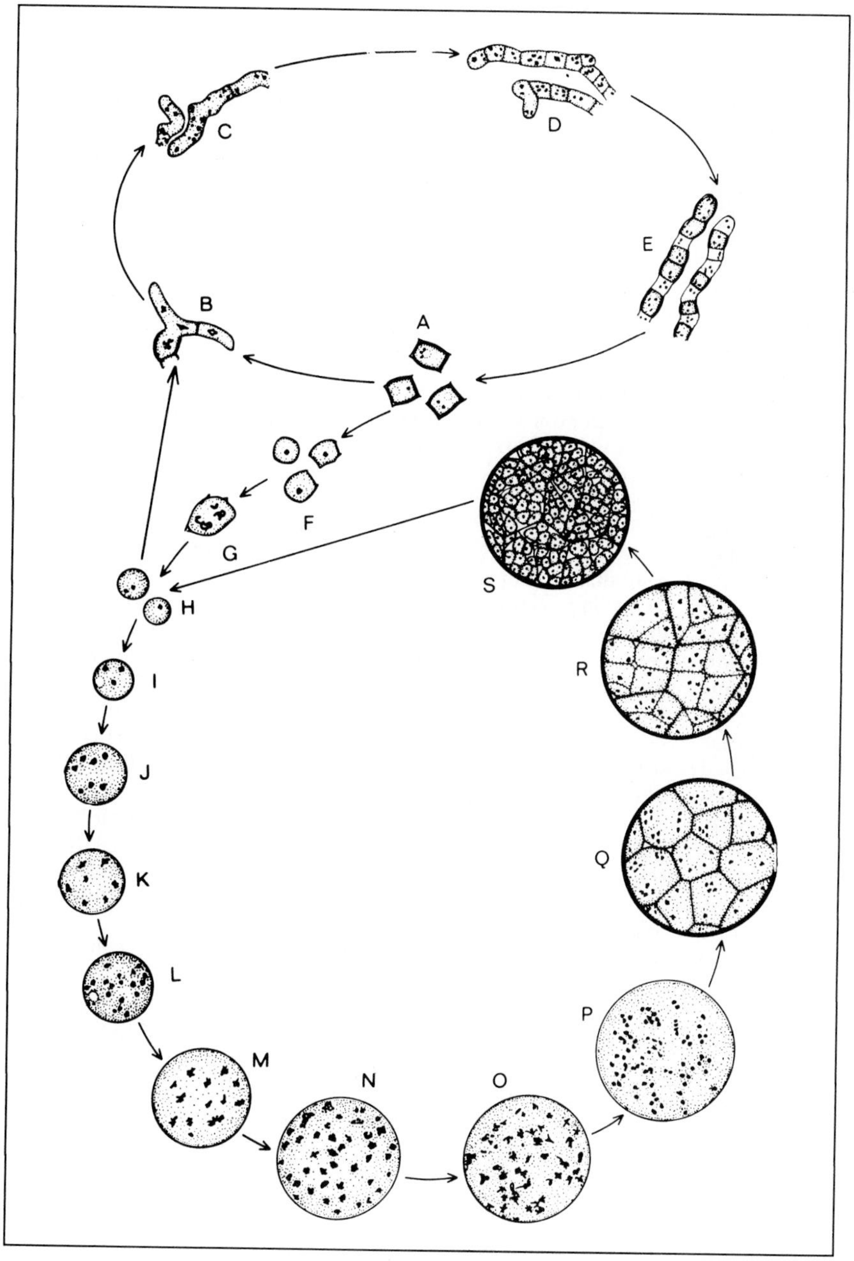

Fig. 82–1. *Coccidioides immitis.* Life cycle in saphrophytic (A–E) and parasitic (F–S) phases. **A.** Arthroconidia (3 × 6 μm). **B–E.** Mycelium. **H–S.** Formation of spherule containing endospores. **S.** Mature spherule (usually 30 to 60 μm in diameter) containing endospores (2 to 5 μm). (*From Sun and Huppert: Sabouraudia 14:185, 1976.*)

Cultural Characteristics. On routine mycologic media, such as Inhibitory Mold or Sabouraud's agar, at the usual incubation temperature of 25C to 30C, different isolates of *C. immitis* produce a wide variety of colony types. Colonies may be white, gray, or brownish in color, with a powdery, wooly, or cottony texture. Because numerous infectious arthroconidia are produced in culture and are readily aerosolized in the dry state, extreme caution should be exercised in handling cultures of *C. immitis*. Tubes or plates should be tightly sealed and opened only under a safety hood that protects both the laboratory worker and the environment.

Spherules can be produced in the laboratory on a complex medium at 40C under 20% CO_2. However, in vitro growth of the tissue phase, even under the most optimal conditions, is seldom extensive.

Clinical Infection

Ecology and Epidemiology

In the United States, the geographic areas endemic for coccidioidomycosis and from which *C. immitis* can be isolated from the soil correspond to the Lower Sonoran life zone. These areas are characterized by a semiarid climate, alkaline soil, and characteristic indigenous desert plants and rodents. The endemic foci in Mexico, Argentina, and other scattered areas

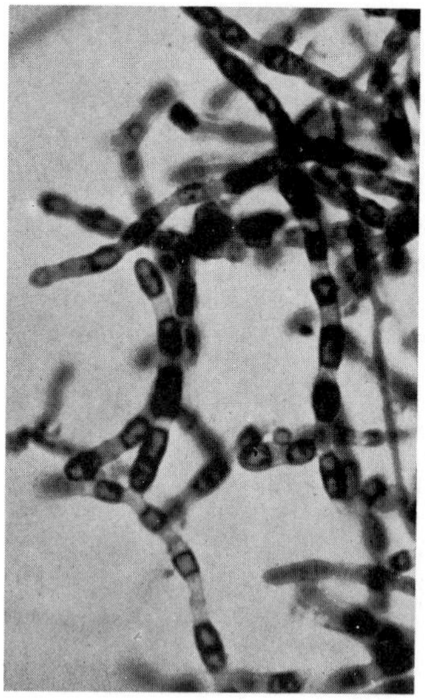

Fig. 82–2. *Coccidioides immitis.* Typical arthroconidia formation in hyphae. From Sabouraud's glucose agar at room temperature. × 736.

of Central and South America are ecologically very similar. Although *C. immitis* grows in the laboratory over a wide range of temperature, pH, and salt concentration and requires only glucose and ammonium salts to grow, it has never become established in soils outside the endemic area, in spite of transmission to other regions by infected animals and fomites. Studies have shown that *C. immitis* is inhibited by other microorganisms, cultivated soil, or treatment with various chemicals. However, none of these factors explains its restricted habitation. The mycelia, which can be found several inches beneath the soil surface, are recovered at the surface after the spring rains. As the weather becomes hot and dry, the mycelia convert to infectious arthroconidia, and this accounts for the peak infection rate during the summer. In the endemic area, natural infectious occur among animals (e.g., desert rodents, dogs, and cattle).

Virtually everyone who inhales the arthroconidia of *C. immitis* becomes infected and acquires a positive delayed-type hypersensitivity response. Approximately half the infections are benign, and most of the others are symptomatic but self-limited. Approximately 1% of these cases will disseminate. Some persons are at increased risk of developing disseminated disease after primary infection. These include persons in certain racial groups, namely, African-Americans, Filipinos, Latin Americans, and Native Americans. This racial predilection for severe disease may be confirmed by correlation with human genetic markers, such as HLA type. In addition to race, males, women in the third trimester of pregnancy, persons with a cellular immunodeficiency (including AIDS), and persons at the age extremes are more susceptible to severe disease.

The areas of endemicity defined by case reports and by isolation of *C. immitis* from soil have been confirmed by skin test surveys with coccidioidin. Within the endemic areas, which include portions of California, Arizona, New Mexico, Nevada, Utah, and Texas, the percent reactivity varies; some of the highest rates are found in Phoenix and Tucson, Arizona, and in Kern County, California. Isolated cases of coccidioidomycosis that occur outside the established areas of endemicity are attributed to fomite transmission of the arthroconidia or to the patient's travel through the endemic area.

Outbreaks of primary infection have been reported among persons simultaneously exposed to a heavy aerosol of arthroconidia. Coccidioidomycosis is therefore considered an occupational hazard for construction workers, archaeology students, and others who disrupt the soil in the endemic areas. In a similar manner, many cases of acute disease developed subsequent to a severe wind storm in California in 1977, when contaminated soil was blown from the San Joaquin Valley far north and west, exposing large populations of unsensitized persons.

Pathogenesis

The cell wall of the infectious particle, the arthroconidium, has several layers. The outer layer represents the original wall of the hypha from which each of these thallic conidia develop. Beneath the outer wall lies a thin layer of fibrous rodlets and a thick inner wall. The outer and rodlet layers contain more mannan, protein, and lipid than the inner layer or the readily solubilized components between the inner and outer layers. The composition of the inner layer includes chitin and 3-*O*-methyl mannose, which has not been found in other pathogenic fungi. Potent antigens associated with all three regions—the outer and inner wall layers and the intermediate zone—are released in vivo when the arthroconidia develop into spherules. At 37C, physiologic levels of CO_2 are sufficient to stimulate arthroconidia to convert to endosporulating spherules.

Although arthroconidia and endospores are readily engulfed within phagosomes by alveolar macrophages, the intracellular fusion of lysosomal granules with the phagosomes is inhibited and neither form of *C. immitis* is killed. However, after activation of macrophages with either immune T cells or lymphokines, phagosome-lysosome fusion and killing are enhanced.

Many of the patients in whom disseminated coccidioidomycosis develops have depressed cell-mediated immunity. There is a marked inverse relationship between the antibody titer (see below) and specific cell-mediated immunity, as measured by skin test and, in vitro, by the numbers of CD4 and CD8 T cells, the responsiveness of T cells to mitogens or antigens, and the production of lymphokines. In severe coccidioidomycosis, patients have elevated antibody titers, circulating immune complexes, and depressed cellular immunity. Recovery often leads to restoration of immune functions. The impaired cellular immune responses are probably due to the documented increase in the population of suppressor cells, although blocking factors, immune complexes, and impaired lymphocyte circulation may also be contributing factors. (This immunoregulation may also involve anti-idiotype or clonal anergy mechanisms.) In vitro experiments by Cantanzaro indicate that certain adherent cells from patients with active dissemination are able to suppress T cell activity by localized enhancement of prostaglandin production. Immune complexes are detected in serum of patients with coccidioidomycosis and correlate with the severity of disease. Evidence suggests that immune complexes may contribute to the immunopathology by at least two mechanisms; deposition of the complexes may lead to local inflammatory reactions, and immunosuppression may result from the binding of complexes to cells bearing Fc receptors. In the mouse model of experimental coccidioidomycosis, specific anergy is correlated with the amount of coccidioidal antigen present.

Clinical Manifestations

Primary Coccidioidomycosis. With the rare exception of cutaneous inoculation, the primary form follows inhalation of arthroconidia, and in most persons the infection causes no symptoms. Others may have fever, chest pain, cough, or weight loss. Radiographic examination often reveals discrete nodules in the lower lobes. Primary pulmonary coccidioidomycosis has an incubation period of 10 to 16 days and usually resolves without complication in 3 weeks to 3 months. A small percentage of patients retain cavities, nodules, or calcifications, but endogenous reactivation of residual pulmonary lesions is rare.

Up to 20% of patients with primary coccidioidomycosis manifest allergic reactions, usually erythema nodosum or erythema multiforme, which appear with the primary symptoms, are very painful, and persist for approximately 1 week. These allergic manifestations are associated with strong immunity and a good prognosis.

Disseminated Coccidioidomycosis. Disseminated or secondary coccidioidomycosis usually develops within a few months as a complication of the primary form. The numerous forms of secondary coccidioidomycosis include chronic and progressive pulmonary disease, single or multiple extrapulmonary dissemination, or generalized systemic infection. Chronic pulmonary coccidioidomycosis usually involves a single, thin-walled cavity, but patients may have enlarging or multiplying nodules or cavities.

Dissemination may be fulminant or chronic, with periods of remission and exacerbation. Extrapulmonary lesions most frequently involve the meninges, skin, or bone. Chronic cutaneous coccidioidomycosis develops from initial lesions that usually appear on the face or neck and that, over a period of years, evolve into thick, raised, verrucous lesions with extensive epithelial hyperplasia. Bone involvement may accompany generalized systemic disease. Both osteomyelitis of long bones, vertebrae, and other bones and arthritis may develop. Draining sinus tracts may evolve from subcutaneous and osseous lesions.

Skin Test

As noted above, coccidioidin, which is a crude toluene extract of a mycelial culture filtrate, is used for skin testing. A delayed-type hypersensitivity reaction is elicited, and a positive test is defined as induration exceeding 5 mm in diameter. Another *C. immitis* antigen, prepared from cultured spherules and termed *spherulin*, is more sensitive but less specific than coccidioidin. Skin testing with either antigen does not induce or boost an immune response. The skin test becomes positive within 2 weeks after the onset of symptoms and before the appearance of precipitins and complement-fixing antibodies and often remains positive indefinitely. A positive reaction has no diagnostic significance without a history of conversion, but a negative test can be used to exclude coccidioidomycosis, except in patients with severe disseminated coccidioidomycosis who may have become anergic. Indeed, a negative skin test in confirmed cases is associated with a grave prognosis. Conversely, a positive test in healthy subjects implies immunity to symptomatic reinfection.

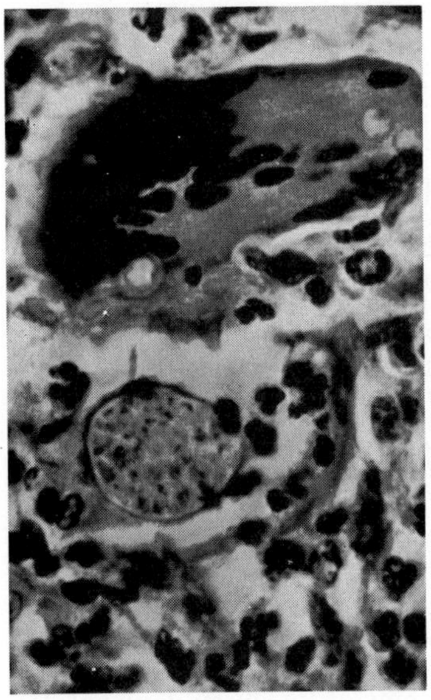

Fig. 82–3. *Coccidioides immitis.* Section of lung showing mature spherule and giant cell containing immature cells. × 736.

Laboratory Diagnosis

Direct Examination. A definitive diagnosis of coccidioidomycosis requires the finding of spherules of *C. immitis* in sputum, draining sinuses, or tissue specimens (Figs. 82–3 and 82–4). Clinical exudates should be examined directly in 10% to 20% potassium hydroxide (KOH) or calcofluor white preparations, and tissue obtained from biopsy can be stained with hematoxylin and eosin or special fungal stains (Chap. 81). Direct microscopic examination of cutaneous or deep tissue specimens, either in calcofluor or KOH preparations or histologic sections, yields positive results in approximately 85%

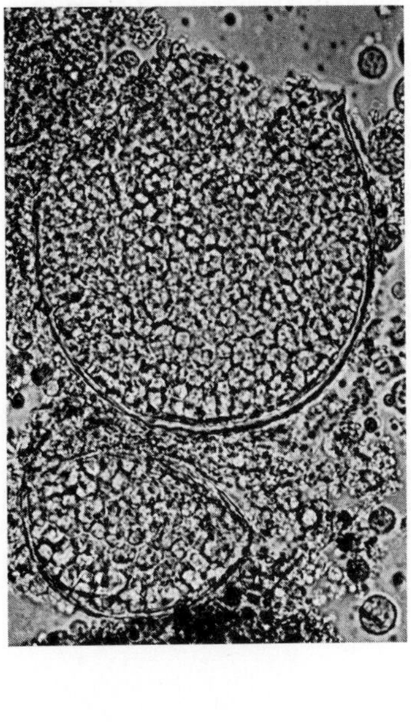

Fig. 82–4. *Coccidioides immitis.* Large spherules with endospores in pus. × 315. (*From Smith: Am J Med 2:594, 1947.*)

TABLE 82-2. SPECIES-SPECIFIC EXOANTIGENS FOR THE IDENTIFICATION OF SYSTEMIC DIMORPHIC FUNGAL PATHOGENS

Fungus	Exoantigens[a]
Coccidioides immitis	HS, F, HL
Histoplasma capsulatum	h, m
Blastomyces dermatitidis	A
Paracoccidioides brasiliensis	1, 2, 3

From Kaufman and Standard: Ann Rev Microbiol 41:209, 1987
[a] Exoantigens are detected by precipitin lines of identity in immunodiffusion tests of concentrated culture supernatant fluids versus reference antigens and antisera.

of proven cases. However, sputum specimens are positive by direct examination or culture in fewer than half of the cases.

Culture. Clinical specimens are cultured on Inhibitory Mold, Sabouraud's agar, or other routine fungal media (Chap. 81). Inhibitory Mold agar is a complex medium designed for optimal recovery of pathogenic fungi. Sabouraud's agar, the standard medium used for morphologic descriptions of pathogenic fungi, is composed of 4% glucose, 1% neopeptone, and agar. A modified Sabouraud's agar, containing 2% glucose, has been recommended as a more effective isolation medium. For the culture of nonsterile specimens, such as sputum, skin, or urine, antibiotics (usually cycloheximide and chloramphenicol or gentamicin) are included in the media to inhibit saprophytic fungi and bacterial contaminants. Inhibitory Mold agar contains all three additives. Colonies of *C. immitis* develop within 1 or 2 weeks and are examined microscopically for the production of characteristic arthroconidia. Microscopic preparations of mycelia should always be prepared under a safety hood.

The identification of *C. immitis* may be confirmed by the production of spherules in vitro by incubation in a complex medium at 40C with 20% CO_2 or by animal inoculation (e.g., intraperitoneal injection of mice or intratesticular inoculation of guinea pigs). An easier method of confirmation involves an immunodiffusion test to demonstrate the presence of a specific antigen(s) in a concentrated overnight, aqueous extract of the colony on solid medium or the supernatant fluid of a short-term broth culture of the isolate. The formation of a precipitin line of identity with reference antisera and control antigen identifies the specific *exoantigen*(s) extracted from the isolate. Production of exoantigen F confirms the identity as *C. immitis*. This method is rapid and is applicable to nonsporulating cultures. As indicated in Table 82–2, the technique has also been expanded to identify other dimorphic pathogens.

With the exception of tissue scrapings, biopsy specimens, and surgical specimens, cultures are more often positive than are direct examinations of clinical material. However, use of both procedures will optimize the opportunity to establish a diagnosis. Between 25% and 50% of sputa, bronchial washes, spinal fluids, and urine specimens yield positive cultures. Positive blood cultures are infrequent but significantly associated with acute, disseminated coccidioidomycosis and high mortality.

Serologic Tests. Fortunately, because of the time required for identification and the hazards involved in working with cultures of *C. immitis*, serologic tests are extremely helpful. Table 82–3 summarizes the useful antibody responses to coccidioidomycosis and other systemic mycoses. Precipitins (IgM) are produced early and assist in the diagnosis of primary infections. They are detected by a sensitive tube test that becomes positive in 90% of patients within 2 weeks after the appearance of symptoms and disappears in most cases within 4 months (Fig. 82–5). Therefore a positive tube precipitin (TP) test indicates active primary (or reactivation) coccidioidomycosis. Results obtained with the original TP method correlate quite well with those obtained with the more rapid and convenient latex particle agglutination test; the latter procedure is more sensitive but less specific than the TP test. The TP antigen, a component of coccidioidin, is heat stable at 60C, whereas the antigen detected in the complement-fixation (CF) test is heat labile.

The CF test for antibodies (IgG) to coccidioidin is a powerful diagnostic and prognostic tool. Because the CF test becomes positive more slowly and persists longer, the presence of CF antibodies may reflect either active infection or the recovery stage. The CF titer correlates with the severity of disease. In most patients with secondary coccidioidomycosis a titer of 1:16 or higher develops, whereas in nondisseminated cases the titer is almost invariably lower. Therefore, a critical titer of 1:32 or higher reflects active, disseminated disease. However, a lower titer does not exclude disseminated disease, because in many patients, such as those with single extrapulmonary lesions (e.g., coccidioidal meningitis), do not develop high titers.

Multiple serum specimens are most helpful because a change in the CF titer reflects the prognosis. The CF titer declines with recovery and eventually disappears. A rising titer indicates active, uncontrolled infection and a poor prognosis. A stable or fluctuating titer often indicates the presence of a recalcitrant or stabilized lesion. An exceptional situation is coccidioidal meningitis, in which only half of the patients have a titer of 1:32 or higher. However, most of these patients will have a positive CF test in their spinal fluid, which is equally valuable.

The immunodiffusion (ID) method can be used to detect both TP and CF antibodies by using reference antisera and

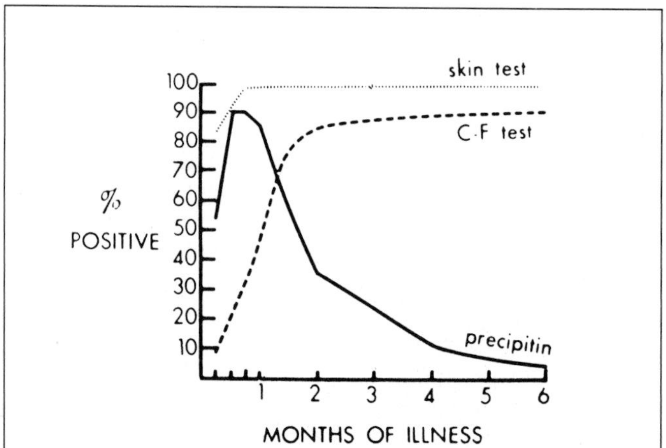

Fig. 82–5. Frequency of serologic reactivity after exposure to *Coccidioides immitis*. (*From Huppert: Mycopathologia 41:107, 1970.*)

TABLE 82-3. SUMMARY OF MYCOSERIOLOGY FOR SYSTEMIC MYCOSIS (ABRIDGED)

Mycosis	Test	Antigen	Sensitivity and Value: Diagnosis	Sensitivity and Value: Prognosis	Limitation/Specificity
Coccidioido-mycosis	TP	C	Early primary infection; 90% cases positive	None	None
	CF	C	Titer ≥1:32 = secondary disease	Titer reflects severity (except in meningeal disease)	Rarely cross-reactive with H
	ID	C	More than 90 cases positive (i.e., F and/or HL band)		More specific than CF test
Histoplasmosis	CF	H	Up to 83% of cases positive (titer ≥1:8)	Fourfold change in titer	Cross-reactions in patients with blastomycosis, coccidioidomycosis, cryptococcosis, aspergillosis; titer may be boosted by skin test with H
		Y	Up to 94% of cases positive (titer ≥1:8)	Fourfold change in titer	Less cross-reactivity than with H
	ID	H(10X)	Up to 85% of cases positive (i.e., m or m and h bands)	Loss of h	Skin test with H may boost m band; more specific than CT test
Blastomycosis	CF	By	Less than 50% of cases positive; reaction to homologous antigen only is diagnostic	Fourfold change in titer	Highly cross-reactive
	ID	Bcf	Up to 80% of cases positive (i.e., A band)	Loss of A band	None; more specific and sensitive than CF test
	EIA	A	Up to 90% of cases positive (titer ≥1:16)	Change in titer	92% specificity
Paracoccidioido-mycosis	CF	P	80%–95% of cases positive (titer ≥1:8)	Fourfold change in titer	Some cross-reactions at low titer with aspergillosis and candidiasis sera
	ID	P	98% of cases positive (bands 1, 2, and/or 3)	Loss of bands	None; band 3 and band m (to H) are identical

Tests: CF, complement fixation; ID, immunodiffusion; TP, tube precipitin; EIA, enzyme immunoassay.
Antigens: C, coccidioidin; H, histoplasmin; Y, yeast phase of *Histoplasma capsulatum*; By, yeast phase of *Blastomyces dermatitidis*; Bcf, culture filtrate of *B. dermatitidis* yeast phase; A, antigen A of *B. dermatitidis*; P, culture filtrate of *Paracoccidioides brasiliensis* yeast phase.

heated (TP only) and unheated antigen. Antibodies to two specific heat-labile antigens, termed F (or CF) and HL, may be detected.

Other methods. Some laboratories recommend direct animal inoculation of specimens as an additional method of primary isolation.

Treatment

Symptomatic treatment is usually adequate for the patient with primary coccidioidomycosis. However, if the primary infection is severe or if there is evidence of dissemination, amphotericin B should be administered (Chap. 81). The chronicity of the disseminated disease usually requires prolonged therapy, increasing the risk of undesirable side effects. Miconazole has also been used extensively, and many, but not all, patients respond well to it. Chronic coccidioidal meningitis often requires intrathecal administration of chemotherapy. Successful treatment with ketoconazole may require continuous administration for more than a year. The oral triazole, fluconazole, offers promise because of its superior penetration into the central nervous system (Chap. 81).

Histoplasmosis

Histoplasmosis, the most prevalent pulmonary mycosis of humans and animals, is caused by the thermally dimorphic fungus, *Histoplasma capsulatum* (teleomorph = *Ajellomyces capsulatus*). Infection, which is initiated by inhalation of the fungus, occurs worldwide. The incidence varies considerably, being negligible in many parts of the world but pronounced in local regions wherein most of the population have been infected. Ninety-five percent of the infections are inapparent and are detected only by the manifestation of residual lung calcification(s), delayed hypersensitivity to *H. capsulatum*, or both. As one of the more common primary mycoses throughout history, its existence has been inferred on the basis of descriptions of the pathogenesis and natural history of disease.

Around the turn of the century the cause of histoplasmosis was discovered by Dr. Samuel Darling, who was a pathologist in the Canal Zone when he described the histopathologic characteristics of infected tissue. He observed intracellular organisms that resembled encapsulated protozoa and named the organism *Histoplasma capsulatum*. Darling's accurate description of the disease led to the recognition of other cases. The fungal origin of histoplasmosis was not established until 1929 by Dr. William de Monbreun, and even though *H. capsulatum* is neither a parasite nor encapsulated, the misleading name, by precedence and taxonomic custom, remains. Dr. K.J. Kwon-Chung discovered the teleomorphic state, and *H. capsulatum* was transferred from the subdivision Deuteromycotina to the family Gymnoascaceae within the subdivision Ascomycotina (Chap. 80). With taxonomic reclassification, the organism was initially renamed *Emmonsiella capsulata* to honor Dr. Chester Emmons, an eminent mycologist whose contributions included many pioneering investigations on the ecology of medically important fungi. Because of the similarity between the sexual reproductive structures of the teleomorphs of *H. capsulatum* and *Blastomyces dermatitidis*, whose teleomorph, *Ajellomyces dermatitidis*, had been discovered earlier, *E. capsulata* was subsequently transferred to that genus as *Ajellomyces capsulatus*. The name *H. capsulatum* is retained by common usage and remains appropriate as the fungus is isolated in its anamorphic state. Recent molecular evolutionary studies have confirmed the close relationship between *H. capsulatum* and *B. dermatitidis*.

The extent of inapparent infection was not appreciated until the 1940s. During extensive skin test surveys for tuberculosis in student nurses from various parts of the country, radiologists observed small calcifications in the lungs of many apparently healthy persons who were nonreactive to old tuberculin (OT). Subsequent skin testing with *histoplasmin*, an antigen from *H. capsulatum* analogous to OT, revealed a very strong correlation between delayed skin test reactivity and pulmonary calcifications in tuberculin-negative persons. The availability of skin test antigens for histoplasmosis has provided a very useful epidemiologic tool.

Morphologic and Cultural Characteristics

Two colonial forms of the mycelial phase of *H. capsulatum* have been described—the A or albino type and the B or brown type. Both phenotypes produce identical yeast and tissue forms. Primary isolates are often brown and become white with prolonged cultivation. If grown in the dark, the B type can be maintained. Type B strains are more pathogenic for mice and rabbits and produce more macroconidia (but fewer microconidia) than type A.

Dimorphism. *H. capsulatum* is a thermally dimorphic fungus. At temperatures below 35C, it grows as a mold, often white or brown in color, and at 37C, it grows as a yeast with small, heaped, and pasty colonies. *H. capsulatum* characteristically grows slowly. Under optimal conditions, the mold colony develops after 1 or 2 weeks, and conidia are produced shortly thereafter. However, cultures of clinical specimens sometimes require incubation periods of 8 to 12 weeks before there is detectable growth.

Both microconidia and macroconidia are produced at temperatures below 35C. The microconidia are borne singly on short conidiophores; they are globose and 1 to 5 μm in diameter. Their small size enables the microconidia to transmit the infection. On dehydration, the conidia are easily dislodged by air currents and aerosolized. The macroconidia, or tuberculate chlamydospores, are very distinctive. Mature forms are large (8 to 16 μm in diameter), spherical, thick-walled structures with projections radiating from the cell wall (Figs. 82–6 and 82–7). Young macroconidia are smooth walled, and the echinulations develop as the conidia mature.

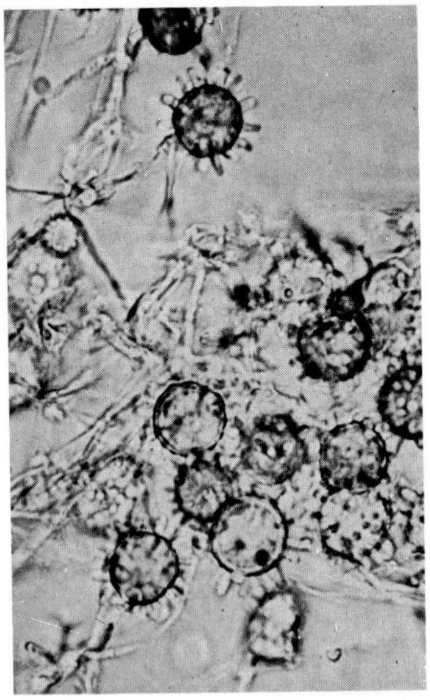

Fig. 82–6. *Histoplasma capsulatum.* Typical tuberculate macroconidia from Sabouraud's glucose agar culture. × 658. (*From Smith: Am J Med 2:594, 1947.*)

At 37C, the mold converts to growth as a small, budding yeast (Fig. 82–8). Conversion is often difficult to effect in vitro but is enhanced by a rich, complex medium, such as brain-heart infusion agar. Hyphal cells may form buds directly at 37C or develop enlarged, transitional cells that subsequently produce buds. Microconidia may also convert to budding yeast cells. The yeast cells are small, ellipsoidal, approximately 1 to 3 μm by 3 to 5 μm in size, and virtually identical to the yeasts observed in vivo within phagocytes (Fig. 82–9).

Comparison of the yeast and mycelial forms of *H. capsu-*

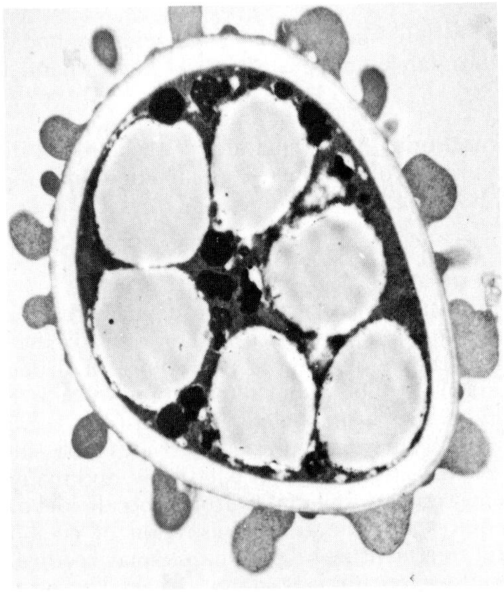

Fig. 82–7. *Histoplasma capsulatum.* Transmission electron photomicrograph of tuberculate macroconidium. × 12,000. (*Courtesy of Dr. J. Spahr.*)

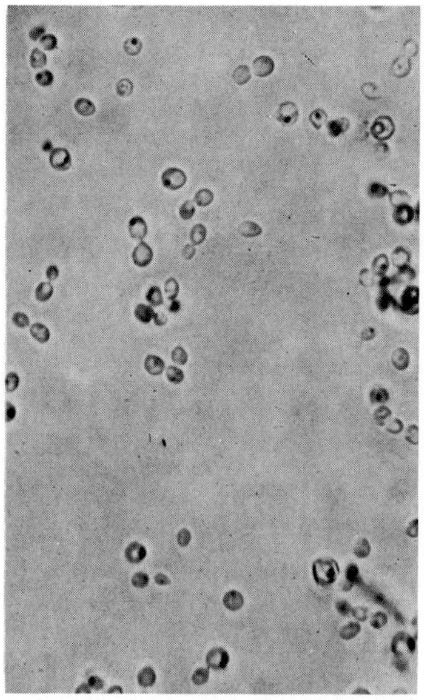

Fig. 82–8. *Histoplasma capsulatum.* Yeast cells from blood agar culture at 37C. × 700.

latum have detected significant differences in chemical composition of the cell walls. On the basis of differences in the relative amounts of chitin, α-glucan, and β-glucan, cell wall chemotypes for each form have been defined. The three RNA polymerases in each growth form are also different.

Molecular aspects of morphogenesis in *H. capsulatum* have been studied extensively by Drs. George S. Kobayashi and Gerald Medoff and their colleagues. In a synthetic medium, conversion between the mycelial form and the yeast form is temperature-dependent:

$$\text{Mold} \underset{25C}{\overset{37C}{\rightleftharpoons}} \text{Yeast}$$

The molecular basis for morphogenesis in *H. capsulatum* involves a protein, histin, isolated from the cytoplasm of the mycelial form. Histin inhibits RNA polymerase and may help to regulate the temperature-dependent control of transcription. It is plausible that an inhibitor, such as histin, may be operative in the mycelia, because protein synthesis is considerably reduced during mycelial growth.

In studying the crucial mycelium to yeast conversion at 37C, Maresca et al. confirmed the importance of cysteine. This conversion proceeds in three stages: (1) During the first 40 hours at 37C, respiration gradually decreases and the intracellular amino acid pools become almost depleted; (2) the cells remain dormant for 4 to 6 days; and (3) concentrations of intracellular cysteine and other amino acids then increase and respiration is restored. Cystine and cysteine are essential for the transition to yeast cells. These compounds and other reducing agents appear to stimulate the mitochondrial electron transport chain, probably via a unique cysteine oxidase. This mycelium-to-yeast conversion is inhibited by elevated cyclic AMP, which may also be regulated intracellularly by the action of sulfhydryl agents.

In recent studies of virulent strains, the sulfhydryl blocking agent, *p*-chloromercuriphenylsulfonic acid (PCMS), irreversibly inhibited the conversion of mycelium to yeast at 37C, but mycelial growth continued at 37C. PCMS-treated mycelia also failed to infect mice. Therefore mycelium-to-yeast transformation appeared necessary for pathogenicity but not for growth at 37C. PCMS-treated mycelia may provide a vaccine for histoplasmosis and indicate the essential changes for transformation.

Sexual Reproduction. As noted, discovery of its sexual reproductive cycle led to reclassification of the anamorph *H. capsulatum* to the teleomorph *A. capsulatus,* which closely resembles the teleomorph of *B. dermatitidis. A. capsulatus* is heterothallic: strains of two opposite (compatible) mating types are necessary for sexual reproduction. Although the mating types, designated "+" and "−", are equally prevalent among soil isolates, almost 90% of infections are caused by the "−" type. Only the asexual, anamorphic state is observed in clinical isolates.

Biotypes. After treatment of DNA extracts of *H. capsulatum* with restriction endonucleases, strains have been subspeciated or biotyped by analysis of the resulting restriction fragment length polymorphisms (RFLP). Biotyping may facilitate epidemiologic studies. Several strains of *H. capsulatum* from patients with AIDS were recently shown to have the same RFLP pattern of mitochondrial DNA, which differed from the RFLP patterns of strains from patients without AIDS.

Determinants of Pathogenicity

Both mating types of *A. capsulatus* can be isolated from soil with a comparable frequency. However, one allele is predominantly recovered from clinical material and is therefore associated with human pathogenicity. The genotype may be linked to virulence or to increased conidiation or conidial survival in nature.

All clinical forms are believed to evolve from the same natural history. Microconidia are inhaled from an exogenous source and penetrate to the alveoli, where they convert to small, budding yeast cells. This temperature-sensitive morphogenesis is related to the virulence of strains of *H. capsulatum.* The yeasts are readily phagocytized by alveolar macrophages. At this stage, the yeast-laden macrophages may be cleared through the upper respiratory tract. They may dis-

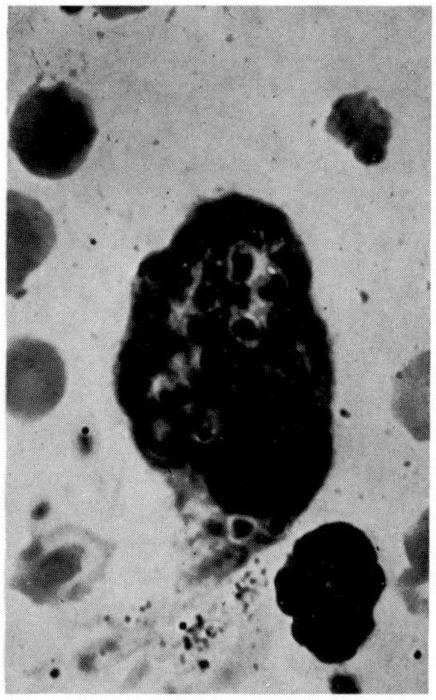

Fig. 82–9. *Histoplasma capsulatum.* Yeast cells within mononuclear cell in peripheral blood smear. × 1540.

seminate by the bloodstream, spreading the yeasts to other reticuloendothelial organs, or they may invoke a tissue response in situ. The tissue reaction may involve an early infiltration of neutrophils and lymphocytes, but the pyogenic inflammatory response gives way to epithelioid cell tubercle formation. In the course of these various possible reactions, the intracellular yeasts may or may not be inactivated by the phagocytes (see below).

The conversion of *H. capsulatum* to the yeast form at 37C appears to be essential for pathogenicity; as noted above, treatment of the mycelial form with PCMS blocks morphogenesis and reduces virulence but does not inhibit survival at 37C. Keath and associates have identified several yeast-specific genes and shown that the expression of one gene in different strains was correlated with virulence for mice and thermal tolerance.

Clinical Infection

Epidemiology

Ecology. In nature, *H. capsulatum* grows in soil with a high nitrogen content and is associated with bat and avian habitats. *H. capsulatum* has been isolated many times from bird roosts, chicken houses, bat caves, and similar environments. Conidia, when dry, are easily airborne and are spread by wind currents as well as by birds and bats.

The fungus is most prevalent in the natural environment in areas where the disease is most endemic, namely, in the Ohio-Mississippi Valley—in Missouri, Kentucky, Tennessee, Indiana, Ohio, and southern Illinois. This area also has the highest population of starlings, which tend to congregate in large numbers. The excrement from these birds provides a superlative medium for the enrichment of *H. capsulatum*. In South America, the chief reservoir appears to be chicken coops and bat caves.

The survival of *H. capsulatum* in soil appears to depend on strict temperature and humidity requirements. It survives best in moist soil (95% to 100% humidity) at temperatures at or below 37C. In dry soil, the vegetative cells rapidly dehydrate and lyse, whereas the microconidia and macroconidia will remain viable for some time. However, with prolonged desiccation, only the macroconidia survive. Similarly, only the macroconidia may be able to survive in moist soil at temperatures above 40C.

It was empirically observed, and subsequently proved in the laboratory, that soil supplemented with fecal extracts from bats and several kinds of birds (starlings, chickens, and blackbirds) provided a much better environment for the growth of *H. capsulatum* than soil alone. Aged feces contain the highest amounts of growth-stimulating components, nitrogenous compounds, phosphates, and cations, and less of the toxic ammonium salts and uric acid.

Both *H. capsulatum* and a stable variant, *H. capsulatum* var. *duboisii*, have been isolated from cases of histoplasmosis in Africa. Infections elsewhere are due to the global variety, *H. capsulatum* var. *capsulatum*. *H. capsulatum* var. *duboisii* causes African histoplasmosis, which is distinguished from the usual infection by (1) a greater frequency of skin and bone lesions, (2) diminished pulmonary involvement, (3) pronounced giant cell formation, and (4) larger, thick-walled yeast cells in tissue. Although these clinical features are unique and reproducible, *H. capsulatum* var. *duboisii* cannot be reliably differentiated in vitro from the type species on the basis of morphology, physiology, and antigenic composition. Indeed, Kwon-Chung has proved that the agents of both forms of histoplasmosis are the same species, as *H. capsulatum* var. *duboisii* mates with *H. capsulatum* var. *capsulatum*, and its sexual form is identical to *A. capsulatus*.

Histoplasmin Skin Test. The antigen, histoplasmin, is produced by growing the mycelial phase of *H. capsulatum* in the same asparagine broth medium used for preparing OT. The filtrate from the culture is dialyzed, the concentration is standardized, and 0.1 mL of the appropriate dilution (usually a 10^{-2} or 10^{-3} dilution of the original material) is injected intradermally. A positive reaction is indicated by induration ≥ 5 mm in diameter after 48 hours.

A positive test, if specific, denotes previous sensitization to the fungus. Without a history of prior negativity, the positive test has no diagnostic significance. Histoplasmin is a crude, polyvalent mixture of antigens, only some of which are specific for *H. capsulatum*. Because some antigenic determinants are shared by other pathogenic fungi, cross-reactions can occur. For example, some persons who are sensitive to *B. dermatitidis* or *C. immitis* will give a false-positive reaction to histoplasmin. Therefore, epidemiologists routinely administer, along with histoplasmin, a battery of skin test antigens, including coccidioidin and blastomycin in the United States and paracoccidioidin in South America. A reaction to a single antigen is generally considered specific. Reactions to two antigens may be caused by sensitization to one or both, although the larger reaction is often considered more specific. In comparing the specificity of the systemic fungal skin test antigens, the decreasing order of specificity (i.e., least likely to be cross-reactive) is coccidioidin, paracoccidioidin, histoplasmin, and blastomycin.

Incidence. Much of the knowledge concerning the prevalence of histoplasmosis has been derived from extensive skin test surveys conducted since the 1950s all over the world. The region with the highest level of reactivity is the central United States, along the valleys of the Ohio, Mississippi, St. Lawrence, and Rio Grande rivers, where in some locales 80% to 90% of the population may be skin-test positive by the age of 20 years. Foci of high reactivity exist elsewhere in the world, such as southern Mexico, Indonesia, the Philippines, and Turkey. In the United States alone, projections based on skin-test surveys have led to estimations that more than 40 million people have been exposed with 500,000 new infections every year. Perhaps 55,000 to 200,000 of these will have symptoms, 1500 to 4000 will require hospitalization annually, and 25 to 100 will die. These projections were made before 1980 and do not include the increasing incidence of opportunistic histoplasmosis in patients with AIDS.

Transmission. In addition to humans, many animals, both wild and domestic, are susceptible to histoplasmosis. Some animals, including the bat, may act as vectors to disseminate the organism in nature.

Outbreaks or epidemics of acute respiratory histoplasmosis result from the simultaneous exposure of a large number of people. These epidemics are *not* caused by direct spread among humans or animals. The experience of youths on Earth Day, 1970, in Delaware, Ohio, is more ironic than most but otherwise typical of these epidemic outbreaks. The young people gathered to reclaim an abandoned park and, in so doing, overturned several truckloads of soil, which was enriched with starling feces and contaminated with an enormous quantity of *H. capsulatum* conidia. Several cases of acute respiratory histoplasmosis followed inhalation of heavy inocula of aerosolized microconidia. Many similar episodes have been documented; the sudden release leads to multiple exposure of a heavy inoculum that has accumulated in a dormant environment. Silos, air-conditioning units contaminated with bird droppings, and accumulations of guano in caves, attics, or parks have all been implicated as fungous reservoirs in outbreaks of this type. Perhaps the largest outbreak occurred in Indianapolis between September 1978 and August 1979. It is estimated that more than 100,000 persons were infected during this time, with more than 300 people hospitalized and at least 15 deaths. The incidence of disseminated histoplasmosis and the fatality rate were unusually high. The environmental source of the fungus was not determined. Indeed, *H. capsulatum* was not recovered from any of the soil samples collected at the most likely site, where an abandoned amusement park had been recently dismantled.

Males develop symptomatic histoplasmosis more often than females, and approximately 75% of all cases occur in males. Before puberty, the attack rate for males and females is identical, and the percentage of positive skin-test reactors is the same for both sexes at all ages. These epidemiologic data suggest that either adult males are inherently more susceptible to the disease or females are more resistant. Severity of disease and mortality are greater at the age extremes, in infancy and beyond the fifth decade of life.

Pathogenesis

After being phagocytized, the yeast cells of *H. capsulatum* are killed by neutrophils, but they are able to survive and multiply within macrophages. The yeast cells do not stimulate superoxide production by macrophages. However, macrophages from immunized animals, as well as normal macrophages activated by immune lymphocytes or lymphokines, restrict the growth of intracellular yeasts. In an experimental model of self-limited murine histoplasmosis, Bullock and associates have demonstrated that various parameters of cell-mediated immunity are suppressed during the height of antigen (yeast) burden, suppressor T cells and macrophage-like suppressor cells are detected, and production of IL-1 and IL-2 is impaired. Concomitant with resolution of the infection, the number of suppressor cells in the spleen diminishes and the number of T helper cells increases. These correlations of competent cell-mediated immune responses with resistance to infection are supported by the clinical data.

Clinical Manifestations

The manifestations of infection with *H. capsulatum* are protean. Several clinical classifications have been devised, but none is completely satisfactory or universally accepted. The abbreviated scheme presented in Table 82–4 is one of the most useful. The initial pulmonary episode may be acute or chronic, or dissemination may occur by hematogenous or lymphatic spread from the lungs to other organs.

Most normal persons contain the infection. The granulomas that form may undergo fibrosis, and residual scars may remain in the lungs or the spleen. Resolution appears to confer some immunity to reinfection. This process occurs asymptomatically in 95% of all persons with acute primary histoplasmosis, whether disseminated or confined to the lung.

TABLE 82-4. CLINICAL FORMS OF HISTOPLASMOSIS

	Acute	Chronic
Pulmonary	Asymptomatic Mild Moderate Severe	Pneumonic or cavitary (anatomic defect)
Disseminated	Benign Progressive	Progressive (mucocutaneous)

Acute Pulmonary Histoplasmosis. Patients with acute pulmonary histoplasmosis manifest symptoms ranging from a mild flulike illness that clears spontaneously to a moderate or severe disease. In healthy hosts, the degree of involvement and symptoms is roughly proportional to the size of the inoculum inhaled. In the previously sensitized person, such reinfection exposure results in a shorter and milder infection with minimal histopathologic change. The incubation period varies from one to several weeks. A moderate disease is characterized by cough, chest pain, dyspnea, and hoarseness. In more severe cases, fever, night sweats, and weight loss also develop. Occasionally, yeast cells may be observed in the sputum. Radiologic examination may reveal multiple lesions scattered throughout the lungs, and in patients with active disease hilar lymphadenopathy is usually present.

The differential diagnosis includes tuberculosis, bacterial bronchiectasis, and lymphoblastoma. Indeed, because there are so many similarities among the different forms of histoplasmosis and the various stages of tuberculosis, it is imperative to establish the diagnosis. Pulmonary lesions due to *H. capsulatum* resolve slowly. Healing may be complete or with fibrosis, but typically calcification occurs.

An experienced radiologist can differentiate between the calcifications of histoplasmosis and tuberculosis. Calcifications produced by *H. capsulatum* are more regular, with halos, and may be found in the liver and spleen as well as in the lungs. Miliary calcifications may also occur. Calcifications are produced more rapidly in children than in adults. Single, solitary, uncalcified lesions, known as coin lesions, are also produced and are similar to those seen in tuberculosis. As these resemble neoplasms, they are often removed surgically. Another tuberculosis-like pulmonary manifestation usually found in the adult lung is a *histoplasmoma*. The histoplasmoma, which may be 2 to 3 cm in diameter, contains a central necrotic area encased in a fibrotic capsule. Calcification begins in the center of the lesion and is followed by the development of concentric rings of fibrosis and calcification.

Chronic Pulmonary Histoplasmosis. The chronic pulmonary form is seen most often in adult males. It is considered to be an opportunistic complication of underlying chronic obstructive lung disease with emphysema and abnormal pulmonary spaces.

With small emphysematous air spaces, transient penumonitis develops, and infection of large bullous spaces may result in cavitary histoplasmosis. Symptoms of the latter may be indistinguishable from those of chronic cavitary tuberculosis. The chronic form is secondary to the underlying pulmonary disease. It may develop immediately after primary inhalation or after years of apparent quiescence. Pathologic and immunologic evidence suggests that the late onset results from reactivation of an old lesion rather than exogenous reinfection. Chronic pulmonary histoplasmosis is usually apical. Patients have a low-grade fever, a productive cough, progressive weakness, and fatigue. Chest films show centrilobular or bullous emphysema. Prognosis depends on control of the underlying disease as much as on treatment of histoplasmosis.

Disseminated Histoplasmosis. The gamut of clinical forms and pathology observed in pulmonary histoplasmosis can also occur in any other part of the body. The yeast cells are probably disseminated throughout the body while inside macrophages. The most common sites of involvement, after the lung, are the reticuloendothelial tissues of the spleen, liver, lymph nodes, and bone marrow. However, lesions have been documented in almost every organ. Dissemination may be completely benign and inapparent except for the presence of calcified lesions, usually in organs of the reticuloendothelial systems.

Alternatively, disseminated histoplasmosis may be acute and progressive. In such cases, the pulmonary symptoms are insignificant, and patients may have splenomegaly and hepatomegaly, weight loss, anemia, and leukopenia. Granulomatous lesions and macrophages packed with yeast cells can be observed throughout the liver, spleen, marrow, and, quite often, the adrenals. Acute progressive histoplasmosis is often fulminant and rapidly fatal. Ultimately every organ can become diseased. This form of histoplasmosis is an opportunistic disease associated with compromised cell-mediated immunity, as in patients with AIDS, those receiving immunosuppressive drugs, and those with underlying lymphomatous neoplasia. In some cases, the compromising condition may have reactivated an old, dormant lesion that was originally acquired years before. Within the endemic area, infants with histiocytosis may develop disseminated histoplasmosis that is characteristically fulminant. Chronic disseminated histoplasmosis may evolve from protraction of the acute disease. This form is progressive, with eventual involvement of every organ, especially the mucocutaneous areas around the eye, tongue, and anus.

Other Forms. Very rarely, chronic disseminated histoplasmosis develops following primary inoculation of the skin or mucocutaneous tissue. The lungs are not involved in these cases, as the organisms are typically introduced after the contamination of a traumatic wound. Such infections may be anatomically localized, as with some ocular cases, or they may chronically progress with involvement along the draining lymphatics.

Another clinical condition, probably unrelated to *H. capsulatum*, is presumed ocular histoplasmosis syndrome (POHS). Patients with POHS exhibit characteristic choroidal lesions, macular subretinal membranes, and peripapillary atrophy. Although POHS is usually associated with a positive histoplasmin skin test, its cause is unknown. Patients with histoplasmosis may have ocular lesions, but POHS is not seen in patients with active histoplasmosis.

Laboratory Diagnosis

Microscopic Examination. The diagnosis of histoplasmosis is confirmed when the yeast cells are found in clinical materials. Suitable specimens include sputa, tissue material obtained from biopsy or surgery, spinal fluid, and blood. The buffy coat of a blood specimen may reveal yeast-filled macrophages. Bone marrow obtained when patients are febrile may contain yeast cells. Smears of infected sputum, blood, marrow, or tissue that have been fixed with methanol and stained with Wright or Geimsa stain will reveal the characteristically small, ellipsoidal yeast cells (approximately 2 by 4 μm) inside macrophages. With either stain, the larger end of the yeast cell contains an eccentric, red-staining mass (Fig. 82–9).

Culture. Sputum specimens should be collected early in the morning, and purulent or sanguineous portions of the sputum should be selected for culture. A bronchial wash is even more likely to be positive. Nonsterile specimens (e.g., sputum, skin, or urine) should be cultured on a blood-enriched medium and inhibitory mold or Sabouraud's agar with antibiotics (cycloheximide and chloramphenicol or gentamicin) and incubated for at least 4 weeks at 25C or 30C. Because *H. capsulatum* may grow very slowly, cultures should be incubated as long as 12 weeks, if possible, before being discarded as negative. If a sporulating mold develops, *H. capsulatum* can be identified by the presence of its characteristic macroconidia (Fig. 82–6) and by conversion to the yeast phase by growth on an enriched medium at 37C (Fig. 82–8). Alternatively, conversion to the yeast may be effected by growth in tissue cultures, such as HeLa cells, or by animal inoculation, such as intraperitoneal injection into mice. Occasional isolates of *H. capsulatum* will not produce conidia, but it may be possible to identify these variants by conversion to the yeast phase or by the detection of *H. capsulatum*–specific exoantigens (Table 82–2).

In endemic areas or in cases where histoplasmosis is suspected, specimens should be inoculated on at least four media: (1) Sabouraud's agar without antibiotics at 25C to 30C; (2) Sabouraud's agar with antibiotics (cycloheximide and chloramphenicol, gentamicin, or penicillin and streptomycin) at 25C to 30C; (3) brain-heart infusion agar with 5% sheep blood and antibiotics at 25C to 30C; and (4) brain-heart infusion agar with 5% sheep blood without cycloheximide at 37C. The pH of these media should be near neutrality, since *H. capsulatum* is inhibited below pH 6.

In disseminated cases, the lysis-centrifugation method is recommended for culturing blood, although transient fungemia may be observed in patients with acute pulmonary histoplasmosis. Blood volumes of 10 ml are added to a tube containing a mixture of anticoagulants and reagents to lyse the blood cells; the tubes are then centrifuged, and the pellet, which contains any yeast cells in the blood, is inoculated onto plates of Inhibitory Mold agar and other media. Lysis-centrifugation has proved to be the most sensitive and rapid method to recover fungi, especially *H. capsulatum*, from blood.

Skin Test. The skin test antigen, histoplasmin, is a valuable epidemiologic tool. Within 2 weeks after infection, most persons become skin test positive, and this reactivity usually persists for many years. The diagnostic value of the skin test is minimal. A negative reaction can be used to rule out active histoplasmosis in the immunocompetent subject, but patients with anergy may be falsely negative. Without a history of a negative skin test, a positive reaction is meaningless except in infants, in whom a positive test can be presumed to result from recent or current infection. With most patients, only a history of conversion from negative to positive is diagnostic.

Because of its limited diagnostic value and the possibility that the skin test may confound the antibody titration (see below), skin testing with histoplasmin should be avoided in most patients.

Serology. Specific antibodies to *H. capsulatum* antigens can be detected during infection. Two serologic tests are now widely accepted because of their convenience, availability, and utility: the measurement of antibodies by complement fixation (CF) and the immunodiffusion (ID) test for precipitins. Both tests may be helpful in the diagnosis and prognosis of histoplasmosis, provided the results are properly interpreted (Table 82–3).

COMPLEMENT-FIXATION TEST. The CF test is routinely performed under standard conditions for measuring fixation of complement by the classic pathway. Sensitized sheep red cells are the indicator system, and two antigens are usually employed: histoplasmin and a standardized suspension of killed *H. capsulatum* yeast cells. Because of the possibility of cross-reactivity, patient serum is also tested at the same time against other fungal antigens, such as coccidioidin, spherulin, *B. dermatitidis*, or *Paracoccidioides brasiliensis*. Serum antibodies specific for *H. capsulatum* antigens can be detected by the CF test 2 to 4 weeks after exposure. Most laboratories perform the CF test on twofold dilutions of patient serum, beginning with a dilution of 1:8. With resolution of the infection, the antibody titer gradually declines and disappears (i.e., titer < 1:8), in most cases within 9 months. The CF test with either *H. capsulatum* yeast or mycelial (histoplasmin) antigen is very sensitive, and 90% of patients are positive (i.e., titer ≥1:8). A titer of 1:32 that persists or rises over the course of several weeks indicates active disease in patients with an established diagnosis of histoplasmosis. Unfortunately, in sensitive patients the skin-test antigen may boost the CF antibody titer to histoplasmin, and the elevated titer may remain for as long as 3 months. Obviously, the CF test, which can deliver results as rapidly as the skin test, is preferable for diagnostic purposes. However, a positive CF test, even in high titer, is not by itself diagnostic, as the results can be caused by cross-reacting antibodies. If a patient's serum is reactive to more than one fungous antigen or if it is anticomplementary, the ID test should be conducted.

IMMUNODIFFUSION TEST. Precipitins can be detected by double diffusion of serum and antigen in agarose gel. The antigen is histoplasmin in 10 times the concentration used for the CF test. The ID test becomes positive in up to 80% of patients with histoplasmosis by the third or fourth week of infection. This test, while less sensitive and requiring a longer time to become positive, is more specific than the CF test. Precipitin lines or bands specific for *H. capsulatum* are detected by the formation of lines of identity with reference serum. Kaufman and associates defined two specific precipitin bands, m and h. The m line, which is observed more frequently, appears soon after infection and may persist in the serum up to 3 years after recovery. The h band, which forms closer to the serum wells, is more transient. Because it disappears soon after the disease, the presence of serum antibodies to the h antigen is better correlated with active infection. As with the CF titer, the m band may be boosted by the administration of the histoplasmin skin test, and the boosting effect may last up to 3 months.

Other serologic tests for antibodies to *H. capsulatum* that are in current use include the direct fluorescent antibody test and counterimmunoelectrophoresis. Tests for circulating polysaccharide antigen are being developed that promise in the future to be more specific and probably more indicative of progressive disease.

Treatment

Most cases of histoplasmosis remain undetected and require no treatment. With symptomatic, progressive disease, the treatment of choice is amphotericin B. The regimen is similar to that applied to other systemic mycoses (Chap. 81), and a total dose of 1.5 g amphotericin B is recommended. Recovery after treatment with amphotericin B is generally faster, and fewer relapses occur than are experienced with blastomycosis and coccidioidomycosis Arrested pulmonary lesions are often removed surgically. Less severe cases in nonimmunocompromised patients may be treated with ketoconazole.

Blastomycosis

Blastomycosis is a chronic infection characterized by granulomatous and suppurative lesions initiated by inhalation of a thermally dimorphic fungus, *Blastomyces dermatitidis* (teleomorph = *Ajellomyces dermatitidis*). From the lung, dissemination may occur to any organ, preferentially to the skin and bones. The disease was called North American blastomycosis because initial cases were confined to the United States, Canada, and Central America. Although the prevalence continues to be highest on the North American continent, blastomycosis has been documented in Africa, South America, and Asia. It is endemic for humans and dogs in the eastern United States.

Blastomycosis was first described in its chronic cutaneous form in the 1890s by Gilchrist. As early case reviews included a large number of cases from Chicago, blastomycosis became known as Gilchrist's or Chicago disease. Many early case descriptions were undoubtedly confused with coccidioidomycosis, cryptococcosis (European blastomycosis), and paracoccidioidomycosis (South American blastomycosis) until Benham firmly established the cause of blastomycosis in 1934. A complete understanding of the relationship between the cutaneous and systemic manifestations of the disease was not available until 1951, when Schwarz and Baum presented evidence derived from pathogenic specimens that both forms originate in the lung. Blastomycosis is primarily a pulmonary infection characterized by secondary spread to the skin and other parts of the body. However, the respiratory episode may be completely subclinical. Primary cutaneous infection has been demonstrated only rarely.

Morphologic and Cultural Characteristics

Cultural Characteristics. Blastomycosis is caused by a single dimorphic species, *B. dermatitidis*. At temperatures below 35C, the organism grows as a mold, producing a colony of uniform, hyaline, septate hyphae and conidia. On Sabouraud's glucose agar at 25C, different isolates of *B. dermatitidis* vary in their rate of growth, colony appearance, and degree and type of conidiation. Usually, however, colonies require at least 2 weeks for full development. Many strains produce a white,

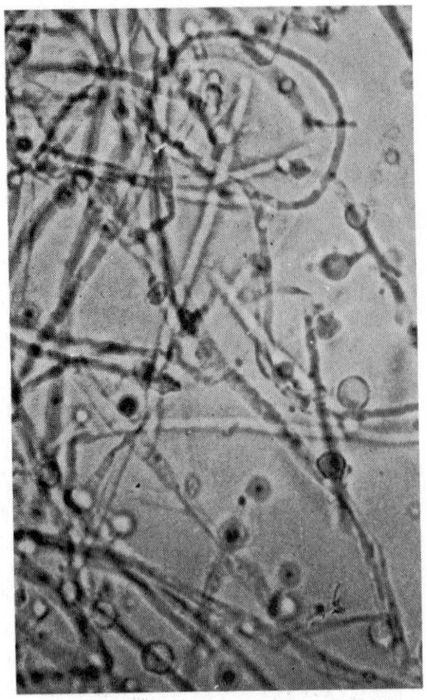

Fig. 82–10. *Blastomyces dermatitidis.* Mycelium and conidia from culture of Sabouraud glucose agar at room temperature. × 736.

cottony mycelium that becomes tan to brown with age. On enriched media at 37C, *B. dermatitidis* grows as a yeast with colonies that are folded, pasty, and moist.

Microscopic Appearance. The mycelial form produces abundant conidia from the aerial hyphae and lateral conidiophores (Fig. 82–10). The conidia are spherical, ovoid, or pyriform in shape and are 3 to 5 μm in diameter. Thick-walled chlamydospores, 7 to 18 μm in diameter, may also be observed. Because the colony and conidia of *B. dermatitidis* may be confused with those of many other fungi, identification must be confirmed by conversion to the characteristic yeast form. This conversion can be accomplished by in vitro cultivation at 37C or by animal inoculation. Under these conditions, the *B. dermatitidis* grows as a thick-walled spherical yeast that usually produces single buds (Fig. 82–11). The bud and the parent yeast have a characteristically wide base of attachment, and the bud often enlarges to a size equal to that of the parent cell before becoming detached. Yeasts normally range in size from 8 to 15 μm, although some cells reach a diameter of 30 μm.

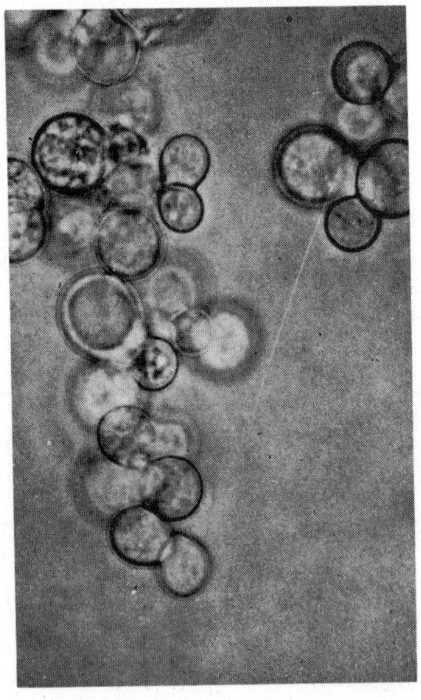

Fig. 82–11. *Blastomyces dermatitidis.* Budding yeast cells from culture on blood agar at 37C. × 700. (*From Conant et al: Manual of Clinical Mycology, ed 3. Saunders, 1971.*)

Sexual Reproduction. The teleomorphic state of *B. dermatitidis* was discovered by McDonough and Lewis. As the sexual progeny are produced within an ascus, the fungus is an ascomycete, a member of the subdivision Ascomycotina (Chap. 80). Because of its sexual apparatus, *B. dermatitidis* has been renamed *Ajellomyces dermatitidis* and classified in the family Gymnoascaceae in the same genus as the teleomorph of *H. capsulatum A. dermatitidis* is heterothallic, requiring two compatible (opposite) mating types for sexual reproduction. Although the two mating types have different antigens, they are similar in many other respects, including pathogenicity. Mating compatibility has been used to confirm that a single species is responsible for blastomycosis among dogs and humans and probably also for cases in North America and Africa.

Determinants of Pathogenicity

Strains of *B. dermatitidis* vary in their virulence for experimental animals, but an explanation of this difference is lacking. Murine virulence has been correlated with lipid content and the ability of the alkali-soluble cell wall fraction of the yeast cells to induce granulomas after intracutaneous injection. Also, a unique chemotactic factor for leukocytes is elaborated by yeast cells of *B. dermatitidis*. The fungal properties and host responses that determine which organs will be most involved are not known.

Clinical Infection

Epidemiology

Ecology. The natural habitat of *B. dermatitidis* is unresolved. Assuming that most cases of blastomycosis are acquired by inhalation of exogenous, infectious particles, the fungus should grow and produce airborne cells in nature. However, with few exceptions, attempts to isolate this agent from the environment have failed. Denton and DiSalvo isolated *B. dermatitidis* in Georgia from 10 of 356 soil samples collected on two occasions almost a year apart; subsequent samplings were negative. The positive samples were collected from a rural environment, including a chicken house, a cattle crossing, and an abandoned shack. More recently, positive samples were collected in Wisconsin from a beaver dam associated with a large outbreak of blastomycosis and from a fishing site at another outbreak. Additional outbreaks of blastomycosis, without recovery of *B. dermatitidis* from environmental samples, have been associated with river banks. Although suggesting an association with fresh water and soil, the ecologic niche occupied by *B. dermatitidis* cannot be defined by these meager findings.

The ecology of *B. dermatitidis* must be highly specialized. There is no evidence that an animal reservoir exists to perpetuate the organism. The fungus probably exists in nature during most of the year in a protected and dormant state but is stimulated by suitable climate or other specific but transient environmental conditions to propagate and to become airborne and infectious.

Geographic Distribution. Because *B. dermatitidis* is not readily recoverable from nature and an adequate skin-test antigen is not available for conducting population surveys of exposure, the geographic distribution of blastomycosis has been estimated from reports of human and animal cases. The endemic area extends roughly east from states that border the Mississippi River. Blastomycosis is endemic in southern Canada east of Manitoba and, in the United States, in Illinois, Wisconsin, Minnesota, Ohio, the Atlantic Coast states, and the southeastern states, with the exception of Florida. The occurrence of cases in New England and elsewhere in the United States is rare. The incidence is highest in Arkansas, Kentucky, Illinois, Louisiana, Mississippi, North Carolina, Tennessee, and Wisconsin. Within these areas, local pockets of high endemicity have been identified.

Clinical reports have also documented autochthonous cases in Africa, both north (Tunisia, Morocco) and south (Uganda, Tanzania, Zimbabwe), as well as in India, Israel, Mexico, and Venezuela. Reports of the infection occurring elsewhere are dubious, because of either a questionable diagnosis or a history of travel to or contact with fomites from an endemic area. Blastomycosis is also a disease of dogs and may occur more frequently in them than in humans. Canine cases follow the same endemic pattern as those of humans.

Eleven outbreaks of blastomycosis have been documented. Table 82–5 summarizes these episodes. Each consisted of a cluster of cases that occurred at approximately the same place and time. All but one area (Westmont, Illinois) are rural. Seven outbreaks occurred during the fall and winter, and four in the summer. These outbreaks have provided helpful insights regarding the ecology of *B. dermatitidis* and the natural history of blastomycosis.

Incidence. In several compilations of case reports, blastomycosis has been reported to occur more frequently during middle age and in males. Although the disease can occur at any age, in a review of 1114 human and 247 canine cases, Furcolow and associates reported that 60% of the human cases occurred in persons between the ages of 30 and 60 years. Only 3.4% of these patients were under 20 years of age, and only four (0.9 percent) were under 10 years of age. In reviewing more recent cases, Steele and Abernathy calculated that 3.5% of cases occurred in children (≤16 years old). Striking exceptions to this age spectrum were observed in the outbreaks, where two thirds of the patients whose ages were given (73 of 109 cases) were children (Table 82–5).

The male-to-female ratios reported in several surveys involving hundreds of patients vary from 6:1 to 15:1, but lower ratios have been reported in small studies and the overall sex ratio of outbreak cases is approximately 1 (Table 82–5). Perhaps both sexes are equally susceptible to acute blastomycosis, but males are more susceptible to chronic or disseminated disease. The other three systemic mycoses caused by exogenous, dimorphic fungi also occur more often in males (Table 82–1), and male animals are more susceptible (or less resistant) than females to challenge with *B. dermatitidis*. Blastomycosis may also resemble histoplasmosis in that children

TABLE 82-5. REPORTED OUTBREAKS OF BLASTOMYCOSIS

Site	No. of Cases[a]	Dates of Onset	No. of Cases		Diagnosis[b]			Skin Test		Field Samples
			Men	<16 y	Smear	Culture	CF[c]	B	H	
Grifton, NC	11	Oct 1953–March 1954	5	7	9/10	10/10	3/8	5/10	0/10	0
Bigfork, Minn	12	Oct–Nov 1972	7	4	4/4	4/4	4/12	10/12	1/12	0/28
Westmont, Ill	5	Aug 1974–April 1975	3	0	?	5/5	2/5	ND	ND	0
Sioux Lookout, Ontario	4	Oct 1974–March 1975	?	?	?	4/4	?	?	?	?
Enfield, NC	5	Nov 1975–Jan 1976	1	3	1/1	5/5	1/1	ND	ND	0/50
Trenton, NC	3	July 1976	2	0	3/3	3/3	ND	ND	ND	ND
Haywood, Wis	7	July 1979	5	2	5/7	5/7	0/5	ND	ND	0
Southampton Co., Va	4	March 1984	4	2	3/3	3/4	2/4	ND	ND	0/17
Eagle River, Wis	48	June 1984	16	46	ND	9/48	4/47	9/48	19/48	2/45
Tomorrow River, Wis	7	May 1985	3	3	ND	4/6	0/6	ND	ND	1/19
Crystal River, Wis	7	June 1985	7	6	5/7	1/3	2/7	ND	ND	0/15

From Furcolow et al: MMWR 25:205, 1976; Kitchen et al: Am Rev Respir Dis 115:1063, 1977; Smith et al: JAMA 158:641, 1955; Tosh et al: Am Rev Respir Dis 109:525, 1974; Goldthorpe, Butler: Can Dis Wkly Rep 1–13:49, 1975; Baron, unpublished observations; Cockerill et al: Chest 86:688, 1984; Armstrong et al: J Infect Dis 155:568, 1987; Klein et al: N Engl J Med 314:529, 1986; Klein et al: J Infect Dis 155:262, 1987; Klein et al: Ann Rev Resp Dis 136:1333, 1987.

CF, complement fixation; ND, not done; ?, data unknown.

Skin test antigen: B, *Blastomyces* vaccine (Grifton) or blastomycin lot KCB-26 (Bigfork and Eagle River); H, histoplasmin.

Additional skin tests: three of the Grifton cases had a positive skin test to 1:1000 old tuberculin, and none of nine tested reacted to coccidioidin. None of 11 Bigfork cases tested reacted to intermediate-strength purified protein derivative. At Eagle River, 36 of 47 patient sera had antibody titers ≥1:8 to antigen A, as detected by an enzyme immunoassay; 7 of 89 control sera (including 4 of 19 histoplasmosis patient sera) were false-positive. Titers ≥1:16 were detected in 31 outbreak patient sera and 1 control serum. Two of 6 patients at Tomorrow River and all 7 at Crystal River had titers ≥1:8.

[a] All 51 patients in the first eight outbreaks and 13 of the last two outbreaks had abnormal radiographs; the 39 culture-negative patients at Eagle River had abnormal chest films, positive skin tests, serology, or lymphocyte transformation. The associated canine cases consisted of four in Trenton and four in Southampton County.

[b] No. positive/No. tested. Specimens were sputum, lung tissue, bronchial washing, or gastric washing. Smear refers to direct microscopic examination of specimens for yeast cells (see Figs. 82–12 and 82–13).

[c] A positve serum CF antibody test to yeast phase antigen of *Blastomyces dermatitidis* is defined as a titer ≥1:8. Only 7 of the 16 positive patients had CF titers greater than 1:8 (three had 1:16, three had 1:32, and one had 1:128). At least four of these CF-positive patients also had a positive CF test for the yeast phase antigen of *Histoplasma capsulatum*.

are equally susceptible to infection and disease, but the sex-related differences are manifested after puberty.

Racial differences in attack rates have not been confirmed. Socioeconomic and occupational data have associated blastomycosis with squalid housing, malnutrition, manual labor, agriculture, construction work, and exposure to dust and wood. Blastomycosis rarely occurs in immunocompromised patients.

Pathogenesis

Almost all cases of blastomycosis originate in the lung. In the alveoli, *B. dermatitidis* induces an inflammatory response characterized by the infiltration of both macrophages and neutrophils and the subsequent formation of granulomas. The accumulation of neutrophils presents a suppurative component that is uncharacteristic of most mycoses and other chronic diseases. Both conidia and yeast cells are susceptible to the oxidative killing mechanisms of neutrophils and the fungicidal activity of macrophages. Neutrophils and cell-mediated immunity cooperate to produce effective resistance to blastomycosis. Unlike histoplasmosis and coccidioidomycosis, blastomycosis is rare in patients with cellular immunodeficiencies.

If the pathogenesis of blastomycosis is similar to that of histoplasmosis and coccidioidomycosis, most infections may be subclinical and resolve spontaneously. Without specific and sensitive skin-test antigens, the extent of exposure to *B. dermatitidis* in the general population has not been determined. Also, as calcification is uncommon, there is little radiologic or histopathologic evidence of residual blastomycotic lesions. The best evidence of the existence of subclinical blastomycosis is derived from the Bigfork and Eagle River outbreaks, where specific skin-test reactivity was used to document exposure to *B. dermatitidis* in the absence of symptoms.

An alternative theory of the pathogenesis of blastomycosis was advanced by Furcolow and Smith. On the basis of the apparent scarcity of *B. dermatitidis* in nature and the marginal evidence of subclinical infections, they postulated that blastomycosis is a rare and unusually serious disease. Studies of experimental canine blastomycosis tend to support this hypothesis. In humans, the primary pulmonary lesion may be inapparent to severe. If inapparent, dissemination to the skin and bones may follow. If the pulmonary episode is severe, the generalized systemic disease may develop, with potential involvement of multiple organs.

Clinical Manifestations

Two classic forms of blastomycosis are recognized—pulmonary, often disseminated blastomycosis and the chronic cutaneous form. In a Veterans Administration Cooperative Study of 198 patients, the most common symptoms that initially led patients to seek medical attention were cough, weight loss, chest pain, skin lesions, fever, hemoptysis, and localized swelling. No characteristic pattern of symptoms was apparent, as other complaints were also documented by patients, albeit less frequently.

Pulmonary Blastomycosis. Primary pulmonary blastomycosis may be asymptomatic or may occur as acute or subacute pneumonia. Cases associated with outbreaks have now confirmed that spontaneous recovery can follow primary blastomycosis. However, the possibility of subsequent reactivation cannot be excluded.

The primary pulmonary infection may also persist locally or spread to any organ. In some patients the initial pulmonary infection causes symptoms of mild respiratory infection. In others the pulmonary lesion heals by fibrosis and resorption. Unlike tuberculosis and histoplasmosis, blastomycotic lesions rarely caseate or calcify. In patients whose pulmonary lesions have resolved, hematogenous, lymphatic, or macrophage-borne dissemination may already have occurred, generally to the skin. The aforementioned Veterans Administration study recognized pulmonary blastomycosis in 60% of the patients, including dissemination in 39%. Of the case total, 35% had involvement in both lung and skin, whereas 19% had infection only in the skin. Alternatively, in some patients the pulmonary focus becomes more severe and is accompanied by pleuritis. An acute to chronic lung infection may develop. The most common forms of pulmonary involvement are infiltration, cavitation, pneumonia, or nodules.

A wide variety of symptoms, pathology, and radiographic appearance may be observed, and the extent of these manifestations tends to reflect the severity of the disease. Because of the tremendous variation in symptoms, blastomycosis is quite often misdiagnosed as some other infection, sarcoid, or cancer and is too often diagnosed by accident or by a process of elimination.

Chronic Cutaneous Blastomycosis. In chronic cutaneous blastomycosis, the initial skin lesion appears as one or more subcutaneous nodules that eventually ulcerate. Lesions are most common on exposed skin surfaces, such as the face, hands, wrists, and lower legs. Spread may occur by extension to the trunk or other areas, and it may take weeks or months for the ulcerative process to evolve. If untreated, elevated, granulomatous lesions with advancing borders will develop in time. The yeast cells can be found in microabscesses near the dermis. Extensive, often verrucous, epithelial hyperplasia overlying the abscesses may develop and resemble carcinoma. These extensive cutaneous lesions are characteristically discolored and crusty, and they tend to heal and scar in the central, older areas. The active microabscesses found at the leading edge of the lesion can be aspirated or biopsied, and the typical yeast cells of *B. dermatitidis* can be observed on direct microscopic examination (Fig. 82–12).

Disseminated Blastomycosis. Dissemination may be widespread in blastomycosis. The most frequently involved extra-

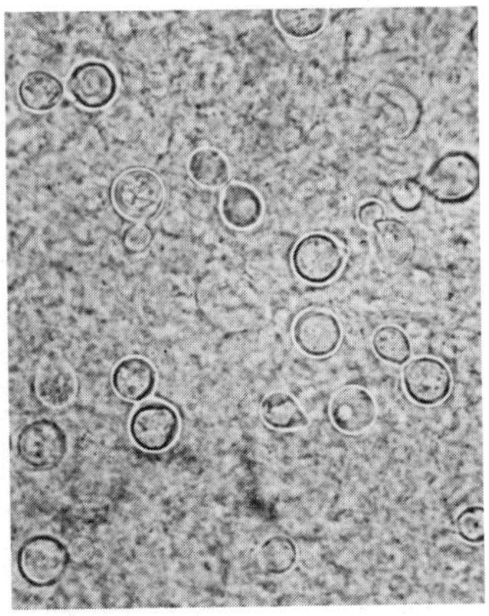

Fig. 82–12. *Blastomyces dermatitidis.* Budding yeast cells in pus. × 762. (*From Conant et al: Manual of Clinical Mycology, ed 3. Saunders, 1971.*)

pulmonary sites are the skin, bones, genitourinary tract, central nervous system, and spleen. Less frequently, the liver, lymph nodes, heart, and other viscera are infected. The progressive systemic form of blastomycosis develops in patients with unresolving pulmonary infection, but the degree of pulmonary involvement is not related to the extent of dissemination. This infection may be chronic, with few organisms present, or multiple pulmonary foci may be demonstrable at the time generalized systemic disease develops.

From the lungs, the yeasts disseminate throughout the body, with a characteristic predilection for the skin and bones. Skin lesions may be more severe than those in chronic cutaneous blastomycosis and are seen in about 75% of the patients. Overall skeletal involvement is observed in approximately 33% of the cases. Osteomyelitis and, in some cases, draining sinuses to the skin, develop and should be examined for the presence of characteristic yeast cells. Because of the frequency of bone involvement and because almost any bone can be affected, a total-body radiographic examination is advisable on diagnosis of blastomycosis. Arthritis may develop by extension from infected bone or by direct dissemination from the lung without bone infection. In up to 22% of the patients, the urogenital tract is involved, especially the male genitalia, kidney, and adrenals. Metastasis to the central nervous system, with resultant meningitis or brain abscess, occurs in up to 10% of patients.

Primary Cutaneous Blastomycosis. Primary cutaneous blastomycosis is initiated by traumatic autoinoculation or contamination of an open wound with the infectious material. The symptoms, pathology, and pathogenesis of this form differ considerably from the other forms of blastomycosis. The lymphatics and regional lymph nodes are involved, but the infection remains localized and often resolves without treatment.

Laboratory Diagnosis

Microscopic Examination. In calcofluor white or KOH preparations of pus, exudate, sputum, or other specimens, a diagnosis can be made by detection of the characteristic yeast cells of *B. dermatitidis*. The yeasts are large (8 to 15 μm in diameter) and typically have thick walls. The cell wall is highly refractile and often resembles a double wall. Budding usually occurs singly. The bud is attached to the parent cell by a broad base and enlarges to the size of the parent yeast before it is detached. These features, as depicted in Figures 82–12 and 82–13, are pathognomonic for blastomycosis and permit an immediate diagnosis to be made. Unsuspected cases of blastomycosis are occasionally diagnosed from Papanicolaou-stained sputum specimens. In tissue stained with hematoxylin and eosin, the yeast cytoplasm stains darkly and the cell wall appears colorless. The cells may be multinucleated. The yeasts are often abundant in cutaneous lesions, and these specimens are often positive on direct examination. If the yeasts are sparse, fungal cell wall stains, such as periodic acid–Schiff or methenamine silver, are helpful.

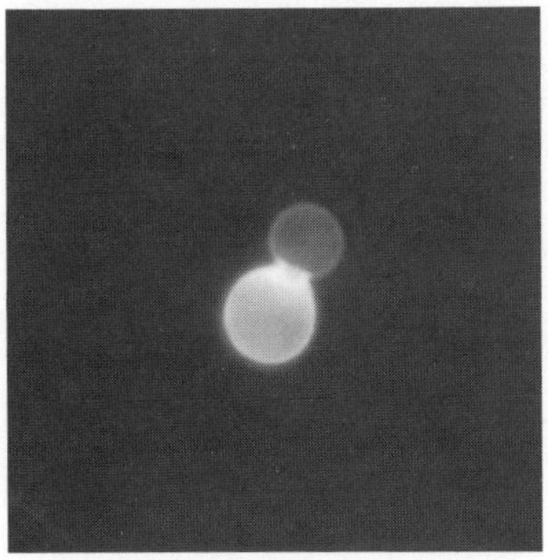

Fig. 82–13. *Blastomyces dermatitidis*. Budding yeast cell in calcofluor white preparation of sputum.

Rarely, small forms of *B. dermatitidis* are seen in tissue. These cells are typical in shape and budding but are only 2 to 5 μm in diameter. Their multinucleation may help to differentiate them from *Cryptococcus neoformans* and *H. capsulatum* var. *duboisii*.

Culture. Specimens should also be cultured on Inhibitory Mold or Sabouraud's agar and sheep blood–enriched media. If the specimen is not normally sterile, media with antibiotics should also be used (Chap. 81). Cultures should be incubated at room temperature for at least 4 weeks. Colonies are white to brown, variably textured, and produce potentially infectious conidia. The identification is confirmed by detection of the A exoantigen (Table 82–2) or by subculture on an enriched medium, such as brain-heart infusion blood agar or Kelly's medium at 37C, for subsequent conversion to the yeast form (Fig. 82–11).

Some laboratories use direct animal inoculation as a method of rapidly isolating and identifying *B. dermatitidis*. Mice are injected intraperitoneally with the clinical specimen, and their peritoneums are examined for typical yeast cells 1 to 2 weeks later.

Skin Test. Delayed-type hypersensitivity to *B. dermatitidis* has been detected by skin tests with both whole cell and culture filtrate antigens (blastomycin). In most cases, the skin test has no diagnostic value. False-negative results are often observed in patients, and false-positive cross-reactions occur in many persons sensitized to other fungi. Reactivity is transient and disappears with time. In persons who are doubly reactive to blastomycin and histoplasmin, the blastomycin reaction is considered specific if it is equal to or greater than the response to histoplasmin. In the Bigfork and Eagle River epidemics (Table 82–5), blastomycin was extremely valuable, as a significant number of the infections were detected by monospecific reactions, whereas the background level of reactivity in the population was negligible.

Other antigen preparations have been shown in animals and in in vitro assays of the cell-mediated immune responses of human lymphocytes to be considerably more specific and sensitive than blastomycin. These improved antigens are not available for routine human skin testing. Nevertheless, results of a study that tested lymphocytes from persons in an endemic area support the occurrence of subclinical exposure to *B. dermatitidis*.

Serology. Measurement of CF antibodies to various antigen preparations of *B. dermatitidis* has not proved reliable. Sera from patients with blastomycosis may react with higher CF titer to heterologous antigens, especially histoplasmin, than to blastomycin. The yeast phase of *B. dermatitidis* provides a more specific antigen, but only 30% to 50% of patients have positive test reactions.

The most useful serologic procedure is an ID test for

specific precipitins. As indicated in Table 82–3, the ID test is more sensitive and more specific than the CF test. With the use of a yeast form filtrate antigen and positive reference sera, antibodies to a specific precipitin line, designated A, can be detected. Although other precipitin lines may occur, apparently only sera from patients with blastomycosis develop antibodies to antigen A, which do not cross-react with the specific precipitin lines formed to antigens of other systemic fungal pathogens (Table 82–2). It is not known how soon after infection the ID test becomes positive, but the precipitin lines disappear within a few months after successful treatment.

An enzyme immunoassay for antibodies to antigen A was recently evaluated. The sensitivity and specificity of this test were 77% and 92%, respectively. The titers reflected severity of disease.

Treatment

Amphotericin B is effective against blastomycosis. A total dose of at least 2 g is required to eradicate all the organisms, as the relapse rate is significant if 1.5 g or less is administered. The protocol for administration of amphotericin B and monitoring of renal functions is the same as for other mycoses (see Table 81–8). Amphotericin B is clearly recommended for treating more severe cases of blastomycosis, such as patients with life-threatening disease, dissemination to the central nervous system, renal failure, or respiratory insufficiency.

Reports of ketoconazole for the treatment of blastomycosis have been mixed but promising. The usual regimen is a 6-month course of 400 mg per day. However, higher doses (800 mg per day) for longer periods, where tolerated, may be required in some cases. Patients treated with ketoconazole should be closely followed for compliance as well as for relapse. Ketoconazole may be recommended for less severe cases, noncavitary pulmonary blastomycosis, and cases involving only lung, skin, or both. Other azole drugs may prove more effective in the future.

Paracoccidioidomycosis

Paracoccidioidomycosis or South American blastomycosis is a systemic mycotic infection caused by a thermally dimorphic fungus, *Paracoccidioides brasiliensis*. The infection is confined to Central and South America. It is a chronic, granulomatous disease that begins with a primary, pulmonary, usually inapparent infection that disseminates to produce ulcerative granulomas in the mucosal surfaces of the nose, mouth, and gastrointestinal tract. Internal organs, as well as the skin and lymph nodes, may become infected.

Morphologic and Cultural Characteristics

On Sabouraud's glucose agar at 25C to 30C, colonies of *P. brasiliensis* grow very slowly, reaching a diameter of 1 to 2 cm after 2 or 3 weeks of incubation. The macroscopic features are variable and nonspecific.

Various conidia are produced by *P. brasiliensis*, including chlamydospores, arthroconidia, and singly borne conidia. In the absence of conidia, which may not be produced for 10 weeks, the mycelia and colony may be indistinguishable from *B. dermatitidis* or many saprophytes. By growth on a rich medium at 35C to 37C, the yeast form can be induced. The yeasts are readily identified by their unique appearance. As seen in Figure 82–14, they produce multiple buds, and each is attached to the parent yeast by a narrow base. The yeasts are large (up to 30 μm in diameter) and have thinner walls than the yeasts of *B. dermatitidis*. These forms have been called pilot wheels.

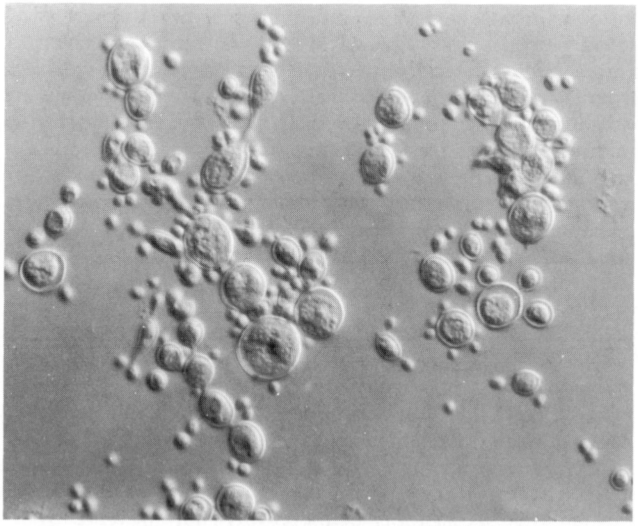

Fig. 82–14. *Paracoccidioides brasiliensis.* Multiply budding yeast cells from 2-week culture on brain-heart infusion blood agar at 37C. Normarski. × 400. (*From McGinnis: Laboratory Handbook of Medical Mycology. Academic Press, 1979.*)

The yeast cells of *P. brasiliensis* die after approximately 2 weeks in broth cultures. Death is attributed to the accumulation of a toxic phenolic metabolite in the medium.

Determinants of Pathogenicity

P. brasiliensis, like *C. immitis*, *H. capsulatum*, and *B. dermatitidis*, causes disease in males more frequently than in females (Table 82–1), although skin-test surveys have revealed comparable reactivity between both sexes, implying equal exposure. Limited studies indicate that physiologic concentrations of sex hormones do not directly inhibit these fungi. Sex-linked differences may be associated with the generally more potent cellular immunity of females. A protein from the mycelial cytosol of *P. brasiliensis* has been shown to bind estrogen but not testosterone or other hormones. Binding prevents conversion of the mycelium to yeast at 37C and may explain the resistance of females to paracoccidioidomycosis.

Once yeast cells of *P. brasiliensis* have developed in the lung, yeast cell wall polysaccharides, such as α-glucan, are associated with virulence and the ability to stimulate granulomas.

Clinical Infection

Epidemiology. The natural habitat of *P. brasiliensis* is not known but is presumed to be soil. The organism has been recovered only sporadically and irreproducibly from soil in Venezuela and Argentina. Like *B. dermatitidis*, its natural existence and life cycle in nature are unknown. There is no evidence of its transmission or of an animal vector. Natural disease does not occur in either wild or domestic animals, although experimental infections can be established in mice and bats after inhalation of an infectious inoculum. Infections are presumed to follow exposure to the organisms from an exogenous source.

Thousands of cases of paracoccidioidomycosis have been reported from Brazil and lesser numbers from Venezuela, Colombia, Argentina, Ecuador, and other South and Central American countries, with the exception of Chile and the Caribbean nations. Discrete endemic foci exist within this broad area of geographic distribution. However, all cases are isolated, and clusters of cases have not been observed. The endemic zones are associated with moderate temperatures (14C to 30C) and rainfall, elevation of 500 to 6500 feet, subtropical forests, and river valleys, but not all areas fitting this description have paracoccidioidomycosis.

Skin test surveys have been conducted with various antigens derived from *P. brasiliensis*. These *paracoccidioidins* exhibit cross-reactivity with histoplasmin, and it is difficult to interpret double reactions of equal size in the same person. As with the skin test antigens of the other dimorphic, systemic pathogens, paracoccidioidin elicits a delayed, indurative reaction that indicates previous exposure. The percentage of reactivity in endemic areas varies from 5% to 25% and occurs equally in both men and women. The highest percentage of reactors occurs among workers in agriculture, specifically coffee, sugar cane, and cattle workers.

Most patients are males (>90%), agricultural workers, often malnourished, and usually 30 to 60 years of age.

Clinical Manifestations. The clinical classification of paracoccidioidomycosis is presented in Table 82–6. Devised by Restrepo and associates, this classification relates the clinical forms of infection to the natural history. The initial form refers to the first contact with *P. brasiliensis* by inhalation. The episode is inapparent, and the organism becomes quiescent for an indefinite period, which may be several decades in some persons, or the lesion may resolve, perhaps with scarring. This asymptomatic infection results in conversion to a positive delayed skin test reaction to paracoccidioidin. The eventual development of symptomatic disease depends on the host-fungal interaction, namely, the integrity of the cell-mediated immunity of the individual, environmental conditions (e.g., temperature, nutrients), host conditions (e.g., age, sex, state of nutrition), and the virulence of the strain of *P. brasiliensis*.

JUVENILE TYPE. Patients under 30 years of age may have an acute, progressive infection characterized by lymphonodular lesions in the lung. This form is rare. The yeasts may disseminate to the reticuloendothelial tissue, lymph nodes, liver, spleen, skin, bone, joints, or other organs. The severity and duration of the illness depend on the extent of organ involvement, but it may be fatal within a period of several weeks or months.

TABLE 82–6. CLINICAL FORMS OF PARACOCCIDIOIDOMYCOSIS

Asymptomatic infection
Initial form
Latent or residua form
Symptomatic disease
Juvenile type or acute/subacute progressive form
Adult type or chronic progressive form
Pulmonary
Disseminated
Initial symptomatic form

Adapted from Restrepo et al: Am J Med 61:33, 1976

ADULT TYPE. More than 90% of the cases are of this type and develop from the latent form, usually after several years. Lesions may be localized in the lung, or metastasis may occur from the lung to other organs, particularly the skin and mucocutaneous tissue, lymph nodes, spleen, liver, adrenals, and combinations thereof. Mucocutaneous, often petechial, lesions frequently develop on the corners of the mouth, lips, gingiva, or tongue. Pulmonary lesions are granulomatous nodules that may cavitate but rarely calcify.

The initial symptomatic form of the disease develops shortly after infection, without a pronounced latent period. Rare cases of primary cutaneous inoculation are also placed in this category.

Laboratory Diagnosis

MICROSCOPIC EXAMINATION. Sputum, tissue, or scrapings of mucocutaneous lesions may reveal the multiply budding yeast cells that are pathognomonic for *P. brasiliensis* (Fig. 82–14).

CULTURE. Specimens should be cultured at 25C to 30C on Inhibitory Mold agar, Sabouraud's agar with antibiotics, Sabouraud's agar without cycloheximide, and brain-heart infusion blood agar at 35C to 37C. The yeast form often grows better at 35C or 36C than at 37C.

SEROLOGIC TESTS. The ID test is extremely useful. As indicated in Table 82–3, nearly 100% of patients have at least one of three specific precipitin lines (designated 1, 2, and 3) detected by identity with reference serum. The ID test also has prognostic value, as the bands disappear with clearing of the infection, and the number of bands is somewhat correlated with the severity of the disease.

The CF test is quantitative and useful for assessing prognosis, but cross-reactions occur with other fungi.

Treatment. Some of the initial clinical trials with ketoconazole demonstrated its efficacy against paracoccidioidomycosis, and ketoconazole is the drug of choice. Amphotericin B is also effective against paracoccidioidomycosis. The total dose usually required is 2 g or less. Nonhospitalized patients may also be given sulfa drugs, such as sulfamethoxypyridazine, at 1 g per day for 3 to 6 months and 0.5 g per day thereafter. Serologic specimens checked every few months to monitor the effectiveness of treatment. Successful cure requires treatment for approximately 2 years.

FURTHER READING

COCCIDIOIDOMYCOSIS

Ampel NM, Ryan KJ, Carry PJ, et al: Fungemia due to *Coccidioides immitis*: An analysis of 16 episodes in 15 patients and a review of the literature. Medicine 65:312, 1986

Ampel NM, Widen MA, Galgiani JN: Coccidioidomycosis: Clinical update. Rev Infect Dis 11:897, 1989

Bayer AS, Yoshikawa TT, Calpin JE, et al: Unusual syndromes of coccidioidomycosis: Diagnostic and therapeutic considerations. Medicine 55:131, 1976

Beaman L, Banjamini E, Pappagianis D: Activation of macrophages by lymphokines: Enhancement of phagosome-lysosome fusion and killing of *Coccidioides immitis.* Infect Immun 39:1201, 1983

Bouza E, Dreyer JS, Hewitt WL, et al: Coccidioidal meningitis—An analysis of 31 cases and review of the literature. Medicine 60:139, 1981

Bronnimann DA, Galgiani JN: Coccidioidomycosis. Eur J Clin Microbiol Infect Dis 8:466, 1989

Catanazro A: Suppressor cells in coccidioidomycosis. Cell Immunol 64:235, 1981

Catanzaro A, Spitler LE, Moser KM: Cellular immune response in coccidiodomycosis. Cell Immunol 15:360, 1975

Cole GT: Models of cell differentiation in conidial fungi. Microbiol Rev 50:95, 1986

Cole GT, Kirkland TN, Sun SH: An immunoreactive water-soluble conidial wall fraction of *Coccidioides immitis.* Infect Immun 55:657, 1987

Cole GT, Sun SH: Arthroconidium-spherule-endospore transformation in *Coccidioides immitis.* In Szaniszlo PJ (ed): Fungal Dimorphism with Emphasis on Fungi Pathogenic for Humans. New York, Plenum Press, 1985, p 281

Cox RA: Immunosuppression by cell wall antigens of *Coccidioides immitis.* Rev Infect Dis 10:5415, 1988

Cox RA: Coccidioidomycosis. In Cox RA (ed): Immunology of the Fungal Diseases. Boca Raton, CRC Press, 1989, p 165

Cox RA, Pope RM, Stevens DA: Immune complexes in coccidioidomycosis. Correlation with disease involvement. Am Rev Respir Dis 126:439, 1982

Cox RA, Vivas JR: Spectrum of in vivo and in vitro cell-mediated immune responses in coccidioidomycosis. Cell Immunol 31:130, 1977

DeFelice R, Galgiani JN, Campbell SC, et al: Ketoconazole treatment of nonprimary coccidioidomycosis: Evaluation of 60 patients during three years of study. Am J Med 72:681, 1982

Deresinski SC, Stevens DA: Coccidioidomycosis in compromised hosts: Experience at Stanford University Hospital. Medicine 54:377, 1975

Deresinski SC, Galgiani JN, Stevens DA: Miconazole treatment of human coccidioidomycosis: Status report. In Ajello L (ed): Coccidioidomycosis: Current Clinical and Diagnostic Status. Miami, Symposia Specialists, 1977, p 267

Deresinski SC, Applegate RJ, Levine HB, Stevens DA: Cellular immunity to *Coccidioides immitis*: In vitro lymphocyte response to spherules, arthrospores, and endospores. Cell Immunol 32:110, 1977

Diamond RD, Bennett JE: A subcutaneous reservoir for intrathecal therapy of fungal meningitis. N Engl J Med 288:186, 1973

Drutz DJ, Catanzaro A: Coccidioidomycosis. Parts I and II. Am Rev Respir Dis 117:559, 727, 1978

Edwards PQ, Palmer CE: Prevalence of sensitivity to coccidioidin, with special reference to specific and nonspecific reactions to coccidioidin and to histoplasmin. Dis Chest 31:35, 1957

Einstein HE, Catanzaro A (eds): Coccidioidomycosis. Proceedings of 4th International Conference. Washington, National Foundation for Infectious Diseases, 1985

Fish DG, Ampel NM, Galgiani JN, et al: Coccidioidomycosis during human immunodeficiency virus infection: A review of 77 patients. Medicine 69:384, 1990

Flynn NM, Hoeprich PD, Kawachi MM, et al: An unusual outbreak of windborne coccidioidomycosis. N Engl J Med 301:358, 1979

Galgiani JN, Ampel NM: Coccidioidomycosis in human immunodeficiency virus-infected patients. J Infect Dis 162:1165, 1990

Graham AR, Sobonya RE, Bronnimann DA, et al: Quantitative pathology of coccidioidomycosis in acquired immunodeficiency syndrome. Hum Pathol 19:800, 1988

Graybill JR, Stevens DA, Galgiani JN, et al: Itraconazole treatment of coccidioidomycosis. Am J Med 89:282, 1990

Hobbs ER: Coccidioidomycosis. Dermatol Clin 7:227, 1989

Huppert M: Serology of coccidioidomycosis. Mycopathologia 41:107, 1970

Huppert M, Krasnow I, Vukovich KR, et al: Comparison of coccidioidin and spherulin in complement-fixation test for coccidioidomycosis. J Clin Microbiol 6:33, 1977

Klotz SA, Drutz DJ, Huppert M, et al: The critical role of CO_2 in the morphogenesis of *Coccidioides immitis* in cell-free subcutaneous chambers. J Infect Dis 150:127, 1984

Knoper SR, Galgiani JN: Systemic fungal infections: Diagnosis and treatment. I. Coccidioidomycosis. Infect Dis Clin North Am 2:861, 1988

Levine HB, Restrepo A, Ten Eyck DR, et al: Spherulin and coccidioidin: Cross-reactions in dermal sensitivity to histoplasmin and paracoccidioidin. Am J Epidemiol 101:512, 1975

Minamoto G, Armstrong D: Fungal infections in AIDS: Histoplasmosis and coccidioidomycosis. Infect Dis Clin North Am 2:447, 1988

Nelson AR: The surgical treatment of pulmonary coccidioidomycosis. Curr Probl Surg 11:1, 1974

Pappagianis D: Epidemiology of coccidioidomycosis. Curr Top Med Mycol 2:199, 1988

Pappagianis D, Zimmer BL: Serology of coccidioidomycosis. Clin Microbiol Rev 3:247, 1990

Rea TH, Einstein H, Levan NE: Dinitrochlorobenzene responsitivity in disseminated coccidioidomycosis: An inverse correlation with complement-fixing antibody titers. J Invest Dermatol 66:34, 1976

Smith CE: Coccidioidomycosis. Med Clin North Am 27:790, 1943

Smith CE, Saito MT, Beard RR, et al: Serological tests in the diagnosis and prognosis of coccidioidomycosis. Am J Hyg 52:1, 1950

Smith CE, Whiting EG, Baker EE, et al: The use of coccidioidin. Am Rev Tuberc 57:330, 1948

Standard PG, Kaufman L: Immunological procedure for the rapid and specific identification of *Coccidioides immitis* cultures. J Clin Microbiol 5:149, 1977

Stevens DA (ed): Coccidioidomycosis: A text. New York, Plenum, 1980

Stobo JD, Paul S, Van Scoy RE, et al: Suppressor thymus-derived lymphocytes in fungal infection. J Clin Invest 57:319, 1976

Tucker RM, Galgiani JN, Denning DW, et al: Treatment of coccidioidal meningitis with fluconazole. Rev Infect Dis 12(suppl 3):S380, 1990

Walsh TJ, Mitchell TG: Dimorphic fungi causing systemic mycoses. In Balows A, Hausler WJ, Herrmann KL, et al (eds): Manual of Clinical Microbiology, ed 5. Washington, DC, American Society for Microbiology 1991, p 630

Woodruff WW, Buckley CE, Gallis HA, et al: Reactivity to spherule-derived coccidioidin in the southeastern United States. Infect Immun 43:860, 1984

HISTOPLASMOSIS

Ajello L, Chick EW, Furcolow ML (eds): Histoplasmosis, Springfield, Ill, Charles C Thomas, 1971

Berliner MD, Biundo N: Effects of continuous light and total darkness on cultures of *Histoplasma capsulatum.* Sabouraudia 11:48, 1973

Boguslawski G, Kobayashi GS, Schlessinger D, et al: Characterization of an inhibitor of ribonucleic acid polymerase from the mycelial phase of *Histoplasma capsulatum.* J Bacteriol 122:532, 1975

Brodsky AL, Gregg MB, Lowenstein MS, et al: Outbreak of histoplasmosis associated with the 1970 Earth Day activities. Am J Med 54:333, 1973

Christie A, Peterson JC: Pulmonary calcification in negative reactors to tuberculin. Am J Public Health 35:1131, 1945

Darling STA: A protozoan general infection producing pseudotubercules in the lungs and focal necrosis in the liver, spleen, and lymph nodes. JAMA 46:1283, 1906

de Monbreun WA: The cultivation and cultural characteristics of Darling's *Histoplasma capsulatum*. Am J Trop Med 14:93, 1934

Dijkstra JW: Histoplasmosis. Dermatol Clin 7:251, 1989

Dismukes WE, Cloud GA, Bowles C, et al: Treatment of blastomycosis and histoplasmosis with ketoconazole: Results of a prospective randomized clinical trial. Ann Intern Med 103:861, 1985

Domer JE, Moser SA: Histoplasmosis—A review. Rev Med Vet Mycol 15:159, 1989

Eisenberg LG, Goldman WE: *Histoplasma capsulatum* fails to trigger release of superoxide from macrophages. Infect Immun 55:29, 1987

Goodman NL, Larsh HW: Environmental factors and growth of *Histoplasma capsulatum* in soil. Mycopath Mycol Appl 33:145, 1967

Goodwin RA, Des Prez RM: Histoplasmosis. Am Rev Respir Dis 117:929, 1978

Goodwin RA, Loyd JE, Des Prez RM: Histoplasmosis in normal hosts. Medicine 60:231, 1981

Graybill JR: Histoplasmosis and AIDS. J Infect Dis 158:623, 1988

Kaufman L, Terry AT, Schubert JH, et al: Effects of a single histoplasmic skin test in the serological diagnosis of histoplasmosis. J Bacteriol 94:1798, 1967

Keath EJ, Painter AA, Kobayashi GS, Medoff G: Variable expression of a yeast-phase-specific gene in *Histoplasma capsulatum* strains differing in thermotolerance and virulence. Infect Immun 57:1384, 1989

Kurtin PJ, McKinsey DS, Gupta MR, et al: Histoplasmosis in patients with acquired immunodeficiency syndrome: Hematologic and bone marrow manifestations. Am J Clin Pathol 93:367, 1990

Kwon-Chung KJ: Sexual stage of *Histoplasma capsulatum*. Science 175:326, 1972

Kwon-Chung KJ: Perfect state (*Emmonsiella capsulata*) of the fungus using large-form African histoplasmosis. Mycologia 67:980, 1975

Larsh HW: Histoplasmosis. In DiSalvo AF (ed): Occupational Mycoses, Philadelphia, Lea & Febiger, 1983, p 29

Maresca B, Kobayashi GS: Dimorphism in *Histoplasma capsulatum*: A model for the study of cell differentiation in pathogenic fungi. Microbiol Rev 53:186, 1989

Maresca B, Lambowitz AM, Kumar VB, et al: Role of cysteine in regulating morphogenesis and mitochondrial activity in the dimorphic fungus *Histoplasma capsulatum*. Proc Natl Acad Sci USA 78:4596, 1981

McGinnis MR, Katz B: *Ajellomyces* and its synonym *Emmonsiella*. Mycotaxon 8:157, 1979

Medoff G, Kobayashi, Painter A, Travis S: Morphogenesis and pathogenicity of *Histoplasma capsulatum*. Infect Immun 55:1355, 1987

Nickerson DA, Havens RA, Bullock WE: Immunoregulation in disseminated histoplasmosis: Characterization of splenic suppressor cell populations. Cell Immunol 60:287, 1981

Nightingale SD, Parks JM, Pounders SM, et al: Disseminated histoplasmosis in patients with AIDS. South Med J 83:624, 1990

Palmer CE: Nontuberculous pulmonary calcification and sensitivity to histoplasmin. Public Health Rep 60:513, 1945

Prechter GC, Prakash UB: Bronchoscopy in the diagnosis of pulmonary histoplasmosis. Chest 95:1033, 1989

Schwarz J: Histoplasmosis. New York, Praeger, 1981

Sptizer ED, Keath EJ, Travis SJ, et al: Temperature-sensitive variants of *Histoplasma capsulatum* isolated from patients with acquired immunodeficiency syndrome. J Infect Dis 162:258, 1990

Taylor ML, Diaz S, Gonzalez PA, et al: Relationship between pathogensis and immune regulation mechanisms in histoplasmosis: a hypothetical approach. Rev Infect Dis 6:775, 1984

Tewari RP, Berkhart FJ: Comparative pathogenicity of albino and brown types of *Histoplasma capsulatum* for mice. J Infect Dis 125:504, 1972

Watson SR, Schmitt SK, Hendricks DE, Bullock WE: Immunoregulation in disseminated histoplasmosis: Disturbances in the production of interleukins 1 and 2. J Immunol 135:3487, 1985

Wheat LJ: Diagnosis and management of histoplasmosis. Eur J Clin Microbiol Infect Dis 8:480, 1989

Wheat LJ, Connolly-Stringfield PA, Baker RL, et al: Disseminated histoplasmosis in the acquired immune deficiency syndrome: Clinical findings, diagnosis and treatment, and review of the literature. Medicine 69:361, 1990

Wheat LJ, French MLV, Kohler RB, et al.: The diagnostic laboratory tests for histoplasmosis: Analysis of experience in a large urban outbreak. Ann Intern Med 97:680, 1982

Wheat LJ, Slama TG, Norton JA, et al: Risk factors for disseminated or fatal histoplasmosis: Analysis of a large urban outbreak. Ann Intern Med 96:159, 1982

Wu-Hsieh BA, Howard DH: Gamma interferon and experimental murine histoplasmosis. In Ayoub EM, Cassell GH, Branche WC, Henry TJ (eds): Microbial determinants of virulence and host response. Washington DC, American Society for Microbiology, 1990, p 133

Wu-Hsieh B, Howard DH: Histoplasmosis. In Cox RA (ed): Immunology of the Fungal Diseases. Boca Raton, CRC Press, 1989, p 199

BLASTOMYCOSIS

Armstrong CW, Jenkins SR, Kaufman L, et al: Common-source outbreak of blastomycosis in hunters and their dogs. J Infect Dis 155:568, 1987

Baker RD: Tissue reactions in human blastomycosis: An analysis of tissue from twenty-three cases. Am J Pathol 18:479, 1942

Benham RW: Fungi of blastomycosis and coccidioidal granuloma. Arch Dermatol 30:385, 1934

Bradsher RW: Development of specific immunity in patients with pulmonary or extrapulmonary blastomycosis. Am Rev Respir Dis 129:430, 1984

Bradsher RW: Systemic fungal infections: Diagnosis and treatment, I. Blastomycosis. Infect Dis Clin North Am 2:877, 1988

Bradsher RW, Rice DC, Abernathy RS: Ketoconazole therapy for endemic blastomycosis. Ann Intern Med 103:872, 1985

Brass C, Volkmann CM, Klein HP, et al: Pathogen factors and host factors in murine pulmonary blastomycosis. Mycopathologia 78:129, 1982

Brummer E, Sugar AM, Stevens DA: Enhanced oxidative burst in immunologically activated but not elicited polymorphonuclear leukocytes correlates with fungicidal activity. Infect Immun 49:396, 1985

Busey JF, Baker L, Birch L, et al: Blastomycosis. I. A review of 198 collected cases in Veterans Administration hospitals. Am Rev Respir Dis 89:659, 1964

Carman WF, Frean JA, Crewe-Brown HH, et al: Blastomycosis in Africa. A review of known cases diagnosed between 1951 and 1987. Mycopathologia 107:25, 1989

Cockerill FR, Roberts GD, Rosenblatt JE, et al: Epidemic of pulmonary blastomycosis (Namekagon fever) in Wisconsin canoeists. Chest 86:688, 1984

Cox RA, Mills LR, Best GK, Denton JF: Histologic reactions to cell walls of an avirulent and a virulent strain of *Blastomyces dermatitidis*. J Infect Dis 129:179, 1974

Davies SF, Sarosi GA: Blastomycosis. Eur J Clin Microbiol Infect Dis 8:474, 1989

Deepe GS: Blastomycosis. In Cox RA (ed): Immunology of the Fungal Diseases. Boca Raton, CRC Press, 1989, p 139

Deepe GS, Taylor CL, Bullock WE: Evaluation of inflammatory response and cellular immune responses in a murine model of disseminated blastomycosis. Infect Immun 50:183, 1985

Denton JF, DiSalvo AF: Isolation of *Blastomyces dermatitidis* from natural sites of Augusta, Georgia. Am J Trop Med Hyg 13:716, 1964

Drutz DJ, Frey CL: Intracellular defenses of human phagocytes against *Blastomyces dermatitidis* conidia and yeast. J Lab Clin Med 105:737, 1985

Duttera M, Osterhout S: North American blastomycosis: A survey of 63 cases. South Med J 62:295, 1969

Furcolow ML, Chick EW, Busey JF, et al: Prevalence and incidence studies of human and canine blastomycosis. I. Cases in the United States, 1885–1968. Am Rev Respir Dis 102:60, 1970

Furcolow ML, Smith CD: A new hypothesis on the epidemiology of blastomycosis and the ecology of *Blastomyces dermatitidis*. Trans NY Acad Sci, Ser II 34:421, 1973

Furcolow ML, Smith C, Gallis H, et al: Blastomycosis—North Carolina. MMWR 25:205, 1976

Gilchrist TC: A case of blastomycetic dermatitis in man. Johns Hopkins Hosp Rep 1:269, 1896

Goldthorpe WG, Butler KF: Blastomycosis outbreak in Sioux Lookout Zone. Can Dis W Rep 1–13:49, 1975

Kaufman L, McLaughlin DW, Clark MJ, et al: Specific immunodiffusion test for blastomycosis. Appl Microbiol 26:244, 1973

Kitchen MS, Reiber CD, Eastin GB: An urban epidemic of North American blastomycosis. Am Rev Respir Dis 115:1063, 1977

Klein BS, Vergeront JM, Kaufman L, et al: Serological tests for blastomycosis: Assessments during a large point-source outbreak in Wisconsin. J Infect Dis 155:262, 1987

Klein BS, Vergeront JM, DiSalvo AF, et al: Two outbreaks of blastomycosis along rivers in Wisconsin. Isolation of *Blastomyces dermatitidis* from riverbank soil and evidence of its transmission along waterways. Am Rev Respir Dis 136:1333, 1987

Klein BS, Vergeront JM, Weeks RJ, et al: Isolation of *Blastomyces dermatitidis* in soil associated with a large outbreak of blastomycosis in Wisconsin. N Engl J Med 314:529, 1986

Kunkel WM, Weed LA, McDonald JR, et al: North American blastomycosis—Gilchrist's disease; clinicopathologic study of ninety cases. Int Abst Surg 99:1, 1954

Lowry PW, Kelso KY, McFarland LM: Blastomycosis in Washington Parish, Louisiana, 1976–1985. Am J Epidemiol 130:151, 1989

Martin DS, Smith DT: Blastomycosis. I. A review of the literature. Am Rev Tuberc 39:275, 1939

McDonough ES: Blastomycosis: Epidemiology and biology of its etiologic agent *Ajellomyces dermatitidis*. Mycopathol Mycol Appl 41:195, 1970

McDonough ES, Lewis AL: *Blastomyces dermatitidis*: Production of the sexual stage. Science 156:528, 1967

Mitchell TG: Blastomycosis. In Feigin RD, Cherry JD (eds): Textbook of Pediatric Infectious Diseases, ed 3. Philadelphia, WB Saunders, 1991

Miyaji M, Nishimura K: Granuloma formation and killing functions of granuloma in congenitally athymic nude mice infected with *Blastomyces dermatitidis* and *Paracoccidioides brasiliensis*. Mycopathologia 82:129, 1983

Mycoses Study Group: Treatment of blastomycosis and histoplasmosis with ketoconazole: Results of a prospective randomized clinical trial. Ann Intern Med 103:861, 1985

Sarosi GA, Davies SF: Blastomycosis. Am Rev Respir Dis 120:911, 1979

Sarosi GA, Davies SF, Phillips JR: Self-limited blastomycosis: A report of 39 cases. Sem Respir Infect 1:40, 1986

Sarosi GA, Hammerman KJ, Tosh FE, et al: Clinical features of acute pulmonary blastomycosis. N Engl J Med 290:540, 1974

Schwarz J, Baum GL: Blastomycosis. Am J Clin Pathol 21:999, 1951

Schwarz J, Salfelder K: Blastomycosis: A review of 152 cases. Curr Top Pathol 65:165, 1977

Sheflin JR, Campbell JA, Thompson GP: Pulmonary blastomycosis: Findings on chest radiographs in 63 patients. Am J Roentgenol Radium Ther Nuc Med 154:1177, 1990

Smith JG, Harris JS, Conant NF, et al: An epidemic of North American blastomycosis. JAMA 158:641, 1955

Steck WD: Blastomycosis. Dermatol Clin 7:241, 1989

Tenenbaum M, Greenspan J, Kerkering TM: Blastomycosis. CRC Crit Rev Microbiol 9:139, 1982

Thurmond LM, Mitchell TG: *Blastomyces dermatitidis* chemotactic factor: Kinetics of production and biological characterization evaluated by a modified neutrophil chemotaxis assay. Infect Immun 46:87, 1984

Tosh FE, Hammerman KJ, Weeks RJ, et al: A common source epidemic of North American blastomycosis. Am Rev Respir Dis 109:525, 1974

Vaaler AK, Bradsher RW, Davies SF: Evidence of subclinical blastomycosis in forestry workers in northern Minnesota and northern Wisconsin. Am J Med 89:470, 1990

PARACOCCIDIOIDOMYCOSIS

Franco M: Host-parasite relationships in paracoccidioidomycosis. J Met Vet Mycol 25:5, 1987

Giraldo R, Restrepo A, Gutierrez F, et al: Pathogenesis of paracoccidioidomycosis: A model proposed on the study of 46 patients. Mycopathologia 58:63, 1976

Greer D, D'Acosta D, Agredo L: Dermal sensitivity to paracoccidioidin and histoplasmin in family members of patients with paracoccidioidomycosis. J Trop Med Hyg 23:87, 1974

Jimenez-Finkel B, Restrepo A: Paracoccidioidomycosis. In Cox RA (ed): Immunology of the Fungal Diseases. Baco Raton, Fla., CRC Press, 1989, p 227

Paracoccidioidomycosis. PAHO Publ. No. 254, 1972

Restrepo A: Paracoccidioidomycosis. Acta Med Colombiana 3:33, 1978

Restrepo A: The ecology of *Paracoccidioides brasiliensis*: A puzzle still unresolved. Sabouraudia 23:323, 1985

Restrepo A, Moncada LH: Characterization of the precipitin bands detected in the immunodiffusion test for paracoccidioidomycosis. Appl Microbiol 28:138, 1974

Restrepo A, Robledo M, Giraldo R, et al: The gamut of paracoccidioidomycosis. Am J Med 61:33, 1976

Restrepo A, Salazar ME, Cano LE, et al: Estrogens inhibit mycelium-to-yeast transformation in the fungus *Paracoccidioides brasiliensis*: Implications for resistance of females to paracoccidioidomycosis. Infect Immun 46:346, 1985

San-Blas G: *Paracoccidioides brasiliensis*: Cell wall glucans, pathogenicity, and dimorphism. Curr Top Med Mycol 1:235, 1985

Stevens DA: The interface of mycology and endocrinology. J Med Vet Mycol 27:133, 1989

Stover EP, Schar G, Clemons KV, et al: Estradiol-binding proteins from mycelial and yeast-form cultures of *Paracoccidioides brasiliensis*. Infect Immun 51:199, 1986

Sugar AM: Paracoccidioidomycosis. Infect Dis Clin North Am 2:913, 1988

CHAPTER 83

Subcutaneous Mycoses

All of the mycoses discussed in this chapter are caused by exogenous fungi that normally reside in nature, and most are associated with soil or vegetation. The fungi enter the skin or subcutaneous tissue by traumatic inoculation with contaminated material. The natural history of the subcutaneous mycosis that develops depends on the pathogenetic potential of the fungus and the defenses of the host. Individual fungi may present a distinctive mycosis, such as sporotrichosis, rhinosporidiosis, lobomycosis, rhinoentomophthoromycosis, or subcutaneous phycomycosis. In other subcutaneous mycoses, several fungi may cause a single disease, as in chromomycosis, phaeohyphomycosis, or mycetoma.

Although these mycoses are usually confined to the subcutaneous tissues, they may rarely become systemic and produce life-threatening disease. Furthermore, some of the related fungi discussed in this chapter are clearly capable of causing primary, systemic infections.

Sporotrichosis

Sporotrichosis is a chronic infection of the cutaneous and subcutaneous tissue and lymphatics caused by the thermally dimorphic fungus, *Sporothrix schenckii*. The infection is initiated by traumatic inoculation of the organisms into the skin. Secondary spread may follow, with involvement of the draining lymphatics, lymph nodes, and, rarely, the underlying muscle and bone. Occasionally, dissemination occurs to internal organs, such as the lungs, central nervous system, or genitourinary tract.

The clinical forms and etiology of sporotrichosis were first described in the early part of this century. A massive epidemic among gold miners in South Africa clarified the natural history of the infection. During a 2-year period, almost 3000 cases were diagnosed. The epidemic was caused not by transmission among the infected laborers but by exposure of large numbers of susceptible miners to a common source of the infectious particles. The fungus was found growing saprophytically on the timber supporting the mine shafts and tunnels. As the miners brushed against the contaminated wood, the skin of their exposed arms and shoulders was abraded, and spores of hyphal fragments of *S. schenckii* were implanted under the skin. Once the source was discovered, the epidemic was controlled by treating the timber with fungicides to eradicate the organisms.

In nature, *S. schenckii* occurs in association with plant life and in the soil. The infection, which is acquired in the course of outdoor activities, follows traumatic implantation of the fungus into the skin. Patients frequently recall a history of trauma. The primary nodule often develops at the site of a previous wound caused by a thorn or splinter, by brushing against tree bark, or by handling of reeds and grasses. Some cases have resulted from skin injury caused by metal objects or animals bites contaminated with soil containing the organism. There is evidence that the fungus may grow on biting insects, such as ants and fleas, and inoculation may occur in this manner. Exposure and infection may possibly follow contact with patients or their contaminated dressings.

Sporothrix schenckii

Morphologic and Cultural Characteristics. On Sabouraud's agar at room temperature, colonies of *S. schenckii* develop in 3 to 5 days. At first, they are usually blackish and shiny but become fuzzy with age as aerial hyphae are produced. The colony appearance of different strains varies considerably. In some strains, colonies are initially yeastlike but convert later to the mycelial form. The colonies of some isolates are white instead of black or gray.

Microscopic examination of the colony reveals thin, branching septate hyphae and small (approximately 3 by 5 μm) conidia that are delicately attached to the distal, tapering ends of slender conidiophores. These conidia usually become detached in a teased preparation, but in a microculture that permits examination in situ, conidia are arranged in flowerlike clusters (Fig. 83–1). Conidiation is sympodial and increases with age. In addition to the characteristic florets, some strains also produce larger, darkly pigmented conidia directly from the hyphae.

S. schenckii is dimorphic. Conversion to the yeast form may be accomplished in vitro by cultivating the organisms on a rich medium, such as brain-heart blood infusion agar at 35C to 37C. Some strains grow poorly at 37C but convert nicely at 35C. Sometimes, the mycelial growth persists, and the yeast cells develop only at the periphery of the colony.

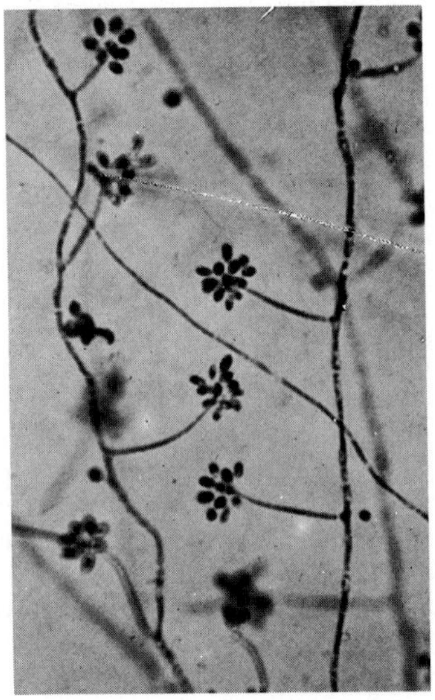

Fig. 83–1. *Sporothrix schenckii.* Mold form. Clusters of pyriform conidia (2 to 3 μm by 3 to 6 μm) formed sympodially from the tips of distally tapering conidiophores. × 650. *(From Conant et al: Manual of Clinical Mycology, ed 3. Saunders, 1971.)*

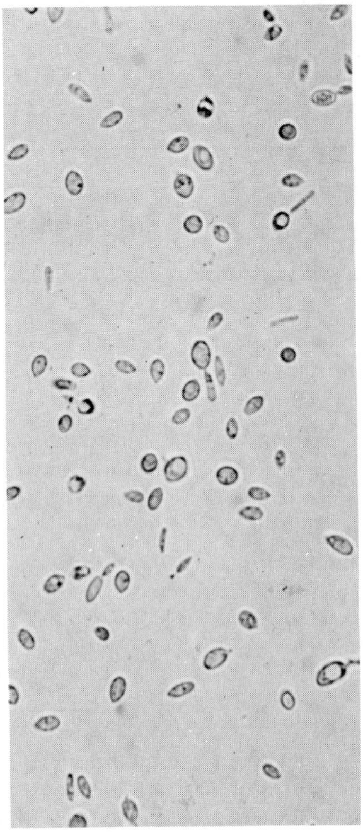

Fig. 83–2. *Sporothrix schenckii.* Yeast form. Fusiform, spherical, and ellipsoidal cells from culture on brain-heart infusion blood agar at 37C. × 790. *(From Conant et al: Manual of Clinical Mycology, ed 3. Saunders, 1971.)*

Yeast colonies are pasty and grayish. Yeast cells from these colonies are variable in shape but often fusiform, approximately 1 to 3 μm by 3 to 10 μm, with multiple buds (Fig. 83–2). As an alternative to in vitro conversion, animal inoculation can be used to induce the yeast phase.

Etiology of Sporotrichosis. The possibility that sporotrichosis may be caused by more than one species is based on tenuous and circumstantial evidence. Several species of *Sporothrix* and *Ceratocystis* are phytopathogens or closely associated with vegetation. A number of these species are difficult to separate. In fact, *S. schenckii* may be morphologically indistinguishable from *Ceratocystis stenoceras.* Because these anamorphic species occupy the same habitat and closely resemble each other, it has been suggested that more than one species might be pathogenic for humans, which would account for the considerable variation in some of the early morphologic descriptions. Species of *Sporothrix* and *Ceratocystis* are similar in cell wall composition and antigenicity. Sera from patients with sporotrichosis contain antibodies to epitopes present in both genera. One such determinant, a rhamnomannan moiety, is also present in the streptococcal cell envelope. The presence of antibodies or delayed hypersensitivity to both *Sporothrix* and *Ceratocystis* presumably results from cross-reactivity. However, experimental infection with *Ceratocystis* has been reported.

Another observation that is compatible with the concept of multiple agents is the contrasting conditions during which the infection is most prevalent in the endemic areas. Although found worldwide, sporotrichosis is endemic in parts of Brazil, Uruguay, South Africa, and Zimbabwe. In these areas, most cases occur during the hot, rainy season. Conversely, in

Mexico, where the disease is also endemic, the peak incidence occurs during the cool, dry season. These differences in seasonal incidence may reflect population differences in host defense or exposure or possibly different etiologic strains. The epidemiology of sporotrichosis also varies in different regions (see below).

Determinants of Pathogenicity. The usual explanation for the subcutaneous nature of sporotrichosis invokes the temperature sensitivity of the organism. The temperature of the skin and subcutaneous tissue is slightly lower than that of deeper tissue. In support of this theory, clinical reports describe the therapeutic effects of fever and the application of hot packs.

The maximal temperature at which most strains of *S. schenckii* will grow in vitro is 38C, and many soil isolates fail to grow at 37C. Passage through mice appears to enhance the virulence of strains, perhaps by selecting thermotolerant cells. Temperature is an important determinant of murine pathogenicity. When mice are inoculated intravenously with comparable inocula of yeast cells of *S. schenckii* and subsequently housed at different temperatures, mice kept at 13C to 17C develop lesions only in the muscle tissue of the legs, whereas mice housed in the cold (ambient temperatures of 2C to 5C) develop miliary lesions in the liver as well as in the extremities. However, intrathoracic inoculation of mice with yeast cells results in a disseminated form of the disease. Isolates of *S. schenckii* from nonlymphangitic (fixed) lesions grow less well at 35C and 37C (both in vitro and in vivo) than isolates obtained from cases of lymphocutaneous sporotrichosis.

At temperatures below 37C, both *Sporothrix* and *Ceratocystis* produce neuraminidase. As neuraminic acid is only found in mammalian tissue and some microorganisms but not in plants, this finding suggests a possible mechanism for tissue tropism and toxicity.

Clinical Infection

Epidemiology. Sporotrichosis occurs globally among persons of all ages. Although 75% of the patients are males, it is not known whether this preference is attributable to sex-linked susceptibility or to increased exposure. The incidence is higher among agricultural workers and persons who live or work around vegetation. Indeed, sporotrichosis must be considered an occupational disease of forest rangers, horticulturists, and similar workers.

Animals, both wild and domestic, are susceptible to *S. schenckii* infection. The disease is similar to that which occurs in humans and has been especially well documented in horses. The highest incidence in the world is in Mexico, where sporotrichosis is the second most common fungal infection. Most cases occur among rural, often malnourished peasants in the endemic areas of Mexico, Central America, and Brazil. Infections are most pronounced in debilitated or malnourished patients, which may partially explain the high incidence in the underdeveloped countries. In developed countries, such as the United States, Canada, and France, cases of sporotrichosis are less frequent and are associated with gardening soil and horticulture. The occurrence in the United States among affluent, middle-aged, white males who may have a history of alcoholism has been described as the alcoholic rose-gardener syndrome.

Occasionally, a cluster of cases follows exposure of several individuals to a common source at the same time, similar to the outbreak among the gold miners of South Africa. Such an outbreak occurred among Mississippi Forestry Commission workers, who developed sporotrichosis of the upper extremities after planting pine seedlings that were packed in sphagnum moss contaminated with *S. schenckii.* A fight among college students who threw contaminated bricks at each other also precipitated a cluster of cases.

Host factors related to nutrition, alcohol, or sex may predispose certain individuals to infection. Experimentally, the presence of cell-mediated immunity to *S. schenckii* restricts the infection. In the endemic areas of Mexico, where relatively fewer cases are lymphangitic, there is a high level of reactivity among the population to the skin test antigen, *sporotrichin*, which reflects delayed hypersensitivity.

Clinical Manifestations

LYMPHOCUTANEOUS SPOROTRICHOSIS. Seventy-five percent of the cases of sporotrichosis are lymphocutaneous, with lesions first appearing in the cutaneous or subcutaneous tissue and progressively involving the draining lymphatics. The classic history begins with the traumatic implantation of the organisms into the skin. The incubation period is highly variable, ranging from a few days to several months, with an average of about 3 weeks. The duration is governed by such factors as the host defenses, virulence of the strain, size of the inoculum, and depth of its inoculation. Initially, a small, movable, nontender, subcutaneous nodule develops. If the organisms are more epidermal than subcutaneous, a small ulcer may develop. The subcutaneous nodule becomes discolored, and the overlying skin darkens to a reddish color and eventually blackens. This necrotic lesion subsequently erupts through the skin surface to form an ulcer or sporotrichotic chancre. After a few weeks, the primary lesion heals, and new ones develop nearby.

CHRONIC SPOROTRICHOSIS. Following the primary nodule, multiple subcutaneous nodules develop along the lymphatic channels, and they become hard and cordlike. The process is the same. A movable nodule forms, which then becomes attached to the overlying skin, discolors due to suppuration, and ulcerates. The initial lesion is more exudative and less gummatous than the secondary ones. Untreated, sporotrichosis usually becomes chronic, but it may heal spontaneously.

FIXED SPOROTRICHOSIS. Fixed sporotrichosis refers to the presence of only one lesion. The infection is restricted and less progressive, and although the lesion may alternately wax and wane, it may resolve completely. It is confined, and the lymphatics are not involved. The lesion may be ulcerative or appear as a plaque or rash. Because the appearance is so variable, a positive culture is required to differentiate sporotrichosis in these cases from a number of other bacterial and mycotic skin lesions and carcinomas. The fixed lesion is more common in highly endemic areas, where this limited pathogenicity may be related to the overall high frequency of delayed hypersensitivity.

OTHER FORMS. Infection may spread to mucocutaneous areas, including the eyes. The most common sites of dissemination are the bones and joints, usually following a negligible, primary skin lesion, and appearing as chronic arthritis. Metastasis to deeper tissues, such as the meninges, occurs rarely.

Primary pulmonary sporotrichosis results from inhalation of the infectious particles rather than secondary dissemination from a superficial location. Pulmonary sporotrichosis can be opportunistic and has been observed in compromised patients in urban hospitals. Patients with systemic sporotrichosis usually have impaired cell-mediated immunity. This rare form of the disease may present a spectrum of manifestations. It can be chronic and mimic cavitary tuberculosis. It can also be acute and rapidly progressive, with lymphadenopathy.

Laboratory Diagnosis

MICROSCOPIC EXAMINATION. Calcofluor white or KOH preparations can be made of smears of biopsy material or exudates from ulcerative lesions. The histopathology of sporotrichotic lesions resembles that of epithelioma. Sections of biopsied specimens yield very few organisms. The yeast cells are so sparse in most infected tissues that even with special stains, such as the periodic acid-Schiff or methenamine silver stain, they are usually difficult to locate. Fluorescent antibody stains can be used to locate the rare yeast cells in tissue.

When yeasts are observed in tissue, they are usually spherical, multiply budding cells 3 to 5 μm in diameter. Some of the yeast cells may be fusiform, elongated, or cigar-shaped. They may appear to be encapsulated, but this is an artifact caused by shrinkage of the cytoplasm from the cell wall during fixation. When present, the asteroid body is characteristic of sporotrichosis The asteroid body consists of the central, basophilic yeast cell surrounded by radiating extensions of eosinophilic material that may be as thick as 10 μm. The rays contain antigen-antibody complexes, complement, and tissue components and probably constitute an immunologic reaction to the organism. Asteroids are not specific for *S. schenckii*, since they can also be formed during infection with other fungi, especially *Aspergillus*, as well as bacteria.

CULTURE. The most reliable method of diagnosis is culture, and isolates of *S. schenckii* grow on a variety of media. Suitable specimens for culture include aspirated fluid, pus, exudative material, or biopsy tissue. Specimens are streaked on inhibitory mold or Sabouraud's agar containing antibacterial antibiotics and incubated at 25C to 30C. Identification is confirmed by growth at 35C and conversion to the yeast form.

SEROLOGY. Because specific antibodies are usually not present in the early stages of infection, serologic study is of little help in establishing the diagnosis. Perhaps the most useful of several tests that have been described in the yeast cell agglutination test. Agglutinins to the yeast cells can be used to monitor the course of infection. Patients with active sporotrichosis have an agglutinating antibody titer of 1:160 or greater. Titers up to 1:40 can be found in recovered patients, healthy individuals, or those with cross-reactive antibodies. Therefore, only titers above 1:80 are significant.

Sporotrichin will elicit delayed skin test reactions in sensitive persons. Positive reactions are observed in many healthy individuals in endemic regions, and the presence of delayed hypersensitivity has been associated with less severe infections.

Treatment. Neither lymphocutaneous nor fixed sporotrichosis is a debilitating infection. The lesions are chronic and may persist without treatment for years, with periods of improvement and regression, and they may heal spontaneously. The prognosis for disseminated sporotrichosis is grave. With this form of disease, spontaneous cures never occur, since the infection is progressive, and the organisms are numerous.

Since 1912, the treatment of choice for cutaneous sporotrichosis has been the administration of an oral solution of saturated potassium iodide (SSKI). This can also be administered topically. A typical regimen consists of SSKI in milk or juice. Dosage is increased daily at 0.5 to 1.0 mL increments from 1 mL three times per day to 4 to 6 mL three times per day. Adverse side effects may be indigestion, rash, cardiac arrhythmias, lacrimation, salivation or swelling of salivary glands. Treatment is tapered off if these occur. Most patients tolerate SSKI, and treatment is continued for at least 4 weeks after resolution of the clinical symptoms. Surface lesions can be treated topically with 2% KI in 0.2% iodine.

The mode of action of iodide therapy is unclear. In vitro, *S. schenckii* is resistant to 10% KI. In vivo, iodides cause resolution of granulomata and abscesses, which is probably the basis for the therapeutic effect. After partial disruption of the tissue response, the organisms are exposed to the host's immunologic defenses.

Except in cases of severe disseminated disease, SSKI should always be tried first. If this fails, amphotericin B may be employed. Case reports have supported the use of other antifungals, including ketoconazole, dihydroxystilbamidine, griseofulvin, and flucytosine. Reports of the use of itraconazole are encouraging. The application of heat to cutaneous lesions is a useful adjunct. With ulcerative lesions, it may also be necessary to treat superinfecting bacteria with appropriate antibiotics.

Chromomycosis and Phaeohyphomycosis

Chromomycosis and phaeohyphomycosis are caused by *dematiaceous fungi*, which are imperfect fungi that produce varying amount of melanin-like pigments (Chap. 80). These pigments are found in the conidia or hyphae or both and give the organism an olive green, brown, or black color. Taxonomic characterization of the dematiaceous fungi is controversial and ever changing. Experimental infections in mice with wild-type and melanin-deficient mutants suggest that melanin production by dematiaceous fungi is associated with virulence.

Chromomycosis (or chromoblastomycosis) is caused by traumatic implantation of any one of several dematiaceous fungal species into the subcutaneous tissue. The infection is chronic and characterized by the slow development of verrucous, cutaneous vegetations. Species generally recognized as agents of chromomycosis are *Fonsecaea pedrosoi*, *Phialophora verrucosa*, *Cladosporium carrionii*, *Rhinocladiella aquaspersa*, and *Fonsecaea compacta*. The natural reservoir of these fungi is soil and plant debris.

Related dematiaceous species cause phaeohyphomycosis, which may be systemic as well as subcutaneous. As the name indicates, pigmented hyphae are observed in tissue.

Dematiaceous fungi cause several other diseases besides chromomycosis and phaeohyphomycosis, as summarized in Table 83–1. Mycetoma may be caused by a variety of fungi, including the dematiaceous species *Exophiala jeanselmei*, *Madurella grisea*, and *Madurella mycetomatis*. Mycetomas are de-

TABLE 83–1. MYCOSES CAUSED BY DEMATIACEOUS FUNGI AND SOME REPRESENTATIVE AGENTS (ABRIDGED)

Mycosis	Etiology
Chromomycosis	*Fonsecaea pedrosoi, Phialophora verrucosa, Cladosporium carrionii, Fonsecaea compacta, Rhinocladiella aquaspersa*
Phaeohyphomycosis	
Phaeomycotic cyst	*Exophiala jeanselmei, Wangiella dermatitidis, Exophiala spinifera, Phialophora hoffmannii, Phialophora parasitica, Phialophora repens, Phialophora richardsiae, Tetraploa aristata, Bipolaris spicifera,* and others
Subcutaneous	*Bipolaris spicifera, Alternaria alternata, Alternaria chlamydospora, Phialophora richardsiae, Exophiala jeanselmei, Exophiala moniliae, Hormonema dematioides*
Systemic (including CNS invasion)	*Alternaria alternata, Bipolaris spicifera, Exserohilum rostratum, Aureobasidium pullulans, Dactylaria constricta, Rhinocladiella atrovirens, Cladosporium devriesii, Curvularia lunata, Curvularia geniculata, Wangiella dermatitidis*
Brain abscess	*Xylohypha bantiana, Bipolaris spicifera, Exserohilum rostratum, Curvulata lunata*
Mycetoma	*Exophiala jeanselmei, Madurella mycetomatis, Madurella grisea, Curvulata lunata,* and others; also nondematiaceous fungi
Keratitis	*Phialophora hoffmannii, Phialophora verrucosa, Bipolaris spicifera, Curvulata lunata,* and others; also nondematiaceous fungi
Sinusitis	*Bipolaris spicifera, Bipolaris hawaiiensis, Curvularia lunata, Exserohilum rostratum, Alternaria alternata;* also nondematiaceous fungi
Tinea nigra	*Phaeoannellomyces werneckii*

scribed in the next discussion. Tinea nigra and keratomycosis are discussed in Chapter 84. In addition to the species of dematiaceous fungi listed in Table 83–1, many others have been encountered in rare infections but are not discussed in detail. Indeed, there is an emerging awareness of the numerous dematiaceous species that are capable of causing a variety of infections in normal as well as compromised hosts. Sinusitis, caused by an increasing number of dematiaceous species, has been recognized more frequently in both immunocompetent and immunocompromised individuals.

Dematiaceous Fungi

In addition to the classic morphologic methods of identifying dematiaceous fungi, new procedures have been developed. The value of these other methods varies with the taxa under study, and they include biochemical reactions, assimilation of

TABLE 83–2. CONIDIA PRODUCTION BY PATHOGENIC GENERA OF DEMATIACEOUS FUNGI

Genus	Type of Conidiogenous Cells
Cladosporium	Blastoconidia (in chains)
Phialophora	Phialides with collarettes
Exophiala	Annellides
Wangiella	Phialides without collarettes
Fonsecaea	Sympodulae, also phialides and blastoconidia

sugars, production of enzymes, detection of specific exoantigens, and comparison of DNA similarities.

Cultural Characteristics. The dematiaceous fungi are similar not only in their pigmentation but also in their antigenic determinants, morphology, and physiologic properties. In culture, the colonies are usually indistinguishable. They are compact, deep brown to black, and develop a velvety, often wrinkled surface (Fig. 83–5A). Dematiaceous yeast species are usually pleomorphic and produce a dark, moist colony that becomes mycelial with age.

Microscopic Appearance. The generic criteria are based on the type and ontogeny of conidiation (Chap. 80). Table 83–2 presents one classification. *Cladosporium* species produce chains of branching conidia by acropetalous (distal) budding. The length of the chains and conidial size differ with individual species. *Phialophora* species produce conidia from flask-shaped phialides with cup-shaped collarettes (Figs. 83–3 and 83–4).

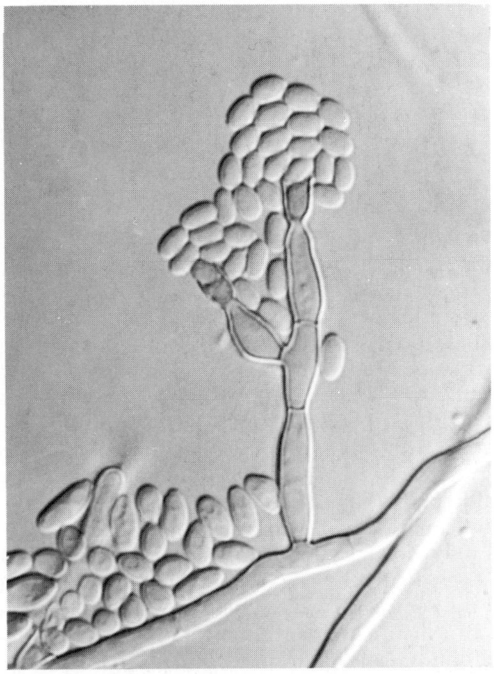

Fig. 83–3. *Phialophora verrucosa.* Phialide with cup-shaped collarette and mass of conidia, from 2-week culture on potato-dextrose agar at 30C. Nomarski. × 1200. *(From McGinnis: Laboratory Handbook of Medical Mycology. Academic Press, 1979.).*

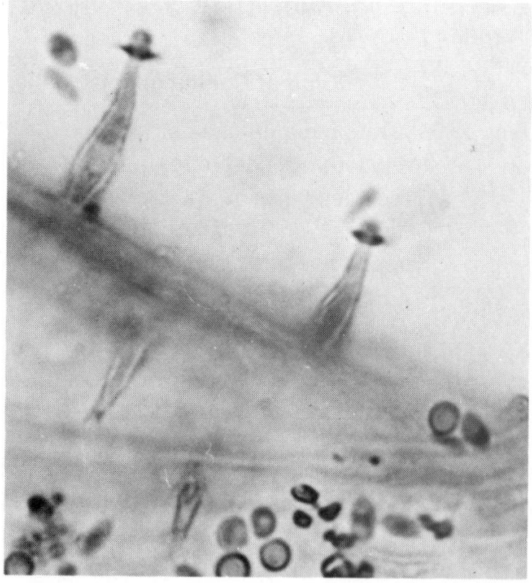

Fig. 83–4. *Phialophora richardsiae.* Phialide with terminal, saucer-shaped collarette. × 1387. *(From Conant et al: Manual of Clinical Mycology, ed 3. Saunders, 1971.)*

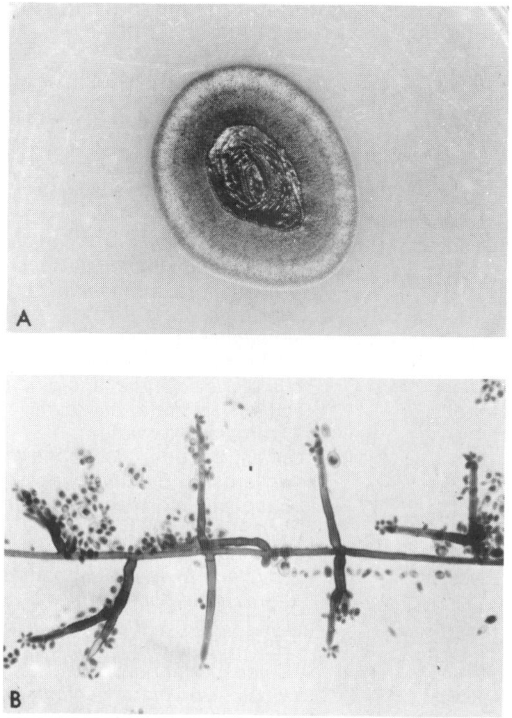

Fig. 83–5. *Exophiala spinifera.* **A.** Typical dematiaceous, darkly pigmented colony from culture on cornmeal agar at 30C. **B.** Deeply pigmented, rigid annellides on cornmeal agar. × 450. *(From Conant et al: Manual of Clinical Mycology, ed 3. Saunders, 1971.)*

Mature conidia are extruded from the phialide and usually accumulate around it. In *Exophiala*, the conidiogenous cells are annellides, which produce conidia from a tapered, ringed tip (Fig. 83–5B). The end of the annellide increases in length and in the number of annellations, with the development of successive conidia from the tip. *Wangiella dermatitidis* is dimorphic and produces conidia by phialides that lack collarettes. *Fonsecaea* is a polymorphic genus. It may exhibit *Phialophora*-type or *Cladosporium*-type sporulation. It also produces lateral or terminal conidia from a lengthening conidiogenous cell. This process is described as sympodial and is typical of the genus *Rhinocladiella*.

Clinical Infection

Clinical Manifestations

CHROMOMYCOSIS. The fungi that cause chromomycosis, of which *F. pedrosoi* is the most common, produce a similar disease and possess a low level of virulence. The localized infection, which usually occurs on the exposed lower extremities, forms a primary sore that is discolored. A mononuclear cellular infiltrate and satellite lesions develop over a period of months or years. With time, these lesions become raised 1 to 3 mm and appear scaly and dull red or grayish in color. The pathology typically consists of granulomatous nodules and epithelial hyperplasia. After several years, elevated (1–3 cm), verrucous cauliflower lesions develop. Patients experience minimal discomfort. Systemic invasion is extremely rare, but when it does occur, the organisms are neurotropic and tend to infect the central nervous system. A recent survey of HLA types in Brazilian patients with chromomycosis and matched controls found a correlation with HLA type A29, suggesting a genetic predisposition to chromomycosis, although only 28% of patients had this HLA type.

PHAEOHYPHOMYCOSIS. The term *phaeohyphomycosis* refers to infections characterized by the presence of darkly pigmented, septate hyphae in tissue (Fig. 83–6). Both cutaneous and systemic phaeohyphomycotic infections are recognized. The clinical forms vary from solitary encapsulated cysts in the subcutaneous tissue to brain abscesses (Table 83–1). The phaeomycotic cyst usually develops on the extremities and may enlarge to several centimeters. The skin and tissue surrounding the cyst are relatively normal.

Approximately half of more than 50 reported cases of phaeohyphomycotic brain abscess were caused by *Xylohypha bantiana* (*Cladosporium bantianum* or *Cladosporium trichoides*). Most patients have headache followed by fever and hemiparesis. However, patients have a variety of underlying conditions and specific symptoms that reflect the size and location of the lesion. The frontal lobes are the most common site, and encapsulated abscesses filled with brown hyphae are present in neurosurgical biopsies or autopsy specimens. *X. bantiana* has been isolated from wood, but the source of infection is uncertain, as patients lack cutaneous and pulmonary lesions. This species is clearly neurotropic.

In pansinusitis and cerebral phaeohyphomycosis, computed tomography (CT) is especially helpful in assessing the extent of involvement before and after surgical excision.

Laboratory Diagnosis. The appearance of the fungi in potassium hydroxide (KOH) preparations or tissue specimens is characteristic for each type of dematiaceous mycosis. Chromomycotic lesions contain spherical, pigmented cells (4 to 12 μm), called *muriform* or *sclerotic bodies*, that exhibit transverse septations. The dark pigment of the sclerotic cells is evident

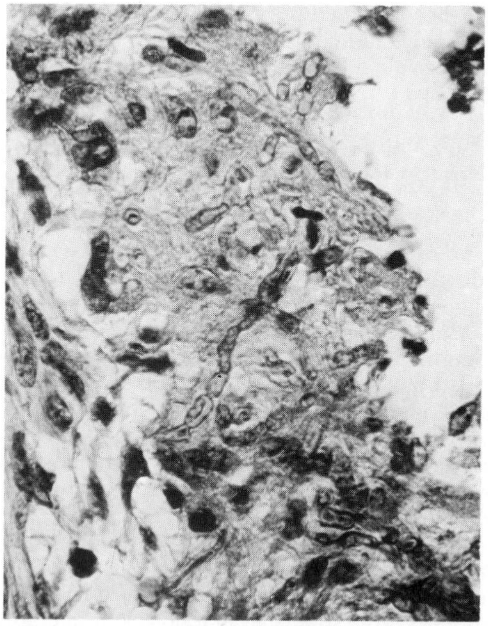

Fig. 83–6. *Phialophora richardsiae.* Pigmented hyphae seen in wall of abscess.

in direct preparations and in stained tissue sections. With phaeohyphomycosis, irregular dark hyphae, as well as yeasts and pseudohyphae, are seen in tissue (Fig. 83–6).

Specimens from chromomycosis and phaeohyphomycosis should be cultured on Sabouraud's agar with and without antibiotics, since some of the agents are susceptible to cycloheximide. In general, dematiaceous saprophytes have active proteolytic enzymes capable of digesting gelatin or Loeffler's serum agar. Pathogenic dematiaceous fungi tend to grow more slowly than saprophytic species, and most pathogens, unlike saprophytes, grow at 37C. *X. bantiana* is capable of growth at 42C. Speciation within the pathogenic genera is based on the mode(s) of conidiation (Table 83–2) and the size, shape, and arrangement of conidia. A commercial system that identifies yeasts (Chap. 85) by testing the assimilation of various sugar substrates also is helpful in identifying many dematiaceous species. Procedures for the extraction and detection of specific exoantigens (Chap. 82) have been developed for the identification of *F. pedrosoi, P. verrucosa, S. bantiana, Bipolaris* species, and *Exserohilum* species, among others.

Treatment. Treatment of these infections is often challenging and complex because isolates of dematiaceous species (Table 83–1) may vary in susceptibility and response to amphotericin B, flucytosine, the azoles, and other drugs. Flucytosine has achieved the most success, but treatment typically requires 6 months to a year. Chromomycosis can be complicated by secondary bacterial infection, which may be more threatening than the fungal infection. Advanced cases have been treated by surgical management and topical compounds. Recent studies have reported success treating chomomycosis and phaeohyphomycosis with itraconazole. In one compilation, 19 patients with phaeohyphyomycosis caused by seven different genera and involving skin, soft tissue, sinuses, bone, joints, or lung were given 50 to 600 mg itraconazole per day. Although most had previously failed treatment with amphotericin B, ketconazole, miconazole, or combinations of these, 9 of the patients responded to itraconazole.

Even with surgical removal of the cerebral abscess and treatment with amphotericin B, most patients with brain lesions have died within a few months. However, surgery and itraconazole have successfully treated brain abscess due to *X. bantiana*. Phaeomycotic cysts are managed by excision.

Mycetoma

Mycetoma (Madura foot, maduromycosis) is a chronic, subcutaneous infection induced by traumatic inoculation with any of several saprophytic fungus species. The clinical features that define mycetoma are local tumefaction and interconnecting, often draining, sinuses that contain granules, which are microcolonies of the agent embedded in tissue material. In addition to being caused by several species of fungi, mycetoma can also be caused by various actinomycetes (Chap. 32), which generally produce a more severe infection. Both fungal and actinomycetous agents of mycetoma are normally found in the soil.

A frequent agent of mycetoma, *Pseudallescheria boydii,* has also been documented as a rare cause of opportunistic systemic infection in compromised patients. Pseudallescheriasis, which indicates a nonmycetomal *P. boydii* infection, is similar to invasive aspergillosis (Chap. 85). In addition to systemic and pulmonary disease, *P. boydii* may cause sinusitis, keratitis, and otomycosis.

Etiologic Agents

Cultural Characteristics. The fungal agents of mycetoma include *P. boydii, E. jeanselmei, Madurella mycetomatis, Madurella grisea, Acremonium falciforme* (*Cephalosporium falciforme*), *Leptosphaeria senegalensis,* and several other species. *P. boydii,* the most common cause of mycetoma in the United States, and *L. senegalensis* are homothallic ascomycetes and may produce cleistothecia or perithecia, respectively, in culture. The colony of *P. boydii* is grayish, and those of *E. jeanselmei, Madurella* species, and *L. senegalensis* are darkly pigmented. *A. falciforme* develops a white to pinkish colony.

Microscopic Appearance. The identification of these fungi is based largely on morphologic differences. *P. boydii* produces both conidia (Fig. 83–7) and ascospores, which are contained within asci in large, pigmented cleistothecia (Chap. 80). The anamorphic state of *P. boydii* is *Scedosporium apiospermum, E. jeanselmei* produces annellides and annelloconidia. *Madurella* species may not produce any characteristic conidia, but several physiologic tests are available to assist in their identification. *A. falciforme* produces characteristic crescent-shaped one- and two-celled conidia that accumulate at the tips of phialides.

Clinical Infection

Mycetoma develops after traumatic inoculation with soil contaminated with one of the etiologic agents. The feet, lower extremities, hands, and exposed areas are most often involved, but any part of the skin can become infected. The disease and

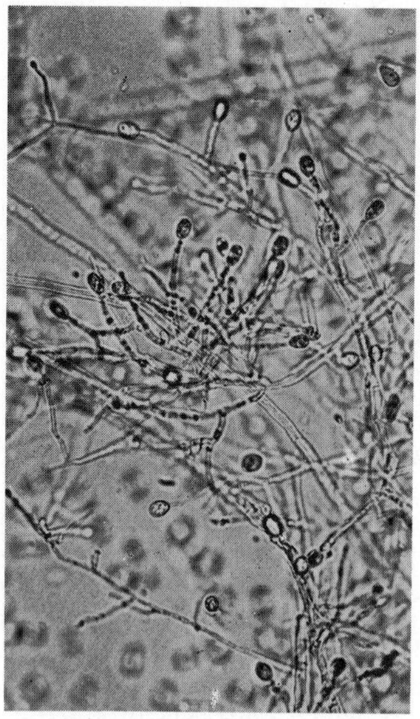

Fig. 83–7. *Scedosporium apiospermum*, anamorph of *Pseudallescheria boydii.* Each conidium is produced at the tip of a short conidiophore. × 305. *(From Conant et al: Manual of Clinical Mycology, ed 3. Saunders, 1971.)*

most of the agents are prevalent worldwide, but the incidence is highest in tropical climates (Table 83–3).

Regardless of the agent, the pathology is characterized by suppuration and abscess formation, granulomata, and the formation of draining sinuses containing granules or microcolonies of the fungi packed with tissue debris. Tumefaction and deformation of the tissue develop slowly. The infections are chronic, and the risk of dissemination is minimal.

Laboratory Diagnosis. The granule color, texture, size, and presence of hyaline or pigmented hyphae are helpful in determining the etiology (Table 83–3). As shown in Figure 83–8, a mycetomatous granule in tissue is grossly similar to an actinomycotic granule (Chap. 32).

Treatment. The management of mycetoma is difficult. Amphotericin B is recommended for *Madurella* infections, although ketoconazole has been used. Topical nystatin and potassium iodide are used in the treatment of *P. boydii* infections, and flucytosine is recommended for *E. jeanselmei.* Surgery may be necessary in protracted cases, since the drugs frequently do not penetrate the infected tissue well enough to reach the fungal pathogens. Invasive infections with *P. boydii* have been treated successfully with amphotericin B; however, in vitro and clinical data suggest that the best drug may be miconazole.

Rhinosporidiosis

Rhinosporidiosis is a chronic infection characterized by the development of polypoid masses of the nasal mucosa. The etiologic agent, which has only recently been recovered from infected tissue, is *Rhinosporidium seeberi.* Since the first report from Argentina by Seeber in 1900, over 2000 cases have been recognized. Approximately 90% of these are from India and Sri Lanka. It is more common in children and young adults, and over 90% of the cases occur in males. Natural infection occurs in horses, cattle, dogs, and other animals. Occasional human and animal infections are diagnosed in the United States, usually in the southeast.

Rhinosporidium seeberi. The etiologic agent of rhinosporidiosis has puzzled mycologists and clinicians for years. *R. seeberi* produces large spherules in lesions and in epithelial cell tissue cultures but has not been grown in vitro on culture media. It stimulates proliferation of epithelial cells in vitro, as in the host. *R. seeberi* is presumed to have a natural reservoir from which patients become infected. In Asia, this habitat has been associated with water, fish, or aquatic insects, and many patients are divers.

Clinical Infection. Lesions are most often found on the mucosa of the nose, nasopharynx, or soft palate, but many other mucocutaneous sites may become infected, including the conjunctiva, skin, larynx, genitalia, or rectum. Lesions are initially flat but develop into discolored, cauliflower-type polypoid masses varying in size up to 20 g. Regardless of location, these characteristic, pedunculated lesions are formed. In the nasal area, respiration may be blocked, and there is a profuse seropurulent discharge. Sporangia may be grossly visible as small white spots on the lesion.

LABORATORY DIAGNOSIS AND TREATMENT. Histologic examination of infected tissue reveals epithelial hyperplasia and a cellular infiltrate of neutrophils, lymphocytes, plasma cells, and giant cells. Also present are the large, thick-walled sporangia. The sporangia enlarge in size to a diameter of 200 to 300 μm and are packed with thousands of endospores (6 to

TABLE 83–3. COMMON AGENTS OF MYCETOMA

Species	Granule		Predominant Geographic Distribution
	Color	Size (mm)	
Pseudallescheria boydii	White	<2	Worldwide, tropical, North America
Madurella mycetomatis	Dark red to black	0.5–2	Worldwide, tropical
Madurella grisea	Black	0.3–0.6	Central and South America
Acremonium falciforme	White	0.5–1.5	Worldwide, tropical
Exophiala jeanselmei	Brown to black	0.2–0.3	Worldwide (very rare)
Leptosphaeria senegalensis	Black	0.5–2	West Africa

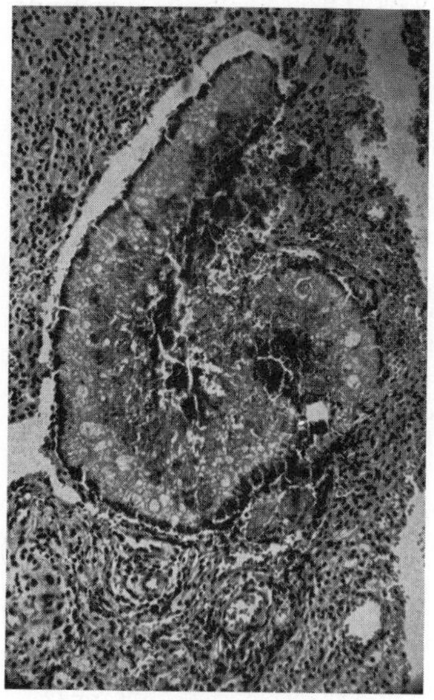

Fig. 83–8. Mycetoma. Section of tissue from foot showing granule. × 112. *(From Fineberg: Am J Clin Pathol 14:239, 1944.)*

7 μm) (Fig. 83–9). At maturity, the cell wall thins, and a pore develops for release of the endospores, which then continue the cycle. The cell wall of the spherule is multilayered and stains with mucicarmine. By contrast, the spherules of *Coccidioides immitis* (Chap. 82) rarely exceed a diameter of 100 μm, rupture to release the endospores, and do not stain with mucicarmine. Rhinosporidial antigen is detectable in patient sera, and the frequency of antigenemia increases with the duration of infection.

Rhinosporidiosis has been treated topically, surgically, and by local injection of ethylstilbamidine.

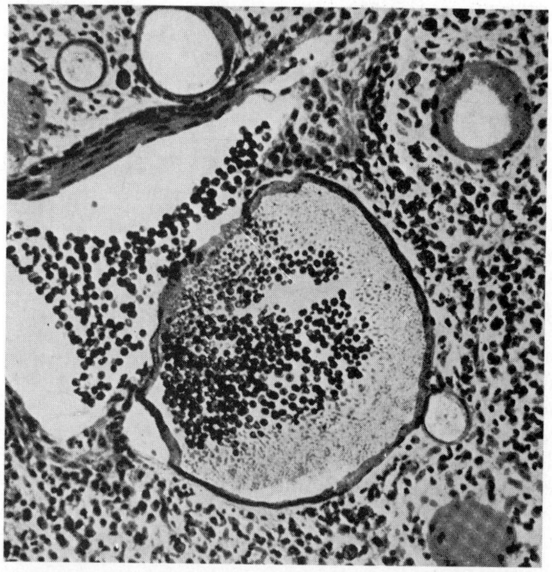

Fig. 83–9. Rhinosporidiosis. Section of nasal polyp showing mature and immature spherules. × 175. *(From Conant et al: Manual of Clinical Mycology, ed 3. Saunders, 1971.)*

Lobomycosis

Loboa loboi. Lobomycosis is a chronic subcutaneous infection of humans and dolphins caused by a fungus named *Loboa loboi* (*Paracoccidioides loboi*). Since its description in 1931 by Lobo, more than 100 additional cases have been reported. Most human cases have occurred in the region of the Amazon River basin among the Caiabi Indians. Most patients have been adults, and almost all have been males. Natural infection has been described in Atlantic bottle-nose dolphins off the coasts of Florida and South America.

Clinical Infection

CLINICAL MANIFESTATIONS. The initial lesions are small, hard subcutaneous nodules usually appearing on the extremities, face, or ear, presumably as a result of traumatic inoculation of the etiologic agent. Lymph nodes are not involved. The infection is chronic and progressive; lesions do not resolve spontaneously but continue to expand gradually over a period of years. There is one case of 50 years' duration. The lesions, which are not painful, may become verrucose or ulcerative and resemble, depending on the duration and tissue response, chromomycosis, mycetoma, or carcinoma.

LABORATORY DIAGNOSIS AND TREATMENT. Lobomycosis is diagnosed by direct, microscopic examination of skin scrapings, biopsies, or wet preparations of exudative lesions. The fungus appears in tissue as large, spherical, or oval yeasts (approximately 10 μm in diameter) that exhibit multiple budding and characteristically form short chains of three to six or more yeast cells. They are multinucleated and thick-walled. Unlike *Paracoccidioides brasiliensis* (Chap. 82), which also produces large, multiply budding yeast cells in tissue, the buds and parent cells of *L. loboi* are the same size. Tissue sections reveal granulomatous nodules and occasional asteroid bodies. The yeasts stain with periodic acid-Schiff or methenamine silver reagents and may be seen inside macrophages. Infected tissues stained with fluorescent antibodies have demonstrated cross-reactions with antigens of many other pathogenic fungi.

The fungal agent of lobomycosis has not been successfully cultured in the laboratory, although it has been maintained in mice by subcutaneous injection of clinical material.

Lobomycosis has been treated with sulfa drugs and surgical excision.

Rhinoentomophthoromycosis

Rhinoentomophthoromycosis (or entomophthoromycosis conidiobolae) is a rare infection of the nasal mucosa caused by *Entomophthora coronata* (*Conidiobolus coronatus*). This fungus is a soil saprophyte and an insect parasite that has been isolated worldwide. *E. coronata* is a zygomycete within the order Entomophthorales (Chap. 80). The first human infection was described in 1965, and since then, over 30 cases have been recognized in Nigeria, elsewhere in Africa, India, and southeast Asia.

Entomophthora coronata. On Sabourand's agar, *E. coronata* produces a fast-growing colony that is flat, glabrous, and colorless or gray to yellow; radial folds and thin aerial hyphae develop. Large, spherical conidia (10 to 20 μm) with hairlike appendages are borne singly on the tips of conidiophores and forcibly ejected at maturity.

Clinical Infection. The disease is confined to the abovementioned tropical areas. Infections are more prevalent among young adult males. Eighty-three percent of the reported cases have occurred in males. Sixty percent of patients have been in their 20s, and only 10% were younger. Rhinoentomophthoromycosis also occurs in horses.

The disease begins with an initial swelling in the nasal area. Hard, subcutaneous nodules develop, and an acute or chronic inflammatory response may ensue. Severe edema of the nose may block the passage of air. The swelling continues to expand, and a large, disfiguring tissue mass develops.

LABORATORY DIAGNOSIS AND TREATMENT. Diagnosis is established by histologic examination of infected tissue and culture. In tissue, numerous branching hyphae approximately 4 to 10 μm in width are observed. These hyphae stain eosinophilically due to the deposition of tissue elements or immune complexes on the walls. An eosinophil infiltrate is often seen, but unlike other zygomycetous pathogens, the blood vessels are not invaded. Specimens are cultured on media without cycloheximide at 25C or 37C. A serologic test for precipitins to *E. coronata* has been reported to be highly specific and sensitive.

Treatment has included surgery, potassium iodide, and amphotericin B.

Subcutaneous Phycomycosis

Subcutaneous phycomycosis (entomophthoromycosis basidiobolae) is a chronic self-limiting infection of the subcutaneous tissue caused by *Basidiobolus haptosporus*. Since the first two cases were described in Indonesia children in 1956, over 100 cases have been reported from Africa (Uganda, Nigeria, Kenya), India, and Indonesia.

Basidiobolus haptosporus. *B. haptosporus*, like the related nonpathogen *Basidiobolus ranarum*, can be isolated from the intestinal tract of beetles, frogs, lizards, and similar creatures. The colony is colorless or brownish, thin, flat, and glabrous. Radial folds develop and become covered with short, white aerial mycelium. The hyphae are 8 to 20 μm wide and produce chlamydospores, forcibly ejected spores, and spherical, smooth-walled zygospores (30 to 50 μm). The zygospores of *B. ranarum* have an undulating wall quite distinct from *B. haptosporus*.

Clinical Infection. This infection is most prevalent in Africa. The highest incidence is among children 5 to 9 years old, and 75% of patients are less than 15 years of age. Seventy to eighty percent of patients are males.

Infection begins on the torso or limb with a small, firm, movable nodule in the subcutaneous tissue. The nodule enlarges, and edema develops and may become massive, involving an entire leg or shoulder. The skin is generally intact but may become very rough. The lesions are not painful; they persist for several months and then resolve spontaneously.

LABORATORY DIAGNOSIS AND TREATMENT. Direct examination of tissue biopsies reveals multiple granulomata, giant cells, and eosinophils. The vasculature is not invaded. Broad, hyaline, branching hyphae (5 to 18 μm wide) with infrequent septa are surrounded by a sheath of eosinophilic material. Specimens are cultured at 25C or 37C on Sabouraud's agar without cycloheximide, and within 2 to 3 days, colonies should appear. An immunodiffusion test has been developed that measures specific precipitins in patient sera.

Potassium iodide is an effective treatment, and the prognosis is very good.

FURTHER READING

Sporotrichosis

Altner PC, Turner RR: Sporotrichosis of bones and joints. Review of the literature and report of six cases. Clin Orthop 68:138, 1979

Auld JL, Beardmore GL: Sporotrichosis in Queensland: A review of 37 cases at the Royal Brisbane Hospital. Aust J Dermatol 29:14, 1979

Beardmore GL: Recalcitrant sporotrichosis: A report of a patient treated with various therapies including oral miconazole and 5-fluorocytosine. Aust J Dermatol 20:10, 1979

Bulmer SO, Kaufman L, Kaplan W, et al: Comparative evaluation of five serological methods for the diagnosis of sporotrichosis. Appl Microbiol 26:4, 1973

Charoenvit Y, Taylor RL: Experimental sporotrichosis in Syrian hamsters. Infect Immun 23:366, 1979

Dellatome DL, Latlanard A, Buckley HR, et al: Fixed cutaneous sporotrichosis of the face. Successful treatment and review of the literature. J Am Acad Dermatol 6:97, 1982

Kaplan W, Invens MS: Fluorescent antibody staining of *Sporotrichosis schenckii* in cultures and clinical material. J Invest Dermatol 35:151, 1961

Kedes KH, Siemienski J, Braude AI: The syndrome of the alcoholic rose gardner: Sporotrichosis of the radial tendon sheath. Ann Intern Med 61:1139, 1964

Kwon-Chung KJ: Comparison of isolates of *Sporothrix schenckii* obtained from fixed cutaneous lesions with isolates from other types of lesions. J Infect Dis 139:424, 1979

Latapi F: Sporotrichose an Mexique. Local Med 34:732, 1963

MacKinnon JE: Ecology and epidemiology of sporotrichosis. In Proceedings of the International Symposium on Mycoses. Washington, DC, Pan Am Health Organization, 1970, p 169

Mariat F: Variant, non-sexue de *Ceratocystis* sp. pathogenic pour-le-hauster. R Acad Sci 260:2329, 1969

Mariat F: Observations sur l'ecologie de *Sporothrix schenckii* et de *Ceratocystis stenoceras* en corse et en Alsace; provinces Francaises indemnes de sporotrichose. Sabouraudi 13:217, 1975

Muller HE: Uber das Vorkommen von Neuraminidase bei *Sporothrix schenckii* und *Ceratocystis stenoceras* und ihre Bedentang fur die Okologie und den Pathomechanismus dieser Pilze. Zentralbl Bakteriol 232:365, 1975

Plouffe JF, Silva J, Fekety R, et al: Cell-mediated immune response in sporotrichosis. J Infect Dis 139:152, 1979

Pluss JL, Opal SM: Pulmonary sporotrichosis: Review of treatment and outcome. Med 65:143, 1986

Powell KE, Taylor A, Phillips BJ, et al: Cutaneous sporotrichosis in forestry workers. JAMA 240:232, 1978

Proceedings of the Transvaal Mine Medical Officers Association: Sporotrichosis infection on mines of the Witwaterstrand, Transvaal Chamber Mines, Johannesburg, 1947

Sanders E: Cutaneous sporotrichosis: beer, bricks, and bumps. Arch Intern Med 127:482, 1971

Sethi KK: Experimental sporotrichosis in the normal and modified host. Sabouraudi 10:66, 1972

Shaw JC, Levinson W, Montanaro A: Sporotrichosis in the acquired immunodeficiency syndrome. J Am Acad Dermatol 21(suppl):1145, 1989

Travassos LR: Antigenic structures of *Sporothrix schenckii*. In Kurstak E (ed): Immunology of Fungal Diseases. New York, Marcel Dekker, 1989, p 193

Travassos LR, Lloyd KO: *Sporothrix schenckii* and related species of *Ceratocystis*. Microbiol Rev 44:683, 1982

Wada R: Studies on mode of action of potassium iodide upon sporotrichosis. Mycopathology 34:97, 1968

Walbaum S, Duriez T, Dujardin L, et al: Etude d'un extrait de *Sporothrix schenckii* (forme levure). Analyse electrophoretique et immunoelectrophoretique; characterisation des activities enzymatiques. Mycopathology 63:105, 1978

Welsh RD, Dolan CT: Sporothrix whole yeast agglutination test. Am J Clin Pathol 59:82, 1973

Wilson DE, Mann JJ, Bennett JE, et al: Clinical features of extracutaneous sporotrichosis. Medicine (Balt) 46:265, 1967

Chromomycosis, Phaeohyphomycosis, Sinusitis, and Opportunistic Mycoses due to Dematiaceous Fungi

Adam RD, Paquin ML, Petersen EA, et al: Phaeohyphomycosis caused by the fungal genera *Bipolaris* and *Exserohilum*. A report of 9 cases and review of the literature. Medicine 65:203, 1986

Alcorn JL: The taxonomy of "*Helminthosporium*" species. Annu Rev Phytopathol 26:37, 1988

Anaissie EJ, Bodey GP, Rinaldi MG: Emerging fungal pathogens. Eur J Clin Microbiol Infect Dis 8:323, 1989

Anaissie E, Bodey GP, Kantarjian HM, et al: New spectrum of fungal infections in patients with cancer. Rev Infect Dis 11:369, 1989

Bansal AS, Prabhakar P: Chromomycosis: A twenty-year analysis of histologically confirmed cases in Jamaica. Trop Geogr Med 41:222, 1989

Bartynski JM, McCaffrey TV, Frigas E: Allergic fungal sinusitis secondary to dermatiaceous fungi—*Curvularia lunata* and *Alternaria*. Otolaryngol Head Neck Surg 103:32, 1990

Connor DH, Gibson DW, Ziefer A: Diagnostic features of three unusual infections: Micronemiasis, pheomycotic cyst, and protothecosis. In Majno G, Cotran RS, Kaufman N (eds): Current Topics in Inflammation and Infection. Baltimore, Williams & Wilkins, 1982, p 205

de Hoog GS, McGinnis MR: Ascomycetous black yeasts. In de Hoog GS, Smith MTh, Weijman ACM (eds): The Expanding Realm of Yeast-like Fungi. Amsterdam, Elsevier Scientific, 1987, p 187

del Palacio-Hernanz A, Moore MK, Campbell CK, et al: Infection of the central nervous system by *Rhinocladiella atrovirens* in a patient with acquire immunodeficiency syndrome. J Med Vet Mycol 27:127, 1989

Dixon DM, Shadomy JH, Shadomy S: Dematiaceous fungal pathogens isolated from nature. Mycopathology 70:153, 1980

Dixon DM, Walsh TJ, Merz WG, McGinnis MR: Infections due to *Xylohypha bantiana* (*Cladosporium trichoides*). Rev Infect Dis 11:515, 1989

Ellis MB: Dematiaceous Hyphomycetes. Kew, Surrey, UK, Commonwealth Mycology Institute, 1971

Ellis MB: More Dematiaceous Hyphomycetes. Kew, Surrey, UK, Commonwealth Mycology Institute, 1976

Espinel-Ingroff A, Shadomy S, Dixon DM, et al: Exoantigen test for *Cladosporium bantianum, Fonsecaea pedrosoi*, and *Phialophora verrucosa* J Clin Microbiol 23:305, 1986

Fader RC, McGinnis MR: Infections caused by dematiaceous fungi: Chromoblastomycosis and phaeohyphomycosis. Infect Dis Clin NA 2:925, 1988

Fukushiro R: Chromoblastomycosis and phaeohyphomycosis. In Kukita A, Seiji M (eds): Proc 16th Internat Cong Dermtol, Tokyo Univ Press, 1983, p 133

Heney C, Song E, Kellen A, et al: Cerebral phaeohyphomycosis caused by *Xylohypha bantiana*. Eur J Clin Microbiol 8:984, 1989

Hohl PE, Holley HP, Prevost E, et al: Infections due to *Wangiella dermatitidis* in humans: Report of the first documented case from the United States and a review of the literature. Rev Infect Dis 5:854, 1983

Kawasaki M, Ishizaki H, Nishimura K, et al: Mitochondrial DNA analysis of *Exophiala jeanselmei* and *Exophiala dermatitidis*. Mycopathology 110:107, 1990

Kotylo PK, Israel KS, Cohen JS, et al: Subcutaneous phaeohyphomycosis of the finger caused by *Exophiala spinifera*. Am J Clin Pathol 91:624, 1989

Kwon-Chung KJ, Wickes BL, Plaskowitz J: Taxonomic clarification of *Cladosporium trichoides* Emmons and its subsequent synonyms. J Med Vet Mycol 27:413, 1989

Maskin SL, Fetchick RJ, Leone CR, Jr et al: *Bipolaris hawaiiensis*-caused phaeohyphomycotic orbitopathy. A devasting fungal sinusitis in an apparently immunocompetent host. Ophthalmology 96:175, 1989

Matsumoto T, Matsuda T: Chromoblastomycosis and phaeohyphomycosis. Semin Dermatol 4:249, 1985

McGinnis MR: Chromoblastomycosis and phaeohyphomycosis: New concepts, diagnosis, and mycology. J Am Acad Dermatol 8:1, 1983

McGinnis MR, Rinaldi MG, Winn RE: Emerging agents of phaeohyphomycosis: Pathogenic species of *Bipolaris* and *Exserohilum*. J Clin Microbiol 24:250, 1986

McGinnis MR, Salkin IF, Schell WA, Parasell L: Dematiaceous fungi. In Balows A, Hausler WJ, Herrmann KL, et al: Manual of Clinical Microbiology, 5th ed. Washington, DC, Am Soc Microbiol, 1991, p 644

Middleton FG, Jurgenson PF, Utz JP, et al: Brain abscess caused by *Cladosporium trichoides*. Arch Intern Med 136:444, 1976

Milam CP, Fenske NA: Chromoblastomycosis. Dermatol Clin 7:219, 1989

Pasarell L, McGinnis MR, Standard PG: Differentiation of medically important isolates of *Bipolaris* and *Exserohilum* with exoantigens. J Clin Microbiol 28:1655, 1990

Polak A: Melanin as a virulence factor in pathogenic fungi. Mycoses 33:215, 1990

Rinaldi MG: Emerging opportunists. Infect Dis Clin North Am 3:65, 1989

Rinaldi MG, Phillips P, Schwartz JG, et al: Human *Curvularia* infections. Report of five cases and review of the literature. Diagn Microbiol Infect Dis 6:27, 1987

Rippon JW: Symposium on medical mycology. The new opportunistic fungal infection: Diagnosis, isolation, identification and impact on mycology. Fear of fungi. Mycopathology 99:143, 1987

Sharkey PK, Graybill JR, Rinaldi MG, et al: Itraconazole treatment of phaeohyphomycosis. J Am Acad Dermatol 23:577, 1990

Terreni AA, DiSalvo AF, Baker AS Jr, et al: Disseminated *Dactylaria gallopava* infection in a diabetic patient with chronic lymphocytic leukemia of the T-cell type. Am J Clin Pathol 94:104, 1990

Tsuneto LT, Arce-Gomez B, Petzl-Erler ML, et al: HLA-A29 and genetic susceptibility to chromoblastomycosis. J Med Vet Mycol 27:181, 1989

Tuffanelli L, Milburn PB: Treatment of chromoblastomycosis. J Am Acad Dermatol 23:728, 1990

Vollum DI: Chromomycosis: A review. Br J Dermatol 96:454, 1977

Other Subcutaneous Mycoses

Baruzzi RG, Marcopito LF, Vicente LS, et al: Jorge Lobo's disease (keloidal blastomycosis) and tinea imbricata in Indians from the Xingu National Park, Central Brazil. Trop Doctor 12:13, 1982

Berenguer J, Diaz-Mediavilla J, Urra D, et al: Central nervous system infection caused by *Pseudallescheria boydii*: Case report and review. Rev Infect Dis 11:890, 1989

Bhawan J, Bain RW, Purtilo DT, et al: Lobomycosis. An electron microscopic, histochemical and immunologic study. J Cutan Pathol 3:5, 1976

Chitravel V, Sundararaj T, Subramanian S, et al: Detection of circulating antigen in patients with rhinosporidosis. Sabouraudi 20:185, 1982

Clark BM: The epidemiology of phycomycosis. In Wolstenholme GE, Porter R (eds): Symposium on Systemic Mycoses. Boston, Little, Brown, 1968, p 179

Fuchs J, Milbrandt R, Pecher SA: Lobomycosis (keloidal blastomycosis): Case reports and overview. Cutis 46:227, 1990

Jaramillo D, Cortes A, Restrepo A, et al: Lobomycosis. Report of the eighth Colombian case and review of the literature. J Cutan Pathol 3:180, 1976

Joe LK, Njo-Injo TE, Kjokronegro S, et al: *Basidiobolus ranarum* as a cause of subcutaneous phycomycosis in Indonesia. Arch Dermatol 74:378, 1956

Kaufman L, Mendoza L, Standard PG: Immunodiffusion test for serodiagnosis subcutaneous zygomycosis. J Clin Microbiol 28:1887, 1990

Lasser A, Smith HW: Rhinosporidiosis. Arch Otolaryngol 102:308, 1976

Levy MG, Meuten DJ, Breitschwerdt EB: Cultivation of *Rhinosporidium seeberi* in vitro: Interaction with epithelial cells. Science 234:474, 1986

Lobo J: Um caso de blastomicose produzida por uma especie nora, encontrada em Recife. Rev Med Pernambuco 1:763, 1931

Lutwick LI, Galgiani JN, Johnson RH, et al: Visceral fungal infections due to *Petriellidium boydii*. Am J Med 61:632, 1976

Mahgoub ES: Mycetoma. Semin Dermatol 4:230, 1985

Mariat F, Destombes P, Segretain G: The mycetomas: Clinical features, pathology, etiology and epidemiology. Contrib Microbiol Immunol 4:1, 1977

Martinson FD, Clark BM: Rhinophycomycosis entomophthorae in Nigeria. Am J Trop Med Hyg 16:40, 1967

McGinnis MR, Fader RC: Mycetoma: A contemporary concept. Infect Dis Clin North Am 2:939, 1988

Schell WA, McGinnis MR: Molds involved in subcutaneous infections. In Wentworth BB (ed): Diagnostic Procedures for Mycotic and Parasitic Infections, ed 7. Washington, DC, Am Public Health Assoc, 1988, p 99

Schwartz DA, Amenta PS, Finkelstein SD: Cerebral *Pseudallescheria boydii* infection: Unique occurrence of fungus ball formation in the brain. Clin Neurol Neurosurg 91:79, 1989

Seeber GR: Un neuvo esporozuario parasito del hombre. Dos casos encontrades en polipos nasales. Tesis. Univ Nat de Buenos Aires, 1900

Sesso A, Baruzzi RG: Interaction between macrophage and parasite cells in lobomycosis. The thickened cell wall of *Paracoccidioides loboi* exhibits apertures to the extracellular milieu. J Submicrosc Cytol Pathol 20:537, 1988

Travis LB, Roberts GD, Wilson WR: Clinical significance of *Pseudallescheria boydii*: A review of 10 years' experience. Mayo Clin Proc 60:531, 1985

Vanbreuseghem R: Rhinosporidiose: Klinischer Aspekt, Epidemiologic and ultrastrukturelle Studien von *Rhinosporidum seeberi*. Dermatol Monatsschr 162:512, 1976

Yangco GB, Nettlow A, Ikafor JI, et al: Comparative antigenic studies of species of *Basidiobolus* and other medically important fungi. J Clin Microbiol 23:674, 1986

Yoo D, Lee WHS, Kwon-Chung KJ: Brain abscesses due to *Pseudallescheria boydii* associated with primary non-Hodgkins lymphoma of the central nervous system: a case report and literature review. Rev Infect Dis 7:272, 1985

CHAPTER 84

Dermatophytosis and Other Cutaneous Mycoses

Dermatophytosis

Dermatophytosis is an infection of the skin, hair, or nails by any of a group of keratinophilic fungi called *dermatophytes*. Dermatophytes parasitize the nonliving, cornified integument. They secrete keratinases, which are proteolytic enzymes that digest keratin, the structural protein of hair, nails, and epidermis. Species of dermatophytes, of which 40 to 50 are recognized, are relatively similar in their morphology, physiology, and biochemical composition. They cause a variety of specific clinical conditions. A single species may be able to produce several types of distinctive skin diseases, and, conversely, several dermatophyte species may be etiologic agents of the same disease.

Dermatophytoses are among the most prevalent infections in the world. Though they are extremely annoying and millions of dollars are spent annually in their treatment, with few exceptions they are not debilitating or life threatening. The incidence varies considerably. The attack rate is higher in institutions and under crowded living conditions. Among military personnel in the United States and England, there is a prevalence of 17% to 24%, but the incidence among service personnel in the tropics increases to 60% to 80%.

Because dermatophytes produce visible lesions, these infections have been observed throughout history and recorded since antiquity. Dermatophyte, or ringworm, infections were the first recognized infectious diseases of humans. During the 1840s, several European physicians independently recognized that ringworm infections were caused by fungi that could be cultivated on artificial media and that these fungi could produce similar infections in healthy skin. These observations represent the first documentation of Koch's postulates some 40 years before Koch formulated them!

Dermatophytes are highly specialized for the infection of skin. If animals are infected by the parenteral route, systemic infection does not occur. This restriction is probably related both to host defenses (e.g., serum growth inhibitor) and fungal properties (e.g., affinity for keratin, inhibition of growth at 37C). The fungistatic property of normal serum has been attributed to transferrin, which chelates iron, an essential growth requirement for fungi, and which may also inhibit fungi by a more direct mechanism.

For more than 100 years, dermatophytes have been isolated and identified. Their speciation, geographic distribution, and clinical manifestations have been subjected to many investigations. Three genera and 42 species of dermatophytes are recognized by most taxonomists: 22 species of *Trichophyton*, 18 species of *Microsporum*, and 2 species of *Epidermophyton*.

Dermatophytes

Biologic Properties

The dermatophytes are unique in several respects. Most pathogenic fungi are acquired exogenously. With the exception of certain yeasts, pathogenic fungi are predominantly saprophytes that live in nature and accidently cause infection—that is, infection represents a transient alteration in the normal life cycle, transmission does not occur, and infection is not advantageous for the fungus. However, dermatophytes appear to be evolving a more permanent and benign host-parasite relationship.

Taxonomy. The genera *Trichophyton*, *Microsporum*, and *Epidermophyton* are all classified within the subdivision Deuteromycotina (Chap. 80). Since 1959, the teleomorph, or sexual reproductive, state of a number of specific dermatophytes has been discovered. Such species subsequently have been reclassified and renamed, but because of common usage, the old names have been retained. All of the species of *Trichophyton* for which a teleomorph has been discovered have been reclassified within the new genus *Arthroderma*. The teleomorph of *Microsporum* species was represented by the genus *Nannizzia*, but these species are not also included in the genus *Arthroderma*, which further reflects the close relationships among the dermatophytes. Since *Arthroderma* produces ascospores inside a cleistothecium (Chap. 80), it is placed within the family Gymnoascaceae in the subdivision Ascomycotina. This family also contains the etiologic agents of histoplasmosis and blastomycosis. The teleomorph has been described for at least 23 species of dermatophytes.

Sexual Reproduction. To observe the teleomorph in the laboratory, two compatible (opposite) mating types of the

TABLE 84–1. DISTINGUISHING MORPHOLOGIC AND PHYSIOLOGIC CHARACTERISTICS OF COMMON DERMATOPHYTES

Species	Culture[a]	Micromorphology
Epidermophyton floccosum	Slow growth; surface fluffy to powdery to velvety, flat or folded, tan to olive-green, reverse yellow to tan	Macroconidia: clavate, 2–4 cells, thin, smooth walls, borne in clusters; no microconidia
Microsporum audouinii	Slow growth; flat, silky; surface cream to brown, reverse red-brown; on rice, no growth but brown color	Conidia rare, chlamydospores
Microsporum canis var *canis*	Rapid growth; surface cottony white, reverse deep yellow	Macroconidia; spindle shaped, more than 6 cells, thick, rough wall
Microsporum canis var *distortum*	Surface white to yellow, folded or flat; good growth on rice	Macroconidia: highly distorted, thick, rough wall
Microsporum cookei	Rapid growth; surface flat, powdery, and white to yellow or pink, reverse red	Macroconidia; 6–8 cells, thick, rough wall; many microconidia
Microsporum ferrigineum	Slow growth; surface smooth, folded, and yellow	No conidia; distorted hyphae
Microsporum gallinae	Rapid growth; surface whitish, reverse pigment diffusible red	Macroconidia: clavate, 2–10 cells
Microsporum gypseum	Rapid growth; surface powdery, tan	Macroconidia: 3–9 cells, thin, rough wall; microconidia: rare, clavate
Microsporum nanum	Rapid growth; surface powdery white, yellow, or pinkish, reverse pink to brown	Macroconidia: 1–2 cells, thin, rough wall; microconidia: clavate
Microsporum vanbreuseghemii	Rapid growth; surface fluffy or powdery, tan, reverse colorless to yellow	Macroconidia: cylindrical, 5–12 cells, thick, rough wall; microconidia: pyriform
Trichophyton ajelloi	Rapid growth; surface flat; cream to tan, reverse colorless to red to black	Macroconidia: numerous, 5–12 cells, thick, smooth wall; microconidia; pyriform
Trichophyton equinum	Rapid growth; surface flat to fluffy, reverse yellow to brown, diffusible; requires nicotinic acid	Microconidia: small, pyriform; macroconidia: rare
Trichophyton megninii	Slow growth, nondiffusible red pigment; requires histidine	Microconidia: pyriform; macroconidia: rare
Trichophyton mentagrophytes	Surface flat; white to yellow, either cottony and downy (var. *interdigitale*) or powdery and granular (var. *mentagrophytes*)	Microconidia: numerous, single or in clusters, spherical; macroconidia: rare, 2–5 cells, spiral hyphae common
Trichophyton rubrum	Slow growth; surface fluffy, white, reverse deep red, nondiffusible pigment; rare isolates yellow powdery	Microconidia: pyriform, small; macroconidia: rare, pencil-shaped, 3–5 cells
Trichophyton schoenleinii	Slow growth; surface compact, white to tan, folded; 37C growth	Conidia: rare; chlamydospores; swollen, knobby hyphae (chandeliers)
Trichophyton tonsurans	Slow growth; surface flat, powdery to velvety, reverse yellow to brown-red; requires thiamine	Microconidia: mostly elongate; macroconidia: rare
Trichophyton verrucosum	Slow growth; surface heaped, wrinkled; requires thiamine and inositol; 37C growth	Conidia: rare; distorted hyphae; chlamydospores in chains at 37C
Trichophyton violaceum	Slow growth; surface heaped, folded; purple; requires thiamine	Conidia: rare

[a] Growth on Sabouraud's dextrose agar at 25C for 2 weeks.

species are required. These mating types are designated "+" and "−", and when they are mixed together on a suitable medium (e.g., moist, sterile soil and hair), they will develop characteristic cleistothecia containing asci and ascospores. The sexual state provides an epidemiologic marker because each species has two mating types. Furthermore, because mating occurs only within the species, sexual reproduction may be used to identify the isolates that undergo sexual reproduction.

Morphology and Physiology. As might be expected from their close taxonomic relatedness, the dermatophytes are very similar in their physiology, growth requirements, morphology, antigenicity, and infectivity. The most distinctive physiologic property of the dermatophytes is their ability to digest keratin. Only a few insects and certain other microorganisms have this capability. Differences in the nutritional requirements of the various dermatophyte species are few, but the differences that do exist, such as a requirement for thiamine or histidine, are used in their identification. Dermatophytes also share a number of surface antigens, both within this group and with several saprophytic fungi. However, despite these marked similarities, subtle but important differences do exist among these fungi, such as the specificity for keratinaceous substrates and the types of conidia produced.

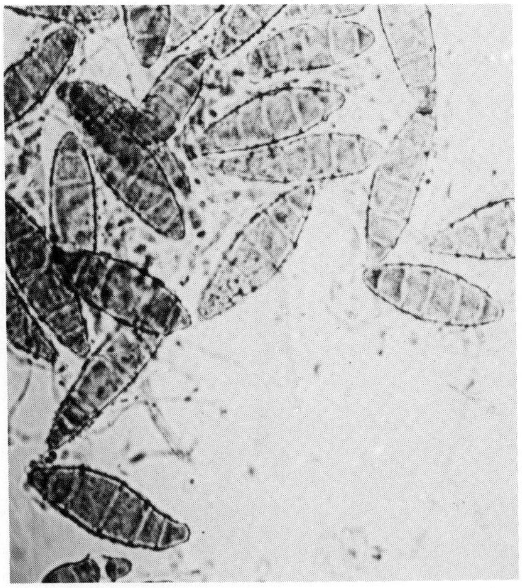

Fig. 84–2. *Microsporum gypseum.* Typical rough, thin-walled macroconidia. × 1000.

Identification. The common dermatophytes are identified on the basis of their colonial appearance and microscopic morphology, as indicated in Table 84–1. *Microsporum* species tend to produce distinctive holothallic, multicellular macroconidia with echinulate or rough walls (Figs. 84–1 and 84–2). *Trichophyton* species develop cylindrical, smooth-walled macroconidia, and characteristic microconidia (Figs. 84–3 and 84–4). Both types of conidia are borne singly in these genera. *Epidermophyton floccosum* produces only macroconidia, which are smooth-walled and clavate; they are produced in groups of two or three (Fig. 84–5). A few nutritional tests are also useful. For example, *Trichophyton tonsurans*, *Trichophyton violaceum*, and *Trichophyton verrucosum* require thiamine, and most strains of *T. verrucosum* also require inositol. Strains of some species can be quite similar in morphology and may be distinguished with specialized tests, such as growth on rice grains (*Microsporum canis* vs *Microsporum audouinii*), in vitro hair perforation (*Trichophyton mentagrophytes* vs *Trichophyton rubrum*), and enhanced growth at 37C (*T. verrucosum* vs *Trichophyton schoenleinii* and *T. tonsurans*).

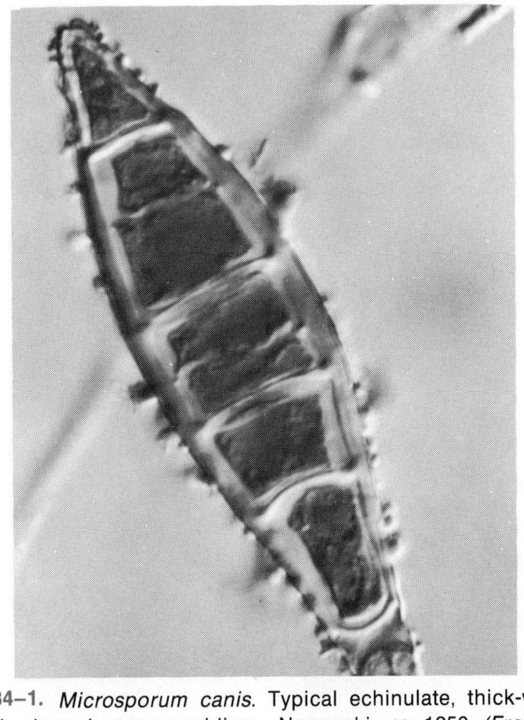

Fig. 84–1. *Microsporum canis.* Typical echinulate, thick-walled, spindle-shaped macroconidium. Nomarski. × 1250 *(From McGinnis: Laboratory Handbook of Medical Mycology. Academic Press*, 1979.)

Clinical Infection

Epidemiology and Ecology. The natural reservoirs of most of the dermatophytes that have been implicated in human infection are given in Table 84–2. Dermatophytes are classified as geophilic, zoophilic, or anthropophilic, depending on whether their usual habitat is soil, animals, or humans. Many dermatophytes whose natural reservoir is soil or animals are still able to cause human infection. Evidence supports the concept that dermatophytes have evolved from geophilism to zoophilism to anthropophilism. In general, as species evolve from habitation in soil to a specific human or animal host, a decrease in both sporulation (asexual and sexual) and host toxicity occurs. Anthropophilic species tend to produce relatively mild and chronic infections in humans, whereas zoophilic dermatophytes cause infections that are more inflammatory and acute. The latter respond better to treatment and usually do not recur. Some anthropophilic species (e.g., *M. audouinii*) apparently survive exclusively by transmission from one human to another. Other dermatophytes not listed in Table 84–2 have been recovered from soil and never implicated in human or animal infection. About 11 species are responsible

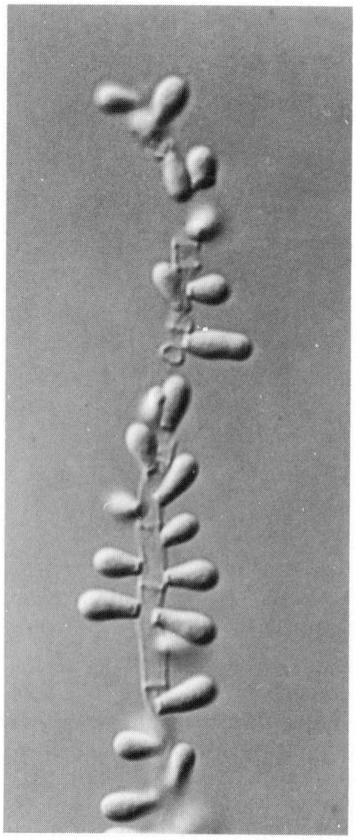

Fig. 84–3. *Trichophyton rubrum.* Typical pyriform and clavate microconidia. Nomarski. × 1250. *(Courtesy of Dr. Michael R. McGinnis.)*

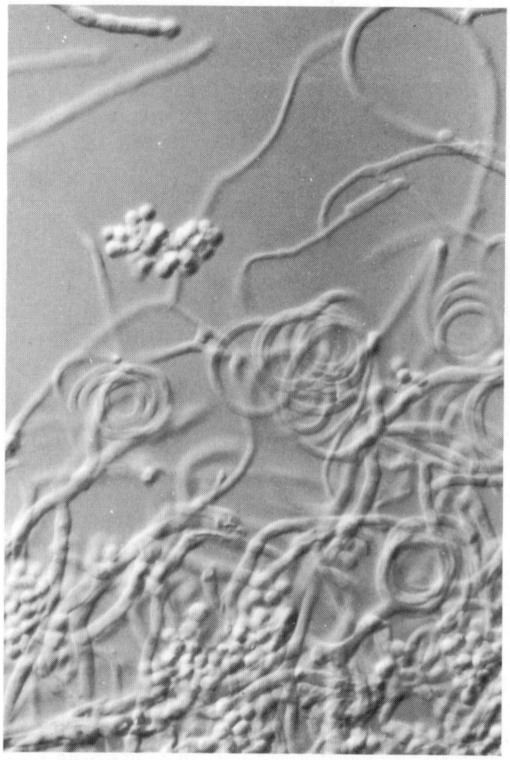

Fig. 84–4. *Trichophyton mentagrophytes.* Clusters of spherical microconidia and coiled hyphae. Nomarski. × 500. *(Courtesy of Dr. Michael R. McGinnis.)*

for the majority of human dermatophytoses throughout the world, and only about 6 species are endemic in the United States. The distribution of dermatophyte species in specific environments and the specialization for certain host species or tissues present a fascinating balance between pathogen and host.

An understanding of the particular evolution and diversity among dermatophytes provides useful clinical information of prognostic value, such as (1) the duration of the infection, (2) the probability of recurrence, (3) the severity of the infection, and (4) the source of the dermatophyte. For example, if a child develops tinea capitis caused by the anthropophilic dermatophyte *M. audouinii*, the infection will probably be self-limiting but will spread to the child's siblings. If the agent is *M. canis*, the lesion will be more inflammatory, and the family dog or cat should be treated to prevent recurrent infections.

Pathogenesis and Immunity. Certain etiologic agents are endemic only in specific geographic areas (Table 84–2). Exposure to geophilic and zoophilic species follows contact with dermatophytes in soil or on animals, respectively. Anthropophilic species may be transmitted by direct contact or fomites.

Dermatophyte infections begin in the cutaneous tissue after contact and trauma. Various studies have shown that host susceptibility may be enhanced by moisture, warmth, specific skin chemistry, composition of sebum and perspiration, youth, heavy exposure, and genetic predisposition. The incidence is higher in hot, humid climates and under crowded

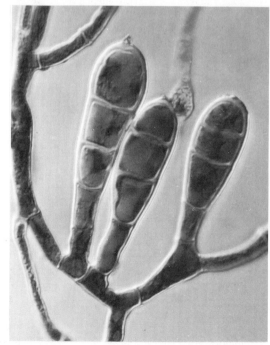

Fig. 85–5. *Epipermophyton floccusum.* Typical clavate macroconidia. Nomarski. × 1250. *(From McGinnis: Laboratory Handbook of Medical Mycology. Academic Press, 1979.)*

TABLE 84–2. ECOLOGY OF HUMAN DERMATOPHYTE SPECIES

Anthropophilic	Zoophilic	Geophilic
Species Found Worldwide		
Epidermophyton floccosum *Microsporum audouinii* *Trichophyton mentagrophytes* var *interdigitale* *Trichophyton rubrum* *Trichophyton schoenleinii* *Trichophyton tonsurans* *Trichophyton violaceum*	*Microsporum canis* (dogs, cats) *Microsporum gallinae* (fowl) *Microsporum nanum*[a] (pigs) *Microsporum persicolor* (moles) *Trichophyton equinum* (horses) *Trichophyton mentagrophytes* var *mentagrophytes* (rodents) *Trichophyton verrucosum* (cattle)	*Microsporum gypseum* *Microsporum fulvum* *Microsporum nanum*[a] *Trichophyton ajelloi* *Trichophyton terrestre*
Rare and Geographically Limited Species		
Microsporum ferrugineum, Far East, Africa, Asia, Europe *Trichophyton concentricum,* Far East, Central and South America *Trichophyton gourvillii,* Africa *Trichophyton megninii,* Europe, Africa *Trichophyton soudanense,* Africa, Europe *Tricohphyton yaoundei,* Africa	*Microsporum distortum* (monkeys), Australia, New Zealand *Trichophyton mentagophytes* var *erinacei* (hedgehogs), Europe, Australia, New Zealand *T. mentagrophytes* var *quinckaenum* (mice), Europe, Australia *Trichophyton simii* (monkeys), India	*Microsporum rademosum,* Europe, North and South America *Microsporum vanbreuseghemii,* Africa, Europe, North America

[a] *Microsporum nanum* can be isolated from human, animal (pigs), and soil habitats.

living conditions. Patients with genetic or acquired cellular immunodeficiency and patients with familial endocrinopathies (e.g., Cushing's syndrome) are predisposed to chronic dermatophytosis.

Several studies have documented poor cell-mediated immune responses to dermatophytic antigens in patients who develop chronic, noninflammatory dermatophyte infections (Table 84–3). Most *trichophytins* are prepared from mycelial extracts, culture filtrates, or both and contain mixtures of unpurified polysaccharides, proteins, and glycoproteins with multiple epitopes. These patients often have immediate skin test reactivity to dermatophytic antigens, elevated IgE, and multiple allergies. Reactions to heterologous antigens are normal. Sera from patients with chronic infections inhibit cell-mediated immunity, perhaps because of the presence of immune complexes or other blocking factors. Patients with acute dermatophytosis have normal immune responses, and both types of patients develop normal IgG antibody titers to dermatophytic antigens.

In the normal host, immunity to dermatophytosis is relative. Data from animal studies suggest that infection confers increased resistance to reinfection. Subsequent infections require a larger inoculum and have a shorter duration.

Clinical Manifestations. The clinical forms of dermatophytoses were erroneously termed *ringworm* or *tinea* because of the raised circular lesion (Table 84–4). Tinea capitis is dermatophytosis of the scalp and hair, which appears as dull, gray, circular patches of alopecia, scaling, and itching. Species of *Microsporum* or *Trichophyton* may cause tinea capitis. Zoophilic species may induce a severe combined inflammatory and hypersensitivity reaction, called a *kerion.* Epidemic tinea capitis in prepubescent children is self-limiting and caused by *T. tonsurans* or, now rarely, *M. audouinii* in the United States.

TABLE 84–3. CLINICAL AND IMMUNOLOGIC COMPARISON OF ACUTE AND CHRONIC DERMATOPHYTOSES

Feature	Acute Infection	Chronic Infection
Etiology	Geophilic or zoophilic species	Anthropophilic species
Inflammation	Severe	Mild
Signs and symptoms	Erythema, vesicles, pruritus, pain	Erythema, scaling, pruritus
Spread of lesions	Usually limited	Often extensive
Duration	Weeks	Months to years
Incidence of skin test reactivity to trichophytin		
Type I immediate	Low	High
Type IV delayed	High	Low
T cell responses in vitro		
To trichophytin	High	Low
To other antigens	Normal	Normal
Incidence of atopy or elevated IgE	Normal (8–10%)	High (ca. 50%)
Prognosis (response to therapy)	Good	Poor
Recurrence	Rare	Frequent

TABLE 84–4. CLINICAL CLASSIFICATION OF THE DERMATOPHYTOSES

Clinical Name	Site of Lesions	Organisms Most Frequently Isolated
Tinea capitis, epidemic	Scalp	*Trichophyton tonsurans, Microsporum audouinii* (US), *Trichophyton violaceum, Microsporum ferrugineum* (outside US)
Tinea capitis, nonepidemic	Scalp	*Microsporum canis, Trichophyton verrucosum, Microsporum gypseum* (rare)
Tinea favosa (favus)	Scalp, torso	*Trichophyton schoenleinii, Trichophyton violaceum*
Tinea barbae	Beard	*Trichophyton rubrum, Trichophyton verrucosum*
Tinea corporis	Arms, legs, torso	*Trichophyton rubrum, Microsporum canis, Trichophyton mentagrophytes*
Tinea cruris	Genitocrural folds	*Trichophyton rubrum, Trichophyton mentagrophytes, Epidermophyton floccosum*
Tinea pedis and manus	Feet, hands	*Trichophyton rubrum, Trichophyton mentagrophytes*
Tinea unguium	Nails	*Trichophyton rubrum, Trichophyton mentagrophytes, Epidermophyton floccosum*
Tinea imbricata	Torso	*Trichophyton concentricum*

Favus is an acute inflammatory infection of the hair and follicle caused by *T. schoenleinii* and similar dermatophytes.

Tinea barbae, tinea corporis, and tinea manum are caused by *T. rubrum* (80%), *T. mentagrophytes* var *interdigitale* (10%), or *E. floccosum* (5%). Classic lesions on glabrous skin are annular and scaly, and they may be embellished with erythema, vesicles, or allergic reactions. The thickness and duration of the lesion and extent of the inflammatory response are determined by the nature of the dermatophyte-host interaction (keratinases, toxins, antigens). Tinea cruris, or jock itch, is caused by the same three dermatophytes. Most cases (99%) occur in males as a dry expanding lesion in the groin.

Tinea pedis (athlete's foot) occurs as a chronic involvement of the toe webs. Other forms are vesicular, ulcerative, or moccasin type, with hyperkeratosis of the sole.

Tinea unguium, or onychomycosis, is most often caused by *T. rubrum* or *T. mentagrophytes*. Nails may show white, patchy, or pitted lesions on the surface. Hyphal invasion beneath the nail results in digestion, discoloration, and deformation of the nail.

A *dermatophytid*, or id, reaction is an allergic response to fungal antigens. A dermatophyte infection in one area (e.g., tinea pedis) elicits an allergic reaction elsewhere (e.g., the hands).

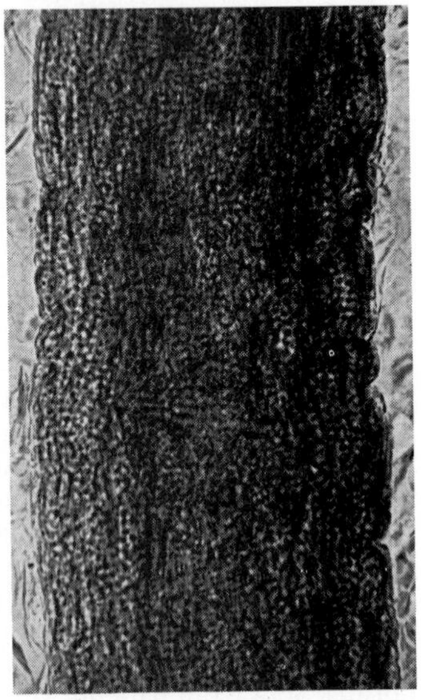

Fig. 84–6. Endothrix involvement of hair caused by *Trichophyton tonsurans*. Arthroconidia are formed inside the hair. × 170. *(From Conant et al: Manual of Clinical Mycology, ed 3. Saunders,* 1971.)

Laboratory Diagnosis

DIRECT EXAMINATION. Cases of suspected tinea capitis should be examined under Wood's light (365 nm), where hairs infected with *Microsporum* species or *T. schoenleinii* exhibit a greenish fluorescence. Hairs can be examined directly under the microscope for *endothrix* involvement, the formation of arthroconidia within the hair shaft (Fig. 84–6), or *ectothrix* infection, a sheath of spores around the shaft (Fig. 84–7). *T. tonsurans* and *T. violaceum* produce endothrix infections, whereas other hair infections are of the ectothrix type. Favic hairs present characteristic air spaces in the hair (Fig. 84–8).

Skin and nail infections may be diagnosed by dissolving skin scrapings or nail clippings in 10% or 20% potassium hydroxide (KOH) and looking for hyaline, branched, septate hyphae among the squamous epithelial cells (Fig. 84–9). Calcofluor white will also stain the fungi within hair, skin, or nail.

The id reaction is diagnosed on the basis of a negative

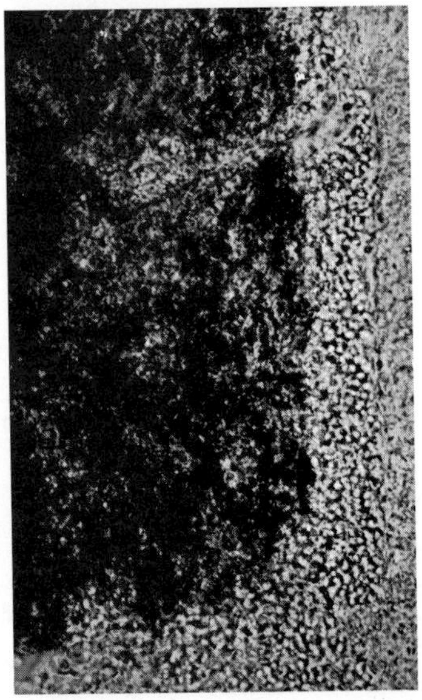

Fig. 84–7. Ecothrix involvement of hair caused by *Microsporum audouinii*. Conidia are around the partially digested hair shaft. × 350.

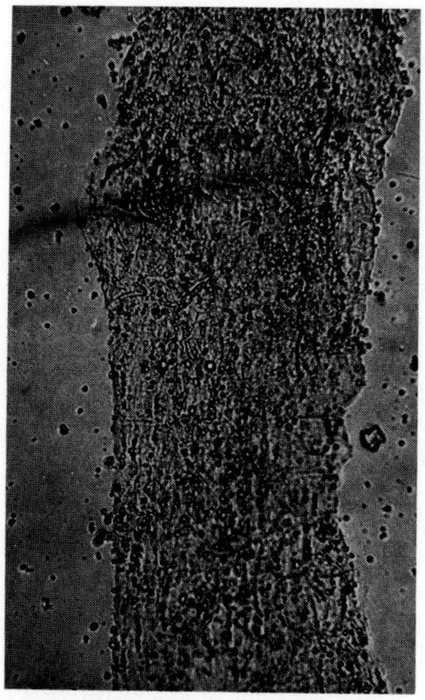

Fig. 84–8. Favic involvement of hair by *Trichophyton schoenleinii*. Hyphae and air spaces in hair shaft. × 170.

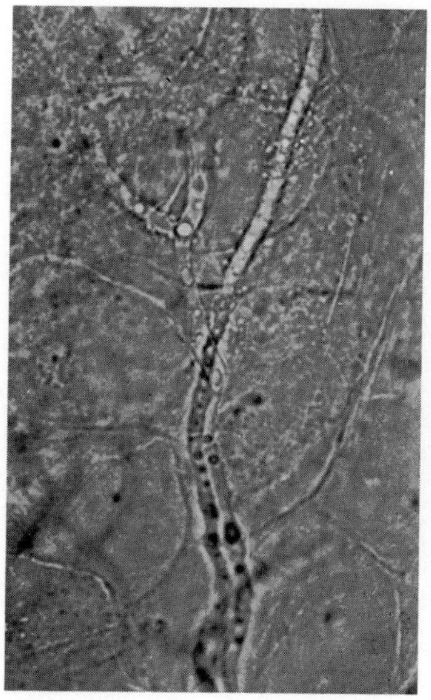

Fig. 84–9. Dermatophytosis. Branching hypha seen in potassium hydroxide preparation of the skin. × 275.

microscopic and cultural examination of the site and finding of dermatophytosis elsewhere on the body.

CULTURE. Hair, skin, or nail specimens should be cultured at 25C to 30C on Inhibitory Mold or Sabouraud's agar with antibiotics. Isolates are identified on the basis of colony appearance (growth rate, surface texture, obverse and reverse pigmentation) and morphology of reproductive structures (Table 84–1). Although designed as a selective medium for dermatophytes, the formulation dermatophyte test medium, which contains antibiotics and a pH indicator, is not specific for dermatophytes.

Treatment. Dermatophytoses of the skin may be treated with multiple daily applications of topical antibiotics, such as cream preparations of tolnaftate, miconazole nitrate, haloprogin, clotrimazole, econazole, or ciclopirox. The most effective antibiotic is griseofulvin, which is given orally for long periods. This poorly absorbed drug is concentrated in the stratum corneum, where it inhibits hyphal growth. The adult dosage is 250 to 500 mg per day of the ultramicrosized form. Scalp and nail infections require griseofulvin. Tinea corporis or tinea capitis is usually cleared with a 2 to 6 week course of griseofulvin. Nail infections may require a year or longer. Recent trials have confirmed that oral ketoconazole is highly effective in some patients.

Pityriasis Versicolor

Pityriasis versicolor (or tinea versicolor) is a chronic and nonirritating superficial infection of the stratum corneum caused by *Malassezia furfur (Pityrosporum orbiculare)*. Invasion of the cornified skin and the host responses are both minimal. Discrete, serpentine, hyperpigmented or depigmented maculae occur on the skin, usually on the chest, upper back, arms, or abdomen. *M. furfur* may also cause folliculitis, opportunistic fungemia, and possibly seborrheic dermatitis or dandruff.

Malassezia furfur. Lipid fractions of *M. furfur* contain high concentrations of C_9 to C_{14} dicarboxylic acids, which are competitive inhibitors of tyrosinase in vitro and may explain the depigmentation of lesions.

P. orbiculare and *Pityrosporum ovale* are lipophilic yeasts and part of the normal microbial flora of the skin and scalp. Originally isolated by Gordon on Sabouraud's medium supplemented with olive oil, *Pityrosporum* can use a variety of fatty acids. Colonies have a yeastlike consistency. Microscopically, *P. orbiculare* produces spherical cells and *P. ovale* produces ovoid or cylindrical cells. The name originally applied to the fungus observed in lesions of pityriasis versicolor was *M. furfur*. The consensus is the *M. furfur* and *P. orbiculare* are identical, as suggested by indirect fluorescent antibody studies of infected skin scales and by experimental infections. *P. orbiculare* and *P. ovale* are probably a single species also.

Clinical Infection. The incidence of pityriasis versicolor increases where the climate is hot and humid and is highest in the tropics. Several studies have indicated a physiologic predisposition to this infection (e.g., excessive perspiration, corticosteroids, malnutrition, and heredity). Its occurrence has been related to the presence of certain amino acids and hydrophobic compounds on the skin, as well as to a decrease in the epithelial turnover in the stratum corneum.

The lesions occur as macular patches of discolored skin that may enlarge and coalesce, but scaling, inflammation, and irritation are usually minimal. Patients seek medical care for cosmetic reasons. The affected skin does not suntan well, and therefore the lesions become more pronounced in the summer.

Two more severe infections due to *M. furfur* are recognized. Variously compromised patients are prone to a more inflammatory folliculitis. Second, lipid emulsions used for parenteral nutrition are an excellent growth medium for *M. furfur*. Both infants and adults receiving this treatment have acquired systemic infections with *M. furfur* resulting from contamination of the lipid emulsion or intravenous catheter.

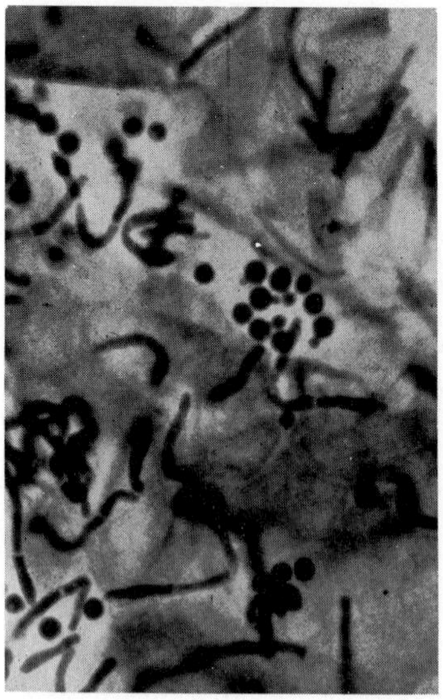

Fig. 84–10. *Malassezia furfur.* Clusters of spherical cells and short hyphae in skin scrapings from pityriasis versicolor. × 736.

Patients were treated by removal of the catheter and, in some cases, with amphotericin B. A related species *Malassezia pachydermatis*, which is distinguished by not requiring added lipid for growth, may similarly cause fungemia.

LABORATORY DIAGNOSIS AND TREATMENT. Diagnosis of pityriasis versicolor is established by direct microscopic examination of skin scrapings of the infected skin, which has been digested with 10% KOH or stained with calcofluor white or both. The finding of short unbranched hyphae and spherical cells is diagnostic of pityriasis versicolor (Fig. 84–10). Because the clinical appearance and microscopic examination are so characteristic, cultures on a medium with lipid substrate are not required to establish the diagnosis. Indeed, the meaning of a positive culture of *M. furfur* is dubious, as it can also be recovered from normal skin. A golden yellow fluorescence extending beyond the periphery of the lesions may be observed under Wood's light.

The usual treatment is topical application of 2.5% selenium sulfide for 10 minutes daily for 7 days. Lesions may remain clear for a year or longer. Lesions have also resolved with topical miconazole and ketoconazole and oral ketoconazole or itraconazole. Folliculitis can be treated with oral ketoconazole.

Tinea Nigra

Tinea nigra (or tinea nigra palmaris) is a superficial, chronic, and asymptomatic infection of the stratum corneum caused by the dematiaceous yeast, *Phaeoannellomyces werneckii* (previously, *Exophiala werneckii*). This fungus, which is a ubiquitous saprophyte in nature, is dimorphic. It converts from yeast to mycelial growth with age, although both forms are usually observed.

Phaeoannellomyces werneckii. *P. werneckii* is a dematiaceous fungus (Chap. 83). The colony initially is shiny, moist, and often white to gray in color. Within a few days, the colony darkens and becomes olive to black. Later, mycelium develops, and the colony appears dull and fuzzy. Microscopically, *P. werneckii* initially produces budding yeasts and chains of yeast cells. Hyphae then develop, and a mixture of variably pigmented hyphae and yeasts is common. Conidia are produced by annellides.

Clinical Infection. Tinea nigra is most frequently found in tropical areas. It is prevalent in Florida and other warm, coastal regions. Approximately 95% of cases occur in teenagers, and 75% are in women. Lesions usually consist of a solitary, innocuous macule with sharply defined margins, which spreads by expansion. The brownish color of the lesion is darkest at the advancing periphery, where most of the actively growing organisms are located. Although many cases involve the palms, other areas of glabrous skin may also be infected, including the fingers and face. The lesions resemble a faded silver nitrate stain. As tinea nigra may also resemble melanoma and other types of skin cancer, it is important to establish a diagnosis.

Diagnosis is easily confirmed by direct KOH or calcofluor white examination and culture of skin scrapings from the periphery of the lesions. Microscopic examination of skin scales reveals brown-pigmented, branched, septate hyphae and budding yeast cells (1 to 5 μm in diameter). The hyphae may be distorted, but the brown color excludes a diagnosis of dermatophytosis, candidiasis, or pityrasis versicolor. Culture of skin on Sabouraud's medium with and without antibiotics should recover *P. werneckii.*

Tinea nigra responds well to topical keratolytic solutions of sulfur, salicylic acid, or tincture of iodine. Recurrence is thought to be due to reinfection.

Mycotic Keratitis

Mycotic keratitis (or keratomycosis) refers to fungous infections of the cornea. Many patients have a history of trauma leading to inoculation of the eye with a fungus. The etiologic agent is introduced from an exogenous source, and most are normally saprophytic fungi, although *Histoplasma capsulatum* and other frankly pathogenic fungi have been known to cause primary keratomycosis. Conversely, endophthalmitis usually represents the ocular manifestations of a systemic mycosis and occurs not infrequently with systemic candidiasis, histoplasmosis, and other systemic mycoses.

Many cases of keratomycosis in the United States are caused by *Fusarium solani.* Others are attributed to other *Fusarium* species and related saprophytes, including dematiaceous fungi (e.g., *Alternaria*) and yeasts (e.g., *Candida*).

Keratomycosis occurs more often in males and individuals below the age of 50 years. Lesions appear as raised corneal ulcers with occasional satellite lesions, plaques, or hypopyon. Diagnosis is established by direct examination of corneal scrapings or surgical specimens for the presence of hyphae. *Fusarium* species grow rapidly in Sabouraud's or enriched media, and most specimens yield positive culture.

The treatment of choice is pimaricin, a tetracene antibiotic, administered topically in 5% solution every few hours. Treatment is decreased with clearance of the lesions. Both keratoplasty and other antibiotics (e.g., nystatin, amphotericin B) have also been used.

FURTHER READING

Dermatophytosis

Ahmed AR: Immunology of human dermatophyte infections. Arch Dermatol 118:521, 1982

Ajello L: Natural history of the dermatophytes and related fungi. Mycopathologia 53:93, 1974

Apodaca G, McKerrow JH: Regulation of *Trichophyton rubrum* proteolytic activity. Infect Immun 57:3081, 1989

Artis WM, Patrusky E, Ragtinejad F, Duncan RL: Fungistatic mechanism of human transferrin for *Rhizopus oryzae* and *Trichophyton mentagrophytes*: Alternative to simple iron deprivation. Infect Immun 41:1269, 1983

Calderon RA: Immunoregulation of dermatophytosis. CRC Crit Rev Microbiol 16:339, 1989

Cox FW, Stiller RL, South DA, et al: Oral ketoconazole for dermatophyte infections. J Am Acad Dermatol 6:455, 1982

Frankel DH, Rippon JW: *Hendersonula toruloidea* infection in man. Index cases in the non-endemic North American host, and a review of the literature. Mycopathologia 105:175, 1989

Green F, Weber JK, Balish E: The thymus dependency of acquired resistance to *Trichophyton mentagrophytes* dermatophytosis in rats. J Invest Dermatol 81:31, 1983

Hashimoto T, Blumenthal HJ: Survival and resistance of *Trichophyton mentagrophytes* arthrospores. Appl Environ Microbiol 35:274, 1978

Hashimoto T, Wu CDR, Blumenthal HJ: Characterization of L-leucine-induced germination of *Trichophyton mentagrophytes* microconidia. J Bacteriol 112:967, 1972

Hay RJ, Shennan G: Chronic dermatophyte infections. II. Antibody and cell-mediated immune responses. Br J Dermatol 106:191, 1982

Hay RJ, Clayton YM, Moore MK, et al: Itraconazole in the management of chronic dermatophytosis. J Am Acad Dermatol 23:561, 1990

Howard DH: Ascomycetes: The dermatophytes. In Howard DH (ed): Fungi Pathogenic for Humans and Animals. Part A. Biology. New York, Marcel Dekker Inc, 1983, p 113

Howell SA, Moore MK, Mallet AI, Noble WC: Sterols of fungi responsible for superficial skin and nail infection. J Gen Microbiol 136:241, 1990

Kaaman T: Dermatophyte antigens and cell-mediated immunity in dermatophytosis. Curr Top Med Mycol 1:117, 1985

Meinhof W (ed): Oral Therapy in Dermatomycosis: A Step Forward. Oxford, Medicine Publ Fdn, 1985

Padhye AA, Young CN, Ajello L: Hair perforation as a diagnostic criterion in the identification of *Epidermophyton, Microsporum* and *Trichophyton* species. Proceedings of the 5th International Conference on Mycoses. Sci Publ no. 396. Washington, DC, Pan American Health Organization, 1980, p 115

Philpot CM: The use of nutritional tests for the differentiation of dermatophytes. Sabouraudia 15:141, 1977

Rebell G, Taplin D: Dermatophytes. Their Recognition and Identification. Coral Gables, Fla, University of Miami Press, 1974

Rippon JW: Medical Mycology, ed 3. Philadelphia, Saunders, 1988

Salzman RS, Jones HE: Ringworm, In Warren KS, Mahmoud AAF (eds): Tropical and Geographical Medicine. New York, McGraw-Hill, 1984, p 949

Summerbell RC, Kane J, Krajden S: Onychomycosis, tinea pedis and tinea manuum caused by non-dermatophytic filamentous fungi. Mycoses 32:609, 1989

Summerbell RC, Rosenthal SA, Kane J: Rapid method for differentiation of *Trichophyton rubrum, Trichophyton mentagrophytes*, and related dermatophyte species. J Clin Microbiol 26:2279, 1988

Van Cutsem J: Animal models for dermatomycotic infections. Curr Top Med Mycol 3:1, 1989

Vincent J: The importance of fatty acids in the pathogenesis of dermatophytosis. Curr Ther Res 22:83, 1977

Weitzman I, McGinnis MR, Padhye AA, Ajello L: The genus *Arthroderma* and its later synonym *Nannizza*. Mycotaxon 25:505, 1986

Pityriasis Versicolor

Back O, Faergemann J, Hornqvist R: *Pityrosporum* folliculitis: A common disease of the young and middle-aged. J Am Acad Dermatol 12:56, 1985

Belew PW, Rosenberg EW, Jennings BR: Activation of the alternative pathway of complement by *Malassezia ovalis* (*Pityrosporum ovale*). Mycopathologia 70:187, 1980

Burke RC: Tinea versicolor: Susceptibility factors and experimental infection in human beings. J Invest Dermatol 36:389, 1961

DaMert GI, Kirkpatrick CH, Sohnle PG: Comparison of antibody responses in chronic mucocutaneous candidiasis and tinea versicolor. Int Arch Allergy Appl Immunol 63:97, 1980

Delescluse J: Itraconazole in tinea versicolor: A review. J Am Acad Dermatol 23:551, 1990

Faergemann J, Fredriksson T: Tinea versicolor: Some new aspects on etiology, pathogenesis, and treatment. Int J Dermatol 21:8, 1982

Hill MK, Goodfield MJD, Rodgers FG, et al: Skin surface electron microscopy in *Pityrosporum* folliculitis: The role of follicular occlusion in disease and the response to oral ketoconazole. Arch Dermatol 126:181, 1990

Keddie FM, Shadomy S: Etiological significance of *Pityrosporum orbiculare* in tinea versicolor. Sabouraudia 3:21, 1963

Kieffer M, Bergbrant I-M, Faergemann J, et al: Immune reactions to *Pityrosporum ovale* in adult patients with atopic and seborrheic dermatitis. J Am Acad Dermatol 22:739, 1990

Klotz SA, Drutz DJ, Huppert M, Johnson JE: *Pityrosporum* folliculitis. Its potential for confusion with skin lesions of systemic candidiasis. Arch Intern Med 142:2126, 1982

McGinley KJ, Leyden JJ, Marples RR, et al: Quantitative microbiology of the scalp in nondandruff, dandruff, and seborrheic dermatitides. J Invest Dermatol 64:401, 1975

Nazzaro-Porro M, Passi S: Identification of tyrosinase inhibitors in cultures of *Pityrosporum*. J Invest Dermatol 71:205, 1978

Nazzaro-Porro M, Passi S, Caprilli F, et al: Induction of hyphae in cultures of *Pityrosporum* by cholesterol and cholesterol esters. J Invest Dermatol 69:531, 1977

Redline RW, Redline SS, Boxerbaum B, Barrat-Dahms B: Systemic *Malassezia furfur* infections in patients receiving intralipid therapy. Hum Pathol 16:815, 1985

Richet HM, McNeil MM, Edwards MC, et al: Cluster of *Malassezia furfur* pulmonary infections in infants in a neonatal intensive-care unit. J Clin Microbiol 27:1197, 1989

Roberts SOB: *Pityrosporum orbiculare*: Incidence and distribution on clinically normal skin. Br J Dermatol 81:264, 1969

Salkin IF, Gordon MA: Polymorphism of *Malassezia furfur*. Can J Microbiol 23:471, 1977

Shek YH, Tucker MC, Viciana AL, et al: *Malassezia furfur*—Disseminated infection in premature infants. Am J Clin Pathol 92:595, 1989

Sohnle PG, Collins-Lech C: Relative antigenicity of *P. orbiculare* and *C. albicans*. J Invest Dermatol 75:279, 1980

Sternberg TH, Keddie FM: Immunofluorescence studies of tinea versicolor. Arch Dermatol 84:999, 1961

Van Cutsem J, Van Gerven F, Fransen J, et al: The in vitro antifungal activity of ketoconazole, zinc pyrithione, and selenium sulfide against *Pityrosporum* and their efficacy as a shampoo in the treatment of experimental pityrosporosis in guinea pigs. J Am Acad Dermatol 22:993, 1990

Tinea Nigra

Carrion AL: Yeastlike dematiaceous fungi infecting human skin. Arch Dermatol Syph 61:996, 1950

Castellani A: Tinea nigra. Mycopath Mycol Appl 30:193, 1966

McGinnis MR, Schell WA, Carson J: *Phaeoannellomyces* and the phaeococcomycetaceae, a new dermatiaceous blastomycete taxa. J Med Vet Mycol 23:179, 1985

Mok YK: Nature and identification of *Exophiala werneckii*. J Clin Microbiol 16:976, 1982

Vaffee AS: Tinea nigra palmaris resembling malignant melanoma. N Engl J Med 283:1112, 1970

Van Velso H, Singletary M: Tinea nigra. Arch Dermatol 90:59, 1964

Mycotic Keratitis

Bulmer C: The ocular mycoses. Contr Microbiol Immunol 4:56, 1977

DeVoe AG, Silva-Hutner M: Fungal infections of the eye. In Locatcher-Khorazo D, Seegal BC (eds): Microbiology of the Eye. St. Louis, Mosby, 1972, p 208

Forster RK, Rebell G: The diagnosis and management of keratomycosis, Parts I and II. Arch Ophthalmol 93:975, 1134, 1975

Forster RK, Rebell G, Wilson LA: Dermatiaceous fungal keratitis. Br J Ophthalmol 59:372, 1975

Gugnani HC, Talwar RS, Njoku-Obi ANU, et al: Mycotic keratitis in Nigeria. A study of 21 cases. Br J Ophthalmol 60:607, 1976

Jones BR: Principles in management of oculomycosis. Trans Am Acad Ophthalmol Otolaryngol 79:15, 1975

Jones BR: Fungal keratitis. In Duane T (ed): Clinical Ophthalmology, vol IV. Hagerstown, Md, Harper & Row, 1978

CHAPTER 85

Opportunistic Mycoses

Modern medicine has managed to prolong the lives of many patients with severely debilitated antimicrobial defenses. Patients who receive corticosteroids, cytotoxic drugs, irradiation, or broad-spectrum antibacterial antibiotics for the management of cancer, organ transplantation, other surgical procedures, immunologic disorders, or chronic infections are predisposed to opportunistic infections. Patients with all forms of leukemia, acquired immunodeficiency syndrome (AIDS), Hodgkin's disease, neutropenia, other hematologic diseases, and endocrinopathies, including diabetes, are particularly susceptible to fungal infections. In general, conditions or treatments that reduce the number or function of phagocytes or impair cell-mediated immunity increase susceptibility to opportunistic mycoses.

These compromised patients are at risk for systemic candidiasis, cryptococcal meningitis, invasive aspergillosis, and rhinocerebral or thoracic mucormycosis. Avoiding exposure to the agents of these mycoses is almost impossible because they are either ubiquitous in the environment or are part of the normal microbial flora. Opportunistic mycoses are life-threatening and the most frequently encountered of the systemic fungal infections. In recent years, the incidence of opportunistic mycoses has continued to increase at an alarming rate.

In addition to their role in opportunistic disease, species of *Candida* and *Aspergillus* also cause other clinical entities.

The mechanisms of host resistance to fungal infection as the determinants of fungal pathogenicity remain to be elucidated for each of the mycoses. Nevertheless, some generalizations can be suggested about the crucial host-fungus interactions in opportunistic mycoses and the distinction between primary and opportunistic fungal pathogens (Chap. 81). Clinical data, experimental infections, and in vitro studies indicate that the fungicidal activity of the neutrophil is essential for normal defense against systemic candidiasis, invasive aspergillosis, and mucormycosis. The tissue forms—the yeast cells of *Candida albicans* and the hyphae of *C. albicans*, *Aspergillus fumigatus*, and *Rhizopus arrhizus*—are killed by neutrophils. Patients who are neutropenic or have neutrophils with impaired killing capacity, such as those with leukemia or chronic granulomatous disease, are susceptible to these fungi. Conversely, neutrophils are relatively ineffective in killing the tissue forms of primary pathogens—the spherules and endospores of *Coccidioides immitis* and the yeast cells of *Histoplasma capsulatum*, *Blastomyces dermatitidis*, and *Paracoccidioides brasiliensis*. Intact cell-mediated immunity and activated macrophages are crucial for adequate defense against these fungi (Chap. 82) and against *Cryptococcus neoformans*. Cell-mediated immunity does not seem to influence the course of systemic candidiasis, invasive aspergillosis, or mucormycosis. Antibodies and other humoral factors are not protective against either primary or opportunistic fungi. This differential susceptibility to neutrophilic killing is not related to the extent of phagocytosis but may reflect fungal susceptibility to oxidative killing mechanisms, degree of phagosome-lysosome fusion, fungal production of catalase and superoxide dismutase, fungal elaboration of neutrophil inhibitors, or other factors.

The importance of neutrophils for defense against opportunistic mycoses and the requirement of T cell–dependent immunity defense against primary pathogens is more complex. Cell-mediated immunity is essential for resistance to cutaneous and mucosal candidiasis, whereas neutrophils are necessary for protection against systemic candidiasis. Resistance to cryptococcosis requires functional cell-mediated immunity. For example, AIDS patients have altered CD4/CD8 T cell ratios and are susceptible to cryptococcal meningitis and mucosal candidiasis, as well as opportunistic coccidioidomycosis and histoplasmosis.

Candidiasis

Several species of the yeast *Candida* are capable of causing candidiasis. These organisms are members of the normal flora of the skin, mucous membranes, and gastrointestinal tract. *Candida* species colonize the mucosal surfaces of all humans during birth or shortly thereafter. The risk of endogenous infection is clearly ever present. Indeed, candidiasis occurs worldwide and is the most common systemic mycosis.

Of more than a hundred species of *Candida*, several are part of the normal flora and are potential pathogens. *C. albicans* causes most infections, followed by *Candida tropicalis*, but at least seven other *Candida* species have also been encountered.

Morphology and Physiology

Dimorphism

C. albicans is capable of producing yeast cells, pseudohyphae, and true hyphae (Chap. 80), as indicated in Figure 85–1. As part of the normal flora, *C. albicans* grows as a budding yeast; hyphal forms are produced only during tissue invasion. Although a number of environmental stimuli are known to trigger or block conversion in vitro from yeast to hyphal growth, regulation of morphogenesis in *C. albicans* remains

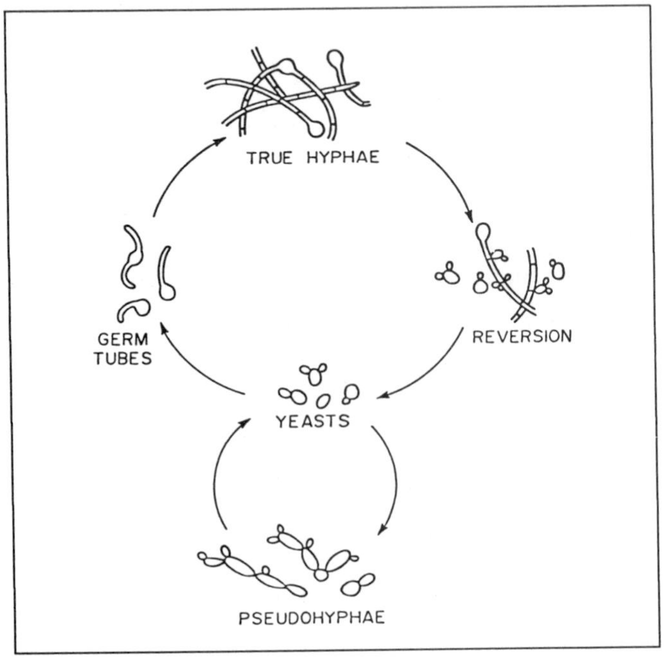

Fig. 85–1. The morphogenesis of *Candida albicans*. (Courtesy of Dr. M. Manning-Zweerink.)

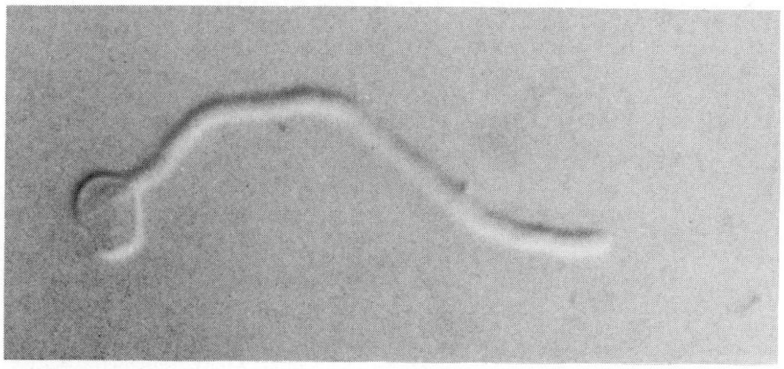

Fig. 85–2. *Candida albicans.* Germ tube formed in normal serum at 37C. × 970. *(Courtesy of W. Schell.)*

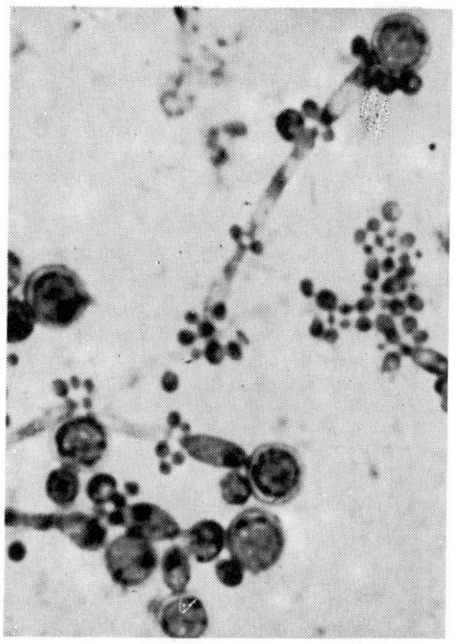

Fig. 85–3. *Candida albicans.* Budding yeast cells (blastoconidia), pseudohyphae, and large, spherical chlamydospores produced on cornmeal agar. × 790. *(From Conant: Am Rev Tuberc 61:696, 1950.)*

inconclusive. One unquestionable stimulant is normal serum. After 90 minutes in serum at 37C, *C. albicans* begins to form true hyphae. This reaction is manifested by the appearance of a germ tube, an elongated appendage, growing out from and about half as wide and more than twice as long as the yeast cell (Fig. 85–2). Germ tubes are distinct from pseudohyphae and are formed only by *C. albicans* and some isolates of *Candida stellatoidea* (Table 85–1). Incubation of an isolate in serum at 37C provides a rapid, presumptive identification of *C. albicans*, but confirmation of *C. albicans* or identification of other *Candida* species requires a battery of physiologic tests (Table 85–2). Germ tubes possess antigens not present on yeast cells, as well as quantitative differences in other cell wall components.

Cultural Characteristics

On most media, *Candida* species cannot be differentiated on the basis of their colony appearance. They produce within 24 to 48 hours raised, cream-colored, opaque colonies about 1 to 2 mm in diameter. After several days on agar medium, hyphae can be observed penetrating the agar.

Microscopic Appearance

Candida species produce ellipsoidal or spherical budding yeasts about 3 to 6 μm in size. Multiple buds and pseudohyphae are routinely formed on medium deficient in readily metabolizable substrates, such as cornmeal agar. Unlike other species, *C. albicans* produces characteristic chlamydospores on this medium (Fig. 85–3). *C. albicans* is capable of producing true hyphae of uniform width that grow by apical elongation and form septa at right angles with membrane-lined pores. Pseudohyphae are formed by budding cells that elongate and remain connected. Such cells are wider than true hyphae and are constricted where they are attached. The differential features of the two forms are compared in Table 85–3. Both hyphae and pseudohyphae may revert to yeast growth, and all three forms may be seen in cultures or in tissue (Fig. 85–1).

Subspeciation

Two serotypes of *C. albicans*, designated A and B, can be recognized with adsorbed polyclonal antisera. Isolates of serotype A are more common and more frequently susceptible

TABLE 85–1. KEY MORPHOLOGIC AND PHYSIOLOGIC CHARACTERISTICS OF COMMONLY ISOLATED YEASTS

Taxa	Growth at 37C	Pseudo/true Hyphae	Chlamydospores	Germ Tubes	Glucose Fermentation	Capsule	Phenol Oxidase	Urease	Ascospores
Candida albicans/C. stellatoidea	+	+	+	+	+	−	−	−	−
Other *Candida* species	+	+	−	−	+[a]	−	−	−[a]	−
Torulopsis glabrata	+	−	−	−	+	−	−	−	−
Cryptococcus neoformans	+	−[a]	−	−	−	+	+	+	−
Other *Cryptococcus* species	−[a]	−	−	−	−	+[a]	−	+	−
Rhodotorula species	+	−	−	−	−	−[a]	−	+	−
Saccharomyces species	+	−[a]	−	−	+	−	−	−	+[a]
Trichosporon species	+[a]	+	−	−	−	−	−	+[a]	−
Blastoschizomyces capitatus	+	+	−	−	−	−	−	−	−
Geotrichum species	+[a]	+	−	−	−	−	−	−	−
Hansenula species	+[a]	−[a]	−	−	+	−	−	−	+[a]

+, presence of characteristic; −, absence.
[a] Variation among species or strains.

TABLE 85–2. BIOCHEMICAL CHARACTERISTICS OF YEASTS ROUTINELY ISOLATED FROM CLINICAL SPECIMENS

Species	Assimilation												Fermentation				
	Glu[a]	Mal	Suc	Lac	Gal	Mel	Cel	Ino	Xyl	Raf	Tre	Dul	Glu	Mal	Suc	Lac	Gal
Candida albicans	+	+	+*	–	+	–	–	–	+	–	+	–	F	F	–	–	F
C. guilliermondii	+	+	+	–	+	+	+	–	+	+	+	+	F	–	F	–	F*
C. kefyr	+	–	+	+	+	–	+*	–	+*	+	–*	–	F	–	F	F*	F
C. krusei	+	–	–	–	–	–	–	–	–	–	–	–	F	–	–	–	–
C. lipolytica	+	–	–	–	–	–	–	–	–	–	–	–	–	–	–	–	–
C. lusitaniae	+	+	+	–	+	–	+	–	+	–	+	–	F	–	F	–	F
C. parapsilosis	+	+	+	–	+	–	–	–	+	–	+	–	F	–	–	–	–
C. rugosa	+	–	–	–	+	–	–	–	+*	–	–	–	–	–	–	–	–
C. stellatoidea	+	+	–	–	+	–	–	–	+	–	+	–	F	F	–	–	–
C. tropicalis	+	+	+	–	+	–	+	–	+	–	+	–	F	F	F	–	F
Torulopsis glabrata	+	–	–	–	–	–	–	–	–	–	+	–	F	–	–	–	–
Cryptococcus neoformans	+	+	+	–	+	–	+	+	+	+*	+	+	–	–	–	–	–
C. albidus	+	+	+	+*	+*	+	+	+	+	+	+	+*	–	–	–	–	–
C. gastricus	+	+	+*	–	+	–	+	+	+	–	+	–	–	–	–	–	–
C. laurentii	+	+	+	+	+	+*	+	+	+	+*	+	+	–	–	–	–	–
C. luteolus	+	+	+	–	+	+	+	+	+	+	+	+	–	–	–	–	–
C. terreus	+	+*	–	+*	+*	–	+	+	+	–	+	–*	–	–	–	–	–
C. uniguttulatus	+	+	+	–	–*	–	–*	+	+	+*	–*	–	–	–	–	–	–
Rhodotorula glutinis	+	+	+	–	+*	–	+	–	+	+	+	–	–	–	–	–	–
R. rubra	+	+	+	–	+	–	+*	–	+	+	+	–	–	–	–	–	–
Saccharomyces cerevisiae	+	+	+	–	+	–	–	–	–	+	+*	–	F	F	F	–	F
Trichosporon beigelii	+	+	+	+	+*	+*	+*	+	+	+*	+*	+*	–	–	–	–	–
T. pullulans	+	+	+	+*	+	+*	+	+*	+*	+*	+	–	–	–	–	–	–
Geotrichum candidum	+	–	–	–	+	–	–	–	+	–	–	–	–	–	–	–	–
Blastoschizomyces capitatus	+	–	–	–	+	–	–	–	–	–	–	–	–	–	–	–	–
Hansenula anomala	+	+	+	–	+	–	+	–	+	–	+	–	F	F*	F	–	F

From Warren and Shadomy: In Balows et al (eds): Manual of Clinical Microbiology, ed 5. American Society for Microbiology, 1991, p 619.
+, growth greater than negative control; –, neither growth over control nor fermentation; *, strain variation; F, fermentation with gas production; Glu, glucose; Mal, maltose; Suc, sucrose; Lac, lactose; Gal, galactose; Mel, melibiose; Cel, cellobiose, Ino, inositol; Xyl, Xylose; Raf, raffinose; Tre, trehalose; Dul, dulcitol.

to flucytosine than are isolates of serotype B. Monoclonal antibodies have been produced to these mannan antigens, and additional reagents have been developed that permit further discrimination of *C. albicans* and routinely isolated species of *Candida*.

TABLE 85–3. COMPARISON BETWEEN THE APPEARANCE OF HYPHAE AND PSEUDOHYPHAE

Feature	Hyphae	Pseudohyphae
Growth process	Apical elongation	Budding
Terminal cell	Longer; cylindrical	Shorter; spherical
Cell walls	Parallel	Constricted at septa
Septa	Straight; perpendicular	Curved or pinched
Origin of branches	No constriction; septum not required	Constricted and septated

Several novel schemes for biotyping *Candida* species have been developed for subspecies identification and tracking individual strains. Biotypes are based on differences in antigens, biochemical (enzymatic) profile, patterns of resistance to a set of chemical reagents, susceptibility to killer toxins produced by other yeasts, analysis of karyotypes, or DNA polymorphisms detected by patterns of restriction enzyme digests or by probing digests with cloned DNA fragments. Some of the methods that have been developed are indicated in Table 85–4. On defined medium and growth conditions, some strains of *C. albicans* display different colonial morphologies. Some strains exhibit high-frequency switching among various colonial phenotypes, and this phenomenon has been exploited by Soll and associates to track strains from different body sites.

Although most of these procedures are still investigational, it is evident that strains of *C. albicans* vary greatly, this variation can be monitored, and particular strains may be associated with individuals, body sites, and virulence factors.

Determinants of Pathogenicity

Strains of *C. albicans* and species of *Candida* have long been recognized to vary in animal pathogenicity. Hyphal production and resistance to phagocytic killing are associated with virulence. High doses of extracts of *C. albicans* exhibit endotoxin-like activity, but this activity is not a prominent feature of its pathogenicity.

Cells of *C. albicans* are able to attach to epithelial cell membranes by a specific ligand-receptor interaction, and germ tubes are more adhesive than yeast cells. *C. albicans* and other *Candida* species adhere to gastrointestinal, vaginal, and buccal mucosal cells, corneocytes, vascular endothelial cells, and fibrin-platelet matrices. This adherence and penetration of host cells are associated with pathogenicity. The yeast adhesin appears to be a mannan or glycoprotein component. Yeast cells of *Candida* species also adhere to plastic surfaces, which would facilitate attachment to catheters and prosthetic devices. This adherence is based on hydrophobic and electrostatic forces between the yeast cell and plastic surfaces. Surface hydrophobicity varies considerably among isolates of *C. albicans* and has been correlated with attachment to mammalian cells and virulence for mice.

Most strains of *C. albicans* secrete inducible protease(s) capable of digesting host immunoglobulins and other substrates. Murine virulence of strains somewhat correlates with proteinase production, as well as adherence to epithelial cells. Other interactions between *C. albicans* and host factors are intriguing and probably influence inflammation and pathogenicity. For example, whole cells or cell walls of *C. albicans*, as most pathogenic fungi, activate the alternative pathway of complement. In addition, *C. albicans* has a surface receptor, similar to the CR3 receptor on human cells, that binds iC3b. *C. albicans* also possess a cytoplasmic protein that is able to bind corticosterone and related steroid hormones and resembles the mammalian glucocorticoid receptor.

Another provocative aspect of *C. albicans* is its immunomodulating activity. The most bioreactive fractions are cell wall glycoproteins. Depending on the route and fraction administered, either immunoadjuvant or immunosuppressive activity can be observed in experimental animals.

TABLE 85–4. METHODS OF BIOTYPING *CANDIDA ALBICANS*

- Analysis of colony morphology types and frequency or pattern of colony switching
- Analysis of proteins (including isoenzymes) separated by one- or two-dimensional polyacrylamide gel electrophoresis
- Serotype; detection of surface antigens
- Combinations of various physiologic phenotypes; schemes involve patterns of assimilation of different substrates, detection of specific enzymes, and resistance to chemicals, flucytosine, or conditions of growth, such as low pH (<2.0) or high salt
- Sensitivity to yeast killer toxins
- Comparison of chromosomes by pulsed-field electrophoresis (electrophoretic karyotype)
- Restriction endonuclease analysis of chromosomal DNA, cloned or amplified sequences
- Hybridization (of whole-cell DNA preparations, amplified sequences, or restriction fragments) with DNA probes

TABLE 85–5. FACTORS PREDISPOSING TO CANDIDIASIS

Cutaneous and Mucosal Candidiasis

- Physiologic
  - Pregnancy
  - Old age
  - Infancy
- Traumatic
  - Maceration
  - Burns
  - Other infection
- Hematologic
  - Cellular immunodeficiency
  - Acquired immunodeficiency syndrome (AIDS)
- Endocrine
  - Diabetes mellitus
- Iatrogenic
  - Antibacterial antibiotics
  - Birth control pill

Systemic Candidiasis

- Iatrogenic
  - Immunosuppression
  - Organ transplantation
  - Surgery
  - Steroid treatment
  - Cytotoxic drugs
  - Antibacterial antibiotics
  - Catheters
  - Hyperalimentation
  - Artificial heart valves
- Hematologic
  - Chronic granulomatous disease
  - Aplastic anemia
  - Agranulocytosis
  - Leukemia, lymphoma, Hodgkin's disease
- Other
  - Other malignancy
  - Malnutrition
  - Trauma
  - Intravenous drug abuse
  - Peritoneal dialysis

Chronic Mucocutaneous Candidiasis

- Hematologic
  - Cellular immunodeficiency
- Endocrine
  - Hypoparathyroidism
  - Iron metabolic disorders
- Other
  - Thymoma
  - Heredity
  - Hypovitaminosis A

Clinical Infection

Epidemiology

Many conditions predispose to opportunistic *Candida* infection (Table 85–5). Certain physiologic changes in otherwise healthy individuals provide the setting for opportunistic candidiasis. The risk factors for the three categories of candidiasis are somewhat different. However, some factors, such as the use of broad-spectrum antibacterial antibiotics, may predispose to both mucosal and systemic candidiasis.

Cutaneous and Mucosal Candidiasis. In nonpregnant women, the incidence of candidal vaginitis is between 10% and 17%, but this incidence approximately doubles during pregnancy. Vaginal candidiasis also is increased among diabetics and women taking oral contraceptives, hormones, or antibacterial antibiotics. The physiologic changes in the cervical and vaginal mucosa that result in overgrowth of *Candida* may relate to the following changes: (1) increase in moisture and carbohydrate substrates on the mucosal surface, (2) decrease or dilution of local transferrin, which would lead to increased levels of available iron, an essential growth requirement for *Candida*, (3) increased secretion of steroids that might promote candidiasis indirectly by reducing local host defenses, such as phagocytosis, (4) decrease in the concentration of specific IgA secretory component, although the protective value of this antibody has not been established, and (5) stimulation of germ tubes with increased adherence to vaginal epithelial cells.

Infants are especially at risk if they are heavily exposed to *Candida* before the normal microbial flora of the gastrointestinal tract and skin has been established. Normally, the attack rate of candidiasis among infants is approximately 4%, but this is increased if the mother has candidal vaginitis. Infants usually develop oral thrush, perianal and genital infections, gastroenteritis with severe diarrhea, or prolonged and painful diaper rash. Spread of the infection from one infant to another by nursery attendants has resulted in epidemics.

Although the intact adult epithelium is normally impervious to *Candida* invasion, certain conditions increase the opportunity for superficial candidiasis. Any trauma, burn, abrasion, or break in the epithelial integrity of skin or gut provides an opportunity for *Candida* to penetrate the skin, mucosa, or subcutaneous tissue. Excessive moisture and warmth increase the numbers of *Candida* on the skin. Cutaneous infections are an occupational disease of dishwashers, bartenders, fruit pickers, and similar workers. Warmth, moisture, and friction result in intertriginous candidal infections of the skin folds, toe webs, groin, or under the breasts, especially in the obese. *Candida* may also secondarily invade lesions or epithelium damaged by other infections.

Mucocutaneous candidiasis is also prevalent in patients with impaired cell-mediated immunity, such as those with hematologic malignancies, receiving corticosteroids, cytotoxic or immunosuppressive drugs, or radiation therapy, or with AIDS. Patients with AIDS are highly susceptible to candidiasis, especially involving the mucosal surfaces of the esophagus and oropharynx. Fifty to seventy percent of patients with AIDS have mucosal candidiasis, usually oral thrush, esophagitis, or both. Indeed, oral candidiasis is one of the criteria for the diagnosis of AIDS and AIDS-related complex. The depression of cell-mediated immunity in these patients is often manifested as abnormally low numbers of T helper/inducer cells and an inversion of the normal T helper to T suppressor/cytotoxic cell (CD4/CD8) ratio. The immunologic defect in patients with AIDS is consistent with the evidence that competent cell-mediated immunity is essential for resistance to both mucocutaneous candidiasis and cryptococcosis.

Endocrinologic disturbances, such as diabetes mellitus, hypoparathyroidism, and Addison's disease, result in an increased incidence of candidiasis, but a reason for the increased incidence has not been found. In many cases, *Candida* infection precedes by several years the open manifestations of diabetes. Patients with decreased parathyroid hormone secretion or adrenal insufficiency (Addison's disease) manifest developmental abnormalities that may involve the skin and mucosa and are prone to cutaneous and mucocutaneous candidiasis.

Systemic Candidiasis. Many blood dyscrasias predispose patients to systemic candidiasis, as does cellular or, less frequently, humoral immunodeficiency. A decrease in numbers or functional capacity of neutrophils lowers resistance to *Candida*, resulting in recurrent systemic infections. Neutrophils from patients with leukemia or chronic granulomatous disease exhibit subnormal in vitro phagocytosis or killing.

Ironically, many medical procedures designed to prolong life also increase the likelihood of life-threatening opportunistic infections. Patients who are treated with such medications and whose host defenses are unduly compromised are especially at risk if they are iatrogenically exposed to *Candida*. Immunosuppressive treatment, as an adjunct to transplantation or anticancer therapy, decreases resistance to *Candida*. As many as 30% of leukemia patients acquire systemic candidiasis. Bone marrow transplant patients are highly susceptible to both systemic candidiasis and invasive aspergillosis, and about 25% acquire opportunistic mycoses.

The probability of postoperative systemic candidiasis is related to the length of the operation and is caused not only by contamination with yeasts during surgery but also by diverse postoperative procedures, such as indwelling catheters or the use of prophylactic antibacterial antibiotics. An additional risk is imposed by prosthetic devices, such as artificial heart valves or intravenous lines, which provide a foreign body that can be colonized by *Candida* in the bloodstream. Similarly, any trauma to the heart valves may induce vegetations that can provide a nidus for *Candida* attachment.

Many patients who develop systemic candidiasis present a history of having received corticosteroids before the infection. Among the many and uncertain effects of corticosteroids are depression of phagocytic activity and cell-mediated immunity. Cortisone-treated animals are less resistant to challenge with *Candida* and other fungi. Antibacterial antibiotics predispose to candidiasis by reducing the competing bacterial flora and perhaps by impairing neutrophil activity. Contamination of intravenous lines, especially at the point of entry, is an unfortunate and too frequent source of candidemia. The skin around injection sites must be scrupulously cleaned and monitored to minimize this source of yeasts. Contamination of Foley catheters may lead to infection of the urinary tract and bladder.

Chronic Mucocutaneous Candidiasis. Defective T cell immunity is evident in most patients with chronic mucocutaneous candidiasis. Other patients have pronounced endocrinopathy, thymoma, genetic predisposition, or other constitutional problems.

Pathogenesis

The pathogenesis of cutaneous and mucosal candidiasis requires (1) an increase in the local, surface census of *C. albicans* and (2) a compromise in the integrity of the epidermal or epithelial surface. Thereafter, intact cell-mediated immunity is essential for adequate resistance. Colonization of epithelial surfaces with *Candida* is higher among patients than in the healthy population. The intact or physiologically normal epithelium is usually resistant to *Candida* invasion. However, *Candida* may invade if there is a marked increase in the number of *Candida* present or if the skin and mucosa are traumatized or are hormonally altered or if *Candida* attachment to endothelial cells is enhanced.

The pathogenesis of systemic candidiasis generally involves (1) the introduction of yeasts into the circulation, either a heavy or light candidemia, and (2) a compromise in the host defenses, especially the neutrophils. Iatrogenic candidemia and candiduria, induced by catheters, surgery, or hyperalimentation, are often successfully managed by the normal host defense mechanisms. However, the ability of patients with hormonal imbalances, immunodeficiencies, and malignancies to control invasion of the deeper tissues is limited. In compromised individuals, *C. albicans* and *C. tropicalis* are able to cross the intestinal mucosa by persorption and enter the circulation.

The host defenses against candidiasis are both specific and nonspecific, cellular and humoral. Serum components, such as opsonins, complement, and transferrin, may inhibit either directly or indirectly the survival of *Candida*. Specific antibodies to *Candida* have a minimal direct effect but may

(1) inhibit the normal clumping of yeasts by serum, (2) affect yeast morphogenesis or respiration, (3) function as opsonins, or (4) mediate antibody-dependent cellular cytotoxicity. Cellular host defenses against *Candida* involve neutrophils, which kill 30% to 50% of the ingested yeasts by both oxidative and nonoxidative mechanisms. The latter include the defensins, which are small (<4000 kDa) cationic proteins in the azurophil granules with potent candidacidal and antibacterial activity. Macrophages are also candidacidal and variously stimulated by *Candida* cell wall components.

Once allowed to grow and develop hyphal forms, *C. albicans* factors may promote pathogenesis by mechanisms that enhance attachment or further compromise the host defenses. For example, secretion of serine proteinase is correlated with virulence. The initial hyphal cells, called *germ tubes*, are more hydrophobic and express more surface receptors for attaching to host cells and binding opsonins than do yeast cells. These properties have been correlated with virulence.

Clinical Manifestations

Candidiasis may be grouped broadly into three categories: cutaneous and mucosal, systemic, and chronic mucocutaneous candidiasis. Table 85–6 lists most of the forms in these categories. Allergic reactions to *Candida* antigens may also occur. However, the concept known as *candidiasis hypersensitivity syndrome* and ascribed to a variety of ill-defined ailments, ranging from general fatigue and depression to gastrointestinal symptoms, is speculative and unproven. Although this syndrome is attributed by some clinical ecologists to *C. albicans*, there is no evidence to support this, and the recommended treatment of long-term oral antifungals may be hazardous.

TABLE 85–6. CLINICAL CLASSIFICATION OF CANDIDIASIS (ABRIDGED)

Cutaneous and Mucosal Candidiasis
Thrush (oral, vaginal)
Stomatitis
Intertriginous candidiasis (groin, axillary, interdigital)
Onychomycosis
Esophagitis
Severe diaper rash
Balanitis
Systemic Candidiasis
Esophagitis
Intestinitis
Infant diarrhea
Bronchopulmonary candidiasis
Pyelonephritis
Cystitis
Endocarditis
Myocarditis
Endophthalmitis
Meningitis
Arthritis
Osteomyelitis
Peritonitis
Macronodular skin lesions
Chronic Mucocutaneous Candidiasis

Cutaneous Candidiasis. Infection of the skin, mucous membranes, and nails by endogenous *Candida* species can be caused by conditions that result in chronic maceration of these areas, physiologic changes in the host, or a compromised immune status.

Candidiasis of the mucous membranes is often referred to as thrush. Oral thrush is most commonly associated with AIDS, infants, patients with chronic mucocutaneous candidiasis, and adults undergoing treatment with steroids, cytotoxic drugs, or antibacterial antibiotics. The lesions may be singular, patchy, or confluent, and a whitish pseudomembrane composed of yeasts and pseudohyphae may cover the tongue, soft palate, and oral mucosa. The diagnosis is confirmed by direct microscopic and cultural examination of scrapings from the lesions.

Vaginal thrush occurs more often in pregnant women, diabetics, and women receiving antibacterial or hormonal treatment, including birth control pills. Patches of gray-white pseudomembrane develop on the vaginal mucosa, and a yellow-white discharge may accompany the infection. From the mucous membranes, infection and inflammation may spread to the adjacent skin. Typical yeasts and pseudohyphae abound in these lesions. Infants develop similar lesions in the perianal region, which may persist as a diaper rash of the genital, perianal, and groin areas. Scratching may spread the infection to other skin sites. In addition to *C. albicans*, *C. tropicalis*, *C. stellatoidea*, and *Candida pseudotropicalis* also may cause vaginitis.

Candida species may cause chronic nail infections and paronychia. The skin around the nail becomes swollen, erythematous, and painful, unlike dermatophytosis of the nail (tinea unguim). *Candida parapsilosis*, *C. tropicalis* and *Candida guilliermondii* are also associated with onychomycosis.

Systemic Candidiasis. Numerous systemic manifestations of candidiasis may follow introduction of *Candida* into the bloodstream. Candidemia may result from contamination of indwelling catheters, surgical procedures, trauma to the skin or gastrointestinal tract, persorption, or aspiration. The extent and severity of the infection that follows are determined by the inoculum size, the virulence of the organisms, and, most importantly, the host defenses.

The scope of systemic candidiasis is protean. Some of the more recognized syndromes are listed in Table 85–6. Clinical indications of occult systemic candidiasis include candiduria (in the absence of catheterization and an imbalanced flora), candidal endophthalmitis, and maculonodular skin lesions. Although *C. albicans* is the most common agent of candidiasis, *C. guilliermondii*, *C. parapsilosis*, and *C. tropicalis* are frequent causes of endocarditis. Overall, *C. tropicalis* is second to *C. albicans* in pathogenetic potential.

Chronic Mucocutaneous Candidiasis. A unique set of predisposing conditions and clinical manifestations is associated with the entity, chronic mucocutaneous candidiasis (CMC). This condition is defined as infection, invariably with *C. albicans*, of any or all of the epithelial surfaces of the body: the skin, oral mucosa, upper respiratory tract, gastrointestinal, urinary, and genital epithelium. Invasion of the bloodstream or deeper tissues in unusual. *C. albicans* apparently attaches to and penetrates the plasma membrane of viable epithelial

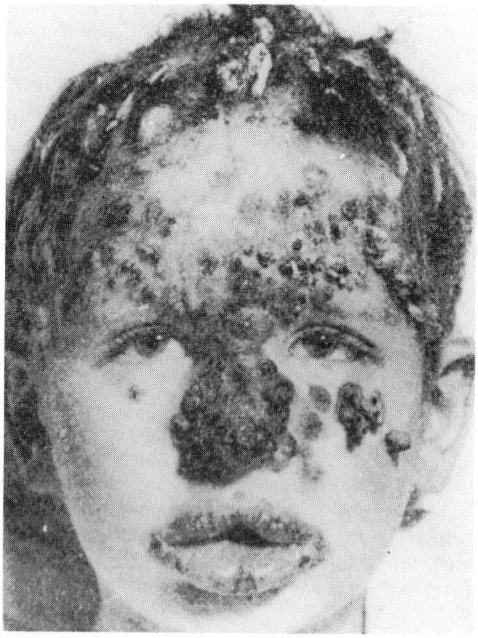

Fig. 85–4. Child with chronic mucocutaneous candidiasis.

cells, causes considerable distortion of these cells, and exists as an intracellular parasite. The onset of CMC begins early in life and often persists for a lifetime. The degree of involvement of the epithelium and mucous membranes varies with different patients and with individual patients at different times. Although some children develop total skin involvement that only minimally recedes with treatment, others have limited but persistent lesions. Some patients respond temporarily to therapy, sometimes for years, but permanent cures rarely, if ever, occur. The classic lesions, as seen in Figure 85–4, are verrucous and warty, with hornlike projections growing out from the skin. These lesions appear at an early age and become chronic, with the development of extensive epithelial hyperplasia.

Several underlying conditions have been correlated with CMC. Most patients have a deficiency in their cell-mediated immunity, but the precise defect has not been defined. Immunologic analyses of CMC patients have revealed no consistent deficiency. Some patients have single and others have multiple defects. It now seems probable that any of several T-dependent immunodeficiency syndromes may provide the setting for CMC. Individual patients may be deficient in any or all of the following ways: (1) delayed skin test anergy and lack of in vitro lymphocyte responsiveness to antigens, (2) unresponsiveness to mitogens, and (3) failure to produce lymphokines.

Many patients with CMC have normal neutrophils, immunoglobulin levels, and numbers of T and B lymphocytes. Some have defective neutrophils (chronic granulomatous disease), whereas others apparently have no immunologic dysfunction. Transfer factor therapy appears to be effective, although it has not been administered without concomitant chemotherapy. The available data would suggest defective macrophage processing, T lymphocyte responsiveness, excessive T suppressor activity, or humoral blocking factors.

Some patients with CMC have other dominant underlying conditions. Endocrinopathies, especially hypoparathyroidism, are present in some patients. In others, abnormalities in iron metabolism have been described, usually iron deficiency, or hypovitaminosis A. CMC has been observed in patients with leukemia, thymoma, and other blood diseases. The mechanism of pathogenesis of CMC remains unclear. Some of the conditions mentioned could result in abnormal physiologic changes in the epithelium, and others may relate to available iron or compromised host defenses. An autosomal genetic predisposition to CMC and its underlying conditions has also been documented.

Three groups of CMC have been delineated by Kirkpatrick and Windhorst based on the time of onset. With early onset, the predisposing defect or defects in cell-mediated immunity are apparently inherited. These patients are subdivided into those with or without endocrinopathy. Onset between the ages of 10 and 30 years offers the best prognosis because the defects in cell-mediated immunity in these patients are often restored after therapy. Adult onset CMC occurs after the age of 40 years, and most, if not all, patients have an associated thymoma.

Laboratory Diagnosis

Microscopic Examination. The appearance in tissue of pseudohyphae or true hyphae along with budding yeast cells is pathognomonic for invasive candidiasis. The presence of hyphal forms in freshly examined skin scrapings, vaginal exudate, and specimens of sputum, centrifuged urine, spinal fluid, or joint fluid also indicates candidiasis. Typical forms seen in a fresh preparation are depicted in Figure 85–5.

Culture. Because *Candida* species are so prevalent, positive cultures are invariably suspect. Specimens from normally sterile sites can be cultured on bacteriologic media. Otherwise, inhibitory mold or Sabouraud's agar containing antibiotics should be employed. Germ tube production provides tentative identification of *C. albicans*. A germ tube-negative yeast that produces pseudohyphae and lacks a capsule and arthroconidia

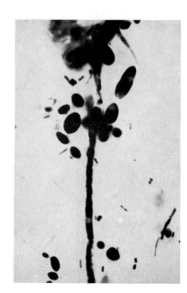

Fig. 85–5. *Candida albicans*. Gram stain of sputum smear showing budding cells of pseudohyphae. × 1175.

may be *Candida* and should be speciated according to the physiologic pattern detailed in Table 85–2.

Candida isolated from normally sterile specimens is significant and should be evaluated in terms of the patient's clinical history. For example, a positive blood culture in a postsurgical patient may reflect a self-limiting transient candidemia, and additional specimens should be cultured. Unfortunately, less than half of patients with systemic candidiasis yield positive blood cultures. Positive cultures from sputum have no diagnostic value. Cultures from surface specimens (skin, vaginal mucosa) should confirm the etiology of clinical lesions. A census of 10^4 to 10^5 colonies per milliliter from a properly obtained urine specimen without indwelling urethral catheter is considered indicative of infection.

Serology. Because of the difficulty of establishing a diagnosis of systemic candidiasis by direct examination or culture, the need for a reliable, diagnostic serologic test is most urgent. Various antigens and methods have been applied to the detection of diagnostic levels of antibodies. Since everyone develops an immune response to *Candida*, these serologic tests are limited to discriminating between normal and disease levels of antibodies. Although not definitive, the detection of precipitins to cytoplasmic antigens by immunodiffusion is probably the most acceptable, readily available test. By itself, a positive test is not diagnostic but must be interpreted with other clinical data. Table 85–7 summarizes the prevailing serologic tests for diagnosis of candidiasis and other opportunistic mycoses.

More specific tests for *Candida* antigen are currently under development. Both *Candida* surface mannan and cytoplasmic proteins have been detected in sera by sensitive methods, such as enzyme immunoassay, radioimmunoassay, quantitative immunofluorescence, or latex particle agglutination. The mannan test usually require pretreatment of sera to dissociate antigen from patient antibody. Mannan and arabinitol, a *Candida* metabolite, can also be measured in sera by gas-liquid chromatographic methods. The detection of circulating *Candida* antigens or metabolites appears to be specific and diagnostic for systemic candidiasis. However, some patients with mucosal candidiasis or transient candidemia give false positive results. The tests for *Candida* antigenemia are also limited by

TABLE 85–7. SUMMARY OF MYCOSEROLOGY FOR OPPORTUNISTIC MYCOSES (ABRIDGED)

			Sensitivity and Value		
Mycosis	**Test**	**Antigen**	**Diagnosis**	**Prognosis**	**Limitations/Specificity**
Candidiasis (systemic)	AG	Ca	60%–75% of cases positive, paired sera and fourfold titer rise required	Fourfold change in titer	Many healthy persons positive
	CIE	HS or S	90%–100% of cases positive; one or more precipitin bands	Titer change or loss of bands	Patients with superficial candidiasis or transient candidemia may also be positive
	ID	HS or S	88% of cases positive	Loss of bands	More specific, less sensitive than CIE test
Cryptococcosis	LA		Detect capsular antigen in serum or spinal fluid; 92% of cases positive (in spinal fluid)	Titer reflects severity	Proper controls eliminate false positives due to rheumatoid factor; cross-reaction with *Trichosporon*
	AG	Cn	38% of cases serum positive; i.e., titer ≥ 1:2; usually positive early and/or posttreatment	May become positive with recovery	Few cross-reactions
	CPA	CP	Titer ≥ 1:4 considered positive	As above	Few cross-reactions; more sensitive, less specific than AG test
Aspergillosis (invasive)	ID	Acf	Sensitivity highly variable; 3–4 bands indicative of invasive aspergillosis or aspergilloma	Number of bands reflects severity	80%–100% of cases with allergic bronchopulmonary aspergillosis and more than 90% with aspergilloma are positive; cross-reactions with other fungi and C-reactive protein
Mucormycosis	ID	Zs	73% cases positive	Unknown	None

From Mitchell: In Wentworth (ed): Diagnostic Procedures for Mycotic and Parasitic Infections, ed 7. American Public Health Association, 1988, p 303; Kaufman and Reiss: In Ross et al (eds): Manual of Clinical Laboratory Immunology, ed 3. American Society for Microbiology, 1986, p 446.

Tests: AG, yeast agglutination; CIE, counterimmunoelectrophoresis; ID, immunodiffusion; LA, latex agglutination, latex particles coated with rabbit anti-*C. neoformans* globulin; CPA, charcoal particle agglutination.

Antigens: Ca, killed yeast cells of *Candida albicans;* HS, Hollister-Steir commercial *Monilia* antigen; S, cytoplasmic antigen of *C. albicans* yeast cells; Cn, killed yeast cells of *Cryptococcus neoformans;* CP, charcoal particles coated with capsular antigen; Acf, pool of culture filtrate of 3 to 5 *Aspergillus* species; Zs, pool of cytoplasmic antigens of 11 zygomycetous species.

low sensitivity. Because the antigen levels are often low or transient, many patients do not develop positive tests until late in disease. A serologic test for early diagnosis of systemic candidiasis is still needed.

Treatment

Cutaneous candidiasis can be treated with topical antibiotics (ketoconazole, nystatin, miconazole) or chemical solutions (gentian violet). For the treatment of systemic candidiasis, amphotericin B flucytosine or both are recommended. Unfortunately, many clinical isolates of *C. albicans* develop resistance to flucytosine. Chronic mucocutaneous candidiasis has been treated with flucytosine, amphotericin B, miconazole, topical chemical solutions, and transfer factor. Ketoconazole has produced dramatic resolution of lesions in many patients. The response of individual patients is highly variable, but resolution of lesions is associated with improved immunocompetance. However, both responses are often only temporary.

Prophylaxis

Prophylaxis of patients at risk for systemic candidiasis has been attempted in several clinical trials using oral ketoconazole or nystatin or a low dose or short course of amphotericin B, often coupled with antibacterial antibiotics. Controlled studies have usually resulted in lower incidences of candidiasis in treated patients, but a proven and standard regimen has not been established.

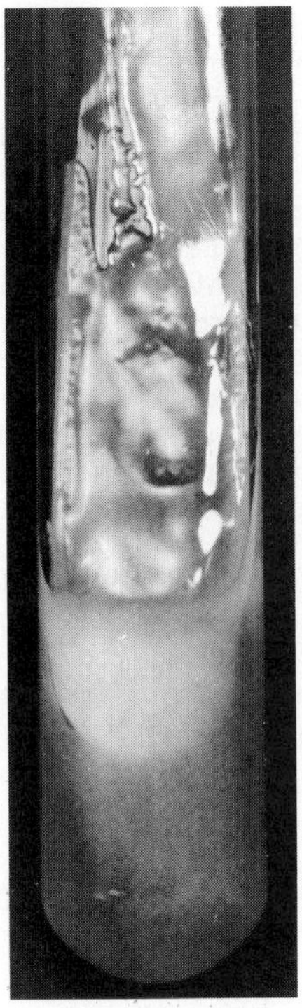

Fig. 85–6. *Cryptococcus neoformans*. Mucoid colony on Sabouraud's glucose agar at room temperature for 10 days.

Cryptococcosis

Cryptococcosis is caused by infection with the encapsulated yeast, *Cryptococcus neoformans*. Outdated synonyms for cryptococcosis include torulosis, European blastomycosis, and torula meningitis. The natural reservoir for *C. neoformans* is the soil and the avian feces, and infection follows airborne exposure and inhalation of the yeasts. In nature, the yeast cells are minimally encapsulated, small, dry, and easily aerosolized. From the lungs, the yeasts may metastasize to virtually any organ in the body, but they preferentially invade the central nervous system.

Although *C. neoformans* is ubiquitous in nature, the incidence of cryptococcosis is relatively low. Therefore, it is likely that many more persons inhale the yeast cells than become ill. Indeed, an intact cell-mediated immune system and competent phagocytes provide strong defense against cryptococcal disease. The actual extent of subclinical exposure is unknown because a good skin test antigen has not been developed for population surveys.

Morphology and Physiology

Cultural Characteristics

Visible colonies of *C. neoformans* develop on routine laboratory media within 36 to 72 hours. They are white to cream colored, opaque, and may be several millimeters in diameter. Colonies may develop sectors that differ in pigmentation. Colonies are typically mucoid in appearance, and the amount of capsule produced can be judged by the degree of colony wetness (Fig. 85–6). Highly encapsulated colonies will actually run down a slant to pool in the bottom of the tube, or they may drip off the medium of inverted plates.

Microscopic Appearance

Most clinical isolates are spherical, budding, encapsulated yeast cells in both tissue and culture. Rarely, short hyphal forms are also observed, and filamentous variants have been isolated. The yeast cells vary in size from 5 to 10 μm in diameter and exhibit both single and multiple budding. The hallmark of *C. neoformans* is its capsule, which may be twice the width of the cell (Fig. 85–7). Considerable variation exists in the size of the capsule, which is determined both by inherent strain differences and conditions of growth. Elevated glucose, CO_2, or temperature enhances capsule formation. Some strains characteristically produce large capsules, medium capsules, or minimal capsules. However, most strains, even those that are consistently small-capsuled in vitro, develop large capsules during infection. In a few rare cases, nonencapsulated cells of *C. neoformans* have been found in tissue.

C. neoformans was shown by Kwon-Chung to represent the anamorphic form of the basidiomycetous species, *Filobasidiella neoformans*. The sexual life cycle of *F. neoformans* is depicted in Figure 85–8. Among clinical and natural isolates of *C. neoformans* (which are fertile and heterothallic), more than 95% belong to only one of the two mating types of *F. neoformans*. Only the anamorph is isolated from clinical or natural samples.

Properties of the Capsule. During infection or immuni-

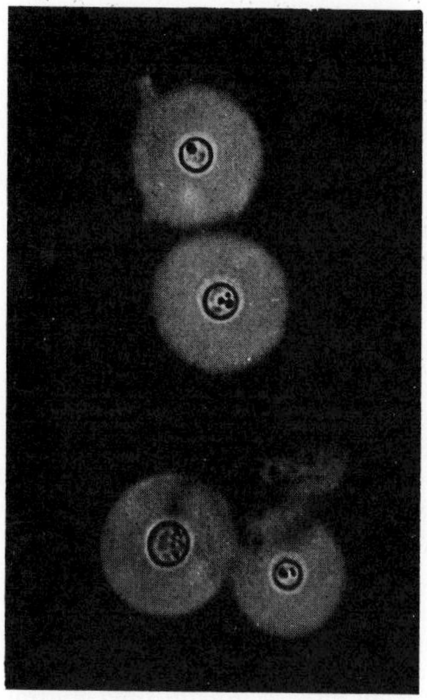

Figure 85–7. Encapsulated yeast cells in *Cryptococcus neoformans*. India ink preparation of spinal fluid. × 736.

zation with whole yeast cells, antibodies are formed to the capsule. By cross-adsorption of rabbit antisera, four different antigenic determinants have been detected in the capsular material of *C. neoformans* and designated A through D. Kwon-Chung has shown that isolates of serotypes A and D and isolates of serotypes B and C represent two distinct varieties. One variety, *C. neoformans* var *neoformans* represents serotypes A and D and is the anamorph of *F. neoformans* var *neoformans*. *C. neoformans* var *gattii* corresponds with serotypes B and C and *F. neoformans* var *bacillispora*.

These capsular serotypes can also be correlated with differences in ecology and prevalence of disease. Strains of serotype A can be isolated worldwide and are the most frequent cause of cryptococcosis. Type D is more common in Europe. Serotypes A and D have been isolated from soil and avian, especially pigeon, feces. Serotypes B and C have only recently been isolated from nature in association with eucalyptus trees in Australia, and infections cause by these two serotypes are concentrated in tropical and subtropical regions, including Australia, and in the United States in southern California.

During growth in vitro or in vivo, the capsule is solubilized and can be precipitated from the culture supernatant fluid or detected in body fluids. The purified capsular material is a high-molecular-weight polysaccharide. Hydrolysis of capsular polysaccharide from cells of serotype A yields mannose, xylose, and glucuronic acid. Chemical studies support an α-1,3-linked polymannose backbone with β-linked monomeric branches of xylose and glucuronic acid. This *glucuronoxylomannan* (GXM) is the major capsular polysaccharide of *C. neoformans*. The structures of the GXMs of the other serotypes differ in the degree of mannosyl substitution. GXM resembles a T cell–independent antigen. It is poorly immunogenic by itself, but if it is conjugated to a protein carrier, a strong antibody response develops, as occurs when the whole cell is the immunogen. GXM exhibits several biologic properties and is a virulence factor (see below).

Culture filtrates of *C. neoformans* also yield smaller amounts of another polysaccharide, a galactoxylomannan, and a mannoprotein, which appears to be the immunodominant antigen for evoking cell-mediated immunity and delayed-type hypersensitivity. In the murine model, Murphy has shown that the mannoprotein can function as an immunomodulator

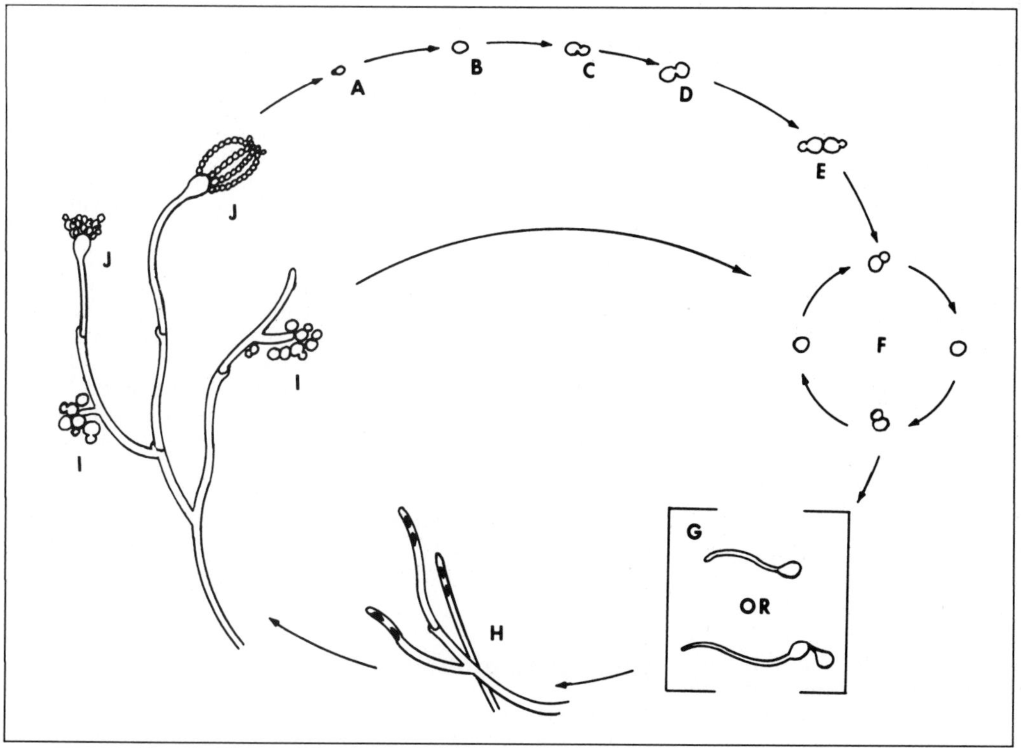

Fig. 85–8. Life cycle of *Filobasidiella neoformans*. **A** to **E.** Swelling of haploid basidiospore and subsequent budding. **F.** Asexual yeast cell cycle (*Cryptococcus neoformans*). **G.** Initiation of hyphal formation by sexually compatible yeast cells. **H.** Dikaryotic hyphae with clamp connections. **I.** Budding yeast cells. **J.** Basidia and basidiospores formed at hyphal tips. *(From Erke: J Bacteriol 128:455, 1976.)*

and elicit a cascade of suppressor cells, which may explain the observation that many patients acquire and retain specific immunosuppression to *C. neoformans*.

Physiology

Of the several species of *Cryptococcus*, only *C. neoformans* and some strains of other species are able to grow at 37C. *C. neoformans* is inhibited or killed at 41C, and this temperature restriction may be an important determinant of its pathogenicity. *C. neoformans* produces a unique phenoloxidase(s) that converts a variety of hydroxybenzoic substrates, including catecholamines such as 3,4-dihydroxyphenylalanine, into brown or black pigments, which impart a dark color to colonies or the medium. This reaction has been used for the rapid identification of *C. neoformans*.

All *Cryptococcus* species are nonfermentative, hydrolyze starch, assimilate inositol, and produce urease. These characteristics distinguish them from other clinically important yeasts. Tables 85–1 and 85–2 summarize some useful physiologic reactions for the most frequently isolated species of *Cryptococcus* and compares them with other common yeasts.

Physiologic tests have been developed to distinguish the two varieties of *C. neoformans*. On appropriate media, more than 85% of isolates of serotypes B and C assimilate glycine and malate and are resistant to concentrations of cycloheximide or canavanine that inhibit isolates of serotypes A and D. Most isolates of the latter pair of serotypes are unable to use malate as a source of carbon or glycine as a sole carbon and nitrogen source. Both varieties use creatinine and are induced to synthesize creatinine deaminase, but only in isolates of A and D is this enzyme repressed by the ammonia by-product. Selective media containing creatinine, glucose, and pH indicators have been devised that exploit this difference to differentiate the two varieties. Serotypes B and C are less susceptible to flucytosine than are serotypes A and D.

Determinants of Pathogenicity

Virulence of *C. neoformans* requires growth at 37C, capsule formation, and production of diphenoloxidase. Different strains of *C. neoformans* serotype A have been shown to vary considerably in both murine virulence and in vitro capsule size. However, these two properties are not directly correlated. Nevertheless, the capsule is a crucial virulence factor. The purified GXM has been shown, under the appropriate conditions, to specifically inhibit both phagocytosis of the yeast and the production of antibody to it.

Differences in virulence among strains of serotype A have been correlated in vitro with resistance to killing by alveolar macrophages, but not with differences in capsular size or the extent of phagocytosis.

Genetic analyses support the association of virulence with phenoloxidase production. Since this enzyme can use natural catecholamines (e.g., norepinephrine, dopamine) as substrates for melanogenesis, it may somehow relate to the unexplained neurotropism of *C. neoformans*. Polacheck and associates recently showed that a mutant lacking phenoloxidase was killed by the epinephrine oxidative system in the presence of a transition metal ion and hydrogen peroxide. The wild type was resistant, which suggests that phenoloxidase may consume epinephrine and protect *C. neoformans* from this system in the central nervous system.

Clinical Infection

Epidemiology

Cryptococcosis is a sporadic infection with a worldwide distribution. *C. neoformans* is ubiquitous in the soil and in avian fecal material, such as pigeon droppings, which apparently provide a reservoir of organisms. Although spontaneous infections occur in animals, no spread of infection among animals or humans has been reported. Although infrequently isolated from the respiratory tracts of healthy individuals, *C. neoformans* is not a part of the normal flora of humans or animals. Cryptococcosis definitely occurs in patients who are not apparently compromised; however, most patients have a preexistent underlying condition or disease.

The underlying conditions that most frequently predispose to opportunistic cryptococcosis are AIDS, leukemia, lymphoma, Hodgkin's disease, sarcoidosis, systemic lupus erythematosus, and immunosuppression. The risk factor having the highest correlation with opportunistic cryptococcosis is treatment with steroids.

Patients with AIDS have a marked depression of cell-mediated immunity and, as might be predicted, are highly susceptible to cryptococcosis, as well as other opportunistic infections. Many of the AIDS patients with cryptococcal meningitis have extremely high antigen titers in both spinal fluid and serum. The microscopic examination of spinal fluid often reveals large numbers of yeast cells and few, if any, leukocytes. Cryptococcosis occurs in up to a third of patients with AIDS.

Cryptococcosis occurs equally in both sexes. Curiously, despite large numbers of children at risk, the incidence of cryptococcosis in patients below the age of puberty is unaccountably rare.

Pathogenesis

The high prevalence of *C. neoformans* in nature and the relatively low frequency of disease suggest that many persons are probably exposed without developing symptoms. The frequency of subclinical infection is unknown because there is no adequate skin test antigen with which to assess exposure, and the primary pulmonary infection does not usually calcify or leave marked residua. The few reports of human skin testing with experimental antigens or measuring antibodies with enzyme immunoassays indicate a high level of reactivity.

Cryptococcosis is initiated in the lung after inhalation of yeast cells of *C. neoformans*. Small ($\leq$5 μm in diameter), minimally encapsulated yeast cells of *C. neoformans* have been isolated from air and soil. The predominance of yeasts of a single mating type among both clinical and natural isolates, including airborne isolates, almost certainly excludes the basidiospore ($\approx$3 μm) as a routine source of infection. In the alveolar spaces, the yeast cells are initially confronted by the alveolar macrophages. Whether active infection and disease follow this interaction depends on the competence of the host cellular defenses and the numbers and virulence of the yeast cells inhaled. Cellular immune mechanisms normally mediate a successful host response through activation of macrophages. The capsular polysaccharide, the mannoprotein and perhaps other yeast components are also capable of subverting the host responses.

Clinical Manifestations

Pulmonary Cryptococcosis. The primary pulmonary infection may evolve in any portion of the lung, mimic an influenza-type respiratory infection, and then resolve spontaneously. Pulmonary cryptococcosis is rarely fulminant, and hilar lymphadenopathy, calcification, and cavitation are seldom observed. Patients may have no symptoms, or a minority may experience cough, sputum production, weight loss, or fever. The tissue response is usually minimal or granulomatous.

Disseminated Cryptococcosis. *C. neoformans* is neurotropic and disseminates to the central nervous system. Meningitis may be acute or chronic. The usual progression of symptoms—fever, headache, stiff neck, and disorientation—are accompanied by spinal fluid that typically is clear, increased opening pressure, presence of cells (predominantly mononuclear), elevated protein, and normal or reduced chloride and sugar. In addition to the central nervous system, dissemination may occur to the skin and viscera.

Laboratory Diagnosis

Microscopic Examination. Spinal fluid, aspirates from skin lesions, sputum, tissue, and other appropriate specimens should be examined directly in an India ink preparation for the presence of yeast cells with capsules (Fig. 85–9). Encapsulated yeasts in tissue sections appear to be surrounded by large empty spaces because of the poor staining of the capsular polysaccharide and distortion resulting from sectioning. The capsule can be stained with mucicarmine. In histologic sections, the cells of *C. neoformans* often appear collapsed and distorted.

Culture. *C. neoformans* can be isolated on most laboratory media, but media containing cycloheximide should not be used because the organism is sensitive to this agent. Most *Cryptococcus* species are encapsulated, are similar in microscopic and colony morphology, and produce extracellular starch and urease, and all are nonfermentative (Table 85–2). *C. neoformans* is unique in its pathogenicity, its ability to grow at 37C, and its production of phenoloxidase, which is demonstrated by a brown pigment when grown on Staib's birdseed agar or caffeic acid medium. Spinal fluid cultures are frequently positive, but blood cultures are often negative except in severe cases.

Serology. The mycoserology for the diagnosis of cryptococcosis is very specific and sensitive. During infection, capsular material is solubilized in the body fluids, and being an antigen, it can be titered with a specific rabbit anti-*C. neoformans* antiserum. The most commonly employed method is a latex agglutination test (Table 85–3). Latex particles are coated with the specific rabbit immunoglobulin and mixed with dilutions of patient serum or spinal fluid. Controls include latex coated with normal rabbit globulin to check for nonspecific agglutination, which occurs with rheumatoid factor. A positive agglutination is diagnostic for cryptococcosis. The serum or spinal fluid titer can be used prognostically. A rising or constant titer indicates a poor prognosis due to active or stabilized infection. With recovery, the antigen titer drops and disappears. Diagnosis by antigen detection is more sensitive than diagnosis by either India ink or culture. The antigen in serum of patients with AIDS is cleared slowly and may persist at high titer despite prolonged therapy.

Antibodies to *C. neoformans* are usually not detectable in the active disease state. Capsular polysaccharide in the serum may combine with circulating antibody, as well as inhibit its synthesis. However, with recovery the serum may be positive for antibody.

Treatment

Cryptococcosis is treated with both amphotericin B and flucytosine, according to a combined therapy protocol. Resistance to flucytosine occurs. Cryptococcosis in patients with AIDS does not respond to the routine combined therapy of amphotericin B and flucytosine. Patients with AIDS often require maintenance therapy for long periods to suppress the infection. Fluconazole has excellent penetration into the central nervous system, and in a controlled study, maintenance therapy with fluconazole prevented recurrence of cryptococcal meningitis.

Aspergillosis

Aspergillosis refers to a spectrum of diseases that may be caused by a number of *Aspergillus* species. Species of *Aspergillus* are ubiquitous in nature, and aspergillosis occurs worldwide. Inhalation of *Aspergillus* conidia or mycelial fragments may elicit in certain people an immediate hypersensitivity response without fungal growth. In allergic bronchopulmonary aspergillosis, there is actual infection by an *Aspergillus* species, and the fungus grows within the bronchial tree. Invasive aspergillosis occurs in certain types of compromised patients and involves actual invasion of the tissue. In other patients, aspergillosis is characterized by a noninvasive colonization of exposed tissue, such as the pulmonary cavity, external ear canal, sinuses, nail plate, or cornea. Certain secondary metabolites produced by species of *Aspergillus* are toxic and carcinogenic.

Some 150 different species and subspecies of *Aspergillus* have been recognized. They can be isolated from vegetation, especially nuts and grains, during their growth or storage, from decaying matter, soil, and air. Many species are pathogenic for plants, and some infect insects, birds, and domestic animals.

A. fumigatus is the most common pathogenic species for humans, although many other species have been known to produce infection. Considering the overall prevalence of pathogenic species and the constant exposure of humans and animals, the incidence of infection is relatively rare. Clearly, a high degree of natural resistance exists in the healthy host. However, when the exposure is overwhelming, as in the occurrence of extrinsic allergic alveolitis among malt workers exposed to the conidia of *Aspergillus clavatus*, or when the host defenses are compromised, as in the case of leukemic patients, a form of aspergillosis may develop.

Morphology and Physiology

Cultural Characteristics

Aspergillus species grow rapidly on many natural substrates and laboratory media. The abundant aerial mycelium becomes powdery and pigmented as conidia, which are characteristic of each species, are produced. Although *A. fumigatus* is the most common pathogenic species, more than a dozen additional species of *Aspergillus* have been known to cause infection.

Some properties of the most frequent clinical isolates are compared in Table 85–8.

Microscopic Appearance

All species of *Aspergillus* are characterized by conidiophores, which expand into large vesicles at the end and are covered with phialides that produce long chains of conidia (Fig. 85–9). Phialides may arise directly from the vesicle (uniseriate) or from metulae, which are attached to the vesicle (biseriate). Species are identified primarily on the basis of the conidial structures, namely, the size, color, and shape of the conidiophore, conidia, and phialides (Table 85–8).

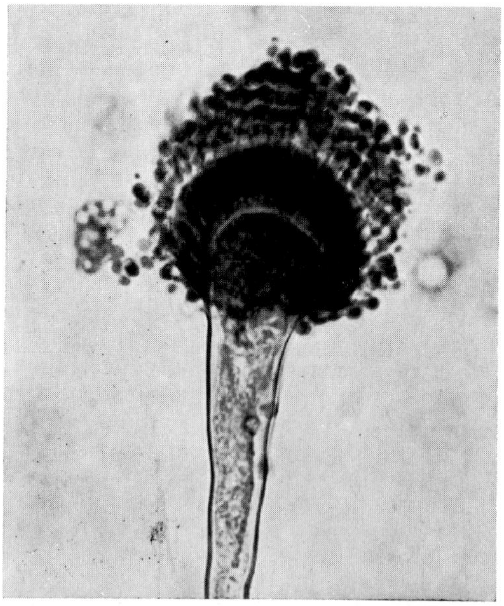

Fig. 85–9. The typical conidiophore of *Aspergillus fumigatus* expands into a vesicle from which phialides arise directly (uniseriate) to produce basipetal chains of conidia. *(From Conant et al: Manual of Clinical Morphology, ed 3. Saunders, 1971.)*

Clinical Infection

Epidemiology

Certain host factors clearly predispose some individuals to invasive aspergillosis. In general, the risk factors of invasive aspergillosis are similar to those associated with systemic candidiasis. There is a significant correlation of invasive aspergillosis with hematologic malignancy (especially acute or chronic leukemia, lymphoma, or Hodgkin's disease), granulocytopenia, therapy with corticosteroids, antibacterial antibiotics, or cytotoxic drugs, or combinations of these conditions. For example, 17 cases of precipitous, invasive aspergillosis in cancer patients inadvertently exposed to a heavy environmental contamination of *Aspergillus* was documented by Aisner and associates. Twelve of these patients had acute nonlymphocytic leukemia, and all 17 displayed some degree of neutropenia. Similar environmental contamination of an air filtration system in a bone marrow transplant unit caused seven fatal cases of invasive aspergillosis. As a result of these experiences, patients with neutropenia, leukemia, or other associated risk are protected with filtered air, positive pressure rooms, limited access, and other precautions to minimize exposure to *Aspergillus*. The allergic forms occur more often in atopic individuals and those who are exposed frequently to massive doses of the conidia. Indeed, aspergillosis is an occupational disease of agricultural workers and whiskey distillery workers exposed to numerous conidia in malting barley. Aspergilloma occurs in individuals who have preexisting pulmonary cavities.

Pathogenesis

Most cases of aspergillosis develop in individuals who have structural abnormalities within the lung or who have severely impaired resistance to infection because of metastatic cancer, leukemia, or lymphomatous diseases or because of the therapy used in combating these diseases. In vitro studies support the clinical evidence that leukocytes are essential in the host defense against aspergillosis. Healthy macrophages are able to contain conidia, and hyphae but not conidia are susceptible to neutrophil and monocyte killing mechanisms. *Aspergillus* products have been described that inhibit activation of the alternative pathway of complement. Allergic forms of aspergillosis involve specific immunopathology without fungal invasion.

Clinical Manifestations

Several classifications of the clinical types of aspergillosis have been proposed. Table 85–9 presents a current view and the associated immune response.

Allergic Forms. Inhalation of antigens associated with *As-*

TABLE 85–8. CHARACTERISTICS OF COMMON PATHOGENIC *ASPERGILLUS* SPECIES

Species	Conidiophore Length	Vesicle Width (μm)	Phialides	Conidia Color	Conidia Diameter (μm)
A. fumigatus	<300 μm	20–30; only top half conidiogenous	Uniseriate	Gray, green, or blue-green	2.5–3.0
A. flavus	<1 mm	25–45	Uniseriate or biseriate	Yellow to green	3.5–4.5
A. niger	1.5–3.0 mm	45–75	Biseriate	Black	4.0–5.0
A. nidulans	60–130 μm	8–10	Biseriate	Dark green	3.0–3.5
A. terreus	100–250 μm	10–16	Biseriate	Orange to brown	1.8–2.4

Adapted from Raper and Fennell: The Genus Aspergillus. Williams & Wilkins, 1965.

TABLE 85–9. CLINICAL TYPES OF ASPERGILLOSIS

Clinical Forms	Hypersensitivity Types
Allergic Forms	
Atopic host	
Asthma	I only
Allergic bronchopulmonary aspergillosis	I and III
Nonatopic host	
Extrinsic allergic alveolitis	III only, or with I or IV
Noninvasive Colonization	
Aspergilloma	I, II, or none
Nonpulmonary, local infection	
Invasive Aspergillosis	None or any
Pulmonary	
Chronic necrotizing pulmonary	
Disseminated	

pergillus species elicits in certain atopic individuals an immediate, asthmatic reaction, mediated by reaginic antibody or specific IgE. Diagnosis is confirmed by patient history, positive I skin tests (wheal and flare) to *Aspergillus* antigens, and presence of specific IgE antibody. Bronchoconstriction occurs in the absence of both fungal growth and pulmonary consolidation in radiographs of the chest.

Allergic bronchopulmonary aspergillosis is the major and well-characterized allergic form of aspergillosis. Table 85–10 lists major diagnostic criteria: (1) asthma, (2) recurrent pulmonary densities in radiographs of the chest, (3) eosinophilia, and (4) hypersensitivity to *Aspergillus* antigen, as shown by an immediate skin test reaction (type I) followed some hours later by an Arthus reaction (type III). Other criteria include positive culture of *Aspergillus* from sputum, anti-*Aspergillus* precipitins in serum, elevated serum IgE levels, and a history of recurrent pneumonia. In allergic bronchopulmonary aspergillosis, IgE-mediated responses develop, and, in addition, IgG antibodies react with solubilized fungal antigens to form immune complexes. Complement is activated by these complexes, which induces a neutrophilic infiltration and general inflammatory response. As a result, the disease is more protracted, and chronic lung changes may ensue.

TABLE 85–10. ALLERGIC BRONCHOPULMONARY ASPERGILLOSIS: DIAGNOSTIC CRITERIA

Criteria	Percent Positive
Asthma	100
Pulmonary infiltrates	91–100
Eosinophilia (in blood)	80–100
Immune responses to *Aspergillus fumigatus* antigen	
Type I (wheal and flare)	100
Type III (Arthus)	100
Serum precipitins	84–91
Sputum	
Eosinophilia	44–100
History of plugs	74
Culture of *A. fumigatus*	46–83

From Safirstein et al: Am Rev Respir Dis 108:450, 1973; Malo et al: Thorax 32:269, 1977; Khan et al: Scand J Respir Dis 57:73, 1976.

Nonatopic hosts can develop another form of hypersensitivity reaction to *Aspergillus* antigens, *extrinsic allergic alveolitis*. This entity is characterized by the presence of serum precipitins to *Aspergillus* antigens and, on skin testing, an Arthus (type III) reaction that occasionally is preceded by an immediate reaction. Inhalation of the antigen will induce fever, leukocytosis, dyspnea, nonproductive cough, myalgia, and rales after several hours.

Aspergilloma and Extrapulmonary Colonization. The conidia of *Aspergillus* species are able to germinate and colonize the surfaces of open pulmonary cavities, paranasal sinuses, and ear canals. Aspergilloma, or fungus ball, refers to the colonization of a pulmonary cavity that may have been caused originally by bronchiectasis, carcinoma, histoplasmosis, malformation, sarcoidosis, or tuberculosis. This is probably the most common type of pulmonary aspergillosis, and the radiographic appearance of an air space surrounding the cavity is highly characteristic, although not diagnostic, of aspergilloma. Many patients with aspergilloma are asymptomatic. Some have productive cough and hemoptysis, but dyspnea and even pulmonary hemorrhage may also follow the appearance of a fungus ball in the chest radiograph.

Noninvasive colonization may occur in the ears, paranasal sinuses, and nasal cavity, followed by symptoms of chronic otitis and sinusitis. Immunosuppressed patients are particularly susceptible to paranasal sinusitis, which may not respond to amphotericin B. Both allergy and superficial trauma are necessary for the development of ear infections. *Aspergillus niger* is the major cause of otomycosis. Primary localized infections of the conjunctiva, eyelids, cornea, orbit, and intraocular structures with *Aspergillus* species have also been described. Cutaneous lesions have been reported. Onychomycosis can be caused by *Aspergillus flavus*, *Aspergillus nidulans*, and *Aspergillus glaucus*.

Invasive Aspergillosis. Whether localized in the lung or generalized and disseminated, the course of invasive aspergillosis depends largely on the underlying illness. Most cases of invasive pulmonary aspergillosis now occur in patients with acute leukemia, granulocytopenia, lymphoma, or rarely, other malignancies, or in the immunosuppressed state associated with bone marrow or organ transplantation (Table 85–11). For example, in a recent review, Denning and Stevens reported that 14% of heart transplant recipients at Stanford had aspergillosis. In the absence of early treatment, the course is uniformly fatal.

In the rare, otherwise healthy host, the prognosis is much better. Invasion of the lung parenchyma may develop immediately in a compromised patient exposed to an infectious dose of *Aspergillus* conidia, or it may follow as a rare complication of an aspergilloma. Invasion seldom occurs with allergic bronchopulmonary aspergillosis. Patients with long-standing AIDS may develop invasive pulmonary aspergillosis or *obstructing bronchial aspergillosis*. In the latter disease, the bronchial passages are colonized with fungal growth. This condition is different from allergic bronchopulmonary aspergillosis and may precede invasive disease.

The hyphae exhibit a propensity for invading the lumen and walls of blood vessels, causing thrombosis, infarction, and hemorrhage. Dissemination from the lungs may result in generalized aspergillosis involving a number of other organs,

TABLE 85–11. RISK FACTORS FOR ASPERGILLOSIS (ABRIDGED)

Aspergilloma (pulmonary cavity)	***Allergic Bronchopulmonary Aspergillosis***
Tuberculosis	Atopy
Sarcoidosis	Cystic fibrosis
Mycosis	Exposure to conidia
Bullous emphysema	***Invasive Aspergillosis***
Cavitary carcinoma	Hematologic malignancy
Pneumoconiosis	Cytotoxic drugs
Chronic Necrotizing Pulmonary Aspergillosis	Immunosuppression
Pulmonary infarction	Neutropenia
Chronic obstructive lung disease	Chronic granulomatous disease
Inactive mycobacterial infection	Organ transplantation with immunosuppression
Sarcoidosis	Bone marrow transplantation
Pneumoconiosis	Corticosteroid treatment
Low-dose corticosteroid treatment	Broad-spectrum antibacterial antibiotics
Connective tissue disorder	Intravenous drug abuse
Diabetes mellitus	Diabetes mellitus
Malnutrition	Acquired immunodeficiency syndrome (AIDS)

including, most frequently, the gastrointestinal tract, brain, liver, kidney, and many other sites, such as the heart, skin, or eye.

Whereas invasive aspergillosis occurs most often as acute pneumonia in cancer or transplant patients receiving corticosteroids, *chronic necrotizing pulmonary aspergillosis* may develop over a period of months. This milder disease usually occurs in middle-aged patients with other conditions: diabetes mellitus, connective tissue disorders, chronic obstructive lung disease, poor nutrition, low-dose corticosteroids, and so forth (Table 85–11). Patients have cough, sputum production, and a chest film that may resemble cavitary tuberculosis with apical infiltrations. The response to antifungal chemotherapy, with or without surgery, is good.

Laboratory Diagnosis

Microscopic Examination. Fresh sputum should be examined for the presence of branching, septate hyphae of uniform width (4 to 7 μm). Sputum may contain sparse filaments or plugs of mycelium (Fig. 85–10). In the bronchi, *Aspergillus* may produce aerial hyphae and characteristic conidia and conidiophores. Conidia may also form in the air space associated with an aspergilloma. In tissue sections, hyphae are often seen in blood vessels, forming parallel arrays with dichotomous branching at acute angles. The true hyphae found in aspergillosis should not be confused with the yeast cells and pseudohyphae associated with invasive candidiasis (Table 85–3).

Culture. *Aspergillus* species will grow on most routine media, but cycloheximide-containing media should not be used. The developing colonies produce surface mycelia within a few days and become pigmented as conidia develop. Most species are identified by their morphology (Table 85–8 and Fig. 85–9).

Because *Aspergillus* species are common contaminants, the significance of a positive culture is often questionable. Active allergic bronchopulmonary aspergillosis, aspergilloma, and other local colonizations can be diagnosed by direct examination or repeatedly positive, often pure cultures. However, in invasive aspergillosis, direct examination of sputum and culture of sputum are often negative. A single positive culture in a compromised patient may, therefore, be highly significant. Aggressive diagnostic efforts are warranted in patients with leukemia, leukopenia, fever, and pulmonary infiltrates. These include transtracheal aspiration, bronchial brush biopsy, or open lung biopsy to obtain specimens for examination in patients who can tolerate these procedures. Routine nasal and respiratory cultures of patients at risk may be helpful in establishing an early diagnosis of invasive aspergillosis. Blood cultures are invariably negative.

Serology. The immunologic responses detected after exposure to *Aspergillus* can sometimes clarify the pathogenesis, diagnosis, and prognosis. Serologic studies involving hundreds of patients have clearly associated the presence of precipitins to various antigen preparations of *Aspergillus* species, as detected by immunodiffusion, with different forms of aspergillosis (Table 85–7). Eighty to one hundred percent of patients with allergic bronchopulmonary aspergillosis or aspergilloma have one or more serum precipitins to *A. fumigatus*. Unfortunately, sera from patients with invasive aspergillosis are much less frequently positive. False-positive tests are rare but may occur with serum containing cross-reacting fungal antibodies or C-reactive protein. Approximately 30% or more of patients with cystic fibrosis have *Aspergillus* precipitins. In patients with allergic bronchopulmonary aspergillosis, specific

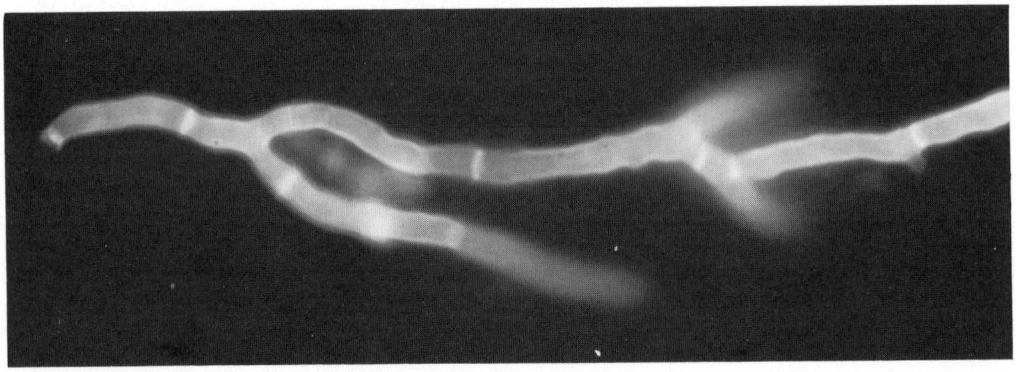

Fig. 85–10. Aspergillosis. Calcofluor white stain of sputum showing uniform, septate hyphae with dichotomous branching typical of *Aspergillus*. × 1000.

IgE antibodies to *A. fumigatus* can be detected by the radioallergosorbent test. Detection of *Aspergillus* antigenemia in patients with invasive aspergillosis is more sensitive and specific than the test for precipitins.

Treatment

Allergic forms of aspergillosis have been treated with corticosteroids and antifungal therapy. Disodium chromoglycate also reduces symptoms but may not prevent recurrence.

The treatment of aspergilloma varies considerably with its severity. Asymptomatic patients may not warrant treatment, whereas other patients may require surgical resection. Both amphotericin B and flucytosine have been recommended, and pulmonary lavage has been suggested to facilitate penetration of the cavity by the drug. Local, superficial aspergillosis is treated with nystatin.

For invasive aspergillosis, aggressive treatment with amphotericin B is initiated as soon as possible. The overall response to amphotericin B is about 50%; however, regardless of therapy, the mortality in patients with bone marrow transplants or cerebral disease is over 90%. Treatment with amphotericin B and flucytosine has been effective in some patients with pulmonary disease. Current clinical trials suggest that itraconazole may be especially effective against *Aspergillus*.

Prophylaxis

As with the prevention of systemic candidiasis in high-risk patients, prophylactic treatment with low-dose amphotericin B or oral itraconazole has been used in patients at risk for invasive aspergillosis. Patients treated with intravenous amphotericin B for proven aspergillosis may be given oral itraconazole to prevent relapse.

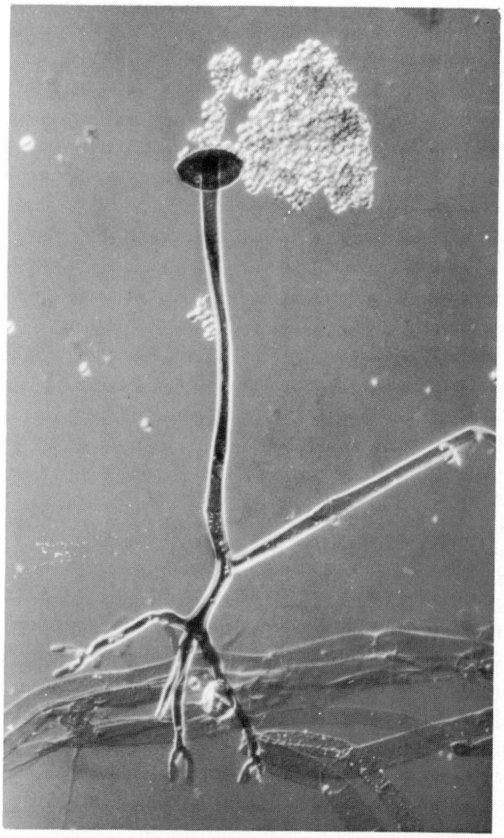

Fig. 85–11. *Rhizopus.* Typical sporangium and rhizoids. Nomarski. × 200. *(From McGinnis: Laboratory Handbook of Medical Mycology. Academic Press, 1980.)*

Mucormycosis

Mucormycosis (synonyms: phycomycosis, zygomycosis) is an opportunistic mycotic infection caused by a number of mold species classified in the order Mucorales of the class Zygomycetes (Chap. 80). These fungi are ubiquitous, thermotolerant saprophytes. Patients with acidosis, leukemias, and immunodeficiencies are particularly at risk from opportunistic mucormycosis.

The etiologic agents of mucormycosis, in an approximate order of their frequency as pathogens, are *Rhizopus arrhizus (Rhizopus oryzae), Rhizopus rhizopodiformis, Absidia corymbifera, Rhizomucor pusillus,* and species of *Rhizomucor, Mucor, Rhizopus, Absidia, Mortierella, Cunninghamella, Saksenaea,* and others. They can be isolated from the air, soil, water, and hospital environments worldwide.

Morphology and Physiology

Cultural Characteristics

These zygomycetes grow rapidly and produce abundant, cottony or fluffy aerial mycelia that often fill the agar test tube or Petri plate. Most genera can be identified on the basis of morphology, but species identification often is difficult.

Microscopic Appearance

Zygomycetes produce broad, sparsely septate hyphae (≈ 10 μm) that often appear twisted and ribbon-like on microscopic examination. They reproduce asexually by the formation of sporangia and sexually with production of a zygospore (Chap. 80). Figure 85–11 depicts the sporangia and characteristic rhizoids of *Rhizopus*.

Clinical Infection

Epidemiology

Patients with ketoacidosis resulting from diabetes mellitus, drugs, or uremia are predisposed to invasive mucormycosis. The disease is also associated with burn patients, leukemia, lymphoma, steroid treatment, and immunosuppression, either natural or induced. Several studies indicate an increase in the frequency of mucormycosis.

Pathogenesis

The sporangiospores apparently germinate and thrive in environments like the nasal, oropharyngeal, or respiratory mucosa of compromised patients. Normal alveolar macrophages inhibit germination of sporangiospores, but alveolar macrophages from diabetic or cortisone-treated mice were unable to prevent spore germination. Artis and associates have demonstrated that in diabetic ketoacidosis, acidosis causes the release of iron from transferrin, which permits the growth of *R. arrhizus*. Hyphae invade the lumen and walls of blood vessels, causing thrombosis, infarction, and necrosis. This process is more rapid than the similar involvement with *Aspergillus* or *Candida*. A suppurative response is elicited, and local necrosis develops.

Clinical Manifestations

Invasive mucormycosis is an acute disease and occurs in two forms, defined by the site of involvement. Local, colonizing infections have occurred in different types of patients.

Rhinocerebral Mucormycosis. With rhinocerebral mucormycosis, invasion begins typically in the nasal region and progresses rapidly to involve the sinuses, eye, brain, and meninges. There is characteristic edema of the involved facial areas, necrosis, and a bloody exudate. The disease can be precipitous, with a terminal outcome in 1 week. Damage to the fifth and seventh cranial nerves, orbital cellulitis, and exophthalmia are frequent manifestations.

Thoracic Mucormycosis. Thoracic mucormycosis follows inhalation of the sporangiospores. The pathology caused by invasion of blood vessels results in profound destruction of lung parenchyma. Pulmonary lesions may be focal or diffuse. The usual course is 1 to 4 weeks from onset to death.

Other Forms. Localized mucormycosis has been described in the kidney after tissue trauma. Cutaneous infection may complicate burn wounds. The application of contaminated bandages for surgical dressings has caused nosocomial infection of the skin.

Laboratory Diagnosis

In specimens of tissue, sputum, or nasal exudate, the hyphae are broad and irregular in width (10 to 15 μm) and exhibit branching, often at right angles. Hyphae are distorted and usually nonseptate (Fig. 85–12).

In systemic cases, blood cultures are invariably negative. Specimens of tissue or drainage should be cultured. If severe disease is not apparent, positive cultures may only be contaminants.

An immunodiffusion test has been described to precipitins in patient sera (Table 85–7).

Treatment

The mortality of invasive mucormycosis has decreased in recent years but remains at approximately 50%. When diagnosis is established antemortem, amphotericin B and surgical debridement are recommended. Recently, adjunctive hyperbaric oxygen has been recommended as well, to stem necrosis and inhibit the fungus. Prognosis depends on control of the underlying disease and is best in patients with underlying diabetes. Survivors usually have permanent changes, such as facial paralysis, loss of an eye, and similar problems.

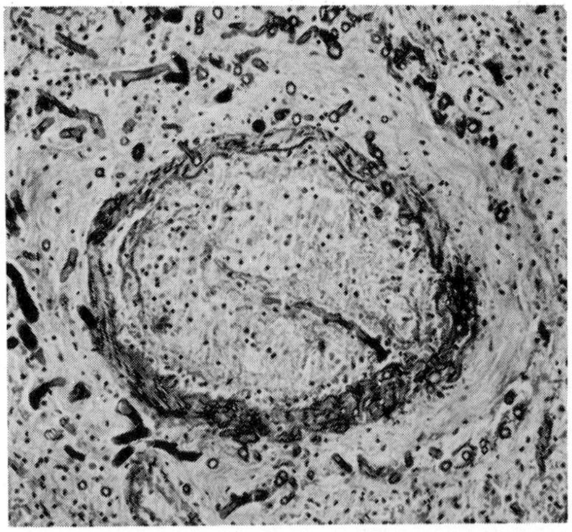

Fig. 85–12. Mucormycosis. Hyphae in wall and lumen of blood vessel and in pulmonary alveoli. × 150. *(From Conant et al: Manual of Clinical Mycology, ed 3. Saunders, 1971.)*

Other Opportunistic Mycoses

Trichosporonosis

Trichosporon beigelii or *Blastoschizomyces capitatus (Trichosporon capitatum)* (Tables 85–1 and 85–2) cause rare but increasing infections in compromised patients. These agents can be isolated from healthy skin and other sites, as well as wood, air and fomites. Trichosporonosis is frequently fatal in patients with hematologic malignancies. Early signs include fever, pneumonia, skin lesions, or positive blood cultures. Patients may have pulmonary infiltrates and *Trichosporon* in the lung or disseminated infection of the spleen, liver, kidney, marrow, brain, eye, or other sites. These fungi are susceptible to amphotericin B, ketoconazole, and miconazole, although most patients with disseminated infection do not survive. Flucytosine in combination with amphotericin B also has been used.

Geotrichosis

Geotrichosis is caused by *Geotrichum candidum*, a fungus found saprophytically in nature and as a commensal in the mouth, gastrointestinal tract, and genitourinary tract. The clinical forms of this rare infection are pulmonary geotrichosis, which mimics tuberculosis in its manifestations, and superficial infections of the skin, oral mucosa, and gastrointestinal tract. Diagnosis is made by culture and identification (Table 85–2). Reported treatments include aerosolized nystatin, iodides, and amphotericin B.

Other Opportunistic Mycoses

Many individuals with compromised host defenses are susceptible to infections by other fungi. Many of the thousands of ubiquitous saprophytic fungi have caused rare infections. Such mycoses occur much less frequently than opportunistic candidiasis, aspergillosis, and mucormycosis because these rare etiologic agents have a low pathogenetic potential due to their weak virulence or high susceptibility to host defenses. In some cases, exposure may be limited by environmental factors.

Humans and other animals are constantly exposed to the hundreds of species of molds that abound in nature. Pulmonary and systemic penicilliosis has been reported sporadically; the most frequent pathogen, *Penicillium marneffei*, is endemic in China. Species of another common saprophyte, *Fusarium*, have infected burn patients. The appearances of *Fusarium*, *Aspergillus*, *Paecilomyces*, and other molds in tissue are indistinguishable, and cultures must be available to establish etiology. Infection with any of these molds is characterized by the presence of hyaline, septate hyphae in tissue and is termed *hyalohyphomycosis*. In contrast, *phaeohyphomycosis* refers to opportunistic infection by a dematiaceous fungus (Chap. 83), such as *Alternaria alternata*, which has been diagnosed in an AIDS patient. The agents of fungal peritonitis in patients receiving peritoneal dialysis include environmental saprophytes, such as *Bipolaris spicifera* and *Rhodotorula rubra*, as well as *Candida* species. Yeasts, such as *Hensenula*, *Rhodotorula*, and *Saccharomyces*, occasionally cause systemic infections.

In the patient with severely compromised host defenses, almost any fungus may become an opportunistic pathogen. To date, several hundred species have been documented as agents of human mycoses. Both the number of opportunistic mycoses and the number of different fungi causing opportunistic mycoses continue to rise.

FURTHER READING

CANDIDIASIS AND FUNGAL OPPORTUNISM

Ahonen P, Myllärniemi S, Sipilä I, et al: Clincial variation of autoimmune polyendocrinopathy-candidiasis-ectodermal dystrophy (APECED) in a series of 68 patients. N Engl J Med 322:1829, 1990

Armstrong D: Problems in management of opportunistic fungal diseases. Rev Infect Dis 11(suppl):S1591, 1989

Bennett JE: Rapid diagnosis of candidiasis and aspergillosis. Rev Infect Dis 9:398, 1987

Bodey GP, Fainstein V (eds): Candidiasis. New York Raven Press, 1985

Bodey GP, Samonis G, Rolston K: Prophylaxis of candidiasis in cancer patients. Semin Oncol 17:24, 1990

Brawner DL, Cutler JE: Oral *Candida albicans* isolates from nonhospitalized normal carriers, immunocompetent hospitalized patients, and immunocompromised patients with or without acquired immunodeficiency syndrome. J Clin Microbiol 27:1335, 1989

Bross J, Talbot GH, Maislin G, et al: Risk factors for nosocomial candidemia: A case-control study in adults without leukemia. Am J Med 87:614, 1989

Calderone RA, Braun PC: Adherence and receptor relationships of *Candida albicans*. Microbiol Rev 55:1, 1991

Caroline L, Rosner F, Kozinn PJ: Elevated serum iron, low unbound transferrin and candidiasis in acute leukemia. Blood 34:441, 1969

Cassone A, Marconi P, Bistoni F: Cell wall of *Candida albicans* and host response. CRC Crit Rev Microbiol 15:87, 1987

Crislip MA, Edwards JE, Jr: Candidiasis. Infect Dis Clin North Am 3:103, 1989

Cutler JE: Acute systemic candidiasis in normal and congenitally thymic-deficient (nude) mice. J Reticuloendothel Soc 19:121, 1976

Cutler JE: Putative virulence factors of *Candida albicans*. Annu Rev Microbiol 45:187, 1991

Datta A, Ganesan K, Natarajan K: Current trends in *Candida albicans* research. Adv Microbial Physiol 30:53, 1989

Davies SF: Diagnosis of pulmonary fungal infections. Semin Respir Infect 3:162, 1988

de Repentigny L, Reiss E: Current trends in immunodiagnosis of candidiasis and aspergillosis. Rev Infect Dis 6:301, 1984

Diamond RD: Fungal surfaces: Effects of interactions with phagocytic cells. Rev Infect Dis 10:S428, 1988

Domer JE: *Candida* cell wall mannan: A polysaccharide with diverse immunologic properties. Crit Rev Microbiol 17:33, 1989

Domer JE, Elkins K, Ennist D, et al: Modulation of immune responses by surface polysaccharides of *Candida albicans*. Rev Infect Dis 10:S419, 1988

Douglas LJ: Adhesion to surfaces. In Rose AH, Harrison JS (eds): The Yeasts. Vol 2: Yeasts and the Environment, Ed 2. London, Academic Press, 1987, p 239

Douglas LJ: *Candida* proteinases and candidosis. Crit Rev Biotechnol 8:121, 1988

Edwards JE, Gaither TA, O'Shea JJ, et al: Expression of specific binding sites on *Candida* with functional and antigenic characteristics of human complement receptors. J Immunol 137:3577, 1986

Eisenberg ES, Leviton I, Soeiro R: Fungal peritonitis in patients receiving peritoneal dialysis: Experience with 11 patients and review of the literature. Rev Infect Dis 8:309, 1986

Ghannoum MA: Mechanisms potentiating *Candida* infections. A review. Mycoses 31:543, 1988

Gold JWM: Opportunistic fungal infections in patients with neoplastic disease. Am J Med 76:458, 1984

Greenfield RA: Pulmonary infections due to higher bacteria and fungi in the immunocompromised host. Semin Respir Med 10:68, 1989

Gupta TP, Ehrinpreis MN: *Candida*-associated diarrhea in hospitalized patients. Gastroenterology 98:780, 1990

Hadfield TL, Smith MB, Winn RE, et al: Mycoses caused by *Candida lusitaniae*. Rev Infect Dis 9:1006, 1987

Hay KD: Candidosis of the oral cavity. Recognition and management. Drugs 36:633, 1988

Hazen KC: Cell surface hydrophobicity of medically important fungi, especially *Candida* species. In Doyle RJ, Rosenberg M (eds): Microbiol Cell Surface Hydrophobicity. Washington, DC, American Society for Microbiology, 1990

Hazen KC, Lay J-G, Hazen BW, et al: Partial biochemical characterization of cell surface hydrophobicity and hydrophilicity of *Candida albicans*. Infect Immun 58:3469, 1990

Holmberg K, Meyer RD (eds): Diagnosis and Therapy of Systemic Fungal Infections. New York, Raven Press, 1989

Hughes WT: Systemic candidiasis: A study of 109 fatal cases. Pediatr Infect Dis 1:11, 1982

Hunter PR, Harrison GAJ, Fraser CAM: Cross-infection and diversity of *Candida albicans* strain carriage in patients and nursing staff on an intensive care unit. J Med Vet Mycol 28:317, 1990

Jones JM: Laboratory diagnosis of invasive candidiasis. Clin Microbiol Rev 3:32, 1990

Keller MA, Sellers BB, Melish ME, et al: Systemic candidiasis in infants—Case presentation and literature review. Am J Dis Child 131:1260, 1977

Khardori N: Host-parasite interaction in fungal infections. Eur J Clin Microbiol Infect Dis 8:331, 1989

Kirkpatrick CH: Chronic mucocutaneous candidiasis. Eur J Clin Microbiol Infect Dis 8:448, 1989

Kirsch DR, Kelly R, Kurtz MB (eds): The Genetics of *Candida*. Boca Raton, Fla, CRC Press, 1990

Klein RS, Harris CA, Small CB, et al: Oral candidiasis in high-risk patients as the initial manifestation of the acquired immunodeficiency syndrome. N Engl J Med 311:354, 1984

Komshian SV, Uwaydah AK, Sobel JD, et al: Fungemia caused by *Candida* species and *Torulopsis glabrata* in the hospitalized patient:

Frequency, characteristics, and evaluation of factors influencing outcome. Rev Infect Dis 11:379, 1989
Lehrer RI, Ganz T, Szklarek D, et al: Modulation of the in vitro candidacidal activity of human neutrophil defensins by target cell metabolism and divalent cations. J Clin Invest 81:1829, 1988
Lew MA: Diagnosis of systemic *Candida* infections. Annu Rev Med 40:87, 1989
Lindblad R, Alobaidy A, Mobacken H, et al: Diagnostically usable skin lesions in *Candida* septicemia. Mycoses 32:416, 1989
Manning M, Mitchell TG: Analysis of cytoplasmic antigens of the yeast and mycelial phases of *Candida albicans* by two-dimensional electrophoresis. Infect Immun 30:484, 1980
Manning-Zweerink M, Maloney CS, Mitchell TG, Weston M: Immunoblot analyses of *Candida albicans*-associated antigens and antibodies in human sera. J Clin Microbiol 23:46, 1986
Mason MM, Lasker BA, Riggsby WS: Molecular probe for identification of medically important *Candida* species and *Torulopsis glabrata*. J Clin Microbiol 25:563, 1987
Matthews R, Burnie J: Assessment of DNA fingerprinting for rapid identification of outbreaks of systemic candidiasis. Br Med J 298:354, 1989
Merz WG: *Candida albicans* strain delineation. Clin Microbiol Rev 3:321, 1990
Meunier F: Prevention of mycoses in immunocompromised patients. Rev Infect Dis 9:408, 1987
Meunier F: Candidiasis. Eur J Clin Microbiol Infect Dis 8:438, 1989
Meunier F: Fluconazole treatment of fungal infections in the immunocompromised host. Semin Oncol 17:19, 1990
Mitchell TG: Serodiagnosis of mycotic infections. In Wentworth BB (ed): Diagnostic Procedures for Mycotic and Parasitic Infections. Washington, DC, Am Public Health Assoc, 1988, p 303
Musial CE, Cockerill FR, Roberts GD: Fungal infections of the immunocompromised host: Clinical and laboratory aspects. Clin Microbiol Rev 1:349, 1988
Odds FC. *Candida* and Candidosis, 2nd ed. London, Bailliere Tindall, 1988
Poulain D, Hopwood V, Vernes A: Antigenic variability of *Candida albicans*. CRC Crit Rev Microbiol 12:223, 1985
Reagan DR, Pfaller MA, Hollis RJ, et al: Characterization of the sequence of colonization and nosocomial candidemia using DNA fingerprinting and a DNA probe. J Clin Microbiol 28:2733, 1990
Reiss E: Molecular Immunology of Mycotic and Actinomycotic Infections. New York, Elsevier, 1986
Rogers TJ, Balish E: Immunity to *Candida albicans*. Microbiol Rev 44:660, 1980
Schaffner A, Davis CE, Schaffner T, et al: In vitro susceptibility of fungi to killing by neutrophil granulocytes discriminates between primary pathogenicity and opportunism. J Clin Invest 78:511, 1986
Scherer S, Magee PT: Genetics of *Candida albicans*. Microbiol Rev 54:226, 1990
Schmid J, Voss E, Soll DR: Computer-assisted methods for assessing strain relatedness in *Candida albicans* by fingerprinting with the moderately repetitive sequence Ca3. J Clin Microbiol 28:1236, 1990
Shepherd MG: Cell envelope of *Candida albicans*. CRC Crit Rev Microbiol 15:7, 1987
Shepherd MG, Poulter RJM, Sullivan PA: *Candida albicans*. Biology, genetics, and pathogenicity. Annu Rev Microbiol 39:579, 1985
Sobel JD: Epidemiology and pathogenesis of recurrent vulvovaginal candidiasis. Am J Obstet Gynecol 152:924, 1985
Stein DK, Sugar AM: Fungal infections in the immunocompromised host. Diagn Microbiol Infect Dis 12:S221, 1989
Stevens DA, Odds FC, Scherer S: Application of DNA typing methods to *Candida albicans* epidemiology and correlations with phenotype. Rev Infect Dis 12:258, 1990
Thaler M, Pastakia B, Shawker TH, et al: Hepatic candidiasis in cancer patients: The evolving picture of the syndrome. Ann Intern Med 108:88, 1988
Valdimarsson H, Higgs JM, Wells AS, et al: Immune abnormalities associated with chronic mucocutaneous candidiasis. Cell Immunol 6:348, 1973
Vanden Bossche H, Mackenzie DWR, Cauwenbergh G, et al (eds): Mycoses in AIDS Patients. New York, Plenum, 1990
Warren NG, Shadomy HJ: Yeasts of medical importance. In Lennette EH, Balows A, Hausler WJ, et al (eds): Manual of Clinical Microbiology, Ed 5. Washington, DC, American Society for Microbiology, 1991, p 617

CRYPTOCOCCUS

Behrman RE, Masci JR, Nicholas P: Cryptococcal skeletal infections: Case report and review. Rev Infect Dis 12:181, 1990
Bennett JE, Kwon-Chung KJ, Howard DH: Epidemiologic differences among serotypes of *Cryptococcus neoformans*. Am J Epidemiol 105:582, 1977
Bhattacharjee AK, Bennett JE, Glandemans CPJ: Capsular polysaccharides of *Cryptococcus neoformans*. Rev Infect Dis 6:619, 1984
Bindschadler DD, Bennett JE: Serology of human cryptococcosis. Ann Intern Med 69:45, 1968
Bolaños B, Mitchell TG: Phagocytosis and killing of *Cryptococcus neoformans* by rat alveolar macrophages in the absence of serum. J Leukocyte Biol 46:521, 1989
Bozzette SA, Larsen RA, Chiu J, et al: A placebo-controlled trial of maintenance therapy with fluconazole after treatment of cryptococcal meningitis in the acquired immunodeficiency syndrome. N Engl J Med 324:580, 1991
Bulmer GS, Sans MD: *Cryptococcus neoformans*. III. Inhibition of phagocytosis. J Bacteriol 95:5, 1967
Chaskee S, Tyndall RL: Pigment production by *Cryptococcus neoformans* from *para-* and *ortho*-diphenols: Effect of nitrogen source. J Clin Microbiol 1:509, 1975
Chechani V, Kamholz SL: Pulmonary manifestations of disseminated cryptococcosis in patients with AIDS. Chest 98:1060, 1990
Cherniak R: Soluble polysaccharides of *Cryptococcus neoformans*. Curr Top Med Mycol 2:40, 1988
Chuck SL, Sande MA: Infections with *Cryptococcus neoformans* in the acquired immunodeficiency syndrome. N Engl J Med 321:794, 1989
Clark RA, Greer D, Atkinson W, et al: Spectrum of *Cryptococcus neoformans* infection in 68 patients infected with human immunodeficiency virus. Rev Infect Dis 12:768, 1990
Denning DW, Tucker RM, Hanson LH, et al: Itraconazole in opportunistic mycoses: Cryptococcosis and aspergillosis. J Am Acad Dermatol 23:602, 1990
Diamond RD, Bennett JE: Prognostic factors in cryptococcal meningitis. Ann Intern Med 80:176, 1974
Diamond RD, Root RK, Bennett JE: Factors influencing killing of *Cryptococcus neoformans* by human leukocytes in vitro. J Infect Dis 125:376, 1972
Dismukes WE: Cryptococcal meningitis in patients with AIDS. J Infect Dis 157:624, 1988
Dismukes WE, Cloud GA, Gallis HA, et al: Treatment of cryptococcal meningitis with combination amphotericin B and flucytosine for four as compared with six weeks. N Engl J Med 317:334, 1987
Dykstra MA, Friedman L, Murphy JW: Capsule size of *Cryptococcus neoformans*: Control and relationship to virulence. Infect Immun 16:129, 1977
Ellis DH, Pfeiffer TJ: Ecology, life-cycle and infectious propagule of *Cryptococcus neoformans*. Lancet 336:923, 1990
Eng RHK, Bishburg E, Smith SM, Kapilla R: Cryptococcal infections

in patients with acquired immune deficiency syndrome. Am J Med 81:19, 1986
Erke KH: Light microscopy of basidia, basidiospores, and nuclei in spores and hyphae of *Filobasidiella neoformans (Cryptococcus neoformans).* J Bacteriol 128:445, 1976
Gal AA, Koss, MN, Hawkins J, et al: The pathology of pulmonary cryptococcal infections in the acquired immunodeficiency syndrome. Arch Pathol Lab Med 110:502, 1986
Gordon MA, Lapa E: Charcoal particle agglutination test for detection of antibody to *Cryptococcus neoformans*: A preliminary report. Am J Clin Pathol 56:354, 1971
Grant IH, Armstrong D: Fungal infections in AIDS. Cryptococcosis. Infect Dis Clin North Am 2:457, 1988
Griffin FM: Roles of macrophage Fc and C3b receptors in phagocytosis of immunologically coated *Cryptococcus neoformans.* Proc Natl Acad Sci USA 78:3853, 1981
Henderson DK, Bennett JE, Huber MA: Long-lasting, specific immunologic unresponsiveness associated with cryptococcal meningitis. J Clin Invest 69:11185, 1982
Hernandez AD: Cutaneous cryptococcosis. Dermatol Clin 7:269, 1989
Jong SC, Bulmer GS, Ruiz A: Serologic grouping and sexual compatibility of airborne *Cryptococcus neoformans.* Mycopathologia 79:185, 1982
Kerkering TM, Duma RJ, Shadomy S: The evolution of pulmonary cryptococcosis. Clinical implications from a study of 41 patients with and without compromising host factors. Ann Intern Med 94:611, 1981
Kovacs JA, Kovacs AA, Polis M, et al: Cryptococcosis in the acquired immunodeficiency syndrome. Ann Intern Med 103:533, 1985
Kozel TR, Pfrommer GST, Guerlain AS, et al: Role of the capsule in phagocytosis of *Cryptococcus neoformans.* Rev Infect Dis 10:S436, 1988
Kwon-Chung KJ: Filobasidiaceae—A taxonomic survey. In de Hoog GS, Smith MTh, Weijman ACM (eds): The Expanding Realm of Yeast-like Fungi. Amsterdam, Elsevier Scientific 1987, p 75
Kwon-Chung KJ, Bennett JE: Epidemiologic differences between the two varieties of *Cryptococcus neoformans.* Am J Epidermiol 120:123, 1984
Littman ML: Cryptococcosis (torulosis). Current concepts and therapy. Am J Med 27:976, 1959
McDonnell JM, Hutchins GM: Pulmonary cryptococcosis. Hum Pathol 16:121, 1985
Miller MF, Mitchell TG: Killing of *Cryptococcus neoformans* strains by human neutrophils and monocytes. Infect Immun 59:24, 1991
Murphy JW: Influence of cryptococcal antigens on cell-mediated immunity. Rev Infect Dis 10:S432, 1988
Murphy JW: Immunoregulation in cryptococcosis. In Kurstak E (ed): Immunology of Fungal Diseases. New York, Marcel Dekker, 1989, p 319
Patterson TF, Andriole VT: Current concepts in cryptococcosis. Eur J Clin Microbiol Infect Dis 8:457, 1989
Perfect JR: Cryptococcosis. Infect Dis Clin North Am 3:77, 1989
Polacheck I, Platt Y, Aronovitch J: Catecholamines and virulence of *Cryptococcus neoformans.* Infect Immun 58:2919, 1990
Rhodes JC, Polacheck I, Kwon-Chung KJ: Phenoloxidase activity and virulence in isogenic strains of *Cryptococcus neoformans.* Infect Immun 36:1175, 1982
Shadomy HJ, Wood-Helie S, Shadomy S, et al: Biochemical serogrouping of clinical isolates of *Cryptococcus neoformans.* Diagn Microbiol Infect Dis 6:131, 1987
Small JM, Mitchell TG: Strain variation in antiphagocytic activity of capsular polysaccharides from *Cryptococcus neoformans* serotype A. Infect Immun 57:3751, 1989
Stamm AM, Diasio RB, Dismukes WE, et al: Toxicity of amphotericin B plus flucytosine in 194 patients with cryptococcal meningitis. Am J Med 83:236, 1987
Sugar AM, Stern JJ, Dupont B: Overview: Treatment of cryptococcal meningitis. Rev Infect Dis 12(suppl): S338, 1990
Utz, JP, Garrigues IL, Sande MA, et al: Therapy of cryptococcosis with a combination of flucytosine and amphotericin B. J Infect Dis 132:368, 1975
Weinke T, Rogler G, Sixt C, et al: Cryptococcosis in AIDS patients: Observations concerning CNS involvement. J Neurol 236:38, 1989
Young RC, Bennett JE, Geelhoed GW, et al: Fungemia with compromised host resistance. A study of 70 cases. Ann Intern Med 80:605, 1974

ASPERGILLOSIS

Aisner J, Schimpff SC, Wiernik PH: Treatment of invasive aspergillosis: Relation of early diagnosis and treatment to response. Ann Intern Med 85:539, 1977
Aisner J, Schimpff SC, Bennett JE, et al: *Aspergillus* infections in cancer patients. Association with fireproofing material in a new hospital. JAMA 235:411, 1976
Al-Doory Y, Dawson JF (eds): Mould Allergy. Philadelphia, Lea & Febiger, 1984
Al-Doory Y, Wagner GE (eds): Aspergillosis. Springfield, Ill, Charles C Thomas, 1985
Binder RE, Faling LJ, Pugatch RD, et al: Chronic necrotizing pulmonary aspergillosis: A discrete clinical entity. Medicine 61:109, 1982
Bodey GP, Vartivarian SE: Aspergillosis. Eur J Clin Microbiol Infect Dis 8:413, 1989
Cox JN, Di Dió F, Pizzolato G-P, et al: *Aspergillus* endocarditis and myocarditis in a patient with the acquired immunodeficiency syndrome (AIDS). A review of the literature. Virchows Arch A 417:255, 1990
De Beule K, De Doncker P, Cauwenbergh G, et al: The treatment of aspergillosis and aspergilloma with itraconazole, clinical results of an open international study (1982–1987). Mycoses 31:476, 1988
Denning DW, Stevens DA: Antifungal and surgical treatment of invasive aspergillosis: Review of 2,121 published cases. Rev Infect Dis 12:1147, 1990
Denning DW, Follansbee SE, Scolaro M, et al: Pulmonary aspergillosis in the acquired immunodeficiency syndrome. N Engl J Med 324:654, 1991
Denning DW, Tucker RM, Hanson LH, et al: Treatment of invasive aspergillosis with itraconazole. Am J Med 86:791, 1989
Diamond RD, Clark RA: Damage to *Aspergillus fumigatus* and *Rhizopus oryzae* hyphae by oxidative and nonoxidative microbicidal products of human neutrophils in vitro. Infect Immun 38:487, 1982
Diamond RD, Huber E, Haudenschild CC: Mechanisms of destruction of *Aspergillus fumigatus* hyphae mediated by human monocytes. J Infect Dis 147:474, 1983
Gerson SL, Talbot GH, Lusk E, et al: Invasive pulmonary aspergillosis in adult acute leukemia: Clinical clues to its diagnosis. J Clin Oncol 3:1109, 1985
Greenberger PA: Allergic bronchopulmonary aspergillosis and fungoses. Clin Chest Med 9:599, 1988
Khan ZU, Sandhu RS, Randhawa HS, et al: Allergic bronchopulmonary aspergillosis: A study of 46 cases with special reference to laboratory aspects. Scand J Respir Dis 57:73, 1976
Levitz SM, Diamond RD: Mechanisms of resistance of *Aspergillus fumigatus* conidia to killing by neutrophils in vitro. J Infect Dis 152:33, 1985
Meyer RD, Young LS, Armstrong D, et al: Aspergillosis complicating neoplastic disease. Am J Med 54:6, 1973
Nalesnik MA, Myerowitz RL, Jenkins R, et al: Significance of *Aspergillus*

species isolated from respiratory secretions in the diagnosis of invasive pulmonary aspergillosis. J Clin Microbiol 11:370, 1980

Paulose KO, Al Khalifa S, Shenoy P, et al: Mycotic infection of the ear (otomycosis): A prospective study. J Laryngol Otol 103:30, 1989

Pauwels R, Stevens EM, vander Straeten M: IgE antibodies in bronchopulmonary aspergillosis. Ann Allergy 37:195, 1976

Peterson DE, Schimpff SC: *Aspergillus* sinusitis in neutropenic patients with cancer: A review. Biomed Pharm 43:307, 1989

Phillips P, Bryce G, Shepherd J, et al: Invasive external otitis caused by *Aspergillus*. Rev Infect Dis 12:277, 1990

Raper KB, Fennel DI: The Genus *Aspergillus*. Baltimore, Williams & Wilkins, 1965

Rogers AL, Kennedy MJ: Opportunistic hyaline hyphomycetes. In Lennette EH, Balows A, Hausler WJ, et al (eds): Manual of Clinical Microbiology, ed 5. Washington, DC, American Society of Microbiology, 1991, p 659

Rogers TR, Barnes RA: Prevention of airborne fungal infection in immunocompromised patients. J Hosp Infect 11:15, 1988

Rinaldi MG: Invasive aspergillosis. Rev Infect Dis 5:1961, 1983

Safirstein BH, D'Souza MF, Simon G, et al: Five-year follow-up of allergic bronchopulmonary aspergillosis. Am Rev Respir Dis 108:450, 1973

Schaffner A, Douglas H, Braude A: Selective protection against conidia by mononuclear and against mycelia by polymorphonuclear phagocytes in resistance to *Aspergillus*: Observations on these two lines of defense in vivo and in vitro with human and mouse phagocytes. J Clin Invest 69:617, 1982

Soltanzadeh H, Wychulis AR, Fauraokh S, et al: Surgical treatment of pulmonary aspergilloma. Ann Surg 186:13, 1977

Timberlake WE: Molecular genetics of *Aspergillus* development. Annu Rev Genet 24:5, 1990

Varkey B, Rose HD: Pulmonary aspergilloma. A rational approach to treatment. Am J Med 61:626, 1976

Viollier AF, Peterson DE, Jongh CA, et al: *Aspergillus* sinusitis in cancer patients. Cancer 58:366, 1986

Washburn RG, Hammer CH, Bennett JE: Inhibition of complement by culture supernatants of *Aspergillus fumigatus*. J Infect Dis 154:944, 1986

Young RC, Bennett JE, Vogel CL, et al: Aspergillosis. The spectrum of the disease in 98 patients. Medicine 49:147, 1970

Yu VL, Muder RR, Poorsattar A: Significance of isolation of *Aspergillus* from the respiratory tract in diagnosis of invasive pulmonary aspergillosis. Results from a three-year prospective study. Am J Med 81:249, 1986

MUCORMYCOSIS

Abramson E, Wilson D, Arby RA: Rhinocerebral phycomycosis in association with diabetic ketoacidosis. Ann Intern Med 66:735, 1967

Artis WM, Fountain JA, Delcher HK, Jones HE: A mechanism of susceptibility to mucor mycosis in diabetic ketoacidosis: Transferrin and iron availability. Diabetes 37:1109, 1982

Blitzer A, Lawson W, Meyers BR, et al: Patient survival factors in paranasal sinus mucormycosis. Laryngoscope 90:635, 1980

Boelaert JR, van Roost GF, Vergauwe PL, et al: The role of desferrioxamine in dialysis-associated mucormycosis: Report of three cases and review of the literature. Clin Nephrol 29:261, 1988

Espinel-Ingroff A, Oakley LA, Kerkerint TM. Opportunistic zygomycotis infections. A literature review. Mycopathologia 97:33, 1987

Ferguson BJ, Mitchell TG, Moon R, et al: Adjunctive hyperbaric oxygen for treatment of rhinocerebral mucormycosis. Rev Infect Dis 10:551, 1988

Fisher J, Tuazon CU, Geelhoed GW: Mucormycosis in transplant patients. Am Surg 46:315, 1980

Ingram CW, Sennesh J, Cooper JN, et al: Disseminated zygomycosis: Report of four cases and review. Rev Infect Dis 11:741, 1989

Keys TF, Haldorson RN, Rhodes KM, et al: Nosocomial outbreak of *Rhizopus* infections associated with Elastoplast wound dressings. Minnesota. MMWR 27:33, 1978

Kurrasch M, Beumer J, Kagawa T: Mucormycosis: Oral and prosthodontic implications. A report of 14 patients. J Prosthetic Dent 47:422, 1982

Lehrer RI, Howard DH, Sypherd RS, et al: Mucormycosis. Ann Intern Med 93:93, 1980

Marchevsky AM, Bolton EJ, Geller SA, et al: The changing spectrum of disease, etiology, and diagnosis of mucormycosis. Hum Pathol 11:467, 1980

Meyer RD, Rosen P, Armstrong D: Phycomycosis complicating leukemia and lymphoma. Ann Intern Med 77:871, 1972

Morduchowicz G, Shmneli D, Shapira Z, et al: Rhinocerebral mucormycosis in renal transplant recipients: Report of three cases and review of the literature. Rev Infect Dis 8:441, 1986

Partrey NA: Improved diagnosis and prognosis of mucormycosis. A clinicopathologic study of 33 cases. Medicine 65:113, 1986

Pillsbury HC, Fischer ND: Rhinocerebral mucormycosis. Arch Otolaryngol 103:600, 1977

Rex JH, Ginsberg AM, Fries LF, et al: *Cunninghamella bertholletiae* infection associated with deferoxamine therapy. Rev Infect Dis 10:1187, 1988

Scholer HJ, Muller E, Schipper MAAA: Mucorales. In Howard DH (ed): Fungi Pathogenic for Humans and Animals. Part A. Biology. New York, Marcel Dekker, 1983, p 9

Straatsma BR, Zimmerman LE, Gass JDM: Phycomycosis. A clinicopathologic study of fifty-one cases. Lab Invest 11:963, 1962

Waldorf AR, Ruderman N, Diamond RD: Specific susceptibility to mucormycosis in murine diabetes and bronchoalveolar macrophage defence against *Rhizopus*. J Clin Invest 74:150, 1984

Virmani R, Connor DH, McAllister HA: Cardiac mucormycosis. A report of five patients and review of 14 previously reported cases. Am J Clin Pathol 78:42, 1982

OTHER OPPORTUNISTIC MYCOSES

Aisner J, Schimpff SC, Sutherland JC, et al: *Torulopsis glabrata* infections in patients with cancer. Am J Med 61:23, 1976

Anaissie E, Bodey GP, Kantarijian HM, et al: New spectrum of fungal infections in patients with cancer. Rev Infect Dis 11:369, 1989

Anaissie EJ, Bodey GP Sr, Rinaldi MG: Emerging fungal pathogens. Eur J Clin Microbiol Infect Dis 8:323, 1989

Armstrong D: Life-threatening opportunistic fungal infection in patients with the acquired immunodeficiency syndrome. Ann NY Acad Sci 544:443, 1988

Berenguer J, Diaz-Mediavilla J, Urra D, et al: Central nervous system infection caused by *Pseudallescheria boydii*: Case report and review. Rev Infect Dis 11:890, 1989

Bodey GP: The emergence of fungi as major hospital pathogens. J Hosp Infect 11(suppl):411, 1988

Buchta V, Otcenase M: *Geotrichum candidum*—An opportunistic agent of mycotic disease. Mycoses 31:363, 1988

Guého E, deHoog GS, Smith MJ, Meyer SA: DNA relatedness, taxonomy, and medical significance of *Geotrichum capitatum*. J Clin Microbiol 25:1191, 1987

Hoy J, Hsu KC, Rolston K, et al: *Trichosporon beigelii* infection: A review. Rev Infect Dis 8:959, 1986

Klein AS, Tortora GT, Malowitz R, et al: *Hansenula anomala*: A new fungal pathogen. Two case reports and a review of the literature. Arch Intern Med 148:1210, 1988

Martino P, Venditti M, Micozzi A, et al.: *Blastoschizomyces capitatus*: An emerging cause of invasive fungal disease in leukemia patients. Rev Infect Dis 12:570, 1990

McGinnis MR: Laboratory Handbook of Medical Mycology. New York, Academic Press, 1980

Merz WG, Karp JE, Hoagland M, et al: Diagnosis and successful treatment of fusarisosi in the compromised host. J Infect Dis 158:1046, 1988

Musial CE, Cockerill FR III, Roberts GD: Fungal infections of the immunocompromised host: Clinical and laboratory aspects. Clin Microbiol Rev 1:349, 1988

Phillips P, Wood WS, Phillips G, et al: Invasive hyalohyphomycosis caused by *Scopulariopsis brevicaulis* in a patient undergong allogeneic bone marrow transplant. Diagn Microbiol Infect Dis 12:429, 1989

Smith JMB. Opportunistic Mycoses of Man and other Animals. Wallingford, UK, CAB Intl Mycol Inst, 1989

Tawfik OW, Papasian CJ, Dixon AY, et al: *Saccharomyces cerevisiae* pneumonia in a patient with acquired immune deficiency syndrome. J Clin Microbiol 27:1689, 1989

Travis LB, Roberts GD, Wilson WR: Clinical significance of *Pseudallescheria boydii*: A review of 10 years' experience. Mayo Clin Proc 60:531, 1985

Walsh TJ, Pizzo PA: Nosocomial fungal infections. A classification for hospital-acquired fungal infections and mycoses arising from endogenous flora or reactivation. Annu Rev Microbiol 42:517, 1988

Walsh TJ, Melcher GP, Rinaldi MG, et al: *Trichosporon beigelii*, an emerging pathogen resistant to amphotericin B. J Clin Microbiol 28:1616, 1990

Wiest PM, Wiese K, Jacobs MR, et al: *Alternaria* infection in a patient with acquired immunodeficiency syndrome: Case report and review of invasive *Alternaria* infections. Rev Infect Dis 9:799, 1987

Young CN, Meyers AM: Opportunistic fungal infection by *Fusarium oxysporum* in renal transplant patients. Sabouraudia 17:219, 1979

SECTION VII

MEDICAL PARASITOLOGY

CHAPTER 86

Introduction to Medical Parasitology

- **Introduction**
- **Definitions**

Introduction

Many clinicians in the United States and in other developed countries fail to realize the impact of diseases caused by parasitic protozoa and worms on human populations. This is due largely to the fact that people living in developed countries are reasonably well-nourished, have high standards of sanitation, benefit from a temperate climate, and enjoy the absence of certain vectors of disease. On a global basis, however, and even after relatively successful campaigns against such infections as malaria, hookworm, and blood fluke in many parts of the world, parasitic infection in association with malnutrition is still the primary cause of morbidity and mortality. In fact, 15 million, or one half of the 30 million children younger than 5 years of age who die from all causes each year, die from a combination of malnutrition and parasitic infection. These 15 million thus represent one fourth of the total 60 million annual worldwide adult and child deaths from all causes. Summaries of worldwide prevalence of selected infections show the following figures:

Infectious Agent	No. Infected
Ascaris	1000 million
Hookworm	900 million
Trichuris	500 million
Giardia	200 million
Schistosoma	275 million
Malaria	150 million

Although parasite-induced diseases are relatively uncommon, they do exist in the United States and are still far from being eradicated. Some estimates place the number of people infected with parasites in the United States at over 50 million. Most of these infections were acquired in the United States, but some, like schistosomiasis and malaria, are constantly being imported by travelers and immigrants. During the last 10 years physicians in the United States caring for patients with acquired immunodeficiency syndrome (AIDS) and others who are either immunodeficient or immunosuppressed, have come to realize that many infectious agents, including some protozoa and worms, may cause serious and even lethal infections.

The recent increased interest in medical parasitology is due to a number of factors, including intensified travel to endemic areas, the "back-to-nature" trend within the United States, the development of drug resistance by some parasites, the AIDS epidemic and the concomitant parasitic infection of such patients, and the wider use of immunosuppressive therapy, which permits the exacerbation of chronic, low-level infection and a general decrease in resistance to infection. Case histories of deaths in the United States due to fulminating strongyloidiasis after kidney transplantation, due to pneumocystosis during immunosuppressive therapy for leukemia, and due to drug-resistant malaria are no longer reported only as medical curiosities in American medical journals. One also reads case histories of homosexual men in Africa dying because of the association between pneumocystosis and Kaposi's sarcoma, as well as rapid deaths due to brain damage caused by a normally free-living ameba found in freshwater swimming holes, lakes, and pools.

It is incumbent upon the medical profession to help dispel the notion that people in the United States are free of infection caused by protozoa and worms. This illusion results from a variety of reasons, including (1) the topic rarely is discussed by "refined" people, (2) the media are reluctant to disseminate such information, (3) poor people usually are the ones most seriously affected, and (4) travel agents and tourist bureaus are both reluctant and inadequately prepared to give travelers an accurate picture of the health hazards that may be encountered abroad. Also, many physicians are inadequately trained and fail to consider parasites as a possible cause of symptoms and disease. Indeed, many curricula in medical schools today offer medical students no, or very little, instruction in this group of infectious agents. Thus in many situations there is no diagnosis or a misdiagnosis, resulting in unnecessary suffering, economic loss, and even death.

Parasitology is the science or study of parasitism, that is, the relationship between parasites and the organisms (hosts) that harbor them. In the fields of medicine and public health, the subject matter of parasitology is usually limited to parasitism in humans. In a broad sense, parasitism involves the study of all organisms parasitic on or within the human body. This comprehensive consideration includes five specialized fields: medical bacteriology, virology, mycology, entomology, and parasitology. In medical parasitology the most important parasites of humans belong to four groups: the Protozoa (eucaryotic protists, i.e., single-celled microorganisms with a true, membrane-bound nucleus); the Nematoda, or true roundworms; the Platyhelminthes, or flatworms; and the Arthropoda, which include not only the true insects but also ticks, mites, and others. Although arthropods affect the health of humans in many ways, they are considered here only where they serve as vectors.

Furthermore, only the more common parasites of the four groups selected are discussed, especially those endemic or indigenous (i.e., present and being transmitted at all times) within the United States. Space, however, is also given to selected exotic or imported (i.e., of foreign origin and not being transmitted in the United States) forms because of their ever-increasing prevalence, especially in travelers to, and immigrants from, endemic areas. Two forms discussed—malarial parasites and blood flukes—produce diseases now considered to be the most important infectious diseases in the world. In this global context, it is worth noting that along with the diseases produced by these two agents, there are three other parasitic diseases (trypanosomiasis, leishmaniasis, and filariasis, including onchocerciasis) singled out by the World Health Organization and the United Nations Development Program as initial target areas in a special program aimed at the acceleration of health and economic betterment in underdeveloped countries. Leprosy is the remaining disease chosen for initial attack.

In presenting the material of this section, an attempt is made to coordinate the medical and biologic approaches to the subject, that is, to give proper attention to both the host and the parasite. The life cycle of the parasite is given, followed by a brief consideration of the principal damage produced in the host and the striking signs and symptoms resulting therefrom. After these discussions for each infection, information on the epidemiology, diagnosis, and treatment is given. Because the emphasis is on important host-parasite relationships, rather than certain factors concerned only with the host or the parasite, the reader should be better able to gain an appreciation and understanding of these infections. In following this approach, however, the space customarily given to details of classification, morphology of the parasite, pathology, and so forth is necessarily limited.

Definitions

Before the information outlined above is presented, a few definitions will help the reader's understanding of the sections on protozoan and helminthic infections that follow.

Most medically oriented parasitologists consider *symbiology* to be a study of the relationship that exists between two dissimilar organisms that live together in close association. When both of these partners benefit in the association, it is spoken of as *mutualism*. When one partner benefits and the other partner neither benefits nor is harmed, the association is known as *commensalism*. However, when one partner harms the other, or in some sense lives at the expense of the other without killing it immediately, the association is known as *parasitism*. In a mutualistic relationship, both partners are called *mutuals*; in a commensalistic relationship, the partner that benefits is called a *commensal* and the other the *host*. In a parasitic relationship, the harmful agent is the *parasite* and the partner that is harmed is the *host*.

A parasite that lives on the surface of its host is called an *ectoparasite*; if it lives in the tissues or gastrointestinal tract, it is an *endoparasite*. A parasite that must spend all or part of its life in or on its host is called an *obligatory parasite*. An organism that is not normally parasitic but does become so when, for example, it is accidentally eaten or enters a wound or natural body orifice, is called a *facultative* or *opportunistic parasite*.

Hosts are also of different kinds. A *final* or *definitive host* is one in which the parasite reaches sexual maturity. If no sexual reproduction occurs in the life cycle of the parasite, such as with many protozoa, the organism arbitrarily deemed the most important is called the final or definitive host. An *intermediate host* is one in which some development of the parasite occurs, but sexual maturity is not reached. Finally, a *reservoir host* is an animal other than a human that is normally infected with a parasite that also is infective for humans. When a parasite can develop only in one or two species of hosts, it is spoken of as manifesting a high degree of *host specificity*. A parasite, such as that causing trichinosis, can infect almost any warm-blooded vertebrate and is spoken of as exhibiting loose host specificity.

FURTHER READING

There are many excellent references dealing with all phases of medical parasitology. The few listed below are considered among the best.

Beaver PC, Jung RC, Cupp EW: Clinical Parasitology, ed 9. Philadelphia, Lea & Febiger, 1984

Binford CH, Connor DH (eds): Pathology of Tropical and Extraordinary Diseases: An Atlas, vols 1 and 2. Washington, DC, Armed Forces Institute of Pathology, 1976

Brown HW, Neva FA: Basic Clinical Parasitology, ed 5. New York, Appleton-Century-Crofts, 1982

Manson-Bahr PEC, Apted FIG: Manson's Tropical Diseases, ed 18. London, Balliere Tindall, 1982

Markell EK, Voge MJ, John DT: Medical Parasitology, ed 6. Philadelphia, WB Saunders Co, 1986

Strickland GT: Hunter's Tropical Medicine, ed 7. Philadelphia, WB Saunders Co, 1990

Warren KS, Mahmoud AF: Tropical and Geographical Medicine, ed 2, New York, McGraw Hill Information Services Co, 1990.

CHAPTER 87

Medical Protozoology

Protozoa are eucaryotic, unicellular organisms composed of a nucleus, or nuclei, and cytoplasm. The cytoplasm is differentiated into an outer layer (the ectoplasm), and an inner layer (the endoplasm). Locomotion, if accomplished, is carried out by special ectoplasmic organelles. Four groups of Protozoa contain important parasites of humans: (1) Rhizopoda (amebae), (2) Mastigophora (flagellates), (3) Ciliophora (ciliates), and (4) Sporozoa. The amebae locomote by means of pseudopodia, the flagellates by flagella, the ciliates by cilia, and the sporozoans lack definite organelles of locomotion. Parasitic protozoa usually reproduce by means of an asexual process called *fission*. Some, however, such as the sporozoans, have both sexual and asexual means of reproduction.

In the presentation of the material of this chapter, the protozoa are grouped according to their usual location within the body of humans. The groups to be considered are the intestinal, urogenital, blood, and tissue protozoa.

Intestinal Protozoa

Amebae

Amebae are common in the environment, and many are parasitic in invertebrate and vertebrate animals. Relatively few species parasitize humans (Table 87–1), and only one, *Entamoeba histolytica*, is known to cause intestinal pathology. *Dientamoeba fragilis*, although known to be a member of the Mastigophora (flagellates), exists only in the ameboid form. Because of its morphologic similarity to the amebae, for convenience it will be presented as an ameba.

Entamoeba histolytica

Entamoeba histolytica, although often living as a harmless inhabitant in the large intestine, has the capacity to colonize on and penetrate the intestinal tissues and to cause ulceration. After penetrating the intestinal tissues, it may spread by metastasis to other tissues and organs.

It is estimated that 10% of all the world's population is infected with *E. histolytica*. Annual deaths are estimated to be between 40,000 and 100,000. In the United States, 1% to 5% of the people are thought to harbor the ameba. Prevalence rates are highest in tropical areas, especially where crowding and poor sanitation exist. Infection, however, is cosmopolitan, being present literally from pole to pole. Fortunately, clinical disease is seen in only a small fraction of those infected. There is increasing evidence for the existence of a variety of strains, and this may partially account for differing pathogenicity. Recent studies have indicated that pathogenic and nonpathogenic strains have differing isoenzyme patterns (zymodemes). Some studies, however, indicate that the bacterial flora may somehow convert a nonpathogenic to a pathogenic strain. This conversion is known to occur under culture conditions; there is no proof that these changes occur in the human intestine.

Life Cycle. The life cycle of *E. histolytica* is comparatively simple, involving the trophozoite (actively metabolizing and motile) and cyst stages (Fig. 87–1). The parasite is passed in the stools of infected individuals. If the specimen is dysenteric or diarrheal or has been obtained after purgation, trophozoites will predominate. Few cysts are observed in such specimens because, presumably, evacuation is too rapid for encystment. Therefore, cysts are usually found only in normal stools, which are formed, at least in part. Cysts will remain viable only if kept moist and if other favorable conditions exist, because they are readily destroyed by desiccation, sunlight, and heat.

Reinfection of the same individual or infection of a new host may occur directly, by contaminated fingers (hand-to-mouth infection), or indirectly, chiefly through contaminated food and water. Waterborne epidemics have occurred in the United States and elsewhere. Sexual transmission through anal intercourse, especially within the male population, is well known. Contaminated apparatus used in colonic irrigation is known to be a mode of transmission.

Ingested cysts pass through the stomach and excyst in the lower small intestine. An ameba containing the four cystic nuclei emerges from each cyst. Before cytoplasmic division the tetranucleate trophozoite undergoes mitosis, giving rise,

TABLE 87–1. INTESTINAL AMEBAE OF HUMANS

Name	Transmission	Pathology	Size (μm) Trophozoite	Size (μm) Cyst	Remarks
Dientamoeba fragilis[a]	Ingestion of trophozoite (?)	Diarrhea	5–25	None	May be transmitted inside pinworm eggs
Endolimax nana	Ingestion of cyst	None	6–15	4–14	
Entamoeba coli	Ingestion of cyst	None	15–40	10–35	
Entamoeba hartmanni	Ingestion of cyst	None	5–12	4–10	Some consider this as a small race of *E. histolytica*
Entamoeba histolytica	Ingestion of cyst; anal intercourse	Diarrhea, dysentery, abscess in extraintestinal tissues (e.g., liver, brain)	12–60	10–20	Most often lives as a harmless commensal
Entamoeba polecki	Ingestion of cyst	None	10–20	5–10	Rare in humans; probably of animal origin
Iodamoeba bütschlii	Ingestion of cyst	None	6–25	6–20	

[a] Actually a flagellate

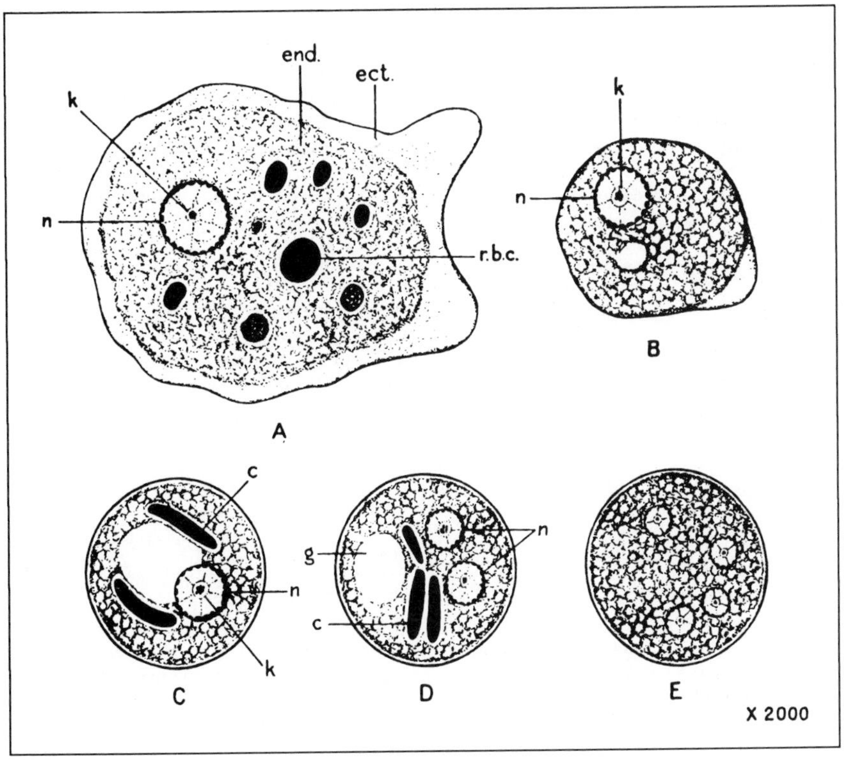

Fig. 87–1. Schematic representation of *Entamoeba histolytica*. **A.** Trophozoite containing red blood cells undergoing digestion. **B.** Precystic ameba devoid of cytoplasmic inclusions. **C.** Young uninucleate cyst. **D.** Binucleate cyst. **E.** Mature quadrinucleate cyst. c, chromatoid bodies; ect., ectoplasm; end., endoplasm; g, glycogen vacuole; k, karyosome; n, nucleus; r.b.c., red blood cells. *(From Belding: Textbook of Clinical Parasitology, ed 2. Appleton-Century-Crofts, 1952.)*

after cytoplasmic division, to eight small, uninucleate metacystic trophozoites. These pass downward to the large intestine where they soon feed and grow to full size. Hence, cysts provide for reproduction as well as transmission.

The trophozoites pass along the intestinal canal until conditions are favorable for colonization, which occurs as the result of rapid and repeated binary fission. This usually occurs first at the cecal area but may take place at a lower level of the large intestine. Tissue invasion is probably accomplished by both lytic and physical means. After the trophozoites enter the tissue, lytic digestion of host cells provides food for the ameba, allowing it to advance. Under certain conditions, some of the trophozoites may metastasize to the liver and other extraintestinal sites. When trophozoites are extruded into the intestinal lumen, they begin their passage from the body. If this passage is not too rapid, they pass first through a precystic stage and occur in the stool as cysts.

There has been support for the opinion that a small, nonpathogenic strain of *E. histolytica* exists. However, it is now generally accepted that it is a separate species named *E. hartmanni*. It is known that geographic strains vary in pathogenicity and that the bacterial flora of the intestine, the resistance, and the nutritional status of the host all are factors in determining whether demonstrable pathology results from a given infection. Thus it would seem wise, until final proof has been established, to consider all strains capable of damaging the host.

Pathology and Symptomatology. Clinically, amebiasis usually presents as an intestinal disease or as an amebic abscess of the liver. The incubation period, after the ingestion of cysts, is generally 3 to 4 weeks in duration but may be as short as 5 days or as long as several months. The severity of the disease varies, but the majority of those infected are symptom-free cyst passers (carriers).

The intestinal pathology of amebiasis is most commonly observed in the cecal area, followed by the sigmoidorectal area, but lesions may occur at any point from the lower ileum downward. The process begins with a small lesion produced at the site of entry into the tissue, usually in the interglandular epithelium, where the shedding of intestinal cells normally takes place. A minute cavity is formed from lytic necrosis. As viewed from the surface, these small lesions are surrounded by a raised yellowish ring and are separated by mucosa that appears normal. These lesions usually show little evidence of inflammatory reaction—hence they fail to suggest the degree of subsurface damage, which may be considerable. As the colony of amebae increases, abscesses are formed, and often, in time, a narrow channel is formed to the base of the mucosa. There, probably because of the greater resistance of the muscularis mucosae, the lesion enlarges and forms an early, characteristic, flask-shaped or teardrop ulcer. This appears to be a critical stage, determining whether extensive damage will be produced and it may, therefore, be thought of as an expression of the degree of adaptation between the parasite and the host. If the organisms are unable to penetrate this layer, repair may keep pace with the damage, and in some cases the amebae may be eliminated. If, however, the organisms erode a passage through the muscularis mucosae into the submucosa, they usually spread out radially and produce an enlarged, ragged ulcer. The mucosa surrounding this is rolled and elevated as a result of the undermining. Secondary infections usually are not observed in these early lesions, despite extensive necrosis, and there is minimal tissue reaction present. Later, the surface of the ulcer sloughs off, exposing shaggy, overhanging edges. At this time, secondary infections are common, and the ulcer is infiltrated with neutrophilic leukocytes and other wandering cells, tending to thicken the overhanging edges. In severe cases, the organisms may spread from the submucosa through the muscular coats into the serosa, where they are likely to cause perforation. Amebomas—granulomatous formations that resemble malignant tumors—are sometimes seen in chronic cases. The differentiation between an ameboma and a malignant tumor is difficult. Many cases are not correctly identified until after surgery.

From the intestinal wall, the amebae may enter the portal venules or, less commonly, the lymphatics and be carried to the liver and other organs. Liver involvement is most common, followed by involvement of the lungs, which is usually by direct extension from the liver abscess. Lesions outside the intestinal tract are always secondary to those in the intestine. Extraintestinal amebiasis bears no relationship to the severity of the intestinal infection, and these conditions do not necessarily coincide. It is important to note that immunosuppressive therapy may cause rapid progression of an *E. histolytica* infection, with resulting liver abscess and increased intestinal damage. As is noted below, other parasites may produce fulminating infections in patients being treated with various immunosuppressants. Increased mortality occurs during pregnancy and puerperium.

The pathology of amebic liver abscess results from the establishment and multiplication of trophozoites in that organ. The early abscess is small, with a grayish brown matrix of necrosed hepatic cells. Connective tissue does not appear to be destroyed by the lytic property of the amebae. As the abscess increases in size, the center liquefies, the wall thickens, and in most cases the contents become a viscid (creamy) yellow, gray, or chocolate-colored mass. At all stages of abscess formation, the amebae are seen invading marginal tissue. Abscesses occur more frequently in the right lobe (right upper quadrant) than in the left and tend to be single rather than multiple. It is important to emphasize that liver abscess may be a sequela of chronic as well as acute intestinal amebiasis (amebic dysentery). In fact, liver abscess without evidence of intestinal involvement and without organisms being seen in the stool is not unusual. When properly treated, lesions caused by the invasive amebae almost invariably heal without the formation of scar tissue. This is especially striking in the liver, where scarring is the usual consequence of infection with other infectious agents.

Cutaneous lesions and abscesses also occur. They usually result from an extension of rectal amebiasis to perianal skin and vulva. Abdominal wall skin lesions also occur as extensions of a hepatic abscess, and penile skin infections as a result of anal intercourse are not rare.

Epidemiology. The life cycle outlined above is simple and does not involve intermediate hosts or nonhuman reservoirs. Cysts may remain viable for days if mild environmental conditions prevail. Fecal contamination of food and water occurs as a result of poor sewage disposal and personal hygiene. Thus travelers from the West should drink only bottled water and avoid ice cubes, salads, and fruits that cannot be peeled by the person eating them. If bottled water is not available, boiled or iodinated water may prevent infection. Laboratory observations indicate that a rapid transmission of parasites from human to human enhances pathogenicity, and this may partly account for the minor clinical significance of amebiasis in the United States. Recent reports, however, incriminate oral-anal sex practices for its alarming resurgence among the homosexual population.

TABLE 87–2. CLASSIFICATION OF AMEBIASIS

Classification	Characteristics
Asymptomatic Intestinal Infection	Colonization without tissue invasion
Symptomatic Intestinal Infection	Invasive infection
Amebic dysentery	Fulminant ulcerative intestinal disease
Nondysentery colitis	Ulcerative intestinal disease
Ameboma	Proliferative intestinal granuloma
Complicated intestinal amebiasis	Perforation, hemorrhage, fistula
Postamebic colitis	Mechanism unknown
Extraintestinal Amebiasis	
Nonspecific hepatomegaly	No demonstrable invasion accompanies intestinal infection
Acute nonspecific infection	Amebae in liver but without abscess
Amebic abscess	Focal structural lesion
Amebic abscess complicated	Direct extension to pleura, lung, peritoneum, pericardium
Amebiasis cutis	Direct extension to skin
Visceral amebiasis	Metastatic infection of lung, spleen, or brain

Diagnosis. A variety of classification schemes for the clinical syndromes caused by *E. histolytica* have been proposed. The one adopted by the World Health Organization is presented in Table 87–2.

In intestinal amebiasis, there often is no definite pattern of symptoms. In fact, the disease may manifest clinically in a deceptive fashion. In acute amebiasis (amebic colitis), the individual usually is acutely ill, feverish (100F to 102F), complains of general abdominal discomfort and tenderness, and passes numerous, malodorous stools, which in most cases are dysenteric. The symptoms are usually referable to the cecal areas and may resemble appendicitis or various other conditions. In subacute infections, the picture is similar but less striking.

Considering the number of cases involved and the difficulty of diagnosis, the major problem is chronic amebiasis. The symptoms in this case exhibit even greater latitude. Some patients may have periodic bouts of diarrhea or, less commonly, dysentery, but longer periods of bowel normalcy or constipation are characteristic. Others are without distinctive signs and symptoms and may complain of a low fatigue threshold, moderate loss of weight, mental dullness, and the like. In many such cases, tenderness can be demonstrated in the right lower quadrant. Last, some infected individuals have been entirely symptom-free.

The symptomatology of amebic liver abscess is characterized by hepatomegaly, tenderness over the liver and referred pain around the right scapula, bulging and fixation of the right leaf of the diaphragm, moderate leukocytosis, and a low-grade, inconstant fever. Blood chemistry studies are not helpful. Liver enzyme levels may be mildly elevated, especially alkaline phosphatase, and serum protein levels are usually depressed. Mild anemias are common. Other diseases to consider during differential diagnosis are appendicitis, diverticulitis, ulcerative colitis, idiopathic colitis, Crohn's disease, bacillary dysentery, and other parasitic diseases.

Definitive diagnosis of amebiasis depends on the demonstration of amebae in stool or in material aspirated from lesions and abscesses. Various methods are used, depending on the type of specimen and other factors. If the specimen is dysenteric or diarrheic or has been obtained by proctoscopic swabbing or after purgation, it is likely to contain only trophozoites (12 to 60 μm). If possible, it should be examined immediately because the trophozoites may soon lose their characteristic features. A fecal smear should be prepared on a microscope slide. The smear is made by emulsifying a bit of the specimen in a drop of tepid physiologic salt solution. A coverglass is placed on the preparation, and the emulsion is carefully examined under the low power and high dry power of a compound microscope. If, in suspected cases of amebiasis, such direct examinations fail to reveal the organisms and especially if Charcot-Leyden crystals have been noted, it is worthwhile to culture a stool specimen.

If the fecal specimen is formed, or at least semiformed, it is likely to contain mostly cysts (10 to 20 μm) rather than trophozoites. Again, direct examination should be made with a dual preparation. In this case, one smear is made in the salt solution, especially to observe the refractive cyst wall, and the other is made in D'Antoni's iodine solution, which will stain the cyst, making the internal structure visible. A third type of smear, that of saline and methylene blue, is helpful in differentiating cysts from leukocytes. The leukocytes take up the blue dye, whereas the cysts do not. If direct examination fails to reveal cysts, a concentration method should be used. The correct identification of *E. histolytica* requires considerable expertise. The most common error made by diagnosticians is that host leukocytes are identified as amebae.

E. histolytica must be differentiated from the other intestinal amebae (Fig. 87–2). The single character that is most diagnostic is the structure of the nucleus (Fig. 87–3). All four species of the genus *Entamoeba* have conspicuous peripheral chromatin on the inner surface of the nuclear membrane, whereas such material is lacking or is not conspicuous in the others. In *E. histolytica*, the nuclear membrane is delicate, and the chromatin on the inner surface appears as fine beads. The karyosome (nucleolus) is small and usually central. In *Entamoeba coli* the membrane is thicker, and the chromatin on the inner surface is in the form of coarse plaques; the karyosome is much larger than that of *E. histolytica* and is located eccentrically. The striking feature of the nucleus of *Endolimax nana* is the large karyosome located in the center or slightly off center. In the case of *Iodamoeba bütschlii*, the karyosome is also large but is surrounded by a ring of achromatic granules, giving a halo effect around the karyosome. It must be emphasized that considerable variation of nuclear morphology of all species of amebae does occur.

Proctoscopic aspirates are occasionally submitted for direct examination and culturing. These should be examined as soon as possible. In a fresh specimen, a variety of host tissue cells are usually present, so it is important to observe the typical motility of the trophozoites before making a definitive diagnosis. A diagnosis of *E. histolytica* can easily be made when the trophozoite stage contains ingested red blood cells; no other species of amebae are known to ingest erythrocytes.

In the direct diagnosis of amebic liver abscess, the aspirated specimen should be treated with streptococcal DNase to

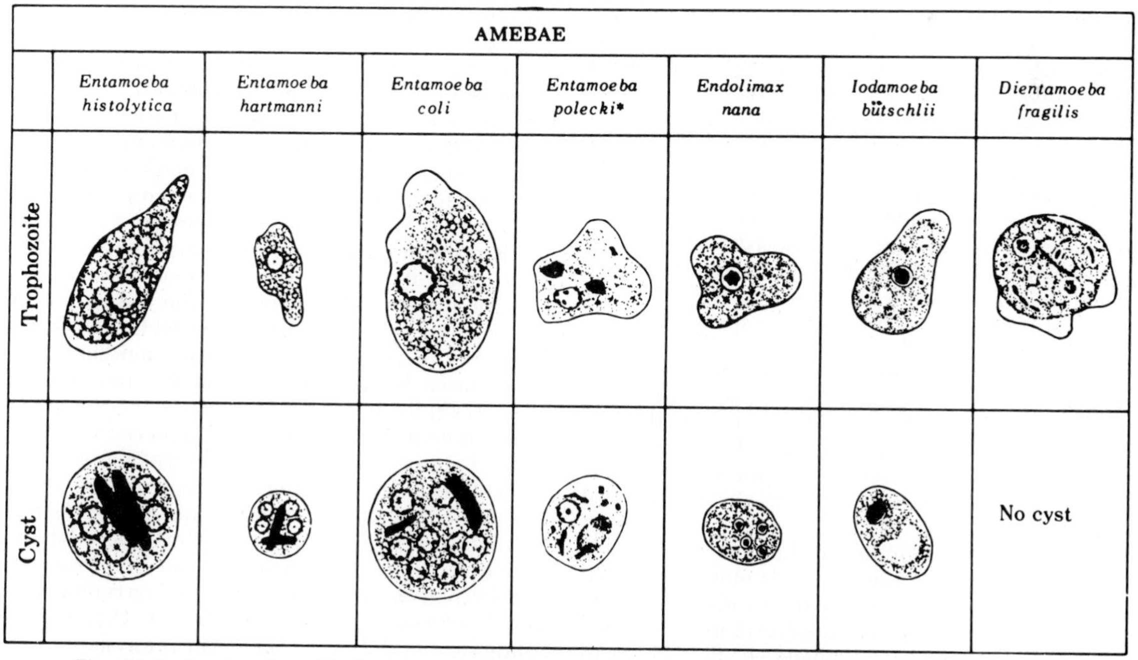

Fig. 87–2. Amebae found in human stool specimens. *Rare, probably of animal origin. *(From Brooke and Melvin: Morphology of Diagnostic Stages of Intestinal Parasites of Man. Public Health Service Publication No. 1966, 1969.)*

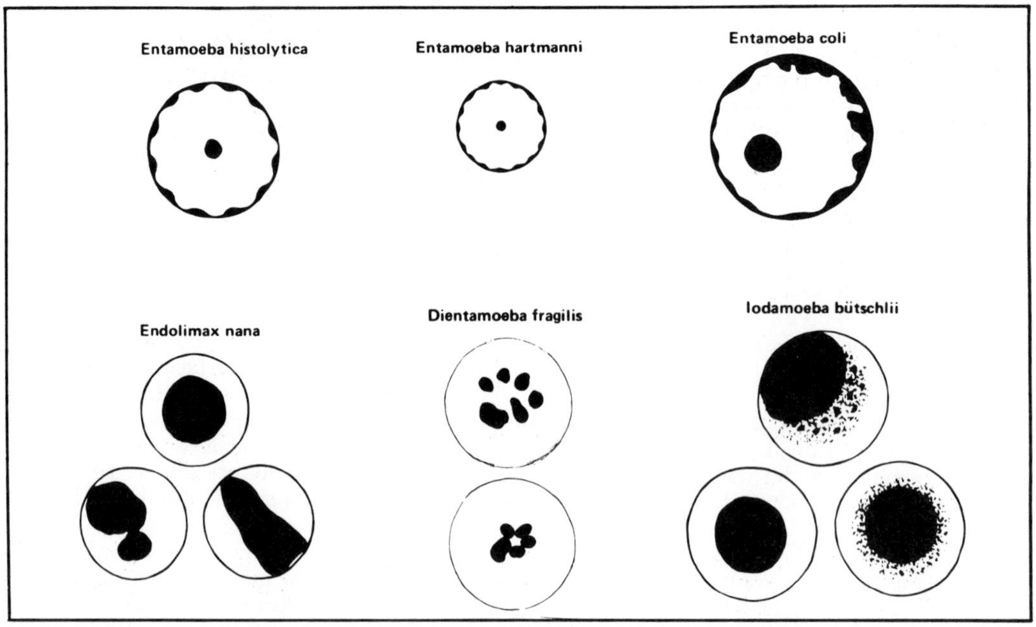

Fig. 87–3. Diagrammatic representation of the various types of nuclei in the amebae of humans. *(From Brooke and Melvin: Morphology of Diagnostic Stages of Intestinal Parasites of Man. Public Health Service Bulletin No. 1966, 1969.)*

free the trophozoites from the coagulum. After this, some of the material should be examined in unstained smears, and some should be placed in culture media. Many investigators have come to rely on the indirect hemagglutination (IHA) test as one means of diagnosis. This test appears to be more sensitive than the complement fixation (CF), indirect immunofluorescence (IIF), and immunodiffusion (ID, or gel diffusion) tests that are available. The enzyme-linked immunosorbent assay (ELISA) holds considerable promise. A skin test is available and, perhaps, will be most useful in epidemiologic studies.

A direct diagnosis made using aspirated material from a suspected lesion in the liver, or elsewhere, is now rarely done. Instead, liver imaging techniques (sonography or computed tomography are preferred) will detect 75% or 95% of the cases. In less well-equipped clinics, roentgenograms are useful adjuncts to diagnosis. If a space-occupying lesion is noted, an appropriate serologic test should be performed.

Laboratory diagnosis of chronic amebiasis, especially in children, is often difficult. Both the clinician and the laboratory worker should be aware that the best results will be obtained from a battery of tests on a series of suitable specimens.

Treatment. Treatment depends on drug therapy, and prevention requires the proper disposal of human wastes and good personal hygiene. Sometimes combination drug therapy is necessary for the treatment of intestinal amebiasis, and even then treatment is not always effective. In contrast, extraintestinal abscesses respond quite well to a variety of individual drugs.

For the treatment of asymptomatic intestinal amebiasis, a large number of antiamebic drugs given by mouth are available. Excellent results have been obtained with iodoquinol. For symptomatic intestinal as well as hepatic infection, metronidazole plus iodoquinol is recommended. For the treatment of liver abscess, dehydroemetine followed by chloroquine phosphate (Aralen), plus iodoquinol, is an alternative therapy.

In acute amebiasis with severe dysentery, emetine HCl, an alkaloid, usually affords prompt relief of symptoms. However, because emetine HCl is ineffective for eliminating the amebae, the usual treatment procedure is first to control the dysentery with emetine and then use one of the above treatments. Because emetine may be highly toxic, it is recommended only for hospitalized patients; it should also be noted that an equally effective but less toxic drug, dehydroemetine, can be obtained on an investigational basis from the Parasitic Diseases Division, Centers for Disease Control (CDC), in Atlanta. Another drug for treating amebiasis, also available from the CDC, is diloxanide furoate, a lumenal amebicide that is highly effective for treating asymptomatic and mildly symptomatic amebiasis in patients who are passing cysts. Diloxanide furoate, therefore, fills a void in the spectrum of amebicidal drugs available to American physicians. As is noted below, additional drugs not on the market in the United States are recommended and may be obtained from the CDC. Table 87–3 lists all such recommended drugs.

Parasitic infections are now encountered throughout the world. With increasing travel, increased use of immunosuppressive drugs and techniques, the spread of AIDS, and continued emigration of people to the United States from less well-developed countries, physicians anywhere may see infections caused by previously unfamiliar parasites. Table 87-3 lists first-choice and alternative drugs. In every case, the need for treatment must be weighed against the toxicity of the drug. A decision to withhold therapy may often be correct, particularly when the drugs can cause severe adverse effects. When the first-choice drug is initially ineffective and the alternative is more hazardous, it may be advisable to try a second course of treatment with the first drug before using the alternative. Several of the drugs recommended in Table 87-3 have not been approved by the U.S. Food and Drug Administration. When a physician prescribes an unapproved drug, or an approved drug for an unapproved indication, it may be advisable to inform the patient of the investigational status and possible adverse effects of the drug.

TABLE 87–3. RECOMMENDED THERAPY FOR PARASITIC INFECTIONS

Infection	Drug of Choice	Alternative Drug
Amebiasis (*Entamoeba histolytica*)		
Asymptomatic	Iodoquinol	Diloxanide furoate and paromomycin
Mild to moderate intestinal disease	Metronidazole followed by iodoquinol	Paromomycin
Severe intestinal disease	Metronidazole followed by iodoquinol	Dehydroemetine followed by iodoquinol, or emetine followed by iodoquinol
Hepatic abscess	Metronidazole followed by iodoquinol	Dehydroemetine followed by chloroquine PO_4 plus iodoquinol; or emetine followed by chloroquine PO_4 plus iodoquinol
Amebic meningoencephalitis, primary		
Naegleria sp	Amphotericin B	
Acanthamoeba sp	No satisfactory therapy	
Ascaris lumbricoides (roundworm)	Mebendazole	Pyrantel pamoate
Balantidium coli	Tetracycline	Iodoquinol or metronidazole
Coccidiosis (*Isospora belli*)	Trimethoprim-sulfamethoxazole	
Cryptosporidiosis (*Cryptosporidium*)	No satisfactory therapy	
Cutaneous larva migrans (creeping eruption)	Thiabendazole	
Dientamoeba fragilis	Iodoquinol	Tetracycline or Paromomycin
Enterobius vermicularis (pinworm)	Pyrantel pamoate	Mebendazole
Filariasis		
Wuchereria bancrofti, Brugia malayi, Mansonella perstans, Loa loa	Diethylcarbamazine	Mebendazole for *M. perstans*
Onchocerca volvulus	Ivermectin	
Flukes, hermaphroditic		
Clonorchis sinensis (Chinese liver fluke)	Praziquantel	
Fasciolopsis buski (intestinal fluke)	Praziquantel	Niclosamide
Paragonimus westermani (lung fluke)	Praziquantel	Bithionol
Giardiasis (*Giardia lamblia*)	Quinacrine HCl	Metronidazole; furazolidone
Hookworms (*Ancylostoma duodenale, Necator americanus*)	Mebendazole	Pyrantel pamoate
Leishmaniasis		
L. braziliensis (American mucocutaneous)	Stibogluconate Na	Amphotericin B
L. mexicana (American cutaneous)	Stibogluconate Na	Amphotericin B
L. donovani (kala-azar, visceral leishmaniasis)	Stibogluconate Na	Pentamide isethionate
L. tropica, L. major (oriental sore, cutaneous leishmaniasis)	Stibogluconate Na	
Malaria		
Plasmodium falciparum, P. ovale, P. vivax, P. malariae		
Suppression or chemoprophylaxis of disease while in endemic area[a]	Chloroquine PO_4	Amodiaquine
Prevention of attack after departure from *P. vivax* and *P. ovale* endemic areas	Primaquine PO_4	
Treatment of uncomplicated attack[a]	Chloroquine PO_4	
Treatment of severe illness[a]	Quinine dihydrochloride or chloroquine HCl[b]	
Prevention of relapses by *P. vivax* and *P. ovale* only ("radical" cure after "clinical" cure)	Primaquine PO_4	
P. falciparum (chloroquine-resistant)		
Suppression or chemoprophylaxis	Chloroquine PO_4 (low-risk areas); chloroquine PO_4 plus pyrimethamine: sulfadoxine	Doxycycline
Treatment of uncomplicated attack	Quinine SO_4 plus pyrimethamine plus sulfadiazine	Quinine SO_4 plus tetracycline
Treatment of severe illness	Quinine dihydrochloride (parenteral dosage)	Quinidine gluconate
Pneumocystis carinii	Trimethoprim-sulfamethoxazole	Pentamidine isethionate
Schistosomiasis		
S. haematobium	Praziquantel	
S. japonicum	Praziquantel	
S. mansoni	Praziquantel	Oxamniquine
Strongyloides stercoralis	Thiabendazole	
Tapeworms (adult or intestinal stage)		
Diphyllobothrium latum (fish tapeworm), *Taenia saginata* (beef tapeworm), *Taenia solium* (pork tapeworm)	Niclosamide or praziquantel	Paromomycin
Hymenolepis nana (dwarf tapeworm)	Praziquantel	Niclosamide
Tapeworms (larval or tissue stage)		
Echinococcus granulosus	Albendazole	
Echinococcus multilocularis	Mebendazole (high dose)	
Cysticercus cellulosae	Praziquantel	Albendazole
Toxoplasmosis (*Toxoplasma gondii*)	Pyrimethamine plus trisulfapyrimidines	Spiramycin
Trichinosis (*Trichinella spiralis*)	Steroids for severe symptoms plus mebendazole	
Trichomonas vaginalis	Metronidazole	
Trichuris trichiura (whipworm)	Mebendazole	
Trypanosomiasis		
T. cruzi (South American trypanosomiasis, Chagas' disease)	Nifurtimox	Benznidazole
T. gambiense, T. rhodesiense (African trypanosomiasis, sleeping sickness)		
Hemolymphatic stage	Suramin	Pentamidine isethionate
Late disease with CNS involvement	Melarsoprol	Tryparsamide plus suramin
Visceral larva migrans	Thiabendazole or diethylcarbamazine	Mebendazole

[a] All *Plasmodium* except chloroquine-resistant *P. falciparum*.

[b] Parenteral dosage only if oral doses cannot be administered, regardless of severity.

Dientamoeba fragilis

D. fragilis is an ameboid parasite that inhabits the large intestine. Although this organism is placed with the amebae in most medical texts because of its appearance, careful study shows it to be a trichomonad flagellate. This organism was originally considered to be a commensal, but it is now known to cause a disturbing gastroenteritis. Although generally thought to be an uncommon parasite, recent surveys show that it is worldwide in distribution; incidence rates as high as 27% have been reported. In the United States a prevalence rate of more than 2% has been proposed.

Life Cycle. *D. fragilis* lacks a cyst stage and thus differs from the true amebae. Although the mode of transmission is unknown, it has been suggested that it may be carried inside the shells of pinworm eggs. Others suggest that the portal of entry is ingestion of the trophozoite, which somehow escapes being killed by the digestive juices of the stomach.

Pathology and Symptomatology. Once the ameba is in the large intestine, it lives in the crypts of the colon where it multiplies by binary fission. This organism is not known to be invasive; it is a lumen dweller. The pathogenesis is unknown, but it is thought that increased mucus production through irritation of the mucosa is a possibility. Diarrhea and abdominal pain are common symptoms. Fibrosis of the appendix has frequently been reported.

Epidemiology. It is very unlikely that the naked trophozoite is the infective stage, because gastric juices are known to be lethal to amebae. If it is proved to be transmitted through pinworm eggs or larvae, this would help explain the lack of association between *D. fragilis* and the other protozoan species that are usually transmitted by fecally contaminated food and water. Infection is seen most often in children younger than 13 years of age. Infections seem to be most common in summer and fall months.

Diagnosis. Gastrointestinal (GI) symptoms include abdominal pain, diarrhea, sometimes alternating with constipation, nausea, anorexia, and flatulence. Common systemic complaints are fever, weight loss, headache, and irritability. Occasionally blood is seen in the stool. The symptoms may continue for 1 month or more if untreated.

A definitive diagnosis is made upon demonstrating the unique, binucleate trophozoite (5 to 15 μm in diameter) in the stool (Figs. 87–2 and 87–3). Because no cyst stage has been seen, routine concentration techniques are of no value. Thus, direct or stained fecal smears are essential for diagnosis, and oil immersion techniques are necessary for correct identification. Of all the intestinal protozoa, *D. fragilis* is probably the most commonly overlooked organism.

Although unusual with protozoan infections, a mild eosinophilia is present in the majority of those proved to be infected. Other blood value criteria have no diagnostic value.

Treatment. Iodoquinol is currently the recommended treatment; tetracycline and paromomycin may be used as alternate drugs.

Flagellate: *Giardia lamblia*

Giardia lamblia is recognized as an important cause of acute gastroenteritis in human beings. Waterborne outbreaks are being reported with increasing frequency, and backpackers have become ill after drinking water from mountain streams. Giardiasis frequently occurs among travelers to foreign countries. Person-to-person transmission occurs in mental institutions, day-care centers, and among male homosexuals. Finally, recent evidence has shown that fecally contaminated food can also be a vehicle for transmission. Infection occurs throughout the world and is most common in children. At least half of those who are infected are asymptomatic. Data show that 2% to 20% of the U.S. population harbors this parasite.

Life Cycle. *G. lamblia* is found in the small intestine; it has both trophozoite and cyst stages. The trophozoites are usually found in the intestinal crypts at the duodenal level, where they are firmly attached to the epithelial surface. At times, they are also found at lower levels of the intestine and in the common bile duct and gallbladder. As revealed by electron microscopy, trophozoites also may occur within epithelial cells, but this is thought to be rare. Multiplication is by longitudinal binary fission, which may result in myriad organisms. Because of their location, trophozoites are not seen in the stool unless the individual has been given a saline cathartic or has persistent diarrhea. Therefore, cysts are usually the only stage found. These occur intermittently and may be numerous. Under moist conditions, the cysts may remain viable for long periods. They presumably reach the mouth of the same person or others by the avenues of transmission discussed for *E. histolytica*. They pass unharmed through the stomach, and excyst in the upper portion of the small intestine. Two trophozoites are produced by each cyst, and thus, this stage provides for reproduction as well as for transmission.

Pathology and Symptomatology. Symptomatic giardiasis may present with any of a variety of signs and symptoms, including epigastric pain, diarrhea or loose stools, flatulence, abdominal cramps, malaise, weight loss, and steatorrhea. In more severe cases, malabsorption and a celiac-like syndrome may occur. Gallbladder irritation and blunting of villi have been noted. It has been suggested that those with severe disease may be immunodeficient with respect to IgA production.

Epidemiology. Asymptomatic infection appears to occur more frequently and may be more important epidemiologically than symptomatic giardiasis. Individuals with asymptomatic infections are much less likely to be detected or to seek treatment than are those with symptomatic infections and therefore are more likely to serve as carriers or disseminators of the disease. The *Giardia* carrier may excrete cysts for months or years. At present, giardiasis is the most frequently identified intestinal parasite in public health laboratories in the United States. Recent interest has centered on the transmission of *Giardia* cysts in drinking water, because epidemics have occurred in various cities of the United States. Because chlorination of water for drinking purposes does not kill the cysts, safe water purification procedures, including filtration, are necessary to eliminate cysts. Another problem has arisen among outdoor enthusiasts who camp in remote, uninhabited areas and drink water from mountain streams and other surface waters long assumed to be safe for human consumption. The source of outbreaks of giardiasis among members of such groups is not known, but it is likely to be cysts excreted by wild animals. *Giardia* must now be included among those organisms that may be transmitted by sexual contact. Although evidence that suggests disease spread in this fashion has been encountered thus far principally among male homosexuals, the possibility of its spread among heterosexuals should not be overlooked.

Diagnosis. Clinically, giardiasis is characterized by severe diarrhea alternating with constipation. During bouts of diarrhea, stools are exceedingly foul-smelling and steatorrheic. Clinical signs are abdominal discomfort, hypoproteinemia, weight loss, and protein malabsorption. These symptoms are also suggestive of peptic ulcer. Infection is common in those who have hypogammaglobulinemia or IgA-selective deficiency. Symptomatic patients are sometimes deficient in folic acid and fat-soluble vitamins.

Definitive diagnosis is made by the finding of cysts or trophozoites in diarrheal specimens or of cysts in formed stools. The trophozoite (10 to 18 μm by 6 to 11 μm) is bilaterally symmetrical, with two nuclei and four pairs of flagella (Fig. 87–4). Living trophozoites on a direct smear have a characteristic flutter, falling-leaf type of movement. It has no oral opening, but on the ventral surface near the anterior end there is a characteristic adhesive disc. The cyst (8 to 14 μm by 6 to 10 μm) is ovoid, and the wall is relatively thickened (Fig. 87–4). When the cyst is stained, two, four, or occasionally more nuclei can be seen, as well as curved fibrils.

At times no cysts are excreted in stools. Alternative methods of diagnosis include intestinal aspiration, biopsies, or the use of a string test (Enterotest). No serologic tests are routinely used, although ELISA, counterimmunoelectrophoresis (CIE), and immunofluorescence tests have been developed.

A number of other nonpathogenic flagellates often inhabit the human intestine. These, such as *Trichomonas hominis* and *Chilomastix mesnili* (Fig. 87–4), must be differentiated from *G. lamblia*. There is some evidence, however, that these organisms, when present alone or together in large numbers, may irritate the intestine and play a role in persistent diarrhea, because the condition often subsides upon their eradication.

Treatment. Quinacrine hydrochloride (Atabrine) is considered the drug of choice. Metronidazole is also effective. Both drugs cause adverse side effects, and caution in their use must be exercised. It appears that none of the drugs currently available will cure all infections, and this raises the possibility of drug-resistant strains, which further complicates the epidemiologic picture.

Ciliate: *Balantidium coli*

B. coli is the only ciliated protozoan infective for humans. Infection is known as balantidiasis, ciliary dysentery, or balantidial dysentery. The infection, although rare in the United States, is distributed worldwide; the general epidemiologic rule is that wherever there are pigs, there are likely to be infections in humans. The precise relationship between the *Balantidium* in humans and the one in pigs is subject to considerable debate and needs to be clarified.

Life Cycle. Both trophozoites and cysts are present in the life cycle (Fig. 87–4). Humans become infected when cysts are ingested, either in contaminated water or through fecal-oral contamination. *B. coli* normally colonizes the large intestine but at times is also present in the cecum and terminal ileum.

Pathology and Symptomatology. *B. coli* usually occurs in the cecal area but may be found at both higher and lower levels of the large intestine. The trophozoites feed on bacteria

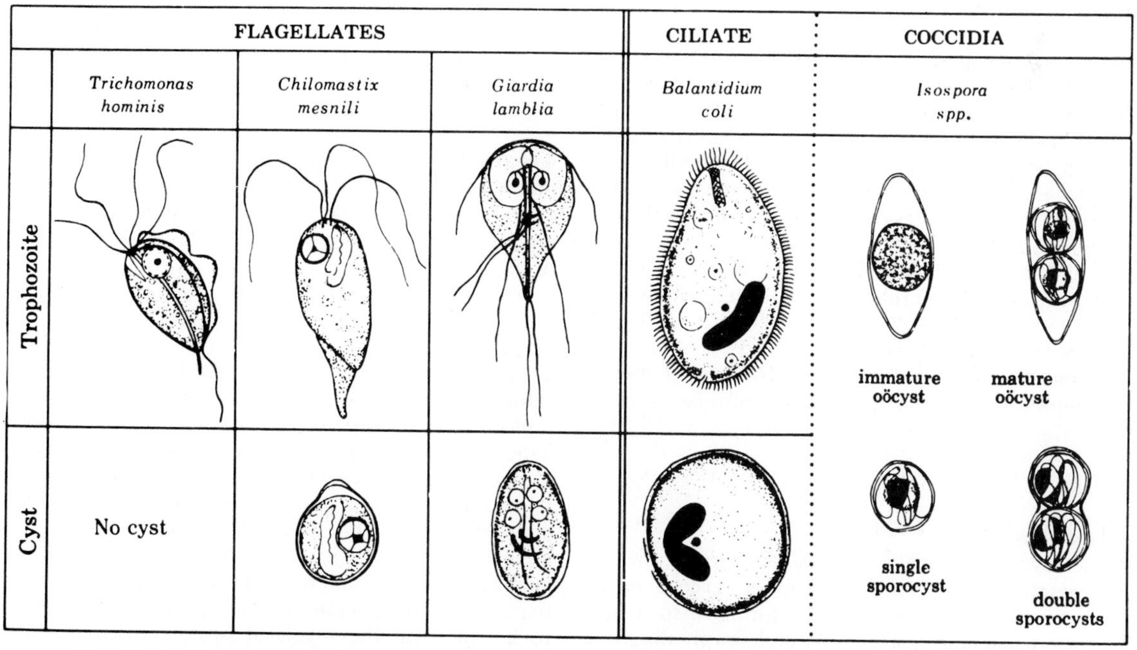

Fig. 87–4. Flagellate, ciliate, and sporozoan protozoa found in stool specimens. *(From Brooke and Melvin: Morphology of Diagnostic Stages of Intestinal Parasites of Man. Public Health Service Publication No. 1966, 1969).*

and other substances in the lumen but take in host cells after they enter the tissues. They reproduce by transverse binary fission, and in certain hosts they may become numerous. The mucosal layer appears to be penetrated both by boring action and by the action of the enzyme hyaluronidase. Because of the large size of the organism, the opening is much larger than that produced by *E. histolytica*. Having gained entrance into the mucosa, the organism has little difficulty in passing through the muscularis mucosae into the submucosa, where it spreads out radially and may cause considerable destruction. Unlike *E. histolytica*, it apparently invades the muscular layers only on rare occasions, and although observed in lymphatics, it is only rarely found in extraintestinal sites. The ulcers produced may occur at all levels of the large intestine but are most common in the cecal and sigmoidorectal areas. They often resemble those produced by *E. histolytica*, especially after bacteria invade them. When this occurs, extensive inflammatory reactions are noted around the organisms, as is a diffuse infiltrate throughout the tissue.

Epidemiology. Although rare in humans, *B. coli* is common in hogs throughout the world. Infections are most prevalent in the tropics where pigs share habitation with people. The pig is usually considered the source of human infection, but attempts to infect humans with the porcine strain have not been successful. Once established, however, person-to-person transmission may occur. This factor becomes significant in environments in which group hygiene may be poor, such as mental hospitals and other places of confinement.

Diagnosis. Many people harboring *B. coli* are symptom-free, but others show symptoms ranging from mild to profuse diarrhea and even fulminating, fatal dysentery. Laboratory diagnosis is usually made by finding the characteristic trophozoites in the stool. Because of their great size, these are easily detected (Fig. 87–4). The trophozoites vary considerably in size (30 to 150 μm by 40 to 70 μm or even larger), are ovoid in shape, and are covered entirely with short, constantly moving cilia. A funnel-shaped peristome (mouth) leads into the cytostome (gullet). One or two contractile vacuoles may be seen within the cytoplasm, as may two nuclei, a large, kidney-shaped macronucleus, and, usually within its concavity, a small micronucleus. The cyst, observed less frequently than the trophozoite, is smaller (45 to 65 μm in diameter) and is almost spherical in shape. Stained cysts reveal clearly the nuclear components.

Anemia and a mild leukocytosis may occur in some patients with symptoms. No serologic or other diagnostic tests are available.

Treatment. Balantidiasis can be treated effectively with tetracycline. Iodoquinol and metronidazole can also be used.

Sporozoans

Isospora species

Isospora species are the cause of a gastroenteritis known as isosporosis or coccidiosis. Taxonomists cannot agree as to the number of species that may be found in humans, so it may be best to take a conservative approach and simply diagnose such infections as being caused by *Isospora*. However, more frequent use of the name *I. belli* as the species that infects humans is seen. Human isosporosis, once considered a rare disease, is now known to be cosmopolitan in distribution. It is seen most often in the warm regions of the world, especially in parts of South America, Africa, and southeast Asia; it appears to be rare in the United States.

Life Cycle. The life cycle is complex. Although it is known for some of the *Isospora* infections in animals other than humans, the life cycle in humans is poorly understood. Infection is considered to begin when a person ingests the oocyst stage in fecally contaminated food or water. Inside the oocysts are eight banana-shaped forms known as *sporozoites*. Once released from the oocysts, the sporozoites invade epithelial cells of the intestine. Division of the parasite occurs within the epithelial cells, and the progeny of this division are released to penetrate other epithelial cells. Eventually some of these progeny become sex cells, unite, and become oocysts, which are shed in the feces. Oocysts are immature when passed and require 24 to 48 hours to become infective.

Pathology and Symptomatology. Isosporosis is usually a mild, self-limiting infection characterized by diarrhea and colicky pains. The pathogenic mechanisms by which *Isospora* organisms cause the gastrointestinal symptoms are not known. Sometimes, however, it may manifest as a chronic infection, with acute episodes of fever, severe diarrhea, and steatorrhea. Such severe cases are most often seen in patients with acquired immunodeficiency syndrome (AIDS) and in infants and children who do not have AIDS. Some mortality has been reported.

Diagnosis. Diagnosis is made by finding the oocysts (20 to 33 μm by 10 to 20 μm) in the stool (Fig. 87–4). Their transparent appearance may cause them to be overlooked by unskilled microscopists. Oocysts are usually present in small numbers, even in diarrheal stools. As a result, a concentration technique, such as the zinc sulfate or formalin-ether technique, should be used. Oocysts of *Isospora* are acid-fast and can easily be distinguished from *Cryptosporidium* organisms on the basis of morphologic characteristics; detection can also be accomplished using the fluorescent auramine dye. No serologic tests are available.

Treatment. Trimethoprim-sulfamethoxazole is the combination drug of choice. Patients with AIDS have a high frequency of recurrence, and thus, some are often kept on a maintenance regimen of the drugs indefinitely at a lower dose.

Cryptosporidium species

Cryptosporidia are protozoan parasites closely related taxonomically to the coccidian parasites *Isospora* and *Toxoplasma*. Unlike these latter two genera, however, infection with *Cryptosporidium* parasites in immunocompetent humans is restricted to the epithelial cells of the microvillous border of the intestinal tract. However, in patients with AIDS and in other immunosuppressed humans. *Cryptosporidium* has been detected in almost all parts of the alimentary canal, the lungs, the biliary system, and the pancreas, and lymphocytic infiltration has been reported. Human infections, until recently, were thought to be rare and the result of opportunistic infections. Hosts normally associated with intestinal cryptosporidosis are numerous and include calves, lambs, guinea pigs, and mice; intestinal and respiratory infections occur in turkeys, chickens, and various reptiles. Since 1980, numerous reports have appeared in the literature and the concept of cryptosporidosis has changed from that of a rare and mainly asymptomatic infection to an important cause of diarrhea and enterocolitis in several species of animals, including humans.

Two events have brought human infection with this agent to the attention of the medical community. The first of these is related to AIDS. It has been found that one of the opportunistic pathogens in these patients is *Cryptosporidium*. The other event is the development of better diagnostic techniques and the demonstration of both asymptomatic and symptomatic infection in immunocompetent hosts. Most recently, it has been shown that zoonotic infection occurs, with transmission from diarrheal calves to humans.

Life Cycle. In general, the life cycle of *Cryptosporidium* follows that of other enteric coccidia. The infective stage is an oocyst containing sporozoites. Upon ingestion, the sporozoites are released from the oocyst and become associated with epithelial cells of the bowel, most often the small intestine. Sporozoites undergo division to form a schizont containing numerous forms known as *merozoites*. These are released from the host epithelial cell, become associated with other epithelial cells, and by the process of gametogenesis eventually form oocysts. The oocyst is released from the epithelial cell and is passed in an undeveloped state in the feces. It should be noted that the question of whether the parasite ought to be considered as intracellular or extracellular is no longer in question. Electron micrographic findings have shown that all developmental stages in the immunocompetent human host are actually intracellular, with the outer layer covering the organisms being of host-cell origin. This fact establishes the relationship of *Cryptosporidium* to the other enteric coccidia.

Pathology and Symptomatology. Symptomatic infection in immunocompetent hosts is usually self-limiting (3 to 14 days) and is characterized by copious, watery diarrhea accompanied by vomiting, weight loss, abdominal cramping and pain, and flatulence. In AIDS and other immunocompromised hosts, a prolonged and severe diarrhea that may last for months is seen. In these cases, malabsorption would be expected. Histologic examinations of intestinal biopsy specimens have shown varying degrees of mucosal damage, including crypt lengthening, partial villous atrophy, and cellular inflammation of the lamina propria.

Epidemiology. Twenty species of animals are known to be susceptible to *Cryptosporidium*, half of which have demonstrated some degree of illness. Ruminants, in general, usually manifest diarrhea if infected at an early age. Several human cases show that the infection may be transmitted from calves and that therefore it is indeed a zoonotic disease. Serologic surveys indicate that infection is not uncommon among the mammalian species examined so far. Although our understanding of this infection in humans is unclear, it is suggested that immunodeficient persons should not work around young animals such as calves, lambs, goats, and pigs. Recent evidence strongly suggests that the organisms infective for humans and cattle are identical; thus *Cryptosporidium parvum* could appropriately be used to identify the organism in human infections.

Diagnosis. Histologic demonstration of the organisms (2 to 4 μm in diameter) attached to the brush border of epithelial cells of the small bowel is a means of diagnosis and has been most widely used in the past. Noninvasive new techniques have been developed, including the modified zinc sulfate centrifugal flotation. Giemsa-stained fecal smears, modified Ziehl-Neelsen carbolfuchsin staining, and Sheather's sugar flotation. Most recently, a sensitive and specific direct fluorescent antibody stain using a murine monoclonal antibody directed against the oocyst wall has been developed and is commercially available. The duodenal string test (Enterotest) has also proved to be a useful technique in diagnosis. Oocysts in feces are 4 to 5 μm in diameter and contain one to six granules.

Treatment. Several antibiotic antiprotozoal, and even anthelmintic agents have been tested against *Cryptosporidium*. None of those tested appears to be effective in treating human disease, but spiramycin may hold some promise. Fluid and electrolyte replacement is of prime importance in both AIDS and non-AIDS patients who are experiencing acute and copious diarrhea.

Urogenital Tract Protozoan: *Trichomonas Vaginalis*

The urogenital tract is, under normal conditions, a rather hostile environment to most parasites because of its acidity and mechanical barriers such as mucus and cilia. When, however, the normal environment is altered by, for example, an increase in pH, organisms such as *Trichomonas vaginalis* can reproduce and flourish.

Trichomoniasis is one of the most common sexually transmitted diseases. In the United States in some areas, incidence among females is reported to be 50%; incidence among males is considerably less. Depending on the population examined and the diagnostic criteria, 20% to 50% of infected women have no symptoms; the majority (50% to 90%) of infected males are without symptoms.

Life Cycle. In females, the organism primarily infects vaginal epithelium and, less commonly, the endocervix. In chronic infection, however, it may invade the urethra, Bartholin's gland, and Skene's gland; bladder infections, as well as rare extravaginal infections, have been reported. In males, the organisms colonize the urethra and prostate gland. There is no cyst stage, and trichomoniasis is therefore essentially a venereal disease. Because the trophozoite can survive a few hours under warm and moist conditions, infection by means of contaminated towels, toilet seats, and underwear is theoretically possible. Newborn infants of both sexes may acquire infection from their infected mothers. The vaginal pH of the newborn is alkaline and, therefore, suitable for colonization. Although a slight vaginal discharge may be present in female infants born of infected mothers, the typical infection is asymptomatic and, in the absence of treatment, self-cure results in 3 to 4 weeks.

Pathology and Symptomatology. In males with nongonorrheal urethral discharge found to be infected with *T. vaginalis*, the symptoms usually are mild until the infection is aggravated by secondary bacterial invasion, after which the condition becomes a purulent urethritis and prostatovesiculitis. In females, trichomoniasis does not always result in a complaint of symptoms, but the vaginal secretions are altered invariably. In typical cases of *T. vaginalis* vaginitis, the normal pH of the vagina (3.8 to 4.4 during sexual maturity) becomes more alkaline, and the glycogen stores of the vaginal mucosa, especially in the superficial layers, are reduced greatly. The normal processes of cellular destruction make the glycogen available to the Döderlein bacillus, an inhabitant of the normal vagina, which metabolizes glycogen and excretes lactic acid. This metabolism maintains the normal acid state of the vagina. In the absence of normal stores of glycogen, the numbers of this organism are reduced, and in severe cases they may be eliminated. When these events occur, the physiologic protection offered by the normal vaginal acidity is altered, and the growth of *T. vaginalis* and other organisms is encouraged. Patients with *T. vaginalis* infection usually have a profuse, watery leukorrheal discharge that produces a chafing of the vagina, vulva, and perineum. Pruritus vaginae and vulvae can be distressing in some.

Epidemiology. In the United States, trichomoniasis occurs in all age-groups. Highest infection rates are in women 30 to 40 years of age, with an estimated 3 to 4 millions new cases each year. It is estimated that prevalence rates range from 5% to 10% among the general female population to as high as 50% to 70% in prostitutes. Women with multiple sex partners, poor personal hygiene, and of low socioeconomic status are at risk of infection. There is also a greater prevalence among black women, multiparous women, women married at an early age, and during pregnancy. Also, those infected with other sexually transmitted diseases are often coinfected with trichomoniasis; for example, up to 50% of women known to have gonorrhea also have trichomoniasis. Although peak incidence is between 16 and 35 years of age, a second peak of incidence has recently been reported in postmenopausal women.

Diagnosis. Clinical diagnosis is based on subjective complaints and evidence of infection. The complaints of discomfort range from irritation and itching to severe vulval pruritus with intense pain. A purulent exudate from the genitalia of both sexes may be seen. Differential diagnosis includes gonorrhea, candidiasis, endometritis, staphylococcal infection, and pelvic inflammatory disease.

Diagnosis is best accomplished by the examination of a temporary microscopic slide preparation of vaginal exudate or urethral discharge in males for detection of the motile trophozoites. Phase contrast microscopy examination is especially helpful. Organisms are 5 to 20 μm in length, pear-shaped, and have a jerky-type movement. Exudate from women is best collected from the vaginal canal with a vaginal speculum.

If wet preparations cannot be examined almost immediately after collection, a stained smear of the exudate should be made. Papanicolaou, Giemsa, and acridine-orange smears are used. The last stain, although excellent, is not often used because it requires a microscope fitted with fluorescent illumination. Culture in appropriate media is sometimes helpful in those cases in which the organism cannot be found in vaginal smears and urethral discharges. Studies show that using both wet mount preparations and culture in an appropriate medium, a detection rate of 98% can be reached. Finally, *T. vaginalis* may be found in urine, especially when the urethra has been colonized.

Complement fixation, IHA, gel diffusion, and immunofluorescent antibody (IFA) tests have been developed. Despite the potential value of these tests for identifying asymptomatic male and female carriers, none has been adopted for routine use in the laboratory.

Treatment. Metronidazole is the drug of choice, and efforts should be made to treat the sex partner(s) of those found to be infected. There is some indication that resistance or tolerance is developing to the drug. Acidic douching to restore normal pH levels of the vaginal canal is sometimes helpful.

Blood and Tissue Protozoa

Amebae: *Naegleria* and *Acanthamoeba*

Free-living soil amebae of the genera *Naegleria* and *Acanthamoeba* are known to produce infections in humans. Among the various species of *Naegleria*, *Naegleria fowleri* is considered the species that causes an acute, rapidly progressing disease of the central nervous system, primary amebic meningoencephalitis (PAM). With only three exceptions, this infection has always had a fatal outcome. *Acanthamoeba* may also cause PAM but, in addition, may cause subacute and chronic infections of the brain, eye, or skin that resemble viral or mycotic disease. When the brain is involved, investigators have termed infections with this organism *amebic meningoencephalitis* (AM). This separation is partially based on the fact that *Naegleria* infections are usually found in healthy, immunocompetent children and young adults, whereas *Acanthamoeba* infections are usually present in patients with other medical problems characterized by a lowering of resistance and immunity. Separation into the two disease categories is also warranted because there are strong indications that the therapy may differ.

Infections with *Naegleria* have been reported from many parts of the world that have a warm climate. In the United States, cases have occurred in 14 states, most of which are located in the eastern and southwestern parts of the country. *Acanthamoeba* infection is not known to be related to any geographic factor or area. Although fewer cases of *Acanthamoeba* infection than of *Naegleria* have been reported on a worldwide basis, infections of *Acanthamoeba* in the United States have been reported from Arizona, Texas, Louisiana, Florida, Virginia, Pennsylvania, and New York.

Life Cycles. Both amebae are normally free-living and ubiquitous in nature and may be found in freshwater lakes, ponds, puddles, swimming pools, and brackish water. Both have trophozoite and cyst stages. In addition, the trophic stage of *Naegleria* not only occurs as an ameba but also, under certain conditions, may change into a flagellated stage. In humans, however, *Naegleria* occurs only in the amebic, nonflagellated form. Infection is thought to occur as a result of diving or swimming underwater, when water containing the amebic stage is forced into the nasal passage, allowing the amebae to invade the mucosa.

Some infections with *Acanthamoeba* probably occur in a similar manner. However, studies have shown that the amebae also exist in the cyst form in nasal secretions and in tissue. In addition to the meningoencephalitis caused by *Acanthamoeba*, upper respiratory, skin, and eye lesions are known. This indicates that the mode of infection and transmission may indeed be quite different for the two organisms.

Pathology and Symptomatology. For infections with *Naegleria*, which resemble bacterial meningitis, the portal of entry is considered to be the nasal mucosa overlying the cribriform plate. The clinical course is dramatic. Prodromal symptoms of headache and fever are followed by rapid onset of nausea and vomiting, accompanied by signs and symptoms of meningitis, with involvement of the olfactory, frontal, temporal, and cerebellar areas of the brain. Involvement of the olfactory area, with disturbances in the sense of smell early in the course of the disease, is characteristic in most patients. Irrational behavior, coma, and death within 2 to 3 days are usual. Spinal puncture reveals a cloudy, purulent, or sanguinopurulent fluid with high leukocyte cell counts (mostly neutrophils), and motile amebae with lobate or blunt, not filiform or spinelike, pseudopodia.

Infection with *Acanthamoeba* is thought to be spread throughout the body by the circulatory system after the ameba invades the nasal mucosa, skin, or lungs. Infections of the brain resemble a brain abscess, and death usually results in 2 to 3 weeks. When, however, the brain is infected directly from the nasal mucosa, as with *Naegleria* organisms, death may result in 2 to 3 days. The incubation period is thought to be about 10 days, and a more prolonged illness results. Infection may be acute, subacute, or chronic, characterized by abscesses or granulomas, or both. Thrombosis and hemorrhage are seen, which clinically resemble mycotic or chronic viral disease. *Acanthamoeba* organisms have also been found in and around corneal ulcers and in the conjunctival fluid. The amebae appear to play a primary role in these eye lesions, and clinicians should consider acanthamebic keratitis when eye lesions fail to respond to bacterial, fungal, and viral therapy.

Epidemiology. *Naegleria* infections have been reported from many areas of the world having warm climates; *Acanthamoeba* infection is not known to be related to any geographic or climatic factor. *Naegleria* infections occur primarily in healthy children, whereas *Acanthamoeba* infections are most common in persons who have some deficiency of the immune or resistance mechanisms.

Cystic forms of the amebae are quite resistant, surviving both freezing temperatures and chlorination of water. Bacteria normally serve as food for the tropic forms, and, thus, thermal pollution of recreational waters presents a serious potential public health hazard. There is also some evidence that *Naegleria* can survive in hospital hydrotherapy pools. It has been suggested that amebae in air conditioning equipment may serve as vectors of *Legionella*. Trophozoites that have ingested *Legionella* may become encysted and then serve as a source of infection for humans via airborne particles.

Diagnosis. The onset of PAM is sudden and resembles acute meningococcal meningitis. Before actual neurologic involvement, fever, neck rigidity, nausea, vomiting, and headache may develop. Within 1 to 2 days after symptoms appear, the patient will become comatose. At this time the sense of taste may be lost, and the sense of smell may be altered. Death usually occurs within 1 week from cardiorespiratory failure and severe cerebral edema.

Diagnosis is difficult because of the nonspecific symptoms and the rapidity with which the disease develops. Sediment from central nervous system fluid should be examined for amebae; use of phase contrast microscopy is recommended. Amebae are usually found in the spinal fluid of persons infected with *Naegleria*; amebae have not been detected in the spinal fluid of those who have brain infections caused by *Acanthamoeba*. Blood cell counts show a leukocytosis, and there is no eosinophilia. Fluid from the central nervous system may be hemorrhagic.

Patients with AM have signs and symptoms very much like those with PAM. However, there is no prior history of swimming. The incubation period is thought to be 10 days or more, and the illness is more prolonged than in PAM. Unlike PAM, in which only the trophozoite is present in human fluids and tissues, both cysts and trophozoites can be demonstrated in brain tissue, nasal secretions, and skin and eye scrapings. Differential diagnosis for both PAM and AM should include bacterial meningitis, cerebral amebiasis, toxoplasmosis, viral encephalitis, and tick fever.

Treatment. The usual drugs for the treatment of intestinal amebiasis are not effective. Amphotericin B therapy has been used in mouse studies, and there are indications it may be beneficial in infections with *Naegleria*. No satisfactory therapy exists for *Acanthamoeba* infections. In vitro studies suggest that flucytosine, polymyxin B, and certain sulfas may eventually prove to be helpful. With the ocular infections, a variety of agents have been used with limited success. It is recommended that the CDC's Parasitic Diseases Division be consulted for the treatment of any proved case.

Flagellates

The flagellates discussed here differ greatly from those reviewed above. In addition to having an entirely different structure, the blood and tissue flagellates are found in various tissues in humans and require a bloodsucking insect to complete their life cycles. Many species are involved, three in the genus *Trypanosoma (T. brucei rhodesiense, T. brucei gambiense*, and *T. cruzi*) and many species of *Leishmania (L. mexicana* complex, *L. braziliensis* complex, *L. tropica, L. donovani, L. major*, and *L. aethiopica*). Aside from a few reported cases of *T. cruzi* and cutaneous leishmanial infections suspected of being acquired in the United States, these various species of so-called hemoflagellates have an exotic origin.

African Trypanosomes

Two morphologically identical species of trypanosomes cause new infections in thousands of people each year on the African continent, which result in considerable mortality and morbidity. One species, *T. b. gambiense*, causes a chronic disease known as Gambian sleeping sickness and is endemic in west and central Africa. The other species, *T. b. rhodesiense*, causes a more acute type of illness called Rhodesian sleeping sickness and is endemic in east and central Africa. At one time, Gambian trypanosomiasis was considered primarily a disease of humans, whereas Rhodesian trypanosomiasis was considered a zoonotic disease, with numerous wild and domestic animals serving as potential reservoir hosts for humans. *T. b. gambiense* has recently been shown by isoenzyme analysis to exist in a variety of wild and domestic animals. Such data challenge the long-held view that transmission was exclusively person to person. Both parasites are transmitted to humans by the bite of infected tsetse flies of the genus *Glossina*.

It is estimated that 1 million Africans are infected at any given time, despite control efforts and chemoprophylactic activities. Although endemic only in Africa, it is well to remember that thousands of citizens of the United States travel to and from Africa each year, and numerous Africans visit the United States for pleasure, business, and education.

Life Cycle. The transmission cycle begins when a tsetse fly feeds on blood from an infected human or animal reservoir. Once inside the vector, the trypomastigotes (Fig. 87–5) pass through the proventriculus into the midgut, where multiplication by longitudinal binary fission results in the production of slender forms. These finally make their way into the salivary glands, where multiplication results in the production of epimastigote forms (Fig. 87–5). Later, these transform into infective-stage trypomastigotes (metacyclic trypomastigotes), which accumulate in the ducts of the salivary glands of the tsetse fly. The entire development within the fly requires about 2 to 3 weeks.

Pathology and Symptomatology. Gambian trypanosomiasis is a chronic disease that eventually gives rise to the torpor and then coma that are characteristic of classic sleeping sickness. Untreated patients usually die as a result of malnutrition and concurrent infection. Soon after inoculation of trypanosomes by an infected tsetse fly, an inflammatory lesion (trypanosomal chancre) may develop at the bite site. There usually are three progressive stages of tissue involvement: (1) parasitemia, when the parasites are numerous in the blood, (2) lymphadenitis, when they are concentrated in the lymph nodes, and (3) central nervous system involvement, when the parasites are numerous in the brain substance and arachnoid spaces. Lymphadenitis is most pronounced in the posterior cervical triangle (Winterbottom's sign). Physical weakness and mental lethargy follow invasion of the central nervous system. Sleepiness develops and becomes progressively pronounced until, in the advanced stage, the patient sleeps continuously. It is thought that the condition may have an autoimmune basis, because antibodies against myelin have been demonstrated. Histologically, a demyelinating encephalitis is noted in advanced cases.

Disease caused by *T. b. rhodesiense* is subacute or acute and is associated with irregular febrile paroxysms, edema, anemia, weight loss, and myocarditis. Although death may occur before the central nervous system is involved, when the disease does progress to central nervous system involvement, behavioral changes and decreased activity are noted. Once the central nervous system is involved, a patient will become progressively

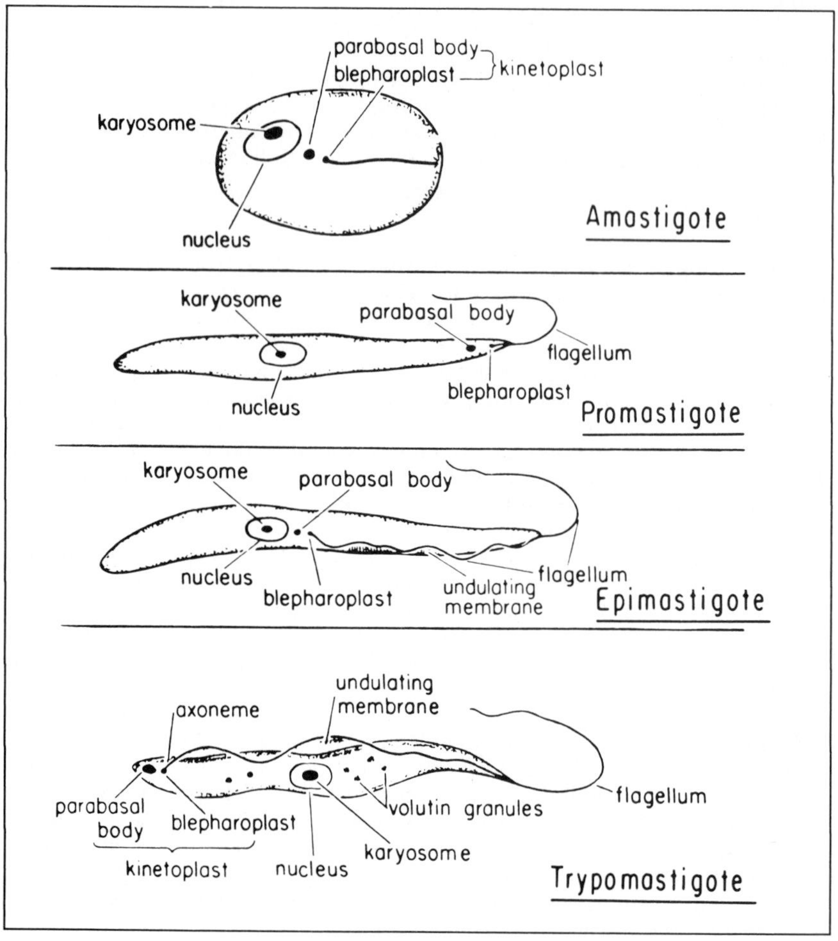

Fig. 87–5. Schematic representation of morphologic forms in the genera *Trypanosoma* and *Leishmania*. *(Modified from Mackie et al: A Manual of Tropical Medicine, ed 2. WB Saunders, 1954.)*

weaker and anemic and within 1 year may die of myocarditis or secondary infection, such as pneumonia.

Epidemiology. *T. b. brucei*, a natural parasite of wild game animals in Africa, especially the antelope, is considered to be the ancestral form of the two human forms. Many domesticated animals are also susceptible to infection, and this leads to a disease known as *nagana*. Both human trypanosomiasis and nagana seriously inhibit the economic development of the continent.

Tsetse flies bite during the day. The species that transmit Rhodesian trypanosomiasis inhabit the open savannah, whereas the species of *Glossina* that transmit the Gambian form are present in riverine areas. Both sexes of tsetse flies ingest blood, are long-lived, and have a wide flight range.

African trypanosomes can change their antigenic composition and thereby evade a host's immune response. This changing antigenicity, known as *antigenic variation*, makes it very difficult to develop long-term protective substances, such as vaccines.

Diagnosis. The clinical picture, although having some common features, differs in the rapidity with which the diseases develop. In general, the Rhodesian form evolves more rapidly to a fatal outcome and many times does not involve the central nervous system. The Gambian form, in contrast, can take several years to develop into the typical sleeping sickness syndrome.

Trypomastigotes of both forms occur in the circulating blood during febrile episodes and sometimes can be demonstrated in thick blood smear preparations. Lymph node aspirates, however, contain a larger concentration of the organisms and are more useful for laboratory diagnosis. After involvement of the central nervous system, examination of spinal fluid may yield positive results. For the reason explained above, this method applies only to *T. b. gambiense* infections. If these various methods fail to establish the diagnosis, susceptible laboratory animals (guinea pigs, white rats, and others) may be inoculated intraperitoneally with some of the patient's blood and later examined at intervals for the parasites.

Both IFA and IHA tests have been developed and used. ELISA and a direct agglutination test have also been developed. Although the IFA test may be helpful in diagnosing an early infection, the ELISA, in conjunction with a demonstration of increased IgM levels by radial immunodiffusion represents the best method for determining the status of infection.

The laboratory finding most suggestive of trypanosomiasis is a marked increase in the IgM level; it may be 10 times the normal value in the Gambian form of the disease and somewhat less in the Rhodesian form. Anemia, increased erythrocyte sedimentation rate (ESR), and elevated protein levels in the fluid of the central nervous system, as well as cells in the spinal fluid, are seen in most cases.

Treatment. During the hemolymphatic stage of both forms of the disease, suramin is the drug of choice. Once the central nervous system is involved, melarsoprol is recommended. Pentamidine isethionate is an alternative drug for the hemolymphatic phase, and tryparsamide plus suramin are used as an alternative for the cases in which central nervous system involvement has occurred.

American Trypanosome

American trypanosomiasis, or Chagas' disease, has been reported in almost all countries of the Americas, including the southern United States. Its main foci, however, are the poorer, rural areas of Latin America. Unfortunately, this infection can be a severely debilitating disease for which there is no known effective curative drug.

Even though suitable vectors and reservoir animals are widely distributed in the southern United States, only a few autochthonous cases in California and Texas have been reported. However, the clinician should pay close attention to the travel history of any patient with symptoms who has returned from an endemic area.

Life Cycle. *Trypanosoma cruzi*, the flagellate that causes Chagas' disease, differs from the African trypanosomes in that it has an intracellular phase involving cells not only of the lymphoid-macrophage system but also those of the muscular system (especially the myocardium), the endocrine glands, and the glial cells of the brain. In this phase, the parasite is a typical amastigote (leishmanial) form (Fig. 87–5), being ovoid in shape, and 1.5 to 3 μm in diameter. No true flagellum or undulating membrane is present. When freed from the host cell, the organism at this stage enters the bloodstream, where it transforms into a C-shaped trypomastigote stage, about 20 μm long, which is the stage taken by the vector. The vectors, in this case, are triatomid (cone-nosed) bugs of the genera *Triatoma, Rhodnius,* and *Panstrongylus.* Many species of these bugs have been found infected naturally. When taken into the bug, the trypomastigote stage of the parasite is carried into the midgut, where it transforms into the epimastigote stage. Later, after multiplication in the hindgut, the infective-stage trypomastigotes are formed, which pass out in the liquid feces of the bug when it is taking a blood meal or immediately thereafter. This usually occurs at night, and the pruritus produced by the bite often results in an infection caused by rubbing into the wound, or nearby skin or mucous membrane, the excrement containing the infective parasites. The entire cycle in the bug requires about 2 weeks.

Pathology and Symptomatology. The disease course varies according to virulence of the strain of *T. cruzi*; host factors such as sex, age, and immune status; and geographic distribution. The acute phase of the disease occurs during the first 6 months, and when symptoms occur, they are usually severe. An infected person has fever; enlargement of the lymph glands, liver, and spleen; and, most important, damage to the heart. Children are particularly susceptible, and death may occur in 10% of those infected. The chronic disease follows the development of the parasite in several visceral organs. Here they multiply as amastigotes, destroying the host cells and bringing about inflammatory reactions in the involved tissues. The principal pathologic changes are noted grossly in the heart and brain, and the predominant symptoms are those of cardiac failure. The spleen and liver are enlarged and congested in relation to the degree of cardiac failure. The brain is congested and edematous and often contains scattered petechial hemorrhages. Collections of organisms may be associated with glial nodules.

Careful study has shown that many infected persons, although manifesting few if any clinical signs and symptoms, do not escape damage to the heart. There is evidence of damage to the heart muscle cells by the invading and reproducing amastigotes. Toxinlike materials affect the nerves that regulate the heartbeat, and autoantibodies may also play an additional role in the destruction of heart tissue. Heart failure may follow.

Megacolon and megaesophagus are rare manifestations of chronic Chagas' disease. It is thought that the neurons serving these organs are damaged by toxinlike materials (or autoantibodies), and the loss of nerve control leads to flaccidity, loss of peristaltic action, and eventually distention of the toneless colon or esophagus.

Epidemiology. *T. cruzi* is a zoonotic infection, infecting not only humans but also many reservoir hosts. Armadillos and opossums are often infected, but cats and dogs may be more important sources for domestic transmission.

Transmission is related to the environment and to habits of both humans and the vectors. The disease is most common where people live in adobe mud huts, where the vectors make their homes in the cracks and crevices of the mud walls. The vectors are night feeders and are able to feed undisturbed, frequently on the conjunctiva of the eye. The fact that there is considerable sylvatic infection in the United States but little human infection attests to the importance of improved housing and living conditions.

Because *T. cruzi* can cross the placental barrier, there have been reports of newborn infants with advanced Chagas' disease. Infections caused by blood transfusion, hypodermic needle contamination, and laboratory accidents are also known.

Diagnosis. An early, almost constant sign of acute *T. cruzi* infection, especially in infants, is edema of the face and eyelids (Romana's sign). The acute form predominates in younger age groups, is usually of short duration, and has a high case fatality rate if untreated. A nodular lesion containing inflammatory cells, called a *chagoma*, may develop at the site of the vector's bite. Fever, edema, diarrhea, adenopathy, hepatosplenomegaly, myocarditis, and sometimes meningoencephalitis may be noted.

T. cruzi also may be found in the circulating blood during febrile periods, but the trypomastigotes are never numerous and, therefore are difficult to demonstrate even in thick blood film preparations. Another trypanosome, *T. rangeli*, occurs in the blood of humans in the same geographic areas as does *T. cruzi*, and it may be misdiagnosed. This species is not pathogenic, has no extravascular stages, and is easily differentiated from *T. cruzi*, being nearly twice as long.

Laboratory animals may be inoculated with blood from suspected cases. A widely used xenodiagnostic test is available and involves the use of parasite-free, laboratory-raised triatomids, which are allowed to take blood from the patient. Examination of the feces or intestinal contents of the bugs after 30 to 50 days will usually reveal trypanosomes if they were present in the blood of the patient. The organisms can be found in stained tissue aspirates and also may be cultivated on various media, e.g., Novy-MacNeal-Nicolle (NNN), Chang's, and in tissue cultures, all of which reveal the epimastigote and trypomastigote forms. Finally, CF, IFA, and IHA tests are available to assist in the diagnosis of latent and chronic cases of the disease.

A lymphocytosis may occur during the acute phase of the disease. Unlike African trypanosomiasis, there is usually no elevation of the IgM level. However, a slight increase in the IgG level may occur during the chronic phase. Heterophile antibody to rat and sheep erythrocytes may appear early in acute infection.

Treatment. Nifurtimox is used for the treatment of Chagas' disease. This eliminates the trypomastigotes from the circulating blood and will improve the clinical condition. However, it does not destroy amastigotes in the tissues, and relapses do occur. As a result, there is no satisfactory treatment for either the acute or chronic forms of the infection.

Leishmania Species

Although leishmania belong to the same major taxonomic group as the trypanosomes, they differ in two major respects. First, instead of being flagellated protozoans that swim freely in the blood of humans, leishmania are small (1 to 3 μm; Fig. 87–5), aflagellated organisms that live inside macrophages. Second, leishmania are transmitted to humans by the bite of small flies of the genera *Phlebotomus* and *Lutzomyia* (sandflies), instead of the larger tsetse flies and triatomids that transmit the various species of *Trypanosoma*.

The taxonomy of the genus *Leishmania* is not well understood at this time. Morphologically, all species are indistinguishable, and, as a result, speciation is based on the clinicopathologic picture, antigen relationships, and geographic distribution. Traditionally, and based on these factors, infections have been separated into three main types (Table 87–4). More complete taxonomic schemes include at least three subspecies within the *L. mexicana* complex (New World cutaneous), five subspecies within the *L. braziliensis* complex (New World mucocutaneous), *L. donovani* (Old World visceral), and an assortment of at least five more species. Such complex taxonomic schemes are based on isoenzyme analysis, DNA probe studies, and clinical and epidemiologic factors.

Life Cycle. Several species of small biting flies called *sandflies* are mainly responsible for transmission to humans and reservoirs. The flies ingest the amastigote form directly from the infected skin or from blood or tissue juices. After being ingested, the parasites develop into the promastigote stage in

TABLE 87–4. *LEISHMANIA* OF HUMANS

Type	Species	Site of Lesions	Geographic Distribution
Visceral	*Leishmania donovani*	Macrophages of the deep viscera (liver, spleen, bone marrow)	India, China, Euro-Asia, Mediterranean basin, Middle East, Africa, and South America
Dermal	*Leishmania tropica* *Leishmania mexicana* *Leishmania peruviana*	Macrophages surrounding skin lesions	Asia, Middle East, India, China, Central Africa, Mediterranean basin, Mexico, and South America
Mucocutaneous	*Leishmania braziliensis*	Macrophages of the nose and pharynx	South America

the midgut (Fig. 87–5). They multiply rapidly, and within a few days many have migrated into the pharynx and mouth parts. In this location, they are ready to be injected into the skin of the next individual when the fly takes another blood meal.

Pathology and Symptomatology. *L. donovani*, agent of kala-azar, causes hyperplasia of the cells of the lymphoid-macrophage system, especially of the spleen, liver, and bone marrow. Both the liver and spleen become enlarged. The usual signs and symptoms include an undulant-type fever, loss of weight (which may be masked by edema), abdominal protuberance, visible pulsation of the carotid arteries, bleeding of the gums, lips, and nares, anemia, and hemorrhage from the intestinal mucosa. The case fatality rate in some areas may be as high as 90% in untreated individuals. In India, post-kala-azar dermal leishmaniasis may develop in about 10% of patients who are fully recovered from kala-azar. This condition is characterized by numerous parasite-laden nodules on the skin. Once a nodule regresses, it may leave a hypopigmented area. *L. tropica* and *L. braziliensis* infections produce local lesions that appear first as a macule, then as a papule with a slightly raised center over a crater. Later the lesion opens at the center to discharge necrotic material. The *L. tropica* ulceration usually occurs late, after which rapid healing is the rule, always with the formation of a scar. Secondary infections, however, may occur, slowing the healing process and causing more extensive scarring. The lesion produced by *L. braziliensis* develops more rapidly, and ulceration and secondary infection usually occur early in the disease. After extension to the mucous membranes, destruction of tissue is usually considerable, and even if healing occurs, the scars are disfiguring to the extent of causing deformity of the face. A variant clinical form of *L. tropica* that occurs in both the New and Old World forms is diffuse cutaneous leishmaniasis (DCL). Although it starts as a typical cutaneous lesion, it progresses to involve many sites as non-ulcerative nodules or plaques on the cooler areas of the body. Ulceration of lesions may occur on those overlying bony prominences.

Epidemiology. Two different types of transmission of visceral leishmaniasis (kala-azar) are seen. In an urban situation, transmission is primarily human to human. In the rural type, infection is epizootic in rodents and other wild animals, and humans are somewhat accidental hosts. Clinical variants of the infection have been described and are considered by some to be due to different strains or subspecies. These variants range from being the classic form of kala-azar in India to a form in Kenya that may be manifested primarily as skin lesions.

Vaccination by inoculating serum from naturally acquired lesions into a nonimmune person is used in various countries to prevent the development of cutaneous leishmaniasis. It should be emphasized that recently the New World forms that cause cutaneous ulcers generally have been referred to as members of the *L. braziliensis* complex, and evidence suggests strongly that the cases confirmed recently in Texas were caused by forms within this complex.

Diagnosis. The onset of visceral leishmaniasis may be sudden or, as is more often the case, gradual. When development is sudden, diarrhea and fever resembling typhoid fever are seen. Hepatosplenomegaly, ascites, and lymphadenopathy may develop during the first few months after infection. Darkening of the skin and other alterations in skin pigmentation may be observed on the forehead, mouth, chest, and legs.

The clinical manifestations of cutaneous leishmaniasis are largely determined by the site of infections. Facial lesions, especially those around the nose and mucous membranes, may be quite extensive and give rise to serious disfigurement. The differential diagnosis of this form of leishmaniasis should include syphilis, yaws, leprosy, tuberculosis, blastomycosis, and skin cancer.

In laboratory diagnosis, *L. donovani* may be demonstrated sometimes in stained blood smears. However, cultivation of the organisms by inoculating the blood into special media (NNN, Chang's, and others) and incubating at 20C to 25C is more likely to be successful. The promastigote stage occurs in cultures (Fig. 87–5). Many workers prefer to prepare stained tissue smears of specimens obtained by biopsy. In the past, spleen and liver specimens were most often used, but today most workers favor the use of a bone marrow specimen from the iliac crest obtained by the van den Bergh technique. A portion of each sample should also be handled aseptically and cultured. If these various methods fail to reveal the amastigotes in suspected cases, hamsters may be inoculated. An immunofluorescence test and a CF test are available and of some value.

L. tropica and *L. braziliensis* may be demonstrated in stained smears made from the crater of an early lesion or, less often, from material obtained from the indurated margin of older lesions. The material can also be cultured, but care must be taken to cleanse the area before taking a sample, because the organisms seldom will grow in the presence of bacteria. A CF test and a skin test (Montenegro) are available for diagnosis of both *L. tropica* and *L. braziliensis*, but the skin test has been more widely used in clinics and in the field to diagnose *L. braziliensis*.

A very large increase in the amount of serum IgG is the most prominent laboratory finding in individuals with visceral leishmaniasis; such an increase is not noted in either the cutaneous or the mucocutaneous forms. Anemia and leukopenia with a relative increase in lymphocytes are also characteristic of the visceral form.

Treatment. Stibogluconate sodium, a drug available from the CDC's Parasitic Diseases Division is the drug of choice for all forms of leishmanial infection. As alternative drugs, amphotericin B can be used to treat the cutaneous and the mucocutaneous forms, and pentamidine isethionate may be used for kala-azar. After secondary bacterial infections of ulcers, the sulfa drugs or antibiotics are used to destroy these agents before specific treatment is given.

Sporozoa

Sporozoa are obligate intracellular protozoa with no organelles of locomotion. Most species produce a spore, which is the infective stage for humans. Infection is either by ingestion or by injection as a result of a biting arthropod. Sexual and asexual generations are present in each species.

Within the Sporozoa are two of the most important and widespread parasites of humans, causing malaria and toxoplasmosis. *Plasmodium*, the genus of malaria organisms, comprises four species (one of which has developed drug-resistant strains) that are of major medical and public health importance. In addition, the mosquito that transmits this disease to humans has also developed resistance to various insecticides, thus hampering control efforts. *Toxoplasma*, the agent of toxoplasmosis, is a sporozoan that infects and multiplies in nucleated cells of almost all vertebrate animals. The domestic cat is the definitive host, and humans can become infected in a variety of ways. Although fetal death, congenital infection leading to mental retardation, and blindness are known to be caused by this parasite, it is still poorly understood and, like visceral larva migrans, may eventually be proved to be of even more importance in human morbidity. *Pneumocystis carinii*, the agent of pneumocystic pneumonia seen in more than 50% of AIDS cases, is considered by some to be a sporozoan; others consider it to be a fungus. For the sake of convenience, it will be presented as a sporozoan.

Malaria

The malaria parasites, some of which were once endemic in the United States, are members of the genus *Plasmodium*, and their life cycles involve both an asexual phase (schizogony in humans as the intermediate host) and a sexual phase (sporogony in certain female anopheline mosquitoes as the definitive host). There are four species of human malarial parasites:

1. *Plasmodium vivax*, agent of benign, tertian malaria, is the most widely distributed and on a worldwide basis is the second most prevalent species.
2. *Plasmodium falciparum*, agent of malignant, subtertian malaria, is as prevalent as *P. vivax* in subtropical and tropical regions but fails to establish itself in areas where there are long, cold seasons. This species is responsible for most cases of malaria worldwide.
3. *Plasmodium malariae*, agent of quartan malaria, is limited almost entirely to tropical and subtropical areas, where it is considerably less prevalent than *P. vivax* and *P. falciparum*.
4. *Plasmodium ovale* is the agent of ovale malaria, a tertian-type of malaria, less common than the other types. It has been reported sporadically from widely separated regions in Africa, South America, and Asia and appears to have almost completely supplanted *P. vivax* on the west African coast. The parasite resembles *P. vivax* in certain characteristics and *P. malariae* in others.

Life Cycle. Although there are striking morphologic differences among the four species, the general features of their life cycles are the same. Specific differences are considered below under diagnosis. The cycle in humans begins with the inoculation of infective sporozoites by a female anopheline mosquito. Within 1 hour, the sporozoites disappear from the circulating blood, and no parasites can be demonstrated in red blood cells (RBCs) for many days. It is known that during this negative phase, the parasite is residing in fixed tissue cells of the liver. The various stages of the parasite observed in exoerythrocytic foci resemble those seen later within the RBCs, but the characteristic malarial pigment (hemozoin), derived from the breakdown of hemoglobin, is, of course, not seen. After the parasites develop in exoerythrocytic foci for many days, their density increases, and certain of the progeny enter the bloodstream and initiate erythrocytic infection. It should be added that the exoerythrocytic forms of *P. vivax* and *P. ovale* in the liver may persist long after the eradication of the erythrocytic forms and thus are known to be the cause of later episodes of parasitemia and clinical relapses.

The first stage observed within the RBCs is the trophozoite. The youngest is referred to as a *ring*, which has a central vacuole and a ring of cytoplasm containing a chromatin dot. The growth of the parasite proceeds gradually, the vacuole disappears, and the cytoplasm increases in size. With the increase in volume of the cytoplasm, pigment increases in amount with increasing age of the parasite, because it is a waste product of hemoglobin metabolism. When the single nucleus of the trophozoite stage divides to form two nuclei, the schizont stage is reached. The chromatin continues to divide until the number of chromatin masses characteristic for the species is reached. At this point, the presegmenter has been produced. The segmenter or mature schizont is observed soon thereafter, when each chromatin mass has been provided, after division of the cytoplasm, with an envelope of cytoplasm to form the merozoites. By this time, the pigment, scattered previously, has become clumped, usually near the center of the parasite. The RBC ruptures, and some of the merozoites enter new cells to begin again the asexual cycle. The length of this cycle—from entry of merozoite to the rupture of the host cell—varies with the species of parasite, being 48 hours for *P. vivax* and *P. ovale*, 72 hours for *P. malariae*, and 36 to 48 hours for *P. falciparum*. The cycle of *P. falciparum*, however, has considerably less synchronization than those of the other three species. In addition to trophozoites and schizonts, a third stage, gametocyte, is seen within the RBCs. The gametocytes, male and female sex cells, nearly fill the RBC and have only a single chromatin mass. It is this stage that initiates the sporogenous cycle in the female anopheline. In summary, there are only three distinct stages within the RBCs of humans: the trophozoite, the schizont, and the gametocyte.

After a female anopheline ingests a blood meal containing ripe gametocytes of both sexes, the sexual cycle begins. In the lumen of the midgut, the gametocytes escape from the host cells and soon undergo changes preparatory to fertilization. The female gametocyte (macrogametocyte) extrudes polarlike bodies, indicating that the haploid condition is being assumed. The male gametocyte (microgametocyte), through a process known as *exflagellation*, forms a number of spermlike bodies. The fact that these changes in both cells are noted within about 20 minutes under favorable conditions, suggests that the lining up process within the nucleus of each actually begins in the human bloodstream. In any event, fertilization occurs when a microgamete enters a macrogamete, and a zygote is formed. Being motile, this form is referred to as the *ookinete*. The ookinete penetrates beneath the peritrophic membrane lining the midgut and, after about 24 hours, penetrates through the cells and becomes encysted under the hemocoelic membrane on the outside wall of the midgut. Here the oocyst is formed, which, when mature, contains a large number of sporozoites. The oocyst ruptures into the body cavity after about 2 weeks, and many of the sporozoites eventually find their way into the trilobed salivary glands. After a few days under optimum conditions, the sporozoites become infective and are capable of initiating an infection in a susceptible individual after being inoculated when the mosquito punctures the skin to take a blood meal.

Pathology and Symptomatology. The most characteristic features of the pathology of malaria are anemia, pigmentation of certain organs, and hypertrophy of the liver and, especially, the spleen. The anemia—a microcytic, hypochromic type—may be produced not only by the direct loss of RBCs as a result of their destruction by the parasite but also from interference with hematopoiesis, by increased phagocytosis of RBCs, and as the result of capillary hemorrhages and thrombosis. In acute cases, *P. falciparum* produces the greatest degree of anemia, especially because of the marked loss of RBCs by the growth of the parasite within them. In chronic cases and especially during malarial cachexia, the anemia is particularly outstanding. During the latter cases, leukopenia, with a monocytosis of 20% or more, is considered diagnostic of malaria. The pigmentation noted in the tissues of malaria victims is due to the phagocytosis of hemozoin, the true malarial pigment, released into the blood upon rupture of the host cells at the termination of each asexual cycle. Hemozoin is taken up in large amounts by cells of the lymphoid–macrophage system, especially by the macrophages in the spleen and bone marrow, and the Kupffer cells in the liver. The pigmentation constantly increases with the age of the infection, so that it may be observed grossly at autopsy in cases of chronic malaria. As would be expected from the massive blood destruction, there is also deposition of pigment in the tissues. The liver is enlarged due to congestion during acute malaria, and it increases considerably in size during a chronic infection. The spleen, the organ affected most seriously in malaria, is also enlarged, first as a result of congestion (after cavernous dilatation of the sinusoids) and later as a result of a great increase in macrophage elements, especially in Billroth's cords. With repeated attacks, the enlargement becomes progressively greater, and the organ may reach considerable size, especially in width, in chronic malaria. Fibrosis of Billroth's cords is outstanding here. Splenomegaly in malaria is so characteristic that palpation of this organ has been used for a long time as a rapid and effective means of appraising the malaria problem in communities. Changes in the bone marrow, although much less striking, are similar in character to those in the spleen.

In addition to these changes, which may be expected in any malarial infection, but especially in those of long standing, another important change, capillary occlusions, should be mentioned. These are most characteristic in *P. falciparum* infections and are most dangerous in the brain, leading to cerebral malaria, which may be fatal if left untreated. The parasitized RBCs become sticky (some believe as a result of a specific antibody-antigen reaction), and agglutinate. Such cells marginate at the periphery of the vessel lumen, probably as a result of centrifugal force, and later the capillary becomes occluded. Following this, hemorrhages occur about such vessels, exclusively in the subcortical and paraventricular white matter, producing a ring effect. The tissue immediately surrounding the vessel is necrotic, and the ring hemorrhage is somewhat removed from the vessel. Usually associated with ring hemorrhages are the so-called malarial granulomas, consisting essentially of a rosette of one or several layers of glial cells arranged around the necrotic zone. Anoxia with necrosis of tissue in the immediate vicinity must be the logical consequence of occluded vessels.

Blackwater fever should be mentioned, because it is associated with malarial infections, especially *P. falciparum* infections. The disease is characterized by intravascular hemolysis with hemoglobinemia and hemoglobinuria. Hemoglobinuric casts occur in the distal convoluted tubules in the kidney. Degeneration, and some regeneration, of the tubular epithelium is also seen.

The symptoms of malaria differ between infections caused by *P. vivax*, *P. ovale*, and *P. malariae* and that caused by *P. falciparum*. The typical paroxysm caused by the first three parasites involves, usually after a brief prodromal period, a cold stage (shaking chill), followed by a fever stage (a characteristic remittent-type fever quickly reaching a level of 41C to 42C and, after many hours, returning suddenly to almost normal), and a marked terminal sweating stage resulting from the sudden fall in body temperature. *P. falciparum* paroxysms differ in many ways: the chill stage is less pronounced (there may be only a chilly sensation), the fever stage is more prolonged and intensified (fever tends to be a continuous or only a briefly remittent type), and because the fever fails to remit sharply, the sweating stage is usually absent. *P. falciparum* infection is more dangerous than those of the other three species, as it is often accompanied by pernicious manifestations, such as hyperpyrexia, convulsion, coma, and cardiac failure. *P. falciparum* parasites may localize in any organ, and those organs bearing the brunt of the attack will display the most striking signs and symptoms. Therefore the symptoms of *P. falciparum* malaria may resemble those of many other diseases.

Epidemiology. Malaria is present in almost all tropical and subtropical areas. The Polynesian and Micronesian islands and Australia are about the only such areas free of this disease. At one time malaria was widespread in Europe and the United States; fortunately, as a result of control efforts it has now largely disappeared from the temperate zones. Recent reports show a few autochthonous cases of *P. vivax* in California.

Malaria is a real threat to nonimmune persons who travel or reside temporarily in malarious areas. The recent appearance of drug-resistant strains of *P. falciparum* has increased this threat, and clinicians in the United States should be well aware of the steps that need to be taken to prevent their patients from contracting malaria when they travel abroad to tropical and subtropical countries.

Rainfall, temperature, and vegetation are factors that influence mosquito breeding and thereby affect seasonal transmission. Other epidemiologic factors affecting endemicity are prevalence in the indigenous host population, genetic factors of the host including those controlling the Duffy blood group and sickle cell antigens, parasite species and strains, immunity level of the population, and housing conditions. In endemic areas, children bear the brunt of malarial mortality, with an estimated 1 million deaths each year in Africa alone. Many believe, however, that this figure is much too large. More accurate and current estimates are certainly needed.

Diagnosis. *P. vivax*, *P. ovale*, and *P. malariae* cause an illness characterized by a high fever of a characteristic periodicity in well-established infections, anemia, and splenomegaly. Infections with these species are usually self-limiting and usually do not cause serious illness or death in untreated cases. On the other hand, *P. falciparum* infection is potentially life-threatening, and unless diagnosed and treated promptly it can lead to rapid death. Cerebral disease may be manifested by symptoms that range from headache to convulsions to coma. Kidney and liver dysfunctions are also noted, and, not infrequently, an attack may mimic influenza.

Definitive diagnosis is made by the demonstration of malarial parasites in blood smears. Both thick smears, for the detection of organisms, and thin smears, for speciation, are recommended. Smears should be stained with Giemsa stain as promptly as possible when malaria is suspected. Repeated blood smears should be made in the case of suspected infection when the initial smears show negative results. Comparative information on the four species of malarial parasites in thin

TABLE 87–5. DIAGNOSTIC CHARACTERISTICS OF MALARIAL PARASITES

	Plasmodium vivax	*Plasmodium malariae*	*Plasmodium falciparum*	*Plasmodium ovale*
Other names	Benign tertian malaria	Quartan malaria	Malignant tertian estivoautumnal malaria	Benign tertian or ovale malaria
Incubation period (d)	14 (8–27) (sometimes 7–10 mo)	15–30	12 (8–25)	15 (9–17)
Erythrocytic cycle (h)	48	72	48	48
Persistent EE stages	Yes	No	No	Yes
Parasitemia (mm^3)				
Average	20,000	6,000	50,000–500,000	9,000
Maximum	50,000	20,000	Up to 2,500,000	30,000
Duration of untreated infection (y)	1.5–4.0	1–30	0.5–2.0	Probably 1.5–4.0

blood smears, including the most important differential diagnostic characteristics, is given in Tables 87–5 and 87–6.

IFA and IHA tests are available. However, they are used primarily for epidemiologic purposes and have little application in the clinical laboratory because they will not differentiate between an active and a past infection.

Treatment. The initial aim of treatment should be to eliminate the acute attack as quickly as possible by eliminating the RBC stages of the parasite. At the same time, steps to combat dehydration, renal failure, hypoxia, and so on must be undertaken, especially in *P. falciparum* infection. Chloroquine is currently the drug of choice to accomplish this with all species of malaria. Chloroquine does not, however, eliminate the persisting tissue stages in the liver of those infected with either *P. vivax* or *P. ovale*. Primaquine should be administered for this purpose to minimize the chance of subsequent relapse.

Quinine sulfate plus pyrimethamine are the drugs recommended for the treatment of chloroquine-resistant *P. falciparum*. Resistance is not total, and, as a result, some suppression does occur in drug-resistant strains. Recrudescence, however, will occur in several days to several weeks, reflecting a failure of the chloroquine to eliminate all erythrocytic parasites.

Currently, chloroquine plus Fansidar (sulfadiazine plus pyrimethamine) is the recommended prophylactic treatment for individuals living in nonendemic areas who plan to travel to endemic areas. Fansidar is usually well-tolerated, but severe adverse reactions (erythema multiforme, Stevens-Johnson syndrome, toxic epidermal necrolysis) have been noted. Consequently, physicians should carefully question patients regard-

TABLE 87–6. DIFFERENTIAL DIAGNOSIS OF MALARIAL PARASITES IN STAINED THIN BLOOD SMEARS

Most Striking Differences	*Plasmodium vivax*	*Plasmodium ovale*	*Plasmodium malariae*	*Plasmodium falciparum*
Abundance of parasites	More abundant than *P. malariae*	As for *P. vivax*	Least abundant	Most abundant
Stages of parasite usually observed	Trophozoites, schizonts, gametocytes	As for *P. vivax*	As for *P. vivax*	Young trophozoites, gametocytes
Changes in infected red blood cells	Enlarges (twice normal), malshaped, Schüffner's dots	Enlarged (1½ × normal), 20% or fimbriated or both	Changes not common	Changes not common
Trophozoites ring stage	Small and large (⅓ diameter of RBC) with vacuole and usually one chromatin dot	Much like *P. vivax*	Much like *P. vivax*	Very small (⅙ diameter of RBC) with vacuole, often with two chromatin dots, peripheral forms (accolé) common, multiple infected cells very common
Half grown	Ameboid, irregular with vacuoles, pigment yellow-brown rods	Oval and/or fimbriated (20%) enlarged cell, compact dark brown pigment	Band forms (25%) compact, pigment coarse black granules	Not usually seen
Schizonts (mature)	12–24 merozoites	6–14 merozoites	8–12 merozoites arranged in rosette	Not usually seen
Gametocytes	Large and rounded, fills up red cell, golden brown pigment	Red cell enlarged and/or fimbriated, dark brown pigment	Parasite fills up cell, dark brown pigment	Kidney-bean shape, round or pointed ends

ing sulfonamide intolerance. Table 87–3 lists the drugs currently recommended for the treatment of all types of malaria.

Toxoplasma gondii

Toxoplasmosis, caused by *Toxoplasma gondii*, is a cosmopolitan and common infection afflicting nearly one third of the human race. It has an amazing lack of host specificity, being found, for example, in various primates, carnivores, rodents, birds, and ungulates. Because of the wider use of immunosuppressive treatment that permits exacerbation of latent infection as well as permitting primary infection, toxoplasmosis is now recognized as an important medical and public health problem. Fortunately, most infections are asymptomatic. When overt disease is present, however, it can leave blindness, deformity of newborn infants, mental retardation, and death in its wake.

Life Cycle. Domestic house cats and other felines are the definitive hosts of *T. gondii*. In the definitive host, an asexual cycle, as well as a sexual cycle occurs in the epithelial cells of the small intestine. The result is the production of oocysts, which are passed in the feces. After a few days, these oocysts sporulate, so that each one contains two sporocysts, each with four sporozoites. If these mature oocysts are ingested by an intermediate host (animals other than felines, including humans), infection results, and trophozoites may be produced in many tissues. Thus, human infection can occur not only by ingestion of cysts in undercooked meat, as has been known for years, but by ingestion of mature oocysts as well. Also, recent evidence of an epidemic in army troops on maneuvers in Panama indicates that the infection may be waterborne.

Pathology and Symptomatology. *T. gondii* is an obligate intracellular parasite. The individual cells, known as trophozoites (formerly called tachyzoites) are 4 to 8 μm long and are crescent shaped (Fig. 87–6). They may be found at times within wandering macrophages in peritoneal, pleural, and cerebral exudates, and in circulating blood. The cells of the lymphoid-macrophage system are most often involved, but the parenchymal cells of the liver, lungs, brain, and other tissues may be parasitized. A cyst, 5 to 200 μm or more in size, may be observed under certain conditions. A cyst is formed by aggregate of *Toxoplasma* bradyzoites and has a delicate, delimiting argyrophilic membrane produced by the parasite. Tissue reaction is seldom associated with cysts, which are usually located in the lungs, brain, heart, and skeletal muscle. Thus the cysts are believed to be the basis for the persistence of the organism during chronic and latent infections. The release of bradyzoites from cysts must be responsible in most instances for the fulminating *Toxoplasma* infections reported in immunosuppressed patients. Such reports raise the question of whether suppression similarly affects other previously established protozoan infections. These organisms may give rise to at least five types of infections:

1. A congenital infection with onset in utero
2. An acquired encephalitic infection in older children
3. An acute febrile illness, usually in adults, resembling typhus or spotted fevers and often producing pulmonary involvement (a typical diffuse interstitial pneumonitis), myocarditis, and other disturbances
4. An infection resembling infectious mononucleosis, with such symptoms as lymphadenopathy, rash, fever, and marked weakness
5. A latent infection, in children or adults, which usually can be recognized only by the presence of specific antibodies in the serum

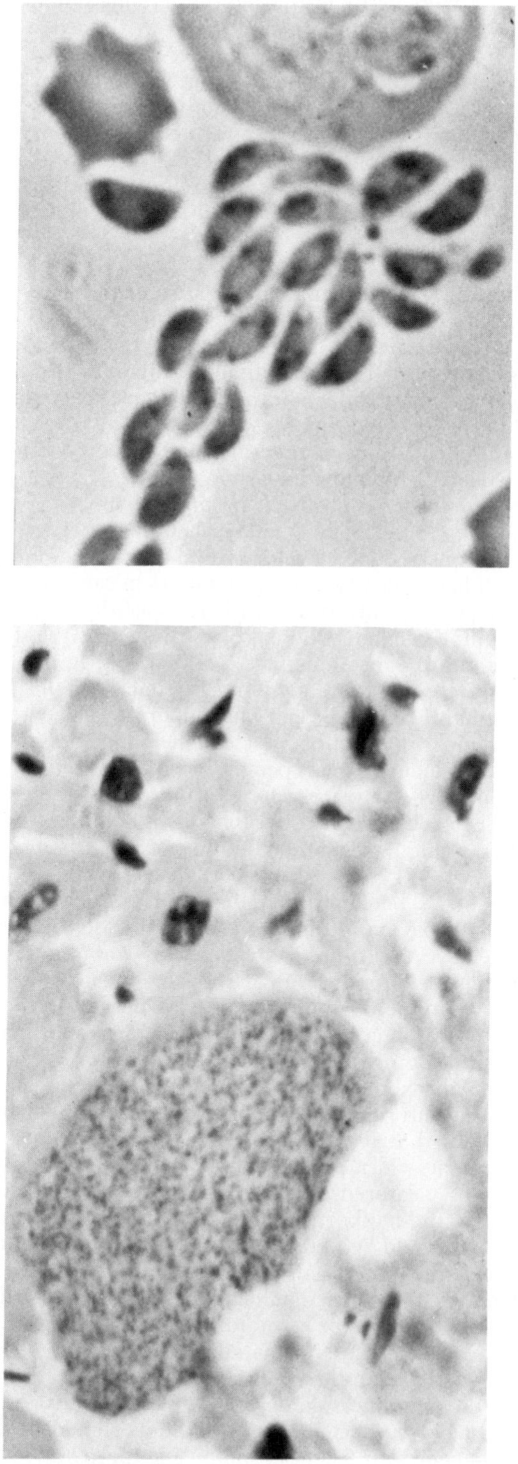

A B

Fig. 87–6. *Toxoplasma gondii*. **A.** Trophozoites. **B.** Cyst containing bradyzoites.

In addition, there is evidence of an association between *Toxoplasma* organisms and unilateral granulomatous uveitis and retinochoroiditis in adults. The congenital infection, with its onset in utero, occurs as a fetal or neonatal encephalomyelitis, which is often fatal soon after birth but which may remain asymptomatic until much later. Marked lesions and necrosis usually occur in the central nervous system and are associated with calcification there and in the eyes. Bilateral retinochoroiditis is common. At times, hydrocephaly or microcephaly and psychomotor disturbances are evident. In infections acquired after birth, lesions in the viscera are more common than those in the central nervous system. In summary, during toxoplasmic infection, the sites most commonly attacked are the lymph nodes, brain, eyes, and lungs. Data indicate that in patients with AIDS the most common cause of necrotic brain lesions is *Toxoplasma*.

Epidemiology. Seroepidemiologic screening surveys have shown that seropositivity may range from 2% to 93% worldwide, depending on the population surveyed. In the United States, rates vary from 17% to 50%. Although toxoplasmosis is usually a latent infection, outbreaks in the United States have been reported since 1969 as a result of eating raw hamburger, inhaling or ingesting oocysts at a riding stable, and drinking contaminated water.

Research has shown that no more than 1% of domestic cats in the United States may be shedding oocysts. Whether cats shed oocysts only once or several times is not known, but research has shown that some immunity in cats does develop.

To prevent infection, which is especially important for nonimmune women who become pregnant, the following precautions are recommended. Meat should be heated to at least 66C before it is eaten, and raw meat should never be fed to cats. If possible, keep cats indoors and change litter in boxes daily, disposing of litter either by burning or flushing down the toilet. When people are working in flower or vegetable gardens, places where cats frequently defecate, care should be exercised to ensure that dirt is not ingested. Finally, children's sand boxes should be kept covered when not in use.

Diagnosis. The clinical manifestations of toxoplasmosis are highly variable and often mimic other diseases. The majority of patients with acquired infection are symptom-free. When symptoms are present, they may mimic pneumonia, myocarditis, hepatitis, and lymphadenitis. Fatigue, chills, fever, headache, and myalgia are sometimes seen. Fatalities may result in immunosuppressed patients.

Ocular toxoplasmosis, either acquired or congenital, usually affects only one eye. It is estimated that 5% of all blindness in the United States is due to retinal involvement. Congenital involvement, which occurs in 30% to 50% of the cases when infection is acquired during pregnancy, may remain asymptomatic in the newborn. When damage does occur, it may be severe. It should be noted that a mother who has transmitted *T. gondii* to her fetus thereafter becomes immune, and no subsequent pregnancies will lead to transplacental infection.

With regard to the laboratory diagnosis, three approaches are available: direct examination, isolation of organisms, and tests for a presumptive diagnosis. For direct examination under the oil-immersion objective, tissue sections and impression films of suspected tissues or fluids should be air-dried and stained with Giemsa stain. The preparations usually examined are tissues taken by biopsy, sputum, vaginal exudates, and the sediment of spinal, pleural, or peritoneal fluids. The organisms can be isolated by intraperitoneal inoculation of white mice with fresh, untreated tissue or fluids most likely to contain these organisms. If organisms are present, a generalized infection will be produced in 5 to 10 days, at which time the organisms usually can be demonstrated easily in the extensive peritoneal exudate. It should be added that this source of organisms is excellent for the preparation of antigens for serologic tests. The animals that die can be examined for *Toxoplasma* organisms by preparing films or sections of the peritoneal fluid, lungs, brain, and other tissues. A presumptive diagnosis can be made by a positive delayed skin reaction or by serologic means. Many serologic tests are available to assist in the diagnosis, including the Sabin-Feldman dye test, which is still used. This test depends on the fact that, in the presence of specific antibodies, the cytoplasm of the living organisms loses its affinity for methylene blue. Newer tests, such as the IHA, IFA, and ELISA, have been reported. Of all tests available, the ELISA appears to be the best.

Treatment. Triple sulfonamides (i.e., equal parts of sulfadiazine, sulfamerazine, and sulfamethazine) and pyrimethamine, which act synergistically, are the treatment of choice for toxoplasmosis. A corticosteroid is suggested for treating eye involvement.

Pneumocystis carinii

Pneumocystis carinii, an organism cosmopolitan in distribution, is generally accepted as a protozoan, but its precise taxonomic position has not been determined. The organism is present in a wide variety of animals and, in humans, causes a diffuse pneumonia in the immunocompromised host. Since 1980 there has been a dramatic increase in the incidence of *Pneumocystis carinii* pneumonia (PCP). This increase coincides with the AIDS epidemic and is the cause of about 60% of the deaths in this population. Even in fatal cases, the organism and the disease usually remain localized to the lung. Recent studies, however, show pneumocystic organisms in a wide variety of autopsy tissues from AIDS-infected humans. Rarely does the disease occur in healthy people.

Life Cycle

The exact life cycle is unknown, but various structural forms have been recognized: (1) a thin-walled trophozoite, (2) a thick-walled cyst that measures 4 to 6 μm in diameter, (3) the intracystic body, a crescent-shaped body within the cyst. As many as eight intracystic bodies may be present in a cyst (Fig. 87–7). Neither the mode of replication nor the mode of transmission is known.

Pathology and Symptomatology

Because the organism is usually found only in lung tissue, it is assumed that the likely mode of transmission is by inhalation. Studies have indicated that the organism does not become intracellular but, rather, attaches to the pneumocyte cell surface during a phase of its replicative cycle. In the vast majority of individuals, the organisms may be dormant and sparsely dispersed, with no apparent damage of host tissue. In others, such as the immunocompromised host, the organisms occur in massive numbers. There is usually a panlobular involvement of the lungs, which are enlarged, of a firm

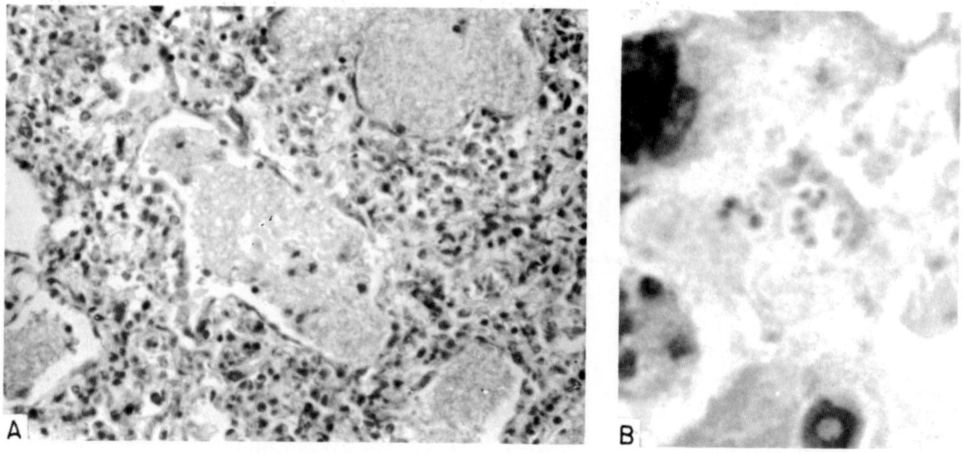

Fig. 87–7. *Pneumocystis carinii* in lungs. **A.** Note ground-glass appearance of exudate. × 250. **B.** Organism showing eight intracystic bodies. *(From Brown and Neva: Basic Clinical Parasitology, ed 5. Appleton-Century-Crofts, 1983.)*

rubbery consistency, and do not collapse when the chest is opened.

In most overt infections, the onset is abrupt. Fever, tachypnea, hypoxia, cyanosis, and asphyxia are common manifestations in acute cases. In debilitated infants, the alveolar septum is thickened with an interstitial plasma cell and lymphocyte infiltration. Illness may last 4 to 6 weeks, and a mortality of 25% to 50% is seen.

Epidemiology

P. carinii has been found in the lungs of rats, rabbits, mice, dogs, sheep, guinea pigs, horses, and a variety of lower animals. Because up to 70% of healthy individuals have humoral antibody to the organisms, subclinical infection must be widespread.

More than 150,000 cases of AIDS have been reported since June 1981. In addition, 500,000 cases of AIDS-related complex (ARC) and 5 to 10 million persons infected with the HIV-1 virus are thought to exist in the world; it is estimated that 2 to 3 million of these symptom-free carriers live in the United States and Europe. There appears to be some relationship between Kaposi's sarcoma in Africa and various opportunistic infections, including *P. carinii*. At present in the United States, nearly 60% of all individuals diagnosed with AIDS also have or have had PCP. In Africa, nearly 40% of patients with AIDS also have PCP.

Diagnosis

Tachypnea and fever are consistent features of *P. carinii* pneumonia. In premature and debilitated infants, onset is subtle, with mild tachypnea. After 1 week, respiratory distress becomes severe, with flaring of the nasal alae and cyanosis. In the immunodeficient child or adult, onset of symptoms is rapid and soon results in death if untreated.

Definitive diagnosis depends on the identification of *P. carinii* in samples taken by transbronchoscopic biopsy, open lung biopsy, or needle aspiration. The most widely used technique today is fiberoptic bronchoscopy, with bronchoalveolar lavage or transbronchial biopsy. Sputum, although not a reliable specimen, should be examined before invasive measures are taken. Cysts and extracystic bodies released from them can be found in smears or sections of lung tissue. Methenamine silver nitrate, toluidine blue, and Giemsa-type stains are used to detect and identify them. A diffuse bilateral alveolar disease is apparent by radiograph. Serum antibody titers are of little diagnostic value. CIE techniques to detect circulating antigen may become a useful diagnostic procedure in the near future. Immunofluorescence correlates well with the use of histologic stains, but attempts to detect soluble antigens of the organism have so far been unsuccessful.

Treatment

Available drugs include pentamidine isethionate, trimethoprim, and sulfamethoxazole, with the latter two drugs being the drugs of choice. Resistance to these two drugs, however, has begun to occur; in the case of such resistance, the drug pentamidine isethionate must be used. Recently, aerosolized pentamidine isethionate was approved for use in AIDS and other patients with PCP. Supportive measures include high oxygen therapy with volume respirator assistance and digitalization to support the myocardium damaged by hypoxia.

CHAPTER 88

Medical Helminthology

In addition to the Protozoa, there are numerous many-celled animals, often referred to as Metazoa, that parasitize humans. *Helminth* is a general term meaning worm and, in the present context, refers to those animals that belong to two groups within the animal kingdom, the Nematoda and the Platyhelminthes. The nematodes are represented by a single group and are commonly called roundworms. The Platyhelminthes are represented by two distinct groups of medical importance, namely, the Cestoda, or tapeworms, and the Trematoda, or flukes. Together, the tapeworms and flukes are commonly called flatworms. In medical literature, helminths are often grouped according to the host organ in which they reside, such as blood flukes, liver flukes, intestinal roundworms, and tissue roundworms. This chapter presents the helminths of humans in the following order: nematodes, cestodes, and trematodes.

Nematodes

The adult nematodes, or roundworms, are characterized by having an elongate, cylindric body that is round in cross section. They are covered with an acellular cuticle and have a complete digestive tract, with mouth and anus, as well as excretory, nervous, and reproductive systems. As in all parasitic worms, sex differences are the most conspicuous. The sexes are separate, and the males are almost invariably smaller than the females (Fig. 88–1). Nematodes vary considerably in size, from forms difficult to see readily by the unaided eye to others many centimeters in length. In order to increase in size, the immature worm (larva) passes through a series of molts, or ecdyses, which are accomplished by shedding the cuticle. The complete stages in the life cycle are as follows: egg, four stages of larvae separated by molts, and adult male or female (Fig. 88–2).

In this section, nematodes are grouped according to the usual location of the adult worms in humans. The main groups to be considered are (1) the intestinal nematodes and (2) the tissue nematodes. All the intestinal nematodes are endemic in the United States, whereas most of the tissue forms are exotic in origin. As an aid to the student, the intestinal nematodes are divided into two groups: (1) those infective for humans in the egg stage, and (2) those infective for humans in a larval stage. Under each grouping, they are presented in increasing order of the complexity of the life cycle.

Intestinal Nematodes Infective for Humans in the Egg Stage

Enterobius vermicularis

The pinworm, sometimes called the seatworm, is probably the most frequently encountered helminth parasite in the United States. Indeed, it is not unreasonable to think that nearly everyone, at one time or another, has had pinworms. Although most infections are thought to be asymptomatic, in some, pruritus ani and occasional bouts of abdominal discomfort in children are the primary manifestations of infection. Although it is rare, most physicians are not aware of the fact that enterobiasis can cause severe, ectopic disease in various parts of the body, especially the urogenital tract of both young girls and young women.

Pinworm is cosmopolitan in distribution and is considered by most to be more prevalent in temperate than in tropical areas. Surveys, however, show that 67% of kindergarten-aged children in Shanghai, 80% in Central Europe, and 70% in West Africa are infected. Thus this concept may change as more data are collected. In the United States, surveys show that 30% to 40% of all white kindergarten-aged children have pinworms; American blacks show about one third this amount. Most often, infection is found in groups of children, such as in families, schools, summer camps, day-care centers, and those who are institutionalized.

Life Cycle. Ingested eggs hatch in the small intestine, each releasing a single larva. These migrate to the large intestine, especially the cecum and colon, where they attach superficially to the mucosa. Many are found down at the base of intestinal crypts. The larvae reach adulthood within 2 to 4 weeks. Infection usually lasts 1 to 2 months, but reinfection is common. No specific immunity seems to develop, but resistance to infection does increase with increasing age of the host.

The gravid females migrate to the anus and emerge at night to extrude their eggs on the perianal and perineal skin. Each female may deposit up to 11,000 to 15,000 eggs before she dies. Eggs have a sticky, albuminous covering and adhere to skin, hair, clothing, and bedding. They become infective for humans in 4 to 6 hours. Occasionally, migrating females may enter the vagina, fallopian tubes, uterus, and even into the peritoneal cavity. Such migrations are rare but can cause serious disease. To a limited extent, eggs on the perineum may hatch prematurely, and the released larvae may reenter

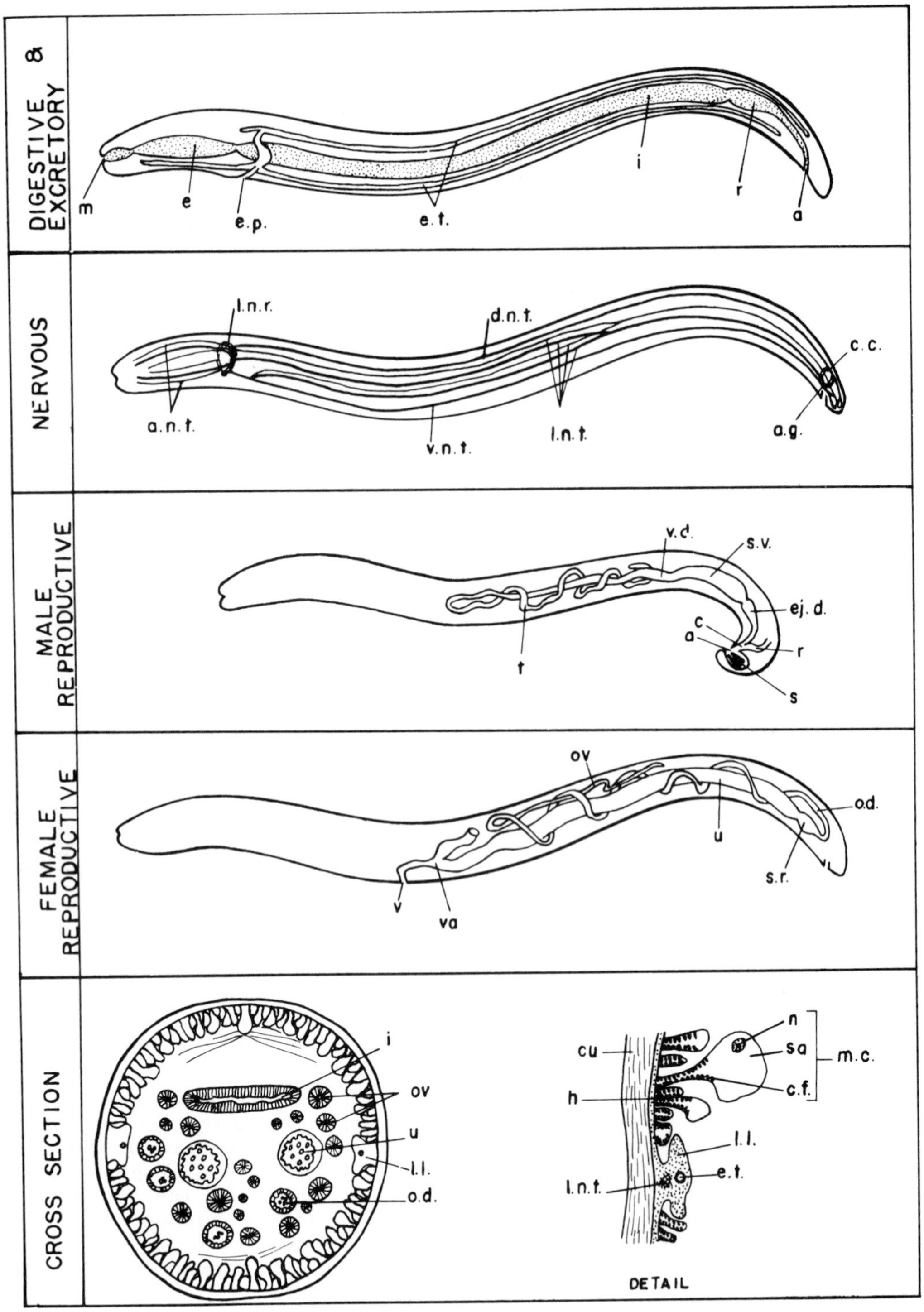

Fig. 88–1. Morphology of a nematode, based on *Ascaris.* a. anus; a.g., anal ganglion; a.n.t., anterior nerve trunks; c, cloaca; cu, cuticle; c.c., circumcloacal commissure (male); c.f., contractile fibers; d.n.t., dorsal nerve trunk; e, esophagus; e.p., excretory pore; e.t., excretory tubules, ej.d., ejaculatory duct; h, hypodermis; i, intestine; l.l., lateral line; l.n.r., circumesophageal ring; l.n.t., lateral nerve trunks; m, mouth; m.c., muscle cells; n, nucleus; ov, ovary; o.d., oviduct; r, rectum; s, spicules; sa., sarcoplasm; s.r., seminal receptacle; s.v., seminal vesicle; t, testis; u, uterus; v, vulva; va, vagina; v.d., vas deferens; v.n.t., ventral nerve trunk. *(From Brown and Neva: Basic Clinical Parasitology, ed 5. Appleton-Century-Crofts, 1983.)*

the intestinal tract (retrofection) through the anus. When this occurs, the cycle may be lengthened considerably.

Pathology and Symptomatology. In those that manifest symptoms, anal pruritus is severe, and the scratching that follows may lead to scarification, which is subject to invasion by bacteria and other infectious agents. Frequently, children manifest insomnia or fretful sleep, irritability, sometimes nausea, nail biting, and pallor. Abdominal discomfort, headache, pallor, and diarrhea have also been reported.

Lower pelvic discomfort in female patients, with or without cystitis and enuresis, has been seen and is due to the abnormal migrations of adult worms. Histologic examination has revealed pelvic peritoneal granulomas around adult worms

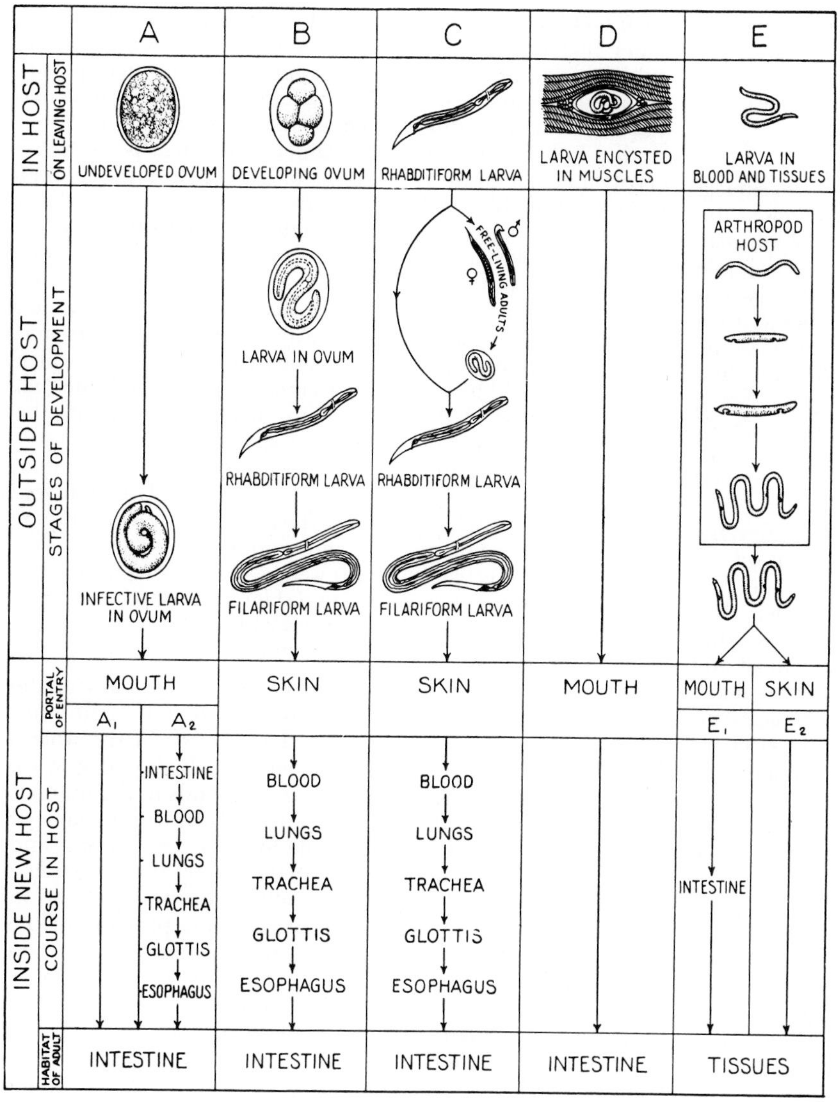

Fig. 88–2. Typical life cycles of important nematodes. **A_1.** *Enterobius vermicularis, Trichuris trichiura.* **A_2.** *Ascaris lumbricoides.* **B.** *Ancylostoma duodenale, Necator americanus.* **C.** *Strongyloides stercoralis.* **D.** *Trichinella spiralis.* **E_1.** *Dracunculus medinensis.* **E_2.** *Wuchereria bancrofti, W. malayi, Loa loa, Acanthocheilonema perstans, Onchocerca volvulus. (From Belding: Basic Clinical Parasitology. Appleton-Century-Crofts, 1958.)*

or ova. Larger nodules, white or yellow, are sometimes recovered at surgery or necropsy and may be confused initially with *Mycobacterium tuberculosis* or metastatic carcinoma.

Mild catarrhal inflammation with small lesions in the large intestine is usually seen. In rare cases, necrosis of the mucosa occurs, and sympathetic nerve endings may be exposed. This, and the absorption of worm metabolites across the intestinal border, may be responsible for the commonly observed nervous symptoms. The worm has been found in both normal and diseased appendixes but is not considered an important factor in appendicitis.

Despite the high prevalence of pinworm infection, the parasite is relatively nonpathogenic. It is estimated that a full third of those who are infected show no symptoms. In addition, symptoms do not occur in most adults who are infected, whereas infected children usually suffer from perianal itching and abdominal discomfort. It is probable that some urinary tract infections are caused by bacteria being passively carried by migrating worms and that some cases of sterility in females are due to pinworm-initiated lesions in the fallopian tubes.

Epidemiology. The intense pruritus produced by the crawling females, and especially by the eggs, results in scratching of the affected areas. In this way, eggs are transferred to the fingertips and may become lodged beneath the nails. Reinfection follows when the fingers or food contaminated by the fingers are placed in the mouth. In addition to direct transfer of eggs, the eggs may reach the mouth of the infected individual and others by one or more indirect routes. The eggs adhere to clothing and bed linen, and some get into air currents to be inhaled or to settle on objects. Thus the household becomes contaminated, and all members sooner or later swallow some of the eggs. Eggs remain viable several weeks under cool and moist conditions. At a temperature above 25C and in dry air, most eggs perish within 1 to 2 days. Good personal hygiene is recommended, but no matter how diligent and meticulous the family is, reinfection usually follows. In the long run, repeated treatment is the only practical solution.

Enterobius vermicularis is the only pinworm that infects humans; there are no animal reservoirs. This is important to remember because many laypeople and physicians alike believe that human infection can result from similar infections in their pet cats and dogs. This does not happen, and veterinarians become justifiably disturbed when this misinformation is promulgated.

Diagnosis. Based on the symptoms discussed above, clinical diagnosis is relatively easy. In the laboratory diagnosis, the characteristic eggs usually are not found in the stool but may be recovered easily from the perianal area by use of a simple cellophane tape or other swab. The tape, sticky side down, is pressed onto the perianal region and then adhered to a microscope slide, where it is examined. It is best to make the cellophane-tape preparation in the morning before the child has bathed or gone to the toilet. Eggs are asymmetrical, being flattened on one side, and range in size from 50 to 60 μm by 20 to 30 μm (Fig. 88–3). A larva is usually contained in each egg and many times can be seen to move when examined microscopically.

At times, and especially at night a few hours after the child has retired, migrating adult worms can be seen on the perianal and perineal tissues. Thus, parents may observe worms by using a flashlight while the child is asleep. Not infrequently, and especially with children still in diapers, adult worms are recovered on a stool. Adult worms are small and whitish, with females being 8 to 13 mm long, whereas males are smaller, being 2 to 5 mm long. Both have a characteristic cephalic swelling (Fig. 88–4). No serologic tests are available for diagnosis, and there are no abnormal hematologic or clinical values.

Treatment. Several drugs are effective in treating enterobiasis; mebendazole and pyrantel pamoate are the most widely used. Because the life span of the infection is approximately 2 months, the major concern should be to prevent reinfection. Unfortunately, meticulous hygienic efforts usually are ineffectual, and repeated treatment is the only recourse. When infection is noted in a family, many physicians treat the entire household. In large families and institutions in which pinworms are perennially present, it is now feasible to deworm the entire population several times a year.

Trichuris trichiura

The nematode *Trichuris trichiura* is commonly known as the whipworm because of its resemblance to a buggy whip. The anterior end is long and narrow, whereas the posterior end is more robust and shorter. Females may reach a length of 50 mm; males are slightly shorter, seldom reaching 40 mm, and can be recognized by the curled tail (Fig. 88–5).

Infection with whipworm occurs extensively throughout the world but is most common in the tropics and subtropics when poor sanitation exists. The World Health Organization has estimated that between 500 and 800 million people are infected, with an 80% incidence in some tropical areas. In the United States, infection is not common but does occur in the warm, moist areas of the South. Areas of high endemicity include the area south of the Piedmont Plateau, the foothills of the southern Appalachian range, and southwest Louisiana. Multiple infections with *Ascaris* and hookworms are not uncommon. In temperate zones, infections are frequently found in mentally retarded persons who are institutionalized, especially those who eat dirt.

Life Cycle. Infection is acquired by the ingestion of food or water that is contaminated with embryonated eggs. The incubation period is 1 to 3 months, and infection may persist as long as 6 years, although 1 year is the norm. When infective eggs are ingested, they hatch in the small intestine. Some studies indicate that the freed larvae enter nearby intestinal crypts and penetrate into glands and stroma. They reenter the lumen of the small intestine from these sites after about 10 days and migrate to the large intestine. Here the anterior ends of the developing adults are sewn into the mucosa of the large intestine, typically of the cecum and appendix. The robust posterior end of each worm hangs freely in the lumen of the intestine. At sexual maturity, copulation occurs and daily egg production of 2000 to 6000 eggs per female worm begins. It should be mentioned that other studies indicate that the freed larvae migrate directly to, or hatch directly in, the cecum without a tissue phase in the small intestine.

Eggs released by the female worms occur in the stool while in the undeveloped (noninfective) stage. Under favorable environmental conditions, which include warm temperature, shade, moisture, and sandy humus soil, eggs develop and become infective in 3 to 6 weeks. *Trichuris* eggs lack the great resistance of *Ascaris* eggs, and their survival is considered to be relatively brief, that is, a matter of weeks.

Pathology and Symptomatology. The worms damage the tissues that they penetrate and may carry bacteria and other infectious agents into these sites. If the heads of the worms penetrate into blood capillaries, petechial hemorrhages are produced. The degree of damage corresponds to the number of worms involved. In light infections, relatively little damage results, but in heavy infections, the mucosa is hyperemic and eroded superficially and may be inflamed extensively. Extreme irritation in the wall of the lower portion of the colon and in the rectum may provoke partial or complete prolapse of the rectum. Depending on the degree of infection and reaction of the individual, the signs and symptoms vary from mild (discomfort in the right lower quadrant, flatulence, loss of appetite and weight) to severe (nausea, vomiting, mucous diarrhea or dysentery, anemia).

Epidemiology. Infections occur most often in areas where humidity is high, temperatures are warm, and soils have good moisture-holding ability. Dooryard pollution and poor sanitation lead to heavy infection. Infections usually coexist with *Ascaris* and, many times, *Entamoeba* and hookworm. Distribution may be more spotty than that of *Ascaris*, however, and this is thought to be due to the lesser resistance of the eggs of *Trichuris*. In general, the severity of infection is correlated with age, nutritional status, and worm burden. Malnourished children are the most severely infected. No animal reservoirs exist.

Diagnosis. Diagnosis based on symptoms is difficult, but parasitologic diagnosis is easily made by finding the characteristic eggs in the feces (Fig. 88–3). These are about 20 to 50 μm in size and are barrel-shaped, having a golden brown color and transparent prominences called *polar plugs* at each end. Eggs may be few in number and difficult to find in fecal smears, in which case it is of assistance to use a concentration method.

Adult worms are rarely seen in the stool because of the firmness with which they are fastened to the intestinal wall.

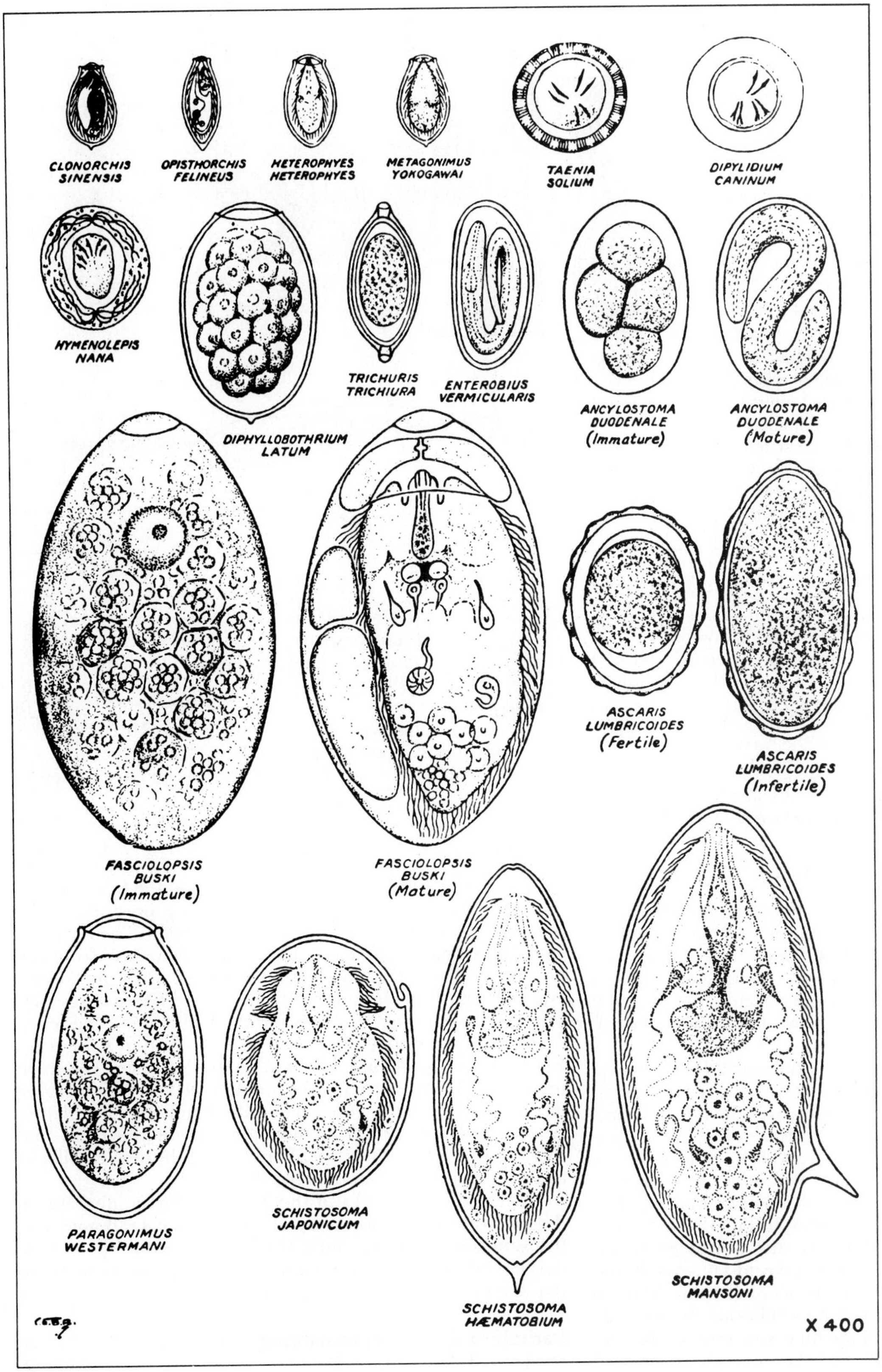

Fig. 88–3. Eggs of the common helminths of humans. The size of this illustration has been increased by one fifth. *(From Belding: Textbook of Clinical Parasitology, ed 2. Appleton-Century-Crofts, 1952.)*

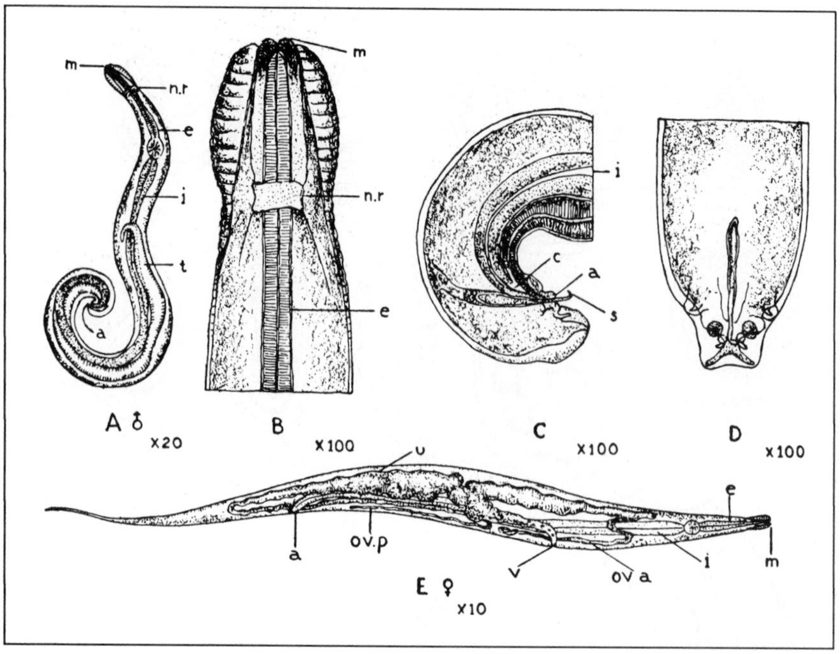

Fig. 88–4. *Enterobius vermicularis.* **A.** Male. **B.** Anterior end of worm. **C.** Posterior end of male, lateral view. **D.** Posterior end of male, ventral view. **E.** Female. a, anus; c cloaca; e, esophagus; i, intestine; m, mouth; n.r., nerve ring; ov. a, anterior ovary; ov.p, posterior ovary; s, spicule; t, testis; u, uterus; v, vulva. *(From Belding: Basic Clinical Parasitology. Appleton-Century-Crofts, 1958.)*

They can be seen, however, in heavy infections when the rectum has prolapsed or as a result of sigmoidoscopy.

Anemia of the microcytic, hypochromic type, reduced hemoglobin concentrations (as low as 3 g), and an eosinophilia of 5% to 20% are sometimes associated with infection. No serologic tests are available.

Treatment. Mebendazole is considered the drug of choice but is not effective in all cases, especially in heavy infections. It is suggested that light, asymptomatic cases not be treated.

Ascaris lumbricoides

Next to pinworm, infection with *Ascaris* (commonly called the large intestinal roundworm) probably is the most common nematode in humans. WHO has estimated that between 800 million and 1 billion people are infected, with most being in the tropics and subtropics. In the United States, infections are most common in the Gulf Coast states and in Appalachia. Coinfection with *Trichuris* is common.

Historically, the domestication of the pig and the bringing of the animal into the home probably account for the development of the strain of *Ascaris* for humans. The role of *Ascaris suum,* the swine ascarid, in human disease has been controversial for many years. Experimental and laboratory accidents have shown that the swine ascarid will infect humans, but naturally occurring infections have been difficult to prove. However, a few cases of children being infected with *A. suum* have been documented. In each case the worms recovered after anthelmintic treatment were shown to be sexually immature; furthermore, worm burdens were light, limited to no more than three worms. There is no doubt that the ingested swine ascarid eggs will hatch in the human intestinal tract and cause a form of visceral larva migrans, with the lungs and liver being most affected. As a result, pediatricians and those family practitioners who practice in rural areas should be aware of the part that pigs may play in human ascariasis.

Life Cycle. Infection begins when the embryonated eggs are ingested with food or drink; water, however, is not thought to be an important source of infection. The parasite then begins its life cycle by the migration of the larvae throughout various tissues of the body. The larvae eventually return to the small intestine, where they mature; 8 to 10 weeks after ingestion of the eggs are required for the larvae to reach maturity. Adults live for about 1 year and then are passed in the feces.

These large nematodes (males 15 to 31 cm and females 20 to 35 cm or more in length) usually live unattached in the lumen of the small intestine (Fig. 88–6). After the worms reach sexual maturity, copulation occurs, and the females soon thereafter begin to lay eggs. The daily egg production per female is phenomenal, averaging about 200,000. The fertilized eggs are still in the one-cell stage when they pass from the host in the feces (Fig. 88–3). Infertile eggs, differing considerably in morphologic detail from the fertilized eggs, are sometimes seen (Fig. 88–3). If the stool containing the fertilized eggs is deposited in a warm, shady, moist area, the eggs will develop. Accidental ingestion of infective eggs results in infection. The eggs hatch in the duodenum, and the emerging larvae penetrate the intestinal wall, enter the circulatory system, and are carried to the right side of the heart and thence to the lungs. They are filtered out of the lung capillaries and later penetrate into the alveoli.

After about 2 weeks in the lungs the larvae migrate up the respiratory tract to the epiglottis and are swallowed into the stomach. Upon reaching the small intestine the worms develop into adult males and females. It should be emphasized that the lung migration is a necessary part of the cycle.

Pathology and Symptomatology. The pathogenesis of ascariasis is related to the life cycle of the parasite. Although some liver damage may occur as a result of the larvae migration, especially in those who either are allergic or have ingested a large number of eggs, the principal damage pro-

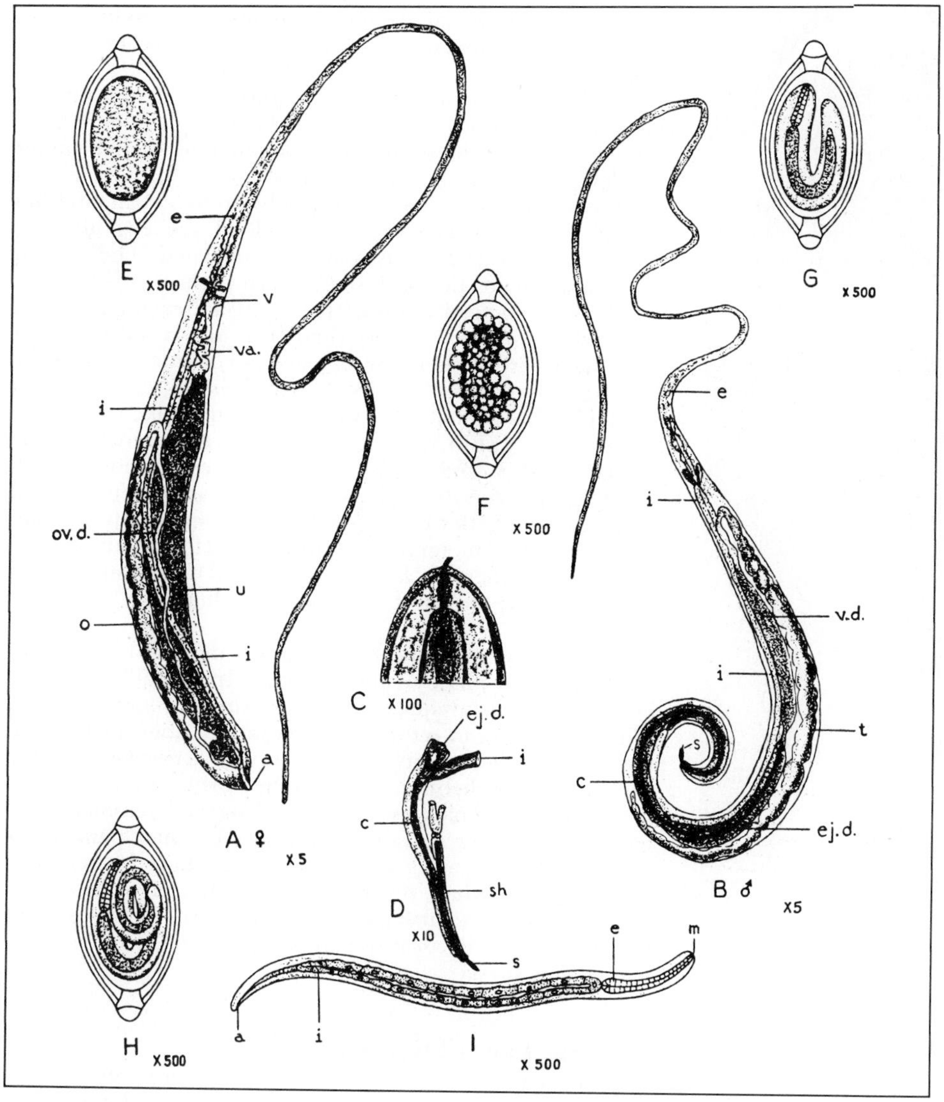

Fig. 88–5. *Trichuris trichiura.* **A.** Female. **B.** Male. **C.** Anterior end showing spear. **D.** Cloaca and copulatory organs of male. **E.** Unicellular stage of egg. **F.** Multicellular stage of egg. **G.** Early larva in egg shell. **H.** Mature larva in egg shell. **I.** Newly hatched larva (**A, B, D–I** adapted from Leuckart, 1876. **C** drawn from photograph by Li, 1933.) a, anus; c, cloaca; e, esophagus; ej.d., ejaculatory duct; i, intestine; m, mouth; o, ovary; ov.d., oviduct; s. spicule; sh, sheath of spicule; t, testis; u, uterus; v, vulva; va., vagina; v.d., vas deferens. *(From Brown and Neva: Basic Clinical Parasitology, ed 5. Appleton-Century-Crofts, 1983.)*

duced by the larvae occurs in the lungs. Petechial hemorrhages are produced after the larvae enter the alveoli. A striking serocellular exudate, in which eosinophils are prominent, will then collect (Löffler's syndrome). Eosinophils are commonly associated with parasitic worms or larvae in tissues, and eosinophilia is characteristic. The cardinal signs and symptoms of *Ascaris* pneumonitis consist of dyspnea, dry cough, fever, and eosinophilia. X-ray findings show scattered mottling of the lungs, suggestive of tuberculosis and other infections.

The adult worms derive most of their nourishment from the semidigested food of the host, and, if the worms are abundant, they may have a detrimental effect on the host's nutrition, especially in infants and young children. Most light infections, however, produce little or no change in the host. Effects from the adult worms are usually noted only in children, who often show loss of appetite and weight, as well as intermittent intestinal colic. Indeed, colicky epigastric or periumbilical pain is the cardinal symptom of ascariasis. The greatest danger from the adult worm results from abnormal migration within the body. They may enter the ampulla of Vater and block the common bile duct or penetrate into the liver parenchyma or the pancreas. They also have been found on rare occasions in other abnormal sites in the body. Sometimes they perforate the intestinal wall, but far more frequently, especially in young children, a mass of tangled worms causes an acute obstruction of the small intestine. Finally there is evidence that absorption of the toxic and allergenic metabolites of the adult worms accounts for various referred symptoms, especially those of a neurologic nature.

Epidemiology. Incidence rates as high as 90% have been reported. The annual global mortality from ascaris infections is estimated to be 20,000, and the annual morbidity, which results primarily from pulmonary and gastrointestinal involvement, is estimated to be 1 million. Disease is endemic in tropical and subtropical countries, but infection and sporadic disease occur worldwide. People living in rural areas where sanitation conditions are poor are most at risk. Adults usually acquire the infection by eating raw vegetables that have been contaminated by feces and human night soil. Children acquire

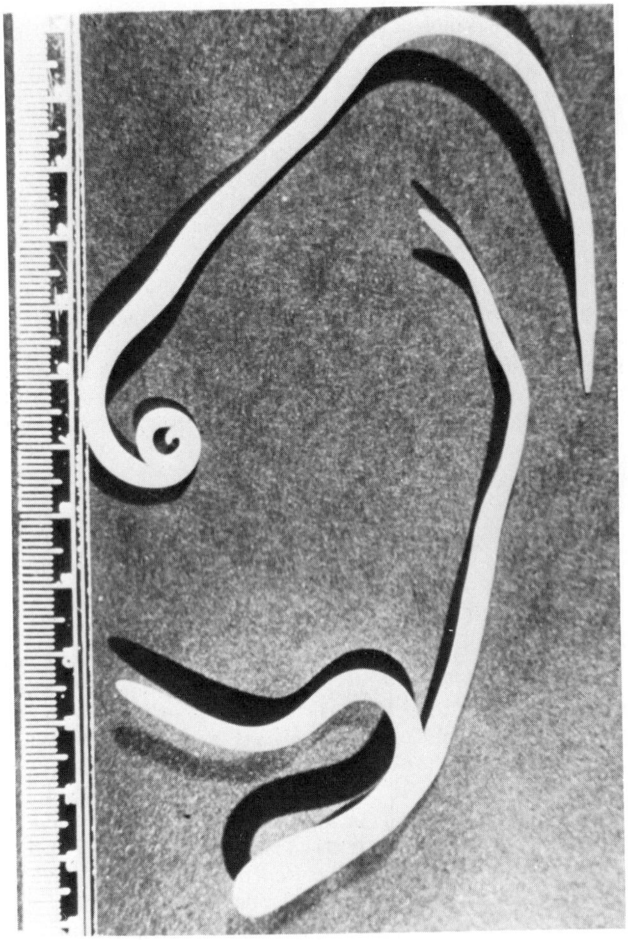

Fig. 88–6. Adult *Ascaris lumbricoides.*

the infection in this manner but also are infected via hand-to-mouth contamination, by pica, or by placing contaminated toys in their mouths.

Eggs are highly resistant to adverse environmental conditions. They develop best in warm, moist soil and, under such conditions, become fully embryonated 2 to 3 weeks after having been passed in human feces. Eggs are also resistant to disinfection, can survive sewage treatment, and remain viable for months or years in night soil. Pollution of wells through improper drainage of surface waters may also result in transmission. Prevention depends on the proper disposal of feces.

Diagnosis. The clinical diagnosis of ascariasis is difficult because pneumonitis, eosinophilia, and intestinal symptoms are similar to those of other intestinal helminthic infections. Diagnosis before eggs appear in the feces and infections with male worms alone is rare. Sometimes, radiologic examination reveals adult worms in the intestine, and, at times, parents will bring to a physician's office the adult worm that was either passed in the feces or actively migrated out the anus. Ascarids are occasionally vomited and can be recovered from the emesis.

A moderate eosinophilia, increased temperature, dyspnea, Charcot-Leyden crystals in the sputum, hemoptysis, coughing, and rales are characteristic of ascaris pneumonitis. Pneumonia, Löffler's syndrome, and asthma must be considered in the differential diagnosis. Patients are often hypersensitive to the worms and display urticaria and other allergic reactions, such as increased serum IgE levels.

Definitive diagnosis usually requires the demonstration of the characteristic egg in the feces. Eggs are present in large numbers and can be found in smears by examination under the low power of the microscope (Fig. 88–3). The egg is bluntly ovoid in shape, 45 to 70 μm by 35 to 50 μm, and has several layers between the single cell of the egg and the outside. The outer layer is coarsely mamillated. The various layers account for the thick shell, which is characteristic.

For serologic diagnosis, the indirect hemagglutination (IHA) test using body cavity fluid from the swine ascarid is sometimes used. Others use this test in conjunction with the bentonite flocculation test (BFT), which is less sensitive than the IHA test but more specific. An enzyme-linked immunosorbent assay (ELISA) using an antigen recovered from the embryonated *Ascaris* egg is reported to be superior in both sensitivity and specificity. Lack of specificity is due to marked cross-reactions with toxocariasis. Finally, complement fixation (CF), agglutination, immunofluorescence (IF), immunodiffusion (ID), and other tests have been used, but none is sufficiently sensitive and specific to be of practical value.

Treatment. Only supportive therapy is indicated during the lung migration phase of the infection. Intestinal obstruction by the adults may require intubation, surgery, and drainage. When adults are in ectopic sites because of abnormal migrations (e.g., peritoneal cavity, liver), surgery is necessary. Saline enemas may be helpful in removing worms from the large bowel during chemotherapy. Many drugs are reasonably effective in treating intestinal ascariasis. Pyrantel pamoate is commonly used, as is mebendazole. It must be stressed, however, that when *Ascaris* coexists with other infectious agents, such as *Trichuris*, it is important to remove the ascarids first. Otherwise, the ascarids may become irritated and migrate into ectopic sites.

Visceral Larva Migrans

Visceral larva migrans (VLM) is a clinical term referring to human infection with the nematode larvae of *Toxocara,* an ascarid of dogs, other canids, and cats. Thus VLM is a zoonotic disease, and humans are an accidental host. VLM is primarily a disease of preschool children, and it is estimated that 10% to 30% of children between the ages of 1 and 6 who have the habit of eating dirt are at risk of being infected. Although the larva of *Toxocara canis* is most often the etiologic agent of VLM, other nematodes of lower animals, such as *Baylisascaris procyonis* (a roundworm of racoons) and *Toxocara cati* (the cat roundworm), are known to be occasionally involved. Some infections that involve the eye are increasing and are referred to as *ocular larva migrans* (OLV). Seldom does infection result in concurrent VLM and OLV.

Life Cycle. Humans become infected when they ingest the developed eggs of the nematode. Subsequent to ingestion, the eggs hatch in the small intestine, and the freed larvae penetrate into the gut wall and enter the circulatory system. Although there are a few reports of larvae returning to the small intestine (typical ascarid life cycle) and becoming adults, it is thought that because humans are accidental hosts, the larvae wander around in the human body and come to rest in any of a variety of organs or body cavities. Reports indicate that the liver, lungs, and eyes are most often the sites of habitation. The exact incubation period is not known but is thought to be at least 1 week in duration. Larvae may remain alive for 2 to 3 years.

Pathology and Symptomatology. The pathogenesis of VLM is related to (1) the number of eggs ingested, (2) the number of larvae that enter the tissue, (3) the amount of larval migration within the host, (4) the location of the larvae in the host, and (5) the host's immune response to the larvae. The larvae for a period of at least several weeks actively migrate through tissues leaving trails of destroyed tissue, resulting in inflammatory and granulomatous lesions. Fortunately, most infected children are symptom-free or only mildly ill. Fatalities do occur, however, and pediatricians should be aware of this possibility. When death does occur, it is due to extensive cardiac or central nervous system involvement.

Symptoms are related to the migration of larvae within tissues and manifest as hepatomegaly, eosinophilia, and hypergammaglobulinemia. Fever, cough, and wheezing are characteristic of pneumonic involvement. Pruritic eruptions and tender nodules on the trunk and lower extremities are sometimes seen. Ocular lesions resembling retinoblastoma are fairly common and may lead to loss of vision and the eye itself. Eye lesions, although usually unilateral and painless, may lead to total retinal detachment.

Epidemiology. *T. canis* is an extremely common parasite of dogs, with more than 80% of all puppies being infected. Surveys show that 30% to 50% of households in the United States include at least one dog, so that the chance for egg transmission is great. Epidemiologic studies also show that the presence of puppies younger than 3 months of age and children in the same house are almost tantamount to infection. Exposure to dogs and cats outside the house (school yards, playgrounds) is not as risky. However, the increased number of infected dogs that are allowed to run free certainly contributes to the increasing incidence of VLM. Control depends on the frequent deworming of puppies and dogs, as well as the proper disposal of dog feces. Unfortunately, once soil has become contaminated with dog feces, it is almost impossible to kill the infective eggs. Thus, geophagia (dirt eating) should be prevented if at all possible.

Diagnosis. Any child with symptoms of hepatomegaly, hypereosinophilia, hypergammaglobulinemia, and a history of geophagia should be suspected of having VLM. These symptoms may last for months or years. In addition, fever and respiratory distress are common, but inconsistent, features.

Laboratory data are sometimes helpful in making a diagnosis because patients with VLM usually manifest an eosinophilia of greater than 10%, increased IgM levels, leukocytosis, and high isoagglutination titers. Aspartate aminotransferase (AST) levels are elevated in 20% of patients. Chest films reveal transient pulmonary infiltrates in many. Differential diagnosis should include a consideration of pulmonary ascariasis, asthma, retinoblastoma, trichinosis, eosinophilic leukemia, tropical eosinophilia, and collagen disease.

Stool examination is of no use in diagnosing VLM because the adult worms do not occur in humans. A definitive diagnosis is made only by the finding of larvae in tissue biopsy specimens. The liver is the preferred source of tissue for biopsy, but because of the small number of worms, the chance of finding larvae is not great. When found, they usually exhibit an eosinophilic granuloma formation (Fig. 88–7).

Serologic testing for VLM disease is increasing. Although far from being completely satisfactory at this time, the IHA, BFT, indirect fluorescent antibody (IFA), and ELISA tests are used. Recent improvements in antigens and the ELISA hold promise for a much better test in the near future. One study showed that the ELISA had a sensitivity of 90% and a specificity of 91% in detecting ocular toxocariasis.

Treatment. Visceral larva migrans is usually a self-limiting disease, and treatment is given only in severe cases. Glucocorticoids and bronchodilators are sometimes used when pulmonary disease is severe. Glucocorticoids are also used to improve vision when endophthalmia occurs. Diethylcarbamazine and thiabendazole have been used by some practitioners. Chemotherapy, however, does not seem to be satisfactory in some cases.

Intestinal Nematodes Infective for Humans in the Larva Stage

Hookworms

Four species are involved in human infections: two of these, *Necator americanus* and *Ancylostoma duodenale,* are true human parasites, and two, *Ancylostoma braziliense* and *Ancylostoma caninum,* are parasites of cats and dogs. The latter two, especially *A. braziliense,* produce a dermatitis (cutaneous larva migrans or creeping eruption) in humans after penetration of the skin by the filariform larvae (see below).

All hookworms have common morphologic characteristics, the most striking being the umbrellalike copulatory bursa of males, the anterior hook or curvature of the body (Fig. 88–8), and thin-shelled eggs. Adults are approximately 1 cm long and reside in the small intestine.

Hookworm disease, once an important and common human condition in the southern United States, although still endemic, is not commonly seen in clinics. *N. americanus* is the only species of importance in human infection throughout the hookworm belt of the southern United States. It is necessary, however, to be alert for *A. duodenale,* which is exotic in origin and occurs in immigrants and others who were infected in endemic areas. The life cycles of these various hookworms are similar.

Life Cycle. The adult worms are usually attached to the upper levels of the small intestine. The head is anchored securely to the intestine, the tip of a villus being drawn into the mouth of the worm, and blood is sucked from the capillaries. After copulation, females lay eggs, which are passed with the feces in an undeveloped state. Under favorable environmental conditions, the eggs develop in 1 to 2 days, and a free-living larval stage (*rhabditiform*) is released. The larvae feed on bacteria and detritus in the feces and soil and eventually metamorphose into the infective (*filariform*) larvae. Filariform larvae do not feed and have a life span of up to 2 weeks. The usual means of human infection is penetration by these larve into the tender skin between the toes of barefooted individuals, but they can penetrate any skin surface. After many hours, the larvae enter the cutaneous blood vessels and are carried through the right side of the heart to the lungs. After a few days, they penetrate from the pulmonary capil-

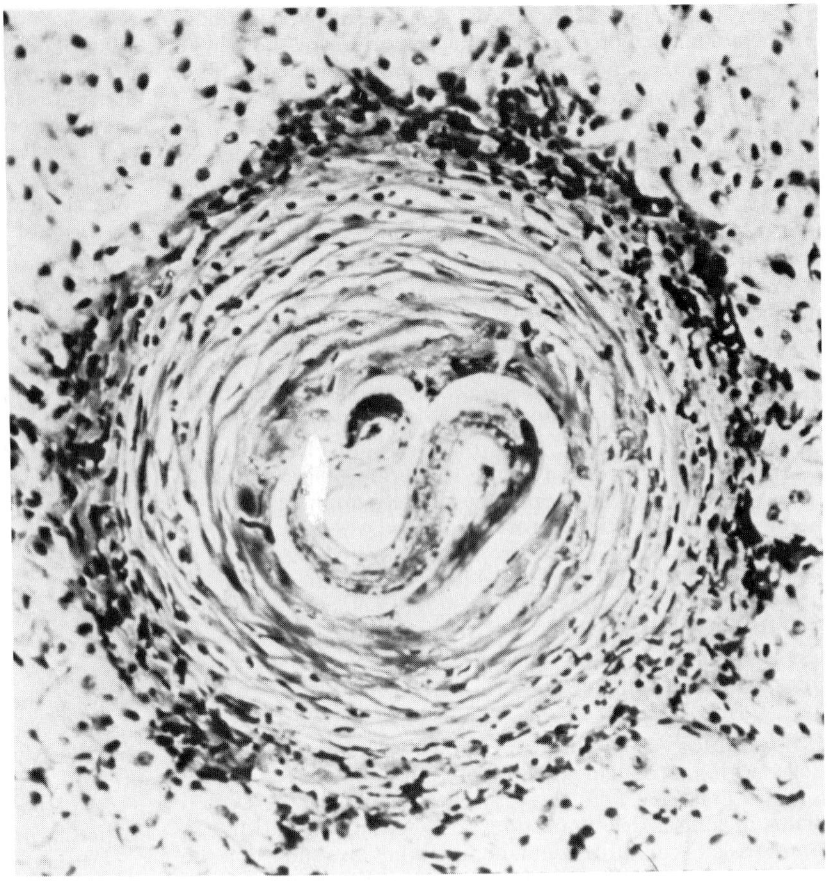

Fig. 88–7. Granuloma formation around larva of *Toxocara.*

laries into the alveoli, ascend the respiratory tract to the epiglottis, and, once they have been swallowed, descend to the upper portion of the small intestine. After attaching to the villi, the young worms grow into sexually mature adults. Recent research suggests that a transmammary infection route is also possible for *A. duodenale.* Although some of the worms in humans may live for 10 to 15 years, most of them will have been lost from the host after 1 year (*A. duodenale*) or from 4 to 5 years (*N. americanus*). The incubation period is about 6 weeks.

Pathology and Symptomatology. At the site of entry of the filariform larvae into the skin, most individuals experience intense itching and burning, followed by edema and erythema. A papule may appear, which transforms into a vesicle. This condition, known as *ground itch,* is more serious in those sensitized by previous infections and in those developing secondary infections. The larvae reaching the lungs produce small focal hemorrhages as they penetrate from the capillaries into the alveoli, but usually only a subclinical pneumonitis is produced. The greatest damage results from the adult worms that are attached to the small intestine. The superficial mucosa of that part of the intestine that is contained within the buccal cavity of the worm becomes denuded, and the surrounding mucosa usually shows a mild inflammatory infiltrate. More important is the blood loss of the host. Blood is sucked from the capillaries of the villi and passes through the digestive tract of the worm. Apparently only certain products are removed, the remainder being extruded through the anus in a wasteful fashion. This blood loss, which may average 0.03 mL/d per worm for *N. americanus* and 0.26 mL/d for *A. duodenale,* is increased by changes in the site of attachment. The former wound continues to ooze blood for a time after the worm has released the tissue. Blood loss from the intestinal wall constitutes the greatest damage from hookworm infection. This loss, unless there is adequate compensation, will give rise to a microcytic, hypochromic anemia. Whether an individual with hookworm infection develops hookworm disease depends, in general, on the number of worms harbored and the host's nutritional status. Even moderately heavy infections may fail to produce a significant anemia if the individual has been receiving an adequate, well-balanced diet rich in animal proteins, iron and other minerals, and vitamins. In heavy infections, however, even with a highly fortified diet, the hematopoietic mechanism is unable to keep pace with the great loss of red blood cells (RBCs). Moderate blood decompensation causes anemia, heart palpitations, and lassitude.

In some areas where hookworm is endemic, the natives are infected repeatedly from early childhood. Thus, chronic hookworm disease is most characteristic. Common signs and symptoms are anemia, epigastric burning, flatulence, sallow skin, tender abdomen, irritability, alternating diarrhea and constipation, dry skin, and blurred vision. When the condition finally produces marked physical weakness, the individual is unfit for any type of manual labor. This accounts for the early term *lazy disease.* Cardiomegaly and cardiac symptoms are

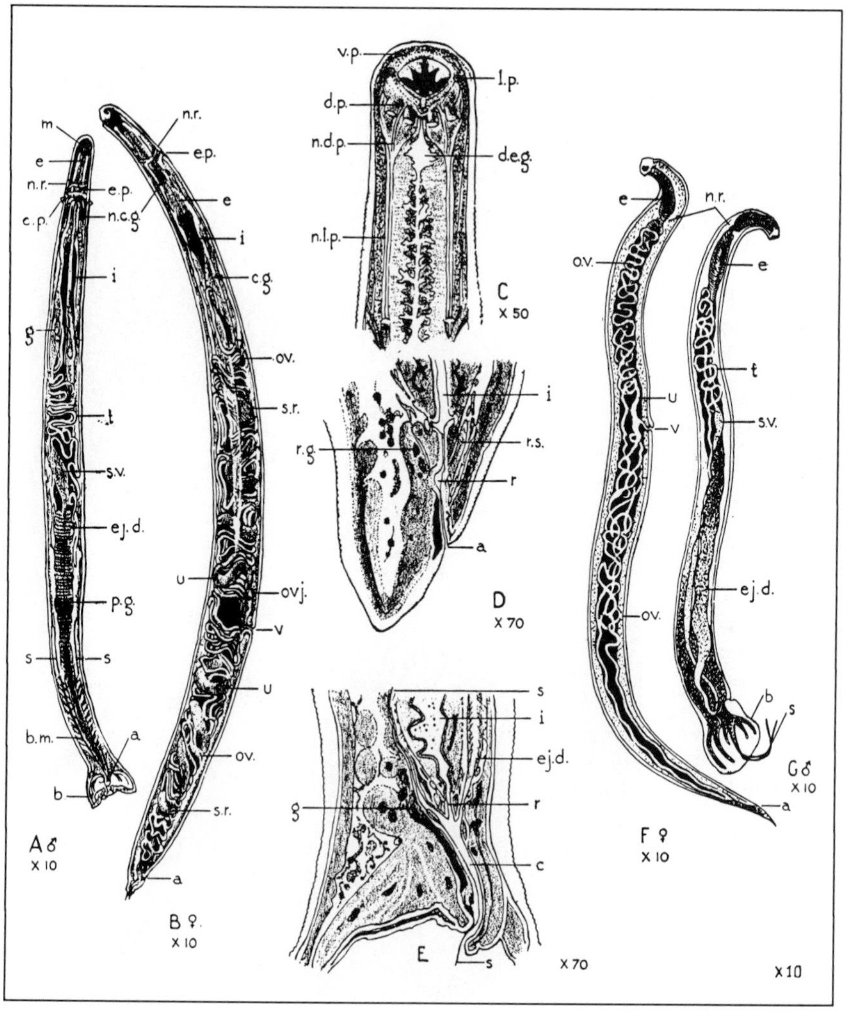

Fig. 88–8. Important hookworms of humans. **A.** Adult male *Ancylostoma duodenale* from ventral side. **B.** Young adult female *A. duodenale* from right side. **C.** Anterior end of *A. duodenale* from dorsal side. **D.** Longitudinal section through end of female *A. duodenale*, somewhat diagrammatic. **E.** Longitudinal section through end of male *A. duodenale*, not quite median. **F.** Female *Necator americanus*. **G.** Male *N. americanus*. a, anus; b, bursa; b.m., bursal muscles; c, cloaca; c.g., cervical gland; c.p., cervical papilla; d.e.g., dorsal esophageal gland; d.p., dorsal papilla; e, esophagus; e.p., excretory pore; ej.d., ejaculatory duct; g, gubernaculum; i, intestine; l.p., lateral papilla; m, mouth; n.c.g., nucleus of cephalic gland; n.d.p., nerve of dorsal papilla; n.l.p., nerve of lateral papilla; n.r., nerve ring; ov., ovary; ovj., ovijector; p.g., prostatic glands; r, rectum; r.g., rectal ganglion; r.s., rectal sphincter; s, spicules; s.r., seminal receptacle; s.v., seminal vesicle; t, testis; u, uterus; v, vulva; v.p., ventral papilla. *(From Belding: Basic Clinical Parasitology. Appleton-Century-Crofts, 1968.)*

evident in many instances; in severe cases, death may result from cardiac failure. Physical (including sexual) stunting is characteristic in children, and many are also retarded mentally.

Epidemiology. Both species occur predominantly in the tropics and subtropics between 36 degrees north and 30 degrees south latitudes. WHO estimates that between 700 and 900 million people are infected worldwide. All races and ages are susceptible. Occupation plays an important role because those who come in contact with soil are more likely to be exposed. The wearing of shoes and the proper disposal of feces will markedly reduce the incidence of infection. As evidence of this, surveys show that in rural areas of certain parts of Asia and Africa, prevalence rates of 60% to 80% are not unusual, whereas in the rural areas of the southern United States, it is rare to find areas where rates exceed 10%.

Temperatures between 25C and 35C and a shady, sandy, or loamy soil are optimum conditions for egg development. It is doubtful that important reservoirs for human infection exist, but it is known that pigs are occasionally infected with *A. duodenale* and some nonhuman primates with *N. americanus.*

Diagnosis. Clinically, the signs and symptoms of disease usually include weakness, pallor, and fatigue. The infection is generally chronic, and the manifestations of infection are related to worm burden and nutritional status as described above.

Ground itch, a sign of acute infection, is characterized by itching, erythema, vesiculation, and secondary infections. Coughing, sore throat, and bloody sputum are pulmonary manifestations and occur within a few days to a week after exposure. Intestinal symptoms arise 2 weeks after infection, and anemia of the microcytic, hypochromic type does not appear for 10 to 20 weeks. Differential diagnosis should include the following:

1. For ground itch—allergic dermatitis and fungal infections
2. For pulmonary phase—asthma and atypical pneumonia
3. For the intestinal phase—enteritis and other types of iron deficiency anemias

Laboratory diagnosis depends on the demonstration of thin-shelled eggs (40 by 60 μm) in a stool specimen (Fig. 88–3). At times, when the stool examination has been delayed, the eggs may have developed and hatched, releasing the rhabditiform larvae. These must be differentiated from *Strongyloides stercoralis*, another intestinal nematode of humans.

Stools from heavily infected patients may be viscous and tarry. These, as well as those from less heavily infected patients, often are positive for occult blood. Decreased hemoglobin and serum iron levels are common. Eosinophilia of 5% to 15% may occur in the early phase of infection, although normal levels of eosinophils are usually present in the chronic stage. In hypersensitive individuals, eosinophilia of 70% has been reported. No practical and useful serologic tests are available.

Treatment. Hookworm infections may be difficult to eradicate because reinfection usually occurs. Available anthelmintics include mebendazole and pyrantel pamoate. Most clinicians agree that if the patient is anemic, the hemoglobin level should be restored by diet and iron supplement to at least 50% of normal value before treatment. If *A. lumbricoides* coexists with the hookworms, the ascarids should be removed first.

Cutaneous Larva Migrans

Cutaneous larva migrans (CLM), sometimes referred to as creeping eruption, is due primarily to the filariform larvae of dog and cat hookworms (*A. caninum* and, especially, *A. braziliense*) penetrating the human skin and subcutaneous tissues. CLM can also be caused by hookworm larvae of other nonhuman hookworms such as *Uncinaria* and *Bunostomum*, parasites of domestic animals. These hookworms are unable to mature in humans, but the larvae are capable of living for long periods in subcutaneous tissues.

CLM is a condition seen worldwide, wherever there are cats and dogs and wherever warm, moist climatic factors prevail. In the United States the infection occurs from Texas to New Jersey, primarily in the southern states, with Florida and Georgia reporting the most cases.

Life Cycle. The life cycles of cat and dog hookworms are the same as that of the human hookworms. It must be emphasized that cat and dog hookworm larvae, although capable of penetrating the human skin, do not mature to the adult stage in humans.

Pathology and Symptomatology. An intensely pruritic eruption caused by the migrating larvae is the primary symptom. At each point of entry into the skin, an itching, reddish papule is produced, followed by a vesicle. After a few days, each larva has developed a serpiginous tunnel in the epidermis as it proceeds (usually at the rate of several millimeters a day). Edema and then a raised inflammatory tract with a crusty opening are characteristic. There is also a striking cellular infiltration, especially of eosinophils. Over a period of weeks or months, this results in extensive skin involvement (Fig. 88–9). At times, severe systemic illness may result. These movements, limited to the skin of humans, and the resulting irritation produce an intense pruritus. This leads to scratching and often opens the lesions to pyogenic organisms.

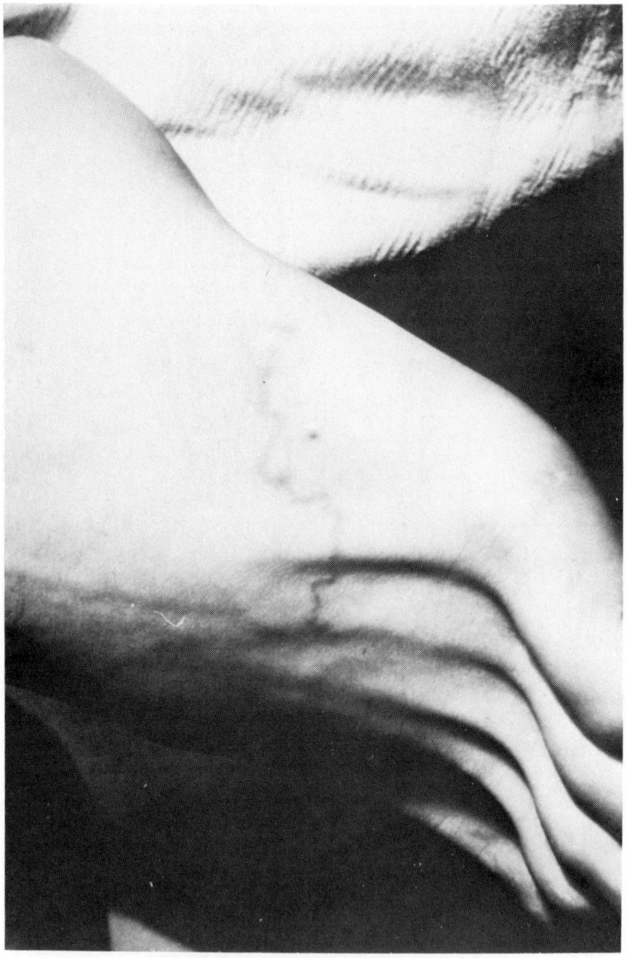

Fig. 88–9. Creeping eruption.

Epidemiology. CLM is an occupational disease of plumbers, construction workers, duck hunters, and others who are exposed to infected soil under buildings, crawlways, and around hunting blinds. Children are often infected at beaches, park play areas, and in home sandboxes. Plastic sheeting to protect workers from exposure to infected soil, covering for sandboxes, and the frequent deworming of cats and dogs would help to control CLM, as would limiting access of cats and dogs to public beaches and park areas.

Diagnosis. Clinicians usually make a presumptive diagnosis on the basis of patient history, signs, and symptoms. Although not routinely done, biopsy of a specimen from the leading edge of a serpiginous tract may show the larva. There are no laboratory values or findings that are helpful in diagnosis. A low-grade eosinophilia might be expected in those who are repeatedly infected. No serologic tests are indicated.

Treatment. Treatment is aimed at killing the larvae and reducing the pruritis. Oral or topical treatment of the lesions with thiabendazole is effective. Lesions may be treated by freezing the leading edge of the larva's tunnel with ethyl chloride.

Strongyloides stercoralis

Along with two protozoan infections of humans, toxoplasmosis and pneumocystosis, strongyloidiasis has recently received an added degree of notoriety because the strongyloid worm is capable of producing an overwhelming and often fatal disseminated infection in the immunologically compromised host.

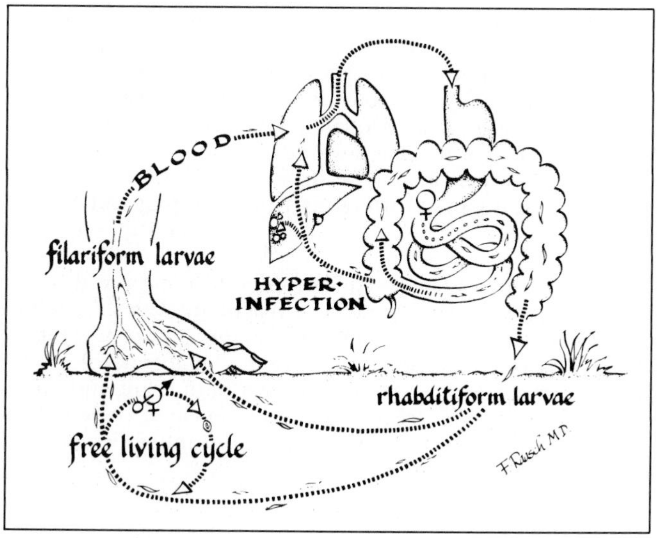

Fig. 88–10. Most common life cycles of *Strongyloides stercoralis*. (AFIP photograph No. 70–73312–2. Artist, Frank Raasch, MD.)

This parasitic helminth is unusual because multiplication and autoinfection occur within the infected person. This accounts for persistence of the infection, which is known to be as long as 40 years in the untreated individual.

The geographic distribution is primarily tropical and subtropical but is generally parallel to that of hookworms, because the environmental conditions of warmth, shade, moisture, sand, and loamy soil, and indiscriminate defecation apply to both parasites. Within the temperate regions of the world, strongyloidiasis is rare in Europe, but in the United States, endemic foci in Appalachia and the southeastern states are well known. WHO estimates on a worldwide basis that 50 to 100 million people are infected. Cats and dogs are known to be susceptible to infection, but they are most likely unimportant reservoirs. In Africa and, perhaps, New Guinea, human infection with *Strongyloides fulleborni* is common in selected loci.

Life Cycle. The life cycle or, more accurately, life cycles are highly complex and unique among the nematode parasites of humans. There are two forms of sexually mature adults: one is a parasite within the tissues of the intestine, and the other is a free-living worm that can live in the soil. *S. stercoralis* is the only nematode whose adults can increase in numbers entirely within a human host.

The direct cycle (Fig. 88–10) is the most common. The parasitic females are slender, filariform worms about 2 mm in length. They usually reside among the epithelial and glandular cells or in the tunica propria in the upper levels of the small intestine. Here, apparently in the absence of males, they lay several dozens of eggs daily. As the eggs filter through the mucosa toward the lumen, they develop and hatch, freeing the larvae. These make their way to the lumen and are passed in the stool. Under favorable conditions and after further development to the infective filariform stage, they enter exposed human skin to initiate a new infection. Their migration to the lungs and then to the small intestine is similar to that described above for the hookworm larvae. After reaching the tissues of the small intestine, the larvae develop into mature females in about 25 days, and these worms may live for several years. They probably are parthenogenetic.

A second type of cycle, common only in the tropics, involves the interpolation of one or more free-living generations. This is the indirect cycle. In this case, the larvae in the stool develop into free-living males and females. These mate, and, eventually, some of the resultant rhabditiform larvae develop into filariform larvae to begin the parasitic cycle. The intrahuman cycle is the same as that of the direct cycle.

The third type of cycle is that known as internal autoreinfection or hyperinfection. In this case, the larvae, while still in the intestinal lumen, molt into the filariform larvae, which after entering the intestinal wall and blood circulation migrate through the tissues of the body (known as disseminated strongyloidiasis). Some reach the lungs, as in the other cycles, and return to the small intestine, but many find their way into various other tissues, where considerable damage may result. Larvae in skin tunnels (*larva currens*) migrate rapidly, covering centimeters per day. This cycle is most common in patients with severe protein-calorie malnutrition or immune deficiencies, and the outcome may be fatal. The fourth type of cycle results from external autoreinfection when precociously developed filariform larvae on fecally contaminated areas penetrate the skin, usually in the perianal area.

Pathology and Symptomatology. When large numbers of larvae penetrate into the skin, a pruritis or ground itch usually develops. A severe pneumonitis may be produced by the larvae in the lungs, somewhat similar to that caused by *Ascaris* larvae. Damage is also produced in the wall of the small intestine by the females, eggs, and rhabditiform larvae. Mechanical and perhaps lytic damage is produced, especially by the females, which move about considerably. Cellular infiltration, often striking, consists chiefly of eosinophils, lymphocytes, and epitheloid cells. Panmucosal duodenitis is characteristic; that is, there is involvement throughout large areas of the mucosa, and it is not, therefore, limited to areas adjacent to the worms. The affected tissue becomes increasingly nonfunctional, and at times sloughing of the tissue down to the muscularis mucosae occurs. There is evidence of systemic damage, consisting of sensitization and probably toxic reactions. As stated above, autoreinfection may produce severe damage in various tissues, with striking signs and symptoms. The most characteristic symptoms of the usual direct type of infection, however, are midepigastric nonradiating pain, a watery mucous diarrhea, and eosinophilia.

Epidemiology. The pattern of transmission is similar to that of hookworms. Although coexisting with hookworm infection around the world, strongyloidiasis is more spotty in distribution and not nearly as prevalent. Autoreinfection accounts for the persistence of the parasite in an individual for as long as 40 years after having left an endemic area.

Diagnosis. Half of those infected are free of symptoms, and the majority of those who have symptoms do not usually have severe clinical manifestations. The development of hyperinfection and disseminated strongyloidiasis and their attendant severe clinical manifestations are probably due to a decreased resistance brought about by a variety of debilitating diseases, malnutrition, and immunosuppressive therapy.

Macular eruptions of the skin due to larval penetration may be noted. Perianal inflammation is sometimes seen when external autoreinfection takes place. Pulmonary signs and symptoms resemble those of hookworm infection. During the intestinal phase, there may be pain, nausea, vomiting, and diarrhea alternating with constipation. Midepigastric pain and an eosinophilia are the hallmarks of this stage, and the symptoms mimic those of peptic or duodenal ulcers. Because of rather nonspecific signs and symptoms, differential diagnosis should include enteritis, allergies, VLM, colitis, hepatitis, cholecystitis, and malnutrition, with or without malabsorption.

A definitive diagnosis depends on the demonstration of larvae in the feces (Fig. 88–11). In general, the presence of larvae in freshly passed feces strongly suggests *Strongyloides;* the presence of thin-shelled eggs suggests hookworm. The formalin-ether concentration technique is highly effective in concentrating larvae for diagnosis. In cases when no larvae can be found in the stool but strongyloidiasis is still suspected, duodenal aspirates, the Entero-test (string test), and sputum or urine examinations may be helpful.

The most consistent laboratory finding is an eosinophilia of 5% to 40%. Many immunocompromised hosts, however, do not show an eosinophilia and may even show eosinopenia. Serum protein and potassium levels may be abnormally low in severe infections. AST and alanine aminotransferase (ALT) levels may be increased. Stools vary in character, from normal to diarrheal and mucoid; some may be steatorrheic. A CF test has been used, but its poor sensitivity and specificity do not merit its routine use. However, an ELISA test has been developed that is both adequately sensitive and specific. It is particularly useful for diagnosis of chronic strongyloidiasis, a condition in which it may be difficult to find larvae in the stool; the test does not differentiate between past and current infection.

Treatment. *Strongyloides* has been one of the more difficult helminthic infections to treat. The risk of autoreinfection and its consequences requires elimination of all worms, rather than just a reduction in worm burden. Thiabendazole is the drug of choice and is effective against both adult and larval worms. If necessary, treatment can be repeated. When autoreinfection is suspected, broad-spectrum antibiotics may be given to control bacterial infections.

Trichinella spiralis

Infection with trichina worms now has a prevalence of 1% to 4% in the United States. Forty years ago, 15% to 20% of all

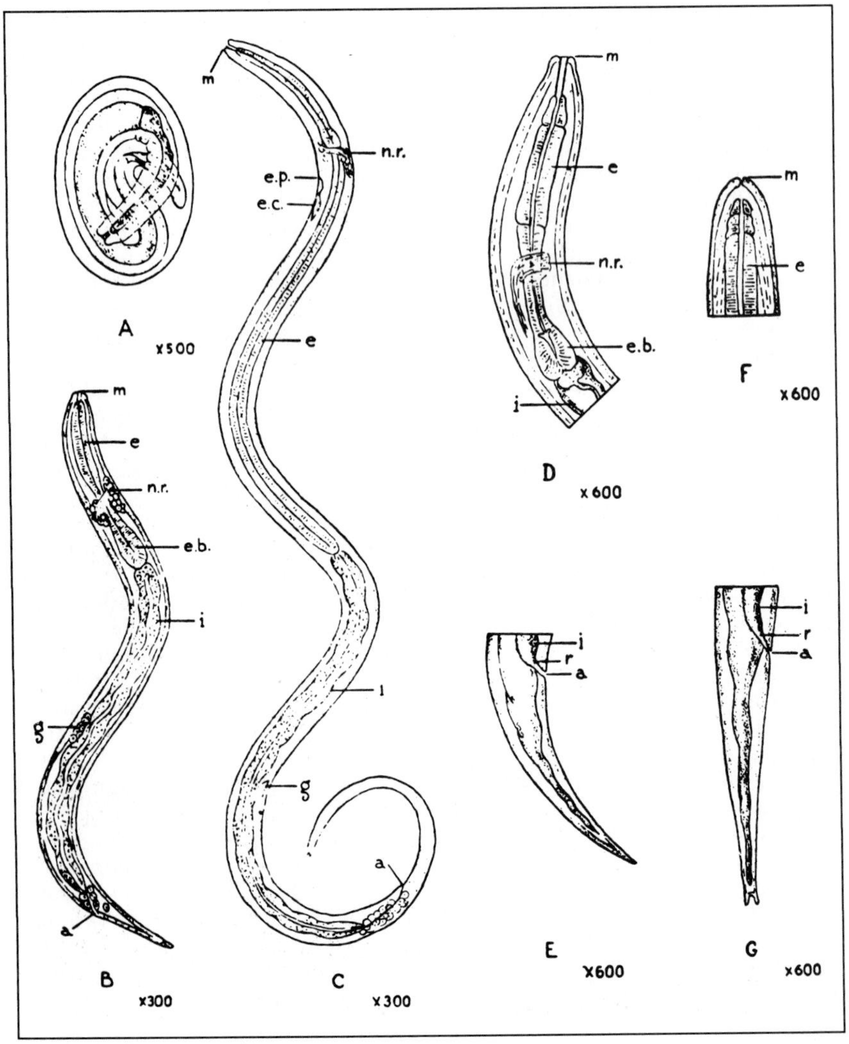

Fig. 88–11. Larvae of *Strongyloides stercoralis.* **A.** Egg containing mature larva of *S. simiae.* **B.** Rhabditiform larva. **C.** Filariform larva. **D.** Anterior end of rhabditiform larva. **E.** Posterior end of rhabditiform larva. **F.** Anterior end of filariform larva. **G.** Posterior end of filariform larva. a, anus; e, esophagus; e.b., esophageal bulb; e.c., excretory cell; e.p., excretory pore; g, genital rudiment; i, intestine; m, mouth; n.r., nerve ring; r, rectum. *(From Belding: Textbook of Clinical Parasitology, ed 2. Appleton-Century-Crofts, 1952.)*

Americans were infected. The cooking of the garbage fed to pigs, widespread commercial and home freezing, better pig-rearing methods, and the inspection of pork for transportation across state lines has greatly reduced the chance of infection. However, undercooked or raw meat, especially pork, can still be hazardous, so thorough cooking should still be encouraged. The United States government is currently monitoring pig herds and hopes to eradicate trinchinosis in swine in the 1990s. In 1930, 10% of swine, in 1970 1%, and now, it is thought, less than 1% of all hogs in commercial operations are infected.

Currently, the highest prevalence rates are in temperate and Arctic regions. In Arctic regions the pig is replaced by bears, seals, and walruses as the sources of human infection. Recent data show that 95% of all Eskimos in northern Canada are infected. Within the United States, and excluding Alaska, trichinosis remains a health hazard primarily because the infection is still enzootic among domesticated pigs. Surveillance shows that in the United States, 75% of infections are due to consumption of pork or pork products, with most of the remainder due to eating improperly cooked ground beef that has been adulterated with pork.

Life Cycle. *T. spiralis* is unusual because in its life cycle it has no external phase, either as free-living larvae or in a vector. Both the adults and larvae are present in an infected host. Humans are infected by ingesting infective larvae (Fig. 88–12) that are encysted in striated muscles of a reservoir host. Gastric digestion frees most of the larvae. They soon enter the small intestine and penetrate into the mucosa. Within 2 days they have reached the adult stage. Copulation occurs and the females (2 to 4 mm in length), after burrowing more deeply into the mucosa or even to lower levels, begin to give off larvae. The release of larvae begins about 5 days after

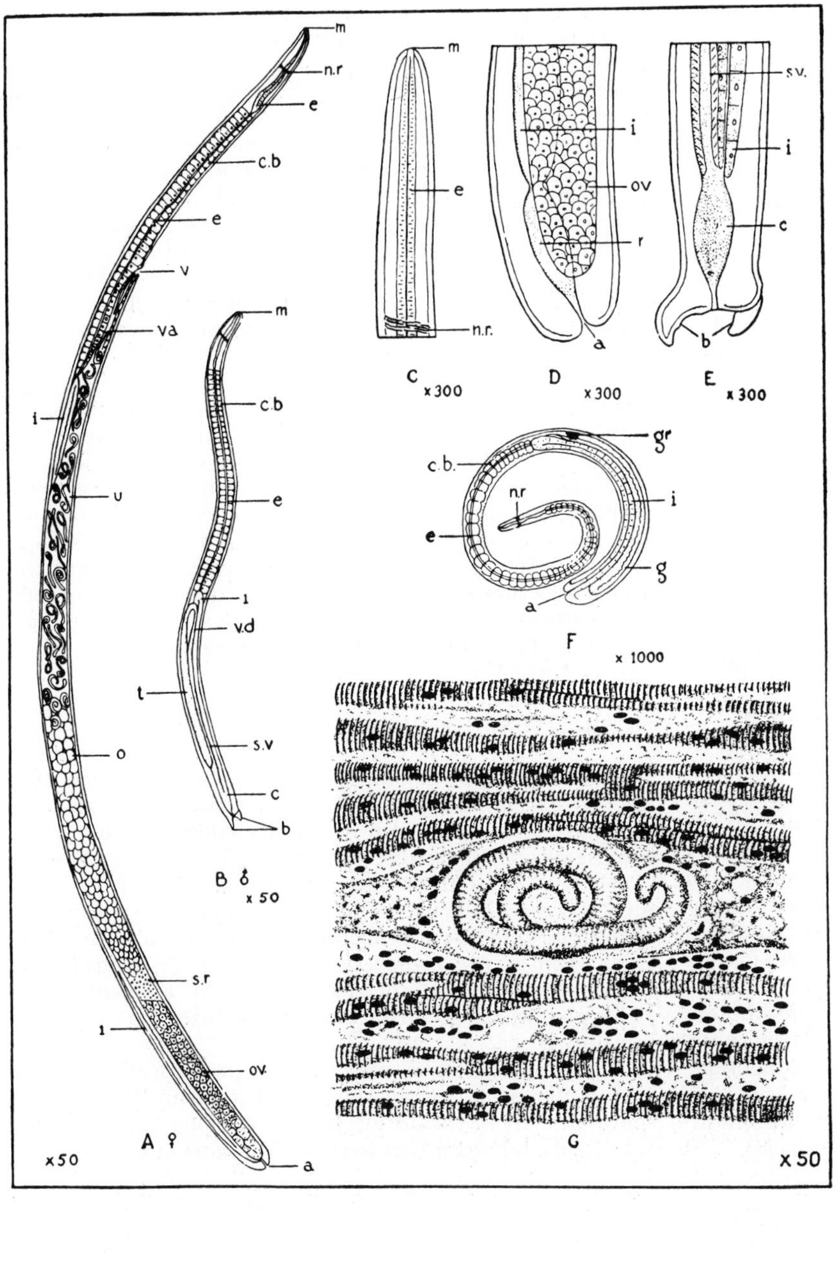

Fig. 88–12. Schematic representation of *Trichinella spiralis*. **A.** Adult female. **B.** Adult male. **C.** Anterior end of worm. **D.** Posterior end of female. **E.** Posterior end of male. **F.** Young larval worm. **G.** Early encysted larva in muscle. (**C** adapted from Leuckart, 1868). a, anus; b, bursa; c, cloaca; c.b., cell bodies; e, esophagus; g, gonads (anlage); gr, granules; i, intestine; m, mouth; n.r., nerve ring; o, ova; ov., ovary; r, rectum; s.r., seminal receptacle; s.v., seminal vesicle; t, testis; u, uterus containing larvae; v, vulva; va, vagina; v.d., vas deferens. *(From Brown and Neva: Basic Clinical Parasitology, ed 5. Appleton-Century-Crofts, 1983.)*

infection, and most of the larvae appear in the circulating blood within 7 to 14 days. The total number of larvae released by each female over a period of several weeks is 500 or more. These larvae are small, about 100 by 6 μm. They enter the circulation and are distributed throughout the body. However, only those entering striated muscles are capable of further development. Here, within 3 weeks after infection, encapsulation begins. This host reaction, initiated by infiltration primarily by lymphocytes and eosinophils, results in the formation of a double-walled, adventitious capsule (Fig. 88–12). The larvae contained within grow to about 0.8 mm in length and become tightly coiled. The larvae are infective for a new host a few days after encapsulation has begun. Some remain viable within cysts for many years, despite the fact that calcification of the cyst is usually observed after 6 months. Stray larvae that invade the myocardium and other tissues, such as the central nervous system, cause damage, but cyst formation does not occur.

Pathology and Symptomatology. The vast majority of infections are asymptomatic. When symptoms are present, trichinosis has been confused with many other diseases, because the parasite may damage many different tissues of the body. For a clear understanding of the disease, it is necessary to consider in turn the various stages involved. During the first stage, the adult worms are becoming established in the mucosa of the small intestine. Because of extensive burrowing, tissue is destroyed and an intense panmucosal and submucosal inflammatory reaction results. Nausea, vomiting, diarrhea, and fever may be experienced. These and other signs and symptoms resemble salmonellosis and other enteric infections; thus trichinosis is not suspected. This stage usually lasts for about 10 days and overlaps the second stage.

The second stage, set arbitrarily between 7 and 14 days after infection, involves most of the larvae in the circulation. The fever usually reaches a peak (41C), and there is characteristic edema, especially around the eye(s), splinter hemorrhages under the fingernails, and eosinophilia. In addition, dyspnea, difficulty in mastication and speech, and petechial hemorrhages, especially in the conjunctivae and retinal vessels, may be noted. Myocarditis with congestive heart failure, as well as neurologic signs and symptoms, is often noted. It should be remembered that any organ may be damaged by the migrating larvae. The features of this stage are most pronounced during the second week but continue throughout the period when larvae are released.

The third stage, after 14 days, is a culmination of the traumatic, allergic, and toxic effects of the infection, and symptoms may continue for 5 to 8 weeks or longer. Myositis is prominent, and muscular pains are usually the chief complaint. The edema, especially around the eyes, persists, as does the hypereosinophilia, which reaches a peak about 21 days after infection. Cachexia may be profound. Many fatal cases have demonstrable congestive heart failure due to myocardial lesions, respiratory paralysis, and anaphylaxis. It is noteworthy that eosinophilia is characteristically absent in such patients. Other than during epidemics, most cases are relatively asymptomatic, presumably because of the consumption of small numbers of larvae. It should be kept in mind, however, that death will result inevitably if large numbers are ingested.

The differential diagnosis should include other causes of gastroenteritis, asthma, rickettsial diseases, VLM, brucellosis, dengue, myositis, myocarditis, and meningoencephalitis.

Epidemiology. In the United States, trichinosis is most often seen clinically among members of ethnic groups who enjoy eating raw pork. Some recent outbreaks occurred among new immigrants who did not understand the need either to cook or to freeze American pork. In the southern United States the custom of tasting raw homemade sausage for flavor during the addition of spices is a significant cause of infection. The entire zoonotic picture of this infection is unknown because, in addition to most carnivores and omnivores, horse and mutton have also been known to be the source of infection. In addition, there is some evidence that marine fish and crabs can serve as transport hosts.

Diagnosis. Myalgia, high eosinophilia, facial edema, and fever should lead a physician to suspect trichinosis, especially if there is a recent history of eating raw meat, mainly pork. Similar symptoms of others eating at the same place further substantiate the presumptive diagnosis.

A direct (specific) means of diagnosis is provided by a small biopsy specimen from the deltoid or other muscle. The larvae may be demonstrated by pressing the tissue firmly between two microscope slides and then examining them microscopically or by recovering the larvae after digestion in artificial gastric juice. To relate the presence of larvae to the current illness, it is important to consider the stage of cyst formation. For example, the finding of calcified cysts alone could not be related to an illness of recent origin. A negative biopsy result, however, does not exclude the possibility of infection. Various serologic tests are available, but the BFT is considered the best for detection of acute infections. An intradermal test is available. Finally, the degree of and changes in the eosinophilic response (as high as 80%), although not specific and not always striking, are of assistance and should be charted.

Treatment. In general, only palliative and supportive measures are of value. Cortisone and related drugs, however, are of great assistance during the larval encystment period. Allergic reactions to and/or toxic effects from the metabolites of the worms often show amelioration after use of cortisone, and on occasion this drug has appeared to be lifesaving. Mebendazole is effective against the adult worms, but the diagnosis is almost always delayed until after most, if not all, of the migrating larvae—the agents of toxic and allergic reactions—have been released by the female worms.

Tissue Nematodes

The tissue nematodes comprise eight species of filariae. *Dracunculus medinensis,* the agent of guinea worm infection, although not a filarial worm, is also included with this group because of its morphologic similarity. All are exotic in origin (Table 88–1) and all are characterized by the following features: (1) the adults live in the tissues, (2) female worms give birth to larvae known as microfilariae that circulate in blood and lymph or are present in tissues, and (3) transmission requires the ingestion of microfilariae by a bloodsucking arthropod, which, in turn, transmits the infection to another human.

Filariasis is a major public health problem involving up to half the adult human population in many tropical and subtropical areas. Incubation periods are long (6 months to a year), and adult worms can live for 15 or more years. Diagnosis

TABLE 88–1. FILARIAE AND *DRACUNCULUS MEDINENSIS*

Parasite	Disease	Location of Adults in Humans	Location of Microfilariae in Humans	Arthropod Intermediate Hosts
Wuchereria bancrofti	Bancroft's filariasis	Lymphatics	Blood	Mosquitoes, especially *Anopheles, Culex, Aedes* sp.
Brugia malayi	Malayan filariasis	Lymphatics	Blood	Mosquitoes, *Mansonia, Anopheles* sp.
Brugia timori	Timorian filariasis	Lymphatics	Blood	*Anopheles* sp., mosquitoes
Onchocerca volvulus	Onchocerciasis	Subcutaneous nodules	Skin tissues	*Simulium* sp., blackflies
Loa loa	Loiasis	Subcutaneous tissues	Blood	*Chrysops* sp., deerflies
Mansonella perstans	Perstans filariasis	Body cavities, especially perirenal tissues	Blood	*Culicoides* sp., biting midges
Mansonella streptocerca	Streptocerciasis	Skin, especially of the trunk	Skin	*Culicoides* sp., biting midges
Mansonella ozzardi	Ozzard's filariasis	Body cavities, especially mesentery fat	Blood	*Culicoides* sp., biting midges
Dracunculus medinensis	Dracontiasis	Visceral connective tissues, in subcutaneous tissues	No microfilarial stage; female discharges rhabditiform larvae	*Cyclops* sp., small crustaceans

is usually made upon recovering the microfilariae from blood or skin. Among those listed in Table 88–1, *Wuchereria bancrofti, Brugia malayi,* and *Onchocerca volvulus* account for most of the pathologic effects associated with these infections and thus are of greatest medical importance.

Wuchereria bancrofti

W. bancrofti, which causes Bancroft's filariasis and elephantiasis, is spotty in distribution throughout the tropics and subtropics; at one time it was endemic in Charleston, South Carolina. The infection occurs primarily in coastal areas and islands with long periods of high humidity and heat. In the western hemisphere, it is found in the West Indies, along the coast of South America from Brazil to Colombia, and at a focus along the Atlantic Coast of Costa Rica. In the United States, the infection is most frequently seen in immigrants, military veterans, and missionaries.

Life Cycle. The adults, usually coiled together, live within the human lymphatic system. The males are about 4 cm long, and the females are about 9 cm. Both sexes are threadlike, being no more than 0.3 mm in diameter. After copulation, the female gives birth to living microfilariae. These ultimately find their way into the bloodstream. In most strains, they circulate in the blood in largest numbers at night and are said to have nocturnal periodicity. In certain other strains, either no particular periodicity is noted or there is a tendency for the occurrence of the largest numbers at dusk. The circulating microfilariae, 125 to 320 μm in length, develop only in certain mosquitoes. Thus, pathologic effects will not occur if blood containing them is transfused into a recipient. Female mosquitoes of various genera (especially *Culex, Aedes,* and *Anopheles*) serve as necessary intermediate hosts for this parasite. When the mosquitoes feed on an infected individual, they ingest the microfilariae from the peripheral bloodstream. The microfilariae pass into the midgut and invade the intestinal wall. Within 24 hours, most of the microfilariae find their way to the thoracic muscles, where they undergo metamorphosis to infective larvae in 1 to 3 weeks. This stage is active and migrates to the tip of the proboscis sheath, from which it penetrates into the skin of the human host at the time the mosquito takes the next blood meal. The larva probably enters the wound made by the mosquito. After entering the skin, these larvae pass to the lymphatic system and grow to maturity. In most cases this probably requires at least 1 year. The adult worms may live for many years in certain individuals.

Pathology and Symptomatology. In endemic areas, most of those who are infected are more or less symptom-free, demonstrating what appears to be an excellent host-parasite adjustment. The host will experience little or no disturbance, and the parasite is able to develop normally, which results in the release of large numbers of microfilariae. These individuals therefore are the main source of infection for the mosquito host, as humans are the only known definitive hosts. In those patients showing clinical evidence of the infection, two distinct stages are evident. In the acute stage there is a characteristic and often profound lymphatic inflammation in response to trapped worms or their metabolites, or both. Tissue changes tend eventually to constrict the wall of the lymphatic vessel or other affected parts of the system. This partial obstruction results in lymph stasis and edema. The cardinal manifestation is a recurrent lymphangitis, usually with an associated lymphadenitis. Some patients experience a low-grade fever, usually of short duration. The location of the obstruction determines the part of the body affected, the external genitalia of both sexes being the most common. In the absence of reinfection, there is usually steady improvement in the individual, each relapse being milder than the former. Thus, even without specific therapy, this condition is self-limiting and presumably will not become chronic in those acquiring the infection during a brief sojourn in an endemic area. It is important to note that microfilariae are difficult to demonstrate during the acute phase, indicating a pronounced disturbance in the host-parasite equilibrium. Sectioning of a biopsy specimen reveals the worms and the characteristic reaction, consisting of a necrotic zone around the worms and a palisaded area of foreign body giant cells, epithelioid cells, and eosinophils.

There is good evidence that the advanced chronic type of filariasis, known as elephantiasis, develops in only a small percentage of highly reactive individuals infected repeatedly for many years. After lymphatic obstruction, striking proliferative changes occur, and the worms die and are absorbed or become calcified. The edema, soft at first, becomes fibrotic after the growth of connective tissue in the area. The redundant skin, being nourished poorly, cracks and becomes fissured and is often secondarily infected with pyogenic or mycotic organisms. This resemblance to elephant skin accounts for the term *elephantiasis* being applied to this chronic, disfiguring condition. Although microfilariae may appear in the blood of chronic cases, because of new, active infection superimposed upon the older ones, they are not often demonstrated. Thus it appears that the more reactive the host, the less likely is the development of the worms and the release of embryos.

Tropical pulmonary eosinophilia (Weingartner's syndrome) is a form of occult filariasis caused by human and nonhuman filarial parasites. It is characterized by an immunologic hyperresponsiveness with a marked increase in IgE and IgG antiparasite antibodies, as well as a hypereosinophilia. Sometimes paroxysmal nocturnal coughing, breathlessness, and wheezing are characteristic of infection. At other times, lymphadenopathy and hepatosplenomegaly are seen. Microfilariae are rarely present in blood, but remnants of them are found in eosinophilic granulomas in the spleen, liver, lymph nodes, and lungs.

Various syndromes are known to coexist with filariasis or are found in filarial endemic regions and have been suggested as being manifestations of infection. These include arthritis, endomyocardial fibrosis, tenosynovitis, dermatosis, lateral popliteal nerve palsy, and others. Further study is necessary to determine the precise role that filariae play, if any, in the above syndromes.

Epidemiology. To date, no naturally infected reservoirs other than humans have been identified. Several species of monkeys can be experimentally infected, however.

Dense populations living in tropical areas where mosquitoes breed unhampered offer ideal conditions for transmission. Reduction in mosquito populations will aid in control, but some vectors have now acquired resistance to almost all the residual insecticides. WHO estimates that 250 million people are infected, with 400 million at risk. No prophylactic drugs are available. Consequently, travelers to endemic areas should avoid being bitten by mosquitoes. Repellants and mosquito netting for those sleeping outdoors are advised.

Diagnosis. The acute clinical manifestations of filariasis are characterized by recurrent attacks of fever and lymphadenitis, sometimes precipitated by hard physical exertion. Although lymphadenitis commonly occurs in the inguinal regions, male genitalia are frequently involved, leading to funiculitis, epididymitis, and orchitis. The whole acute clinical course of an episode of fever and lymphadenitis may last from 3 weeks to 3 months and can result in prolonged inability to work.

The clinical course of chronic infection occurs after prolonged residence in an endemic area. Thus, when symptomatic disease does occur, patients should be reassured that the prognosis is good and advised that elephantiasis is a rare complication that is limited to persons from endemic areas who have had constant exposure to the infected mosquitoes for years.

In the laboratory a direct diagnosis is made by demonstrating the microfilariae, usually in thick blood smears or blood filtrates. Membrane filtration techniques are the most sensitive methods currently available. In most areas of the world, microfilariae are present in appreciable numbers only at night, usually with greatest frequency between 10 PM and 2 PM. Microfilariae are also sometimes seen in urine and in chylous and hydrocoele fluids. It should be remembered that microfilariae cannot be demonstrated during the incubation period and usually not during the acute phase of the infection. In the absence of microfilariae, a presumptive diagnosis can be made on the basis of the history of exposure, clinical evidence of the disease, and positive serologic test results (IHA and BFT) or a positive intradermal test reaction. Lymph node biopsy, during clinical quiescence only, often will reveal adult or immature worms. This, however, is a research tool and should not be used except in unusual circumstances and then only by adhering to strict surgical techniques.

The differential diagnosis of filariasis should include hernia, venous thrombosis, obstructive lesions of the lymphatics, multiple lipomatosis, heart failure, and gonococcal infection.

Treatment. Patients with acute disease resulting from recent primary exposure should be removed from the endemic area, if possible. Bed rest and supportive measures, such as hot and cold compresses, are of assistance in reducing the edema. Psychotherapy is often necessary, especially for young men with scrotal involvement. Although surgical excision of lymph nodes is rarely indicated, and usually not successful, surgical removal of elephantoid breast, vulva, or scrotum is successful. Administration of antibodies for patients with secondary bacterial infections and analgesics as well as anti-inflammatory agents during the painful, acute stage is helpful.

Diethylcarbamazine is the drug of choice. It should be remembered that chemotherapy is of little value during advanced disease, because the worms may already be dead and irreversible tissue damage has already occurred.

Onchocerca volvulus

Onchocerciasis is the term used to describe an infection with *O. volvulus*. Geographically, it occurs in the tropical zone of Africa and Central and South America. A small focus has recently been discovered in the Yemen Arab Republic.

The infection has emerged as a major health problem, with more than 20 million people being infected and 2 million of these blinded by the worm. Depending on the region of the world, it is known as river blindness, blinding filarial disease, gale filarienne, Robles' disease, and craw-craw.

Life Cycle. Filamentous females, 23 to 70 cm in length, and 3 to 6 cm long dwarf males live in subcutaneous tissues. Here they are either coiled up within fibrous nodules the size of a pea or walnut or remain free. Microfilariae produced by the female worms migrate to the upper layers of the skin and other parts of the body, including the eye. It is thought that females may live for up to 20 years and microfilariae for up to 2.5 years.

Blackflies of the genus *Simulium* ingest microfilariae when they ingest blood. Within the vector, metamorphosis to the infective larval stage takes place in 6 to 8 days. When the infected *Simulium* feeds, the larvae enter the subcutaneous tissues and mature into the adult form in 6 to 9 months.

Pathology and Symptomatology. The disease may be arbitrarily divided into three forms: dermatologic, nodular with its associated lymphadenitis, and ocular. The dermatologic and nodular forms usually occur simultaneously. Adult worms are most likely rather innocuous, whereas the microfilariae can cause severe pathologic effects.

Itching and scratching, with subsequent development of dermal lesions in the form of papular rashes, are usually the first signs of infection. Altered pigmentation of the skin usually follows. Skin may be mottled (*leopard skin*), scaly and wrinkled (*lizard skin*), or hyperpigmented (*sowda*). Skin changes result because the normal architecture of the dermis is lost and is replaced by a toneless, thickened, pachydermlike layer. In some African patients, skin and lymph node involvement in the inguinal region leads to the loss of tissue elasticity, resulting in a *hanging groin.* It has been postulated that immune complexes are formed because of the antigenicity of the living and dead microfilariae. These complexes trigger a chronic inflammatory response with subsequent perivascular fibrosis and obstructive lymphadenitis. This form of the disease is similar to the elephantoid form of wuchereriasis.

Nodules are usually visible, palpable, firm, rounded, and nontender masses varying in size from 0.5 to 10 cm in diameter. Nodules may be single or may occur in clusters and resemble a tumor. Nodules tend to be located over bony prominences, such as skull, elbow, and scapula. In Africa, nodules tend to be on the lower portion of the body along the iliac crest, groin, knees, thighs, and spine. In Central America, more than half the nodules are on the head.

Ocular onchocerciasis frequently climaxes as visual impairment or blindness before the infected patient reaches adulthood. This form of the disease should be regarded as a hypersensitive type, because symptoms do not appear until the microfilariae begin to die. The other forms of the disease (nodular and dermal) may precede or occur simultaneously with the ocular form. In the early stage, microfilariae are present in the anterior chamber and cornea. Cellular accumulations occur around the dead microfilariae, causing punctate keratitis. With larger numbers of microfilariae and with greater hypersensitivity, a severe sclerotic keratitis, often with an anterior uveitis, may end in blindness. Iridocyclitis, cataracts, secondary glaucoma, and postneuritic optic atrophy may also occur.

Epidemiology. Onchocerciasis occurs in the environment containing fast-running streams where the blackflies breed. The flies have a limited flight range, and as a result, infection is most prevalent along streams. This has created "ghost villages" in Africa, when entire populations have moved inland to get away from the blindness that accompanies chronic infection. Humans are the only known host. There is some evidence, however, that the horse and other domestic animals may serve as reservoirs.

Diagnosis. The living and dying microfilariae produce an intense itching and pruritis. In time, the skin pigmentation is altered, and it becomes toneless and thickened. It has been said that onchocerciasis makes young people look old, and old people look like lizards. Nodules and corneal opacities should, of course, suggest onchocerciasis in those from endemic areas.

Diagnosis is best made by obtaining superficial skin snips. Skin removed near a nodule affords the best chance of finding the microfilariae. The removed skin is teased apart in a drop of saline and examined microscopically. At times, microfilariae have been demonstrated in urine and sputum. A recent advance in diagnosis has been the membrane filter concentration technique. In this technique, skin is teased apart in saline, allowed to stand 6 to 12 hours, and then expressed through a Nucleopore or Millipore membrane of 5 μm porosity. The membrane is then removed, stained, and examined.

Ocular involvement can be detected by slit-lamp examination. Histologic sections of removed skin or nodules may also demonstrate adults and microfilariae. It should be remembered that blood examinations are of no value because the microfilariae do not circulate in the blood.

Low to moderate eosinophilia is common in onchocerciasis. Serum IgG, IgM, and IgA levels may be increased twofold higher than normal values. Various skin and serologic tests are available. At present, the best test is the IFA test.

Treatment. Diethylcarbamazine (DEC) and suramin have been used until recently. Microfilariae die rapidly after DEC treatment, and frequently the treated person will respond with a severe hypersensitive reaction (pruritis and erythema). To minimize this reaction, such anti-inflammatory agents as aspirin, antihistamines, and corticosteroids are prescribed. Ivermectin, a newly developed drug, is not associated with these complications and is now, in conjunction with suramin, the drug of choice. Nodules, especially those on the face and near the eyes, should be removed surgically before chemotherapy is started.

Cestodes

Cestodes, or tapeworms, are so named because the adult stage resembles a measuring tape. Anatomically, the adult tapeworm is composed of a joined chain (*strobila*) of segments (*proglottids*). Each mature proglottid contains a complete set of male and female reproductive organs (Fig. 88–13). No digestive tract is present, and all nutrients are absorbed through the body wall (tegument). At the most anterior end is a hold-fast or attachment organ known as a *scolex* that may bear hooks, suckers, or suckerlike grooves (bothria). Immediately posterior to the scolex is a short germinal center (neck) from which new proglottids arise. Maturation of proglottids proceeds toward the posterior end of the worm. Thus, groups of proglottids from anterior to posterior are termed *immature, mature,* and *gravid* (proglottids that are full of eggs). Many times, gravid proglottids will detach from the strobila and pass in the stool.

Even though some tapeworms are large (up to 10 m in length) the adult forms in the human intestine are generally well tolerated. In most instances, major complaints are absent until the patient observes proglottids that have been passed during defecation or have emerged from the anus at other times. In general, the patient's attitude to infection with adult tapeworms is either undue alarm or indifference. Both attitudes are to be discouraged, but certainly, any intestinal tapeworm infection should be treated.

The life cycles of most tapeworms infecting humans are

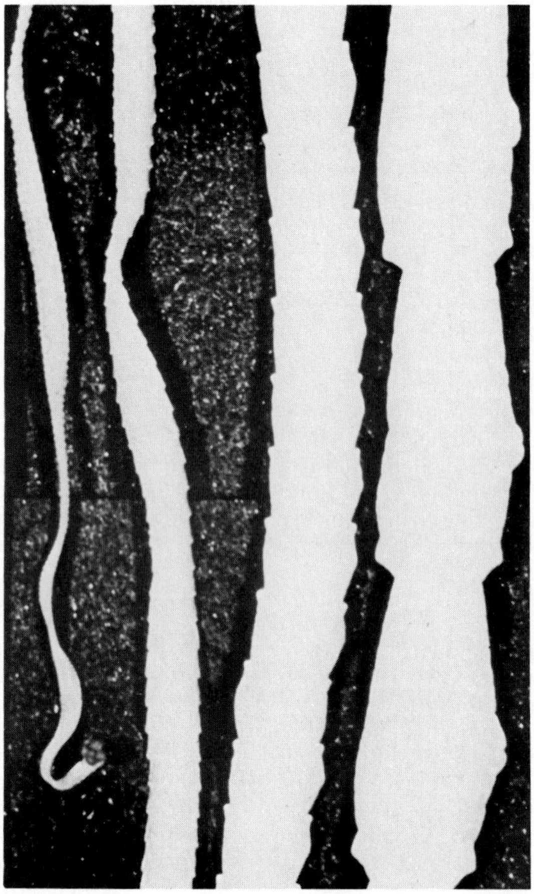

Fig. 88–13. Adult tapeworm.

complicated and involve one or more intermediate hosts. The larvae in these intermediate hosts are usually cystlike or bladderlike forms. In a few instances, humans can serve as hosts for the larval stage, and this can lead to severe disease and even death.

In the material that follows, the cestodes are grouped according to their common habitats in the body—the intestinal tract and various tissues. The intestinal cestodes live as adults in humans, whereas the tissue cestodes occur as larvae.

Intestinal Cestodes

Only the four most common intestinal cestodes of humans are presented: *Diphyllobothrium latum* (fish or broad tapeworm), *Taenia saginata* (beef tapeworm), *Taenia solium* (pork tapeworm), and *Hymenolepis nana* (dwarf tapeworm). All are endemic in the United States, but *T. solium* appears to be uncommon. In the adult stage, the first three are very large, ranging in length from 2 to 10 m or more, whereas the fourth is, by comparison, a dwarf, being 45 mm or less.

Diphyllobothrium latum

D. latum is called the broad or fish tapeworm of humans: "broad" because the individual proglottids are wider than they are long, and "fish" because humans acquire the infection by ingesting raw or improperly cooked fish of certain species. *D. latum* is the largest of the human tapeworms, frequently reaching 10 m or more in length.

Although worldwide in distribution (9 million infected), it is most common in north temperate areas where pickled or raw freshwater fish are eaten. Endemic centers include various Scandinavian countries (especially Finland), Canada, Chile, Argentina, and in the United States, the Great Lakes region and Alaska. The prevalence of this infection in the Great Lakes region is much lower now than in previous decades, and some consider it now a rare infection. Bears, dogs, cats, seals, and walruses are known to be infected and may serve as reservoirs for human infection.

Life Cycle. *D. latum* differs from other human tapeworms, both in structure and the complexity of its life cycle. The scolex is spatulate and is provided with median ventrally and dorsally grooved suckers (Fig. 88–14). The proglottids are broad (10 to 20 mm), and the centrally located uterus has a characteristic rosette arrangement. Eggs within the fully developed uterus are discharged continuously in large numbers from the uterine pore (Figs. 88–3 and 88–14). These are undeveloped when passed in the stool and will embryonate only upon reaching cool, fresh water. A ciliated embryo (coracidium) escapes from the shell and swims about actively. When this stage is ingested by one of the first intermediate hosts (copepods), the embryo burrows into the body cavity and transforms into a mature first larva stage (procercoid). Ingestion of the first intermediate host containing these mature larvae by the second intermediate host (many different species of fish) continues the cycle. The larvae migrate into the flesh, often between the muscle fibers of the fish, and then metamorphose within several weeks into a third larva stage (plerocercoid, also known as a sparganum). Larger, edible fish acquire the infection from eating their infected young or infected smaller species. Human consumption of fish flesh containing mature plerocercoid larvae completes the cycle. The worm, usually limited to one per infection in the United States, develops to maturity in the small intestine in 3 to 5 weeks and may live for many years.

Pathology and Symptomatology. Only about half of those people infected exhibit symptoms. Those with symptoms usually complain of vague abdominal discomfort, nausea, diarrhea, vomiting, and weight loss. When several worms are present, their bulk can cause blockage of the intestine. In some persons, when the worm or worms are attached to the proximal portion of the small intestine, a pernicious anemia of the megaloblastic type may result. The anemia is associated with the worm's ability to compete with the host for vitamin B_{12}, which it readily absorbs from the intestinal chyme.

Epidemiology. In the United States, uncooked or pickled pike and walleyes are the usual sources of human infection. These fish are considered choice ones in the preparation of gefilte fish, and tasting for seasoning before cooking is not uncommon. The pollution of streams and lakes is a major factor in the infection cycle.

At one time only freshwater fish were considered to be suitable intermediate hosts. Recent evidence indicates, however, that marine fish also harbor the larvae that may infect humans. Thus Japanese sushi and sashimi, Latin American

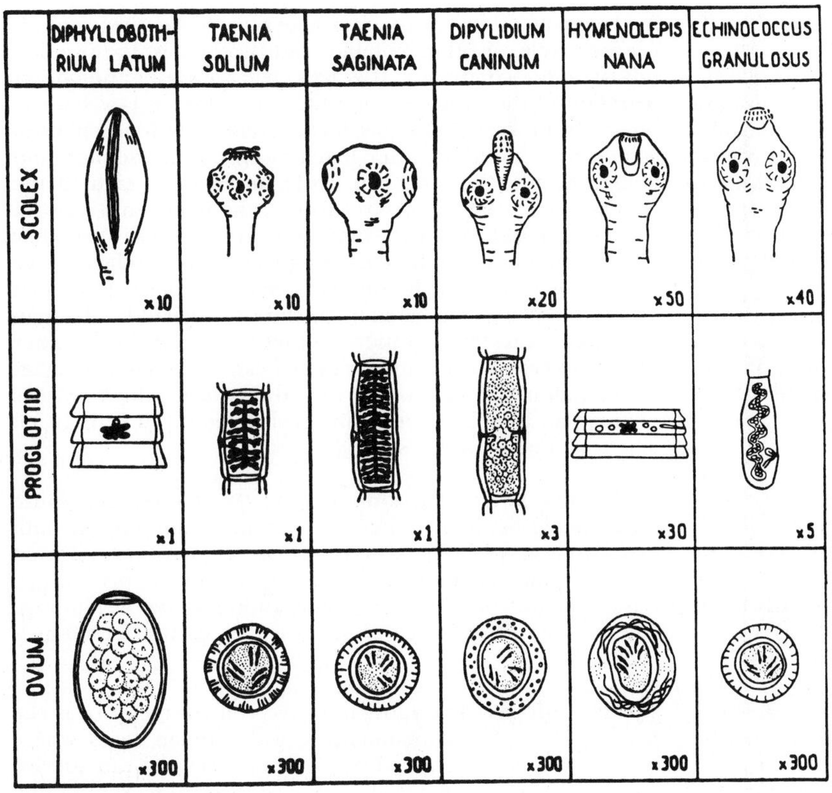

Fig. 88–14. Differential characteristics of common tapeworms of humans. *(From Belding: Textbook of Clinical Parasitology, ed 3. Appleton-Century-Crofts, 1965.)*

ceviche, and Dutch green herring are potential sources of infection.

Diagnosis. Infection is usually benign and often asymptomatic. Clinical symptoms such as abdominal discomfort with diarrhea, vomiting, and nausea are not uncommon. A travel history and questions concerning eating habits will help in diagnosis.

The gravid proglottids usually disintegrate before being passed, and consequently, only eggs are found in the stool. The eggs measure 45 by 70 μm, are thin-shelled, ovoid, and yellow-brown. An operculum (lid) is at one end and a small, knoblike protuberance may be present at the other end (Figs. 88–3 and 88–14). As for all operculated eggs, concentration must be done by a sedimentation technique, such as the formalin-ether method.

Laboratory findings that usually accompany infection are a low to moderate eosinophilia, slight leukocytosis, and a low serum vitamin B_{12} level. If tapeworm-induced anemia is present, it is typical of the pernicious type. No serologic test is available.

Treatment. Yomesan (niclosamide) is the drug of choice. This drug is a nonabsorbed oxidative phosphorylation inhibitor that kills the scolex and anterior segments on contact, after which the worm is expelled. Those patients with megaloblastic anemia should also receive vitamin B_{12} therapy. Praziquantel is reported as being equally effective.

Hymenolepis nana

H. nana, the dwarf tapeworm, is the most common tapeworm in humans in the United States, being most prevalent in the southeastern states where it is estimated that 3% of all children younger than 8 years of age either are or have been infected. On a worldwide basis, it is cosmopolitan in distribution, with highest infection rates being in the tropics. Worldwide, *H. nana* is the most prevalent cestode infection of humans with an estimated 45 to 50 million cases; two thirds of those infected live in Asia.

Life Cycle. Unlike the large tapeworms affecting humans, where only a single worm is present in an infection, numerous *H. nana* adults are usually present. An adult worm, 2 to 4 cm in length, attaches to the mucosa of the small intestine. Its life cycle is unique in that eggs can be directly infective for humans, without the necessity of an intermediate host. In the direct cycle, eggs initiate infection upon ingestion. Such infections may be of a direct hand-to-mouth type or of an indirect type via contaminated foods or fluids. The eggs hatch in the duodenum, and the liberated embryos penetrate into nearby villi. The resulting larval stage (cysticercoid) matures in about 4 days, returns into the intestinal lumen, attaches to the mucosa, and develops in about 2 weeks into the adult worm. Adults live for months. In the indirect cycle, arthropods, especially certain beetles, serve as intermediate hosts. Accidental ingestion of those containing the mature larvae (cysticercoids) results in infection.

Pathology and Symptomatology. Variability in clinical manifestations is common in mild to moderate infections. Some infections are asymptomatic, whereas others produce diarrhea, abdominal discomfort, and anorexia. In heavy infections, symptoms are usually more pronounced and include profuse diarrhea, abdominal pain, pruritis, nervous disorders, and apathy. Generalized toxemia may develop in some heavily infected children.

Epidemiology. Although humans themselves are the most important source of human infection, rats and mice may also be involved. The accidental ingestion of rodent feces (direct cycle) that contain *H. nana* eggs is thought to be more important in contributing to the prevalence of the disease than is the ingestion of infected beetles (indirect cycle). Infection seems to be as common in urban settings as in rural areas, which is unusual for helminthic infections.

Infection is usually confined to children younger than 8 years old. Autoreinfection does occur and may account for infection with hundreds of worms within a single host. Proper hygiene and rodent and vermin control are essential in preventing infection.

Diagnosis. Clinical symptoms are rather vague, and diagnosis depends on the laboratory demonstration of the typical egg (Figs. 88–3 and 88–14) as proof of infection. Proglottids are not usually found in or on the stool because these disintegrate in the intestine before being passed. The egg, 50 μm in diameter, is slightly oval, with a thin, colorless outer shell. Within the egg is another membrane enclosing the six-hooked larva (*oncosphere*). Between the outer shell and the membrane surrounding the oncosphere are eight to ten threadlike polar filaments. Adult worms, when recovered, can be identified on the basis of their size and the presence of a baseball bat–shaped scolex that bears four suckers and a circlet of hooks on the rostellum. About one third of those infected will have an eosinophilia of 5% or more. No serologic tests are available.

Treatment. On a comparative basis, *H. nana* is difficult to eradicate. Both niclosamide (Yomesan) and praziquantel have proved to be effective. Praziquantel is the drug of choice, however.

Taenia saginata

The beef tapeworm (*T. saginata*) and the pork tapeworm (*T. solium*) are large worms that may occur in humans when raw or insufficiently cooked meat is eaten. Both infections are known as taeniasis, but it is imperative that a species diagnosis be made because the pathologic consequences of *T. solium* can be severe, whereas those of the beef tapeworm are rather innocuous.

The beef tapeworm may be found wherever beef is eaten. Areas of high prevalence are Kenya, Ethiopia, Taiwan, the Philippines, and Iran. Infection in these areas is associated with eating raw beef, poor sanitation, and the practice of allowing cattle on pastures fertilized by sewage sludge. In addition to cattle, several other ungulates such as camels and antelope may serve as sources of infection. Humans are the only host infected with the adult tapeworm. In the United States, infection is seen infrequently, but meat inspection records show that 10,000 to 15,000 beef animals are slaughtered each year that harbor the larva stage. As a result, there may be more human infections than is generally realized.

Life Cycle. The adult tapeworm, usually only one worm per infection in the United States, is attached to the mucosa of the small intestine by the scolex. The distal most gravid proglottids become separated from the strobila and actively migrate out of the anus or are evacuated in the stool. If grazing cattle, or other suitable ungulates, ingest the proglottids or, more commonly, the eggs that are freed after disintegration of the proglottids on moist earth or in raw sewage, the cycle proceeds. The six-hooked embryos (oncospheres) escape from the eggs, after hatching in the duodenum, and penetrate into the intestinal tissue, ultimately reaching the circulation. They are carried through the blood, and most of them reach skeletal muscles or the heart. In these sites, they transform in 60 to 75 days into a typical cysticercus larva stage (*Cysticercus bovis*), which contains a scolex, similar to that of the adult worm, invaginated into a fluid-filled bladder. Human infection occurs by ingestion of these larvae in beef, either raw or processed inadequately. The head of the larva attaches to the wall of the ileum, and the adult worm, which reaches maturity in 8 to 10 weeks, can reach a length of 5 to 10 m. The worm may live for several years.

Pathology and Symptomatology. Most infections cause little discomfort and, indeed, are usually symptomless until proglottids have been passed and detected by the infected person. Some patients complain of abdominal discomfort, hunger pains, episodes of diarrhea, anorexia, and weight loss. There is ample evidence to suggest that gastric secretion is reduced.

Epidemiology. The most effective control measure is the prevention of soil contamination with human feces where cattle are likely to graze. Eggs are resistant and can survive for months in soil. Chemical treatment of soil and even routine sewage plant treatment does not kill the eggs. The thorough cooking of beef and the freezing of meat before consumption will also disrupt the cycle.

Diagnosis. Clinical signs and symptoms are either absent or very vague and indicate some kind of gastric and digestive disturbance. As previously noted, most infected individuals are unaware of the infection until proglottids are noticed in the stool or, more alarmingly, crawl out of the anus and down the leg.

Definitive diagnosis depends on the recovery of the typical rhomboidal scolex, equipped with four suckers, but without hooks (Fig. 88–14). The egg, about 35 μm in diameter and characterized by a striated shell containing the six-hooked oncosphere, may be detected microscopically. The eggs, however, are indistinguishable from those of *T. solium.* More commonly, the gravid proglottids are used for making a diagnosis. When passed, proglottids, each approximately 1 to 2 cm long, are creamy white. When pressed gently between two glass slides and held in front of a bright light, 15 to 20 main lateral branches of the uterus on each side can be seen (Fig. 88–14). Abnormal laboratory values rarely occur. Sometimes a mild eosinophilia is seen, as are lymphocytosis and anemia.

Treatment. Niclosamide and praziquantel are the drugs of choice.

Taenia solium

The major differences between *T. solium*, the pork tapeworm, and the beef tapeworm are (1) infection is acquired by eating raw or improperly cooked pork and (2) humans can serve as the intermediate host as well as the definitive host. The fact that humans can be infected with the egg of *T. solium* and can harbor the larva stage (cysticercus) makes this infection a serious and often a life-threatening condition.

Pork tapeworm infection occurs wherever pigs are raised, sanitation is poor, and pork is eaten raw or is insufficiently cooked. Fortunately, human infection in the United States is rare. However, it is endemic in Mexico, Latin America, tropical Africa, southeast Asia, the Philippines, and in the Indian subcontinent. Prevalence rates of 1% to 3% have been reported from Spain, Hungary, and Czechoslovakia.

Life Cycle. Attachment of the adult tapeworm to the mucosa of the small intestine is by means of the scolex. In addition to the four cup-shaped suckers there are 22 to 32 small hooklets on the rostellum. The length of the worm is shorter (2 to 8 m) than that of *T. saginata,* and the structure of the proglottids differs in the two species (Fig. 88–14). The life cycles of the two species are similar, except that the hog is the usual intermediate host for *T. solium.* The scolex of the larval stage (*Cysticercus cellulosae*) is provided with four suckers and a crown of hooklets. This stage may also occur in humans and cause serious injury (see below). For this reason, *T. solium* has greater medical and public health importance than has *T. saginata.*

Pathology and Symptomatology. The clinical manifestations of a *T. solium* infection with adult worms are the same as those induced by *T. saginata.* The clinical manifestations due to infection with the larval stage are discussed below.

Epidemiology. In addition to swine, other animals, such as camels, dogs, sheep, and deer, can serve as intermediate hosts. Although humans are the only known definitive host, the incidence of human infection is rare in some areas compared to the prevalence of cysticercosis in hogs (*measly pork*). Fecally contaminated slop and the foraging of swine on fecally contaminated forage result in an incidence of cystercercosis of 25% in some regions. Thorough cooking of pork is, obviously, essential in prevention of infection.

Diagnosis. Clinical symptoms due to the adult stage are the same as those of *T. saginata.* Because it is important to know whether the infected person has *T. solium* or *T. saginata,* either the recovered scolex with its crown of hooks (Fig. 88–14) or the gravid proglottid must be recovered, because the eggs of both species are identical. The pork tapeworm proglottid, when pressed between two glass slides and held in front of a bright light, will show 7 to 13 main lateral branches of the median stem of the uterus (Fig. 88–14).

Treatment. Niclosamide and praziquantel are the drugs of choice. Because internal autoreinfection is possible (see below), it is suggested that a purge be done after therapy to prevent reverse peristalis. Nausea and vomiting during therapy should also be avoided because this could lead to the backwash of eggs and possible internal autoreinfection.

Tissue Cestodes

Sparganosis

Sparganosis is a tissue infection of humans with the plerocercoid larva stage of *Diphyllobothrium*-like tapeworms. In most cases, the genus involved is *Spirometra,* a tapeworm of cats and dogs. Although worldwide in distribution, it is most common in the Orient. As a result of the immigration of large numbers of Asians into the United States within the past few years, sparganosis is now occasionally seen.

Spargana are whitish and elongated (a few millimeters to centimeters long), and have a wrinkled appearance. They enter human tissues during treatment of wounds or sores with poultices of plerocercoid-infected frog or snake flesh. When the poultice application is near the eye, ocular sparganosis may occur. Infection may also be acquired by the ingestion of raw plerocercoid-infected flesh of snakes, birds, amphibians, and mammals. The ingested plerocercoids migrate to subcutaneous tissue or eyelids or remain in the intestinal tissue. Humans may also develop sparganosis by drinking water containing infected water fleas (*Cyclops*). The procercoids within *Cyclops* invade the human gut wall and usually migrate to subcutaneous tissues. The migratory phase is usually asymptomatic.

When migration stops, a painful inflammatory reaction develops; encystation does not occur, but a fibrous nodule about 2 cm in diameter is formed by the host around the larva. Periorbital edema and ocular ulcers develop as a result of ocular sparganosis. A rare budding type of sparganum (*Sparganum proliferum*) has been reported, and this is known to cause death.

Diagnosis is made only after surgical removal of the sparganum. Leukocytosis and eosinophilia are usually seen. There is no satisfactory drug therapy, but both mebendazole and praziquantel have been used to treat *S. proliferum.*

Cysticercosis

Cysticercosis in humans most often is caused by the larvae of *Taenia solium* (i.e., *Cysterіcus cellulosae*), which have a predilection for skeletal muscles and the nervous system. The egg stage initiates human infection. A patient harboring the adult worm may become infected by transferring mature eggs from the anus to the mouth on fingertips (*external autoinfection*), or these may be transferred indirectly to another person (*heteroinfection*). A third type of infection, *internal autoreinfection,* is thought to occur when detached gravid proglottids are transferred by reverse peristalsis into more proximal parts of the small intestine, where some of the eggs become liberated. In all instances the eggs hatch in the small intestine, and the larvae (oncospheres) are carried to the tissues via the blood circulation.

Cysticerci reach a size of 2 cm and may occur in various human tissues, but the greatest concern is the common involvement of the eyes and the brain. Ocular cysticercosis may result in uveitis, dislocation of the retina, and other conditions. Pain, flashes of light, grotesque figures in the field of vision, and other complaints have been noted. Cerebral cysticercosis usually follows involvement of the meninges, with jacksonian (rolandic) epilepsy as the most characteristic consequence. Infection of the third and fourth ventricles, with hydrocephalus, headache, and diplopia, are also noteworthy. Cysticerci may live for 3 to 5 years before they die, degenerate, and become calcified. Cysts in skeletal muscle, liver, lungs, kidneys, and heart may cause symptoms. Virtually no inflammation results from the living larvae, but dead larvae precipitate an acute cellular inflammation.

Cysticercosis is common in regions where taeniasis due to *T. solium* is endemic, such as Mexico, Thailand, and eastern Europe. Often a patient will remember a previous tapeworm infection, and physicians should be aware that symptoms of cysticercosis may not occur until several years after infection. A recent report shows neural cysticercosis in 2% of all autopsies performed in Mexico.

Infections of tissues other than neural tissue are usually asymptomatic. At the time of death of the cysticercus, however, there is the liberation of the cyst's fluid contents, which appear to be toxic and allergic.

The diagnosis of cerebral cysticercosis is primarily clinical and may be quite difficult. Symptoms include headache, vomiting, impaired vision, and convulsions.

Various laboratory values are of limited use. Blood chemistry and hematologic data are not distinctive, although central nervous system fluid may show pleocytosis, increased protein levels, decreased glucose values, and eosinophils. Radiologic data are especially helpful because vascular changes and calcified cysticerci are readily seen in muscle and soft tissues. Computed tomography (CT) is also a useful diagnostic tool.

Until recently, there was no satisfactory chemotherapy, and surgical removal of those cysts in operable sites was the only treatment possible. However, use in clinics of praziquantel appears to be effective. This drug has not been completely evaluated, but it does hold considerable promise. Epileptic-like symptoms are treated with anticonvulsant drug therapy.

A variety of serologic tests that strongly indicate infection are available in the United States. Cross-reactions and false-negative results do occur, however; thus caution in interpretation must be exercised.

Hydatidosis

Hydatidosis is a zoonotic infection in which humans harbor the larval stage of the canine tapeworms, *Echinococcus granulosus* and *Echinococcus multilocularis.* Domestic dogs, wolves, foxes, and coyotes are the normal definitive hosts. A wide range of animals, including sheep, moose, field mice, and voles, are the normal intermediate hosts. Humans become infected by ingesting eggs of either species.

After ingestion of the eggs, the hatched oncospheres invade the mucosa of the intestine and enter the hepatic portal system. In the circulation, they may be filtered out in the liver, but if not, they may eventually come to reside in the lungs, brain, bones, spinal column, or other visceral organs. The incubation period is extended, being from several months to years. Infections are frequently symptomless and chronic.

Infection with the larval stage of *E. granulosus* (known as unilocular hydatid disease) is cosmopolitan in distribution. Its greatest incidence is in areas of the world where sheep raising is an important industry, such as Australia, South America, and the Mediterranean. In the United States, endemic foci are in the Southwest and Utah, Colorado, and California. *E. multilocularis,* agent of alveolar or multilocular hydatid disease, is endemic in northern, temperate climates, including Canada and northern United States. It is primarily a sylvatic disease, with the typical life cycle involving the fox and vole, whereas *E. granulosus* has a typical cycle involving the dog and sheep. Sheep raisers are those most often infected with larvae of *E. granulosus,* and hunters and trappers are most often infected with *E. multilocularis.*

As stated above, human infection is through the inadvertent ingestion of eggs. In the case of *E. granulosus,* any organ or tissue may be involved, but the liver and lungs are the most common sites. By a remarkable process of asexual reproduction, the embryos metamorphose into hydatid cysts. These vacuolated larval cestodes are called unilocular hydatid cysts. Cysts in soft tissues, such as liver and lungs, are somewhat similar, but the type in bone tends to elongate as it flows into and erodes the body canal. The unilocular hydatid cyst of the liver is the most common in humans. It consists typically of a central fluid-filled cavity lined with a germinative, protoplasmic layer, surrounded by a cuticular, protective layer that tends to become laminated. It is usually many years before the cyst reaches a large size. In time, it becomes covered with a fibrous host-tissue capsule. Arising from the germinative layer, internal buds (brood capsules) are produced (Fig. 88–15). When full size, each forms vesicles along its inner margin. Typically, each vesicle (10 to 20 or more) develops into a small protoscolex, usually invaginated, which serves to protect the 20 to 30 rosteller hooklets, and a short neck region. Thus a large mature cyst containing thousands of these protoscolices produces a heavy infection of adult worms when eaten by a definitive host.

After ingestion of the egg of *E. multilocularis,* the released larval stage penetrates the gut wall and is carried to the liver or, less often, other visceral sites, where it grows by exogenous budding to form another larval stage, the alveolar hydatid cyst. The alveolar cyst in humans lacks a strong protective layer, which appears to encourage branching formations or cavities, with little fluid and few, if any, protoscolices. The liver is most often involved, and the damage resembles that produced by a large amebic liver abscess. The liver disease is almost always fatal.

The hydatid cysts of *E. granulosus* are usually single, but they may be multiple. Their size and contour depend on the site of implantation and the age of the cysts. Because of the slow growth of cysts, vital processes are usually not sufficiently disturbed to cause concern to the patient until many years after infection. Ultimately, however, there may be tissue destruction and striking signs and symptoms. The type and degree of this damage and the resulting clinical manifestations correspond to the exact location and size of the cyst(s). It should be added that systemic intoxication or sensitization often occurs in those with a unilocular hydatid cyst having a vascularized wall that permits leakage of sensitizing fluids. Sensitized individuals exhibit marked eosinophilia, and in some, urticaria or angioneurotic edema is evident. Anaphylaxis may be precipitated by the sudden release of hydatid fluid, as in the case of spontaneous rupture of a large intra-abdominal cyst or rupture following a severe blow to the area.

Both infections usually are diagnosed by indirect means, such as roentgenograms, and intradermal and serologic tests. Ultrasonic echotomography has been of great advantage in detecting hydatid cysts.

In treatment, surgical intervention is limited to those patients with unilocular cysts in operable sites. Because of the probability of causing anaphylaxis, meticulous care must be taken to prevent spillage of the cyst contents into the operative cavity. Cetrimide is usually injected into the cyst to kill the germinative membrane and protoscolices, inasmuch as their release from the cyst can result in the formation of new hydatid cysts.

Mebendazole in high doses has been used with some success. This drug appears to cause regression of cyst size, as verified by echotomographic examination, and also destroys the cyst's contents before surgery. Mebendazole has also been used when a cyst either ruptured before or during surgery.

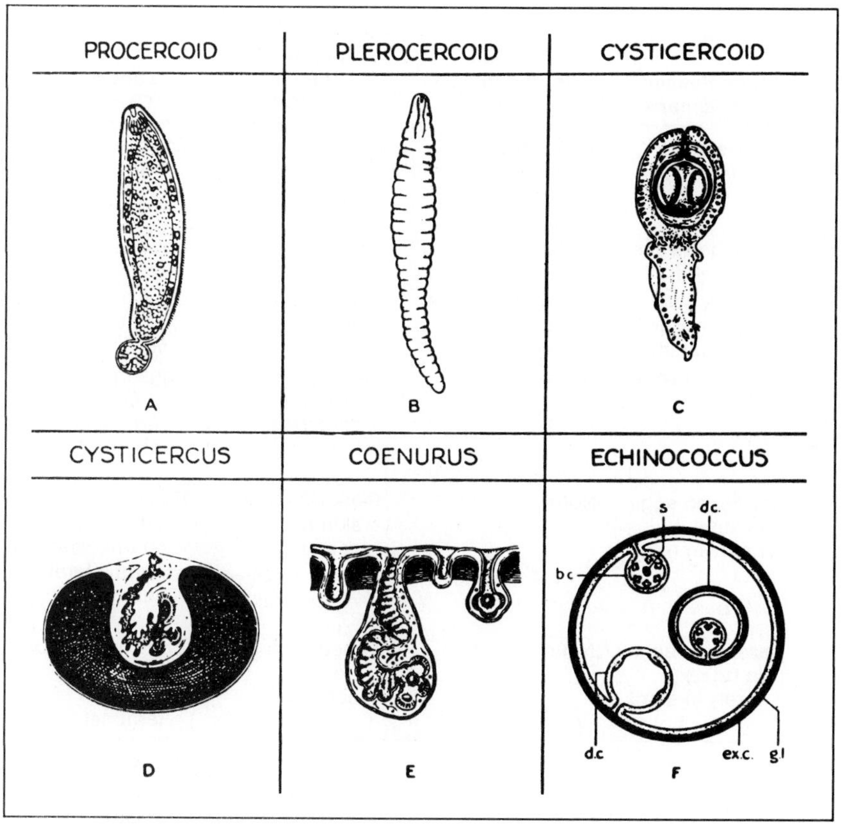

Fig. 88–15. Larval forms of tapeworms, b.c., brood capsule; d.c., daughter cyst; ex.c., external laminated cuticle; g.l., germinal or inner nucleated layer; s, scolex. *(From Belding: Textbook of Clinical Parasitology, ed 2. Appleton-Century-Crofts, 1952.)*

Trematodes

Trematodes, or flukes, as these parasitic flatworms are called, have unique life cycles; sexual reproduction occurs in vertebrate hosts and asexual reproduction occurs in snails, which are intermediate hosts. Adult trematodes are usually flat, elongated, and leaf-shaped. They vary considerably in size, from less than 1 mm to several centimeters in length. Characteristic external features include an oral and, in most species, a ventral sucker, the acetabulum. The principal internal organs include a blind, bifurcated intestinal tract, an excretory system, prominent reproductive organs, and a primitive nervous system. The arrangement, shape, and site of these various structures are characteristic for different species.

Unlike the tapeworms discussed above, none of the trematodes of humans is endemic in the United States. Because of immigration, however, trematode infections, especially the blood flukes, occur in large numbers in new residents in the United States.

With the exception of the blood flukes (*schistosomes*), all trematodes are hermaphroditic. Eggs that are produced are passed from humans in either a developed or an undeveloped stage. When fully developed, the larval stage within (*miracidium*) must take up residence within the tissues of an appropriate species of snail where prodigious asexual reproduction occurs. Eventually, *cercariae* are produced, and these leave the snail and either pass to the next intermediate host where they encyst and become metacercariae or actively swim and penetrate the skin of the definitive host. As a result of ingestion of the *metacercaria* or the penetration of vertebrate skin by the cercaria, the larva develops to the adult worm stage after a prepatent period that is characteristic of the species.

Information concerning the most commonly found trematodes of humans in the United States and the infections they cause is listed in Table 88–2. The schistosomes are of the greatest medical and public health importance and are thus discussed in greater detail than the others. It should be remembered that there are other trematode infections of humans, but these are only rarely encountered in the United States and are, therefore, not discussed here.

Schistosomes or Bloodflukes

Schistosomes differ in many ways from the other trematodes. The important differences include the presence in schistosomes of separate sexes, nonoperculated eggs with spines, fork-tailed cercariae, and the absence of a true metacercarial stage in the life cycle. As noted in Table 88–2, three species occur commonly in humans: *Schistosoma japonicum, Schistosoma mansoni,* and *Schistosoma haematobium.* Although the other two species lack important natural reservoirs, *S. japonicum* has numerous mammalian reservoirs (cats, dogs, cattle, water buffalos). Humans however, are usually the most important source of eggs of all three species. The adult worms occur characteristically in pairs in mesenteric veins (*S. japonicum* and *S. mansoni*) and vesical veins (*S. haematobium*) on the outside wall of the intestines or urinary bladder. The male attaches

TABLE 88–2. IMPORTANT TREMATODES OF HUMANS

Parasite	Disease	Location of Adults Where Eggs Are Laid	Stage Passed from Humans	Second Intermediate Host[a]	Means of Human Infection	Laboratory Diagnosis
Fasciolopsis buski	Fasciolopsiasis	Small intestine	Undeveloped eggs in stool	Water caltrop, cetain other freshwater plants	Ingestion of metacercariae	Eggs in stool (140 × 80 μm)
Clonorchis sinensis	Clonorchiasis	Distal bile ducts of liver	Developed eggs in stool	Certain freshwater fishes	Ingestion of metacercariae	Eggs in stool (30 × 16 μm)
Paragonimus westermani	Paragonimiasis	In lung capsules	Undeveloped eggs in stool and sputum	Certain freshwater crabs and crayfishes	Ingestion of metacercariae	Eggs in stool and sputum (85 × 50 μm)
Schistosoma japonicum	Schistosomiasis japonica	Venules of superior and inferior mesenteric veins	Developed eggs in stool	None	Penetration of skin by cercariae	Eggs in stool (89 × 66 μm with rudimentary lateral spine)
Schistosoma mansoni	Schistosomiasis mansoni	Venules of inferior, and at times superior, mesenteric veins	Developed eggs in stool, rarely in urine	None	Penetration of skin by cercariae	Eggs in stool or urine (150 × 60 μm, with large lateral spine)
Schistosoma haematobium	Schistosomiasis hematobium	Venules of vesical and pelvis plexuses	Developed eggs in urine, rarely in stool	None	Penetration of skin by cercariae	Eggs in urine or stool (150 × 60 μm, with large terminal spine)

[a] Certain snails are the first intermediate host.

to the wall of the blood vessel, holding the female in a ventral groove, the gynecophoral canal. The female is able to extend its anterior end into the smaller venules where the eggs are discharged.

WHO has stated that this infection is second only to malaria in causing morbidity and mortality in the tropics. Widespread over three continents, it affects an estimated 200 million people. *S. mansoni,* the agent of Manson's bloodfluke infection, is common throughout most of tropical Africa, especially in the Nile Delta, and in the Western Hemisphere in Brazil, Venezuela, the West Indies, and Puerto Rico. It is estimated that 250,000 infected persons live in the United States, many of whom are Puerto Ricans. Little risk of transmission is involved, however, because appropriate snails are lacking, and sanitation is generally good. *S. japonicum,* agent of the Oriental bloodfluke infection, is confined to the Far East. *S. haematobium,* agent of urinary bloodfluke infection, coexists with *S. mansoni* in much of tropical Africa and is also endemic in the Near East, India, and Portugal. Other species, such as *Schistosoma mekongi* (Far East), *Schistosoma intercalatum* (Zaire), and a variety of cattle bloodflukes, also occur in humans but are of minor importance when compared with the others.

Life Cycle. The adults (Fig. 88–16) of *S. japonicum* and *S. mansoni* are found normally in the tributaries of the superior and inferior mesenteric veins, respectively, whereas those of *S. haematobium* find the venous plexus of the bladder the optimum location. Although these are the usual locations, it should be remembered that the worms may be found in other sites. Perhaps most important in this connection is the well-known fact that after infection with *S. haematobium* a small percentage of the worms fail to reach the normal site and remain in the rectal vessels. Thus some of the eggs released may occur in the stools rather than in the urine, as expected in this infection. After copulation, the female flukes give off a considerable number of eggs over a long period of time. These are undeveloped when laid but usually contain a fully developed ciliated larva (miracidium) after they have succeeded in passing through the wall of the intestine or bladder to occur in the stools or urine (Fig. 88–13). Upon reaching freshwater, the eggs hatch and the miracidium swims about. If appropriate intermediate hosts are present in the immediate vicinity, the miracidium will penetrate the soft tissues. The intrasnail cycle lasts for several weeks and involves three distinct stages: the first (mother) and second (daughter) generations of sporocysts and cercariae. The latter, with characteristic forked tails, escape from the snail at intervals and swim about in the water. When they come into contact with the skin of humans or other susceptible definitive hosts, they discard their tails and penetrate the skin. These larvae, now called *schistosomula,* reach the bloodstream and are carried through the right side of the heart to the lungs. Here they pass the capillary filters and are carried to the left side of the heart and thence into the large arterial vessels. From the superior mesenteric artery, where most of them are carried, they pass through the capillaries into the intrahepatic portal blood. They feed and grow in this site, and when sexual maturity approaches (after about 16 days of residence), they migrate against the portal blood flow to the areas where egg laying is to occur. *S. haematobium* is thought to pass from the rectal veins through hemorrhoidal anastomoses into the pudendal vein to reach ultimately the vesical venous plexus. Several weeks are required for the maturation of the adult worms (4

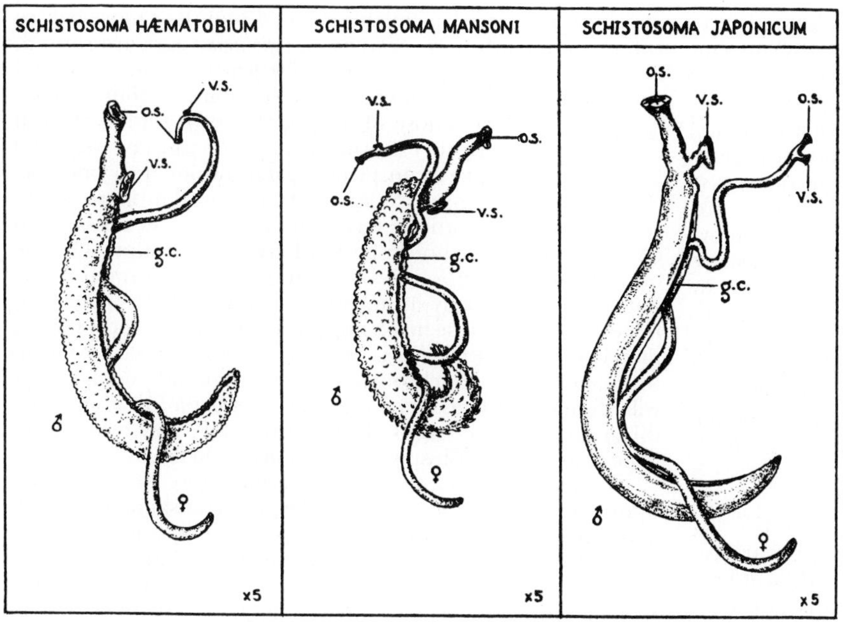

Fig. 88–16. Schematic representation of important schistosomes of humans. g.c., gynecophoric canal; o.s., oral sucker; v.s., ventral sucker. *(From Belding: Textbook of Clinical Parasitology, ed. 3. Appleton-Century-Crofts, 1965.)*

to 5 weeks for *S. japonicum,* 6 to 7 weeks for *S. mansoni,* and 10 to 12 weeks after skin penetration in the case of *S. haematobium*), and they may live for many years.

Pathology and Symptomatology. For all three species, penetration of the skin by the cercariae produces small hemorrhages. After the schistosomula break out of the capillaries in the lungs, they cause an acute inflammatory reaction predominated by eosinophils. Upon their arrival in the intrahepatic portal blood, an acute hepatitis may follow, as well as systemic intoxication and sensitization, all due presumably to the toxic and/or allergenic metabolites released. Many patients exhibit toxic manifestations, such as fever and sweats, epigastric distress, and pain in the back, groin, or legs. Others develop giant urticaria and toxic diarrhea. Eosinophilia is common. These reactions may continue long after the worms have migrated to the area of oviposition. The penetration of the cercariae and the migrations of the schistosomula, and, later, the movements of the developing worms usually produce detrimental effects. The main agents of pathology in schistosomiasis, however, are the eggs released from the females.

The period of egg deposition and extrusion from the body is usually referred to as the acute stage, or as Katayama fever. In the instance of the two intestinal forms, *S. japonicum* and *S. mansoni,* the events of this stage are, in general, similar. It is important, however, to add that the females of *S. japonicum* release considerably more eggs and therefore the damage is proportionately greater. In both species the intestinal tissue is the first to be damaged—usually the small intestine in the case of *S. japonicum* and the colon in the case of *S. mansoni.* Considerable trauma and hemorrhage are produced by the eggs as they are filtered through the perivascular tissues into the lumen. An allergen released by the developing miracidium escapes through pores in the egg shell and causes a striking cell-mediated response in the affected areas. Eggs trapped in these sites are walled off, usually individually, by an eosinophilic abscess, which later transforms into a characteristic granuloma (pseudotubercle). The egg or its shell alone usually is surrounded by a peripheral ring of connective tissue and then by eosinophils, plasma cells, and lymphocytes. Fibrous nodules and scarring result. The acute stage begins with diarrhea or dysentery and the appearance of eggs in the stools. Daily fever, anorexia, loss of weight, severe abdominal pain, and anemia are common. Many of the eggs are swept into the intrahepatic portal vessels, where they provoke granuloma formation. Liver involvement is more rapid and severe in *S. japonicum* infections. The liver becomes tender and enlarged. Coarse bands of dense connective tissue, chiefly about the large radicals of the portal vein, have been responsible for the term *Symmer's clay pipestem fibrosis,* associated with schistosomiasis japonica and mansoni. Blockage causes portal hypertension, and opening of a secondary circulatory shunt leads to varices in esophageal and gastric veins, ascites, and gross hepatosplenomegaly. It should be added that nests of *S. japonicum* eggs often also occur in ectopic sites, such as the brain and heart.

The chronic stage of schistosomiasis is one of tissue proliferation and repair. The intestinal wall becomes thickened by fibrosis, and the lumen may be reduced considerably. Anal polyps are common, as are papillomas and fistulas. Hemorrhoids may be the first indication of the infection, resulting from portal obstruction. The liver may become increasingly damaged because of extensive periportal fibrosis, and there may be a compensatory congestive enlargement of the spleen, especially in *S. japonicum* infections. Thus, in many patients, there is a rapidly developing dysfunction of the intestinal wall and periportal tissues. In the late stages of the disease in those with heavy infections, emaciation is severe and many patients die of exhaustion or of a concurrent infection, such as salmonellosis.

In infection with *S. haematobium,* the acute stage involves primarily the wall of the urinary bladder, but the lungs also may be involved. The latter involvement is due to eggs and, at times, worms that are probably carried via the common iliac vein, the inferior vena cava, and right heart to reach the pulmonary arterioles. Here, granulomas are produced as described above, and as a result fibrosis of arterioles and pulmonary hypertension may develop. In time, heart disease (cor pulmonale) may follow. The damage produced in the wall of the urinary bladder is similar to that described above for the wall of the intestine. Hematuria is usually the first evidence of infection. As time passes, the bladder wall becomes thickened by dense fibrosis of the muscular and submucous coats, and multiple urinary polyps, papillomas, and fistulas are common. The superficial mucosa of the bladder may show metaplasia, an intense inflammatory infiltrate, and eggs (many calcified). Fever, suprapubic tenderness, and difficulty in urination are common. Bladder colic is a cardinal symptom. In addition to the bladder, other parts of the genitourinary system often become involved. Finally, it is worth noting that in some areas there is a close association between chronic schistosomiasis of the bladder and squamous cell carcinoma, because eggs in capillaries are seen in the midst of an infiltrating carcinoma. In fact, the term *Egyptian irritation cancer* is well known.

Epidemiology. Schistosomiasis, also known as bilharziasis or snail fever, is present in many countries and afflicts at least 250 million people. Unfortunately, the infection is spreading in association with implementation of water resource projects in most developing countries. As an example of this increase, the prevalence rose from 10% to 100% among the inhabitants around Volta Lake, Ghana, within 5 years of water impoundment.

Although it is unlikely that schistosomiasis can be eradicated, it is possible to reduce its incidence and prevalence, as well as the accompanying morbidity and mortality. To this end, advances are being made in (1) the treatment of affected persons so they do not pass eggs, (2) the prevention of eggs in feces and urine from reaching water, (3) the control of snail hosts, and (4) the development of vaccines and other prophylactic treatment.

Diagnosis. Schistosomiasis usually manifests as a long-term, chronic illness and, in large measure, is an immunologic disease due to cell-mediated granulomatous reactions around the eggs. Acute disease is rare in the United States and is associated with a primary infection acquired by persons living within endemic areas such as Puerto Rico, Africa, and the Philippines. Clinical signs and symptoms of each of the three phases of infection—penetration, acute, and chronic—are discussed above. It is important to remember that a history of travel or residence in an endemic area is an important consideration in diagnosis. The differential diagnosis of acute disease should include a consideration of amebic or bacterial dysentery, hepatitis, and typhoid fever.

With regard to the laboratory diagnosis, in most cases *S. haematobium* eggs can be demonstrated in the sediment that settles out of urine. In some instances, a small bladder biopsy specimen will reveal the eggs when they cannot be demonstrated in urine. If these measures fail in suspected cases, stool examinations and/or rectal biopsies should be considered, because these worms may involve the rectum as well. The mature eggs (Fig. 88–3) range from 110 to 170 μm in length by 40 to 70 μm in width (average 150 by 60 μm). Intradermal and serologic tests, although available, are usually not needed to provide evidence of infection.

The eggs of *S. japonicum* and *S. mansoni* can usually be recovered from the stools of patients during the acute stage, but they tend to be released in clutches, making it necessary to perform repeated examinations for 1 month or more before ruling out the infection. *Schistosoma japonicum* eggs are rotund, measure 70 to 100 μm by 50 to 70 μm (average 89 by 66 μm), and have a rudimentary lateral spine within a hook cavity (Fig. 88–3). Those of *S. mansoni* are rounded at both ends, measure 115 to 175 μm by 45 to 70 μm (average 150 by 60 μm), and have a conspicuous lateral spine near one pole (Fig. 88–3). The eggs of *S. japonicum* are more numerous and tend to be mixed with the feces, and therefore a cross-section of the fecal bolus should be used for examination. On the other hand, eggs of *S. mansoni* tend to be concentrated in the outer layer, especially in mucus or blood. In both infections, but especially in those involving *S. mansoni*, simple fecal smears may fail to reveal the eggs, necessitating the use of a concentration technique. In chronic cases, rectosigmoid punch biopsy will often reveal eggs when they have not been found in many different stool specimens. Intradermal, CF, and other serologic tests with schistosome antigen are available.

Other laboratory findings are a moderate to high eosinophilia during the acute stage, elevated transaminase levels, abnormal liver function test results, anemia, and increased levels of IgG, IgM, and IgE. If eggs have been largely confined to the intestine, there are few abnormal values. Even in some patients with hepatosplenic involvement, blood and chemistry values may be near normal. These have been termed *compensated cases.*

Treatment. The treatment of schistosomiasis has undergone rapid change, with praziquantel now being the drug of choice for all three species. Before this time the optimal therapy varied according to the species and geographic strain. For example, *S. mansoni* infection in the New World was treated with oxamniquine whereas hycanthone was used in Africa. Because praziquantel's use has been limited and of short duration, it is recommended that the current literature and the Parasitic Diseases Division of the Centers for Disease Control be consulted when cases in the United States are discovered.

Schistosome Dermatitis

Many birds and mammals are infected with their own peculiar species of schistosomes, and the life cycles are similar to those of species normally parasitic in humans. As a result of birds or mammals defecating in bodies of water, the infected snails may shed cercariae that can penetrate the skin of humans who come in contact with the water. In these cases, humans are abnormal hosts, and the cercariae are walled off in the skin and evoke an acute inflammatory response characterized by a leukocyte infiltration and edema. Severe itching follows, and thus the condition is popularly called *swimmer's itch.* Papules, hemorrhagic rash, and pustules may last 1 week or longer, and secondary infections due to scratching are common.

Schistosome dermatitis is a plague of swimmers during the summer season in the northern lakes of the United States and in southern Canada. Similar outbreaks are seen along the saltwater beaches of the eastern coasts. Some of the beaches in the Gulf States, California, and Hawaii are also involved. Topical ointments to relieve the itching and edema are recommended.

Clonorchis sinensis

Infection with *C. sinensis* is known as clonorchiasis, Oriental liverfluke infection, biliary distomiasis, and biliary trematodiasis. In addition to *C. sinensis,* various species of *Opisthorchis, Fasciola,* and *Dicrocoelium* are also liverflukes of humans. Because treatment may vary for each species, it is important to determine which fluke is involved.

WHO estimates 20 million people are infected, with endemic centers being in the Far East. The fluke is being seen more frequently in the United States because of the recent immigration of thousands of Indochinese.

Life Cycle. The hermaphroditic adults, up to 2 cm in length, usually live in the distal bile ducts but have also been found throughout the biliary passages, gallbladder, and pancreatic duct. Eggs are shed in the feces, and a typical intrasnail cycle occurs when suitable snails ingest the eggs. Cercariae leave the infected snails and seek out suitable freshwater fish, which are used as the second intermediate host. The cercariae encyst in the muscles of the fish, and humans become infected by eating raw or improperly cooked fish. After ingestion, the excysted metacercaria migrates up the ampulla of Vater and enters the biliary tract. The incubation period varies, but most worms become mature in 1 month and live for more than 20 years.

Pathology and Symptomatology. Many times clonorchiasis is an asymptomatic infection. When symptoms are present, their severity will depend on worm burden, duration of infection, and the number of reinfections suffered by the host. Pathogenesis seems to be related to the mechanical actions and toxic products of the worms. Epidemiologic data indicate a possible relationship between clonorchiasis and adenocarcinoma of the liver in patients in endemic areas.

Pathologic changes include biliary hyperplasia, connective tissue hyperplasia, fatty degeneration of liver parenchyma, and fibrosis, which may lead to portal cirrhosis. A pancreatitis may develop when worms have invaded the pancreatic duct.

Diagnosis. The signs and symptoms of infection may include epigastric pain, anorexia, diarrhea, ascites, and hepatomegaly. In heavy and chronic infections, progressive hepatic dysfunction is common. Malignancies, hepatitis, and cirrhosis due to other causes need to be considered in a differential diagnosis. There are few, if any, abnormal laboratory values in asymptomatic and mild infections. Moderate to heavy infections may show eosinophilia, anemia, and elevated serum alkaline phosphatase and bilirubin values. Numerous serologic tests have been developed, but none is of practical use in the clinic laboratory setting.

A definitive diagnosis depends on the demonstration of the typical small, operculated, brownish egg that measures 30 by 15 μm (Fig. 88–3). In difficult cases, duodenal aspirates are sometimes of value.

Treatment. Before 1984, there did not appear to be any drug of real value for liverfluke infection. Aralen had been used extensively and provided some relief of symptoms but did not kill the adult worms. Praziquantel is now the drug of choice.

Paragonimus westermani

P. westermani is the cause of paragonimiasis, or endemic hemoptysis. Human infections are common in the Far East, especially in China, Korea, Japan, Taiwan, and the Philippines. Other endemic foci are in Africa and India, and unidentified species are reported in Mexico, Central America, Peru, and Ecuador. Cases are being detected among Indochinese (Laotian) refugees in the United States.

The adult flukes, about 1 cm long, live in the parenchyma of the lung. Other tissues and organs are sometimes involved, including the central nervous system and skin. Humans become infected by ingesting raw freshwater crabs or crayfish that harbor the infective larval stage. After ingestion, the excysted larva penetrates the intestinal wall, migrates in the peritoneal cavity, and eventually passes through the diaphragm and into the lungs.

There are usually no or few signs and symptoms during the migration phase. Once the larvae are in the lungs, hemoptysis with brown or red sputum occurs, as does pleurisy. Paragonimiasis mimics tuberculosis, and because of the high rate of tuberculosis among Indochinese refugees, diagnosis is sometimes difficult; in some patients, fluke infection and tuberculosis coexist. Hemoptysis and cough in the absence of a reaction to tuberculin should increase suspicion of paragonimiasis.

Diagnosis is based on finding the characteristic egg (Fig. 88–3) in the sputum or feces. CF tests may aid in diagnosis but should not be the sole basis for treatment. Radiographic films may also show cysts in lung, brain, and other sites. Treatment should be administered when diagnosis is confirmed. Praziquantel seems to be very effective and has been widely used in endemic areas.

Fasciolopsis buski

In addition to *F. buski,* other species such as *Metagonimus yokogawai* and *Heterophyes heterophyes* are intestinal flukes of humans. All are endemic in the Far East and have numerous reservoir hosts.

F. buski, known as the giant intestinal fluke (up to 8 cm in length), lives in the small intestine and attaches to the mucosa. Humans become infected by ingesting the encysted metacercariae that are present on water plants, such as caltrop, water bamboo, and water hyacinth. Mature flukes are present 3 months after ingestion of the infective larvae.

Adult worms cause ulceration, inflammation, and hypersecretion of mucus around attachment sites. In heavy infections, worms may inhabit the stomach and colon. Diarrhea, edema of face and legs, and marked anemia may be seen. In a comparison of infected humans, children usually are more severely affected than are adults. Mature worms may live 20 to 30 years. Death is usually attributable to cachexia and intercurrent infection.

Definitive diagnosis depends on finding the large operculated egg (Fig. 88–3). Laboratory findings include anemia and eosinophilia. Praziquantel is the drug of choice.

Index

Page numbers followed by *f* refer to illustrations.
Page numbers followed by *t* refer to tables.